Cardiovascular Imaging

OTHER VOLUMES IN THE
EXPERT RADIOLOGY SERIES

Abdominal Imaging

Head and Neck Imaging

Imaging of the Chest

Imaging of the Musculoskeletal System

Imaging of the Spine

Image-Guided Interventions

FORTHCOMING VOLUMES IN THE
EXPERT RADIOLOGY SERIES

Breast Imaging

Gynecologic Imaging

Imaging of the Brain

Pediatric Neuroimaging

Obstetric Imaging

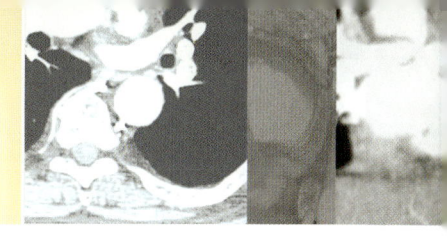

Cardiovascular Imaging

Volume I

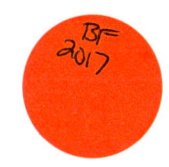

Vincent B. Ho, MD, MBA, FAHA

Fellow, American Heart Association
Professor, Uniformed Services University of the Health Sciences
President, North American Society for Cardiovascular Imaging
Guest Researcher, National Institutes of Health
Editorial Board, *Circulation: Cardiovascular Imaging*
Bethesda, Maryland

Gautham P. Reddy, MD, MPH

Professor of Radiology
Vice Chair for Education
Director of Thoracic Imaging
Department of Radiology
University of Washington School of Medicine
Seattle, Washington

ELSEVIER
SAUNDERS

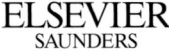

3251 Riverport Lane
St. Louis, Missouri 63043

CARDIOVASCULAR IMAGING　　　　　　　　　　　　　　　　　ISBN: 978-1-4160-5335-4

Copyright © 2011 by Saunders, an imprint of Elsevier Inc.

No part of this publication may be reproduced or transmitted in any form or by any means, electronic or mechanical, including photocopying, recording, or any information storage and retrieval system, without permission in writing from the publisher. Details on how to seek permission, further information about the Publisher's permissions policies and our arrangements with organizations such as the Copyright Clearance Center and the Copyright Licensing Agency, can be found at our website: www.elsevier.com/permissions.

This book and the individual contributions contained in it are protected under copyright by the Publisher (other than as may be noted herein).

Notices

Knowledge and best practice in this field are constantly changing. As new research and experience broaden our understanding, changes in research methods, professional practices, or medical treatment may become necessary.

Practitioners and researchers must always rely on their own experience and knowledge in evaluating and using any information, methods, compounds, or experiments described herein. In using such information or methods they should be mindful of their own safety and the safety of others, including parties for whom they have a professional responsibility.

With respect to any drug or pharmaceutical products identified, readers are advised to check the most current information provided (i) on procedures featured or (ii) by the manufacturer of each product to be administered, to verify the recommended dose or formula, the method and duration of administration, and contraindications. It is the responsibility of practitioners, relying on their own experience and knowledge of their patients, to make diagnoses, to determine dosages and the best treatment for each individual patient, and to take all appropriate safety precautions.

To the fullest extent of the law, neither the Publisher nor the authors, contributors, or editors, assume any liability for any injury and/or damage to persons or property as a matter of products liability, negligence or otherwise, or from any use or operation of any methods, products, instructions, or ideas contained in the material herein.

The opinions or assertions contained herein are the private views of the authors and are not to be construed as official or reflecting the views of the Department of Defense or the Uniformed Services University of the Health Sciences.

Library of Congress Cataloging-in-Publication Data
Cardiovascular imaging / [edited by] Vincent B. Ho, Gautham P. Reddy.—1st ed.
　　p. ; cm.
　Includes bibliographical references and index.
　ISBN 978-1-4160-5335-4
　1. Cardiovascular system—Diseases—Diagnosis.　2. Diagnostic imaging.　I. Ho, Vincent B.
II. Reddy, Gautham P.
　[DNLM: 1. Cardiovascular Diseases—diagnosis.　2. Diagnostic Imaging—methods.　3. Diagnostic Techniques, Cardiovascular.　WG 141 C2686 2010]
　RC670.C364 2010
　616.1′075—dc22
　　　　　　　　　　　　　　　　　　　　　　　　　　　　　　　　2010021017

Publishing Director: Linda Duncan
Acquisitions Editor: Rebecca Gaertner
Developmental Editor: Jennifer Shreiner
Publishing Services Manager: Patricia Tannian
Project Manager: Fran Gunning
Project Manager: Carrie Stetz
Design Direction: Steve Stave

Printed in China

Last digit is the print number:　9　8　7　6　5　4　3　2　1

Working together to grow libraries in developing countries
www.elsevier.com | www.bookaid.org | www.sabre.org
ELSEVIER　BOOK AID International　Sabre Foundation

*To our families, mentors, colleagues, fellows, residents, and students—
this book is for you.*

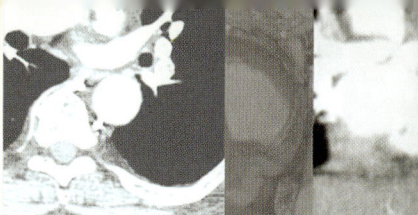

Contributors

Theodore P. Abraham, MD, FACC, FASE
Associate Professor of Medicine
Johns Hopkins University;
Vice-Chief of Cardiology
Co-Director, Echocardiography
Director, Johns Hopkins Hypertrophic
   Cardiomyopathy Clinic
Director, Translational Cardiovascular Ultrasound
   Laboratory
Baltimore, Maryland

Christopher J. Abularrage, MD
Assistant Professor of Surgery
Attending Surgeon
Division of Vascular Surgery and Endovascular
   Therapy
The Johns Hopkins University School of Medicine
Baltimore, Maryland

Mouaz H. Al-Mallah, MD, MSc, FACC, FAHA, FESC
Associate Professor of Medicine
Wayne State University
Detroit, Michigan;
Consultant Cardiologist and Division Head, Cardiac
   Imaging
King Abdul-Aziz Cardiac Center
King Abdul-Aziz Medical City (Riyadh)
National Guard Health Affairs
Saudi Arabia

Mehran Attari, MD
Assistant Professor
Internal Medicine, Cardiology
University of Cincinnati College of Medicine;
Director
Electrophysiology Laboratory
University of Cincinnati Medical Center
Cincinnati, Ohio

Jonathan Balcombe, MD
Radiologist
Imaging On Call
Poughkeepsie, New York

Sanjeev Bhalla, MD
Associate Professor of Radiology
Washington University
Mallinckrodt Institute of Radiology;
Chief, Cardiothoracic Imaging Section
Barnes Jewish Hospital
St. Louis, Missouri

Kostaki G. Bis, MD, FACR
Clinical Professor
Oakland University William Beaumont School of
   Medicine
Rochester Hills, Michigan;
Associate Director, Body Imaging
Department of Radiology
William Beaumont Hospital
Royal Oak, Michigan

Michelle M. Bittle, MD
Assistant Professor
University of Washington
Harborview Medical School
Seattle, Washington

Ron Blankstein, MD
Instructor in Medicine
Harvard Medical School
Brigham and Women's Hospital
Boston, Massachusetts

Thorsten Bley, MD
Assistant Professor
Department of Radiology
University Medical Center Hamburg-Eppendorf
Hamburg, Germany

David A. Bluemke, MD, PhD
Director
Radiology and Imaging Sciences
National Institutes of Health
Bethesda, Maryland

Contributors

Jamieson M. Bourque, MD, MHS
Fellow in Cardiovascular Disease and Advanced Cardiovascular Imaging
University of Virginia Health System
Charlottesville, Virginia

Lawrence M. Boxt, MD
Professor of Radiology
Albert Einstein College of Medicine;
Director of Cardiac CT and MR Imaging
Division of Cardiology
Montefiore Medical Center
Bronx, New York

Lynn S. Broderick, MD
Professor
Department of Radiology
University of Wisconsin-Madison
Madison, Wisconsin

Thomas G. Brott, MD
Professor, Department of Neurology
Associate Dean for Research
Mayo Clinic
Jacksonville, Florida

Allen Burke, MD
Associate Professor of Pathology
University of Maryland School of Medicine
University of Maryland Medical System
Baltimore, Maryland

Alexander Bustamante, MD
Cardiology Staff
National Naval Medical Center
Bethesda, Maryland

Hugh Calkins, MD
Professor
Medicine and Cardiology
Director, Electrophysiology
Director, ARVD Program
Johns Hopkins Hospital
Baltimore, Maryland

Jeffrey P. Carpenter, MD
Professor and Chief
Department of Surgery
UMDNJ-Robert Wood Johnson Medical School
Camden, New Jersey;
Vice President for Perioperative Services and Chief of Surgery
Cooper Health System
Voorhees, New Jersey

James C. Carr, MD, FFR RCSI
Associate Professor of Radiology and Medicine
Northwestern University Feinberg School of Medicine;
Director of Cardiovascular Imaging
Northwestern Memorial Hospital
Chicago, Illinois

Frandics P. Chan, MD, PhD
Associate Professor of Radiology
Stanford University School of Medicine
Department of Radiology
Stanford, California

Joseph Jen-Sho Chen, MD
Radiology Resident
University of Maryland Medical Center
University of Maryland School of Medicine
Baltimore, Maryland

Bennett Chin, MD
Associate Professor of Radiology
Duke University School of Medicine
Associate Professor of Radiology
Duke University Medical Center
Durham, North Carolina

Jonathan H. Chung, MD
Fellow and Clinical Assistant, Cardiothoracic Imaging
Harvard Medical School
Massachusetts General Hospital
Boston, Massachusetts

William R. Corse, DO
Director of Cardiovascular MRI
Doylestown Hospital
Doylestown, Pennsylvania

Carlos Cuevas, MD
Assistant Professor
Department of Radiology, Body Imaging Section
University of Washington School of Medicine
Assistant Professor
University of Washington Medical Center
Seattle, Washington

Zelmira Curillova, MD
Division of Cardiology
Department of Medicine
VA Boston Healthcare System
West Roxbury, Massachusetts

Ricardo C. Cury, MD
Consulting Radiologist
Massachusetts General Hospital
Harvard Medical School
Boston, Massachusetts;
Director of Cardiac MRI and CT
Baptist Cardiac and Vascular Institute
Miami, Florida

David H. Deaton, MD, FACS
Chief, Endovascular Surgery
Associate Professor of Surgery
Georgetown University Hospital
Washington, DC

Subrato J. Deb, MD, FCCP
Assistant Professor of Surgery
Uniformed Services University
F. Edward Hébert School of Medicine
Bethesda, Maryland;
Cardiovascular and Thoracic Surgeon
Western Maryland Regional Medical Center
Cumberland, Maryland;
Cardiothoracic Surgeon
National Naval Medical Center;
Captain, United States Navy
Naval Reserve, National Naval Medical Center
Bethesda, Maryland

Patrick J.H. de Koning, MSc
Researcher, Image Processing
Leiden University Medical Center
Department of Radiology, Division of Image Processing
Leiden, The Netherlands

J. Kevin DeMarco, MD
Associate Professor
Michigan State University
East Lansing, Michigan;
Attending Radiologist
Lansing, Michigan

Albert de Roos, MD
Professor of Radiology
Leiden University Medical Center
Leiden, The Netherlands

Swati Deshmane, MBBS, DMRD
Research Volunteer
Cardiovascular Imaging
University of California Los Angeles
Los Angeles, California

Lisa M. Dias, MD
Diagnostic Radiology Resident
Department of Radiology
William Beaumont Hospital
Royal Oak, Michigan

Marcelo F. Di Carli, MD, FACC, FAHA
Director, Noninvasive Cardiovascular Imaging Program
Chief, Division of Nuclear Medicine and Molecular Imaging
Brigham and Women's Hospital
Boston, Massachusetts

Manjiri Dighe, MD, DMRE
Assistant Professor
University of Washington Medical Center
Seattle, Washington

Vasken Dilsizian, MD
Professor of Medicine and Radiology
University of Maryland School of Medicine
Chief, Division of Nuclear Medicine
Director, Cardiovascular Nuclear Medicine and PET Imaging
University of Maryland Medical Center
Baltimore, Maryland

Vikram S. Dogra, MD
Professor of Radiology, Urology, and Biomedical Engineering
Director of Ultrasound and Radiology Residency
University of Rochester School of Medicine
Rochester, New York

Jeremy C. Durack, MD
Assistant Professor of Radiology
University of California San Francisco
San Francisco, California

James P. Earls, MD
Medical Director
Cardiovascular CT and MRI
Fairfax Radiological Consultants PC
Fairfax, Virginia

Frederick K. Emge, MD
Departments of Surgery, Radiology, Pediatric Cardiology, and Cardiothoracic and Vascular Surgery
Geisinger Medical Center
Danville, Pennsylvania

A. Sanli Ergun, PhD
Assistant Professor
TOBB-University of Economy and Technology
Ankara, Turkey

Elif Ergun, MD
Instructor in Radiology
Ankara Training and Research Hospital
Ankara, Turkey

Stanford Ewing, MD, FAAP, FRCP(C)
Clinical Assistant Professor
University of Pennsylvania;
Attending Pediatric Cardiologist
Children's Hospital of Philadelphia
Philadelphia, Pennsylvania

Peter Faulhaber, MD, MA
Associate Professor of Radiology
Case Medical Center
Case Western Reserve University;
Director
Clinical PET
University Hospitals Case Medical Center
Cleveland, Ohio

Elliot K. Fishman, MD
Professor of Radiology and Oncology
Johns Hopkins University School of Medicine;
Director, Diagnostic Imaging and Body CT
Johns Hopkins Hospital
Baltimore, Maryland

Mark A. Fogel, MD, FACC, FAHA, FAAP
Associate Professor of Pediatrics and Radiology
Director of Cardiac MRI
University of Pennsylvania School of Medicine;
Children's Hospital of Philadelphia
Philadelphia, Pennsylvania

Thomas K.F. Foo, PhD
Assistant Professor
Department of Radiological Sciences
Uniformed University of the Health Sciences
Bethesda, Maryland;
Manager, MRI Lab
GE Global Research
Niskayuna, New York

Aletta Ann Frazier, MD
Associate Professor of Diagnostic Radiology
University of Maryland School of Medicine
Baltimore, Maryland;
Biomedical Illustrator in Radiologic Pathology
Armed Forces Institute of Pathology
Washington, DC

Tamar Gaspar, MD
Faculty of Medicine
Technion-Israel Institute of Technology;
Head of Cardiovascular Imaging
Carmel Medical Center
Haifa, Israel

Eva Maria Gassner, MD
Department of Radiology
University Hospital Innsbruck
Innsbruck, Austria

Jon C. George, MD
Adjunct Research Instructor
Cardiovascular Research Center
Temple University School of Medicine
Philadelphia, Pennsylvania

Thomas C. Gerber, MD, PhD
Professor of Medicine and Radiology
Mayo Clinic College of Medicine
Rochester, Minnesota;
Consultant in Cardiology
Mayo Clinic
Jacksonville, Florida

Christian L. Gilbert, MD, FACS
Associate Medical Director
The International Children's Heart Foundation
Memphis, Tennessee

Robert C. Gilkeson, MD
Associate Professor
Case Western Reserve University;
Section Chief, Cardiothoracic Imaging
University Hospitals Case Medical Center
Cleveland, Ohio

James F. Glockner, MD, PhD
Assistant Professor
Consultant
Mayo Clinic
Rochester, Minnesota

Michael B. Gotway, MD
Clinical Associate Professor of Diagnostic Radiology and Biomedical Imaging and Pulmonary/Critical Care Medicine
University of California
San Francisco, California;
Scottsdale Medical Imaging, Ltd., an affiliate of Southwest Diagnostic Imaging
Scottsdale, Arizona

Curtis E. Green, MD
Professor of Radiology and Medicine
University of Vermont College of Medicine;
Staff Radiologist
Fletcher Allen Healthcare
Burlington, Vermont

S. Bruce Greenberg, MD
Professor of Radiology
Arkansas Children's Hospital
University of Arkansas for Medical Sciences
Little Rock, Arkansas

Heynric B. Grotenhuis, MD, PhD
Pediatric Cardiologist
Leiden University Medical Center
Leiden, The Netherlands

Martin L. Gunn, MB, ChB, FRANZCR
Assistant Professor
Department of Radiology
University of Washington
Seattle, Washington

Sandra Simon Halliburton, PhD
Adjunct Professor of Chemical and Biomedical Engineering
Cleveland State University;
Cardiac Imaging Scientist
Cleveland Clinic
Cleveland, Ohio

Ulrike Hamper, MD
Professor of Radiology, Urology, and Pathology
Johns Hopkins University School of Medicine
Baltimore, Maryland

Christopher J. Hardy, PhD
Principal Scientist
GE Global Research
Niskayuna, New York

Jeffrey C. Hellinger, MD
Assistant Professor of Radiology
The Children's Hospital of Philadelphia
Philadelphia, Pennsylvania

Miguel Hernandez-Pampaloni, MD, PhD
Assistant Professor of Radiology
Chief, Nuclear Medicine
University of California San Francisco
San Francisco, California

Charles B. Higgins, MD
Professor of Radiology
University of California San Francisco
San Francisco, California

Vincent B. Ho, MD, MBA, FAHA
Fellow, American Heart Association
Professor, Uniformed Services University of the Health Sciences
President, North American Society for Cardiovascular Imaging
Guest Researcher, National Institutes of Health
Editorial Board, *Circulation: Cardiovascular Imaging*
Bethesda, Maryland

Maureen N. Hood, MS, RN, RT(R)(MR)
Assistant Professor
Department of Radiology and Radiological Sciences
Uniformed Services University of the Health Sciences
F. Edward Hébert School of Medicine
Bethesda, Maryland

Michael D. Hope, MD
Assistant Professor of Radiology
University of California San Francisco
San Francisco, California

Thomas A. Hope, MD
Resident in Radiology
University of California San Francisco
San Francisco, California

Jiang Hsieh, PhD
Adjunct Professor
Medical Physics Department
University of Wisconsin-Madison
Madison, Wisconsin;
Chief Scientist
GE Healthcare
Brookfield, Wisconsin

W. Gregory Hundley, MD
Professor
Wake Forest University School of Medicine
Winston-Salem, North Carolina

John Huston 3d, MD
Professor of Radiology
Mayo Clinic College of Medicine
Rochester, Minnesota

Neil R.A. Isaac, MD
Radiologist
North York General Hospital
Toronto, Ontario

Benjamin M. Jackson, MD, MS
Assistant Professor of Surgery
Division of Vascular Surgery and Endovascular Therapy
University of Pennsylvania
Philadelphia, Pennsylvania

Aditya Jain, MBBS, MPH
Research Fellow
Johns Hopkins Hospital
Baltimore, Maryland

Olga James
Nuclear Medicine Resident
Duke Hospital
Durham, North Carolina

Cylen Javidan-Nejad, MD
Assistant Professor
Mallinckrodt Institute of Radiology
Washington University;
Fellowship Director
Section of Cardiothoracic Imaging
Mallinckrodt Institute of Radiology
St. Louis, Missouri

Jean Jeudy, MD
Assistant Professor
Department of Diagnostic Radiology and Nuclear Medicine
University of Maryland, School of Medicine
Baltimore, Maryland

Saurabh Jha, MBBS, MRCS
Assistant Professor of Radiology
University of Pennsylvania
Philadelphia, Pennsylvania

Pamela T. Johnson, MD
Assistant Professor
Johns Hopkins University School of Medicine
Assistant Professor of Radiology
Johns Hopkins Hospital
Baltimore, Maryland

Praveen Jonnala, MD
Radiologist
Interventional Radiologist and Cardiac Imager
Long Beach Memorial Medical Center
Long Beach, California

Wouter J. Jukema, MD, PhD
Professor, Cardiology
Leiden University Medical Center
Department of Radiology, Division of Image Processing
Leiden, The Netherlands

Bobby Kalb, MD
Assistant Professor
Emory University School of Medicine
Atlanta, Georgia

Sanjeeva P. Kalva, MD
Assistant Professor of Radiology
Harvard Medical School
Assistant Radiologist
Massachusetts General Hospital
Boston, Massachusetts

John A. Kaufman, MD, FSIR
Radiologist
Professor of Radiology
Chief, Vascular Interventional Radiology
Dotter Interventional Institute
Oregon Health Sciences University
Portland, Oregon

Aoife N. Keeling, MD, FFR RCSI
Fellow
Cardiovascular and Interventional Radiology
Northwestern Memorial Hospital
Chicago, Illinois

Danny Kim, MSE, MD
Assistant Professor of Radiology
New York University School of Medicine
New York University Langone Medical Center
New York, New York

Sooah Kim, MD
Assistant Professor of Radiology
New York University School of Medicine
New York University Langone Medical Center
New York, New York

TaeHoon Kim, MD
Associate Professor of Radiology
Yunsei University College of Medicine;
Associate Professor
Department of Radiology
Gangnam Serverance Hospital, College of Medicine
Seoul, Korea

Amy Kirby, MD
Medical Director
Ponca City Regional, Logan Medical Center
Kingfisher Regional Medical Center
Oklahoma City, Oklahoma;
Eagle Eye Radiology
Reston, Virginia

Jacobo Kirsch, MD
Section Head
Cardiopulmonary Radiology
Cleveland Clinic Florida
Weston, Florida

Jonathan D. Kirsch, MD
Assistant Professor, Diagnostic Radiology
Associate Chief, Section of Ultrasound
Yale University School of Medicine
Yale-New Haven Hospital
New Haven, Connecticut

Pieter H. Kitslaar, MSc
Researcher, Image Processing
Leiden University Medical Center
Department of Radiology, Division of Image Processing
Leiden, The Netherlands

Michael V. Knopp, MD, PhD
Professor of Radiology
Director, Wright Center of Innovation in Biomedical Imaging
Novartis Chair of Imaging Research
The Ohio State University
Columbus, Ohio

Marc Kock, MD
Department of Radiology
Albert Schweitzer Hospital
Dordrecht, The Netherlands

Maureen P. Kohi, MD
Clinical Fellow
University of California San Francisco
San Francisco, California

Gerhard Koning, MSc
Researcher, Image Processing
Leiden University Medical Center
Department of Radiology, Division of Image Processing
Leiden, The Netherlands

Christopher M. Kramer, MD
Professor
Department of Radiology and Medicine
Director
Cardiovascular Imaging Center
University of Virginia Health System
Charlottesville, Virginia

Mayil S. Krishnam, MD, MRCP, DMRD (UK), FRCR (UK), ABR
Associate Clinical Professor
University of California Irvine
Irvine, California;
Director, Cardiovascular and Thoracic Imaging
UCI Medical Center
Orange, California

Rajesh Krishnamurthy, MBBS
Clinical Assistant Professor of Radiology and Pediatrics
Baylor College of Medicine;
Radiologist
EB Singleton Department of Pediatric Radiology
Texas Children's Hospital
Houston, Texas

Lucia J.M. Kroft, MD, PhD
Radiologist
Leiden University Medical Center
Leiden, The Netherlands

Rahul Kumar, MD
Clinical Cardiology Fellow
Wake Forest Baptist Medical Center
Winston-Salem, North Carolina

Raymond Kwong, MD, MPH, FACC
Assistant Professor of Medicine
Harvard Medical School;
Director, Cardiac Magnetic Resonance Imaging
Brigham and Women's Hospital
Boston, Massachusetts

Brajesh K. Lal, MD, FACS
Associate Professor, Departments of Vascular Surgery,
   Physiology, and Bioengineering
University of Maryland
Baltimore, Maryland

Warren Laskey, MD
Professor of Medicine
Chief, Division of Cardiology
University of New Mexico School of Medicine;
Chief, Division of Cardiology
University of New Mexico Hospital
Albuquerque, New Mexico

Vivian Lee, MBA, MD, PhD
Vice-Dean for Science
Chief Scientific Officer
Professor of Radiology
New York University Medical Center
New York, New York

Christianne Leidecker, PhD
Scientific Collaboration Manager
Siemens Medical Solutions USA, Inc.
Malvern, Pennsylvania

Tim Leiner, MD, PhD
Associate Professor of Radiology
Utrecht University Medical Center
Department of Radiology
Utrecht, The Netherlands

Rachel Booth Lewis, MD
Assistant Professor of Radiology
Uniformed Services University of Health Sciences;
Staff Radiologist
National Naval Medical Center
Bethesda, Maryland;
Chief of Gastrointestinal Radiology
Armed Forces Institute of Pathology
Washington, DC

Jonathan Liaw, MD, MRCP, FRCR
Assistant Professor of Diagnostic and Interventional
   Imaging
University of Texas Houston Medical School;
Assistant Radiologist
Memorial Hermann Hospital
Houston, Texas

Harold Litt, MD, PhD
Assistant Professor of Radiology and Medicine
University of Pennsylvania School of Medicine;
Chief, Cardiovascular Imaging Section
Hospital of the University of Pennsylvania
Philadelphia, Pennsylvania

Derek G. Lohan, MD
Consultant Radiologist
Galway University Hospitals;
Department of Radiology
Hospital Ground, Merlin Park Hospital
Galway, Republic of Ireland

Roi Lotan, MD
Faculty
Robert Wood Johnson University Hospital
New Brunswick, New Jersey

Amit Majmudar, MD
Nuclear Medicine/PET Specialist
Diagnostic Radiology
Radiology, Inc.
Powell, Ohio

Amgad N. Makaryus, MD
Assistant Professor of Clinical Medicine
New York University School of Medicine
New York, New York;
Director of Cardiac CT and MRI
Department of Cardiology
North Shore University Hospital
Manhasset, New York

Jeffrey H. Maki, MD, PhD
Department of Radiology
University of Washington School of Medicine
Puget Sound VA Health Care Service
Seattle, Washington

Neil Mardis, DO
Assistant Professor of Radiology
University of Missouri;
Pediatric Radiologist
The Children's Mercy Hospital and Clinics
Kansas City, Missouri

Henk A. Marquering, PhD
Assistant Professor, Cardiovascular Image Processing
Amsterdam Medical Center
Department of Biomedical Engineering and Physics
Amsterdam, The Netherlands

Diego Martin, MD, PhD
Professor of Radiology
Director of MRI
Emory University School of Medicine
Atlanta, Georgia

Alison Knauth Meadows, MD, PhD
Assistant Professor of Radiology and Pediatrics
University of California San Francisco
San Francisco, California

Lina Mehta, MD
Assistant Professor of Radiology
Associate Dean for Admissions
Case Western Reserve University
University Hospitals Case Medical Center
Cleveland, Ohio

Kristin Mercado, MD
Fellow in Cardiovascular Imaging
Harvard Medical School
Brigham and Women's Hospital
Boston, Massachusetts

Steven A. Messina, MD
Resident
Diagnostic Radiology and Nuclear Medicine
Department of Radiology
University of Florida College of Medicine
Gainesville, Florida

Cristopher A. Meyer, MD
Professor
University of Wisconsin School of Medicine and Public Health
Madison, Wisconsin

Mariana Meyers, MD
Resident
University Hospitals Case Medical Center
Cleveland, Ohio

Donald L. Miller, MD
Professor of Radiology and Radiological Sciences
Uniformed Services University of the Health Sciences;
Interventional Radiologist
Department of Radiology
National Naval Medical Center
Bethesda, Maryland

Edward J. Miller, MD, PhD
Assistant Professor
Uniformed Services University of the Health Sciences;
Staff Cardiologist
National Naval Medical Center
Bethesda, Maryland

Tan-Lucien Mohammed, MD
Residency Program Director, Imaging Institute
Fellowship Program Director, Section of Thoracic Imaging
Staff Radiologist, Section of Thoracic Imaging
Cleveland Clinic
Cleveland, Ohio

Phillip Moore, MD, MBA
Professor of Clinical Pediatrics
University of California San Francisco Medical School;
Director, Pediatric and Adult Congenital Cardiac Catheterization Laboratory
University of California San Francisco
San Francisco, California

Mariam Moshiri, MD
Clinical Assistant Professor
University of Washington
Clinical Assistant Professor
Director of Body Imaging Fellowship
University of Washington Medical Center
Seattle, Washington

Gaku Nakazawa, MD
CV Path Institute
Gaithersburg, Maryland

Gautam Nayak, MD
Department of Cardiology
National Naval Medical Center
Bethesda, Maryland

Kenneth J. Nichols, PhD
Associate Professor of Radiology
Hofstra University
Hempstead, New York;
Senior Medical Physicist
Division of Nuclear Medicine & Molecular Imaging
North Shore-Long Island Jewish Medical Center
Manhassett & New Hyde Park, New York

Jonathan A. Nye, PhD
Assistant Professor
Department of Radiology
Emory University
Atlanta, Georgia

James K. O'Donnell, MD
Professor of Radiology
School of Medicine
Case Western Reserve University;
Director of Nuclear Medicine
Case Medical Center
University Hospitals of Cleveland
Cleveland, Ohio

Karen G. Ordovas, MD
Assistant Professor of Radiology
University of California San Francisco
San Francisco, California

Hideki Ota, MD, PhD
Research Fellow
Michigan State University
East Lansing, Michigan

Jaap Ottenkamp, MD, PhD
Pediatric Cardiologist
Leiden University Medical Center
Leiden, The Netherlands

Maitraya K. Patel, MD
Assistant Professor of Radiology
David Geffen School of Medicine at UCLA
Los Angeles, California

Smita Patel, MBBS, MRCP, FRCR
Associate Professor of Radiology
University of Michigan Medical School
University of Michigan Medical Center
Ann Arbor, Michigan

Aurélio C. Pinheiro, MD, PhD
Post-Doctoral Research Fellow
Adult Echocardiography Laboratory
Johns Hopkins University
Baltimore, Maryland

Benjamin Pomerantz, MD
Instructor of Radiology
Harvard Medical School;
Assistant Radiologist
Massachusetts General Hospital
Boston, Massachusetts

Martin R. Prince, MD, PhD
Professor
Weill Cornell Medical Center;
Professor
Columbia College of Physicians and Surgeons
New York, New York

Joan C. Prowda, MD, JD
Associate Clinical Professor of Radiology
Columbia University College of Physicians and Surgeons;
Associate Attending
New York Presbyterian Hospital
New York, New York

Chirapa Puntawangkoon, MD
Research Fellow
Wake Forest University School of Medicine
Winston-Salem, North Carolina

Steven S. Raman, MD
Associate Professor of Radiology
David Geffen School of Medicine at UCLA
Los Angeles, California

Gautham P. Reddy, MD, MPH
Professor of Radiology
Vice Chair for Education
Director of Thoracic Imaging
Department of Radiology
University of Washington School of Medicine
Seattle, Washington

Johan H.C. Reiber, PhD
Head, Division of Image Processing
Leiden University Medical Center
Department of Radiology, Division of Image Processing
Leiden, The Netherlands

Justus E. Roos, MD
Assistant Professor
Stanford University;
Assistant Professor
Department of Radiology
Medical Center Stanford University
Stanford, California

Stefan G. Ruehm, MD, PhD
Associate Professor and Director, Cardiovascular CT
Director, Cardiovascular Imaging
Santa Monica Hospital
University of California Los Angeles;
Department of Radiology
Medical Center and Orthopedic Hospital
David Geffen School of Medicine at UCLA
Los Angeles, California

Raymond R. Russell, MD, PhD
Associate Professor of Medicine and Diagnostic Radiology
Yale University School of Medicine
New Haven, Connecticut

Marcel Santos, MD, PhD
Attending Radiologist
University Hospital of the School of Medicine of Ribeirao Preto
Sao Paulo, Brazil

U. Joseph Schoepf, MD, FAHA, FSCBT-MR, FSCCT
Professor of Radiology and Medicine
Director of Cardiovascular Imaging
Medical University of South Carolina
Charleston, South Carolina

Leslie M. Scoutt, MD
Professor of Diagnostic Radiology
Yale University School of Medicine;
Chief, Ultrasound Service
Yale-New Haven Hospital
New Haven, Connecticut

Laureen Sena, MD
Clinical Instructor
Harvard Medical School;
Staff Radiologist
Children's Hospital
Boston, Massachusetts

Nidhi Sharma, MD
Fellow, Section of Molecular and Functional Imaging
Cleveland Clinic
Cleveland, Ohio

Rajesh Sharma, MD
Department of Radiodiagnosis
Government Medical College Hospital
Jammu, India

Matthew J. Sharp, MD
Staff Radiologist
Portland Veterans Affairs Medical Center
Adjunct Professor, Oregon Health and Sciences University
Portland, Oregon

John J. Sheehan, MD, MRCSI, FFRRCSI
Assistant Professor of Radiology
The University of Chicago, Pritzker School of Medicine;
Director of Cardiovascular Imaging
NorthShore University Health System
Chicago, Illinois

Mark Sheldon, MD
Assistant Professor of Medicine
University of New Mexico, School of Medicine;
Assistant Professor
University of New Mexico Health Sciences Center
University of New Mexico Hospital
Albuquerque, New Mexico

Marilyn J. Siegel, MD
Professor of Radiology and Pediatrics
Washington University School of Medicine
St. Louis, Missouri

Albert J. Sinusas, MD
Professor of Medicine and Diagnostic Radiology
Director, Animal Research Laboratories, Section of Cardiovascular Medicine
Director, Cardiovascular Nuclear Imaging and Stress Laboratories
Yale University
New Haven, Connecticut

Ting Song, PhD
Assistant Professor
Department of Radiology
Uniformed Services University of the Health Sciences;
Scientist
GE Healthcare
Bethesda, Maryland

Anand Soni, MD
Cardiac Imaging Fellow
Massachusetts General Hospital
Harvard Medical School
Boston, Massachusetts

William Stanford, MD
Professor Emeritus
Roy T. and Lucille A. Carver College of Medicine
The University of Iowa;
Professor Emeritus
Department of Radiology
The University of Iowa Hospitals and Clinics
Iowa City, Iowa

Alexander B. Steever, MD
Assistant Clinical Professor of Radiology
Columbia University Medical Center
Harlem Hospital
New York, New York

Robert M. Steiner, MD
Professor of Radiology and Medicine
Temple University School of Medicine
Philadelphia, Pennsylvania;
Clinical Professor of Radiology
Stanford University School of Medicine
Stanford, California;
Chief, Thoracic Radiology
Temple University Hospital
Philadelphia, Pennsylvania

Jadranka Stojanovska, MD
Clinical Lecturer
Department of Radiology
University of Michigan Medical School
University of Michigan Medical Center
Ann Arbor, Michigan

Harikrishna Tandri, MD
Assistant Professor of Cardiology
Johns Hopkins Hospital
Baltimore, Maryland

Shawn D. Teague, MD
Associate Professor of Clinical Radiology
Indiana University School of Medicine
Indianapolis, Indiana

John S. Thurber, MD
Assistant Professor of Surgery
Uniformed Services University of the Health Sciences
F. Edward Hébert School of Medicine;
Integrated Chief of Cardiothoracic Surgery
Attending Cardiothoracic Surgeon
Captain, Medical Corps
United States Navy
National Naval Medical Center
Bethesda, Maryland;
Walter Reed Army Medical Center
Washington, DC

Ahmet T. Turgut, MD
Associate Professor in Radiology
Ankara Training and Research Hospital
Ankara, Turkey

Rob J. van der Geest, MSc
Assistant Professor, Image Processing
Leiden University Medical Center
Department of Radiology, Division of Image Processing
Leiden, The Netherlands

Ronald van 't Klooster, MSc
Researcher, Image Processing
Leiden University Medical Center
Department of Radiology, Division of Image Processing
Leiden, The Netherlands

Jens Vogel-Claussen, MD
Assistant Professor
Johns Hopkins University;
Department of Radiology
Tübingen University
Tübingen, Germany

John R. Votaw, PhD
Professor and Vice Chair for Research
Department of Radiology
Emory University
Atlanta, Georgia

Thomas G. Vrachliotis, MD, PhD
Director of Interventional Radiology
Henry Dunant Hospital
Athens, Greece

Dharshan Raj Vummidi, MRCP, FRCR
Acting Instructor and Senior Fellow in Cardiothoracic Imaging
University of Washington
Seattle, Washington

Stephen Waite, MD
Assistant Professor of Clinical Radiology and Internal Medicine
Chief of Cardiovascular Radiology
SUNY Downstate
Brooklyn, New York

T. Gregory Walker, MD
Instructor in Radiology
Harvard Medical School
Associate Radiologist
Fellowship Director, Vascular Imaging and Intervention
Massachusetts General Hospital
Boston, Massachusetts

Gaby Weissman, MD
Assistant Professor of Medicine
Georgetown University;
Cardiac Imaging
Washington Hospital Center
Washington, DC

Charles S. White, MD
Professor of Radiology
Director of Thoracic Imaging
Department of Radiology
University of Maryland
Baltimore, Maryland

Kevin K. Whitehead, MD, PhD
Assistant Professor of Pediatrics
University of Pennsylvania School of Medicine;
Noninvasive Imaging
Children's Hospital of Philadelphia
Philadelphia, Pennsylvania

Oliver Wieben, PhD
Assistant Professor
Departments of Medical Physics and Radiology
University of Wisconsin
Madison, Wisconsin

Eric E. Williamson, MD
Assistant Professor, Cardiovascular Radiology
Mayo Clinic Rochester
Rochester, Minnesota

Priscilla A. Winchester, MD
Associate Professor of Clinical Radiology
Weill Cornell Medical College
New York Presbyterian Hospital
New York, New York

Carol C. Wu, MD
Clinical Instructor
Harvard Medical School
Assistant Radiologist
Massachusetts General Hospital
Boston, Massachusetts

Louis Wu, MD, CM
Director, MRI
Department of Radiology
Lakeridge Health Oshawa
Oshawa, Ontario, Canada

Vahid Yaghmai, MD, MS
  Associate Professor
  Northwestern University;
  Medical Director CT
  Northwestern Memorial Hospital
  Chicago, Illinois

Douglas Yim, MD
  Assistant Professor of Radiology and Radiologist Sciences
  Uniformed Services University of the Health Sciences;
  Chief, Interventional Radiology
  National Naval Medical Center
  Bethesda, Maryland

Phillip M. Young, MD
  Assistant Professor of Diagnostic Radiology
  Mayo Clinic College of Medicine;
  Senior Associate Consultant in Diagnostic Radiology
  Mayo Clinic
  Rochester, Minnesota

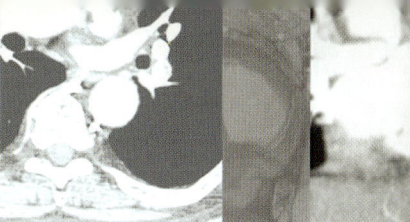

Preface

The ability to image the cardiovascular system has improved exponentially over the past 20 years. This project began rather modestly but quickly ballooned to a two-volume book of 119 chapters as we began to lengthen our list of the most important cardiovascular imaging techniques and common conditions. We were fortunate to have enlisted an excellent group of highly dedicated experts from the best universities and cardiovascular centers in the world.

Our book consists of two volumes: Cardiac Imaging (Volume I) and Vascular Imaging (Volume II). Section 1 of Volume I begins with an introduction to normal cardiac embryology, anatomy, and physiology. Section 2 reviews the physics and technical considerations for the various cardiac imaging techniques ranging from plain film, echocardiography, and invasive catheterization to advanced cardiac CT, MR, SPECT, and PET/CT. This section is supplemented by special discussions on CT dose reduction strategies, CT and MR contrast agents, MR safety, radiopharmaceuticals, and pharmacologic stress agents. Section 3 is dedicated to cardiac interventions, covering both percutaneous as well as open procedures. In Section 4, coronary artery imaging is reviewed with detailed discussions of imaging of coronary artery calcium, congenital coronary anomalies, obstructive coronary disease, coronary artery aneurysms, and coronary revascularization procedures. Section 5 reviews the wide variety of acyanotic and cyanotic congenital heart disease with special mention of coarctation of the aorta as well as vascular rings and slings. In Section 6, the pathologic basis for ischemic heart disease is reviewed and followed by detailed discussions of myocardial perfusion, function, and viability as determined by CT, MR, and radionuclide imaging. Valvular heart disease is reviewed in Section 7. Section 8 details the various forms of cardiomyopathy (i.e., dilated, restrictive, and hypertrophic), including chapters on arrhythmogenic right ventricular dysplasia and myocarditis. Section 9 provides a brilliant pictorial of cardiac tumors. In Section 10, pericardial diseases are discussed.

Volume II is devoted to vascular imaging and begins with Section 11, which reviews normal arterial and venous anatomy in the thorax, abdomen, pelvis, and extremities. Section 12 provides a technical and clinical discussion of vascular ultrasound, CT angiography (CTA), MR angiography (MRA), CTA/MRA image postprocessing, and vascular applications of nuclear medicine. Section 13 provides a review of the various arterial percutaneous and open procedures. Noninvasive imaging of atherosclerotic plaque ("plaque imaging") is reviewed in Section 14. In Section 15, carotid artery disease and imaging using ultrasound, CTA, and MRA are reviewed. Section 16 discusses common vascular thoracic conditions such as thoracic aortic aneurysm, acute aortic syndrome, aortic trauma, aortitis, pulmonary thromboembolism, pulmonary arterial hypertension, pulmonary edema and pulmonary hemorrhage, and vasculitis. This is followed by Section 17, which explores imaging considerations for the various abdominal vascular conditions such as abdominal aortic disease, endograft arterial repair, open surgical arterial repair, renal artery hypertension, renal and central venous conditions, hepatic transplantation, and renal and pancreatic transplantation. In Section 18, peripheral arterial disease and lower extremity imaging are described, with inclusion of newer techniques for peripheral CTA and MRA. In Section 19, upper extremity vascular imaging applications, including hemodialysis fistulas, are discussed.

This project is the culmination of many years of experience from a multitude of contributors with a variety of backgrounds. We hope that readers will enjoy reading the chapters as well as appreciate the expert recommendations provided by our contributors.

In addition to the contributing authors, we would like to thank many people at Elsevier—notably Rebecca Gaertner for entrusting this most important portion of the *Expert Radiology* collection to us, Jennifer Shreiner for providing critical and timely editorial guidance and assistance, and Fran Gunning and Carrie Stetz for providing terrific closure for this project.

Vincent B. Ho, MD, MBA, FAHA
Bethesda, Maryland

Gautham P. Reddy, MD, MPH
Seattle, Washington

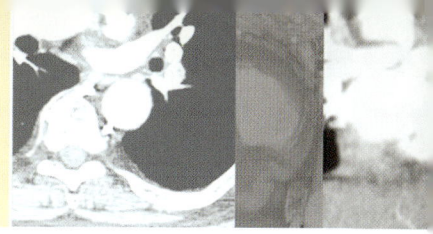

Contents

VOLUME I

PART ONE: AN INTRODUCTION TO THE HEART

CHAPTER 1 Embryologic Basis and Segmental Approach to Imaging of Congenital Heart Disease   3
Rajesh Krishnamurthy

CHAPTER 2 Cardiac Anatomy   30
Dharshan Raj Vummidi and Gautham P. Reddy

CHAPTER 3 Coronary Anatomy   38
Jadranka Stojanovska and Smita Patel

CHAPTER 4 Physiology of the Heart   57
Phillip M. Young and Thomas C. Gerber

PART TWO: CARDIAC IMAGING TECHNIQUES

CHAPTER 5 Radiology of the Heart: Plain Film Imaging and Diagnosis   71
Robert M. Steiner

CHAPTER 6 Echocardiography   98
Theodore P. Abraham and Aurélio C. Pinheiro

CHAPTER 7 Diagnostic Coronary Angiography   123
Curtis E. Green

CHAPTER 8 Physics of Cardiac Computed Tomography   133
Christianne Leidecker

CHAPTER 9 Clinical Techniques of Cardiac Computed Tomography   143
Shawn D. Teague

CHAPTER 10 Radiation Dose Reduction Strategies in Cardiac Computed Tomography   150
Sandra Simon Halliburton

CHAPTER 11 Contrast Agents and Medications in Cardiac Computed Tomography   156
Justus E. Roos

CHAPTER 12 Image Postprocessing in Cardiac Computed Tomography   167
Elliot K. Fishman and Pamela T. Johnson

CHAPTER 13 Methods for Cardiac Magnetic Resonance Imaging   180
Thomas K.F. Foo and Christopher J. Hardy

CHAPTER 14 Clinical Techniques of Cardiac Magnetic Resonance Imaging: Morphology, Perfusion, and Viability   201
Louis Wu and Gautham P. Reddy

CHAPTER 15 Clinical Techniques of Cardiac Magnetic Resonance Imaging: Function   215
Rahul Kumar and W. Gregory Hundley

CHAPTER 16 Clinical Techniques of Cardiac Magnetic Resonance Imaging: Functional Interpretation and Image Processing   227
Chirapa Puntawangkoon and W. Gregory Hundley

CHAPTER 17 Magnetic Resonance Evaluation of Blood Flow   239
Michael D. Hope, Karen G. Ordovas, Thomas A. Hope, Alison Knauth Meadows, Charles B. Higgins, and Gautham P. Reddy

CHAPTER 18 Contrast Agents in Magnetic Resonance Imaging   251
Michael V. Knopp

CHAPTER 19 Magnetic Resonance Imaging Safety   261
Maureen N. Hood

CHAPTER 20 Physics and Instrumentation of Cardiac Single Photon Emission Computed Tomography   270
Edward J. Miller and Raymond R. Russell

CHAPTER 21 Clinical Single Photon Emission Computed Tomography Cardiac Protocols   281
Miguel Hernandez-Pampaloni

CHAPTER 22 Radiopharmaceutical Single Photon Emission Computed Tomography Imaging Agents   298
Alexander Bustamante and Gautam Nayak

CHAPTER 23 Physics and Instrumentation of Cardiac Positron Emission Tomography/Computed Tomography 304
John R. Votaw and Jonathan A. Nye

CHAPTER 24 Clinical Techniques of Positron Emission Tomography and PET/CT 325
Marcelo F. Di Carli and Mouaz H. Al-Mallah

CHAPTER 25 Radiopharmaceuticals and Radiation Dose Considerations in Cardiac Positron Emission Tomography and PET/CT 339
Gaby Weissman and Albert J. Sinusas

CHAPTER 26 Pharmacologic Stress Agents 352
Alexander Bustamante and Gautam Nayak

PART THREE: CARDIAC INTERVENTIONS

CHAPTER 27 Congenital Percutaneous Interventions 363
Phillip Moore

CHAPTER 28 Congenital Cardiac Surgery 383
Frederick K. Emge and Christian L. Gilbert

CHAPTER 29 Percutaneous Catheter-Based Treatment of Coronary and Valvular Heart Disease 393
Mark Sheldon and Warren Laskey

CHAPTER 30 Surgery for Acquired Cardiac Disease 412
John S. Thurber and Subrato J. Deb

CHAPTER 31 Imaging of Atrial Fibrillation Intervention 442
Cristopher A. Meyer and Mehran Attari

PART FOUR: CORONARY ARTERY IMAGING

CHAPTER 32 Coronary Calcium Assessment 457
William Stanford

CHAPTER 33 Congenital Coronary Anomalies 466
James P. Earls

CHAPTER 34 Indications and Patient Selection in Obstructive Coronary Disease 477
Eva Maria Gassner and U. Joseph Schoepf

CHAPTER 35 Interpretation and Reporting in Obstructive Coronary Disease 493
Tamar Gaspar

CHAPTER 36 Coronary Artery Aneurysms 509
Jon C. George, Mariana Meyers, and Robert C. Gilkeson

CHAPTER 37 Imaging of Coronary Revascularization: Coronary Stents and Bypass Grafts 515
Jean Jeudy, Stephen Waite, and Joseph Jen-Sho Chen

PART FIVE: CONGENITAL HEART DISEASE

CHAPTER 38 Coarctation of the Aorta 535
Marilyn J. Siegel

CHAPTER 39 Vascular Rings and Slings 542
Marilyn J. Siegel

CHAPTER 40 Magnetic Resonance Imaging of the Aorta and Left Ventricular Function in Inherited and Congenital Aortic Disease 549
Heynric B. Grotenhuis, Jaap Ottenkamp, Lucia J.M. Kroft, and Albert de Roos

Section One: Acyanotic Heart Disease with Increased Vascularity

CHAPTER 41 Atrial Septal Defect 563
Amgad N. Makaryus and Lawrence M. Boxt

CHAPTER 42 Ventricular Septal Defect 572
Amgad N. Makaryus and Lawrence M. Boxt

CHAPTER 43 Patent Ductus Arteriosus 583
Cylen Javidan-Nejad

Section Two: Cyanotic Heart Disease with Increased Vascularity

CHAPTER 44 Transposition of the Great Arteries 601
Frandics P. Chan

CHAPTER 45 Truncus Arteriosus 616
Frandics P. Chan

CHAPTER 46 Anomalous Pulmonary Venous Connections and Drainage 625
Laureen Sena and Neil Mardis

CHAPTER 47 Tetralogy of Fallot 640
S. Bruce Greenberg

CHAPTER 48 Ebstein Anomaly 654
Jeffrey C. Hellinger

CHAPTER 49 Complex Congenital Heart Disease 656
Kevin K. Whitehead, Stanford Ewing, and Mark A. Fogel

CHAPTER 50 Magnetic Resonance Imaging in the Postoperative Evaluation of the Patient with Congenital Heart Disease 689
Alison Knauth Meadows, Karen G. Ordovas, Charles B. Higgins, and Gautham P. Reddy

PART SIX: ISCHEMIC HEART DISEASE

CHAPTER 51 Atherosclerotic Coronary Artery Disease 705
Allen Burke, Gaku Nakazawa, and Charles S. White

CHAPTER 52 Acute Coronary Syndrome 715
Joseph Jen-Sho Chen and Charles S. White

CHAPTER 53 **Magnetic Resonance and Computed Tomographic Imaging of Myocardial Perfusion** 726
Ricardo C. Cury, Anand Soni, and Ron Blankstein

CHAPTER 54 **Nuclear Medicine Imaging of Myocardial Perfusion** 738
Olga James, Kenneth J. Nichols, and Bennett Chin

CHAPTER 55 **Magnetic Resonance and Computed Tomographic Imaging of Myocardial Function** 752
Kristin Mercado and Raymond Kwong

CHAPTER 56 **Nuclear Medicine Imaging of Ventricular Function** 771
Bennett Chin and Kenneth J. Nichols

CHAPTER 57 **Magnetic Resonance Imaging of Myocardial Viability** 781
Zelmira Curillova and Raymond Kwong

CHAPTER 58 **Nuclear Medicine Imaging of Myocardial Viability** 790
Steven A. Messina and Vasken Dilsizian

CHAPTER 59 **Postoperative Imaging of Ischemic Cardiac Disease** 810
Praveen Jonnala, Swati Deshmane, and Mayil S. Krishnam

PART SEVEN: VALVULAR HEART DISEASE

CHAPTER 60 **Aortic and Mitral Valvular Disease** 827
Roi Lotan and Jens Vogel-Claussen

CHAPTER 61 **Tricuspid and Pulmonary Valvular Disease** 839
Jeffrey C. Hellinger

PART EIGHT: CARDIOMYOPATHIES AND OTHER MYOCARDIAL DISEASES

CHAPTER 62 **Dilated Cardiomyopathy** 851
James F. Glockner

CHAPTER 63 **Restrictive Cardiomyopathy** 861
James F. Glockner

CHAPTER 64 **Hypertrophic Cardiomyopathy** 874
Gautham P. Reddy, Matthew J. Sharp, and Karen G. Ordovas

CHAPTER 65 **Arrhythmogenic Right Ventricular Dysplasia** 884
Aditya Jain, Harikrishna Tandri, Hugh Calkins, and David A. Bluemke

CHAPTER 66 **Myocarditis** 896
Carol C. Wu and Mayil S. Krishnam

PART NINE: TUMORS AND MASSES

CHAPTER 67 **Cardiac Tumors** 905
Aletta Ann Frazier and Rachel Booth Lewis

PART TEN: PERICARDIAL DISEASE

CHAPTER 68 **Pericardial Effusion** 941
Lynn S. Broderick

CHAPTER 69 **Acute Pericarditis** 945
Lynn S. Broderick

CHAPTER 70 **Constrictive Pericarditis** 949
Lynn S. Broderick

VOLUME II

PART ELEVEN: VASCULAR ANATOMY AND CIRCULATION/ARTERIAL ANATOMY

CHAPTER 71 **Arterial Anatomy of the Thorax** 955
Amy Kirby, Jacobo Kirsch, and Eric E. Williamson

CHAPTER 72 **Arterial Anatomy of the Abdomen** 969
Jeremy C. Durack and Maureen P. Kohi

CHAPTER 73 **Arterial Anatomy of the Pelvis and Lower Extremities** 978
Douglas Yim and Donald L. Miller

CHAPTER 74 **Arterial Anatomy of the Upper Extremities** 989
Douglas Yim and Donald L. Miller

CHAPTER 75 **Venous Anatomy of the Thorax** 996
Jacobo Kirsch, Amy Kirby, and Eric E. Williamson

CHAPTER 76 **Venous Anatomy of the Abdomen and Pelvis** 1005
Jeremy C. Durack and Maureen P. Kohi

CHAPTER 77 **Venous Anatomy of the Extremities** 1019
Jeffrey C. Hellinger

PART TWELVE: NONINVASIVE VASCULAR IMAGING TECHNIQUES

CHAPTER 78 **Vascular Ultrasonography: Physics, Instrumentation, and Clinical Techniques** 1033
Elif Ergun, Ahmet T. Turgut, A. Sanli Ergun, and Vikram S. Dogra

CHAPTER 79 **Physics of Computed Tomography** 1047
Jiang Hsieh

CHAPTER 80 **Computed Tomographic Angiography: Clinical Techniques** 1055
John J. Sheehan, Aoife N. Keeling, Vahid Yaghmai, and James C. Carr

CHAPTER 81 **Magnetic Resonance Angiography: Physics and Instrumentation** 1078
Oliver Wieben and Thorsten Bley

CHAPTER 82 **Magnetic Resonance Angiography: Clinical Techniques** 1102
Stefan G. Ruehm and Derek G. Lohan

CHAPTER 83 **Basic Three-Dimensional Postprocessing in Computed Tomographic and Magnetic Resonance Angiography** 1120
Ting Song, William R. Corse, and Vincent B. Ho

CHAPTER 84 **Advanced Three-Dimensional Postprocessing in Computed Tomographic and Magnetic Resonance Angiography** 1128
Rob J. van der Geest, Pieter H. Kitslaar, Patrick J.H. de Koning, Ronald van 't Klooster, Wouter J. Jukema, Gerhard Koning, Henk A. Marquering, and Johan H.C. Reiber

CHAPTER 85 **Nuclear Medicine: Extrathoracic Vascular Imaging** 1144
Amit Majmudar and James K. O'Donnell

PART THIRTEEN: CATHETER ANGIOGRAPHY AND INTERVENTIONS

CHAPTER 86 **Percutaneous Vascular Interventions** 1155
Jonathan Liaw, Benjamin Pomerantz, and Sanjeeva P. Kalva

CHAPTER 87 **Vascular Surgery** 1172
Christopher J. Abularrage and David H. Deaton

PART FOURTEEN: ATHEROSCLEROSIS

CHAPTER 88 **Noninvasive Imaging of Atherosclerosis** 1193
Jamieson M. Bourque and Christopher M. Kramer

PART FIFTEEN: THE CAROTID ARTERIES

CHAPTER 89 **Carotid Artery Disease** 1217
Brajesh K. Lal and Thomas G. Brott

CHAPTER 90 **Ultrasound Evaluation of the Carotid Arteries** 1227
Leslie M. Scoutt, Jonathan D. Kirsch, and Ulrike Hamper

CHAPTER 91 **Magnetic Resonance and Computed Tomographic Angiography of the Extracranial Carotid Arteries** 1251
J. Kevin DeMarco, John Huston 3d, and Hideki Ota

PART SIXTEEN: THE THORACIC VESSELS

CHAPTER 92 **Thoracic Aortic Aneurysms** 1271
Saurabh Jha and Harold Litt

CHAPTER 93 **Acute Aortic Syndrome** 1288
TaeHoon Kim and Harold Litt

CHAPTER 94 **Thoracic Aortic Trauma** 1306
Jonathan Balcombe and Harold Litt

CHAPTER 95 **Thoracic Aortitis** 1314
Neil R.A. Isaac and Harold Litt

CHAPTER 96 **Subclavian Steal Syndrome** 1326
Dharshan Raj Vummidi and Gautham P. Reddy

CHAPTER 97 **Acute Pulmonary Thromboembolic Disease** 1332
Nidhi Sharma and Tan-Lucien Mohammed

CHAPTER 98 **Chronic Pulmonary Embolism** 1344
Sanjeev Bhalla

CHAPTER 99 **Pulmonary Hypertension** 1353
Michael B. Gotway

CHAPTER 100 **Pulmonary Edema** 1373
Michael B. Gotway

CHAPTER 101 **Pulmonary Hemorrhage and Vasculitis** 1383
Michael B. Gotway

PART SEVENTEEN: THE ABDOMINAL VESSELS

CHAPTER 102 **The Abdominal Aorta** 1397
Martin L. Gunn, Jonathan H. Chung, Michelle M. Bittle, and Jeffrey H. Maki

CHAPTER 103 **Postendograft Imaging of the Abdominal Aorta and Iliac Arteries** 1420
Thomas G. Vrachliotis, Kostaki G. Bis, and Lisa M. Dias

CHAPTER 104 **Open Repair of Abdominal Aortic Aneurysms and Postoperative Assessment** 1439
Lisa M. Dias, Kostaki G. Bis, and Thomas G. Vrachliotis

CHAPTER 105 **Magnetic Resonance Imaging of Vascular Disorders of the Abdomen** 1451
Marcel Santos, Bobby Kalb, and Diego Martin

CHAPTER 106 **Renal Artery Hypertension** 1471
Tim Leiner

CHAPTER 107 **Renal Arteries: Computed Tomographic and Magnetic Resonance Angiography** 1483
Danny Kim, Sooah Kim, and Vivian Lee

CHAPTER 108 **Renal Artery Scintigraphy** 1492
Lina Mehta, James K. O'Donnell, and Peter Faulhaber

CHAPTER 109 **Sonography of the Renal Vessels** 1497
Rajesh Sharma and Vikram S. Dogra

CHAPTER 110 **Inferior Vena Cava and Its Main Tributaries** 1524
Carlos Cuevas, Manjiri Dighe, and Mariam Moshiri

CHAPTER 111 **Vascular Imaging of Hepatic Transplantation** 1544
Maitraya K. Patel and Steven S. Raman

CHAPTER 112 **Vascular Imaging of Renal and Pancreatic Transplantation** 1559
Alexander B. Steever, Martin R. Prince, Priscilla A. Winchester, and Joan C. Prowda

PART EIGHTEEN: THE LOWER EXTREMITY VESSELS

CHAPTER 113 **Peripheral Artery Disease** 1573
Benjamin M. Jackson and Jeffrey P. Carpenter

CHAPTER 114 **Lower Extremity Operations and Interventions** 1585
T. Gregory Walker, Sanjeeva P. Kalva, and John A. Kaufman

CHAPTER 115 **Computed Tomographic Angiography of the Lower Extremities** 1610
Saurabh Jha and Harold Litt

CHAPTER 116 **Peripheral Magnetic Resonance Angiography** 1628
Tim Leiner

PART NINETEEN: THE UPPER EXTREMITY VESSELS

CHAPTER 117 **Vascular Diseases of the Upper Extremities** 1643
Tim Leiner and Marc Kock

CHAPTER 118 **Venous Sonography of the Upper Extremities and Thoracic Outlet** 1661
Jonathan D. Kirsch, Ulrike Hamper, and Leslie M. Scoutt

CHAPTER 119 **Hemodialysis Fistulas** 1672
Tim Leiner

Index I-1

PART ONE

An Introduction to the Heart

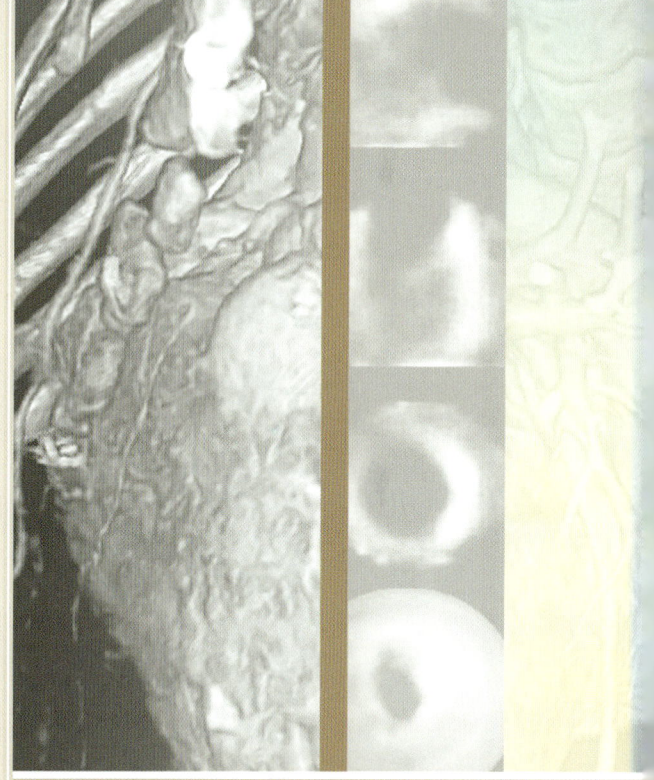

CHAPTER 1

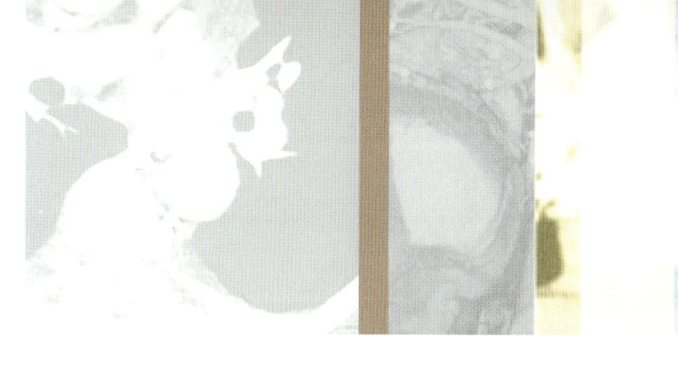

Embryologic Basis and Segmental Approach to Imaging of Congenital Heart Disease

Rajesh Krishnamurthy

There is incredible diversity in the types of human hearts. The first step to accurate diagnosis and management of congenital heart disease is a standardized and logical approach to not only understanding, but also describing, the disease process. This is called the *segmental approach* to heart disease,[1-3] first proposed by Richard Van Praagh in 1972, and later modified by others.[4] It is strongly rooted in embryologic principles, and follows a logical sequence from evaluation of morphology and physiology of the heart to decision making regarding treatment. This chapter will summarize the key events of cardiac development and link them to the developmental pathology of the common congenital heart diseases. The discussion of embryology will follow a morphologic approach, and will lay the groundwork for understanding the segmental approach to heart disease by cross-sectional imaging. The molecular genetic basis of cardiac development and congenital heart disease is beyond the scope of this chapter.

CARDIAC EMBRYOLOGY

Formation of the Heart Tube

During the first 2 weeks of embryonic life, there is no heart or vascular system. Cell-to-cell diffusion provides nutrient and oxygen supply to the fetus. As the fetus grows, the stored food supply in the yolk sac is unable to support fetal life, and the cardiovascular system must develop to transfer nutrition from the maternal umbilical cord. The heart develops from two simple epithelial tubes that fuse to form a single-chambered heart that is efficiently pumping blood by the fourth week of embryonic development. The origins of the heart tube are clusters of angiogenic cells that are located in the cardiogenic crescent. The cardiogenic crescent is derived from splanchnopleuric mesoderm, and is located cranial and lateral to the neural plate. These angiogenic cell clusters coalesce to form right and left endocardial tubes.[5] Each tube is continuous cranially with a dorsal aorta, its outflow tract, and caudally with a vitello-umbilical vein, its inflow tract. The lateral and cranial folding of the embryo forces the tubes into the thoracic cavity. As a result, these tubes come to lie closer to each other and begin to fuse in a cranial to caudal direction. At approximately day 21, they are completely fused. The splanchnic mesoderm around the heart tube thickens and forms the myoepicardial mantle (future myocardium and epicardium).

Components of the Heart Tube

From caudal to cranial, the following components of the newly formed heart tube (Fig. 1-1) are:

Sinus venosus: consists of right and left horns. Each horn receives blood from three important veins: the umbilical vein, the common cardinal vein, and the vitelline vein.
Paired primitive atria: will later fuse to form a common atrium
Atrioventricular sulcus: divides the common atrium and the primitive ventricle
Primitive ventricle: becomes the left ventricle

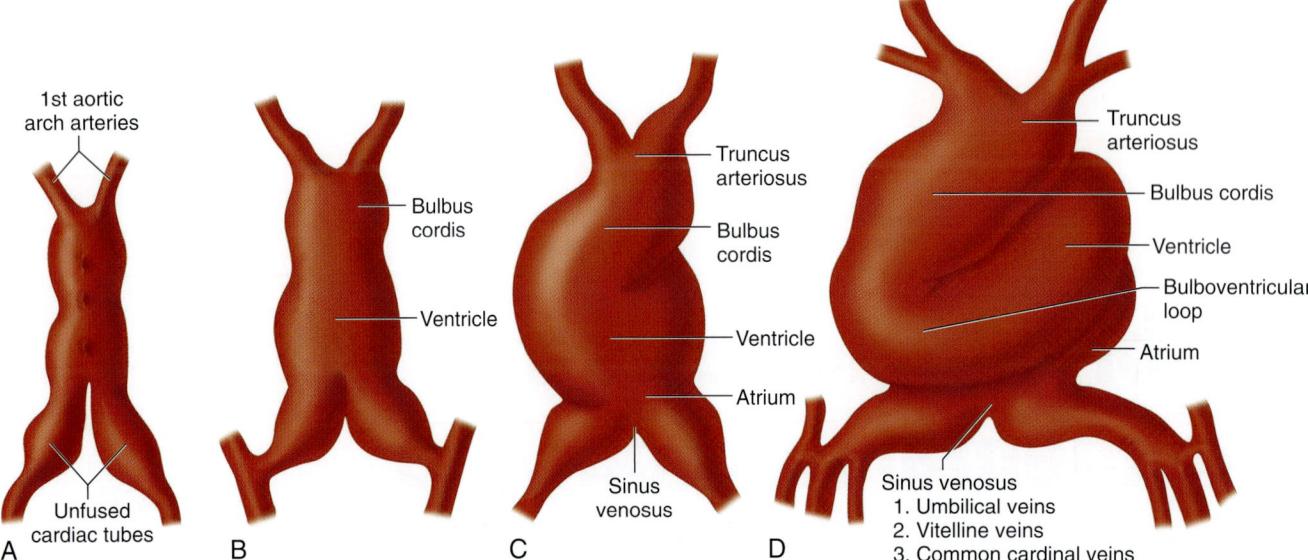

FIGURE 1-1 Development of the primitive heart tube. **A,** Paired cardiac tubes fuse in cephalad to caudad direction. **B,** Fused cardiac tube with beginning of chamber differentiation. **C,** Bulboventricular looping to the right. **D,** Heart tube after completion of bulboventricular looping. Various chambers of the heart are well delineated. *(Adapted from Gedgaudas E, Moller JH, Castaneda-Zuniga WR, Amplatz K. Embryology and anatomy of the heart. In Gedgaudas E, Moller JH, Castaneda-Zuniga WR, Amplatz K [eds]. Cardiovascular Radiology. Philadelphia, WB Saunders, 1985, pp 1-23.)*

Interventricular sulcus: divides the primitive ventricle and the bulbus cordis

Bulbus cordis: This may be divided as follows: the proximal one third gives rise to the body of the right ventricle. The distal-most section is called the *truncus arteriosus*, which develops into the aortic root and part of the ascending aorta. The remaining mid-portion is called the *conus cordis* and connects the primitive right ventricle to the truncus arteriosus. The conus cordis partitions to form the outflow tracts of the right and left ventricles.

Aortic sac: will give rise to the aortic arches

Bulboventricular Looping and Formation of the Ventricles

Whereas the two ends of the heart tube remain relatively fixed, rapid growth of the middle section results in the development of a large S-shaped curve called *the bulboventricular loop* (Fig. 1-2). As the heart tube grows and becomes longer, it usually bends to the right, termed by Van Praagh as *D-looping*.[1,3] D-looping is responsible for the proximal bulbus cordis (RV) lying anterior and to the right of the primitive ventricle (LV). If the heart tube loops to the left, termed *L-looping*, the RV will lie anterior and to the left of the LV. The mechanisms underlying normal looping are still being studied, but they are under strong genetic control.[6-8] Failure of normal looping (i.e., looping of the heart tube to the left) is a very early embryologic defect,[9] and it is not surprising that associated defects of septation and valve formation are the rule rather than the exception.

Formation of the Ventricles and Interventricular Septum

In the newly formed bulboventricular loop, the primitive right and left ventricles appear as expansions in the heart tube. The interventricular sulcus/ridge separates the right and left ventricles (Fig. 1-3). Both ventricles will continue to expand until the late 7th/early 8th week. The growth of the ventricles is due to the centrifugal growth of the myocardium and the diverticulation of the internal walls, which gives the ventricle its trabeculated appearance. The development of the interventricular septum begins around the 27th day of gestation. It develops from three embryonic components: the endocardial cushions, the conus cushions, and the muscular septum (Fig. 1-4). The fusion of the opposing ventricular walls gives rise to the muscular interventricular septum. The endocardial cushions divide the inflow tracts from the ventricles. The conus cushions divide the outflow region of the ventricles.

Developmental Pathology

Failure of ventricular septation causes various forms of ventricular septal defects (VSD). If the interventricular ridge does not form, the result is a single ventricle. If portions of the ventricular ridge do not fuse, multiple muscular defects are the result. A lack of contribution of endocardial or conal tissue results in a high inlet, an outlet, or a membranous type VSD.

Division of the Atrioventricular Canal

Because the proximal bulbus cordis gives rise to the RV, blood flows in series from the primitive atrium to the left

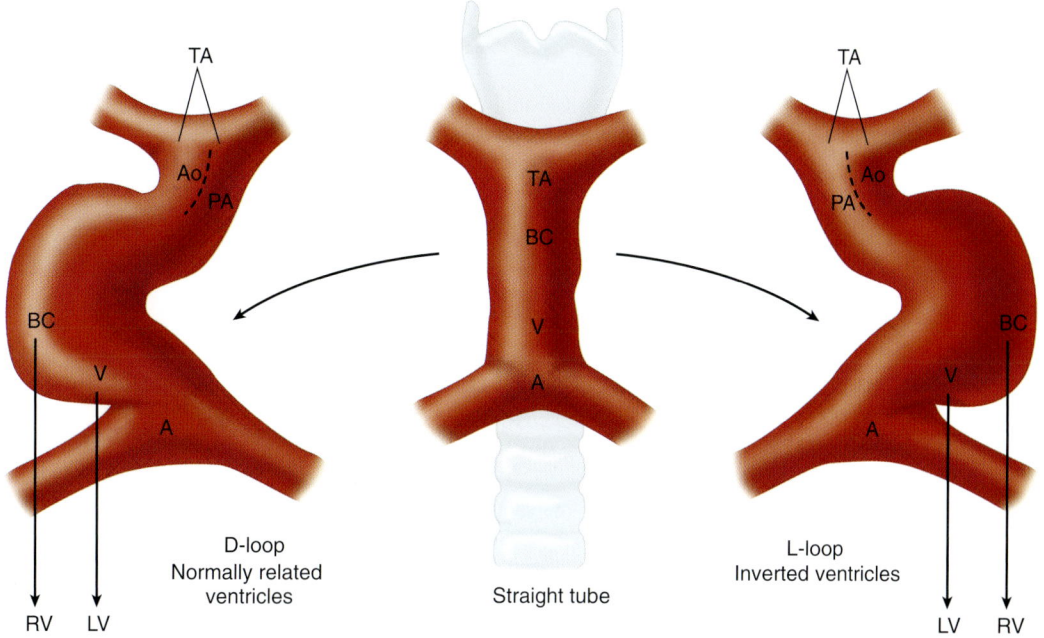

FIGURE 1-2 Bulboventricular looping of the primitive heart tube may occur to the right (D-looping) or to the left (L-looping). A, primitive atrium; V, primitive ventricle; BC, bulbus cordis; TA, truncus arteriosus; Ao, aorta; PA, pulmonary artery. *(Adapted from Van Praagh R, Weinberg PM, Matsuoka R, Van Praagh S. Malposition of the heart and the segmental approach to diagnosis. In Adams FH, Emmanouilides GC [eds]. Moss' Heart Diseases in Infants, Children and Adolescents, 3rd. ed. Baltimore, Williams and Wilkins, 1983, pp 422-458.)*

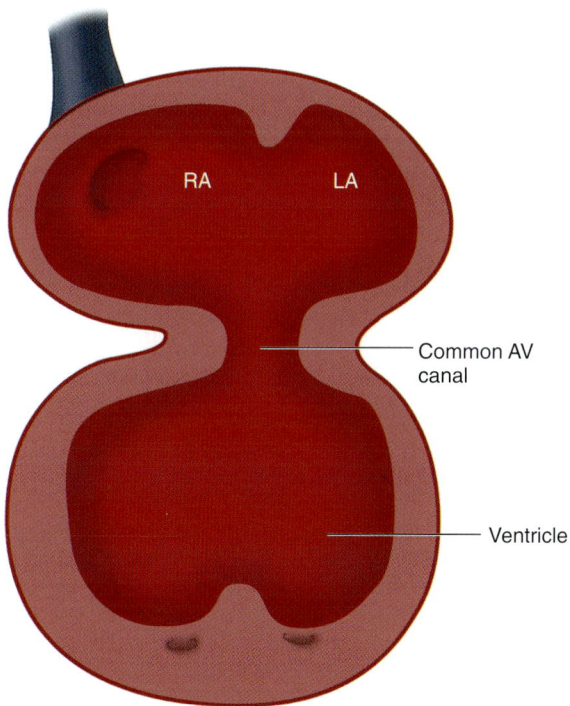

FIGURE 1-3 Development of the atrioventricular (AV) canal. At this stage, the AV canal connects the left side of the common atrium to the left side of the common ventricle.

ventricle, and then to the RV (see Fig. 1-1). There is no direct communication between the atria and the RV—even after the formation of the bulboventricular loop. The atrioventricular canal must shift to the right to achieve communication to the right ventricle in addition to the left ventricle (see Fig. 1-3). Swellings of mesenchymal tissue, the endocardial cushions, appear on the borders of the atrioventricular canal. There are four cushions: inferior and superior (ventral and dorsal), left and right. These are the precursors of the atrioventricular valves and they function during this early development as primitive valves. The endocardial cushions grow toward each other and fuse at approximately day 42, separating the atrioventricular canal into two openings which will eventually become the tricuspid and mitral valves (Fig. 1-4). The fused endocardial cushions are also responsible for the closure of the ostium primum by fusing with the free edge of the septum primum.

Developmental Pathology

Failure of the endocardial cushions to form will produce an AV canal defect (also known as an *endocardial cushion defect*). Incomplete endocardial cushion formation leads to variations of primum atrial septal defect, AV valve malformations, and/or inlet ventricular septal defect. Failure of the endocardial cushion tissue to shift over both ventricles can result in both AV valves entering the primitive left ventricle, forming a double inlet left ventricle. Failure of the endocardial cushions to shift to their normal position over the ventricles, combined with problems in ventricular septation, can also produce an "unbalanced AV canal" with a large single valve situated primarily over one ventricle.[10]

The tricuspid and mitral valves are formed by the endocardial cushion tissue. Stenosis of the atrioventricular valves is probably the result of partial fusion, whereas atresia of the atrioventricular valves probably results from complete fusion of the tissue.[5]

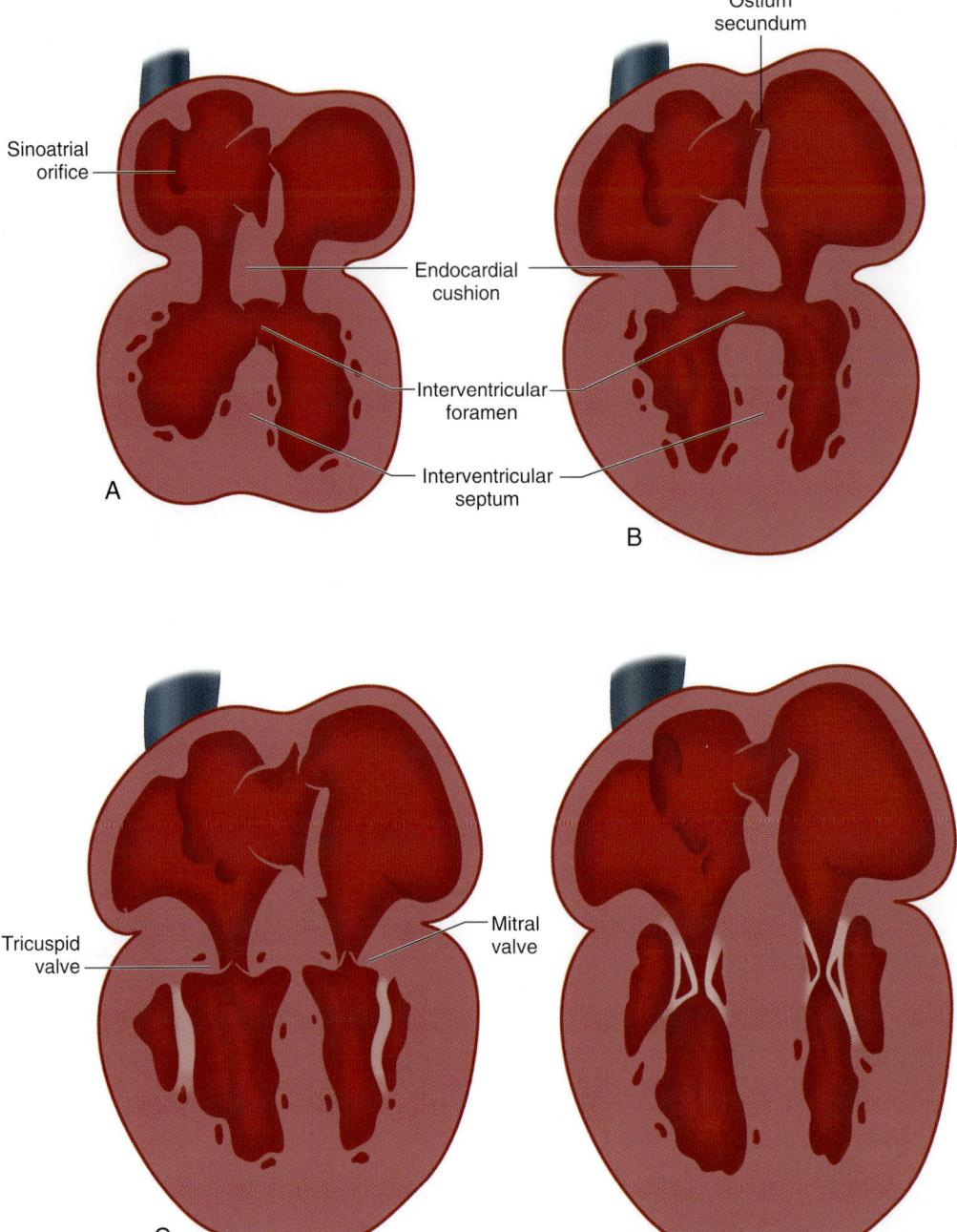

FIGURE 1-4 Further development of the AV canal. **A,** Endocardial cushions split the common AV canal. Continued growth of the endocardial cushions. **B,** Ostium secundum ASD and inlet VSD are visualized. **C,** Ventricular septum is sealed. Endocardial cushions begin to differentiate into valvular tissue. **D,** Endocardial cushions complete differentiation into septa and septal leaflets of the AV valves. *(Adapted from Gedgaudas E, Moller JH, Castaneda-Zuniga WR, Amplatz K. Embryology and anatomy of the heart. In Gedgaudas E, Moller JH, Castaneda-Zuniga WR, Amplatz K [eds]. Cardiovascular Radiology. Philadelphia, WB Saunders, 1985, pp 1-23.)*

Formation of the Ventricular Outflow Tracts and Septation of the Truncus Arteriosus

In the heart tube stage, the primitive LV and the proximal bulbus cordis (primitive RV) are separated from the truncus arteriosus (which gives rise to both great arteries) by the conus or infundibulum (Fig. 1-5). This fact is fundamental to the understanding of the conotruncal malformations, which are due to abnormal development of the conus. The conus consists of the subpulmonary and subaortic conus cushions. Normally, there is expansile growth of the subpulmonary conus, causing it to protrude anteriorly on the left, carrying the pulmonary valve anteriorly, superiorly, and to the left of the aortic valve. There is resorption of the subaortic conus. Hence, the aortic valve lies posterior, inferior, and right-sided, in direct fibrous contiguity with the mitral valve (Fig. 1-6). Anterior protrusion of the pulmonary conus also twists the developing great arteries because they are fixed distally by the arterial arches. Spiral twisting of the growing tissue and a shift of

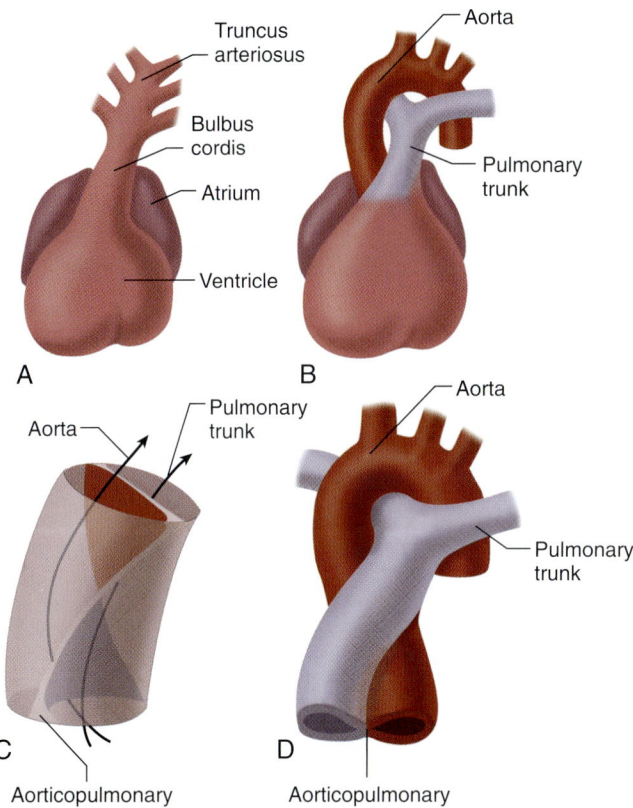

FIGURE 1-5 Development of ventriculoarterial (V-A) connections and great arteries. **A,** The bulbus cordis separates the primitive ventricles from the common outflow tract, the truncus arteriosus, which gives rise to the aortic arches. **B,** Development of the conus cordis results in alignment of the RV with the developing pulmonary artery and the LV with the aorta (see text). **C,** Separation of the truncus arteriosus by ingrowth of a spiral septum that develops cephalad to caudad. **D,** Separation of the aorta and pulmonary artery is complete. *(Adapted from Gedgaudas E, Moller JH, Castaneda-Zuniga WR, Amplatz K. Embryology and anatomy of the heart. In Gedgaudas E, Moller JH, Castaneda-Zuniga WR, Amplatz K [eds]. Cardiovascular Radiology. Philadelphia, WB Saunders, 1985, pp 1-23.)*

the conal base to the middle causes the outflow tracts to align with the nearest ventricle (see Fig. 1-5). The anterior pulmonary artery arises above the anterior ventricle (RV) and leads to the posterior sixth arterial arch, which forms the branch pulmonary arteries. The posterior aorta originates above the posterior LV, and leads to the anterior fourth arterial arch (which forms the aortic arch). Recent investigation has shown that this normal partitioning of the conus involves migration of mesenchymal cells from the neural crest.[11]

By the 28th day of development, the truncus arteriosus divides by means of a bisecting spur that protrudes from both the aorta and pulmonary artery. The resultant aorticopulmonary septum continues in a spiral fashion toward the conus cordis until the two vessels are completely separated, giving rise to the aortic and pulmonary channels (see Fig. 1-5). The truncal cushions meet the conal cushions to complete the closure of the base of the respective outflow tracts.[5] At the level of the conus cordis, the truncal swellings develop into pulmonary and aortic valve cusps and form two of the three cusps in each valve. A third swelling, the intercalated swelling, forms the third cusp.

Developmental Pathology

Abnormal conal development can result in tetralogy of Fallot or abnormal connections between the great vessels and the ventricles such as truncus arteriosus, transposition of the great arteries, double outlet RV, or double outlet LV (see Fig. 1-6).

Tetralogy of Fallot occurs when anterior displacement of the conal septum results in a narrowed pulmonary outflow tract, subsequent RV hypertrophy, an inability of the ventricular septum to close, and an abnormally placed aorta, overriding the VSD.[5]

Truncus arteriosus occurs when there is atresia of the subpulmonary conus, with absence of the pulmonary valve, resulting in a common vessel through which blood flows out of the heart to both pulmonary and systemic circulations.[12] Because the absent or hypoplastic truncal cushions cannot meet the conal tissue, an obligatory VSD is present.

Transposition of great arteries was previously thought to be related to a failure of spiral twisting of the aorticopulmonary septum. But now, it is believed to result from variations in differential growth of the aortic and pulmonary conus.[13] For instance, the most common form, D-transposition, is due to persistence and overgrowth of the subaortic conus and resorption of the subpulmonary conus. This elevates the aortic valve superiorly, protrudes it anteriorly above the RV, and causes aortic-tricuspid valve fibrous discontiguity. The pulmonary valve stays posterior and inferior, above the posterior LV, and in direct fibrous contiguity with the mitral valve.

The **double outlet right ventricle** results from variable development of both the subaortic and subpulmonary conus, and failure of the conus to shift to the center, with both great vessels arising from the primitive bulbus cordis (eventually the RV).[5]

The semilunar valves are formed from three small tubercles of tissue. A failure to develop one of the tubercles causes **bicuspid** aortic or pulmonary valves. Fusion of two or all three of the valve leaflets produces **stenosis** or **atresia** of the valve.[5]

Formation of the Interatrial Septum

By the time the heart tube has formed the bulboventricular loop, the primitive right and left atria have fused to form a common atrium, which lies cranial to the primitive ventricle and dorsal to the bulbus cordis (see Fig. 1-1D). The truncus arteriosus lies on the roof of the common atrium causing a depression and indicates where septation of the atrium will occur (see Fig. 1-5A). The interatrial septum forms between the 27th and the 37th day of development and occurs in conjunction with the development of the ventricular septum and separation of the truncus arteriosus.

A crest of tissue known as the *septum primum* grows from the dorsal wall of the atrium toward the endocardial cushions (Fig. 1-7). The ostium (opening) formed by the free edge of septum primum is the ostium primum. Before

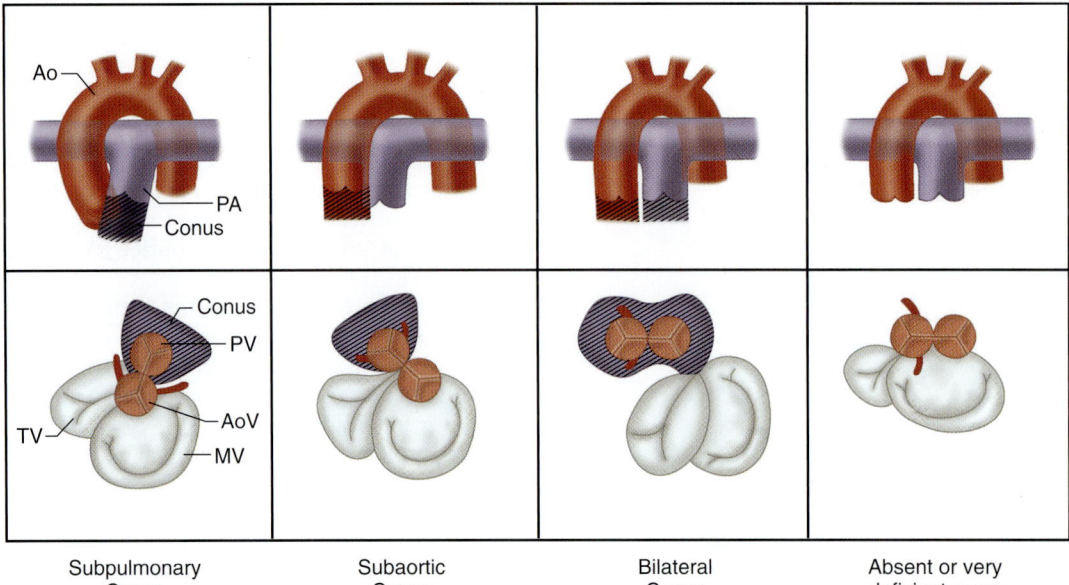

■ **FIGURE 1-6** Normal and abnormal conal development (*see text*). **A**, Subpulmonary conus seen in normally related great arteries. **B**, Subaortic conus in typical transposition of the great arteries. **C**, Bilateral conus, as in double outlet right ventricle. **D**, Absent or deficient conus, as in double outlet left ventricle. On the side of the conus, the semilunar valve sits atop the muscular infundibulum, and there is no direct fibrous contiguity between the semilunar valve and the AV valve. On the side of the deficient conus, there is usually direct fibrous contiguity between the AV valve and the semilunar valve. *(Adapted from Van Praagh R, Weinberg PM, Matsuoka R, Van Praagh S. Malposition of the heart and the segmental approach to diagnosis. In Adams FH, Emmanouilides GC [eds]. Moss' Heart Diseases in Infants, Children and Adolescents, 3rd. ed. Williams and Wilkins, Baltimore, 1983, pp 422-458.)*

the septum primum fuses with the endocardial cushions, perforations appear in the upper portion of the septum primum. These perforations will coalesce to form the ostium secundum. Another muscular ridge of tissue known as the *septum secundum* arises from infolding of the dorsal wall of the atrium, to the right of the septum primum, and covers the ostium secundum. Its free edge forms the foramen ovale. The left venous valve and the septum spurium, located on the dorsal wall of the right atrium, fuse with the septum secundum as it grows.

At the end of the seventh week the human heart has reached its final stage of development. Because the fetus does not use its lungs, most of the blood is diverted to the systemic circulation by right-to-left shunting across the foramen ovale. At birth the child will use its lungs for the first time and consequently more blood will flow into the pulmonary circulation. The pressure increase in the left atrium will force septum primum to be pushed up against septum secundum. Shortly thereafter the two septa fuse to form a common atrial septum.

Developmental Pathology

If the septum secundum fails to form and cover the perforations in the septum primum, the result is a **secundum atrial septal defect** (ASD). If the very last portion of the septum primum fails to meet with endocardial cushion tissue (coming from lower in the heart), a **primum ASD** is formed. Embryologists also speculate that if the septum primum perforations fail to form or close prematurely, the diminished right-to-left flow and diminished left-sided volume in utero result in underdevelopment of the left-sided structures, producing **hypoplastic left heart syndrome**.[14]

Formation of the Right Atrium, Coronary Sinus, and Systemic Veins

Unlike the atria, the sinus venosus remains a paired structure with right and left horns. Each sinus venosus receives blood from the yolk sac via the vitelline veins, from the chorionic villi via the umbilical veins, and from the cranial region of the embryo and body via the anterior and posterior cardinal veins. The fate of each structure is as follows (Fig. 1-8):

The left horn of the sinus venosus becomes partially obliterated leaving behind the oblique vein of the left atrium and the coronary sinus.
The right horn of the sinus venosus becomes enlarged.
The right anterior cardinal vein becomes the superior vena cava.
The right vitelline vein becomes the inferior vena cava.
The right umbilical vein is obliterated.

Gradually the sinoatrial orifice shifts to the right until the sinus venosus communicates with only the right atrium via the sinoatrial orifice. Further into development, the right sinus horn is incorporated into the expanding right atrium. As the atrium expands, the smooth tissue of the sinus venosus displaces the trabeculated tissue of the primitive right atrium anteriorly and laterally where it becomes the right atrial appendage (auricle). The smooth tissue forms part of the atrium called the *sinus venarum*.

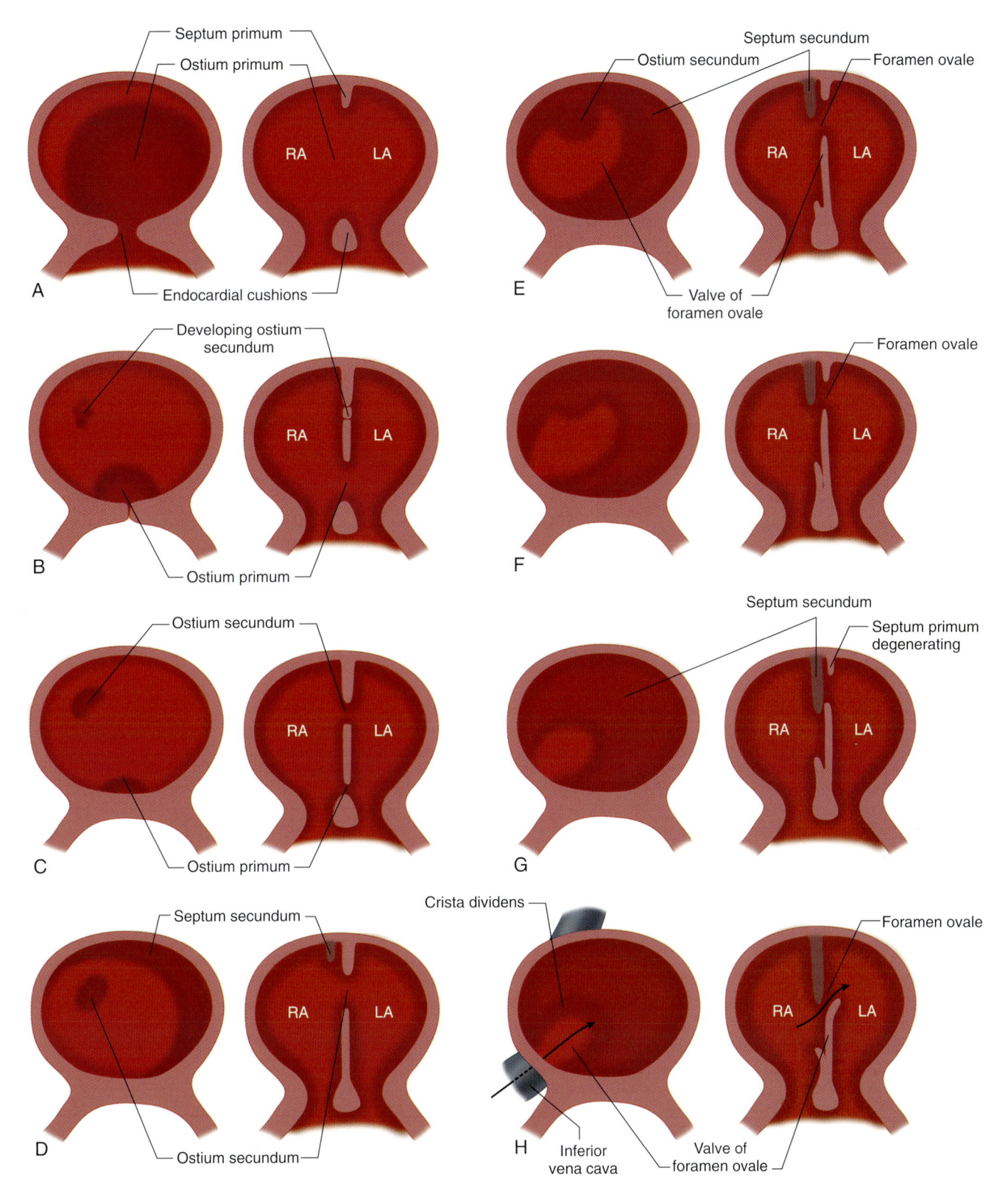

FIGURE 1-7 Development of the atrial septum, right lateral and anterior views. **A-H,** show progressive growth of the septum primum (pink) and septum secundum (gray) and closure of the ostium primum and ostium secundum. The final image shows completed development, with flow of blood from right-to-left across the foramen ovale. *(Adapted from Gedgaudas E, Moller JH, Castaneda-Zuniga WR, Amplatz K. Embryology and anatomy of the heart. In Gedgaudas E, Moller JH, Castaneda-Zuniga WR, Amplatz K [eds]. Cardiovascular Radiology. Philadelphia, WB Saunders, 1985, pp 1-23.)*

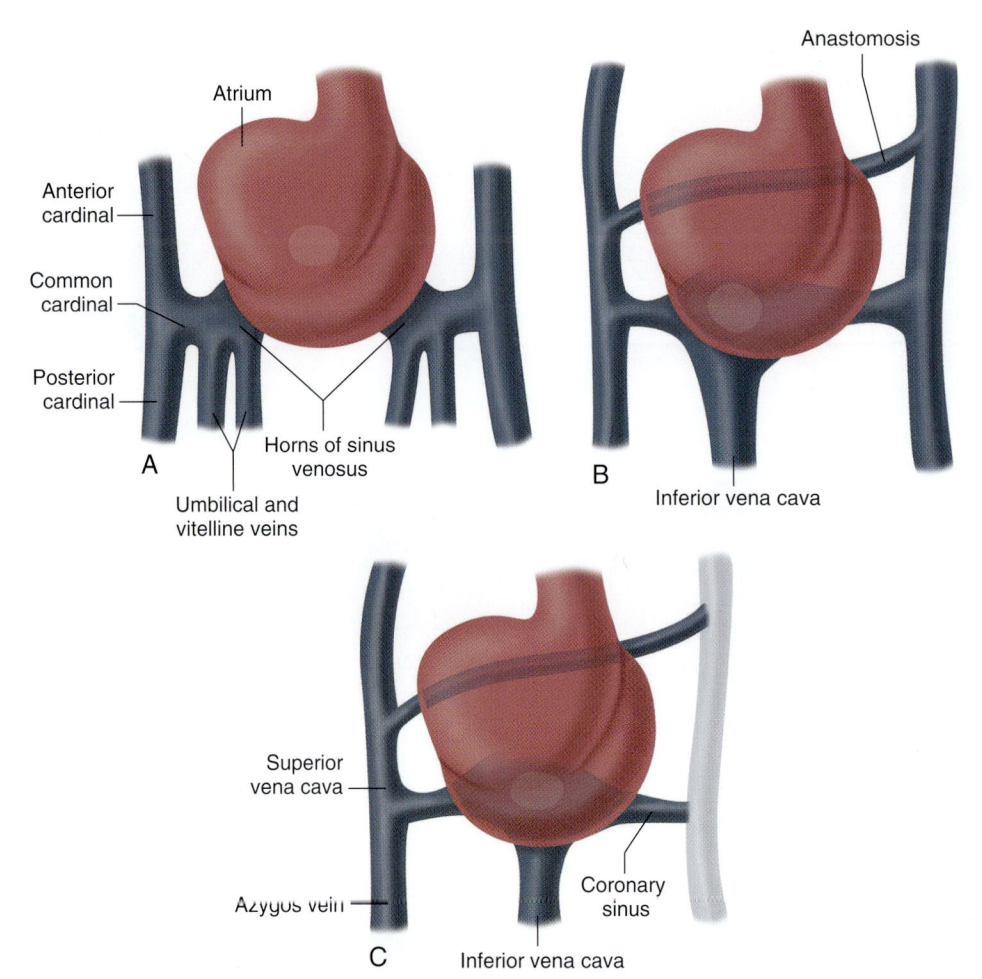

■ **FIGURE 1-8** Development of the sinus venosus and systemic veins. On each side, the anterior and posterior cardinal veins join to form the common cardinal vein, which, along with the umbilical vein from the placenta, and vitelline vein from the yolk sac, join the sinus venosus. Development of the SVC, IVC, and azygos vein. The left horn of the sinus venosus involutes, leaving behind the coronary sinus. *(Adapted from Gedgaudas E, Moller JH, Castaneda-Zuniga WR, Amplatz K. Embryology and anatomy of the heart. In Gedgaudas E, Moller JH, Castaneda-Zuniga WR, Amplatz K [eds]. Cardiovascular Radiology. Philadelphia, WB Saunders, 1985, pp 1-23.)*

The crista terminalis is a ridge of tissue located to the right of the sinoatrial orifice, which forms the boundary between the auricle and the sinus venarum.

Formation of the Left Atrium and Pulmonary Veins

Development of the left atrium occurs concurrently with that of the right atrium. During the early part of the fourth week, a single pulmonary vein develops as an outgrowth from the back of the left atrium (Fig. 1-9), grows toward the developing lungs, and connects to the blood vessels growing out of the lungs to form pulmonary venous drainage.[10] As the left atrium expands, it incorporates both the vein and, eventually, the four connecting pulmonary vessels. As the atrial wall expands, the smooth tissue of the pulmonary veins is incorporated into the wall of the atrium and displaces the trabeculated tissue anteriorly and laterally which will then form the left atrial appendage.

Developmental Pathology

Anomalous pulmonary venous return occurs when the single pulmonary vein fails to fuse with the developing intrapulmonary vessels, either because of lack of development or because of early involution.[5] If the intrapulmonary vessels do not connect to the pulmonary vein, they can connect to other "alternative" vessels, such as the superior vena cava, inferior vena cava, the right atrium, the coronary sinus, or other vascular structures.[15]

Development of the Aortic Arches

In embryonic vascular development, ventral and dorsal aortae are connected by six pairs of aortic/branchial arches. As normal cardiovascular development proceeds, a patterned regression and persistence of the various arches and right-sided dorsal aorta occur,[16] ultimately resulting in the mature configuration of the thoracic aorta and its branches (Fig. 1-10). Normally, the first, second, and fifth arches involute, the left fourth arch becomes the aortic arch, the proximal right fourth arch contributes to the innominate artery, the distal left sixth arch becomes the ductus arteriosus, the proximal sixth arches bilaterally contribute to the proximal branch pulmonary arteries, the left dorsal aorta becomes the descending thoracic aorta,

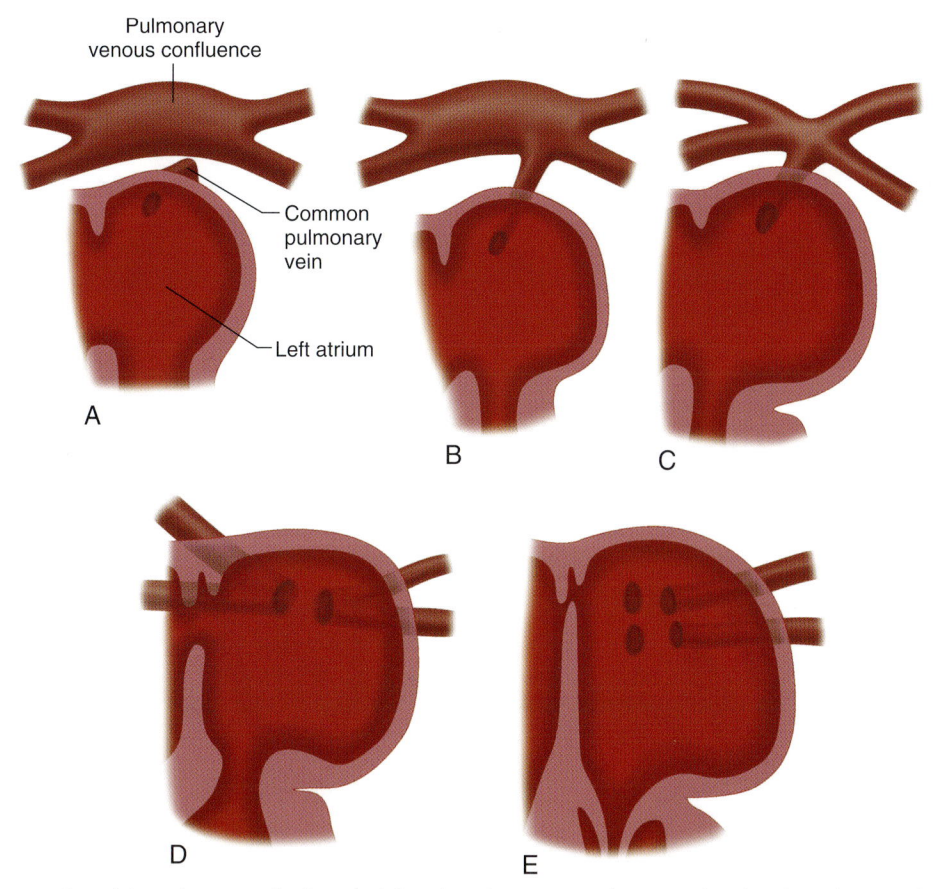

■ **FIGURE 1-9** Incorporation of the pulmonary veins into the left atrium. A common pulmonary vein arises from the posterior wall of the left atrium (**A**) and makes contact with the pulmonary venous confluence (**B**). **C-E**, show progressive incorporation of the pulmonary vein confluence, ultimately resulting in separate insertion of the pulmonary veins into the posterior wall of the left atrium. *(Adapted from Gedgaudas E, Moller JH, Castaneda-Zuniga WR, Amplatz K. Embryology and anatomy of the heart. In Gedgaudas E, Moller JH, Castaneda-Zuniga WR, Amplatz K [eds]. Cardiovascular Radiology. Philadelphia, WB Saunders, 1985, pp 1-23.)*

and the seventh dorsal intersegmental arteries bilaterally become the subclavian arteries.

Developmental Pathology

Vascular rings are formed when this process of regression and persistence does not occur normally, and the resulting vascular anatomy completely encircles the trachea and esophagus.[16,17] If bilateral fourth arches persist, a **double aortic arch** is formed. If the right fourth arch persists, and the proximal left fourth arch involutes, a **right aortic arch with an aberrant left subclavian artery** results. The ductus/ligamentum arteriosus travels from the origin of the left subclavian artery to the pulmonary artery, completing the ring. A number of normal variants may occur without forming a complete vascular ring. If the proximal right fourth arch regresses, a **left arch with an aberrant right subclavian artery** is formed. If the right fourth arch persists, and the distal left fourth arch involutes, a **right aortic arch with mirror image branching** is formed. In this setting, the ligamentum usually travels from the left innominate artery to the left pulmonary artery without forming a vascular ring. If the left ligamentum travels from the pulmonary artery to the descending thoracic aorta, a vascular ring results.

Embryologic Basis for the Segmental Approach to Heart Disease

The segmental approach involves the analysis of the three major cardiac segments: atria, ventricles, and great arteries, and the two connecting segments: the atrioventricular canal and the conotruncus. These segments of the heart can be distinguished in the very early embryo.

The development of the suprahepatic portion of the inferior vena cava is closely linked to the growth of the liver, so that the anatomic right atrium and the liver almost invariably develop on the same side of the body. This concept of visceroatrial situs is fundamental to the segmental approach.

Another important concept underlying the segmental approach is the recognition that the ventricular looping is independent of the visceroatrial situs. This gives rise to the concept of concordance (RA-RV and LA-LV) and discordance (RA-LV and LA-RV).

Bulboventricular looping is responsible for the relative position of the ventricles. With D-looping, the proximal bulbus cordis (RV) lies anterior and to the right of the primitive ventricle (LV). With L-looping, the RV will lie anterior and to the left of the LV.

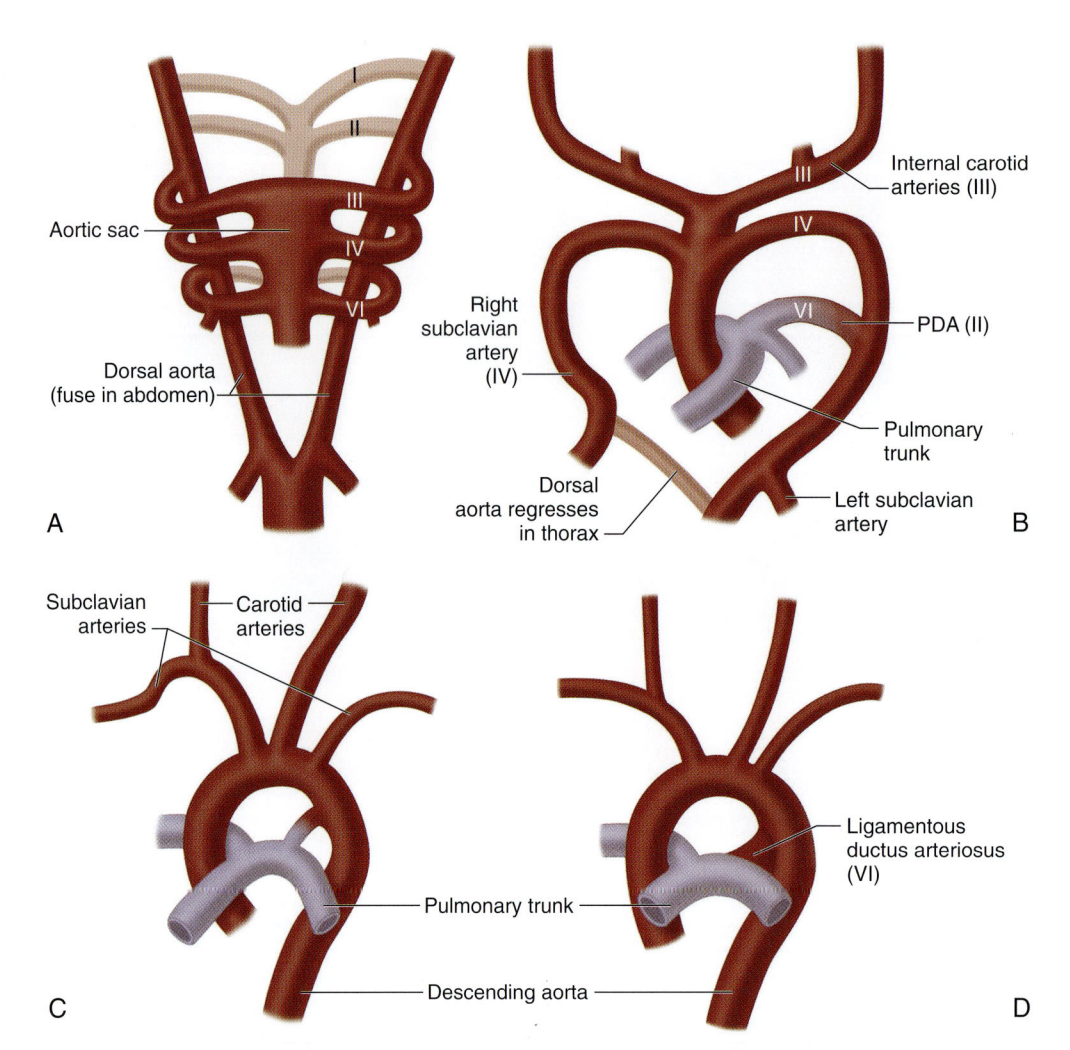

FIGURE 1-10 Development of the aortic arches. The first, second, and fifth arches involute; the third arches form the carotid arteries bilaterally; the left fourth arch becomes the aortic arch; the proximal right fourth arch contributes to the innominate artery; the distal left sixth arch becomes the ductus arteriosus; the proximal sixth arches bilaterally contribute to the proximal branch pulmonary arteries; the left dorsal aorta becomes the descending thoracic aorta; and the seventh dorsal intersegmental arteries bilaterally become the subclavian arteries. *(Adapted from Gedgaudas E, Moller JH, Castaneda-Zuniga WR, Amplatz K. Embryology and anatomy of the heart. In Gedgaudas E, Moller JH, Castaneda-Zuniga WR, Amplatz K [eds]. Cardiovascular Radiology. Philadelphia, WB Saunders, 1985, pp 1-23.)*

Similarly, ventricular looping and great arterial relationship are independent entities. The ventricles and great arteries do not connect directly due to the interposition of the conus or infundibulum. Abnormal development of the subpulmonary and subaortic conus cushions is responsible for the wide spectrum of outflow tract malformations.

The direction of bulboventricular looping, and the development of the conotruncus is responsible for the ultimate relationship of the great arteries to each other, and to the underlying ventricles and atrioventricular valves.

The Segmental Approach to Diagnosis and Management of Congenital Heart Disease

Any imaginable combination of visceral, atrial, ventricular, and great vessel morphology can and does occur in congenital heart disease. A simple, logical, step-by-step approach to diagnosis and decision-making and a standardized nomenclature go a long way in advancing patient care by ensuring that different caregivers have similar understanding of the disease and are speaking the same language. This approach is known as the *segmental approach* to heart disease, first described by Richard Van Praagh in 1972.

One can think of the heart as a three-level house (Fig. 1-11). The first level is the visceroatrial situs, the middle level is the ventricular loop, and the third level is the conotruncus. To describe it simply, the three levels are the atria, ventricles, and great arteries. There are two separating walls with doors: the atrioventricular junction and the ventriculoarterial junction. There are two entrances: the systemic veins and the pulmonary veins. The levels represent the major cardiac segments. The connecting doors represent the connecting segments.

The segmental approach to heart disease comprises the following steps:[18]

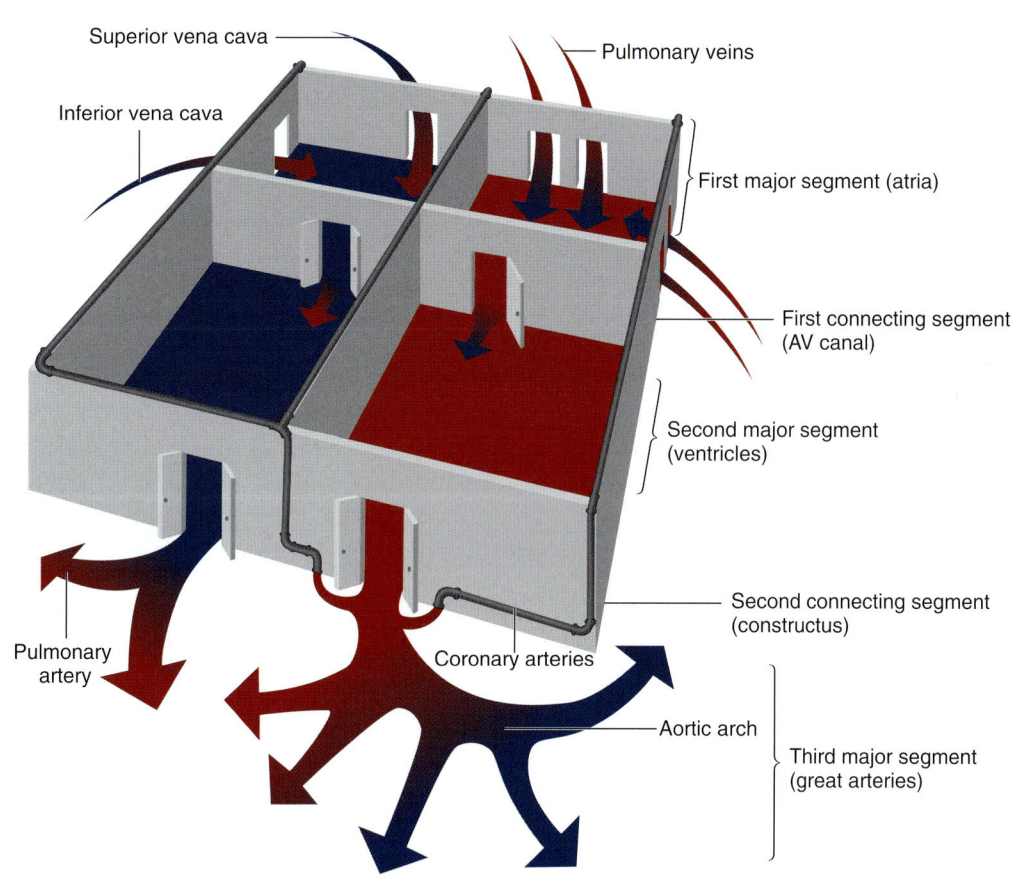

FIGURE 1-11 The 'house' model of the heart. The three levels (major cardiac segments) are the atria, ventricles and great arteries. There are two connecting walls with doors (connecting segments): the atrioventricular junction and the ventriculoarterial junction. There are two entrances: the systemic veins and the pulmonary veins. *(Adapted from the website of Dr. Hasan Abdallah, The Children's Heart Institute, Va.)*

1. What is the anatomic type of each of the three major cardiac segments: the atria, the ventricles and great arteries?
2. How is each segment connected to the adjacent segment?
3. What are the associated anomalies involving the valves, atrial and ventricular septum, and the great vessels?
4. How do the segmental combinations and connections, with or without the associated malformations, function?

The first three steps in the segmental approach are concerned with morphology, whereas the last step determines physiology.

Van Praagh used a segmental set to provide a shorthand description of the floor-plan of the heart. The first letter stands for the visceroatrial situs, the second for the ventricular loop, and the third for the great arterial relationship. In a person with *situs solitus* of the viscera and atria, *D-looping* of the ventricles, and *solitus* relationship of the great arteries, the segmental set is expressed as {S,D,S}.

Identification of the Major Cardiac Segments

Reliable identification of the cardiac chambers based on specific morphologic features is the first step in the segmental approach to heart disease. It is important to remember that right and left do not refer to the side of the body on which the chamber lies, but to specific morphologic criteria that identify each component of the heart. For instance, right atrium does not refer to the atrium that is on the right side of the body, but to the atrium that receives the insertion of the IVC and the coronary sinus, and has a triangular appendage with a broad base. Hence, the morphologic right atrium will be on the right side of the body in situs solitus, and on the left side in situs inversus.

Atrial Identification

The defining features of the morphologic right atrium (systemic venous atrium) and left atrium (pulmonary venous atrium) are based on their venous connections as well as their appendage and pectinate muscle morphology. Use of venoatrial connections for atrial identification is based on the fact that the sinus venosus, which carries the systemic venous return, is an integral part of the morphologic right atrium.[19] Hence, the morphologic right atrium receives the inferior and superior vena cavae, and orifice of coronary sinus. However, the SVC and coronary sinus have a high incidence of variation, which can be a source of diagnostic confusion. These variations include left SVC to an unroofed coronary sinus, and bilateral SVC

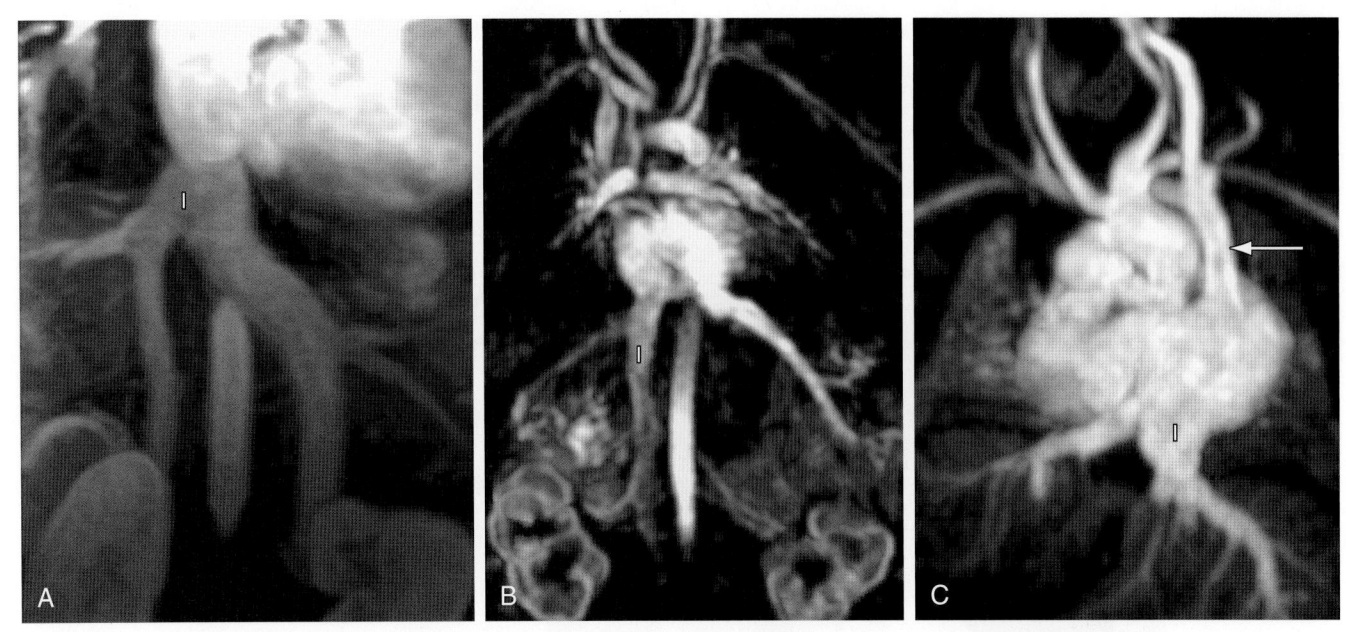

FIGURE 1-12 The IVC as a marker of the morphologic right atrium. **A,** Bilateral IVC which fuse prior to entering the right atrium. **B,** Right hepatic vein enters the IVC, which drains into the right atrium, whereas the remaining hepatic veins drain separately into the left atrium. **C,** Left-sided interrupted IVC with azygos continuation. There is a suprahepatic segment of the IVC (I), which drains into the left-sided right atrium in this patient with atrial situs inversus. A left SVC is also present (*arrow*).

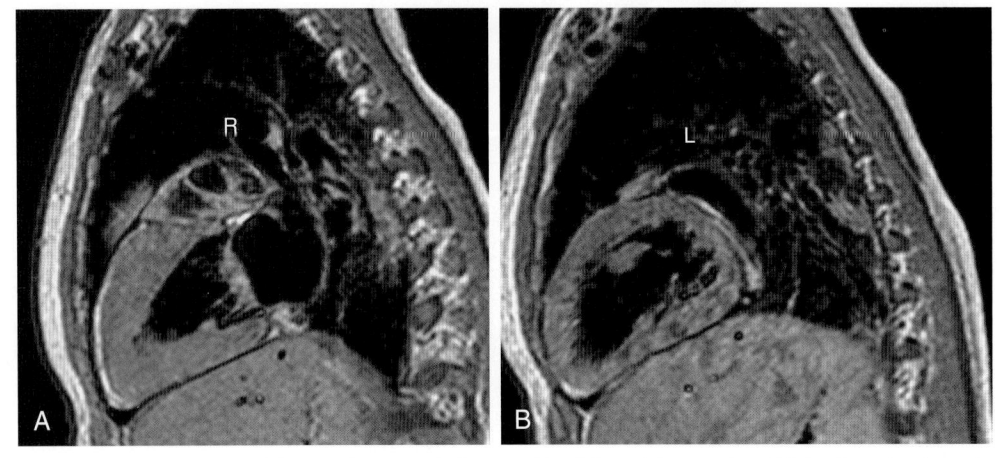

FIGURE 1-13 Atrial identification using atrial appendage morphology. **A,** The right atrial appendage (R) is triangular shaped with a broad base and is heavily trabeculated. **B,** The left atrial appendage (L) is tubular with a narrow base and has a smooth contour.

with the left SVC draining to an unroofed coronary sinus. In these cases, the SVC would appear to drain into the left atrium. In rare instances, even the IVC may drain into the coronary sinus, which may be unroofed, or the coronary sinus septum may be absent. In spite of this rare exception, the most reliable means of identifying the morphologic right atrium by cross-sectional imaging is by recognizing its connection to the IVC (Fig. 1-12). Even in the setting of an interrupted IVC, a suprahepatic segment of the IVC is present entering the right atrium, allowing accurate identification.

The morphologic left atrium is defined as the atrium that receives all or half of the pulmonary veins, and none of the systemic veins (except an SVC to an unroofed coronary sinus). The left atrium is also the chamber that may receive no veins at all (in the setting of total anomalous pulmonary venous return). When all systemic veins and part or all of the pulmonary veins drain into one atrium, this atrium represents the morphologic right atrium.

Anderson has described the morphologic right atrium (systemic atrium) as being characterized by the presence of a triangular appendage with a broad junction (Fig. 1-13), and by the recognition of pectinate muscles extending to the atrioventricular junction. The morphologic left atrium is characterized by a tubular narrow-based appendage, and lack of pectinate muscle extension to the atrioventricular junction. Because determination of pectinate muscle morphology is beyond the resolution of MRI or CT, atrial identification is performed by recognition of venoatrial connections and morphology of the appendages. If this analysis fails to yield a confident identification of the right and left atrium, then a diagnosis of atrial situs ambiguous is made. Even in the setting of visceral situs ambiguous, reliable identification of atrial situs may be made in more than 80% of the cases.

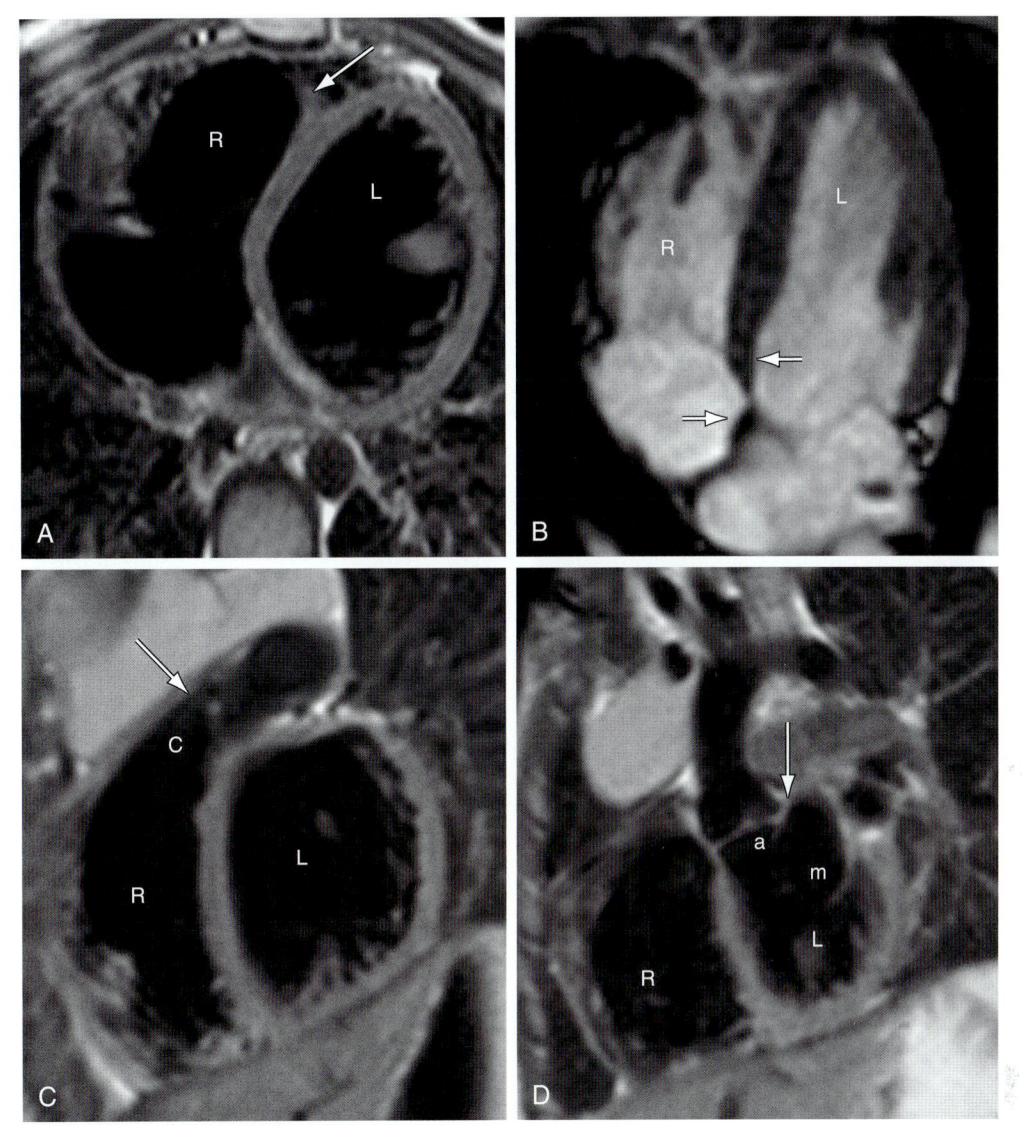

FIGURE 1-14 Ventricular identification: **A,** Moderator band of the RV. **B,** The AV valve of the RV (tricuspid valve) is more apically displaced (*arrow*) than the AV valve of the LV (mitral valve). **C,** The conus (C) is a marker of the RV. It is a muscular cone of tissue that separates the AV valve from the semilunar valve on the same side. **D,** The LV does not have a conus, resulting in mitral (m) to aortic (a) fibrous contiguity (*arrow*).

Ventricular Identification

Ventricles are defined by their morphologic features, not by their spatial relationships. The morphologic right ventricle is defined by the following features:

1. Muscular connection between the free wall and the interventricular septum (moderator band) (Fig. 1-14A).
2. The septal attachment of the AV valve of the RV (tricuspid valve) is more apically placed relative to the LV (see Fig. 1-14B).
3. Presence of a conus/infundibulum. The infundibulum is identified as a muscular cone of tissue that separates the atrioventricular valve from the semilunar valve on the same side, resulting in lack of fibrous contiguity between the two valves (see Fig. 1-14C and Fig. 1-15A).

The morphologic LV is identified by the following features:

1. Smooth surface of the interventricular septum without any muscular attachments to the free wall (see Fig. 1-15B).
2. The septal attachment of the AV valve of the LV (mitral valve) is more cranially located relative to the RV (see Fig. 1-14B).
3. Absence of a conus/infundibulum, resulting in fibrous contiguity between the atrioventricular valve and the semilunar valve on that side (see Fig. 1-14D).

The atrioventricular valves follow the ventricle, rather than the atrium. Thus, the tricuspid valve is related to the morphologic right ventricle and the mitral valve to the morphologic left ventricle. The tricuspid valve typically has papillary muscle attachments to the right ventricular septal surface (septophilic valve), whereas the mitral valve is septophobic and attaches only to the free wall of the left ventricle.

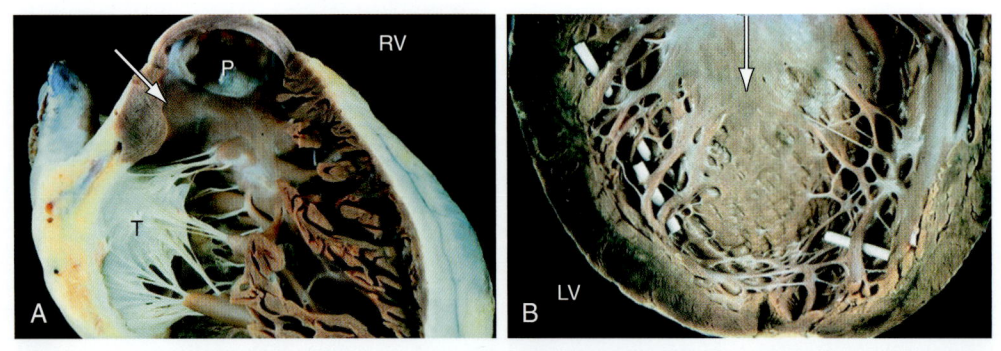

FIGURE 1-15 Gross specimens of the RV (**A**) and LV (**B**). The conus of the RV (*arrow* in **A**) is noted separating the tricuspid valve (T) from the pulmonary valve (P). The *arrow* in **B** shows the smooth septal surface of the LV without any muscular attachments. *(Courtesy of William D. Edwards, MD. From Crawford MH, DiMarco JP, Paulus WJ [eds]. Cardiology, 3rd. ed. London, Mosby, 2010.)*

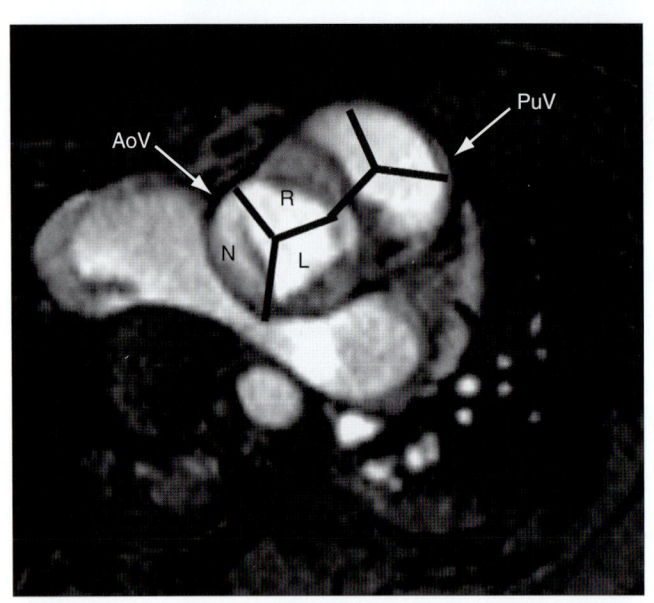

FIGURE 1-16 Solitus (normal) relationship of the great arteries. The aortic valve annulus (AoV) lies posterior and to the right of the pulmonary valve annulus (PuV). The intercoronary commissure of the aortic valve is pointed toward the right-left commissure of the pulmonary valve.

Neither the shape of the ventricle nor the degree of trabeculation or hypertrophy is considered a reliable marker for ventricular identification because they are frequently affected by pressure or volume changes in the ventricle.

Great Arterial Identification

The pulmonary artery gives rise to branches to the lungs, and no branches to the body. The aorta gives rise to branches to the body as well as the coronary arteries. A common vessel arising from the ventricles that gives rise to the coronaries, branches to the body as well the lungs and is termed a *common arterial trunk* or *truncus*, and a segmental relationship is not assigned (labeled 'X' for undetermined). On transverse cross-sectional imaging at the level of the outflow tract, the coronary artery origin is used to identify the aortic annulus. The intercoronary commissure of the aortic valve is pointed toward the right-left commissure of the pulmonary valve and is an important landmark for determining great arterial relationship (Fig. 1-16). In solitus relationship of the great arteries, the aortic valve annulus lies posterior and to the right of the pulmonary valve annulus.

Analysis of the Three Major Cardiac Segments

First Major Segment: Visceroatrial Situs

Situs refers to the position of the atria and viscera relative to the midline. There are three types of situs: solitus (S), inversus (I), and ambiguous (A) (Fig. 1-17). Heterotaxy is synonymous with situs ambiguous and is simply defined as 'situs other than solitus or inversus'.

Visceral situs solitus is characterized by the presence of a right-sided liver, a single or dominant left-sided spleen, three-lobed right lung with an eparterial bronchus, and a two-lobed left lung with a hyparterial bronchus. Atrial situs solitus is characterized by the presence of the systemic venous atrium on the right, and the pulmonary venous atrium on the left. Situs inversus is defined as the "mirror-image" of situs solitus. Hence, visceral situs inversus is characterized by a left-sided liver, a single or dominant right-sided spleen, three-lobed left lung with an eparterial bronchus, and a two-lobed right lung with a hyparterial bronchus. Atrial situs inversus is characterized by the presence of the systemic venous atrium on the left and the pulmonary venous atrium on the right. Although the location of the cardiac apex and the stomach is usually on the left in situs solitus, and on the right in situs inversus, they are not considered reliable markers of visceral situs due to the high incidence of variation in the setting of normal situs.

Because heterotaxy is defined as "situs other than solitus or inversus", it is not a specific disease, but a constellation of cardiac, vascular, and visceral abnormalities, including situs ambiguous of the viscera, lung symmetry, atrial appendage symmetry, anomalous systemic venous return, anomalous pulmonary venous return, and associated intracardiac defects. No single finding is pathognomonic. Although there are three syndromes, there is a tendency toward clustering of defects into two syndromes based on the predominance of right-sided or left-sided structures (Fig. 1-18):

CHAPTER 1 • Embryologic Basis and Segmental Approach to Imaging 17

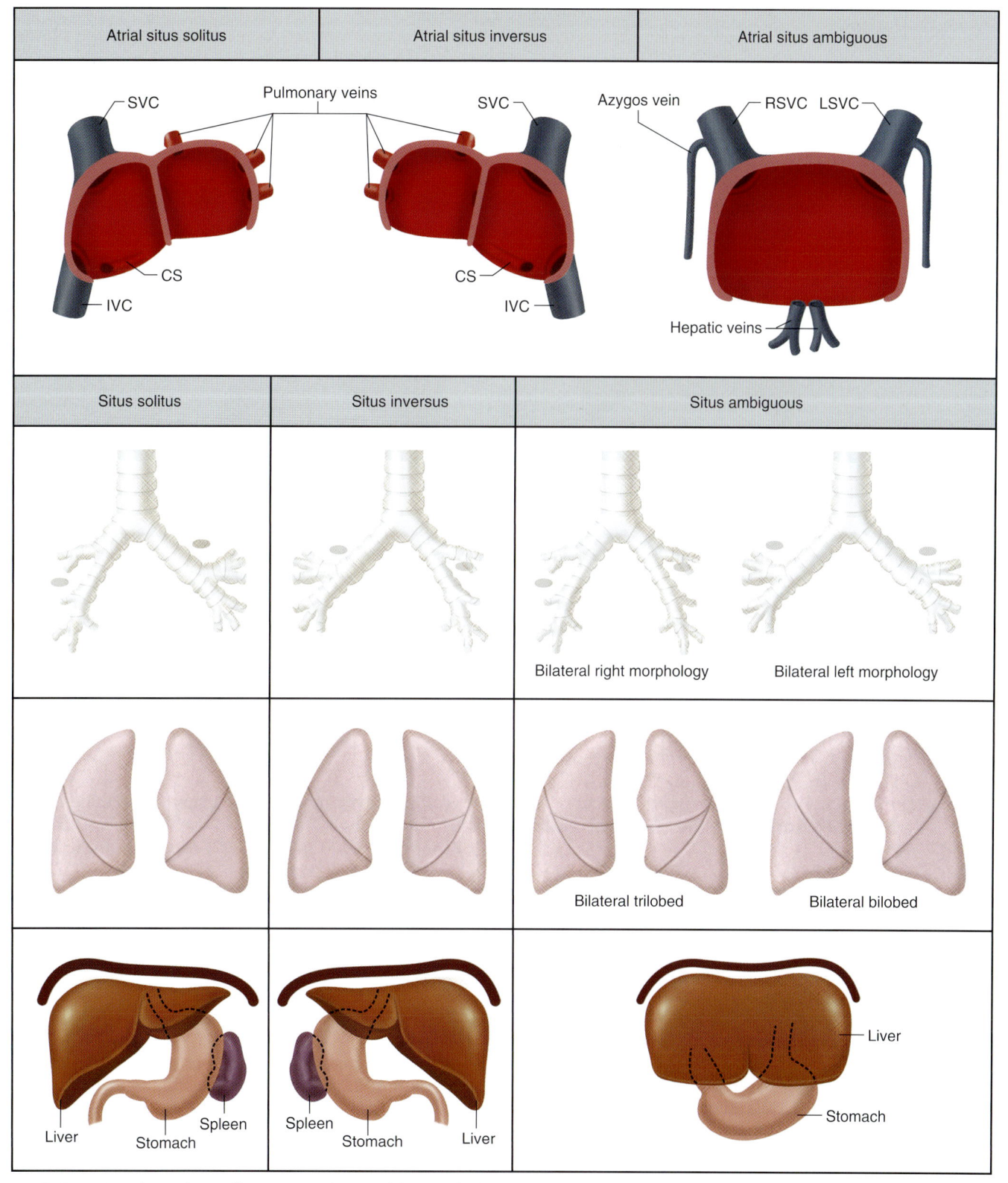

■ FIGURE 1-17 First major cardiac segment: Visceroatrial situs. The three types of visceroatrial situs: situs solitus, situs inversus, and situs ambiguous. (Adapted from Van Praagh R, Weinberg PM, Matsuoka R, Van Praagh S. Malposition of the heart and the segmental approach to diagnosis. In Adams FH, Emmanouilides GC [eds]. Moss' Heart Diseases in Infants, Children and Adolescents, 3rd. ed. Williams and Wilkins, Baltimore, 1983, pp 422-458.)

Heterotaxy Syndromes

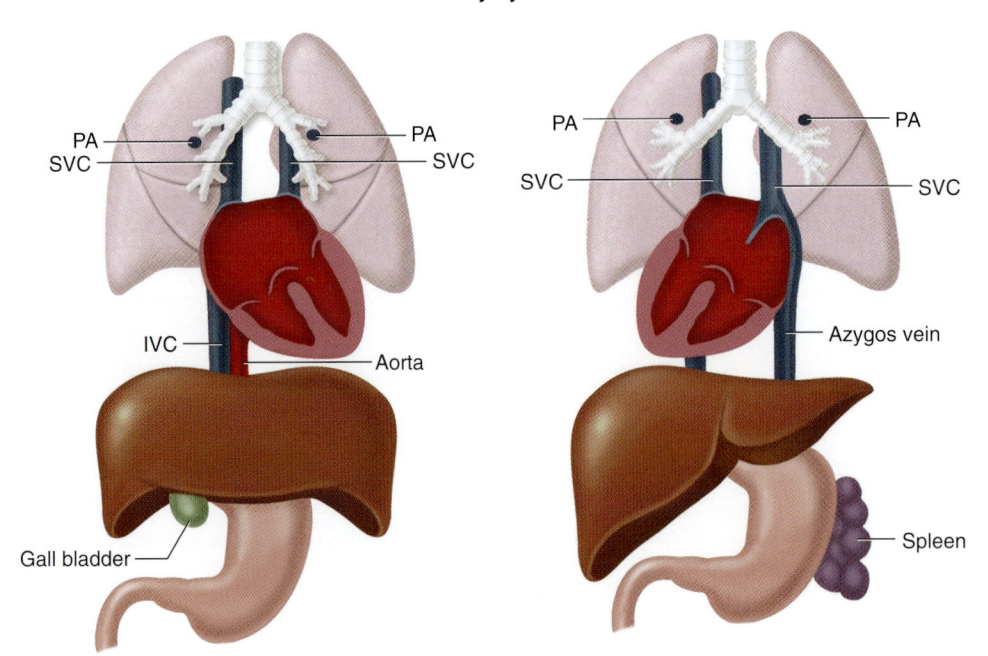

FIGURE 1-18 Syndromic approach to heterotaxy, with asplenia complex on left and polysplenia complex on right. This approach has been discarded in favor of a segmental approach in which there is an independent assessment of every involved organ system without any preconceived notions. *(Adapted from Hashmi A, Freedom RM, Yoo SJ: The syndrome of isomeric right atrial appendages and visceroatrial heterotaxy, often associated with congenital asplenia. In Freedom RM, Yoo SJ, Mikalian H, Williams WG [eds]: The Natural and Modified History of Congenital Heart Disease. New York, 2004, Futura, p 424.)*

1. Asplenia complex—Manifestations include bilateral three-lobed lungs with eparterial bronchi, transverse or symmetric liver, bilateral SVC, and bilateral triangular broad-based atrial appendages. The spleen is absent.
2. Polysplenia complex—Manifestations include bilateral two-lobed lungs with hyparterial bronchi, transverse liver, multiple splenic fragments, and bilateral tubular atrial appendages. The renal to hepatic segment of the IVC is frequently absent, with associated azygos continuation.
3. Van Praagh has added a third syndrome of heterotaxy manifested by levocardia with a single right-sided spleen. Features of this syndrome are similar to that of right isomerism.

The usage of the terms *atrial isomerism, bilateral right-sidedness* or *left-sidedness* as substitutes for the syndromes of situs ambiguous is discouraged because they are semantically inaccurate representations of the anatomy found in these patients.

In an autopsy series of 109 cases of heterotaxy syndrome by Van Praagh, 53% were asplenia, 42% polysplenia, and 5% single right-sided spleen with levocardia.[20] There is a relatively high incidence of discordance between the different components of visceral situs as well atrial situs. Hence, the syndromic approach to heterotaxy has been discarded in favor of a segmental approach in which there is an independent assessment of every involved organ system without any preconceived notions.[21] Determining visceral situs by chest radiography is challenging and can be achieved by recognizing the bronchial branching pattern (Fig. 1-19). A symmetric branching pattern is a common manifestation of heterotaxy. The cardiac apex and stomach position are not used for determining visceral situs because of the high incidence of discordance.[22] For accurate determination of visceral situs, cross-sectional imaging by ultrasound, CT, or MRI is required for evaluating the status of the liver and spleen.

Second Major Segment: Ventricular Loop

Depending on the direction of ventricular looping during development, the right ventricle may be located spatially on the right or left side of the heart (Fig. 1-20). If the bulboventricular loop occurs to the right, it is termed a *D-loop*, and the morphologic RV lies anterior and to the right of the morphologic LV. If the bulboventricular loop occurs to the left, it is termed an *L-loop*, and the morphologic RV lies anterior and to the left of the morphologic LV.

Third Major Segment: Great Arterial Relationship

Normally, the aortic annulus lies posterior, inferior, and to the right of the pulmonary valve annulus. This position is called *solitus (S)* (Fig. 1-21A). In situs inversus, the aorta lies posterior and to the left of the pulmonary valve, termed *inversus (I)* (see Fig. 1-21B). Any other position of the aorta and pulmonary artery other than solitus or inversus is termed *malposition*. If the aorta lies to the right of the PA, it is called *D-malposition* (see Fig. 1-21C). If the aorta lies to the left of the PA, it is termed *L-malposition* (see Fig. 1-21D). In rare cases, the aorta lies straight—anterior to the pulmonary artery, and is referred to as *A* according to segmental nomenclature. If the aorta lies straight—posterior to the pulmonary artery, it is termed *P*.

CHAPTER 1 • *Embryologic Basis and Segmental Approach to Imaging* 19

Different Types of Human Hearts

The segmental possibilities at each level are as follows:

Atria: Solitus (S), inversus (I) and ambiguous (A)
Ventricles: D and L
Great arteries: solitus (S), inversus (I), D malposition, and L malposition

Based on the various permutations and combinations of atrial, ventricular, and great arterial relationships, as well as on the anatomy of the conus, Van Praagh provided an overview of the diversity that exists in human hearts (Fig. 1-22).[18] It becomes immediately apparent that a pattern-based approach or an approach based on connections or the direction of flow of blood will not do justice to the complexity of the disease process. The segmental approach not only takes into account the morphologic variations at each level, but it also provides structural landmarks to distinguish the variations from each other and to determine their impact on physiology, thereby allowing informed decision-making regarding management.

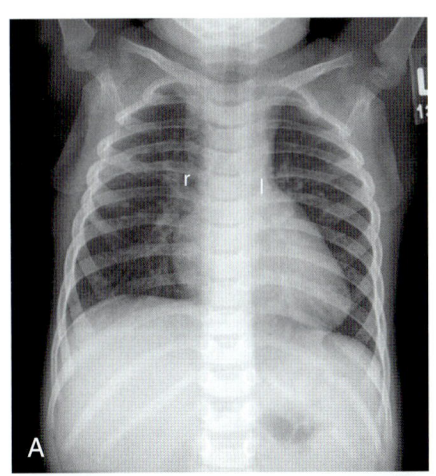

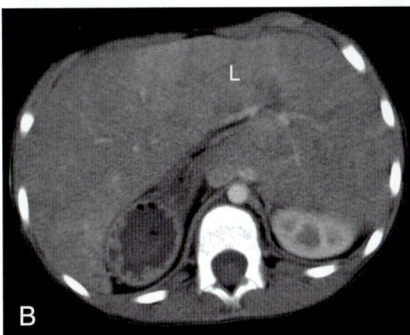

Analysis of the Connecting Segments

First Connecting Segment: Atrioventricular Junction

The anatomic possibilities at the atrioventricular junction level may be classified based on the number of ventricles as follows:

1. Biventricular AV connections
2. Univentricular AV connections

The types of biventricular AV connections (Fig. 1-23) include the following:

1. Concordant AV connections (RA-RV and LA-LV)
2. Discordant AV connections (RA-LV and LA-RV)
3. Straddling AV valve, in which there is abnormal attachment of the tensor apparatus of the valve to the opposite ventricle
4. Overriding AV valve, in which the AV valve annulus crosses the interventricular septum and partly overlies the opposite ventricle
5. Overriding and straddling AV valve

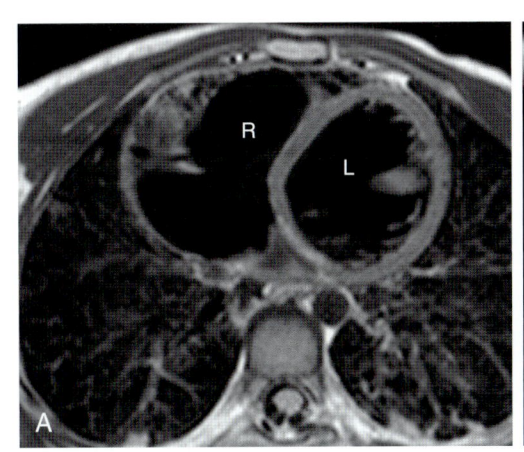

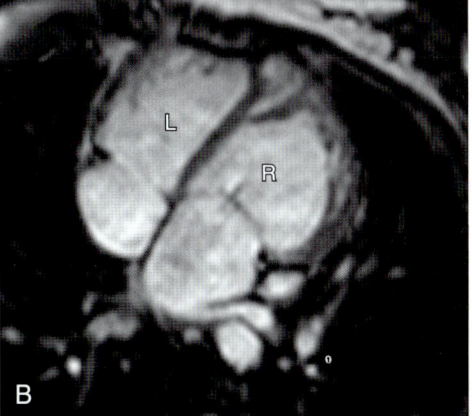

■ **FIGURE 1-19** **A,** Determining visceral situs by chest radiography may be achieved by studying the bronchial branching pattern. r and l indicate the symmetric eparterial upper lobe bronchi in this patient with asplenia complex. The cardiac apex and stomach position are not reliable indicators of visceral situs. **B,** Cross-sectional imaging by ultrasound, CT or MRI is needed for reliable determination of visceral situs by evaluating the status of the liver and spleen. This patient has a transverse liver (L) with asplenia.

■ **FIGURE 1-20** The second major cardiac segment: Ventricular looping. **A,** D-looping with the RV lying anterior and to the right of the LV. **B,** L-looping, with the RV lying anterior and to the left of the LV. The RV is identified by the moderator band, apical displacement of the AV valve, and the conus (*not shown*).

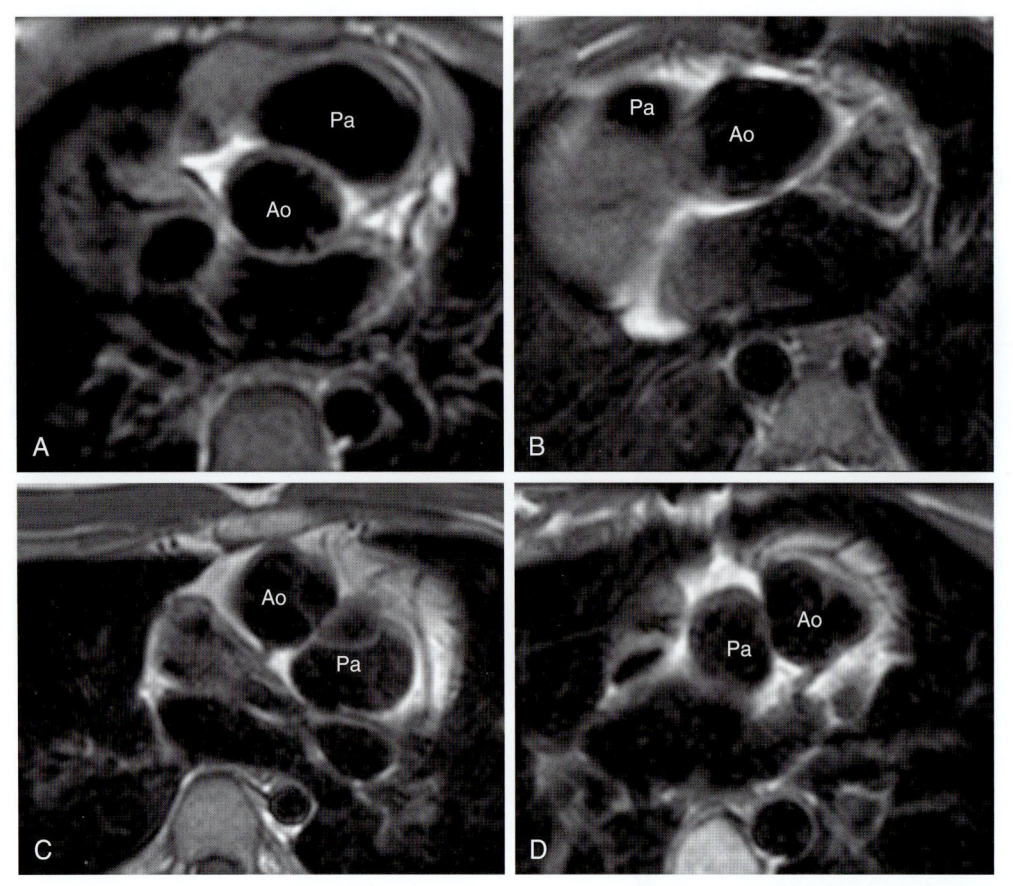

■ **FIGURE 1-21** The third major cardiac segment. Great arterial relationship. **A,** Solitus (S): the aortic annulus (Ao) lies posterior, inferior, and to the right of the pulmonary valve annulus (Pa). **B,** Inversus (I): the aorta lies posterior and to the left of the pulmonary valve. **C,** D-malposition: the aorta lies anterior and to the right of the PA. **D,** L-malposition: the aorta lies anterior and to the left of the PA.

6. Balanced common AV canal with two symmetric-sized ventricles

The types of univentricular AV connections (Figs. 1-24 and 1-25) include the following:

1. Unilateral left AV valve atresia (mitral atresia)
2. Unilateral right AV valve atresia (tricuspid atresia)
3. Double inlet LV
4. Double inlet RV
5. Left dominant unbalanced common AV canal
6. Right dominant unbalanced common AV canal

In the setting of univentricular AV connections, one of the AV valves is atretic, or both AV valves open partly or wholly into the same ventricle. The second ventricular chamber is subsequently very small or just an outflow chamber, and is of little functional use, apart from serving as a conduit for one of the great arteries. The segmental approach may be applied even in the setting of such functional single ventricles (see Fig. 1-25). Single ventricles may be of a left ventricular, right ventricular, or indeterminate morphology.[23] The functional single LV is characterized by the presence of a bulboventricular foramen, which connects the LV chamber to the small anteriorly located infundibular outlet chamber of the RV. The RV sinus (inflow portion) is typically absent. A functional single RV is characterized by the presence of a septal band, and in some cases, by a rudimentary posterolaterally located LV chamber.

Twisted atrioventricular connections: Van Praagh[24] introduced the concept of atrioventricular alignment as an independent entity from atrioventricular connections mainly to describe the spectrum of conditions with twisted or crossed atrioventricular connections, variably described as criss-cross, or topsy-turvy hearts.[25] These are hearts with discordance between atrioventricular alignment and atrioventricular connection. For instance, Figure 1-26 shows a 3-D volume rendered image of a patient with situs solitus of the atria and viscera, criss-cross atrioventricular relationship, and L-malposition of the great arteries. The RV lies superior and slightly to the left of the LV. But, because of the crossed atrioventricular connections, this patient has concordant atrioventricular connection, with the right atrium connecting to the left-sided RV. The base to apex axis of the heart spirals almost 180 degrees, with the two atrioventricular blood streams crossing each other. The physiology is that of uncorrected transposition. Because of the presence of associated straddling, AV valve, and severe pulmonary stenosis, a single ventricle repair was performed with a Fontan procedure.

CHAPTER 1 • *Embryologic Basis and Segmental Approach to Imaging*   21

Types of Human Hearts:
Segmental Combinations and Connections

Normal	{S,D,S}		{I,L,I}	
Isolated ventricular discordance	{S,L,S}		{I,D,I}	
Isolated atrial noninversion	{S,L,I}			
Transposition of the great arteries	{S,D,D}	{S,L,L}	{I,L,L}	{I,D,D}
Anatomically corrected malposition of the great arteries	{S,D,L}	{S,L,D}	{I,L,D}	{I,D,L}
Double outlet right ventricle	{S,D,D}	{S,L,L}	{I,L,L}	{I,D,D}
Double outlet left ventricle	{S,D,D}	{S,L,L}	{I,L,L}	{I,D,D}

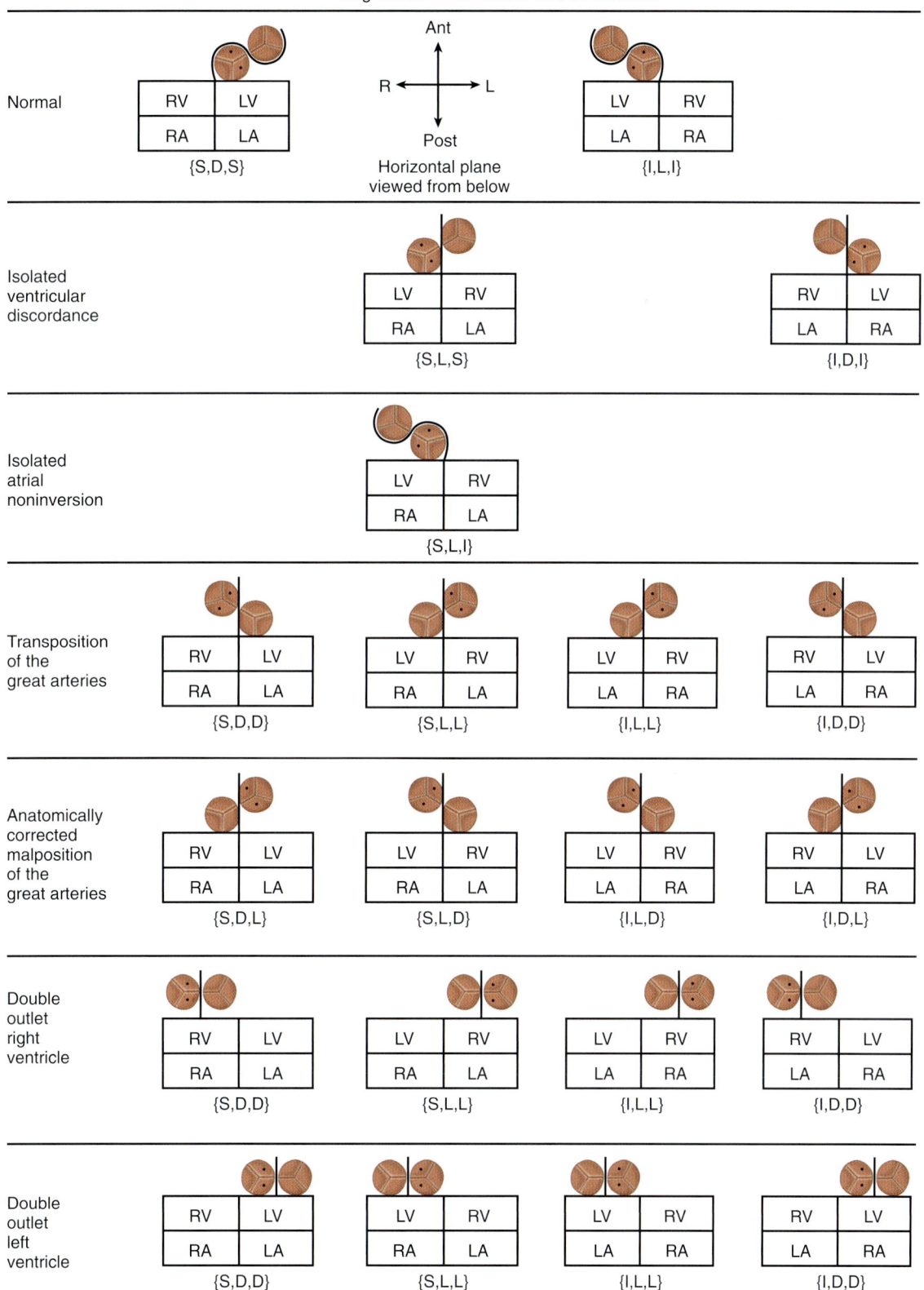

Orientation key: Ant / Post, R ↔ L. Horizontal plane viewed from below.

■ **FIGURE 1-22** Van Praagh's types of human hearts, based on segmental combinations of visceroatrial situs, ventricular looping, and great arterial situs. The segmental combination is expressed as a set, within braces. For instance, a normal heart would be expressed as {S,D,S} for visceroatrial situs solitus, D-looping of the ventricles, and solitus relationship of the great arteries. The segmental connections and associated anomalies are expressed outside the braces. For instance, physiologically corrected transposition would be expressed as {S,L,L} transposition of the great arteries for solitus atria, L-looped ventricles, and L-malposition of the great arteries. If this patient also had straddling AV valve and an inlet VSD, it would be expressed as {S,L,L} TGA, straddling tricuspid valve, inlet VSD. *(Adapted from Van Praagh R, Weinberg PM, Matsuoka R, Van Praagh S. Malposition of the heart and the segmental approach to diagnosis. In Adams FH, Emmanouilides GC [eds]. Moss' Heart Diseases in Infants, Children and Adolescents, 3rd. ed. Williams and Wilkins, Baltimore, 1983, pp 422-458).*

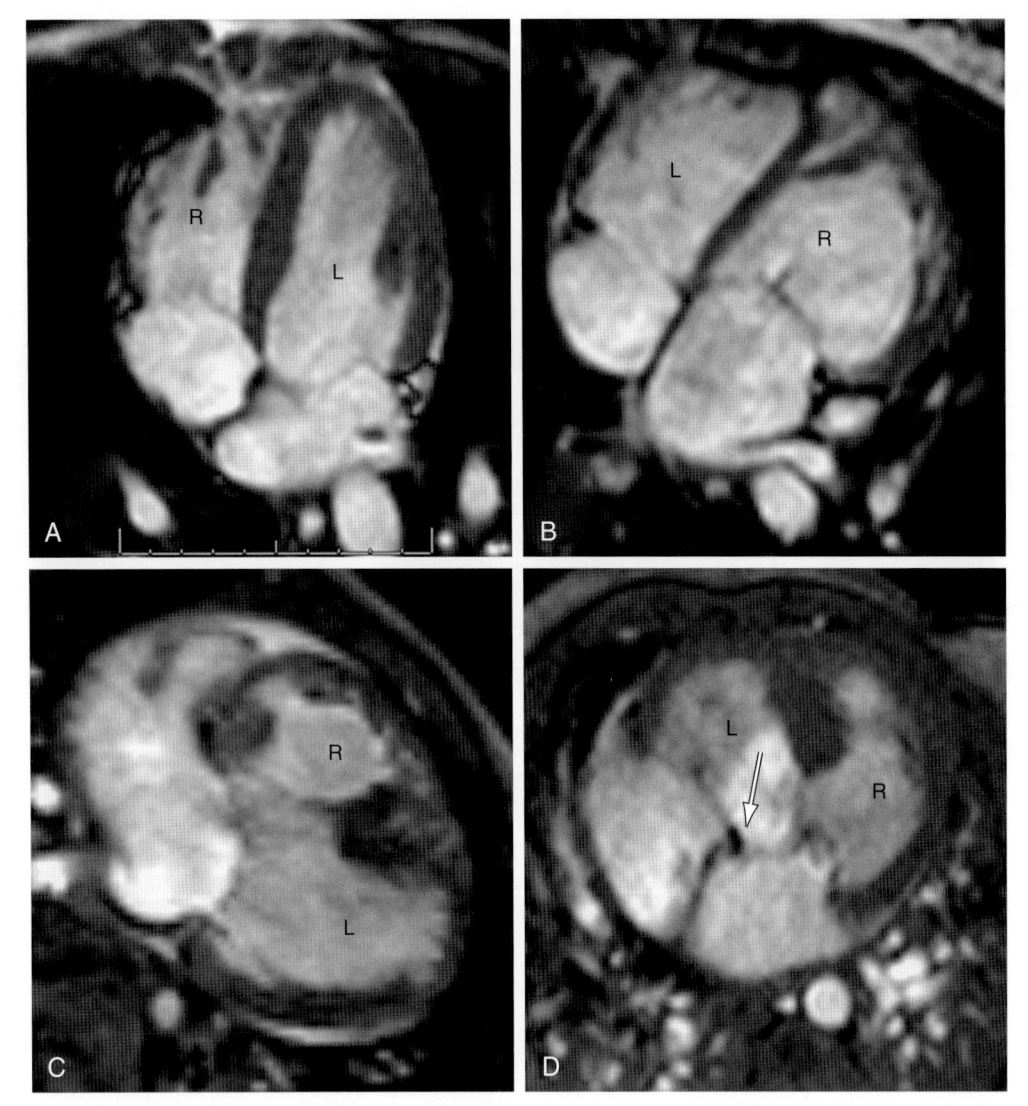

FIGURE 1-23 Types of biventricular AV connections. **A,** R: right ventricle; L, left ventricle; concordant AV connections (RA-RV and LA-LV). **B,** Discordant AV connections (RA-LV and LA-RV). **C,** Balanced common AV canal with two symmetric-sized ventricles. **D,** Straddling and overriding tricuspid valve (*arrow*), in a patient with L-looped ventricles.

Second Connecting Segment: Conotruncus or Ventriculoarterial Junction

The development of the conotruncus is the most important variable in the genesis of outflow tract anomalies. The differential growth of the subpulmonary and subaortic conus cushions largely determines the relationship between the semilunar valves, between the semilunar valves and the ventricles, and between the semilunar valves and the atrioventricular valves. It also determines the presence of distal infundibular stenosis and the location of the VSD in outflow tract anomalies. Based on conal development, the following anatomic types of conus (Fig. 1-27) may be recognized[26]:

1. Development of subpulmonary conus and resorption of the subaortic conus results in ventriculoarterial concordance and normal relationship of great arteries. The aorta lies posterior and to the right in a D-loop heart (solitus), and posterior and to the left in an L-looped heart (inversus).

2. Development of the subaortic conus and resorption of the subpulmonary conus results in ventriculoarterial discordance and transposition of the great arteries. Transposition means that the left ventricle is connected to the main pulmonary artery and the right ventricle to the aorta. The aorta lies anterior and to the right in a D-looped heart (D-malposition) (Fig. 1-28), and anterior and to the left in an L-looped heart (L-malposition).

3. Persistence and development of both the subaortic and subpulmonary conus leads to double outlet RV. Double outlet right ventricle means that both great vessels arise predominantly from the RV. There may be variable development of the pulmonary and aortic conus resulting in variable location of the VSD in relation to the great arteries.

Univentricular AV connections

Double inlet right ventricle

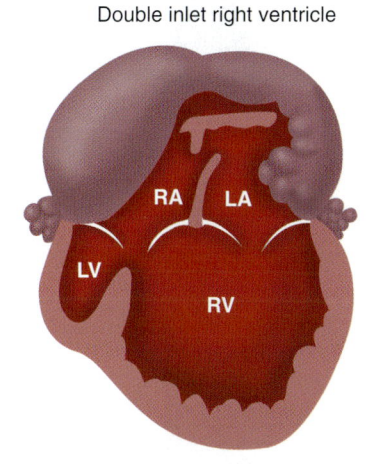

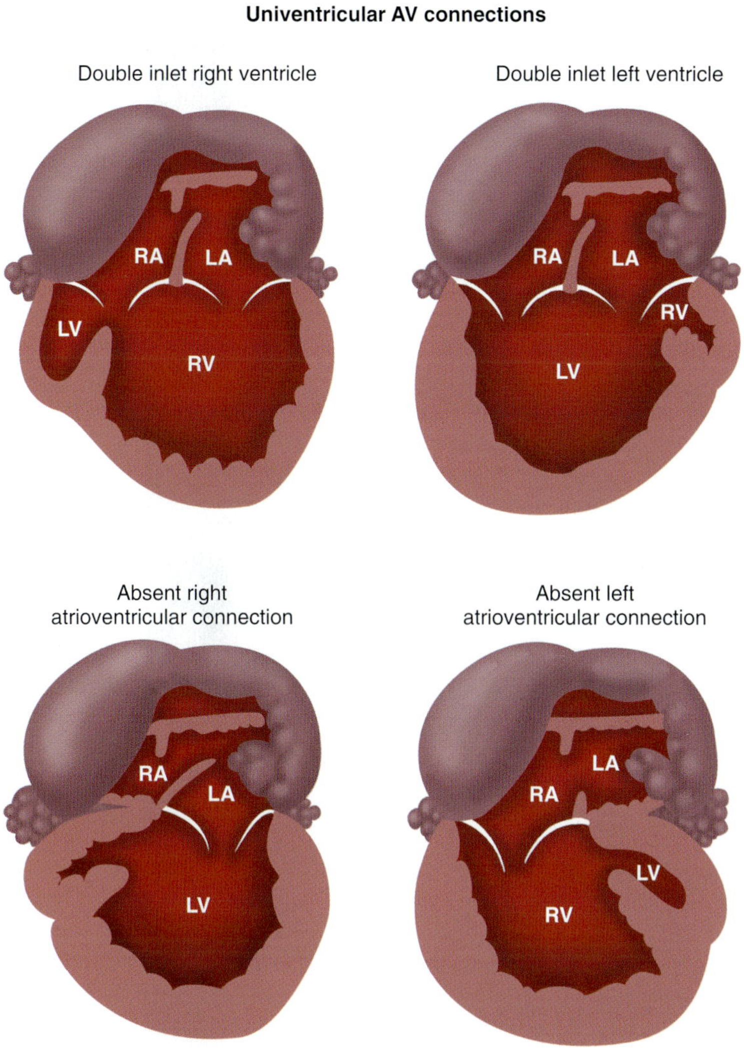

Double inlet left ventricle

Absent right atrioventricular connection

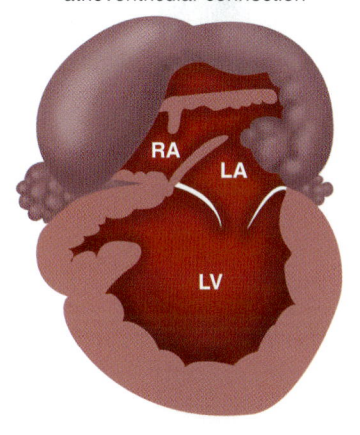

Absent left atrioventricular connection

■ **FIGURE 1-24** Univentricular AV connections: Double inlet RV and double inlet LV (illustrated in the setting of L-looped ventricles in the figure), as well as unilateral AV valve atresia result in underdevelopment of the affected ventricle and a functional single ventricle situation. The segmental approach may still be used for ventricular identification in these situations. *(Adapted from The segmental and sequential approach to heart disease. In Freedom RM, Mawson JB, Yoo SJ, Benson LN [eds]: Congenital Heart Disease: Textbook of Angiocardiography, Armonk, NY, 1997, Futura, p 109.)*

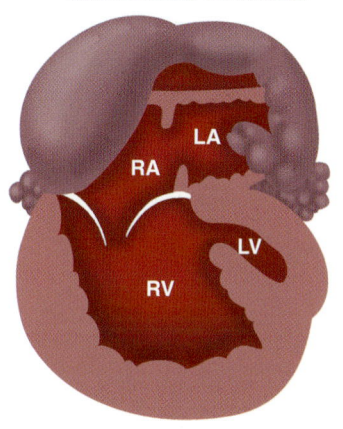

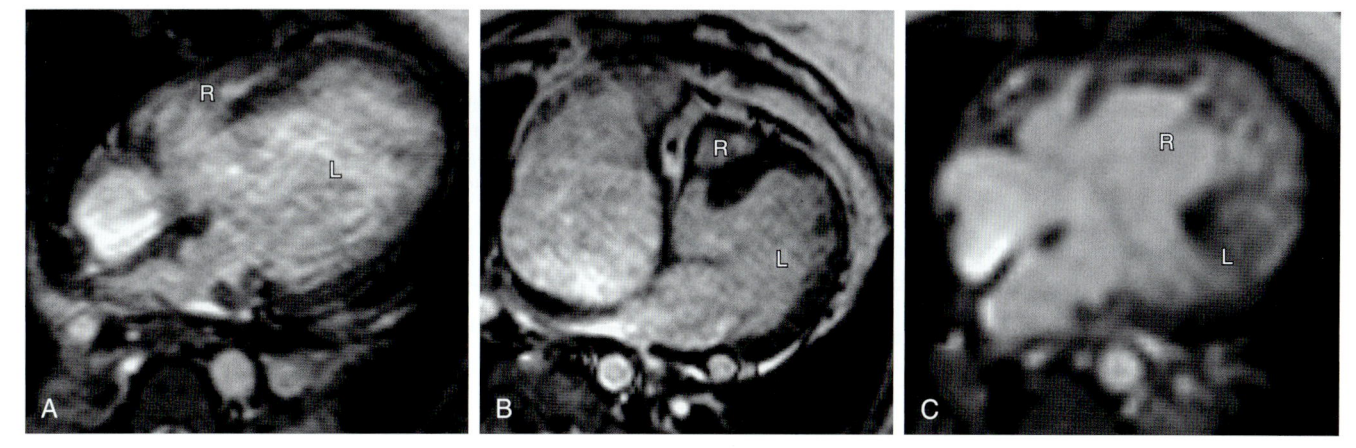

■ **FIGURE 1-25** Types of univentricular AV connections. **A,** Double inlet LV. **B,** Tricuspid atresia. **C,** Right dominant unbalanced common AV canal.

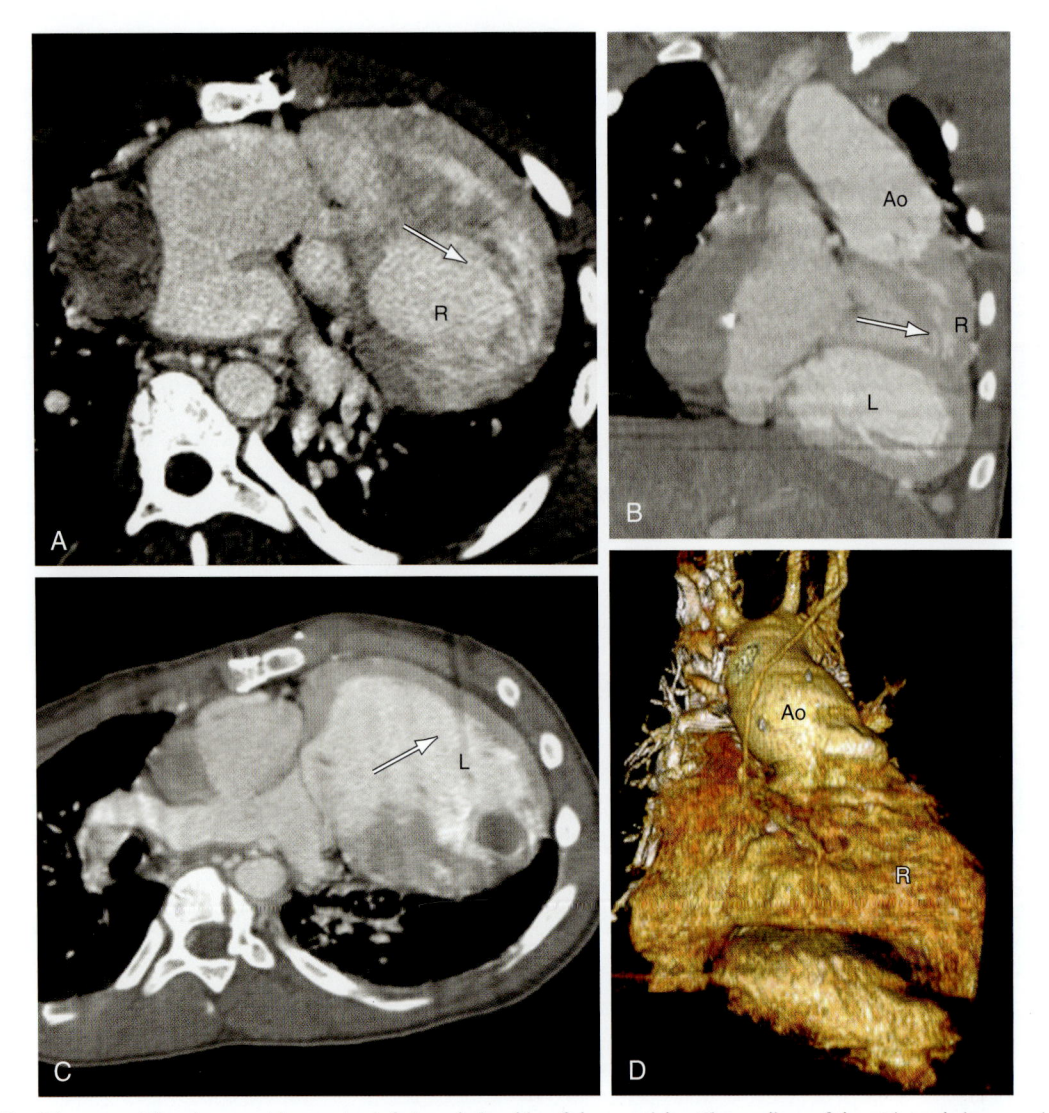

FIGURE 1-26 Criss-cross AV pathways with superior-inferior relationship of the ventricles. Situs solitus of the atria and viscera, criss-cross atrioventricular relationship, and L-malposition of the great arteries. The base to apex axis of the heart spirals nearly 180 degrees, with the two atrioventricular blood streams crossing each other (*arrows* in **A-C**). The physiology is that of uncorrected transposition. A thrombus is noted in the LV apex in **C**. **D** is a 3D-volume rendered image from the CT angiogram showing the crossing RA-RV pathway, and the L-malposed aorta arising from the RV.

4. Resorption of both the subpulmonary and subaortic conus results in double outlet LV. Double outlet LV means that both vessels arise predominantly from the LV.

A rare form of conal maldevelopment is anatomically corrected malposition of the great arteries in which there is origin of the malposed aorta above the LV, and origin of the malposed pulmonary artery above the RV.[27] Malalignment of the conal septum is also the cause of infundibular obstruction in tetralogy of Fallot (anterior malalignment) and subaortic stenosis with interrupted aortic arch (posterior malalignment).

Evaluation of Associated Anomalies

The presence of associated anomalies involving the atrial and ventricular septum, the atrioventricular and semilunar valves, aorta, pulmonary arteries, pulmonary veins, and systemic veins (Fig. 1-29) plays an important part in the functional outcome of the patient, and screening for these conditions is an integral part of the segmental approach to heart disease.

Evaluation of Function

The final step in the segmental approach to heart disease is to determine how the segmental combinations and connections, with the associated anomalies, function (Case Study 1, Fig. 1-30). Broadly, abnormal function of the congenitally malformed heart may be classified into the following subgroups:

1. Pressure overload, related to valvular stenosis, coarctation, branch pulmonary artery stenosis, etc.

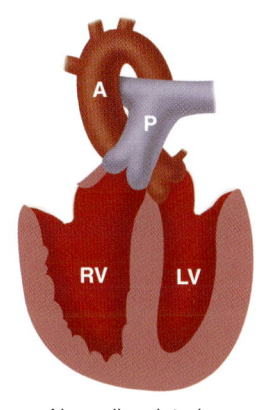

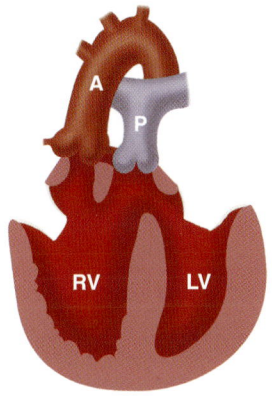

CHAPTER 1 • Embryologic Basis and Segmental Approach to Imaging

Ventriculoarterial Connections

- Normally related great arteries
- Double-outlet right ventricle
- D-TGA
- Double-outlet left ventricle

FIGURE 1-27 Types of ventriculoarterial connections based on conal development. *(Adapted from The segmental and sequential approach to congenital heart disease. In Freedom RM, Mawson JB, Yoo SJ, Benson LN [eds]: Congenital Heart Disease: Textbook of Angiocardiography. Armonk, NY, 1997, Futura, p 111.)*

2. Volume overload, related to valvular regurgitation, left-to-right shunts, etc.
3. Intermixing, in which there is mixing of oxygenated blood with deoxygenated blood before entering the systemic circulation. This typically occurs in the setting of a common chamber, vessel or valve, or in a right-to-left shunt.
4. Poor contractility of the myocardium related to cardiomyopathy, ischemia, etc.

When all relevant information regarding morphology and function has been collected, decisions regarding management may be made, which may be in the form of medical therapy, surgical therapy, or both.

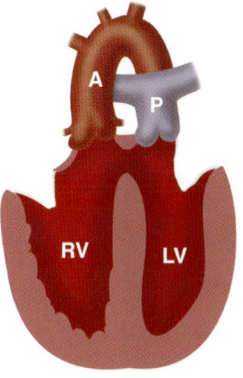

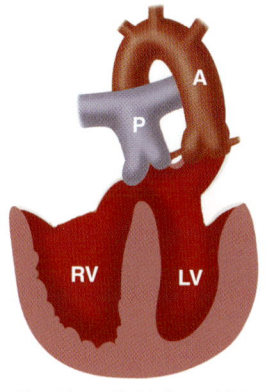

KEY POINTS

- The segmental approach to heart disease provides an elegantly simple method to break down the complexity of congenital heart disease on cross-sectional imaging.
- It creates a template for standardizing nomenclature in CHD, thereby ensuring that caregivers from different specialties understand each other.
- It is firmly rooted in embryologic principles and is, therefore, fairly intuitive to the beginner in the field. MRI and CT almost rival pathologic evaluation of specimens in the detail that they provide on cardiovascular morphology.
- MRI provides unique information regarding function, flow, and tissue characterization that decreases the need for more invasive means of diagnosis.

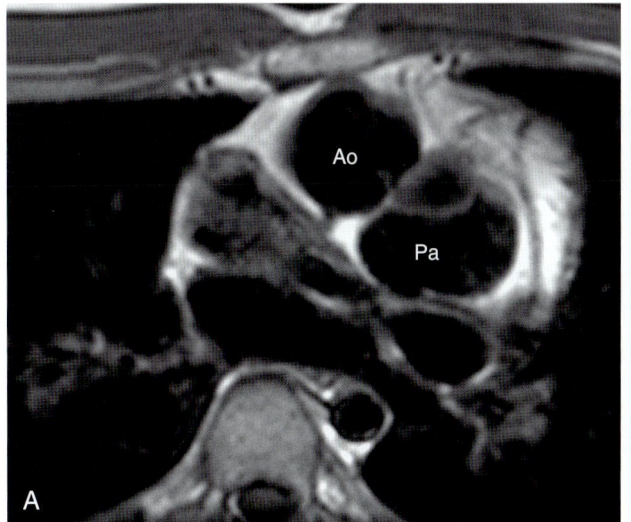

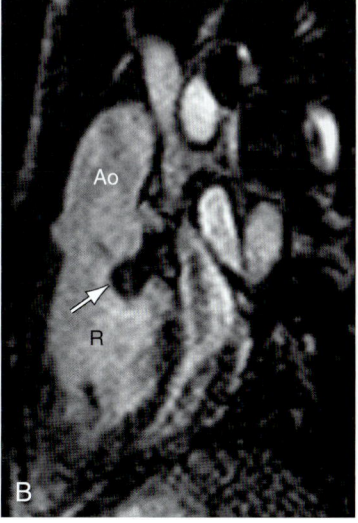

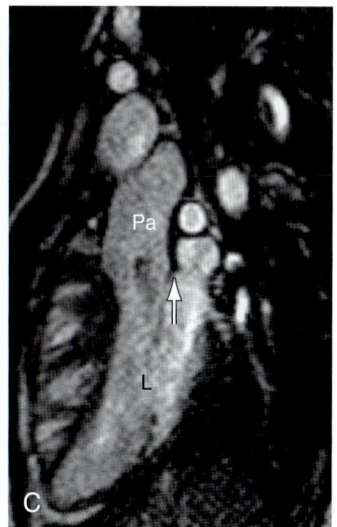

FIGURE 1-28 Conus in D-TGA. **A,** The aorta lies anterior and to the right of the pulmonary artery (D-malposition). **B,** The right ventricle (R) is connected to the aorta (Ao) by a muscular infundibulum (*arrow*), resulting in lack of fibrous contiguity between the tricuspid valve and the aortic valve. **C,** The left ventricle (L) is connected to the main pulmonary artery (Pa) with absence of an intervening conus, resulting in direct fibrous contiguity between the aortic and pulmonary valves.

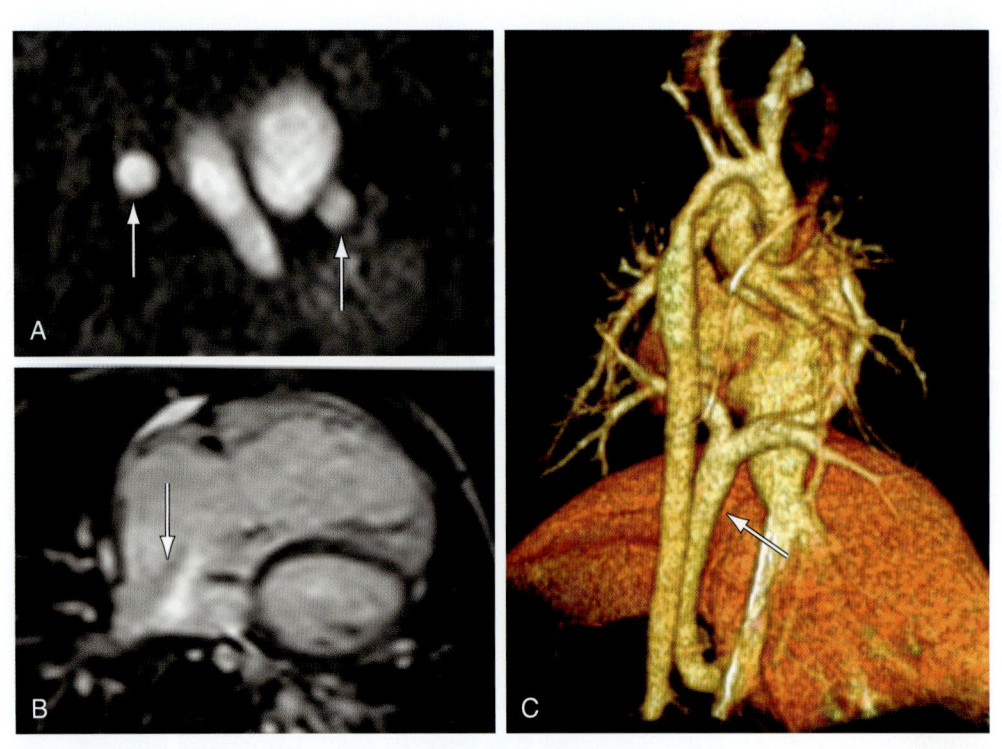

FIGURE 1-29 Evaluation of associated anomalies. **A,** Bilateral SVC without a connecting vein. **B,** Large secundum atrial septal defect. **C,** Infradiaphragmatic total anomalous pulmonary venous return to the main portal vein (*arrow*), and aortic coarctation.

CHAPTER 1 • Embryologic Basis and Segmental Approach to Imaging 27

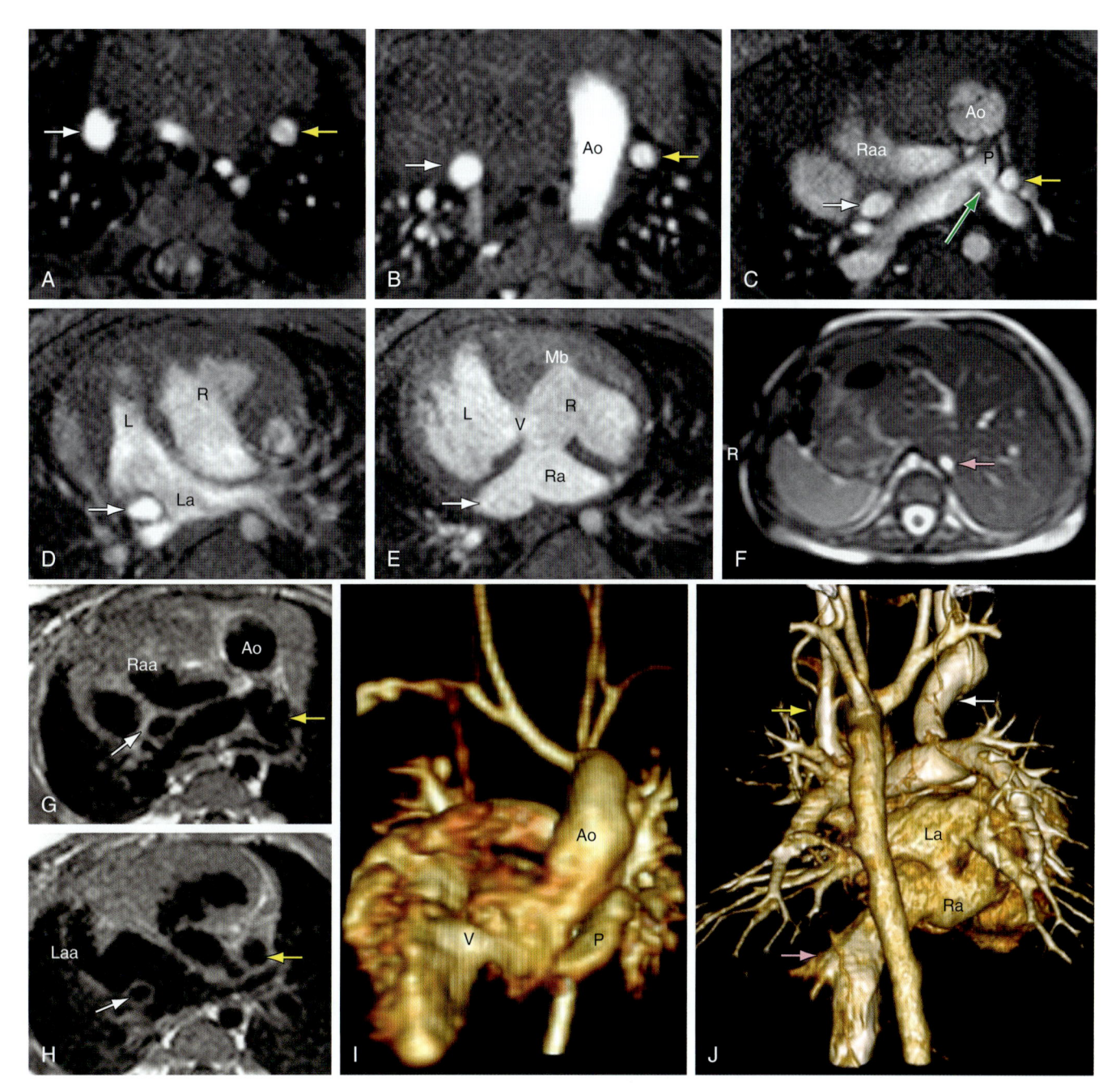

■ **FIGURE 1-30** Case Study 1. The segmental approach to heart disease is illustrated on a cardiac MRI study on a 4-day-old male with double outlet right ventricle (I,L,D): *white arrow*: right SVC; *yellow arrow*: left SVC; *pink arrow*: IVC; Ra: morphologic right atrium; La: morphologic left atrium; Raa: right atrial appendage; Laa: left atrial appendage; R: morphologic right ventricle; Mb: moderator band; L: morphologic left ventricle; V: inlet VSD; Ao: aorta; Pa: pulmonary artery.

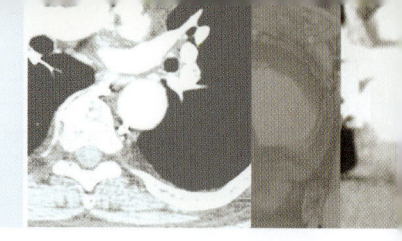

CASE STUDY

Chapter 1 Embryologic and Segmental Approach to Imaging of Congenital Heart Disease

CASE STUDY 1 (see Figure 1-30)

- Visceroatrial situs: there is visceral and atrial situs inversus. A left-sided liver and single right-sided spleen are noted in Figure 1-30F, right-sided left atrium receiving pulmonary veins (Fig. 1-30D), left-sided IVC entering left-sided right atrium (Figs. 1-30F and 1-30J).
- Ventricles: L-loop. The right ventricle is located anterior and to the left of the left ventricle (Figs. 1-30D and 1-30E). Note moderator band within left-sided RV and smooth septal surface of the LV.
- Great arteries: D-malposition (aortic valve is anterior and slightly to the right of the pulmonary valve, in Figs. 1-30C, 1-30G, and 1-30I).
- Atrioventricular connection: Concordant (LA connected to LV and RA connected to RV) in Figures 1-30D and 1-30E.
- Ventriculoarterial connection: Double outlet right ventricle. Both subpulmonary and subaortic conus are present. Both great arteries are remote from the VSD (Fig. 1-30I).
- Associated anomalies: (1) large inlet VSD, which is remote from both great arteries (Figs. 1-30E and 1-30I); (2) hypoplastic pulmonary valve annulus and moderately severe left pulmonary artery stenosis (Figure 1-30C); (3) bilateral SVC, with the right SVC draining via the coronary sinus (Fig. 1-30E); (4) right juxtaposition of the atrial appendages (Figs. 1-30G and 1-30H).
- Physiology: Well balanced pulmonary circulation at birth due to the presence of moderate pulmonary stenosis. Progressive cyanosis developed at 6 months of age because of increasing pulmonary stenosis.
- Treatment decision: Although he had two normal-sized ventricles, he was not a candidate for two ventricle repair due to the remote location of the VSD with respect to the aorta and the presence of severe pulmonary stenosis. At 6 months of age, he underwent staged single-ventricle palliation with a bilateral bidirectional Glenn procedure and left pulmonary artery augmentation with a pericardial patch with anticipated Fontan completion at 18 months of age.

SUGGESTED READINGS

Clark EB, Van Mierop LHS: Development of the cardiovascular system. In Adams FH, Emmanouilides GC, Riemenschneider TA (eds): Moss' Heart Disease in Infants, Children, and Adolescents. Baltimore, Williams & Wilkins, 1989, pp 2-15.

Freedom RM, Yoo SJ, Mikalian H, Williams WG (eds): The Natural and Modified History of Congenital Heart Disease. New York, Futura, 2004.

Krishnamurthy R, Chung T: Current imaging status: pediatric MRI. In Lucaya J, Strife JL (eds): Pediatric Chest Imaging. 2nd ed. Berlin, Springer, 2007.

The segmental and sequential approach to congenital heart disease. In Freedom RM, Mawson JB, Yoo SJ, Benson LN (eds): Congenital Heart Disease: Textbook of Angiocardiography. Armonk, NY, Futura, 1997, pp 95-120.

Van Mierop LHS, Kutsche LM: Embryology of the heart. In Hurst JW (ed): The Heart. 7th ed. New York, McGraw-Hill, 1990.

Van Praagh R: The segmental approach to understanding complex cardiac lesions. In Eldridge WJ, Gberg H, Lemole GM (eds): Current Problems in Congenital Heart Disease. New York, SP Medical and Scientific Books, 1979, pp 1-18.

REFERENCES

1. Van Praagh R: The segmental approach to diagnosis in congenital heart disease. Birth Defects: Original Article Series 8:4-23, 1972.
2. Van Praagh R: The segmental approach to understanding complex cardiac lesions. In Eldredge WJ, Gberg H, Lemole GM (eds): Current Problems in Congenital Heart Disease. New York, 1979, Medical and Scientific Books, pp 1-18.
3. Van Praagh R: Diagnosis of complex congenital heart disease: morphologic-anatomic method and terminology. Cardiovasc Intervent Radiol 1984; 7:115-120.
4. Shinebourne EA, Macartney FJ, Anderson RH: Sequential chamber localization-logical approach to diagnosis in congenital heart disease. Br Heart J 1976; 38:327-340.
5. Van Mierop LHS, Kutsche LM: Embryology of the heart. In Hurst JW (ed). The heart, 7th ed. New York, 1990, McGraw-Hill Information Services Company.
6. Brueckner M, D'Eustachio P, Horwich AL: Linkage mapping of a mouse gene, *iv*, that controls left-right asymmetry of the heart and viscera. Proc Natl Acad Sci USA 1989; 86:5035-5038.
7. Burn J: Disturbance of morphological laterality in humans. Ciba Foundation Symposium 1992; 282-300.
8. Hanzlik AJ, Binder M, Layton WM, et al: The murine situs inversus viscerum (*iv*) gene responsible for visceral asymmetry is linked tightly to the Igh-C cluster on chromosome 12. Genomics 1990; 7:389-393.
9. Layton WM, Jr, Manasek FJ: Cardiac looping of early *iv/iv* mouse embryos. In Van Praagh R, Takao A (eds): Etiology and Morphogenesis of Congenital Heart Disease. Mount Kisco, NY, Futura, 1980, pp 109-126.
10. Anderson RH. Another look at cardiac embryology. In Yu PN, Goodwin JF (eds). Progress in Cardiology. Philadelphia, Lea & Febiger, 1978, pp 1-53.
11. Clark EB, Van Mierop LHS: Development of the cardiovascular system. In Adams FH, Emmanouilides GC, Riemenschneider TA (eds). Moss' Heart Disease in Infants, Children, and Adolescents. Baltimore, Williams and Wilkins, 1989, pp 2-15.
12. Calder L, Van Praagh R, Van Praagh S, et al: Truncus arteriosus communis. Clinical, angiocardiographic, and pathologic findings in 100 patients. American Heart J 1976; 92(1);22-38.
13. Van Praagh R, Perez-Trevino C, Lopez-Cuellar M, et al: Transposition of the great arteries with posterior aorta, subpulmonary conus and fibrous continuity between aortic and atrioventricular valves. Am J Cardiol 1971;28(6):894-904.
14. Reller MD, McDonald RW, Gerlis LM, Thornburg, KL. Cardiac embryology: Basic review and clinical correlations. J Am Soc Echocardiog 1991;4:519-532.
15. Neill CA: Development of the pulmonary veins. With reference to the embryology of anomalies of pulmonary venous return. Pediatrics 1956;18:880-887.
16. Edwards JE: Anomalies of derivatives of aortic arch system. Med Clin North Am 1948; 32:925-949.
17. Stewart JR, Kincaid OW, Edwards JE: An atlas of vascular rings and related malformation of the aortic arch system. Springfield, Charles C. Thomas, 1964.
18. Van Praagh R. Terminology of congenital heart disease. Glossary and commentary. Circulation 1977;56:139-143.
19. Huhta JC, Smallhorn JF, Macartney FJ, et al: Cross-sectional echocardiographic diagnosis of systemic venous return. Br Heart J 1982;48:388-403.
20. Van Praagh S, Kreutzer J, Alday L, Van Praagh R: Systemic and pulmonary venous connections in visceral heterotaxy, with emphasis on the diagnosis of the atrial situs: a study of 109 postmortem cases. In Clark E, Takao A (eds). Developmental Cardiology, Morphogenesis and Function. Mt. Kisco, NY, Futura, 1990, pp 671-721.
21. Machado-Atias I, Anselmi G, Machado-Hernandez I, Febres C: Discordances between the different types of atrial arrangement and the positions of the thoraco-abdominal organs. Cardiol Young 2001;11(5):543-550.
22. Van Praagh R, Vlad P: Dextrocardia, mesocardia, and levocardia: the segmental approach to diagnosis in congenital heart disease. In Keith JD, Rowe RD, Vlad P (eds). Heart disease in Infancy and Childhood. New York, NY, Macmillan, 1978, pp 638-695.
23. Colvin EV: Single ventricle. In Garson A Jr., Bricker JT, McNamara DG (eds). The Science and Practice of Pediatric Cardiology. Philadelphia, Lea and Febiger, 1990, pp 1246-1279.
24. Van Praagh R: When concordant or discordant atrioventricular alignments predict the ventricular situs wrongly. I. Solitus atria, concordant alignments, and L-loop ventricles. II. Solitus atria, discordant alignments, and D-loop ventricles. J Am Coll Cardiol 1987; 10:1278-1279.
25. Geva T, Van Praagh S, Sanders SP, et al: Straddling mitral valve with hypoplastic right ventricle, criss-cross atrioventricular relations, double outlet right ventricle and dextrocardia: Morphologic, diagnostic and surgical considerations. J Am Coll Cardiol 1991;17:1603-1612.
26. Van Praagh S, Layton WM, Van Praagh R: The morphogenesis of normal and abnormal relationships between the great arteries and the ventricles: pathologic and experimental data. In Van Praagh R, Takao A, (eds). Etiology and Morphogenesis of Congenital Heart Disease. Mt. Kisco, NY, Futura, 1980, pp 271-316.
27. Van Praagh R, Weinberg PM, Smith SD, et al: Malpositions of the heart. In Adams FH, Emmanouilides GC, Riemenschneider TA (eds). Moss' Heart Disease in Infants, Children, and Adolescents. Baltimore, Williams and Wilkins, 1989, pp 530-580.

ized by the paper-thin smooth walls into which the venae cavae and coronary sinus drain. The triangle of Koch is an important landmark formed by the coronary sinus, tendon of Todaro, and septal tricuspid leaflet. This landmark identifies the atrioventricular node and helps to avoid injury during surgery.[5] The right atrial appendage is a triangular structure that projects laterally and overlaps the right side of the aortic root. The ostium of the right atrial appendage is wide and, unlike the left atrial appendage, is not a site of thrombus formation.[6] The right atrium is connected to the right ventricle through the tricuspid valve, which has three cusps. Partial absence of the pericardium exposes a portion of the right atrium to the pleural cavity, and a herniation through the defect may resemble a right atrial mass on imaging.

CHAPTER 2

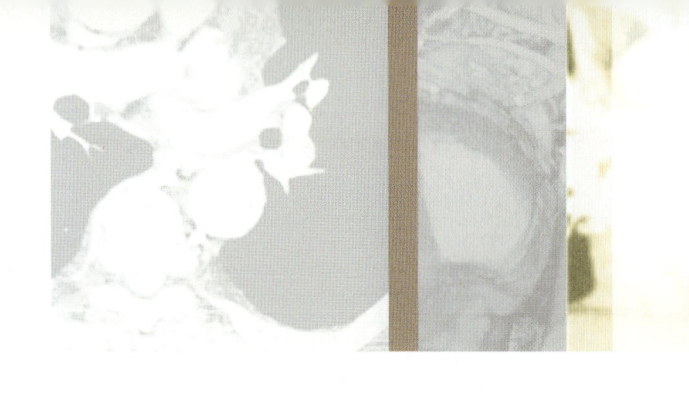

Cardiac Anatomy

Dharshan Raj Vummidi and Gautham P. Reddy

The heart is a muscular pump in the mediastinum weighing approximately 250 to 350 g. It extends obliquely from the second to the fifth ribs and is positioned against the diaphragm, flanked by the lungs on either side. It has a broad base directed toward the right shoulder and a narrow apex pointing inferolaterally toward the left hip. In the older individual, the heart has a more horizontal position, with a laterally pointing apex.

The heart has four chambers, two superior atria and two inferior ventricles. A fibrous interatrial septum divides the atria and a muscular interventricular septum divides the ventricles (Figs. 2-1 and 2-2). The heart is enveloped in a serous membrane, the pericardium, which has a visceral and parietal layer that contains a minimal amount of fluid.

The right atrium of the heart receives desaturated blood from the inferior and superior vena cava and the left side receives oxygenated blood through the four pulmonary veins. The right ventricle pumps the deoxygenated blood through the pulmonary arteries into the lungs. The left ventricle pumps oxygenated blood through the aorta into the systemic circulation.

Multidetector computed tomography (CT) and magnetic resonance imaging (MRI) have revolutionized cardiac imaging. The multiplanar capability of cross-sectional imaging enables the accurate diagnosis of cardiac pathology and function, and a thorough knowledge of cardiac anatomy is essential to interpret these examinations correctly. This chapter reviews cardiac anatomy, with an emphasis on the perspective of CT and MRI. Coronary artery anatomy will be covered in Chapter 3.

NORMAL ANATOMY

General Anatomic Descriptions

Pericardium

The pericardium is a two-layered membrane that envelops all four cardiac chambers and the origins of the great vessels. It consists of parietal and visceral layers separated by a small amount of serous fluid—normally, about 15 to 50 mL—that is mainly an ultrafiltrate of plasma. The pericardium limits the spread of infection and inflammation from adjacent mediastinal structures, prevents excessive dilation of the heart, and reduces friction between the heart and surrounding structures.[1]

CT and MRI are excellent modalities for imaging the pericardium. The normal pericardium is less than 2 mm thick and requires the presence of epicardial fat or pericardial fluid to distinguish it from the myocardium.[2] The pericardium is visible over the right atrium and right ventricle but the lateral and posterior walls of the left ventricle are often bare (Fig. 2-3). Left atrial enlargement is attributed to its partial coverage by pericardium. Several pericardial recesses may be visible on CT and MRI scans. Small amounts of fluid may be present in these structures in healthy individuals. The superior pericardial recess, a curvilinear structure wrapped around the right wall of the ascending aorta, may be mistaken for an aortic dissection, mediastinal mass, lymph node, or thymus. The transverse pericardial sinus, which is dorsal to the ascending aorta, sometimes may be mistaken for aortic dissection or lymphadenopathy (Fig. 2-4). The oblique pericardial sinus, which is situated behind the left atrium, may be misinterpreted as esophageal lesions or bronchogenic cysts. Knowledge of the locations of these recesses can help the imaging specialist differentiate them from abnormal lesions.[3]

Atria

Right Atrium

The atria are divided into a venous component, vestibule of the atrioventricular valve, septal component, and appendage. The right atrium is embryologically derived from the sinus venosus and primitive auricle, with the former evolving into the venous component and the latter into the appendage. These corresponding parts are separated internally by a muscular band called the *crista terminalis* (Fig. 2-5), which could be misinterpreted as a right atrial mass.[4] The posterior part of the atrium is

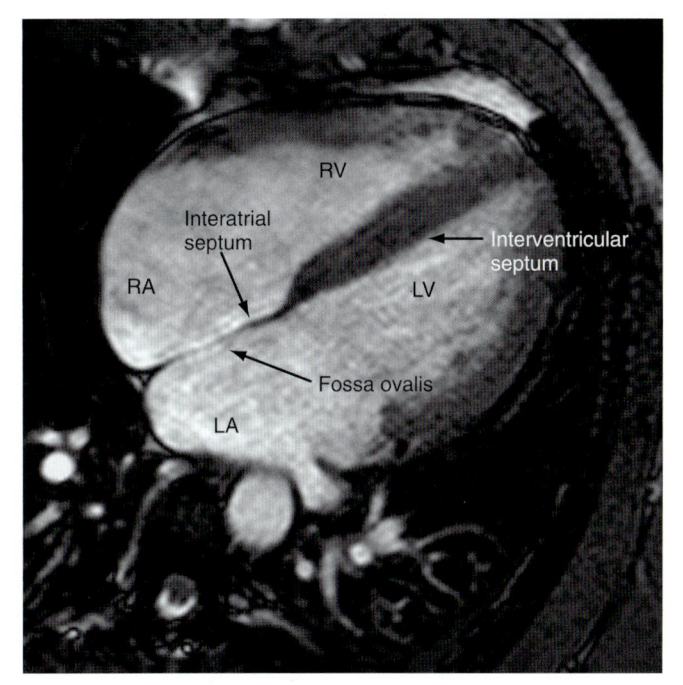

CHAPTER 2 • *Cardiac Anatomy* 31

■ **FIGURE 2-1** Axial bSSFP (balanced steady-state free precession) white blood image demonstrating the four chambers of the heart, interatrial and interventricular septa.

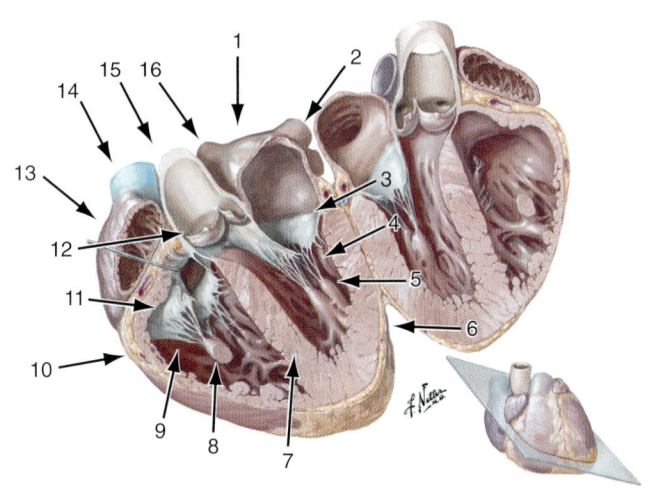

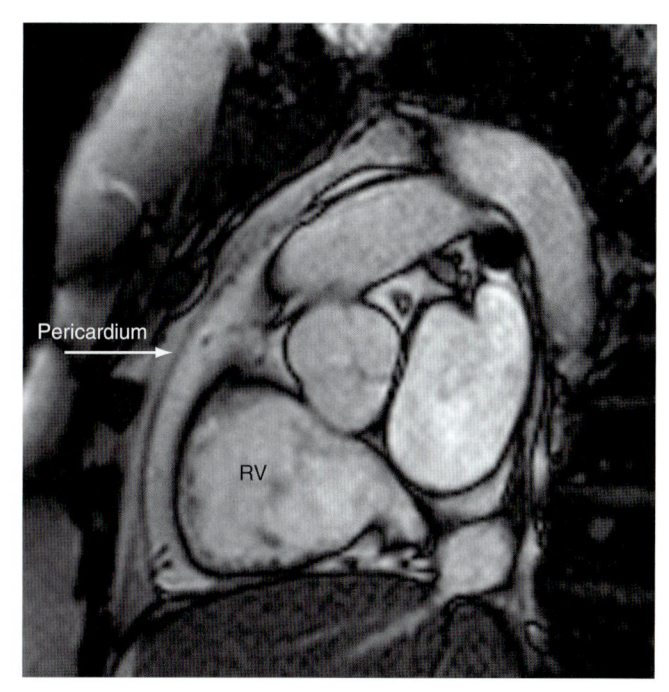

■ **FIGURE 2-3** Short-axis bSSFP image illustrating the normal pericardium anterior to the right ventricle.

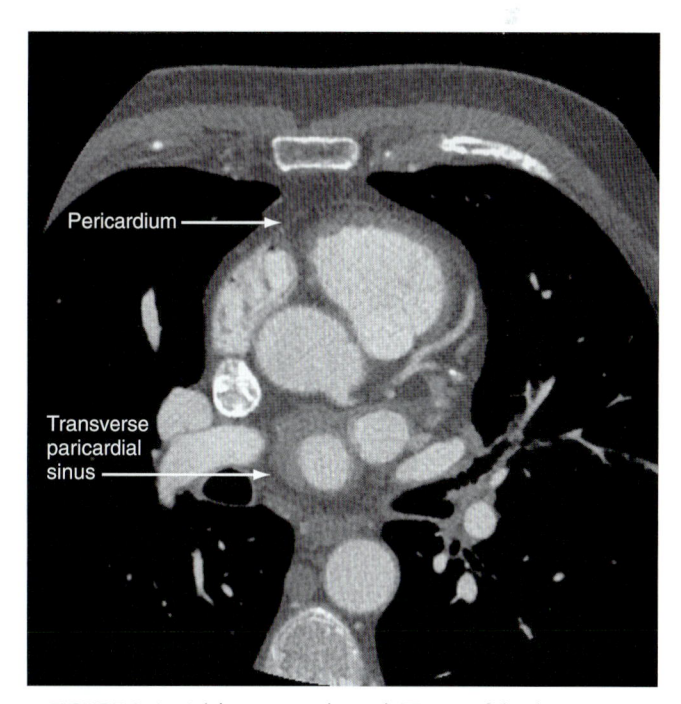

1. Left atrium
2. Left superior pulmonary vein
3. Mitral valve
4. Chordae tendinae
5. Papillary muscle
6. Left ventricle
7. Interventricular septum
8. Papillary muscle
9. Chordae tendinae
10. Right ventricle
11. Tricuspid valve
12. Aortic valve
13. Right atrium
14. Superior vena cava
15. Aorta
16. Right superior pulmonary vein

■ **FIGURE 2-2** Atria, ventricles, and interventricular septum section through the heart showing the structure of all chambers of the heart. (From Netter Illustration Collection at www.netterimages.com © Elsevier Inc. All Rights Reserved. The author has added new labels to this image that are not part of the original image.)

■ **FIGURE 2-4** Axial contrast-enhanced CT scan of the thorax illustrating the normal pericardium and transverse pericardial sinus.

derived from the sinus venosus and has a smooth interior, whereas the appendage, derived from the primitive auricle, has trabeculations and pectinate muscles that branch from the crista terminalis at right angles (Fig. 2-6). The venous component of the right atrium receives the superior and inferior vena cavae on its posterior surface and the coronary sinus at its junction with the septal component, just above the posterior interventricular groove (Fig. 2-7). The right atrial appendage has a triangular appearance and is best appreciated ventral to the junction of the superior vena cava (SVC) and right atrium. The smooth-walled vestibule incorporates the attachments for the tricuspid valve. The right atrium forms the right lateral border of the heart on a chest radiograph and enlargement of the appendage may be seen in the retrosternal space.

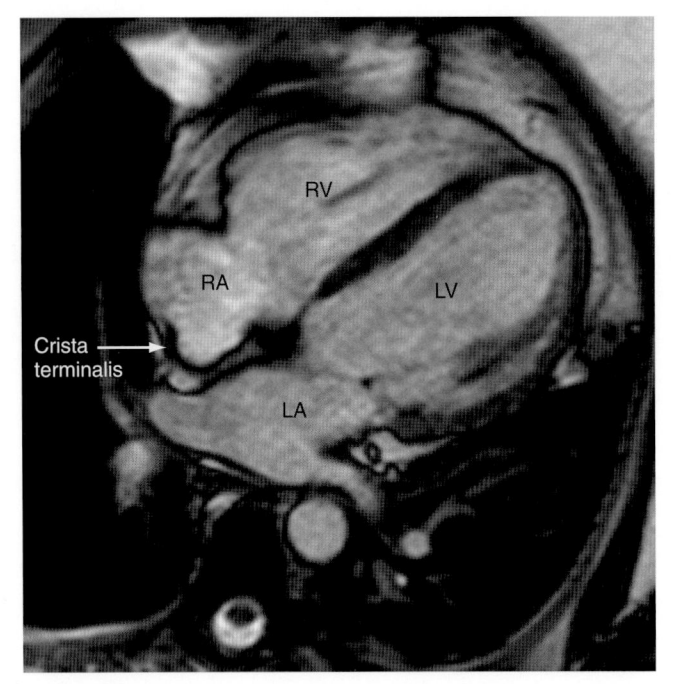

■ **FIGURE 2-5** Axial bSSFP image demonstrating the four chambers of the heart and the crista terminalis dividing the right atrium into the venous component and the appendage.

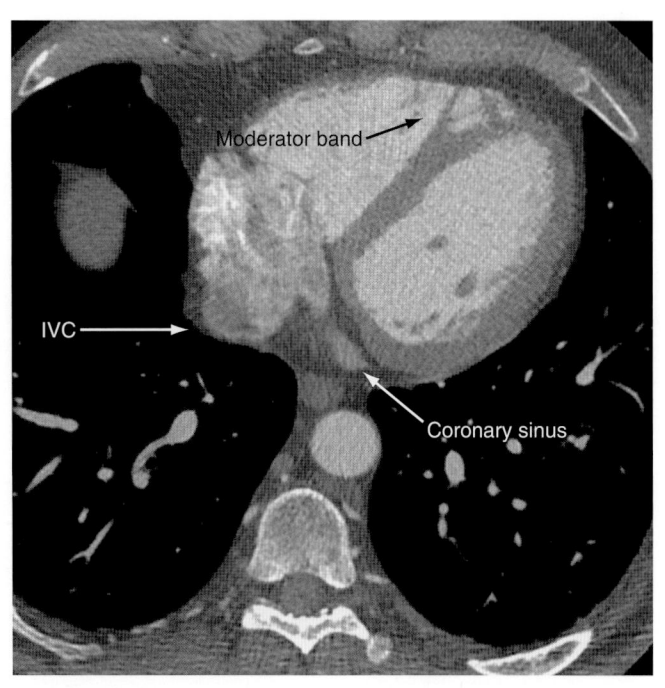

■ **FIGURE 2-7** Axial contrast-enhanced CT scan of the thorax illustrating the inferior vena cava (IVC), with the coronary sinus draining into the right atrium. The moderator band is a defining feature of the right ventricle and carries the right bundle branch.

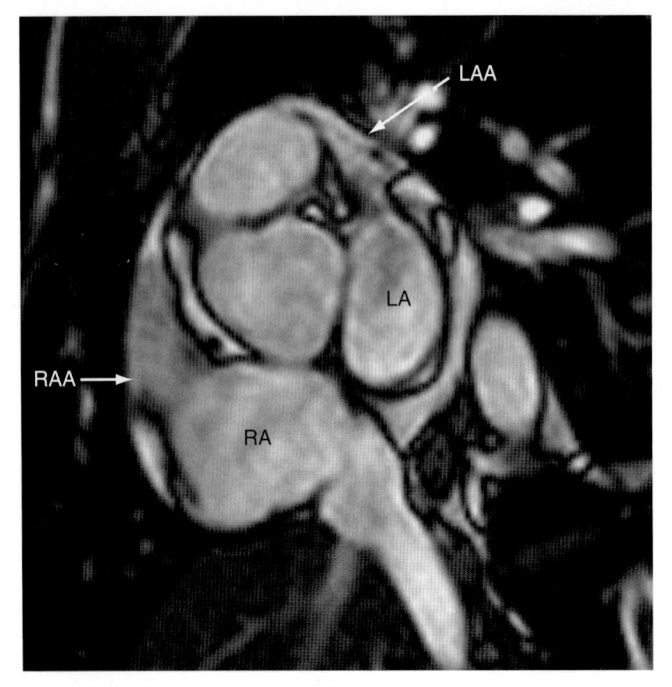

■ **FIGURE 2-6** Short-axis bSSFP image of the heart illustrating the atria and their respective appendages with pectinate muscles. The triangular right atrial appendage (RAA) has a wide mouth and the rectangular left atrial appendage (LAA) has a narrow mouth.

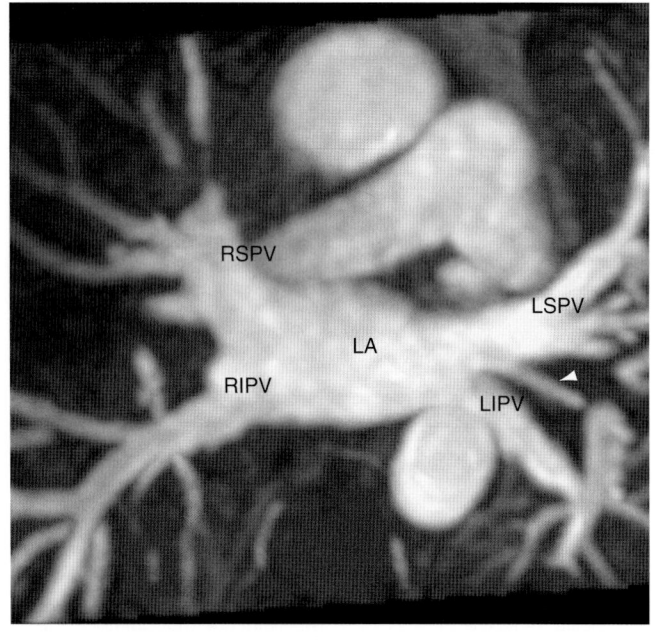

■ **FIGURE 2-8** Maximum intensity projection (MIP) image from an axial contrast-enhanced MR of the pulmonary veins demonstrating the pulmonary veins. Note the early branch from the left superior pulmonary vein (*arrowhead*).

Left Atrium

The left atrium forms the upper posterior heart border on chest radiographs and lies just beneath the carina anterior to the esophagus. This latter characteristic makes it an ideal window in transesophageal echocardiography. The left atrium is also derived from the sinus venosus and the primitive auricle, with similar components. The posteriorly located smooth-walled venous component receives the four pulmonary veins (Fig. 2-8). The vestibule is also smooth-walled and supports the leaflets of the mitral valve.

The left atrial appendage is long and tubular in shape, with pectinate muscles that measure more than 1 mm (see

Fig. 2-6).[5] These can be mistaken for clots and are less prominent than those in the right atrium. The appendage contributes to the left cardiac contour on chest radiographs and is ventral to the left atrioventricular (AV) groove and left circumflex artery. Knowledge of the pulmonary venous anatomy and description of any accessory veins is important because of their propensity to form ectopic arrhythmogenic foci, and the multiplanar capability of CT and MRI is particularly useful for mapping the left atrial anatomy.[6] Enlargement causes posterior displacement of the esophagus on the lateral radiograph and widening of the carinal angle on the frontal radiograph.

Atrial Septum

The atria are separated by the interatrial septum. Atrial septation is a complex process involving many components.[7] The true septum is composed of the fossa ovalis, which is a remnant of the septum primum. The septum secundum, the superior rim of the fossa ovalis, is an enfolding of the atrial wall between the SVC and pulmonary vein. The atrial septum is visualized on MRI as a hypointense line, but the foramen ovale can sometimes be almost imperceptible and thus mistaken for an atrial septal defect (see Fig. 2-1). The fusion of the foramen ovale with the septum occurs in the first 2 years of life; incomplete fusion results in a patent foramen ovale in 25% of the population. Multidetector CT is a powerful tool for the demonstration of the patent foramen ovale.[8] A patent foramen ovale can be associated with atrial septal aneurysms and Chiari networks, which are implicated in cryptogenic strokes.[9]

Ventricles

Right Ventricle

The right ventricle is the most anterior chamber in a normal heart, contributing to the inferior border. It has a characteristic external pyramidal shape and is supplied by the right coronary artery (Fig. 2-9). The left anterior descending artery in the anterior interventricular groove demarcates it from the left ventricle. The right ventricle (RV) has an inlet with the valvular apparatus, an apical trabecular component, and a subpulmonic outflow tract. The unique distinguishing features of the right ventricle are septal chordae tendinae for the septal leaflet of the tricuspid valve, a feature that is absent in the morphologic left ventricle. Coarse apical trabeculations and the moderator band, a continuation of the right bundle branch that extends from the interventricular septum to the free anterior ventricular wall, are other unique features (see Fig. 2-7).[10] The pulmonary and tricuspid valves lack fibrous continuity, unlike on the left, and are separated by an infolding of the roof called the *supraventricular crest*. The more numerous papillary muscles are less prominent and are found on septal and free walls. The infundibulum is incorporated into the RV and forms the outflow tract. These characteristic features are integral to the recognition the morphologic right ventricle in congenital heart disease.[10] The right ventricle is a thin-walled chamber normally measuring approximately 3 mm in thickness that

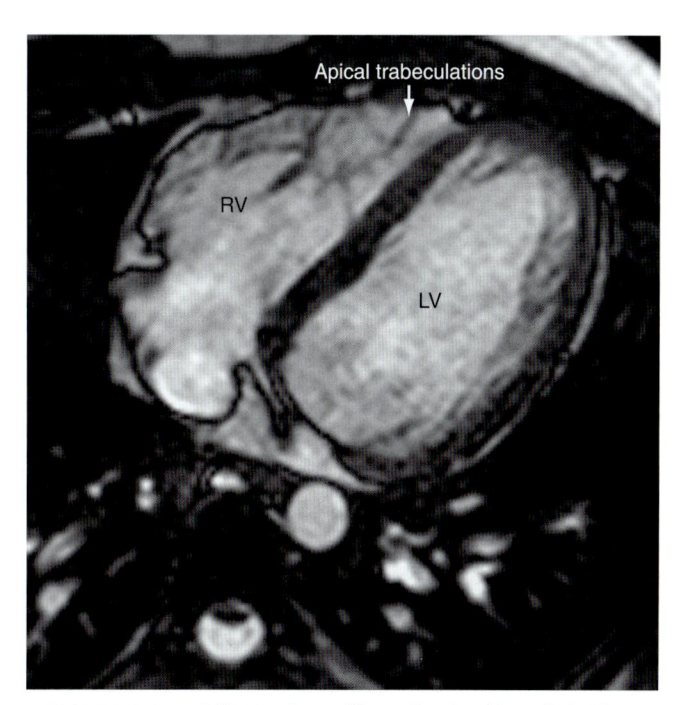

■ **FIGURE 2-9** Axial bSSFP image illustrating the thin-walled right ventricle with apical trabeculations (*white arrow*) and thicker left ventricle.

pumps deoxygenated blood into the low-pressure pulmonary arterial bed (25 mm Hg). The physiologic apical thinning of the RV free wall must not be confused with arrhythmogenic right ventricular dysplasia (ARVD).

The right ventricle enlarges anteriorly, reducing the retrosternal clear space laterally and causing leftward displacement of the apex lifting off the hemidiaphragm. RV enlargement on cross-sectional imaging measured at the plane of the tricuspid valve is a sign of right heart strain in acute pulmonary embolism when the RV/LV ratio is more than 1.[11]

Left Ventricle

The morphologic left ventricle pumps oxygenated blood to the systemic circulation through the aorta and its branches. It is the most imaged chamber of the heart as a result of the consequences of its failure. It is a thick-walled conical chamber (see Fig. 2-9) that pumps blood when the pressure exceeds 120 mm Hg (the systemic peripheral resistance).

The left ventricle is characterized by the same chambers as the right—the inlet, apical, trabecular, and outlet. The inlet extends from the atrioventricular junction to the attachments of the papillary muscle and contains the mitral valve. The mitral valve, which has fibrous continuity with the aortic valve, has two cusps, anterior and posterior, with no septal attachments. The corresponding large papillary muscles are well seen on cross-sectional imaging (Fig. 2-10). The apex has fine trabeculations and the septum is smooth, thus distinguishing it from the morphologic right ventricle. The ventricular outlet is short and is deficient in conal muscles, in contrast to the right.

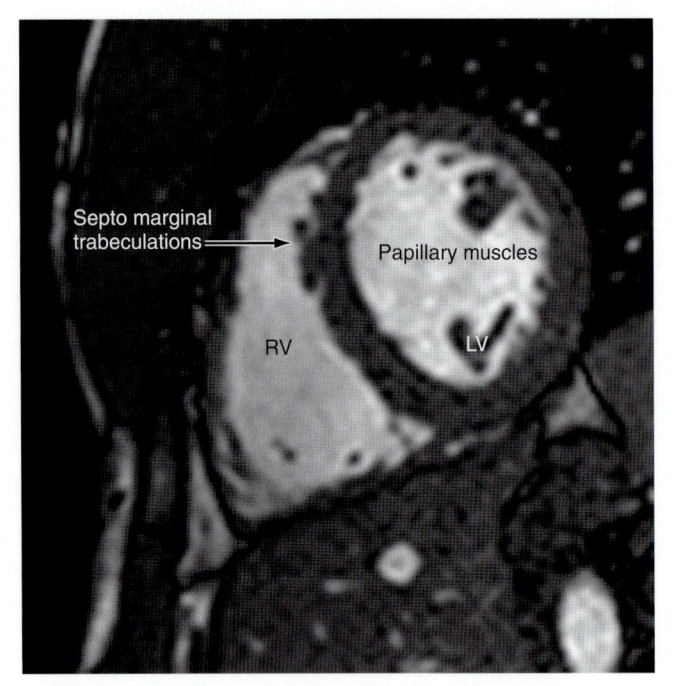

FIGURE 2-10 Short-axis bSSFP image demonstrating the smooth left ventricular septal surface with large papillary muscles and the trabeculated septal surface of the right ventricle.

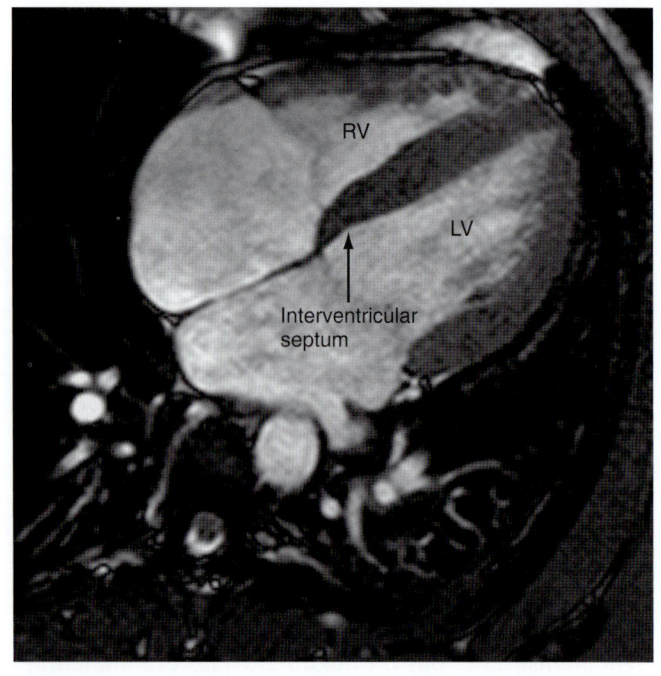

FIGURE 2-11 Axial bSSFP image reveals the thick-walled interventricular septum.

The left ventricular wall is not uniform in thickness. This is most accentuated in the longitudinal direction, toward the apex, where gradual wall thinning is noticed. The lateral wall segment thickness measures 7 to 8 mm in women and 9 mm in men. The apex can measure 3 mm. The circumferential wall thickness nonuniformity is less pronounced.[12] Left ventricular enlargement tends to be in a leftward and inferior direction.

Interventricular Septum

The ventricles are separated by a thick-walled muscular layer, the septum. In the subaortic region, where the septum thins out, it is referred to as the membranous portion. Muscle fibers from the free ventricular walls contribute to the septum. The septum is normally slightly convex toward the right ventricle because of the higher pressure on the left, which is maintained throughout the cardiac cycle. This feature is best appreciated on short-axis and horizontal long-axis images (Figs. 2-11 and 2-12). Physiologic flattening of the septum in early diastole is called ventricular coupling. Pathologic flattening, or leftward bowing, is seen in constrictive pericarditis, cor pulmonale, and atrial septal defects.[13]

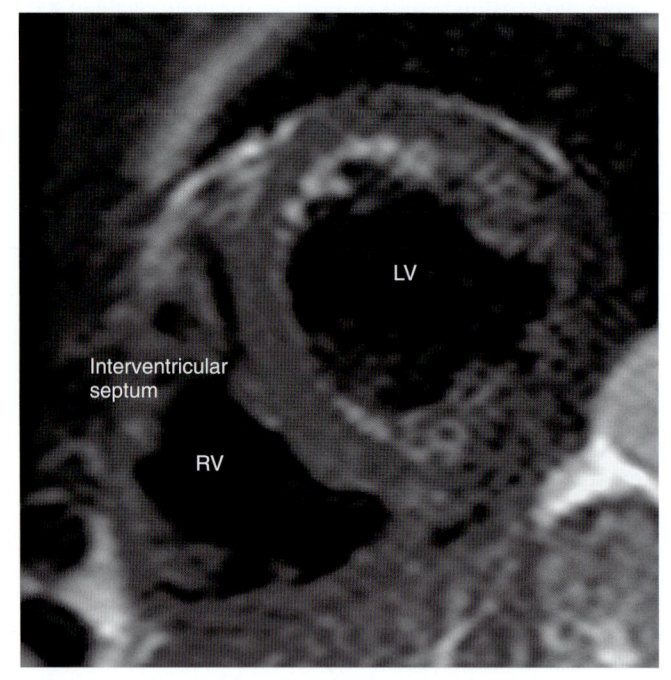

FIGURE 2-12 Short-axis T2-weighted black blood MRI image illustrates the interventricular septum, which is slightly convex toward the right ventricle.

Valves

The AV valves form the conduit from the atria to the ventricle. The tricuspid on the right and mitral on the left are so named because the right sided AV valve has three cusps and the left-sided bicuspid valve resembles a bishop's miter (Fig. 2-13). The mitral valve (MV) is composed of an anterior and posterior leaflet. The MV and aortic valve share fibrous continuity (Fig. 2-14). The MV annulus embedded in the myocardium is part of the cardiac skeleton.[14] Calcification of the MV annulus is a common abnormality that makes identification of the difficult to visualize annulus possible with cardiac CT angiography. The papillary muscles (see earlier), with their chordae tendinae, are also a component of the MV apparatus (Fig. 2-15). The mitral valve has no septal attachments, thus distinguishing it from the tricuspid valve.

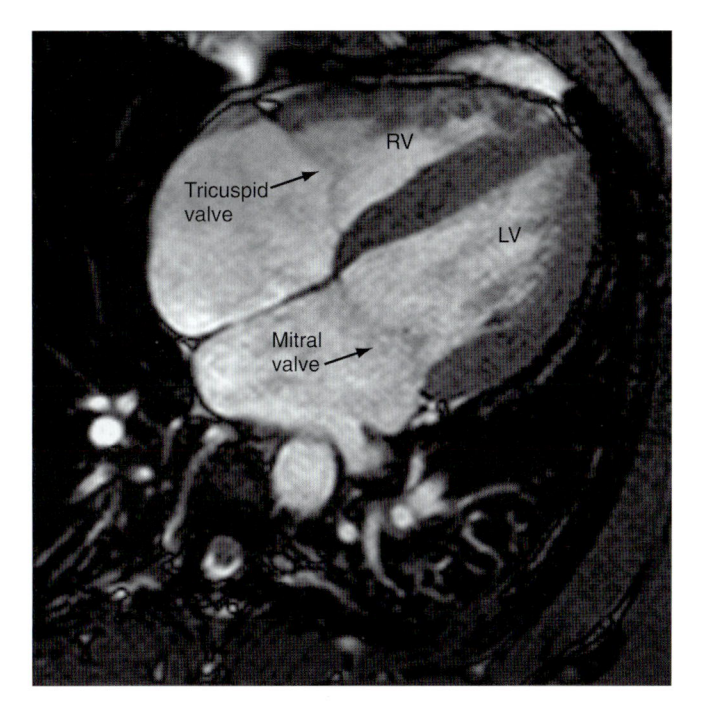

■ **FIGURE 2-13** Axial bSSFP image shows the mitral and tricuspid valves.

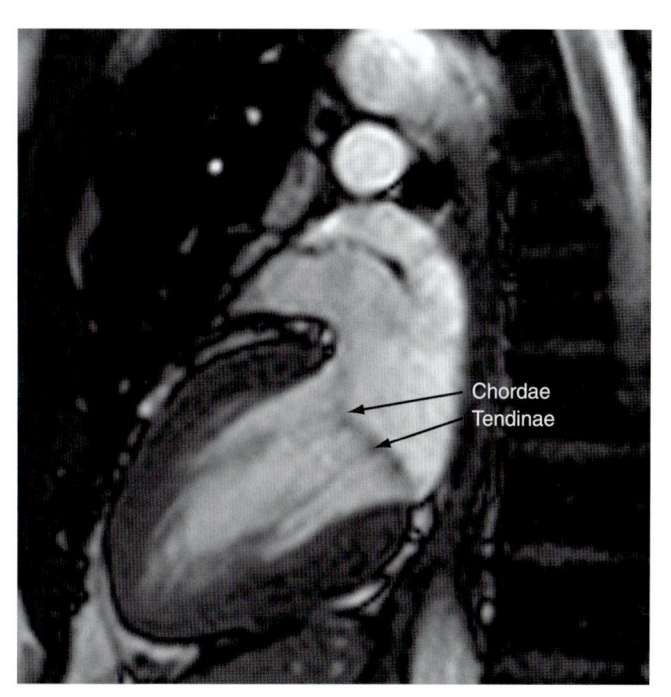

■ **FIGURE 2-15** This bSSFP vertical long-axis image shows the chordae tendinae, which attach the papillary muscle to the mitral valve leaflets.

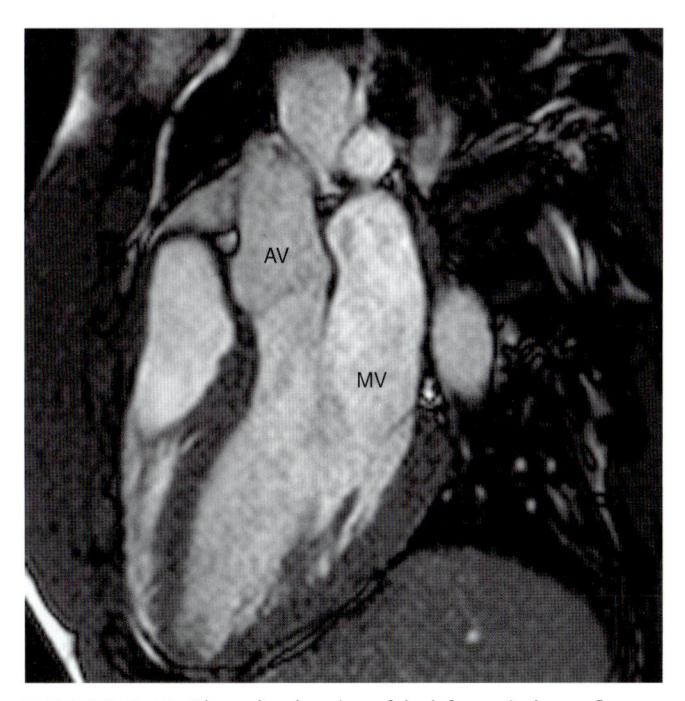

■ **FIGURE 2-14** Three-chamber view of the left ventricular outflow tract illustrating the fibrous continuity of the mitral and aortic valves.

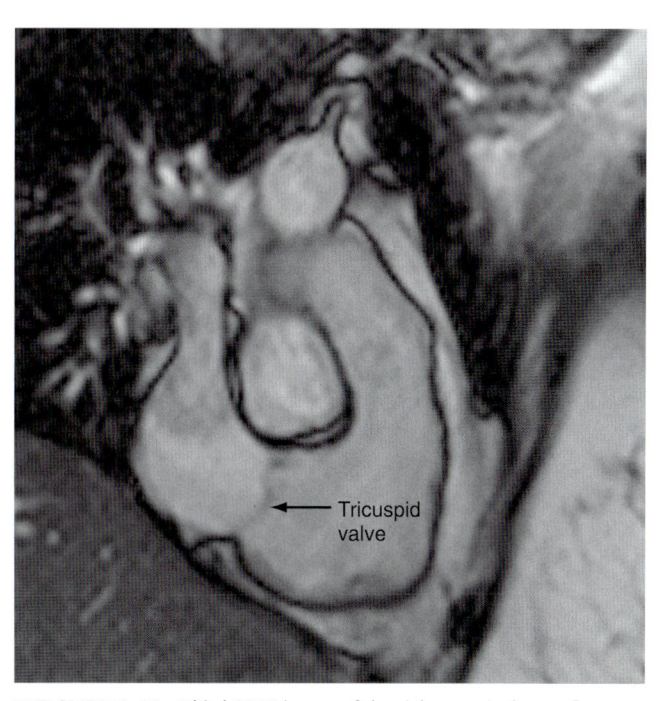

■ **FIGURE 2-16** This bSSFP image of the right ventricular outflow tract illustrates the tricuspid valve. Note the well-developed right ventricular outflow tract.

The tricuspid valve separates the right atrium (RA) from the RV and is composed of the same structures as the MV—leaflets, annulus, commissures (sites where two leaflets come together to attach to the aortic wall), papillary muscles, and chordae tendinae. It is normally connected to the morphologic RV (Fig. 2-16). As its name implies, the tricuspid valve is a trileaflet valve (anterior, posterior, and septal leaflets) and is separated from the pulmonary valve by the crista supraventricularis, a muscular ridge, unlike the MV, which is contiguous with the aortic valve. The tricuspid valve is more apically located.

The aortic valve separates the LV outflow tract from the ascending aorta. It is composed of an annulus, cusps, and commissures. No papillary muscles or chordae tendinae are associated with the aortic valve. The three cusps (right, left, and posterior or noncoronary) of the aortic

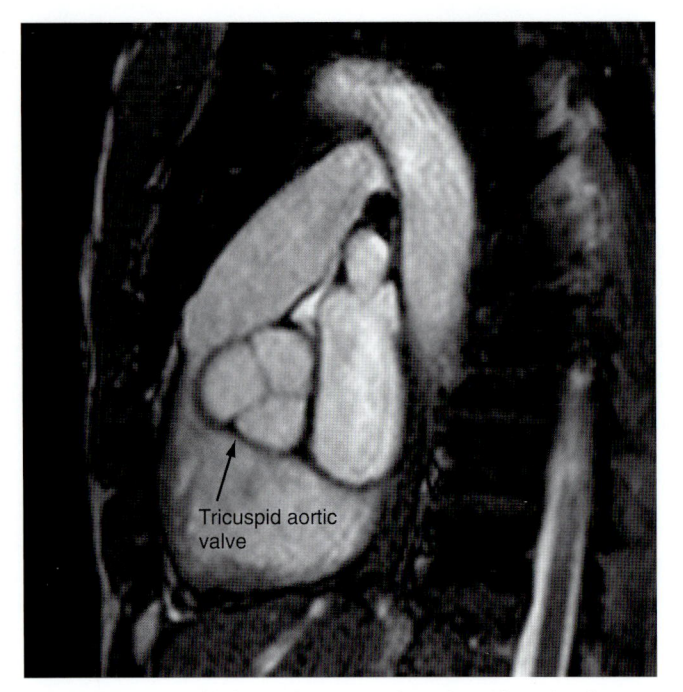

FIGURE 2-17 This bSSFP image reveals a tricuspid aortic valve from a right ventricular long-axis stack.

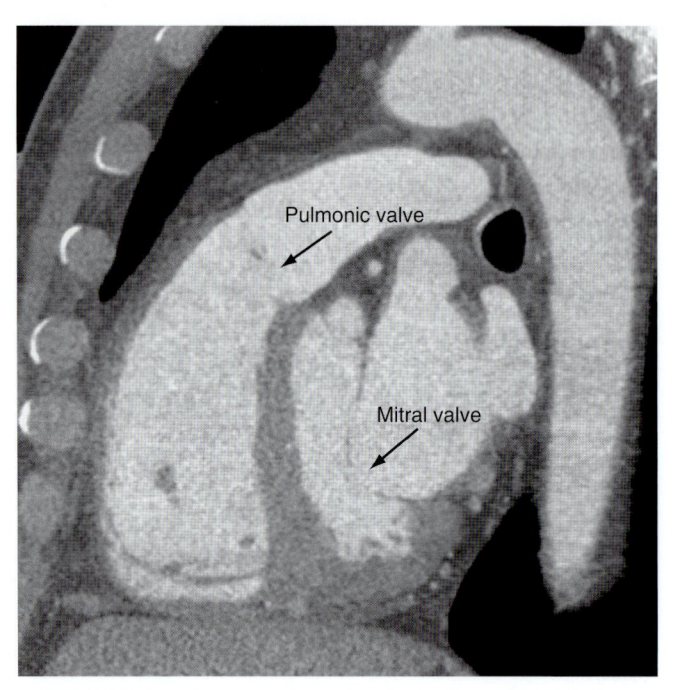

FIGURE 2-18 Contrast-enhanced sagittal reformation of the heart reveals the pulmonic valve and the mitral valve.

valve form pocket-like outpouchings that are designed to direct blood into the sinuses of Valsalva during diastole and flatten against the aorta during systole (Fig. 2-17).[14]

The pulmonic valve separates the RV outflow tract from the main pulmonary artery but lacks fibrous continuity with the tricuspid valve (Fig. 2-18). It is otherwise essentially identical to the aortic valve, with right, left, and posterior leaflets.

Cardiac Veins

The anatomy of the cardiac venous system is variable. The coronary sinus is the most constant structure running in the left AV groove and emptying into the right atrium (see Fig. 2-7).[14] The coronary sinus continues as the great cardiac vein, which courses in the left atrioventricular groove with the left circumflex artery and then becomes the anterior interventricular vein in the anterior ventricular groove adjacent to the left anterior descending artery.

The first branch is the middle cardiac vein or posterior interventricular vein, running in the eponymously named groove from base to apex along with the posterior descending artery.[13] The other two branches that are often variants are the posterior vein of the left ventricle and the left marginal vein, with the former being absent in up to 55% of individuals. Knowledge of their variant anatomy is important because the LV pacer lead of the implantable cardioverter defibrillator for the treatment of heart failure is inserted into one of these two veins.[16]

KEY POINTS

- This chapter reviews cardiac anatomy from the perspective of CT and MRI.
- Knowledge of cardiac anatomy is essential for the interpretation of imaging studies of the heart.

SUGGESTED READINGS

Malouf JF, Edwards WD, Tajik AJ, Seward JB. Functional anatomy of the heart. In Fuster V, Alexander RW, O'Rourke RA, et al (eds). Hurst's the Heart, 11th ed. New York, McGraw-Hill, 2005.

O'Brien JP, Srichai MB, Hecht EM, et al. Anatomy of the heart at multidetector CT: what the radiologist needs to know. Radiographics 2007; 27:1569-1582.

REFERENCES

1. Spodick DH. The normal and diseased pericardium: current concepts of pericardial physiology, diagnosis and treatment. J Am Coll Cardiol 1983; 1:240-251.
2. Sechtem U, Tscholakoff D, Higgins CB. MRI of the abnormal pericardium. AJR Am J Roentgenol 1986; 147:245-252.
3. M Levy-Ravetch YA, Rubenstein WA, Whalen JP, Kazam E. CT of the pericardial recesses. AJR Am J Roentgenol 1985; 144:707-714.
4. Menegus M, Greenberg M, Spindola-Franco H, Fayemi A. Magnetic resonance imaging of suspected atrial tumors. Am Heart J 1992; 123:1260-1268.

5. Veinot J, Harrity P, Gentile F, et al. Anatomy of the normal left atrial appendage: a quantitative study of age-related changes in 500 autopsy hearts: implications for echocardiographic examination. Circulation 1997; 96:3112-3115.
6. Jongbloed M, Dirksen M, Bax J, et al. Atrial fibrillation: multi-detector row CT of pulmonary vein anatomy prior to radiofrequency catheter ablation—initial experience. Radiology 2005; 234:702-709.
7. Anderson R, Brown N, Webb S. Development and structure of the atrial septum. Heart 2002; 88:104-110.
8. Saremi F, Attai S, Narula J. 64 multidetector CT in patent foramen ovale. Heart 2007; 93:505.
9. Mügge A, Daniel W, Angermann C, et al. Atrial septal aneurysm in adult patients. A multicenter study using transthoracic and transesophageal echocardiography. Circulation 1995; 91:2785-2792.
10. Choe Y, Kim Y, Han B, et al. MR imaging in the morphologic diagnosis of congenital heart disease. Radiographics 1997; 17:403-422.
11. Ghaye B, Ghuysen A, Bruyere P, et al. Can CT pulmonary angiography allow assessment of severity and prognosis in patients presenting with pulmonary embolism? What the radiologist needs to know. Radiographics 2006; 26:23-39.
12. Bogaert J, Rademakers F. Regional nonuniformity of normal adult human left ventricle. Am J Physiol Heart Circ Physiol 2001; 280:H610-H620.
13. Higgins CB. Acquired heart disease. In Higgins CB, Hricak H, Helms CA (eds). Magnetic Resonance Imaging of the Body. Philadelphia, Lippincott-Raven, 1997, pp 409-460.
14. Malouf JF, Edwards WD, Tajik AJ, Seward JB. Functional anatomy of the heart. In Fuster V, Alexander RW, O'Rourke RA, et al (eds). Hurst's the Heart, 11th ed. New York, McGraw-Hill, 2005.
15. Van de Veire N, Schuijf J, De Sutter J, et al. Non-invasive visualization of the cardiac venous system in coronary artery disease patients using 64-slice computed tomography. J Am Coll Cardiol 2006; 48:1832-1838.
16. Bax JJ, Abraham T, Barold SS, et al. Cardiac resynchronization therapy. II. Issues during and after device implantation and unresolved questions. J Am Coll Cardiol 2005; 46:2168-2182.

CHAPTER 3

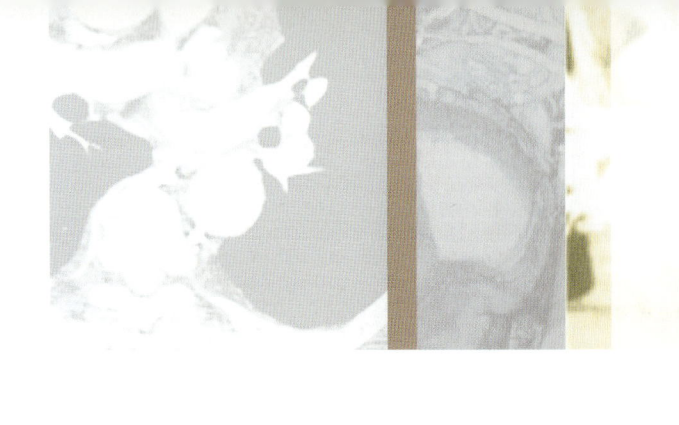

Coronary Anatomy

Jadranka Stojanovska and Smita Patel

Multidetector CT has become an important tool for noninvasive evaluation of cardiovascular structures.[1] With advances in multidetector CT technology, the role of imaging has progressed from detection and quantification of the calcium score on noncontrast CT to detection of luminal stenoses, and detection and characterization of plaque composition on coronary CT angiography.[2,3] Basic knowledge of the normal coronary arterial anatomy is essential for evaluation and interpretation of cardiac CT studies. Properly performed, coronary CT angiography provides high spatial resolution, three-dimensional data for detailed visualization of the coronary arteries, which are typically small, and rapidly moving, and have tortuous and complex anatomic arrangements. The anatomy of the coronary arteries and their normal variants is well described using conventional coronary angiography. The cross-sectional nature of CT has the benefit, however, of more precisely displaying the spatial relationship of coronary arterial and venous anatomy with respect to adjacent cardiac structures.

CT clearly displays the anatomy of the coronary arteries, in terms of their origin from the aorta, course and number of branches, bifurcation angles, and normal variants and anomalies. The volumetric data set can be viewed on dedicated cardiac software platforms using postprocessing techniques that display the coronary arteries as oblique multiplanar reformats with long-axis and orthogonal short-axis views, curved multiplanar reformats, maximum intensity projection (MIP), stretched out lumen view, volume rendered coronary tree images, or volume rendering of the heart. Volume rendering allows excellent surface display of the coronary arteries and their relationship to adjacent structures, and is particularly useful to show bypass graft anatomy; origin, termination, and course of anomalous coronary arteries; and tortuous collateral vessels.

Multidetector CT is a continually evolving technique that in recent years has been mainly used to evaluate the coronary arteries. Less attention has been paid to the coronary venous system until more recently.[4,5] Evaluation of the cardiac venous anatomy is important for preprocedural planning of percutaneous resynchronization therapy and treatment of resistant ventricular arrhythmias. In this chapter, we discuss the detailed normal anatomy of the coronary arteries and their normal variants and the anatomy of the cardiac veins.

CORONARY ARTERIES

The coronary network is composed of coronary arteries, capillaries, and coronary veins. In end diastole, oxygenized blood from the aorta flows through the epicardial coronary arteries and into the myocardium. The blood advances through the network of capillaries into the coronary veins, which drain most of the cardiac venous return into the right atrium. The coronary arteries are the network of blood vessels that carry oxygen-rich and nutrient-rich blood to the cardiac muscle to enable the heart muscle to contract and relax continuously. They progressively branch into smaller vessels. Their major branches are located predominantly on the epicardial surface of the heart surrounded by fat, with the exception of the septal perforators, which run in the ventricular septum and are surrounded by muscle. The smaller branches penetrate the heart muscle.

The definition of the abnormal versus normal anatomy of the coronary arteries presents a complex problem. Angelini and colleagues[6,7] have proposed the following terms to define these categories: *normal*—any morphologic feature observed in greater than 1% of an unselected population; *normal variant*—an alternative, relatively unusual, morphologic feature seen in greater than 1% of the population; and *anomaly*—a morphologic feature (e.g., number of ostia, proximal course, termination) rarely encountered (<1%) in the general population. The normal coronary arteries and their variations can be described in terms of their ostia (with respect to their number, location, size, and angle of origination), the size and length of the coronary arteries, their proximal and

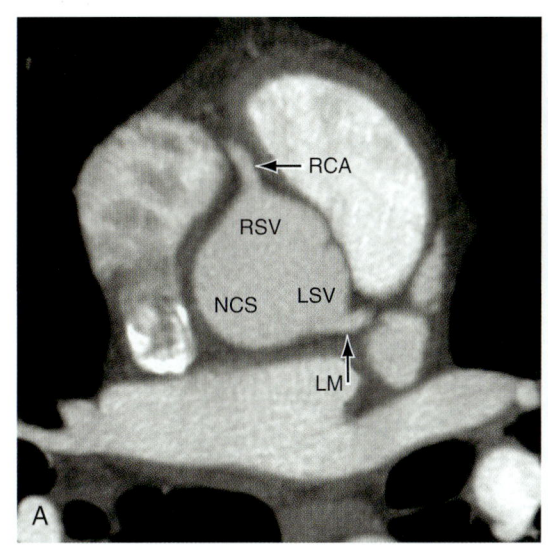

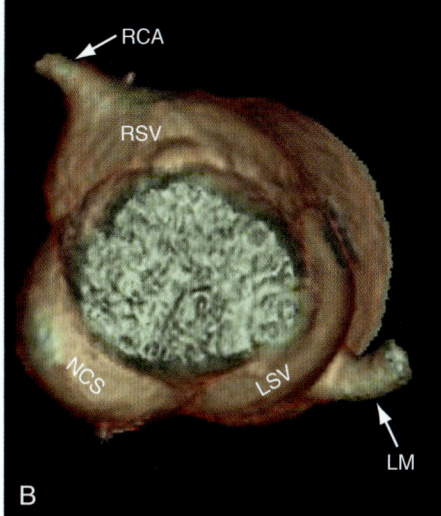

FIGURE 3-1 Origins of the left main (LM) coronary artery and right coronary artery (RCA) from their respective sinuses of Valsalva. **A**, Axial maximal intensity projection (MIP) image. **B**, Volume rendered image. LSV, left sinus of Valsalva; NCS, noncoronary sinus; RSV, right sinus of Valsalva.

mid course (intramyocardial bridging), arteriolar ramifications, and terminations.

NORMAL CORONARY ARTERY ANATOMY

There are two coronary arteries, the right coronary artery (RCA) and left coronary artery (LCA), which originate from their respective sinuses of Valsalva—the RCA from the right sinus of Valsalva and the LCA from the left sinus of Valsalva (Fig. 3-1). The right sinus of Valsalva is located anteriorly and the left sinus of Valsalva posteriorly and to the left. The third sinus of Valsalva, located posteriorly and to the right, does not give rise to a coronary artery, and is referred to as "noncoronary cusp/sinus." There may be variations in the number, shape, and location of coronary ostia or origins of the coronary arteries, most of which are of no clinical significance.

The coronary ostia are usually located in the upper third of the respective sinus of Valsalva. Ostia located near the aortic valve commissures, ostia located in the posterior (noncoronary) sinus, and ostia showing a high takeoff are considered abnormal. The high takeoff of the coronary artery may reduce diastolic coronary artery blood flow, and the patient may become symptomatic.[8] High takeoff of a coronary artery may result in a long intramural course which could be potentially pathologic (Fig. 3-2).

In terms of the number of the coronary ostia, two ostia are considered normal, one in the respective sinus for the RCA and LCA; however three or four are considered as normal variants, such as a separate origin of a conal branch from the aorta (prevalence 11.6%)[9] or absence of the left main (LM) coronary artery with the left anterior descending artery (LAD) and left circumflex artery (LCX) having separate origins from the aorta. An absent LM is considered a benign anomaly. A separate origin of the sinus node artery from the aorta has a prevalence of 0.2%.[9] The single coronary artery and ectopic origin of the coronary arteries from the aorta and pulmonary artery are considered as anomalous and are discussed in Chapter 33.

Right Coronary Artery

On axial images, the RCA arises from the right sinus of Valsalva, inferior to the origin of the LCA (Fig. 3-3). It courses anteriorly and inferiorly under the right atrial appendage along the right atrioventricular (AV) groove, toward the acute margin of the heart, where it turns posteriorly and inferiorly toward the crux of the heart and divides into the posterior descending coronary artery

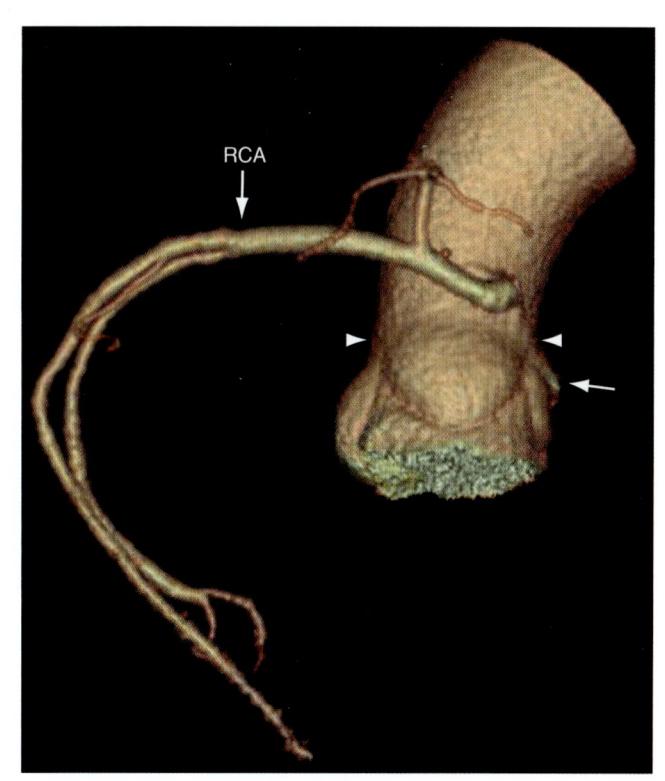

FIGURE 3-2 High takeoff. Three-dimensional volume rendered coronary tree CT image shows the right coronary artery (RCA) arising (15 mm) above the sinotubular junction (*arrowhead*). The *short arrow* depicts the normal location of the left coronary artery ostium.

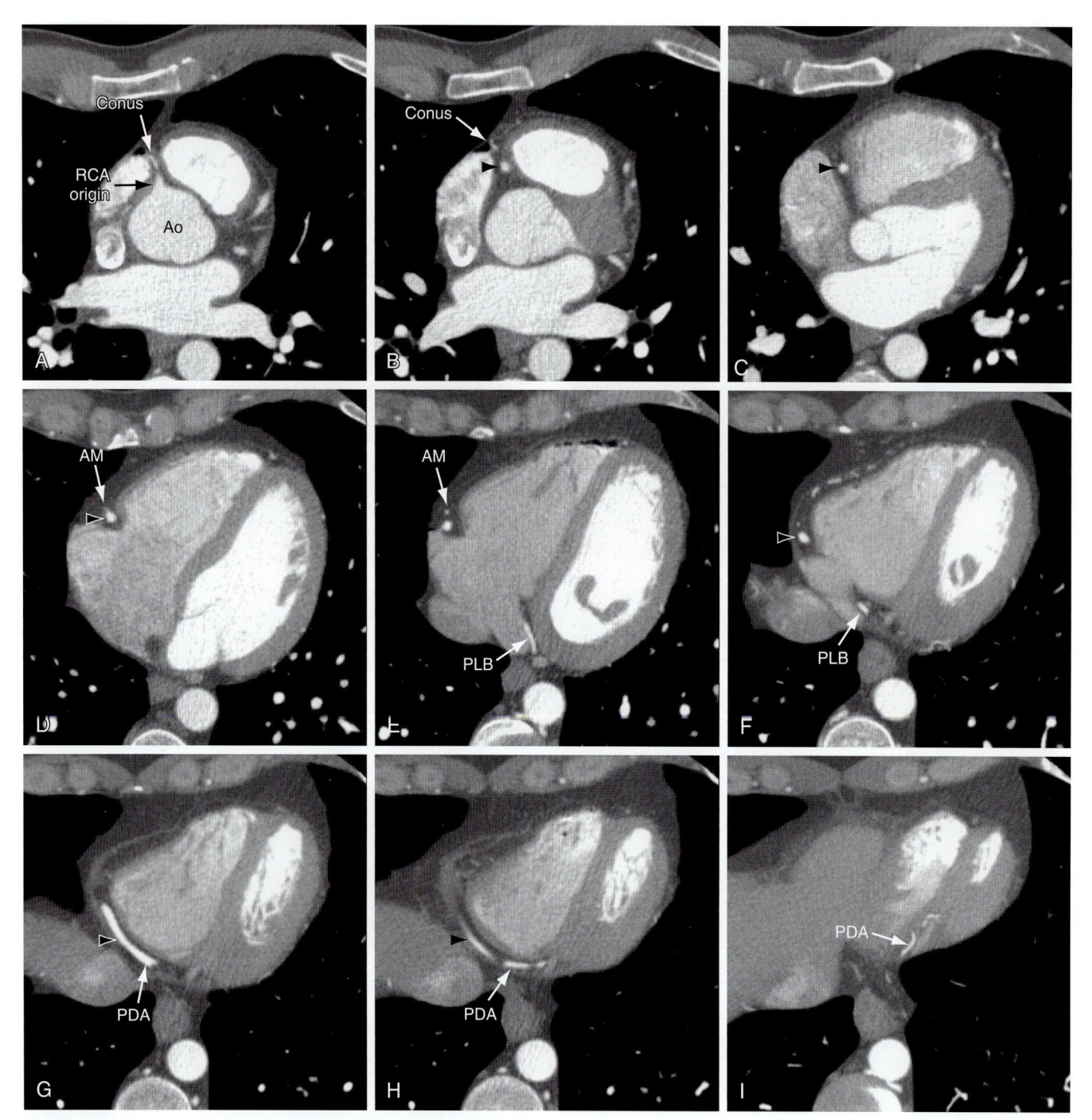

FIGURE 3-3 Normal axial anatomy of the right coronary artery (RCA) on 64-slice CT coronary angiography at 0.625-mm collimation. *Black arrowheads* denote the RCA. **A**, RCA arising from the right sinus of Valsalva. Conus branch arises from proximal RCA. **B** and **C**, Proximal RCA in anterior atrioventricular groove. **D**, Acute marginal (AM) branch origin from RCA at the acute margin of the heart. **E** and **F**, Mid RCA at the acute margin of the heart; the posterolateral branch (PLB), a branch of the distal RCA, crosses the crux of the heart and runs in the left posterior AV groove. **G-I**, Horizontal portion of the distal RCA is seen in the posterior right AV groove. The posterior descending coronary artery (PDA) comes off the RCA and is running in the posterior interventricular septum alongside the middle cardiac vein.

(PDA) and the posterolateral ventricular branch (PLB) (Fig. 3-4; see Fig. 3-3). The RCA supplies the right atrium, right ventricle, posterior third of the interventricular septum, and sinoatrial and AV nodes.

In 50% to 64% of the population, the conus branch arises as the first branch of the RCA (Fig. 3-5A).[9] The conus may arise from the ostial RCA in 22.3% or separately from the aorta in 11.6% of the population (Fig. 3-5B).[9] The conus branch courses anteriorly and to the right and supplies the pulmonary outflow tract. Rarely, this branch can arise from the LCA.

The sinoatrial nodal artery is the second branch that arises from the proximal RCA in 65.4%, immediately distal to the RCA origin (Fig. 3-6A). In 16.6% of cases, the sinoatrial nodal artery arises from the LCX (Fig. 3-6B); in 9.2%, it arises from the RCA and the LCX; in 0.2%, it arises from

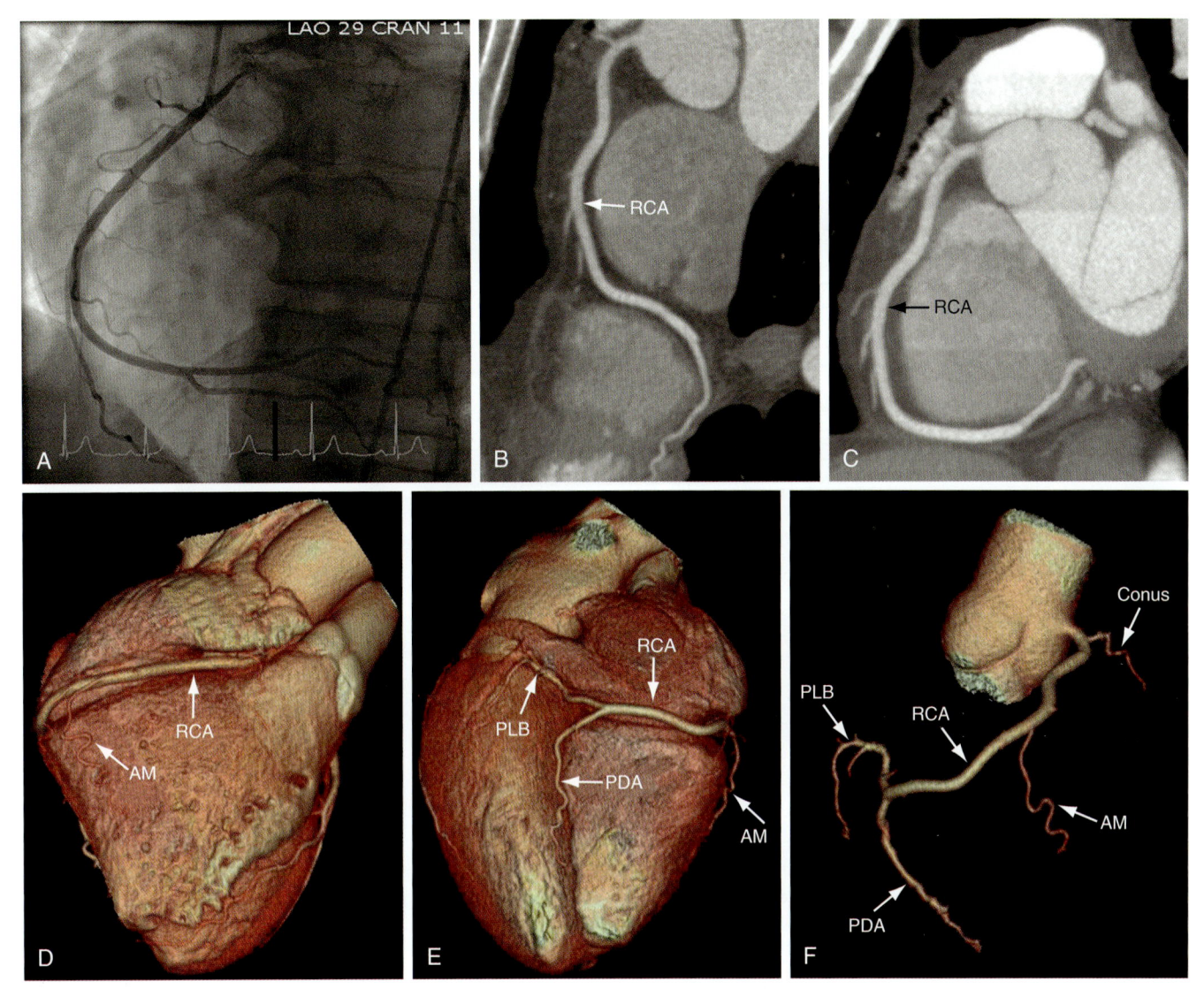

FIGURE 3-4 A-C, Normal right coronary artery (RCA) at selective coronary catheterization showing RCA and its branches (A), curved multiplanar reformat (B), and long-axis MIP (C). D-F, Normal RCA origin and course in the right atrioventricular groove and its major branches on volume rendered images (D and E) and volume rendered coronary tree image (F). AM, acute marginal; PDA, posterior descending coronary artery; PLB, posterolateral branch.

the LCX and the pulmonary artery; and in 0.2%, it arises directly from the aorta.[9] This artery courses toward the superior vena cava near the cranial aspect of the interatrial septum.

The next branches of the RCA are the marginal branches that supply the right ventricular myocardium (see Figs. 3-3 and 3-4). The acute marginal artery comes off the acute margin of the heart and courses anteriorly and to the right, anterior to the right ventricle. The acute marginal branches supply the free wall of the right ventricular myocardium. In 10% to 20% of patients, an acute marginal branch runs on the diaphragmatic surface of the heart to supply the distal posterior interventricular septum. After the RCA gives off the acute marginal branches, it continues in the right AV groove toward the diaphragmatic aspect of the heart. At the crux of the heart, the RCA makes a U-turn and branches into the PDA and PLB (see Fig. 3-4).

The PDA is of variable size and runs along the diaphragmatic surface in the posterior interventricular groove toward the inferior septum. Short septal branches arising perpendicularly from the PDA supply the posterior third of the septum and can connect with the septal branches from the LAD to form a collateral circulation. The PLB runs in the posterior left AV groove and gives off multiple branches that supply the posterior and inferior wall of the left ventricle (see Fig. 3-4). The average angle between the PDA and PLB is 53 ± 27 degrees.[10] Within 1 to 2 cm of the crux, the PLB runs on the diaphragmatic surface of the left ventricle parallel to the PDA to supply the posterolateral diaphragmatic surface of the left ventricle. Here the RCA can serve as a collateral for an occluded LCX. Also close to the crux of the heart, just distal to the PDA origin, the RCA gives rise to a small AV nodal artery that supplies the AV node of the conduction system (Fig. 3-7). The AV nodal artery arises from the LCX in a left dominant system.

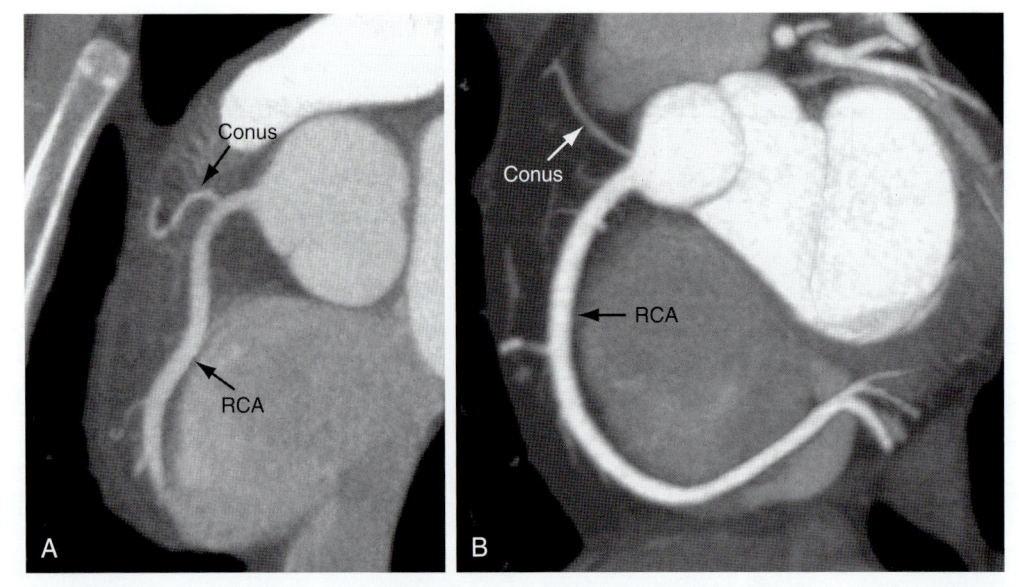

FIGURE 3-5 Conus branch origins. **A** and **B,** Curved multiplanar reformats show conus branch arising from proximal right coronary artery (RCA) (**A**), and conus branch arising from right coronary cusp (**B**).

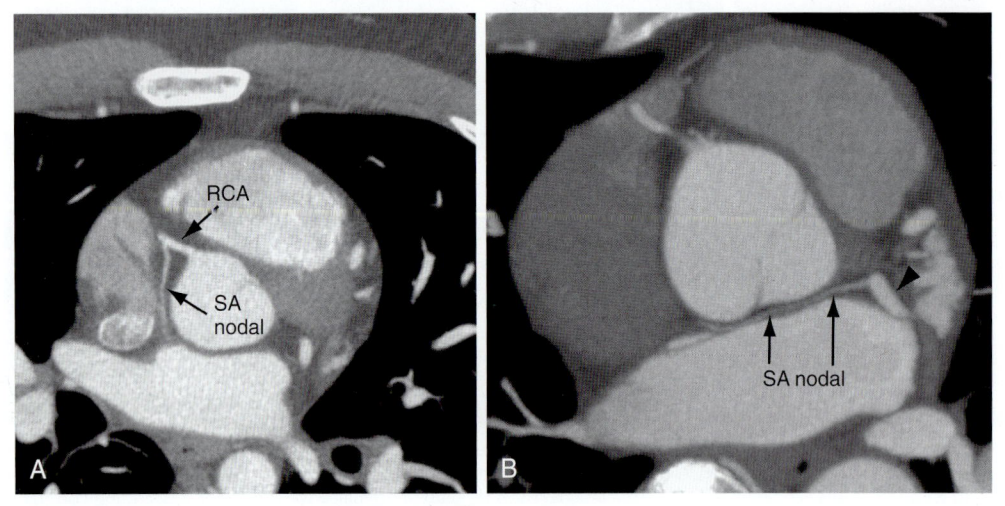

FIGURE 3-6 Oblique axial MIP images show sinoatrial (SA) nodal branch origins. **A,** SA nodal branch arising from proximal right coronary artery (RCA). **B,** SA nodal branch arising from the left circumflex artery (*arrowhead*).

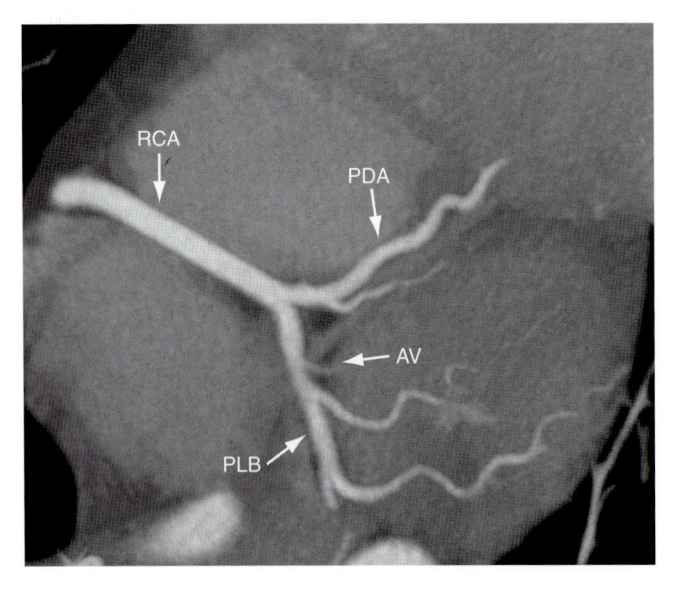

FIGURE 3-7 Atrioventricular (AV) nodal artery. Oblique MIP showing the AV nodal artery coming off the right coronary artery (RCA) after the posterior descending coronary artery (PDA) takeoff. PLB, posterolateral branch.

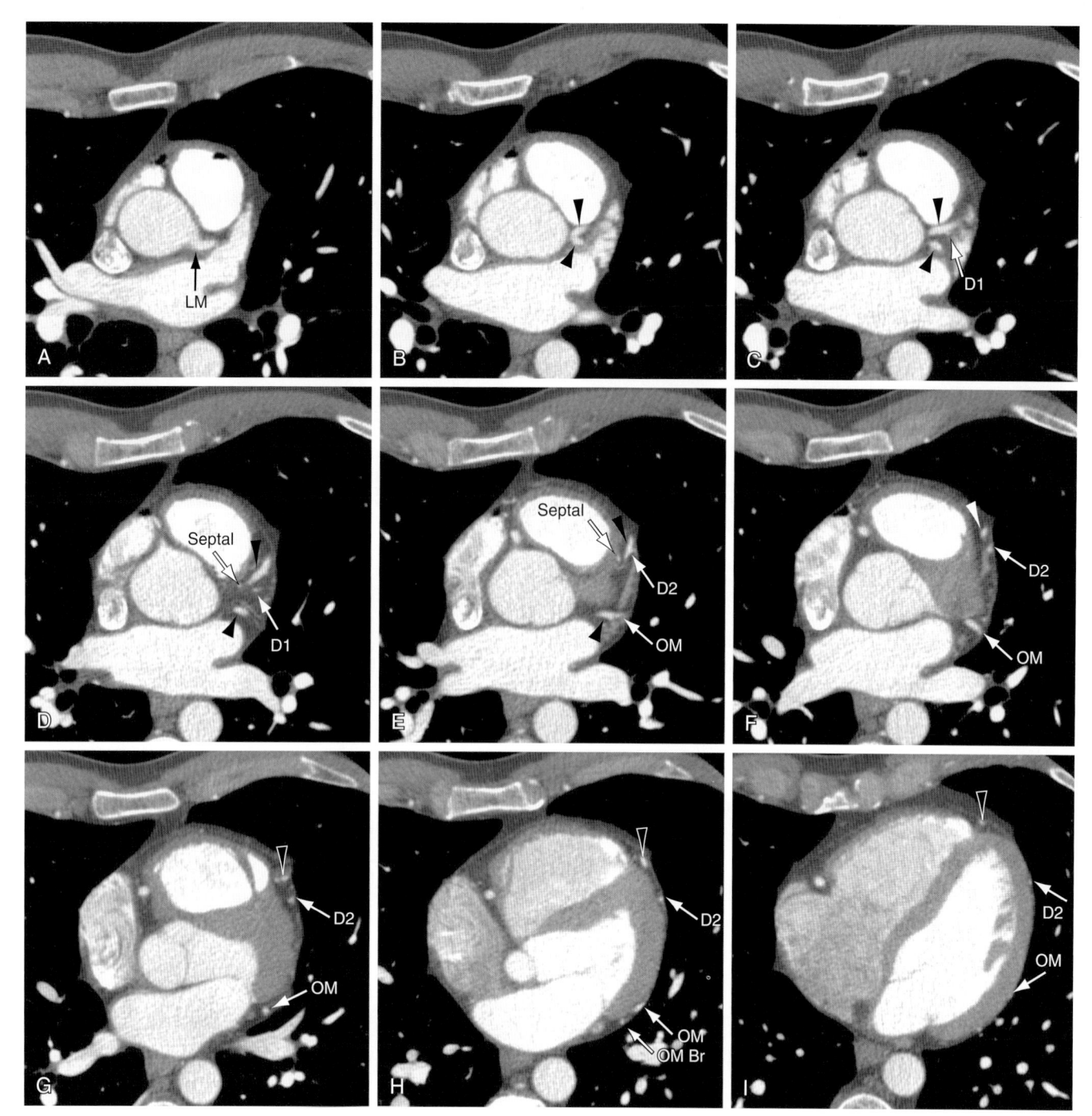

■ **FIGURE 3-8** Normal axial anatomy of the left main (LM) coronary artery, left anterior descending artery (LAD) and its branches, and left circumflex artery (LCX) and its branches on 64-slice CT coronary angiography at 0.625-mm collimation. *Long thin arrowhead* denotes the LAD, and *short thick arrowhead* denotes LCX. **A,** LM origin from left sinus of Valsalva. **B,** LM branches into LAD and LCX. **C-I,** LAD runs in the anterior interventricular groove to the apex of the heart and gives rise to septal perforators and diagonal branches (D1, D2). LCX runs in the left atrioventricular groove, and at the obtuse margin (OM) of the heart gives rise to the OM, which branches (OM Br) early and runs along the posterolateral margin of the heart.

Left Coronary Artery

On axial images, when scrolling from the cranial to caudal direction, the LCA or LM is the first coronary artery that is seen arising from the left sinus of Valsalva (Fig. 3-8). It courses to the left, beneath the left atrial appendage and posterior to the right ventricular outflow tract, before branching into the LAD and the LCX (Fig. 3-9). The LM varies in length from 5 to 25 mm (mean 13.5 mm), and its diameter ranges from 2 to 5.5 mm (mean 4 mm) (Fig. 3-10).[7,11] In 543 patients, Cademartiri and colleagues[9] reported a length of less than 1 cm in 41.6%, 1 to 2 cm in 47.3%, and greater than 2 cm in 7% of patients. Pflederer and coworkers[10] examined average angles of coronary bifurcations in 100 patients at four branch points: LAD/LCX, LAD/first diagonal branch, LCX/first obtuse marginal branch (OM1), and PDA/right posterolateral branch. The average LAD/LCX angle was reported as 80 ± 27 degrees.

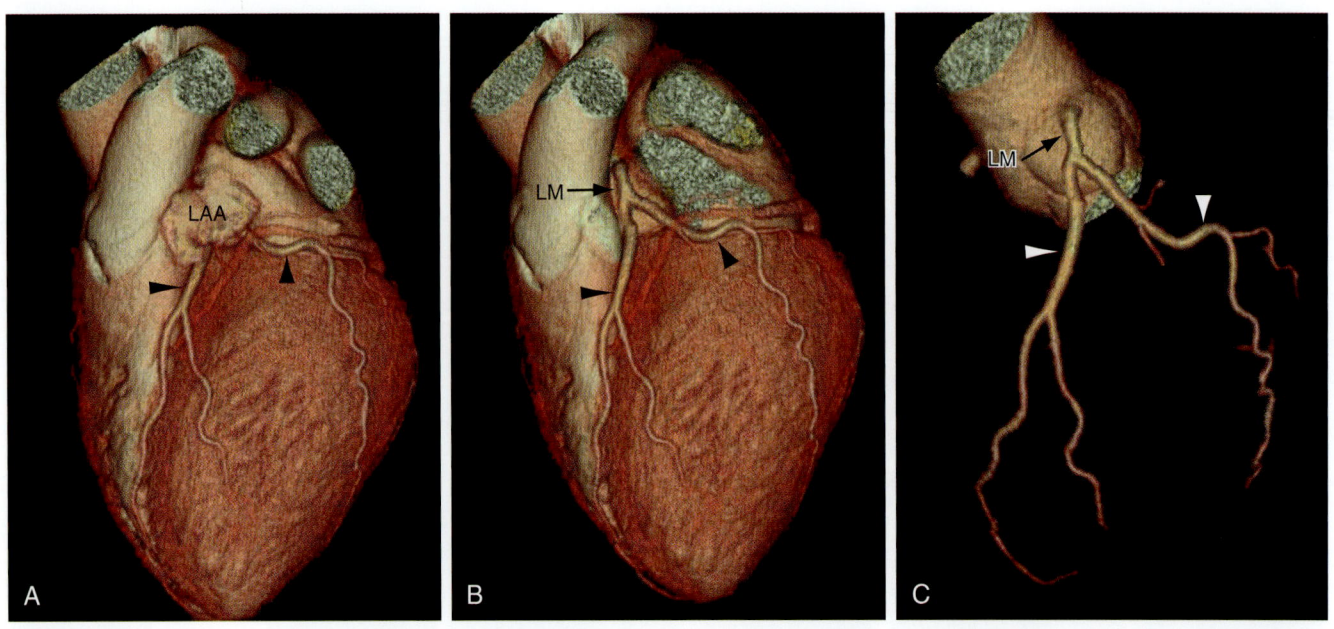

■ **FIGURE 3-9** **A-C,** Left main (LM) coronary artery courses behind the left atrial appendage (LAA) (**A**) and divides into the left anterior descending artery and left circumflex artery. *Long thin arrowhead* denotes the left anterior descending artery, and *short thick arrowhead* denotes left circumflex artery. Volume rendered surface display (**A** and **B**), and volume rendered coronary tree images (**C**).

The interobserver variability of bifurcation angle measurements by contrast-enhanced 16-slice multidetector CT was significantly better ($r = 0.91$) than invasive angiography ($r = 0.62$).[10] A normal variation in the anatomy is a true trifurcation of the LM, when the middle branch between the LAD and LCX is called the ramus intermedius (RI).[9,12] The LM may be absent in fewer than 1% of the population; in these cases, the LAD and LCX arise separately from the aorta.[7]

Left Anterior Descending Artery

The LAD runs anteriorly and inferiorly in the anterior interventricular groove to the apex of the heart, and supplies the anterior and anterolateral wall of the left ventricular myocardium and the anterior two thirds of the interventricular septum (Figs. 3-11 and 3-12; see Fig. 3-10). In approximately 82% of cases, the LAD curves around the cardiac apex to supply part of the inferior wall of the left ventricle. In 7%, it may not reach the apex of the heart, and in about 11% of cases, the LAD terminates in the distal anterior interventricular groove or even more proximally.[13] In such cases, the distal territory may be supplied by an unusually long diagonal branch or by RCA branches that traverse the posterior interventricular groove or the inferior surface of the heart, a normal variant.[14] This is one of the potential collateral routes if either the RCA or the LAD is occluded.

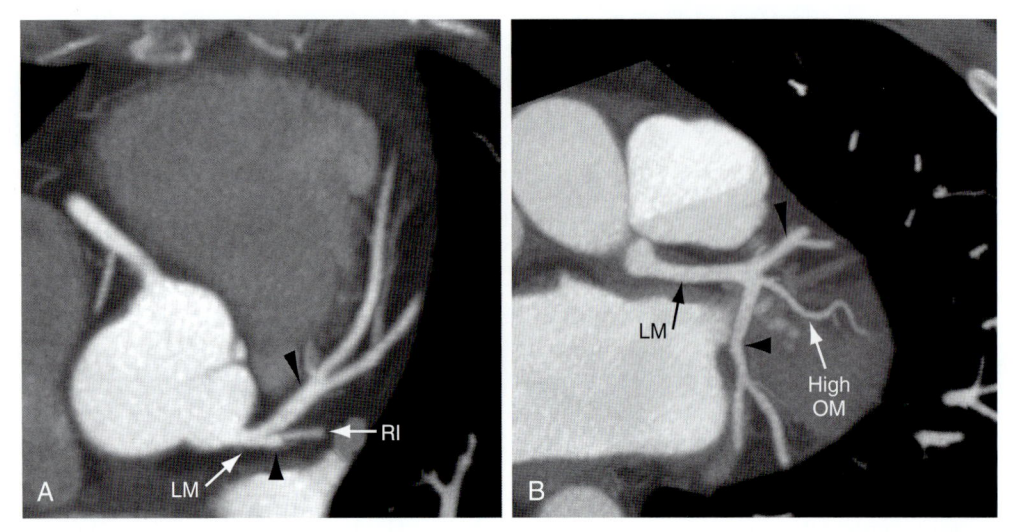

■ **FIGURE 3-10** Varying lengths of the left main (LM) coronary artery on oblique multiplanar reformats. **A,** LM less than 1 cm. **B,** LM measuring 2 cm. Note high takeoff of the first obtuse marginal (OM) from the left circumflex artery. *Long thin arrowhead* denotes the left anterior descending artery, and *short thick arrowhead* denotes left circumflex artery. RI, ramus intermedius.

CHAPTER 3 • Coronary Anatomy 45

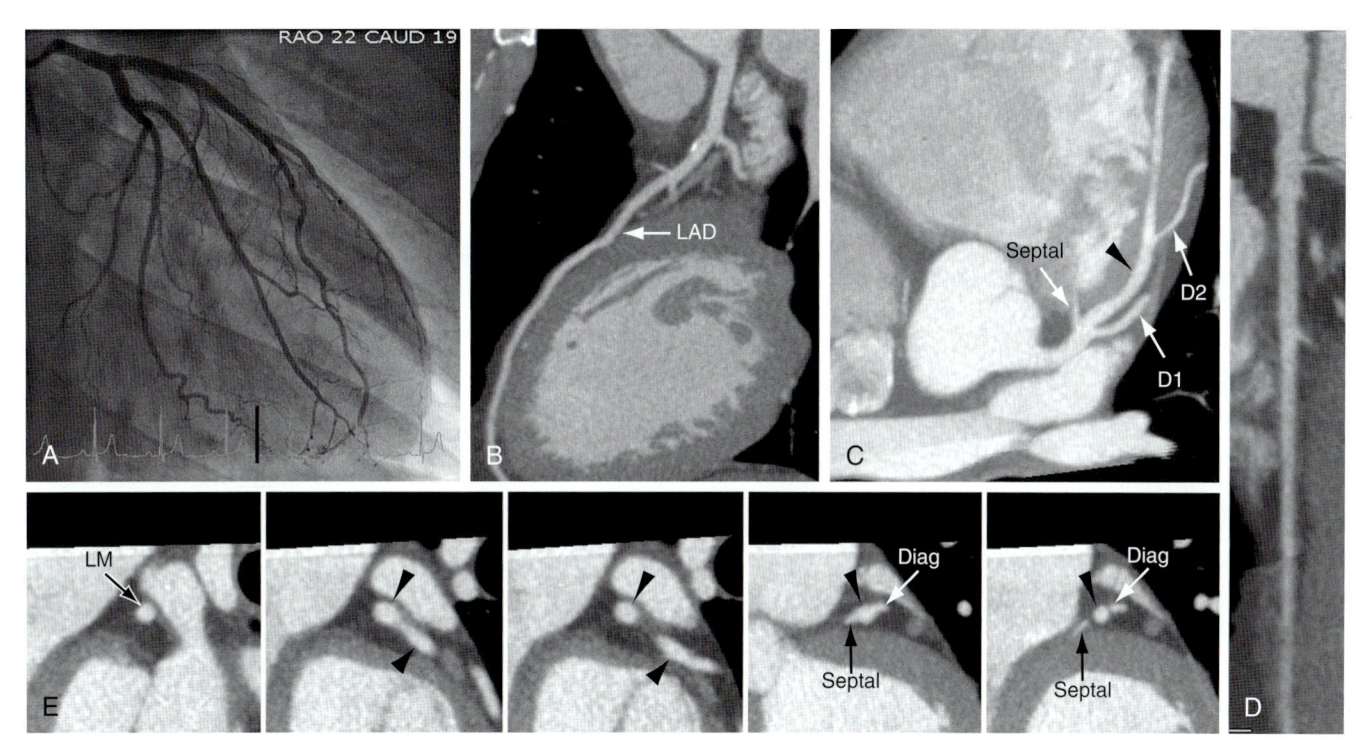

FIGURE 3-11 Left anterior descending artery (LAD) and its branches. *Long thin arrowhead* denotes the LAD, and *short thick arrowhead* denotes left circumflex artery. **A,** Selective injection of the left coronary at cardiac catheterization shows the LAD and left circumflex artery and their branches. **B,** Curved reformat of the LAD, which courses down to the apex of the heart. **C,** Oblique MIP of the LAD and its branches, the septal perforators and the diagonals, which are numbered sequentially as they arise (D1, D2). **D,** Lumen view image of left main (LM) and LAD. **E,** Cross-sectional orthogonal views of the LM and proximal LAD. Note septal perforator origin and course in the anterior interventricular septum. The first diagonal (Diag) arises at the same level.

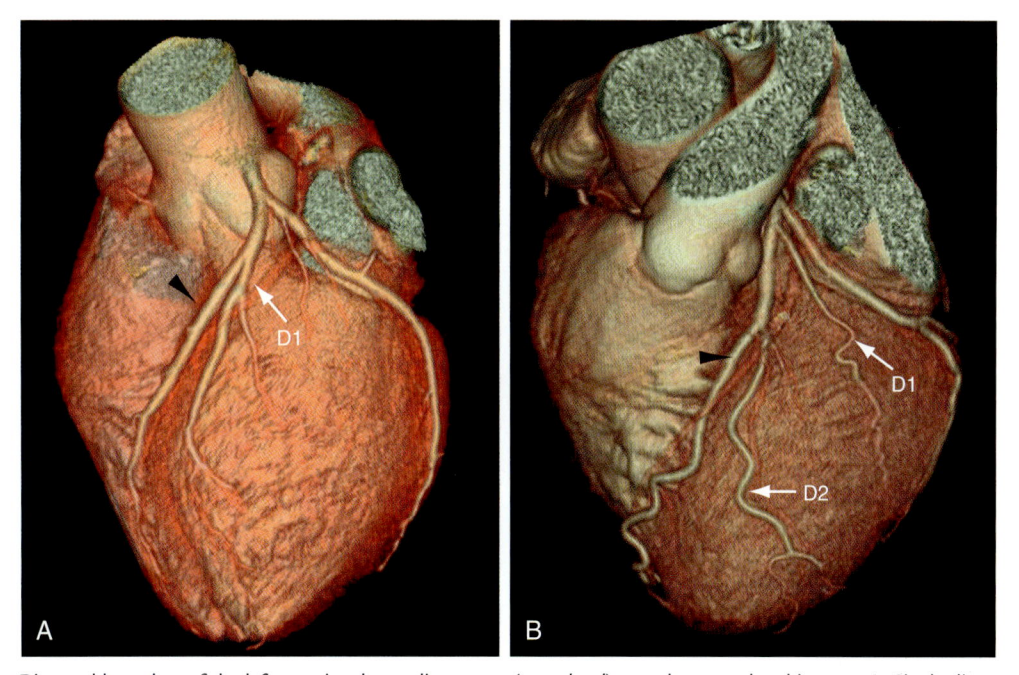

FIGURE 3-12 Diagonal branches of the left anterior descending artery (*arrowhead*) on volume rendered images. **A,** Single diagonal. The left anterior descending artery gives off a single large diagonal (D1) that bifurcates early and runs on the anterolateral epicardial surface of the heart. **B,** Two diagonals. A high large-caliber D1 and a large-caliber D2 come off the left anterior descending artery to supply the anterolateral surface of the heart.

The LAD gives off septal perforators and diagonal branches (see Figs. 3-11 and 3-12). The diagonal branches course along and supply the anterior and anterolateral wall of the left ventricular myocardium (see Figs. 3-11 and 3-12). They can vary in size and number, and are sequentially numbered as they arise from the LAD. In a series of 543 consecutive patients who underwent 64-detector coronary CT angiography, Cademartiri and colleagues[9] reported variable numbers of diagonal branches: a single diagonal branch in 136 cases (25%), two diagonal branches in 270 cases (49.7%), and more then two branches in 130 cases (24%) (see Figs. 3-11 and 3-12). Diagonal branches were absent in seven cases (1.3%). The septal perforator branches arise at right angles from the LAD and supply the anterior two thirds of the interventricular septum. They are numbered sequentially as they arise from the LAD and are of smaller caliber then diagonal branches and vary in number (one to five) and distribution. The first septal branch is more constant in position than the first diagonal. It may branch early with both branches running parallel within the septum. Occasionally, a septal branch runs parallel to the LAD within the myocardium of the septum. The average angle between the LAD and the first diagonal has been reported as 46 ± 19 degrees.[10]

Left Circumflex Artery

The LCX runs posteriorly and to the left in the left AV groove (Fig. 3-13). It gives rise to obtuse marginal branches that are also numbered sequentially as they arise from the LCX (OM1, OM2, and OM3) (Fig. 3-14). Cademartiri and colleagues[9] reported the prevalence of the number of the marginal branches arising from the LCX as 35.2% for one obtuse marginal branch, 46.2% for two obtuse marginal branches, and 18% for more than two obtuse marginal branches. The average angle between LCX/OM1 is 48 ± 24 degrees.[10] Marginal branches of the LCX are observed in 99.4% (n = 540).[9] The LCX and its branches supply the lateral and posterolateral wall of the left ventricle. Additional branches of the LCX are small atrial branches that supply the lateral and posterior regions of the left atrium.

Ramus Intermedius Artery

The RI is the most common variation of LCA anatomy, occurring when the LM trifurcates; the branch between the LAD and the LCX is the RI (Fig. 3-15). The RI can supply the myocardial territory of the diagonal branch or the obtuse marginal branch depending on whether it supplies the anterior wall or the lateral wall of the left ventricular myocardium.[9,15] When large, the RI perfuses a significant portion of the myocardial territory of the diagonal branch and OM1. An RI was seen in approximately 21.9% of the cases reported by Cademartiri and colleagues.[9] When the RI supplied vascularization to the anterolateral wall of the left ventricle, a decreased number of diagonal branches was observed: no diagonals in 3.4%, a single diagonal in 38.6%, two diagonals in 43.7%, and more than two diagonals in 14.3%.[9] The first diagonal not only may be small, but also may arise more distally from the LAD than from the proximal third of the LAD (see Fig. 3-15A).

Coronary Artery Dominance

The artery that supplies the inferior portion of the posterior interventricular septum is considered to be the dominant artery. In 80% to 85% of cases, the RCA is dominant; when at the crux of the heart, it gives rise to the PDA and PLB (Fig. 3-16A). In a left dominant system, the LCX

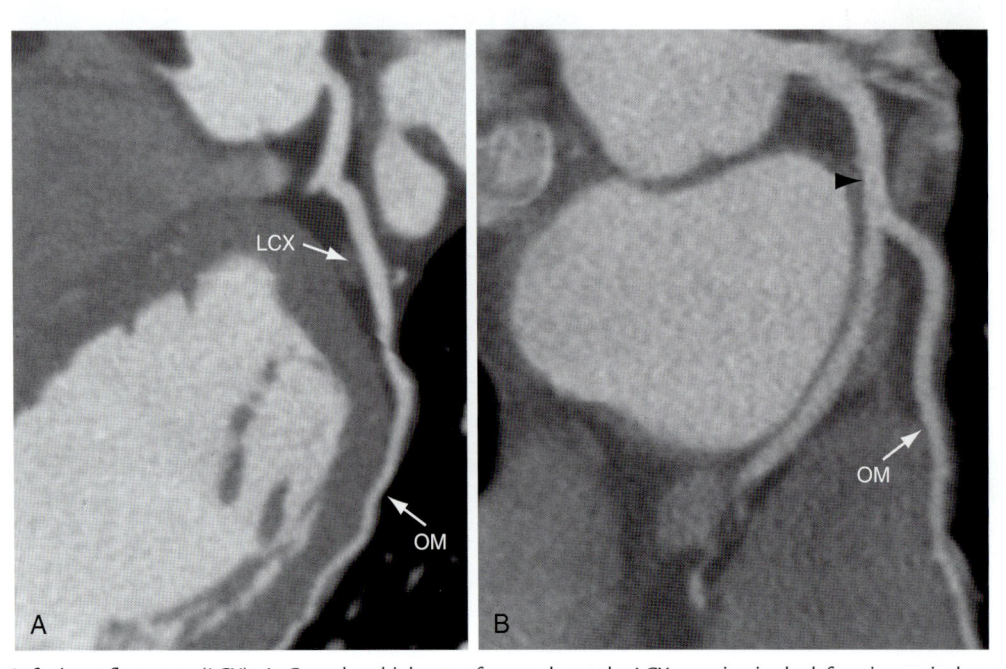

■ **FIGURE 3-13** Left circumflex artery (LCX). **A,** Curved multiplanar reformat shows the LCX coursing in the left atrioventricular groove on the posterior epicardial surface of the heart. **B,** A large-caliber obtuse marginal (OM) branch comes off the LCX (*arrowhead*).

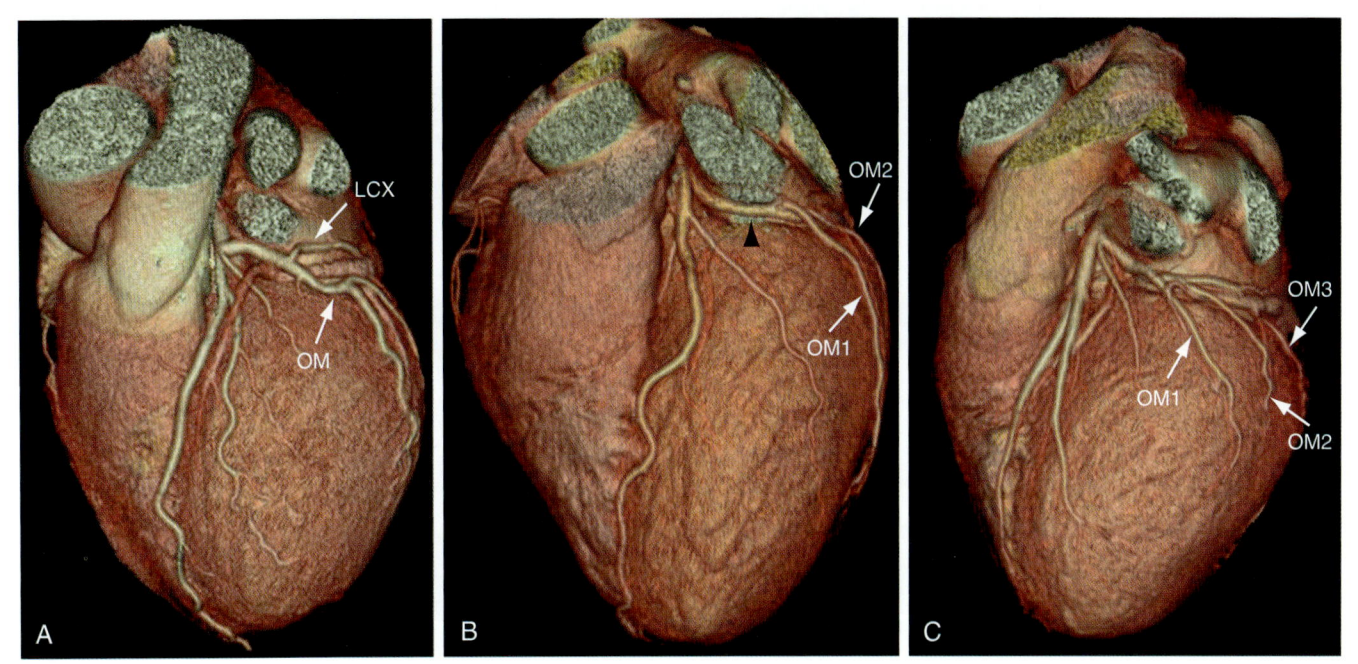

■ **FIGURE 3-14** Obtuse marginal branches (OM) of the left circumflex artery (LCX) on volume rendered images. **A,** Single OM. The LCX gives off a single large OM that runs on the posterolateral epicardial surface of the heart. **B,** Two OMs. A large-caliber OM1 and a slightly smaller caliber OM2 come off the LCX (*arrowhead*). **C,** Three OMs. Three OMs of varying caliber (OM1, OM2, OM3) arise from the LCX.

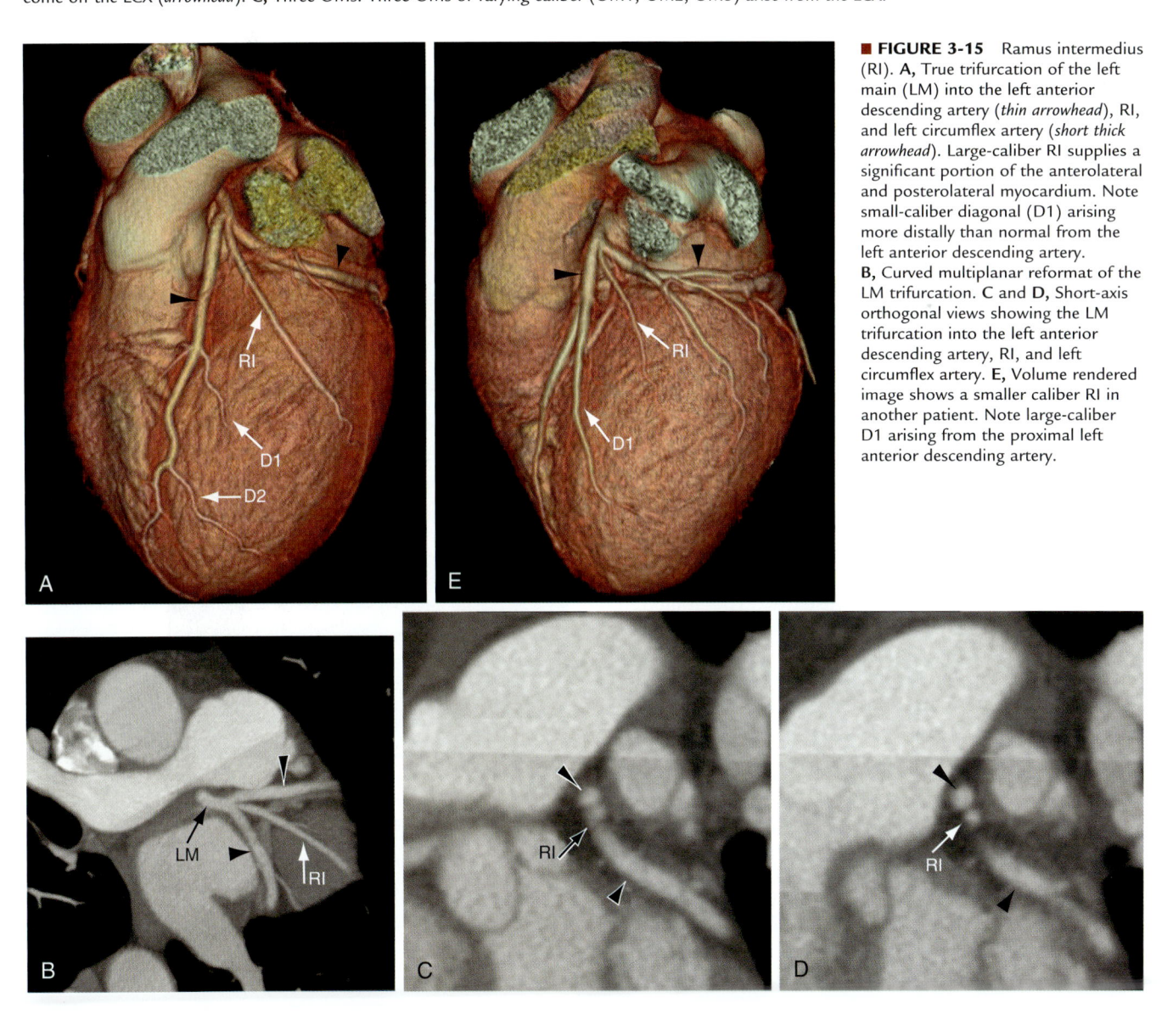

■ **FIGURE 3-15** Ramus intermedius (RI). **A,** True trifurcation of the left main (LM) into the left anterior descending artery (*thin arrowhead*), RI, and left circumflex artery (*short thick arrowhead*). Large-caliber RI supplies a significant portion of the anterolateral and posterolateral myocardium. Note small-caliber diagonal (D1) arising more distally than normal from the left anterior descending artery. **B,** Curved multiplanar reformat of the LM trifurcation. **C** and **D,** Short-axis orthogonal views showing the LM trifurcation into the left anterior descending artery, RI, and left circumflex artery. **E,** Volume rendered image shows a smaller caliber RI in another patient. Note large-caliber D1 arising from the proximal left anterior descending artery.

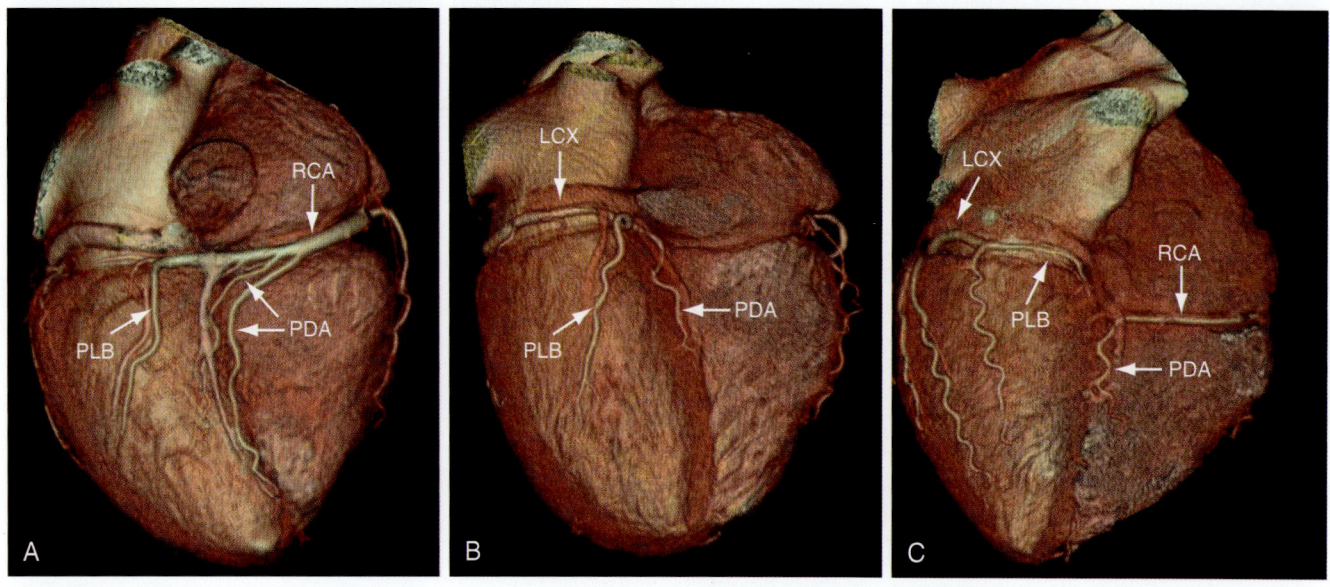

FIGURE 3-16 Volume rendered CT shows dominance. **A,** Right dominant system. The posterior descending coronary artery (PDA) and posterolateral branch (PLB) come off the right coronary artery (RCA). The patient has a dual PDA. **B,** Left dominant system. The PDA and PLB come off the left circumflex (LCX). **C,** Codominant system. The PDA comes off the RCA, and the PLB comes off the LCX.

continues in the posterior left AV groove and gives rise to the PDA and PLB; this is seen in 7% to 8% of the population (see Fig. 3-16B). In the remaining 7% to 8%, there is a codominant system or balanced circulation in which the RCA gives rise to the PDA and terminates in the posterior interventricular groove; the LCX may also give rise to a PDA with two PDAs running parallel in the interventricular septum, or the LCX may give rise to all posterolateral branches (see Fig. 3-16C).[12,15] The nondominant artery is usually smaller in size and terminates early in its respective AV groove.

NORMAL VARIANTS OF CORONARY ARTERIAL ANATOMY

Duplication of the coronary arteries is rare and can be seen with the LAD, RCA, or PDA. With LAD duplication, one branch (short LAD) terminates in the proximal aspect of the anterior interventricular sulcus (AIVS), and the second, longer branch has a variable course outside the AIVS and returns to the AIVS distally.[14] The long LAD usually arises from the LAD; however, it rarely can arise from the RCA and enter the distal AIVS. Four subtypes of dual LAD have been described. In all subtypes, the short LAD terminates in the proximal AIVS. The long LAD takes one of four courses before entering the distal AIVS. In type 1, the long LAD courses to the left of the AIVS over the left ventricular myocardium (Fig. 3-17). In type 2, the long LAD courses to the right of the AIVS over the left ventricular myocardium. Type 3 is extremely rare with the proximal long LAD taking an intramyocardial course before entering the distal AIVS. Type 4 dual LAD is a distinct type in which the long LAD originates from the RCA, takes an anomalous course, and enters the anterior interventricular groove. Recognition of these variants is important for correct surgical identification of the short and long LADs

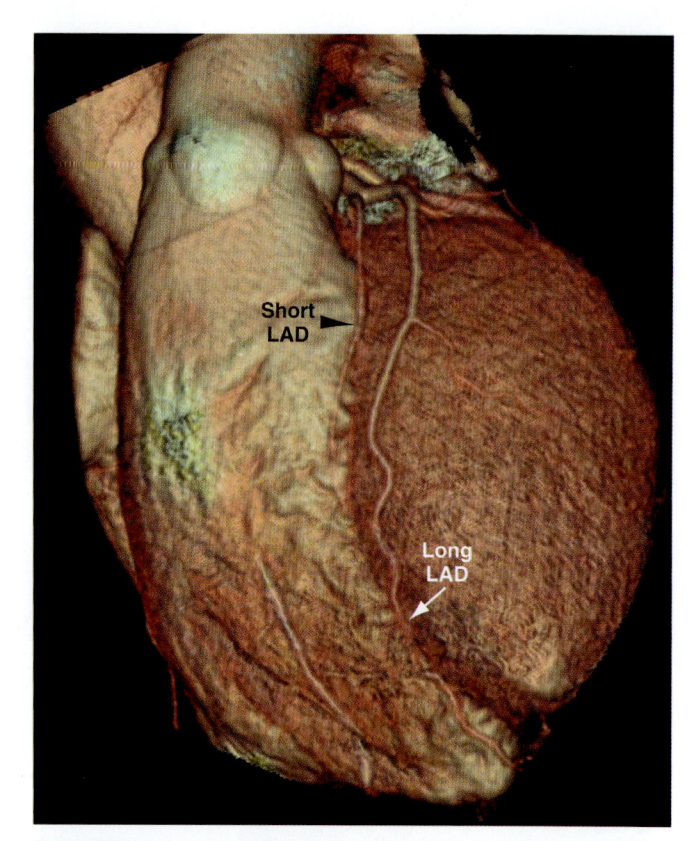

FIGURE 3-17 Dual left anterior descending artery (LAD). Three-dimensional volume rendered CT image of the heart shows a short LAD that courses and terminates in the mid septum. The long LAD courses to the left of the anterior interventricular groove and enters the distal septum running inferiorly, to the apex of the heart.

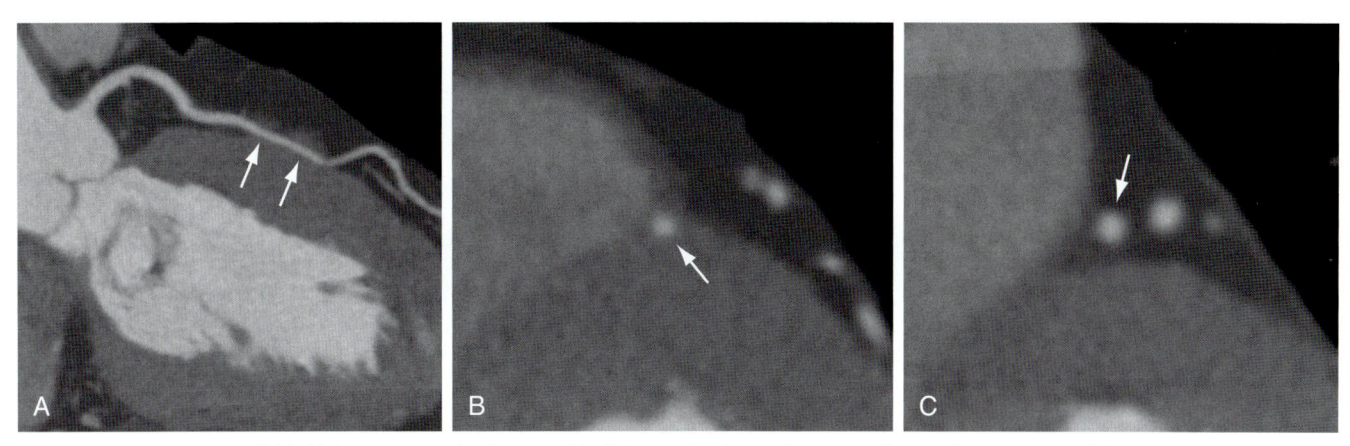

■ **FIGURE 3-18** Myocardial bridging. **A,** Curved reformat of the left anterior descending artery shows a long segment of the mid left anterior descending artery with an intramyocardial course (*arrows*). **B** and **C,** On the cross-sectional orthogonal MIP view (**B**), the tunneled artery (*arrow*) is surrounded by muscle, and the artery proximal to it is surrounded by epicardial fat (**C**).

for revascularization purposes or correct placement of an arteriotomy.[14]

Myocardial Bridge

Extramural arteries are expected to plunge into the myocardium only once, at their distal end. An exception to this is an intramural/intramyocardial course of the coronary artery, or "myocardial bridging," which is considered an anomaly of aberrant course of the involved coronary artery. Myocardial bridging is most commonly seen in the LAD, predominantly in the mid LAD (Fig. 3-18). Konen and associates[16] reported a mid LAD myocardial bridge in 27 of 47 (57%) cases and a distal LAD myocardial bridge in 7 of 47 (15%). Three patterns of myocardial bridging were observed: superficial septal in 10 of 34 (29.4%), deep septal in 14 of 34 (41.1%), and right ventricular type in 10 of 34 (29.4%), with the length of the intramuscular segment ranging from 13 to 40 mm.[16] Multiple segments of myocardial bridging can be seen in a single vessel, and several vessels in a single patient can show myocardial bridging. If data are available in diastole and systole, the tunneled segment can be evaluated for potential narrowing during systole—the so-called milking effect that has been described on conventional catheter angiography.

Reported prevalence of intramuscular coronary arteries ranges from 5% to 86% at autopsy and 0.8% to 4.9% at coronary angiography.[16-18] The incidence of myocardial bridging as reported in the study from Konen and associates[16] is 30.5%. Intramuscular coronary arteries can cause technical problems during coronary artery bypass surgery, including inadvertent perforation of the right ventricle.[16] Myocardial bridging also occurs in the diagonal branches (23.4%), obtuse marginal branches (19.1%), and RCA.[18]

CORONARY ARTERY SEGMENTAL ANATOMY

Nomenclatures for segmental anatomy of the coronary arteries that have been developed and modified by the American Heart Association (AHA) are used predominantly for research purposes.[19,20] In 1975, Austen and coworkers[19] developed a 15-segment coronary arterial model by dividing the coronary arteries into multiple segments. The proximal RCA segment commences from the ostium to the acute marginal, the mid segment curves around the acute margin of the heart, and the distal segment runs along the posterior AV groove. Segments 1 through 4 denote the RCA and its branches—1, proximal RCA; 2, mid RCA; 3, distal RCA; 4a, PDA; and 4b, PLB. Segment 5 denotes the LM.

For practical catheterization or coronary CT reports, the LAD is divided into proximal, mid, and distal segments using the origins of septal perforators or diagonals as follows: the proximal segment starts from the origin of the LAD to either the first diagonal or the first septal perforator, the mid segment commences from that point to the second diagonal, and the distal segment commences distal to that point.[19] The proximal, mid, and distal LAD segments correspond to segments 6, 7, and 8, and the first and second diagonals correspond to segments 9 and 10.

Regarding the LCX, the proximal segment is from the origin to OM1, and the distal segment is distal to that point. The LCX and its branches correspond to segments 11 through 15. More recently, a 17-segment model has been suggested (Fig. 3-19). Other modifications include the Bypass Angioplasty Revascularization Investigation (BARI) classification, used for revascularization procedures.[20]

Segmentation of the Left Ventricle

All cardiac imaging modalities should define, orient, and display the heart using the long axis of the left ventricle and selected planes oriented at 90-degree angles relative to the long axis that provide precise localization of the coronary distribution and link the segments to known coronary arterial topography by using anatomic landmarks.[21] The AHA has standardized the nomenclature of cardiac planes generated by cardiovascular magnetic resonance (CMR), single photon emission tomography (SPECT), positron emission tomography (PET), and cardiac CT. The nomenclature *short-axis, vertical long-axis,* and *horizontal long-axis views* (Fig. 3-20) is used and corresponds to the nomenclature *short-axis, apical two-*

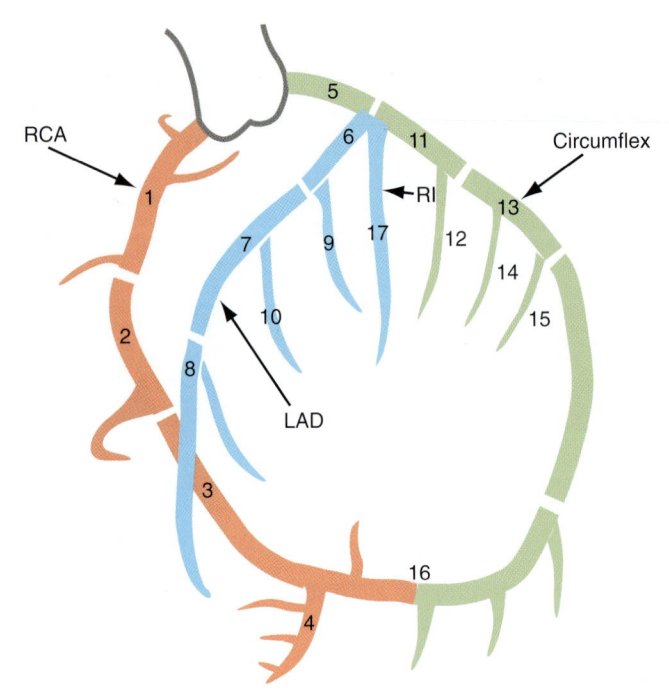

FIGURE 3-19 Segmental anatomy of the coronary arteries—modified AHA 17-segment model. LAD, left anterior descending artery; RCA, right coronary artery; RI, ramus intermedius.

chamber, and *apical four-chamber planes* traditionally used with two-dimensional echocardiography.[21]

Despite the tremendous variability in the coronary artery blood supply to the ventricular myocardial segments, it is important to assign myocardial segments to specific coronary artery territories. A standard 17-segment model was established using the precise data on mass and size of the myocardium from autopsy studies.[22] These segments correlate with the segments proposed and used in echocardiography. On this 17-segment model, a distribution of myocardial mass of 35%, 35%, and 30% for the basal, mid-cavity, and apical thirds of the heart, respectively, reflects the autopsy data closely. This model does not include the true apical myocardial segment.[23]

The myocardial segments are named and localized with reference to the long axes of the left ventricle and the 360-degree circumferential locations on the short-axis views. With regard to the circumferential location, the basal and mid-cavity slices are divided into six segments of 60 degrees each,[21] and the apical slice is divided into four segments (Fig. 3-21). Segment 17, the left ventricular apex, is represented on the vertical and horizontal long-axis views (see Fig. 3-21); this leads us to the recommended 17 segments that are represented on a bull's-eye display. The circumferential locations at the base and mid-cavity level are the anterior, anteroseptal, inferoseptal, inferior, inferolateral, and anterolateral myocardial segments. Segments 1 and 7 correspond to the anterior wall at the base and mid-cavity levels. The appropriate nomenclature for these segments is *basal anterior* and *mid-anterior segments.* The septum, delineated by the attachment of the right ventricle, is divided into anterior and inferior segments. Segments 2 and 3 are basal anteroseptal and basal inferoseptal. Segment 4 is the basal inferior, segment 5 is the basal inferolateral, and segment 6 is the basal anterolateral segment. Similar names are used for the six segments (numbers 7 through 12) at the mid-cavity level. Only four segments represent the left ventricular apical myocardium as the left ventricle tapers at the apex. Segments 13 through 16 represent the apical anterior, apical septal, apical inferior, and apical lateral myocardium. Segment 17 represents the extreme tip of the ventricle, the ventricular apex, where the left ventricular cavity is no longer seen.[21]

The greatest variability in the myocardial blood supply occurs at the extreme apex, or segment 17, which can be supplied by any of the three arteries, RCA, LCX, or LAD. Segments 1, 2, 7, 8, 13, 14, and 17 are assigned to the LAD distribution; segments 3, 4, 9, 10, and 15 are assigned to the RCA distribution; and segments 5, 6, 11, 12, and 16 are assigned to the LCX distribution.[21] The anteroseptal and anterior segments of the basal, mid-cavity, and apical segments are assigned to the LAD; the inferoseptal and inferior segments of the basal, mid-cavity, and inferior apical segments are assigned to the RCA; and the inferolateral and lateral segments of the basal, mid-cavity, and lateral apical segments are assigned to the LCX. Knowledge of the correlation between the segments of the left ventricle and the corresponding coronary artery distribution is crucial to detect corresponding coronary artery disease. Abnormalities of wall motion are usually reported using the descriptive anatomic locations of the myocardium such as anterior, septal, lateral, or inferior wall abnormalities at the three levels, although some institutions use the 17-segment model.

CORONARY VENOUS ANATOMY

The coronary venous system is increasingly used for diagnostic and therapeutic electrophysiologic procedures, such as percutaneous transcatheter therapy for cardiac resynchronization, ablation of various supraventricular arrhythmias, and therapy of mitral regurgitation by percutaneous mitral annuloplasty. The cardiac venous anatomy is not as well known to clinicians as the coronary arterial anatomy. Comprehensive knowledge of the cardiac venous system and its relationship to the surrounding structures is essential for preprocedural guidance of catheter or lead placement in a tributary of the coronary sinus.[4,5]

There are two major epicardial cardiac venous systems: the coronary sinus (CS) and its tributaries, which drain the major portion of the heart, and the anterior cardiac veins, which drain the anterior right ventricle and the right cardiac border. Additional small thebesian veins open directly into any of the four cardiac chambers.

The CS is a wide venous channel about 2 cm in length, located in the posterior part of the coronary sulcus covered by muscular fibers from the left atrium. It extends from the valve of Vieussens to its orifice in the right atrium (Fig. 3-22), which is between the opening of the inferior vena cava and the AV aperture; the orifice is guarded by a semilunar valve, the valve of the CS (thebesian valve). The diameter of the CS ranges from 7.3 to 18.9 mm, with the anteroposterior diameter reported as 11.5 mm and the superoinferior diameter reported as 12.6 mm, resulting in an oval-shaped ostium.[24] The CS is larger

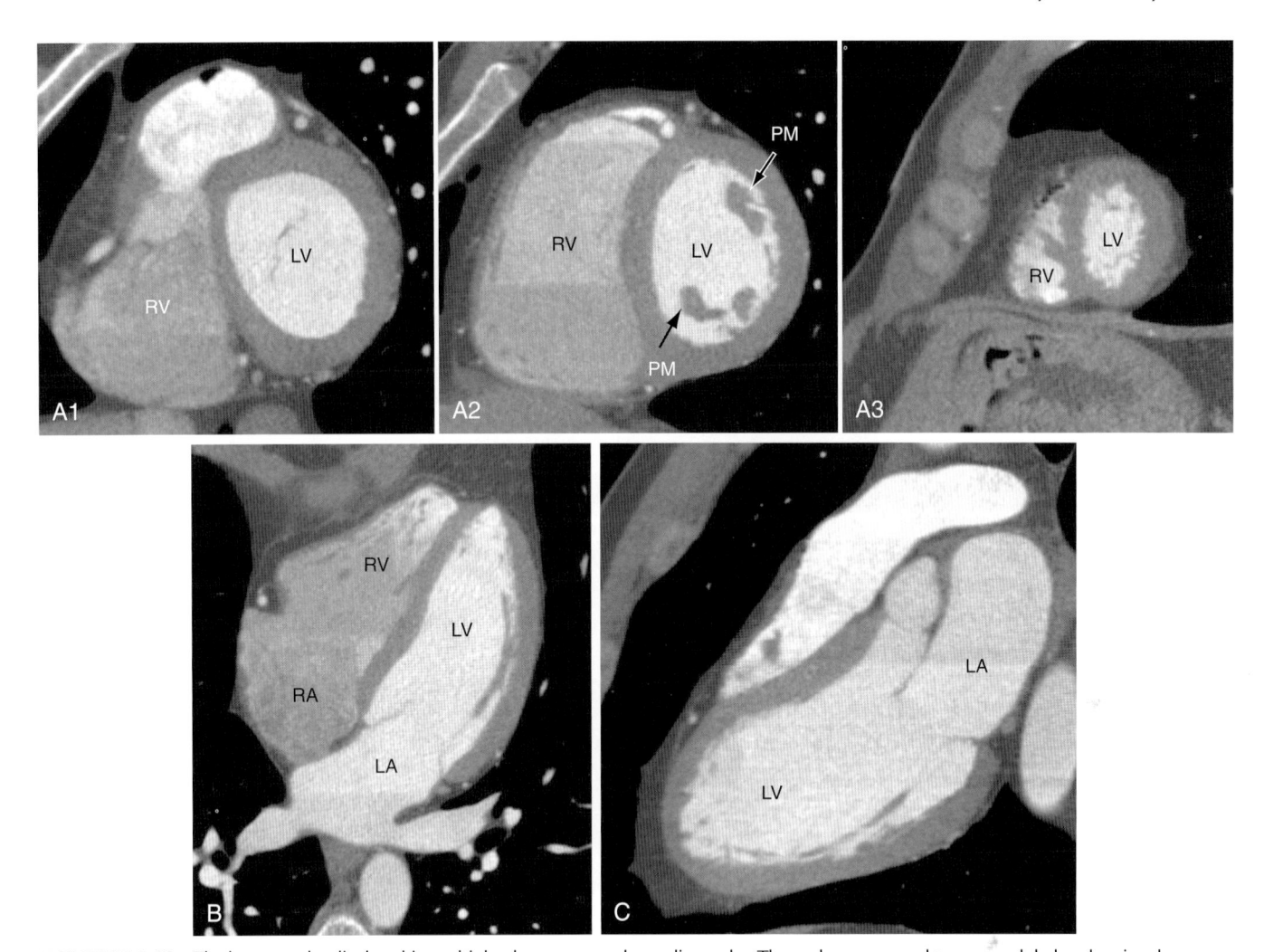

FIGURE 3-20 The heart can be displayed in multiple planes as on echocardiography. These planes are used to assess global and regional wall motion. **A-C,** Left ventricle (LV). **A1-A3,** Short-axis view at the level of the base, mid body, and apex of the LV. **B,** Horizontal long-axis or four-chamber view. **C,** Vertical long-axis or two-chamber view. LA, left atrium; PM, papillary muscle; RA, right atrium; RV, right ventricle.

in men than in women and in patients with ischemic cardiomyopathy compared with patients with nonischemic cardiomyopathy. The RCA is inferior to the CS at the crux of the heart.

The tributaries of the CS are the great, small, and middle cardiac (posterior interventricular) veins; the posterior vein of the left ventricle; and the oblique vein of the left atrium, all of which have a valve at their orifices except for the oblique vein of the left atrium (see Fig. 3-22). The diameter of the tributaries also varies from 1.3 to 10.5 mm.[24] An acute takeoff angle from the CS, a small diameter, and a tortuous course are anatomic characteristics that make cannulation of the vein difficult. Blendea and colleagues[24] reported an acute takeoff in 27% of posterior veins and 25% of lateral veins. In principle, the veins run parallel to the arteries.

The anterior interventricular vein originates in the lower or middle third of the anterior interventricular groove, runs parallel to the LAD, connects with diagonal veins, and drains the lateral and anterolateral portions of the left ventricle and receives blood from the anterior two thirds of the interventricular septum (Fig. 3-23). It continues to run vertically and upward in the anterior interventricular groove, and as it turns posteriorly at the AV groove and courses horizontally it becomes the great cardiac vein (GCV) or left coronary vein. The GCV is the main tributary of the CS and is the longest venous channel of the heart that runs in the left AV groove, to reach the back of the heart, draining into the left side of the CS (Figs. 3-24 and 3-25; see Figs. 3-22 and 3-23). It receives tributaries from the left atrium and from both ventricles, and one of the tributaries, the left marginal vein, is of considerable size and ascends along the left margin of the heart (see Fig. 3-24). At the origin of the LAD, the GCV crosses over the LAD and LCX arteries, where it forms the base of the triangle of Brocq and Mouchet, and then turns into the left AV groove, running parallel to the circumflex artery.

The distance from the GCV and the LM is variable (0 to 7 mm), and sometimes the GCV touches the LM and turns with a very sharp angle to the left AV groove, crossing under the branches of the LM coronary artery. The LCX is covered by the GCV in 60% of cases so that the underlying anatomy of the LCX is obscured or inadequately visualized, especially on volume rendered images (see Fig.

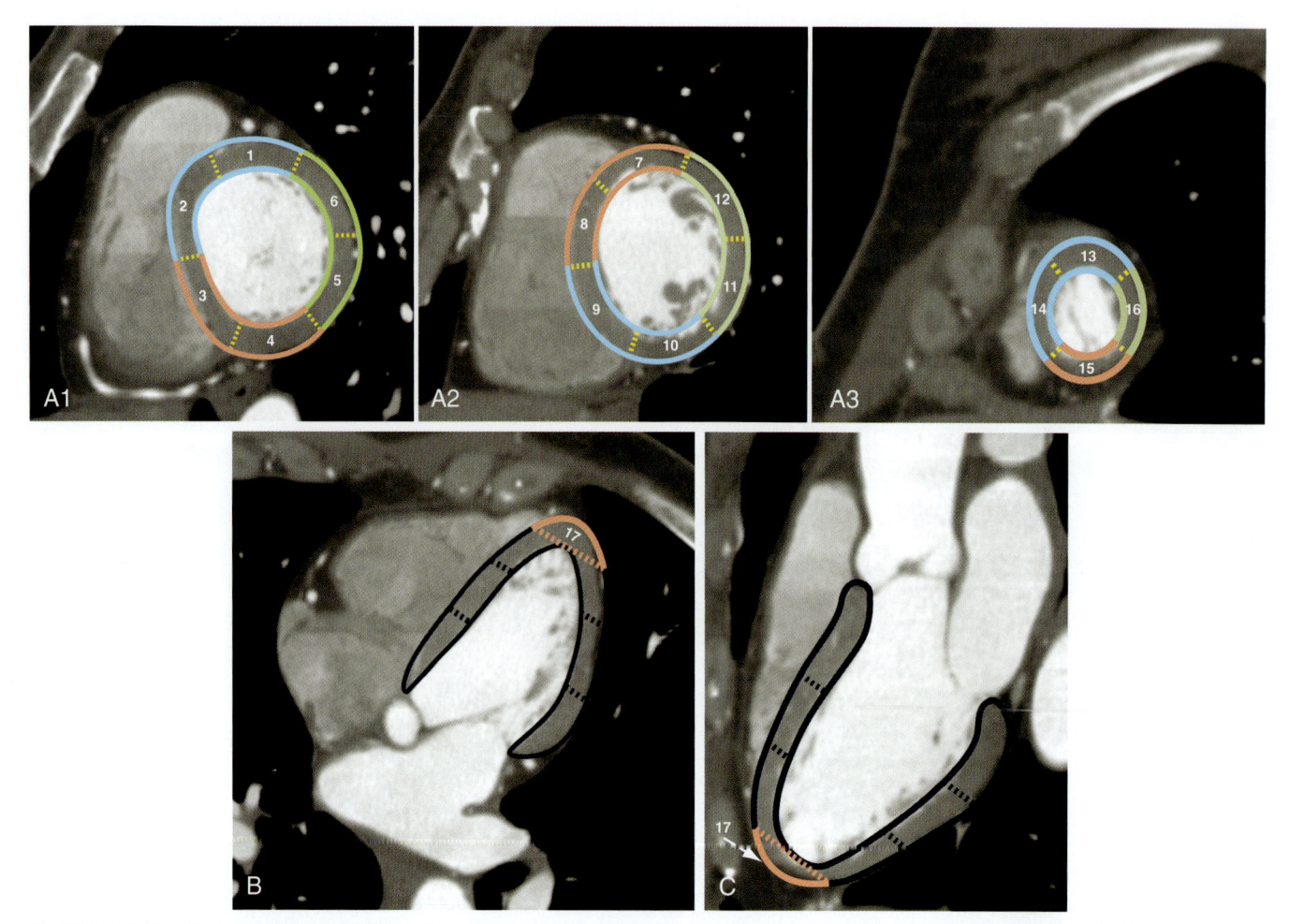

FIGURE 3-21 AHA 17-segment left ventricular segmentation model. *Orange* indicates the right coronary artery, *blue* indicates the left anterior descending artery, and *green* indicates the left circumflex artery on short-axis views at the base, mid-cavity, and apex. **A1-A3,** Segments 1-16. **B** and **C,** Segment 17 is represented on the horizontal long-axis (**B**) and vertical long-axis (**C**) views. With the understanding that there is great variability in the blood supply especially to the apex, the individual segments are assigned to representative coronary artery territories as follows: left anterior descending artery = 1, 2, 7, 8, 13, 14, 17; right coronary artery = 3, 4, 9, 10, 15; left circumflex artery = 5, 6, 11, 12, 16.

3-23). The proximal diameter of the GCV is 7.2 ± 1.4 mm, and the distal diameter is 4.9 ± 1.1 mm.[25] Christiaens and coworkers[4] reported an angle of greater than 90 degrees between the lateral marginal vein and GCV in 12% of cases, 60 to 90 degrees in 22%, and less than 60 degrees in 58%. The GCV becomes the CS at the entrance site of the left atrial oblique vein of Marshall. In cases where the left atrial oblique vein of Marshall is not present, the CS begins at the valve of Vieussens. The GCV and CS encircle most of the left AV conduction system and are frequently used for location of assessorial electrical pathways that are present in Wolff-Parkinson-White syndrome.

The tributaries of the CS that originate off the lateral wall are referred to as marginal veins. These marginal veins are defined further by the location of the veins as they empty into the GCV in the left anterior oblique projection—anterolateral marginal, lateral marginal, and inferolateral marginal (see Fig. 3-24). The prevalence of the lateral marginal vein is 73% to 88%, whereas the prevalence of the posterolateral marginal vein varies from 13% to 80% of cases.[25-27] The diameters of posterolateral and lateral marginal veins have been documented as 3.8 ± 0.7 mm and 3.1 ± 0.8 mm.[25] The lateral veins are less prevalent in patients with a history of lateral myocardial infarction than in patients without such a history (33% vs. 96%)[24] and (27% vs. 71%).[25]

The posterior lateral ventricular vein (PLVV) drains the inferior (posterior) aspect of the left ventricle. The PLVV is often confused with the posterolateral marginal vein because of their similar location. The PLVV is usually larger in caliber than the posterolateral marginal vein, and sometimes drains into the middle cardiac vein. The PLVV runs on the diaphragmatic surface of the left ventricle to the CS, but may end in the great cardiac vein. (see Fig. 3-25).

The middle cardiac vein originates near the cardiac apex, runs in the posterior interventricular groove, and drains either directly into the right atrium or into the CS in 87% of cases just before the CS drains into the right atrium (see Figs. 3-22, 3-24, and 3-25). The middle cardiac vein receives blood from the posterior third of the septum, and runs parallel to and stays to the left of the PDA. It crosses over the PLB branch of the RCA, and when the LCX is dominant, it drains blood from the inferior wall of

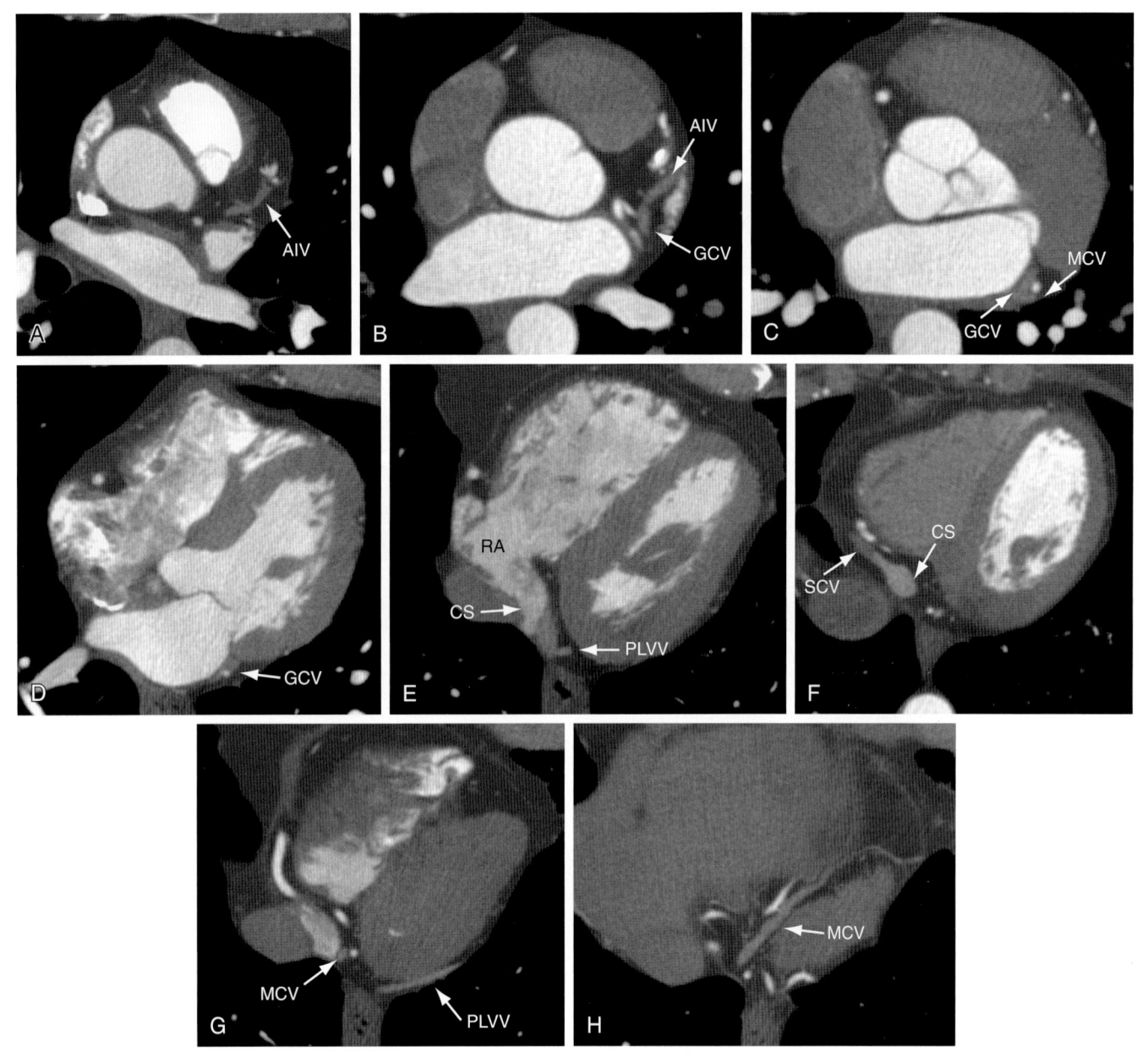

FIGURE 3-22 Normal axial anatomy of the coronary sinus (CS) and its tributaries. **A,** The anterior interventricular vein (AIV) in the anterior interventricular groove alongside the left anterior descending artery. **B,** The anterior interventricular vein runs from the AIV groove to the left atrioventricular groove where it continues as the great cardiac vein (GCV). **C,** The left marginal vein draining into the GCV in the left atrioventricular groove. Note obtuse marginal branch of left circumflex artery adjacent to left marginal vein. **D,** The GCV in the atrioventricular groove alongside the left circumflex artery. **E,** The posterior left ventricular vein (PLVV) draining into the GCV in the posterior left ventricular groove. The CS empties into the right atrium (RA). **F,** The small cardiac vein (SCV) seen in the right posterior atrioventricular groove as it drains into the CS. **G,** The middle cardiac vein (MCV) at the crux of the heart adjacent to the posterior descending coronary artery. The PLVV runs along the posterolateral diaphragmatic surface of the left ventricle. **H,** The MCV in the posterior interventricular groove alongside the posterior descending coronary artery.

the left ventricle and crosses over the artery before entering the CS.

Additional coronary veins drain the lateral wall of the left ventricle and enter the CS between the GCV and middle cardiac vein. The largest of these are used for implantation of the second lead of biventricular pacemakers. These lateral veins cover the area of the heart that is depolarized in the presence of a left ventricular bundle branch block, which makes it the most effective site for additional left ventricular pacing.

The small cardiac vein (vena cordis parva; right coronary vein) is present in only 36% of cases; it runs in the right AV groove, and opens into the right side of the CS, but may drain into the middle cardiac vein or directly into the right atrium. It receives blood from the back of the right atrium and ventricle. The most frequent anatomic variant observed (52%) is a connection of the small cardiac vein to the CS at the crux cordis (Fig. 3-26).

The oblique vein of the left atrium or oblique vein of Marshall is a small vessel that descends obliquely on the

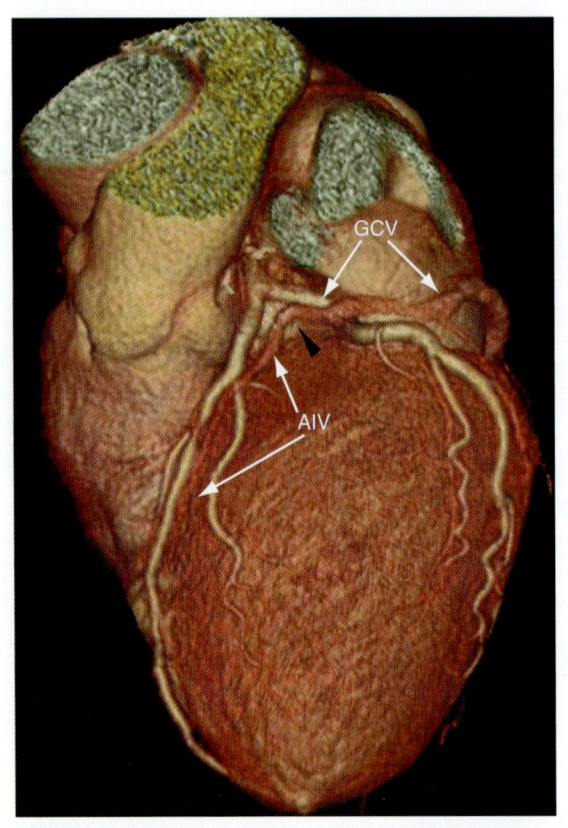

■ **FIGURE 3-23** The anterior interventricular vein (AIV) and the great cardiac vein (GCV). Volume rendered image shows AIV running parallel to the left anterior descending artery in the proximal and mid anterior interventricular sulcus. The AIV becomes the GCV when it makes an angle to enter the left atrioventricular groove (*arrowhead*).

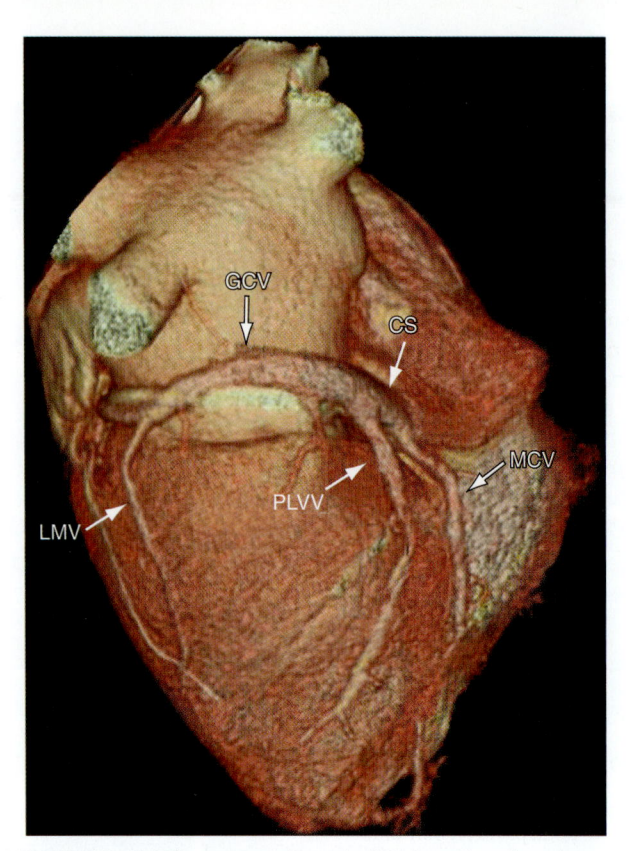

■ **FIGURE 3-25** The great cardiac vein (GCV) and its tributaries. Volume rendered image shows a large posterior left ventricular vein (PLVV) and a small left marginal vein (LMV) emptying into the GCV.

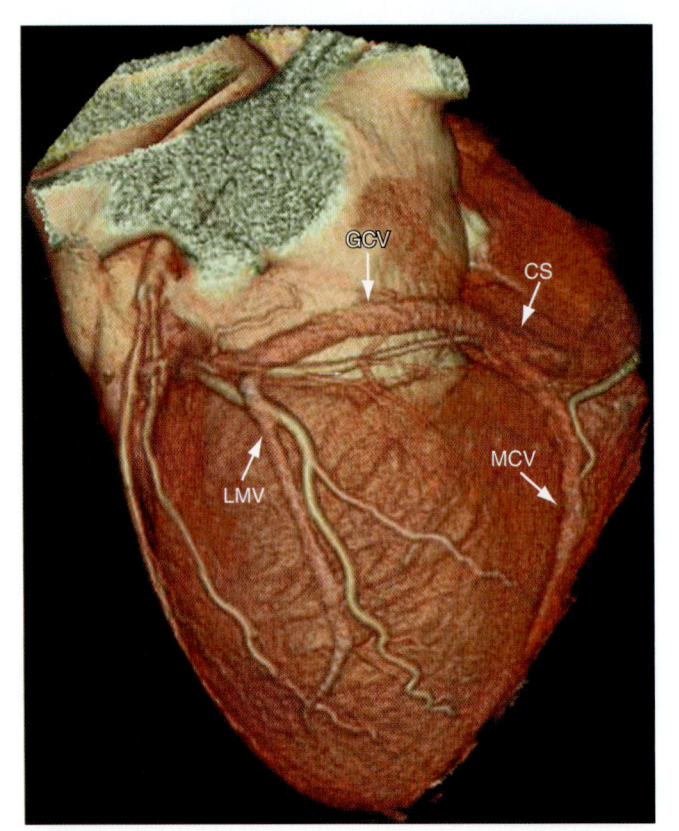

■ **FIGURE 3-24** The great cardiac vein (GCV) and its tributaries. Volume rendered image shows a large marginal vein emptying into the GCV. Note a small posterior left ventricular vein. The middle cardiac vein (MCV) runs in the posterior interventricular groove along with the posterior descending coronary artery and empties into the coronary sinus (CS).

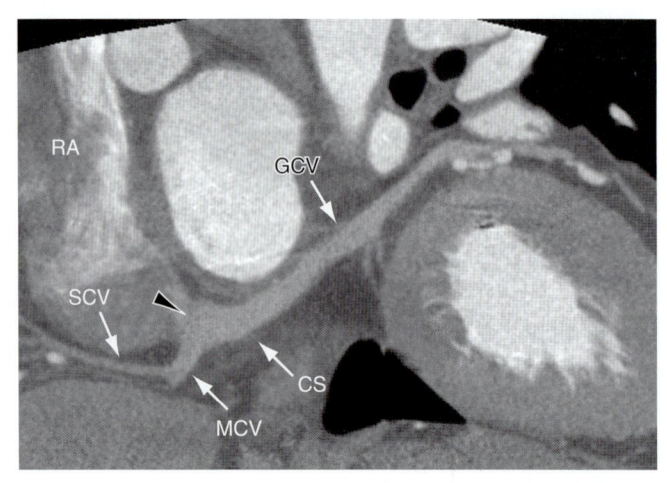

■ **FIGURE 3-26** Oblique MIP shows the small cardiac vein (SCV) in the right posterior atrioventricular groove draining into the middle cardiac vein (MCV) and not the coronary sinus (CS). *Arrowhead* denotes the valve of the CS (thebesian valve) at the entrance site of the CS into the right atrium (RA). See the great cardiac vein (GCV) in the AV groove.

back of the left atrium and drains into the CS near its left edge. This vein was identified in 37 of 51 patients included in the study by Blendea and colleagues[24] with diameters of 1.7 ± 0.5 mm and takeoff angles of 154 ± 15 degrees, which makes the vein accessible for cannulation for ablation procedures for atrial fibrillation.[28]

Cardiac veins that do not drain into the CS are the anterior cardiac veins, comprising three or four small vessels that collect blood from the front of the right ventricle and open into the right atrium via atrial sinuses. The sinus coronarius atrii dextri is so large that it can be confused with the RCA. The right marginal vein opens into the right atrium, and is regarded as belonging to this group. The smallest cardiac veins (thebesian veins) consist of numerous minute veins arising in the muscular wall of the atria and ventricles and draining into their respective chambers.[5,29,30]

CONCLUSION

This chapter reviews and illustrates detailed coronary arterial and venous anatomy. A thorough knowledge of the coronary arterial anatomy and coronary arterial and left ventricular segmentation is required for evaluation of suspected coronary artery disease, diagnosis of variant and anomalous coronary arterial anatomy, and evaluation of structural abnormalities of the heart. Newer therapeutic options for resynchronization therapy and resistant atrial and ventricular arrhythmias mandate detailed anatomic knowledge of the coronary venous system.

SUGGESTED READINGS

Achenbach S. Computed tomography coronary angiography. J Am Coll Cardiol 2006; 48:1919-1928.

Angelini P. Coronary artery anomalies: an entity in search of an identity. Circulation 2007; 115:1296-1305.

Scanlon PJ, Faxon DP, Audet AM, et al. ACC/AHA guidelines for coronary angiography. A report of the American College of Cardiology/American Heart Association Task Force on practice guidelines (Committee on Coronary Angiography). Developed in collaboration with the Society for Cardiac Angiography and Interventions. J Am Coll Cardiol 1999; 33:1756-1824.

REFERENCES

1. Achenbach S. Computed tomography coronary angiography. J Am Coll Cardiol 2006; 48:1919-1928.
2. Hamon M, Morello R, Riddell JW, et al. Coronary arteries: diagnostic performance of 16- versus 64-section spiral CT compared with invasive coronary angiography—meta-analysis. Radiology 2007; 245:720-731.
3. Knollmann F, Ducke F, Krist L, et al. Quantification of atherosclerotic coronary plaque components by submillimeter computed tomography. Int J Cardiovasc Imaging 2008; 24:301-310.
4. Christiaens L, Ardilouze P, Ragot S, et al. Prospective evaluation of the anatomy of the coronary venous system using multidetector row computed tomography. Int J Cardiol 2008; 126:204-208.
5. Jongbloed MRM, Lamb HJ, Bax JJ, et al. Noninvasive visualization of the cardiac venous system using multislice computed tomography. J Am Coll Cardiol 2005; 45:749-753.
6. Angelini P. Coronary artery anomalies: an entity in search of an identity. Circulation 2007; 115:1296-1305.
7. Angelini P, Velasco JA, Flamm S. Coronary anomalies: incidence, pathophysiology, and clinical relevance. Circulation 2002; 105:2449-2454.
8. Burck H. High and funnel-like origin of the coronary arteries. Beitr Pathol Anat 1963; 128:139-156.
9. Cademartiri F, La Grutta L, Malago R, et al. Prevalence of anatomical variants and coronary anomalies in 543 consecutive patients studied with 64-slice CT coronary angiography. Eur Radiol 2008; 18:781-791.
10. Pflederer T, Ludwig J, Ropers D, et al. Measurement of coronary artery bifurcation angles by multidetector computed tomography. Invest Radiol 2006; 41:793-798.
11. Sos TA, Sniderman KW. A simple method of teaching three-dimensional coronary artery anatomy. Radiology 1980; 134:605-606.
12. Patel S. Normal and anomalous anatomy of the coronary arteries. Semin Roentgenol 2008; 43:100-112.
13. Paulin S. Coronary angiography: a technical, anatomic and clinical study. Acta Radiol (Diagn) (Stockh) 1964; 233(Suppl):1.
14. Spindola-Franco H, Grose R, Solomon N. Dual left anterior descending coronary artery: angiographic description of important variants and surgical implications. Am Heart J 1983; 105:445-455.
15. Kini S, Bis KG, Weaver L. Normal and variant coronary arterial and venous anatomy on high-resolution CT angiography. AJR Am J Roentgenol 2007; 188:1665-1674.
16. Konen E, Goitein O, Sternik L, et al. The prevalence and anatomical patterns of intramuscular coronary arteries: a coronary computed tomography angiographic study. J Am Coll Cardiol 2007; 49:587-593.
17. Mohlenkamp S, Hort W, Ge J, et al. Update on myocardial bridging. Circulation 2002; 106:2616-2622.
18. De Rosa R, Sacco M, Tedeschi C, et al. Prevalence of coronary artery intramyocardial course in a large population of clinical patients detected by multislice computed tomography coronary angiography. Acta Radiol 2008; 49:895-901.
19. Austen WG, Edwards JE, Frye RL, et al. A reporting system on patients evaluated for coronary artery disease. Report of the Ad Hoc Committee for Grading of Coronary Artery Disease, Council on Cardiovascular Surgery, American Heart Association. Circulation 1975; 51:5-40.
20. Scanlon PJ, Faxon DP, Audet AM, et al. ACC/AHA guidelines for coronary angiography. A report of the American College of Cardiology/American Heart Association Task Force on practice guidelines (Committee on Coronary Angiography). Developed in collaboration with the Society for Cardiac Angiography and Interventions. J Am Coll Cardiol 1999; 33:1756-1824.
21. Cerqueira MD, Weissman NJ, Dilsizian V, et al. Standardized myocardial segmentation and nomenclature for tomographic imaging of the heart: a statement for healthcare professionals from the Cardiac Imaging Committee of the Council on Clinical Cardiology of the American Heart Association. Circulation 2002; 105:539-542.
22. Edwards WD, Tajik AJ, Seward JB. Standardized nomenclature and anatomic basis for regional tomographic analysis of the heart. Mayo Clin Proc 1981; 56:479-497.
23. Henry WL, DeMaria A, Gramiak R, et al. Report of the American Society of Echocardiography Committee on Nomenclature and Standards in Two-dimensional Echocardiography. Circulation 1980; 62:212-217.
24. Blendea D, Shah RV, Auricchio A, et al. Variability of coronary venous anatomy in patients undergoing cardiac resynchronization

therapy: a high-speed rotational venography study. Heart Rhythm 2007; 4:1155-1162.
25. Van de Veire NR, Schuijf JD, De Sutter J, et al. Non-invasive visualization of the cardiac venous system in coronary artery disease patients using 64-slice computed tomography. J Am Coll Cardiol 2006; 48:1832-1838.
26. Mao S, Shinbane JS, Girsky MJ, et al. Coronary venous imaging with electron beam computed tomographic angiography: three-dimensional mapping and relationship with coronary arteries. Am Heart J 2005; 150:315-322.
27. Meisel E, Pfeiffer D, Engelmann L, et al. Investigation of coronary venous anatomy by retrograde venography in patients with malignant ventricular tachycardia. Circulation 2001; 104:442-447.
28. de Oliveira IM, Scanavacca MI, Correia AT, et al. Anatomic relations of the Marshall vein: importance for catheterization of the coronary sinus in ablation procedures. Europace 2007; 9:915-919.
29. Gerber TC, Sheedy PF, Bell MR, et al. Evaluation of the coronary venous system using electron beam computed tomography. Int J Cardiovasc Imaging 2001; 17:65-75.
30. Singh JP, Houser S, Heist EK, et al. The coronary venous anatomy: a segmental approach to aid cardiac resynchronization therapy. J Am Coll Cardiol 2005; 46:68-74.

CHAPTER 4

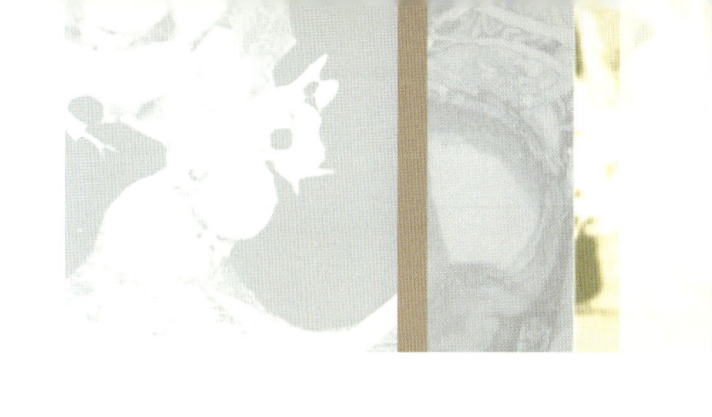

Physiology of the Heart

Phillip M. Young and Thomas C. Gerber

The regular contraction of the beating heart relies on a complex but closely interconnected cascade of electrical, chemical, and mechanical events. To understand basic cardiac physiology, one must consider events at the cellular and ultrastructural tissue levels, and the dynamics of the mechanical action of the myocardium and of blood flow. This chapter reviews basic cardiac physiology and function with an emphasis on the physiologic abnormalities underlying diseases that are commonly evaluated with cardiac imaging.

CARDIAC ELECTROPHYSIOLOGY

Orderly, sequential contraction of the cardiac chambers is driven by electrical impulses originating at the sinoatrial (SA) node, which is located in the wall of the right atrium near its confluence with the superior vena cava. Under normal circumstances, the SA node, with regulatory input from the autonomic and neuroendocrine systems, periodically generates electrical impulses that travel along a specialized cellular conduction system (CS) and determine the heart rate. Although CS cells in locations other than the sinus node can also spontaneously depolarize, the SA node normally has the fastest rate of spontaneous depolarization and drives the electrical cycle. Myocytes can also trigger depolarization and contraction of myocardial cells, but this typically occurs only under pathologic conditions.

Conduction of the electrical impulse is mediated by rapid changes of an electrical potential across cell membranes secondary to varying intracellular and extracellular concentration of sodium, calcium, and potassium ions. A sodium/potassium exchange pump creates, in the intracellular space, a low concentration of sodium ions and a high concentration of potassium ions, creating a baseline electrochemical potential across the membrane. A sudden increase in membrane permeability to sodium ions, mediated through sodium ion channels, causes rapid influx of sodium into the cell, depolarizing the electrical potential. Eventually, repolarization occurs through activation and deactivation of other transmembrane ion channels, and the baseline transmembrane gradient necessary to initiate a new episode of electrical depolarization is re-established. The depolarization propagates along the cells of the conduction system, spreads through the adjacent myocardium, and triggers electrochemical mechanisms that stimulate myocyte contraction.

Electrical depolarization initiated by the SA node first travels through the CS of the atria. This part of the electrical cycle is represented on the ECG by the P wave. Figure 4-1 is a diagram depicting the functional anatomy of the conduction system. The normal ECG appearance is shown in Figure 4-2.

A second regulatory event occurs when the impulse reaches the atrioventricular (AV) node and bundle of His, where the atrial CS converges at the anatomic junction of the atrial and ventricular septa. Here the speed of propagation of the electrical impulse is slowed, allowing for a temporal delay between atrial and ventricular systole. This delay optimizes pressure differentials between the chambers and allows optimal ventricular filling with the help of atrial systole ("atrial kick"). The alternating pressure differences between the atria, ventricles, and great vessels drive the opening and closing of the cardiac valves.

Distal to the bundle of His, the ventricular CS organizes into discrete right and left "bundle branches," which drive depolarization and contraction of the right and left ventricles. The left bundle branch divides further into anterior and posterior fascicles. As depolarization advances from the bundle of His into the right and left bundle branches, contraction of myocytes is initiated by electrical wave fronts spreading through ventricular myocardium, resulting in ventricular systole. The electrical depolarization of the left ventricular myocardium initiated by the right and left bundle branches is represented by the QRS complex on the ECG. The left bundle branch depolarizes earlier than the right bundle branch, and normal left ventricular

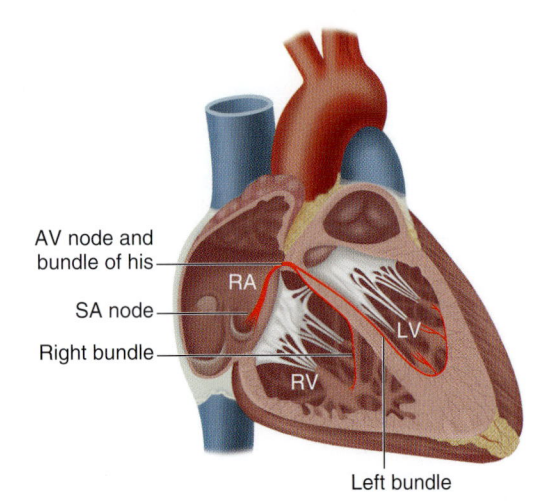

FIGURE 4-1 Conduction system of the heart. AV, atrioventricular; LV, left ventricle; RA, right atrium; RV, right ventricle; SA, sinoatrial.

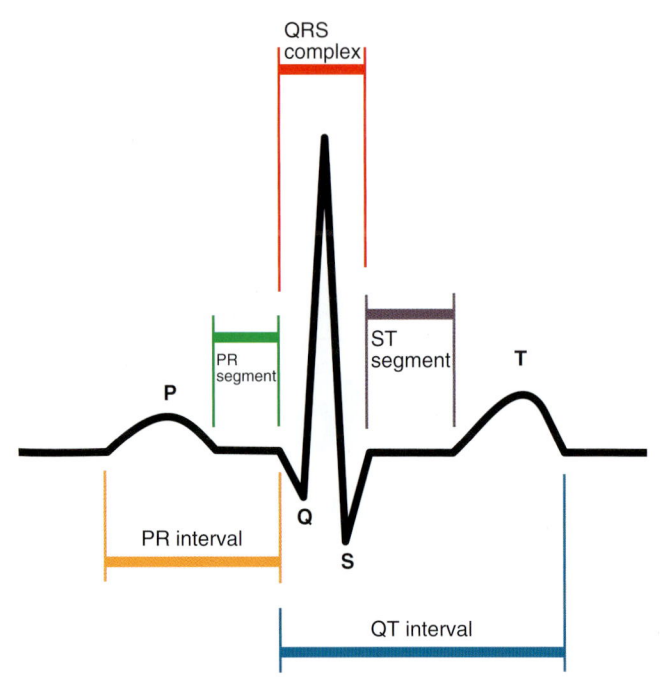

FIGURE 4-2 Schematic representation of a normal ECG sequence.

depolarization proceeds from the septum anteroapically, with the posterior base activated last.

As in the atria, repolarization must occur before another signal can be transmitted. Ventricular repolarization is represented by the T wave on the ECG. Because atrial repolarization temporally coincides with the much larger QRS complex, it is not detectable on the typical 12-lead surface ECG.

Atrial Fibrillation

Atrial fibrillation is a common impulse generation and conduction abnormality in which disorganized and irregular electrical activation of the atrial myocardium results in ineffective atrial systole. In this setting, the heart rate is typically irregular because activation of the AV node occurs by random synergistic confluence of atrial signals. Tachycardia invariably occurs if AV nodal function is normal. For this reason, negatively chronotropic medications, such as β receptor–blocking agents or calcium channel–blocking agents, are typically given to patients with atrial fibrillation to depress AV nodal conduction. A ventricular rate of less than 100 beats/min in patients with atrial fibrillation in the absence of negatively chronotropic medications implies CS disease. The irregularly irregular ventricular rate in atrial fibrillation is a common problem for gating cardiac CT and MRI studies.

Left Bundle Branch Block

Left bundle branch block, another common abnormality of electrical impulse generation and conduction that is relevant to cardiac imaging, can be idiopathic, but it often occurs in the setting of myocardial disease. In this condition, the left bundle branch conducts transmitted impulses with delay or not at all. Instead, ventricular depolarization begins via the right bundle branch only, and left ventricular myocardium depolarizes without the help of the CS, causing the left ventricle to contract later than the right ventricle. As a result, the interventricular septum moves and contracts in atypical, "paradoxical" fashion. This common abnormality of ventricular septal contractility must (and can) be differentiated from other causes of abnormal septal motion.

MYOCARDIAL AND VALVULAR FUNCTION

Cardiac myocytes are linked with each other by a network of extracellular matrix. The matrix consists primarily of collagen and proteoglycans synthesized by fibroblasts and smooth muscle cells. Individual myocytes are linked to the extracellular matrix by molecules called *integrins*. When triggered by electrical membrane depolarization, a rapid intracellular increase in calcium causes sequential contraction of the sarcomere through actin/myosin interactions (Fig. 4-3). Coordinated contraction of individual myocytes, connected to each other through the extracellular matrix, results in ventricular systole and propulsion of blood through the cardiac chambers.

Several variables or parameters can be used to quantify myocardial function. *Stroke volume* is defined as the difference between end-diastolic and end-systolic volumes (the volume ejected from the ventricular cavity between the beginning and end of systole). Dividing the stroke volume by the end-diastolic volume gives the ejection fraction (EF), the percentage of end-diastolic volume ejected. The EF is the most commonly used measure of systolic function.[1]

Sequential flow of blood through the cardiac chambers is driven by myocardial contraction and opening and closing of the cardiac valves (Fig. 4-4). The cardiac valves are one-way valves that open and close passively in response to pressure differences between the chambers they connect. Under normal circumstances, the cardiac

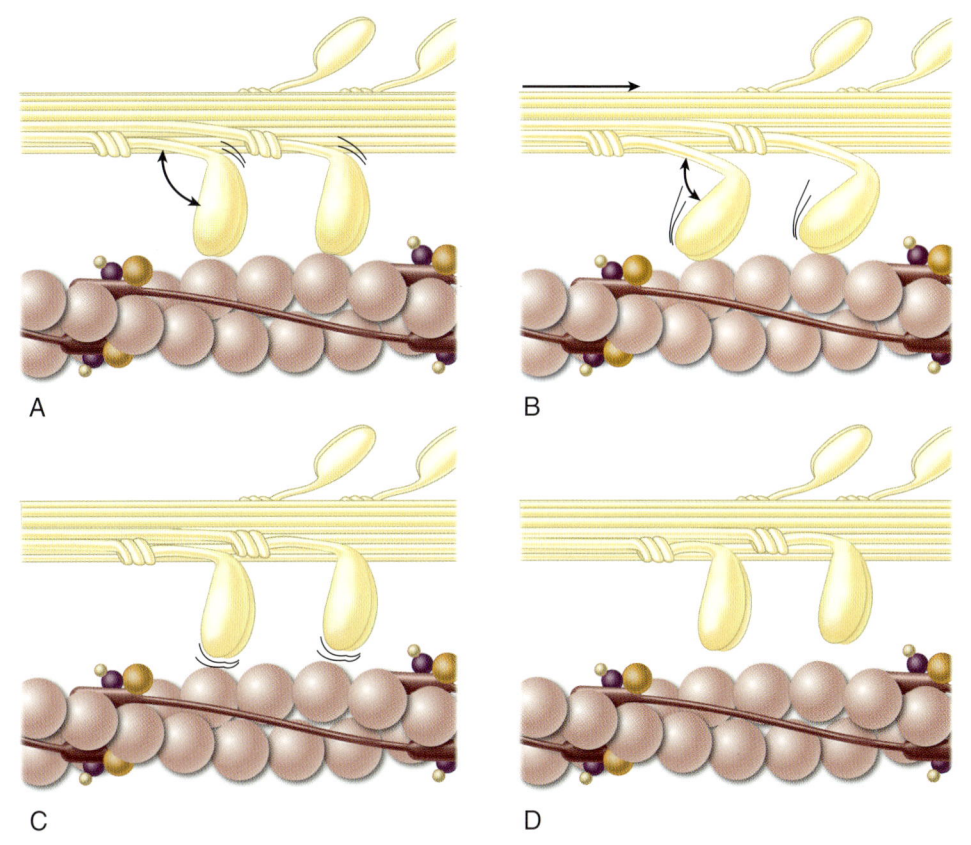

■ **FIGURE 4-3** A-D, Sequential illustrations show the interaction of actin and myosin causing sequential myocyte contraction. **A,** Actin and myosin filaments are cross-linked. **B,** Myosin chain translocates with respect to the actin filament by shortening the angle of its lever arm, a process powered by hydrolysis of ATP. **C** and **D,** Release of myosin from actin filament, allowing relaxation of the muscle fiber.

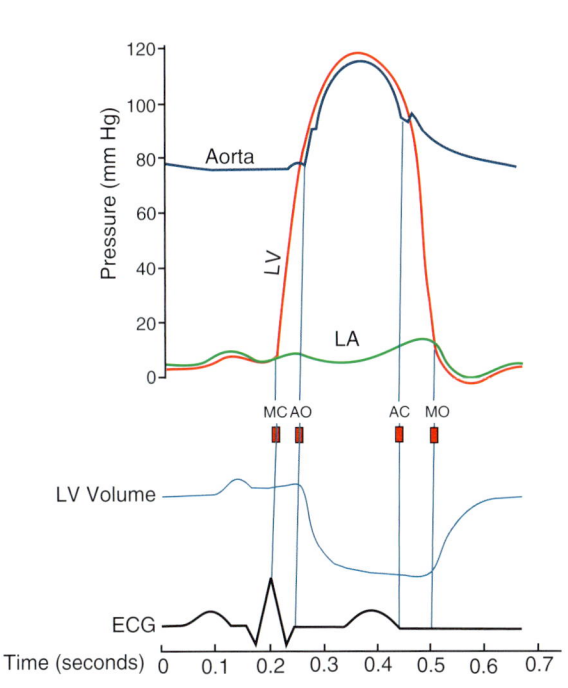

■ **FIGURE 4-4** Graphic representation of pressure-volume relationships in the left ventricle (LV), correlated temporally with an ECG tracing. The period of isovolumetric contraction occurs between mitral valve closure (MC) and aortic valve opening (AO). The isovolumetric relaxation phase occurs between aortic valve closure (AC) and mitral valve opening (MO). LA, left atrium.

valves permit forward flow only and prevent backward flow of blood.

During ventricular diastole, pressure in the ventricles decreases to less than the pressure in the atria, causing opening of the AV valves and inflow of blood from the atria into the ventricles. Near the end of diastole, ventricular filling is augmented by atrial contraction. This "atrial kick" increases preload by distending the ventricular cavity at end-diastole, increasing the effectiveness of systolic contraction as a result of the Frank-Starling mechanism.[2] At the beginning of ventricular systole, the rapid increase of pressure within the ventricular cavity causes closure of the AV valves. After a brief period of isovolumic contraction, pressure within the ventricular cavity exceeds the aortic and pulmonary arterial pressures, resulting in opening of the aortic and pulmonic valves and forward flow of blood into the aorta and pulmonary artery.

ATHEROSCLEROTIC CORONARY DISEASE

Coronary artery disease (CAD) is the largest contributor to cardiac mortality in developed countries, and was the cause of one of every four deaths in the United States in 2005.[3] The morbidity and mortality of CAD can manifest in two forms: (1) chronically with reduction of coronary flow or flow reserve resulting from stenoses of the coronary arteries, and (2) acutely with atherothrombotic occlusion of a coronary artery. The stages of development

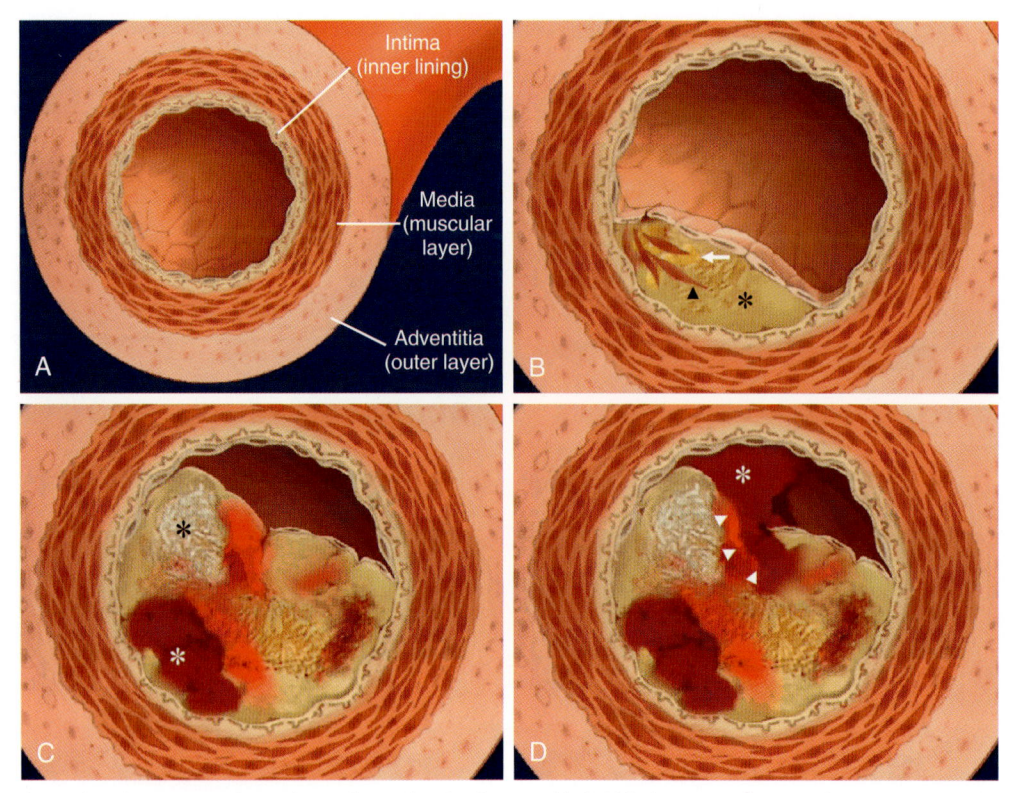

FIGURE 4-5 Atherosclerosis. **A,** Normal vessel. **B,** Atherosclerotic plaque, with lipid-laden macrophages (*white arrow*), smooth muscle proliferation (*black arrowhead*), and extracellular matrix (*asterisk*). **C,** Marked luminal narrowing from plaque growth. Variable amounts of collagen (*black asterisk*) and intraplaque hemorrhage (*white asterisk*) are present within the plaque. **D,** Plaque rupture (*arrowheads*) resulting in intravascular thrombosis (*asterisk*). (*Images courtesy of Dr. Amir Lerman, Mayo Clinic, Rochester, MN.*)

of atherosclerosis and the mechanisms of disease manifestation are briefly reviewed.

Vascular Biology of Atherosclerosis

The normal blood vessel wall consists of three distinct layers—intima, tunica media, and tunica adventitia. The innermost layer, the intima, is the site where atherosclerosis first manifests (Fig. 4-5). The intima consists mainly of endothelial cells, whereas the media contains smooth muscle cells, macrophages, mast cells, and extracellular matrix (primarily collagen and proteoglycans). The adventitia is composed primarily of extracellular connective tissue, but it also contains the vasa vasorum (vascular supply to the blood vessel wall itself) and nerve fibers involved in vasoregulation.

In areas of low shear stress (e.g., at vessel bifurcations or near the ostia of side branches), the endothelial layer may thicken (often eccentrically). These areas of thickened endothelium often show early findings of atherosclerosis.[4] The earliest atherosclerotic manifestation is the "fatty streak," characterized by intimal deposition of lipid-laden macrophages and T lymphocytes.[5] Fatty streaks occur in areas of intimal thickening because of multifactorial endothelial dysfunction and denudation, allowing intraintimal deposition of serum lipoproteins. Toxic damage from tobacco smoking and oxidative damage from very-low-density lipoproteins can be contributory factors. This initial endothelial injury incites an inflammatory response mediated by vascular cell adhesion molecules, selectins, and cytokines. The inflammatory response leads to ingestion of the lipoproteins by monocytes and macrophages, producing characteristic lipid-laden macrophages ("foam cells") on histology.[6]

Over time, demise and disintegration of lipid-laden macrophages and further deposition of serum lipoproteins lead to accumulation of extracellular lipid in the growing "plaque." Connective tissue, with varying portions of smooth muscle, collagen, and other extracellular proteins, also proliferates. As the plaque grows in size, the lumen of the vessel can become narrowed, although adaptive, positive remodeling of the vessel lumen by outward expansion of the vessel wall with an increase of vessel cross-section area (see Fig. 4-5) may initially prevent stenosis.[7] Paradoxically, positive remodeling may occur in an effort to resist endothelial shear stress, but the lower shear stress created by positive remodeling may lead to further lipid accumulation.[4] Vascular remodeling can be examined well with cross-sectional imaging modalities that show lumen and vessel wall (Fig. 4-6). On invasive, selective coronary angiography, the vessel wall is not imaged, and plaque "hidden" by positive remodeling may not be recognized.

Calcification frequently occurs in atherosclerotic plaque, and can occur in lipid-rich and predominantly fibrotic plaques. The quantity of coronary calcification is nonlinearly proportional to overall atherosclerotic burden. Coronary calcification represents approximately 20% of plaque volume.[8] The location of calcification does not predict the location of high-grade stenosis or plaque prone

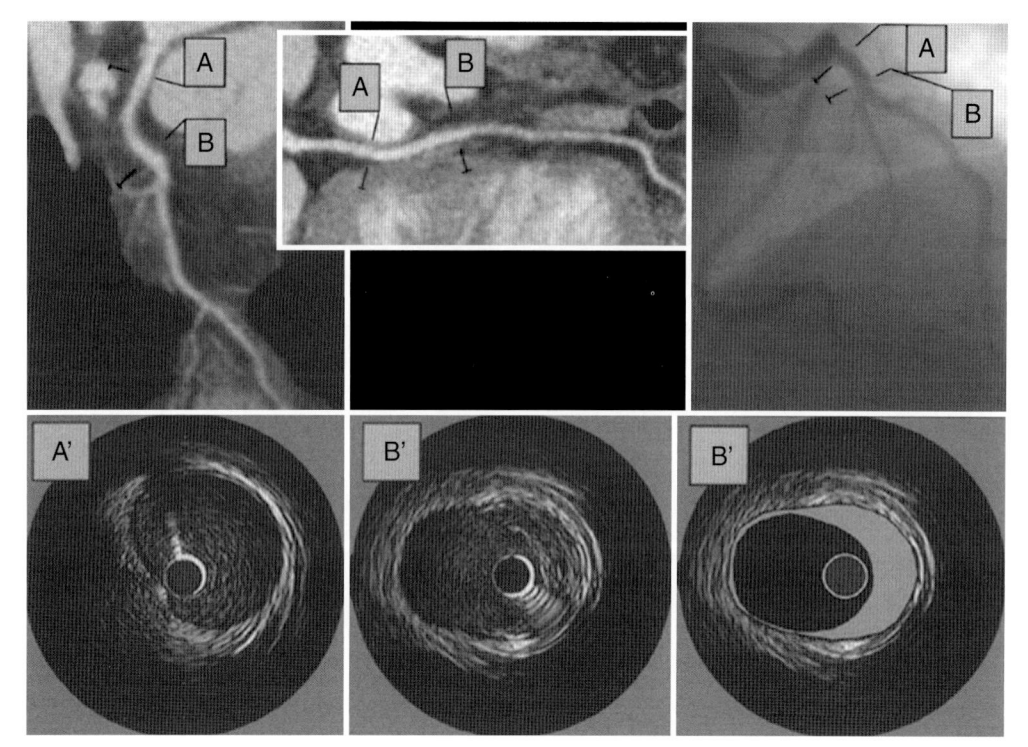

■ **FIGURE 4-6** Correlation of coronary CT angiography (*upper left*), selective coronary angiography (*upper right*), and intravascular ultrasound (*lower panel*). Caliber of the proximal left anterior descending artery on selective coronary angiography is normal at two locations (*A, B*) where CT and intravascular ultrasound show presence of noncalcified atherosclerotic plaque. (From Schoenhagen P, Tuzcu EM, Stillman AE, et al. Non-invasive assessment of plaque morphology and remodeling in mildly stenotic coronary segments: comparison of 16-slice computed tomography and intravascular ultrasound. Coron Artery Dis 2003; 14:459-462.)

to rupture. The relationship between coronary calcification and overall atherosclerotic burden provides the rationale for the practice of coronary artery calcium screening for risk stratification.[9]

The plaque core eventually becomes hypoxic as it outstrips the nutrient supply by the vascular network within the blood vessel wall, the vasa vasorum. Subsequent hypoxia-induced cellular death within the plaque core and recruitment of fragile, immature neovasculature predisposes to intraplaque hemorrhage. Necrosis of the plaque core and intraplaque hemorrhage are the key contributors to plaque growth at later stages and eventually to rupture of the "unstable" plaque. When the plaque ruptures, the exposed lipid-rich core triggers platelet aggregation and intravascular thrombosis.[10]

Plaque Rupture and Acute Coronary Syndromes

Counterintuitively, plaque rupture leading to acute cardiac events is more likely to occur in coronary segments with low-grade stenoses than in segments with high-grade coronary stenoses. An analysis of factors associated with progression of CAD in 2938 coronary segments in 298 patients who had not undergone coronary bypass from the Coronary Artery Surgery Study (CASS) showed that although individual segments with high-grade stenoses were more likely to become occluded than individual segments with low-grade stenoses, occlusion was overall much more likely to occur in segments with low-grade stenoses because low-grade stenoses are much more common.[11]

The acute interruption of coronary blood flow, typically by plaque rupture, without adequate compensatory mechanisms to maintain oxygen supply to the myocardium results in myocardial infarction, defined as myocyte necrosis. The diagnostic criteria for myocardial infarction include prolonged severe chest discomfort of acute onset; elevation of the ST segment on the ECG; and elevated blood concentrations of enzymes specific for myocyte demise, such as the MB-fraction of creatine kinase or the troponins.[12] Infarction occurs within minutes to hours from the inciting event. Because myocardial oxygen is supplied from the epicardial vessels toward the subendocardial perforators, the subendocardial myocardium is the layer affected first as the end-vessel territory. With prolonged severe ischemia, myocyte necrosis spreads transmurally from the endocardium toward the mesocardial and epicardial layers. The treatment of choice is revascularization by percutaneous coronary intervention within 4 to 6 hours of symptom onset if available. Intravenous administration of thrombolytic agents, such as recombinant tissue plasminogen activator (rTPA), is an acceptable alternative.[13]

Chronic Coronary Artery Disease

In the setting of chronic CAD with progressive narrowing of the coronary lumen but without sudden complete occlusion, the typical clinical feature is chronic stable angina. "Typical" angina is defined as retrosternal discomfort that is provoked by exertion and relieved by rest or administration of nitroglycerin. Episodes of typical angina last less than 30 minutes. It can be difficult to determine with anatomic imaging modalities such as coronary CT or MRI whether a stenosis caused by plaque is "significant"—severe enough to limit oxygen delivery and be the cause of angina or myocardial dysfunction (see later section on myocardial viability) or both. At rest, the myocardial oxygen extraction rate is approximately 60%.[14] An increase in oxygen consumption, such as occurs with physical activity, requires an increase in oxygen delivery, which is accomplished by vasodilation under normal circumstances. The ability of the coronary vasculature to increase coronary blood flow, expressed as the ratio of maximal coronary flow to resting flow, is referred to as *coronary flow reserve*.[15] In the presence of coronary stenosis, vasodilation to improve blood flow distal to the narrowed segment occurs at rest. This vasodilation decreases coronary flow reserve because the compensatory mechanism is already employed at baseline. The ability to elicit and document abnormal coronary flow reserve is the basic principle underlying stress testing as a functional means for assessing CAD.[16]

Although numerous studies have shown a correlation between percent stenosis and decrease in coronary flow reserve, the correlation is nonlinear. Functional severity of a given percent stenosis may vary among patients, depending on many factors, including coronary perfusion pressure, narrowest lumen diameter, and number and length of stenoses. Although it is generally accepted that stenoses greater than 70% reduce coronary flow reserve to a clinically relevant degree, the clinical "significance" of stenoses of intermediate severity (50% to 70%) can be difficult to ascertain. Qualitative or quantitative assessment of myocardial perfusion during stress and at rest using nuclear medicine techniques or MRI can provide information that is complementary to arterial illustration using conventional x-ray or CT angiography, and has important implications for patient management.[17,18]

When chronic ischemia occurs in the presence of a coronary stenosis, numerous compensatory mechanisms are activated in addition to chronic vasodilation. Among these is the development of collaterals from other coronary artery perfusion territories. The precise mechanism of collateral development is unclear, but probably involves recruitment and enlargement of existing coronary anastomoses and generation of new connections by neovascularization.

Myocardial infarction in the setting of chronic CAD with preexisting high-grade coronary stenoses can occur (1) as a consequence of plaque rupture, or (2) in situations where myocardial oxygen demand exceeds the oxygen supply that is limited by coronary stenosis, such as during unusual physical exertion or other physiologic stress, including high-risk surgery or severe systemic illness. The latter scenario often results in so-called non–ST segment elevation myocardial infarction.[19,20]

MYOCARDIAL DISEASE

Systolic myocardial dysfunction represents decreased ventricular contractility and decreased systolic ejection of ventricular blood into the systemic circulation, resulting from primary or secondary cardiomyopathy. The management of any form of secondary myopathy consists of treatment of the underlying condition (cardiovascular or other).

Ischemic Cardiomyopathy

The most prevalent and important form of secondary cardiomyopathy is ischemic in origin. The key imaging feature distinguishing primary from ischemic cardiomyopathy is the presence of global hypokinesis in the former and of regional wall motion abnormalities in the latter. The regionality of myocardial dysfunction in ischemic cardiomyopathy reflects the fact that coronary arteries are end arteries, each of which, with large variability, supplies a specific myocardial perfusion territory. Chronic severe, diffuse CAD can cause global left ventricular dysfunction, however, which is indistinguishable from primary cardiomyopathy by imaging of myocardial contractile function alone.

Information on the degree of left ventricular dysfunction is crucial for patient management. Poor left ventricular function predicts poor outcome. At an EF of less than 20%, the average 1-year survival is less than 50%. In these patients, ventricular dysrhythmia is at least as important a cause of death as is heart failure. Placement of implantable cardioverter defibrillators can improve survival, and is recommended for prevention of sudden cardiac death in patients with EF less than 30% to 40% and New York Heart Association (NYHA) class II-III heart failure or EF less than 30% to 35% and NYHA class I heart failure.[21]

Myocardial Viability, Stunning, and Hibernation

Assessing the status of the coronary arteries is a key step in the management of newly recognized left ventricular dysfunction. If CAD is present and believed to be the main cause of left ventricular dysfunction, it is important to establish whether coronary revascularization can improve the cardiomyopathy.

In chronic CAD, compensatory changes occur at the myocardial level, such as decreased oxygen demand and increased myocardial oxygen extraction, cell loss, and increased glycogen storage. With more severe chronic ischemia, hemodynamic and functional adaptations, including elevation of end-diastolic pressure, decreased stroke volume, and delayed myocardial contraction and relaxation, help cope further with reduced oxygen delivery. The net effect of these mechanisms representing "myocardial hibernation" decreased systolic function, which may be reversible if adequate oxygen supply is restored by revascularization.[22] Reversible myocardial dysfunction may also result from "stunning" in the setting of acute but transient ischemic events. Stunning may be the only consequence of an acute coronary syndrome or may coexist with irreversible myocyte damage.

The concept of viability imaging is important for decision making in these situations. If dysfunctional myocardium can be shown to have retained metabolic activity, or does not show evidence for fibrosis typical of repair of irreversible myocardial damage, improvement of systolic function after revascularization may reasonably be expected.

Pressure and Volume Overload

The response of the heart to increased work demand is hypertrophy—an increase in myocardial mass accomplished by enlargement of individual myocytes. Hypertrophy can represent a physiologic response to repetitive exercise, and probably plays a role in the normal enlargement of the heart through childhood and adolescence as well as in physiologic states such as pregnancy. The hypertrophic response can result in decompensated hypertrophy, however, in the setting of pressure or volume overload, or when it occurs as a compensatory mechanism after infarction of another coronary perfusion territory. The relationship between pressure and volume can be quite complex, and although the classification into pressure and volume overload is a useful conceptual construct, many patients have elements of both processes and may not fit neatly into one category or the other.[23]

Pressure overload (e.g., as seen in hypertension, left ventricular outflow obstruction, or aortic coarctation) causes increased systolic wall stress, stimulating concentric hypertrophy of the myocardium. Pressure overload causes not only myocyte hypertrophy, but also upregulation of extracellular matrix production, with the effect of increasing the thickness and the stiffness of the myocardium. These patients are prone to have diastolic dysfunction (see later).

A similar pattern is seen in genetically determined hypertrophic cardiomyopathies. These diseases, which are associated with a large variety of mutations in genes that encode for sarcomeric and nonsarcomeric proteins, are characterized phenotypically by myocyte hypertrophy and disarray, and extracellular fibrosis. Hypertrophic cardiomyopathy is one of the most frequent causes of death in young individuals, particularly young athletes. Death may result from the hemodynamic abnormalities in the left ventricular outflow tract or from ventricular arrhythmia, or both.

Volume overload, which may result from valvular disease or intracardiac or extracardiac shunting of blood, typically results in dilative, eccentric hypertrophy. There are also genetically determined primary forms of dilated cardiomyopathy that respond poorly to treatment other than pharmacologic management of heart failure or, eventually, may require heart transplantation. In pure dilated cardiomyopathies of all types, the common gross morphologic feature is a characteristic dilated, thin-walled chamber.

PHYSIOLOGY OF DIASTOLE

Diastolic dysfunction can result from myocardial or pericardial disease and results in diminished passive filling during early diastole and increased dependence of preload on atrial contraction in late diastole. Diastolic dysfunction is synonymous with "restrictive physiology." So-called "constrictive physiology" is a subform of restrictive physiology.

Diastolic dysfunction resulting from myocardial disease occurs in the setting of increased myocardial stiffness. Increased myocardial stiffness may be due to myocardial fibrosis at preserved left ventricular wall-to-cavity ratio or due to left ventricular hypertrophy. Left ventricular hypertrophy (see earlier) most often results from long-standing hypertension, but may also be due to infiltrative diseases such as amyloidosis or primary genetic disorders. Diastolic dysfunction is probably under-recognized in many settings. Although there is controversy about the clinical importance of diastolic dysfunction, its presence seems to increase mortality.[24]

PERICARDIAL DISEASE

The pericardium is a sac of fibrous tissue composed of visceral and parietal layers. It surrounds the heart and the proximal great vessels, and typically contains a physiologic small amount of fluid (Fig. 4-7). In normal patients, the pericardium does not play a significant role in cardiac physiology; patients with complete or partial congenital absence of the pericardium rarely have clinical signs or symptoms attributable to abnormal diastolic function.[25] The pericardium or its contents can impede normal diastolic and systolic function, however. The two principal manifestations of pericardial disease are tamponade and constriction.

Tamponade

Tamponade is a pathophysiologic state in which pericardial effusion alters the filling pressures of the heart.

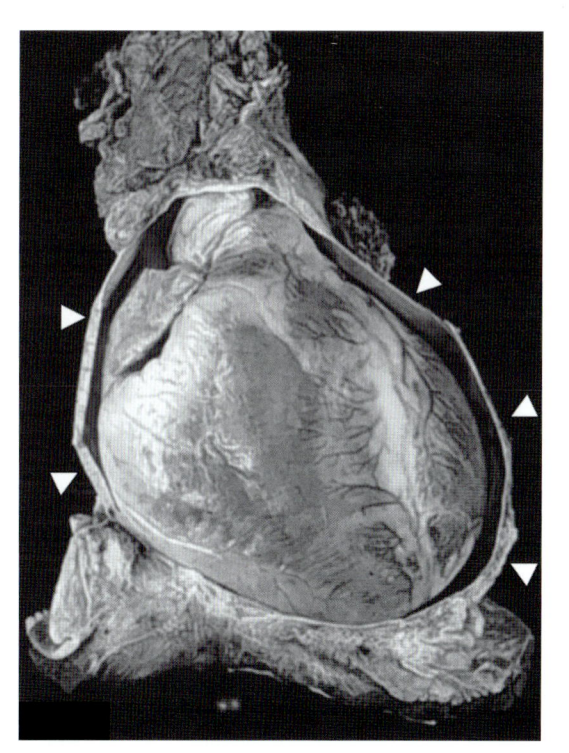

■ FIGURE 4-7 Autopsy specimen showing the location and anatomy of the pericardium (*arrowheads*) relative to the heart and the great vessels. (*From Breen JF. Imaging of the pericardium. J Thorac Imaging 2001; 16:47-54.*)

TABLE 4-1 Causes of Cardiac Tamponade and Constrictive Pericarditis

Causes of Cardiac Tamponade		Causes of Constrictive Pericarditis
Acute	**Chronic**	
Trauma	Heart failure	Postoperative
Iatrogenic	Uremia	Trauma
Infection	Metastasis	Radiation
Myocardial infarction with rupture	Infection	Infection (particularly tuberculosis)
	Radiation	

Because of its stiff fibrous makeup, the pericardium cannot accommodate rapid increases in pericardial fluid. Even with small but rapidly accumulating pericardial effusions, intrapericardial pressure may increase sufficiently to equal the pressures in the cardiac chambers, and any further increase in volume of pericardial fluid occurs at the expense of the chamber volumes. As a result of decreased chamber volumes and diastolic compliance, venous return is first shifted from systole and early diastole to systole only. Eventually, venous return may decrease sufficiently that the decrease in ventricular preload affects cardiac output and results in profound systemic hypotension, often resulting in exacerbated pulse weakening during inspiration (a phenomenon known as *pulsus paradoxus*). Pulsus paradoxus occurs because the increased venous return during inspiration expands the right ventricle at the expense of the left ventricle.

Acute cardiac tamponade is a medical emergency. The treatment of choice is emergent pericardiocentesis, preferably under echocardiographic guidance if available. Chronic tamponade can have numerous causes (Table 4-1). Because the pericardium can gradually expand to accommodate slowly growing effusions, however, the volume of pericardial effusion can be large (2 L), and is generally less important than the rate of increase for determining the physiologic consequences (Fig. 4-8). In this situation, removal of even small amounts of fluid can result in impressive improvement of diastolic filling and cardiac output.

Constrictive Pericarditis

Constrictive pericarditis results from pericardial scarring, which often has a nodular and calcified appearance on imaging (Fig. 4-9). Constrictive pericarditis can occur secondary to many causes, all of which functionally eliminate the pericardial space and "constrict" the volume of the heart (Table 4-2). In contrast to tamponade, early diastolic filling not only is unimpeded by pressure equalization, but also is even more rapid than usual. Mid-diastolic and late diastolic filling is decreased, however, when the volume of the heart approaches the fixed volume of the constricting pericardium.

As a feature distinguishing the physiologies of tamponade and constrictive pericarditis, systemic venous return does not increase during inspiration in the latter. Clinically, patients often present with findings of venous con-

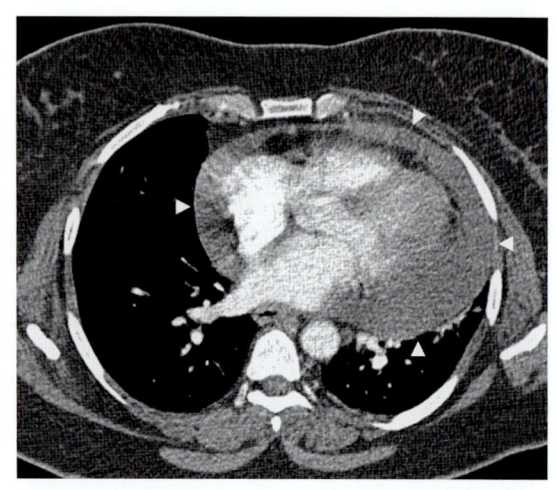

■ **FIGURE 4-8** Large effusion without tamponade. CT shows large pericardial effusion (*arrowheads*) in a patient who had undergone total thyroidectomy and had not received thyroid hormone replacement therapy. Despite the large size of the effusion, Doppler echocardiography showed no evidence of tamponade.

gestion and severe right heart failure, which can mimic hepatic failure. As might be expected, the clinical presentation is similar to restrictive cardiomyopathy. In contrast to restrictive cardiomyopathy, constrictive pericarditis can generally be treated successfully with a pericardial resection. It is important to distinguish constrictive from merely restrictive physiology when diastolic dysfunction is present. Imaging can be useful to confirm the presence of pericardial thickening or calcifications to support a diagnosis of pericardial constriction. The most compelling data for the clinician are determined by cardiac catheterization; specific patterns of the left ventricular pressure curve, equalization of diastolic pressure in all chambers, and greatly increased "ventricular interdependence" during respiration are features diagnostic of constrictive pericarditis.[26]

VALVULAR DYSFUNCTION

Dysfunction of the cardiac valves primarily manifests as insufficiency or stenosis. *Insufficiency,* also referred to as *regurgitation,* is characterized by insufficient valve closure, allowing inappropriate retrograde flow of blood through the AV valves during systole or the semilunar valves during diastole. *Stenosis* is characterized by inadequate valve opening, creating an obstacle to antegrade flow across the valve and increasing flow velocity through the valve orifice. Left-sided (mitral or aortic) valvular dysfunction is more common and more relevant to clinical practice than right-sided valvular dysfunction. The left-sided valvular abnormalities encountered most frequently are mitral insufficiency and aortic stenosis.[27]

Mitral Valve Disease

The principal causes of mitral insufficiency are abnormalities of the mitral valve (e.g., mitral valve prolapse) or the mitral valve annulus, defective tensor apparatus (papillary muscles and chordae), and altered left atrial or ventricular size or geometry (dilative or hypertrophic cardiomyopa-

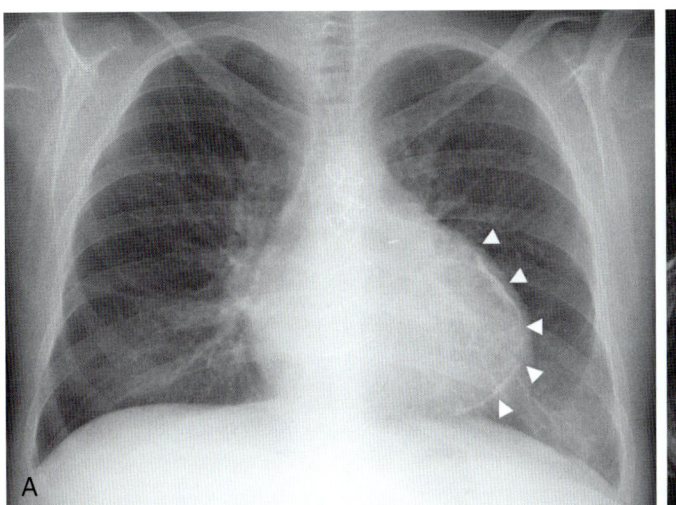

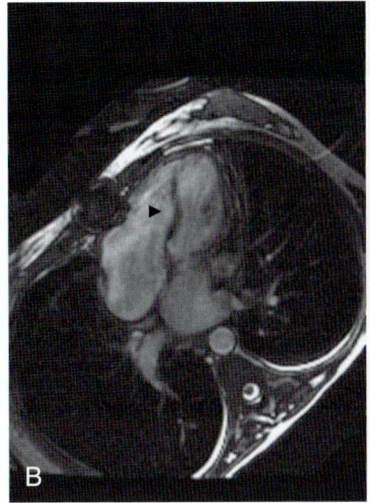

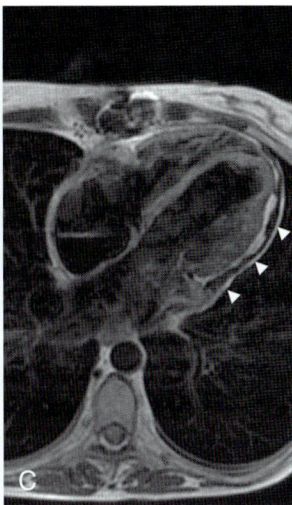

FIGURE 4-9 Constrictive pericarditis. **A,** Posteroanterior chest radiograph shows pericardial calcifications (*arrowheads*) in a patient with constrictive pericarditis after coronary artery bypass graft surgery. **B,** MRI horizontal long-axis steady-state free precession sequence shows bowing of the septum into the left ventricular cavity during diastole (*arrowhead*). **C,** Double inversion recovery fast spin-echo sequence shows nodular pericardial thickening, compatible with constrictive pericarditis (*arrowheads*).

thies). In addition, chronic elevation of end-systolic pressure from hypertension and obesity may contribute to mild, asymptomatic valvular regurgitation in many patients. Physical examination shows a systolic murmur, often holosystolic or preceded by a "mid-systolic click," depending on the mechanism of mitral insufficiency. Because of the chronic volume overload resulting from continuous back-and-forth flow of blood across the insufficient valve, the left atrium and left ventricle enlarge, and stroke volume and EF are supranormal. The treatment of choice is valve repair (where possible) or valve replacement. Optimal timing of surgery is when mitral regurgitation is "severe" (stage 4) while the patient is still asymptomatic.[28] Acute mitral regurgitation can occur as a complication of myocardial infarction, endocarditis, or trauma, and often causes severe hemodynamic instability and congestive heart failure. This group of patients requires aggressive management and early surgery.

Mitral stenosis is currently rare in the Western world. The principal cause is rheumatic fever. Dyspnea and exercise intolerance are initial symptoms. Classic findings on cardiac auscultation are an "opening snap" followed by a "diastolic rumble." Left atrial enlargement and atrial fibrillation are common. Pulmonary hypertension and right ventricular failure are irreversible late consequences of mitral stenosis. Timing of surgery depends on severity symptoms and the diastolic gradient across the mitral valve. In many scenarios, clinical guidelines now favor transcutaneous balloon valvotomy over surgical management.

Aortic Valve Disease

Aortic stenosis can be subvalvular (which is different from the dynamic outflow tract obstruction in hypertrophic cardiomyopathy), valvular, or supravalvular. The valvular form is most common, and the most common cause is senile degeneration. Rarer causes of aortic stenosis include congenitally bicuspid valve and rheumatic fever. Physical examination is remarkable for a systolic murmur, the characteristics of which vary and can provide important clues to distinguishing aortic stenosis from hypertrophic cardiomyopathy. The increased afterload leads to compensatory left ventricular hypertrophy (which serves to normalize wall stress.) Chamber size is typically normal until compensatory mechanisms are exhausted, and left ventricular dilation and dysfunction occur. The proximal aorta may show typical "poststenotic" dilation. The treatment of choice is valve replacement. Valve replacement is indicated for all patients with "critical" aortic stenosis (pressure gradient between left ventricular outflow tract and thoracic aorta >80 mm Hg or aortic valve area <0.7 cm^2). Traditionally, severe aortic stenosis (pressure gradient >40 mm Hg or aortic valve area <1 cm^2) was an indication only for patients symptomatic with dyspnea, chest pain, or syncope. More recent studies of the natural history of severe aortic stenosis suggest, however, that asymptomatic patients with severe aortic stenosis should also undergo valve replacement.[29]

Imaging Assessment of Valve Disease

Echocardiography is the mainstay of assessing heart valve disease noninvasively. Physiologic and hemodynamic

TABLE 4-2 Normal Ventricular Values

Normal Ventricular Pressures in Recumbent Adults:

	Right Ventricle	Left Ventricle
Diastole	0-8 mm Hg	5-12 mm Hg
Systole	15-28 mm Hg	90-120 mm Hg

Basic parameters of function:
Ejection fraction = (stroke volume/end diastolic volume)/end diastolic volume
Stroke volume = end diastolic volume − end systolic volume

Normal Values	Male	Female
Ejection fraction (%)	56-78	56-78
Stroke volume (mL)	51-133	33-97

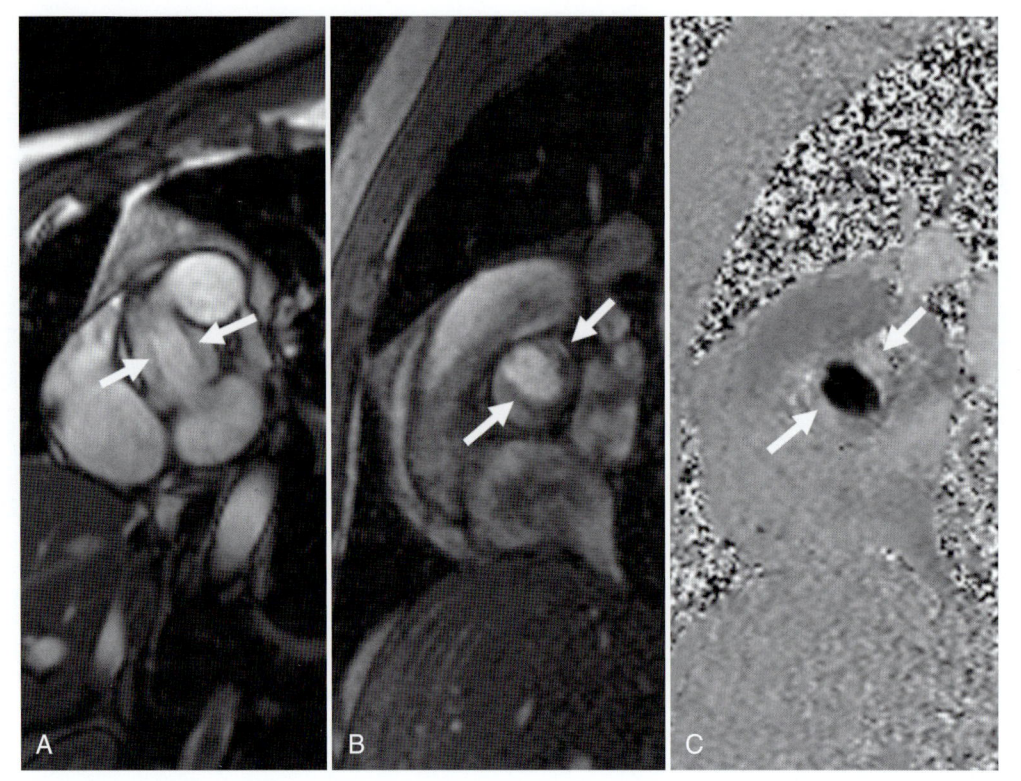

FIGURE 4-10 MRI of bicuspid aortic valve. **A-C,** Steady-state free precession (SSFP) images of the left ventricular outflow tract, perpendicular (**A**) and parallel (**B**) to the aortic valve plane, and phase contrast image parallel to the valve plane (**C**), showing the flow through a bicuspid aortic valve that appears like a "lens" or open "fish mouth." Note dephasing from the turbulent flow across the valve leaflets on the SSFP sequences and retrograde flow lateral to the valve leaflets on the phase contrast sequence (*arrows*).

measurements obtained by Doppler sonography are at least as important as visualization of the diseased valve or assessing heart chamber size. Invasive, catheter-based hemodynamic assessment of valvular disease is reserved for patients in whom symptoms and physical examination are inconsistent with echocardiographic findings, or if hemodynamic assessment can be combined with therapy (balloon valvulotomy for mitral stenosis).

Clinically, MRI is increasingly used to evaluate valvular function in various clinical scenarios.[30] These examinations classically are performed using phase-contrast sequences that allow quantification of flow (Fig. 4-10). Even in the absence of such dedicated sequences, many "bright blood" gradient-echo sequences show intravoxel dephasing from turbulent flow. These findings can provide important clues to valvular abnormalities on conventional MRI examinations, on which the valve leaflets themselves are often seen only partially or not at all (Fig. 4-11). Assessment of valvular disease by CT is currently not part of routine clinical practice.

CONCLUSION

To provide meaningful guidance to the clinician, the practitioner of cardiac imaging must have a basic understanding of the mechanisms underlying normal and abnormal perfusion of the body tissues. Effective delivery of oxygen and other metabolites to the body tissues requires coordination of electrical, chemical, and mechanical events that occur on the molecular, cellular, and ultrastructural tissue levels. The mechanisms underlying the coordinated atrial and ventricular contractions are complex, but the resulting pressure differentials cause orderly antegrade flow of blood through the cardiac chambers and valves.

CAD is one of the most important etiologies of left ventricular function manifesting as heart failure. Other clinically relevant hemodynamic disturbances that can affect the ability of the heart to supply metabolic substrates to the rest of the body may occur from primary abnormalities of the myocardial tissue, the cardiac valves, or the pericardium.

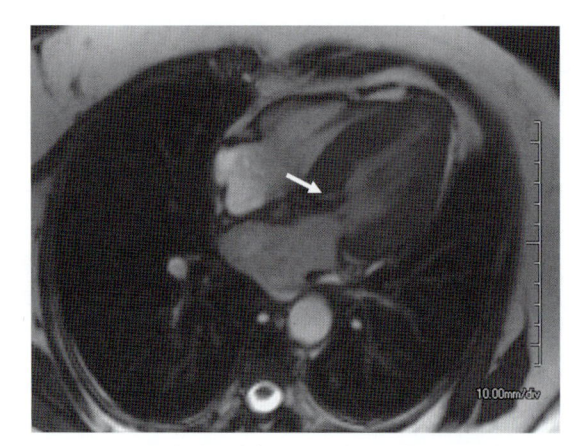

FIGURE 4-11 Patient with hypertrophic cardiomyopathy and systolic anterior motion of the anterior mitral valve leaflet on MRI, causing subaortic stenosis (*arrow*) on bright blood imaging.

KEY POINTS

- Cardiac physiology comprises a complex interplay of biochemical, electrical, and mechanical events that normally occur in orderly and sequential fashion.
- The fundamental physiologic principles of normal cardiac physiology include sequential generation and conduction of electrical impulses, efficient contraction of the myocardium, delivery of oxygen and nutrients to the myocardium through the coronary arteries, and antegrade propulsion of blood through the cardiac chambers, driven by changes in chamber pressures and geometry, and effective, timely opening and closing of the cardiac valves.
- When any of the fundamental functions of cardiovascular system performance fail to execute normally, characteristic clinical syndromes and physiologic patterns can occur.
- Imaging can be used to characterize or quantify the anatomic and physiologic features underlying normal and pathologic function of the cardiovascular system.
- Understanding normal and abnormal physiologic mechanisms of cardiovascular function is essential to understanding the principles of cardiac imaging and to interpreting clinical images.

SUGGESTED READINGS

Chatzizisis YS, Coskun AU, Jonas M, et al. Role of endothelial shear stress in the natural history of coronary atherosclerosis and vascular remodeling. J Am Coll Cardiol 2007; 49:2379-2393.

Fowler SJ, Narula J, Gurudevan SV. Review of noninvasive imaging for hypertrophic cardiac syndromes and restrictive physiology. Heart Fail Clin 2006; 2:215-230.

Gilkeson RC, Markowitz AH, Balgude A, et al. MDCT evaluation of aortic valvular disease. AJR Am J Roentgenol 2006; 186:350-360.

Glockner JF, Johnston DL, McGee KP. Evaluation of cardiac valvular disease with MR imaging: qualitative and quantitative techniques. RadioGraphics 2003; 23:e9.

Raggi P, Berman DS. Computed tomography coronary calcium screening and myocardial perfusion imaging. J Nucl Cardiol 2005; 12:96-103.

Vogel-Claussen J, Pannu H, Spevak PJ, et al. Cardiac valve assessment with MR imaging and 64-section multi-detector row CT. RadioGraphics 2006; 26:1769-1784.

Wang ZJ, Reddy GP, Gotway MB, et al. CT and MR imaging of pericardial disease. RadioGraphics 2003; 23:S167-S180.

REFERENCES

1. Rumberger JA, Behrenbeck T, Bell MR, et al. Determination of ventricular ejection fraction: a comparison of available imaging methods. The Cardiovascular Imaging Working Group. Mayo Clin Proc 1997; 72:860-870.
2. Hanft LM, Korte FS, McDonald KS. Cardiac function and modulation of sarcomeric function by length. Cardiovasc Res 2008; 77:627-636.
3. Kung HC, Hoyert DL, Xu J, et al. Deaths: final data for 2005. Natl Vital Stat Rep 2008; 56:1-120.
4. Chatzizisis YS, Coskun AU, Jonas M, et al. Role of endothelial shear stress in the natural history of coronary atherosclerosis and vascular remodeling: molecular, cellular, and vascular behavior. J Am Coll Cardiol 2007; 49:2379-2393.
5. Stary H. Natural history and histological classification of atherosclerotic lesions: an update. Arterioscler Thromb Vasc Biol 2000; 20:1177-1178.
6. Libby P. Inflammation in atherosclerosis. Nature 2002; 6917:868-874.
7. Schoenhagen P, Tuzcu EM, Stillman AE, et al. Non-invasive assessment of plaque morphology and remodeling in mildly stenotic coronary segments: comparison of 16-slice computed tomography and intravascular ultrasound. Coron Artery Dis 2003; 14:459-462.
8. Sangiorgi G, Rumberger JA, Severson A, et al. Arterial calcification and not lumen stenosis is highly correlated with atherosclerotic plaque burden in humans: a histologic study of 723 coronary artery segments using nondecalcifying methodology. J Am Coll Cardiol 1998; 31:126-133.
9. Rumberger JA, Sheedy PF, Breen JF, et al. Electron beam computed tomographic coronary calcium score cutpoints and severity of associated angiographic lumen stenosis. J Am Coll Cardiol 1997; 29:1542-1548.
10. Virmani R, Burke A, Farb A, et al. Pathology of the vulnerable plaque. J Am Coll Cardiol 2006; 47(8 Suppl):C13-C18.
11. Little WC, Constantinescu M, Applegate RJ, et al. Can coronary angiography predict the site of a subsequent myocardial infarction in patients with mild-to-moderate coronary artery disease? Circulation 1988; 78:1157-1166.
12. Thygesen K, Alpert JS, Ryden L, et al. Myocardial infarction redefined—a consensus document of the joint European Society of Cardiology/American College of Cardiology committee for the redefinition of myocardial infarction. J Am Coll Cardiol 2000; 36:959-969.
13. Antman EM, Anbe DT, Armstrong PW, et al; American College of Cardiology; American Heart Association; Canadian Cardiovascular Society. ACC/AHA guidelines for the management of patients with ST-elevation myocardial infarction—executive summary. A report of the American College of Cardiology/American Heart Association Task Force on Practice Guidelines (Writing Committee to revise the 1999 guidelines for the management of patients with acute myocardial infarction). J Am Coll Cardiol 2004; 44:671-719.
14. Porenta G, Cherry S, Czernin J, et al. Noninvasive determination of myocardial blood flow, oxygen consumption and efficiency in normal humans by carbon-11 acetate positron emission tomography imaging. Eur J Nucl Med 1999;26:1465.
15. Vassalli G, Hess OM. Measurement of coronary flow reserve and its role in patient care. Basic Res Cardiol 1998; 93:339.
16. Fraker TD Jr, Fihn SD; 2002 Chronic Stable Angina Writing Committee; American College of Cardiology; American Heart Association: 2007 chronic angina focused update of the ACC/AHA 2002 guidelines for the management of patients with chronic stable angina: a report of the American College of Cardiology/American Heart Association Task Force on Practice Guidelines Writing Group to develop the focused update of the 2002 guidelines for the management of patients with chronic stable angina. J Am Coll Cardiol 2007; 50:2264-2274.
17. Beanlands RS, Muzik O, Melon P, et al. Noninvasive quantification of regional myocardial flow reserve in patients with coronary atherosclerosis using nitrogen-13 ammonia positron emission tomography: determination of extent of altered vascular reactivity. J Am Coll Cardiol 1995; 26:1465-1475.

18. DiCarli M, Czernin J, Hoh CK, et al. Relation among stenosis severity, myocardial blood flow, and flow reserve in patients with CAD. Circulation 1995; 91:1944-1951.
19. Braunwald E, Antman EM, Beasley JW, et al. ACC/AHA guidelines for the management of patients with unstable angina and non-ST-segment elevation myocardial infarction. A report of the American College of Cardiology/American Heart Association Task Force on Practice Guidelines (Committee on the Management of Patients with Unstable Angina) [published correction appears in J Am Coll Cardiol 2001; 38:294-295]. J Am Coll Cardiol 2000; 36:970-1062.
20. Braunwald E, Antman EM, Beasley JW, et al. ACC/AHA guideline update for the management of patients with unstable angina and non-ST-segment elevation myocardial infarction—2002: summary article. A report of the American College of Cardiology/American Heart Association Task Force on Practice Guidelines (Committee on the Management of Patients with Unstable Angina). Circulation 2002; 106:1893-1900.
21. Zipes DP, Camm AJ, Borggrefe M, et al. ACC/AHA/ESC 2006 guidelines for management of patients with ventricular arrhythmias and the prevention of sudden cardiac death—executive summary. A report of the American College of Cardiology/American Heart Association Task Force and the European Society of Cardiology Committee for Practice Guidelines (Writing Committee to develop guidelines for management of patients with ventricular arrhythmias and the prevention of sudden cardiac death). J Am Coll Cardiol 2006; 48:1064-1108.
22. Camici PG, Prasad SK, Rimoldi OE. Stunning, hibernation, and assessment of myocardial viability. Circulation 2008; 117:103-114.
23. Burkhoff D, Mirsky I, Suga H. Assessment of systolic and diastolic ventricular properties via pressure-volume analysis: a guide for clinical, translational, and basic researchers. Am J Physiol Heart Circ Physiol 2005; 289:501-512.
24. Redfield MM, Jacobsen SJ, Burnett JC Jr, et al. Burden of systolic and diastolic ventricular dysfunction in the community appreciating the scope of the heart failure epidemic. JAMA 2003; 289:194-202.
25. Gatzoulis MA, Munk MD, Merchant N, et al. Isolated congenital absence of the pericardium: clinical presentation, diagnosis, and management. Ann Thorac Surg 2000; 69:1209-1215.
26. Talreja DR, Nishimura RA, Oh JK, et al. Constrictive pericarditis in the modern era. J Am Coll Cardiol 2008; 51:315-319.
27. Supino PG, Borer JS, Preibisz J, et al. The epidemiology of valvular heart disease: a growing public health problem. Heart Fail Clin 2006; 2:379-393.
28. Calvinho P, Antunes M. Current surgical management of mitral regurgitation. Expert Rev Cardiovasc Ther 2008; 6:481-490.
29. Brown ML, Pellikka PA, Schaff HV, et al. The benefits of early valve replacement in asymptomatic patients with severe aortic stenosis. J Thorac Cardiovasc Surg 2008; 135:308-315.
30. Stork A, Franzen O, Ruschewski H, et al. Assessment of functional anatomy of the mitral valve in patients with mitral regurgitation with cine magnetic resonance imaging: comparison with transesophageal echocardiography and surgical results. Eur Radiol 2007; 12:3189-3198.

PART
TWO

Cardiac Imaging Techniques

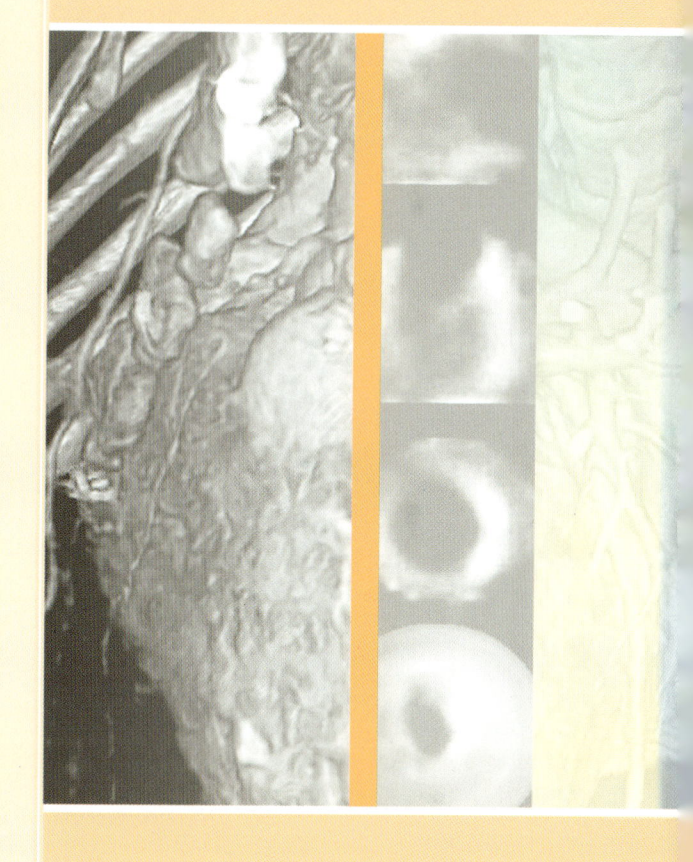

CHAPTER 5

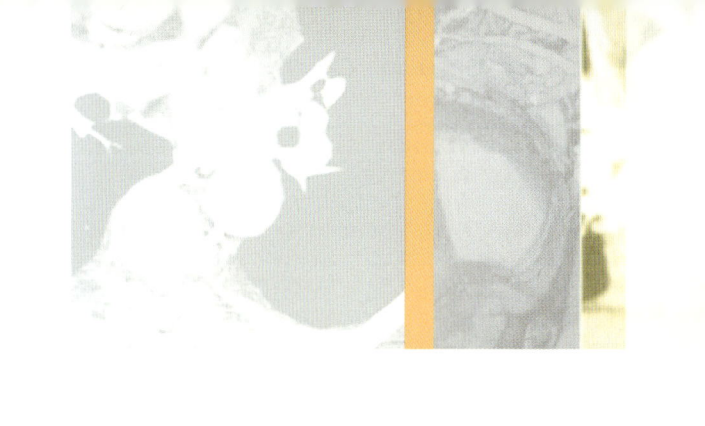

Radiology of the Heart: Plain Film Imaging and Diagnosis

Robert M. Steiner

INTRODUCTION

Imaging of the heart and the great vessels with plain film radiography dates to the earliest days of radiology. Since that time, more advanced technologies including fluoroscopy, kymography, and more recently nuclear imaging, echocardiography (ECHO), computed tomography (CT) and magnetic resonance (MRI) have revolutionized cardiac imaging.

All of these newer modalities yield anatomically detailed images of the heart and great vessels not possible with plain film radiography alone. However, the chest radiograph continues to provide valuable and often unique information concerning the structure and function of the cardiovascular system. The chest radiograph presents an opportunity to recognize subtle and/or overlooked abnormalities such as cardiac chamber enlargement, clinically important calcifications, and evidence of right and left heart dysfunction. Because the pulmonary arteries and veins are visualized in exquisite detail on a well-performed posterior-anterior (PA) and lateral chest radiograph, over and under pulmonary circulation as well as the findings of pulmonary arterial and venous hypertension can be appreciated. Adult onset congenital heart disease, often misdiagnosed or overlooked clinically, can often be identified on a plain film chest radiograph.[1,2]

The portable chest radiograph, usually performed in the anterior-posterior (AP) supine or erect position is the imaging modality of choice for the evaluation and monitoring of patients with cardiopulmonary disease in the intensive care unit (ICU) including postoperative cardiac patients and in those with implanted cardiovascular devices.[3,4]

In this chapter, the role of plain film chest imaging including alterations of cardiovascular anatomy in a variety of disorders is discussed.

NORMAL AND ABNORMAL CARDIAC BORDERS

Chest Radiograph

The chest radiograph has the advantage of allowing predictable and precise definition of the air-filled lung and soft tissues, thereby permitting the pulmonary arteries, veins, and fissures to be clearly visualized. For this reason, the PA chest film is the ideal screening examination for the evaluation of the vascular structures, the pulmonary parenchyma, and the pleural surfaces. The heart and other mediastinal structures appear as a sharply delineated but featureless opaque silhouette. The coronary arteries, great vessels, cardiac valves and other mediastinal structures cannot be separately identified because they have similar attenuation characteristics as the remainder of the mediastinum. The goal for the image interpreter is to appreciate the normal and abnormal patterns of the cardiac silhouette in a variety of normal and abnormal states. A significant depth of training and experience is needed to recognize the range of patterns of the cardiac silhouette in both normal and abnormal patients and to use that information to establish a clinical diagnosis or suggest additional studies needed to further clarify the findings appreciated on the plain film radiograph.

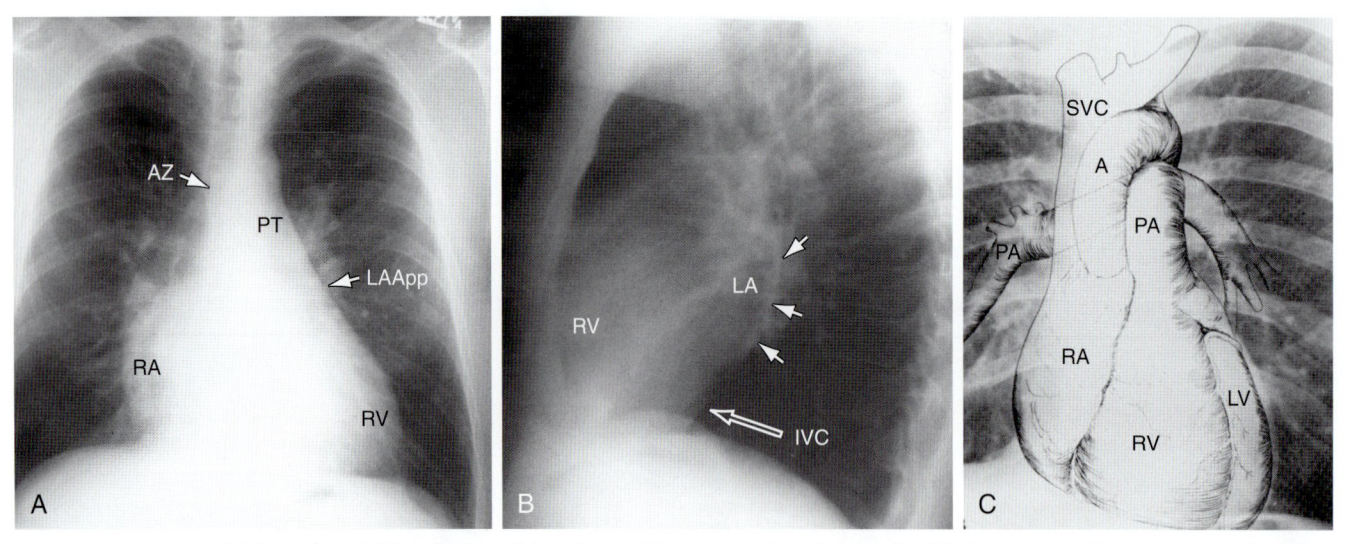

FIGURE 5-1 Frontal (**A**) and lateral (**B**) projection of the left and right heart borders. Line drawing (**C**) demonstrates the anatomic relationships of the cardiac chambers. *(From Van Houten FX, Adams DF, Abrams HL: Radiology of valvular heart disease. In Sonnenblick E, Lesch M [eds]: Valvular Heart Disease. New York, Grune & Stratton, 1974.)*

It is important also to appreciate that an abnormal cardiac border may be due to a nonvascular abnormality such as a pericardial cyst, thymoma or lymphoma, or other solid or cystic masses that may alter the cardiac border. A systematic approach to identify the anatomic landmarks of the heart borders is essential to avoid missing an important, but often subtle, abnormality of the cardiac configuration.

In a well-positioned PA or frontal chest radiograph, the cardiac silhouette and other vascular structures are predictably outlined against the lung as a series of bulges and indentations along the right and left mediastinal borders (Fig. 5-1).

Left Mediastinal Border

In the normal patient, the most superior border-forming structure along the left side of the mediastinum is the left subclavian artery (LSCA). Positioned just above the aortic arch and below the left clavicle, it usually forms a concave border with the lung and lies medial to the aortic arch (see Fig. 5-1). When blood flow through the LSCA is increased, as in a postductal coarctation of the aorta, or when the vessel is tortuous because of atherosclerosis, it will lie at or lateral to the aortic knob or arch—an important clue to the diagnosis of disease. A vertical, straight, or convex, double shadow parallel to the LSCA border is found when a left superior vena cava is present (Fig. 5-2). A cervical aortic arch or the elongated aortic arch of a pseudocoarctation of the aorta may also obscure the normal LSCA border.

Aortic Arch

The aortic arch or "knob" forms a convex segment along the left mediastinal border below the LSCA border and above the main pulmonary artery border. The aortic convexity is the distal posterior portion of the arch measuring 2.0 ± 1 cm in the young adult and 2.5 to 3.5 cm in the normal middle-aged individual. A clue to the location of the medial border of the aortic arch is the right-sided displacement of the tracheal airway at the same level as the arch. Although the aortic arch border usually has smooth margins, a rounded 2 to 3 mm extension or "nipple" may be present. This structure, seen in up to 10% of normal individuals, is the left superior intercostal vein (LSIV) (Fig. 5-3). An enlarged LSIV will suggest obstruction to blood flow in the deep mediastinal venous system such as superior vena caval obstruction. A dilated LSIV is similar in significance to a dilated azygos vein.

The left side of the descending thoracic aorta forms a clearly visualized interface with the left lung behind the left heart border on a well-penetrated frontal chest film (see Fig. 5-4). Pleural effusion and pulmonary masses, left lower lobe pneumonia, and other soft tissue opacities may obliterate the descending aortic border.

The aortic border enlarges in older patients due to a variety of abnormalities such as aortic regurgitation, systemic hypertension, aneurysm, or atherosclerosis. The ascending aorta along the right mediastinal border will also widen and the brachiocephalic arteries may become tortuous and dilate—mimicking a substernal thyroid or other superior mediastinal mass. An aberrant right subclavian artery will also widen the superior right mediastinal border. These right upper mediastinal conditions may require CT scan or MRI for a specific diagnosis.

When the aortic arch border on the left side of the mediastinum is not visible and when the trachea is displaced to the left, the presence of an aortic arch on the right side of the mediastinum will suggest the diagnosis of right aortic arch (RAA) (Fig. 5-4). It is associated in most cases with an aberrant left subclavian artery; however, RAA may occur without an associated aberrant subclavian artery in mirror image RAA with or without associated cyanotic heart disease.

Below the aortic arch segment of the left heart border and above the main pulmonary artery border is a variable-sized concavity or indentation termed the *aorticopulmonary window*. This anatomic landmark is associated with

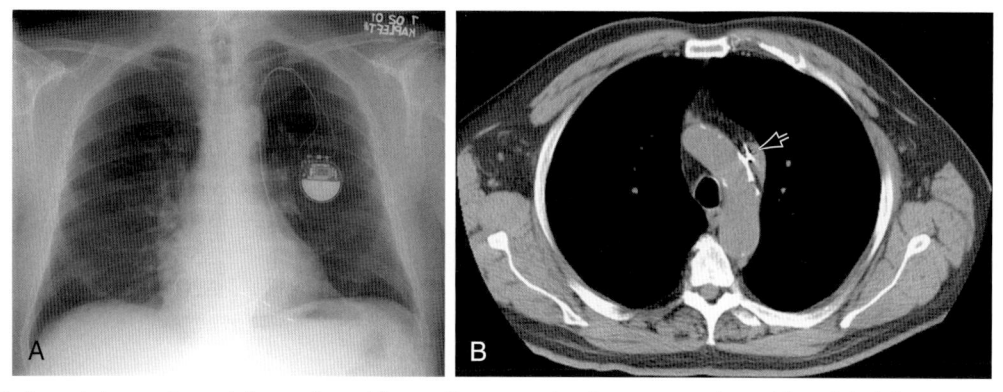

FIGURE 5-2 **A,** Frontal chest radiograph in a patient with a cardiac pacemaker demonstrates the position of the left superior vena cava (LSVC) extending from a position above the aortic arch downward across the medial portion of the left hilum to the region of the coronary sinus. **B,** Axial nonenhanced thoracic CT shows the pacemaker wire in the LSVC, which lies adjacent to the aortic arch (*arrow*).

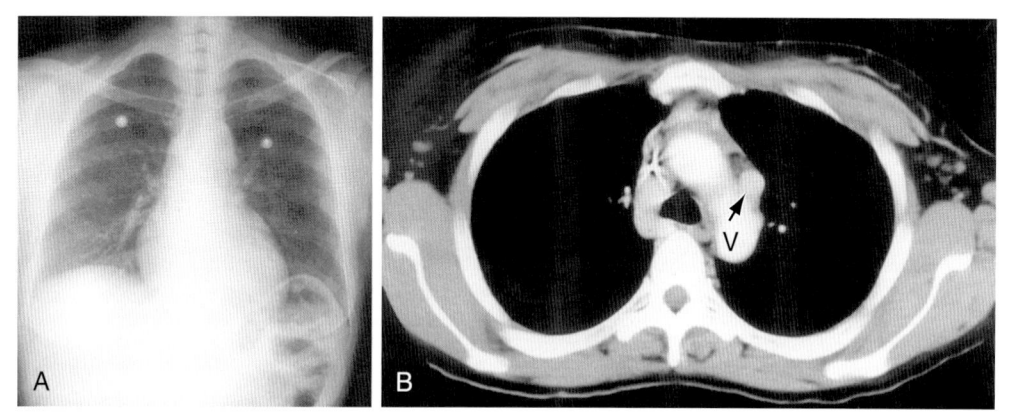

FIGURE 5-3 **A,** small convex bulge or "nipple" is visible along the aortic arch border representing the left superior intercostal vein. This normal anatomic structure is usually 2 to 3 mm in diameter but will enlarge because of increased blood flow secondary to SVC or other deep venous obstruction in the mediastinum. **B,** Contrast-enhanced CT shows the anatomic relationship of the left superior intercostal vein (V) to the aortic arch (**A**). *(From Steiner RM. Radiology of the heart and great vessels. In Braunwald E, Zipes PD, Libby P [eds]. Heart Disease: A Textbook of Cardiovascular Medicine, 6th ed. Philadelphia, Saunders, 2001.)*

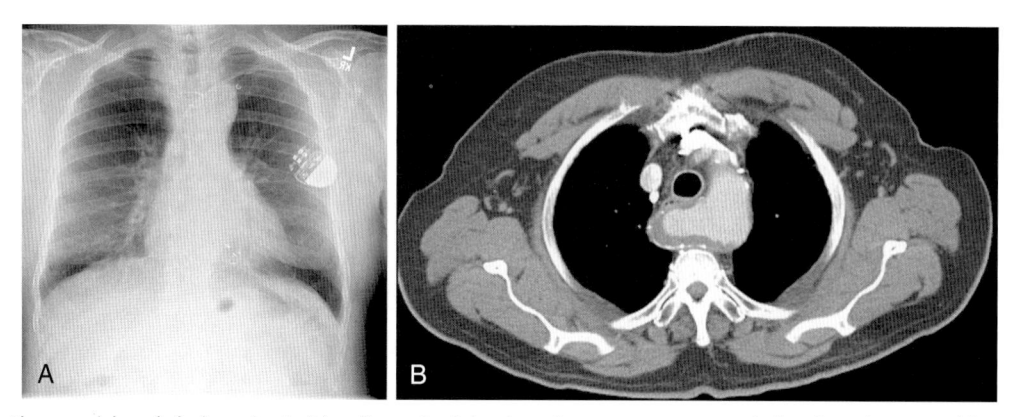

FIGURE 5-4 Aberrant right subclavian vein. **A,** PA radiograph of the chest demonstrates a convex bulge along the upper right mediastinal border due to an aneurysmal aberrant right subclavian artery. **B,** Contrast-enhanced axial CT image demonstrates a partially thrombosed dilated aberrant artery corresponding to the convex bulge on the chest radiograph.

several important structures including the recurrent laryngeal nerve, the ligamentum arteriosum or ductus arteriosus, and the ductus node which drains the lymphatics of the left lung. A convex bulge instead of a concave indentation will suggest important pathology such as an enlarged ductus node due to neoplasm or an inflammatory disorder such as tuberculosis or sarcoidosis. A ductus diverticulum can also create a distinct bulge in the aorticopulmonary window. Left vocal cord paralysis may occur as a result of pressure on the left recurrent laryngeal nerve from intrusion into this confined space from any of these pathologic entities.

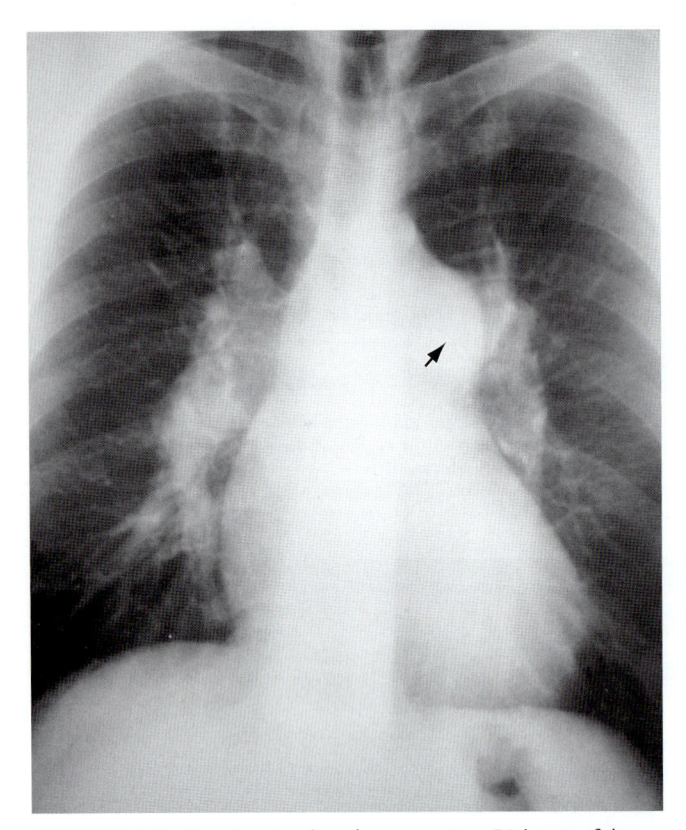

■ **FIGURE 5-5** Prominent main pulmonary artery. PA image of the chest in a 58-year-old man shows a large main pulmonary artery (*arrow*). The heart is enlarged and the peripheral pulmonary vessels are engorged in this patient with ASD and pulmonary hypertension.

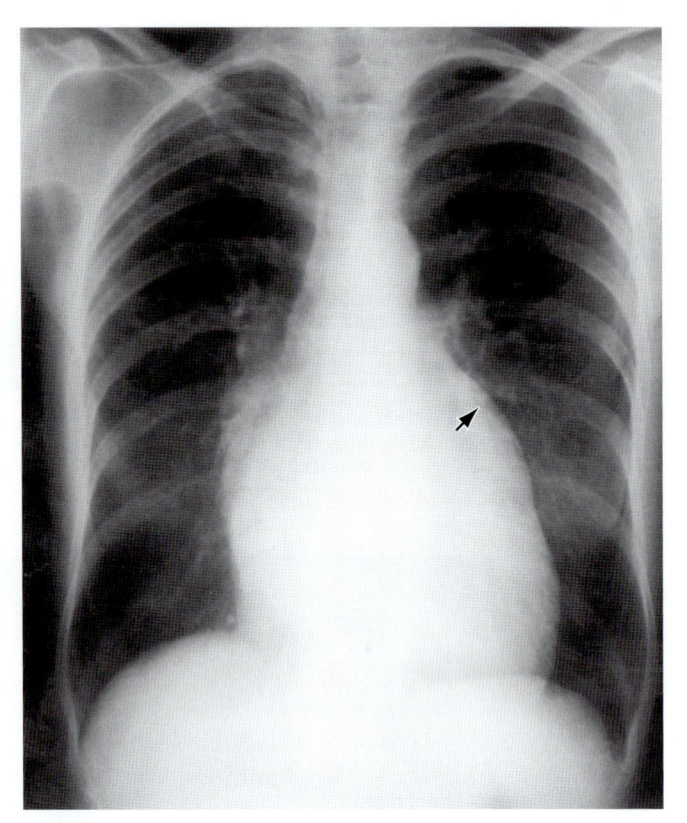

■ **FIGURE 5-6** Prominent left atrial appendage. A patient with mitral stenosis. The left atrial appendage border is convex due to enlargement of the appendage secondary to increased pressure and weakening due to rheumatic carditis (*arrow*).

Main Pulmonary Artery Border (see Fig. 5-1)

The normally convex main left pulmonary artery (LPA) is situated immediately below the aorticopulmonary window and extends posteriorly as it arches over the left bronchus. It will enlarge because of increased pulmonary blood flow due to a left-to-right shunt, increased pulmonary pressure in patients with obliterative lung disease or Eisenmenger physiology, pulmonary valve stenosis, or weakness of the pulmonary arterial wall in an arteritis (Fig. 5-5). The main pulmonary artery (MPA) and LPA will bulge to the left and the pulmonary artery branches will converge at the lateral border of the enlarged vessel. Alternatively, if the pulmonary artery border is flat or concave, the MPA may be absent or stenotic when truncus arteriosus, tetralogy of Fallot, pulmonary atresia, or transposition of the great vessels is present.

Left Atrial Border (LAA)

The LAA lies below the left main-stem bronchus in the frontal projection and is border forming with the lung. The LAA forms a smooth and slightly concave portion of the left heart border (see Fig. 5-1). Atrial enlargement should be suspected when the LAA is convex and prominent (Fig. 5-6) but the LA may enlarge significantly, even when the LAA remains small, so that enlargement of the LA may be suspected by other signs of enlargement including a double right atrial-left atrial border on the right side of the mediastinum, elevation and widening of the carinal angle, and a prominent LA bulge on the lateral projection. Nonvascular pathology may simulate enlargement of the left atrial appendage. For example, a pericardial cyst, lymphoma, thymoma, or other mediastinal or pleural neoplasms may appear as a convexity of the left atrial border (Fig. 5-7). Bulging of the LAA border may also be caused by partial absence of the pericardium.

Left Ventricular Border (LV)

The left ventricular border continues downward seamlessly from the left atrial border. The LV is usually mildly convex in relation to the nearby lung. When the LV is hypertrophic as a result of aortic stenosis or hypertrophic obstructive cardiomyopathy, it may be round and slightly enlarged. When the left ventricle is dilated, as may occur with aortic regurgitation or other causes of decompensation, the apex is displaced downward and laterally (Fig. 5-8). An enlarged right ventricle (RV) may displace the LV border downward, thereby simulating LV dilation or aneurysm.

When the LV dilates because of volume overload as in patients with mitral regurgitation, the dimensions of the LV chamber increase markedly, assuming a globular or water flask appearance similar to a large pericardial effusion. The LV border may extend to the left and can reach the lateral ribs in massive LV dilation. As the LV enlarges, the LA border is obscured. In such circumstances, the left anterior oblique (LAO) projection is helpful to separate

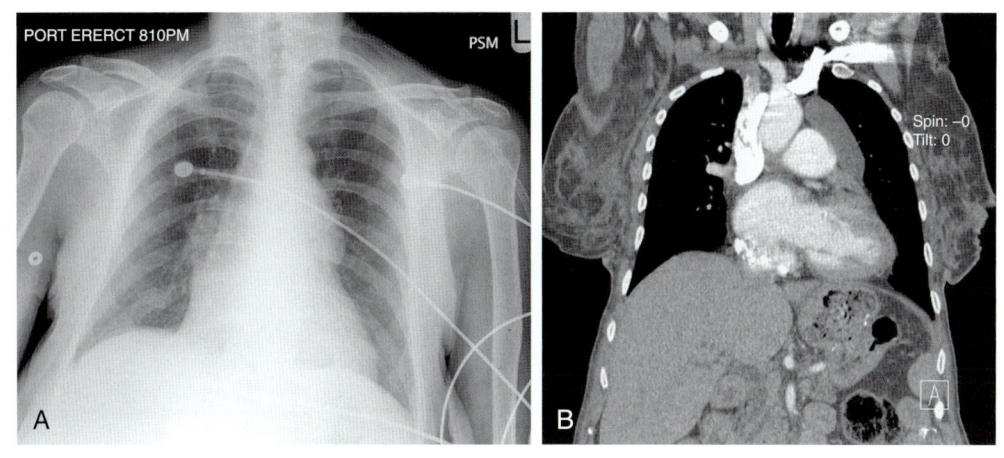

■ **FIGURE 5-7** Pericardial cyst. **A,** A portable erect image demonstrates an abnormal left mediastinal border characterized by a convex opacity extending from the aorticopulmonary window to the area of the left atrial appendage. **B,** A coronal reformatted contrast-enhanced CT image shows the nonenhanced water density structure that conforms to the abnormal left mediastinal border visualized on plain film. The diagnosis of pericardial cyst was entertained.

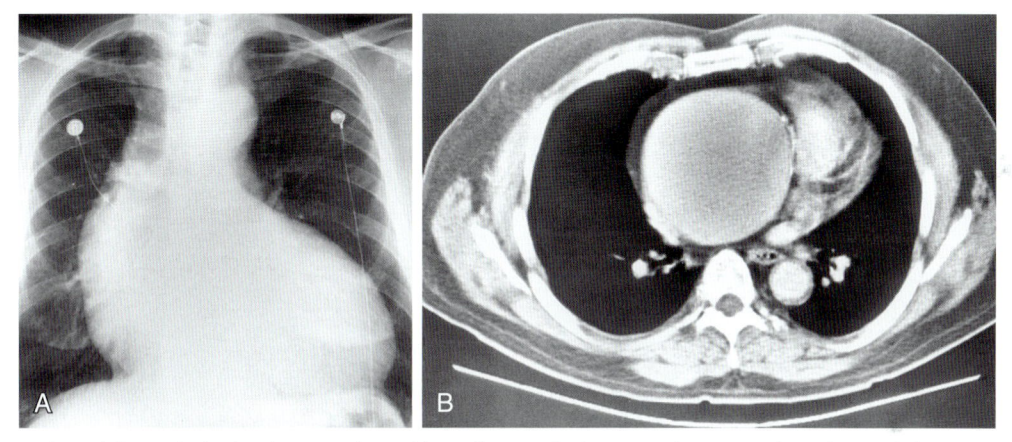

■ **FIGURE 5-8** Prominent left ventricular border. **A,** Patient with aortic regurgitation secondary to annuloaortic ectasia in a patient with Marfan syndrome. **B,** CT shows the massive enlargement of the ascending aorta due to the breakdown of the walls of the vessel.

the two chambers so that their relative sizes can be discerned (Fig. 5-9). Separating the left heart chambers assumes importance when the differential diagnosis lies between ischemic cardiomyopathy (in which case the left ventricle is larger than the left atrium) and mitral regurgitation (in which case the left atrium may be larger than the left ventricle).

Right Mediastinal Border

The right atrial (RA) border is convex in its relationship to the medial segment of the right middle lobe. In the frontal projection, the superior vena cava (SVC) border above the RA is usually straight, and in a good inspiratory film, it can be clearly separated from the RA. The outline of the LA may be visible deep to the RA border as an additional convex shadow and the confluence of the right pulmonary veins directed toward the mid-point of the LA border may also be appreciated. In a well-penetrated film, the LA is also clearly visualized deep to the RA border because of intrusion of lung between the anterior portion of the LA and the more posterior border of the RA. If the LA is markedly enlarged, its border may actually be lateral to the RA. The borders of the right and left atria can be differentiated because the inferior border of the RA blends with the inferior vena cava, whereas the LA crosses the mid-line toward the left side of the heart (Fig. 5-10) The upper right atrial convexity blends superiorly with the SVC, which forms a straight interface with the adjacent lung as it continues into the neck. The RA is considered enlarged when it bulges more than 5.5 cm to the right of the mid-line.

Right Ventricular Border (RV)

Unlike the RA, the RV is usually not border forming in the frontal projection and cannot be directly visualized. However, as the RV dilates, the LV is displaced posteriorly and to the left and the RA is displaced to the right, which causes widening of the cardiac shadow. In cardiac anomalies such as tetralogy of Fallot, the enlarged RV displaces the LV laterally and superiorly, thereby creating a high, round LV border.

Ascending Aortic Border

The ascending aorta is superimposed on the superior vena cava and forms a convex border with the lung above the

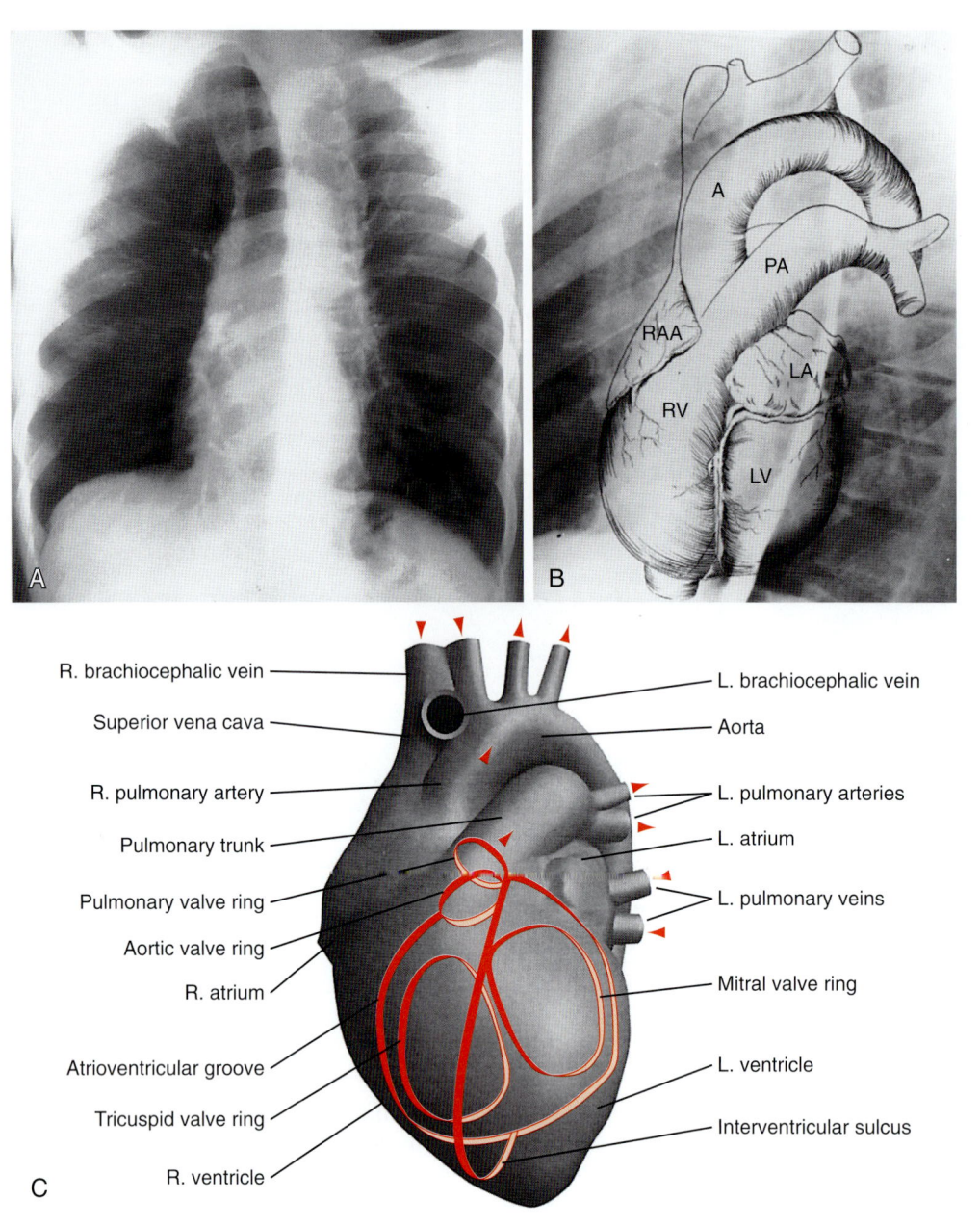

■ **FIGURE 5-9** Left anterior oblique projection. **A,** A frontal chest radiograph in a 60-degree LAO projection. **B,** Superimposed drawing of the ventricular chambers and vessels. **C,** A computer-generated diagram in the LAO projection highlights the valve rings, the atrioventricular groove, and the anatomic relationship of the ventricular chambers. *(From Steiner RM: Radiology of the heart and great vessels. In Braunwald E, Zipes PD, Libby P [eds]. Heart Disease: A Textbook of Cardiovascular Medicine, 6th ed. Philadelphia, Saunders 2001.)*

right atrium. The aortic valve and annulus and the coronary arteries are not visible on plain films, unless they are calcified, because they lie deep to the edge of the mediastinum and their x-ray attenuation characteristics are similar to those of the rest of the heart. These structures and their anatomic relationships with the remainder of the mediastinum are best appreciated by cross-sectional imaging such as CT and MRI.

Azygos Vein

The azygos vein forms an elliptical or teardrop structure at the right tracheobronchial angle (see Fig. 5-1A). It ascends in the right paravertebral sulcus and arches forward over the right mainstem bronchus to enter the back of the SVC. The azygos vein and its left-sided equivalent, the hemiazygos vein, receive intercostal veins and act as an important collateral pathway when the deep mediastinal veins are obstructed. Normally measuring 0.7 ± 0.3 cm across in the erect and 1.0 ± 0.3 cm in the supine position, the azygos vein is a good indicator of changing cardiovascular dynamics. It is enlarged in SVC and IVC obstruction, in the absence of the intrahepatic portion of the inferior vena cava, in portal vein obstruction, and in both left- and right-sided cardiac failure. A change in diameter of the azygos vein from film to film will parallel changes in pulmonary venous pressure, which makes it a useful guide to the development of congestive heart failure on plain film radiographs. An azygos fissure can be found in 3% of the population. When an azygos fissure is present,

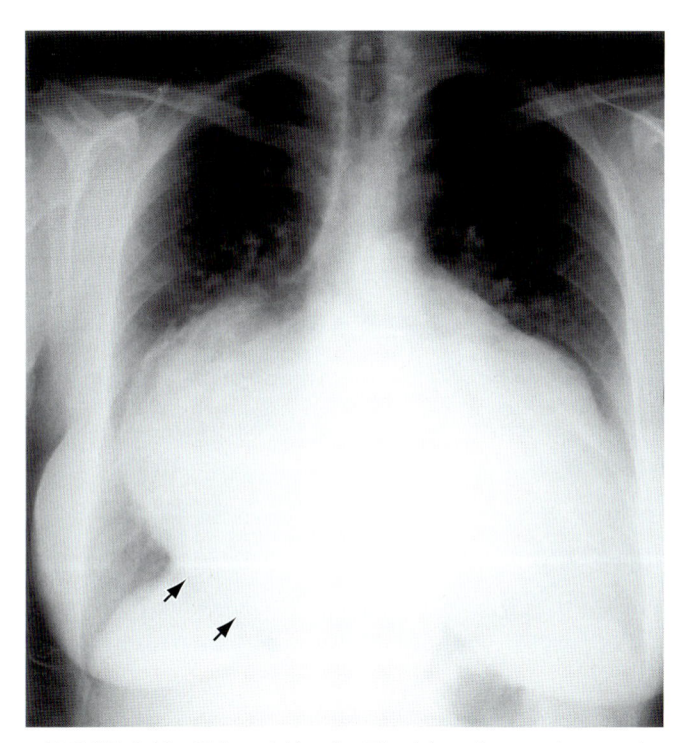

FIGURE 5-10 Right atrial border. The right atrium continues to the inferior vena cava; the inferior margin of the left atrium indents away from the right heart border as it passes to the left side of the heart. In this patient with mitral stenosis both the left atrium and the right atrium are prominent.

the azygos vein is displaced laterally and superiorly and will dilate under the same conditions as a normally positioned azygos vein.

Lateral View of the Thorax

Proper positioning of the patient in the lateral projection is critical for accurate identification of cardiac structures.[5] The need for accurate positioning in the lateral projection is exemplified by the RA. The normal RA is not border forming in this projection, but if the patient is rotated backward, the RA will form part of the lower posterior cardiac border and simulate enlargement. The RV is the border-forming structure in the subxiphoid region and usually extends superiorly about one third the distance between the diaphragm and the suprasternal notch (Fig. 5-11). As the RV enlarges, it encroaches farther into the retrosternal space or lucency. The relationship between the size of the RV and the degree of retrosternal encroachment is affected by the patient's body habitus and lung volume. For example, in a patient with emphysema, right ventricular enlargement may coexist with an expanded retrosternal space.

The anterior margins of the main pulmonary artery and the ascending aorta lie above the RV in the lateral projection; however, because they are adjacent to a broad retrosternal mediastinal fat plane, neither structure is visualized clearly in the lateral projection in the normal patient. In those individuals with severe emphysema, the increased retrosternal lung volume permits the MPA and the ascending aorta to be well outlined. The ascending aorta is usually well defined in normal patients, except where the superior vena cava crosses the aorta and where the brachiocephalic arteries enter the aorta in front of the tracheal airway. The inferior margin of the posterior aortic arch is often visible because of intrusion of lung into the aorticopulmonary window. The semilunar lucency of the aorticopulmonary window also outlines the superior margin of the LPA. The descending aorta is not usually discernible in the normal individual because it lies adjacent to the spine and the posterior mediastinal fat. However, in patients with hyperaeration or in those with a tortuous or calcified aorta, the descending aorta may be well-delineated.

Left Atrial Border in the Lateral Projection

The normal LA forms a shallow convex bulge along the upper aspect of the posterior border of the heart on the lateral view. It may be easily identified because the posterior border of the left atrium lies immediately anterior to the pulmonary venous confluence (see Fig. 5-11).

Left Ventricle in the Lateral Projection

In the lateral projection, the normal LV forms a long convexity along the posteroinferior heart border just above the diaphragm. LV enlargement is suggested by the Hoffman-Rigler sign, a measurement determined by drawing a 2.0 cm vertical line upward along the inferior vena cava from the point where the posterior wall of the left ventricle and inferior vena cava cross in the lateral projection. At this point, a second line is drawn parallel to the vertebral bodies. The distance between the LV border and the vertical line should not exceed 1.8 cm. If it does, LV enlargement is suggested. Although this sign can be helpful, it is often inaccurate because of poor positioning of the patient, which adversely influences this measurement.[6]

Right Anterior Oblique Projection

Chest radiography in the right anterior oblique (RAO) projection (Fig. 5-12) is performed with the patient in a 45-degree obliquity to the film cassette (right shoulder toward the cassette). In this projection, the ventricles are elongated; the long axes of the ventricles are in view, and the atrioventricular groove is in profile, thereby permitting an advantageous view of a calcified mitral or tricuspid valve. This view helps to determine the presence of LA enlargement, a common feature of mitral stenosis or regurgitation. The aortic arch is foreshortened in the RAO projection, so the arch and proximal descending aorta are often superimposed and obscured. The anterior border of the heart in the RAO projection consists of the sinus portion of the right ventricle inferiorly and the right ventricular outflow tract and the main pulmonary artery superiorly. The right-sided or posterior heart border is made up of the right atrium superiorly and the left atrium inferiorly.

Left Anterior Oblique Projection (LAO)

The LAO projection (see Fig 5-9) is performed with the patient positioned in a 60-degree oblique relationship to

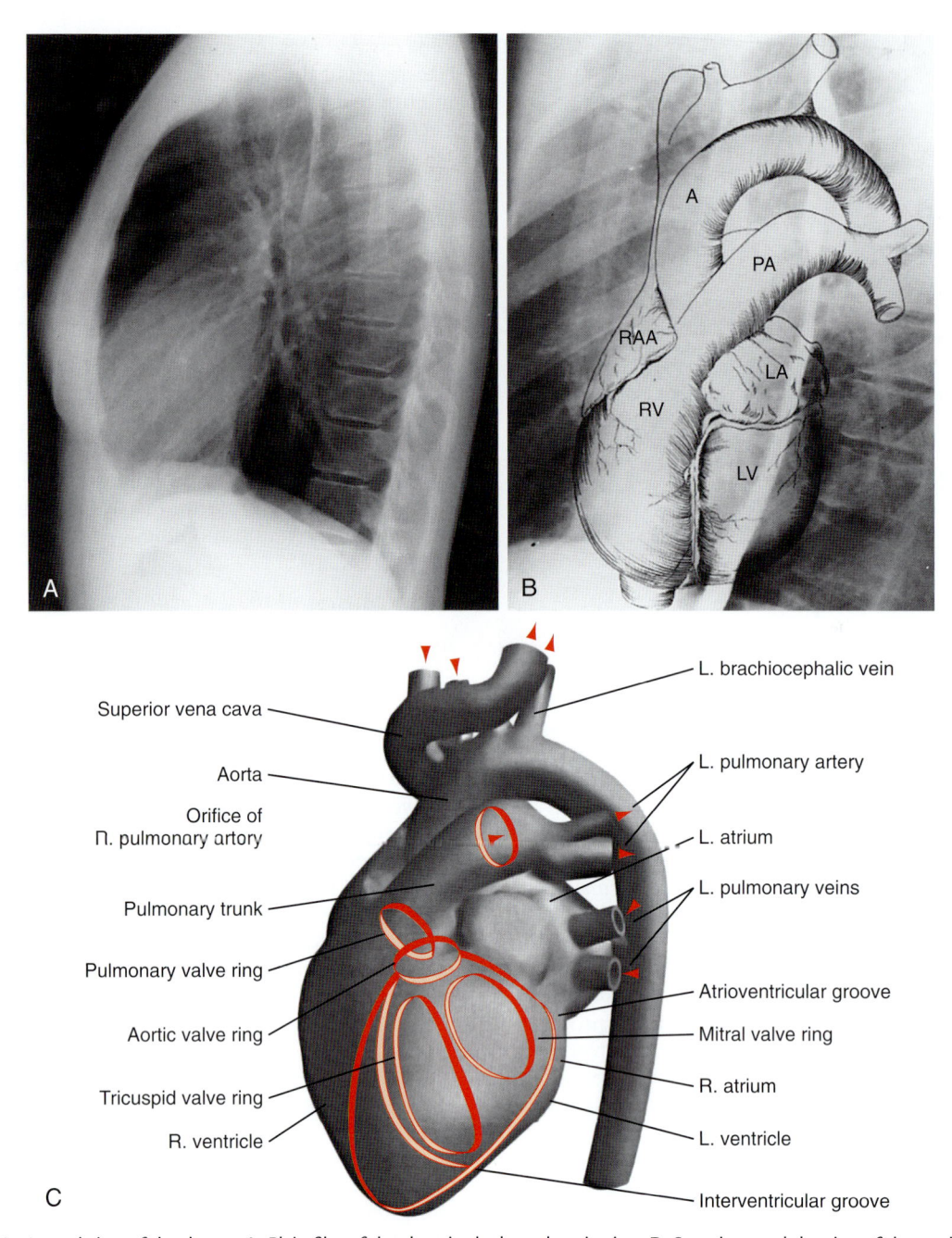

FIGURE 5-11 Lateral view of the thorax. **A,** Plain film of the chest in the lateral projection. **B,** Superimposed drawing of the cardiac chambers and the major vessels. *(From Van Houten FX, Adams DF, Abrams HL: Radiology of valvular heart disease. In Sonnenblick E, Lesch M [eds]: Valvular Heart Disease. New York, Grune & Stratton, 1974.)* **C,** A computer-generated model in the lateral projection demonstrates the valves, chambers, and sulci. *(From Steiner RM: Radiology of the heart and great vessels. In Braunwald E, Zipes PD, Libby P [eds]: Heart Disease: A Textbook of Cardiovascular Medicine, 6th ed. Philadelphia, Saunders, 2001.)*

the cassette. This view is useful to identify the presence of left ventricular enlargement. Because the ventricular septum is in profile in this projection, septal defects and abnormalities of right and left ventricular anatomy can be identified with angiography or with LAO equivalent projection using MR or CT.[7] In this projection, the aortic and pulmonary valves are in profile, so that aortic valve calcifications can be clearly visualized and aortic or pulmonary stenosis or regurgitation can be assessed with angiography or cross-sectional imaging. The aortic arch is also in profile in this projection, making it the ideal view for evaluating the presence or absence of aortic dissection or aneurysm for studying the origins of the head and neck vessels as well as identifying aortic coarctation and patent ductus arteriosus (Fig. 5-13).

MEASURING CARDIAC SIZE

Direct measurement of heart size by plain film radiographs is rarely performed because analysis of cardiac anatomy and chamber volume is available with ECHO, CT scan, and MRI. However, because an enlarged heart on the chest radiograph is abnormal, estimation of the cardiothoracic ratio and changes in cardiac size may be a valuable yard-

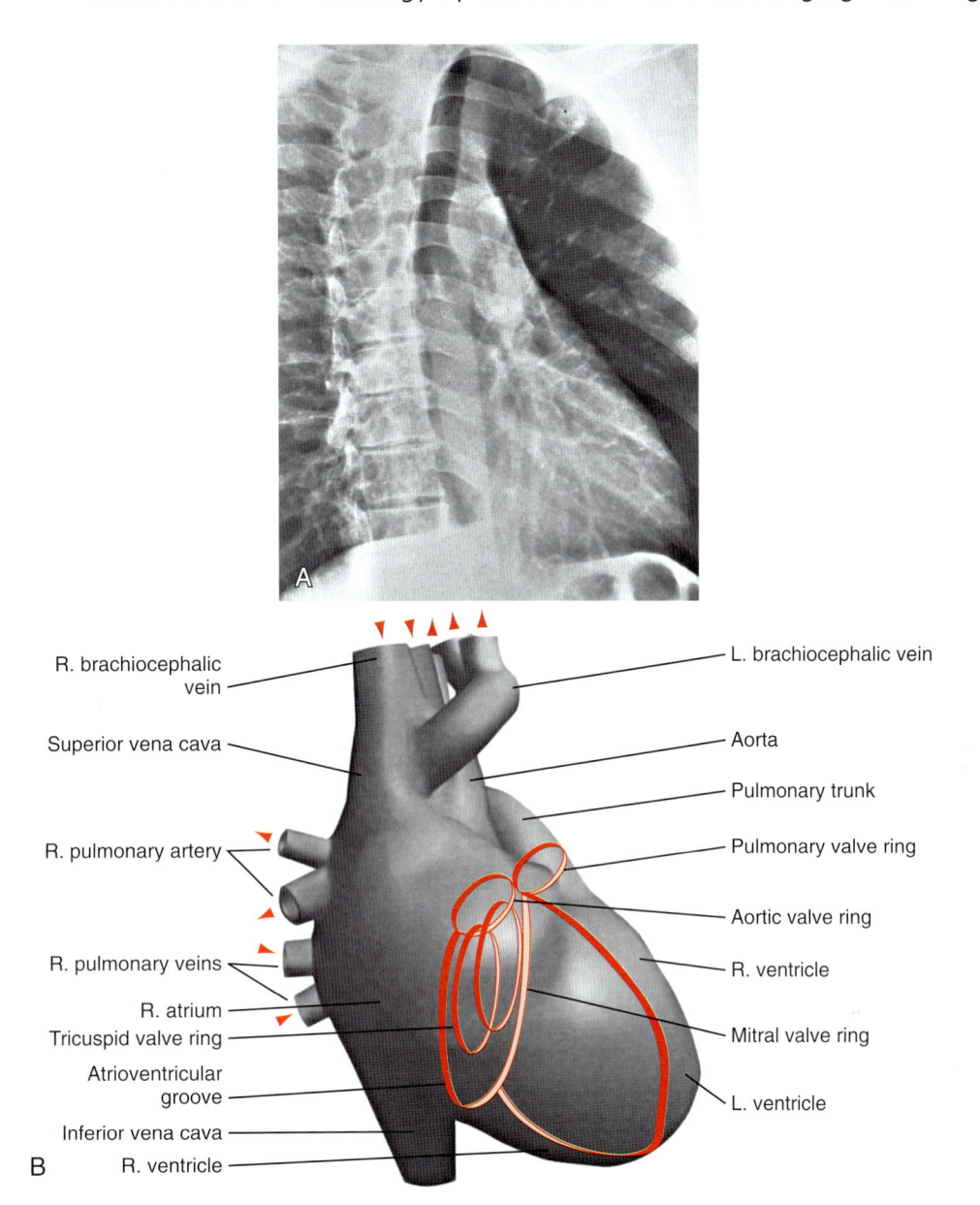

■ **FIGURE 5-12** Right anterior oblique projection (RAO). **A,** 45-degree RAO film of the chest in a normal patient. **B,** Computerized image of the heart in the RAO projection demonstrates the anatomic relationships of the cardiac chambers and valves. (**A,** from Van Houten FX, Adams DF, Abrams HL: Radiology of valvular heart disease. In Sonnenblick E, Lesch M [eds]: Valvular Heart Disease. New York, Grune & Stratton, 1974; **B,** from Steiner RM: Radiology of the heart and great vessels. In Braunwald E, Zipes PD, Libby P [eds]: Heart Disease: A Textbook of Cardiovascular Medicine, 6th ed. Philadelphia, Saunders, 2001.)

stick to assess anatomic changes coinciding with adverse cardiac events. This assessment may be done subjectively by estimating whether a heart is normal in size, enlarged, or grossly enlarged on the basis of an average cardiothoracic ratio of 0.50. The cardiothoracic ratio may also be derived by measuring the ratio between the maximum transverse diameter of the heart divided by the maximum width of the thorax. The transverse cardiac measurement is based first on creating a vertical line on the radiograph through the mid-point of the spine from the sternum to the diaphragm. The transverse cardiac diameter is obtained by adding the widest distance of the right heart border from the mid-line and the left heart border to the mid-line.[8] This diameter is then divided by the maximum transverse diameter of the thorax. The normal range of the transverse cardiac measurement is 10 cm in a small, thin individual to 16.5 cm in a tall, heavy person. A measurement 10 percent beyond these values represents the upper limits of normal.

A normal heart may appear larger in the frontal projection when the anterior-posterior dimension is small related to a pectus excavatum deformity or straight back. A large heart may appear smaller than it really is because of a downward displaced cardiac apex in patients with aortic regurgitation or in an elderly patient with a large AP diameter caused by a severe spinal curvature. The cardiac outline will be truly small in patients with Addison disease or anorexia nervosa because of the absence of brown fat. Because of cardiac magnification on AP films (including portable radiographs), visual correction must be made to avoid the over-diagnosis of heart enlargement. A reduction in the calculation of heart size by 10% to 12.5%, depending on the anode-to-tube distance, will correct this

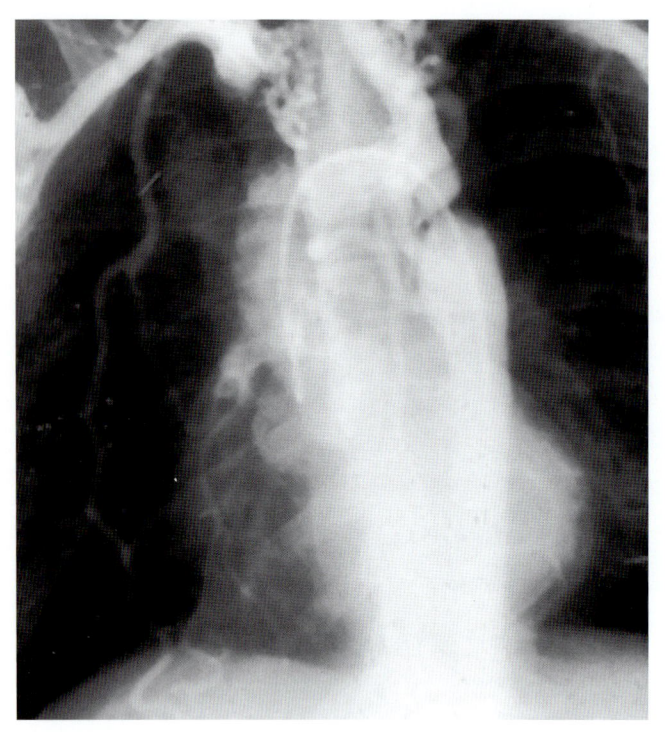

FIGURE 5-13 Aortography in the LAO plane in this patient with coarctation of the aorta demonstrates to best advantage the full expanse of the aortic arch—a useful projection for the diagnosis of aortic aneurysm, dissection, tubular hypoplasia, and patent ductus arteriosus.

discrepancy.[9,10] In practice, these calculations are of historical interest and are seldom performed today because more accurate estimation of cardiac size can obtained with cross-sectional techniques.

PERICARDIUM

The incidence of pericardial disease parallels the frequency of cardiac surgery, thoracic irradiation, multisystem inflammatory disease, and the administration of medications that adversely affect the pericardium.[11]

The Normal Pericardium

Normal pericardium is frequently identified on the lateral chest film as a thin linear opacity separating the anterior mediastinal fat from the subepicardial fat (Fig. 5-14) The pericardium may also be visualized occasionally on the frontal chest film as a lucent stripe paralleling the left heart border. The normal and abnormal pericardium is best appreciated on CT and MRI because of the superior contrast resolution of both techniques. With both CT and MRI, the anterior, lateral, and posterior portions of the pericardium are clearly separated from mediastinal fat, and even subtle areas of pericardial widening may be clearly delineated. One pitfall of both MRI and CT is that pericardial recesses may be confused with aortic dissection or mediastinal lymphadenopathy.

Pericardial Effusion

Pericardial effusions may be a transudate or may be hemorrhagic, gaseous, or chylous, and are due to a wide variety of causes. When a large fluid collection accumulates in the pericardial sac, the cardiac silhouette assumes a flask-like or globular silhouette (Fig. 5-15). The normal indentations and prominences along the left and right heart borders are effaced, so the shape of the cardiac silhouette becomes smooth and featureless. Because the pericardium extends up to the pulmonary bifurcation, when a large pericardial effusion is present, the hilar structures are draped and obscured by the distended pericardial cavity. This radiographic appearance should help distinguish a large pericardial effusion from massive cardiomegaly, which will not obscure the hilar vessels.

In the lateral chest radiograph in a patient with pericardial effusion, the retrosternal space is typically narrowed or obliterated by the expanding cardiac silhouette. Normally, the low-density subepicardial fat merges imperceptibly with the mediastinal fat because the two fat planes are separated by only the 2 mm-thick stripe of the pericardium. When pericardial effusion is present, the subepicardial fat is displaced posteriorly by the higher density fluid, which may be visible as a wide, opaque vertical band between the anterior border of the heart and the mediastinum. This "epicardial fat pad sign" is best visualized on the lateral projection and is highly specific for pericardial effusion.[11]

Although pericardial effusion may be suggested by plain film findings, ECHO is the most sensitive modality for the detection of pericardial effusion and/or thickening. ECHO has the advantage of ease of performance at the bedside in critically ill patients, is noninvasive, and emits no ionizing radiation when constriction, neoplasm, or hemorrhage is present. If ECHO is inconclusive, CT can be helpful in detecting pericardial thickening, diffuse or loculated effusion, calcification, and adjacent mediastinal and pulmonary disease, as well as neoplasm. MRI not only can clearly detect pericardial effusion with great sensitivity, but also can characterize thrombus, tumor, fibrosis, and hemorrhage. Pericardial fibrosis is characterized by a medium-intensity signal on T1-weighted or dark signal intensity on T2-weighted images. Intrapericardial masses, cysts, and diffuse thickening are well demonstrated with MRI.[11]

Pericardial Constriction

Pericardial constriction may complicate viral or tuberculous pericarditis, hemopericardium, pericarditis associated with radiation, and postpericardiotomy syndrome. In patients with chronic pericardial constriction, the overall heart size is large when the pericardium is thickened to 2 cm or more; otherwise, the cardiac silhouette remains normal or small. The right atrial border is flattened, and pulmonary vascular redistribution may be observed.

Small-to-large pleural effusions are found in 60% of patients with pericardial constriction, and enlargement of the azygos vein and left atrium will be seen in up to 20% of cases of constriction. Pericardial calcification is best appreciated along the anterior and inferior cardiac borders or in the atrioventricular groove. Although it is important to appreciate that the presence of pericardial calcification indicates chronic pericarditis, it does not of itself establish a diagnosis of pericardial constriction.

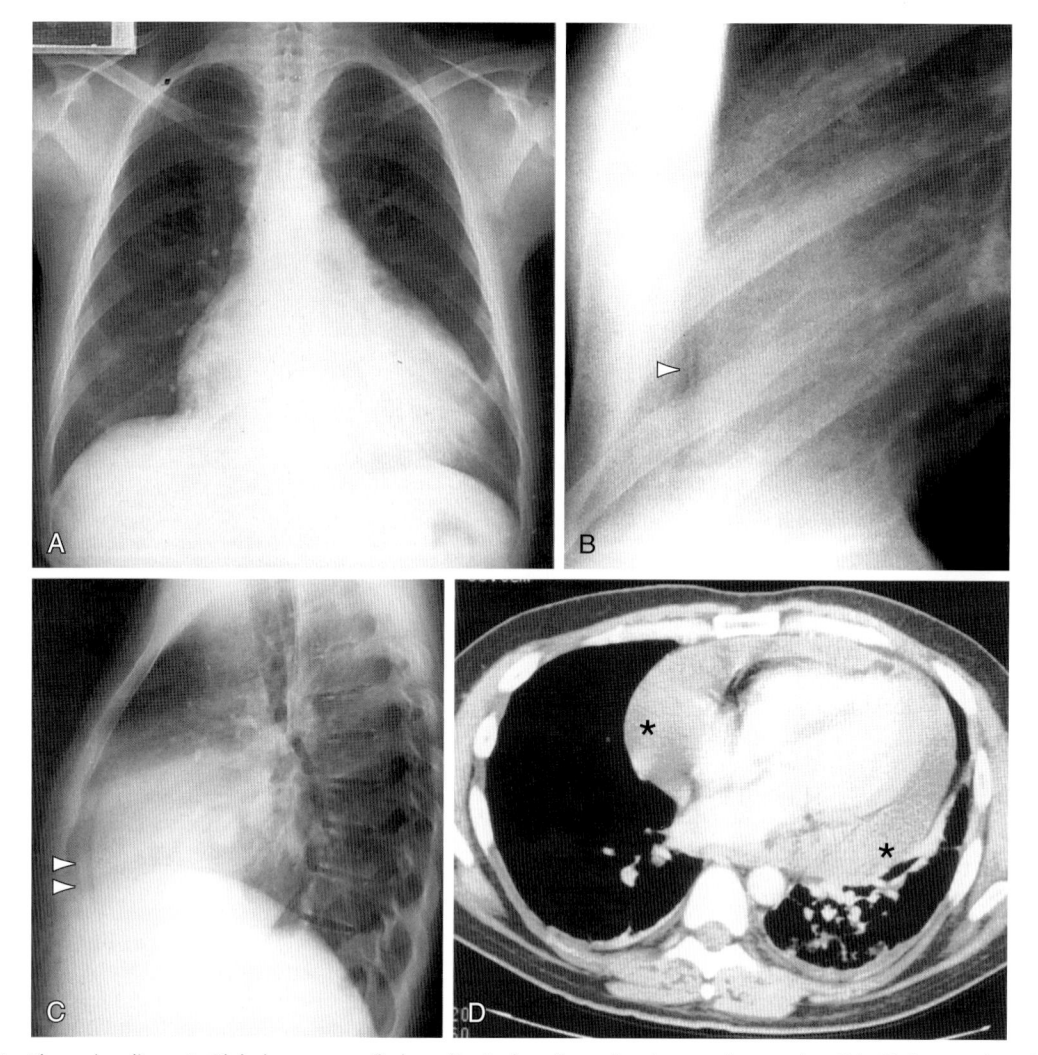

■ **FIGURE 5-14** The pericardium. **A,** Globular or water flask mediastinal configuration due to a large pericardial effusion. **B,** The subepicardial fat stripe (*arrowhead*) in the normal patient is separated from the anterior mediastinal fat by the 2 to 4 mm line or band representing the normal width of the pericardium. **C,** When a pericardial effusion is present, the soft tissue stripe is widened because of the presence of increased fluid in the pericardial sac (*arrowheads*). **D,** A contrast-enhanced CT scan shows a wide band of water density enveloping the heart due to a large effusion (*asterisks*). *(From Steiner RM: Radiology of the heart and great vessels. In Braunwald E, Zipes PD, Libby P [eds]: Heart Disease: A Textbook of Cardiovascular Medicine, 6th ed. Philadelphia, Saunders, 2001.)*

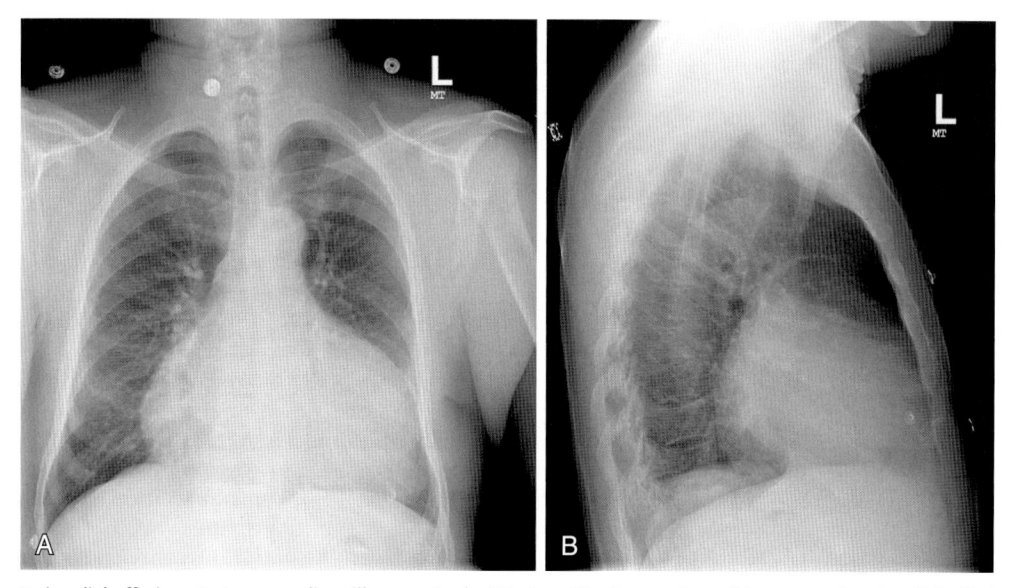

■ **FIGURE 5-15** Pericardial effusion. **A,** Large cardiac silhouette in the PA chest film in a patient with suspected pericardial effusion. **B,** A wide pericardial stripe is visible on the lateral view confirming the pericardial abnormality.

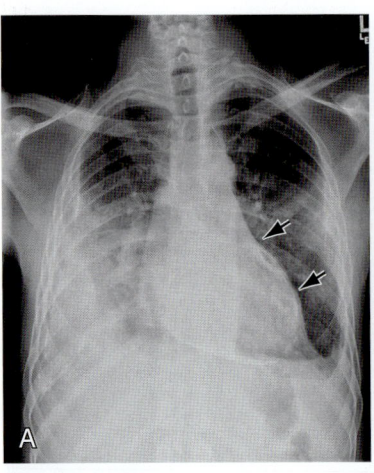

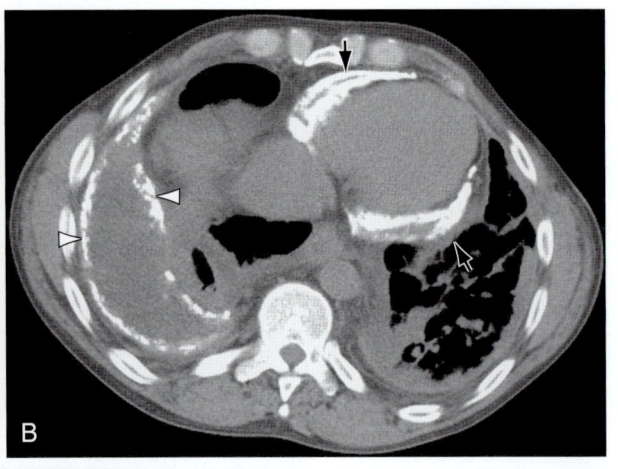

■ FIGURE 5-16 Pericardial calcification. **A,** PA chest film shows the extensive pericardial calcification (*arrows*) as well as calcification of the right pleural surfaces. **B,** CT in the axial plane confirms the pericardial (*arrows*) and pleural calcification (*arrowheads*) in this patient with a history of tuberculous pleuritis and pericarditis.

Pericardial constriction is often confused with restrictive cardiomyopathy, and MRI and CT are helpful in differentiating these two conditions. The pericardium in patients with restrictive cardiomyopathy is normal in thickness and is free of calcification. In addition, diffuse limitation of global cardiac excursion in systole and diastole is present, together with myocardial thickening in hearts with restrictive cardiomyopathy.[12]

Pericardial Calcification

Pericardial calcification is most often associated with previous inflammation or with blunt cardiac or pericardial trauma. Common causes include viral illness, especially coxsackievirus or influenza infection, tuberculosis, and histoplasmosis. Calcification following trauma or hemopericardium followed by calcification is a frequent scenario (Fig. 5-16).

Pericardial masses such as intrapericardial teratomas and cysts may calcify. In constrictive pericarditis, calcification is found in up to 50% of patients. Calcification helps distinguish pericardial constriction from restrictive cardiomyopathy, which although similar hemodynamically, is not associated with pericardial calcification. Extensive calcification without the signs of restriction may occur and myocardial calcifications involving the myocardial walls or coronary arteries may be confused with pericardial calcification. Pericardial calcification may be distinguished from myocardial calcification by differences in distribution. Pericardial calcification is most common along the RA and RV borders and in the region of the atrioventricular groove. Alternatively, the pericardium adjacent to the left ventricle is most often free of calcification, probably related to its vigorous pulsations. Calcification rarely occurs along the posterior LA border because of the absence of pericardium behind the left atrium. Myocardial calcification is most often found in the LV and is much less common in the right heart. To identify calcification on plain film radiography, over-penetrated films may be helpful and certainly CT may demonstrate calcium not seen on plain chest films.

Pericardial Cyst

A pericardial cyst appears as a smooth convex bulge along the lower right heart border near the cardiophrenic sulcus in 80% of cases of pericardial cysts. However, 20% of pericardial cysts lie along the left heart border, sometimes mimicking a prominent left atrial appendage or left ventricular aneurysm (see Fig. 5-7). Pericardial cysts rarely calcify and do not communicate with the pericardial sac, unlike pericardial diverticula which do communicate with the pericardial sac. Their clinical importance lies in the need to differentiate pericardial cysts from other masses with a similar appearance on plain films, such as thymoma, lymphoma, and postoperative hematoma. Pericardial cysts are best diagnosed by ECHO, CT, or MRI as smoothly marginated, fluid-filled structures adjacent to the right heart border (Fig. 5-17).

NORMAL PULMONARY VASCULATURE

The pulmonary veins and arteries are clearly distinguished on the plain chest film. As a result, normal, increased, decreased, redistributed and asymmetric blood flow may be identified and correlated with other indications of cardiovascular disease.

Normal Pulmonary Vascular Anatomy

The main pulmonary artery (MPA) divides within the mediastinum into the left and right main pulmonary arteries. The LPA passes to the left and posterior just above the left main-stem bronchus. Its lateral borders are visible just above the middle of the left hilum. The RPA follows a horizontal course within the mediastinum forming a round or elliptical opacity in front of the right main-stem bronchus on the lateral projection (Fig. 5-18). The LPA, in the lateral view, lies posterior to the airway and parallels the aortic arch. The RPA divides within the mediastinum proximal to the right hilum into the upper branch or truncus anterior and the inferior or interlobar branch. Within the

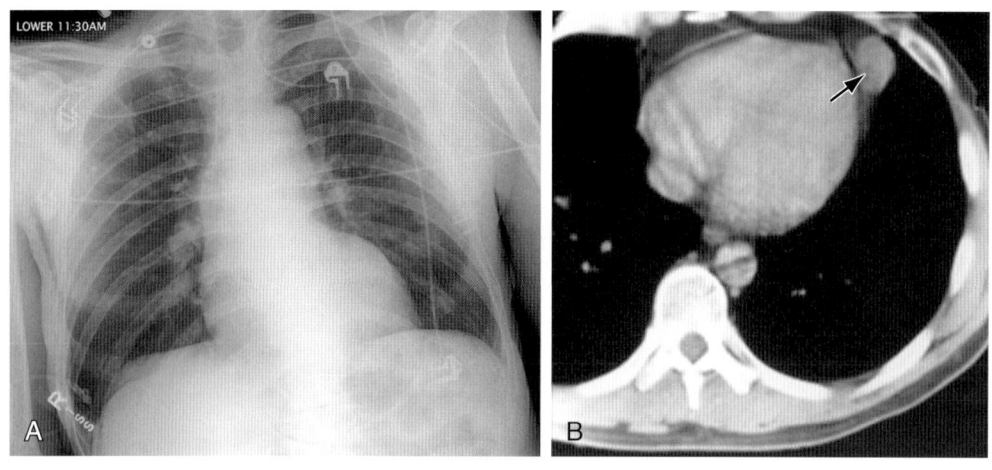

■ **FIGURE 5-17** Pericardial cyst. **A,** A bulge along the left heart border on the PA chest film. **B,** The abnormality is confirmed on CT as a water-density filled sharply marginated structure along the left side of the mediastinum compatible with the diagnosis of pericardial cyst (*arrow*).

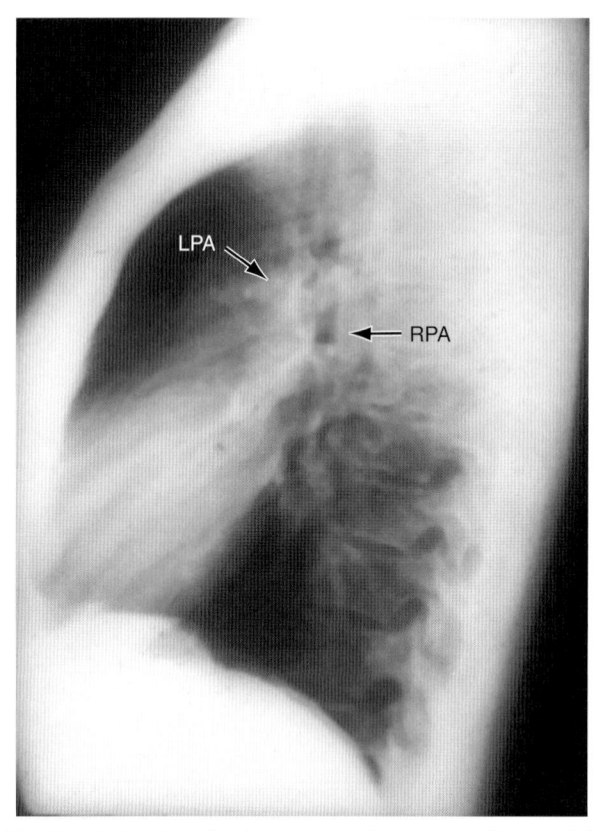

■ **FIGURE 5-18** Normal pulmonary vasculature. Lateral image of the chest shows the normal anatomy of the left and right pulmonary arteries in the lateral projection The RPA follows a horizontal course within the mediastinum producing an elliptical opacity. The LPA lies behind the airway and assumes a "shepherd's crook" configuration parallel to the descending thoracic aorta.

lungs, the pulmonary arteries parallel the bronchi and divide in an orderly manner gradually tapering toward the lung periphery. The bronchi and the pulmonary artery in the same pulmonary segment are approximately the same diameter at any one level with a ratio of about 1.2 to 1.0. Knowledge of this relationship is important to help determine the presence of increased redistributed or reduced blood flow.

In the erect position, pulmonary blood flow is greater to the lower lobes than to the upper lobes. In part, this is because of the effect of gravity and because the lower lobes are substantially larger than the upper lobes, requiring a greater pulmonary blood supply. The normal distribution of pulmonary blood flow is also affected by the difference in alveolar pressure between the upper lung zones or zone 1 which has a higher intra-alveolar pressure compared to the lower lung zones (zone 2 and zone 3) which have a lower intra-alveolar pressure.

On the chest radiograph in the supine and prone positions, blood flow appears equal in the upper and lower lung zones, but actually blood flow is greatest in the most dependent position, (zone 3) or the posterior third of each lung in the supine position and the anterior third of each lung in the prone position.

In the normal patient, the pulmonary vessels in the outer third of the lung are too small to be identified on the PA chest radiograph. Central pulmonary arteries can usually be distinguished from pulmonary veins because they follow different pathways. Pulmonary veins course within the interlobar septa and converge as horizontal vascular structures into the posterior aspect of the left atrium. The pulmonary arteries radiate outward from the left and right hila several centimeters above the pulmonary venous confluence. Veins to the upper lobes are usually lateral to or are superimposed on their companion pulmonary arteries. For the most part, the veins are larger than their neighboring arteries and branch less frequently. In a normal erect individual, the vessels in the upper lung zones are smaller than vessels at the base of the lungs because of important gravitational differences between the apex and the lung base, causing increased distribution of blood to the base of the lung (Fig. 5-19).

In most individuals there are two major pulmonary veins on each side—an anterior-superior branch and a posterior-inferior branch. Arrhythmias such as atrial fibrillation are related to abnormal electrical impulses emanating at the junction of the pulmonary veins and the left atrium. The anatomic relationships of these branches and the electrical pathways of the heart are important to determine the site for catheter ablation. For this reason, MRI

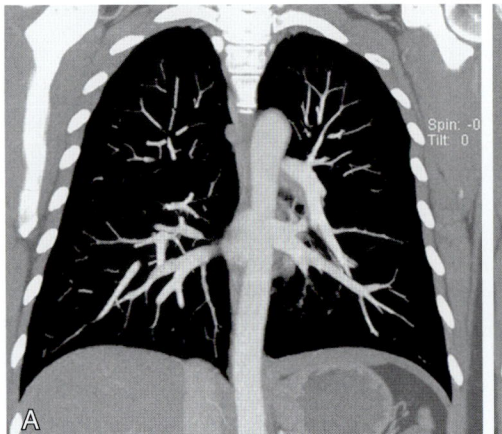

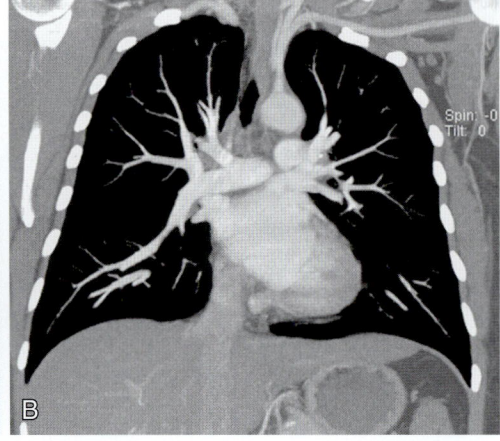

FIGURE 5-19 Pulmonary vasculature. Two contrast-enhanced CT images with maximum intensity projection (MIP) illustrates to best advantage the relationships between the pulmonary veins and arteries in the lower and upper lung zones.

or CT is often performed to map the relationship between the pulmonary veins and the left atrium before an invasive procedure.

Abnormal Pulmonary Blood Flow

Increased Pulmonary Flow

The diameter of the pulmonary arteries in the normal patient is proportional to the pulmonary blood volume, so when cardiac output is increased, the pulmonary branches will dilate up to the reserve of the pulmonary vascular bed. When the reserve of the pulmonary vascular bed is exceeded—and this usually occurs at eight times the normal flow—the size of the vessels will enlarge because of the combination of increased blood flow and increased pressure or because of pressure alone. The pulmonary veins also may enlarge as pulmonary arterial blood flow increases.

Enlarging pulmonary branches are found in a variety of conditions including left-to-right intercardiac shunts such as atrial septal defect (ASD), admixture lesions such as total anomalous pulmonary venous return, and situations that increase cardiac output such as pregnancy or chronic anemia (Fig. 5-20). As pulmonary blood flow increases, radiographs will demonstrate enlarged vessels clearly seen to the edge of the pleura.

Decreased Pulmonary Blood Flow

When pulmonary outflow tract obstruction or a right-to-left cardiac shunt is present, pulmonary blood flow is reduced and both veins and arteries are smaller in size. The central vessels narrow and the peripheral vessels are not visible. When the reduced blood flow is generalized or diffuse and when cyanosis is also present, tetralogy of Fallot or other causes of pulmonary outflow tract obstruction should be considered. When the restricted blood flow is regional, other diagnostic possibilities, such as pulmonary embolism, emphysema, tumor invasion, and vasculitis are more likely possibilities (Fig. 5-21). When pulmonary perfusion is significantly reduced, as in pulmonary atresia or extensive thromboembolism, the bronchial

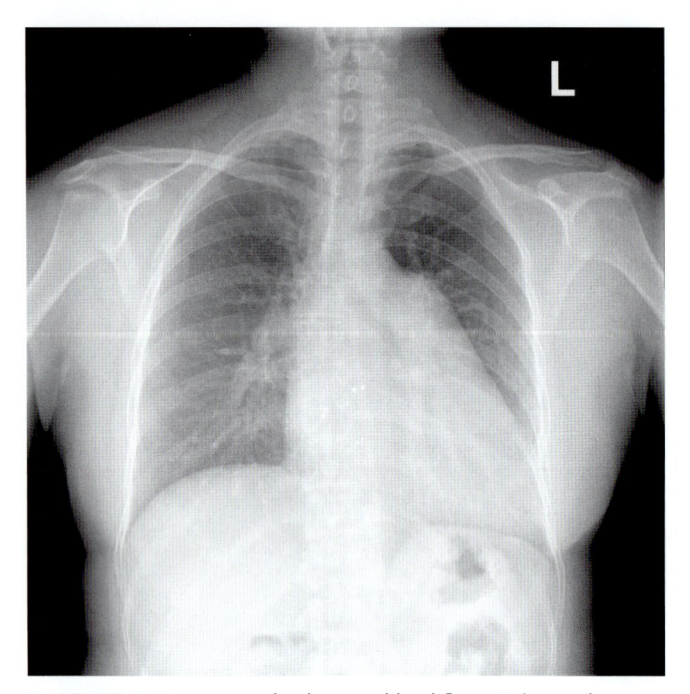

FIGURE 5-20 Increased pulmonary blood flow. PA image shows increased size of the central and peripheral pulmonary vasculature in a patient with atrial septal defect.

and other collateral arteries may increase in size. On a plain chest radiograph, bronchial vessels tend to be tortuous and nontapered, and because they emanate from the descending aorta, they do not radiate from the hilum. Normal-sized or small pulmonary arteries and veins may contribute to pulmonary vascularity in lungs with significant bronchial circulation because pulmonary arteries and bronchial arteries interconnect and blood flow preferentially passes from the higher pressure systemic bronchial arteries to the lower pressure pulmonary arterial bed.

Pulmonary Arterial Hypertension

When the pulmonary vascular reserve is recruited by increased blood flow or is reduced by vasoconstriction, the pressure within the pulmonary circulation will rise.

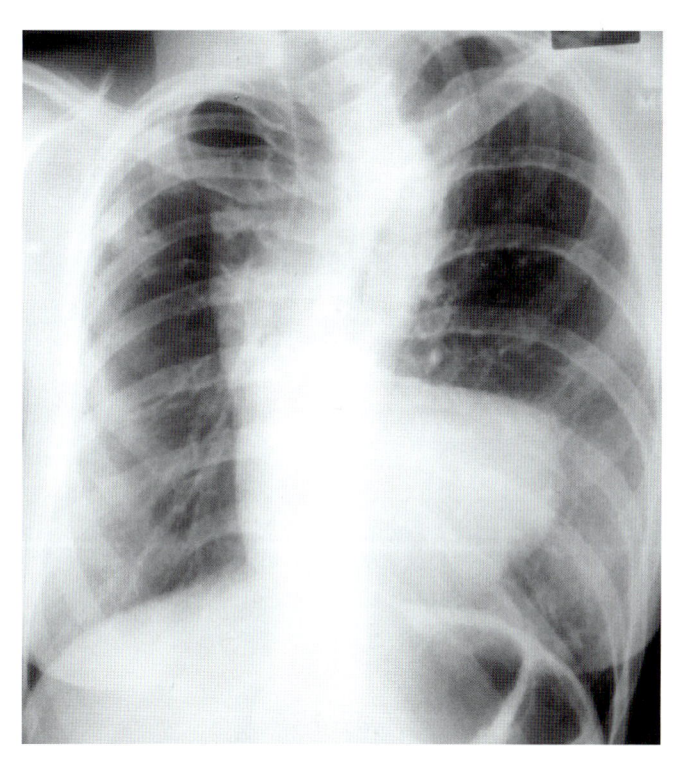

FIGURE 5-21 Decreased pulmonary vasculature. An adult patient with flattening of the MPA border and a high, rounded left ventricular border owing to right ventricular enlargement. The peripheral pulmonary vasculature is markedly reduced. The result is a classic boot-shaped heart in this patient with tetralogy of Fallot.

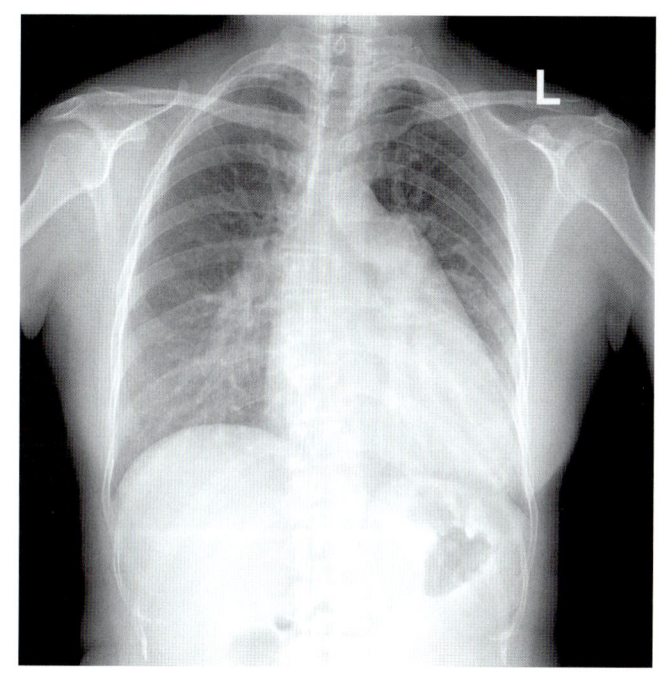

FIGURE 5-22 Pulmonary arterial hypertension. The MPA is markedly enlarged in this patient with Eisenmenger physiology due to a reversed intercardiac shunt.

Accompanying increased pressure is vasospasm, vessel wall thickening, and peripheral vasoconstriction. Ultimately, peripheral blood flow is reduced and the outer third of the lungs may appear hyperlucent. In pulmonary arterial hypertension (Fig. 5-22), the central elastic pulmonary arteries will enlarge including the main and central branching vessels. In long-standing and severe pulmonary arterial hypertension, pericardial infusion, abnormal pulmonary parenchymal mosaic perfusion patterns, and calcification of the main pulmonary artery and its proximal branches may be seen.[13] Pulmonary arterial hypertension may be primary, particularly in women in the childbearing age group, but is more likely secondary to a variety of systemic disorders, such as chronic hypoxia, collagen vascular disease, chronic pulmonary emboli, sleep apnea syndrome, or cardiovascular causes such as Eisenmenger physiology.[13]

Pulmonary Venous Hypertension

An increase in pulmonary venous pressure above the normal range of 8 to 12 mm Hg may occur with mitral stenosis, pulmonary venous obstructive disease, obstructing left atrial myxoma, and left ventricular failure. When pressure within the left atrium rises to the level of 12 to 18 mm Hg, pulmonary blood flow is redirected into the upper lobes in the erect position and anteriorly in the supine position, so the normal differences in size between the smaller zone 1 and larger zone 3 vessels are reversed. Enlargement of the mediastinal vessels leads to widening of the mediastinal contour or "vascular pedicle".[14] When there is a further increase of pulmonary venous pressure above 18 mm Hg, pulmonary interstitial edema occurs. When the pulmonary venous pressure rises above 25 mm Hg, alveolar flooding or edema will ensue.

Cephalization or redistribution of pulmonary venous and arterial flow to the upper lobes (zone 1) is one of the earliest signs of pulmonary venous hypertension. One clue to redistributed flow is the diameter of blood vessels at the first anterior costal interspace. Normally, blood vessels at the level of the first anterior interspace measure no more than 3 mm in diameter; however, if they are larger, increased or redirected flow may be the source. The chest radiograph is particularly useful in distinguishing significant from mild pressure elevations, but more precise grading of pulmonary venous pressure levels by plain film radiographs is rarely possible. The exact mechanism of vascular redistribution remains unclear, but one theory has been proposed by several authors. With a pulmonary venous pressure increase, fluid leaks from the pulmonary veins into the surrounding interlobular spaces first in the lower lobes because of gravitational effects. Then fluid leaks from the interlobular spaces decreasing pulmonary compliance, increasing the alveolar-capillary interface causing relative ischemia and resulting in vasoconstriction. This interplay will result in restriction of fluid and increase in venous pressure to the lower lobes. As a result, redirection or diversion of blood flow to the upper lobes will occur (Fig. 5-23A).

Pulmonary Alveolar and Interstitial Edema

Normally, fluid continually passes from the pulmonary veins within the interlobular spaces into adjacent interlobular lymphatics, which then returns the fluid to the central pulmonary veins. When the reserve within the

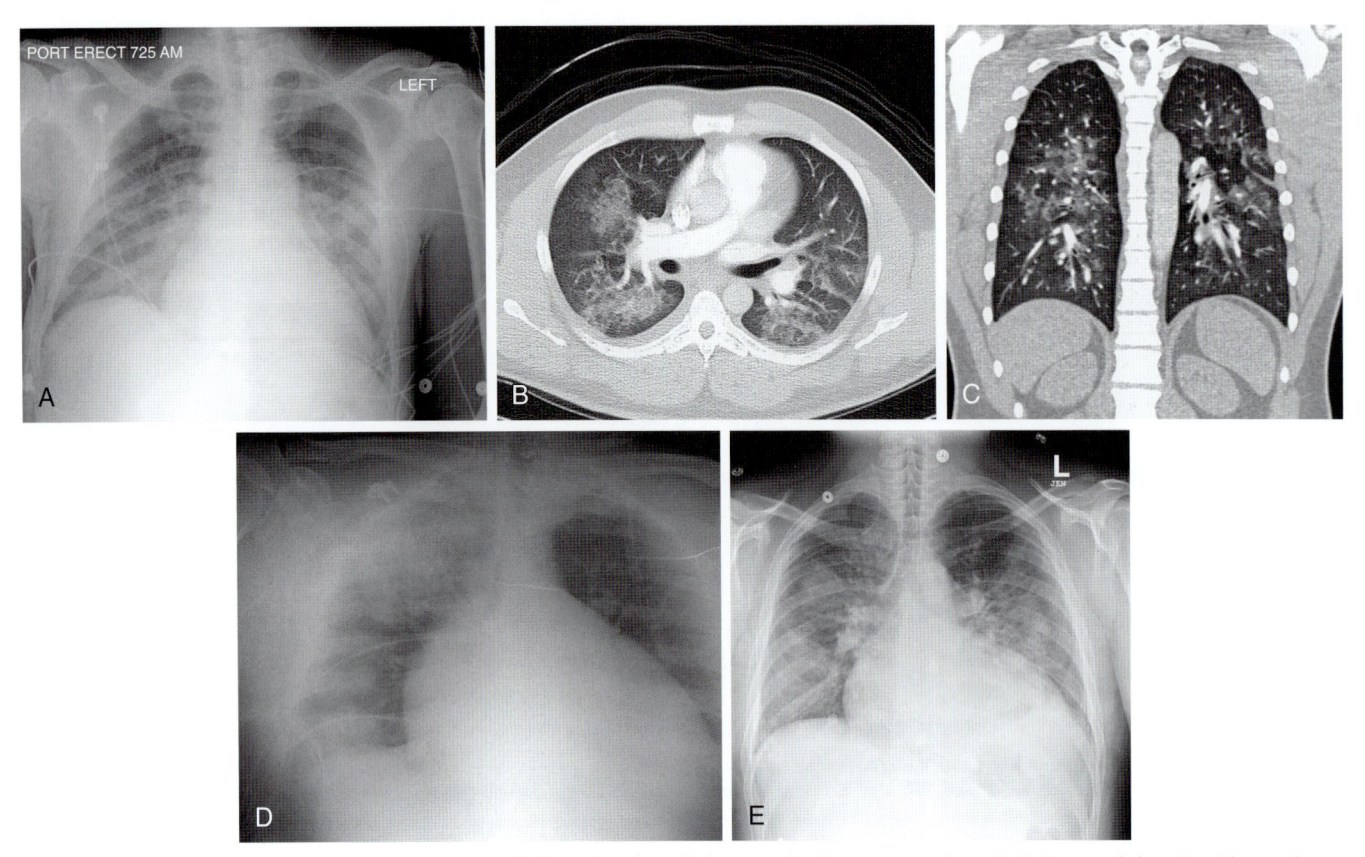

FIGURE 5-23 Pulmonary venous hypertension. **A,** The heart is enlarged, the central pulmonary vessels are indistinct, and there is evidence of cephalization in this patient with left sided heart failure. **B** and **C,** CT scan of the chest in the same patient showing the ground-glass pattern of pulmonary edema. **D,** There is preferential pulmonary edema in the right upper lobe due to acute CHF with mitral regurgitation. The focal right upper lobe pulmonary edema is thought to be due to the orientation of the regurgitant blood flow into the right upper lobe pulmonary veins. **E,** 4 days later the pulmonary edema pattern is symmetric as the pulmonary venous pressure rises in all lung zones.

lymphatic structures is overcome by increased transudate as a result of elevated pulmonary venous pressure, the interlobular septa thicken and become visible radiographically as septal or Kerley lines. Simultaneously, redistribution of blood flow to the upper lung zones or "cephalization" will occur with reduction in compliance and vasoconstriction in the lower lobes paralleling increases in pulmonary venous pressure.

When the pulmonary venous pressure rises to 18 to 25 mm Hg, interlobular septal lines are visible as thin horizontal structures perpendicular to the lateral pleural surface on the frontal chest film. Prominent interstitial opacities throughout the lung reflect increased thickened septal lines. Clear definition of the segmental and subsegmental blood vessels is lost and subpleural effusions occur. When the pulmonary interstitial edema is due to disordered cardiovascular hemodynamics, the heart may be normal or enlarged depending on the chronicity of cardiac decompensation. Prominent interlobular septa may also be found in noncardiac conditions such as lymphatic spread of tumor, asbestosis, interstitial pneumonia, and sarcoidosis.

With further increases in pulmonary venous pressure above 25 mm Hg, the leakage of fluid into the pulmonary alveoli leads to pulmonary edema. Small nodular areas of increased opacity (alveolar nodules) representing fluid in scattered acini or primary lobules are visible followed by coalescence into large confluent areas of opacity (pulmonary edema).

On the plain film radiograph, pulmonary alveolar edema secondary to cardiovascular disease will usually be found in the inner two thirds of the lung producing a "bat-wing" or "butterfly" appearance (see Fig. 5-23). One explanation for the development of the central distribution of pulmonary edema in patients with cardiovascular disease is that the outer third of the lung or the pulmonary cortex has better aeration, superior pumping effect during the respiratory cycle, more efficient lymphatic drainage, and better compliance than the inner two thirds of the lung. As a result, fluid concentrates preferentially in the center portion of each lung. It is sometimes difficult to distinguish pulmonary edema caused by heart disease and "congestive heart failure" from that caused by increased pulmonary permeability edema." In order to distinguish pulmonary edema caused by heart failure from other forms of pulmonary edema, criteria based on heart size, width of the vascular pedicle, blood flow distribution, regional distribution of edema, and interstitial thickening have been developed. In general, cardiovascular pulmonary edema is associated with a large heart, vascular redistribution, septal lines, pleural effusions, increased pulmonary blood volume, and regional distribution of pulmonary edema.[14,15]

In permeability pulmonary edema, there is generally no cardiac enlargement, little to no pleural effusion, absence of septal lines, and the edema is peripheral rather than central in distribution. The heart and vascular pedicle are not enlarged. When asymmetric pulmonary edema is present, it is usually related to an underlying change in the lung itself. Perhaps the most common cause for asymmetric pulmonary edema is emphysema in heavy cigarette smokers or end-stage sarcoidosis. Other causes of asymmetric pulmonary edema include thromboembolism and irradiation. Plain film radiography has been the most frequently used examination for the diagnosis of pulmonary edema. However, the superior resolution of CT has led to a more precise description of the findings in both interstitial and alveolar edema. Computed tomography may also yield additional insights into the cause and distribution of the edema and the presence of associated abnormalities.[16,17]

Cardiac Calcification

Myocardial Calcification

Calcification of the myocardium (Fig. 5-24) is most often due to a large myocardial infarction. Myocardial calcification occurs most frequently in true left ventricular aneurysms located at the left ventricular apex or the anterior lateral aspect of the left ventricular wall. Calcifications within left ventricular aneurysms tend to be curvilinear and are usually located in the periphery of the infarct or aneurysm. Calcification may occasionally be homogeneous when the entire infarcted area is affected. A false left ventricular aneurysm will occur when a tear in the myocardial wall occurs and blood leaks into the pericardium, at which time the blood passing into the pericardium is contained by adhesions or pressure. False aneurysms are most likely to occur along the posterolateral wall of the left ventricle.

Calcification may also be found within the left atrial chamber or in left atrium appendage in patients with rheumatic carditis and may be associated with mitral stenosis or regurgitation. Left atrial calcification is most often found in the endocardial layers of the heart muscle and is found less often within an organized thrombus adherent to the chamber wall. Like left ventricular aneurysms, left atrial calcification is generally thin-walled and curvilinear forming a shell around the circumference of the left atrial appendage. Myocardial calcifications may be appreciated on plain radiographs; however, MRI, CT, ultrasonography, and scintigraphy will add to the information derived from the plain film examination by showing the extent of the aneurysm and overall left ventricular function.

Valvular Calcification

Visible calcifications within a cardiac valve (Fig. 5-25) suggest the presence of a hemodynamically significant stenosis.[18] Calcification in the mitral valve appears thick and irregular or linear, measuring 2 to 4 cm in diameter. It is most frequently caused by rheumatic carditis.

Isolated aortic valve calcifications in patients 40 years of age or younger generally suggests the diagnosis of aortic stenosis owing to bicuspid aortic valve. In older patients, aortic valve calcifications may be related to "senile" sclerosis and degeneration of otherwise normal valve leaflets (Fig. 5-26).

The pattern of the aortic valve calcification may help determine its origin. For example, an irregular, thick, semilunar ring pattern with a central bar or knob is typical of a stenotic bicuspid valve and is seen in more than 50% of patients with congenital aortic stenosis. The distinctive pattern of calcification of a bicuspid valve results from calcification of the valve raphe or dividing ridge and the line of insertion of the shallow conjoint leaflet and the convex unfused leaflet.[18] The abundance of calcification in this entity is thought to be due to constant wear and tear from the abnormal injury-producing motion of the valve leaflets. Occasionally, three-leaflet aortic valves will mimic bicuspid valves because of fusion of two of the three leaflets.

The location of valve calcification on plain films is often confusing. For this reason, several measurements have been suggested as a means of identifying the location of valvular calcification on plain films. A line drawn on the lateral chest film from the junction of the anterior chest wall and the diaphragm through the hilum to the lung apex will separate anterosuperior aortic calcification from posteroinferior mitral calcification.

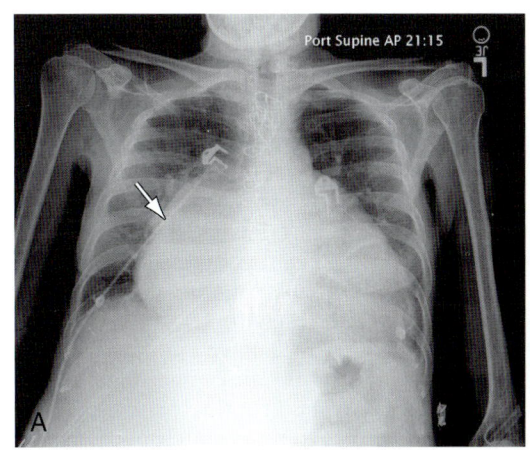

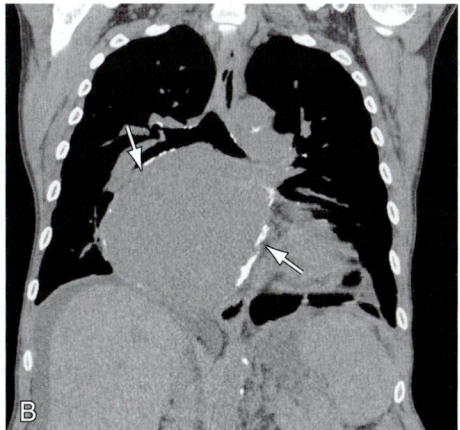

■ **FIGURE 5-24** Myocardial calcification. **A,** Curvilinear-shaped calcification (*arrow*) is visualized along the anterior wall of the LA in this individual with a history of rheumatic heart disease and atrial fibrillation. **A,** PA projection. **B,** coronal CT reformatted image.

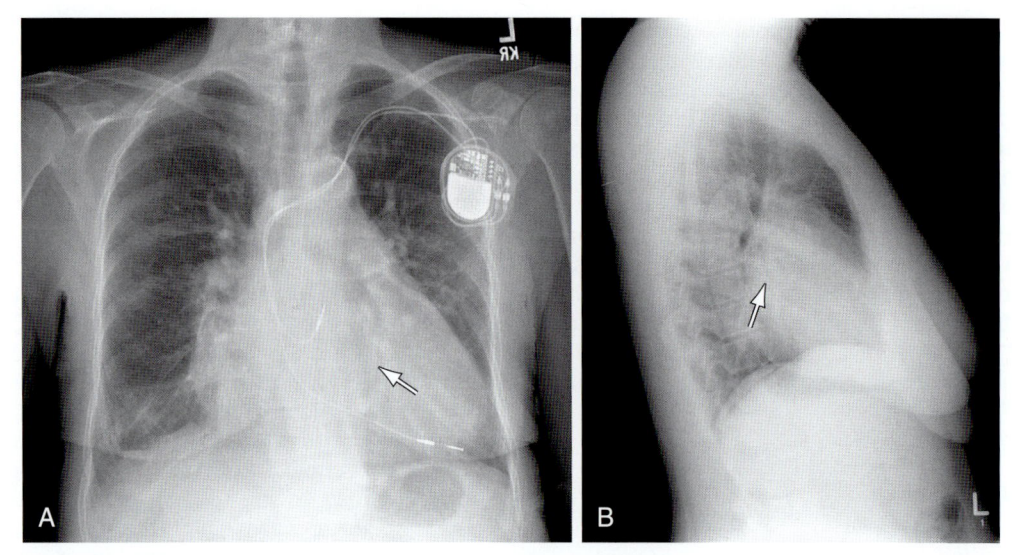

■ **FIGURE 5-25** Mitral valve calcification. PA film of the chest shows calcification in the area of the mitral valve (*arrows*). Valve calcification should not be confused with annular calcification, which is circular, larger, and scalloped. **B,** Lateral projection. *(From Steiner RM: Radiology of the heart and great vessels. In Braunwald E, Zipes PD, Libby P [eds]: Heart Disease: A Textbook of Cardiovascular Medicine, 6th ed. Philadelphia, Saunders, 2001.)*

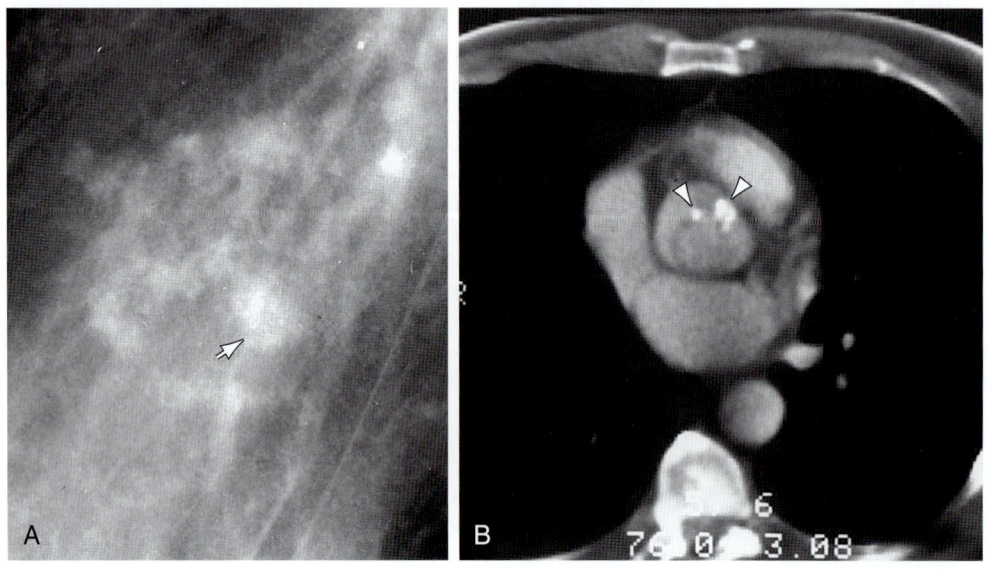

■ **FIGURE 5-26** Aortic valve calcification. Course nodular and linear calcification conforms to the aortic annulus and the fibrotic, partially fused aortic valve leaflets in a patient with aortic stenosis secondary to bicuspid aortic valve. **A,** Coned–down view of the chest film in the lateral projection (*arrow*). **B,** CT in the axial plane in the same patient shows typical calcifications of the aortic valve (*arrowheads*). *(From Steiner RM: Radiology of the heart and great vessels. In Braunwald E, Zipes PD, Libby P [eds]: Heart Disease: A Textbook of Cardiovascular Medicine, 6th ed. Philadelphia, Saunders, 2001.)*

Coronary Artery Calcification

Coronary artery calcification can be detected by a number of imaging modalities, including plain radiography, fluoroscopy, and CT. Of these modalities, MDCT and electron beam CT have been studied most intensively (Fig. 5-27).[19]

The chest film is readily available and relatively inexpensive but has low sensitivity for the detection of coronary calcification when compared with CT. Coronary artery calcifications are most often seen on the lateral chest radiograph, where a calcified left anterior descending artery projects as a double line of calcification along the anterior border of the heart. In the PA projection, the main left coronary artery and its proximal branches may be visible just below the left main-stem branches at the level of the left atrial appendage. Visualization of the coronary arteries by plain chest radiography is severely limited by superimposed structures, low contrast resolution, and motion when compared with other modalities.

Conventional CT is clearly superior to plain film radiography for the detection of coronary calcification. In fact, four times as many patients will be found to have calcified coronary arteries with CT than with plain film. Recent studies with MDCT have emphasized its value as a screening procedure. Because plain film chest radiographs and CT are performed routinely for other disease indications, it is important to make note of coronary calcifications and their distribution on CT to alert the clinician to their presence and significance.[20]

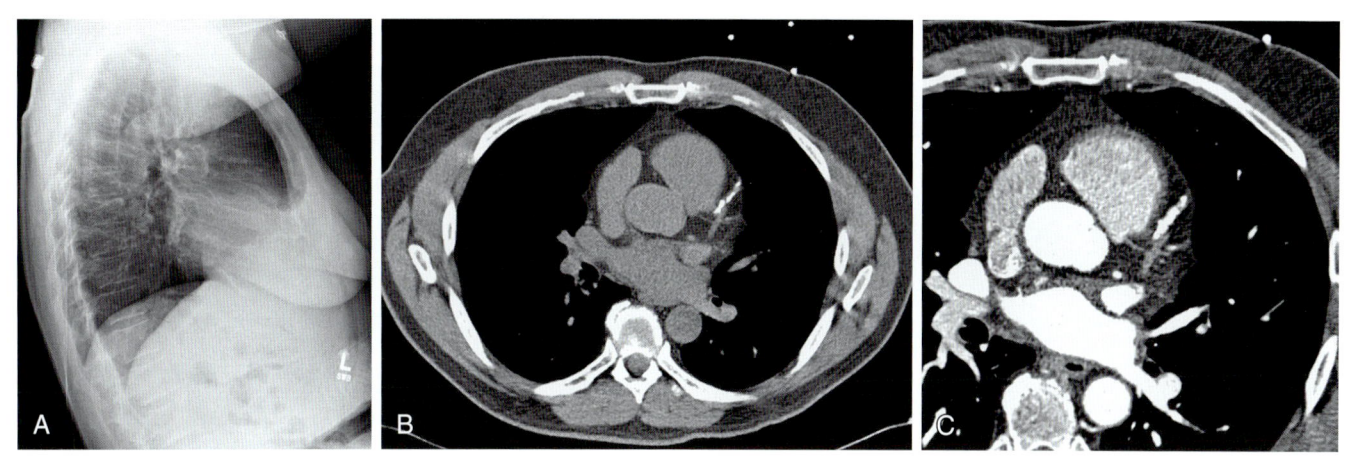

■ FIGURE 5-27 A, Lateral plain film radiograph demonstrates calcification of the left anterior descending artery (LAD) as a "tram track" immediately behind the sternum, indicating externsive calcific coronary atherosclerosis of the LAD. B, Nonenhanced axial CT image shows externsive LAD calcification in the same patient as A. C, An ECG-gated angiogram in the axial plane in another patient shows extensive calcification of the LAD together with opacification of surrounding cardiac structures.

Calcification of the Great Vessels

Aortic calcification, particularly in the region of the arch, is almost ubiquitous in individuals older than 50 years. It is usually noted on chest radiographs as a thin curvilinear opacity near the lateral border of the arch. When the calcification is located deep to the aortic border, dissection may be present (Fig. 5-28).[21] Other causes of aortic calcification are syphilis (usually involving the ascending aorta), sinus of Valsalva aneurysm, calcified ductus arteriosus, and Takayasu arteritis. Calcification of the main pulmonary artery also occurs in severe long-standing pulmonary hypertension.

CONGENITAL HEART DISEASE (CHD) IN THE ADULT

The radiologic manifestations of congenital heart disease in the adult can be classified by the incidence of the abnormalities and by associated findings such as the state of the pulmonary vessels and related skeletal abnormalities, whether the aortic arch is right- or left-sided, and thorax abdominal situs.[22] A history of the presence or absence of cyanosis and the time of onset of the clinical manifestations of the disorder should help to narrow the diagnosis. Several of the common cardiovascular disorders in the older patient found with some frequency are described subsequently.

Coarctation of the Thoracic Aorta (COA)

Coarctation of the aorta (Fig. 5-29; also see Fig. 5-13) is due to a deformity of the aortic intima and media with posterior infolding off the aortic lumen at or near the junction of the arch and descending aorta. Coarctation of the aorta accounts for 5% to 10% of childhood congenital heart defects and as many as 6% of CHD in the adult. Of those who escape diagnosis in early childhood, 25% die by the age of 20 years and nearly 50% die by the age of 30 years. The most common associated anomaly is a bicuspid aortic valve, which occurs in as many as 85% of patients with coarctation of the aorta.

The diagnosis of COA can be established on the PA chest film alone in as many as 92% of patients. The most common finding owing to the diagnosis of COA is widening of the LSCA border, but the most useful radiographic sign is pre- and poststenotic dilation at the site of the coarctation, which may appear as a double bulge above and below the usual site of the aortic knob. This pattern has been described as a "figure 3" sign.[22,23] This pattern is seen in as many as 60% of adults with untreated coarctation. The upper arc of the "3" is the dilated arch proximal to the coarctation and/or a dilated left subclavian artery. The lower bulge represents poststenotic dilation of the aorta immediately below the coarctation. When the esophagus is filled with barium, a reverse "3" or "E" sign, best visualized in the LAO projection, represents a mirror image of the "figure 3" sign. The "3" sign varies in that the upper arc may be small and the lower arc may be large or vice versa. Widening of the upper mediastinum or scalloping of the sternum caused by large internal mammary collateral arteries may be visible in some patients. A prominent left ventricular border often occurs with COA, especially when there is a bicuspid aortic valve associated with aortic stenosis.[23]

Bilateral symmetrical rib notching, readily appreciated on the chest film, is typical of COA. It is due to obstructed blood flow at the aortic coarctation with collateral blood flow through the third to eighth intercostal arteries. Rib notching, unusual in infancy, is present in 75% of adults with COA. The major routes of collateral flow include (1) from the LSCA subclavian artery to the internal mammary artery to the intercostal arteries; (2) transverse cervical and suprascapular arteries to the intercostal arteries; (3) LSCA to the costovertebral trunk to the intercostal arteries.

Computed tomography is diagnostic and demonstrates the site of the coarctation and associated anomalies such as bicuspid aortic valve best seen in the reformatted sagittal oblique images. MRI is particularly valuable to show the site of coarctation, the state of the aortic valve, and with phase-contrast imaging, to calculate the amount of collateral blood flow. CT, MRI, and ECHO are valuable to identify and characterize complications of COA repair

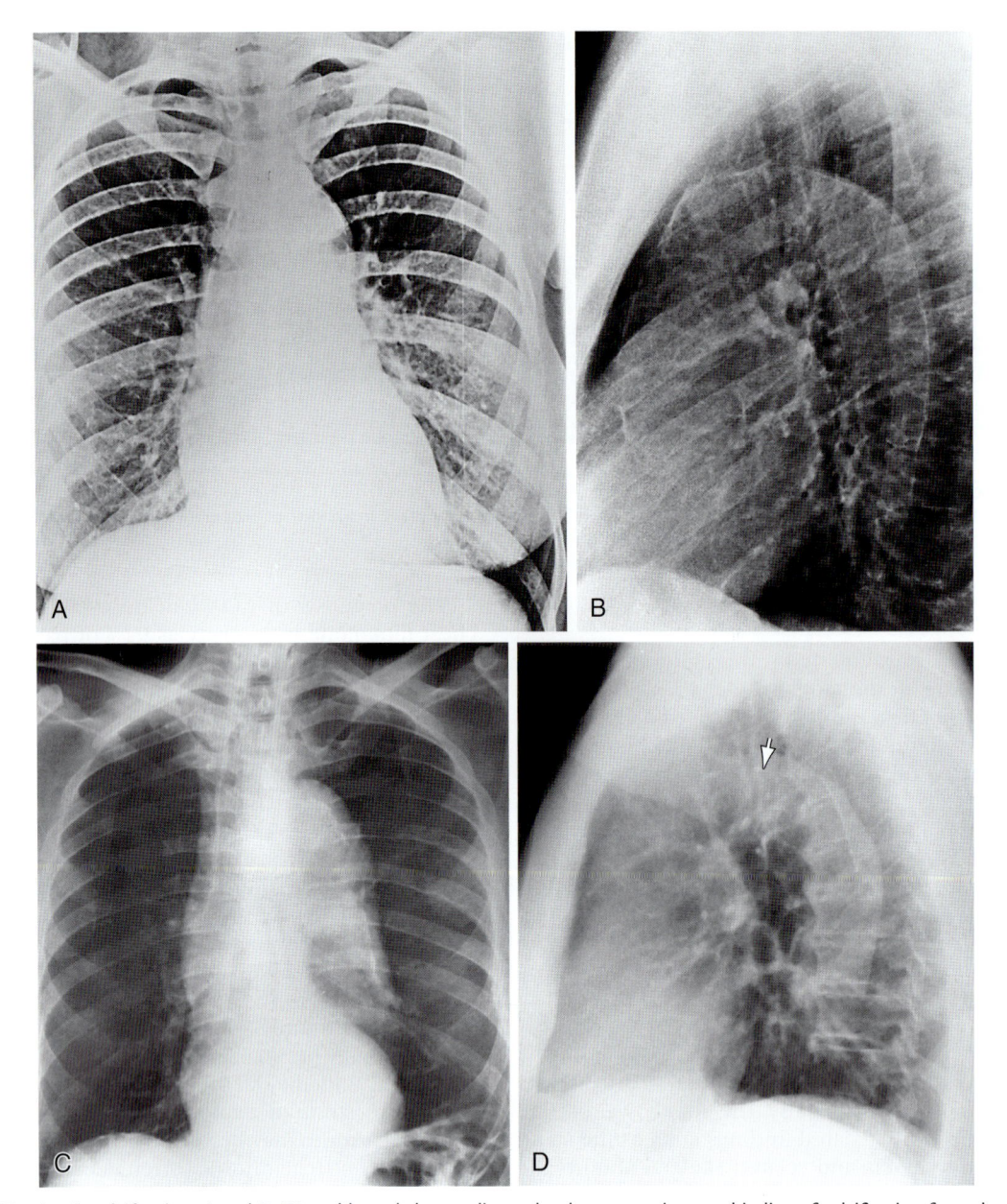

FIGURE 5-28 Aortic calcification. **A** and **B**, PA and lateral chest radiographs show a continuous thin line of calcification from the ascending aorta to the lower descending thoracic aorta in a 24-year-old patient with severe temporal cephalgia. Biopsy of a temporal artery confirmed the diagnosis Takayasu arteritis. **C** and **D**, PA and lateral chest radiographs in a 60-year-old patient with systemic hypertension shows thoracic artery dilation with a rim of calcification deep to the edge of the aortic border. This pattern is compatible with diagnosis of thoracic aortic dissection. *(From Steiner RM: Radiology of the heart and great vessels. In Braunwald E, Zipes PD, Libby P [eds]: Heart Disease: A Textbook of Cardiovascular Medicine, 6th ed. Philadelphia, Saunders, 2001.)*

such as dissection, postoperative pseudoaneurysm, infective endocarditis, and restenosis at the surgical site.[24,25]

Ostium Secundum Atrial Septal Defect (ASD) (Fig. 5-30)

ASD, the most common left-to-right shunt first diagnosed in the adult, occurs in more than 40% of adult congenital heart defects. The chest radiograph may appear normal in a patient with a small shunt, but if the ratio is of 1:2 or more, the MPA and the enlarged peripheral pulmonary branches, the RA, and the RV borders are prominent. It is possible in many patients to differentiate ASD from other causes of intracardiac left-to-right shunts. Less pulmonary artery dilation is usually seen in PDA than in ASD, and both PDA and VSD are associated with enlarged left-sided cardiac chambers. In adults older than 50 years with systemic hypertension or left ventricular failure, the radiographic findings of ASD are often atypical and may include left atrial enlargement, vascular cephalization, and pulmonary edema. In uncomplicated ASD without pulmonary hypertension, the MPA, RA, and RV are prominent but the aorta and left-sided chambers are normal.[23] The size and the location of the ASD can often be visualized—as well as associated abnormalities such as mitral valve prolapse—with MRI; the size and location of the defect can be important for placement of an occluder device.[26]

CHAPTER 5 • *Radiology of the Heart: Plain Film Imaging and Diagnosis* 91

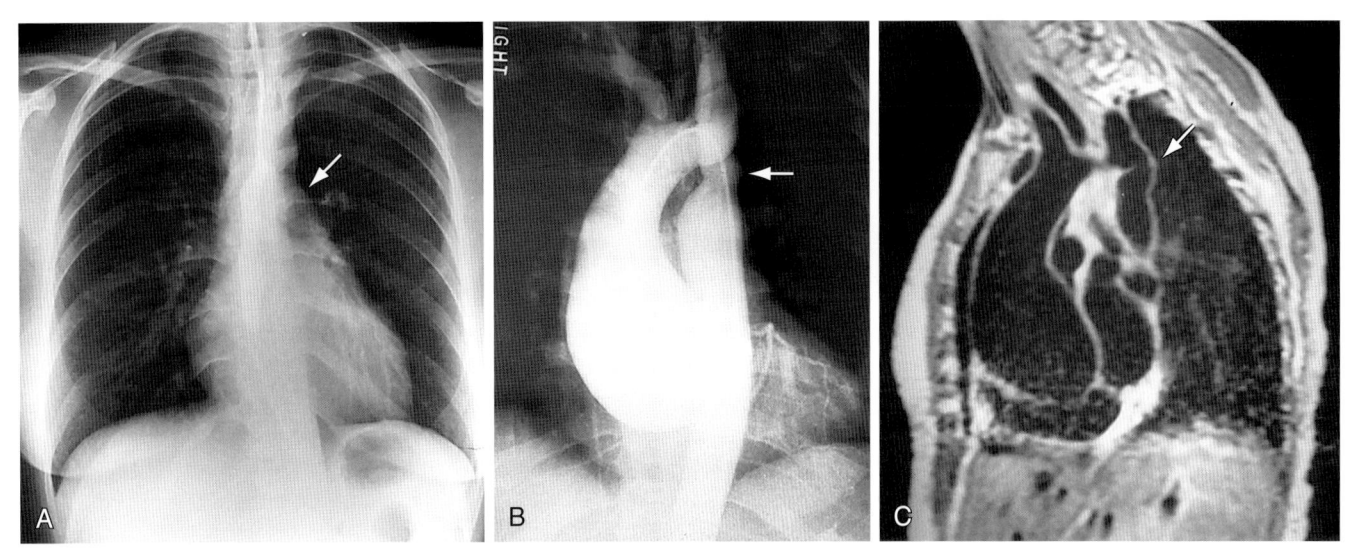

■ **FIGURE 5-29** Coarctation of the aorta. A through C, PA chest radiograph, frontal, angiographic, sagittal MRI images show a zone of narrowing or constriction of the proximal descending aorta in the region of the ligamentum arteriosum—the most frequent site for aortic coarctation. *(From Steiner RM: Radiology of the heart and great vessels. In Braunwald E, Zipes PD, Libby P [eds]: Heart Disease: A Textbook of Cardiovascular Medicine, 6th ed. Philadelphia, Saunders, 2001.)*

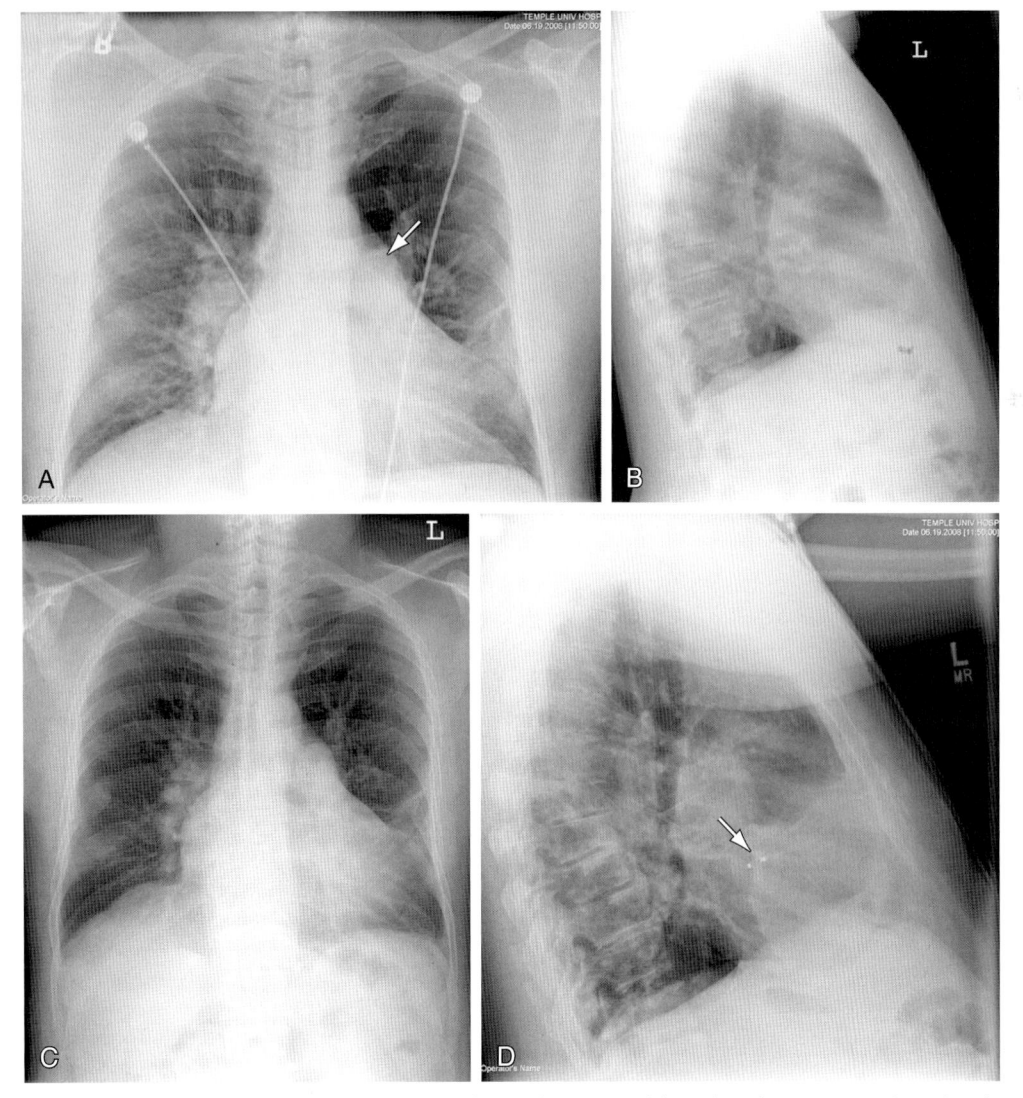

■ **FIGURE 5-30** Atrial septal defect. A and B, PA and lateral views show enlargement of the main pulmonary artery *(arrow)* and prominence of the LPA and RPA in the lateral projection. C and D, Within the cardiac silhouette is the radio-opaque Amplatz ASD occluder device *(arrow)* in the area of the interatrial septum.

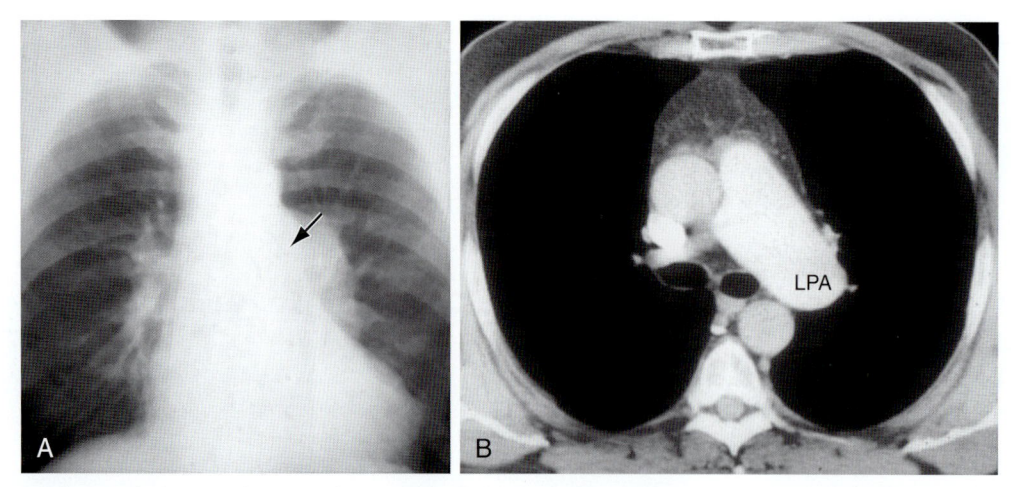

■ **FIGURE 5-31** Pulmonary valvular stenosis. **A,** PA chest radiograph shows prominent MPA (*arrow*). The heart is not enlarged and the LPA is prominent. **B,** CT shows a large pulmonary artery. The LPA is asymmetrically enlarged because the blood flow pattern is directed toward the left pulmonary circulation.

Pulmonary Valvular Stenosis

Pulmonary valvular stenosis (PVS) is usually an isolated anomaly in the adult. Mild-to-moderate enlargement of the MPA is demonstrated because of poststenotic dilation thought to result from the jet effect of blood flow through the narrowed pulmonary valve orifice. As the blood flow is oriented toward the LPA, that vessel is often preferentially enlarged. The differential diagnosis of PVS (Fig. 5-31) includes primary and secondary pulmonary hypertension, idiopathic pulmonary artery dilation, and other causes of pulmonary artery enlargement including left-to-right intracardiac shunts and arteritis.

ACQUIRED HEART DISEASE

The plain film of the chest offers important clues to global or segmental enlargement of the heart by analysis of cardiac border configuration and size. However, cross-sectional imaging modalities have largely supplanted the plain film for the diagnosis and assessment of acquired heart disease.

Valvular Heart Disease

Aortic Stenosis

Congenital bicuspid aortic valve is the most common cause of isolated aortic stenosis. When other valves are also involved, including the tricuspid and mitral valves, rheumatic heart disease should be a major consideration in the differential diagnosis. In addition to bicuspid aortic valve, causes of left ventricular outflow tract narrowing resulting in left ventricular enlargement include hypertrophic cardiomyopathy and supravalvular and subvalvular aortic stenosis.

In patients with aortic valvular disease,[27] the typical radiographic findings include a normal-sized heart with rounding of the left ventricular border or an elongated cardiac silhouette with displacement downward of the cardiac apex as a result of concentric left ventricular hypertrophy. In those patients with aortic stenosis, a characteristic bulge is seen along the right side of the ascending aorta just above the sinus of Valsalva related to poststenotic dilation. Calcification of the leaflets may occur over time so that by the age of 40 years, more than 90% of patients with aortic stenosis caused by a bicuspid valve, will have visible aortic calcification. When aortic stenosis is severe, left ventricular decompensation will occur, enlarging the left ventricular border accompanied by secondary aortic regurgitation.

Subaortic Stenosis

Obstructive and nonobstructive forms of hypertrophic cardiomyopathy are sources of left ventricular enlargement and left ventricular outflow tract obstruction. Unfortunately, the plain films in this condition are, at most, suggestive and a specific diagnosis of hypertrophic obstructive disease, cardiomyopathy is best established with MRI, ECHO, or CT. In this condition, blood flow is normal during ventricular systole, and the ascending aorta does not dilate nor does the aortic valve calcify.

Aortic Regurgitation

Aortic regurgitation may result from a variety of conditions including rheumatic valvulitis, endocarditis, and the sequel of stenotic bicuspid aortic valve. Specific dilation of the aortic annulus is found preferentially in ankylosing spondylitis, psoriatic arthritis, Marfan syndrome, and Reiter syndrome, among others (see Fig. 5-8). In rheumatic heart disease, aortic regurgitation is frequently associated with mitral disease or may, in advanced cases, involve all four cardiac valves. Occasionally, aortic regurgitation will accompany direct trauma to the aortic leaflets or may be found in association with Stanford type A aortic dissection.

The plain film radiograph in patients with aortic regurgitation will show the heart size to be normal or mildly enlarged when the regurgitant fraction is mild. However, when regurgitation is severe, increased dilation of the left ventricle is seen. In severe aortic regurgitation, the entire aorta is diffusely and often massively enlarged, unlike aortic stenosis where the ascending aorta is primarily

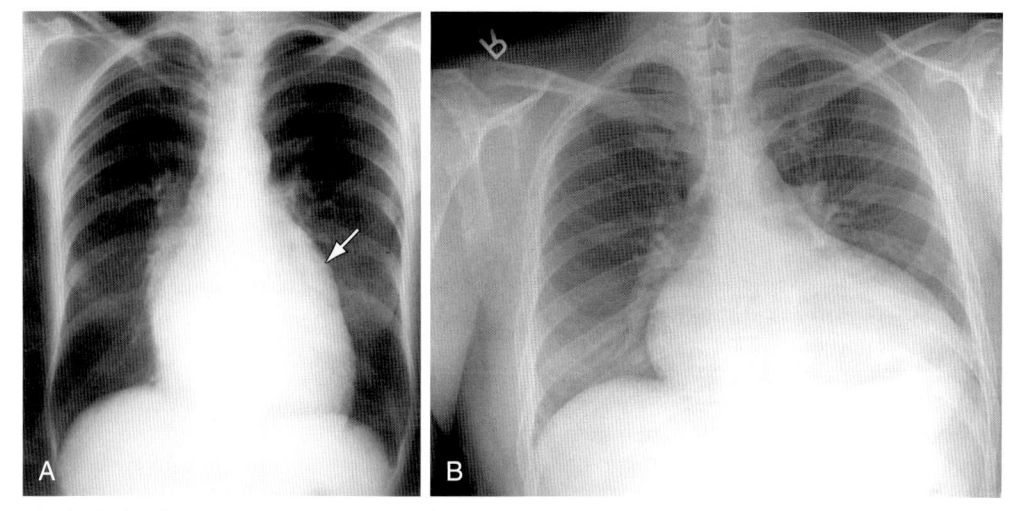

FIGURE 5-32 Mitral valvular disease. **A,** Mitral stenosis: The left atrial appendage (*arrow*) is markedly enlarged in an otherwise normal cardiac silhouette related to the weakening of the LAA owing to rheumatic carditis. **B,** Mitral regurgitation: Large cardiac silhouette is shown in this patient with severe mitral regurgitation.

involved. Where the mitral valve is regurgitant, in addition to aortic regurgitation, the left atrium may be markedly enlarged.

When aortic regurgitation occurs acutely due to infective endocarditis, trauma, or aortic dissection, the left ventricle may remain normal in size, but because end-diastolic left ventricular pressure dramatically increases, pulmonary venous hypertension will occur and pulmonary interstitial or alveolar edema may be identified. Alternatively, in chronic compensated aortic regurgitation, progressive volume overload occurs with left ventricular dilation and an increase in overall cardiac size with normal-appearing lungs.

Mitral Stenosis

Mitral stenosis is defined by a reduction of the valve area from the normal range of 4 to 6 cm^2 to less than 2 cm^2. In patients with rheumatic heart disease, by far the most common cause of mitral stenosis, isolated mitral valve involvement is most frequent. A combination of mitral and aortic valve disease is also a common finding in rheumatic carditis. Left atrial myxoma and congenital mitral disease, as well as calcified mitral annulus with extension into the valve leaflets, may be an additional source for mitral valve obstruction.

The early radiologic signs of mitral stenosis may be subtle and include mild left atrial enlargement characterized by a prominent bulge at the level of the LAA on the PA projection (see Fig. 5-31). In most patients with mitral stenosis, the left ventricular border is normal. With severe mitral stenosis, characterized by a valve area less than 1 cm^2, the LA may increase in size, but there is poor correlation between the degree of stenosis and the size of the LA chamber. In patients with rheumatic carditis, the LAA may be enlarged, but the shape of the appendage may bear no relationship to the degree of absence of associated findings such as thrombosis (Fig. 5-32). As the LA enlarges, the left main-stem bronchus may be displaced upward. The RA is displaced to the right, and pulmonary blood flow is redistributed to the upper lobes because of increased pulmonary venous pressure. The MPA is enlarged related to secondary arterial hypertension and the left ventricle and aorta are usually normal or small. The LA wall and the LAA may be calcified due to carditis or secondary to left atrial thrombus related to atrial fibrillation often found in patients with rheumatic carditis. The findings of pulmonary interstitial edema are common.

Later, hemosiderosis (Fig. 5-33) due to recurrent minute hemorrhages related to elevated capillary pressure may be associated with mitral stenosis. The pattern of pulmonary hemosiderosis is that of interstitial or miliary lung disease, most common in the mid and lower lung zones. Rarely, with chronic pulmonary interstitial edema, small puncture opacities can be found within the alveoli representing islands of bones visible as dense nodules on the chest radiograph.

Mitral Regurgitation

Acute mitral regurgitation may be related to ruptured chordae or papillary muscle dysfunction due to myocardial infarction or infective endocarditis. In acute mitral regurgitation, the heart may not be enlarged, but severe pulmonary edema is frequently visible due to left-sided heart failure. Pulmonary edema due to acute mitral regurgitation is usually symmetric. However, selective right upper lobe pulmonary edema has been described in as many as 9% of patients with either acute or chronic mitral regurgitation.[28] More than likely, this phenomenon is related to selective retrograde blood flow from the mitral valve directly into the right upper pulmonary veins.

When mitral regurgitation is chronic, it may be secondary to mitral valve prolapse, ischemic and hypertrophic cardiomyopathy, or from rheumatic heart disease. Other causes include mitral annulus calcification, collagen vascular disease, and Marfan syndrome The plain film of the chest in chronic mitral regurgitation will demonstrate both LA and LV border enlargement. In fact, the heart may be massive in size because of volume overload and increased intracardiac pressure. As the LA enlarges, it will extend toward the right and may be observed as a double shadow along the right heart border. The RA and RV may also enlarge in the patient with chronic mitral regurgitation owing to tricuspid insufficiency caused by secondary pulmonary arterial hypertension.

ISCHEMIC HEART DISEASE

Invasive coronary arteriography, radionuclide stress studies, stress ECHO, coronary artery CT, and MRI may contribute to the diagnosis of ischemic heart disease. In those patients with ischemic cardiomyopathy, the chest radiograph may be entirely normal, even in patients with severe disease. However, left ventricular enlargement and/or left ventricular aneurysm may be present. It is important to consider that if congestive heart failure persists in spite of treatment, the complications of myocardial infarction including aneurysm, pseudoaneurysm, ventricular wall, papillary muscle rupture, or interventricular septal defect may have developed.

COMPLICATIONS OF MYOCARDIAL INFARCTION

Postmyocardial infarction syndrome (Dressler syndrome) is characterized by an enlargement of the cardiac silhouette caused by pericardial effusion. Unilateral or occasionally bilateral pleural effusions are seen and lower lobe consolidation especially on the left side, may occur in up to 20% of patients. Dressler syndrome usually occurs within 2 to 6 weeks after myocardial infarction and is analogous to the postpericardiotomy syndrome seen following surgery.

Aneurysm will occur in as many as 15% of patients after myocardial infarction. It is most commonly found at the cardiac apex or along the anterior free wall of the left ventricle. The chest film may show a localized bulge along the ventricular wall near the apex and, when chronic, a thin rim of calcification may be present. The differential diagnosis of left ventricular aneurysm will include other deformities of the left heart border produced by pericardial cysts, tumor, or other mediastinal or pleural masses. CT, ECHO, and MRI will show with precision, areas of decreased contractility or paradoxical cardiac motion associated with left ventricular aneurysm.

In 0.2% of patients with a recent ventricular septal infarction, rupture of the septum may occur within 7 to 12 days after the event, leading to cardiomegaly, acute pulmonary edema, and poor myocardial contractility. When a postmyocardial infarction intraventricular septal defect occurs, there is a high mortality rate of up to 71%. An expected increase in pulmonary blood flow may not be appreciated because of superimposed pulmonary edema.

Cardiac rupture is a catastrophic complication following an acute transmural infarction. Most of these patients die immediately, but in a minority of cases, the rupture is enclosed by surrounding extracardiac soft tissues and a pseudoaneurysm develops. Although a new bulge along the left ventricular border may be observed on the plain film, pseudoaneurysms are best seen with ECHO, CT, or MRI and may be characterized by a wide neck and seen most commonly along the left ventricular posterolateral wall.[29]

In 1% of patients following myocardial infarction, papillary muscle rupture may occur. Plain film radiographs demonstrate a variety of findings including normal chest films or cardiac enlargement associated with acute pulmonary edema. MRI or ECHO will demonstrate the flail valve leaflets and estimate the mitral regurgitant.

THE CARDIOMYOPATHIES

Cardiomyopathy includes a variety of myocardial disorders of varying etiology and pathophysiology broadly classified as dilated or congestive, infiltrative, restrictive, hypertrophic, and ischemic cardiomyopathy.

In *congestive, dilated,* and *ischemic cardiomyopathy,* the chest may be normal in size and configuration or may be diffusely enlarged, resembling a large pericardial effusion. Echocardiography will demonstrate decreased ventricular contraction and enlargement of the left atrium and ventricle. MRI may reveal mitral or tricuspid regurgitation caused by dilation of the valve annulus. Left-sided and, later, biventricular failure occurs in most patients, an important predictive indicator of shortened survival time.

The radiographic appearance of *hypertrophic cardiomyopathy* is variable. Chest radiographs may demonstrate a normal heart or enlargement of the left ventricle, which can be focal or diffuse. Congenital hypertrophic cardiomyopathy is an autosomal dominant condition which may be apical, septal, or diffuse in distribution. If mitral regurgitation is present, the left atrium is also enlarged. The diagnosis of hypertrophic cardiomyopathy is usually established by ECHO or MRI, and cardiac catheterization.

Restrictive cardiomyopathy is characterized by myocardial rigidity with poor left ventricular diastolic relaxation. There are no consistent plain film features of restrictive cardiomyopathy. The heart is normal in size or may be moderately or, more rarely, markedly enlarged. The left atrium may also be enlarged when mitral regurgitation is present. Pulmonary congestion occurs in most patients and calcification of the right or left ventricular wall may develop.

INTENSIVE CARE IMAGING

The erect and supine portable chest radiographs are among the most commonly ordered examinations in a typical tertiary care medical center. In postsurgical cardiac patients and in nonsurgical patients with severe cardiac and pulmonary disease, to accurately interpret the portable chest film, special attention must be given to optimization of technique.

Technique

Appropriate film-screen combinations, computed and digital imaging, as well as careful patient positioning, are needed to overcome the effects of poor film-screen geometry, low-capacity portable equipment producing low-kilovoltage technique, and high amounts of scatter radiation and motion artifacts compared with conventional PA and lateral chest radiographs. The use of laser beam-aligned antiscatter featureless grids that require less precise geometric alignment with the x-ray source are approaches to obtain higher quality portable chest films than are possible with nongrid systems. Although conventional analog portable chest x-ray equipment continues to be the "norm," digital images provide a variety of advantages and have largely replaced analog equipment. At present, computed radiology with storage phosphor plates as the radiation detector and laser scanning of conventional film-screen radiographs are the most frequently used methods for producing digital chest images, but fully digital equipment is available and is increasingly used.[31] A major advantage of storage phosphor plates is their sensitivity over a wide range of exposures versus the much narrower exposure range of conventional x-ray film. This difference results in more consistent image quality over a wider range of exposures than is possible with analog systems. The advantage of digital systems is particularly important in portable x-ray equipment where overexposure and underexposure are ubiquitous. This improvement helps increase diagnostic accuracy and reduces the need for repeat films.[30]

When conventional erect PA films are compared with portable radiographs, the differences in cardiac size and configuration and the degree of inspiration between preoperative erect PA and postoperative supine AP films must be taken into account. An 11% increase in cardiac diameter, a 9% increase in the cardiothoracic ratio, and a 15% increase in mediastinal width have been described when an inspiratory PA film is compared with an inspiratory AP chest film. Seriously ill patients may not be able to be positioned properly because orthogonal, lordotic, and oblique films with disturbing motion artifacts along with a host of visually disturbing devices, lines, and catheters, increase conspicuity and blunt the ability of the observer to make an accurate diagnosis.

After cardiac surgery, a daily morning film exposed in the ICU following a predetermined protocol is often taken. It has been suggested that daily films in these subsets of postoperative patients are justified, especially in those with endotracheal (ET) tubes and Swan-Ganz catheters. In the postoperative period, other critical care films, chest radiographs, a myriad of tubes, wires, catheters, and other devices are present in or overlie the postoperative chest (Table 5-1) (Fig. 5-33).[31,32] These devices include ET tube, which should be positioned in the mid-trachea 5 ± 2 cm above the carina to allow excursion with flexion and extension of the neck. If the ET tube lies too close to the carina, flexion of the head or neck may force the distal end of the tube into one of the main-stem bronchi causing varying degrees of atelectasis of the opposite lung and barotrauma if assisted ventilation is used. If the tube is too high, pulmonary aspiration is increased. In spite of close observation, up to 15% of patients have significant malposition of the ET tube following cardiac procedures. It is also important to observe for overinflation of the endotracheal cuff, which may lead to tracheal injury.

The CVP catheter is best positioned between the most proximal valve of the subclavian vein and the RA within

TABLE 5-1 Cardiovascular and Pulmonary Devices and Other Appliances in the ICU Patient

- Amplatz septal occluders
- Arterial stents and grafts
- Central venous pressure catheters
- Implantable pacemakers, generators, and leads
- Interaortic balloon catheters
- Left ventricular assistance devices (LVAD)
- Nasogastric and feeding tubes
- PICC and subclavian catheters
- Prosthetic valves and rings
- Saphenous graft rings
- Sternotomy wires, retention sutures
- Swan-Ganz catheters
- Tracheostomy and endotracheal appliances

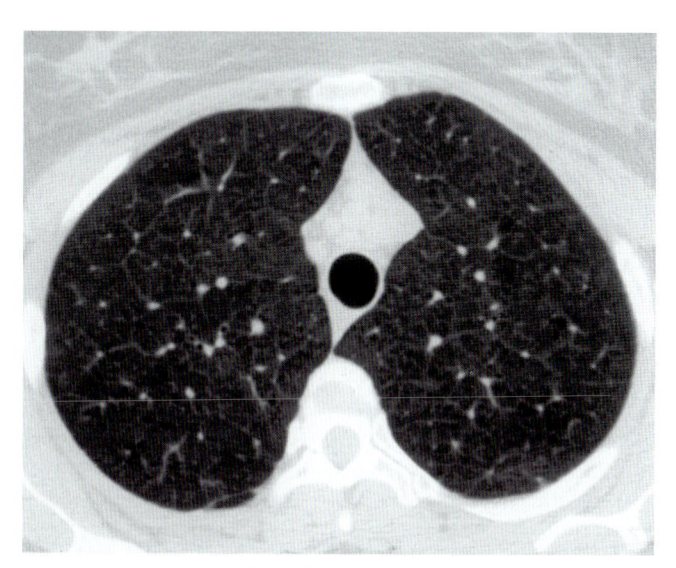

FIGURE 5-33 Nonenhanced axial CT using lung windows demonstrates the lacelike pattern of interstitial lung disease compatible with hemosiderosis of the lung, secondary to long-standing mitral stenosis.

the SVC. When the distal tip is found in the RA, pressure measurements are accurate, but the risk of perforation of the thin-walled cardiac chamber is increased.

Peripherally inserted central catheters (PICC) are frequently introduced after cardiac surgery. They are small-caliber tubes placed under sterile conditions usually in the interventional radiology suite. A major advantage of PICC is that they may be left in place for long periods. A Swan-Ganz catheter is usually placed in either major pulmonary artery (ideally with the tip lying within a proximal pulmonary artery 2 to 3 cm distal to the bifurcation) to monitor pulmonary artery or pulmonary capillary wedge pressure and to obtain mixed venous blood samples. After placement, the tip can be floated distally to a wedged position, whereon the balloon is inflated. If the catheter is too peripheral in position, the inflated balloon near the tip of the catheter may damage the pulmonary artery wall and produce a perforation leading to hemorrhage or pseudoaneurysm.

When circulatory assistance is needed, a sausage-shaped intra-aortic counterpulsation balloon (IACB) is positioned just below the level of the LSCA within the proximal descending aorta. Careful placement of the IACB is critical to avoid occluding the subclavian or renal arteries. Left ventricular assistance device leads, prosthetic valves, and implantable cardioverter-defibrillators are frequently placed in a hospital with a busy cardiac surgical service and careful observation for lead or component malposition, pouch infection, or fracture is necessary. A nasogastric tube is also usually present. It may be inadvertently placed in a bronchus and pass into the lung or even the pleura. When malposition of a nasogastric tube is not quickly recognized, aspiration may occur, causing a chemical pulmonary edema or pneumonia.

Early recognition of the normal and abnormal positions of the large number of catheters, wires, and tubes found on the postoperative chest radiograph requires rapid interpretation by an observer thoroughly familiar with the appearance of the postoperative chest radiograph and the possible complications that may frequently occur.

The Early Postoperative Chest Radiograph

The portable chest film obtained on the first day following cardiac surgery usually exhibits varying degrees of left and right lower lobe atelectasis, mediastinal widening, pulmonary edema, and pleural effusion.[33,34] Unilateral or bilateral lower lobe atelectasis, usually accompanied by small pleural effusions, is the source of the lower lung zone opacities found in almost all cardiac surgery patients within 8 hours after surgery, and these usually clear within 5 to 7 days. Lower lobe atelectasis may be confused with a bacterial pneumonia, but pneumonia is much less common immediately following cardiac surgery.[35] Left lower lobe atelectasis is more common than right-sided atelectasis because of paralysis of the phrenic nerve caused by cardioplegic solutions or crushed ice administered for myocardial preservation or retained secretions. Other causes of postoperative left lower lobe atelectasis include dependent pooling of secretions, preferential suctioning of the right main-stem bronchi, and compression from the cardiac insulation pad used during surgery.[36]

Pleural Effusion

Pleural effusion is manifested radiographically as blunting of the costophrenic angle, loss of sharpness of the diaphragmatic contour, and increased opacity behind the dome of the diaphragm. It may be difficult to identify in a supine film but should be easily recognized on an erect bedside radiograph.[37]

The development of pleural effusions after surgery is probably related to pericardial fluid that leaks into the pleural space through the surgically created pericardial defect or to irritation of the pleura during the procedure. Postpericardiotomy syndrome and congestive heart failure are additional sources of pleural effusion in some patients and increasingly larger or persistent pleural fluid collections may be due to hemomediastinum.

Patchy diffuse consolidation in both lungs after cardiac surgery is usually caused by pulmonary edema. Pulmonary edema from increased capillary permeability or adult respiratory distress syndrome is common after cardiac surgery and is caused by release of vasoactive substances during cardiopulmonary bypass that affect capillary permeability. Pulmonary edema usually occurs within 2 days of surgery and is reversible with supportive therapy, including diuretics. Postperfusion pulmonary edema occurs after cardiopulmonary bypass because of a pooling of fluid in the extravascular space. The mechanism for postperfusion pulmonary edema is thought to be related to the contact of circulating blood with foreign surfaces during the bypass procedure. Cardiac failure following cardiac bypass surgery occurs in patients with poor cardiac output. Typically, vascular redistribution to the upper lobes, septal lines, small bilateral pleural effusions, and the patchy opacities resulting from pulmonary edema are present in patients with heart failure.

Other early radiographic findings following cardiac surgery identified on the AP portable chest radiograph include pneumopericardium, sternal dehiscence, pulmonary embolism pneumothorax, mediastinal hematoma, pneumomediastinum, and subcutaneous emphysema. Rib fractures occur in 2% to 4% of patients, causing chest pain which may be confused with angina, pulmonary embolism, or aortic dissection.[38]

Pneumothorax is often difficult to identify in a supine patient. Unlike pneumothorax in the PA erect film, where the crisp opaque line of the visceral pleura located medial to the rib cage is diagnostic, in the supine position, a pneumothorax appears as a poorly defined lucency overlying the lower lung zones. Decubitus views are helpful in clearly defining the presence of a pleural air collection.

Mediastinal Hemorrhage

Widening of the mediastinum because of postoperative bleeding is common after cardiac surgery. Typically, the mediastinum is widened by up to 35% of the presurgical mediastinal width in comparison with the preoperative PA chest film. Katzberg and associates found that if the mediastinum is widened more than 70%, surgery is usually required to excavate the hematoma.[37] It is important to consider that bleeding may be present without visible mediastinal widening, especially if the patient is undergoing positive end-expiratory pressure support, which may compress the mediastinum. Some patients may have a wide mediastinum but remain hemodynamically stable, have no significant bloody drainage, and do not require reoperation.

KEY POINTS

- Plain film imaging of the heart is particularly helpful for the evaluation of the effects of cardiac disease on the nearby lung and pleura.
- It is essential to appreciate the contour of the mediastinum in both the normal patient and in the patient with a variety of cardiac abnormalities to take full advantage of the plain chest radiograph.
- Recognition of the patterns of calcification of the cardiac valves, the myocardium, the pericardium, great vessels, and coronary arteries will help identify important cardiac disease.

SUGGESTED READINGS

Bettman MA. The chest radiograph. In Braunwald E, Zipes DP, Libby P (eds). Heart Disease: A Textbook of Cardiovascular Medicine, 8th ed. Philadelphia, WB Saunders, 2008, pp 327-343.

Chen JTT. Essentials of Cardiac Imaging, 2nd ed. Philadelphia, Lippin-cott-Raven, 1997.

Gatzoulis M, Webb G, Daubeney P, Diagnosis and Management of Adult Congenital Heart Disease. Churchill Livingstone, London, 2003.

Gowda RM, Boxt L. Calcification of the heart. Radiol Clin North Am 2004;42:603-617.

Jefferson K, Rees S. Clinical Cardiac Radiology, 2nd ed. Butterworth, London, 1980.

Miller SW. The Requisites: Cardiac Radiology, 2nd ed. Mosby-Elsevier. Philadelphia, 2003.

Milne ENC, Pistolessi M. Reading the Chest Radiograph: A Physiologic Approach. St. Louis, Mosby—Yearbook, 1993, pp 9-50.

Perloff JK: Clinical Recognition of Congenital Heart Disease, 5th ed. WB Saunders, Philadelphia, 2003.

Reddy G, Steiner RM. Cardiac Imaging Case Review Series, Philadelphia, Mosby-Elsevier, 2006.

Steiner RM, Rao VM. Radiology of the Pericardium. In Grainger RG, Allison DJ (eds). Diagnostic Radiology, London, Churchill Livingstone, 1991, pp 675-689.

REFERENCES

1. Steiner RM, Gross GW, Flicker S, et al: Congenital heart disease in the adult patient: The value of plain film chest radiology. J Thorac Imaging 1995; 10:1-26.
2. Steiner RM. Radiology of the heart and great vessels. In Braunwald E, Zipes DP, Libby P (eds). Heart Disease: A textbook of Cardiovascular Medicine. 6th ed. Philadelphia, WB Saunders, 2001, pp 237-272.
3. Henry DA. Radiologic evaluation of the patient after cardiac surgery. Radiol Clin North Am 1996; 34:119-135.
4. Henschke C, Yankelevitz DF, Wand A, et al: Accuracy and efficiency of chest radiography in the intensive care unit. Radiol Clin North Am 1996; 34:21-27.
5. Robinson AE: The lateral chest film: Is it doomed to extinction? Acad Radiol 5:322, 1998.
6. Freeman V, Mutatir C, Pretorius M: Evaluation of left ventricular enlargement in the lateral position of the chest using the Hoffman-Rigler sign. Cardiovasc J S Africa 2003; 14:134-136.
7. Morgan PW, Goodman LR, Aprahamian C, et al. Evaluation of traumatic aortic injury: Does dynamic contrast enhanced CT play a role? Radiology 1992; 182:661-666.
8. Kabala JE, Wilde P: Measurement of heart size in the anteroposterior chest radiograph. Br J Radiol 1987; 60:981-985.
9. Van der Jagt EJ, Smits HJ: Cardiac size in the supine chest film. Eur J Radiol 1992; 14:173-176.
10. Rubinowitz A, Siegel M, Tocino I. Thoracic imaging in the ICU. Critical Care Clinics. 2007; 23:539-573.
11. Wang ZJ, Reddy GP, Gotway MB, et al. CT and MR imaging of pericardial disease. Radiographics 2003; 23:S167.
12. Vaitkus P, Kussmaul W: Constrictive pericarditis versus restrictive cardiomyopathy: A reappraisal and update of diagnostic criteria. Am Heart J 1991; 122:1431.
13. Vogel M, Berger F, Kramer A, et al. Incidence of secondary pulmonary hypertension in adults with atrial septal or sinus venosus defects. Heart 1999; 82:30-33.
14. Ely EW, Hoponik EF. Using the chest radiograph to determine intravascular volume status: the role of the vascular pedicle width. Chest 2002; 121:942-950.
15. Ketai LH, Goodwin JD: A new view of pulmonary edema and acute respiratory distress syndrome: state of the art. J Thorac Imaging 1998; 131:147-171.
16. Morgan PW, Goodman LR: Pulmonary edema and acute respiratory distress syndrome. Radiol Clin North Am 1991; 29:943-963.
17. Stern EJ, Muller NL, Swensen SJ, Hartman TE: CT mosaic pattern of lung attenuation: etiologies and terminology. J Thorac Imaging 1995; 10:294-297.
18. Rodan BA, Chen JTT, Halber MD, et al: Chest roentgenographic evaluation of the severity of aortic stenosis. Invest Radiol 1980; 15:416-442.
19. Li J, Galvin HK, Johnson SC, et al. Aortic calcification on plain film radiography increases risk for coronary artery disease. Chest 2002; 121:1468-1471.
20. Feuchtner GM. The utility of computed tomography in the context of aortic valve disease. Int J Cardiovasc Imaging 2009; 6:611-614.
21. Stanford W, Thompson BH: Imaging of coronary artery calcification: Its importance in assessing atherosclerotic disease. Radiol Clin North Am 1999; 37:257-272.
22. Perloff J. Congenital heart disease in the adult: clinical approach. J Thorac Imaging 1994; 9:260.
23. Ferguson EC, Krishnamurthy R, Oldham SAA. Classic imaging signs of congenital cardiovascular abnormalities. Radiographics 2007; 27: 1323-1334.
24. Yuan SM, Raanani I. Late Complications of coarctation of the aorta. Cardiol J 2008; 15:517-524.
25. Greenberg SB, Balsara R, Faerber E. Coarctation of the aorta:diagnostic imaging after corrective surgery. J Thorac Imaging 1995; 10:36.
26. Itoey ET, Gopalan D, Ganesh V, et al. Atrial septal defects: magnetic resonance and computed tomography appearances. J Med Imaging Radiat Oncol 2009; 53:261-270.
27. Boxt LM. CT of valvular heart disease. Int J Cardiovasc Imaging 2005; 21:105-113.
28. Agesilas F, Herblard A, Valentino P, et al. Right upper lobe pulmonary edema as a consequence of mitral regurgitation. Am J Emerg Med 2007; 25:196-197.
29. Oliva P, Hammill S, Edwards WC: Cardiac rupture, a clinically predictable complication of acute myocardial infarction: Report of 70 cases with clinicopathologic correlations. J Am Coll Cardiol 1993; 22:720-726.
30. Nicklason L, Chan H-P, Cascade P, et al. Portable chest imaging: comparison of storage phosphor digital, asymmetric screen-film and conventional screen-film radiography. Radiology 1993; 186:387-392.
31. Krivopal M, Shlobin DA, Schwartzstein RM. Utility of daily portable chest radiographs in mechanically ventilated patients in the medical ICU. Chest 2003; 123:1607-1614.
32. Barge-Caballero E, Estevez-Cid F, Bouzas-Mosquera A, et al. Chest radiography of life supporting interventions. Lancet 2009;374:476.
33. Graham R, Meziane M, Rice J, et al. Postoperative portable chest radiographs: Optimum use in thoracic surgery. J Thorac Cardiovasc Surg 1998; 115:45.
34. O'Brien W, Karski J, Cheng D, et al. Routine chest roentgenography on admission to the intensive care unit after heart operations: Is it of value? J Thorac Cardiovasc Surg 1997; 113:130.
35. Henry D. Radiologic evaluation of the patient after cardiac surgery. Radiol Clin North Am 1996; 34:119.
36. Landay M, Mootz A, Estrera A: Apparatus seen on chest radiographs after cardiac surgery in adults. Radiology 1990; 174:477.
37. Katzberg R, Whitehouse G, deWeese J: The early radiologic findings in the adult chest after cardiopulmonary bypass surgery. Cardiovasc Radiol 1978; I:205.
38. Sommer T, Fehske W, Holzknecht N, et al. Aortic dissection: a comparative study of diagnosis with spiral CT, multiplanar transesophageal echocardiography and MR imaging. Radiology 1996; 199:347-352.

CHAPTER 6

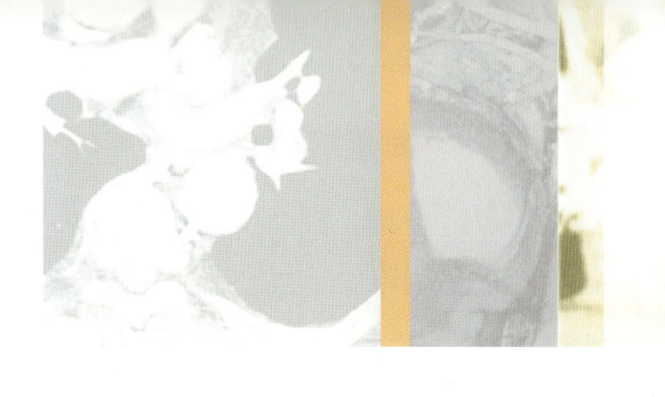

Echocardiography

Theodore P. Abraham and Aurélio C. Pinheiro

INTRODUCTION

Since the first mitral valve movements registered with the use of ultrasound by Edler and Hertz in 1954, echocardiography has reached an amazing technologic improvement and can be considered the main diagnostic imaging modality for cardiac diseases.

The principle of echocardiography analysis is based on the construction of images from the reflected ultrasound waves by normal or abnormal cardiac structures. Ultrasound transducers generate higher frequency sound waves that are inaudible to humans. High frequency transducers (e.g., 5 MHz or 7.5 MHz) are used in the pediatric population because the penetration is shallower and the images are high-resolution quality compared with the 2 MHz or 2.5 MHz typically used in adult patients.

There are two types of ultrasound images: the *fundamental* and the *harmonic*. The first type is generated from reflected ultrasound waves by cardiac structures in the same frequency they were transmitted by the transducer. When specific cardiac structures or other elements such as micro-bubbles (used for specific cardiac diagnostic situations) are imaged, they reflect the ultrasound wave in a different frequency compared to the transmitted one, and certain types of transducers are capable of processing different reflected frequency that improved image quality. Because myocardial tissue can itself reflect in a higher frequency than that transmitted, endocardial border delineation is better using harmonic imaging.

DESCRIPTION OF TECHNICAL REQUIREMENTS

Because the quality of an ultrasound study is operator dependent, it is highly recommended that the operator have a solid knowledge of ultrasound physics and the various options available on the ultrasound equipment used.

Moreover, information such as patient identification, blood pressure measurements, any other specific clinical condition during which the study is recorded (e.g., the use of a specific drug, electrocardiogram tracing) are all necessary for a clear understanding of the problem to be studied. Specific details regarding each of the echocardiography techniques are discussed below.

Techniques

M Mode

The M (for *motion*) mode consists of a graphic in which it is possible to analyze the motion of cardiac structures over time. It is necessary for the correct position of a cursor line along the anatomic cardiac structure to be studied and this cursor line has its origin point at the ultrasound transducer itself. Errors in measurements with M mode are possible because some planes might be in an oblique orientation. This can be corrected with the anatomic M mode, an adjustable cursor line (angle up to 180 degrees), available in actual echocardiograph machines. The M mode is used for cardiac dimensions, subtle cardiac motion abnormalities, and assessment other time-related parameters (Fig. 6-1).

Two-Dimensional Mode (2D Mode)

With the 2D mode it is possible to get real images of the heart in motion and it can be used as a reference for the M mode discussed previously. There are four basic thoracic positions used to get 2D images: parasternal, apical, subcostal, and suprasternal. The parasternal and apical are obtained with the patient in the left lateral position; for the subcostal and suprasternal, the patient lies in supine position. All different planes are obtained with simple tilting and twisting of the probe (Fig. 6-2).

Doppler Echocardiography and Color Flow Imaging

Doppler echocardiography uses ultrasound waves to calculate blood flow velocities based on the way the

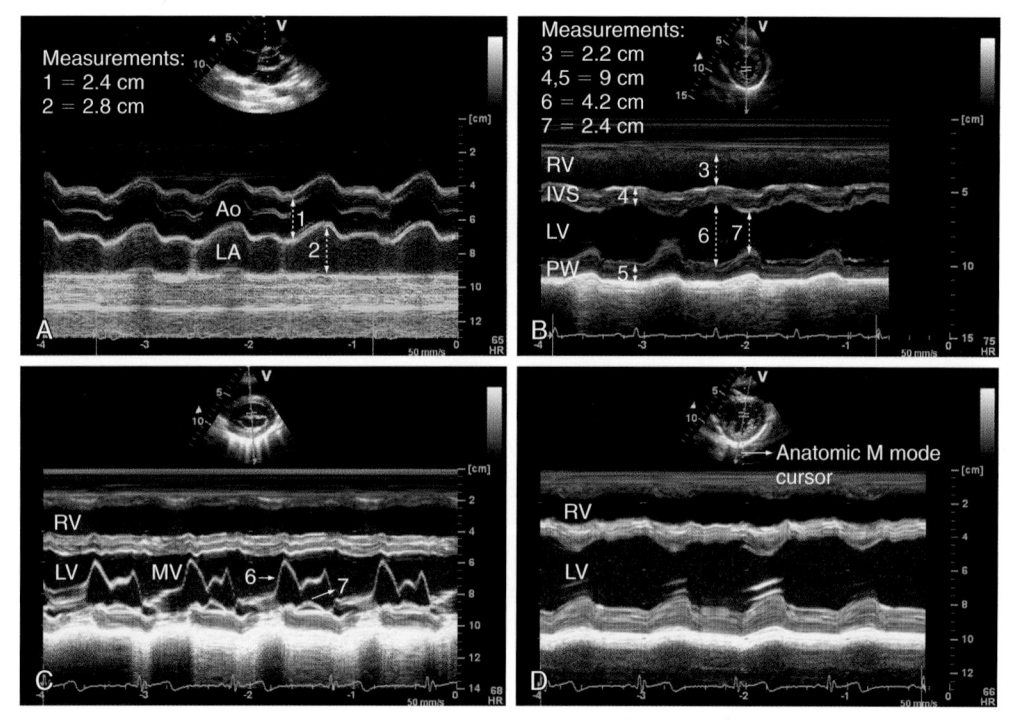

■ **FIGURE 6-1** Pictures of M mode tracings, showing small two dimensional images of short axis view on the top as a reference and the M mode cursor (*green arrow*). **A**, aortic root and left atrial chamber. **B**, left ventricle at mitral valve level. **C**, left ventricle at papillary muscle level (mid level). **D**, mid left ventricle view using anatomic M mode with twisting of the cursor 10 degrees clockwise. Refer to image **B** for references on plane view levels (*white lines*). Left ventricle mass calculation is possible with the interventricular septum and posterior wall thickness and the chamber internal dimensions measured as shown in **B**; in the formula, the numbers are in centimeters LV mass = $0.8 \times \{1.04[(LVDD + PWT + SWT)3 - (LVDD)3]\} + 0.6$ g = $0.8 \times \{1.04 [(4.2 + 0.9 + 0.9)3 - (4.2)3]\} + 0.6 = 242$ g. Ao, aortic root; IVS, interventricular septum; LA, left atrium; RV, right ventricle; LV, left ventricle; LVDD, LV diastolic diameter; MV, mitral valve; PW, posterior wall; PWT, posterior wall thickness; SWT, septal wall thickness; AL and PL, anterior and posterior mitral valve leaflets line tracings.

flowing blood reflects the ultrasound waves. The reflected ultrasound frequency is higher when the blood flows toward the transducer, and the opposite effect is true when it flows away from the transducer. One important aspect of the way Doppler works is the angle of interrogation. The more parallel the reflected waves to the transducer, the higher the reflected sound waves (called Doppler shift) and the peak velocities. *Pulsed* wave Doppler uses only one crystal to transmit and receive the reflected frequency. This kind of Doppler is used to study lower blood flow velocities such as mitral and tricuspid diastolic flows. The *continuous* wave Doppler uses one crystal to send and another one to receive the sound frequency from the blood and it can measure highest velocities along the way of its beam, such as the flow through a stenotic aortic valve. The color flow Doppler uses the same principle as the pulsed wave Doppler, with the difference being for the several sampling sites along multiple ultrasound beams, so it can analyze the blood flow in different velocities, directions, and extent of turbulence. The flow is coded in multiple colors: blue for the flow going away from the transducer and red if it is coming toward the transducer. Properly configured, the green color can also show turbulence and its extent.

Important hemodynamic information can be obtained by using 2D and Doppler techniques but none of them, not even the invasive approach, is perfect, being influenced by several other hemodynamic factors. Flow velocities can be converted to pressure gradients by using the modified Bernoulli equation[1]:

$$\text{Pressure gradient} = 4 \times v^2$$

where v is peak velocity. It is modified because several other elements can be ignored such as the velocity proximal to a fixed orifice and also flow acceleration and viscous friction. The pressure gradient obtained by this equation represents the instantaneous gradient, which is different from the peak-to-peak pressure measurement in the catheterization (cath) lab because those two peaks are not simultaneous. Several pressure measurements can be made using this equation such as: aortic stenosis gradient, right ventricle systolic pressure, pulmonary end-diastolic and mean arterial pressure, left atrial systolic pressure, and left ventricular end-diastolic pressure.

With the use of Doppler, it is also possible to obtain the stroke volume and cardiac output based on the equation that uses the hydraulic orifice formula, which is[1]:

$$\text{Flow rate} = \text{cross sectional area (CSA)} \times \text{flow velocity}$$

The flow velocity is given by the sum of all instantaneous velocities of the curve by Doppler tracings, after tracing the area enclosed by the baseline and the Doppler spectrum. The CSA is given by the assumption that the orifice is a perfect circle so the diameter is measured and applied in the equation:

$$\text{CSA} = (D/2)^2 \times \pi = D^2 \times 0.785$$

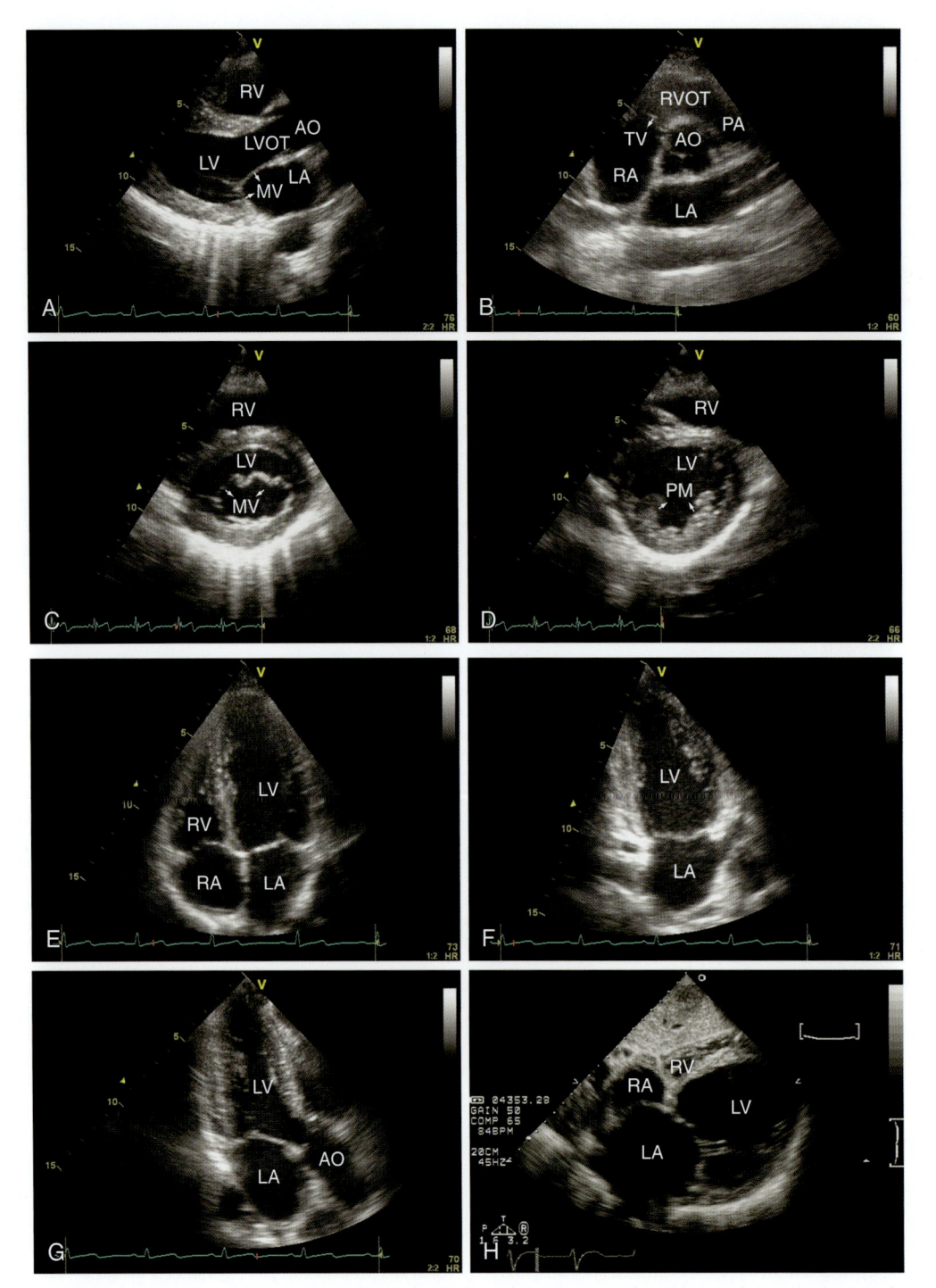

FIGURE 6-2 Basic plane views for transthoracic echocardiography: **A** through **D**: Parasternal position. **A**, long axis view. **B**, short axis view, aortic valve level. **C**, short axis view of basal left ventricle with opened mitral valve. **D**, short axis view of left ventricle, at papillary muscles level (mid left ventricle). **E**, **F**, and **G**: apical view images. **E**, apical four-chamber view. **F**, two-chamber view. **G**, three-chamber view. **H**, subcostal view. AO, aorta; ASC Ao, ascending aorta; DESC Ao, descending aorta; LV, left ventricle; LVOT, LV outflow tract; MV, mitral valve; PA, pulmonary artery; PM, papillary muscles; RV, right ventricle; RVOT, RV outflow tract; TV, tricuspid valve.

in which "D" means diameter. To calculate the systolic volume, the left ventricular outflow tract (LVOT) area is used in the first equation. And then, to get the cardiac output, the systolic volume is multiplied by the heart rate. Any flow across an orifice in the heart can be calculated using this method. Hence, it is possible to get the right ventricular outflow tract (RVOT) flow and, together with the LVOT flow, to get the ratio between pulmonary and systemic flows—important in some quantification of severity in congenital abnormalities. This method is also useful to obtain the regurgitant volume across a heart valve, such as mitral or aortic regurgitation (Fig. 6-3).

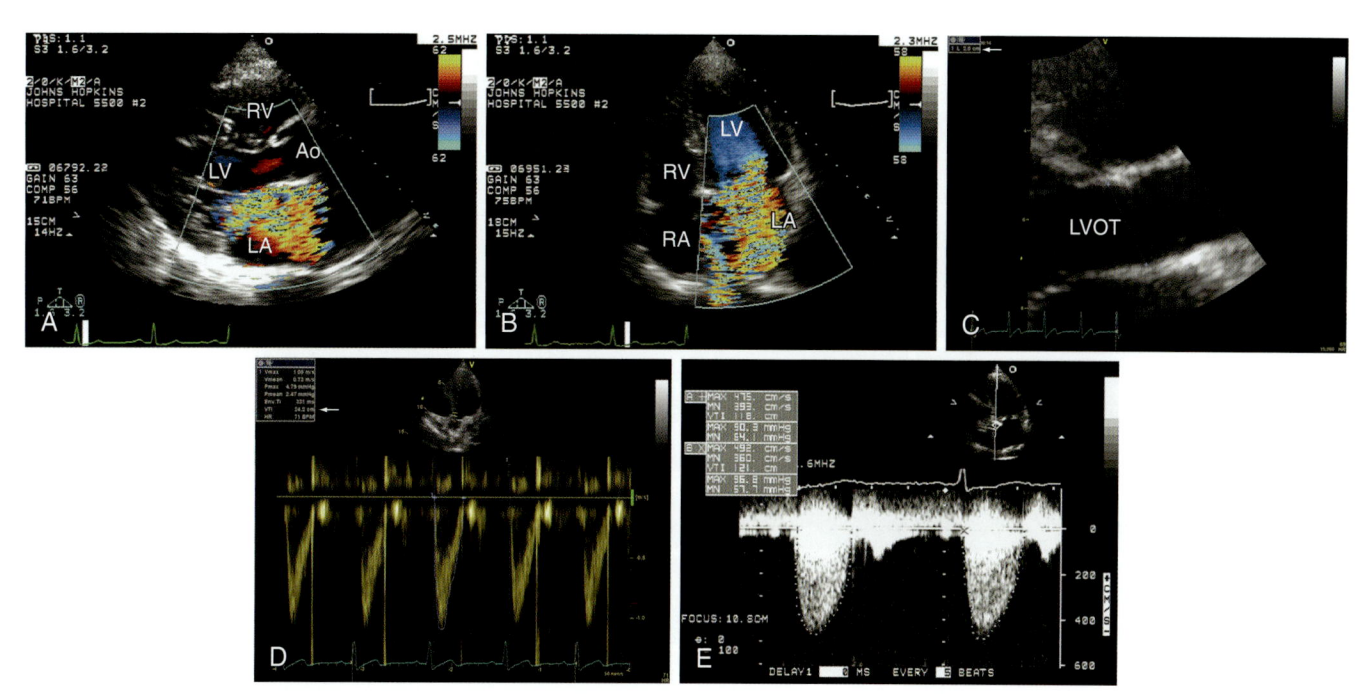

FIGURE 6-3 **A** and **B**, color Doppler images of mitral regurgitation. The predominant *blue* color is the regurgitant jet going toward the anterior left atrial wall in parasternal long axis view (**A**) and filling almost the entire left atrial chamber in the four-chamber view (**B**). **C** and **D**, stroke volume calculations. **C**, left ventricle outflow tract (LVOT) diameter measurement (*white arrow*). **D**, Pulsed wave Doppler curve tracings in LVOT showing velocity-time integral (VTI) value after curve being manually traced (*white arrow*). Using the equation *Flow Rate = Cross Sectional Area × Flow Velocity =* $D^2 \times 0.785 \times VTI = 2.02 \times 0.785 \times 24.2 = 3.14 \times 24.2 = 76$ mL. **E**, pressure gradients calculations using the modified Bernoulli equation in an aortic stenosis gradient curve. Second curve showing 492 cm/s peak velocity or 4.92 m/s. According to the formula *Pressure Gradient* $= 4 \times v^2 = 4 \times (4.92)^2 = 4 \times 24.2 = 96.8$ mm Hg. Ao, aorta; LA, left atrium; LV, left ventricle; RA, right atrium; RV, right ventricle.

Transesophageal Echocardiography (TEE)

Since its first use, TEE has been considered not only an accessory imaging technique but in some circumstances, it is the main imaging modality for cardiac diagnoses, such as mitral valve disease, aortic dissection, endocarditis and its complications, atrial septum defects, cardiac tumors, and electrophysiology studies monitoring. In patients with atrial fibrillation, TEE information can be decisive in the choice of treatment.

The TEE uses a gastroesophageal endoscopy probe modified with a 7 to 10 MHz transducer on the tip. The study technique consists of inserting the probe through the esophagus, making it possible to get high resolution images of the heart. The study is performed in a special room, with emergency-trained personnel, suction and oxygen devices, and all necessary resuscitation equipment. The probe then can be anteflexed and retroflexed, moved from side to side, rotated clockwise and counterclockwise manually and the planes can be moved from 0 to 180 degrees wide with the touch of one button (Fig. 6-4).

Three-Dimensional Echocardiography (3D)

The 3D images are possible with the use of special transducers in which about 3000 elements are enclosed. These transducers can provide a pyramidal image of a heart section with most cardiac structures included. The images are acquired in several heart beats and the patient must hold the breath during image acquisition. With software and hardware improvements, it is possible to change between 2D and 3D modes using the same probe and to get specific views using different reference points for the final image reconstruction. The 3D image set can be used for volume and mass calculations as well as improved evaluation of congenital heart defects, heart valve diseases, and left ventricular (LV) dyssynchrony.

Intracardiac Echocardiogaphy (ICE)

By using small diameter probes, it is possible to get intracardiac images. These probes are inserted until they reach the right atrium, from which all the image planes are made, and because those probes are multifrequency they have capabilities of complete 2D and Doppler study. The great advantage of ICE is for interventional studies such as transcatheter closure device placement for atrial septum defects, including a more detailed study of the defect, its size, and associated congenital defects such as pulmonary vein anatomy, and the margins of the defect—all this information being useful to predict the success of the closure. Ablation procedures, such as pulmonary vein isolation for atrial flutter, with better visualization of the tissue for radiofrequency energy application, avoids complications such as pulmonary valve stenosis owing to inadvertent ablation.

Indications

In the following sections, the most important clinical situations for the use of echocardiography will be discussed, including transthoracic and transesophageal echocardiography, as well as other techniques.

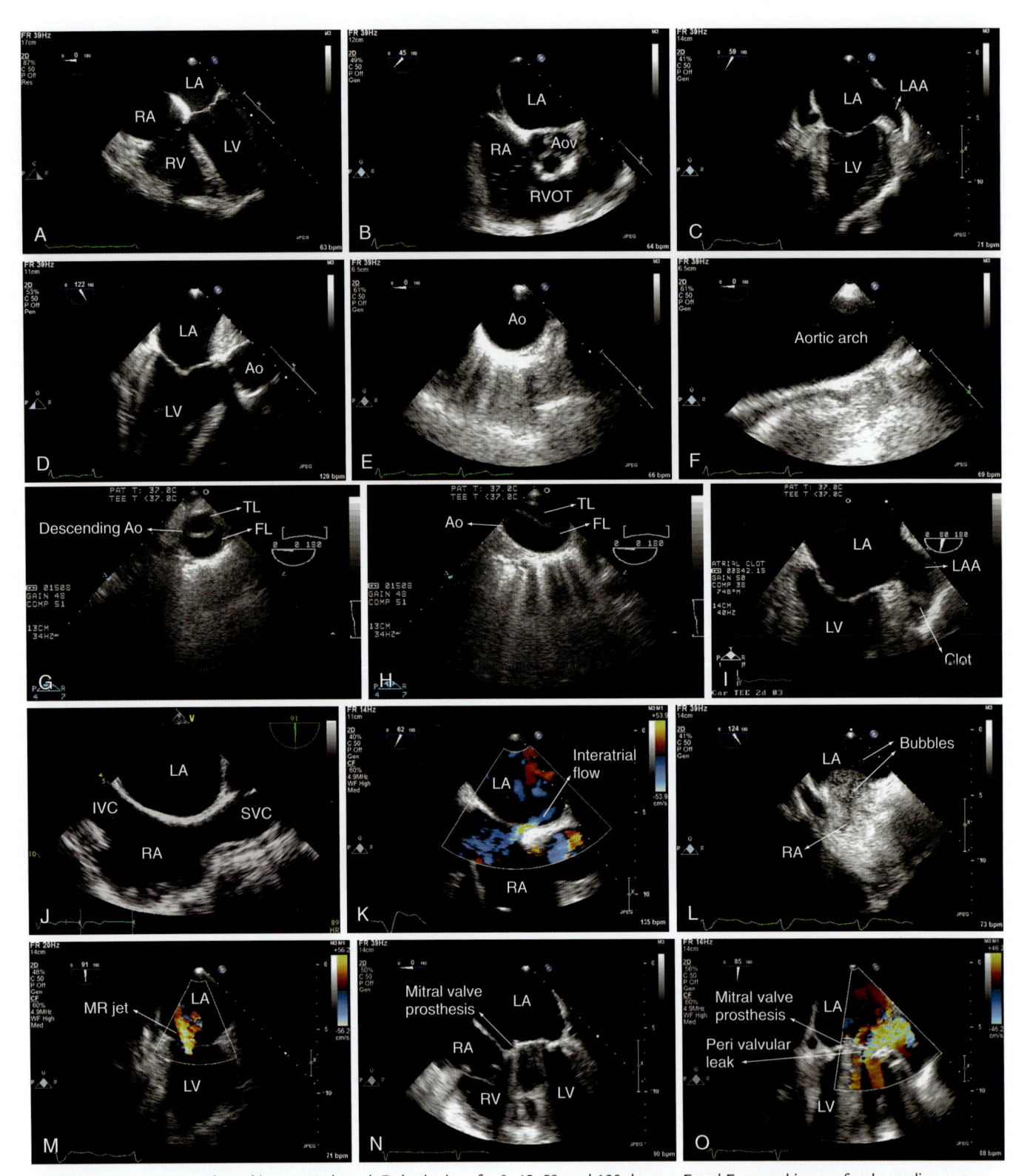

FIGURE 6-4 Transesophageal images. **A** through **D**, basic views for 0, 45, 59, and 120 degrees. **E** and **F**, normal images for descending aorta and aortic arch. **G** and **H**, examples of aortic dissection. **I**, clot in left atrial appendage. **J**, normal view of interatrial septum. **K** and **L**, image of a patent foramen ovale shown in a color Doppler study and after injection of saline contrast, with the bubbles being demonstrated in left atrium just after the contrast fills the right atrium. **M**, image of a mitral regurgitation with the jet in *red/orange* directed toward the left atrium. **N**, image of mitral valve mechanical prosthesis, with the reverberation shadow in the left ventricle. **O**, perivalvular leak in a mitral mechanical valve prosthesis, with the jet in turbulence in *blue* and *yellow* colors. Ao, aorta; AoV, aortic valve; FL, false lumen; IVC, inferior vena cava; LA, left atrium; LAA, left atrial appendage; LV, left ventricle; MR, mitral regurgitation; RA, right atrium; RV, right ventricle; RVOT, right ventricle outflow tract; TL, true lumen.

Systolic Function and Quantification of Cardiac Chambers

The 2D echocardiography is the main tool for the evaluation of systolic function and chamber quantification, even considering the newer techniques such as 3D echocardiography, tissue Doppler, strain and strain rate imaging. With 2D images of the LV it is possible to analyze the thickening of ventricular walls and provide not only a subjective evaluation of LV function but also the quantitative assessment, which can be done by calculating changes in size and volume of the chamber. The systolic function is crucial for guiding the patient's treatment and prognosis; the evaluation of regional contractility is important for patients with suspected or diagnosed coronary heart disease.

Left ventricle. The LV size can be obtained by the 2D image of parasternal short axis view and the M mode for that plane at the level of the papillary muscles or from the long axis view. This method can be used for normal hearts or with no regional wall motion abnormalities and the mass also can be calculated from the measurements of the interventricular septum and posterior wall thickness. LV function is calculated from the diastolic and systolic diameters and also by the Simpson method. From the diameter values, it is possible to calculate the fractional shortening, the percentage change in LV dimensions, by the following formula:

$$\text{Fractional Shortening} = \text{LVEDD} - \text{LVESD}/\text{LVEDD} \times 100\%$$

in which LVEDD means left ventricular end-diastolic diameter and LVESD means left ventricular end-systolic diameter. The Simpson method can be used to obtain LV volumes and then the calculated ejection fraction (EF) by the following formula[2]:

$$\text{Ejection Fraction} = \text{End Diastolic Volume (EDV)} - \text{End Systolic Volume (ESV)}/\text{EDV}.$$

Regional wall motion analysis is the most important tool for the evaluation and diagnosis of patients with suspected or confirmed coronary heart disease. For this purpose, the LV is divided into 16 segments. First into three levels: basal, mid, and apical. The basal and mid levels have six segments: antero-septum, anterior, lateral, posterior, inferior, infero-septum; and the apex is then divided into four segments being the anterior, lateral, inferior, and septum. There was only 1 change for an additional "apical cap" segment by the Association Writing Group on Myocardial Segmentation for Cardiac Imaging with the total of 17 segments.[3] Each segment is scored according to its contractility: 1-normal; 2-hypokinesis; 3-akinesis, 4-dyskinesis, and 5-aneurysmal. Each value of each segment is summed and the total is divided by the number of segments analyzed for the wall motion score index (WMSI), being normal if equal to 1.

Right ventricle (RV). The RV size is best measured from the apical four-chamber view and its thickness from the subcostal view at the peak R on the ECG. RV size is useful to detect volume and/or pressure overload and can be accompanied by RV wall thickness higher than 5 mm, the abnormal value.[2]

Left atrium (LA). The left atrium size is measured from the parasternal long axis view (PLAX) at end systole. This view can provide some underestimation on the chamber size because the LA can enlarge longitudinally. Because of this aspect of LA diameter, the best method is to calculate its volume from two orthogonal apical views using one of the four methods available (Fig. 6-5).[2]

Diastolic Function

With the increase in aging population and the options of treatment of several cardiac diseases, especially hypertension and coronary heart disease, diastolic heart failure is becoming more prevalent and it is important to correctly evaluate those patients. The majority of those patients have symptoms of heart failure but not necessarily systolic dysfunction and this is the reason myocardial relaxation abnormalities must be completely studied with available Doppler techniques. Not only the study of flow velocities through the mitral and tricuspid valves and central veins, but also the additional information on how myocardial tissue changes, by using tissue Doppler tracings, makes the use of echocardiography a powerful option in this setting. Increment value can be included if 2D findings are associated, such as the increase in LA diameter, LV thickness (e.g., hypertension, hypertrophic cardiomyopathy [HCM], obesity).

Mitral inflow velocities. With mitral inflow tracings obtained by the use of pulsed wave Doppler, it is possible to measure peak velocities of early (E wave) and late (A wave) diastolic filling, the time from peak E wave to baseline (deceleration time—DT) and also the isovolumic relaxation time (IVRT), between the aortic valve closure and before mitral valve opening. Usually the DT and IVRT are prolonged in relaxation abnormalities because it takes a longer time for the LV filling pressure, in those cases, to equilibrate the LA pressure. And both are shortened in normal individuals or in situations of a higher filling pressure in the LV (with higher LA pressure).[1]

Mitral annulus velocities. Typical tracings of mitral annulus velocities obtained by tissue Doppler include three waves: one systolic (S′) and two diastolic: an early diastolic wave (E′) and a late diastolic wave (A′). For the purpose of evaluating diastolic function, the most important among those three waves is the E′. It is lower in patients with abnormal relaxation and does not increase with exercise, which is an opposite effect in normal subjects. In general E′ velocity remains lower and E wave velocity increases with higher filling pressures. It has been used as a ratio between those waves to estimate diastolic dysfunction.[1]

Pulmonary vein flow velocities. There are four different waves in tracings of pulmonary vein flow: two systolic, one diastolic velocity and one atrial flow reversal. Among those, the atrial flow reversal component is the most important, especially its size and morphology.[1]

Left atrium. The importance of LA dimension is that with progressing LV diastolic stiffness, the LA volume increases being considered one of the best parameters of chronic diastolic dysfunction and is related to further cardiac events such as atrial fibrillation, heart failure, stroke, and death (Figs. 6-5GH and 6-6).[4]

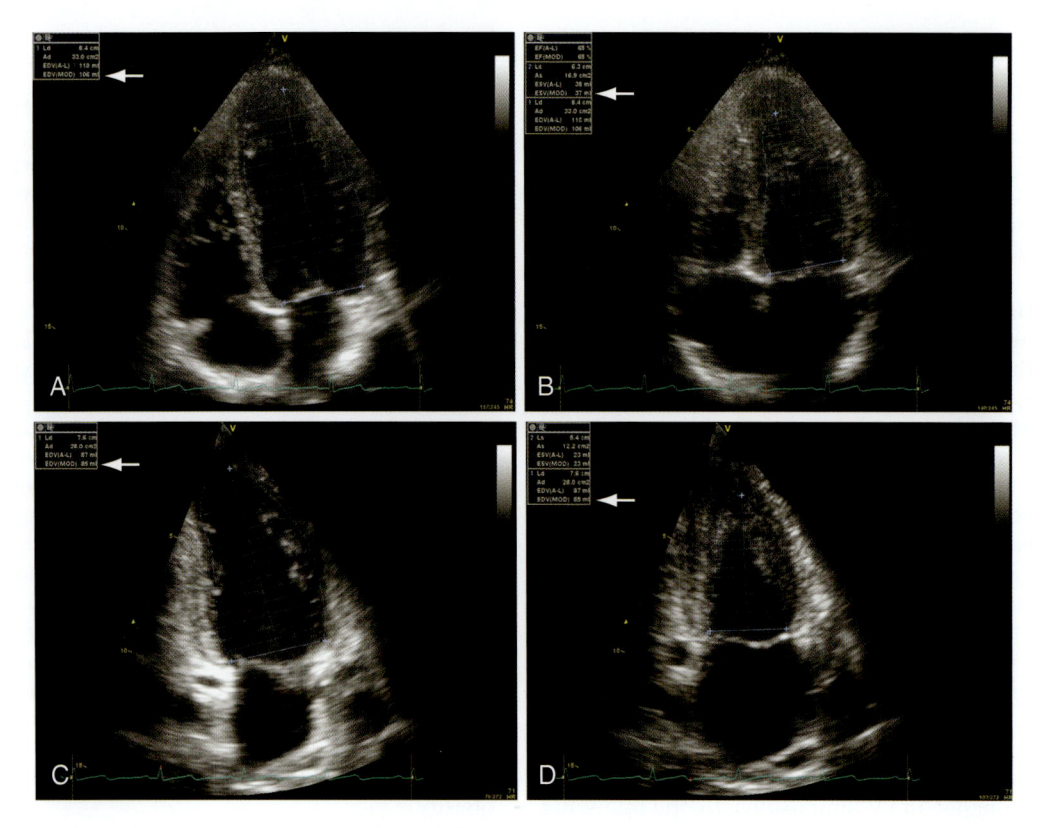

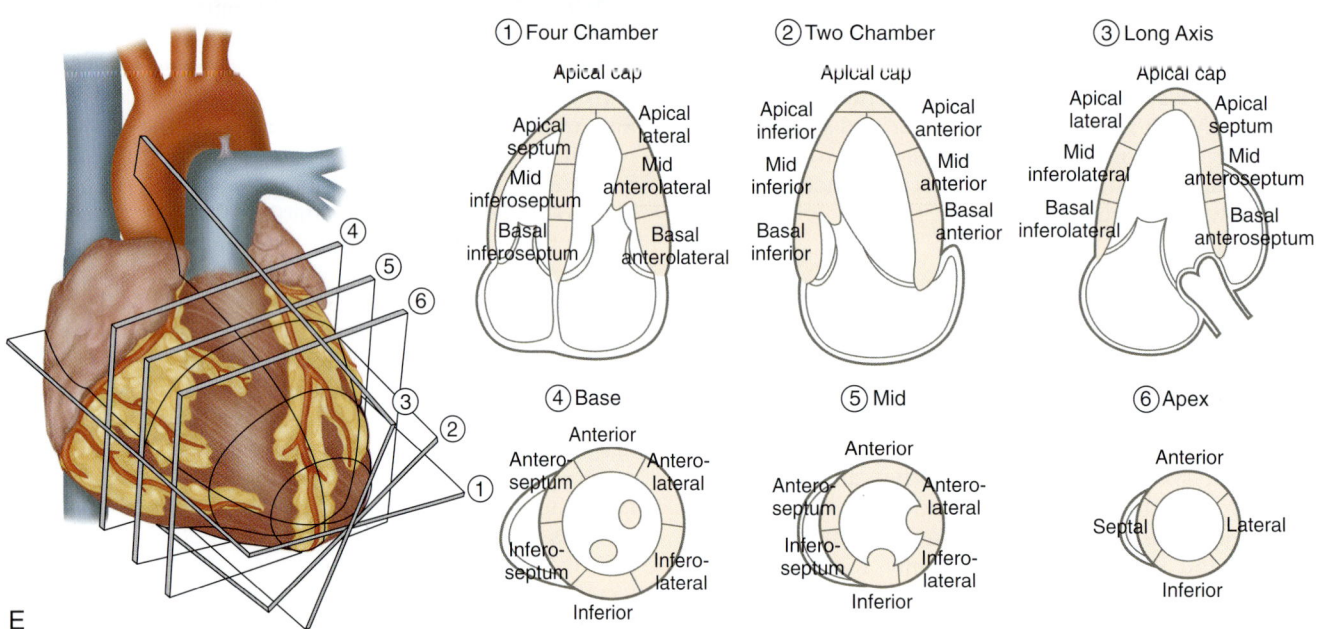

FIGURE 6-5 Ejection fraction (EF) calculation based on the modified Simpson rule, showing left ventricle volumes in diastolic and systolic phases (*white arrows*). **A** and **B**, four-chamber views. **C** and **D**, two-chamber views. The EF for the four-chamber views is EF = end diastolic volume − end systolic volume/end diastolic volume = 106 − 37/106 = 65%. Using the same formula, the EF for the two-chamber view is 73%, and the final EF is then 69%. ESV(Mod), end systolic volume by modified Simpson rule; EDV(Mod), end diastolic volume by modified Simpson rule. **E**, Images of LV segmentation for wall motion analysis. On the *top panel*, the three apical views are shown: four-chamber, two-chamber and three-chamber view or long axis; the *bottom panel* shows three short axis views: basal, mid, and apical levels. These levels are displayed in the heart drawing on the left side of this picture. All wall regions are identified in each view. The apical cap can be used for wall motion analysis but is especially considered for studies such as myocardial perfusion or contrast studies.

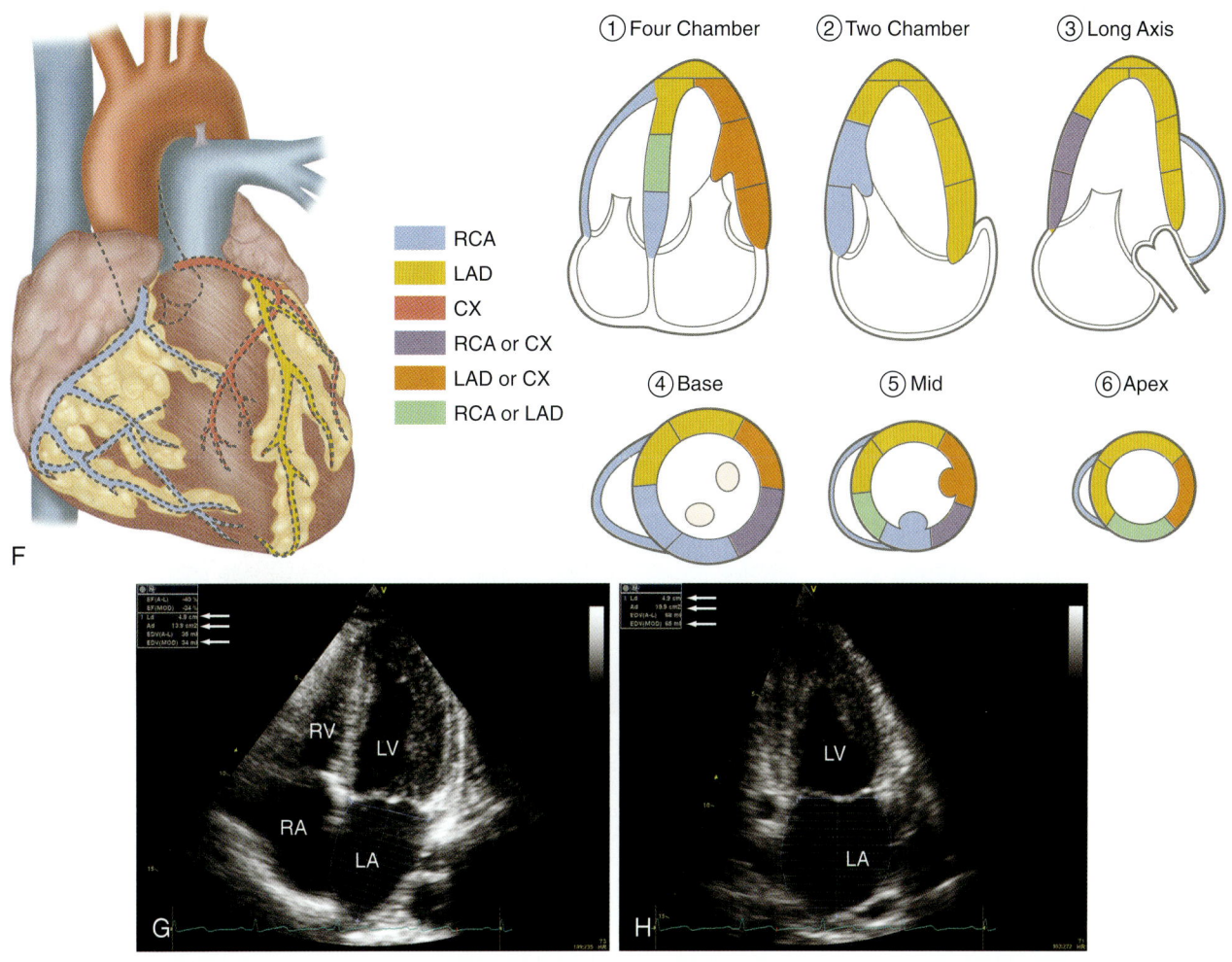

■ **FIGURE 6-5, cont'd** **F**, same arrangement for images is shown: *top panels* for three apical views and *bottom panels* showing three levels of short axis views. In this image, the coronary supply is shown for each wall and region. LV, left ventricle; CX, circumflex artery; LAD, left anterior descending artery; RCA, right coronary artery. **G, H,** left atrial (LA) volume calculations. The LA is shown in two apical views, four-chamber (**G**) and two-chamber (**H**), with measurements displayed on the *top left corner* (*white arrows*). Considering the area-length method: Left atrial volume = $8/3\pi[(A1)(A2)/(L)]$, in which A1 and A2 correspond to the two area numbers (*Ad*) and *L* corresponds to the length (*Ld*) and the highest number is included in the formula; then, $LA = 0.85[(13.9)(19.9)]/(4.9) = 48$ mL. Another method of LA volume calculation is using the modified Simpson rule, the same rule used for left ventricle ejection fraction measurement. The final volume is obtained tracing the endocardial border of the left atrial chamber in the final systole and the final volume is the average of the two orthogonal volumes in the two apical views, which in this case is 49.5 mL, the number comparable with the area-length method (48 mL). LA, left atrium; Ld, length; LV, left ventricle; RA, right atrium; RV, right ventricle. (**F**, Modified from Lang RM, et al. Recommendations for Chamber Quantification: A Report from the American Society of Echocardiography's Guidelines and Standards Committee and the Chamber Quantification Writing Group, Developed in Conjunction with the European Association of Echocardiography, a Branch of the European Society of Cardiology. J Am Soc Echocardiogr 2005; 18:1440-1463.)

Pulmonary Hypertension

It is part of the routine echocardiography to measure the pulmonary artery systolic pressure (PASP) using the tricuspid regurgitation velocity. Pulmonary hypertension is when the PASP is greater than 25 mm Hg at rest. Not only can the PASP be obtained by the Doppler techniques, but also the mean and the diastolic pulmonary artery pressure, associating the tracings of pulmonary regurgitation, as discussed earlier.

It is important to distinguish between acute and chronic pulmonary hypertension. Usually acute pulmonary hypertension is due to pulmonary embolism. Chronic pulmonary hypertension causes are related to cor pulmonale. Important findings in both cases are enlargement of right chambers with the LV being "compressed" by the pressure overloaded RV, and also the RV decreased systolic function. It is possible to find images compatible with thrombi, more related to pulmonary embolism. In some cases, it can be difficult to differentiate the acute and chronic pulmonary hypertension. The presence of increased RV thickness may be found in patients with chronic pulmonary hypertension (Fig. 6-7).

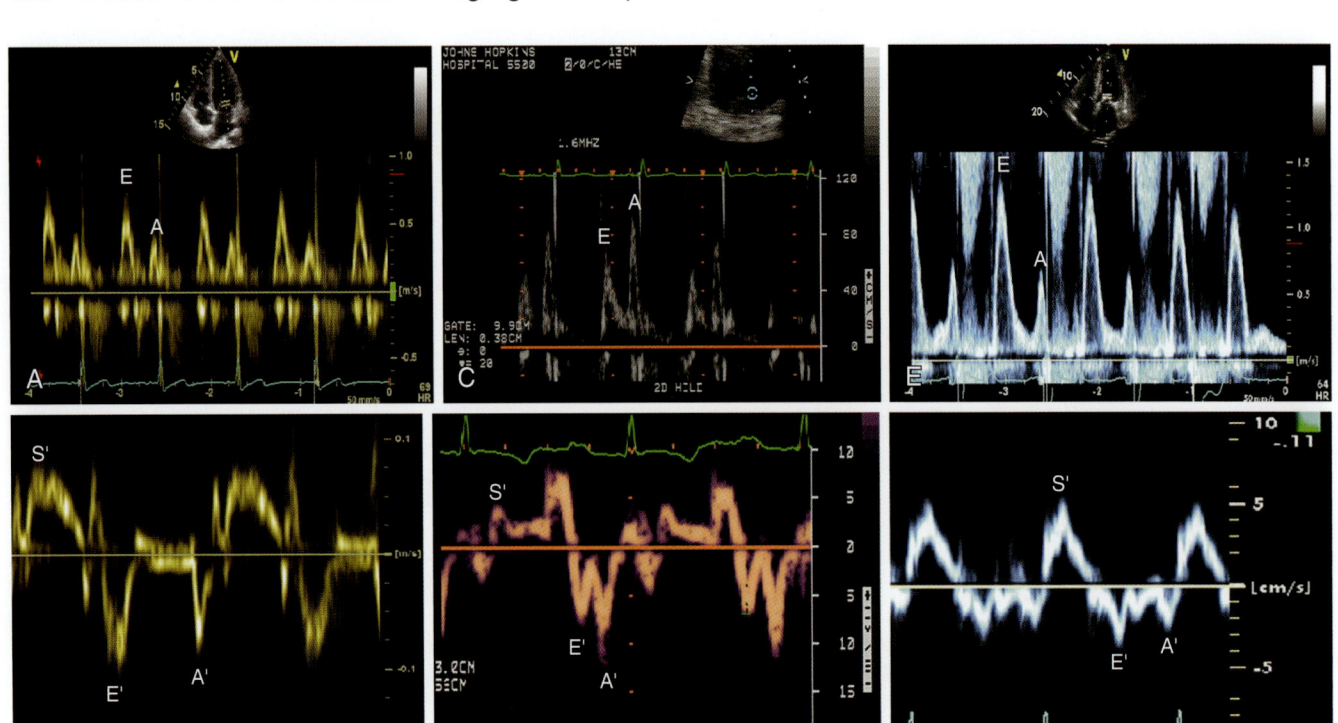

FIGURE 6-6 Images of diastolic filling patterns. *Top panel* shows mitral inflow pulsed wave. Doppler curves with early (E) and late (A) diastolic waves; *bottom panel* shows tissue velocity curves with the systolic (S′), early (E′) and late (A′) diastolic waves. **A, B,** normal filling pattern. **C, D,** mild diastolic dysfunction with abnormal relaxation pattern. **E, F,** severe diastolic dysfunction in a restrictive cardiomyopathy. Note the differences in the proportion between the E and A waves for Doppler curves in the different situations and the low velocity peak numbers in the restrictive cardiomyopathy tissue velocity curve for the diastolic curves (E′ and A′).

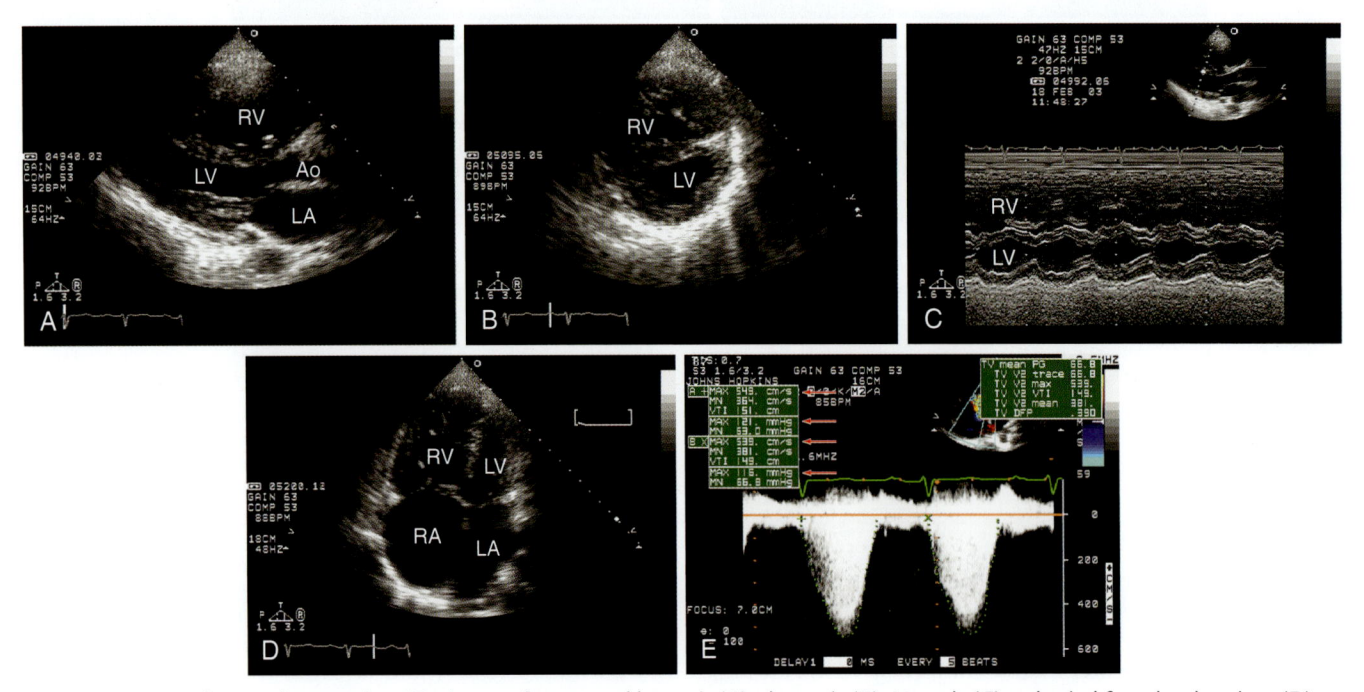

FIGURE 6-7 Pulmonary hypertension: 2D pictures of parasternal long axis (**A**), short axis (**B**), M mode (**C**) and apical four-chamber views (**D**). Note the right ventricle (RV) enlargement in **A, B,** and **C** with the compression of the left ventricle chamber by the RV, and the D letter shape of the left ventricle (**B**) of short axis view. In **E**, a tricuspid regurgitation continuous wave Doppler curve with peak velocity numbers of 5.49 m/seg and 5.39 m/seg and thus, with gradient values of 121 mm Hg and 116 mm Hg (*red arrows*). These gradient numbers must be added to the estimated right atrial pressure varying from 10 mm Hg to 15 mm Hg (or even 20 mm Hg in most cases such as this of pulmonary hypertension) and then the final pulmonary artery systolic pressure values can be as high as 131 mm Hg and 136 mm Hg. Ao, aorta; LA, left atrium; LV, left ventricle; RA, right atrium; RV, right ventricle.

Coronary Artery Disease (CAD)

Echocardiography is one of the best noninvasive tools to evaluate patients with suspected CAD or patients submitted to risk stratification because of CAD. It is already known that quantification of global and regional contractility by echocardiography has a close relation to the patient's short- and long-term prognosis. Evaluation of global LV function by 2D echo was discussed previously. Regional contractility analysis was also addressed previously and what is important to point out in this section is that the higher the wall motion score index, the bigger the infarcted area, which in turn might correlate with a poor prognosis.[5] Another important aspect of the regional contractility analysis is that wall motion changes may occur before any ST-T segment elevation in the electrocardiography (ECG) or even before symptoms. Doppler is useful to analyze diastolic function and the initial abnormality is altered myocardial relaxation with prolonged IVRT, DT, lower E, and higher A waves. The restrictive pattern is associated with severe LV systolic dysfunction. Using tissue Doppler parameters is also useful and the E/E' ratio can be a predictor of survival after acute myocardial infarction (AMI).[6]

Also important about echocardiography in CAD especially in AMI setting, is that not all patients show ECG changes because of low sensitivity of this technique. In patients with prolonged chest pain and no ECG typical findings, echocardiography is used to exclude any other cause of chest pain such as aortic dissection, cardiac tamponade, and pulmonary embolism. In the follow-up of an unstable post-AMI patient, echocardiography is used to evaluate the presence of any complications such as: LV failure, RV infarct, free wall rupture and pseudoaneurysm, ventricular septal rupture, papillary muscle rupture, ischemic mitral regurgitation, true LV aneurysm, and thrombus.

Tako-tsubo cardiomyopathy. This specific kind of myocardial infarction is characterized by usually apical akinesia not associated with coronary obstruction. There is a relation with psychologic and physical stress situations. It is possible to find typical ECG and cardiac marker abnormalities. This group of patients can show unstable hemodynamics, but almost all of them recover fully.[7]

Stress echocardiography. Usually after an AMI episode, patients need to be evaluated regarding risk assessment and myocardial viability. Echocardiography is considered the best imaging technique for that purpose by the stress testing. There are two types of stress testing: exercise and pharmacologic. The exercise test includes the use of treadmill or bicycle—the latter is done in the supine position. In the treadmill exercise stress test, the images are acquired in baseline and right after the peak exercise. In the bicycle exercise test, the images can be acquired even during peak exercise.

For the patients who cannot exercise for any number of reasons, the pharmacologic stress test is used and the drugs used are dobutamine, dipyridamole, and adenosine. Stress echocardiography is capable to detect any of the following findings: worsening of wall motion abnormalities (WMA) and/or development of new ones, which are related to stress-induced ischemia. Specifically for pharmacologic test, myocardial viability can be evaluated if there is an improvement in contractility with low-dose dobutamine and worsening with higher doses of the drug, the so called *biphasic response*. Other findings include: LV dilation and/or decrease in systolic function, which might be related to severe CAD. More detailed information on pharmacologic stress agents can be found in Chapter 26.

Contrast echocardiography. There are two types of contrast agent that can be used to increase the accuracy of echocardiography in diagnosis and quantification of cardiac diseases: gas-filled microbubbles and agitated saline.

The first type of contrast uses artificially made microbubbles small enough to pass through the pulmonary circulation without being destroyed and to make possible LV opacification. This is useful for better definition of endocardial border and thus for LV function measurements using the Simpson method. It is also is better for the WMA and in HCM to distinguish between apical dyskinesia and cases of mid LV or apical hypertrophy.

The microbubbles injected have the capability to reflect the ultrasound signals with twice the frequency transmitted, called the *harmonic signal*, the reason for the enhancement of picture definition in the LV. But at the same time after some specific adjustments on probe used in these studies, the ultrasound signals can be strong enough to destroy the microbubbles and then it is possible to see myocardial perfusion image, after the myocardial tissue is replenished with those bubbles. That is the reason for the great usefulness of this type of contrast in diagnosis and follow-up of patients with CAD.

The other type of contrast agent, agitated saline, consists of 10 mL of saline which is agitated with a three-way stopcock and two syringes five times before the injection in the venous circulation. The bubbles appear first in the right chamber and then in the left side. The main indication for this technique (also known as a "bubble study") is to study right-to-left shunts such as through a patent foramen ovale (PFO). If there is flow through the PFO, the contrast appears immediately in the left atrium right after the right one (see Fig. 6-4). Another indication for this technique is to study intrapulmonary shunts, in which the contrast can also be seen in the left atrium immediately after the injection. Normally it is not possible for the bubbles to be seen before at least three consecutive beats. Another useful situation for this saline contrast is to increase the tricuspid regurgitation signal to measure right ventricular systolic pressure because one third of patients may not show a good tricuspid regurgitation Doppler signal (Fig. 6-8).

Valvular Heart Disease and Prosthetic Valves

The importance of echocardiography for heart valve disease evaluation is unquestionable. All the hemodynamic derived Doppler data make echocardiography a handy and reliable tool for heart valve disease analysis. And, in some situations, echocardiography provides the most accurate hemodynamic information such as the mean transmitral gradient in mitral stenosis. The complete evaluation includes 2D analysis from which the valve morphology is studied and is completed with all Doppler modes such as color, pulsed and continuous wave.

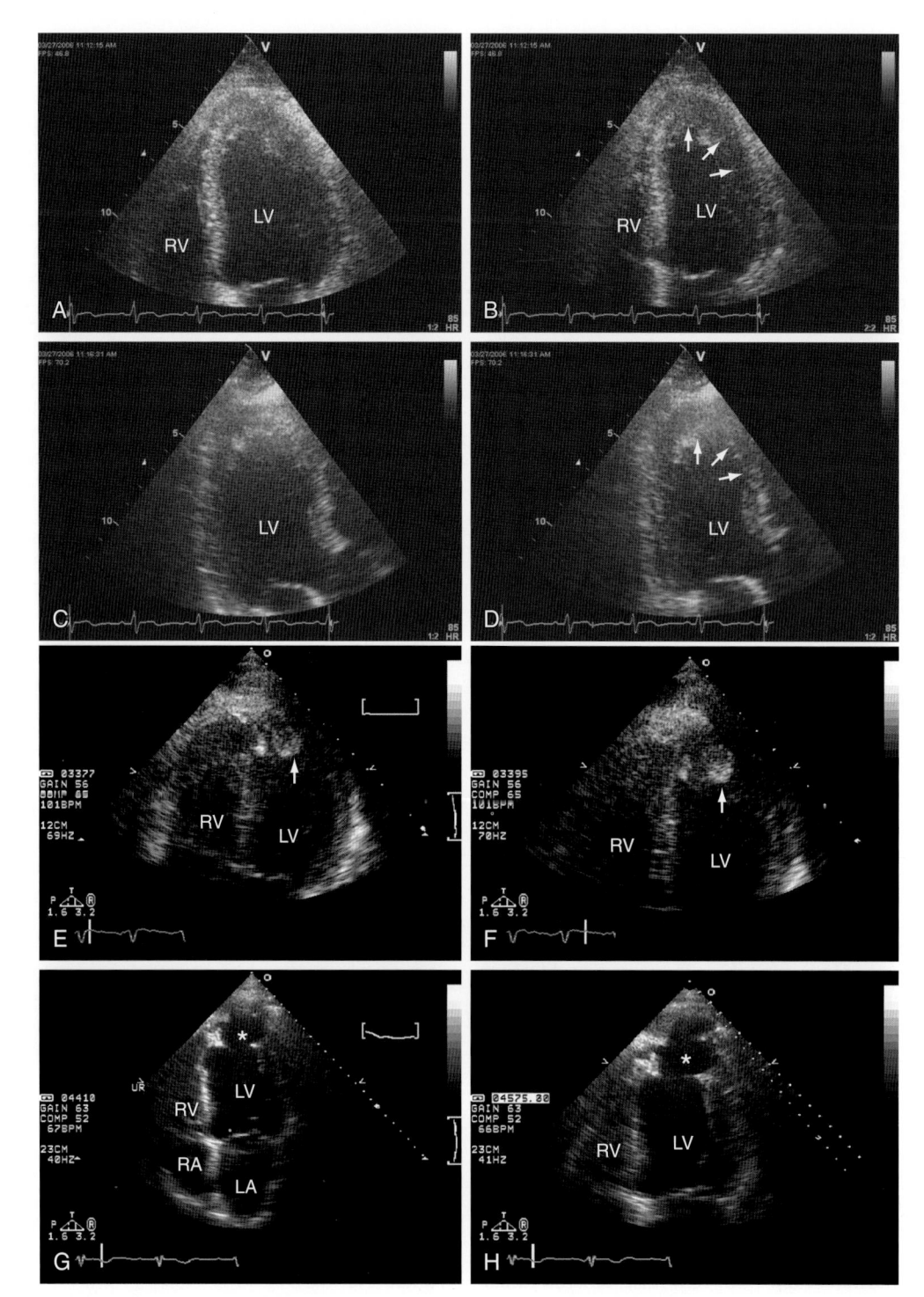

■ **FIGURE 6-8** Myocardial infarction. In **A** and **B**, apical four-chamber views of an anteroapical akinetic area (*white arrows*) in end systole (*red lines in electrocardiography tracings*). **C** and **D**, apical three-chamber views of the same patient showing the akinetic apical region in end systole. LV, left ventricle. Myocardial infarction complications. In **E** and **F**, apical four-chamber views showing a thrombus in an akinetic apical region (*white arrow*) with bright round contour. **G** and **H,** apical four-chamber views showing a left ventricle pseudoaneurysm in apical region (*asterisk*), with a discontinuity of the apical region, due to a tear or rupture of the myocardial wall and thus held the epicardial layer of the pericardium.

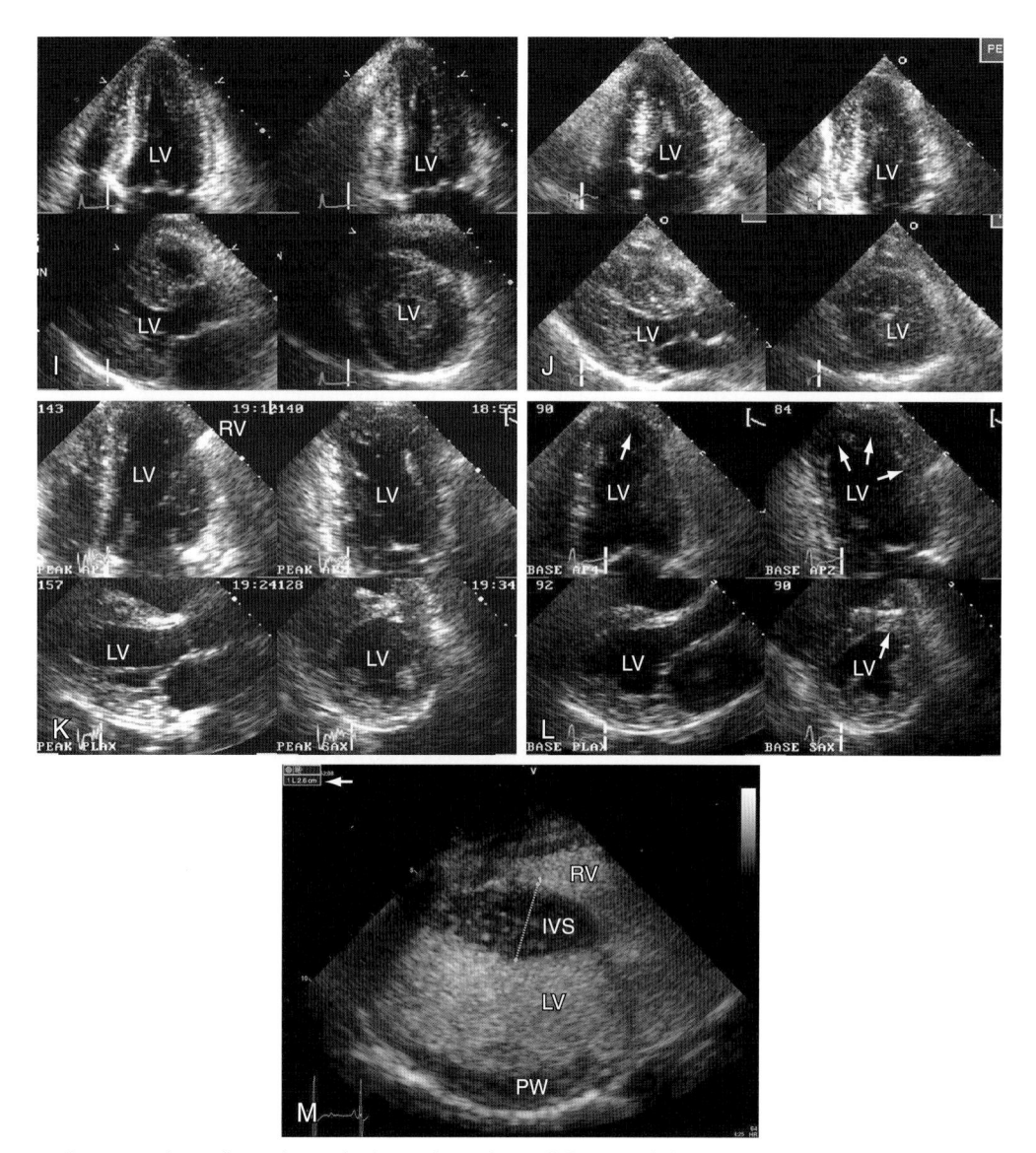

■ **FIGURE 6-8, cont'd** Stress echocardiography. Each picture shows four still frames: (*clockwise*) apical four-chamber; apical two-chamber; parasternal long axis and short axis views. **I,** baseline images in a normal stress study. **J,** peak stress images with hypercontractility of the walls. **K,** baseline of positive stress echocardiography study. **L,** peak stress phase of a positive study showing hypokinesia of apical, anterior, and anteroseptum (*white arrows*). Note that the left ventricle cavity is enlarged compared to the baseline images and to the normal peak stress images at the *top panel*. **M,** left ventricle contrast image with opacification of the cavity in a hypertrophic cardiomyopathy patient. The interventricular septum thickness is best delineated and the measurement is shown. IVS, interventricular septum; LA, left atrium; LV, left ventricle; PW, posterior wall; RA, right atrium; RV, right ventricle.

Aortic Stenosis (AS)

There are two important causes of AS: degenerative and congenital. By using 2D echocardiography, it is possible to study basic features of the aortic valve that can provide the diagnostic cause. Thus in degenerative aortic disease, calcification predominates as the main characteristic. Not much calcification is seen in the congenital valve with AS, particularly in early stages. Still in the 2D mode, it is possible to study the valve opening and some hemodynamic consequences in the heart such as LV mass and function. Doppler echocardiography is the best option to establish the severity of AS. With the peak aortic flow velocity from continuous wave Doppler, it is possible to calculate: peak and mean transaortic pressure gradient, aortic valve area, and LVOT/aortic time-velocity integral (TVI) ratio.[8] It is important to point out that in some patients because of "pressure recovery" the calculated gradients might be higher than those derived from catheter angiography studies. After the blood flow passes through the aortic valve, the kinetic energy can be recovered while in the aorta, making the pressure level in this site higher even if it is away from the valve.

Mitral Stenosis (MS)

The most common cause of MS is rheumatic heart disease. Infrequent causes of MS include degenerative calcification, hypereosinophilia, medication toxicity, and vegetation. 2D echocardiography is extremely useful in MS because it can provide information used to select patients for mitral balloon valvuloplasty in the cath lab. Each morphologic item is given a grade from 0 to 4 and the total sum must be equal or less than 8, which is related to a good result after valvuloplasty procedure (Wilkins-Block score). Doppler echocardiography can reliably measure the pressure gradient across the mitral valve but can sometimes be variable because of its volume relationship. The mitral valve area calculation is a more reliable method for MS evaluation and can be done with one of the three methods: pressure half time (PHT) (Fig. 6-9), the continuity equation, and the proximal iso-velocity surface area (PISA).

Aortic Regurgitation (AR)

There are several causes of AR: congenital, endocarditis, degenerative calcific aortic valve, Marfan syndrome, dilated aortic root, aortic dissection. 2D echocardiography is usually able to visualize those abnormalities. Another important feature of chronic severe AR is LV increased diameter and the "fluttering" of the anterior mitral leaflet because of the proximity with the flow from the AR. With color Doppler it is possible to identify the regurgitant jet in the left ventricle outflow tract and with continuous wave Doppler—to measure the pressure half time (PHT), which is the time from the peak early diastolic gradient until the point it reaches its half level, used for severity quantification.[9]

Mitral Regurgitation (MR)

As in AR, there are several causes for MR: mitral valve prolapse, endocarditis, flail mitral leaflet, ruptured chordae, mitral annulus calcification, papillary muscle dysfunction or rupture, rheumatic disease. 2D echocardiography is used to study the mitral valve anatomy and to establish the etiology of the regurgitation. It is also important to perform LV chamber measurements to obtain ejection fraction and to study the hemodynamic response to the severity of the MR. With color Doppler it is possible to recognize the turbulent regurgitant flow in the left atrial chamber during systole and have an estimation of severity based of the regurgitant jet area inside the LA. Pulsed wave Doppler can be used to identify the regurgitant jet in the systolic phase, but with the continuous wave Doppler, the regurgitant orifice area and volume can be calculated.[9]

Prosthetic Heart Valves

There are basically two types of prosthetic heart valves: made from tissue (biologic) and mechanical. This latter can be a ball-cage or disk valve. The evaluation of prosthetic heart valves starts with 2D echocardiography, by which it is possible to visualize certain abnormalities such as: dehiscence, vegetation, thrombus, and tissue prosthesis degeneration. What is challenging is the fact that it is not always possible to use only transthoracic echocardiography (TTE) for that purpose because of reverberation and reflectance of the prosthetic material, and TEE is necessary for proper evaluation (see Fig. 6-4).

With Doppler echocardiography it is possible to obtain pressure gradients and prosthetic valve area measurements using the same equations considered for the native valve calculations. What is important to notice is that prosthetic heart valves are inherently stenotic, thus velocities and pressure gradients, as well as prosthetic valve areas, are variable and dependent on the type and manufacturer of each one (see Fig. 6-9).

ENDOCARDITIS

Echocardiography is the best imaging tool for analyzing patients with suspected or diagnosed endocarditis with a sensitivity ranging from 60% to 80%. Vegetation found on an echocardiography study is one of two major criteria for the diagnosis of endocarditis. Vegetations are usually highly mobile, linear, or round and are found on the atrial side of atrioventricular valves or ventricular face of semilunar valves. Echocardiography is also important for the detection of endocarditis complications, especially for vegetations greater than 10 mm. TEE has the best accuracy for diagnosis of endocarditis with 95% sensitivity and is usually performed in patients with a nondiagnostic TTE and also to detect complications, especially if aortic valve is involved such as: mitral-aortic intervalvular fibrosa aneurysm and/or perforation with communication into the LA, aortic annular abscess, or perforation of the mitral leaflet (Fig. 6-10).

CARDIOMYOPATHIES

There are five major forms of cardiomyopathies, according to pathophysiologic mechanism or etiologic/pathogenic factor: (1) dilated cardiomyopathy; (2) hypertrophic cardiomyopathy; (3) restrictive cardiomyopathy; (4) arrhythmogenic right ventricular dysplasia or cardiomyopathy; and (5) noncompaction cardiomyopathy.

Dilated Cardiomyopathy (DCM)

This cardiomyopathy can be caused by myocarditis, coronary artery disease, alcohol abuse, hemochromatosis, sarcoidosis, AIDS, sepsis, doxorubicin therapy, and peripartum cardiomyopathy. It is characterized by increased systolic and diastolic diameters and decreased LV function and some patients might present regional wall motion abnormalities. Also found in this cardiomyopathy is enlargement of mitral annulus diameter with associated mitral regurgitation and apical thrombus. Doppler study is useful for the dyssynchrony analysis with tissue velocities and diastolic function evaluation. These patients can have impaired relaxation in compensated situations or even a nonreversible restrictive pattern, which correlates with a poor prognosis.

Hypertrophic Cardiomyopathy (HCM)

The hypertrophy is usually asymmetric in this type of cardiomyopathy. But some other variations may occur such as concentric, apical, and free wall hypertrophy. With 2D mode it is possible to find the basal septum hypertrophy, which is responsible in part for the dynamic LVOT obstruction. The narrowing of the jet in this area is responsible for the so called *Venturi effect*, which in turn brings the anterior mitral leaflet toward the septum, thereby worsening the LVOT obstruction and causing mitral regurgitation. The quantification of LVOT

CHAPTER 6 • Echocardiography 111

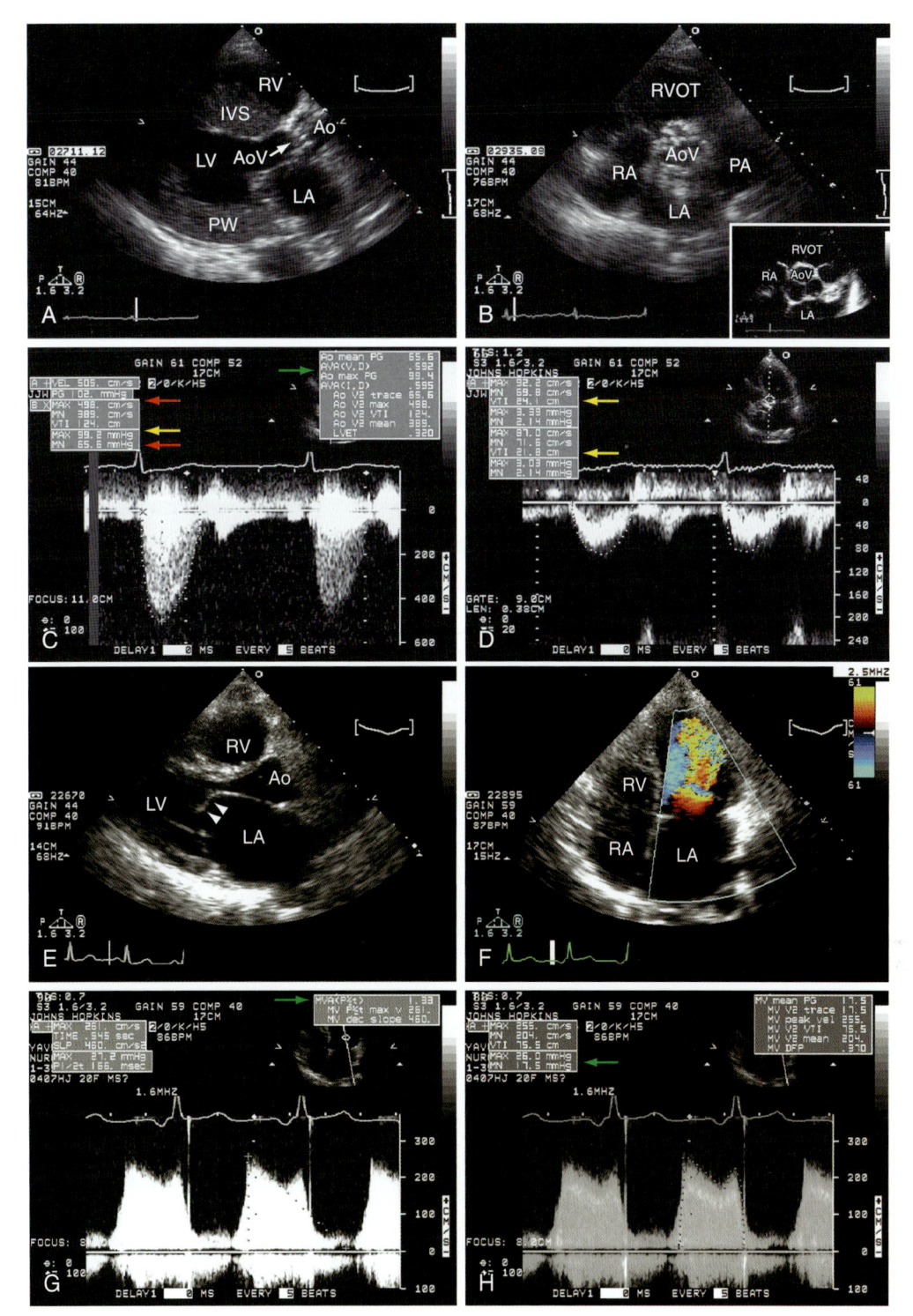

■ **FIGURE 6-9** Heart valve disease—aortic stenosis (AS). **A**, parasternal long axis view of an AS patient showing a calcified aortic valve and left ventricle hypertrophy (thickened septum and posterior wall). **B**, comparison of a calcified aortic valve in short axis view image with a normal aortic valve (*small square image on the bottom right*). **C**, continuous wave Doppler curve with peak transaortic gradient of 102 mm Hg and 99.2 mm Hg (peak velocity of 5.05 m/s and 4.98 m/s, respectively) and a mean gradient value of 65.6 mm Hg (severe if peak velocity ≥ 4 m/s and mean gradient ≥ 40 mm Hg (*red arrows*); time-velocity integral (TVI) of 124 cm (*yellow arrow*); and an aortic valve area (AVA) of 0.6 cm^2 (severe if ≤ 1.0 cm^2) (*green arrow*). **D**, left ventricle outflow tract (LVOT) pulsed wave Doppler curve showing VTI values of 24.1 cm and 21.8 cm (*yellow arrows*). The LVOT/aortic VTI ratio in this case is: 22.95/124 (the first number being the average of 24.1 and 21.8) = *0.18* (severe AS is considered if it is ≤0.25). Mitral stenosis (MS). **E**, parasternal long axis view of an MS case showing an enlarged LA and the "hockey-stick" appearance of the anterior mitral leaflet during the diastolic phase (*white arrowheads*). **F**, apical four-chamber view with the color Doppler showing the turbulence in the diastolic filling from the mitral valve (predominant *yellow and red* color toward the left ventricle) together with an enlarged left atrium. **G**, continuous wave Doppler curve of diastolic flow in a stenotic mitral valve with the calculations for mitral valve area by the pressure half time (PHT) method (*green arrow*). **H**, same curve used for calculations of peak and mean transvalvular gradients (*green arrow*) being 26 mm Hg and 17.5 mm Hg, respectively.

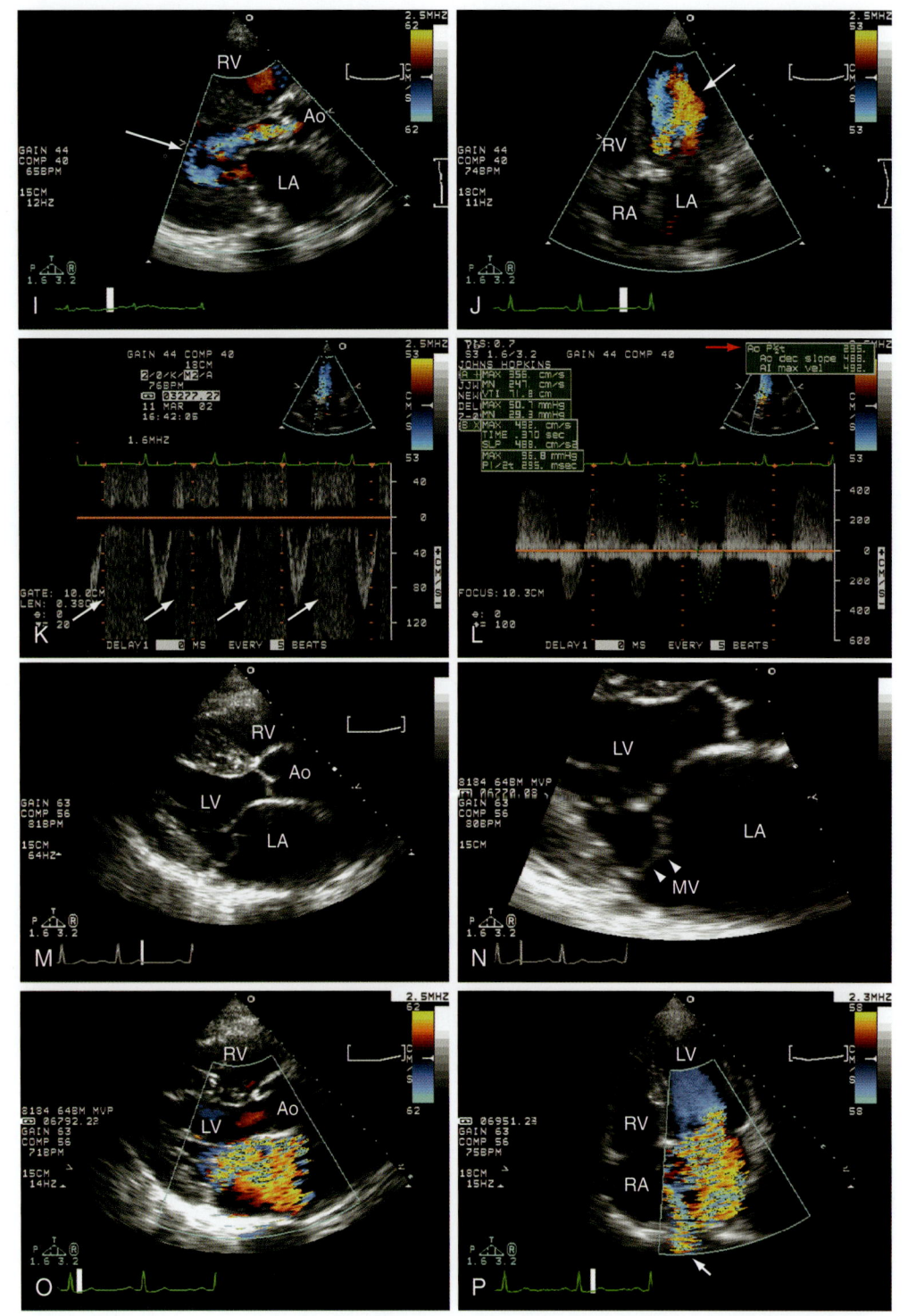

FIGURE 6-9, cont'd Aortic regurgitation. **I**, parasternal long axis view with color Doppler showing a *blue* jet in left ventricle outflow tract (LVOT) directed toward the left ventricle (LV) cavity in diastolic phase. **J**, apical four-chamber view with color Doppler with the regurgitant jet in *red* and *yellow* in the LV cavity during diastolic phase. **K**, pulsed wave Doppler curve for AR with the regurgitant jet being demonstrated during diastolic phase (*white arrows*). Because the regurgitant jet has a higher velocity, it is shown as an aliasing effect, or as a "distortion," if compared with the systolic flow (negative directed curves), due to a low pulsed repetition frequency (PRF), typical feature of pulsed wave Doppler mode. **L**, same patient being studied with the continuous wave Doppler to measure the pressure half time (PHT) (= 295 ms), which is consistent with moderate AR. Ao, aorta; LA, left atrium; RA, right atrium; RV, right ventricle. Mitral regurgitation (MR). **M**, parasternal long axis view showing a protrusion of the posterior leaflet in the left atrial chamber due to mitral valve prolapse (*white arrows* in the zoomed image in N). **O**, parasternal long axis view with color Doppler showing the *blue and yellow* regurgitant jet (high velocity turbulent flow) in the left atrial chamber during systole. **P**, apical four-chamber view showing *blue and yellow* regurgitant jet in the left atrial chamber during systole, reaching the right superior pulmonary vein (*white arrow*). Ao, aorta; Aov, aortic valve; LA, left atrium; LV, left ventricle; MV, mitral valve; PA, pulmonary artery; PW, posterior wall; RA, right atrium; RV, right ventricle; RVOT, right ventricular outflow tract.

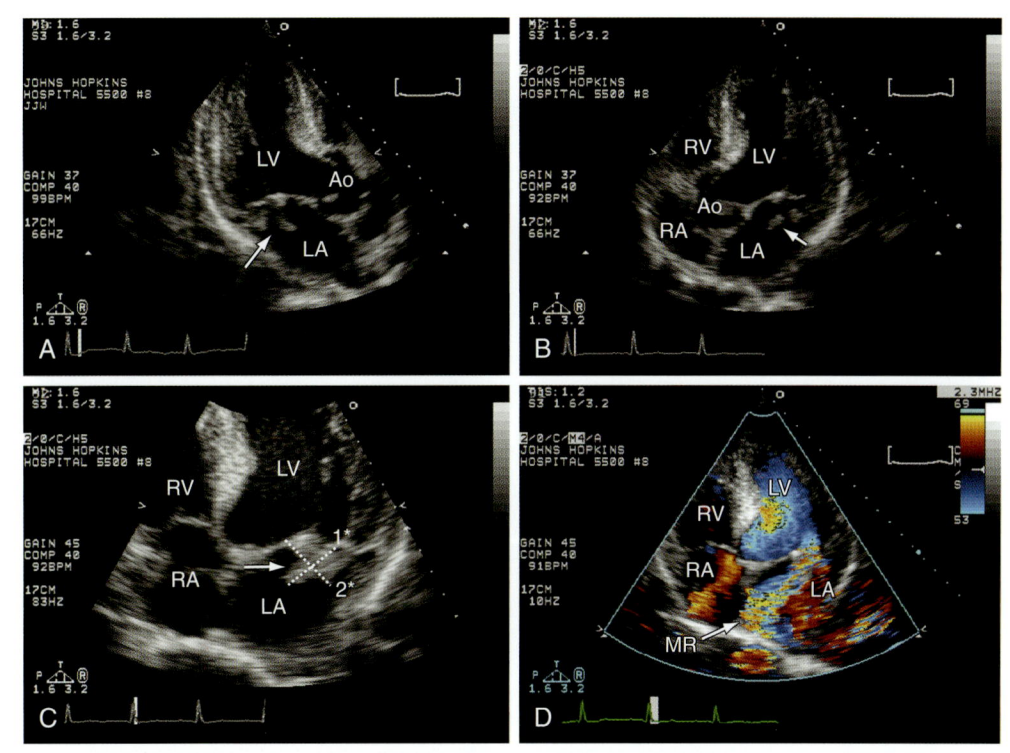

FIGURE 6-10 Mitral valve endocarditis. **A,** apical three-chamber view showing a large mobile mass on the atrial side of the mitral valve *(white arrow)*. **B,** apical four-chamber view with the initial portion of the ascending aorta in the middle (apical five-chamber view) showing the same image *(white arrow)*. **C,** zoomed image of an apical five-chamber view showing the vegetation dimensions *(white arrow)* (1 = 1.8 cm and 2 = 2.5 cm). **D,** apical four-chamber view with color Doppler showing mitral regurgitation (MR) jet in the left atrial chamber in *blue and yellow.* Ao, aorta; LA, left atrium; LV, left ventricle; RA, right atrium; RV, right ventricle.

obstruction is made with continuous wave Doppler and the curve shows a specific feature such as the late peak. Impaired relaxation can evolve to restrictive pattern as the disease progresses.

Restrictive Cardiomyopathy (RCM)

The important characteristics of RCM are preserved LV size and systolic function, normal wall thickness and biatrial enlargement. The restrictive diastolic pattern is usually seen, but what is important to point out is that restrictive filling can be seen in several cardiac diseases. Mitral inflow curves show high peak E velocities with ratio E/A as high as 2; short DT and IVRT; low S′ and E′ in tissue Doppler tracings.

Arrhythmogenic Right Ventricular Dysplasia/Cardiomyopathy

Several RV abnormalities can be found related to this diagnosis such as: increased RVOT and RV inflow diameters, abnormal RV function, and RV regional wall motion abnormalities—mostly apical and anterior wall. Contrast echocardiography can be useful because of better endocardial delineation.

Noncompaction Cardiomyopathy (Isolated Ventricular Noncompaction)

Because of an embryonic defect in the compaction mechanism, the LV wall in this cardiomyopathy can show marked trabeculations and intratrabecular recesses with blood flow mapped by color flow Doppler. Patients with this condition may present during the follow-up with heart failure, thromboembolic events, ventricular tachycardia, and sudden death (Fig. 6-11).

PERICARDIAL DISEASES

Two important pericardial diseases are promptly recognized by echocardiography: pericardial effusion and constrictive pericarditis. In pericardial effusion, if the echo-free space image is seen throughout the cardiac cycle, the amount of effusion is about 25 mL; smaller amounts can be seen only in systole and in posterior localization.

Tamponade

If effusion is big enough to make intrapericardial pressures higher than the systemic venous return to the right atrium, tamponade occurs. Typical signs of tamponade detectable by echocardiography are: the "swinging" motion of heart in the pericardial space; late diastolic collapse of right atrium; early diastolic collapse of right ventricle, and abnormal interventricular septum motion. Doppler findings of tamponade are more sensitive and early compared to previous abnormalities. These are the exaggerated phasic variations in right and left ventricle inflow and outflow. If the variability is higher than 15% for LV inflow, 25% for the RV inflow, and 10% for aortic and pulmonary outflows, it is consistent with tamponade hemodynamics.

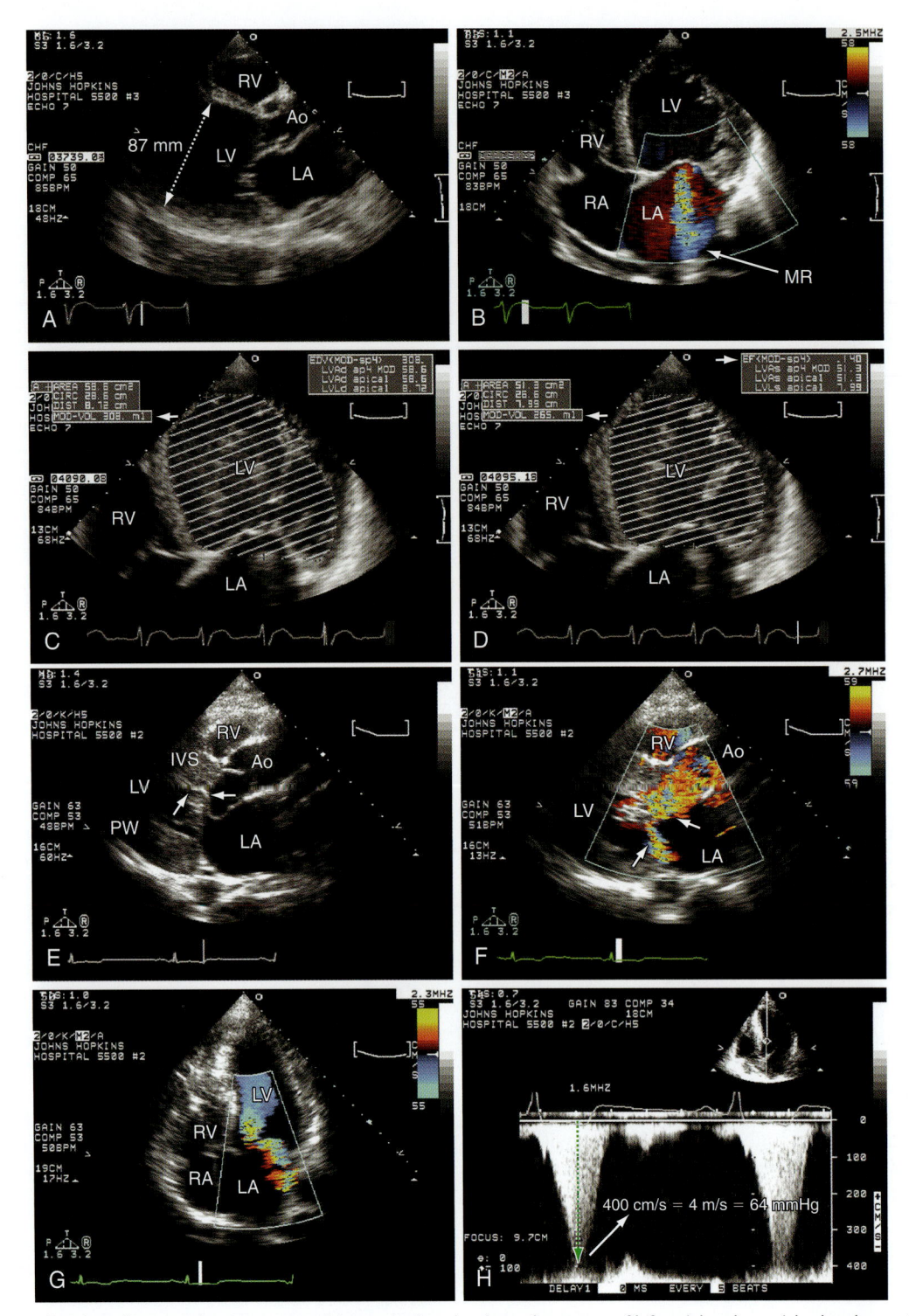

■ **FIGURE 6-11** Dilated cardiomyopathy. **A**, parasternal long axis view showing enlargement of left atrial and ventricle chambers, with diastolic diameter of 87 mm. **B**, apical four-chamber view with color Doppler showing mitral regurgitation (MR) jet in the left atrial chamber in *blue and yellow* in systolic phase, together with the more spherical geometry of the left ventricle. **C** and **D**, apical four-chamber views with measurements of diastolic (308 mL), systolic volumes (265 mL) and ejection fraction (0.14 or 14%) by Simpson modified rule (*white arrows*). Hypertrophic cardiomyopathy (HCM). **E**, parasternal long axis view showing thickened interventricular septum and posterior wall, together with enlargement of the left atrial chamber. Typical feature of HCM is the systolic anterior mitral leaflet motion toward the basal region of interventricular septum during systole and thus contributing to left ventricle outflow tract obstruction (*white arrows*) seen as a predominant *red and yellow* jet flow directed toward the ascending aorta in **F**. **G**, apical four-chamber view with color Doppler showing a mitral regurgitation jet as in *blue* flow inside the left atrial chamber. **H**, because of the interventricular septum hypertrophy and the systolic anterior motion of mitral leaflet, left ventricle outflow tract gradient can be obtained by continuous wave Doppler shown in this image with the 64 mm Hg peak value.

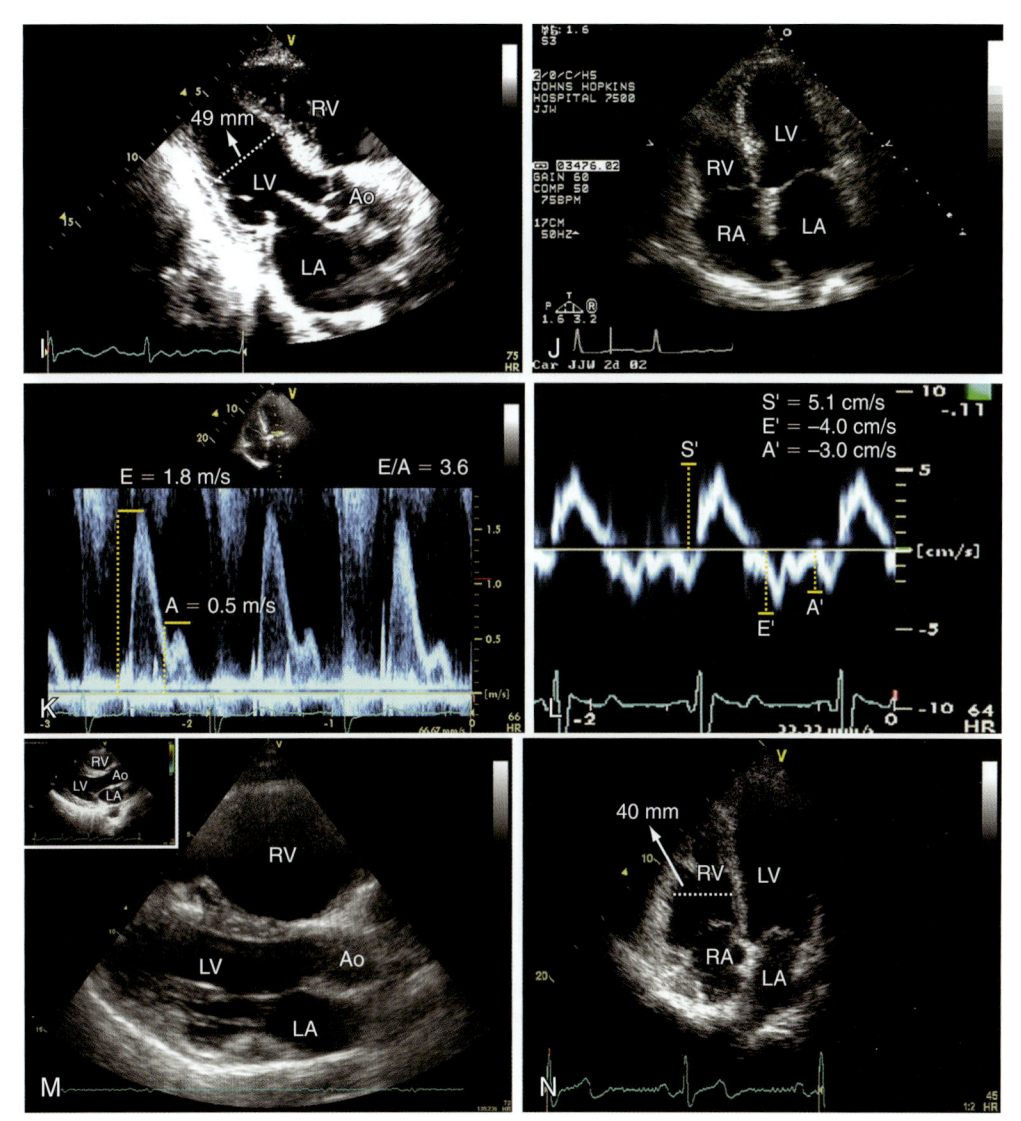

■ **FIGURE 6-11, cont'd** Restrictive cardiomyopathy. **I**, parasternal long axis view showing a normal end diastolic diameter of the left ventricle (49 mm), which can be frequently seen in this kind of cardiomyopathy, and an enlargement of the left atrial chamber. **J**, apical four-chamber view showing enlargement of both atrial chambers, a typical finding in restrictive cardiomyopathy. **K**, mitral inflow pulsed wave Doppler curves on a typical restrictive pattern with an E/A ratio ≥1.5 and tissue Doppler curve with a restrictive pattern with low diastolic velocities (**L**). Tissue Doppler curves: S′, systolic velocity; E′, early diastolic velocity; A′, late diastolic velocity. Arrhythmogenic right ventricular dysplasia/cardiomyopathy. **M**, parasternal long axis view showing a right ventricle enlargement (compare with a normal parasternal image in the small box on the top right). **N**, apical four-chamber view showing the right ventricle end diastolic diameter at the mid region (40 mm) which can be compatible with a moderately abnormal enlargement. Ao, aorta; IVS, interventricular septum; LA, left atrium; LV, left ventricle; PW, posterior wall; RA, right atrium; RV, right ventricle.

Constrictive Pericarditis

Previous cardiac surgery, viral infection, radiation to the chest, tuberculosis and collagen vascular disease can cause the pericardium to be inflamed, thickened, and adherent to the heart; in chronic cases, calcification may be seen. The main hemodynamic event of constrictive pericarditis is impaired diastolic filling. The 2D and M-mode can show some signs of constriction, but they are not specific, such as: thickened pericardium, abnormal interventricular septum motion, and dilated inferior vena cava. Doppler can be more helpful and usually the important changes compatible with constriction are: respiratory variation of the right and left ventricle, restrictive pattern of mitral inflow, hepatic vein flow reversal, superior vena cava with no variation due to respiration, E′ equal or higher than 7 cm/seg. If TTE is not conclusive, TEE can be used to study pulmonary vein flow, especially if there is an associated loculated effusion (Fig. 6-12).

CARDIAC MANIFESTATIONS OF SYSTEMIC ILLNESSES

Amyloidosis

Echocardiographic changes found in patients with amyloidosis are: normal cavity size, thickened walls, granular appearance of myocardium, and diastolic dysfunction. Some patients can show thickening of heart valves with

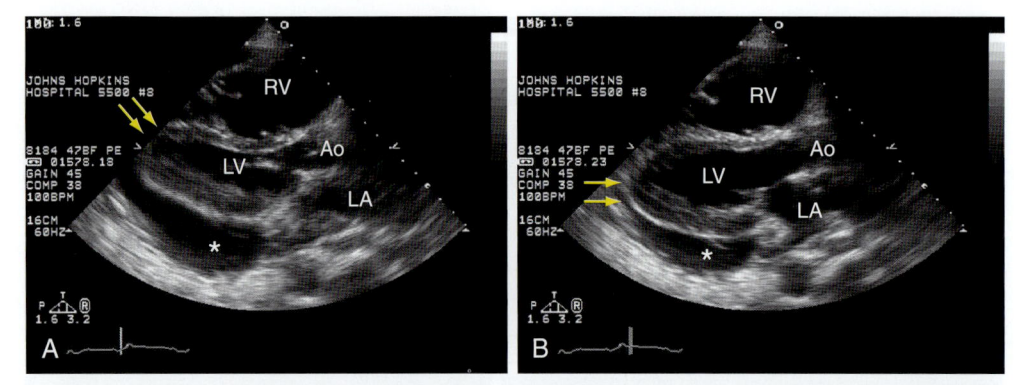

FIGURE 6-12 Pericardial effusion and tamponade. **A** and **B**, parasternal long axis views showing an echo-free space (*asterisk*) in posterior face of the left ventricle. Note the displacement of the apex region comparing the two pictures (*yellow arrows*), a typical finding (*swinging heart*) in pericardial effusion with tamponade. Ao, aorta; LA, left atrium; LV, left ventricle; RV, right ventricle.

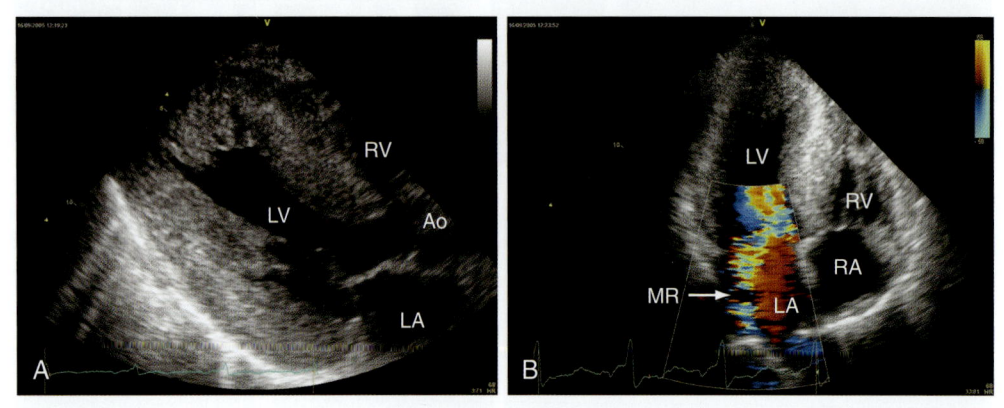

FIGURE 6-13 Amyloidosis. **A**, parasternal long axis view showing the increased thickness of the interventricular septum and the posterior wall with the granular appearance of the myocardial tissue. **B**, apical four-chamber view with color Doppler image showing a mitral regurgitant jet in the left atrial chamber in *blue and yellow* colors. Ao, aorta; LA, left atrium; LV, left ventricle; RA, right atrium; RV, right ventricle.

variable degrees of multivalvular regurgitation. The systolic function can deteriorate as the disease progresses (Fig. 6-13).

TUMORS AND MASSES

Myxoma

It is the most common primary tumor in the heart, and is frequently located in the LA, especially at the interatrial septum, and RA, RV, and LV. The tumor itself can cause some complications, depending on its size and location—causing obstruction in the mitral valve if located in the LA or the outflow tract if it is in the LV cavity. Myxomas can be found isolate or associated with a systemic syndrome such as familial myxoma syndrome, in which the tumors are multiple and can recur after surgery.

Fibroma

Usually found in LV free wall, apical (can be mistaken by apical hypertrophy) or intraventricular septum (IVS), these tumors can grow into LV cavity causing diastolic filling abnormalities, congestive heart failure, or malignant arrhythmias.

Rhabdomyoma

Common in the children with tuberous sclerosis, rhabdomyomas are located in RV, RV outflow tract, and pulmonary artery.

Papillary Fibroelastoma

Frequently found in the aortic, mitral, tricuspid, pulmonary valves, IVS, LV free wall, RV outflow tract, and LA. These tumors have a specific appearance like a "sea anemone" and can cause embolism if in the left chambers.

Malignant Tumors

They are usually angiosarcoma, rhabdomyosarcoma, myxosarcoma, osteosarcoma, fibrosarcoma, and synovial sarcoma; in general, they have a poor prognosis. Metastatic tumors are more frequent than primary tumors and originate from kidney, lungs, breast, liver, lymphoma, melanoma, and osteogenic sarcoma. They can be found in the RA and because of this location, the inferior vena cava should always be scanned.

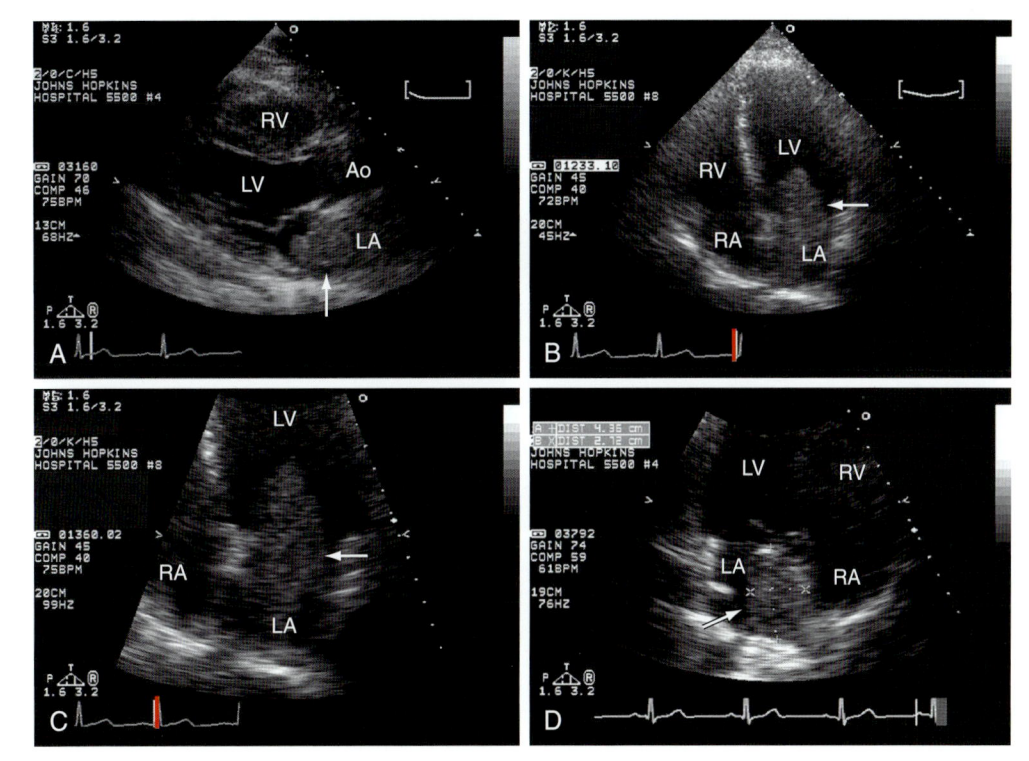

FIGURE 6-14 Myxoma. **A**, parasternal long axis view showing a round shape mass in the left atrial chamber (*white arrow*). **B** and **C**, apical four-chamber view showing the mass protruding into the left ventricle chamber (*white arrow*) in diastolic phase (*red line* on ECG tracing), which can cause obstruction and symptoms similar to mitral stenosis. **D**, apical four-chamber view with a myxoma in the left atrial chamber showing dimensions of 4.36 × 2.72 cm (*white arrow*). Ao, aorta; LA, left atrium; LV, left ventricle; RA, right atrium; RV, right ventricle.

Other Masses

Other masses in the heart can be mistaken by a specific tumor and include left atrial lipomatous hypertrophy, right atrial eustachian valve; pacemaker lead, central line catheter, and thrombi. If TTE is not conclusive for the specific etiology, TEE can be used for that purpose (Fig. 6-14).

DISEASES OF THE AORTA

Echocardiography is extremely valuable for the diagnosis of aortic abnormalities. The finding of atherosclerosis or debris in the aortic images has been related to cerebrovascular events, and they appear as mobile and irregularly shaped images. Aneurysms, frequently found in patients with history of hypertension, atherosclerosis, and Marfan syndrome must be promptly measured, using TTE or TEE because of the risk of rupture with diameters equal to or greater than 5 cm. The risk of rupture is also found in aneurysms of the sinus of Valsalva because of the absence of media layer. This type of aneurysm must be distinguished from aneurysm of membranous ventricular septum and other complications can be present such as embolic events, endocarditis, fistulous communications, and left-to-right shunts.

Other types of aortic disease can also be completely studied by echocardiography. Aortitis, caused by Takayasu disease, giant cell arteritis, ankylosing spondylitis, rheumatoid arthritis, and infection such as syphilis, appears as narrowing or even obstruction of thoracic or abdominal aorta or just thickened aortic wall, which sometimes is hard to distinguish from intramural hematoma. Coarctation of aorta is a narrowing of the descending thoracic portion, after the subclavian artery. Because it is a cause of hypertension in young patients, the study of the descending thoracic section must be done extensively in this group of patients with the use of continuous wave Doppler.

Aortic Dissection

There are several publications that studied the feasibility and accuracy of echocardiography in the diagnosis of aortic dissection. TTE is usually the option for screening and TEE is the imaging technique for a complete study. It is possible to visualize the thoracic aorta and the proximal portion of its abdominal section. The TEE must be detailed enough to find the point of intimal tear, or even an intramural hematoma, which can be the precursor lesion of dissection. Intramural hematoma is an echodense image between the intima and adventitia and it is different from atherosclerotic plaque because the latter has an irregular surface. Also important in aortic dissection is the identification of the true and false lumen, as well as complications such as coronary involvement, hemopericardium, aortic regurgitation, and LV dysfunction (Fig. 6-15).

Congenital Heart Disease

Atrial Septal Defect (ASD)

There are four types of ASD defects: secundum, primum, sinus venosus, and coronary sinus. TTE is usually a

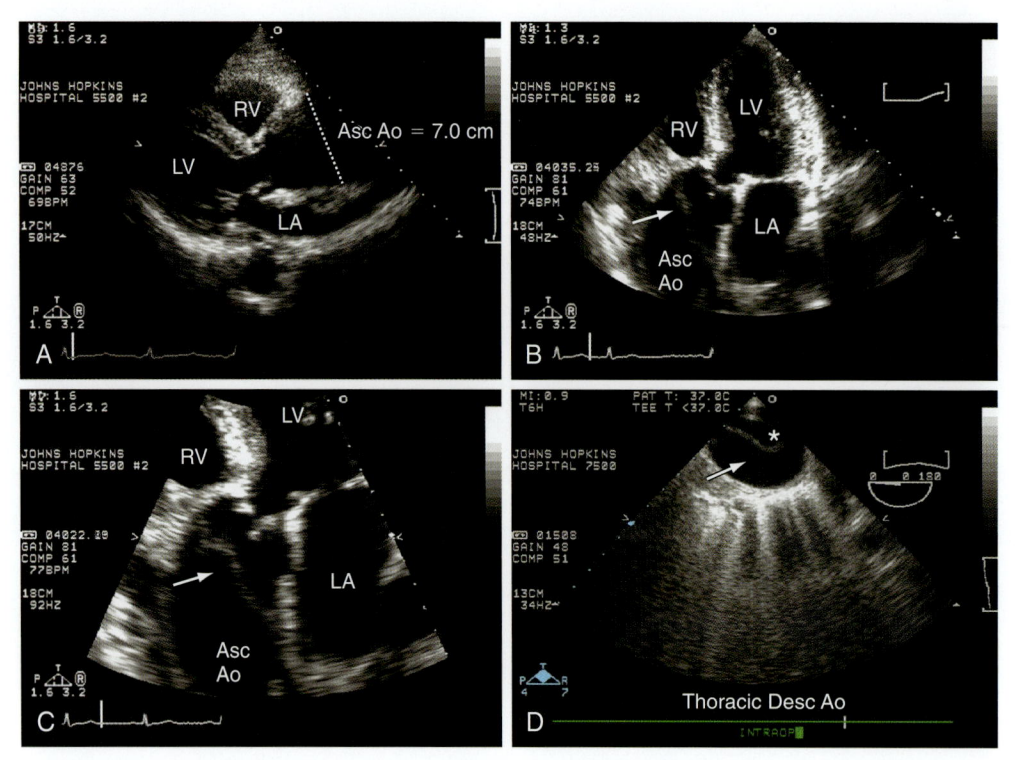

■ **FIGURE 6-15** Aortic diseases. **A**, parasternal long axis view showing an enlargement of the initial portion of the ascending aorta (aneurysm) with diameter of 7.0 cm. **B,**: apical four-chamber view with initial portion of ascending aorta being visualized (apical five-chamber view) showing a flap (*white arrow*) due to aortic dissection and in a zoomed image (**C**). **D**, transesophageal image showing thoracic descending aorta with an intimal flap due to dissection (*white arrow*) with a clear delimitation of the true (*asterisk*) and false lumen (*white arrow*). Ao, aorta; Asc Ao, ascending aorta; LA, left atrium; LV, left ventricle; RV, right ventricle; Thoracic Desc Ao, thoracic descending aorta.

good imaging technique for the first two types of defects. TEE can be used as an option to complete evaluation of these defects. Doppler echocardiography is used to confirm the left-to-right shunts by color flow mapping; 2D analysis is usually enough to confirm overload to right chambers; quantification of the shunt by calculating the systemic-to-pulmonary flow ratio has some pitfalls.

Ventricular Septal Defect (VSD)

This is a common congenital defect. There four types: (1) membranous, located at the thinnest portion of the interventricular septum, next to aortic and tricuspid valves, associated with aortic and tricuspid regurgitation; (2) muscular, usually small and not adjacent to any heart valve; (3) in association with complete AV defects; (4) supracristal (subarterial), located in the outflow tracts of aortic and pulmonary arteries.

Anomalous Pulmonary Venous Connections

There are two types of anomalous pulmonary vein connections: (1) partial, in which some of the veins are involved; (2) total, in which all the four pulmonary veins are involved. The latter is subclassified into three other types according to the position of the connection: (1) supracardiac, when the common pulmonary vein connects to the superior vena cava; (2) cardiac, when the connection is to a cardiac chamber or the coronary sinus; and (3) infracardiac, in which the common pulmonary vein connects to the hepatic circulation.

Anomalous Systemic Veins

The most common is the persistence of left superior vena cava and the enlargement of the coronary sinus is a well known sign of this defect, although not specific.

Patent Ductus Arteriosus (PDA)

This is a communication between the descending aorta and the pulmonary artery. This is best studied with the transducer in the high left parasternal plane view. The complete study is made by Doppler echocardiography which can detect blood flow in the descending aorta and its persistence in the diastolic phase.

Ventricular Outflow Tract Obstruction

This cardiac defect can be congenital, including an aortic and pulmonary stenosis. The appearance is a thickened valve with fusion of commissures. The valve area calculations by Doppler studies are not accurate because of some limitations in the use of small outflow diameters in the continuity equation. The subaortic stenosis can be represented by the discrete type, with a fibromuscular ridge below the aortic valve or the tunnel type, which is a hypoplasia of the LVOT and also can be associated with hypoplasia of the aorta.

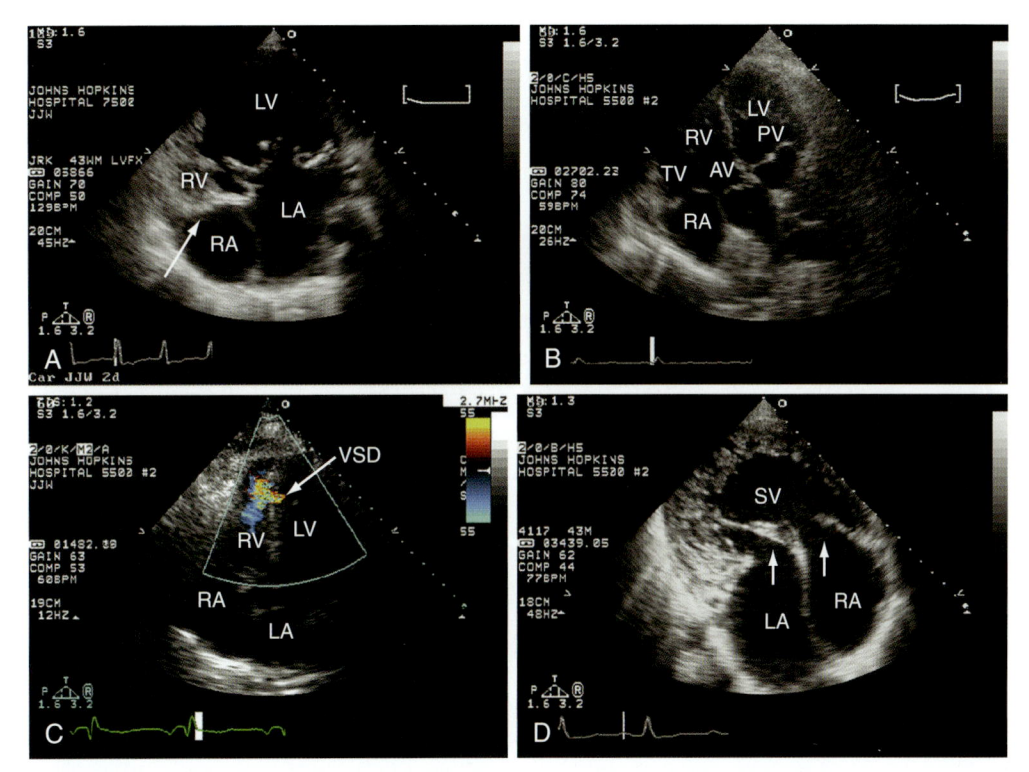

FIGURE 6-16 Congenital heart defects. **A**, apical four-chamber view showing an absent tricuspid valve *(white arrow)* and no communication between right ventricle and right atrium compatible with tricuspid atresia (an atrial septal defect is present in this case but not well seen in the image). **B**, apical plane view showing aortic valve (AV) in the right ventricle outflow tract and the pulmonary valve (PV) in the left ventricle outflow chamber in a congenitally corrected transposition of the great arteries. **C**, apical four-chamber view with color Doppler showing a muscular ventricular septal defect with flow from left ventricle to the right ventricle *(white arrow)*. **D**, apical four-chamber view showing a univentricular atrioventricular (AV) connection with the two AV valves opened *(white arrows)*. Ao, aorta; LA, left atrium; LV, left ventricle; RA, right atrium; RV, right ventricle; SV, systemic ventricle.

Complex Congenital Cardiac Malformations

Ebstein Anomaly

The main defect in this congenital malformation is the apical displacement of septal insertion of the tricuspid valve. It is possible to find tricuspid regurgitation, myocardial dysfunction in the RV, and a possible association with ASD (ostium secundum) or PFO.

Tetralogy of Fallot

The main defect is the misalignment of the infundibular portion of the interventricular septum. There are four classic signs of this syndrome: (1) pulmonary or subpulmonary stenosis; (2) VSD; (3) override aortic valve annulus; (4) RV hypertrophy.

Complete Transposition of Great Arteries

There is a misconnection between the great arteries and the ventricles. The pulmonary artery is connected to the LV and the aorta is connected to the RV. There is a chance for association with PDA, ASD, VSD, and coronary artery anomalies.

Congenitally Corrected Transposition of the Great Arteries

The basic principle in this cardiac defect is that the venous flow reaches the correct great artery through a "misplaced" ventricle. Thus the RV is connected to the LA and pulmonary veins and the LV is connected to the RA and vena cavae.

Univentricular Atrioventricular Connection

In this congenital cardiac syndrome one of the two mechanisms can be found: the small size of one ventricle prevents it to work as a circulatory pump or the association of defects that interfere with a division of the two ventricular chambers such as straddling of an atrioventricular valve (Fig. 6-16).

TISSUE DOPPLER AND STRAIN IMAGING

Conventional Doppler uses the sound reflection capabilities of blood cells to record flow velocities. For tissue velocities, some special adjustments are necessary in Doppler settings. Those adjustments are usually automatically set in commercially available machines, and they include the exclusion of high velocities and low intensity

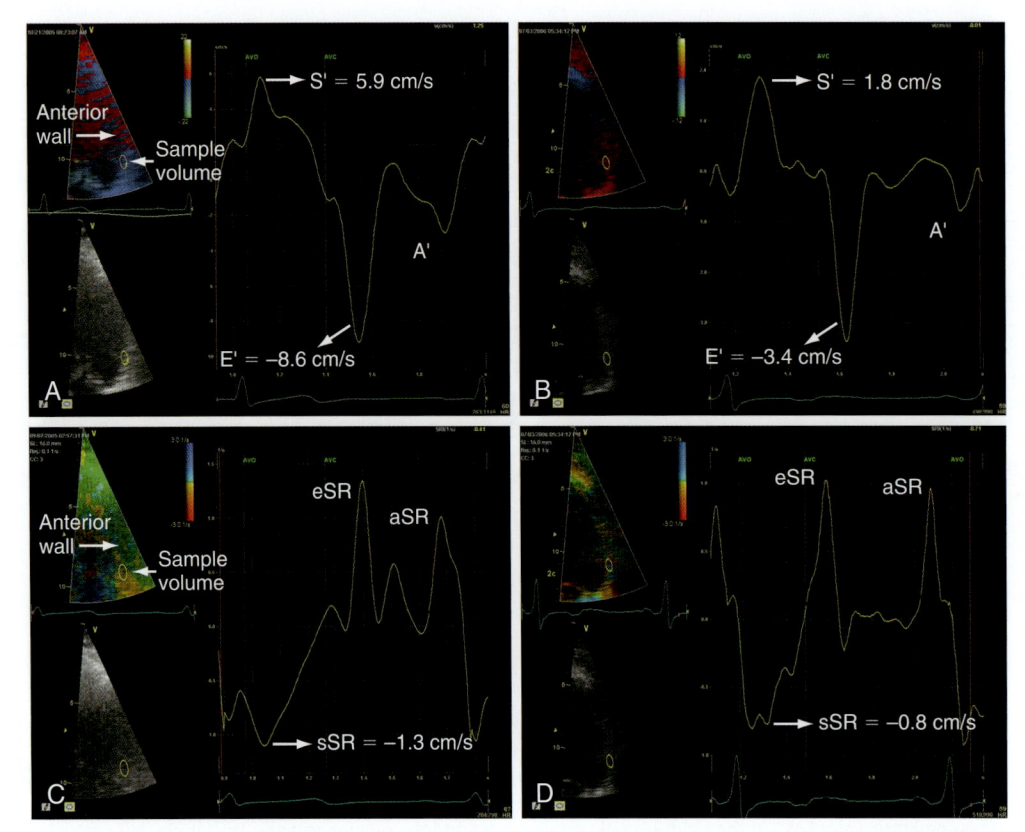

FIGURE 6-17 Tissue velocities. **A**, isolated anterior wall with colored tissue Doppler image and a sample volume placed in the basal region of a normal patient showing a normal tissue velocity curve with systolic velocity (S') of 5.9 cm/s and an early diastolic velocity (E') of −8.6 cm/s. **B**, same image in an anterior myocardial infarction patient showing low values for S' and E' of 1.8 cm/s and −3.4 cm/s, respectively. Strain rate curves. **C**, isolated anterior wall image of a normal patient showing a normal strain rate curve with systolic strain rate (sSR) of −1.3 cm/s. **D**, same image of an anterior myocardial infarction patient with a sSR of −0.8 cm/s.

reflectors, such as the blood cells. Tissue velocities are much lower than blood flow (<30 cm/sec) and it is possible to use color flow mapping to translate different velocities patterns in the same image. The main limitation of tissue Doppler tracings is the fact that in some circumstances the accuracy is low due to the complex movement of the heart (translational movement) and tethering.

Two other contractility parameters can be derived from tissue velocities, used to correct those limitations. *Strain* (e) is the amount of shortening of a myocardial fiber and is expressed in percentage (%) and *strain rate* (ε) is the rate of change in length and is calculated as the difference between two velocities normalized to the distance between them, expressed as *seconds*$^{-1}$ or s^{-1}. Both parameters are expressed as negative numbers for the normal systolic shortening and positive for diastolic or stretching.

The last parameter obtained by tissue Doppler imaging is displacement, which is the distance a region of interest moves relative to its original location. It is calculated as an integration of tissue velocity in a given time.

Another method of obtaining *strain* and *strain rate* and even tissue velocities is to use 2D images, which has the advantage of angle independence, compared to Doppler-derived parameters. The 2D method uses the speckles to track the complex movements of the heart. Speckles are acoustic points or markers in the myocardial tissue produced by the ultrasound and they are used to track movement in a frame-by-frame manner to calculate shortening, stretching, and the complex heart motion such as twisting and rotation.

All these parameters have been used extensively to study global and regional contractility as well as diastolic function; rest and stress studies in coronary heart disease, and left ventricular dyssynchrony (Fig. 6-17).[10-13]

Contraindications

Transesophageal echocardiography in particular must be carefully judged and contraindicated if any esophageal diseases are suspected such as diverticula, tumors, strictures, or even recent surgery.

Pitfalls and Solutions

Pitfalls can be considered when the examiner is not experienced and not familiar with the correct technique, not only for the TTE but for the TEE as well. When a good acoustic quality window is possible, one of the major sources of pitfalls in both TTE and TEE is the blood flow study using Doppler. Taking aortic and mitral stenosis as examples, care must be taken with the source of the high velocity jet as being aortic or mitral regurgitation in origin and the angle between ultrasound beam and the jet. In the evaluation of mitral stenosis, a coexisting

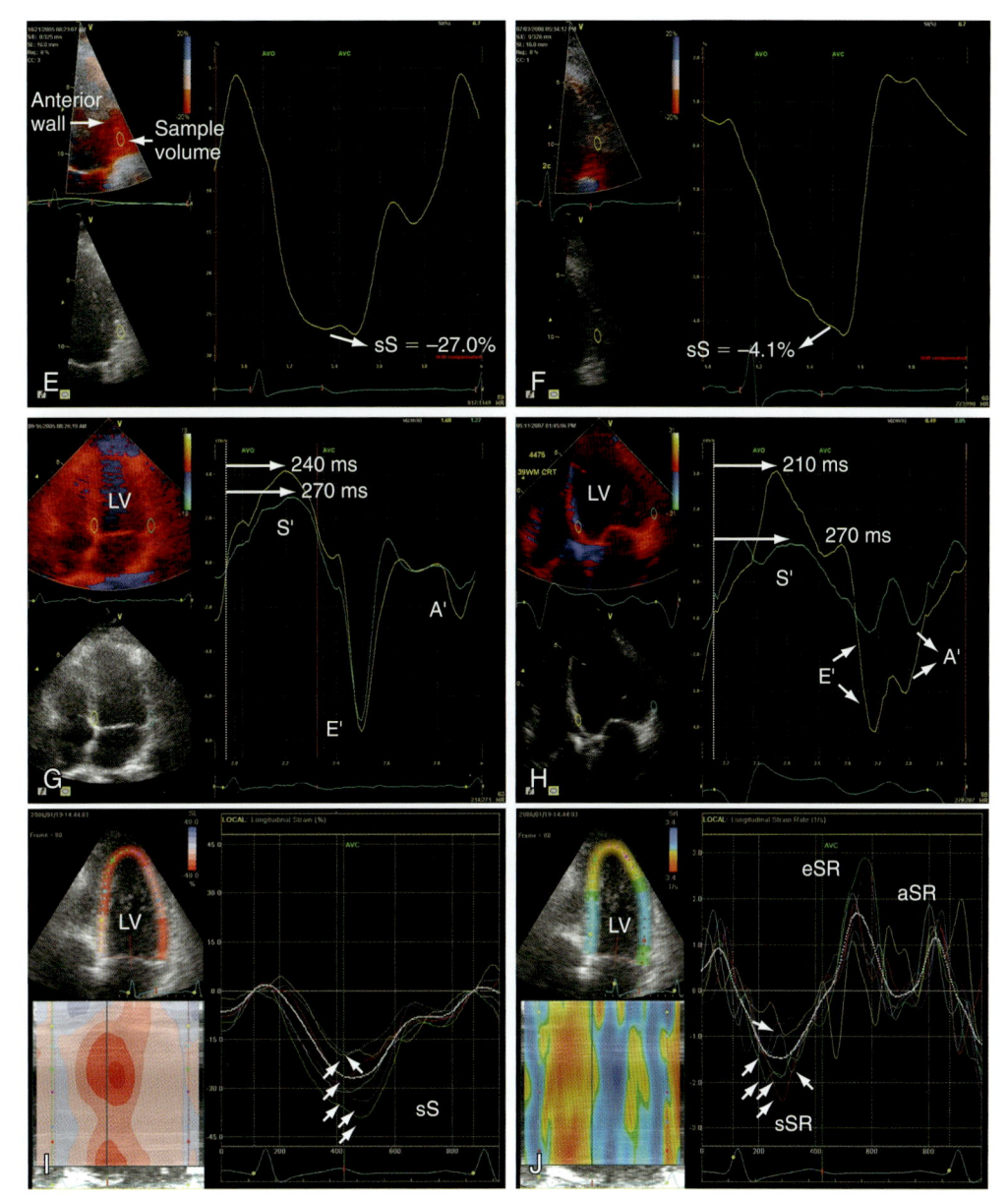

FIGURE 6-17, cont'd Strain curve. **E**, strain image and curve of a normal patient showing a systolic strain (sS) of −27%. **F**, same image of an anterior myocardial infarction patient showing an sS of −4.1%. Tissue velocities in dyssynchrony analysis. **G**, apical four-chamber view with color tissue velocity image. The curves are used to measure the time from the onset of QRS in the electrocardiogram to the peak systolic velocity (time-to-peak) (*dashed white vertical lines and white arrows*) with the comparison between the interventricular septum and the lateral walls. The comparison is based on the difference between the two time-to-peak intervals in the two walls. In this case, the difference is 30 ms in a normal patient. **H**, same image in a heart failure patient, using the same parameters in the same wall regions with a difference in time-to-peak intervals of 60 ms. Bidimensional (2D) strain and strain rate. Apical four-chamber view used for strain (**I**) and strain rate curves (**J**) based on 2D method or speckle tracking. Note the difference in the point for the peak systolic strain curves for each wall (*white arrows*). A′, late diastolic velocity; E′, early diastolic velocity; S′, systolic velocity; sS, systolic strain; sSR, systolic strain rate; eSR, early diastolic strain rate; aSR, late diastolic strain rate; LV, left ventricle.

aortic regurgitation can lead to erroneous measurements of valve area and gradients based on Doppler interrogation.

All measurements made by 2D echocardiography and especially by Doppler can have some variability due to changes in stroke volume related to changes in blood pressure and heart rate, respiratory variation and, considering the examiner's learning curve, an intra- and interobserver expected difference.

Transesophageal echocardiography has several pitfalls that must be considered during the analysis. Many anatomical structures that are not well seen in transthoracic echocardiography can be confused with masses, thrombus (such as pectinate muscles in atria and atrial appendages or surgical sutures of prosthetic valves, or other patch material); the thickened atrial septum in lipomatous hypertrophy can be misinterpreted as a mass such as myxoma; the eustachian valve, in the right atrium at the orifice of the inferior vena cava can appear as a mobile membrane or mass.[14]

The quality of studies of aortic dissection can be compromised due to the existence of artifacts produced by the lungs in the mid-descending aorta and linear artifacts can be confused with dissection flaps. Caution must always be taken when suspected images such as these are found and when the final quality of the images is compromised by air.[14]

All the pitfalls discussed here can be minimized by the use of several planes of view in the transthoracic echocardiography and the use of multiplane probes for the transesophageal echocardiography, and most importantly by the experience of the examiner.[14]

KEY POINTS

- **M Mode Technique**
  - M mode is useful for its higher temporal resolution.
  - Used mainly to measure cardiac chambers dimensions.
- **2D Mode Technique**
  - Bidimensional mode is basic method to study cardiac anatomy and function
  - Used to apply all other methods for echocardiography studies such as M mode and Doppler
  - Always useful to study the human heart in all different planes possible
- **Doppler Echocardiography and Color Flow Imaging**
  - Doppler echocardiography provides graphic and bidimensional information of flow in the heart.
  - Possible to calculate several hemodynamic data.
  - Care with the technique and its own limitations can provide useful diagnostic and prognostic data in many cardiac diseases.
- **Transesophageal Echocardiography**
  - Due to its proximity with the heart, transesophageal echocardiography provides detailed high resolution images.
  - Care should be taken with patients' limitations to the technique.
- **3D Echocardiography**
  - 3D echocardiography shows complete anatomy and function of the heart in many views.
  - It can be used in several cardiac conditions applying all bidimensional and Doppler-derived methods.
- **Tissue Doppler and Strain Imaging**
  - Tissue Doppler and strain imaging are sensitive techniques to study myocardial performance.
  - These techniques can be used in all cardiac diseases.
  - Studies of dyssynchrony and specific cardiomyopathies are the main examples of applicability of tissue Doppler and strain imaging.

SUGGESTED READING

Oh JK, Seward JB, Tajik AJ: The Echo Manual, 3rd ed. Philadelphia, Lippincott Williams & Wilkins, 2006.

REFERENCES

1. Quiñones MA, Otto CM, Stoddard M, et al. Recommendations for quantification of Doppler echocardiography: A report from the Doppler quantification task force of the nomenclature and standards committee of the American Society of Echocardiography. J Am Soc Echocardiogr 2002; 15:167-184.
2. Lang RM, Bierig M, Devereux RB, et al. Recommendations for Chamber Quantification: A Report from the American Society of Echocardiography's Guidelines and Standards Committee and the Chamber Quantification Writing Group, Developed in Conjunction with the European Association of Echocardiography, a Branch of the European Society of Cardiology. J Am Soc Echocardiogr 2005; 18:1440-1463.
3. Cerqueira MD, Weissman NJ, Dilsizian V, et al. Standardized Myocardial Segmentation and Nomenclature for Tomographic Imaging of the Heart: A Statement for Healthcare Professionals From the Cardiac Imaging Committee of the Council on Clinical Cardiology of the American Heart Association. Circulation 2002; 105:539-542.
4. Abhayaratna WP, Seward JB, Appleton CP, et al. Left Atrial Size: Physiologic Determinants and Clinical Applications. J Am Coll Cardiol 2006; 47:2357-2363.
5. Møller JE, Hillis GS, Oh JK, et al. Wall motion score index and ejection fraction for risk stratification after acute myocardial infarction. Am Heart J 2006; 151:419-425.
6. Møller JE, Søndergaard E, Poulsen SH, et al. Color M-mode and pulsed wave tissue Doppler echocardiography: powerful predictors of cardiac events after first myocardial infarction. J Am Soc Echocardiogr 2001; 14:757-763.
7. Tsuchihashi K, Ueshima K, Uchida T, et al. Transient left ventricular apical ballooning without coronary artery stenosis: a novel heart syndrome mimicking acute myocardial infarction. J Am Coll Cardiol 2001; 38:11-18.
8. Otto CM. Valvular Aortic Stenosis: Disease Severity and Timing of Intervention. J American Coll Cardiol 2006; 47:2141-2151.
9. Zoghbi WA, Enriquez-Sarano M, Foster E, et al. Recommendations for evaluation of the severity of native valvular regurgitation with two-dimensional and Doppler echocardiography. J Am Soc Echocardiogr 2003; 16:777-802.
10. Abraham TP, Belohlavek M, Thomson HL, et al. Time to onset of regional relaxation: feasibility, variability and utility of a novel index of regional myocardial function by strain rate imaging. J Am Coll Cardiol 2002; 39:1531-1537.
11. Yip G, Abraham T, Belohlavek M, Khandheria BK. Clinical applications of strain rate imaging. J Am Soc Echocardiogr 2003; 16:1334-1342.
12. Sutherland GR, Di Salvo G, Claus P, et al. Strain and strain rate imaging: a new clinical approach to quantifying regional myocardial function. J Am Soc Echocardiogr 2004; 17:788-802.
13. Yu CM, Zhang Q, Fung JW, et al. A novel tool to assess systolic asynchrony and identify responders of cardiac resynchronization therapy by tissue synchronization imaging. J Am Coll Cardiol 2005; 45:677-684.
14. Khandheria BK, Seward JB, Tajik AJ. Critical appraisal of transesophageal echocardiography: limitations and pitfalls. Crit Care Clin 1996; 12:235-251.

CHAPTER 7

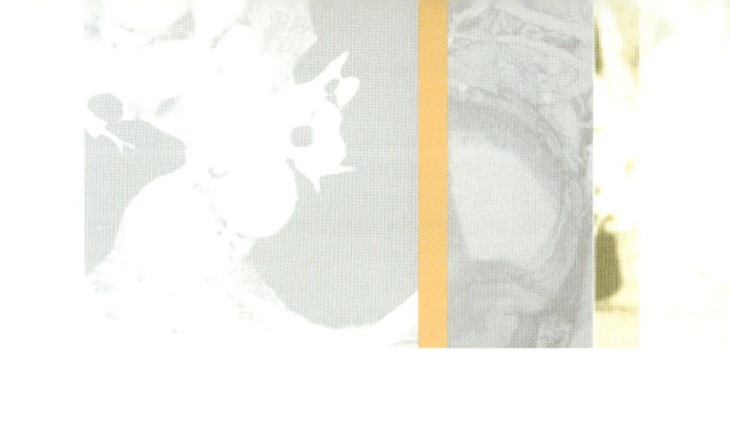

Diagnostic Coronary Angiography

Curtis E. Green

Despite significant advances in coronary CT angiography and MR angiography in the past decade, coronary angiography is the mainstay for the evaluation of coronary artery morphology and disease, and is a mandatory prerequisite for coronary intervention. Therefore, it is useful to have an appreciation for its strengths and limitations relative to coronary CT angiography.

TECHNICAL REQUIREMENTS

High-quality coronary angiography requires excellent quality fluoroscopic and digital imaging and a C-arm capable of three-dimensional rotation. These may be either single plane or biplane. Biplane laboratories are most useful for pediatric angiography and studies where simultaneous biplane fluoroscopy is needed (e.g., electrophysiologic studies). The x-ray tube must have a high heat capacity and small and large focal spots so that large patients can be imaged. Digital image receptors should have multiple magnification modes so that the entire heart can be imaged with a large field of view, and the coronary arteries can be imaged with a smaller field of view at higher spatial resolution. The use of higher magnification modes requires more panning (table movement during angiography) and higher radiation dose. As in static image systems, a grid is placed on the face of the image intensifier to reduce the effect of scatter radiation on the radiographic image. Coronary cineangiograms are typically recorded at 15 frames/sec, 30 frames/sec, or 60 frames/sec depending on the indication for the study.

In the past, images were recorded on 35-mm cine film and viewed on a cine projector. Today, catheterization laboratories use digital recording with viewing on a computer monitor. Although the spatial resolution of cine film is higher, digital recording is so much more convenient that it has become the standard. Digital recording does not require film processing with its inherent requirements for quality control, and the storage space required for cine film and the cost of cine film are enormous compared with digital media storage and cost.

TECHNIQUE

Indications

Although coronary CT angiography has begun to replace diagnostic coronary angiography in some patient groups, conventional coronary angiography is still considered the definitive technique for evaluation of suspected coronary disease. Even in centers where coronary CT angiography is readily available, coronary angiography is the first-choice test in a patient with clear-cut unstable angina or myocardial infarction owing to the benefits of acute intervention in patients with acute myocardial infarction. It is also usually the preferred test in patients with known coronary artery disease who are undergoing coronary artery bypass surgery or cardiac valve replacement. Patients with heavily calcified coronary arteries are also usually more readily imaged with conventional coronary angiography than with CT angiography.

Contraindications

As with all diagnostic tests using radiographic contrast material, renal dysfunction is a relative contraindication to coronary angiography, especially in a patient in whom the suspicion for coronary disease is low. In many patients, angiography can be performed with a low volume of contrast material and any patient with arterial access can be safely studied if necessary.

TECHNIQUE DESCRIPTION

Coronary angiography is almost always performed via puncture of a femoral artery (Judkins' technique). In a few patients, a brachial artery cutdown is performed (Sones' technique). Coronary catheters used for Judkins' technique are preshaped and come in various sizes to make selective cannulation of the left and right coronary arteries simple in most patients. So-called multipurpose catheters are occasionally used and can be directed into either coronary ostium, although with slightly more difficulty. The coronaries must be selectively engaged to obtain diagnostic quality studies with a minimum amount of contrast material.

When performing coronary angiography, the goal is to show optimally each part of each artery in at least two, preferentially orthogonal, projections, free of overlap with other vessels and free of foreshortening. This imaging requires a great deal of attention to radiographic and angiographic technique. Radiographic factors that contribute to the quality of the angiograms include the following:

1. Keeping the image receptor as close to the patient as possible
2. Using as small a focal spot as x-ray tube loading allows
3. Optimal collimation of the x-ray beam

Angiographic factors include the following:

1. Adequate engagement of the coronary ostium
2. Rapid injection of an adequate amount of contrast material
3. Use of properly positioned angiographic views
4. Minimizing table motion (panning) during the cine run.

ANGIOGRAPHIC VIEWS

Various angiographic projections are used to achieve the goal of viewing each coronary segment in at least two projections, free of foreshortening and free of overlap with other vessels. This goal was impossible before the advent of C-arms capable of triaxial motion. With modern equipment, angiographic views are limited only by physical impingement of the x-ray tube or image receptor on the patient or table, and the patient's body habitus. In addition to rotation in the axial plane (generally from about 45 degrees right anterior oblique [RAO] to left lateral), the image receptor must be positioned over the patient's shoulder to produce cranially angulated views and over the hip to produce caudally angulated views to image many coronary artery segments adequately. Cranial or caudal angulation is usually limited to about 25 degrees in most patients.

In most patients, the right coronary artery is best imaged with a combination of left lateral, cranial left anterior oblique (Cr-LAO), RAO, and Cr-RAO views. Although not used by many cardiologists, the lateral view (Fig. 7-1) has several advantages over a standard 60-degree LAO view because it usually allows better visualization of the mid right coronary artery and collaterals to the left anterior descending artery (LAD). The Cr-LAO view is necessary to lay out the posterior descending artery and posterolateral branches arising from the right coronary artery beyond the posterior descending artery (Fig. 7-2). In patients with large posterolateral branches, the Cr-RAO view projects the posterior descending artery and postero-

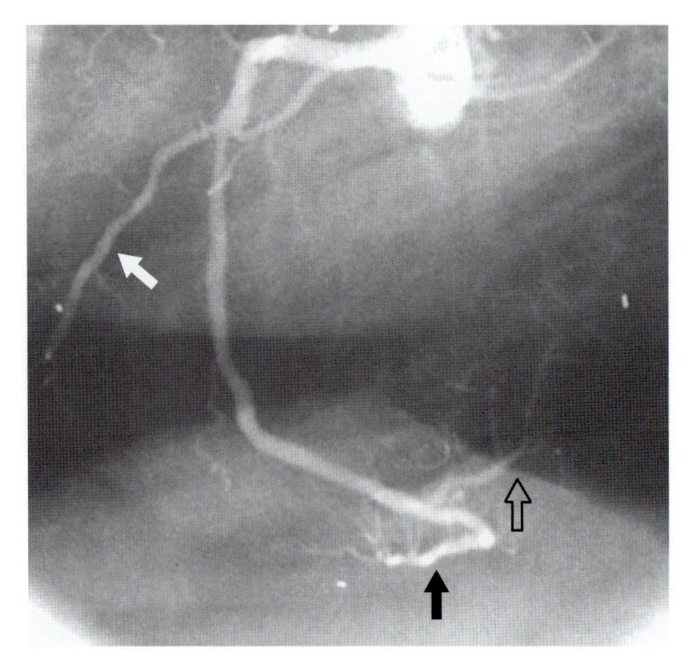

■ **FIGURE 7-1** Lateral view of the right coronary artery showing excellent visualization of most of the vessel and the large acute marginal (*white arrow*). The posterior descending artery (*solid black arrow*) and posterolateral segment artery (*open black arrow*) are foreshortened.

lateral branches clear of each other (Fig. 7-3). Usually, one should not use the Cr-RAO view to the exclusion of the RAO view (Fig. 7-4); however, because the body of the right coronary artery is foreshortened in the Cr-RAO view.

In the average patient, the left main coronary artery is projected at true length in either a posteroanterior or a shallow LAO view (Fig. 7-5). The bifurcation and proximal portions of the LAD and left circumflex artery are usually best seen in the Cr-LAO[1] (Fig. 7-6) and RAO projections. Enough LAO rotation should be used to place the distal LAD between the spine and the diaphragm. In some indi-

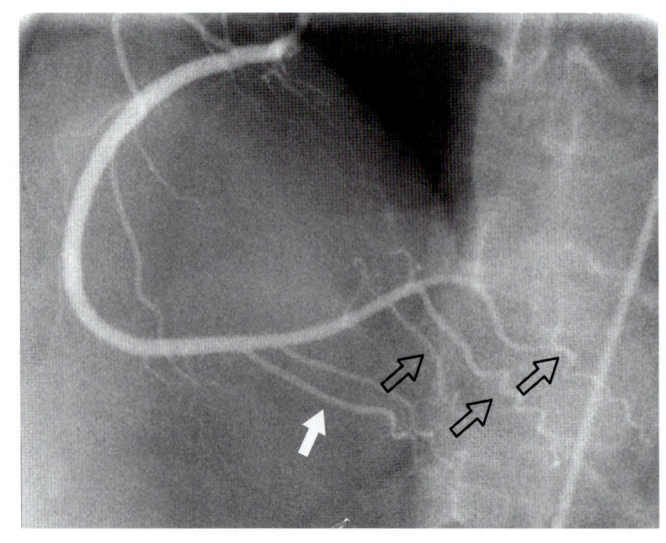

■ **FIGURE 7-2** Cr-LAO view of the right coronary artery. The body of the right coronary artery is foreshortened, but the posterior descending artery (*white arrow*) and posterolateral branches (*open black arrows*) are nicely laid out.

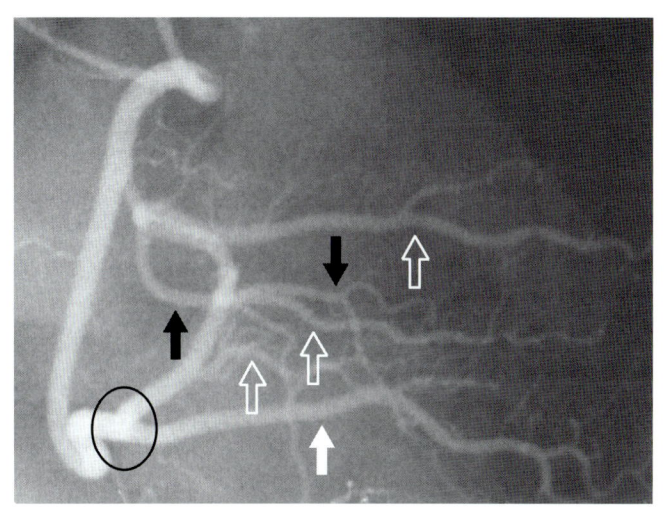

■ **FIGURE 7-3** Cr-RAO view of the right coronary artery shows the origin of the posterior descending artery (*circle*) and projects the posterior descending artery (*white arrow*) clear of the posterolateral branches (*open white arrows*). An acute marginal artery overlaps a posterolateral branch (*black arrow*). The body of the right coronary artery is foreshortened.

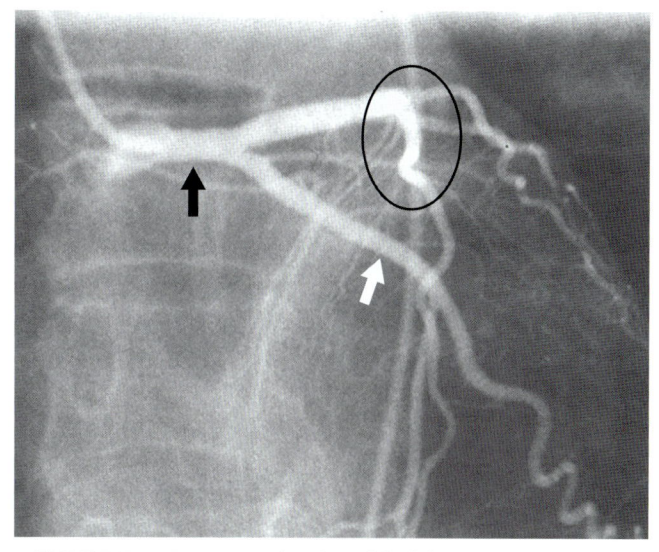

■ **FIGURE 7-5** Posteroanterior view of the left coronary artery shows the major portion of the left main coronary artery (*black arrow*), but does not profile the origin. The mid-body of the left anterior descending artery is foreshortened (*inside oval*). The left circumflex artery (*white arrow*) is well shown.

viduals, the left main coronary artery has an up-going course. This requires using caudal angulation to eliminate foreshortening. The caudal LAO[2] view is the only angiographic view that should be performed with the patient holding his or her breath in expiration (Fig. 7-7). If the patient inspires, the effect of the caudal angulation is negated; this is most common in large patients and requires more exposure than nonangulated views resulting in a degraded image. Because the distal LAD frequently is superimposed on the diaphragm in the Cr-LAO view, a lateral view is often useful (Fig. 7-8).

At least two RAO views should be obtained in almost all patients. Because the proximal portion of the left circumflex artery curves posteriorly, one must use caudal angulation[3] to visualize it and the origins of any proximally arising obtuse marginal branches adequately (Fig. 7-9). With regard to the LAD, the diagonal branches frequently are superimposed on the LAD in the straight RAO view, so cranial angulation of 20 to 25 degrees may be useful

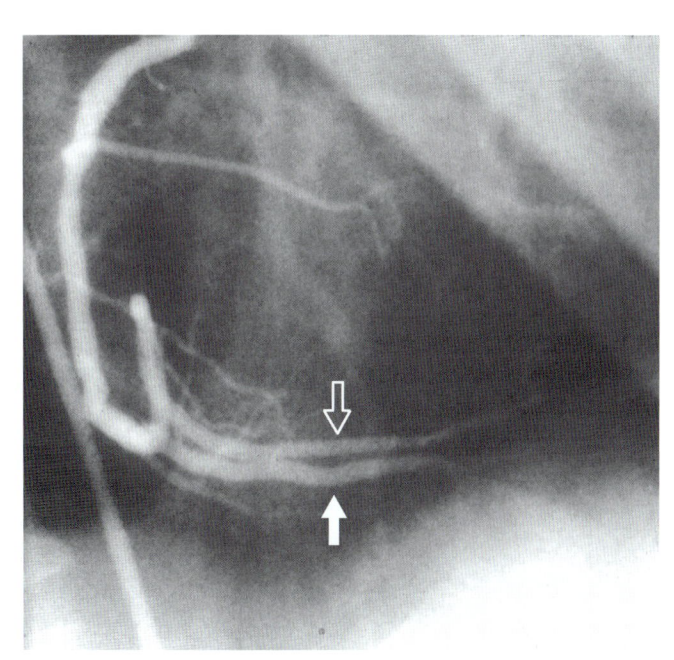

■ **FIGURE 7-4** Straight RAO view of the right coronary artery. The posterior descending artery (*solid arrow*) and posterolateral branch (*open arrow*) nearly overlap.

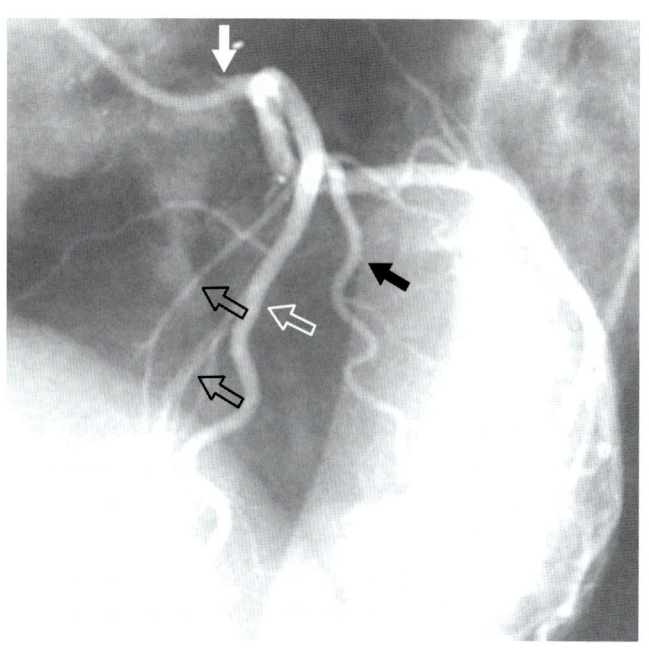

■ **FIGURE 7-6** Cr-LAO view of the left coronary artery shows the origin of the left main coronary artery (*solid white arrow*) and the left anterior descending artery (*open white arrow*), diagonal artery (*solid black arrow*), and septal perforators (*open black arrows*). The left circumflex artery is obscured by the spine, and the distal left anterior descending artery is obscured by the diaphragm.

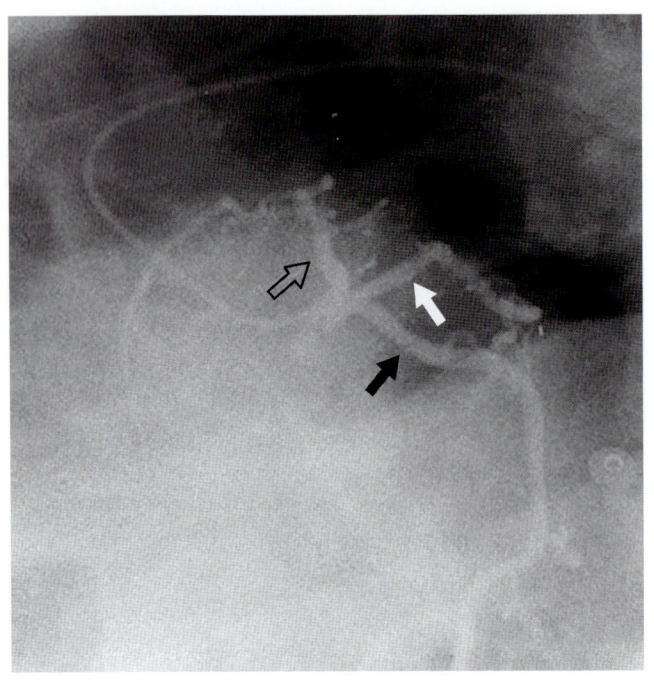

■ FIGURE 7-7 Caudal LAO view of the left coronary artery shows the origins of the left anterior descending artery (*open arrow*), left circumflex artery (*white arrow*), and ramus intermedius (*black arrow*) arteries, but image quality is significantly degraded.

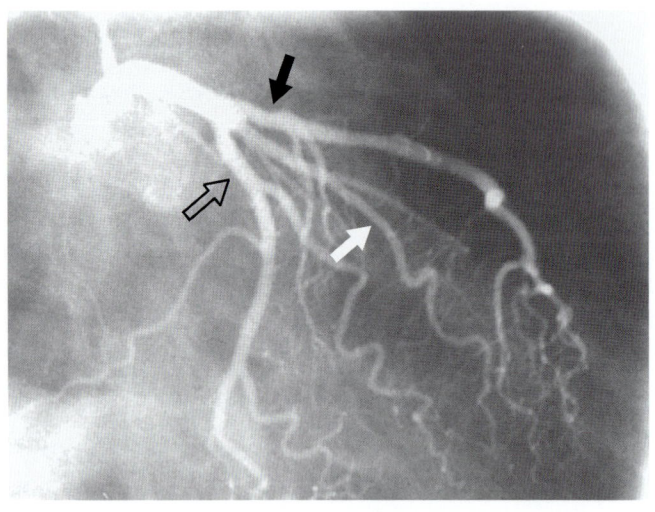

■ FIGURE 7-9 Caudal RAO view of the left coronary artery. The proximal portion of the circumflex artery (*open arrow*) appears longer than in the straight RAO view (see Fig. 7-11). The left anterior descending artery (*solid black arrow*) and ramus intermedius (*solid white arrow*) are also well seen.

(Fig. 7-10).[4] The straight RAO view can be added if the distal LAD is poorly visualized in the other RAO views (Fig. 7-11).

PITFALLS AND SOLUTIONS

Coronary angiography has many advantages over CT angiography and MR angiography of the coronary arteries. Spatial resolution and temporal resolution are superior to CT angiography and MR angiography. High spatial resolution allows one to visualize submillimeter vessels and narrower arterial lumens. High temporal resolution allows for evaluation of arterial filling patterns such as delay in flow, a valuable indicator of severe stenosis, and for assessment of collateral filling of obstructed arteries. Coronary angiography has several disadvantages, however, including the need for arterial puncture and direct cannulation of the coronary ostia, and the fact that the number of views is limited by radiation and contrast dose considerations. Because of limited views, one does not have the ability to look at the arteries from any angle, as one can with coronary CT angiography. Also, similar to all planar angiograms, coronary angiograms are luminograms—one cannot see the wall of the vessel, only the contrast-filled lumen. This becomes important for reasons discussed subsequently.

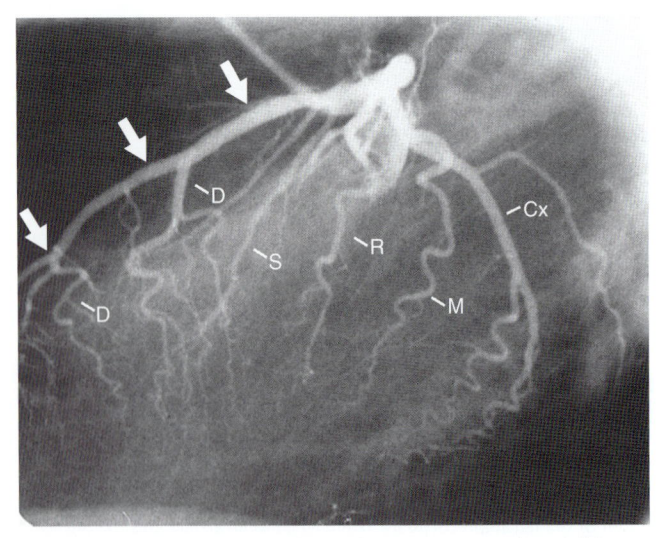

■ FIGURE 7-8 Lateral view of the left coronary artery shows all but the most proximal portion of the left anterior descending artery (*arrows*). Cx, left circumflex; D, diagonal; M, obtuse marginal; R, ramus intermedius; S, septal perforator.

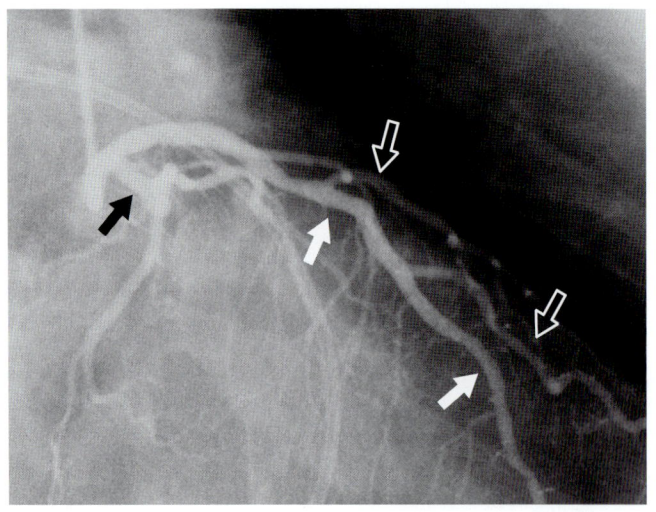

■ FIGURE 7-10 Cr-RAO view of the left coronary artery projects the diagonals (*open arrows*) clear of the left anterior descending artery (*solid white arrows*). The proximal circumflex artery (*black arrow*) is severely foreshortened.

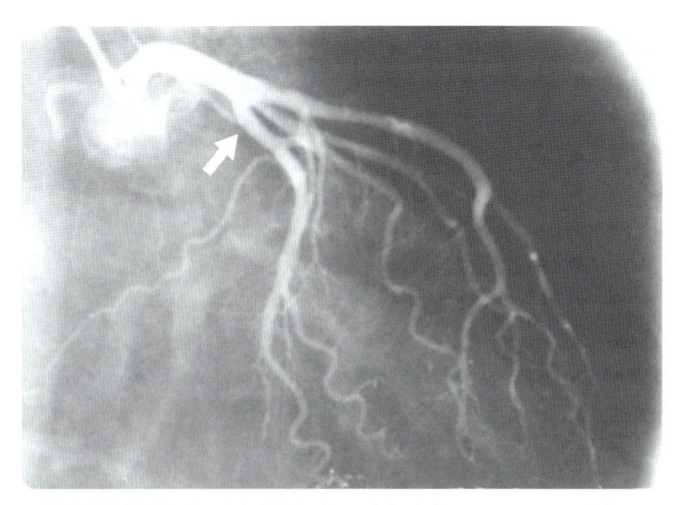

FIGURE 7-11 Straight RAO view of the left coronary artery. The proximal circumflex appears shorter (*arrow*) than in the caudal view from the same patient (compare with Fig. 7-9). In some cases, the foreshortening may hide a lesion in this region.

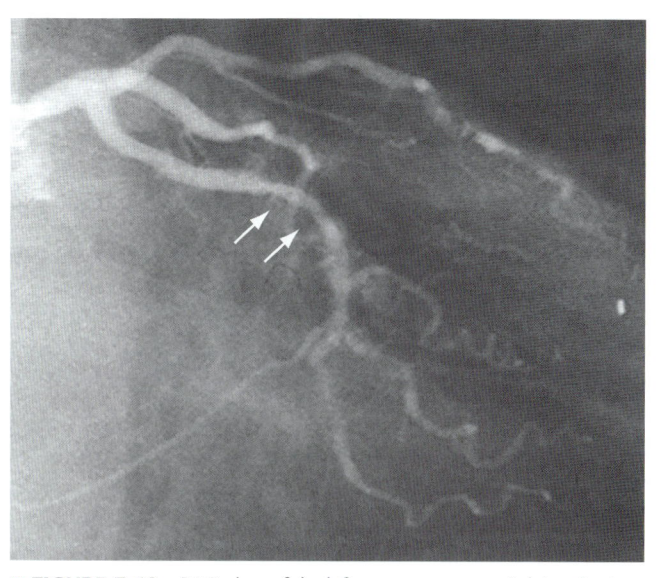

FIGURE 7-12 RAO view of the left coronary artery. Calcium in the wall of the circumflex artery (*arrows*) demarcates the vessel wall and un-narrowed diameter of the lumen at that point.

IMAGE INTERPRETATION

Coronary atherosclerosis is a diffuse process with focal exacerbations.[5] Despite this, the time-honored method of evaluating coronary narrowing is by determination of percent luminal diameter narrowing. This evaluation requires comparing a region of narrowing with that of an adjacent vessel segment that appears to be relatively normal. The normal or reference region may be diffusely narrowed, resulting in underestimation of the degree of stenosis. If there is calcium in the wall of the coronary artery, one may be able to determine the actual diameter of the vessel at that point (Fig. 7-12); however, one still would not know whether that is the true size of the vessel before it became diseased because it may be dilated (see later). Coronary stenoses are rarely concentric, and the severity of narrowing may vary widely in different projections (Fig. 7-13). Some angiographers have tried to circumvent these limitations by calculating percent area narrowing; this still usually requires the assumption that the lesion is concentric, and in my opinion only adds another layer of imprecision to the assessment.

Generally, luminal diameter narrowing of 50% or greater is considered likely to be hemodynamically significant. Resistance through a stenosis is a function of many variables, however, including length and morphology—so this is only a crude gauge, similar to using a cardiothoracic ratio of 50% to identify cardiomegaly on a chest radiograph. Finally, unless one uses some type of caliper, there is a marked tendency to overestimate visually the severity of narrowing; this has been jokingly referred to as the "oculostenotic reflex," but is a very real phenomenon. For these reasons, one should not rely solely on the angiographic appearance of a lesion in determining therapy.

Coronary narrowing can be broadly characterized as either discrete or diffuse. We know that atherosclerosis tends to be a diffuse process with focal exacerbations, so when we use the term *discrete*, it should be understood that we are accepting the limitations of angiography for

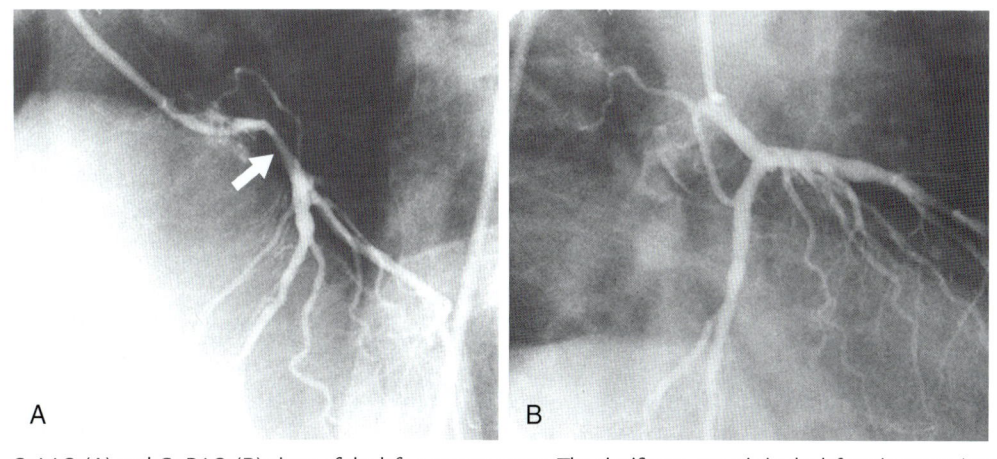

FIGURE 7-13 Cr-LAO (**A**) and Cr-RAO (**B**) views of the left coronary artery. The significant stenosis in the left main artery (*arrow* in **A**) is unapparent in the RAO view (**B**).

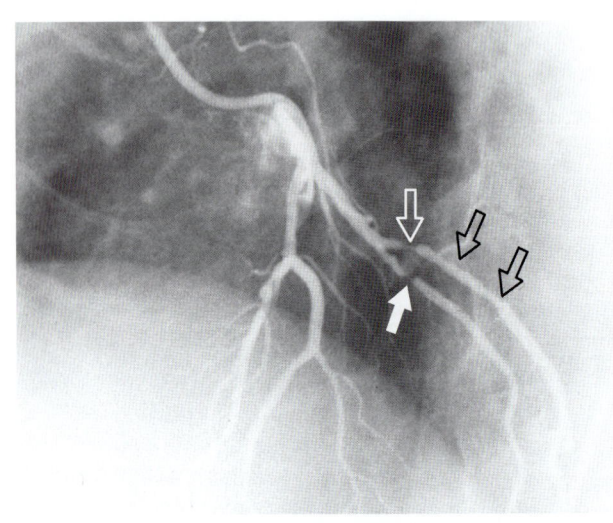

FIGURE 7-14 Cr-LAO view of the left coronary artery. Discrete-appearing stenoses are present in the first obtuse marginal (*solid white arrow*) and mid-circumflex (*open white arrow*). Mild, diffuse narrowing is present in the circumflex artery beyond the stenosis (*open black arrows*).

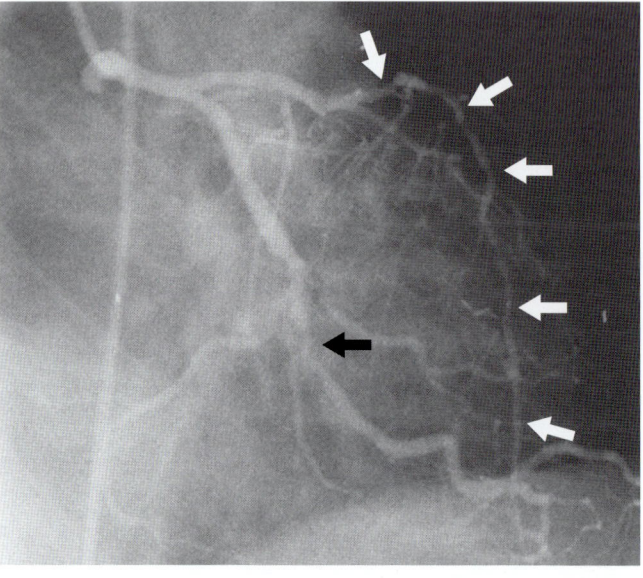

FIGURE 7-16 RAO view of the left coronary artery. Most of the left anterior descending artery is severely narrowed (*white arrows*). A discrete-appearing stenosis is also present in the second obtuse marginal (*black arrow*).

characterizing lesions. Discrete stenoses (Fig. 7-14) tend to occur in the proximal portions of the epicardial coronary arteries. They may have noncalcified (soft) plaque, calcified (hard) plaque, or a mixture of the two. Soft plaque is less stable than hard plaque and accounts for most acute coronary occlusions. Patients with mostly hard plaque are more likely to present with chronic angina. Angiography does a poor job of distinguishing between the two.

Diffuse narrowing is less commonly identified at angiography because of its inability to image the vessel wall. The narrowing may appear to involve only a relatively short distance (Fig. 7-15) or most of a vessel (Fig. 7-16).

In the latter case, one may be unable to give an estimate of percent diameter narrowing. As mentioned previously, diffuse narrowing can cause underestimation of the severity of the relatively discrete stenoses occurring either within the diffusely narrowed area or on either end of it. The ability to see the wall of the coronary artery is one of the great advantages of coronary CT angiography compared with conventional coronary angiography.

In addition to narrowing, atherosclerosis can cause coronary artery enlargement. This enlargement can result from the dilation caused by early remodeling or from atherosclerotic ectasia. With ectasia, the area of dilation may be focal (Fig. 7-17) or diffuse (Fig. 7-18). In either case, it

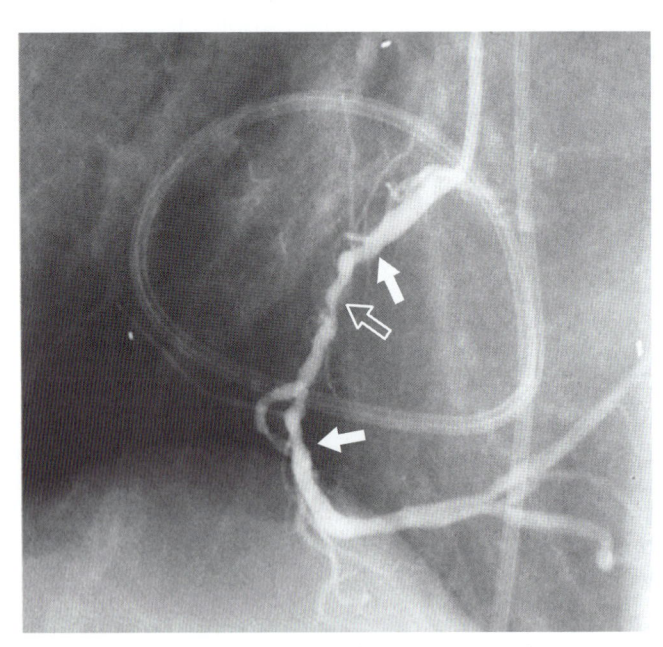

FIGURE 7-15 LAO view of the right coronary artery shows moderate diffuse narrowing of the right coronary (between the *solid arrows*) with a more severe lesion in the mid-body (*open arrow*).

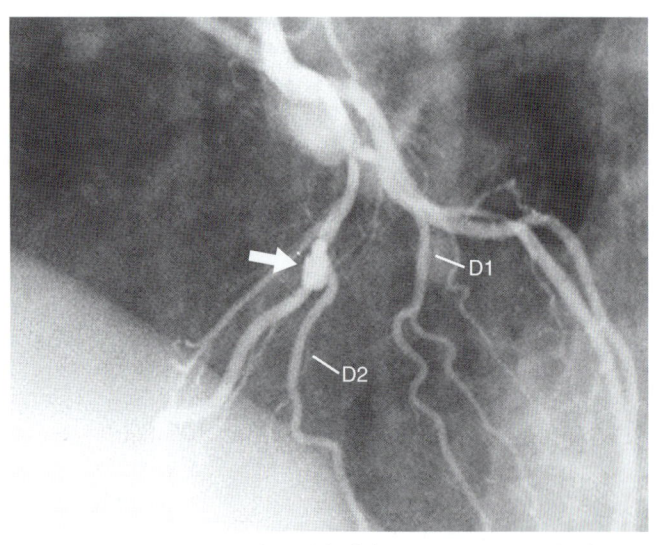

FIGURE 7-17 Cr-LAO view of the left coronary artery. A focal aneurysm (*arrow*) is present in the mid left anterior descending artery at the origin of the second diagonal (D2). D1, first diagonal.

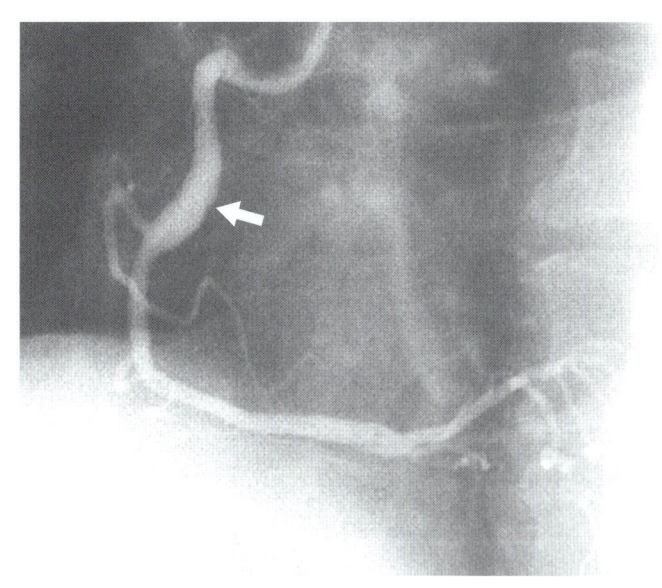

■ **FIGURE 7-18** LAO view of the right coronary artery shows an area of fusiform dilation (*arrow*) in the mid-body.

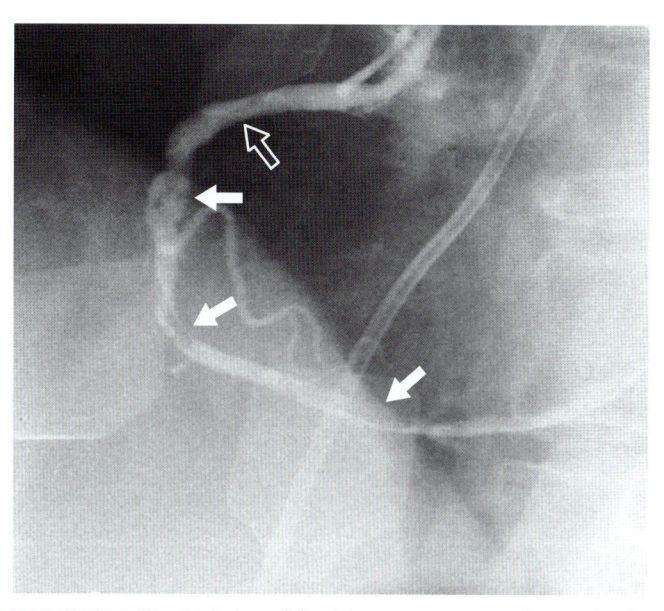

■ **FIGURE 7-20** LAO view of the right coronary artery after proximal right coronary dissection (*open arrow*). There is extensive thrombus (*solid arrows*) throughout the right coronary distal to a high-grade mid-body stenosis.

may harbor thrombus. Another problem caused by coronary dilation is that if the chosen reference segment is actually dilated rather than normal, the reference diameter may be greater than in the predisease state, and can result in overestimation of the severity of narrowing.

Coronary artery dissection can occur spontaneously or as the result of catheter-induced trauma or balloon angioplasty. The findings are similar to findings seen in aortic dissection with an intimal flap within the coronary lumen (Fig. 7-19). In some cases, the coronary artery may occlude, making the identification of dissection difficult in spontaneous cases.

Coronary thrombosis typically results from rupture of soft plaque, although it may be seen during coronary intervention and rarely in other circumstances, such as coronary artery compression by a mass or enlarged pulmonary artery. The clot may result in a filling defect within the lumen (Fig. 7-20) or an abrupt occlusion with a concave-appearing proximal border (Fig. 7-21).

Emboli to the coronary arteries are rare, and may be difficult to detect angiographically. A typical appearance would be that of an abrupt occlusion with a convex proximal border identical to that of a thrombus.

Evaluation of collateral flow to a diseased coronary artery is straightforward at angiography and difficult to impossible with coronary CT angiography. Collateral vessels typically are a consequence of slowly developing

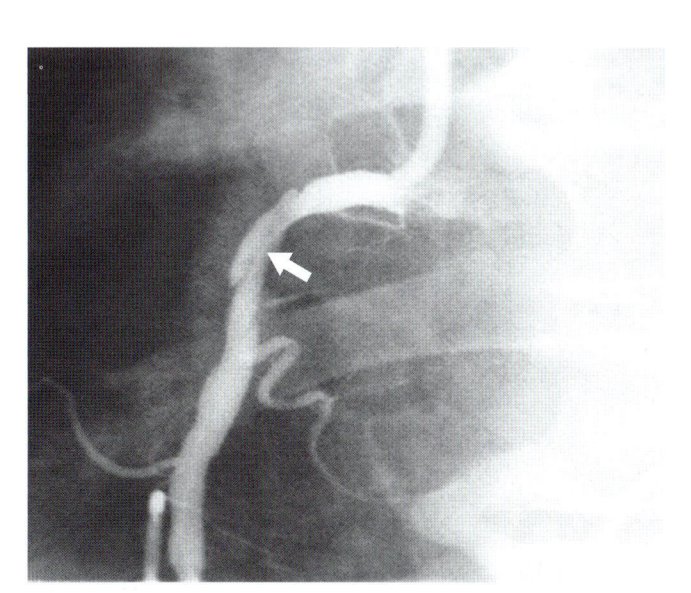

■ **FIGURE 7-19** LAO view of the right coronary artery shows an intimal flap (*arrow*) in the proximal right coronary artery caused by dissection during balloon angioplasty.

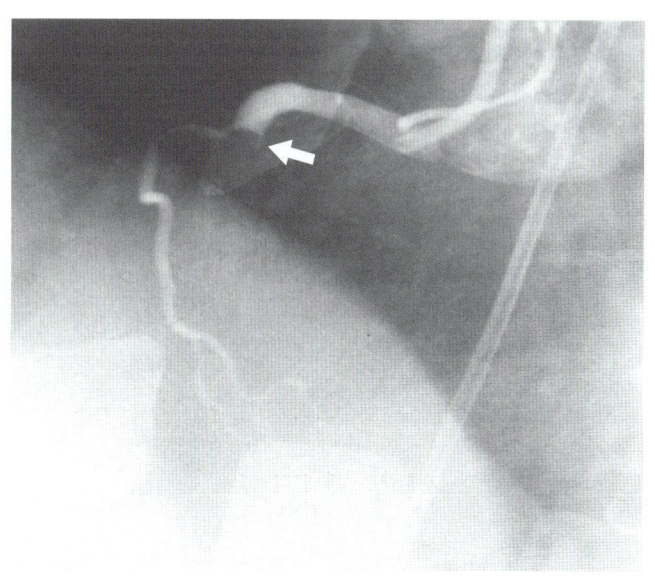

■ **FIGURE 7-21** Cr-LAO view of the right coronary artery shows occlusion of the proximal coronary artery (*arrow*) by thrombus. A coronary embolus would have a similar appearance.

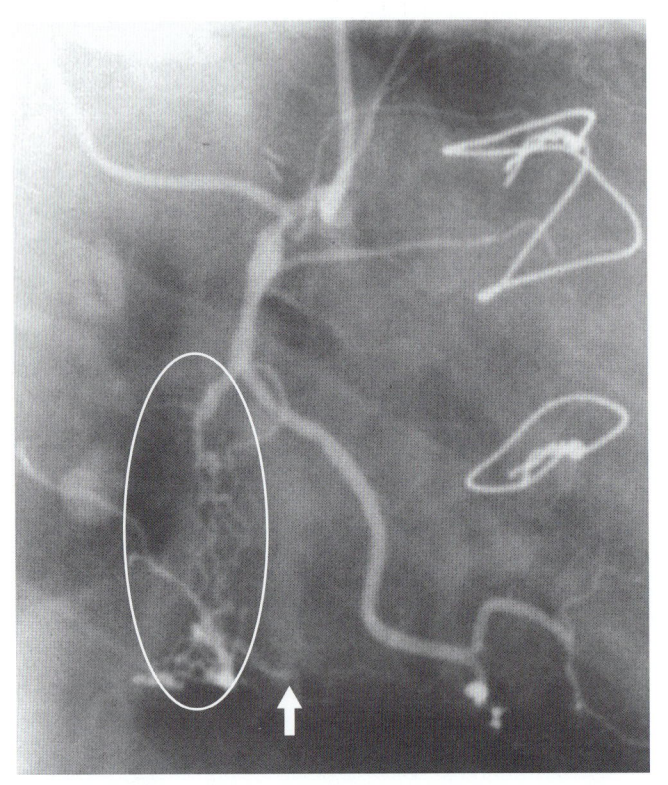

FIGURE 7-22 RAO view of the right coronary artery. Complete occlusion of the mid-coronary is bridged by myriad tiny intracoronary collaterals (*inside oval*). The posterior descending artery (*arrow*) is faintly visualized.

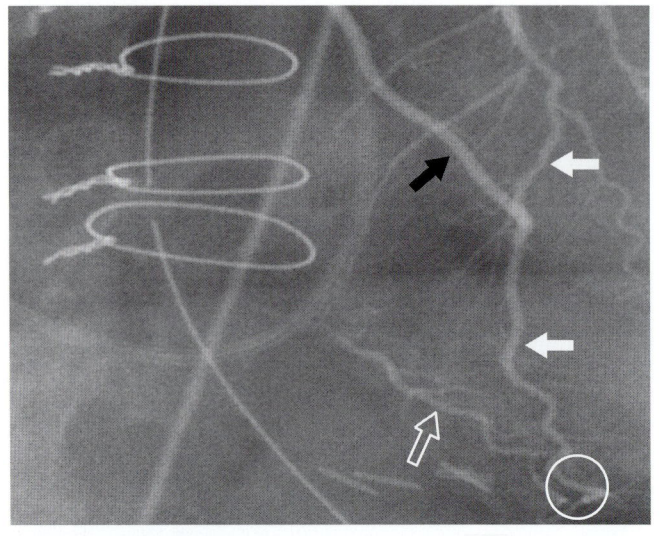

FIGURE 7-23 Extreme Cr-RAO view of the left coronary artery after injection of a bypass graft (*black arrow*) shows a collateral between the left anterior descending artery (*white arrows*) and posterior descending artery (*open arrow*) at the apex (*circle*).

coronary artery stenosis, but can also be seen more immediately. Intracoronary collaterals directly bridge an obstructed coronary artery segment (Fig. 7-22). Intercoronary collateral vessels connect branches of different coronary arteries or branches of the occluded artery. The myriad intercoronary collateral pathways can seem confusing sometimes, but visualization is easier if one realizes that the connections must be made through shared myocardium. Collateral vessels do not course through the middle of chambers or usually cross another coronary artery. Collateral vessels are typically quite tortuous, but may look almost like a normal coronary artery. Common intercoronary collateral pathways are listed in Table 7-1 and shown in Figures 7-23 through 7-28.

TABLE 7-1	Common Coronary Collateral Pathways
LAD to RCA	LAD to PDA around the apex (see Fig. 7-23)
	LAD to acute marginals over RV free wall (see Fig. 7-24) through the interventricular septum (see Fig. 7-25)
	Conus artery to LAD
LCx to RCA	Distal circumflex to distal RCA (AV groove artery) (see Fig. 7-26)
	Obtuse marginals to posterolateral branches (see Fig. 7-27)
RCA to RCA	SA node to AV node through the atrial septum
	Conus artery to acute marginal
	Acute marginal to PDA
LAD to LCx	Diagonal to obtuse marginal (see Fig. 7-28)
	LAD to obtuse marginal at apex
LCx to LCx	Left atrial circumflex artery
	Obtuse marginal to obtuse marginal
LAD to LAD	Septal perforators
	Diagonal to diagonal

AV, atrioventricular; LAD, left anterior descending artery; LCx, left circumflex artery; PDA, posterior descending artery; RCA, right coronary artery; RV, right ventricular; SA, sinoatrial.

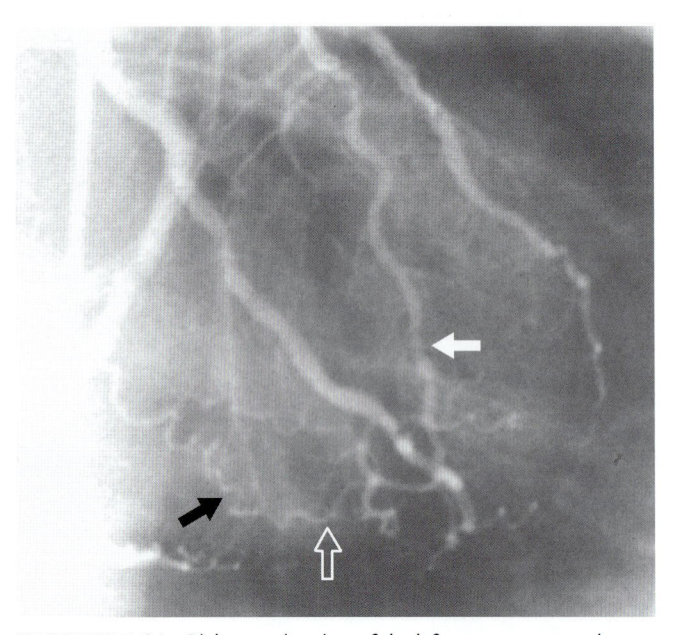

FIGURE 7-24 Right anterior view of the left coronary artery shows a tiny collateral (*open arrow*) connecting the distal left anterior descending artery (*white arrow*) and an acute marginal artery (*black arrow*).

CHAPTER 7 ● Diagnostic Coronary Angiography 131

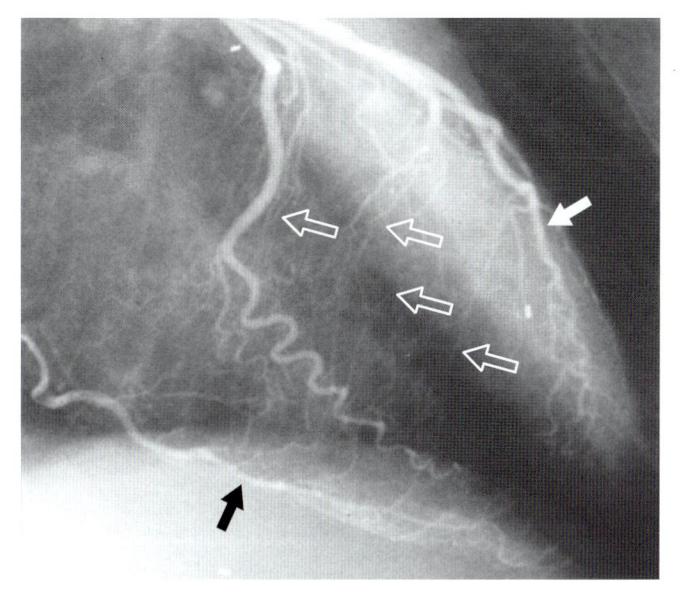

■ **FIGURE 7-25** Right anterior view of the left coronary artery shows septal collaterals (*open arrows*) from the left anterior descending (*white arrow*) to the posterior descending (*black arrow*).

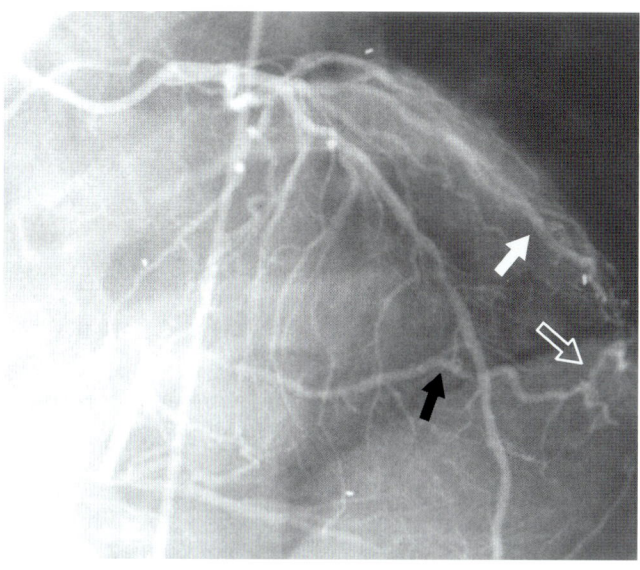

■ **FIGURE 7-27** RAO view of the left coronary artery shows a large collateral vessel (*open arrow*) connecting an obtuse marginal (*solid white arrow*) and the last posterolateral branch of the right coronary artery (*black arrow*).

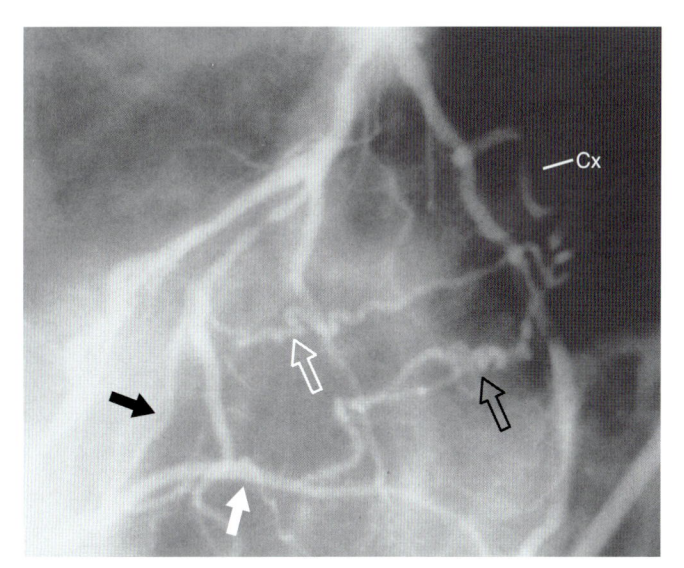

■ **FIGURE 7-26** Cr-LAO view of the left coronary artery shows filling of the distal right coronary artery branches from the circumflex (Cx). The more superior collateral (*open white arrow*) connects the distal Cx to the atrioventricular nodal artery (*solid black arrow*); the more inferior collateral (*open black arrow*) connects the distal Cx to the posterolateral segmental artery (*solid white arrow*) via the atrioventricular groove.

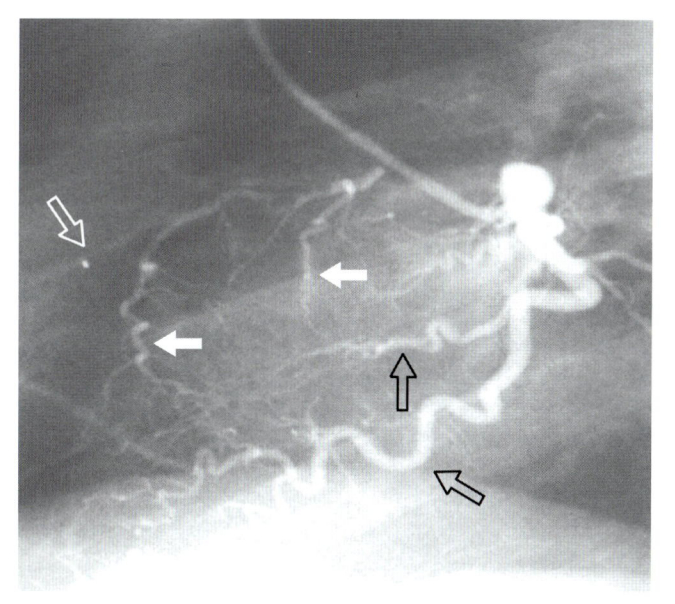

■ **FIGURE 7-28** Lateral view of the left coronary artery in a patient with total occlusion of the left anterior descending artery. Obtuse marginal branches (*open black arrows*) fill diagonal branches (*solid white arrows*), which fill the left anterior descending (*open white arrow*).

KEY POINTS

- Adequate visualization of the coronary arteries requires visualization of each major coronary segment from two, preferably orthogonal, views, free of overlap with other vessels and free of foreshortening.
- Coronary angiograms visualize only the lumen of the coronary artery, and may underestimate the amount of coronary narrowing.
- Atherosclerosis can cause dilation and narrowing of the coronary arteries.

SUGGESTED READING

Green CE. Coronary Cinematography. Philadelphia, Lippincott-Raven, 1996.

REFERENCES

1. Bunnell IL, Greene DG, Tandon RN, et al. The half axial projection: a new look at the proximal left coronary artery. Circulation 1973; 48:1151.
2. Elliott LP, Bream PR, Soto B, et al. The significance of the caudal-left anterior oblique view in analyzing the left main coronary artery and its major branches. Radiology 1981; 139:39.
3. Elliott LP, Green CE, Rogers WJ, et al. The importance of angled right anterior oblique views in improving visualization of the coronary arteries. Part I: caudocranial view. Radiology 1982; 142:631.
4. Elliott LP, Green CE, Rogers WJ, et al. The importance of angled right anterior oblique views in improving visualization of the coronary arteries. Part II: craniocaudal view. Radiology 1982; 142:637.
5. Arnett EN, Isner JM, Redwood DR, et al. Coronary artery narrowing in coronary heart disease: comparison of cineangiographic and necropsy findings. Ann Intern Med 1979; 91:350.

CHAPTER 8

Physics of Cardiac Computed Tomography

Christianne Leidecker

Computed tomography (CT) was first introduced in 1972 and has since become an indispensable tool for noninvasive diagnostic imaging. It is a robust and reproducible technique and its benefit for noninvasive cardiac imaging was soon envisioned and desired. Technical limitations prevented its applicability until the mid-1980s, but it was not until the introduction of multislice CT scanners with subsecond rotation times and higher volume coverage in the early 2000s[1-3] that noninvasive cardiac CT imaging evolved into clinical routine.[4-11] Among its various applications, coronary CT angiography (coronary CTA) has emerged as a valuable tool for imaging the coronary arteries, for which it has been shown to quantify coronary artery stenosis with high accuracy and especially to have a high negative predictive value for coronary artery disease (CAD). Imaging the heart and coronary anatomy poses high demands on spatial and temporal resolution. The small coronary arteries, with diameters typically of 2 to 4 mm, require optimal image quality and maximum resolution for reliable visualization and analysis. Because of their location close to the heart muscle and consequent strong movement during the cardiac cycle, their imaging requires almost freezing the heart to avoid motion artifacts. Finally, the scan time for covering the complete heart volume should be within the time of a single breath-hold to avoid breathing artifacts and limit radiation exposure and amount of contrast administered.

First introduced in 2004,[12] 64-slice CT systems helped establish CT imaging of the heart in clinical routine and were until recently considered state of the art. This section will therefore focus on 64-slice CT because it is still the widest available technology. The most recent developments, such as dual-source CT with high-pitch scanning and volume acquisition CT scanners, are expected to improve cardiac imaging further. These will be discussed at the end of this chapter.

CARDIAC IMAGING REQUIREMENTS

For reliable visualization and analysis of the cardiac anatomy, the imaging modality has to fulfill the requirements of high temporal resolution and high spatial and contrast resolution, which has to be simultaneously optimized with scan time and radiation exposure. Trading off one or more parameters to optimize one performance dimension may not lead to clinical useful results; rather, these conflicting requirements must be fulfilled within the same cardiac scan protocol.

Two goals can generally be defined for cardiac imaging. First, the imaging modality should allow virtual "freezing" of the motion of the heart to avoid motion artifacts. The time interval of the cardiac cycle contributing to an image should be short enough to allow the depiction of at least slow motion heart phases without motion artifacts. Second, the imaging technique should allow the selection of defined heart phases of the cardiac cycle. Because motion intensity varies over the heart cycle, with the slowest motion (usually) present in the diastolic phase, imaging is typically performed during this phase of the cardiac cycle to minimize image blurring caused by motion. A temporal resolution of 250 ms is generally considered sufficient for motion-free imaging for slow to moderate heart rates of up to 65 beats/min, because the length of the diastolic phase shortens with increasing heart rate.[13] However, if imaging is desired for phases other than diastole (e.g., for functional information), more stringent requirements are necessary. Posing very rigorous demands on image quality, such as motion-free imaging in all heart phases, would require a temporal resolution shorter than 50 ms.

IMAGE RECONSTRUCTION TECHNIQUES FOR OPTIMIZED TEMPORAL RESOLUTION

Because of the permanent cardiac motion during the acquisition, standard reconstruction techniques result in images with high artifact content (e.g., blurring) and limited diagnostic use. The aim of dedicated cardiac image reconstruction algorithms is therefore to use only short scan segments and align these with the heart motion pattern so that the motion is frozen in a desired phase.

The optimal temporal resolution is achieved with algorithms that use the minimum amount of required data for image reconstruction.[2,3,14] Generally, CT image reconstruction requires at least a parallel projection data angle range of 180 degrees. As a consequence, the temporal resolution will be on the order of $t_{rot}/2$, where t_{rot} is the time required for a full rotation of the scanner. However, the temporal resolution varies with the position in the scan field of view, which is determined by the temporal interval covered by the data contributing to the reconstruction to a particular image point. In a centered region of the scan field of view, the temporal resolution equals half the rotation time. In clinical practice, the heart should be sufficiently centered during data acquisition to maintain stable temporal resolution of half the rotation time. Half-scan reconstruction techniques preserve the spatial resolution compared with standard reconstructions, but because of less data contributing to an image, the noise is usually increased by a factor of $\sqrt{2}$. Special considerations apply to today's third-generation modern CT scanners, in which data acquisition is performed in fan beam geometry. Data is acquired over a range of 180 degrees plus fan angle and is then transformed to parallel beam geometry using so-called "rebinning techniques." The previously described half-scan reconstruction algorithm is then applied to achieve the best temporal resolution.

With the introduction of multislice helical CT, almost isotropic three-dimensional resolution became feasible. Dedicated reconstruction algorithms are necessary to optimize temporal resolution, helical artifact reduction, and volume coverage. The basic concepts for phase-correlated imaging for multislice CT have been introduced with four-slice systems[1,15] and are used in slightly different forms in today's scanners.

Modern 64-slice CT scanners all offer rotation times of less than 0.5 second and down to 0.3 second. Thus, it is possible to achieve a temporal resolution of 150 ms, which allows for motion-free imaging in the diastolic phase for moderate to high heart rates. As a consequence, the usage of β blockers, intravenous or oral, to slow down the heart rate is common practice.[8] Nevertheless, motion artifacts remain the most important challenge for coronary CTA, even with 64-slice CT systems.

ECG Synchronization

Traditionally, the patient's electrocardiogram (ECG) has been used to correlate acquisition and reconstruction of CT data with heart motion. Data can be acquired in phases with slow motion to minimize motion artifacts; alternatively, the acquisition and reconstruction of different heart phases are possible for functional studies. Usually, the R wave of the ECG is used as a reference point, with the R wave being the most pronounced peak in the ECG. Alternative approaches to derive the motion signal retrospectively have been proposed, using information from CT raw data directly or from the generated images.[16] However, for phase-correlated data acquisition, the ECG signal is used.

The start point of data acquisition or, respectively, data selection for image reconstruction is usually determined relative to the R waves of the ECG signal by a phase parameter. Three phase selection strategies are commonly used (Fig. 8-1)—relative delay (e.g., at 65% of the R-R interval), absolute delay, and absolute reverse (e.g., 400 ms after and before the R wave, respectively). For the relative delay, a temporal delay relative to the start point of the previous R wave is used to determine the start point of the ECG-triggered acquisition or the data reconstruction interval. This delay is determined individually for each heart cycle. For prospective data acquisition, the R-R interval times have to be prospectively estimated based on prior R-R intervals. The absolute delay uses a fixed delay time after onset of the R wave to trigger the data acquisition or start point of the reconstruction. Absolute reverse describes a fixed time prior to the onset of the next R wave for starting data acquisition or the start point of the reconstruction interval. For ECG-triggered data acquisition, the position of the next R wave again has to be estimated from previous R-R interval times.

TECHNICAL PRINCIPLES OF CARDIAC IMAGE ACQUISITION

Until recently, available CT technology did not allow covering the entire heart in one single heartbeat. Therefore, images at consecutive z positions are generated from data acquired in different cardiac cycles to cover the entire heart volume. Phase-consistent synchronization of the data acquisition and reconstruction with the heart motion is necessary; this is achieved by using the simultaneously recorded ECG signal of the individual patient. The heart phase-correlated data acquisition can be subdivided into two techniques, prospective triggering and retrospective gating.

Prospective Triggering

Prospective triggering uses the ECG signal to start the scan (data acquisition and x-ray on time). This technique is typically used with axial scans, meaning that the patient table is at rest during data acquisition. For imaging, the user specifies the delay time after the R wave; usually, the scan delay time is selected so that the data are acquired during the diastole of the heart. For each position, the scanner is continuously rotating until the ECG trigger signal indicates the desired heart phase, when the x-ray is switched on and data are acquired for 180 degrees plus the fan angle. The number of reconstructed images corresponds to the number of detector rows used. With the x-ray then switched off, the table advances to the next position, which typically corresponds to the total detector

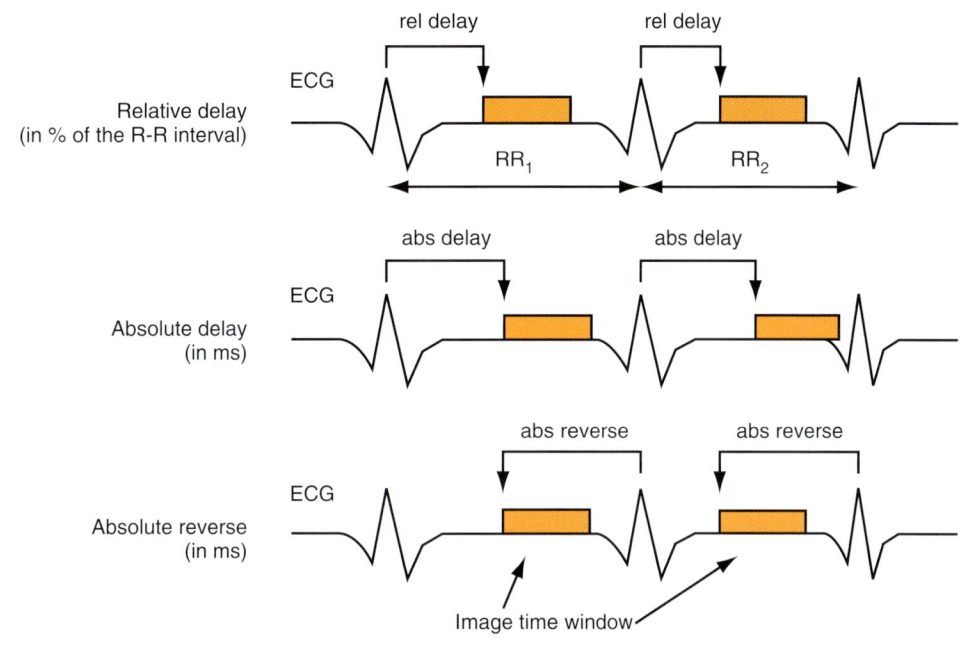

FIGURE 8-1 Strategies for phase definition with ECG-synchronized data acquisition and reconstruction. **Top,** Relative delay, the delay time defined as a fraction of the R-R interval after the previous R wave. **Middle,** Absolute delay, a constant delay time after the previous R wave. **Bottom,** Absolute reverse, a constant time interval prior to the next R wave.

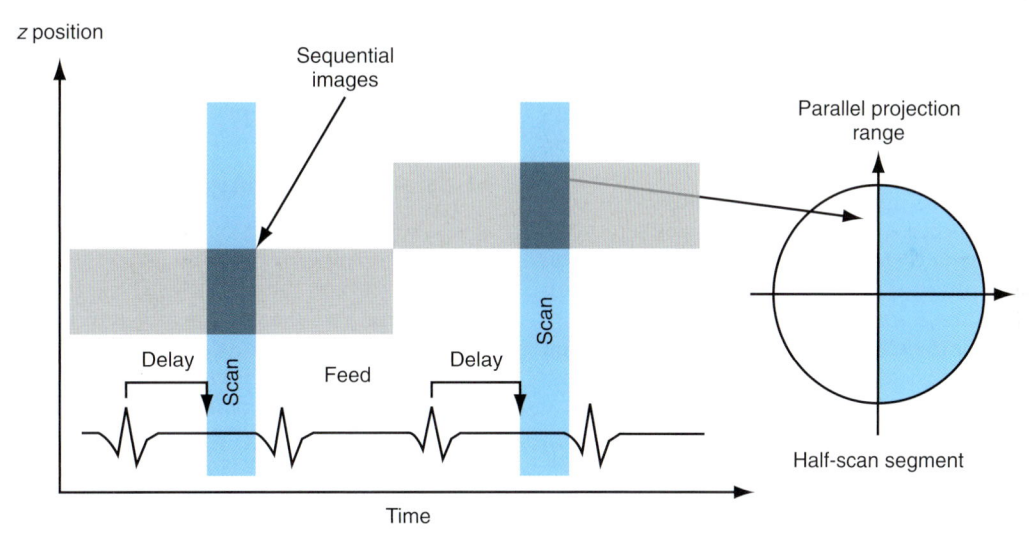

FIGURE 8-2 For cardiac imaging, only data corresponding to a specified heart phase contribute to image reconstruction. With prospective ECG-triggered data acquisition, this phase is determined by a user-specified delay. The patient's ECG signal is schematically shown as a function of time. The width of the data interval determines the temporal resolution. Because the table position has to be advanced between the acquisitions, scanning usually occurs in every other heart cycle.

collimation (slight overlaps are necessary for contiguous volume coverage). This is repeated until the heart range is covered; thus, the technique is commonly referred to as a "step-and-shoot mode" (Fig. 8-2). Image reconstruction is performed with previously described half-scan algorithms, and so the temporal resolution corresponds to half the rotation time.

Prospective triggering has several limitations for clinical use. The sequential nature of data acquisition means that the table has to move between the scans, so that for typical heart rates, a heartbeat has to be skipped between every two scans and the total examination time will depend on the individual heart rate. The heart phase has to be chosen prior to scanning; therefore, irregularities in the heart cycle can lead to limitations of the data set. In a worst case scenario, this might require a further scan to obtain diagnostic images. Because the acquisition typically lasts over several heart cycles and the scan is triggered with respect to a mean length of the heart cycle, scanning can occur in the wrong phase. This can result in severe artifacts, especially in volume representations. The sequential nature of data acquisition means that it does not benefit from the higher image quality that can be achieved with helical CT. For example, the lack of true volumetric coverage can lead to misregistration of anatomic details if the patient moves between two table positions. Finally, prospective trigger techniques do not offer the option of regional or global functional analysis of the heart because the number of reconstructed phases typically covers only a small portion of the cardiac cycle.

However, cardiac CT examinations have recently been subjected to increased scrutiny because of their relatively high radiation dose.[17,18] Prospective triggered data acquisition offers the highest dose savings and hence has experienced renewed interest.[19-21] In addition, improvements in ECG synchronization, such as so-called adaptive triggering or padding techniques, allow the system to react to ectopic beats and allow image reconstruction in a narrow phase range beyond the specified acquisition phase.

Retrospective Gating

Multislice helical CT scanning represented an important step toward true volumetric imaging, with the advantage of reconstructing overlapping image slices to enable isotropic three-dimensional resolution. Retrospective gated helical scanning synchronizes the reconstruction of a true volumetric helical scan to the heart motion by using the ECG signal recorded simultaneously during data acquisition. Only data acquired in a predefined phase of the cardiac cycle, usually the diastolic phase, is then used for image reconstruction. In addition, with continuous data acquisition, retrospective ECG gating can improve the robustness of the ECG synchronization against arrhythmia during the scan.

With submillimeter slice thickness, 64-slice CT offers considerable advantages over earlier technology in terms of spatial resolution and volume coverage. Two different scanner concepts were introduced. The volume concept provides a further increase in volume coverage by increasing the number of detector rows to 64. The resolution concept uses 32 physical detector rows in combination with double sampling in the longitudinal z direction. Thus, 64 overlapping slices are simultaneously acquired to increase longitudinal resolution independently of the pitch and reduce helical artifacts.[12]

With the advent of multislice helical CT scanning, various image reconstruction concepts have been introduced to take full advantage of volumetric ECG-gated data acquisition.[1,14] The reconstruction process typically comprises two steps. The first step generally involves multislice helical interpolation algorithms to compensate for the continuous table movement during data acquisition. The second step uses half-scan reconstruction techniques for the generated transverse data segments to optimize temporal resolution.

Retrospective ECG-gated reconstruction allows reconstruction of the images at an arbitrary phase of the cardiac cycle. The start position for image reconstruction is shifted relative to the R peak and a stack of images can be reconstructed at adjacent z positions, depending on the volume coverage of the scanner. Figure 8-3A shows successive stacks reconstructed in consecutive heart cycles covering the cardiac volume. The entire volume can be reconstructed without gaps in the illustrated heart phases, as well as any other user-selected heart phases. This is a prerequisite for true functional volume imaging of the heart.

An important requirement for continuous and contiguous volume coverage is the restriction that the table feed per heart cycle should not exceed the total collimation width. The maximum table speed depends on the total duration of the heart cycle and therefore on the heartbeat. It can be shown as

Table speed < (total collimation)/(time for a single heartbeat)

or, in symbols,

$$d/t_{rot} < T/(1/f_H)$$

where d is the table feed, t_{rot} is the rotation time, T is the total collimation, and f_H is the heart rate. The maximum pitch (p_{max}) consequently has to fulfill the following condition:

$$p_{max} = d_{max}/T = f_H \cdot t_{rot}$$

This implies that for helical CT of the heart, the pitch is limited to relatively small values. For example, a heart rate of 60 beats/min and a rotation time of 0.33 second results in a maximum pitch of 0.33. As shown in Figure 8-3A, the slope of the detector position is proportional to the pitch that is correctly chosen so as to ensure continuous volume coverage. If the pitch is too high, volume gaps will occur between image stacks reconstructed at different heart cycles (see Fig. 8-3B). Typically, the pitch is set prior to the scan and stays constant throughout the scan, even if the heart rate changes. Therefore, the pitch should be chosen according to the minimum expected heart rate for an individual patient.

Multisegment Image Reconstruction

Dedicated reconstruction techniques can improve the temporal resolution of an image by using data from multiple subsequent heart cycles. Using so-called multisegment image reconstruction, the temporal resolution can be improved up to $t_{rot}/(2N)$ by using data of N subsequent heart cycles.[1] However, for an increasing number of segments used, the achieved improvement in temporal resolution comes at the expense of slower volume coverage because the pitch is no longer only limited by heart rate but also by the number of heart cycles used for reconstruction.

Multisegment techniques assume absolute periodicity of the cardiac cycle because data from several heart beats are combined to reconstruct a single image. However, slight differences in heart cycles occur even for regular heart rates, and images generated from multiple heart cycles represent only an average of the used cardiac cycles. In general, an increase in the number N of used segments compromises the reliability of the technique. The limitations of such techniques are obvious in patients with arrhythmia or changing heart rates during the cardiac cycle.

Finally, with multisegment reconstruction with $N > 1$ segments, the optimal temporal resolution can only be achieved if the patient's heart rate and gantry rotation time of the scanner are properly desynchronized (Fig. 8-4A). Only if the start and end of the segments fit together and form a complete half-scan can the half-scan be subdivided into N segments of equal size and the temporal reso-

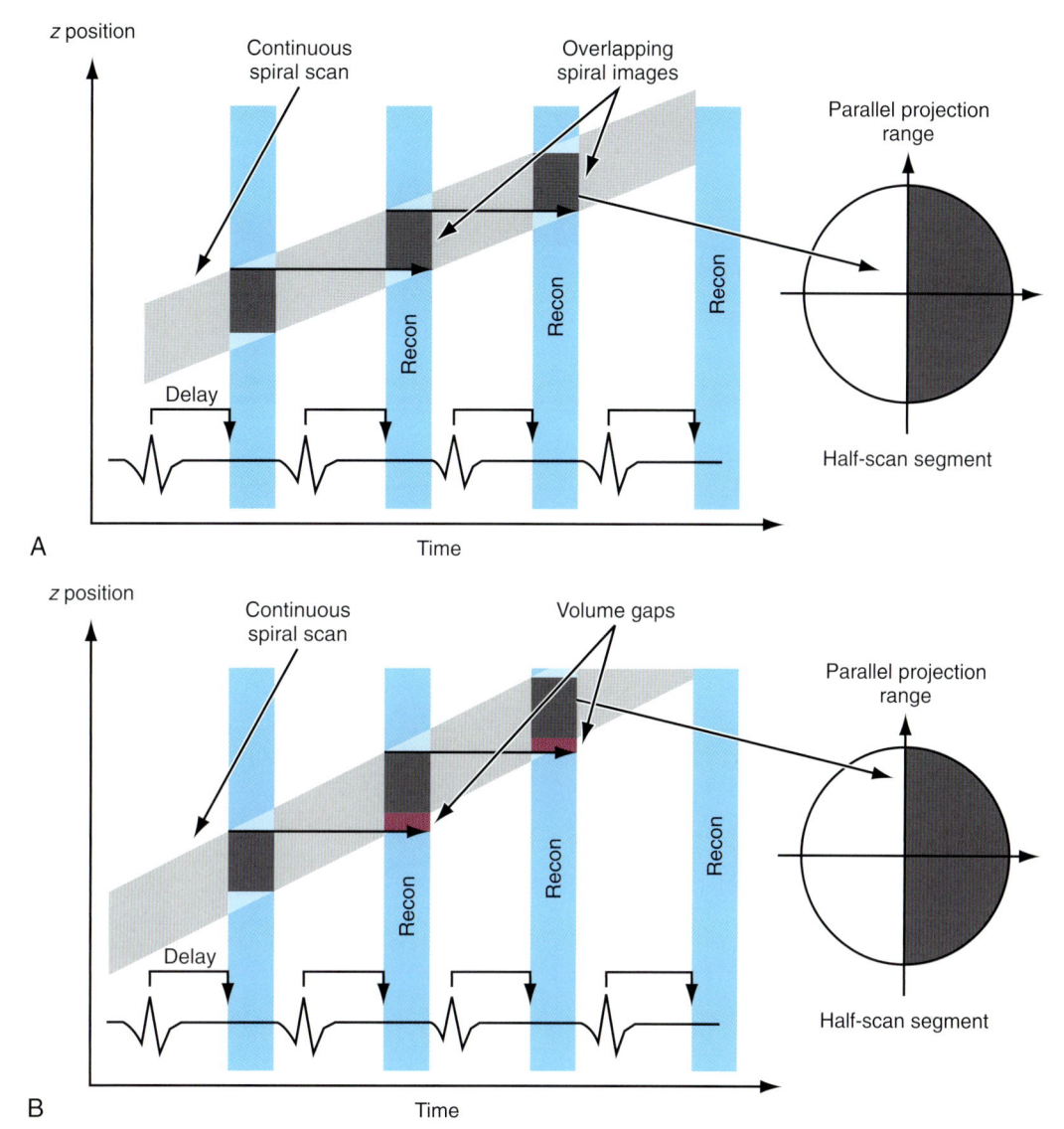

FIGURE 8-3 Retrospective ECG-gated helical scanning with continuous exposure allows the reconstruction of images in every cardiac cycle, with a temporal resolution of half the rotation time. With continuous data acquisition, one can vary the heart phase from reconstruction to reconstruction to optimize image quality. As a prerequisite for gapless volume coverage, the pitch (p) is restricted to values of $p < f_H \cdot t_{rot}$. **A,** The slope of the detector position illustrates a pitch value that has been chosen properly for continuous volume coverage. **B,** If the pitch is too high for the actual heart rate, continuous coverage of the heart is no longer possible and volume gaps are present between the image stacks.

lution be equal to $t_{rot}/(2N)$. If the heart rate and rotation time are (partially) synchronized, the segments cover different temporal data intervals and the temporal resolution is determined by the segment with the longest duration (see Fig. 8-4B). Thus, the benefits of multisegment reconstruction are only available for a few "sweet spots," determined by rotation time and heart rate (Fig. 8-5).

Optimal Reconstruction Phase

An important advantage of retrospective ECG gating is the ability to analyze the ECG trace after the scan for possible modification of the synchronization of the ECG signal and data reconstruction. Particularly for irregular heart rates or inappropriately detected R peaks (e.g., extrasystoles), the editing of the time interval and R peak positions has a beneficial effect.[22]

The intensity of the heart motion varies substantially during the heart cycle, with strong motion during the contraction in systole and slow motion during relaxation in diastole. Generally, the diastolic phase is the most suitable phase for motion-free imaging of the heart, but with increasing heart rate and reduced duration of the diastolic phase, imaging in the systolic phase more frequently yields superior image quality. Additionally, the course of the ECG trace shows variations for the individual patient in addition to its dependency on heart rate. Thus, the prediction of the optimal heart phase for imaging is generally not feasible. It has been common practice to determine the optimal phase adaptively by reconstructing multiple heart phases and analyzing them individually. More recently, automatic algorithms have been introduced to determine the optimal reconstruction phase in a single reconstruction step.[23]

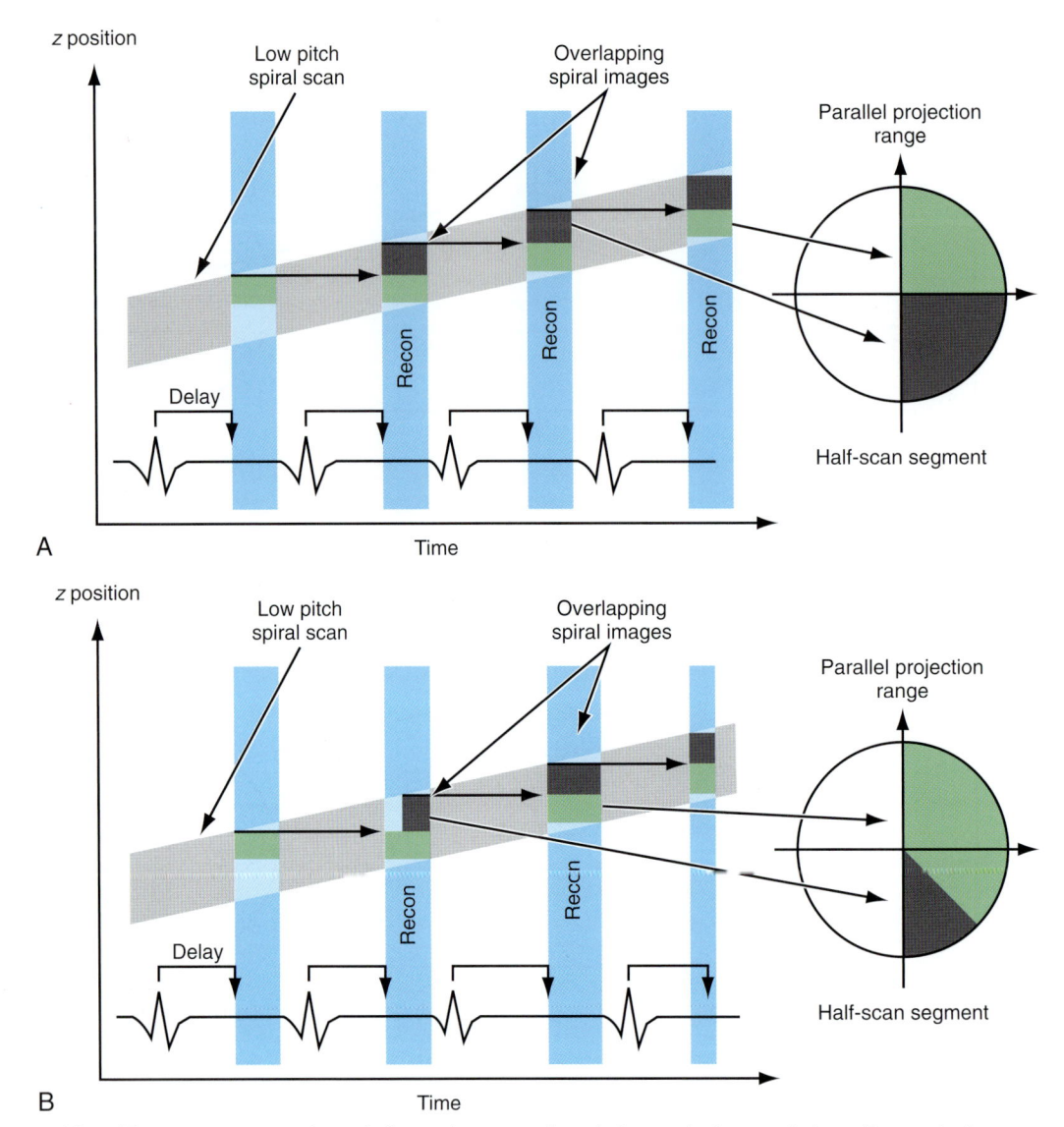

FIGURE 8-4 With multisegment reconstruction techniques, the temporal resolution can be improved, depending on the heart rate and system rotation time. **A,** For optimal desynchronized heart rate and rotation time, a temporal resolution of $t_{rot}/(2N)$ can be achieved, shown here for two segments. **B,** For only partially desynchronized heart rate and rotation time, the segment with the longest temporal data interval determines the temporal resolution.

ECG Tube Current Modulation

Whereas retrospective ECG-gated data acquisition is the more robust acquisition mode compared with ECG-triggered data acquisition, it is also associated with high radiation exposure because of the continuous data acquisition at relatively low pitch. The low pitch is a consequence of the required phase-consistent coverage of the heart; however, coverage of all heart phases is not necessary if only a single heart phase—for example, in diastole—is targeted for image reconstruction. In this case, a significant portion of the acquired data is redundant. ECG-controlled tube current modulation, in which the tube current is reduced during phases of less importance, has been shown to reduce the radiation dose effectively during retrospective ECG-gated cardiac helical CT.[3,18] Algorithms have been developed that restrict the nominal tube current to a predefined time window and reduce the tube current during the remaining time to about 20% of its nominal value (Fig. 8-6). The benefit of not switching off x-ray radiation completely lies in the preserved ability of continuous volume reconstruction in all phases of the cardiac cycle; specifically, functional imaging is still feasible. For images acquired at low dose and used for functional analysis, the image quality in terms of signal-to-noise ratio can be improved by using thick slices in image reconstruction.

Typically, the user can prescribe the position and width of the temporal window within which the nominal tube current is used relative to the heart cycle. This is defined prior to the scan by preliminary estimation of the optimal reconstruction interval based on the patient's individual heart rate.

A limitation of current ECG tube modulation techniques occurs when the patient' heart rate is not stable, because then the optimal reconstruction window might

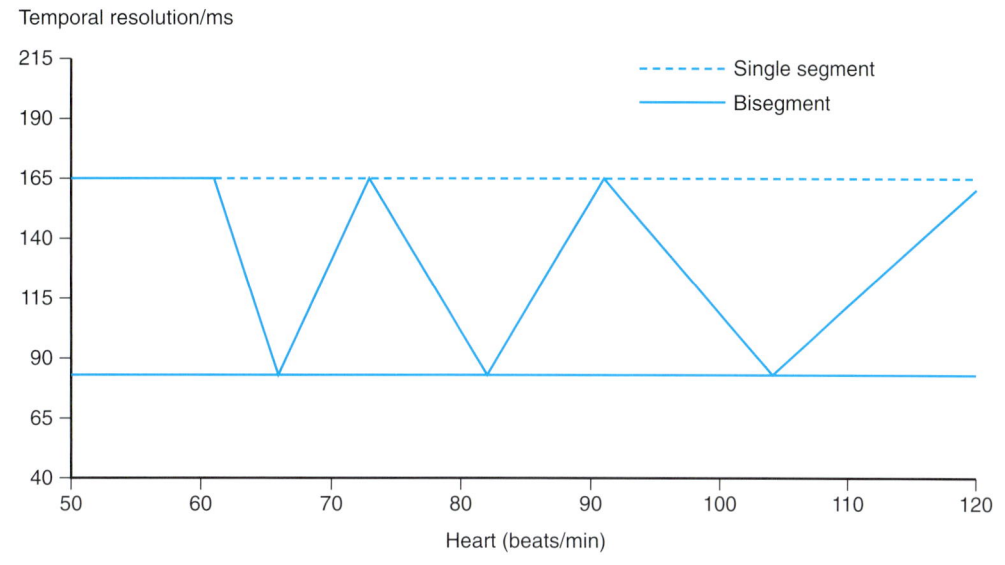

FIGURE 8-5 Temporal resolution as a function of the patient's heart rate for a single-source CT system with a gantry rotation time of 0.33 second. Single-segment reconstruction provides a constant temporal resolution of 165 ms (*dashed blue line*). With two-segment reconstruction, a temporal resolution of 82.5 ms can be achieved for selected heart rates of 66 beats/min, 81 beats/min, and 104 beats/min (*blue line*). However, no better temporal resolution than 165 ms is possible for heart rates of 91 and 72 beats/min.

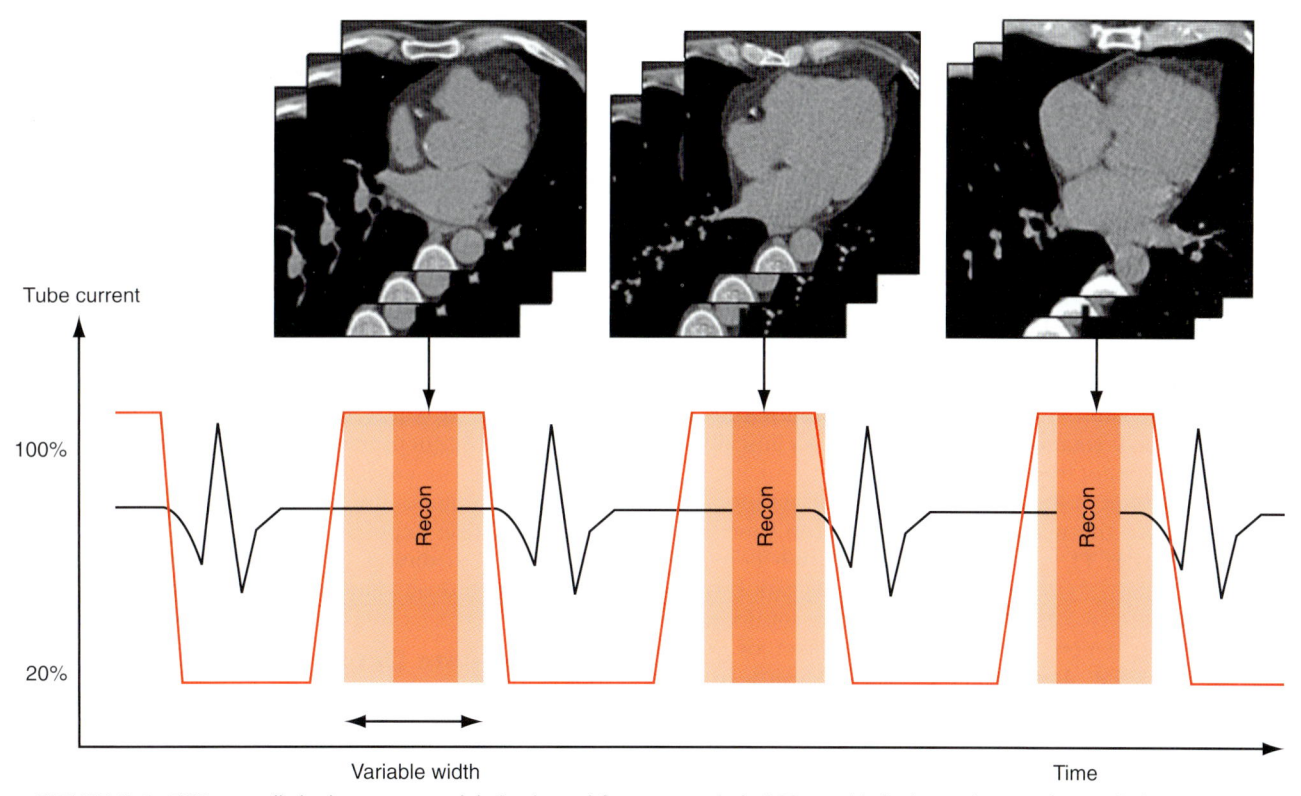

FIGURE 8-6 ECG-controlled tube current modulation is used for retrospectively ECG-gated helical scanning to reduce radiation exposure. The tube current is at a nominal value during targeted heart phases, typically the diastole, and is reduced by 80% during phases with high cardiac motion. The tube current curve has a trapezoidal shape, accounting for ramp up and down times. Whereas the width of the image reconstruction window is defined by the temporal resolution of the system, the total width of the temporal window with nominal tube current can be selected by the user if a larger range of the heart cycles is to be imaged. For high-quality images, the reconstruction window (*dark bars*) should be within the maximum tube current window (*shaded bars*).

occur during the reduced tube current window. An efficient mechanism for ECG tube current modulation is that it has the flexibility to detect and react to ectopic beats and heart rate variations by automatically increasing the tube current to its nominal value when an R-R interval that is significantly different from the previous cycles is recognized.

The relatively high radiation exposure associated with ECG-gated helical data acquisition compared with prospective ECG trigger techniques has resulted in improved modulation techniques; these allow further reduction of the tube current outside the specified heart phase, typically to 4% of its nominal value. Although functional imaging might no longer be possible, it still maintains the advantages of volumetric data acquisition and flexibility to react to heart rate irregularities.[20]

For prospectively gated sequential scanning techniques, the duration of the x-ray is usually set to a predetermined time window based on the R-R interval length of the heart rate prior to beginning the scan. Recently introduced algorithms, referred to as padding or adaptive triggering, use a new technique that includes continuous analysis of the individual heart rate, which thus can vary the location and duration of the scanning window.[19,24]

Although comparable results in terms of image quality and dose savings of up to 70% can be expected for patients with normal heart rhythms, an improved stability of image quality is achieved only with slightly increased exposure. In patients with irregular heartbeats, conventional prospective gating still results in the highest dose savings, but at the expense of reduced image quality. Here, a dynamic length of the nominal tube current window with fast adaptation to changes in the ECG signal offers increased reliability at a relatively low dose.

NEW DEVELOPMENTS IN CARDIAC CT IMAGING

Dual-Source CT

Motion artifacts remain the most important challenge for coronary CTA, even with 64-slice CT systems. Thus, the use of β blockers prior to scanning is an important step of the cardiac CT examination to control the heart rate to values generally below 60 beats/min. If stable imaging at all heart rates is desired, the target temporal resolution is less than 100 ms, independent of the heart rate. For conventional third-generation CT systems, this would require an increased gantry rotation speed to ensure a clinically robust improvement of the temporal resolution.[25] An alternative scanner concept that provides enhanced temporal resolution without the need for a faster rotation time is dual-source CT (DSCT), with two tubes and two corresponding detectors.[26,27] In the first clinical realization of this type of system, two acquisition systems are mounted onto the rotating gantry, with an angular offset of 90 degrees (SOMATOM Definition, Siemens Healthcare, Forchheim, Germany).[28] In the axial plane, one detector covers the entire field of view (50 cm in diameter), whereas the other detector is restricted to a smaller, central field of view (26 cm). The two detectors are equivalent in the longitudinal direction, using the manufacturer's high-resolution concept of providing simultaneous acquisition of 64 overlapping 0.6-mm slices by means of z-flying focal spot technology.

As a practical consequence of the two-tube–detector configuration, DSCT offers improved temporal resolution of 25% of the gantry rotation time. The data acquisition is split up between the two systems, which acquire the data simultaneously in the same relative phase of the patient's cardiac cycle and at the same anatomic level. Using single-segment reconstruction algorithms, the temporal resolution is 25% of the rotation time in a centered region of the scan field of view that is covered by both acquisition systems. Moreover, the temporal resolution is independent of the heart rate; the system achieves 83 ms, with a rotation time of 0.33 second.

An important consequence of the high stable temporal resolution is the optional use of β blockers. Studies have shown that high diagnostic accuracy is achieved in patients with high heart rates without the administration of β blockers.[29,30]

Efforts to reduce radiation dose to the patient are continued in dual-source systems. For retrospective ECG-gated examinations, the table feed can be optimally adapted to the heart rate as a consequence of the single-segment reconstruction approach. Thus, the pitch is significantly increased at elevated heart rates, thereby not only reducing the examination time but also the radiation dose to the patient. For low heart rates, radiation dose values for ECG-gated helical cardiac examinations with DSCT are similar to those obtained with comparable conventional CT systems, and even lower values are achieved for higher heart rates.[31] Finally, ECG-triggered prospective scanning modes are available for patients with sufficiently stable heart rates.[24]

The newest generation of DSCT technology introduces a high-pitch scan mode to acquire a helical CT data set while covering the entire volume of the heart in one cardiac cycle.[32] Prerequisites for the feasibility of such a scan mode were technical improvements, such as a faster rotation time (0.28 second), a larger detector coverage (two 4-cm detectors that acquire 128 slices each), and pitch values up to 3.2 in dual-source scanning. The scan mode is an implementation of the prospective triggered ECG mode; however, with the fast helical scan, the heart is covered within a heartbeat. Images are reconstructed with a temporal resolution that corresponds to 25% of the rotation time (75 ms). With a total acquisition time on the order of 250 ms, it is interesting to note that throughout the data set, subsequent images are reconstructed at later points of time in the cardiac cycle. The immediate advantage of this scan mode, however, is the elimination of the additional radiation exposure that typically occurs during low-pitch gated scanning. Thus, it might be possible to achieve effective dose values of 1 mSv or lower.[33]

CT with Volume Detectors

Technologic advances since the establishment of 64-slice cardiac CT have diverged, with one approach focusing on temporal resolution (DSCT; see earlier) and the second focusing on increasing volume coverage.[34-36] With area detector technology and related cone beam reconstruction techniques, the aim is to allow coverage of the entire cardiac anatomy in a single heartbeat without movement of the table. The first commercially available system was introduced in 2007 (Aquilion ONE, Toshiba Medical Systems, Tustin, Calif). It uses a 320-row detector and 0.5-mm detector elements. Thus, single heartbeat cardiac imaging becomes feasible with prospective ECG-triggered image acquisition. The theoretical advantages of this system is the elimination of stair-step artifacts between slabs of images from different heart cycles, which are inherent to techniques that require multiple gantry rotations to cover the whole heart volume. The diagnostic quality of this one shot that covers the entire heart, however, depends on the available temporal resolution. With a rotation time of 0.35 second, it is necessary to use multisegment reconstruction techniques to achieve temporal resolution beyond 175 ms.[37]

With area detector CT scanners, high-resolution imaging of the cardiac morphology, as well as dynamic and functional assessment through repeated scanning of the same scan range, may become possible.

SUMMARY AND OUTLOOK

Motion artifact–free phase-correlated cardiac imaging requires fast data acquisition and dedicated image reconstruction techniques that allow one to correlate imaging with the heart cycle. For this purpose, the patient's ECG signal is recorded simultaneously with data acquisition and is used for synchronization.

Image reconstruction algorithms can be divided into single-segment and multisegment algorithms. Single-segment reconstruction provides a stable temporal resolution equal to the time required to acquire a range of 180 degrees of projection data, which corresponds to half the rotation time for single-source CT systems. Multisegment approaches collect data from multiple heart cycles and may improve the temporal resolution significantly for stable heart rates that are not in resonance with the scanner's rotation time. Dual-source CT systems have been introduced to improve temporal resolution to 25% of the system's rotation time, independent of the heart rate, and have been shown to provide diagnostic images reliably, even with high heart rates.

Today, use of fast scanner rotation times can routinely result in temporal resolution far below 100 ms. Together with isotropic submillimeter spatial resolution, CT images of the heart provide an image quality of high diagnostic value. In the future, technology will likely focus on further improving spatial and temporal resolution. This requires better detector technology, faster rotation times, and innovative concepts such as multiple sources and area detector technology.

KEY POINTS

- The goal of cardiac CT imaging is to image the heart free of motion artifacts in a specified phase of the cardiac cycle. This requires high temporal and spatial resolution combined with fast volume coverage and minimal radiation dose.
- Data acquisition and image reconstruction are synchronized to the heart motion using the patient's ECG signal.
- State of the art CT technology comprises multislice scanners with subsecond rotation time and isotropic submillimeter spatial resolution.
- With dedicated ECG-synchronized scan and reconstruction techniques (half-scan algorithms), a heart rate independent temporal resolution of 83 ms can be achieved.

SUGGESTED READINGS

Achenbach S, Ropers D, Kuettner A, et al. Contrast-enhanced coronary artery visualization by dual-source computed tomography—initial experience. Eur J Radiol 2006; 57:331-335.

Kopp A, Schröder S, Küttner A, et al. Coronary arteries: retrospectively ECG-gated multidetector row ct angiography with selective optimization of the image reconstruction window. Radiology 2001; 221:683-688.

Kuettner A, Beck T, Drosch T, et al. Diagnostic accuracy of noninvasive coronary imaging using 16-detector slice spiral computed tomography with 188 ms temporal resolution, J Am Coll Cardiol 2005; 45:123-127.

Mollet N R, Cademartiri F, van Mieghem CA, et al. High-resolution spiral computed tomography coronary angiography in patients referred for diagnostic conventional coronary angiography. Circulation 2005; 112:2318-2323.

Nieman K, Cademartiri F, Lemos PA, et al. Reliable noninvasive coronary angiography with fast submillimeter multislice spiral computed tomography. Circulation 2002; 106:2051-2054.

Ropers D, Baum U, Pohle K, et al. Detection of coronary artery stenoses with thin-slice multi-detector row spiral computed tomography and multiplanar reconstruction. Circulation 2003; 107:664-666.

REFERENCES

1. Kachelriess M, Ulzheimer S, Kalender W. ECG-correlated image reconstruction from subsecond multi-slice spiral CT scans of the heart. Med Phys 2000; 27:1881-1902.
2. Taguchi K, Anno H. High temporal resolution for multi-slice helical computed tomography. Med Phys 2000; 27:861-872.
3. Ohnesorge B, Flohr T, Becker C, et al. Cardiac imaging by means of electrocardiographically gated multisection spiral CT—initial experience. Radiology 2000; 217:564-571.
4. Achenbach S, Ulzheimer S, Baum U, et al. Noninvasive coronary angiography by retrospectively ECG-gated multi-slice spiral CT. Circulation 2000; 102:2823-2828.
5. Becker C, Knez A, Ohnesorge B, et al. Imaging of noncalcified coronary plaques using helical CT with retrospective EKG gating. AJR Am J Roentgenol 2000; 175:423-424.
6. Knez A, Becker C, Leber A, et al. Non-invasive assessment of coronary artery stenoses with multidetector helical computed tomography. Circulation 2000; 101:e221-e222.
7. Nieman K, Oudkerk M, Rensing B, et al. Coronary angiography with multi-slice computed tomography. Lancet 2001; 357:599-603.
8. Leber AW, Knez A, von Ziegler F, et al. Quantification of obstructive and nonobstructive coronary lesions by 64-slice computed tomography: a comparative study with quantitative coronary angiography and intravascular ultrasound. J Am Coll Cardiol 2005; 46:147-154.
9. Raff GL, Gallagher MJ, O'Neill WW, Goldstein JA. Diagnostic accuracy of noninvasive coronary angiography using 64-slice spiral computed tomography. J Am Coll Cardiol 2005; 46:552-557.
10. Hendel RC, Patel MR, Kramer CM, et al; American College of Cardiology Foundation Quality Strategic Directions Committee Appropriateness Criteria Working Group; American College of Radiology; Society of Cardiovascular Computed Tomography; Society for Cardiovascular Magnetic Resonance; American Society of Nuclear Cardiology; North American Society for Cardiac Imaging; Society for Cardiovascular Angiography and Interventions; Society of Interventional Radiology. ACCF/ACR/SCCT/SCMR/ASNC/ NASCI/SCAI/SIR

2006 appropriateness criteria for cardiac computed tomography and cardiac magnetic resonance imaging: a report of the American College of Cardiology Foundation Quality Strategic Directions Committee Appropriateness Criteria Working Group, American College of Radiology, Society of Cardiovascular Computed Tomography, Society for Cardiovascular Magnetic Resonance, American Society of Nuclear Cardiology, North American Society for Cardiac Imaging, Society for Cardiovascular Angiography and Interventions, and Society of Interventional Radiology. J Am Coll Cardiol 2006; 48:1475-1497.
11. Hoffmann U, Nagurney JT, Moselewski F, et al. Coronary multidetector computed tomography in the assessment of patients with acute chest pain. Circulation 2006; 114:2251-2260.
12. Flohr T G, Stierstorfer K, Ulzheimer S, et al. Image reconstruction and image quality evaluation for a 64-slice CT scanner with z-flying focal spot. Med. Phys 2005; 32:2536-2547.
13. Hong C, Becker CR, Huber A, et al. ECG-gated reconstructed multi-detector row ct coronary angiography: effect of varying trigger delay on image quality. Radiology 2001; 220:712-717.
14. Flohr T, Ohnesorge B, Bruder H, et al. Image reconstruction and performance evaluation for ECG-gated spiral scanning with a 16-slice CT system. Med Phys 2003; 30:2650-2662.
15. Kachelriess M, Kalender W. Electrocardiogram-correlated image reconstruction from subsecond spiral computed tomography scans of the heart. Med Phys 1998; 25:2417-2431.
16. Kachelriess M, Sennst DA, Maxlmoser W, Kalender WA. Kymogram detection and kymogram-correlated image reconstruction from subsecond spiral computed tomography scans of the heart. Med Phys 2002; 29:1489-1503.
17. Gerber TC, Carr JJ, Arai AE, et al. Ionizing radiation in cardiac imaging: a science advisory from the American Heart Association Committee on Cardiac Imaging of the Council on Clinical Cardiology and Committee on Cardiovascular Imaging and Intervention of the Council on Cardiovascular Radiology and Intervention. Circulation 2009; 119:1056-1065.
18. Hausleiter J, Meyer T, Hermann F, et al. Estimated radiation dose associated with cardiac CT angiography. JAMA 2009; 301:500-507.
19. Earls JP, Berman EL, Urban BA, et al. Prospectively gated transverse coronary CT angiography versus retrospectively gated helical technique: improved image quality and reduced radiation dose. Radiology 2008; 246:742-753.
20. Stolzmann P, Scheffel H, Schertler T, et al. Radiation dose estimates in dual-source computed tomography coronary angiography. Eur Radiol. 2008; 18:592-599.
21. Steigner ML, Otero HJ, Cai T, et al. Narrowing the phase window width in prospectively ECG-gated single heart beat 320-detector row coronary CT angiography. Int J Cardiovasc Imaging 2009; 25: 85-90.
22. Cademartiri F, Mollet NR, Runza G, et al. Improving diagnostic accuracy of MDCT coronary angiography in patients with mild heart rhythm irregularities using ECG editing. AJR Am J Roentgenol 2006; 186:634-638.
23. Ruzsics B, Gebregziabher M, Lee H, et al. Coronary CT angiography: automatic cardiac-phase selection for image reconstruction. Eur Radiol 2009; 19:1906-1913.
24. Stolzmann P, Leschka S, Scheffel H, et al. Dual-source CT in step-and-shoot mode: noninvasive coronary angiography with low radiation dose. Radiology 2008; 249:71-80.
25. Halliburton SS, Stillman AE, Flohr T, et al. Do segmented reconstruction algorithms for cardiac multi-slice computed tomography improve image quality? Herz 2003; 28:20-31.
26. Robb R, Ritman E. High-speed synchronous volume computed tomography of the heart. Radiology 1979; 133:655-661.
27. Ritman E, Kinsey J, Robb R, et al. Three-dimensional imaging of heart, lungs, and circulation. Science 1980; 210:273-280.
28. Flohr TG, McCollough CH, Bruder H, et al. First performance evaluation of a dual-source CT (DSCT) system. Eur Radiol 2006; 16: 256-268.
29. Scheffel H, Alkadhi H, Plass A, et al. Accuracy of dual-source CT coronary angiography: First experience in a high pre-test probability population without heart rate control. Eur Radiol 2006; 16:2739-2747.
30. Achenbach S, Ropers U, Kuettner A, et al. Randomized comparison of 64-slice single- and dual-source computed tomography coronary angiography for the detection of coronary artery disease. JACC Cardiovasc Imaging 2008; 1:177-186.
31. McCollough CH, Primak AN, Saba O, et al. Dose performance of a 64-channel dual-source CT scanner. Radiology. 2007; 243:775-784.
32. Achenbach S, Marwan M, Schepis T, et al. High-pitch spiral acquisition: a new scan mode for coronary CT angiography. J Cardiovasc Comput Tomogr 2009; 3:117-121.
33. Hausleiter J, Bischoff B, Hein F, Feasibility of dual-source cardiac CT angiography with high-pitch scan protocols. J Cardiovasc Comput Tomogr 2009; 3:236-242.
34. Kondo C, Mori S, Endo M, et al. Real-time volumetric imaging of human heart without electrocardiographic gating by 256-detector row computed tomography: initial experience. J Comput Assist Tomogr 2005; 29: 694-698.
35. Mori S, Endo M, Tsunoo T, et al. Physical performance evaluation of a 256-slice CT-scanner for four-dimensional imaging. Med Phys 2004; 31:1348-1356.
36. Mori S, Endo M, Obata T, et al. Properties of the prototype 256-row (cone beam) CT scanner. Eur Radiol 2006; 16:2100-2108.
37. Rybicki FJ, Otero HJ, Steigner ML et al. Initial evaluation of coronary images from 320-detector row computed tomography. Int J Cardiovasc Imaging 2008; 24:535-546.

CHAPTER 9

Clinical Techniques of Cardiac Computed Tomography

Shawn D. Teague

Over the last decade, cardiac computed tomography (CT), and in particular coronary CT angiography (CTA), has undergone significant technical improvements, resulting in a reliable ability to evaluate coronary arteries with a noninvasive technique. There are still many questions to be answered with respect to how this test will be used in specific patient populations and the impact it will have, not only on patient management but also on patient outcomes. This chapter is meant to be an overview of the technical considerations for performing a clinical cardiac CT scan in a routine daily clinical practice.

PATIENT PREPARATION

The patient should be kept NPO for at least 4 hours prior to the scan as a precaution, as is standard for all contrast CT examinations, because of the potential for nausea and vomiting associated with contrast administration. It is extremely important that the patient not consume caffeine for at least 12 hours prior to the examination; this helps with heart rate control, which is critical for optimal image quality. With the newer generation of scanners having improved temporal resolution, high-quality images can be obtained with higher heart rates.

Electrocardiogram (ECG) leads need to be attached, which are used by the scanner to determine data reconstruction and electrocardiographic tube modulation, if used. In addition, this allows monitoring of the patient for absolute heart rate, heart rate variability, and arrhythmias, which are critical in determining the optimum protocol. A good electrocardiographic tracing (Fig. 9-1) is required, especially if using electrocardiographic tube modulation for overall dose reduction, because the x-ray tube modulation is synchronized with the cardiac cycle, using the R wave as a reference. It is important to ensure that the wire leads and ECG patches are outside the scanning field as much as possible, and in particular to ensure that the wires are not coiled on the patient's chest, which can result in significant streak artifact. For someone who is very hairy, good adherence and electrical conductivity of the pads may require shaving a small area. In particular, noisy electrocardiographic tracings (Fig. 9-2) can lead to inappropriate modulation of the tube current, resulting in a poor signal-to-noise ratio at the specific phase of the cardiac cycle required for coronary evaluation. In addition, be sure that the R wave peak is of greater amplitude compared with the T wave to prevent tube current modulation synchronized to the wrong phase of the cardiac cycle. Some scanners allow switching of the lead at the scanner console; if not, manual switching of the lead attachments to the ECG patches on the patient can often correct a situation in which the T wave has a higher peak.

If the patient's baseline heart rate is above an acceptable limit for optimal image quality, the use of β blockers is recommended, provided no contraindications (e.g., asthma, aortic stenosis) are present.[1] This acceptable limit is increasing with the latest generation of scanners. However, with the current generation of 64-slice scanners, a heart rate below 65 beats/min is highly recommended to increase the likelihood of an optimal high-quality scan with the least amount of motion artifact. There are multiple protocols for the administration of β blockers. The two basic protocols include the use of oral administration, both the night before and the morning of the scan, or just the morning of the scan, versus intravenous (IV) administration just prior to the scan.[1] In general, oral administration seems to result in a more predictable result, and it also requires less time and personnel commitment from the support staff. However, IV administration can be effective if the patient did not have prior administration of an oral β blocker or the target heart rate was not achieved after the administration of an oral dose. IV administration tends to have an all or none effect, meaning that usually if there is a noticeable decrease in heart rate with the first dose administered, a desired heart rate can usually be achieved. However, in many patients,

143

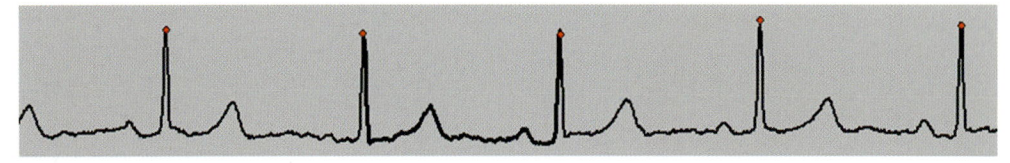

■ FIGURE 9-1 Good electrocardiographic tracing with clean R wave peaks and essentially no baseline noise.

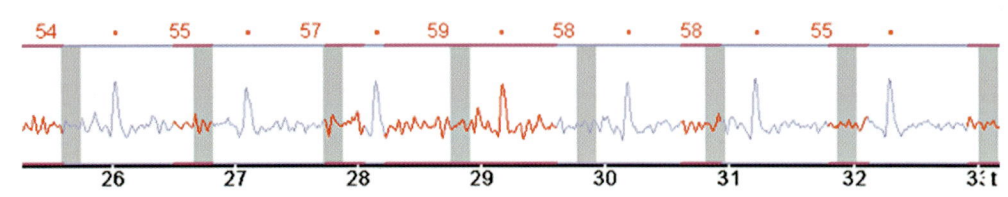

■ FIGURE 9-2 Poor-quality ECG tracing, with very noisy baseline.

the maximum dose (25 mg metoprolol at our institution) is administered without a noticeable change in heart rate. If the patient's heart rate does not reach the target, then the scan can be obtained with the understanding that it will likely be suboptimal, with the potential for nonevaluable segments of the coronary arteries, or the patient can be rescheduled with more aggressive oral β blocker administration prior to the scan.

If the patient has severe arrhythmias, then the patient is generally not a good candidate for cardiac CT and requires management of the arrhythmia prior to a coronary CTA. Usually, this is the obligation of the referring physician unless the performing physician is comfortable with antiarrhythmic medications.

A perfect breath-hold is critical for coronary imaging in particular. This requires the patient to have a steady breath-hold throughout the entire scan and needs to be relaxed—that is, no Valsalva maneuver. Therefore, the patient is coached on the breath-hold technique, which is practiced at least twice with the patient prior to the scan. The patient is instructed to take a breath in and hold the breath, with additional instructions during the breath-hold to be relaxed, not to bear down, and not to let any air out or take any air in once the breath is held. The breath-hold is practiced for approximately 5 seconds longer than the time required for the actual scan being performed.

A baseline heart rate and blood pressure are documented. Then, a brief history is obtained from the patient, including contraindications to the medications that will be administered for the examination, which may include a beta blocker and nitroglycerin. The patient is questioned about history of asthma, heart failure, and heart murmur with respect to β blockers and erectile dysfunction medications, and sildenafil with respect to nitroglycerin. Nitroglycerin is administered to dilate the coronary arteries for optimal visualization.[2] If there are no contraindications, the medications to be administered for the examination include up to 25 mg of metoprolol IV, in 5-mg push increments, and two 0.4-μg sublingual tablets. The onset of action for a sublingual nitroglycerin tablet is 1 to 3 minutes; it reaches maximum effect at 5 minutes, lasting at least 25 minutes. Therefore, these will be administered just prior to the scout and coronary CTA will be performed at approximately 5 to 6 minute after administration.

Additional history, which is collected while administering the β blocker, includes any symptoms, as well as their character and length of duration. Also, risk factors, including smoking, diabetes, lipid profile, hypertension, and family history, are documented. If additional testing has already been performed, these data are collected. especially if the previous testing led to the performance of cardiac CT.

SCANNING TECHNIQUE

The scan can be performed using retrospective electrocardiographic gating or a prospective electrocardiographic triggering (step and shoot) technique. With the retrospective electrocardiographic gating technique, the scan is performed using a standard helical scan acquisition, as for routine chest or abdominal CT scans, except a much smaller pitch, usually around 0.2, is used to ensure adequate data acquisition at all anatomic locations throughout the entire cardiac cycle. At the same time that the helical CT scan is obtained, the electrocardiographic tracing from the patient is recorded. Unless electrocardiographic tube modulation is used to reduce radiation exposure, the electrocardiographic tracing has no effect on the helical CT scan at the time of data acquisition. Rather, the tracing will be used to reconstruct axial source images from the raw data during the predefined portion of the cardiac cycle chosen after the scan. The tracing is used as a reference to determine which data at a specific anatomic location were collected during the defined phase of the cardiac cycle.

Image Quality

There are many factors that affect the image quality of cardiac CT examinations. With each generation of CT scanner release, the image quality has improved, mainly because of two elements—spatial and temporal resolution. Spatial resolution improved significantly with 4-, 16-, and 64-slice scanners. In addition to improvement in the actual spatial resolution of a single detector in the detector array, there is now also the ability to obtain high-resolution images using the entire detector array, resulting in an overall faster scan time. This results in significantly shorter breath-holds required by the patients and therefore better compliance and reproducibility of the scans. Temporal resolution is most affected by the gantry rotation time. With each generation of scanner, the gantry rotation times have improved, currently achieving 270 ms. With slow heart rates, the temporal resolution of the images is approximately half that of one gantry rotation time (e.g., with a 270-ms gantry rotation time, the temporal resolution would 135 ms). As a comparison, electron beam CT (EBCT) has a temporal resolution of 50 to 100 ms,[3] and usually in cardiac MRI, the temporal resolution is less than 50 ms.[4] Cardiac catheterization with a temporal resolution less than 20 ms is the best modality for imaging coronary arteries with respect to temporal resolution.[5] So, even though temporal resolution has significantly improved, there is still a potential for more improvement. The manufacturers, however, have been able to reduce the temporal resolution of images when the heart rate is more than 65 beats/min. By combining data from at least two different detector elements along the detector array from at least two different physical cardiac cycles, but from the same anatomic location and same phase of the cardiac cycle, an image can be created with an improved temporal resolution approaching 35 ms (four-phase reconstruction; gantry rotation = 270 ms). However, combining two different physical cardiac cycles introduces inherent motion artifact.[6] There must be a balance between combining data from different physical heartbeats and trying to improve temporal resolution.

Contrast Administration

The IV contrast is administered through an 18-gauge angiocatheter in the antecubital fossa. IV access is preferably via the right arm, which helps prevent significant streak artifact from the dense inflow of contrast, especially when scanning to the level of the aortic arch for evaluation of aortic pathology or the origin of coronary artery bypass grafts (in particular, the left internal mammary). To ensure adequate IV access, consider training CT technologists to place the angiocatheter under ultrasound guidance. We also use a trapeze, which helps keep the patient's arms straight, thus helping to prevent complications of high-flow injections. We also find it more comfortable for our older patients, who frequently have shoulder disabilities that make it difficult for them to place their arms above their head. The trapeze has 10 pounds of weight at the other end, helping to hold the patient's arms comfortably in an extended position, out of the way of the scan (Fig. 9-3).

The contrast is administered using a test bolus or a track and trigger technique. Briefly, the test bolus system injects a 20-mL bolus of contrast followed by 20 to 40 mL of saline push at the same injection rate planned for the coronary CTA scan. Intermittent low-dose images are obtained at the level of the carina, beginning approximately 10 seconds after the start of injection and are acquired every 1 to 2 seconds, until the peak of contrast has been demonstrated in the ascending aorta.[7] The images are loaded into an analysis software application on the scanner, which determines the time of peak contrast enhancement. The coronary CTA scan is then obtained with the full dose of contrast administered and the scan acquisition timing determined according to peak enhancement. The scan acquisition is usually planned to begin approximately 2 to 4 seconds after the peak enhancement determined from the test bolus to allow stabilization of the enhancement curve prior to scanning. This was an important technique in the past, especially with the slower scanners and longer breath-holds required for coronary CTA examinations (40 seconds on a four-slice scanner). With the faster scanners today having scan times as short as 4 to 5 seconds on a 256-slice scanner, a track and trigger technique can result in excellent opacification, without the need for the additional 20 mL of contrast of the test bolus. Therefore, coronary CTA with the track and trigger technique on the 256-slice scanner can be performed with as little as 50 mL of contrast.

For coronary CTA evaluation, the scan is performed in a craniocaudal direction to allow for washout of dense contrast in the right heart and allow better visualization of the right coronary artery. This scan direction also allows adequate opacification of the distal coronary vessels while minimizing contrast in the coronary veins. A patient who has undergone coronary artery bypass grafting will also be scanned in a craniocaudal direction, beginning at the level of the clavicles to include the origin of the left internal mammary artery. This is a longer total scan time and therefore a larger volume of contrast is required. When performing cardiac CTA for pulmonary vein evaluation, the scan is performed in a caudocranial direction. This allows for washout of dense contrast from the superior vena cava (SVC), which is usually in close approximation to the right

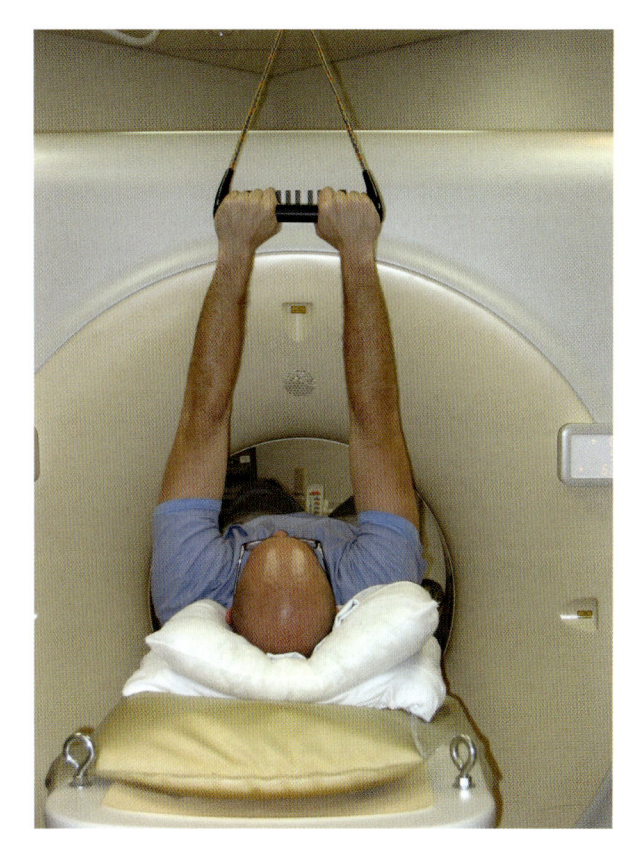

■ **FIGURE 9-3** Trapeze device used to elevate patient's arms during the scan.

superior pulmonary vein, resulting in difficulty evaluating the right superior pulmonary vein because of streak artifacts. It also allows for washout of the pulmonary arterial system, which is very helpful in the postprocessing portion of the examination. To create volume rendered images of the pulmonary veins and left atrium, which are used for an overview of the anatomy, the pulmonary arteries need to be removed. If the pulmonary arteries have been washed out, with a resulting difference of 100 HU (Hounsfield units) or more between the pulmonary arteries and veins, a threshold technique based on Hounsfield units can be used to render the pulmonary arteries invisible, rather than having to cut the vessels out.

The amount of contrast is tailored for each patient and each examination. For injection of contrast, a rate of 5 to 7 mL/sec is recommended, depending on the contrast medium's viscosity and iodine content. It is very important to be sure that the contrast has been warmed to near body temperature to allow easy contrast injection without reaching the pressure limit of the power injector, which can fragment the contrast bolus. Two techniques are currently used for contrast administration—contrast followed immediately by a saline push (two-phase), or contrast followed by a contrast and saline mix followed by saline push (three-phase). The purpose of these techniques is to provide minimal opacification in the right heart to help identify any incidental findings of the right heart, such as a thrombus or mass. However, if there is too much contrast in the right heart, the right coronary artery (RCA) could be obscured by streak artifact or there could be the false appearance of a stenosis caused by a streak artifact. Intracardiac shunts such as patent foramen ovale (PFO), atrial septal defect (ASD), or ventricular septal defect (VSD) may be obscured if there is not enough difference in contrast enhancement between the left and right heart.

To calculate the volume of contrast required for a two-phase technique, the time required to perform the scan needs to be known. If using a track and trigger technique, the time from the point the scan is triggered to the time the scan actually begins (post–threshold trigger delay) needs to be added to the time of the actual scan acquisition. For residual mild enhancement in the right ventricle, an extra 1 to 2 seconds of contrast injection is added. Thus, the total time of contrast injection should be the scan time plus post–threshold trigger delay time plus a 1- to 2-second additional "fudge factor." For example, for a new 256-slice scanner, the scan time is 5 seconds and the time from trigger to the beginning of the scan is 4 seconds, which results in a total of 10 to 11 seconds of contrast injection needed to opacify the right heart minimally. If we use 6 mL/sec, 60 to 66 mL of contrast is needed.

Tube Modulation to Minimize Radiation Dose

If the patient has the desired slow heart rate (<65 beats/min) and is in normal sinus rhythm without arrhythmias, then electrocardiographic tube modulation should be used to minimize radiation dose. This allows the x-ray tube to modulate the tube current (mA) in synchronization with the cardiac cycle. This technique can only be used during a retrospective electrocardiographic gated scan; with an appropriately slow heart rate, it can result in a dose reduction of up to 50%. As the heart rate increases, there is less dose savings, because the tube has less chance to reach minimum output. Once a heart rate of approximately 85 to 90 beats/min is reached, there is no dose savings, because the tube cannot modulate fast enough. The tube will be at maximum current during late diastole and minimum current during systole because in general the best reconstructed phase to evaluate the coronary arteries is a late diastolic phase.[8] If a step and shoot technique is used, the x-ray tube is turned on and off between each step and image acquisition. It is not a helical technique but an axial technique, with data acquired only at discrete anatomic steps and only during predefined portions of the cardiac cycle. This significantly reduces the radiation dose; however, it does not allow for capture of the full cardiac cycle, thus eliminating the data required to evaluate valve and overall cardiac function. It also allows only visualization of the heart during the predefined portion of the cardiac cycle. If based on heart rate, therefore, a systolic reconstruction would result in better images of the RCA,[9] images that would be unavailable using this technique if the predefined phase of scanning were in the late diastolic phase. However, with the retrospective technique, even if electrocardiographic tube modulation were used, the images could be reconstructed at any phase of the cardiac cycle at any anatomic location, even though the images reconstructed during systole would have a poor signal-to-noise ratio.

POSTPROCEDURAL CONSIDERATIONS

Once the scan is complete, if everything has gone well, there will be optimal quality images, resulting in easier interpretation. First, review the electrocardiographic tracing to be sure that no arrhythmias occurred during the scan that will require editing for optimization of the data set. Next, pan and zoom the images to optimize spatial resolution for viewing the coronary arteries. Keep in mind that with a standard 512×512 matrix, the smaller the field of view, the better the spatial resolution will be, which is paramount in coronary artery evaluation. In general, reconstructed axial images should be 0.6 to 0.9 mm thick, with a 50% increment (0.3 to 0.45 mm). If performing stent evaluations, the thinnest possible slice thickness with a 50% increment is recommended, combined with a sharp kernel or filter.[10,11] It is usually helpful to reconstruct three coronary data sets, including the phase of the R-R interval, which is usually optimal, as well as ±5% around this phase of the cardiac cycle. Depending on the scanner manufacturer, this may be 60% to 65% to 70% or 70% to 75% to 80%. It should be noted that there is a difference in manufacturer definition of the percentage of the R-R interval, either defining it based on the beginning of the temporal window or at the center of the temporal window. At a heart rate of 60 beats/min, this results in approximately a 10% shift, depending on how the phase is defined (i.e., 65% vs. 75%). In addition, if there is motion in the right coronary artery, a systolic reconstruction may be beneficial (e.g., 35% or 40%).[9] A multiphase data set of 5% to 95% every 10% is also reconstructed, with a slice thickness of 1.5 mm and increment of 1.5 mm; this is used for valve evaluation and qualitative and quantitative cardiac functional analysis. Finally, a full field of view data set can be created, which includes all soft tissues from skin to skin along the z-axis coverage of the scan, to evaluate for incidental findings, which may be the source of the patient's chest pain. These are reconstructed using a routine chest CT protocol such as 4-mm slice thickness with a 3-mm increment.

With the current generation of software on a dedicated workstation, it is fairly easy and accurate to determine cardiac function using the multiphase data set.[12] Curved multiplanar reconstructions (MPRs) of the coronary arteries are also created and stored on the picture archiving and communication system, which is very helpful in communicating the findings to referring physicians.

As for image interpretation, this is almost exclusively performed on a dedicated workstation. There are multiple software packages and techniques available for image interpretation, but those with the most experience tend to use the full axial data sets combined with interactive MPR and maximal intensity projection (MIP) visualization when a lesion is identified. This has been found by at least one study to be the most accurate method of image interpretation, as opposed to prerendered curved MPRs or vessel view technique.[13] Creating a structured report is highly encouraged.[14] The recommended method of reporting coronary narrowing and stenosis is based on visual inspection without noting specific diameter or area narrowing measurements because generally the CT technique overestimates the narrowing compared with coronary angiography.

Pitfalls and Solutions: Artifacts

Breathing artifacts are easily recognized by stair-step artifacts in the sternum (Fig. 9-4). There are essentially no techniques during postprocessing that will compensate for breathing artifacts. If there is gross movement of the patient during the scan, the sternum and spine will have stair-step artifacts.

If there are stair-step artifacts in the heart but not in the sternum or spine, this is consistent with a synchronization and data reconstruction issue, referred to as *electrocardiographic misregistration* (Fig. 9-5). In this situation, the images can be significantly improved by editing the tagging of the electrocardiographic tracing. This may be a result of an arrhythmic beat, which can be completely ignored (Fig. 9-6), or it may be caused by inappropriate R wave tagging by the scanner either tagging a T wave or putting in false R wave tags caused by a noisy electrocardiographic tracing (Fig. 9-7). Once the ECG has been corrected, the images often are at the least diagnostic and frequently are of high quality.

If there are no problems with the tagging, but there still remains a motion or stair-step artifact in the images, especially those of the RCA, a systolic reconstruction may be very helpful (see earlier).

KEY POINTS

- There are many technical considerations when performing routine cardiac CT, even in a daily clinical practice.
- The time spent to optimize the examination up front, however, will be well rewarded at the time of image interpretation because of the resulting high image quality.

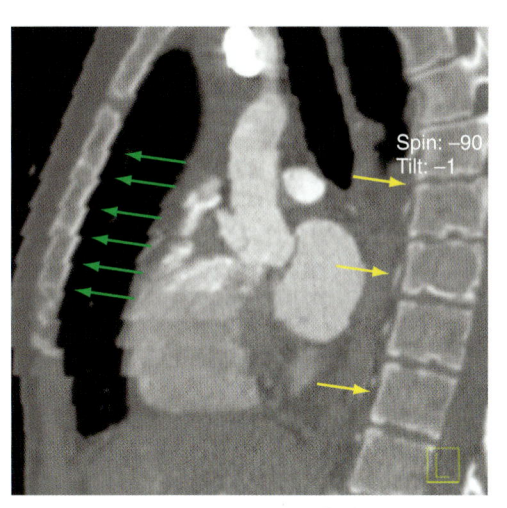

■ **FIGURE 9-4** Stair-step artifact of the sternum (*green arrows*) and soft tissues of the heart and mediastinum secondary to patient breathing during the scan. Notice the lack of artifact in the spine (*yellow arrows*), indicating that this is breathing and not gross patient motion.

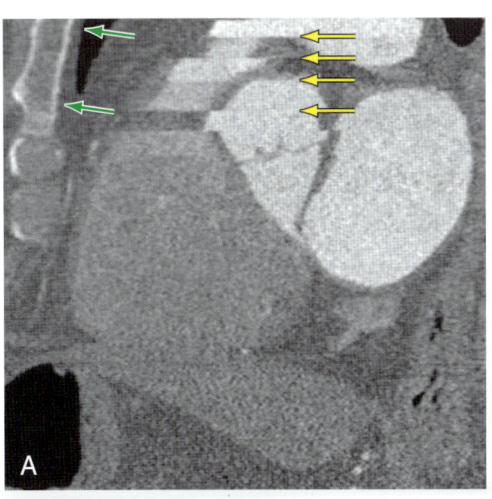

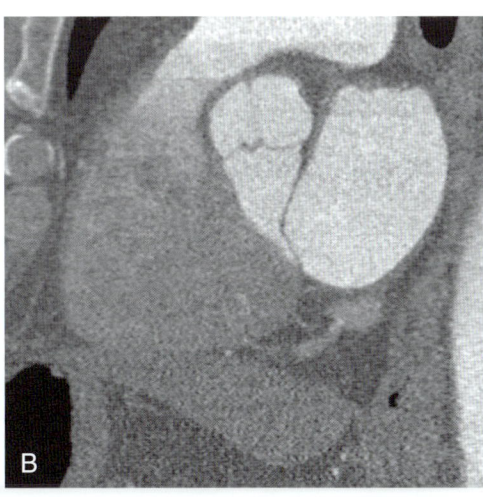

■ **FIGURE 9-5** **A,** Stair-step artifact seen only in the heart (*yellow arrows*) but sparing the sternum (*green arrows*). **B,** Artifact is absent after editing, confirming electrocardiographic misregistration.

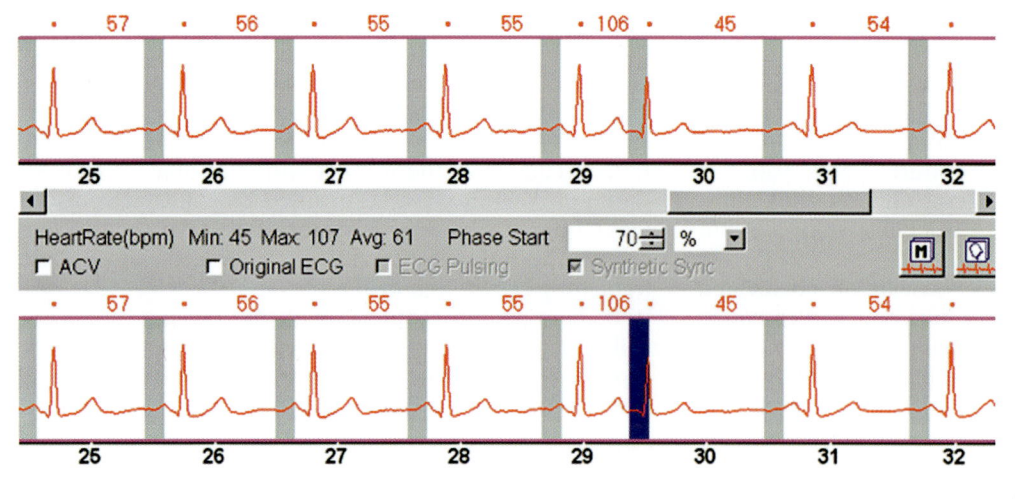

FIGURE 9-6 Electrocardiographic editing in which the premature beat (*highlighted in blue*) is simply ignored when the axial data set is constructed from the raw data.

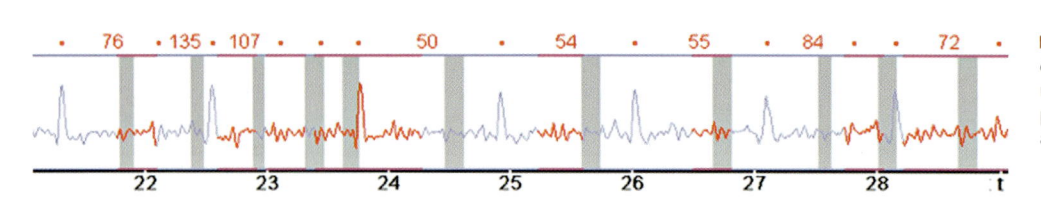

FIGURE 9-7 Poor-quality electrocardiographic tracing, which resulted in extra R-wave tags being placed by the scanner secondary to a noisy baseline.

SUGGESTED READINGS

Desjardins B, Kazerooni EA. ECG-gated cardiac CT. AJR Am J Roentgenol 2004; 182:993-1010.

Flohr TG, Raupach R, Bruder H. Cardiac CT: how much can temporal resolution, spatial resolution, and volume coverage be improved? J Cardiovasc Comput Tomogr 2009; 3:143-152.

Flohr TG, Schoepf UJ, Ohnesorge BM. Chasing the heart: new developments for cardiac CT. J Thorac Imaging 2007; 22:4-16.

Kaira MK, Brady TJ. Current status and future directions in technical developments of cardic computed tomography. J Cardiovasc Comput Tomogr 2008; 2:71-80.

Kerl JM, Hofmann LK, Thilo C, et al. Coronary CTA: image acquisition and interpretation. J Thorac Imaging 2007; 22:22-34.

Lawler LP, Pannu HK, Fishman EK. MDCT evaluation of the coronary arteries, 2004: how we do it—data acquisition, postprocessing, display, and interpretation. AJR Am J Roentgenol 2005; 184:1402-1412.

Lesser JR, Flygenring BJ, Knickelbine T, et al. Practical approaches to overcoming artifacts in coronary CT angiography. J Cardiovasc Comput Tomogr 2009; 3:4-15.

Mayo JR, Leipsic JA. Radiation dose in cardiac CT. AJR Am J Roentgenol 2009; 192:646-653. Erratum 2009; 192:1167.

Pannu HK, Alvarez W Jr, Fishman EK. Beta-blockers for cardiac CT: a primer for the radiologist. AJR Am J Roentgenol 2006; 186:S341-S345.

Ramkumar PG, Mitsouras D, Feldman CL, et al. New advances in cardiac computed tomography. Curr Opin Cardiol 2009; 24:596-603.

REFERENCES

1. Pannu HK, Alvarez W, Jr., Fishman EK. Beta-blockers for cardiac CT: a primer for the radiologist. AJR Am J Roentgenol 2006; 186:S341-S345.
2. Dewey M, Hoffmann H, Hamm B. Multislice CT coronary angiography: effect of sublingual nitroglycerine on the diameter of coronary arteries. Rofo 2006; 178:600-604.
3. McCullough CH. Principles and performance of electron beam computed tomography. In Fowlkes JB (ed). Medical CT and Ultrasound: Current Technology and Applications. Madison, Wis, Advanced Medical, 1995, pp 411-436.
4. Boxerman JL, Mosher TJ, McVeigh ER, et al. Advanced MR imaging techniques for evaluation of the heart and great vessels. Radiographics 1998; 18:543-564.
5. Goldberg HL, Moses JW, Fisher J, et al. Diagnostic accuracy of coronary angiography utilizing computer-based digital subtraction methods. Comparison to conventional cineangiography. Chest 1986; 90:793-797.
6. Halliburton SS, Stillman AE, Flohr T, et al. Do segmented reconstruction algorithms for cardiac multi-slice computed tomography improve image quality? Herz 2003; 28:20-31.
7. Moloo J, Shapiro MD, Abbara S. Cardiac computed tomography: technique and optimization of protocols. Semin Roentgenol 2008; 43:90-99.
8. Herzog C, Arning-Erb M, Zangos S, et al. Multi-detector row CT coronary angiography: influence of reconstruction technique and heart rate on image quality. Radiology 2006; 238:75-86.
9. Kopp AF, Schroeder S, Kuettner A, et al. Coronary arteries: retrospectively ECG-gated multi-detector row CT angiography with selective optimization of the image reconstruction window. Radiology 2001; 221:683-688.
10. Maintz D, Seifarth H, Flohr T, et al. Improved coronary artery stent visualization and in-stent stenosis detection using 16-slice computed-tomography and dedicated image reconstruction technique. Invest Radiol 2003; 38:790-795.

11. Suzuki S, Furui S, Kaminaga T, et al. Evaluation of coronary stents in vitro with CT angiography: effect of stent diameter, convolution kernel, and vessel orientation to the z-axis. Circ J 2005; 69: 1124-1131.
12. Savino G, Zwerner P, Herzog C, et al. CT of cardiac function. J Thorac Imaging 2007; 22:86-100.
13. Ferencik M, Ropers D, Abbara S, et al. Diagnostic accuracy of image postprocessing methods for the detection of coronary artery stenoses by using multidetector CT. Radiology 2007; 243:696-702.
14. Stillman AE, Rubin GD, Teague SD, et al. Structured reporting: coronary CT angiography: a white paper from the American College of Radiology and the North American Society for Cardiovascular Imaging. J Am Coll Radiol 2008; 5:796-800.

CHAPTER 10

Radiation Dose Reduction Strategies in Cardiac Computed Tomography

Sandra Simon Halliburton

Rapid technical advances in CT and increased availability of cardiac-capable CT systems have led to a sharp increase in the number of cardiac CT examinations performed during the last decade. Some technical advances (smaller detectors, faster gantry rotation) have necessitated increased x-ray exposure to the patient to maintain image noise. Concern regarding the resulting increase in radiation dose to the population from cardiac CT and the associated biologic risk has motivated critical assessment of dose-related imaging parameters.

A strategy for reducing radiation dose to the patient undergoing cardiac imaging should be employed particularly for patients at greatest risk for harm from x-ray exposure to the chest, young patients, and female patients.[1] This plan should include educating patients on the risks of exposure to ionizing radiation, seeking alternative studies that do not rely on ionizing radiation (e.g., MRI or ultrasonography) when appropriate, assessing the risk/benefit ratio of CT for the individual patient, and applying the as low as reasonably achievable (ALARA) principle to the selection of CT scan parameters.

TECHNICAL REQUIREMENTS

This chapter focuses on the selection of critical scan parameters directly or indirectly affecting radiation dose. Numerous modifiable scan parameters, including x-ray tube current, peak x-ray tube voltage, pitch (for helical scanning) or image acquisition spacing (for axial scanning), scan length, and, on some systems, scan field of view [SFOV], directly influence radiation dose by altering the number or energy of the x-ray photons interacting with the patient. Other scan parameters, including reconstructed slice thickness, indirectly affect dose by changing image quality and prompting the scanner operator to change parameters directly influencing dose. Strategies for customizing these parameters for the individual patient and minimizing radiation dose are presented in general terms to benefit users of any CT system.

TECHNIQUE TO REDUCE X-RAY TUBE CURRENT

ECG-Based Reduction in Tube Current

Acquisition of data using a lower dose, axial mode is indicated for contrast-enhanced evaluation of the coronary arteries in patients with low, stable heart rates; non–contrast-enhanced evaluation of coronary artery calcium (also known as calcium scoring), and evaluation of less mobile cardiovascular anatomy (e.g., aorta) if the z coverage of the scanner allows a reasonable breath-hold time. Helical data acquisition is typically required for contrast-enhanced coronary evaluation in patients with high or irregular heart rates. Online, ECG-based modulation of the tube current should be used with helical techniques to the extent possible for a given scanner.

Size-Based Reduction in Tube Current

Reduction of the nominal x-ray tube current before scanning is indicated in thin patients imaged with axial or helical techniques to reduce radiation dose. Online, anatomic-based tube current modulation during scanning can be used for all patients imaged with axial and non–ECG-gated, helical techniques.

Technique Description

X-rays used for CT imaging are generated when accelerated electrons strike a tungsten target. The number of electrons striking the target per unit time is described as the x-ray tube current and expressed in units of milliamperes (mA). A decrease in the x-ray tube current decreases

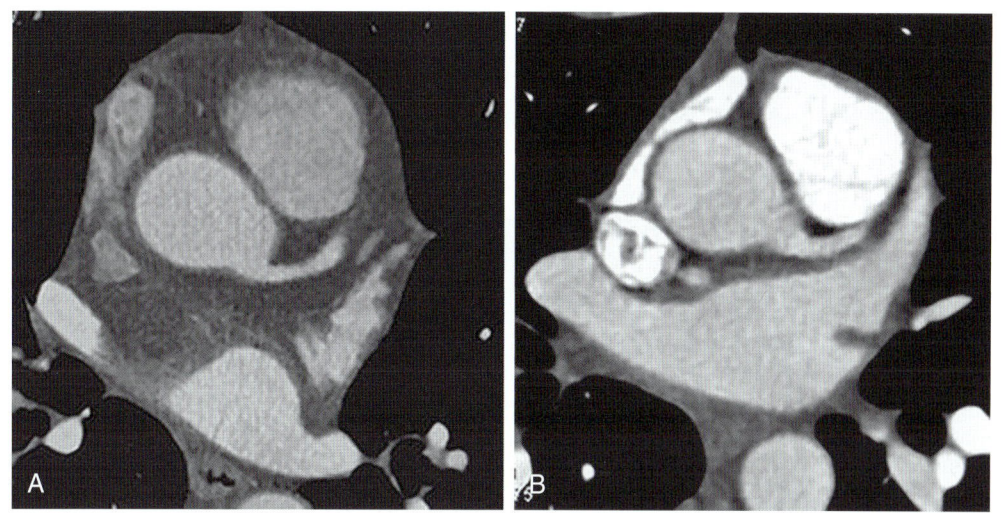

■ **FIGURE 10-1** **A** and **B**, Axial images from a larger patient (lateral width at top of liver 40 cm) (**A**) and a smaller patient (lateral width 27 cm) (**B**). To achieve noise equal to approximately 25 HU, 400 mAs/rotation was required in the larger patient, whereas only 320 mAs/rotation was required to achieve the same noise level in the smaller patient. Data acquisition with a lower tube current and resultant decrease in patient x-ray exposure is acceptable for imaging of smaller compared with larger patients without increasing image noise.

the number of electrons striking the target and, subsequently, the number of x-rays produced per unit time.

Radiation dose decreases linearly with a decrease in tube current such that a 20% reduction in tube current results in a 20% reduction in dose. Dose savings is achieved at the expense, however, of increased image noise because decreasing the number of x-ray photons produced per unit time decreases the probable number of photons penetrating the patient and reaching the detector array. Image noise is proportional to $1/\sqrt{\text{tube current}}$ such that a 20% reduction in tube current results in a 12% increase in image noise.

The parameter manipulated on clinically available CT scanners is often the product of the tube current and the exposure time per rotation with units of milliampere-second (mAs). The tube current × time product determines the number of x-ray photons produced per rotation. Additionally, some manufacturers automatically normalize the tube current × time product to pitch for helical scanning and define the resulting value in units of effective mAs or mAs/slice.

ECG-Based Reduction in Tube Current

During cardiac imaging, the x-ray tube current can be switched off or greatly reduced during systolic phases of the cardiac cycle significantly decreasing radiation dose. In patients with low, stable heart rates, data acquisition can be confined to a limited portion of the RR interval using prospectively ECG-triggered axial techniques. Average effective radiation doses of 2 to 3 mSv have been reported using these techniques to image the coronary arteries.[2,3]

Axial imaging is associated with increased sensitivity to arrhythmia, owing to prospective referencing of the ECG signal, and increased examination times, owing to incrementing the patient table between acquisitions. It is often necessary to acquire data during the entire cardiac cycle using a helical mode and retrospectively reference image reconstruction to a simultaneously recorded ECG signal. Although ECG-gated helical techniques require continuous x-ray exposure, tube current outside the phase of interest can be reduced to decrease patient radiation dose significantly. Effective radiation doses can easily exceed 15 mSv[4] using helical imaging without ECG-based dose modulation, but can be reduced 50% or more depending on patient heart rate,[5] the minimum tube current value,[6] and the duration of the full tube current window.[7]

Size-Based Reduction in Tube Current

The x-ray tube current can be reduced for slimmer patients. Attenuation of the incident x-ray beam decreases with the thickness of the tissue between the x-ray source and the detector such that less radiation exposure is required to penetrate thinner tissues and achieve desired image noise (Fig. 10-1). Patients can be assigned to size categories based on visual inspection, weight, body mass index, or cross-sectional body measurements from scout images,[8] and the tube current can be adjusted manually to a predefined value. Weight-adapted tube current protocols were shown to reduce coronary CT angiography dose by 18% in men and 26% in women[9] at one institution.

Automatic methods of online adaptation of tube current to patient size can also be used to reduce dose. The tube current can be modulated along the x, y, and z directions during scanning based on local tissue thickness without sacrificing image noise. Tube current is reduced at projection angles and table positions requiring less x-ray penetration. Online, anatomic-based tube current modulation has been shown to reduce radiation exposure to the thorax by 20% compared with a fixed tube current while maintaining image noise.[10]

Pitfalls and Solutions

ECG-Based Reduction in Tube Current

Axial imaging is vulnerable to cardiac motion artifacts, particularly in patients with high or irregular heart rates, according to prospective data collection. Some additional data beyond the minimum required for image reconstruction can be acquired (also known as padding) to permit minor retrospective adjustments of the reconstruction window and, potentially, to reduce cardiac motion artifacts.

Helical data acquisition with retrospective ECG gating is less susceptible to cardiac motion artifacts and provides an alternative to axial imaging at high or irregular heart rates. ECG-based tube current modulation is prescribed before scanning, however, so changes in heart rate could result in unintended reduction of the tube current during a desired phase of reconstruction for a given cardiac cycle. Some CT systems allow adjustment of the full tube current duration, increasing the utility of ECG-based tube current modulation for patients with high or irregular heart rates because the optimal reconstruction phase is less predictable.[7] For patients with severe arrhythmia, some systems temporarily suspend or permanently switch off ECG-based tube current modulation if beat-to-beat variation exceeds a threshold value during data acquisition, virtually eliminating the risk of improperly timed downward modulation of the tube current.

Another consideration when employing ECG-based tube current modulation with helical imaging is the availability of multiphase data for functional evaluation because of increased image noise during periods of low tube current. Although reconstruction of thin slices (<1 mm) is confined to a small portion of the cardiac cycle, the reconstruction of thick slices (>5 mm) useful for functional evaluation may still be possible because noise decreases as reconstruction section thickness increases.

Size-Based Reduction in Tube Current

Weight-based approaches to categorizing patients are limited for cardiac imaging because attenuation depends on the thickness of the chest, which can vary substantially among patients of similar weight. Even body mass index cannot always adequately account for differences in chest size, particularly for women. Measurement of cross-sectional body dimensions from scout images or even visual inspection may be more appropriate for size categorization of cardiac patients and determination of the tube current necessary to achieve the desired image noise.

Online, anatomic-based modulation of the tube current in the z-direction is limited in combination with ECG-based modulation. Because position and time change along the z-axis, anatomic-based modulation in this direction competes with ECG-based modulation. In practice, ECG-based tube current modulation is given priority, and anatomic-based modulation serves only to determine the optimal nominal tube current value necessary to achieve the desired noise based on the scout image.

TECHNIQUE TO REDUCE TUBE VOLTAGE

Indications

Selection of a reduced x-ray tube voltage is indicated in thin patients to reduce radiation dose.

Technique Description

Electrons striking a tungsten target are accelerated by applying a potential difference between the positive and negative electrodes of an x-ray tube. The potential difference is described as the x-ray tube voltage in units of kilovolts (kV), and determines the energy of the accelerated electrons. Discrete values for peak x-ray tube voltage, the maximum voltage across the tube, are selectable on clinical CT scanners: 80 kVp, 100 kVp, 120 kVp, 135 kVp, and 140 kVp (specific tube voltages available vary with scanner type). A tube voltage of 120 kVp is standard for cardiac imaging and is suitable for most patients. Decreasing the peak tube voltage (kVp) decreases the energy of electrons striking the target and, subsequently, the energy and number of the x-rays produced.

Radiation dose with CT is approximately proportional to the square of the tube voltage such that a reduction in tube voltage from 120 to 100 kVp results in a 31% reduction in dose—assuming no other changes to dose related parameters are made. An additional benefit of decreased tube voltage is increased image contrast. Within the diagnostic CT energy range, lower energies produce greater differences in attenuation among body tissues. Decreased radiation dose and increased image contrast are achieved at the expense of increased image noise, however, because decreasing the peak tube voltage decreases the probable number of photons penetrating the patient and reaching the detector array. Image noise is proportional to 1/tube voltage such that a reduction in tube voltage from 120 to 100 kVp results in a 20% increase in image noise. In practice, selection of a lower tube voltage typically results in an automatic increase in tube current to minimize the negative impact on image noise, but with a net decrease in x-ray exposure.

As with x-ray tube current, x-ray tube voltage can be reduced according to patient size to avoid unnecessary exposure to slimmer patients, while still achieving acceptable image noise. Size can be assessed as described previously, and tube voltage can be adjusted accordingly. A more recent study showed a tube voltage of 100 kVp could be used to obtain diagnostic quality coronary CT angiography images from patients of normal weight with a 25% decrease in average effective dose compared with a tube voltage of 120 kVp; the average effective dose was decreased by 50% and diagnostic image quality was maintained when tube current was also reduced.[11]

Pitfalls and Solutions

Hounsfield unit (HU)–dependent analysis of cardiac CT images is affected by changes in tube voltage because of associated changes in tissue attenuation characteristics. Automatic bolus timing methods rely on the attenuation of enhanced blood within a specified region of interest to reach a predefined threshold before initiating the scan. Because iodine absorption increases with a decrease in tube voltage, iodinated contrast material appears brighter on 100 kVp images compared with 120 kVp images. This may necessitate a higher threshold with automatic bolus timing to prevent premature initiation of the scan if the contrast injection protocol is unchanged. Alternatively, it may be possible to reduce iodinated contrast media volume at 100 kVp compared with 120 kVp, but maintain blood pool opacification.[12] Additionally, attenuation-based characterization of tissues typically relies on HU thresholds or ranges established with 120 kVp imaging that may not be appropriate at 100 kVp. Affected cardiac applications include, but are not limited to, quantification of coronary artery calcium, characterization of coronary artery plaque, and differentiation of simple fluid and blood products or soft tissue.

TECHNIQUE TO SHORTEN SCAN LENGTH

Indications

Scan length should be optimized for all patients to avoid unnecessary x-ray exposure.

Technique Description

The length of the scan in the z-direction (direction of patient movement) is defined using scout images. Increasing the scan length increases the irradiated portion of the body. Therefore, scan length is directly proportional to patient radiation exposure. Optimization of scan length from the scout image can be inexact, particularly when imaging the chest because of variation in the position of the heart with respiratory state. The scan start can be more accurately determined by performing an additional low-dose, cross-sectional scan before the diagnostic scan to verify anatomic location. The scan end should be carefully specified using standard landmarks on the scout image. If allowed by the scanner, manual stoppage of the scan should be initiated if the desired anatomy is covered before reaching the programmed value for the scan end.

Pitfalls and Solutions

For coronary artery imaging, the scan is typically started just below the tracheal carina. In patients with a large abdomen, the heart may shift upward significantly during a breath-hold, changing its position relative to the carina such that a scan start at the standard location would miss critical anatomy. Minimization of the scan range in these patients may be secondary to ensuring sufficient coverage and avoiding repeat scanning.

TECHNIQUE TO INCREASE BEAM PITCH (FOR HELICAL SCANNING)

Indications

With some CT scanners, an increased beam pitch may be indicated in cardiac patients with higher heart rates to reduce dose.

Technique Development

The spatial distribution of individual scans during helical imaging is described by the beam pitch. Specifically, beam pitch is defined as the table feed per gantry rotation (mm)/beam collimation (mm). An increase in the beam pitch results in less overlap between successive data acquisitions.

Radiation dose is inversely proportional to beam pitch such that a twofold increase in pitch results in a 50% reduction in dose. An increase in beam pitch causes degradation of the slice sensitivity profile and decreased spatial resolution, however, because data are averaged over a greater distance along the z-axis. In addition, increased pitch results in increased noise because of less data sampling. The exception is scanners that normalize tube current values to beam pitch (e.g., effective mAs, mAs/slice). In this case, x-ray flux is changed with beam pitch to maintain image noise, and dose savings is not realized. Some manufacturers fix beam pitch for a given clinical application to ensure image quality standards are maintained.

A low beam pitch (e.g., 0.2) or highly overlapping scans are required for imaging with fast gantry rotation to ensure continuous anatomic coverage with reconstruction of data from successive cardiac cycles. If the pitch is too high for the patient's heart rate, the table moves too far between consecutive cardiac cycles to sample the data adequately, resulting in gaps in the imaged volume. This situation is of particular concern for multisegment reconstruction algorithms that use data from two or more consecutive cardiac cycles (rather than a single cardiac cycle) to reconstruct each image. Higher beam pitch (e.g., 0.2 to 0.5) can be used to image patients with higher heart rates, particularly when single-segment reconstruction algorithms are used.

Pitfalls and Solutions

A decrease in heart rate is sometimes observed after initiation of a breath-hold. If beam pitch is too high for the resulting heart rate, portions of the desired anatomy are missing from the reconstructed images. One solution is to practice breath-holding with the patient and decrease the pitch before scanning if a decrease in heart rate is observed. The pitch should also be lowered below the recommended value for the patient's average heart rate if any heart rate irregularities are noted before scanning or during the practice breath-hold. Selecting a lower pitch results in increased dose, but ensures adequate anatomic coverage.

TECHNIQUE TO INCREASE BEAM FILTRATION

Indications

With some CT scanners, restriction of in-plane x-ray beam dimensions through selection of the SFOV may be indicated in smaller patients to reduce radiation dose.

Technique Development

X-rays generated for CT imaging are filtered before reaching the patient to limit x-ray exposure. Highly attenuating material is placed in the path of the x-ray beam to absorb unhelpful low-energy photons and to restrict the x-ray

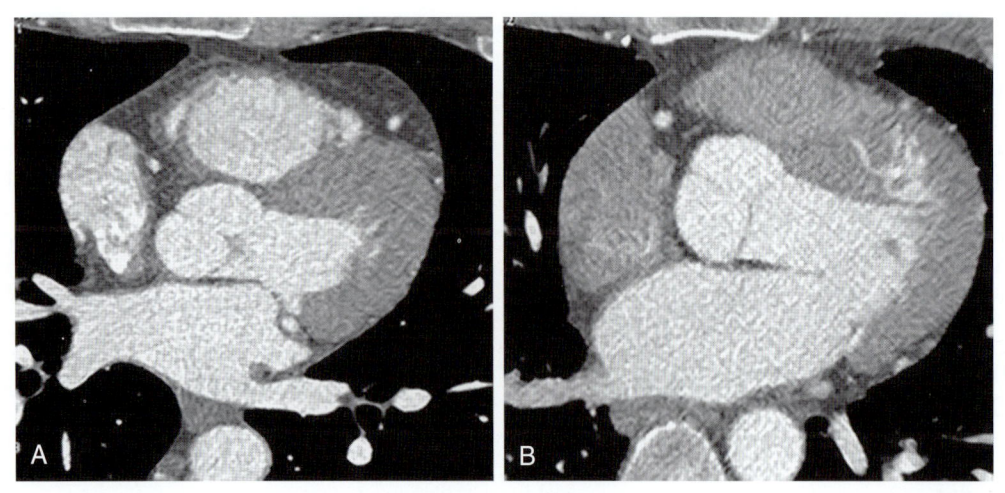

FIGURE 10-2 **A** and **B,** Axial images from two different patients of similar size (lateral width at top of liver 39 cm for both) reconstructed with 0.75 mm slice thickness (**A**) and 1.5 mm slice thickness (**B**). To achieve noise equal to approximately 32 HU, 350 mAs/rotation was required in 0.75 mm thick images, but only 280 mAs/rotation was required to achieve the same noise level in 1.5 mm thick images. Reconstruction of thicker images is acceptable for evaluation of pulmonary vein anatomy, permitting data acquisition with a lower tube current and a resultant decrease in patient x-ray exposure compared with reconstruction of thinner images.

beam to the minimum required spatial dimensions. On some CT systems, additional in-plane beam filtration can be applied by the user through selection of the SFOV. On these systems, smaller SFOV can be selected for smaller patients to reduce radiation dose. With other scanners, data are obtained from the entire field, and FOV is a reconstruction parameter used to control the anatomic area displayed. When FOV is designated as a reconstruction parameter, it has no impact on in-plane beam filtration, and no impact on radiation dose.

Pitfalls and Solutions

If an additional filter is placed between the x-ray beam and the patient by selection of a smaller SFOV, any information outside the SFOV is unavailable for image reconstruction. Care must be taken to ensure that the entire region of interest is included within the SFOV. Lung fields may be excluded with a small SFOV for some cardiac patients.

TECHNIQUE TO INCREASE RECONSTRUCTED SLICE THICKNESS

Indications

The reconstruction of thicker images is indicated for non–contrast-enhanced evaluation of coronary calcium and the evaluation of larger cardiovascular anatomy (e.g., aorta, pulmonary vein). Thicker slices permit a reduction in x-ray tube current and, subsequently, a reduction in patient radiation dose.

Technique Development

The reconstructed slice thickness determines the number of absorbed x-ray photons contributing to the CT image. An increase in the reconstructed slice thickness increases the number of x-ray photons contributing to each image allowing a decrease in the number of absorbed x-ray photons (i.e., decrease in radiation dose) to achieve the same image noise (Fig. 10-2). Noise is proportional to $1/\sqrt{\text{reconstructed slice thickness}}$ such that a 3 mm thick image has 73% less noise than a 1 mm thick image. The decrease in tube current and radiation dose made possible by an increase in reconstructed slice thickness comes at a cost of decreased spatial resolution. The reconstruction of thicker slices is inappropriate for evaluation of small cardiac anatomy such as the coronary arteries.

Pitfalls and Solutions

Increasing reconstructed slice thickness (a reconstruction parameter) has no direct effect on x-ray exposure. It is incumbent on the user also to decrease the x-ray tube current (a data acquisition parameter) to reduce patient radiation dose.

KEY POINTS

- Reducing x-ray tube current is the most straightforward method to reduce radiation dose.
- ECG-based tube current modulation can be used most aggressively in patients with low, stable heart rates.
- The nominal tube current can be reduced for smaller patients before imaging, but anatomic-based, online modulation has limited utility for cardiac imaging.
- Decreasing the tube voltage can reduce radiation dose and is appropriate in smaller patients, but affects the attenuation properties of tissues.
- The scan length should be optimized in all patients to reduce x-ray exposure.
- Beam pitch can be increased for patients with higher heart rates when single-segment reconstruction is employed, but the option is currently available from only one manufacturer.
- An increase in reconstructed slice thickness permits a decrease in x-ray tube current for evaluation of larger cardiac anatomy.

SUGGESTED READINGS

Kalara MK, Maher MM, Toth TL, et al. Strategies for CT radiation dose optimization. Radiology 2004; 230:619-628.

Kubo T, Lin PP, Stiller W, et al. Radiation dose reduction in chest CT: a review. AJR Am J Roentgenol 2008; 190:335-343.

McNitt-Gray MF. AAPM/RSNA physics tutorial for residents: topics in CT. Radiation dose in CT. RadioGraphics 2002; 22:1541-1553.

Paul JF, Abada HT. Strategies for reduction of radiation dose in cardiac multislice CT. Eur Radiol 2007; 17:2028-2037.

Primack AN, McCollough CH, Bruesewitz MR, et al. Relationship between noise, dose, and pitch in cardiac multi-detector row CT. RadioGraphics 2006; 26:1785-1794.

REFERENCES

1. Einstein AJ, Henzlova MJ, Rajagopalan S. Estimating risk of cancer associated with radiation exposure from 64-slice computed tomography coronary angiography. JAMA 2007; 298:317-323.
2. Earls JP, Berman EL, Urban BA, et al. Prospectively gated transverse coronary CT angiography versus retrospectively gated helical technique: improved image quality and reduced radiation dose. Radiology 2008; 246:742-753.
3. Husmann L, Valenta I, Gaemperli O, et al. Feasibility of low-dose coronary CT angiography: first experience with prospective ECG-gating. Eur Heart J 2008; 29:191-197.
4. Hausleiter J, Meyer T, Hermann F, et al. Estimated radiation dose associated with cardiac CT angiography. JAMA 2009; 301:500-507.
5. Jakobs T, Becker CR, Ohnesorge B, et al. Multislice helical CT of the heart with retrospective ECG gating: reduction of radiation exposure by ECG-controlled tube current modulation. Eur Radiol 2002; 12:1081-1086.
6. Stolzmann P, Scheffel H, Schertler T, et al. Radiation dose estimates in dual-source computed tomography coronary angiography. Eur Radiol 2008; 18:592-599.
7. Leschka S, Scheffel H, Desbiolles L, et al. Image quality and reconstruction intervals of dual-source CT coronary angiography: recommendations for ECG-pulsing windowing. Invest Radiol 2007; 42:543-549.
8. McCollough CH, Ulzheimer S, Halliburton SS, et al. A multi-institutional, multi-manufacturer, international standard for the quantification of coronary artery calcium using cardiac CT. Radiology 2007; 243:527-538.
9. Jung B, Mahnken AH, Stargardt A, et al. Individually weight-adapted examination protocol in retrospectively ECG-gated MSCT of the heart. Eur Radiol 2003; 13:2560-2566.
10. Mulkens TH, Bellinck P, Baeyaert M, et al. Use of an automatic exposure control mechanism for dose optimization in multi-detector row CT examinations: clinical evaluation. Radiology 2005; 237: 213-223.
11. Leschka S, Stolzmann P, Schmid FT, et al. Low kilovoltage cardiac dual-source CT: attenuation, noise, and radiation dose. Eur Radiol 2008; 18:1809-1817.
12. Sigal-Cinqualbre AB, Hennequin R, Abada HT, et al. Low-kilovoltage multi-detector row chest CT in adults: feasibility and effect on image quality and iodine dose. Radiology 2004; 231:169-174.

CHAPTER 11

Contrast Agents and Medications in Cardiac Computed Tomography

Justus E. Roos

Earlier generations of multidetector CT scanners provided the foundation for cardiac multidetector CT angiography, and the implementation of 64-multidetector CT technologies made it a reliable tool with a high degree of diagnostic efficacy.[1-3] In contrast to CT angiography applications using intravenous contrast medium (CM) administration elsewhere in the body, adequate cardiac opacification is not always simple to achieve, particularly in light of continuously evolving CT technology, with scan times becoming substantially shorter, but yielding improved spatial and temporal resolution. Empiric injection protocols are no longer adequate because they do not take into account the complexity of all confounding variables that allow consistent, robust cardiac imaging.[4] These confounding variables include the requirement for a controlled and regular heart rate and carefully timed arterial enhancement for optimal cardiac and coronary vessel enhancement during minimal cardiac motion. Physiologic and pharmacokinetic constraints of cardiac enhancement in addition to inherent technical scanner properties have to be considered when building an integrated scanning and injection protocol for cardiac CT angiography.

This chapter reviews the general properties and safety aspects of (1) medications used for patient preparation and of (2) iodinated CM administration with particular relevance to cardiac imaging. Basic principles of arterial enhancement (early CM dynamics) and their impact on successful cardiac imaging, and specific modifications for optimal timing of CM injection and data acquisition for cardiac CT angiography are discussed.

TECHNICAL REQUIREMENTS
Medications for Cardiac Imaging

Although newer generations of multidetector CT scanners have shown a substantial improvement in temporal resolution—and with this, the capability to "freeze" cardiac motion—it is still desirable for most cardiac applications to slow the heart rate for various reasons. Slow heart rates prolong the cardiac phases with the least cardiac motion, specifically end-diastolic relaxation and end-systolic contraction. Best image quality is achieved when the data reconstruction window fits temporally into these phases.[5] Slower heart rates also decrease heart rate variability during data acquisition and allow optimal efficacy of ECG-gated dose modulation techniques to control patient radiation dose.[6]

In our practice, we aim for a target heart rate less than 65 beats/min. To slow the heart rate, β blockers are ubiquitously used, and different means of β blocker administration for cardiac imaging are described, depending on patient, workflow, and logistics-related factors. Knowledge of the pharmacologic properties of the various β blockers is key to ensure safe and efficient patient prescan preparation. First-generation agents, such as propranolol, nonselectively block all β receptors (β_1 and β_2 receptors). Second-generation agents, such as atenolol, metoprolol, acebutolol, and others, have a relative selectivity, when given in low doses, for β_1 (largely cardiac) receptors. The administration of β_1 adrenoreceptor antagonists is favored for cardiac CT because of fewer side effects and fewer contraindications. Table 11-1 summarizes the effects mediated by β_1 and β_2 adrenoreceptors, and Figure 11-1 shows the important effects of nonselective and selective β blockers.

Diverse cardiac CT imaging centers have proposed different protocols of β blocker administration. Some centers routinely use an oral β blocker (e.g., atenolol [Tenormin]) to slow the heart rate and add an intravenous β blocker (e.g., metoprolol tartrate [Lopressor]) only if rate control is unsatisfactory. Other centers performing cardiac CT suggest different medication protocols (i.e., no combination of intravenous and oral β blocker administration)

CHAPTER 11 • Contrast Agents and Medications in Cardiac Computed Tomography

Table 11-1 Effects Mediated by β_1- and β_2-Adrenoreceptors

Tissue	β_1	β_2	Effect
Heart			
SA node	X	X	Heart rate ↑ (+ chronotrop)
AV node	X	X	Conduction velocity ↑ (+ dromotrop)
Atria	X	X	Contractility ↑ (+ inotrop)
Ventricles	X	X	Contractility ↑ (+ inotrop)
Arteries		X	Vasodilatation
Veins		X	Vasodilatation
Skeletal muscle		X	Contractility ↑
Liver		X	Glycogenolysis/gluconeogenesis
Pancreas (β cells)		X	Insulin secretion
Fat cells	X		Lipolysis
Bronchi		X	Bronchodilatation
Kidney	X		Renin release
Gallbladder		X	Relaxation
Urinary bladder		X	Relaxation
Uterus		X	Relaxation
Gastrointestinal		X	Relaxation
Nerves		X	Noradrenalin release
Parathyroid glands	X	X	Parathormone
Thyroid gland		X	T4 → T3 conversion

based on their experience and available operational logistics. Table 11-2 shows the sequence of our routine β blocker administration in the absence of any contraindications. Any patient preparation protocol should include a checklist for contraindications to the use of β blockade. The general contraindications for the therapeutic use of β blockers also apply for a "one-time" use for cardiac CT.

Table 11-3 summarizes the most important contraindications for the drugs involved in cardiac CT. In case of questionable contraindications, the responsible imaging specialist should confer with the referring physician and determine if the administration of a β blocker is justified, or if alternatives should be applied.

Calcium channel blockers embody an alternative heart rate-controlling medication. In patients with contraindications to β blockers (i.e., asthma), an attempt with calcium channel blockers may be worthwhile. There is less experience with calcium channel blockers in the setting of cardiac CT, and the imaging physician should be familiar with the medication, its administration (see Table 11-2), and its contraindications (see Table 11-3). Consultation with the referring physician is suggested to obtain an optimal and safe result.

Organic nitrates are widely used to treat angina and alleviate symptoms of myocardial ischemia through various mechanisms.[7] Intracoronary injection of nitroglycerin has long been used to obtain maximal arterial dilation during conventional coronary angiography.[8] Similarly, oral administration of short-acting nitrates (sublingual nitroglycerin tablets or sublingual nitroglycerin spray) is an accepted practice to dilate the lumen of the coronary arteries during coronary CT angiography.[9] Its vasodilative effect on the coronary arterial bed allows improved visualization of smaller arterial branches.[10] The significant impact on the diameter of coronary arteries seems to be more pronounced in nondiseased/nonstenotic coronary segments when compared with diseased/stenotic coronary segments.[11] This additional pharmacologic end-organ response is a welcome side effect because it accentuates further the difference between diseased and nondiseased

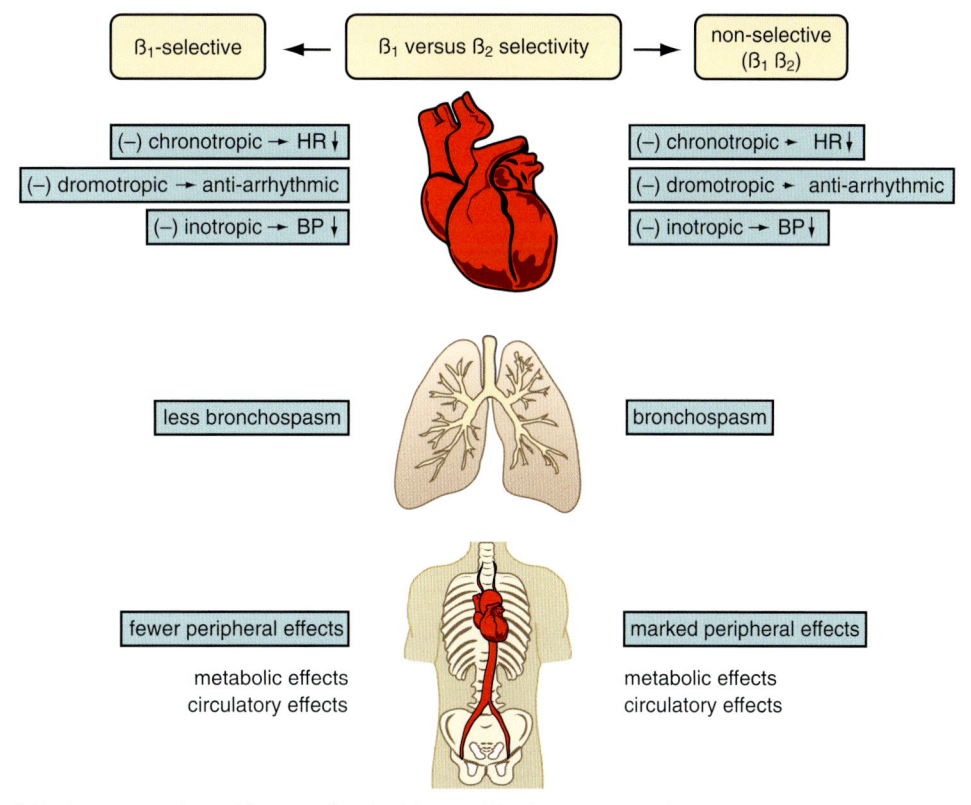

■ **FIGURE 11-1** β-blocker. Comparison of β_1 versus β_2 selectivity. BP, blood pressure; HR, heart rate.

Table 11-2 Sequence of Pharmacological Patient Preparation for Cardiac CT (Stanford Protocol)

		Purpose: Goal:	Decrease HR and R-to-R Variability Steady Heart Rate of 50-65 bpm	Alternatives
A		Questionaire Obtain baseline HR and BP	Rule out contraindications if HR ≤ 65 bpm → [D] if HR > 65 bpm → [B]	CA channel blockers
B		**Oral atenolol (Tenormin)**	100 mg PO 1-2 min before cardiac CT if HR ≤ 65 bpm → [D] if HR > 65 bpm → [C]	Oral diltiazem (Cardizem, regular release): 30 mg PO or doubling oral dose for patients currently taking oral CA channel blockers OR
C		**IV metoprolol (Lopressor)** Injection with patient on the scanner table Wait 3-4 min	5 mg IV slow injection over 1 min if HR ≤ 65 bpm → [D] If HR > 65 bpm → repeat [C] up to two times at 3-4 min intervals Maximal dose: 15 mg metoprolol (Lopressor) if HR ≤ 65 bpm → [D] If HR > 65 bpm → regardless of HR	If systolic BP > 100 and HR > 60, intravenous diltiazem (Cardizem Monovial): 10 mg IV over 2 min, repeat 10 mg IV in every 10 min to maximal dose of 40 mg
D		Purpose Questionnaire Sublingual nitroglycerin (Nitroquick) Wait 5 min	Coronary artery dilation for better visualization Rule out contraindications 0.4 mg tablet → [E]	Sublingual nitroglycerin spray (0.4 mg/L)
E		Scan Postscan monitoring	→ [F] Outpatients: for 30 min	
F		HR and BP Recommendations	Inpatients: on ward Outpatients: do not operate machinery for 3 hours (e.g., driving car)	

Table 11-3 Contraindications for the Use of β Blocker, CA Channel Blockers, and Nitroglycerin for Cardiac CT

	Medication		
	β Blockers (β₁ Selective Blocker e.g., Atenolol, Metoprolol)	CA Channel Blocker (e.g., Verapamil, Diltiazem)	Nitroglycerin
Heart			
Sick sinus syndrome	++	++	0
Severe bradycardia	++	++	0
Second-/third-degree heart block	++	++	0
Hypotension (systolic BP < 100 mm Hg)	++	++	++
Severe aortic stenosis	+	+	+
Early myocardial infarction	+	+	++
Obstructive cardiomyopathy	0	+	++
Constrictive pericarditis	+	+	+
High doses of other agents depressing SA and AV nodes (digoxin, anti-arrhythmics)	++	++	0
Lung			
Asthma	++	0	0
Bronchospasms	++	0	0
Severe COPD	++	0	0
Other			
Severe anemia	0	0	++
Increased intracranial pressure	0	0	++
Migraine sensitive to nitrates			++
Peripheral arterial occlusive disease	+	0	0
Hypersensitivity	++	++	++
Erectile dysfunction treated with nitrate based medications (e.g., Viagra, Cialis, Levitra)			++
Pulmonary arterial hypertension treated with nitrate based medications (e.g., Viagra)			++
Glaucoma			++

++ Absolutely contraindicated; + relatively contraindicated; 0 not contraindicated

coronary segments, and improves depiction of subtle coronary arterial disease. In addition to dilation of the vascular bed, nitroglycerin suppresses potential coronary artery spasm that may mimic stenosis at coronary CT angiography, especially in younger patients.

Our rationale of nitroglycerin administration is summarized in Table 11-2. Because the blood level peaks around 2 minutes, and the half life is around 7 minutes, we suggest waiting approximately 5 minutes after sublingual nitroglycerin administration to ensure maximal effect of coronary artery vasodilation.

The side effects of nitroglycerin are harmful; severe decreases in blood pressure and death have been reported in patients given nitroglycerin within 24 hours because of a pharmacologic interaction with phosphodiesterase type 5 inhibitors (e.g., sildenafil citrate [Viagra] or tadalafil [Cialis]). A careful check for any contraindications before administration of nitroglycerin must be a part of any patient premedication protocol (see Table 11-3).

Contrast Media

CT contrast agents are water-soluble derivates of iodinated benzene rings, which are either charged (ionic contrast agent) or not charged (nonionic contrast agent) monomeric or dimeric chemical structures. The x-ray absorption is proportional to the concentration of the iodine captured within the agent.[12] Other important physicochemical properties of CM are their osmolality (high-osmolar, low-osmolar, iso-osmolar) and viscosity. Higher flow rates are necessary for cardiac CT imaging. Warming the contrast agent to body temperature reduces viscosity and maintains high injection flow rates.[13] The viscosity of CM decreases about 50% by heating it from 20° C to body temperature.

Safety Issues of Contrast Media

Nonionic contrast agents for CT angiography are considered to be very safe with an adverse event rate of approximately 3%.[14] Most adverse effects are mild to moderate, but severe reactions may occur in approximately 0.04%.[15] Non–dose-dependent, (idiosyncratic) allergy-like and dose-dependent (nonidiosyncratic) reactions are the two major categories of adverse effects. Guidelines for patient screening, premedication, and management of acute adverse reactions are available in the literature.[16] There is also a substantial incidence of delayed cutaneous reactions occurring 24 hours or more after CM injection.[17] Because these events tend to recur with reinjection of the same CM, screening and documentation of these reactions is of paramount importance.[17] Another absolute contraindication for iodinated CM is manifest hyperthyroidism (i.e., Graves disease) with the risk of triggering a thyrotoxic crisis.[18]

Important dose-dependent effects include CM extravasation, cardiovascular effects, drug interactions, and contrast-induced nephropathy (CIN). CM extravasation is a well-known problem that occurs with an incidence of approximately 0.2% to 0.6% with the use of mechanical power injectors.[19] Injection flow rates of 5 to 6 mL/s are routinely used for cardiac CT imaging and are considered to be safe.[20] Only large volumes (>30 mL) of CM extravasation are at risk of severe side effects such as skin necrosis, ulceration, or compartment syndrome. Although adverse effects are more common and severe with ionic CM, they have been described to occur occasionally with nonionic agents as well. Conservative management of extravasation injuries (applying warm or cold compresses) is often adequate. For more severe injuries, plastic or hand surgery consultation is recommended to determine optimal treatment. Any adverse effects should be documented for future therapeutic planning.

To avoid any extravasation, intravenous access should be tested for stable and correct cannula position by a preliminary rapid manual injection of saline with the patient's arm in the scanning position. Most extravasation events happen within the first seconds of injection; however, they may also occur later during mid or late phase of injection. Checking the intravenous access during early CM administration does not entirely prevent any extravasation. Extravasation detection devices linked to the power injector provide monitoring during the entire CM administration and may reduce the risk of late extravasation.[21] Their use comes, however, with increased cost and risk of erroneous abortion of CM administration because of false-positive alarms.

Cardiovascular adverse events after intravenous administration of nonionic agents are probably rare; the literature suggests that severe reactions are more likely to be due to cardiopulmonary decompensation than to allergy-like reactions.[22] Rapid injection of CM volume may lead to acute decompensation in patients with preexisting substantial cardiopulmonary compromise. Reducing the CM volume and injection rate seems to be one rational technique to reduce this specific risk.

CIN resulting from nonionic CM is rare (<2%) in the general population, but it may be substantial in the subset of patients at increased risk (>25%).[23] CIN is defined as a greater than 25% increase of serum creatinine from baseline value within 3 days after CM injection in the absence of other causes.[24] Controversy exists currently as to which features of the CM abet the development of CIN. In most cases, CIN is reversible, but it may be associated with considerable morbidity and mortality.[25] Primary risk factors include preexisting renal insufficiency, diabetes, volume depletion, and interaction with nephrotoxic drugs.

Screening for patients at risk and taking subsequent renoprotective measures to reduce the risk of CIN is mandatory in any patients referred for cardiac CT angiography. Different operational logistics between inpatient and outpatient clinics determines the practice of screening. In an outpatient setting, routine measurement of serum creatinine is unnecessary in patients younger than 70 years if a simple questionnaire designed to elicit a history of renal disorders and exclude risk factors for CIN is used.[26] In patients with prior kidney disease (including renal transplantation), patients with diabetes, patients with congestive heart failure, and patients older than 70 years, serum creatinine levels should be obtained. We request a serum creatinine level in all inpatients before CM administration. Because serum creatinine levels only partially reflect renal function, it has been suggested to calculate the patient's estimated glomerular filtration rate based on patient's body surface, age, sex, race, and serum creatinine. Convenient World Wide Web–based calculators are available (e.g., http://www.kidney.org/kls/professionals/gfr_calculator.cfm). Any estimated glomerular filtration rate equal to or less than 60 mL/min/1.73 m^2 indicates a patient at risk for CIN.

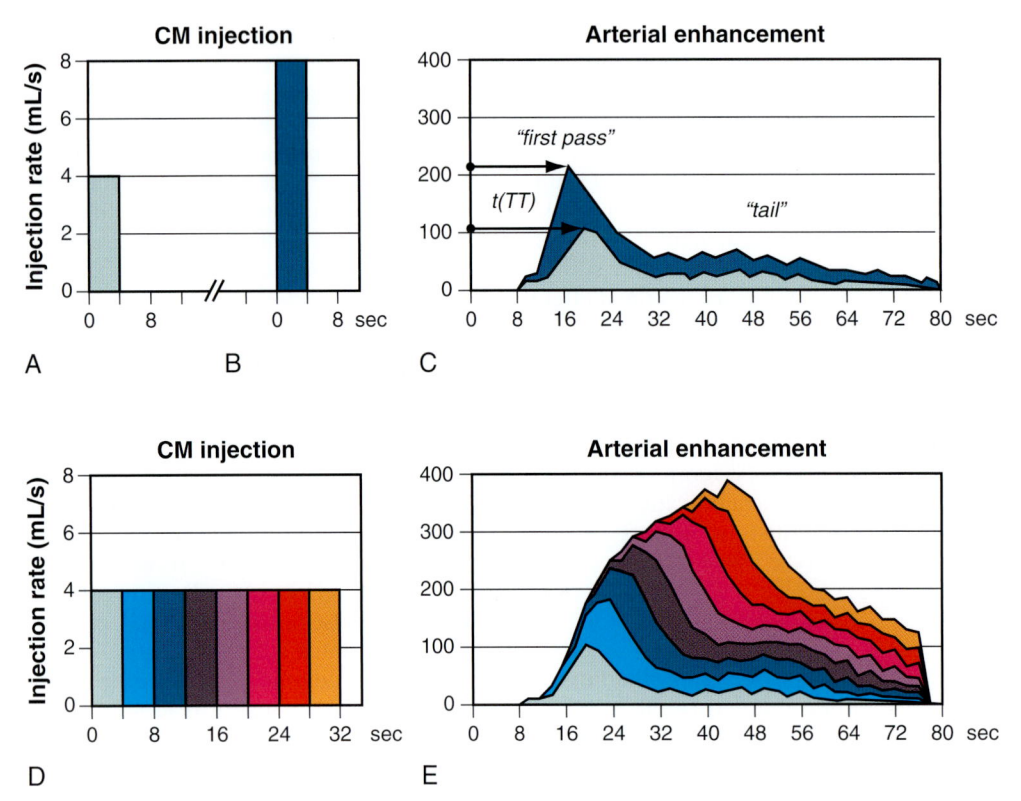

FIGURE 11-2 A-E, The relationship between contrast medium (CM) injection and arterial enhancement. CM injection of one 4-second long bolus (situation A, 16 mL at 4 mL/s) causes an arterial response (situation C), which results in a "first-pass" peak at the CM transit time (t[TT]) and lower "tail" of enhancement, owing to bolus broadening and recirculation. Doubling the injection flow rate (situation B, 32 mL at 8 mL/s) results in approximately twice the arterial enhancement (situation C). A normal bolus (situation D, cumulative bolus of 8 × 16 mL = 128 mL at 4 mL/s) can be regarded as the sum (time integral) of eight enhancement responses (situation E). The asymmetric shape of the single bolus and the recirculation effect results in continuously increasing enhancement over time. *(From Fleischmann D. High-concentration contrast media in MDCT angiography: principles and rationale. Eur Radiol 2003; 13[Suppl 3]:N39-N43.)*

Renoprotective measures in at-risk patients in whom CT angiography is desired include the use of the lowest possible dose of low-osmolar or iso-osmolar nonionic contrast agent, discontinuation of any nephrotoxic drugs (i.e., nonsteroidal anti-inflammatory drugs) 24 hours before the scan, and, importantly, volume expansion with intravenous fluid for several hours before and after the scan.[27] Intravenous hydration with sodium bicarbonate 1 hour before the scan seems to have a similar protective effect,[28] as does oral hydration. Other regimens with various drugs—although with initially very promising results—do not seem to offer consistent protection against CIN. Post–CT angiography serum creatinine levels should be obtained to monitor any change in renal function and with this, the development of CIN.

Interactions with other drugs also have to be expected with the administration of CM and have been addressed in several reports.[29] Nephrotoxic drugs, loop diuretics, interleukin-2, metformin, and hydralazine are some medication categories with known interaction. Most important in the context of cardiac CT angiography is the potential interaction with β blockers. Anaphylactic reactions and reduced effectiveness of epinephrine in a case of shock are more common in patients who received intravenous CM than in matched controls.[16] Effects of CM on coagulation, fibrinolytic drugs, and calcium channel blockers are usually not relevant for cardiac CT angiography.

TECHNIQUES

CM delivery embodies a pivotal part of cardiac multidetector CT. Although CT technology has substantially evolved, the physiology and pharmacokinetics of arterial enhancement remain unchanged. A thorough knowledge of early CM dynamics is a prerequisite to design reliable CM injection protocols for cardiac imaging.

Early Arterial Contrast Media Dynamics

Early arterial enhancement describes the relationship between intravenous CM injection and the corresponding arterial enhancement.[30] Figure 11-2 schematically shows the early arterial enhancement and its dependence on two user-selectable parameters, the administrated iodine flux (IF) and contrast injection duration (ID). Every CM injection results in a "first-pass" peak of enhancement at the CM transit time (TT) and in a lower "tail" of enhancement, owing to bolus broadening and recirculation. The TT is variable among individuals and is an important parameter for scan timing. The bolus broadening occurs within the cardiac and pulmonary circulation and is also due to a recirculation effect of opacified venous blood from highly perfused organs, such as kidney and brain.

Enhancement response is proportional to the administrated IF (milligrams of iodine injected per second [mg I/s]), referred to as the first "primary" injection parameter. IF (mg I/s) is a function of contrast injection flow rate (IR) (mL/s) and iodine concentration (IC) (mg I/mL) of the CM. Doubling the IF approximately doubles the degree of enhancement (HU), whereas the TT does not change substantially.[30]

ID (s) is the second "primary" injection parameter. CM volume (CV)—as we used it intuitively in the past—is just a secondary (dependent) injection parameter and is derived by simple multiplication of IR and ID. The effect of increasing the ID is not proportional to the degree of enhancement (HU) and is less intuitive. The degree of increased enhancement is mainly based on the recirculation phenomena. A schematic based on the assumption of a time-invariant linear system, as shown in Figure 11-2, may help to explain the effect of a prolonged injection (ID) on arterial enhancement (HU). Generally, the arterial enhancement (HU) continuously increases over time with longer ID. The shape of the enhancement curve is characterized by a steep enhancement increase at the TT time, followed by a more gradual increase of enhancement (shoulder) for approximately the ID and finally by a rapid decrease of enhancement. Consequently, shorter ID leads to lower enhancement (HU), and not, as widely believed, to an equal enhancement for a shorter time. Only longer ID increases the arterial enhancement (HU) if the IF is kept constant.[30]

The high variability of arterial enhancement among individuals for a given injection protocol makes it difficult to ensure robust enhancement across the entire patient population. Individual arterial enhancement is mainly based on cardiac output (CO) and central blood volume (CBV). Arterial enhancement varies inversely with CO and to some degree with CBV (CBV influences mainly tissue enhancement and recirculation).[31] Patients with high CO dilute the injected CM more, and have less arterial enhancement (HU), despite their shorter TT time, compared with patients with normal or lower CO.[32] Body weight allows an approximation of CO and CBV in the daily routine.[33] Adjusting the CM IR to the body weight allows reduction in the interindividual differences of arterial enhancement, and should be an integral part in any injection protocol.

Basic rules of early arterial CM dynamics can be summarized as follows:

1. Arterial enhancement (HU) is directly proportional to the IF (mg I/s). IF can be controlled by the IR (mL/s) and the IC of the CM (mg I/mL).
   - *Example*: 50% increase of IF (for a given ID) results in a 50% increase of arterial enhancement (HU) (at cost of 50% more CM volume)
   - *Example*: 23% increase of IC with the use of 370 (mg I/mL) instead 300 (mg I/mL) contrast agent (for a given IR and ID) results in a 23% stronger arterial enhancement (HU)
2. Arterial enhancement continuously increases over time with longer ID (s), owing to the cumulative effects of bolus broadening and recirculation. Increasing the ID also improves vascular opacification.
   - *Example*: see Figures 11-2 and 11-4
3. The strength of an individual's enhancement response to intravenously administered CM is controlled by CO and CBV, and correlates with body weight.

Contrast Media Injection

Cardiac imaging generally requires higher injection flow rates (5 mL/s) and higher concentration contrast agents (350 mg I/mL) than nonvascular CT examinations. Our practice includes CM injection at flow rate of 5 mL/s through a 20-gauge cannula (pink ISO color code) placed in a cubital or antebrachial vein. It is important to warm the contrast agent to decrease the viscosity and improve the achievable flow rate through the cannula. Generally, larger cannulas are required if flow rates greater than 6 mL are anticipated. We generally try to avoid CM injections through central venous catheters for cardiac imaging. Newer types of peripherally inserted central venous catheters are designed to endure pressure limits of 300 psi, which could allow injection at the rates required for cardiac CT angiography.

Mechanical power injectors deliver constant flow rates—required for cardiac CT—up to an injection pressure of approximately 300 psi. Monophasic, biphasic, and multiphasic injection protocols can be administered using commercially available double-barrel injectors. Parallel loading of contrast agent and saline syringes is possible, which allows either a saline "chaser" after the CM bolus or—with newer systems—admixing of the contrast agent with saline to achieve different contrast enhancements in different vascular regions.

Timing of Contrast Media Injection

There are basically two timing issues to be considered when designing a CT angiography injection protocol: ID and scan delay (shown in Fig. 11-3). The scan time itself ultimately depends on the requested anatomic coverage (i.e., only cardiac coverage for coronary artery CT angiography; cardiac and great vessel coverage for coronary artery bypass graft assessment), the scan mode (helical vs. nonhelical technique), and proprietary scanner specifications such as detector bank width or pitch. The scanner console provides the scan time after choosing the above-mentioned parameters. Normal scan times range from 5 to 20 seconds depending on the specific clinical question and type of CT system.

When the scan time is determined, the ID has to be determined to ensure a sufficient contrast filling of the vascular territory of interest (Fig. 11-4). Normally, this time for injection is longer than the effective scan time, which necessitates adding a scan delay to allow for longer CM injection before data acquisition is initiated. This scan delay refers to the time between the start of CM injection and the start of the CT data acquisition, and includes the trigger event to time the start of the data acquisition relative to the patient's individual CM arrival time (TT). TTs are determined by either a test bolus injection or an automatic bolus-triggering technique. The test bolus experiment provides the "time to peak" time by injection of a small test bolus (20 mL) before the final scan, whereas the automated bolus-triggering technique initiates the scan

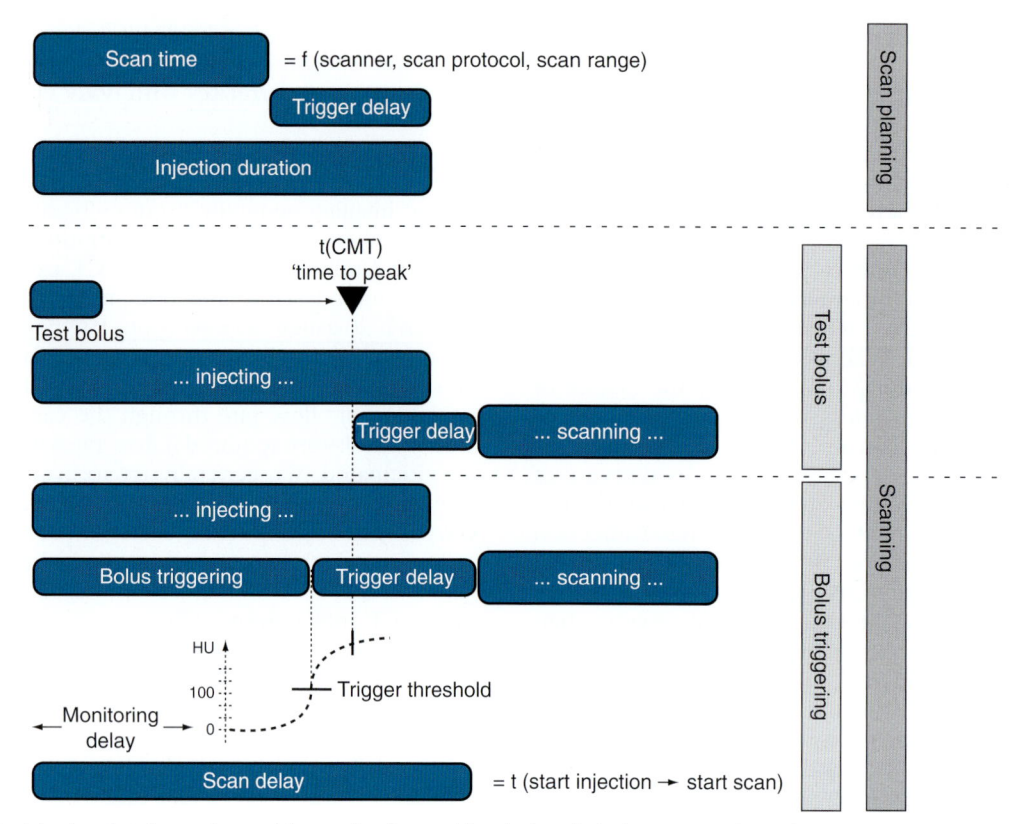

FIGURE 11-3 Injection duration and scan delay need to be considered when designing a CT angiography injection protocol.

automatically after reaching a specific threshold enhancement (e.g., 100 HU) in the target vessel (e.g., the ascending aorta) during the CM injection.

Inherent scanner-specific differences in bolus-triggering techniques exist, and some time elapses from reaching the threshold enhancement to the actual start of the data acquisition. The term *trigger delay* refers to this time period. Other terms such as *diagnostic delay* and *user delay* have been used by different venders for trigger delay. Various tasks, including table translation, collimator switching, and breath-holding commands and maneuvers, occur during the trigger delay. The minimal length of the trigger delay is scanner specific, but the ability to lengthen the delay interactively is an important way to ensure longer ID, and with this ensure stronger arterial enhancement.

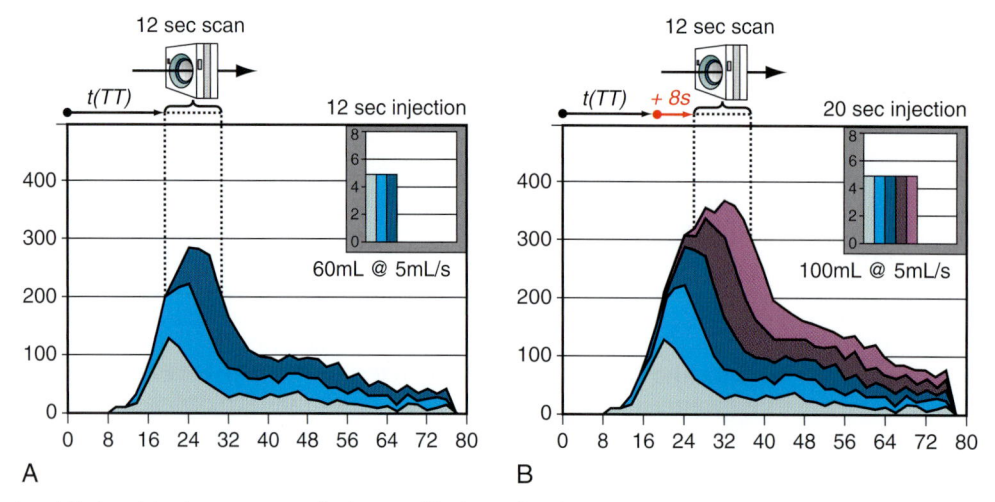

FIGURE 11-4 A and B, Arterial enhancement can be improved by increasing the injection duration by adding some time to the scanning delay. Instead of a 12-second injection (situation A) for a 12-second scan, the injection duration can be increased by adding an additional trigger delay (e.g., +8 seconds) to the scan delay, which results in an injection duration of 20 seconds (situation B). With increasing the scan delay by 8 seconds—the start of the scan is intentionally postponed by 8 seconds—relative to the contrast medium transit time (t[TT]), a stronger enhancement is achieved and the data acquisition is tailored to the peak of the enhancement curve.

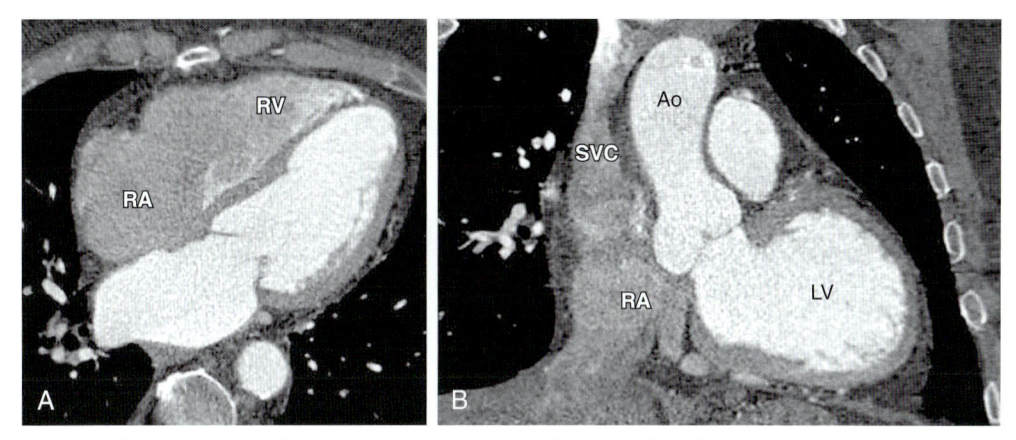

■ **FIGURE 11-5** A 53-year-old business executive status post–coronary artery bypass graft with equivocal stress echocardiography is referred for coronary artery bypass CT angiography (64 × 0.6 mm detector configuration, scan time 16 seconds, trigger delay 5 seconds, injection duration 21 seconds, injection flow rate 5.5 mL/s, contrast volume 116 mL, contrast agent 370 mg/mL, 40 mL saline flushing). **A** and **B**, Four-chamber view (**A**) and modified short-axis view (**B**) show strong enhancement of the left ventricle (LV) and aorta (Ao), whereas the contrast medium in the superior vena cava (SVC), right atrium (RA), and right ventricle (RV) got washed out by the 40-mL saline flush after the contrast medium injection. The lack of contrast medium in the right heart precludes any functional or morphologic assessment of these chambers.

Saline Flushing

Saline flushing allows use of the remaining CM in the upper extremity at the end of the CM injection bolus. Without use of a saline flush, ±15 mL of CM is normally trapped in the arm veins, outside the target imaging field. Probably more importantly, the use of a saline flush reduces the perivenous streak artifacts by "washing out" the superior vena cava and clearing the right atrium and ventricle to reduce the artifacts near the right coronary artery. Initially, complete clearance of the right heart chambers was suggested for coronary CT angiography, but complete lack of CM in the right heart may compromise morphologic and functional analysis of the right heart and potentially left heart (e.g., interventricular septum thickness inaccessible). Newer power injectors allow "splitting" the bolus and admixing contrast agent and saline at the end of the injection. This dilute contrast material (e.g. 30% contrast agent, 70% saline) at the end of the injection significantly reduces the above-mentioned artifacts, but still provides the assessment of the right heart chambers (Figs. 11-5 and 11-6).[34]

Clinical Contrast Media Injection Protocols

Although injection protocols have to take into account inherent scanner-specific properties, basic rules apply for any scanner type. Table 11-4 summarizes clinical injection protocols for coronary CT angiography, coronary artery bypass graft CT angiography, and left atrial and coronary vein mapping.

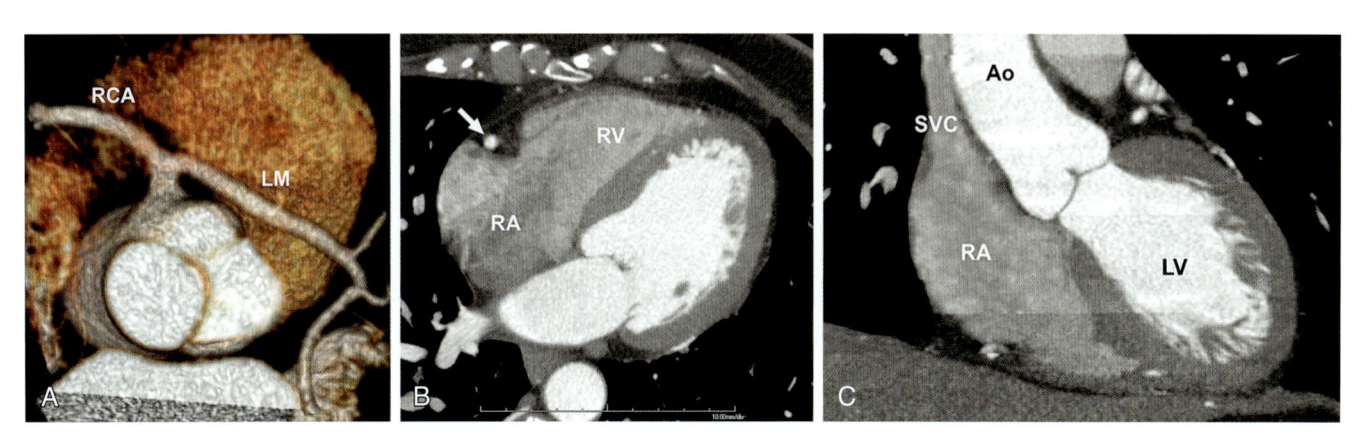

■ **FIGURE 11-6** A 59-year-old administrative associate with chest pain is referred for coronary artery CT angiography after abnormal catheter coronary angiography (64 × 0.6 mm detector configuration, scan time 12 seconds, trigger delay 8 seconds, injection duration 20 seconds, injection flow rate 4.5 mL/s, contrast volume 90 mL, contrast agent 370 mg/mL), flushing with 50 mL diluted contrast material (30% contrast agent/70% saline) followed by 30 mL saline. **A**, Volume rendering view with strong enhancement of the coronary arteries shows anomalous origin of left main (LM) coronary artery taking off the right coronary artery (RCA). **B** and **C**, Four-chamber view (**B**) and modified short-axis view (**C**) show strong enhancement of the left cardiac chambers (left ventricle [LV] and aorta [Ao]). Flushing with a split bolus of diluted contrast material at the end of the injection allows an improved morphologic and functional assessment of the right heart (right atrium [RA], right ventricle [RV]) compared with Figure 11-5. Note the lack of streak artifacts within the superior vena cava (SVC) and over the right atrioventricular groove carrying the RA (*arrow* in **B**).

Table 11-4 Clinical Contrast Media Injection Protocols

A. Injection Protocol for Coronary CTA (CCTA)

	Injection Duration (ID)	18s		20s		22s	
Scan Time (ST)	Trigger Delay (TD)	10s	8s	12s	8s	14s	8s
Flow Rate (mL/s) (IR)	Body Weight (kg)	Contrast Volume (mL)		Contrast Volume (mL)		Contrast Volume (mL)	
4.0	<55	72		80		88	
4.5	55-65	81		90		99	
5.0	65-85	90		100		110	
5.5	85-95	99		110		121	
6.0	>95	108		120		132	
Saline flushing: at flow rate as contrast phase		40		40		40	

Contrast concentration (CC) ≥370 mgI/mL
Contrast volume (CV) = (ST + TD)*IR
Automated bolus timing ROI: Ascending aorta; Threshold: 120 HU

B. Injection Protocol for Coronary Bypass Graft CTA

	Injection Duration (ID)	21s		23s		25s	
Scan Time (ST)	Trigger Delay (TD)	16s	5s	18s	5s	20s	5s
Flow Rate (mL/s) (IR)	Body Weight (kg)	Contrast Volume (mL)		Contrast Volume (mL)		Contrast Volume (mL)	
4.0	<55	84		92		100	
4.5	55-65	95		104		113	
5.0	65-85	105		115		125	
5.5	85-95	116		127		138	
6.0	>95	126		138		150	
Saline flushing: at flow rate as contrast phase		40		40		40	

Contrast concentration (CC) ≥370 mgI/mL
Contrast volume (CV) = (ST + TD)*IR
Automated bolus timing ROI: Ascending aorta; Threshold: 120 HU

C. Injection Protocol for Left Arterial Mapping

	Injection Duration (ID)	21s		23s		25s	
Scan Time (ST)	Trigger Delay (TD)	10s	5s	12s	5s	14s	5s
Flow Rate (mL/s) (IR)	Body Weight (kg)	Contrast Volume (mL)		Contrast Volume (mL)		Contrast Volume (mL)	
3.5	<55	53		60		67	
4.0	55-65	60		68		76	
4.5	65-85	68		77		86	
5.0	85-95	75		85		95	
5.5	>95	83		94		105	
Saline flushing: at flow rate as contrast phase		40		40		40	

Contrast concentration (CC) ≥350 mgI/ml
Contrast volume (CV) = (ST+TD)*IR
Automated bolus timing ROI: Left atrium; Threshold: 150 HU

D. Injection Protocol for Coronary Vein Mapping

Injection duration (ID)	45s	45s	45s
Scan time (ST)	10s	12s	14s
Scan delay (SD); no bolus trigger	50s	50s	50s
Flow rate [mL/s] (IR)	3	3	3
Contrast volume [mL]	3	3	3
Saline flushing: at flow rate as contrast phase	40	40	40

Table 11-4 Clinical Contrast Media Injection Protocols—cont'd

Injection Protocol for Coronary CTA (CCTA); Split Bolus 30%/70%

Scan Time Flow Rate [mL/s] (IR)	Trigger Delay Body Weight [kg]	18s			20s			22s		
Injection Duration (ID)		10s	8s		12s	8s		14s	8s	
			Split Bolus			Split Bolus			Split Bolus	
		Main Bolus	Flushing		Main Bolus	Flushing		Main Bolus	Flushing	
		100%:0%	30%:70%	0%:100%	100%:0%	30%:70%	0%:100%	100%:0%	30%:70%	0%:100%
4.0	<55	72	50	30	80	50	30	88	50	30
4.5	55-65	81	50	30	90	50	30	99	50	30
5.0	65-85	90	50	30	100	50	30	110	50	30
5.5	85-95	99	50	30	110	50	30	121	50	30
6.0	>95	108	50	30	120	50	30	132	50	30

KEY POINTS

- Contrast media administration embodies an integral part in every protocol designed for cardiac CT angiography.
- Only through a good working knowledge of early arterial contrast enhancement, and a broad understanding of the physiology and pharmacokinetic principles involved in contrast media delivery, can one chop and dice the right "ingredients" for a successful injection protocol.
- Contrast media administration has to be optimized for each patient to guarantee safety and to minimize interindividual differences among different patients.

SUGGESTED READINGS

Bae KT, Heiken JP, Brink JA. Aortic and hepatic contrast medium enhancement at CT. Part II: effect of reduced cardiac output in a porcine model. Radiology 1998; 207:657-662.

Fleischmann D. Use of high-concentration contrast media in multiple-detector-row CT: principles and rationale. Eur Radiol 2003; 13(Suppl 5):M14-M20.

Hallett RL, Fleischmann D. Tools of the trade for CTA: MDCT scanners and contrast medium injection protocols. Tech Vasc Interv Radiol 2006; 9:134-142.

Schoepf UJ, Zwerner PL, Savino G, et al. Coronary CT angiography. Radiology 2007; 244:48-63.

REFERENCES

1. Gallagher MJ, Ross MA, Raff GL, et al. The diagnostic accuracy of 64-slice computed tomography coronary angiography compared with stress nuclear imaging in emergency department low-risk chest pain patients. Ann Emerg Med 2007; 49:125-136.
2. Raff GL, Gallagher MJ, O'Neill WW, et al. Diagnostic accuracy of noninvasive coronary angiography using 64-slice spiral computed tomography. J Am Coll Cardiol 2005; 46:552-557.
3. Raff GL, Goldstein JA. Coronary angiography by computed tomography: coronary imaging evolves. J Am Coll Cardiol 2007; 49:1830-1833.
4. Fleischmann D, Hittmair K. Mathematical analysis of arterial enhancement and optimization of bolus geometry for CT angiography using the discrete fourier transform. J Comput Assisted Tomogr 1999; 23:474-484.
5. Giesler T, Baum U, Ropers D, et al. Noninvasive visualization of coronary arteries using contrast-enhanced multidetector CT: influence of heart rate on image quality and stenosis detection. AJR Am J Roentgenol 2002; 179:911-916.
6. Jakobs TF, Becker CR, Ohnesorge B, et al. Multislice helical CT of the heart with retrospective ECG gating: reduction of radiation exposure by ECG-controlled tube current modulation. Eur Radiol 2002; 12:1081-1086.
7. Parker JD, Parker JO. Nitrate therapy for stable angina pectoris. N Engl J Med 1998; 338:520-531.
8. Feldman RL, Marx JD, Pepine CJ, et al. Analysis of coronary responses to various doses of intracoronary nitroglycerin. Circulation 1982; 66:321-327.
9. Schoepf UJ, Zwerner PL, Savino G, et al. Coronary CT angiography. Radiology 2007; 244:48-63.
10. Decramer I, Vanhoenacker PK, Sarno G, et al. Effects of sublingual nitroglycerin on coronary lumen diameter and number of visualized septal branches on 64-MDCT angiography. AJR Am J Roentgenol 2008; 190:219-225.
11. Schnaar RL, Sparks HV. Response of large and small coronary arteries to nitroglycerin, $NaNO_2$, and adenosine. Am J Physiol 1972; 223:223-228.
12. Dawson P, Blomley MJ. Contrast media as extracellular fluid space markers: adaptation of the central volume theorem. Br J Radiol 1996; 69:717-722.
13. Knopp M, Kauczor HU, Knopp MA, et al. [Effects of viscosity, cannula size and temperature in mechanical contrast media administration in CT and magnetic resonance tomography]. Rofo 1995; 163:259-264.

14. Caro JJ, Trindade E, McGregor M. The risks of death and of severe nonfatal reactions with high- vs low-osmolality contrast media: a meta-analysis. AJR Am J Roentgenol 1991; 156:825-832.
15. Katayama H, Yamaguchi K, Kozuka T, et al. Adverse reactions to ionic and nonionic contrast media. A report from the Japanese Committee on the Safety of Contrast Media. Radiology 1990; 175:621-628.
16. Thomsen HS, Morcos SK. Contrast Media Safety Committee of European Society of Urogenital Radiology. Management of acute adverse reactions to contrast media. Eur Radiol 2004; 14:476-481.
17. Webb JA, Stacul F, Thomsen HS, et al. Members of the Contrast Media Safety Committee of the European Society of Urogenital Radiology. Late adverse reactions to intravascular iodinated contrast media. Eur Radiol 2003; 13:181-184.
18. van der Molen AJ, Thomsen HS, Morcos SK. Contrast Media Safety Committee, European Society of Urogenital Radiology (ESUR). Effect of iodinated contrast media on thyroid function in adults. Eur Radiol 2004; 14:902-907.
19. Bellin MF, Jakobsen JA, Tomassin I, et al. Contrast Media Safety Committee of the European Society of Urogenital Radiology. Contrast medium extravasation injury: guidelines for prevention and management. Eur Radiol 2002; 12:2807-2812.
20. Jacobs JE, Birnbaum BA, Langlotz CP. Contrast media reactions and extravasation: relationship to intravenous injection rates. Radiology 1998; 209:411-416.
21. Birnbaum BA, Nelson RC, Chezmar JL, et al. Extravasation detection accessory: clinical evaluation in 500 patients. Radiology 1999; 212:431-438.
22. Cochran ST, Bomyea K, Sayre JW. Trends in adverse events after IV administration of contrast media. AJR Am J Roentgenol 2001; 176:1385-1388.
23. Parfrey PS, Griffiths SM, Barrett BJ, et al. Contrast material-induced renal failure in patients with diabetes mellitus, renal insufficiency, or both: a prospective controlled study. N Engl J Med 1989; 320:143-149.
24. Morcos SK. Contrast media-induced nephrotoxicity—questions and answers. Br J Radiol 1998; 71:357-365.
25. Levy EM, Viscoli CM, Horwitz RI. The effect of acute renal failure on mortality: a cohort analysis. JAMA 1996; 275:1489-1494.
26. Choyke PL, Cady J, DePollar SL, et al. Determination of serum creatinine prior to iodinated contrast media: is it necessary in all patients? Tech Urol 1998; 4:65-69.
27. Morcos SK. Prevention of contrast media nephrotoxicity—the story so far. Clin Radiol 2004; 59:381-389.
28. Merten GJ, Burgess WP, Gray LV, et al. Prevention of contrast-induced nephropathy with sodium bicarbonate: a randomized controlled trial. JAMA 2004; 291:2328-2334.
29. Morcos SK, Thomsen HS, Exley CM. Contrast media: interactions with other drugs and clinical tests. Eur Radiol 2005; 15:1463-1468.
30. Fleischmann D. Use of high-concentration contrast media in multiple-detector-row CT: principles and rationale. Eur Radiol 2003; 13(Suppl 5):M14-M20.
31. Sheiman RG, Raptopoulos V, Caruso P, et al. Comparison of tailored and empiric scan delays for CT angiography of the abdomen. AJR Am J Roentgenol 1996; 167:725-729.
32. Bae KT, Heiken JP, Brink JA. Aortic and hepatic contrast medium enhancement at CT. Part II: effect of reduced cardiac output in a porcine model. Radiology 1998; 207:657-662.
33. Fleischmann D, Rubin GD, Bankier AA, et al. Improved uniformity of aortic enhancement with customized contrast medium injection protocols at CT angiography. Radiology 2000; 214:363-371.
34. Kerl JM, Ravenel JG, Nguyen SA, et al. Right heart: split-bolus injection of diluted contrast medium for visualization at coronary CT angiography. Radiology 2008; 247:356-364.

CHAPTER 12

Image Postprocessing in Cardiac Computed Tomography

Elliot K. Fishman and Pamela T. Johnson

The role of CT in the evaluation of cardiac disease is no longer the subject of possible applications, but more in the realm of determining positive and negative predictive values as cardiac CT angiography becomes a central part of cardiac imaging. Whether the application is to determine coronary artery stenosis in native vessels, to determine patency of bypass grafts or stents, or to detect anomalous anatomy, CT has been shown in many cases to be the study of choice. In the emergency department, the power of a 100% negative predictive value promises to lead to a paradigm shift in emergency department triage for patients with chest pain.[1,2] Similarly, a gated CT acquisition has become the standard of care to evaluate aortic root pathology, including valvular disease, suspected dissection, Marfan syndrome, and Loeys-Dietz syndrome.[3-5] Other applications, such as preoperative assessment and postoperative evaluation in congenital heart disease, are becoming a well-accepted application for CT angiography.[6,7]

Despite more than 400 articles on the subject and a body of literature that continues to grow, few published data have focused on the technical aspects of different processing techniques for the evaluation of the heart and coronary arteries.[8-13] The "how-to" of data acquisition (16 vs. 64 vs. 128 detector scanners)[14-16] is addressed in detail in the literature, as are contrast delivery techniques (test bolus vs. bolus triggering vs. timed injection),[17-19] but the analysis of the resultant CT data has been the topic of only a few articles of note. This chapter provides a systematic approach to data analysis, with emphasis on how to use each postprocessing tool to its greatest advantage (Figs. 12-1 through 12-4), to interpret most accurately an isotropic multidetector CT volume of the heart.

TECHNICAL REQUIREMENTS

With respect to data analysis, the most comprehensive article has been by Ferencik and colleagues.[11] Two important statements from this article are as follows:

- "The evaluation of multidetector CT coronary angiography with interactive image display methods, especially interactive oblique MPRs [multiplanar reformats], permit higher diagnostic accuracy than evaluation of prerendered images (curved MPR, curved MIP [maximum intensity projection], or VRT [volume-rendering technique] images)."
- "Interactive evaluation of multidetector CT coronary angiography data sets on a workstation should thus be the preferred way of interpretation."

The key point made by this article was that the method of data set evaluation (interactive interrogation of the volume by the interpreting physician vs. review of preset images generated by an individual not performing the interpretation) is perhaps even more important than the postprocessing tools used. Interacting with the data set using only axial images and MPRs was more efficacious than review of preset three-dimensional images. When preset images are reviewed, the information seen depends on the skill of the individual (interpreting physician or technologist) who performed the postprocessing. We have found that in nearly every case, errors in postprocessing can result in key mistakes in data interpretation. Interactivity means that the interpreting physician must process the images himself or herself. The following rules are suggested to do this successfully:

1. Interpreting physicians should learn how to use a workstation for cardiac-specific applications.
2. The ideal workstation should have dedicated tools for cardiac evaluation, including but not limited to automated vessel segmentation (with minimal user time), stenosis calculation software, vessel tracking software, four-dimensional motion studies, excellent and easy-to-use filming, archiving, and networking solutions.

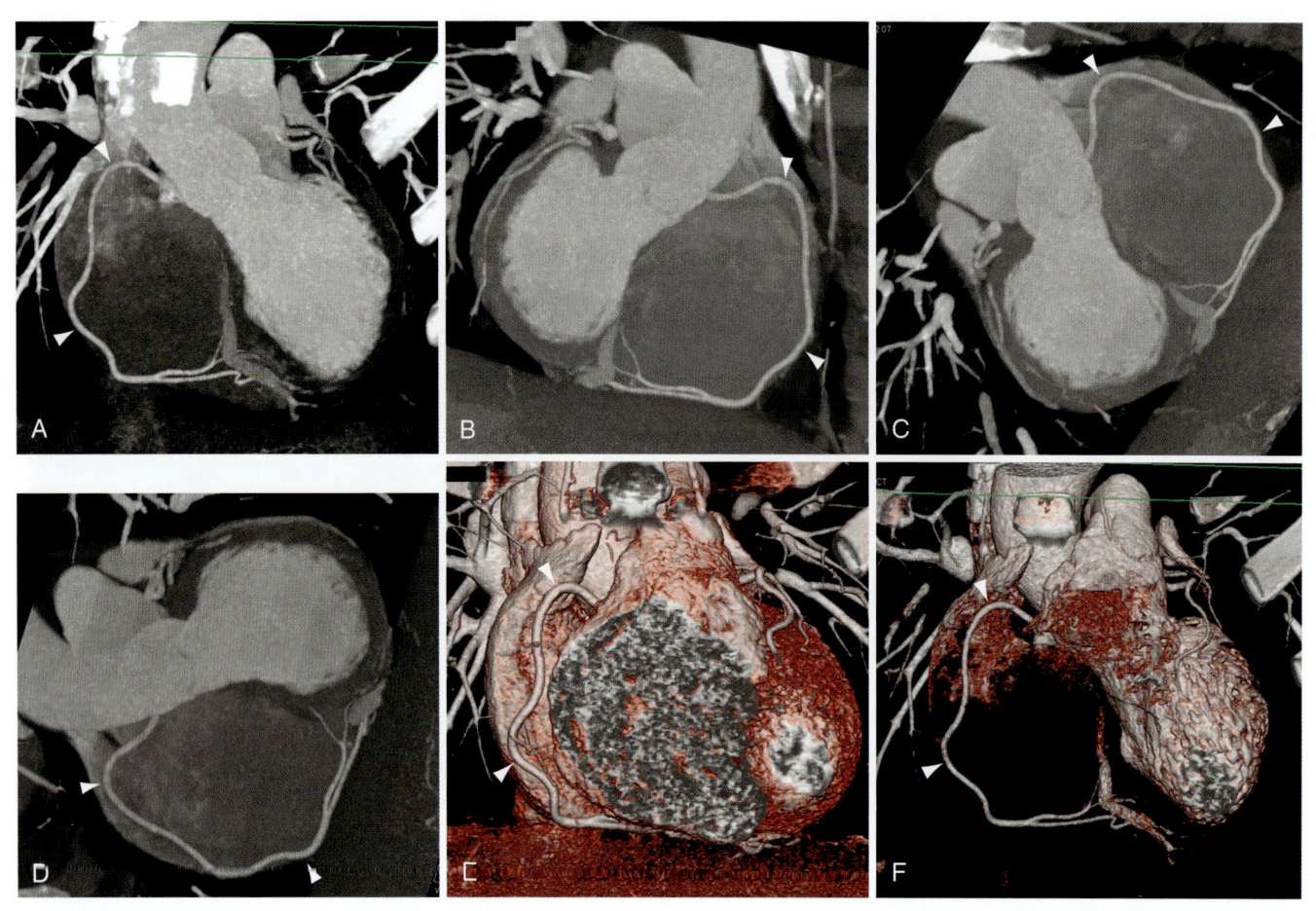

FIGURE 12-1 A-F, This set of images shows the relative utilities of each rendering technique. A-D, The proper study protocol has yielded a clear view of the right coronary artery (*arrowheads*) with MIP imaging, but with MIP it is hard to be certain that one is actually imaging the origin of the right coronary artery. E and F, With VRT, this is not an issue, and the color-coded VRT images provide a better three-dimensional perspective. The VRT images are the same projection, but use different rendering parameters.

3. Interpreting physicians should be involved in the full scope of the imaging process, ranging from protocol design to quality assurance.
4. Interpreting physicians must be familiar with the various rendering techniques, including MPR, MIP, and VRT, and must know how to use these techniques, their advantages, and their disadvantages.
5. Another area of practical concern is the quality of the data set to be analyzed. The ability to acquire routinely a high-quality data set is mandatory to doing a quality interpretation. Although scan protocols are beyond the scope of this chapter, they cannot be overemphasized. The proper gating technique (retrospective or perspective), control of the patient's heart rate, and timing of delivery of contrast material (contrast agent and saline flush) and data acquisition must be optimized.

Let us assume that the patient has been scanned, the data have been processed into the appropriate slice thickness (0.6 to 0.75 mm) and interscan spacing (0.4 to 0.5 mm), and the data have been sent to the workstation. Now what? That question is guided in part by individual preference and by workflow, and partly dictated by the workstation available to the user. Regardless of the workstation specifics, some general principles can be implemented across almost all current platforms.

TECHNIQUE

Axial Images

Although a cardiac CT scan typically is reviewed at least using multiplanar reconstruction and three-dimensional renderings, the axial images (see Fig. 12-3) remain a crucial part of the study workflow. At some sites with highly experienced interpreting physicians, interpretation is typically limited to the axial images with sparing use of additional views in selected cases. On a workstation with a composite display of axial, coronal, and sagittal images combined with a three-dimensional image, our strategy for axial images is to scroll interactively through the data set in what the scanner selects as the optimal phase (0% to 90% of R–R interval on retrospective gated study) for coronary artery visualization. We then do the following:

1. Scroll through the data set to define the quality of the study, including contrast delivery timing, lack of motion

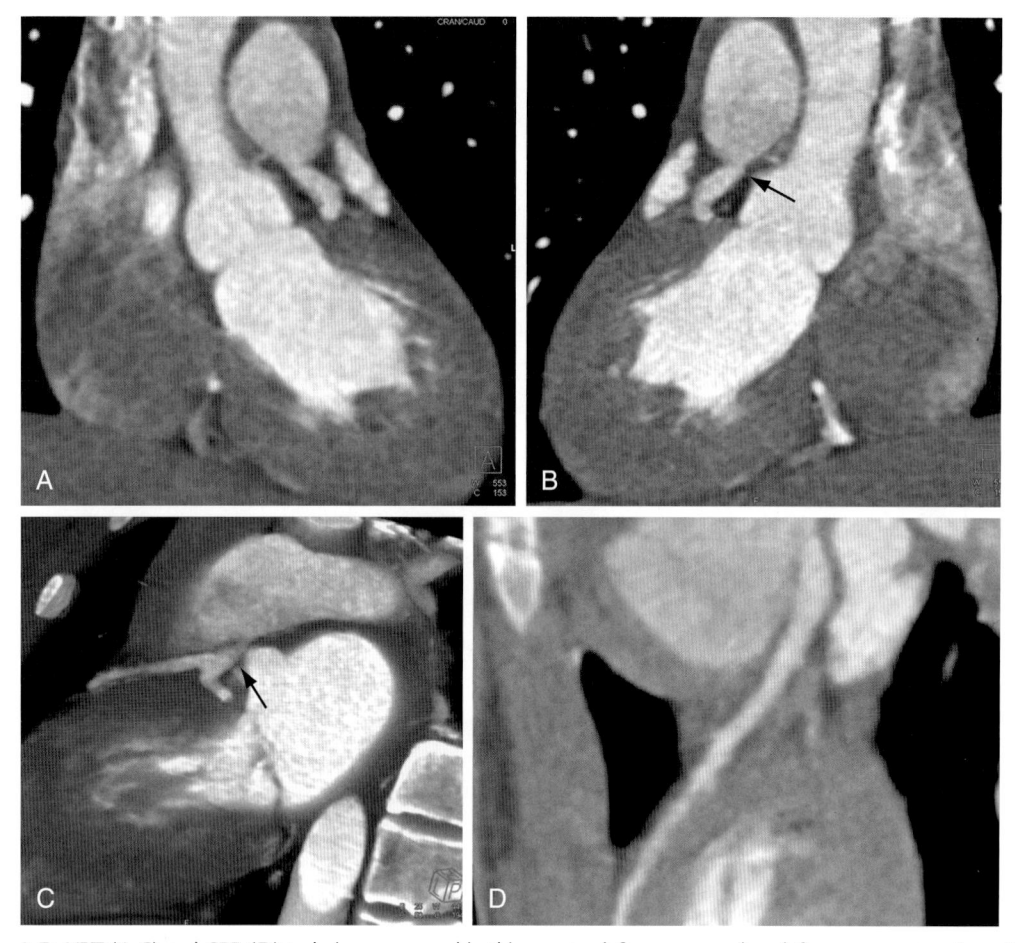

FIGURE 12-2 A-D, VRT (A-C) and CPR (D) techniques are used in this case to define an anomalous left coronary artery (*arrow*) arising off the posterior aspect of the main pulmonary artery. The unusual location was impossible to define on routine axial scans or with routine MPR imaging.

artifact, and coronary artery opacification. Based on a quick look, one can quickly ascertain how good the study is technically. We also ensure that the "optimal" phase was selected because occasionally multiple phases need to be processed and viewed.
2. Scroll through the heart in a global sense with analysis of chamber size, and a look for any abnormalities including the pericardium and the paracardiac regions. We also note the size of the ascending and descending aorta.
3. Scroll through the coronary arteries, and look for the origin of each vessel and its branching pattern. Vessels such as the sinoatrial nodal branch and atrioventricular nodal branch are often best seen on the axial images. We follow each coronary artery to look at lumen diameter and determine the presence or absence of calcified or noncalcified plaque. Axial images often nicely define noncalcified plaque especially when lipid-rich. Axial images also define the presence and extent of calcification, although a wide window often is needed in the presence of extensive calcification.

The limitation of axial images is that one may need to look at 200 to 350 individual slices to get through a single vessel, such as the left anterior descending coronary artery. Vessels with off-axis courses, such as the right coronary artery, are best defined when one is looking beyond the axial plane. A more global presentation of an entire coronary artery is impossible without a curved planar reconstruction (CPR) (see Fig. 12-4) or three-dimensional display.

Our experience is that referring physicians desire three-dimensional maps to correlate with what they typically see on classic catheter angiography. Axial CT images in this regard are not helpful and do not provide similar information.

Although we typically scroll through the classic axial display interactively, other physicians believe that reading studies can be noninteractive, and that there are no data to prove otherwise. This controversy needs to be addressed in a future study. One issue is the lack of a well-designed, controlled study on the use of different techniques for coronary CT angiography analysis. This is in contrast to many articles published on reading techniques (e.g., two-dimensional vs. three-dimensional) for virtual colonoscopy.

Although most physicians review the axial images as slabs in the plane acquired, one helpful hint is to draw a line through the plane of the aortic valve, and scroll up and down through this plane. This practice often provides a perfect en face display of the proximal coronary arteries.

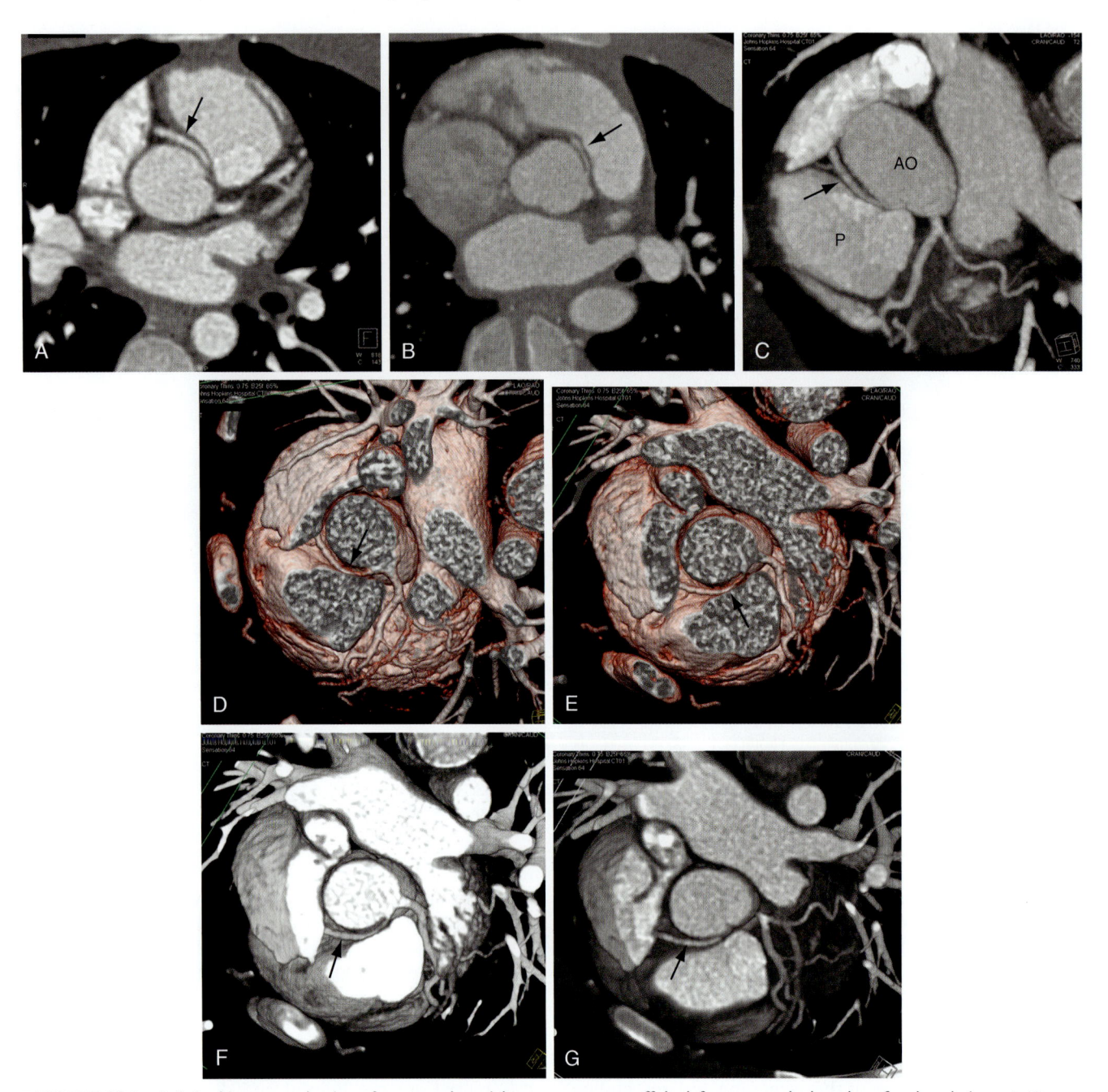

■ **FIGURE 12-3** A-G, In this case, evaluation of an anomalous right coronary artery off the left cusp reveals the value of each technique. **A**, On a single axial image, one can define the vessel (*arrow*), but would need a series of individual images to delineate its course. **B**, With MPR images rendered in the optimal perspective, the origin of the right coronary artery is seen. **C**, MIP images show the vessel coursing between the aortic root (AO) and pulmonary outflow tract (P), but the full course of the vessel is hard to see without use of very thin slabs. **D-G**, VRT is ideal for complex vascular anatomy, and color (**D** and **E**) or gray-scale mapping (**F** and **G**) can be used.

Multiplanar Reconstruction— Coronal and Sagittal Images

The use of coronal and sagittal reconstructions is common in a range of CT applications, and in cardiac CT its role is also defined. With isotropic data, the individual cardiac chambers, aorta, and pulmonary vasculature can benefit from these displays, and they are routinely used. Whether it is for suspected aortic dissection or suspected pulmonary embolism, these displays are essential. On most workstations, the thickness of the reconstruction can be interactively adjusted (Fig. 12-5), but when slabs are reduced to beyond a few millimeters, the images become fuzzy and are of no value. This is in contrast to MIP images, where often less data may prove to be useful for these large-volume applications. One issue with coronal and sagittal reconstruction and evaluation of the coronary arteries is that because the vessels have a nonlinear pathway, only short segments can be analyzed at a time. When the left anterior descending coronary artery is ana-

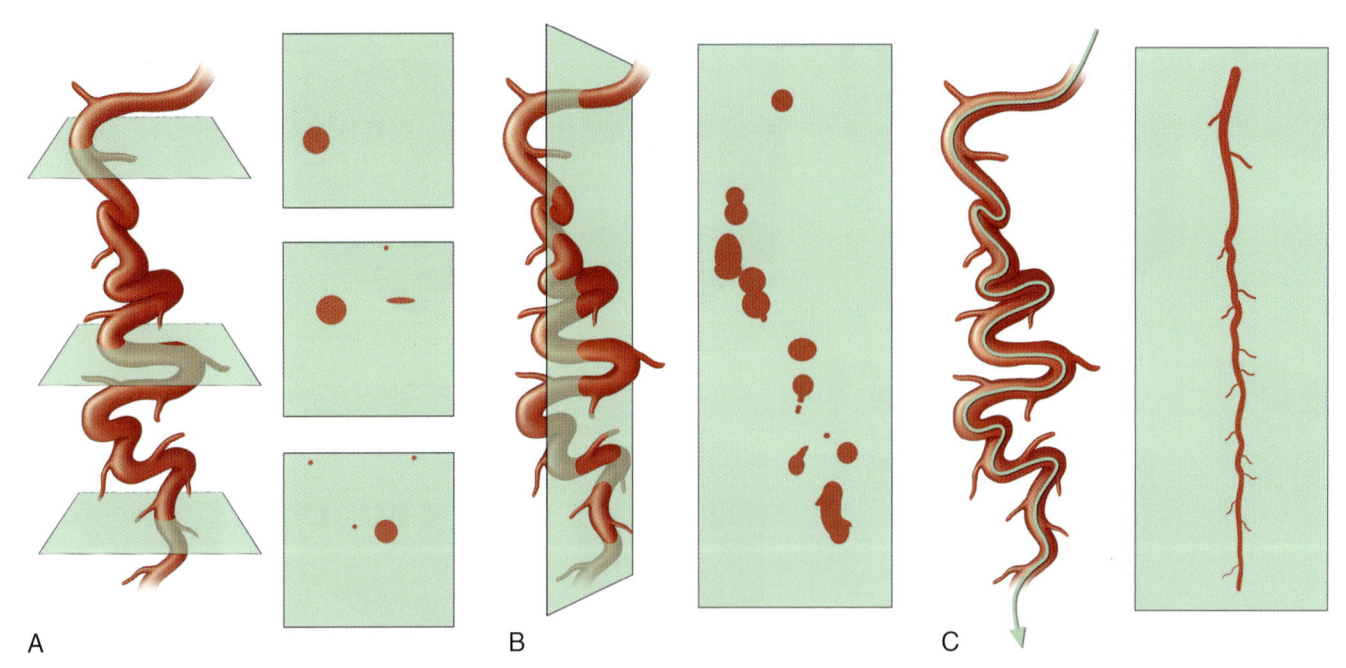

FIGURE 12-4 Schematic representation of the value of CPR in imaging complex vascular anatomy. **A,** Axial sections show only segments of the artery in cross section. **B,** Multiplanar reconstruction in the orthogonal plane displays only various oblique cross sections of the artery. **C,** CPR generated by center-line tracking captures and displays the entire artery.

lyzed with a coronal or axial display, one must constantly change the angle of the reconstruction plane to follow the vessel. Changing the angle can be done interactively, but potentially results in more room for error and less than ideal image displays. For analyzing selected segments of a vessel, this technique might be perfect. If there is a suspect area on the axial views, the coronal or sagittal view may help clarify and quantify this potential narrowing. Key points include the following:

1. Coronal and sagittal imaging may be useful, but it depends on the vessel tracking capabilities of the workstation. Ideally, a specific point is selected, and viewing is adjusted from that perspective.
2. Interactivity is key.
3. The oblique planes are valuable for additional viewing of selected suspicious areas, which often arise after review of the axial images.
4. With coronal, sagittal, and oblique images, one needs to be cautious in grading stenosis and not be fooled by partial averaging. We do not attempt to grade stenosis based only on these images because of this pitfall.
5. We have found that these reconstructions are best for larger vessels, as discussed previously.
6. Many sites now do preprocessed batched coronal and sagittal images at 1- to 3-mm intervals. This may mean a data set of 30 to 120 images that can be scrolled through on a picture archiving and communication system (PACS). Although this technique may be sufficient for routine abdominal or chest CT interpretation, interpreting physicians must recognize the limited utility of this technique for evaluation of the coronary arteries because of the vessel size (typically 3 to 5 mm) and ectatic course of the coronary vessels.

Curved Planar Reconstruction

As discussed, the limitations with coronal and sagittal reconstruction largely involve the inability to track the complex courses of the coronary arteries. CPR addresses the issue directly (Fig. 12-6). CPR is best thought of as a reconstruction plane that perfectly tracks a vessel regardless of the complexity of its course or direction. In the initial versions of CPR, the user would drop multiple points through the path of a vessel, and the computer algorithm would track the points and create a vessel map. Currently, most vendors have designed software that makes the process more robust and easier to use, and requires minimal user interaction.[10,12] On some workstations, there is a program that can be used for tracking the coronary vessels. One simply picks a start and an end point, and the computer automatically tracks the vessel. The vessel is laid out like a string or piece of spaghetti, and the user can rotate the plane to look at the vessel and analyze it from multiple perspectives. The vessel path is calculated as a central line through the vessel, which is also crucial in avoiding errors in analysis. The curved planar images can be viewed in classic soft tissue window or altered to be presented in MIP mode. In cases where there is a gap or stenosis in the vessel, dropping additional seed points can be done to help with vessel tracking.

We use CPR for every coronary artery CT angiography (Figs. 12-7 and 12-8). The ability to lay out a vessel without the worry of partial averaging is important not only when trying to define the presence of stenosis, but also for calculating the degree of stenosis. On some systems, the CPR also serves as the basis for the system to calculate automatically the percent stenosis present. A function that is common on all cardiac-specific software packages and

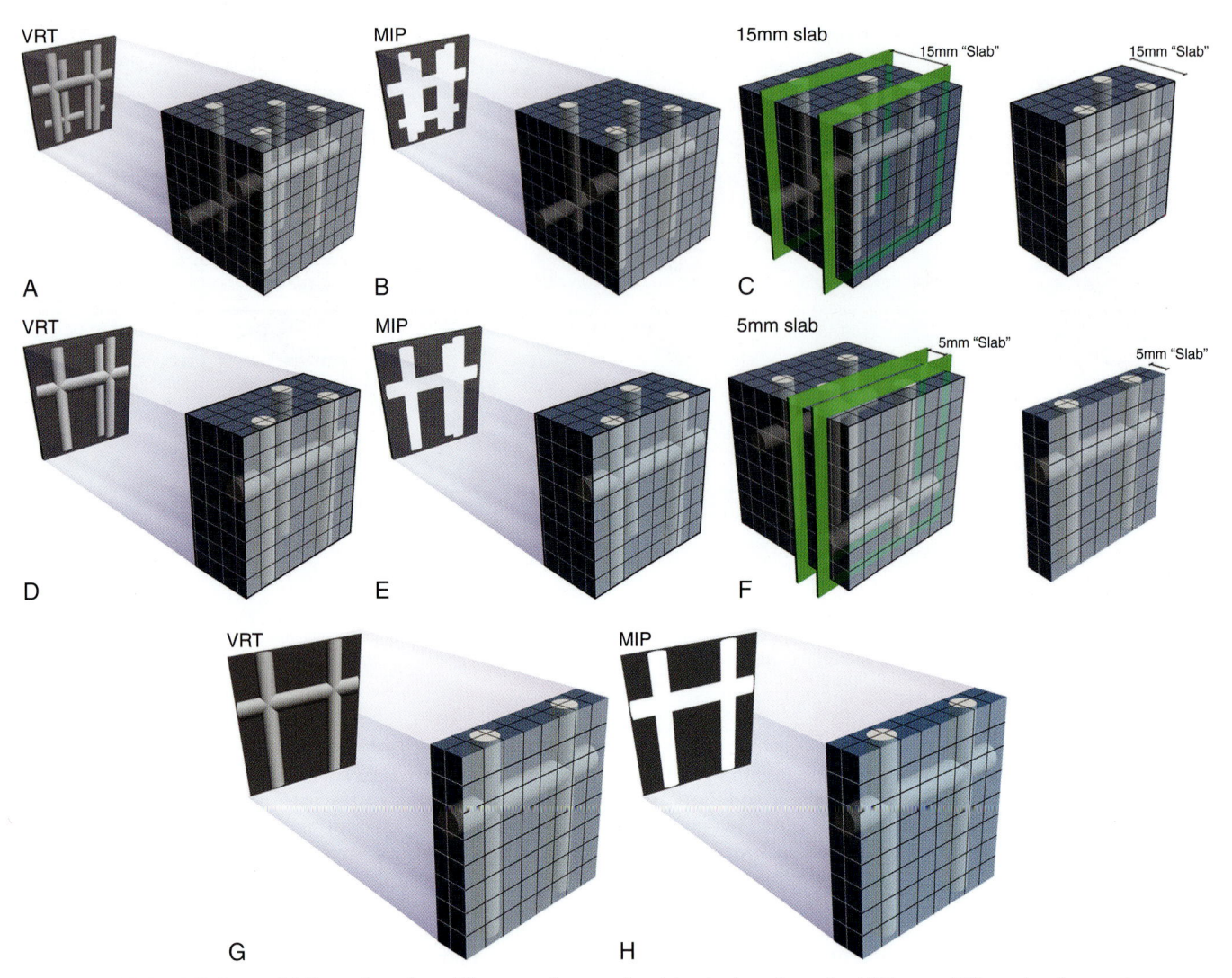

FIGURE 12-5 **A-H,** Sequential illustrations show different requirements for slab selection when using VRT versus MIP, to visualize vessels distinctly within a volume. **A,** When the entire volume is volume rendered, vessels are clearly defined and separated because the three-dimensional relationships are maintained. **B,** With MIP, the vessels are displayed without separation or true spatial orientation. **C-E,** Reduction of the large volume to a 15-mm slab **(C)** removes one vessel and results in continued good spatial discrimination with VRT **(D).** With MIP **(E)** the vessels remain unseparated without spatial orientation. **F-H,** Further narrowing of the slab to 5 mm **(F)** enables VRT **(G)** and MIP **(H)** to show the vessels discretely; MIP remains a flat projection that does not convey three-dimensional relationships. *(From Fishman EK, Ney DR, Heath DG, et al. Volume rendering versus maximum intensity projection in CT angiography: what works best, when, and why. RadioGraphics 2006; 26:905-922.)*

many vessel analysis packages has the user pick the area of concern (usually area with greatest stenosis) and select a point of normal vessel proximal and distal to the stenosis. When selected, the system automatically calculates the percent stenosis. It is important to be careful with these programs because there are many potential sources of error, but at least they are a guide, and in the future they should be more robust. Several key points regarding CPR and some highlights and pitfalls are as follows:

1. The success of CPR depends on the delivery of a well-timed contrast medium bolus with homogeneous enhancement of the vessel. Values of 250 HU and greater are ideal. With poor opacification, automated vessel extraction programs have issues and result in errors of omission and commission.
2. The success of CPR depends on a good center-line definition. In larger vessels such as the aorta, this is fairly simple. In the coronary arteries measuring 2 to 5 mm, if the center-line trace is inaccurate, it could result in the overestimation of stenosis. A center-line error is most likely to occur in the presence of extensive coronary artery calcification.
3. Although dense calcification can potentially throw off the center-line measurement, CPR is especially valuable in defining the degree of stenosis in these cases. With dense calcification, rotation of the vessel 360 degrees helps with determining whether the calcification is mainly eccentric and representing positive remodeling or causing a critical stenosis.
4. Some newer software versions allow the computer to segment the vessels automatically without user interaction. This may work well in selected cases, but careful attention to recognize incorrect tracking is crucial. When a CPR is viewed in MIP mode, it is advisable to make the vessel thicker when looking at the vessel for

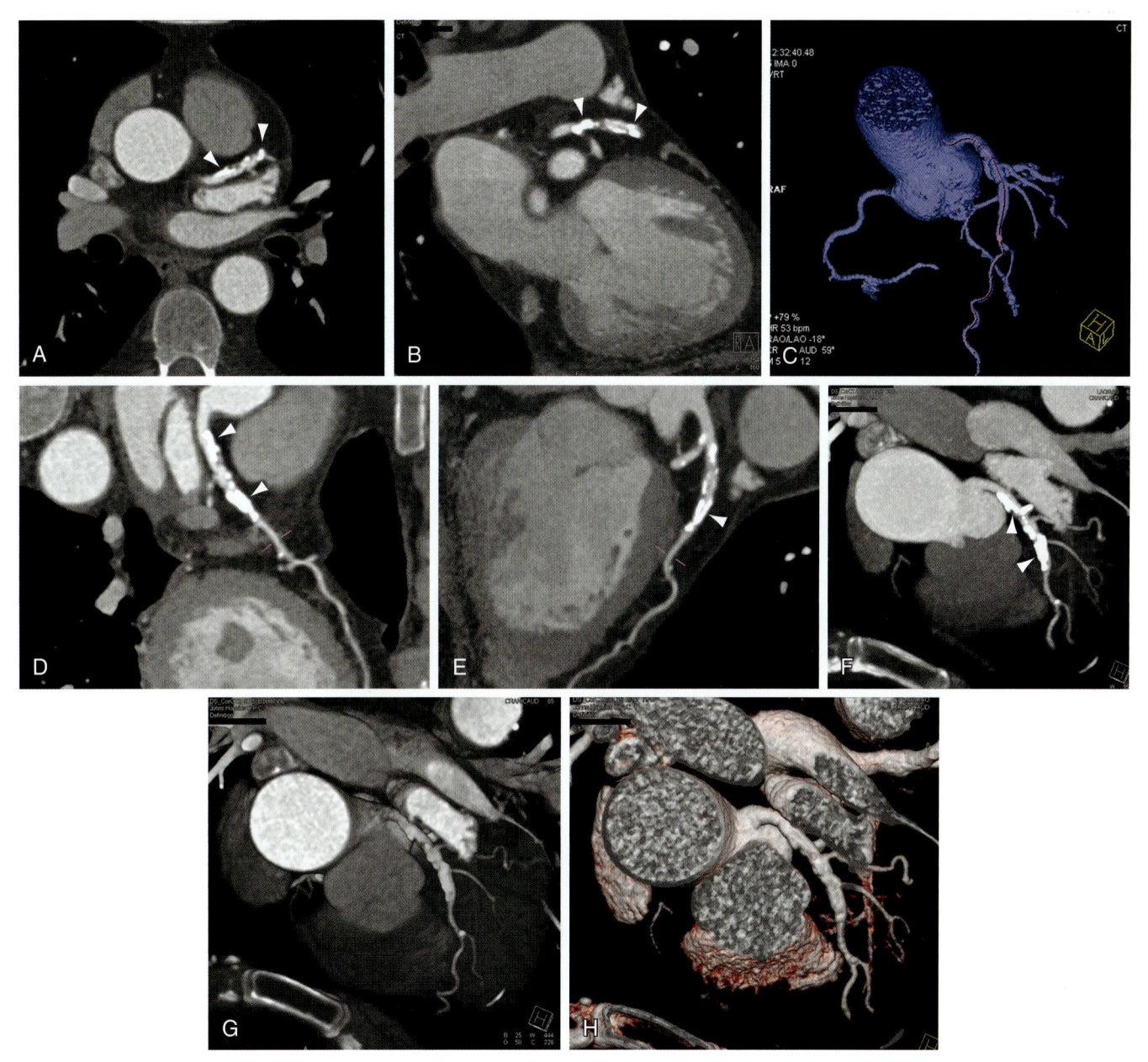

CHAPTER 12 ● *Image Postprocessing in Cardiac Computed Tomography* 173

■ **FIGURE 12-6** **A-H,** Extensive calcification (*arrowheads*), as shown in this case, makes it difficult to determine the degree of stenosis. After analysis using multiple postprocessing tools, we are able to define correctly a greater than 70% stenosis in the left anterior descending artery, which was stented. In these cases, we often find a combination of axial (**A**), MPR (**B**), and CPR (**C-E**) images the most helpful. MIP (**F**) and VRT (**G** and **H**) added little to the final diagnosis, but did give a nice representation of the extent of calcification.

potential stenotic areas. If reviewed in standard soft tissue mode, this would not be helpful.
5. CPR often does not work if the patient has an arrhythmia that may result in step-off artifacts in the data set. Similar problems can occur with breathing-related artifacts.

Maximum Intensity Projection

The role of three-dimensional imaging, using MIP or VRT, still is controversial today. Although most sites use some type of three-dimensional imaging for selected cardiac applications, experts have yet to reach consensus as to whether this practice is mandatory or necessary in all cases. Our experience is just the opposite, however. Postprocessing with three-dimensional imaging is an essential part of every examination, providing crucial information not revealed by other interpretative methods. One caveat is that MIP is most valuable and accurate in a patient without coronary artery calcification. In the presence of small amounts of calcification, MIP images can easily overestimate the presence and extent of stenosis.

In practice, MIP is usually performed with a sliding slab to look at the coronary arteries. The term *sliding MIP* is used to emphasize that it is done interactively at the workstation by the interpreting physician to define the best plane for vessel display. There are numerous tricks of the trade and pitfalls with MIP in general.[20,22] By adjusting the

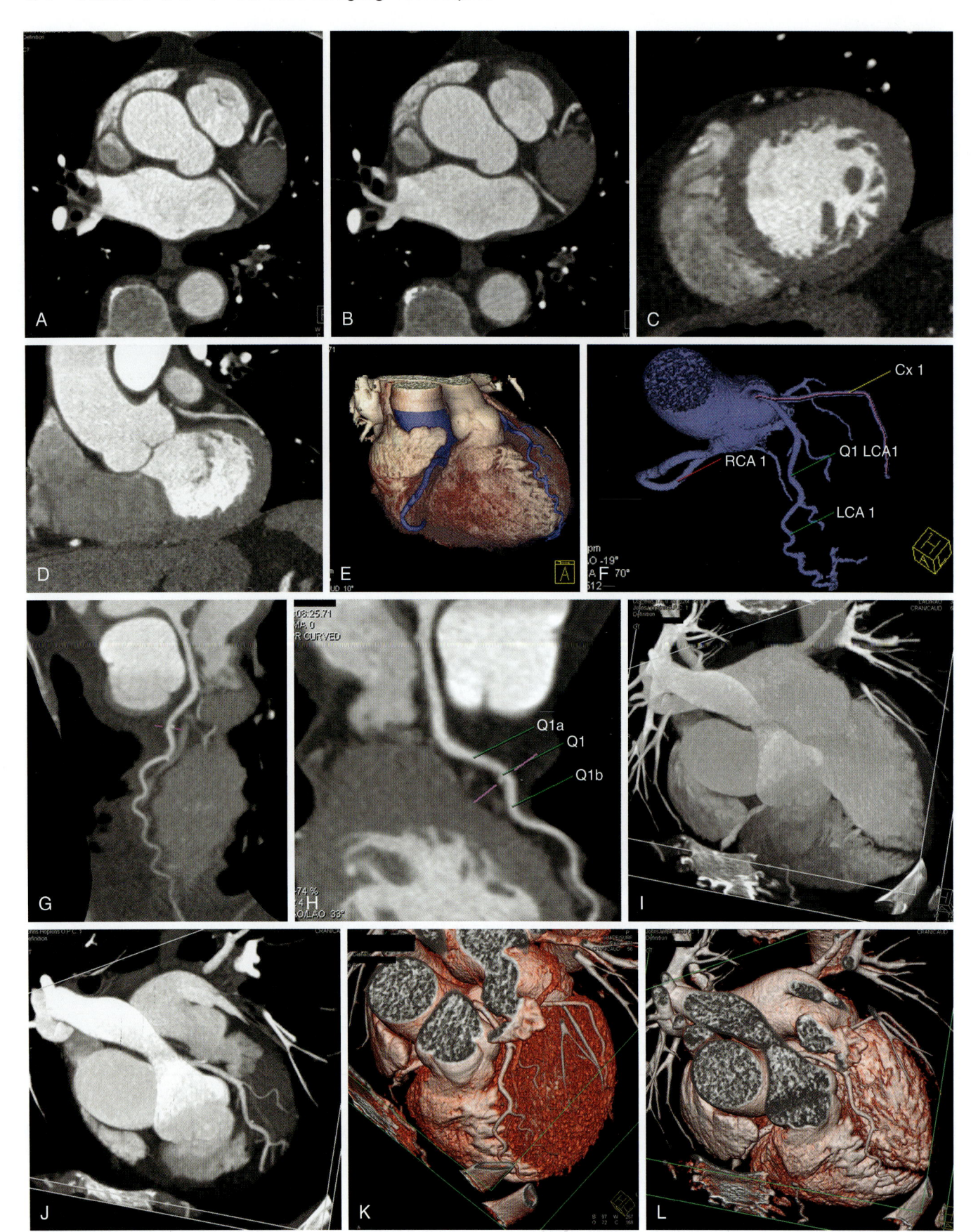

■ **FIGURE 12-7** A-L, Small calcified and noncalcified plaque (*purple line* in **G** and **H**), which do not cause any significant narrowing of the left anterior descending artery, are identified in this case. To supplement the axial images (**A** and **B**), MPRs (**C** and **D**) and CPRs (**E-H**) are ideal for image analysis. The small plaque in the left anterior descending artery is seen on the MIP images (**I** and **J**), but is hard to define prospectively on the VRT images (**K** and **L**). This case also reveals the importance of thin slabs for vessel detection on the MIP images.

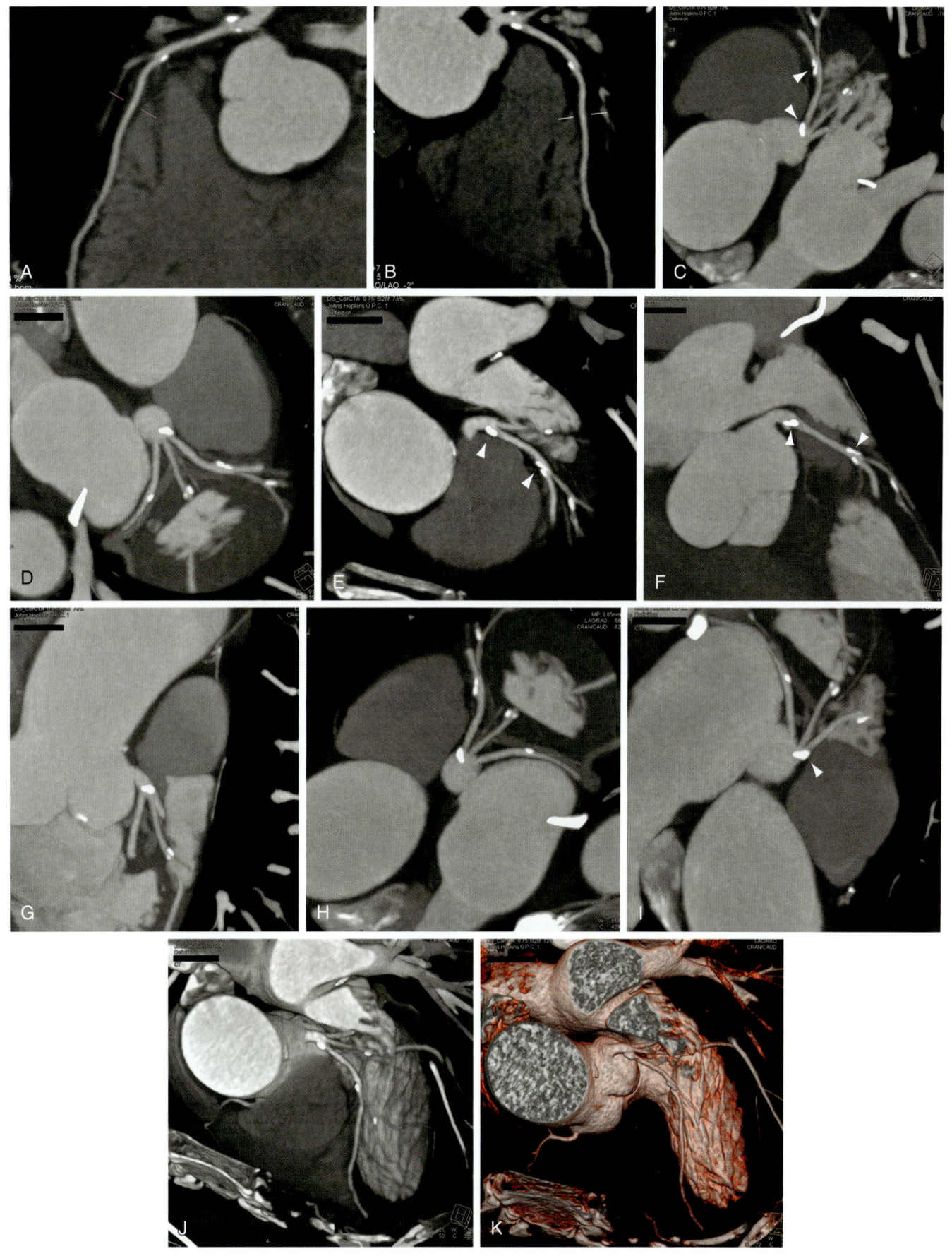

■ **FIGURE 12-8** A-K, A patient with a high calcium score (Agatston >500) but without a critical stenosis. **A** and **B**, CPR images are best for defining the vessel lumen and the positive plaque remodeling. **C-I**, A series of MIP images with varying slab thickness of 1 to 20 mm and varying orientations show how difficult it is to use MIP images in the face of calcification (*arrowheads*). Depending on the view and parameters, the left anterior descending artery, circumflex artery, and ramus intermedius can look occluded or patent. **J** and **K**, VRT images help show the eccentric nature of the plaque burden.

MIP slab thickness (1 to 30 mm), one can interactively vary the size of the segmented volume as needed (see Fig. 12-5), but one always needs to be careful not to edit out crucial parts of the data set. The potential issues with MIP can be seen through a careful understanding of the technique itself. Some key points from a technical perspective are as follows:

1. The displayed pixel intensity represents only the material with the highest intensity (i.e., density in the case of CT) along the projected ray. A high-intensity material, such as calcification, would obscure information from an intravascular contrast agent. This limitation can be partially overcome with use of nonlinear transfer functions or, more practically, through volume editing. Volume editing can take the form of a preprocessing step (e.g., section-by-section or "slab" editing) or an interactive process (e.g., "sliding-slab" MIP).
2. Use of the highest intensity of the image in effect also selects the "noisiest" background voxels, and decreases the visibility of vessels in brightly enhancing structures, such as the cardiac chambers and pulmonary arteries.
3. MIP images cannot be displayed with surface shading or other depth cues, which can make assessment of three-dimensional relationships difficult. MIP images can be misleading, and incorrect interpretation can be a result of viewing only the MIP images. Also, volume averaging (the effect of finite volume resolution) coupled with the MIP algorithm commonly leads to MIP artifacts. A normal small vessel passing obliquely through a volume may have a "string of beads" appearance because it is only partially represented by voxels along its length. The severity of these artifacts depends on the resampling filters used.
4. MIP is probably the easiest technique to master because of its simplicity (it uses window width and level), but in practice has a reasonable robustness for many applications. In our experience, MIP is very useful as an adjunct to VRT, and we routinely use MIP viewing in practice. Because of its limitations, however, we would never use MIP alone without evaluation of axial, MPR, CPR, and VRT images.

In a patient without calcification, MIP can create agreeable images of long segments of the coronary arteries that superficially appear as a comprehensive display. Soft plaque is overlooked, however, unless it creates significant lumen narrowing. Rybicki and coworkers[13] also noticed this issue and issued the following warning:

> "In summary, while thick MIP images are visually appealing and can be used for rapid interpretation algorithms in the emergency setting, they must be used prudently. When the MIP thickness is increased, multiple structures are projected onto the same plane. Distinguishing details between these structures can be lost when the thickness is too large, and, thus, the user must have full understanding of the anatomic detail before MIP images can be safely rendered."

We use MIP in every case because it does add value, especially in terms of speed and for viewing small-caliber distal portions of smaller vessels. Some key points are as follows:

1. When using MIP, the interpreting physician must be careful not to cut away crucial pathology or create a "pseudolesion."
2. MIP works best when there is little or no calcification present. In the presence of calcification, MIP can lead to overestimation of stenosis or misinterpretation of an occlusion.
3. One must adjust the slab thickness carefully to see the vessel in full view, but one must be careful not to overlook lesions, especially very proximal lesions.
4. One must never use MIP as the only rendering technique for interpretation of a case. Even when the study looks normal, another display technique should be used for confirmation.
5. MIP works best when used interactively by the interpreting physician. MIP images generated by technologists or physicians other than the interpreting physician may have several of the pitfalls noted earlier.
6. Because MIP relies on the brightest pixels, proper synchronization of contrast medium injection and data acquisition is crucial to maximize image contrast resolution.
7. In selected cases, one can go directly from the axial images to MIP to generate a vascular map, especially when the axial images suggest a normal study without any plaque burden.

Volume Rendering Technique

VRT has a crucial role in evaluation of cardiac and coronary CT angiography (Fig. 12-9). The role of VRT in the analysis of these cases is based on numerous factors, including the ability of VRT to display large volumes of data accurately, especially from complex data sets. The best way to understand the crucial role of VRT is to remember several of the basics of VRT.[20]

VRT can display data without classifying it into rigid all-or-nothing categories as thresholding does. VRT is most often performed with a method of classification termed *percentage classification*. The key difference between thresholding classification and percentage classification is that, in thresholding, it is assumed that each voxel contains either all or none of a particular tissue type, and no mixtures of tissues. In percentage classification, it is assumed that a voxel can contain one or more tissue types, and the amount of each tissue is a continuum between 0% and 100%. Percentage classification is possible to approximate more closely true voxel content in voxels containing tissue mixtures, or volume averaging. Percentage classification involves examination of each voxel to determine the amounts (percentages) of each tissue type present in the voxel. The resultant classified volume data consist of voxels still representing the percentage of each tissue type initially present.

The most common method used to determine the percentage contents is probabilistic classification involving a trapezoidal approximation. This method for determining

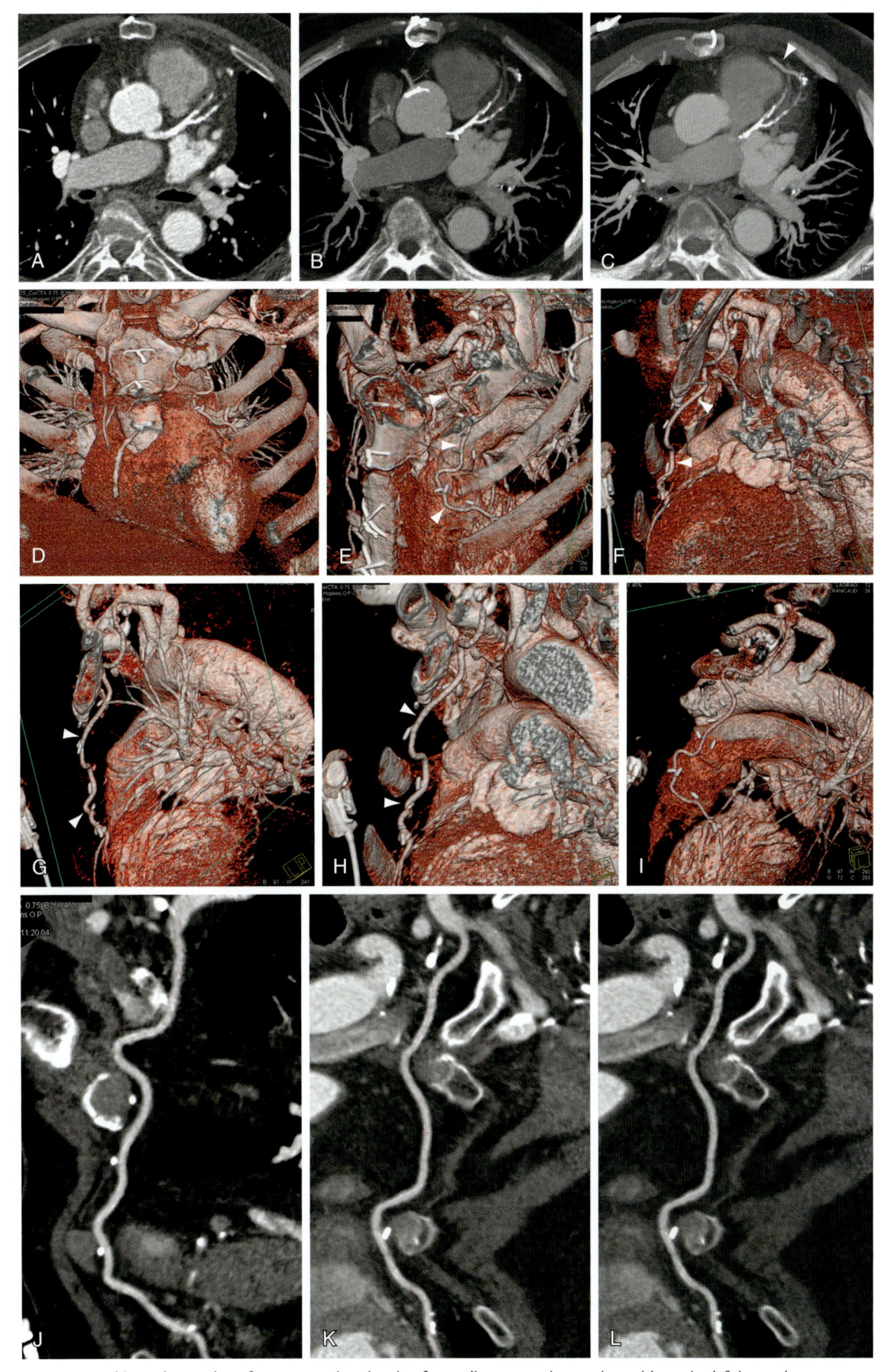

■ **FIGURE 12-9** **A-L,** This study was done for preoperative planning for cardiac surgery in a patient with a prior left internal mammary artery graft. The surgeon wanted to know the location of the graft (*arrowheads* in **E-H**) and relationship to the left anterior descending artery and chest wall. **A-C,** Axial images (**A**) are very limited in this regard, as are MIP images (**B** and **C**). **D-I,** VRT images are ideal, and with interactive editing provide the information the surgeon needed. **J-L,** We supplemented these with CPR images, which define patency of the graft and its touch-down points. The combination of VRT and CPR is excellent in this type of application.

tissue-type percentages works well for CT data. For trapezoidal classification, each tissue type is assigned a nominal value range that theoretically represents that tissue type exactly. A voxel with a signal within that nominal value range is considered to contain 100% of that tissue. Around this ideal nominal value range, another range is defined by choosing a high and low point representing attenuation values at which a voxel would contain none of the designated tissue. Voxels with signal intensities that lie between 0% and 100% are assigned a corresponding percentage between 0% and 100%. A voxel with signal intensity precisely halfway between 0% and 100% would be assigned 50% of that tissue. A voxel with signal intensity three fourths of the way toward 100% would be assigned 75% of that tissue. All values between 0% and 100% represent voxels in which volume averaging is present (i.e., more than one tissue is present). This trapezoidal classification models closely the actual volume averaging in CT voxels.

When the data have been assigned percentages, they must be processed further to form a final image. Each tissue is assigned a color and transparency. Each voxel is assigned a color and transparency by taking a weighted sum of the percentage of each tissue present in the voxel and the color and transparency assigned to those tissues. A final image is produced by casting simulated rays of light through the volume containing the classified and colored voxels. As the simulated rays pass through a voxel, the color and transparency of the voxel modulates the color of the ray.

A few words of caution: although MIP images may seem similar from one workstation to the other, this rule does not hold true with VRT. Each vendor has its own "flavor" of volume rendering. The generic term *volume rendering* simply refers to a method of making three-dimensional images from volume data that allows every voxel in the volume potentially to contribute to the final image. Many different specific methods of volume rendering can produce vastly different results. Which method the vendor uses has a large effect on the resulting images. In addition, for most volume rendering methods, there are many adjustable parameters that change the way the image looks. The simplest parameters are windowing settings (window center and width). VRT has many other parameters, such as color, opacity, and shading. Because there is no standardization in VRT, the parameters from one system do not generally translate well to another system. Image quality also varies among different vendors.

The method of VRT has the biggest effect on image quality. Other factors also come into play, however. Does the system use full 12-bit (−1024 to 3072 HU) input data for rendering? Does it limit the volume size to some maximum so that larger volumes are shrunk when loaded? What is the quality of the video display? All of these factors have an effect on image quality. The interpreting physician must learn the specific capabilities of the available system to be used for image processing.

VRT can help accurately define complex anatomy via what we would describe as global or volume visualization. With this technique, one can view the entire data set or a subset, yet keep the spatial relationships intact. VRT allows for either gray-scale or color mapping; the latter is especially attractive in complex cases. Although techniques such as MIP require careful editing to be able to do routine visualization, VRT provides global viewing of the heart—notably its chambers and coronary arteries, and their relationship to the sternum and chest wall. This global visualization is especially valuable in a patient with complex cardiac anomalies or a patient who has had prior cardiac surgery ranging from bypass grafts to stents to conduits. In contrast to other techniques, VRT tends to create a more global view; several of the conditions in which this is a huge advantage include the following:

1. Cases where the global perspective is needed, such as studies to define bypass grafts or to define location of stents.
2. Cases requiring delineation of anatomic relationships to chest wall, such as in redo procedures where the thoracic surgeon needs landmarks and a good three-dimensional map preoperatively.
3. Cases with complex congenital anomalies before or after repair where a global view of complex anatomy is desired.
4. Cases where anomalies of coronary artery origin are suspected. VRT can help define the course of even the most complex variation. It can provide all of the information in a series of select views or as part of a video or audio-video interleave presentation. As noted by Duran and colleagues,[21] "As a conclusion, our study showed that multidetector CT, especially volume rendering and maximum intensity projection techniques, may be useful for assessment of complex variations, when the conventional angiography may not be sufficient."
5. Cases in which four-dimensional or motion studies are viewed, such as looking at chamber motion, valve motion, or vessel motion.
6. Cases that are reviewed with patients or their families by an interpreting physician or referring physician. The statement "A picture tells a thousand words" is usually true.

Generally, we like to review the VRT images of the heart to get a "lay of the land." Many unsuspected pathologies are seen on these initial overviews. Although VRT images should not be used to grade stenosis, with experience one can recognize stenosis on the images, which may be helpful in further evaluation of the data set. VRT can introduce substantial errors in the volume display, so there is a definite learning curve with this technique.

CONCLUSION

The interpreting physician reviewing cardiac CT imaging needs to master numerous image interpretation skills for optimal viewing and analysis of three-dimensional image data sets. This chapter addresses key points needed for analysis of CT angiography of the coronary arteries and interpretation to assist the reader in daily practice. The interpreting physician needs to use each visualization tool to its maximum advantage and develop a personal workflow that is comfortable and accurate.

KEY POINTS

- The method of data set evaluation (interactive interrogation of the volume by the interpreting physician vs. review of preset images generated by an individual not performing the interpretation) is perhaps even more important than the postprocessing tools used. Interactivity means that the interpreting physicians must process the images themselves.
- When reviewing axial images on a workstation with a composite display of axial, coronal, and sagittal images combined with a three-dimensional image, the interpreting physician should scroll interactively through the data set in the optimal phase for coronary artery visualization.
- CPR is an essential postprocessing tool for evaluating the coronary arteries that addresses the limitations of traditional multiplanar reconstructions. CPR is a reconstruction plane that can track a vessel more optimally, regardless of the complexity of its course or direction.
- Although easy to use, MIP has important limitations that must be recognized. It requires creation of a sliding slab to focus on individual coronary arteries, and is best done interactively at the workstation by the interpreting physician. Care should be taken to define the optimal plane for vessel display, and to avoid inadvertently segmenting portions of the artery from the volume. In addition, MIP is of limited utility in the setting of dense calcification.
- VRT creates a global view that can accurately define complex anatomy by keeping spatial relationships intact; in this regard, color mapping is especially useful for complex cases. VRT can introduce substantial errors in the volume display if parameters are not selected correctly, so there is a learning curve with this technique. Although VRT images should not be used to grade stenosis, with experience one can recognize stenosis on the images, which may be helpful in further evaluation of the data set.

SUGGESTED READINGS

Calhoun PS, Kuszyk BS, Heath DG, et al. Three-dimensional volume rendering of spiral CT data: theory and method. RadioGraphics 1999; 19:745-764.

Dalrymple NC, Prasad SR, Freckleton MW, et al. Informatics in radiology (infoRAD): introduction to the language of three-dimensional imaging with multidetector CT. RadioGraphics 2005; 25:1409-1428.

Fishman EK, Ney DR, Heath DG, et al. Volume rendering versus maximum intensity projection in CT angiography: what works best, when, and why. RadioGraphics 2006; 26:905-922.

REFERENCES

1. Hoffmann U, Nagurney JT, Moselewski F, et al. Coronary multidetector computed tomography in the assessment of patients with acute chest pain. Circulation 2006; 114:2251-2260.
2. Rubinshtein R, Halon DA, Gaspar T, et al. Usefulness of 64-slice cardiac computed tomographic angiography for diagnosing acute coronary syndromes and predicting clinical outcome in emergency department patients with chest pain of uncertain origin. Circulation 2007; 115:1762-1768.
3. Feuchtner GM, Dichti W, Muller S, et al. 64-MDCT for diagnosis of aortic regurgitation in patients referred to CT coronary angiography. AJR Am J Roentgenol 2008; 191:W1-W7.
4. Konen E, Goitein O, Feinberg MS, et al. The role of ECG-gated MDCT in the evaluation of aortic and mitral mechanical valves: initial experience. AJR Am J Roentgenol 2008; 191:26-31.
5. Laissy JP, Messika DZ, Serfaty JM, et al. Comprehensive evaluation of preoperative patients with aortic valve stenosis: usefulness of cardiac multidetector computed tomography. Heart 2007; 93:1121-1125.
6. Leschka S, Oechslin E, Husmann L, et al. Pre- and postoperative evaluation of congenital heart disease in children and adults with 64-section CT. RadioGraphics 2007; 27:829-846.
7. Spevak PJ, Johnson PT, Fishman EK. Surgically corrected congenital heart disease: utility of 64-MDCT. AJR Am J Roentgenol 2008; 191:854-861.
8. Cademartiri F, Mollet N, Alemos PA, et al. Standard versus user-interactive assessment of significant coronary stenoses with multislice computed tomography coronary angiography. Am J Cardiol 2004; 94:1590-1593.
9. Choi JW, Seo JB, Do KH, et al. Comparison of transaxial source images and 3-plane, thin-slab maximal intensity projection images for the diagnosis of coronary artery stenosis with using ECG-gated cardiac CT. Korean J Radiol 2006; 7:20-27.
10. Cordeiro MA, Lardo AC, Brito MS, et al. CT angiography in highly calcified arteries: 2D manual vs. modified automated 3D approach to identify coronary stenoses. Int J Cardiovasc Imaging 2006; 22(3-4):507-516.
11. Ferencik M, Ropers D, Abbara S, et al. Diagnostic accuracy of image postprocessing methods for the detection of coronary artery stenoses by using multidetector CT. Radiology 2007; 243:696-702.
12. Dewey M, Schnapauff D, Laule M, et al. Multislice CT coronary angiography: evaluation of an automatic vessel detection tool. Rofo 2004; 176:478-483.
13. Rybicki FJ, Lu M, Fail P, Daniels M. Utilization of thick (>3 mm) maximum intensity projection images in coronary CTA interpretation. Emerg Radiol 2006; 13:157-159.
14. Dewey M, Hoffmann H, Hamm B. CT coronary angiography using 16 and 64 simultaneous detector rows: intraindividual comparison. Rofo 2007; 179:581-586.
15. Heffernan EJ, Dodd JD, Malone DE. Cardiac multidetector CT: technical and diagnostic evaluation with evidence-based practice techniques. Radiology 2008; 248:366-377.
16. Flohr T, Stierstorfer K, Raupach R, et al. Performance evaluation of a 64-slice CT system with z-flying focal spot. Rofo 2004; 176:1803-1810.
17. Cademartiri F, Luccichenti G, Marano R, et al. Techniques for optimisation of coronary artery opacification in non-invasive angiography with a 16-row multislice computed tomography. Radiol Med (Torino) 2004; 107(1-2):24-34.
18. Cademartiri F, Nieman K, van der Lugt A, et al. Intravenous contrast material administration at 16-detector row helical CT coronary angiography: test bolus versus bolus-tracking technique. Radiology 2004; 233:817-823.
19. Bae KT. Test-bolus versus bolus-tracking technique for CT angiographic timing. Radiology 2005; 235:369-370.
20. Fishman EK, Ney DR, Heath DG, et al. Volume rendering versus maximum intensity projection in CT angiography: what works best, when, and why. RadioGraphics 2006; 26:905-922.
21. Duran C, Kantarci M, Durur S, et al. Remarkable anatomic anomalies of coronary arteries and their clinical importance: a MDCT angiographic study. J Comput Assist Tomogr 2006; 30:939-948.
22. Calhoun PS, Kuszyk BS, Heath DG, et al. Three-dimensional volume rendering of spiral CT data: theory and method. RadioGraphics 1999; 19:745-764.

Methods for Cardiac Magnetic Resonance Imaging

Thomas K.F. Foo and Christopher J. Hardy

Magnetic resonance as an imaging modality provides excellent soft tissue differentiation and the ability to visualize and quantify flow, and is an ideal choice for imaging of the heart. Cardiovascular MRI techniques must meet the twin challenges of synchronizing image acquisition to the cardiac cycle and avoiding the effects of respiratory motion, while providing the contrast necessary to meet the diagnostic need specific to each cardiac application. For cardiac R–R intervals of 500 to 1000 ms (corresponding to heart rates of 120 to 60 beats/min), a temporal resolution between 25 ms and 50 ms is often needed to generate images free of blurring from cardiac motion. MRI must be performed in the shortest time possible to minimize the effects of respiratory motion.

CLINICAL APPLICATIONS

The primary clinical applications of cardiac MRI include the visualization and assessment of the following:

- Ventricular function, including the assessment of cardiac anatomy and morphology. This typically involves the generation of images with T1 or T2 (or T1/T2) contrast at one or more phases of the cardiac cycle. Multiple phases are required for depicting myocardial wall motion.
- Myocardial perfusion, which can be regionally impaired in ischemic cardiac disease. This application targets the imaging of multiple slice locations in the heart to visualize the first pass of contrast media. Typically, images are acquired from only a single cardiac phase.
- Myocardial viability, an application that puts a premium on high spatial resolution and good T1 contrast between healthy and infarcted myocardium. This application usually is used in conjunction with contrast media to enhance the signal intensity differences.
- Coronary artery patency, where a key requirement is clear depiction of the coronary vasculature with high spatial resolution.
- Functional assessment of flow, the ability to quantify flow velocity and flow volumes across vessels or shunt lesions. This includes the ability to visualize the magnitude and direction of blood flow in the heart and associated vascular structures.

TEMPORAL RESOLUTION AND SPATIAL RESOLUTION

Because the heart is in constant motion, the duration of image acquisition (temporal resolution) must be sufficiently brief (<100 ms) to avoid motion blurring artifacts. Single-shot MRI techniques that acquire all necessary k-space data after a single radiofrequency (RF) excitation, such as echo planar imaging (EPI),[1-3] single-shot fast spin-echo (FSE),[4] or spiral imaging methods,[5,6] yield images with insufficient spatial resolution, insufficient signal-to-noise ratio (SNR), or too long an image acquisition window to image the beating heart properly. The necessary MRI (i.e., k-space) data required to reconstruct the image must be acquired in segmented fashion across multiple cardiac cycles.[7] These segmented k-space acquisition techniques incorporate the repeated acquisition of MRI k-space data over a small temporal window in the cardiac R–R interval, after ECG triggering. The acquisition is repeated over multiple cardiac cycles until sufficient k-space data are collected to reconstruct an image.

Because the image spatial resolution is directly proportional to the number of k-space lines acquired, a minimum total image acquisition time is necessary to achieve high image quality. In practice, a tradeoff exists in segmented k-space acquisition between the overall imaging time (number of cardiac cycles) and the image temporal resolution (acquisition window within each cardiac cycle). To achieve high temporal resolution, one must extend the acquisition time across more cardiac cycles; this introduces increased probability of respiratory motion artifacts and adversely affects image quality. Compromises are often made in spatial and temporal resolution to produce image acquisition times corresponding to achievable breath-hold durations in patients (6 to 18 seconds) for segmented k-space techniques.

Similar considerations exist for free-breathing, navigator-gated acquisitions because high spatial resolution imaging requires prolongation of the scanning duration. Navigator-gated acquisitions during tidal respiration greater than 10 minutes is associated with many additional concerns, such as bulk patient motion and respiratory drift of the diaphragm position, which increase motion blurring artifacts and degrade overall image quality.

This chapter describes the various MRI acquisition techniques designed for different cardiac applications that are in current routine clinical use. In addition, methods are described that use new developments in MRI hardware to accelerate image acquisition by reducing the amount of k-space data necessary to produce images of equal spatial and temporal resolution. Advanced MRI techniques that allow for the acquisition of functional data, such as rapid flow, and motion correction techniques are described.

APPLICATION-SPECIFIC CARDIAC MRI METHODS

Ventricular Function: Cine Imaging

For the assessment of ventricular function (e.g., assessment of left ventricular wall motion), images of the heart at multiple time points or phases in the cardiac cycle are acquired. An optimal MRI pulse sequence provides good contrast between the ventricular blood pool and the myocardium, and high spatial and high temporal resolution. Gradient-recalled-echo (GRE) techniques are typically used. A variant of steady-state GRE acquisition, balanced steady-state free precession (SSFP), has gained acceptance as the primary method for cardiac cine imaging at 1.5 T. Gradient-echo imaging is still used at 3.0 T, however, because of the sensitivity of balanced SSFP to off-resonance effects that can cause significant black banding and ghosting image artifacts. The balanced SSFP pulse sequence (depending on MRI scanner manufacturers known as trueFISP, FIESTA, or balanced-FFE) yields the highest image SNR by refocusing all available magnetization at the end of each sequence repetition period (TR).[8,9]

Images acquired at different cardiac time points are played back in a movie loop to enable the assessment of the contractile function of the left ventricle—hence the name *cine* (referring to the motion picture technique). There are several techniques for generating a cine series. Because the imaging pulse sequence is unable to complete image acquisition within the 25- to 100-ms time frame of a phase in the cardiac cycle, the acquisition is segmented over several cardiac cycles. As shown in Figure 13-1A, the number of views, or k-space lines, acquired in a cardiac cycle, or R–R interval, is known as the views-per-segment (vps). Segments are acquired repeatedly throughout the cardiac cycle, with each segment at a different temporal phase, starting from the R wave trigger. This segment acquisition continues until the next cardiac R wave trigger is encountered, at which time the next set of k-space encoding views are updated, and the process is repeated

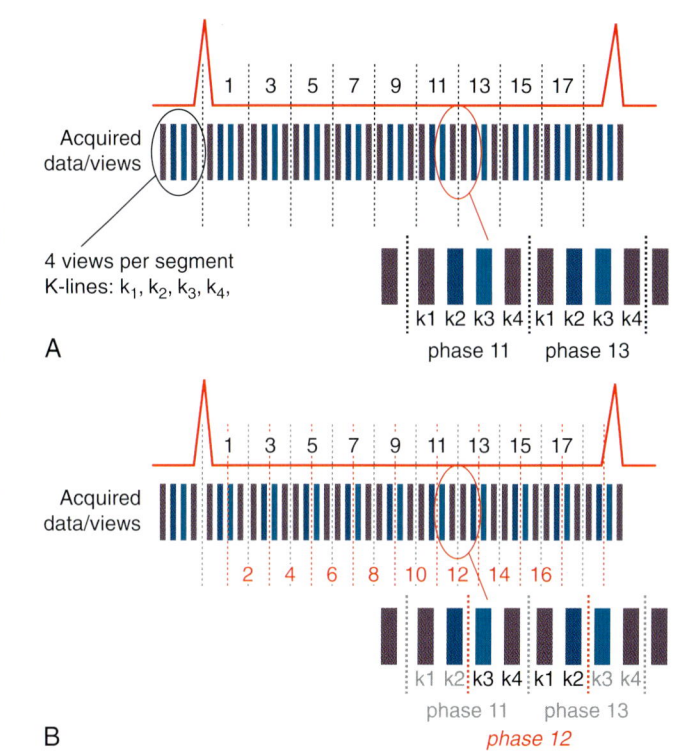

FIGURE 13-1 **A**, In a segmented k-space acquisition, k-space encoding lines are acquired continuously throughout the cardiac cycle. In this example, with 4 vps, only $n = 9$ segments can fit into the R–R interval (segments labeled 1, 3, 5, ... , 17). **B**, To double the number of phases using view sharing effectively, the nearest k-space lines from adjacent segments are combined (shared) to form an intermediate segment that lies midway in time between the acquired segments (2, 4, 6, ... , 16). These new interpolated segments together with the acquired segments now yield $(2n - 1)$ reconstructed cardiac phases.

until all k-space encoding views have been acquired. An acquisition that is prescribed for a phase encoding matrix dimension of 128 requires a total of 128 views and 16 heartbeats to complete, using 8 vps (128 views ÷ 8 vps = 16 segments; 1 segment per heartbeat for a total of 16 heart beats).

All of the data from each segment, when reconstructed, characterize the heart at the corresponding time or cardiac phase within the R–R interval. For segmented acquisitions, it is assumed that the heart is in the same cardiac phase for the same cardiac delay time as measured from the R–R interval, for all cardiac cycles. The acquired temporal resolution (Δt) of the cine sequence is simply:

$$\Delta t = vps \times TR \quad (1)$$

where *TR* is repetition time. The number of acquired cardiac phases that can fit into an R–R interval is limited by the temporal resolution of the acquisition and the patient's heart rate. The number of acquired phases is:

$$n_{phases} = \frac{avail\_RRtime}{vps \times TR} \quad (2)$$

where *avail_RRtime* is the cardiac R–R interval time and is given (in ms) as:

$$\text{avail\_RRtime} = \frac{60 \times 10^3}{\text{heart\_rate}} \times (1.0 - \text{trig\_window}) \quad (3)$$

where the heart rate is given in beats per min and *trig_window* is the fraction of the cardiac R–R interval where data acquisition is disabled to wait for the next cardiac R wave trigger. The number of heart beats that are required to reconstruct an image is given by:

$$\text{scan time} = \frac{\text{yres}}{\text{vps}} \quad (4)$$

where *yres* is the image resolution in the phase-encoding direction and represents the number of k-space lines in the image.

For a heart rate of 80 beats/min, TR = 5 ms, and vps = 12, with a 10% trigger window (*trig_window* = 0.10), 11 phases or segments can be acquired per cardiac interval. For fast heart rates and low temporal resolution, the number of acquired phases is small, and does not allow a smooth depiction of cardiac motion. The effective temporal resolution can be substantially increased, however, using view sharing.[10]

View sharing effectively doubles the number of reconstructed cardiac phases by sharing k-space lines between adjacent acquired data segments to generate an intermediate-phase image. As shown in Figure 13-1B, where a view-sharing factor of 2 is used for a 4-vps acquisition, k-space encoding lines $k1, \ldots, k4$ are acquired in each segment. To generate an intermediate phase image, k-space encoding lines $k3$ and $k4$ from segment n are combined with k-space encoding lines $k1$ and $k2$ lines from segment $n + 1$ to form an intermediate time point or phase image between acquired phases n and $n + 1$.

This nearest neighbor interpolation reconstructs an image at a time point midway between two adjacent acquired phases. Although the acquired temporal resolution is still given by Equation 1, the effective temporal resolution is now doubled to:

$$\Delta t' = (\text{vps} \times \text{TR})/\text{vvs} \quad (5)$$

where *vvs* is the view sharing factor, and typically, *vvs* = 2.

One disadvantage of view sharing or nearest neighbor interpolation is that not all of the cardiac R–R interval is fully imaged. Because of the trigger window at the end of the cardiac interval, visualization of end-diastolic function, such as end-diastolic atrial contraction, is impossible with prospective gating techniques. Another disadvantage of prospective gating with view sharing is that the number of reconstructed phases ($2n_{phases} - 1$) varies according to the heart rate. This variation makes functional assessment of wall motion at different slice locations quite difficult, if the number of phases in each location is different because of changes in the patient's heart rate during the cardiac cine examination.

With the increased speed in computational hardware, imaging of the complete cardiac cycle is now possible, eliminating the dead time at the end of the cardiac R–R interval. This improvement comes with the ability of MRI systems to monitor events in real time and effect a change in the pulse sequence in response. For full R–R coverage, the cardiac R wave trigger event is monitored in each TR

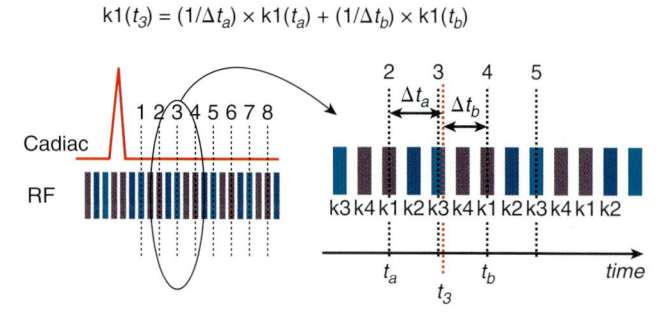

$$k1(t_3) = (1/\Delta t_a) \times k1(t_a) + (1/\Delta t_b) \times k1(t_b)$$

■ **FIGURE 13-2** Diagram illustrating the retrospective reconstruction of cine cardiac phases. In this example with 4 vps, the R–R interval is divided into equal intervals. For the third cardiac phase ($t = t_3$), the closest k1 encoded lines occur at times $t = t_a$ and $t = t_b$. To calculate the k1 encoded line at time $t = t_3$, a linear interpolation is performed between the closest k1 acquired views with an inverse weighting of the time from $t = t_3$ (shown as Δt_a and Δt_b).

interval. If a valid cardiac trigger is detected, the k-space encoding views are updated, and data acquisition continues until all k-space views are collected.

The number of acquired segments for each cardiac R–R interval can change owing to possible variations in the patient's heart rate. These variations in the number of segments and the R–R interval are tracked over time, however, by the MRI scanner's computer or real-time data processor. After data acquisition is complete for each cardiac cycle, the acquired views for each cardiac R–R interval are sorted retrospectively and binned or interpolated into the appropriate cardiac phase.[11] As shown in Figure 13-2, with retrospective gating or sorting, we can choose to reconstruct an arbitrary number of phases for any given number of actual acquired segments. With retrospective interpolation, each cardiac R–R interval is divided into equal time points. The acquired views for each cycle are interpolated to each reconstructed time point using a linear interpolation scheme.

Because the cardiac phase is defined as the fraction (in time) of the cardiac R–R interval, k-space views from different cardiac cycles interpolated to the same cardiac phase regardless of the actual delay time of that time point from the R wave trigger are good representations of the cardiac motion at that phase of the cardiac cycle. The same, fixed number of phases can be acquired for every patient, yielding cine data sets with a standard number of reconstructed cardiac phases, independent of the patient's heart rate. By using this retrospective approach, events over the full cardiac cycle can be easily captured.

Black Blood Imaging

To visualize the cardiac anatomy, black blood imaging, typically a T2-weighted spin-echo pulse sequence, is often used. Because blood returns high signal intensity with T2-weighted pulse sequences, blood suppression techniques are applied to prevent the bright blood signal from masking abnormal structures in the myocardium. As with cine acquisitions, a segmented k-space approach is also used for T2-weighted cardiac imaging. In a segmented k-space FSE acquisition, the primary spin-echo formed after the RF excitation pulse is repeatedly refocused by a

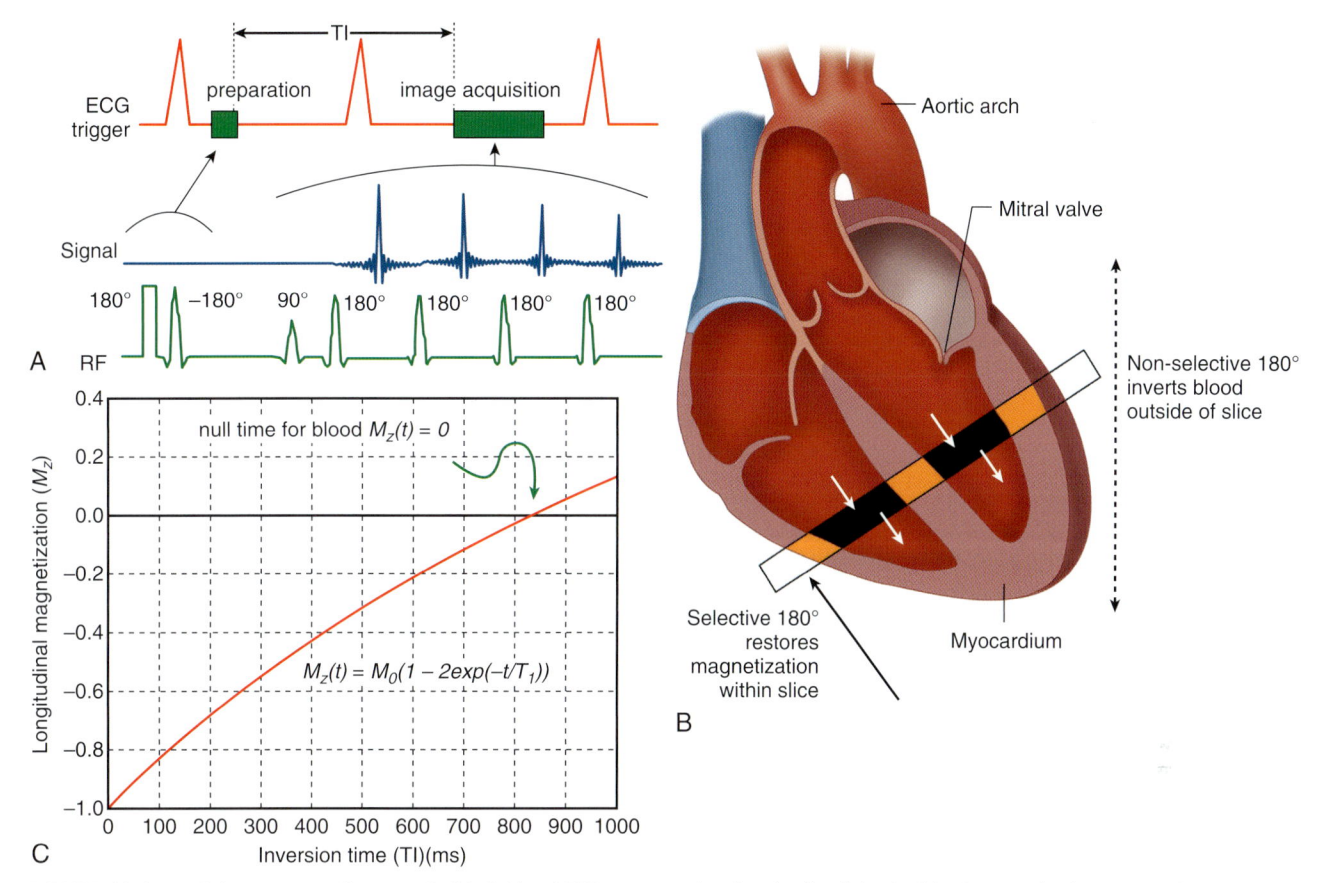

FIGURE 13-3 **A,** Pulse sequence diagram of a black blood FSE sequence showing details of the double IR magnetization preparation segment and the FSE image acquisition segment. **B,** The first nonselective IR pulse inverts the spins everywhere. This is immediately followed by a slice-selective inversion RF pulse that reinverts or restores the perturbed magnetization only in the imaged slice. Following an interval TI, uninverted blood has exited the slice and is replaced by inverted blood. **C,** By choosing the TI time such that the longitudinal magnetization of blood is zero, blood signal within the imaged slice is suppressed.

series of 180-degree RF pulses and forms a train of spin-echoes. Each spin-echo in the train is encoded for a different k-space view. Multiple k-space views are encoded for a single RF excitation pulse. The number of echoes (echo train length [ETL]) acquired per RF excitation pulse is analogous to the vps in cine scans. Strong T2-weighting can be achieved at a fraction of the time required to acquire a conventional spin-echo image. With an ETL = 16, a gated FSE image can be acquired in 8 to 16 heartbeats, depending on the desired in-plane spatial resolution.

Blood suppression is achieved by using a double inversion recovery (IR) technique.[12] As shown in Figure 13-3, a nonselective IR RF pulse inverts all spins in the RF coil volume. This inversion is followed immediately by a slice-selective IR RF pulse to restore the longitudinal magnetization only within the imaged slice. The aim of the reinversion RF pulse is to ensure that the spins within the imaged slice are unperturbed. At an appropriate inversion time (TI), selected so that TI = $TI_{null,blood}$, the point in time where the inverted longitudinal magnetization of blood is zero ($TI_{null,blood} = T_{1,blood} \log_e 2$), the FSE image acquisition is applied. In this TI interval, blood within the imaged slice is replaced with blood from outside the slice (with inverted longitudinal magnetization). At the moment of data acquisition (just after application of the 90-degree RF excitation pulse), the longitudinal magnetization of blood passes through zero resulting in a suppression of blood signal in the imaged slice. Image acquisition usually spans two R-R intervals to allow for a more complete recovery of the longitudinal magnetization (in the second R-R interval), for increased image SNR.

Typical image acquisition parameters for a black blood FSE acquisition are a 256 × 192 acquisition matrix with an ETL = 20 and two R-R intervals per acquisition segment; this translates to an approximate breath-hold time per slice of about 20 seconds (assuming 60 beats/min heart rate). Complete coverage of the heart using black blood FSE requires about 8 to 12 slice locations with separate breath-holds at each location. To further improve the efficiency of the black blood FSE acquisition, the inversion and image acquisition can be compacted into a single R-R interval (e.g., *FSEuno*). By removing the time for recovery of the longitudinal magnetization in the second R-R interval, increased T1-weighting is also achieved. Additionally, the acquisition of four slices in the same time as a single slice in a conventional two R-R interval gated FSE pulse sequence (e.g., *FSEquatro*) can be realized by grouping adjacent slice locations together.[13] As shown in Figure 13-4, two slice locations are acquired in each R-R interval (for four slices in total for a two R-R interval acquisition). Because the slices are adjacent to each other, the slice-

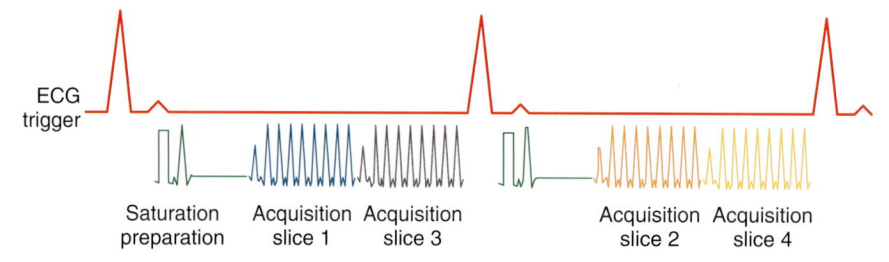

FIGURE 13-4 Diagram illustrating how four slice locations can be acquired in a single acquisition by interleaving. Because each R–R interval has a nonselective IR pulse (from the double-IR saturation preparation at the start of systole) that affects spins over the entire heart, there is less time for recovery of M_z in the imaged slice in segmented k-space acquisitions. The images have a stronger component of T_1 weighting than conventional two R–R black blood imaging sequences. Referred to as FSEquatro, this type of acquisition sequence significantly reduces the overall scan time.

selective reinversion RF pulse now spans two slice locations providing blood suppression for both slices. The number of breath-holds for whole heart coverage is reduced by a factor of 4 (Fig. 13-5), significantly speeding up the cardiac examination and reducing patient fatigue from frequent and repeated breath-holds.

Myocardial Perfusion

Myocardial perfusion imaging identifies regions where there is a blood flow deficit in the myocardium by tracking the first pass of a contrast medium bolus over several cardiac cycles. This tracking requires the use of a fast imaging pulse sequence that repeatedly acquires an image every one to two R–R intervals over 30 to 40 seconds, with sufficiently high image contrast to delineate regional differential uptake of contrast medium. In addition, any changes in image contrast over time must be due only to changes in concentration of the contrast medium in the tissue, and must be immune to variations in heart rate.

To achieve robust image contrast, a 90-degree saturation recovery magnetization preparation segment, followed by a fixed time TI, is used for myocardial perfusion studies. A 90-degree rather than a 180-degree preparation RF pulse is used because the longitudinal magnetization recovers from the same level ($M_z = 0$) during the TI interval for each ECG-gated acquisition during the contrast uptake. With saturation recovery magnetization preparation, the tissue signal intensity is independent of the cardiac R–R interval, eliminating signal variations caused by arrhythmia (Fig. 13-6). The relatively short TI time (100 to 200 ms) of the saturation recovery preparation pulse suppresses signals from long T1-weighted tissues, such as the unenhanced myocardium and blood, while emphasizing tissues with markedly reduced T1 times from contrast medium uptake. With the correct selection of acquisition

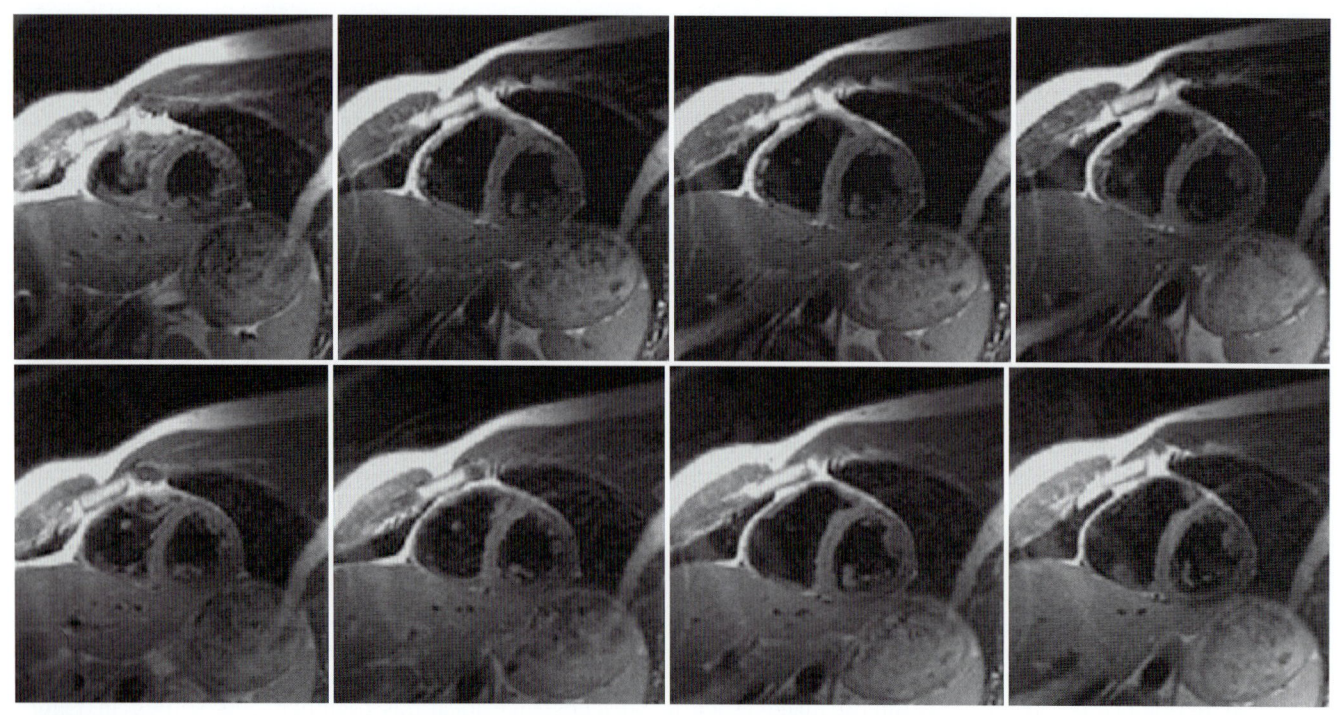

FIGURE 13-5 Comparison between a multislice study using FSEquatro (*top row*) and conventional FSE (*bottom row*). The FSEquatro scheme acquired four slice locations in a single 22-second breath-hold (ETL = 16), whereas the conventional two R–R FSE could acquire only one slice location per breath-hold. Overall, the conventional two R–R FSE acquisition took 4 minutes, allowing the patient to rest between breath-holds. Image quality between the two approaches is equivalent, emphasizing the improved efficiency of current black blood FSE imaging developments.

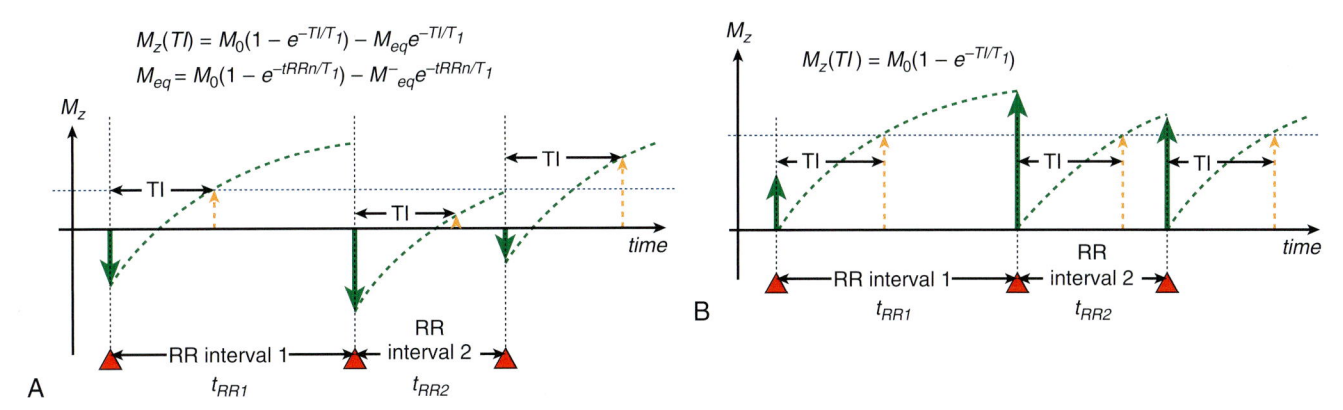

■ **FIGURE 13-6** **A,** Variation in signal intensity, given as $M_z(TI)$, with IR preparation. The signal intensity is a strong function of the longitudinal magnetization at the end of each R–R interval (t_{RRn}). If the patient's heart rate varies during the myocardial perfusion acquisition, there is a strong variation in signal intensity depending on the heart rate changes. **B,** In contrast, if a saturation recovery preparation is used, the signal intensity depends only on the TI time, and is immune to variations in the patient's heart rate. The *solid triangles* indicate the time of a detected cardiac trigger and the point in time when the magnetization preparation pulse is applied. M_{eq}^- is defined as the longitudinal magnetization just prior to the application of the IR pulse in RR interval n (i.e., the longitudinal magnetization at the end of RR interval ($n - 1$)).

parameters and contrast medium dose, saturation recovery magnetization preparation can yield signal intensity changes that are linear with contrast medium concentration, providing an opportunity for quantitative assessment of myocardial perfusion.

To achieve full coverage of the left ventricle during the first pass of the contrast medium, it must be possible to fit an optimal number of acquisition segments (with each segment consisting of the magnetization preparation pulse, TI interval, and data acquisition section) into either one or two R-R intervals. The TI interval section and the data acquisition segment can be optimized to provide the shortest possible time with best possible image quality. Although single-shot EPI (all k-space lines acquired after a single RF excitation pulse) has poor image quality for cardiac perfusion studies, a segmented and interleaved approach accomplishes short scan time and good image quality.[14-16] In interleaved EPI, only a few echoes per RF excitation pulse (ETL = 4) are used, resulting in short (6 ms) TR times; this yields an acquisition approach with high efficiency (time per echo). With improvements in gradient hardware, however, fast gradient echoes (and balanced SSFP) with an ETL = 1 and TR = 2 ms or less have also yielded images with comparable image quality and with equal compactness in time.[17-19]

Effective assessment of myocardial perfusion defects requires maximal tissue contrast, which is obtained from an optimal TI time at typical contrast medium doses of 0.05 to 0.10 mmol/kg.[20] To maximize the number of slice locations that can be acquired per R-R interval, however, the time for each acquisition segment needs to be as compact as possible. By minimizing the TI time, more slice locations can be acquired per R-R interval; however, this leads to compromises in image contrast because there is an inherent tradeoff between TI and image contrast-to-noise ratio (CNR). Several approaches allow for significantly reduced TI times, while maintaining sufficient tissue contrast. By interleaving the saturation recovery RF pulse and image acquisition using a slice-selective notched saturation, longer TI times can be achieved with minimal dead times.[21] Alternatively, the center of k-space in the image acquisition section can be reordered to the end of the acquisition segment, yielding a longer "effective" TI time. Both approaches produce satisfactory image contrast with as compact an acquisition segment as possible.

Sections of the myocardium where there is a regional perfusion deficit are hypointense relative to the normal myocardium because of reduced uptake of contrast medium. By a qualitative assessment of signal intensity changes, myocardial perfusion deficits can be easily identified (Fig. 13-7). A troubling artifact with myocardial perfusion using MRI is the so-called "dark rim" artifact, which is characterized by a transient and distinct hypointense thin region in the endocardium that mimics a perfusion defect (Fig. 13-8).[22] This phenomenon usually occurs immediately after the contrast medium bolus first arrives in the left ventricle, but does not persist over time. Improvements in spatial resolution and substantial reduction in image acquisition times reduce the occurrence of these artifacts, as does requiring positive identification of a defect that spans several slices and persists through multiple frames of the scan.

Myocardial Viability

Myocardial delayed enhancement (MDE) imaging provides an accurate method for determination of myocardial viability.[23,24] On first-pass perfusion imaging, infarcted myocardial tissue does not enhance after gadolinium-chelate contrast agent administration because of its restricted blood flow. Over time, the gadolinium-chelate contrast agent diffuses into the infarcted region. The poor vascular supply to the infarcted region is associated with diminished washout of contrast agent. Infarcted tissue exhibits delayed gadolinium uptake and delayed washout. Normally perfused myocardium has much faster early uptake and brisk washout. Delayed imaging of the left ventricle (beginning 5 to 10 minutes after contrast agent administration) enables optimal differentiation of infarcted from noninfarcted (i.e., normal) myocardium. On delayed imaging, infarcted myocardium appears more enhanced (i.e., "hyperenhanced") relative to that of normal enhancing myocardium (T1 shortening).

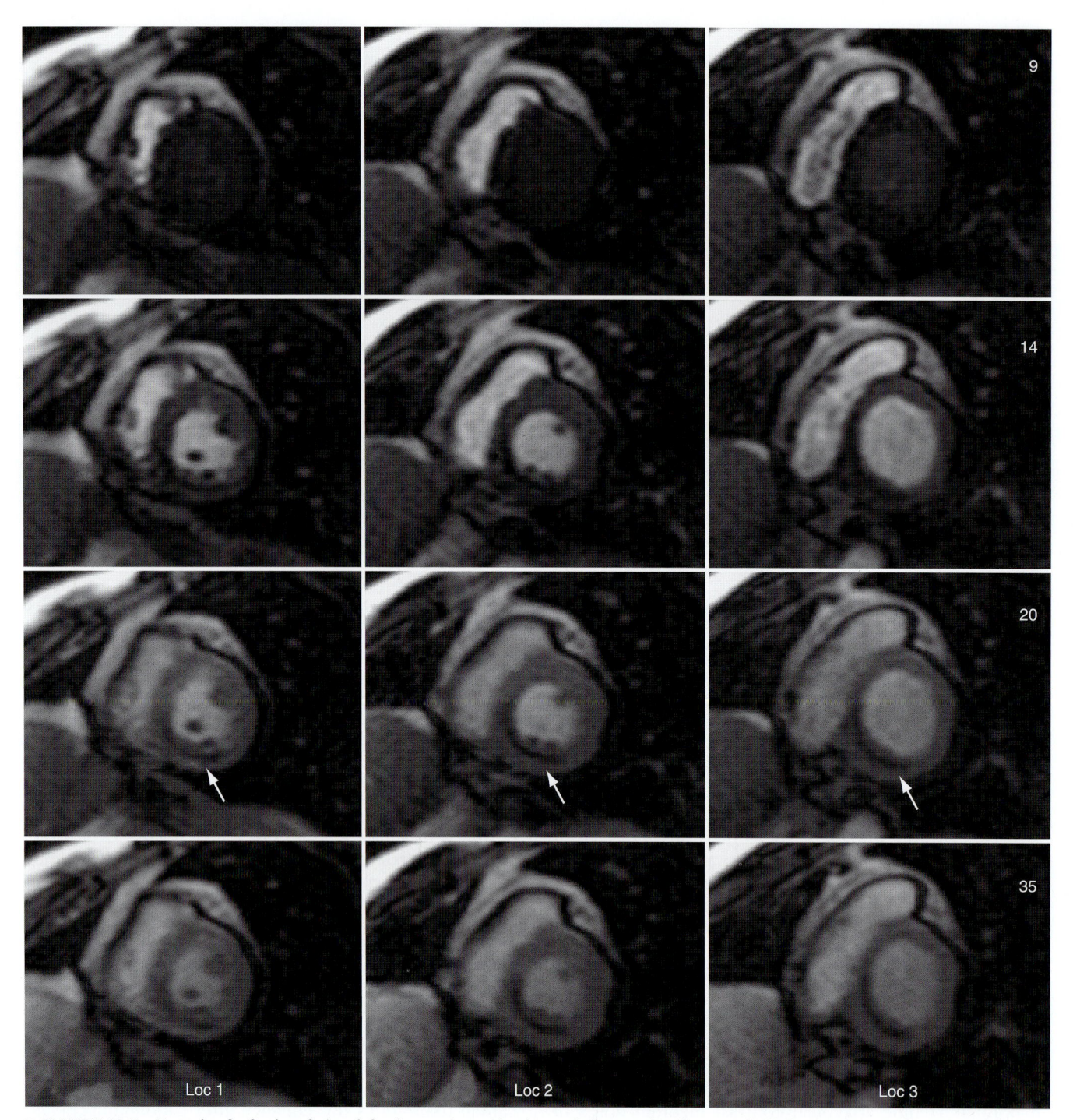

■ **FIGURE 13-7** Example of a fixed perfusion defect in a patient with a known inferoseptal wall myocardial infarction (*arrow*). Three short-axis slices are shown at different time points (*each row*) following a 0.10-mmol/kg contrast bolus. A persistent region of hypointensity observed is indicative of a perfusion deficit and was evident over 20 frames. With a two R–R acquisition, each frame (number) represents two heartbeats.

The best technique for visualizing delayed hyperenhancement is an IR GRE pulse sequence that suppresses signal of the normally enhancing myocardial tissue, while maximizing the signal difference with that of the hyperenhancing infarcted tissue.[25] To maximize the image contrast between normal myocardium and hyperenhancing infarcted tissue, the TI time is selected to null normal myocardial signal during the acquisition of the central k-space view. Because hyperenhancing infarcted tissue has a higher concentration of gadolinium contrast agent, it has a substantially shorter T1 time (approximately 75 ms) relative to normal myocardium (approximately 290 ms). Nulling the signal from normal myocardium yields a high contrast image differentiating the bright infarcted regions from the dark background. The primary image acquisition technique is an ECG-gated, segmented k-space, two-dimensional acquisition where each slice is acquired in a single breath-hold (Fig. 13-9), requiring

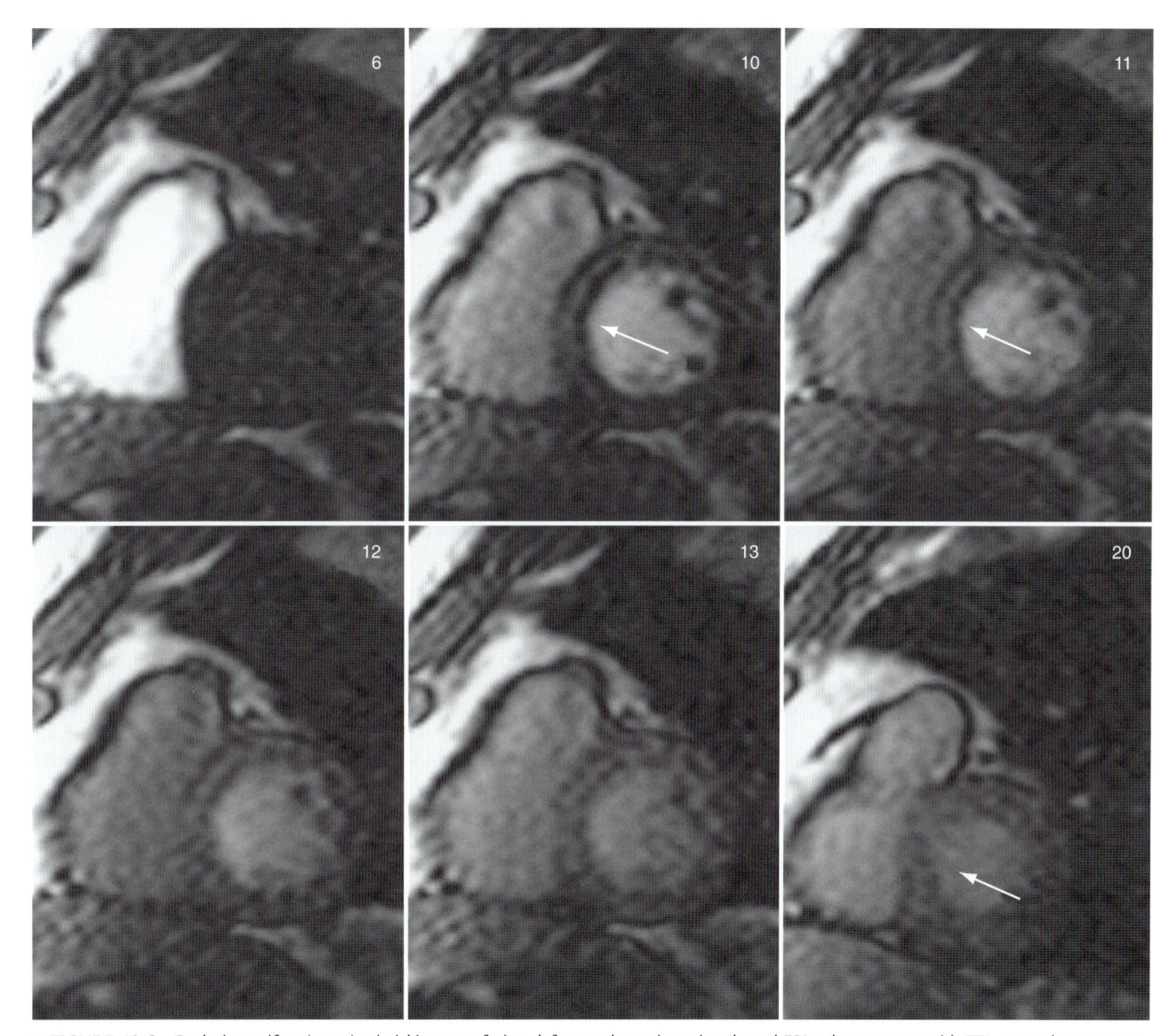

FIGURE 13-8 Dark rim artifact (*arrow*) mimicking a perfusion defect as shown in an interleaved EPI pulse sequence with ETL = 4 and 128 × 128 acquisition matrix. This example shows 6 frames from a 30-frame acquisition. The artifact is evident in *frames 10 and 11* during the first pass of the contrast bolus through the myocardium. This dark rim rapidly diminishes in subsequent heart beats (*frames 12 and 13*) and is completely absent in *frame 20*. Nonpersistent regions of hypointensity that do not span several slice locations are generally classified as image artifacts and are ignored.

multiple breath-holds for complete coverage of the left ventricle.

Although a temporal resolution of about 40 to 50 ms is usually targeted in cine imaging to best visualize motion over the whole cardiac cycle, MDE imaging is able to tolerate temporal resolutions of 150 ms without significant cardiac motion degradation. The number of vps can be substantially increased over a cine scan (see Equation 1), shortening the overall scan time. Typical image acquisition occurs in mid-to-end systole or at a delay of 300 to 400 ms from the cardiac R wave.

To improve image CNR, there are two approaches. With a two R-R interval approach, image acquisition occurs in the first R-R interval, and the second R-R interval is used for more complete magnetization recovery.[24]

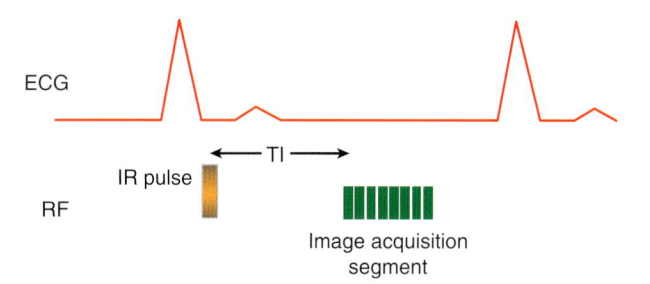

FIGURE 13-9 Diagram illustrating MDE acquisition. The image acquisition section is an ECG-gated segmented k-space gradient-echo pulse sequence that follows a nonselective IR RF pulse. Typically, 20 k-space lines are acquired in each cardiac interval. The subsequent R-R interval either can be repeated for signal averaging or can be used to allow for a more complete recovery of the longitudinal magnetization.

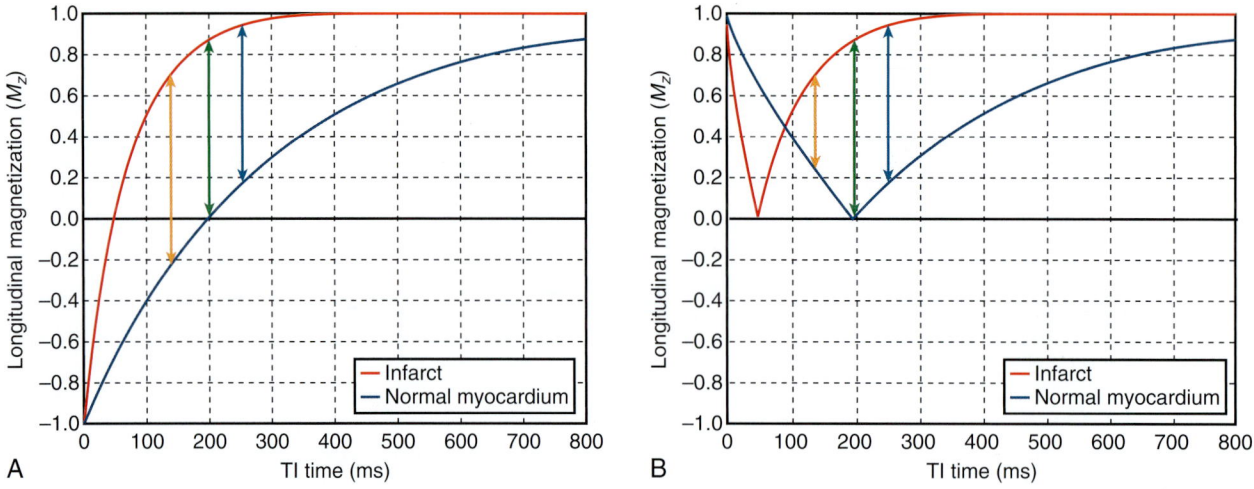

FIGURE 13-10 **A** and **B,** Plot showing the evolution of longitudinal magnetization of normal myocardium (TI = 290 ms) and infarcted tissue (T_1 = 75 ms) with a phase-sensitive IR (**A**) and magnitude IR (**B**) acquisition. As shown in this example, the optimum TI time is at TI = 200 ms, and results in maximum contrast between normal and infarcted myocardium. For TI greater than the optimum TI time (TI > 200 ms), contrast for phase-sensitive IR and magnitude IR is identical. For TI times less than the optimum time (TI < 200 ms), contrast in phase-sensitive IR is maintained, whereas contrast for magnitude IR is diminished. This is because the signal phase is preserved in the phase-sensitive image, whereas magnitude IR has signal intensities greater than zero only. Subsequently, inversion of contrast is possible for short TI times.

An alternative approach is a single R-R acquisition with double the number of excitations. In the latter approach, there is less time for longitudinal magnetization recovery, but by doubling the number of signal averages, some reduction in motion-related artifacts is realized. In both schemes, the overall scan time is the same, where one slice location is acquired in a single breath-hold.

Maximizing image CNR between normal and infarcted myocardial tissue requires a judicious choice of TI times. As noted in Figure 13-10, the contrast at different TI times varies according to whether phase-sensitive inversion recovery (PSIR) or magnitude IR is used. With PSIR, the signal phase is preserved, allowing for negative values of signal intensity (i.e., to account for negative signal intensities when the longitudinal magnetization is <0).[26,27] In magnitude IR, phase information is lost, and all signal intensities are positive (>0). PSIR and magnitude IR provide identical tissue contrast for TI > $t_{null,myo}$, the null point for normal myocardium. The advantage in PSIR occurs when TI is significantly shorter than $t_{null,myo}$, where contrast is maintained between normal and infarcted myocardium, whereas in magnitude IR, contrast diminishes and inverts if the TI time is decreased further. Although PSIR is less sensitive to TI times when TI < $t_{null,myo}$, there is no benefit if TI ≥ $t_{null,myo}$. The optimum TI must still be determined for maximum contrast to avoid setting too long a TI time.

The optimal TI time can be chosen by performing repeated test scans at several different TI times; this can be time-consuming because each acquisition requires a separate breath-hold. As contrast medium concentrations diminish over time, the optimal TI time also changes as a function of time after contrast injection. Alternatively, the appropriate TI time can be determined using a scout acquisition that acquires images at different TI times in a single acquisition. By selecting the best image that has complete suppression of normal myocardium, the corresponding TI time can be used in the MDE acquisition. One such TI scout technique uses a GRE cine pulse sequence with an IR pulse applied immediately at the cardiac R wave trigger.[28,29] This cine IR approach reconstructs images at different times from the IR pulse where each cardiac phase represents a different TI time. Images at multiple TI times can be obtained in a single breath hold acquisition to choose the appropriate TI time (Fig. 13-11).

As with a two-dimensional cine scan, an MDE study can be challenging for a patient because of repeated breath-holding. Single-shot methods using shorter TR gradient-echo or balanced SSFP have longer acquisition windows, but allow multiple slice locations to be acquired in a single breath-hold or in a series of much shorter breath-holds.[30,31] Compared with a conventional MDE study where the acquisition window of 120-150 ms per cardiac cycle is used, single-shot techniques use acquisition windows in the range of 220 to 250 ms. In addition, a much shorter TR with higher receiver bandwidth leads to a reduction in image CNR. By using approximately the same acquisition window per R-R interval, the MDE study can be extended to a three-dimensional acquisition where a $\sqrt{n}$ SNR advantage is realized (where n is the number of slice partitions in the volume scan).[32-34] By trading off some increased motion blurring (that does not compromise diagnosis) against higher SNR, the efficiency of the myocardial viability study can be improved. In addition, variations that include fat suppression allow for assessment of specific patterns of hyperenhancement as may be seen in arrhythmogenic right ventricular dysplasia.[35]

Tagging and Wall Motion Assessment

Although cine MRI allows the assessment of wall motion by visualizing global myocardial contractility, MRI also has the ability to measure regional myocardial wall function directly. The basic approach is to set up a series of grid lines at the start of systole using a magnetization preparation segment consisting of nonselective RF pulses and

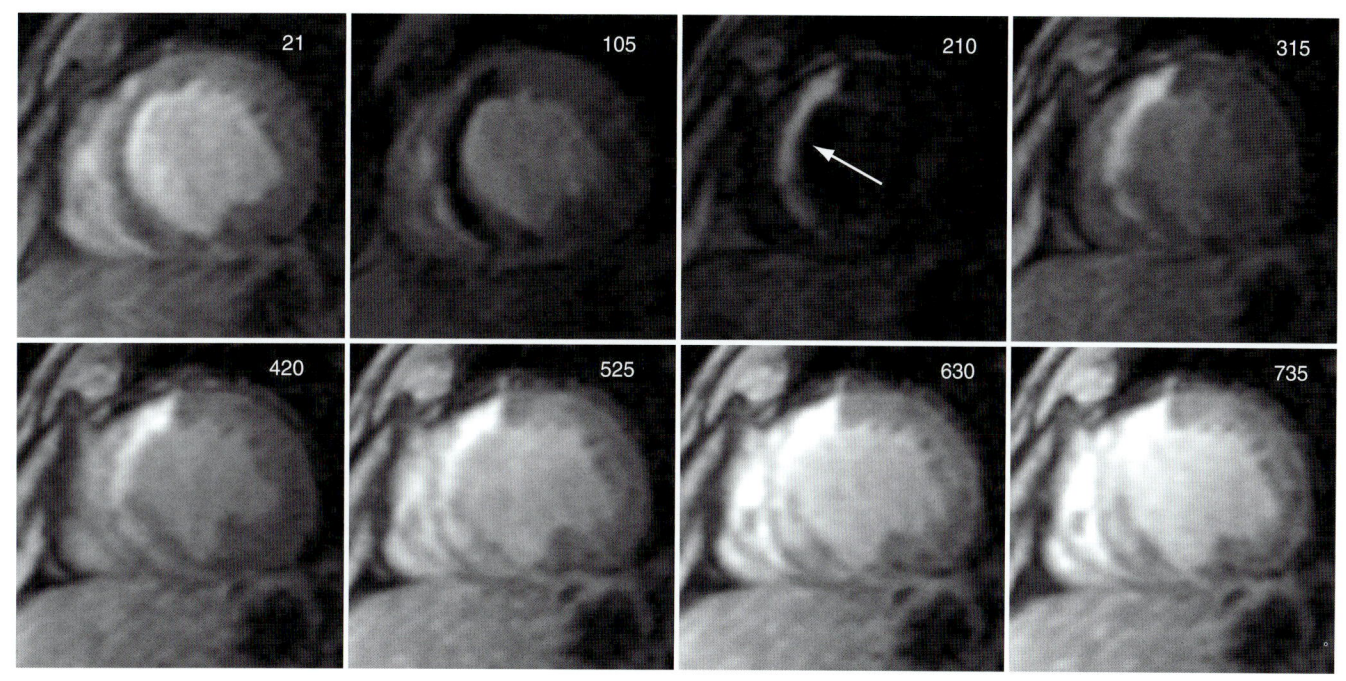

FIGURE 13-11 cine IR images acquired in a single acquisition at equivalent TI times of 21 ms, 105 ms, 210 ms, 315 ms, 420 ms, 525 ms, 630 ms, and 735 ms. This approach acquires 40 phases, with each phase at a different TI time from the IR pulse. By inspecting the reconstructed images, the optimal TI time can be selected and used for the high spatial resolution acquisition. In this case, TI = 210 ms results in maximal suppression of the normal myocardium and high contrast of the large septal infarct (*arrow*) in this patient. At TI < 210 ms, there is an inversion of contrast (dark infarct) in this magnitude reconstruction. At TI > 210 ms, there is reduced contrast as the longitudinal magnetization of the normal myocardium and infarct approach similar thermal equilibrium values.

gradient pulses, and to follow the evolution of these tagged lines through systole.[36,37] Tag lines in the image are applied using a tagging sequence as shown in Figure 13-12. In a simple view with a two-RF pulse tagging sequence, the first RF-excitation pulse tips into the transverse plane all spins within the coil volume. The gradient pulse causes the spins to acquire a relative phase as a function of position. At some time τ, a second RF pulse restores the longitudinal magnetization except for the spins that are aligned along the x'-axis in the rotating frame. Spatial locations that have acquired a relative phase where $\phi = \pi/2, 3\pi/2, \ldots, (2n + 1)\pi/2$ will have minimal signal ($\phi = \int_0^\tau \gamma \vec{G}_r(t) \cdot \vec{r} dt$, where $\vec{G}_r(t)$ is the magnetic field gradient, $\vec{r}$ is the position, τ is the gradient waveform pulse width, and γ is the gyromagnetic ratio).

Because only the component of the transverse magnetization that is perpendicular to the direction of the applied RF excitation field (x'-axis) is restored by the second RF pulse to the longitudinal axis, a range of signal intensities according to position is generated by the tagging sequence. The signal intensity varies as:

$$M_z(\vec{r}) = M_0 \cos\left(\int_0^\tau \gamma \vec{G}_r(t) \cdot \vec{r} dt\right). \quad (6)$$

This results in a sinusoidal variation of signal intensity according to position. Two-dimensional grid tags can easily be applied by first applying the tagging sequence in one direction, followed by the same tagging sequence but with a gradient field in an orthogonal direction. The tag lines can also have better definition (sharpness) by increasing the number of RF pulses and corresponding gradient pulses, and varying the relative amplitudes of the component RF pulses.[38] The tag separation can be controlled

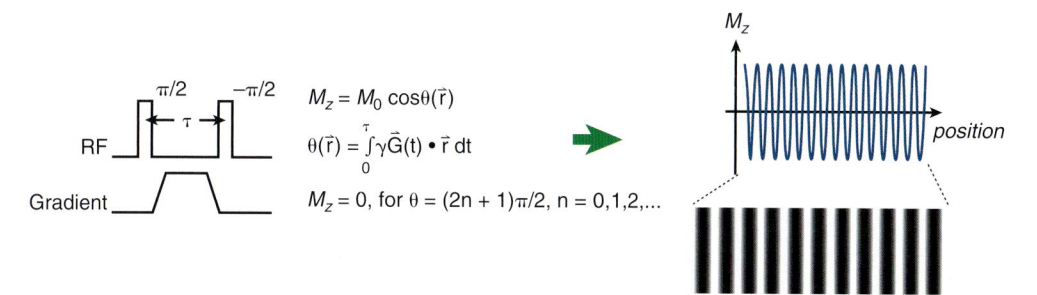

FIGURE 13-12 Diagram illustrating a simple tagging sequence. The two RF excitation pulses and intervening gradient waveform generate a sinusoidally varying intensity in the image. The *dark lines* in the image correspond to $M_z = 0$. Better definition of the tag lines can be achieved by using more RF pulses.

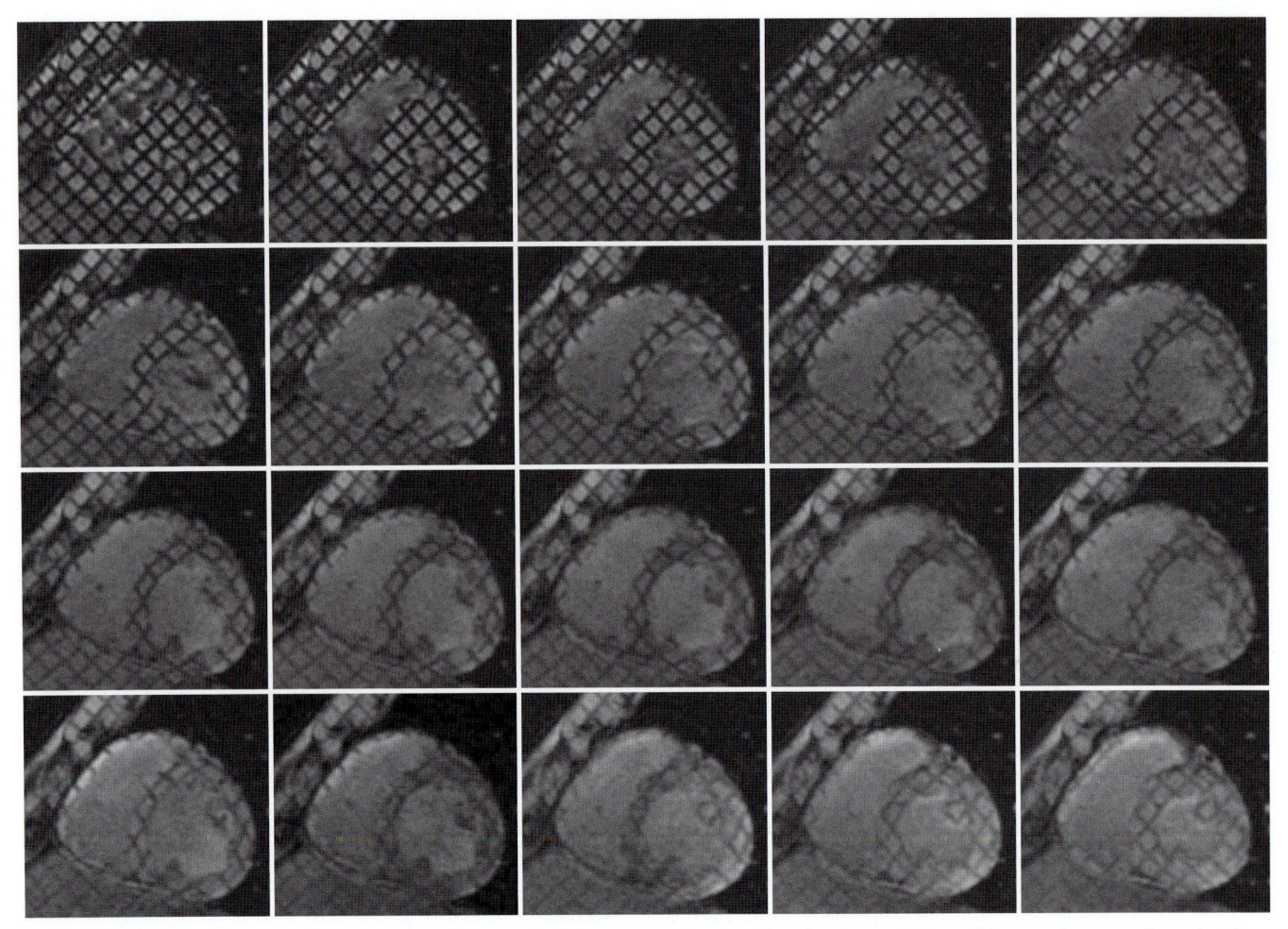

■ **FIGURE 13-13** Twenty phases from a segmented k-space tagging sequence in a healthy volunteer at 3.0 T. In this example, a two-dimensional tagging grid is applied at the cardiac R wave. As the heart contracts in systole and dilates in diastole, the deformation of the regular grid pattern is evident. Uniform deformation of the myocardial tagging grid of the left ventricle is indicative of normal wall motion and function.

better with an increased number of RF and gradient pulses in the tagging sequence.

As the tagged regions evolve over the cardiac cycle, normal myocardial wall motion is seen as a contraction of the pattern of grid lines in systole, followed by separation or relaxation in diastole (Fig. 13-13). Nonfunctioning sections of the myocardium exhibit no such contractility. Quantitative assessment of myocardial strain is possible from analysis of the deforming tag lines. More efficient techniques have been introduced that allow faster computation of myocardial strain by analyzing the phase evolution of the tag lines in k-space.[39,40]

Coronary Artery Imaging

Developments in navigator technology and faster acquisition pulse sequences have resulted in substantial progress in using MRI for coronary artery stenosis assessment. Coronary artery imaging methods can be divided into whole heart imaging[41] and targeted oblique acquisitions.[42,43] In the latter technique, the volume (three-dimensional) acquisition is targeted to specific vessels. Typically, to image the left main coronary artery, left anterior descending coronary artery, right coronary artery, and left circumflex coronary artery, three separate acquisitions are required. For whole heart imaging approaches, the entire heart is imaged in a single acquisition, followed by segmentation of the coronary arteries using postprocessing algorithms available on image analysis workstations.

Short breath-hold three-dimensional techniques[42,44] are most suitable for the targeted approach. With breath-hold times of 20 to 28 seconds, an oblique three-dimensional volume encompassing the coronary artery can be easily and rapidly acquired. Three targeted, breath-hold coronary three-dimensional MR angiography acquisitions that include the left main and proximal segments of the left anterior descending coronary artery, right coronary artery, and left circumflex coronary artery are typically imaged within 5 minutes, assuming the patient is able to tolerate repeated breath-holding. The short scan times allow the coronary artery assessment to be completed immediately after the first-pass perfusion study and before performing the myocardial viability assessment.

Because most patients with cardiac disease are unable to tolerate long breath-holds, free-breathing or respiratory-navigator techniques are employed.[45] In navigator imaging of the coronary arteries, the position of the diaphragm is monitored before data acquisition in each R–R interval.

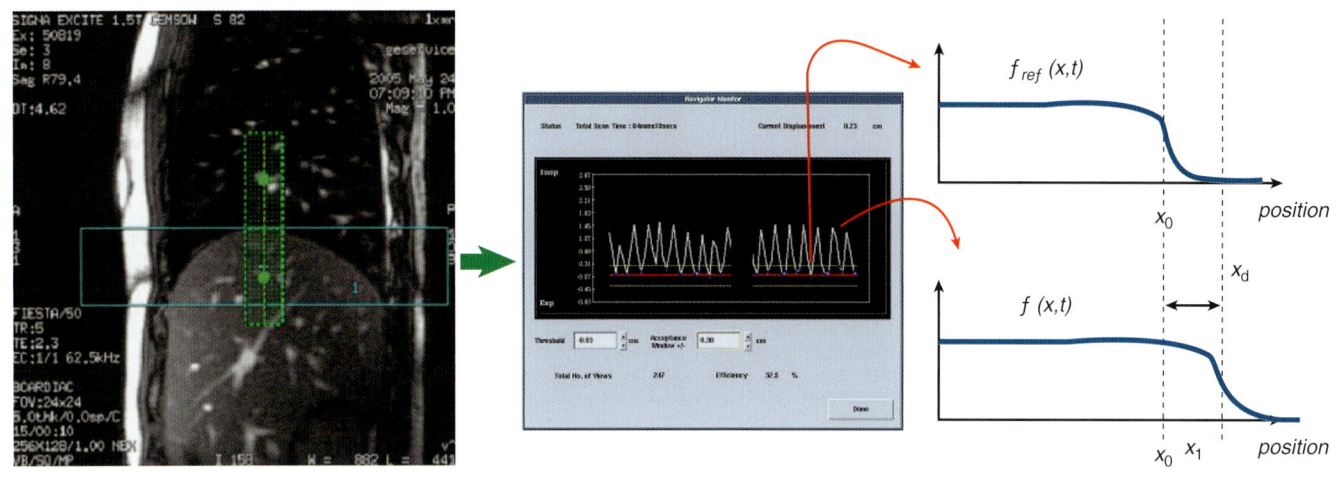

FIGURE 13-14 Principle of navigator-echo gating. A two-dimensional selective excitation is made in the cranial-caudal direction over the right hemidiaphragm. From the projection along the excitation column, an edge detection algorithm detects and displays the position of the diaphragm as a function of time (*center plot*). The displacement relative to a reference position, x_d, is measured using a least-squares fit. From these data, the end-respiratory position (*red line*) can be displayed. If the diaphragm position falls within the acceptance window of the end-respiratory position, the data are accepted.

The navigator acquisition is a two-dimensional slice selective column that is prescribed typically over the right hemidiaphragm in the cranial-caudal direction. The right hemidiaphragm is chosen for tracking diaphragmatic excursion because the lung-liver interface provides an excellent tissue-contrast interface. The placement of the tracker in the right hemithorax places the dark saturation bands related to navigator gating away from the heart. In each R–R interval, the profile along the navigator column is measured and analyzed to track the displacement of the lung-liver interface. A training phase is usually performed to determine automatically the end-expiration position; this is used as a reference profile (Fig. 13-14). During the navigator scan, a least-squares determination of the displacement of the measured profile is made relative to the reference profile (end-expiration). If the position falls within an acceptance window around the end-expiration position, the data are accepted. If not, the same k-space encoding views are repeated until the diaphragm position is noted to fall within the acceptance criteria.[46]

Let $f_{ref}(x_0)$ be the profile along the navigator column that represents the mean end-expiratory position, where x_0 is the reference position in mm. To determine the displacement at time t, the corresponding navigator profile is $f(x',t)$, where x' denotes position of the navigator profile at time t. The relative displacement of x' from x_0 is determined by varying x_d over a range of values such that:

$$|f(x'-x_d,t)-f_{ref}(x_0)|^2 \rightarrow min \quad (7)$$

where x_d is the displacement of the profile from its measured position. The value of x_d is the displacement of the subject navigator profile from the reference profile. This value is plotted as a function of time (as shown in Fig. 13-14) in real time either to accept or to reject that acquisition view.

Specifically for coronary artery imaging, the navigator segment must be integrated with the data acquisition segment and a fat suppression segment (Fig. 13-15). Fat suppression is required because the coronary arteries are embedded in epicardial fat that yields high signal intensities similar to that of blood. The navigator gating sequence synchronizes image acquisition for end-expiration, and enables the extension of the imaging window over many respiratory cycles for improved high spatial resolution, whole heart imaging of the coronary arteries. From the three-dimensional volume, planar reformations or surface rendering can better depict long lengths of the coronary artery.[47]

Free-breathing techniques have disadvantages. In practice, the shorter the scan time, the greater the chances that the scan is successful. There is a normal drift in the location of the diaphragm over time[48] that changes the end-expiration position, resulting in poor performance of the navigator compensation. If the scan time can be shortened (e.g., using parallel imaging), the probability of diaphragm drift can be reduced, improving the image quality. The ongoing development of coronary artery imaging techniques has focused on minimizing the effects of cardiac and respiratory motion, primarily by reducing the overall acquisition time, but also by determining the optimal quiescent period of the heart when there is minimal motion.

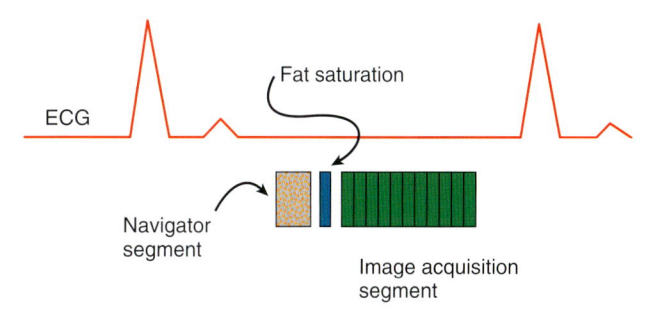

FIGURE 13-15 Navigator-echo gating in a segmented acquisition. In each cardiac R–R interval, a navigator segment is played out followed by the fat suppression magnetization preparation segment and the data acquisition segment. The sequence is repeated until all necessary data for the three-dimensional volume acquisition are acquired.

$$\phi_1 = \gamma v \int_0^{2\tau} tG(t)dt + \phi_{non\text{-}flow}$$

$$\phi_2 = -\gamma v \int_0^{2\tau} tG(t)dt + \phi_{non\text{-}flow}$$

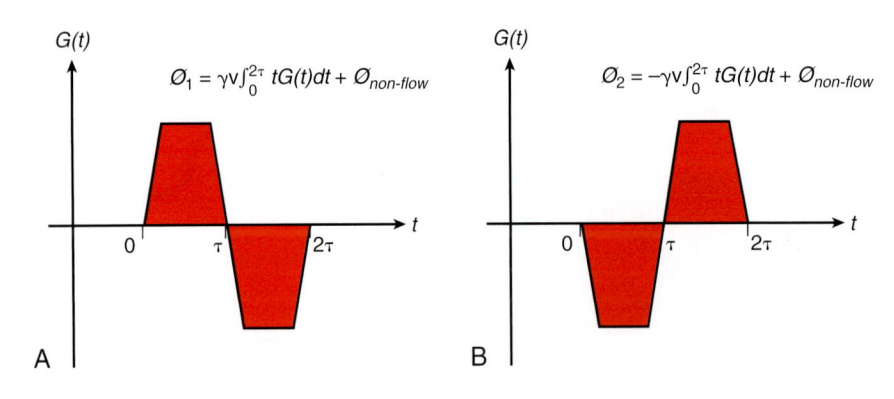

Phase-difference, $\Delta\phi = \phi_1 - \phi_2$
$$= 2\gamma v \int_0^{2\tau} tG(t)dt = \gamma v \Delta M_1$$

■ **FIGURE 13-16** **A,** Bipolar flow-sensitizing gradient waveform. Because the second lobe is identical but of opposite polarity to the first gradient lobe, accumulated phase from stationary spins (i.e., protons) is zero, and the remaining nonzero accumulated phase is due only to motion (moving protons such as flowing blood). However, there may be nonzero phase from nonflow-related sources ($\phi_{nonflow}$). **B,** When a second acquisition is performed with the polarity of the bipolar gradient reversed, the phase from nonflow-related sources is unchanged, but the phase arising from blood flow is the negative of the phase from the first acquisition. Taking the phase difference between the two acquisitions, the nonflow-related phase is canceled, leaving only the phase that is due to blood flow.

Phase Contrast Imaging

In addition to excellent soft tissue visualization, MRI affords the ability to quantify flow in a manner similar to Doppler ultrasonography, but without the restrictions of limited acoustic windows. Phase contrast angiography[49-51] discriminates between flowing spins and stationary tissue by measuring differences in accumulated phase in the direction of a flow-sensitizing gradient. Phase contrast data can provide the velocity of flowing spins (i.e., flowing blood) and the direction of blood flow.

If we consider a magnetic field gradient applied in a specific direction, the phase accumulated by an ensemble of spins moving with a constant velocity, $\vec{v}$, in that direction is:

$$\phi = \int_0^\tau \gamma \vec{G}_r(t) \cdot \vec{r}(t) dt$$
$$= \gamma r_0 \left\{ \int_0^\tau \vec{G}_r(t) dt \right\} + \gamma v \left\{ \int_0^\tau t \vec{G}_r(t) dt \right\} \quad (8)$$
$$= \gamma r_0 M_0 + \gamma v M_1$$

where $\vec{G}_r(t)$ describes the time-varying gradient (direction and amplitude), γ describes the gyromagnetic ratio, and r_0 describes the initial position of the spins. The terms M_0 and M_1 represent the zero and first moments of motion of the spins in the gradient field. If we follow this first gradient waveform with a second waveform that is identical but of opposite polarity, the accumulated phase is then:

$$\phi = \int_0^\tau \gamma \vec{G}_r(t) \cdot \vec{r}(t) dt + \int_\tau^{2\tau} \gamma \left(-\vec{G}_r(t)\right) \cdot \vec{r}(t) dt$$
$$= \gamma r_0 M_0 + \gamma v M_1 + (-\gamma r_0 M_0) + \gamma v M_1' \quad (9)$$
$$= \gamma v M_1'',$$

where M_1'' represents the first gradient moment from the combined bipolar gradient waveform. The phase accumulation from this bipolar gradient waveform (Fig. 13-16) arises only from flowing spins, with the contribution from stationary spins (the r_0 component) canceled out by the gradient lobes of equal amplitude but opposite polarity. Only flowing spins contribute to nonzero phase accumulation, the magnitude and sign of which are directly related to the velocity and direction of flow.

A single acquisition with a bipolar flow-sensitizing gradient ideally provides an image whose phase represents flow in the direction of the applied gradient as given by Equation 9. Residual eddy currents, magnetic field inhomogeneity, and miscentering of the MRI echo in the acquisition window contribute to a spatially varying nonzero phase unrelated to flow or motion (Fig. 13-17A and B). To overcome this problem, two images with bipolar gradients of opposite sign (toggled bipolar gradients) are subtracted. Any nonzero phase in stationary tissue is canceled out, leaving an image with the phase difference accumulated in the two acquisitions owing only to flow (Fig. 13-17C). The phase difference ($\Delta\phi$) from the toggled bipolar flow gradient is then:

$$\Delta\phi = \gamma v \Delta M_1'' \quad (10)$$

with:

$$\Delta M_1'' = \int_0^{2\tau} 2tG(t) dt, \quad (11)$$

where $G(t)$ is the bipolar gradient waveform.

The phase contrast approach to velocity imaging can be applied to cine pulse sequences (see Figs. 13-1 and 13-2) to generate ECG-gated images that depict flow velocities in the heart and blood vessels as a function of the cardiac cycle. With phase contrast cine images, the magnitude and direction of intracardiac shunts and valvular dysfunction (Fig. 13-18) can be easily observed. It is also possible to compute net flow (integrated over the entire cardiac cycle) through vessel cross sections (Fig. 13-19), and the forward and reverse components of flow. Phase contrast cine is an essential tool for flow quantification in patients with atrial septal defects or similar congenital cardiac disease where the measurement of regurgitant volumes or shunt flow is required.[52,53]

ACCELERATED CARDIAC MRI

Although segmentation of the MRI data acquisition across multiple R-R intervals using ECG gating and respiratory navigation allows the synchronization of image acquisition to specific phases of the cardiac and respiratory cycle, long acquisition times leave the possibility of

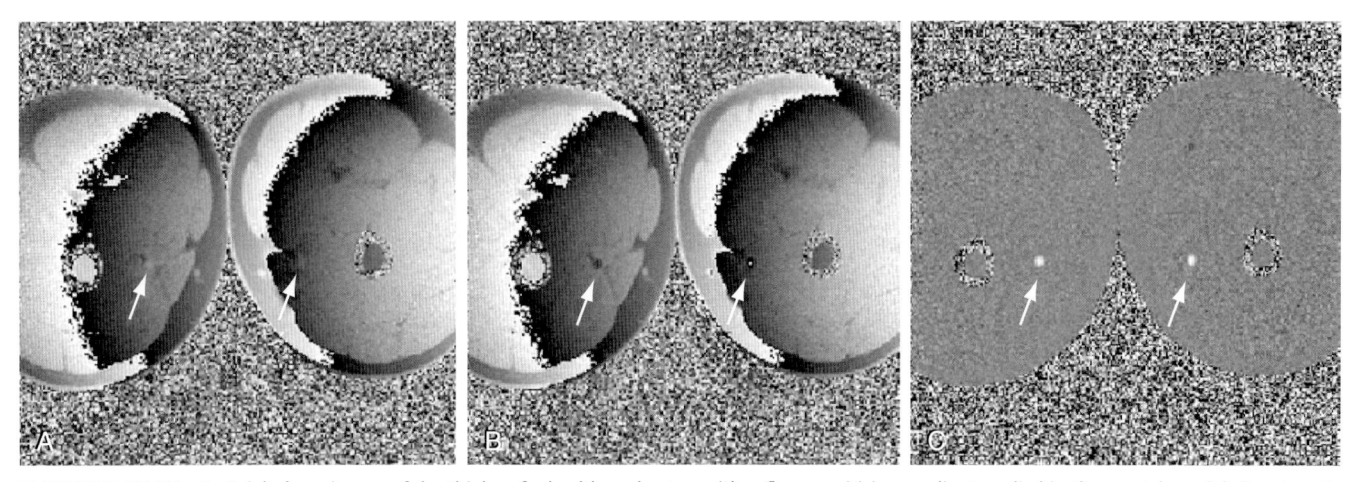

■ **FIGURE 13-17** **A**, Axial phase image of the thighs of a healthy volunteer with a flow-sensitizing gradient applied in the cranial-caudal direction. A spatially varying nonzero phase is observed in the stationary tissue and the arterial and venous structures. **B**, Axial phase image of a second acquisition, but with the polarity of the flow-sensitizing bipolar gradient reversed. Signal in the femoral arteries is now negative (*arrows*) relative to the first acquisition (**A**), but the background phase is unchanged. **C**, Taking the phase difference between the two acquisitions cancels out the nonzero phase unrelated to flow, leaving the phase signal in the femoral arteries clearly depicted. The phase of the stationary background tissue is now zero.

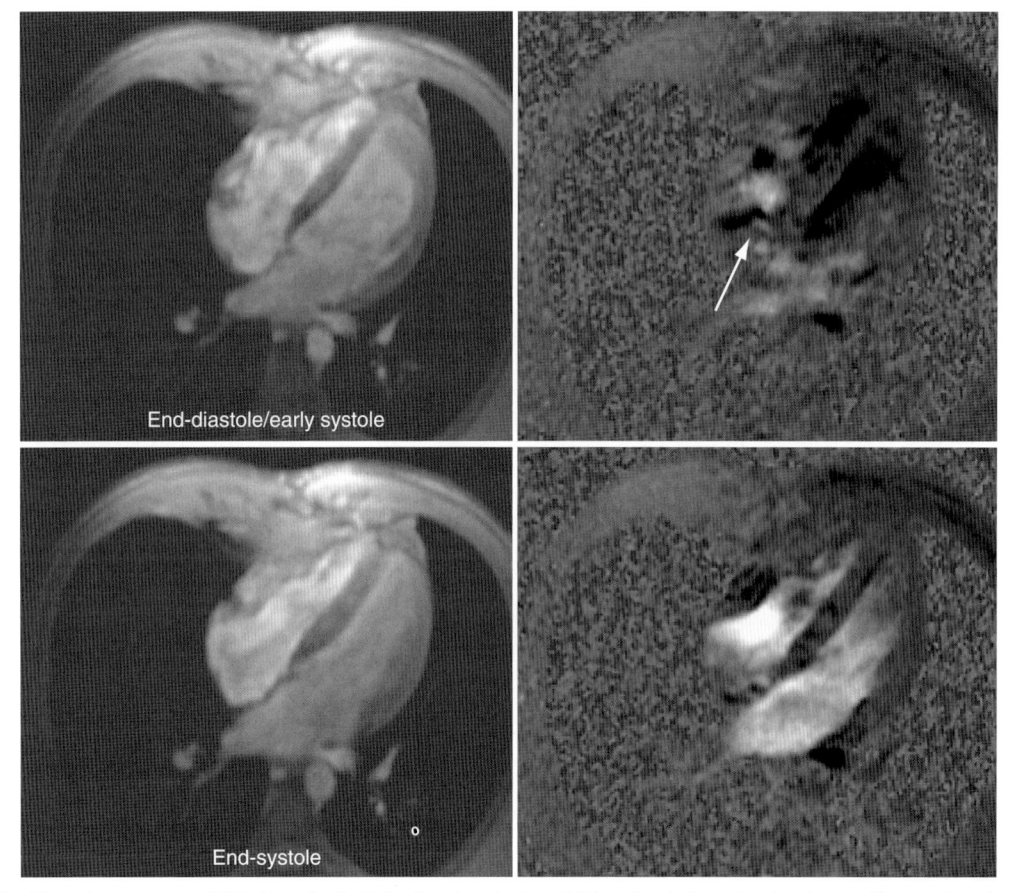

■ **FIGURE 13-18** Cine phase contrast MRI. Magnitude (*left column*) and phase (*right column*) four-chamber images from a cine phase contrast examination in a patient with tricuspid insufficiency. The acquisition was acquired with flow sensitivity in the right-left, anteroposterior, and superoinferior directions. Only the right-left phase-velocity image is shown. There is black flow (*arrow*) on the four-chamber phase velocity map image (*top right image*) signifying left-to-right flow (i.e., regurgitant) into the right atrium during systole; it cannot be seen in the magnitude image. Antegrade flow through the tricuspid valve is seen during diastole as white (bright) signal signifying right-to-left flow direction on the diastolic phase velocity map (*bottom right image*). Direction of blood flow is encoded as either bright or black pixels based on flow direction. On a right-left phase velocity map, right-to-left flow is bright; left-to-right flow is black.

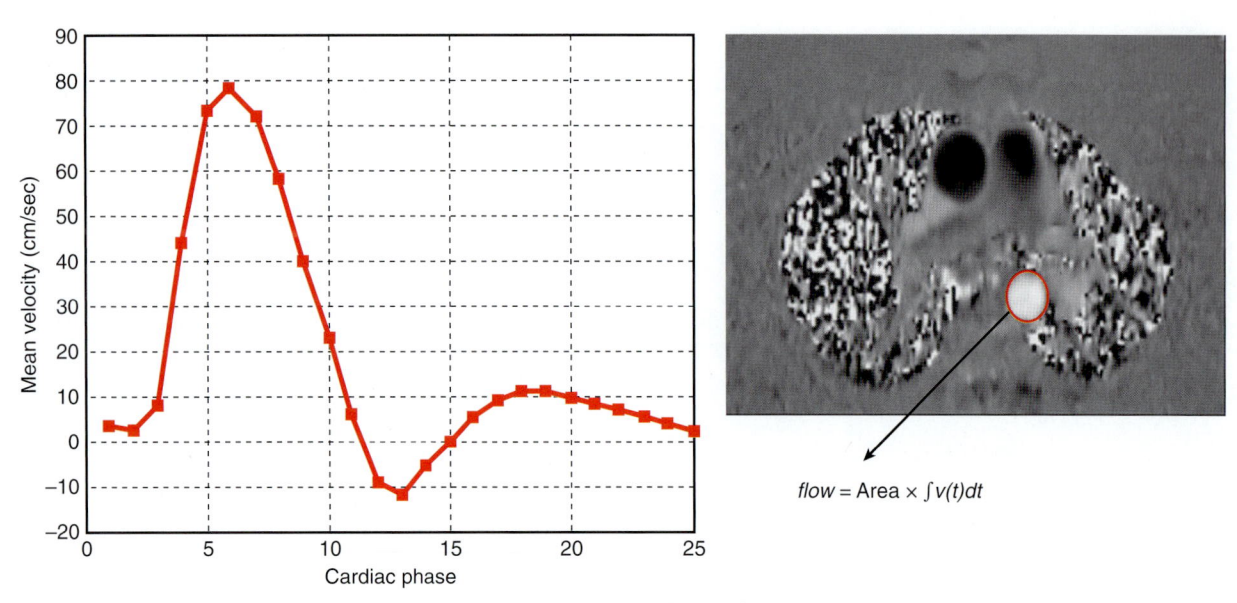

FIGURE 13-19 Measurement of mean flow velocities across a cross-sectional area of the descending aorta as a function of cardiac phase in a cine phase contrast examination. The net flow is computed by integrating the velocity-time curve over the cardiac cycle and multiplying this by the measured cross-sectional area of the vessel.

$flow = Area \times \int v(t)dt$

a transient event or aperiodic motion corrupting the resulting image. It is desirable to have more rapid or accelerated imaging by reducing the data necessary to reconstruct an image and reducing the overall image acquisition time. Significant reduction of overall scan time for any given acquisition scheme produces benefits not only for breath-hold acquisitions, but also for navigator-gated acquisitions in which prolonged acquisition times are prone to diaphragmatic motion drift in the end-expiration position over time.

Apart from the reduction in breath-holding time for the patient, imaging acceleration is also beneficial for imaging patients with poor ECG gating because it provides opportunities for improvements such as in temporal sampling or shortened image acquisition time. Shorter acquisition times also can provide opportunities for better functional perfusion information because data from all slice locations covering the left ventricle can be acquired in each heartbeat for improved characterization of the passage of the MRI contrast agent through the myocardium. Significantly shorter image acquisition times can also afford improved image quality without compromises in temporal or spatial resolution.

Fast Pulse Sequences

A primary method for speeding up imaging of the heart has been the adoption of faster pulse sequences. The first of these to be developed, the echo-planar imaging (EPI) sequence,[1] executes a raster pattern back and forth across all of raw-data space, or "k-space,"[5] after a single RF excitation. This is in contrast to conventional acquisition approaches that acquire a single line of k-space data per excitation (Fig. 13-20). Although this sequence dates from the earliest days of MRI, it did not become practical for cardiac imaging until the advent of improved gradient hardware.[3,54] This improved hardware has also enabled

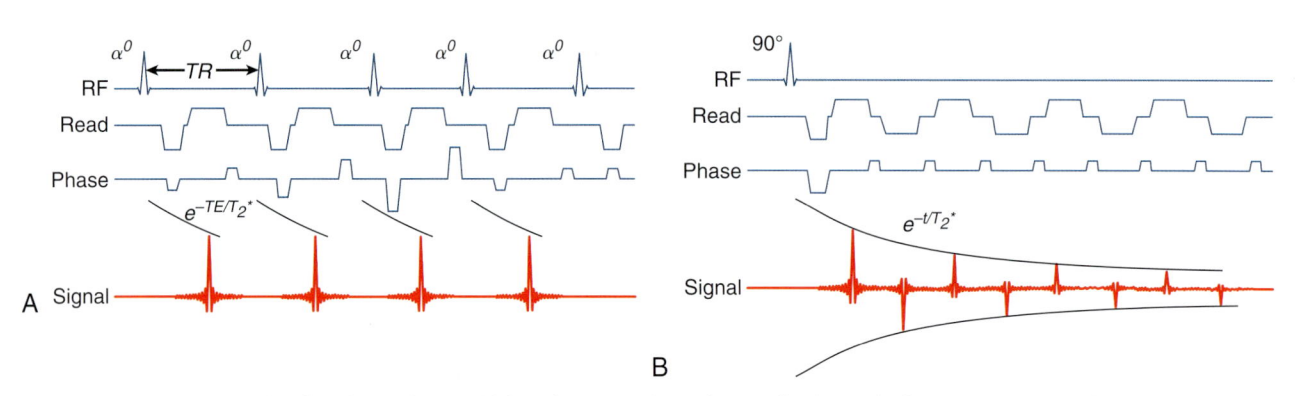

FIGURE 13-20 A, Conventional gradient-echo acquisition where one echo or k-space line is acquired per RF excitation pulse. To maintain higher SNR, a low flip angle ($\alpha < 90$ degrees) is used. B, In contrast, EPI acquires multiple echoes for a single RF excitation pulse. The gradient echo is refocused multiple times by gradient reversal, allowing multiple k-space lines to be acquired, increasing the acquisition efficiency. The echo amplitudes in an EPI train are modulated, however, by T_2^* decay.

real-time[54] EPI movie loops and high-quality phase contrast interleaved EPI images[15] of the heart. Interleaved EPI pulse sequences,[14,15] which employ multiple excitation pulses with interleaved k-space trajectories, were developed later to reduce the ETL, and minimize some of the artifacts associated with EPI sequences.

Improvements in gradient hardware also benefited another class of fast imaging sequence, balanced SSFP.[8,55] This method relies on balanced gradient waveforms and short TR to rewind coherently the magnetization after each readout, and avoid signal saturation effects that degrade other short TR sequences. Balanced SSFP images are characterized by relatively high SNR and bright blood signal, but require TR on the order of 3 ms or less (at 1.5 T) to avoid dark banding artifacts arising from off-resonance effects. The greater the inhomogeneity present, the shorter the TR times required.

Another class of imaging sequence replaces rectilinear k-space trajectories with curved paths that push the gradient slew rate (which can be viewed as the rate of change of motion along the trajectory) more evenly over the entire sequence. The most successful of these arguably has been the spiral trajectory[5,6] and its variants. The spiral trajectory can be traversed at a nonuniform angular rate to produce constant gradient amplitudes or slew rates, and maximize bandwidth.[56] The advantages of reduced echo times gained by interleaving in EPI also hold for interleaved spirals. Spirals have the further benefits of good flow characteristics[57] and relative insensitivity to motion,[58] making them especially useful for cardiac imaging. Off-resonance and susceptibility effects can affect image quality, however, and measures such as automated field-map calculation and correction in the image reconstruction are generally necessary to prevent regional image blurring.[59]

Parallel Imaging

The conventional approach to faster MRI pulse sequences, through reductions in the sequence TR time, is inherently limited by gradient amplitude and slew-rate constraints. These constraints arise partly from hardware limitations, but more fundamentally from the potential for peripheral nerve stimulation. A newer class of methods for speeding up MRI acquisitions, parallel imaging,[60,61] overcomes this limitation by shifting some of the responsibility for spatial encoding from the gradients to an array of RF receiver coils.[62] This shift removes the dependence for shortening scan times on reducing TR by instead reducing the amount of data to be collected.

In parallel imaging, k-space is undersampled (reducing the overall data required to reconstruct an image) to improve imaging speed. Normally, undersampling k-space results in aliased images in which signals from different locations appear (erroneously) to originate from the same pixel. Because the signal from each location is uniquely weighted in each coil element (with each coil element having different spatial sensitivity patterns), however, this feature can be used to distinguish each location's contribution to the aliased pixels, and unwrap the overlapping signals.

This method of undersampling k-space and using spatially arrayed RF coils to reconstruct artifact-free images is termed *parallel imaging*. Parallel imaging techniques fall into two classes: k-space-based techniques such as SMASH (simultaneous acquisition of spatial harmonics)[60] and GRAPPA (generalized autocalibrating partially parallel acquisitions),[63] and image-space–based methods such as SENSE (sensitivity encoding).[61] These techniques typically use either a separate acquisition first to generate spatial sensitivity maps for each coil or autocalibration, in which the center of k-space is fully sampled within an undersampled acquisition, and low-resolution sensitivity maps are generated from that portion of the data.

Early application of parallel imaging to the heart used the SMASH method in coronary MRI, to bring a factor of 2 improvement to breath-hold times, spatial resolution, or time resolution.[64] Soon after this, SENSE imaging with a half-Fourier segmented EPI sequence was applied to breath-hold and real-time imaging to accelerate scanning by factors up to 3.2, resulting in low spatial resolution images in times as short as 13 ms using six-element cardiac phased-array coils.[65,66] Acceleration factors are constrained by the number of spatially arrayed coil elements. The higher the acceleration factor, the greater the undersampling of k-space data, and the greater the reliance on more coil elements for spatial encoding. Exceeding the threshold acceleration factor for the number of coil elements present leads to decreased ability to unwrap aliased pixels.

As channel counts increased, 32-coil torso[67] and cardiac[68] arrays were used for cardiac MRI, enabling acceleration factors of 16 for whole heart imaging. This development allows all three main branches of the coronary tree to be captured in a single breath-hold (Fig. 13-21). Arrays with higher channel counts have also brought improved image quality for accelerated real-time balanced-SSFP imaging at frame rates of 50 frames per second, potentially enabling improved stress testing.[69] An example of real-time cardiac imaging with a 32-channel cardiac array is shown in Figure 13-22. Channel counts have since continued to increase beyond 32 to 128,[70,71] resulting in improved quality for highly accelerated breath-hold cardiac MRI. Cardiac imaging with 128 channels has been shown more recently to yield acceleration rates greater than 12 to 20.[72] Although coil losses and electrodynamics considerations seem to indicate that we may be nearing the useful limits of channel count (at least for field strengths of 1.5 to 3 T), more work remains to be done to explore the best use of high-channel cardiac MRI.

k-t Methods

In some cases, redundancies in the MRI signal acquired at different times in the cardiac cycle can be exploited to accelerate cardiac MRI effectively without the need for stronger gradients or multiple RF coils. In the earliest example of this, a sliding-window reconstruction was used to improve the effective frame rate of real-time fluoroscopic MRI.[73] In this method, as each new line (or group of lines) of k-space is acquired, it is combined with other, most recently acquired lines to compose a complete data

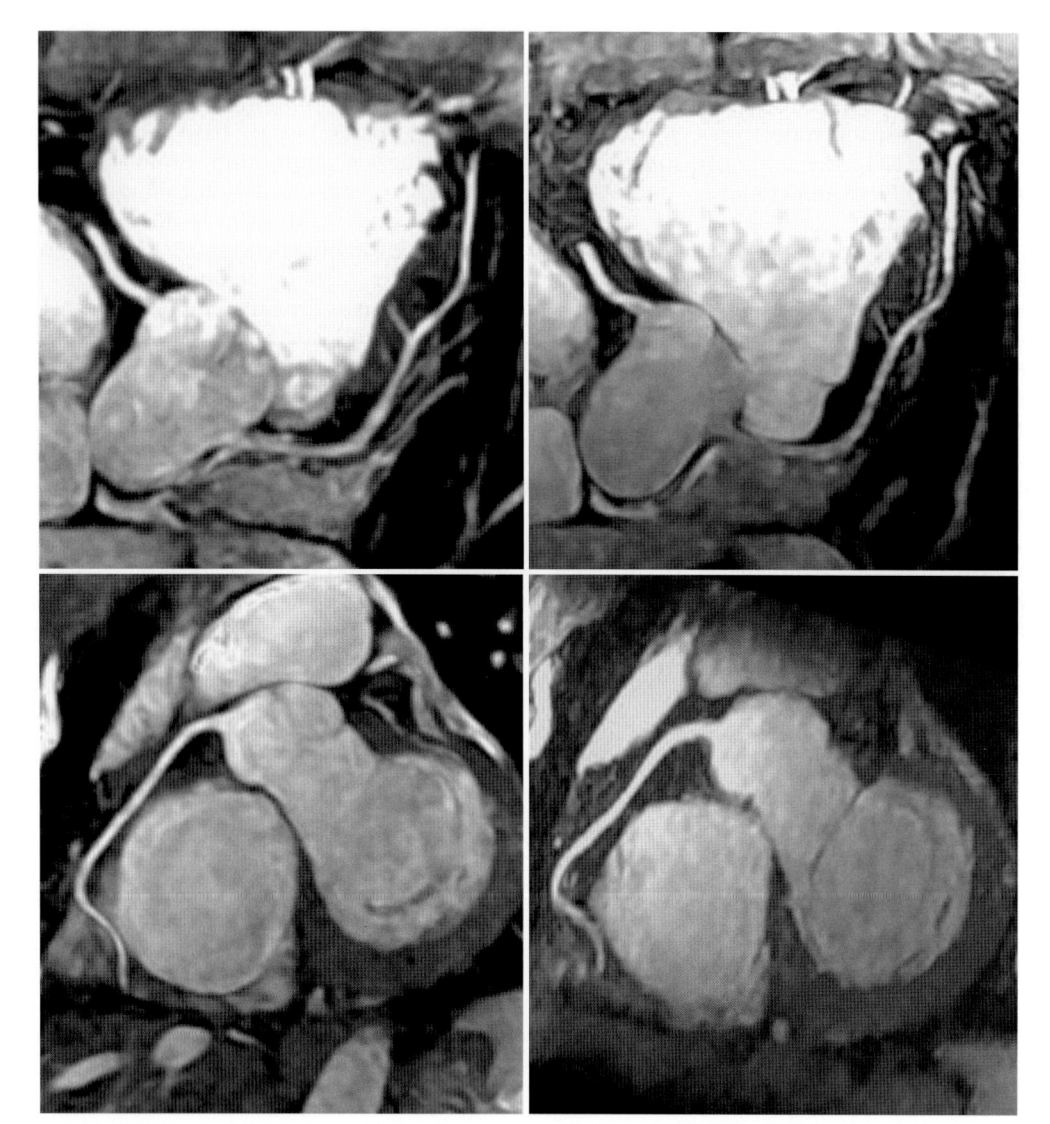

■ **FIGURE 13-21** Planar angiographic reformations of left main and left anterior descending (*top*) and right coronary artery (*bottom*) using conventional thin targeted three-dimensional slab approach (matrix size 256 × 256 × 12) (*left*) and eightfold (4 × 2) accelerated three-dimensional parallel MRI of whole heart (*right*). With an increased number of channels (32), higher acceleration factors can be used, allowing significantly higher spatial coverage (matrix size 256 × 256 × 60) for the same imaging time as for a lower channel count MRI system.

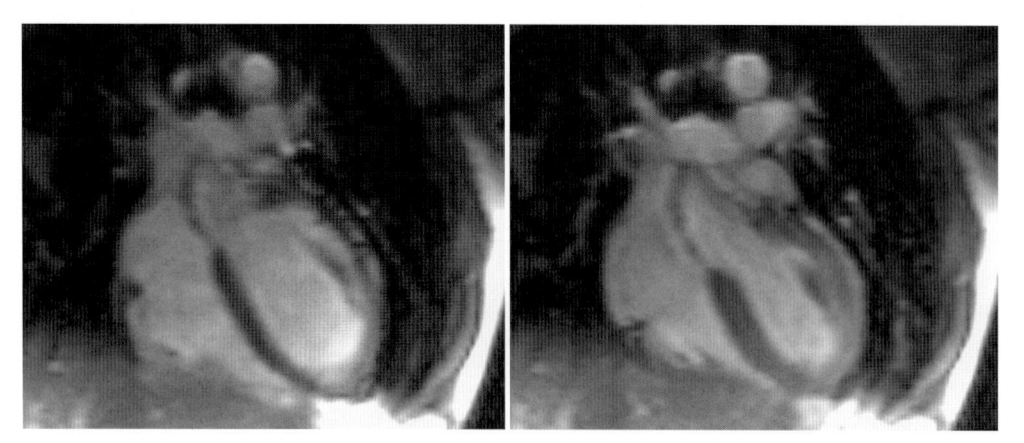

■ **FIGURE 13-22** Diastolic and systolic frames from real-time balanced SSFP four-chamber data set acquired at 22 frames per second. This acquisition used a 32-channel cardiac phased array coil with an acceleration factor of 2 in a 128 × 72 matrix in a 33-cm field of view.

set that is reconstructed to form an image for that point in time. In this way, the image reconstruction window is "slid" along in time, updating different parts of k-space at each new time point. Essentially, only a small but different portion of k-space is acquired at each time point, yielding a sparsely sampled k-t space (a data matrix with k-space along one dimension and time in the other). This method has also been applied to real-time cardiac MRI using interleaved spirals.[58]

In a more recent development called UNFOLD (unaliasing by Fourier-encoding the overlaps using the temporal dimension), data from the dynamic object (the beating heart) are made to populate k-t space in a denser, more efficient manner.[74] Specifically, the data are undersampled by a factor of 2 and acquired in a time series where every odd image in the series uses a sampling function shifted in k-space by half of a line spacing compared with that used for the even images. After reconstructing each undersampled k-space data set at each time point (Fourier transformation in the k-dimension), this results in the signal intensity of aliased pixels alternating in position (shifted by half an image field of view) in each time frame, while unaliased pixels remain constant. When the time frames are played out as in a movie loop, the aliased pixels appear to flicker (i.e., change with high temporal frequency), whereas the unaliased pixels are steady (i.e., they exhibit only low temporal frequencies). After reconstructing the k-t data set to a series of images in time, this yields a pixel (x)-time (t) data set (or x-t data set).

The time series of images can be Fourier transformed in the time domain to generate plots of signal intensity at each pixel (x) versus temporal frequency (f) (i.e., resulting in an x-f space data set). Assuming that the temporal frequency distribution of the aliased and unaliased signals do not overlap, applying a low-pass filter removes the contribution of the high temporal frequency aliased signal, preserving the low temporal frequency unaliased signal. An inverse Fourier transformation back into the time domain (of the low-pass filtered x-f data set) returns flicker-free and unaliased time-series images. An image acceleration factor of 2 can be achieved even if only a single coil element is used. The amount of acceleration that is possible with this technique depends on the frequency spectrum of the cardiac motion. A wider range of cardiac frequencies indicative of the cardiac motion implies the need to use a wider bandwidth low-pass filter, limiting the maximum extent of undersampling. This is because for UNFOLD to work, the high temporal frequency distribution of the aliased pixels must be distinct and separate from the imaged object.

A more generalized k-t approach does not rely on such separation of temporal frequency data. This technique, called k-t BLAST (broad-use linear acquisition speed-up technique),[75] enables much higher acceleration factors than UNFOLD, while similarly not being constrained by the number of coil elements. The principle of k-t BLAST is simple. The time-series MRI data are uniformly undersampled in k-t space (i.e., different parts of k-space are collected at different times to form a sheared grid pattern—"quasi" diamond pattern—in k-t space). On Fourier transformation of this undersampled k-t data set, a replication of objects in the corresponding x-f space is obtained (i.e., pixels are aliased). Fully sampled data would yield x-f space that has fairly localized signal with noise everywhere else (i.e., pixels are not aliased). In the undersampled case, the object in x-f space is replicated throughout, and may overlap. This is in contrast to the case of UNFOLD, where the aliased or replicated objects do not overlap with the primary object. Because the replicated objects may overlap, the use of a low-pass filter as in UNFOLD would also remove data from the unaliased pixels. A much better method to remove the aliased pixels is needed.

The k-t BLAST technique uses a calibration scan or training data set to provide the necessary information to remove the aliased pixels in x-f space. By using a low spatial resolution fully sampled training data set (where there are no replicated objects), the areas of background noise in x-f space can be correctly identified to provide an expected background noise level. By comparing the expected noise level in each pixel in x-f space between that of the undersampled data set and the training data set, a reconstruction approach that minimizes the difference between the expected and measured noise levels effectively unwraps the aliased signals at each point in x-f space.

An inverse Fourier transformation back to k-t space yields an approximation of a fully sampled set that can be reconstructed normally to obtain alias-free images. In this manner, eightfold acceleration for cardiac imaging with reduced artifacts relative to a sliding-window reconstruction has been achieved without the use of multiple element phased-array coils.[75,76]

Real-Time MRI

Rapid imaging pulse sequences are most useful when employed in the context of a system capable of high-speed reconstruction, real-time image display, and interactive scan-plane control. Such a setup was first developed and demonstrated by Wright et al.,[77] who used a workstation and array processor connected to a conventional MRI scanner. Other systems were developed later to enable real-time graphic control of the scan plane, or control by the use of three-dimensional hardware controllers.[78,79] Real-time interactive MRI systems have been applied to coronary MRI,[80] evaluation of left-ventricular function, MRI color flow,[81] and interventional guidance,[82] among other applications in the heart, and commercial real-time MRI systems are now widely available.

Because not all patients are able to maintain short breath-holds repeatedly over an extended time, real-time imaging provides an alternative that allows the completion of a cardiac examination with image quality sufficient for diagnosis. MRI system improvements, including faster imaging techniques and higher receiver channel counts, provide opportunities for real-time acquisition with significant advantages in temporal resolution, while improving spatial resolution. Real-time systems can also be essential enablers for new MR cardiac applications, such as pharmacologic or physical (e.g., bicycle or hand grip exercise) stress testing.

KEY POINTS

- Methods for imaging the heart using MRI are described. Descriptions on how cine images of the heart can be obtained over several cardiac cycles, and the basics for acquiring images that provide information on myocardial viability, perfusion, and cardiac wall motion are provided.
- In addition to soft tissue contrast, functional information can be obtained with MRI. Specifically, MRI is able to acquire images with information on the direction and velocity of flow. This information allows measurements of flow volumes and other physiologic indicators of cardiovascular disease.
- Image acquisition times are currently longer than the periods of cardiac motion. Several cardiac cycles are required to acquire sufficient data to reconstruct images depicting the heart at different cardiac phases. Fast imaging techniques using parallel acceleration that reduce the k-space data requirements for image reconstruction have substantially sped up image acquisition. With a larger number of receiver coils, high acceleration factors permit real-time image acquisition with acceptable spatial resolution; this allows imaging with the patient breathing freely throughout image acquisition, rather than requiring repeated breath-holding.

SUGGESTED READINGS

Earls JP, Ho VB, Foo TK, et al. Cardiac MRI: recent progress and continued challenges. J Magn Reson Imag 2002; 16:111-127.

Lima JAC, Milind DY. Cardiovascular magnetic resonance imaging: current and emerging applications. J Am Coll Cardiol 2004; 44:1164-1171.

Pruessmann KP. Encoding and reconstruction in parallel MRI. NMR Biomed 2006; 19:288-299.

REFERENCES

1. Mansfield P, Pykett I. Biological and medical imaging by NMR. J Magn Reson 1978; 29:355-373.
2. Young I. Nuclear magnetic resonance systems. US patent 4,355,282. 1979.
3. Rzedzian RR, Pykett IL. Instant images of the human heart using a new, whole-body MR imaging system. AJR Am J Roentgenol 1987; 149:245-250.
4. Semelka RC, Kelekis NL, Thomasson D, et al. HASTE MR imaging: description of technique and preliminary results in the abdomen. J Magn Reson Imaging 1996; 6:698-699.
5. Likes R. Moving gradient zeugmatography. US patent 4,307,343 August 1979.
6. Meyer CH, Hu BS, Nishimura DG, et al. Fast spiral coronary artery imaging. Magn Reson Med 1992; 28:202-213.
7. Atkinson DJ, Edelman RR. Cineangiography of the heart in a single breath hold with a segmented turboFLASH sequence. Radiology 1991; 178:357-360.
8. Oppelt A, Graumann R, Barfuss H, et al. FISP—a new fast MRI sequence. Electromedica 1986; 54:15-18.
9. Barkhausen J, Ruehm SG, Goyen M, et al. MR evaluation of ventricular function: true fast imaging with steady-state precession versus fast low-angle shot cine MR imaging: feasibility study. Radiology 2001; 219:264-269.
10. Foo TKF, Bernstein MA, Aisen AM, et al. Improved ejection fraction and flow velocity estimates with use of view sharing and uniform repetition time excitation with fast cardiac techniques. Radiology 1995; 195:471-478.
11. Feinstein JA, Epstein FH, Arai AE, et al. Using cardiac phase to order reconstruction (CAPTOR): a method to improve diastolic images. J Magn Reson Imaging 1997; 7:794-798.
12. Simonetti OP, Finn JP, White RD, et al. "Black blood" T2-weighted inversion-recovery MR imaging of the heart. Radiology 1996; 199:49-57.
13. Saranathan M, Slavin GS. Quadrupled efficiency for black blood imaging using slice-pair interleaving (abstract). Proceedings of the 11th meeting of the International Society of Magnetic Resonance in Medicine, Toronto, Canada, July 2003.
14. McKinnon GC. Ultrafast interleaved gradient-echo-planar imaging on a standard scanner. Magn Reson Med 1993; 30:609-616.
15. McKinnon GC, Debatin JF, Wetter DR, et al. Interleaved echo planar flow quantitation. Magn Reson Med 1994; 32:263-267.
16. Ding S, Wolff SD, Epstein FH. Improved coverage in dynamic contrast-enhanced cardiac MRI using interleaved gradient-echo EPI. Magn Reson Med 1998; 39:514-519.
17. Klocke FJ, Simonetti OP, Judd RM, et al. Limits of detection of regional differences in vasodilated flow in viable myocardium by first-pass magnetic resonance perfusion imaging. Circulation 2001; 104:2412-2416.
18. Schreiber WG, Schmitt M, Kalden P, et al. Dynamic contrast-enhanced myocardial perfusion imaging using saturation-prepared TrueFISP. J Magn Reson Imaging 2002; 16:641-652.
19. Foo TK, Wu KC, Azevedo CF, et al. Partial Fourier steady-state free precession (FIESTA) first-pass perfusion with improved image quality and efficient spatial coverage (abstract). Proceedings of the 12th Annual Meeting International Society of Magnetic Resonance in Medicine, Kyoto, Japan, May 2004.
20. Bertschinger KM, Nanz D, Buechi M, et al. Magnetic resonance myocardial first-pass perfusion imaging: parameter optimization for signal response and cardiac coverage. J Magn Reson Imaging 2001; 14:556-562.
21. Slavin GS, Wolff SD, Gupta SN, et al. First-pass myocardial perfusion MR imaging with interleaved notched saturation: feasibility study. Radiology 2001; 219:258-263.
22. Di Bella EV, Parker DL, Sinusas AJ. On the dark rim artifact in dynamic contrast-enhanced MRI myocardial perfusion studies. Magn Reson Med 2005; 54:1295-1299.
23. Lima JA, Judd RM, Bazille A, et al. Regional heterogeneity of human myocardial infarcts demonstrated by contrast-enhanced MRI: potential mechanisms. Circulation 1995; 92:1117-1125.
24. Kim RJ, Wu E, Rafael A, et al. The use of contrast-enhanced magnetic resonance imaging to identify reversible myocardial dysfunction. N Engl J Med 2000; 343:1445-1453.
25. Simonetti OP, Kim RJ, Fieno DS, et al. An improved MR imaging technique for the visualization of myocardial infarction. Radiology 2001; 218:215-223.
26. Kellman P, Arau AE, McVeigh ER, et al. Phase-sensitive inversion recovery for detecting myocardial infarction using gadolinium-delayed hyperenhancement. Magn Reson Med 2002; 47:272-283.

27. Setser RM, Chung YC, Weaver JA, et al. Effect of inversion time on delayed-enhancement magnetic resonance imaging with and without phase-sensitive reconstruction. J Magn Reson Imaging 2005; 21:650-655.
28. Ho VB, Hood MN, Montequin M, et al. cine inversion recovery (IR): rapid tool for optimized myocardial delayed enhancement imaging (abstract). Proceedings of the 13th Annual Meeting International Society of Magnetic Resonance in Medicine, Miami, May 2005.
29. Setser RM, Kim JK, Chung YC, et al. Cine delayed-enhancement MR imaging of the heart: initial experience. Radiology 2006; 239:856-862.
30. Huber A, Schoenberg SO, Spannagl B, et al. Single-shot inversion recovery TrueFISP for assessment of myocardial infarction. AJR Am J Roentgenol 2006; 186:627-633.
31. Sievers B, Elliott MD, Hurwitz LM, et al. Rapid detection of myocardial infarction by subsecond, free-breathing delayed contrast-enhancement cardiovascular magnetic resonance. Circulation 2007; 115:236-244.
32. Foo TK, Stanley DW, Castillo E, et al. Myocardial viability: breath-hold 3D MR imaging of delayed hyperenhancement with variable sampling in time. Radiology 2004; 230:845-851.
33. Saranathan M, Rochitte CE, Foo TK. Fast, three-dimensional free-breathing MR imaging of myocardial infarction: a feasibility study. Magn Reson Med 2004; 51:1055-1060.
34. Tatli S, Zou KH, Fruitman M, et al. Three-dimensional magnetic resonance imaging technique for myocardial-delayed hyperenhancement: a comparison with the two-dimensional technique. J Magn Reson Imaging 2004; 20:378-382.
35. Tandri H, Saranathan M, Rodriguez ER, et al. Noninvasive detection of myocardial fibrosis in arrhythmogenic right ventricular cardiomyopathy using delayed-enhancement magnetic resonance imaging. J Am Coll Cardiol 2005; 45:98-103.
36. Zerhouni EA, Parish DM, Rogers WJ, et al. Human heart: tagging with MR imaging—a method for noninvasive assessment of myocardial motion. Radiology 1988;169:59-63.
37. Axel L, Dougherty L. MR imaging of motion with spatial modulation of magnetization. Radiology 1989; 171:841-845.
38. Axel L, Dougherty L. Heart wall motion: improved method of spatial modulation of magnetization for MR imaging. Radiology 1989; 172:349-350.
39. Osman NF, Kerwin WS, McVeigh ER, et al. Cardiac motion tracking using cine harmonic phase (HARP) magnetic resonance imaging. Magn Reson Med 1999; 42:1048-1060.
40. Aletras AH, Ding S, Balaban RS, et al. DENSE: displacement encoding with stimulated echoes in cardiac functional MRI. J Magn Reson 1999; 137:247-252.
41. Weben OM, Martin AJ, Higgins CB. Whole-heart steady-state free precession coronary artery magnetic resonance angiography. Magn Reson Med 2003; 50:1223-1228.
42. Wielopolski PA, van Geuns RJ, de Feyter PJ, et al. Breath-hold coronary MR angiography with volume-targeted imaging. Radiology 1998; 209:209-219.
43. Stuber M, Botnar RM, Danias PG, et al. Double-oblique free-breathing high resolution three-dimensional coronary magnetic resonance angiography. J Am Coll Cardiol 1999; 34:524-531.
44. Foo TKF, Ho VB, Saranathan M, et al. High spatial resolution 3D breath-held coronary artery imaging: feasibility of integration with myocardial perfusion and viability studies. Radiology 2005; 235:1025-1030.
45. Ehman RL, Felmlee JP. Adaptive technique for high-definition MR imaging of moving structures. Radiology 1989; 173:255-263.
46. Stuber M, Botnar RM, Danias PG, et al. Submillimeter three-dimensional coronary MR angiography with real-time navigator correction: comparison of navigator locations. Radiology 1999; 212:579-587.
47. Etienne A, Botnar RM, Van Muiswinkel AM, et al. "Soap-Bubble" visualization and quantitative analysis of 3D coronary magnetic resonance angiograms. Magn Reson Med 2002; 48:658-666.
48. Taylor AM, Jhooti P, Wiesmann F, et al. MR navigator-echo monitoring of temporal changes in diaphragm position: implications for MR coronary angiography. J Magn Reson Imaging 1997; 7:629-636.
49. Moran PR. A flow velocity zeugmatographic interlace for NMR imaging in humans. Magn Reson Imaging 1982; 1:197-203.
50. Nayler GL, Firmin DN, Longmore DB. Blood flow imaging by cine magnetic resonance. J Comp Assist Tomogr 1986; 10:715-722.
51. Dumoulin CL, Souza SP, Walker MF. Three-dimensional phase contrast angiography. Magn Reson Med 1989; 9:139-149.
52. Sechtem U, Pflugfelder P, Cassidy MC, et al. Ventricular septal defect: visualization of shunt flow and determination of shunt size by cine MR imaging. AJR Am J Roentgenol 1987; 149:689-692.
53. Beerbaum P, Korperich H, Barth P, et al. Noninvasive quantification of left-to-right shunt in pediatric patients: phase-contrast cine magnetic resonance imaging compared with invasive oximetry. Circulation 2001; 103:2476-2482.
54. Chapman B, Turner R, Ordidge RJ, et al. Real-time movie imaging from a single cardiac cycle by NMR. Magn Reson Med 1987; 5:246-254.
55. Patz S, Hawkes RC. The application of steady-state free precession to the study of very slow fluid flow. Magn Reson Med 1986; 3:140-145.
56. Hardy C, Cline H. Broadband nuclear magnetic resonance pulses with two-dimensional spatial selectivity. J Appl Phys 1989; 66:1513-1516.
57. Nishimura DG, Irarrazabal P, Meyer CH. A velocity k-space analysis of flow effects in echo-planar and spiral imaging. Magn Reson Med 1995; 33:549-556.
58. Kerr AB, Pauly JM, Hu BS, et al. Real-time interactive MRI on a conventional scanner. Magn Reson Med 1997; 38:355-367.
59. Irarrazabal P, Hu BS, Pauly JM, et al. Spatially resolved and localized real-time velocity distribution. Magn Reson Med 1993; 30:207-212.
60. Sodickson DK, Manning WJ. Simultaneous acquisition of spatial harmonics (SMASH): fast imaging with radiofrequency coil arrays. Magn Reson Med 1997; 38:591-603.
61. Pruessmann KP, Weiger M, Scheidegger MB, et al. SENSE: sensitivity encoding for fast MRI. Magn Reson Med 1999; 42:952-962.
62. Roemer PB, Edelstein WA, Hayes CE, et al. The NMR phased array. Magn Reson Med 1990; 16:192-225.
63. Griswold MA, Jakob PM, Heidemann RM, et al. Generalized autocalibrating partially parallel acquisitions (GRAPPA). Magn Reson Med 2002; 47:1202-1210.
64. Jakob PM, Griswold MA, Edelman RR, et al. Accelerated cardiac imaging using the SMASH technique. J Cardiovasc Magn Reson 1999; 1:153-157.
65. Weiger M, Pruessmann KP, Boesiger P. Cardiac real-time imaging using SENSE. SENsitivity Encoding scheme. Magn Reson Med 2000; 43:177-184.
66. Pruessmann KP, Weiger M, Boesiger P. Sensitivity encoded cardiac MRI. J Cardiovasc Magn Reson 2001; 3:1-9.
67. Niendorf T, Hardy CJ, Giaquinto RO, et al. Toward single breath-hold whole-heart coverage coronary MRA using highly accelerated parallel imaging with a 32-channel MR system. Magn Reson Med 2006; 56:167-176.
68. Hardy CJ, Cline HE, Giaquinto RO, et al. 32-element receiver-coil array for cardiac imaging. Magn Reson Med 2006; 55:1142-1149.
69. Hardy CJ, Darrow RD, Marinelli L, et al. 32-channel real-time MRI at ~50 frames per sec for irregular heart motion (abstract). Proceedings of the 14th Annual Meeting International Society of Magnetic Resonance in Medicine, Seattle, May 2006.
70. Schmitt M, Potthast A, Sosnovik DE, et al. A 128-channel receive-only cardiac coil for highly accelerated cardiac MRI at 3 Tesla. Magn Reson Med 2008; 59:1431-1439.
71. Hardy CJ, Giaquinto RO, Piel JE, et al. 128-channel body MRI with a flexible high-density receiver-coil array. J Magn Reson Imaging 2008; 28:1219-1225.
72. Shankaranarayanan A, Fung M, Beatty P, et al. 128-channel highly-accelerated breath-held 3D coronary MR imaging. Proceedings of the 16th annual meeting of ISMRM, Toronto, 2008.
73. Riederer SJ, Tasciyan T, Farzaneh F, et al. MR fluoroscopy: technical feasibility. Magn Reson Med 1988; 8:1-15.
74. Madore B, Glover GH, Pelc NJ. Unaliasing by Fourier-encoding the overlaps using the temporal dimension (UNFOLD), applied to cardiac imaging and fMRI. Magn Reson Med 1999; 42:813-828.
75. Tsao J, Boesiger P, Pruessmann KP. k-t BLAST and k-t SENSE: dynamic MRI with high frame rate exploiting spatiotemporal correlations. Magn Reson Med 2003; 50:1031-1042.

76. Tsao J, Kozerke S, Boesiger P, et al. Optimizing spatiotemporal sampling for k-t BLAST and k-t SENSE: application to high-resolution real-time cardiac steady-state free precession. Magn Reson Med 2005; 53:1372-1382.
77. Wright RC, Riederer SJ, Farzaneh F, et al. Real-time MR fluoroscopic data acquisition and image reconstruction. Magn Reson Med 1989; 12:407-415.
78. Hardy CJ, Darrow RD, Nieters EJ, et al. Real-time acquisition, display, and interactive graphic control of NMR cardiac profiles and images. Magn Reson Med 1993; 29:667-673.
79. Debbins JP, Riederer SJ, Rossman PJ, et al. Cardiac magnetic resonance fluoroscopy. Magn Reson Med 1996; 36:588-595.
80. Hardy CJ, Darrow RD, Pauly JM, et al. Interactive coronary MRI. Magn Reson Med 1998; 40:105-111.
81. Nayak KS, Pauly JM, Kerr AB, et al. Real-time color flow MRI. Magn Reson Med 2000; 43:251-258.
82. Guttman MA, Lederman RJ, Sorger JM, et al. Real-time volume rendered MRI for interventional guidance. J Cardiovasc Magn Reson 2002; 4:431-442.

CHAPTER 14

Clinical Techniques of Cardiac Magnetic Resonance Imaging: Morphology, Perfusion, and Viability

Louis Wu and Gautham P. Reddy

Cardiac magnetic resonance imaging (MRI) is still experiencing the rapid upstroke of its growth phase as novel hardware, software, and processing techniques have brought it to the forefront of imaging cardiac diseases. The information provided by a single examination can include a detailed assessment of morphology, tissue characterization, and quantitative physiology. It is these advances and the validation of the newer techniques that have allowed MRI to move from the realm of a research tool and peripheral clinical use to the primary imaging tool of the heart.

This chapter will introduce some of these technical advances in software. The discussions will highlight indications and common techniques as well as some practical information; more detailed information will follow in chapters dedicated to perfusion and viability imaging.

TECHNICAL REQUIREMENTS: MOTION COMPENSATION

The ability to compensate for motion, both cardiac and respiratory in origin, is critical to successful MR imaging of the heart. As newer generations of cardiac scanners, with software and hardware advances, have become increasingly available, the motion obstacle can be better resolved. One of the most important obstacles for MRI to overcome has been the ability to image quickly enough to overcome the limited window of opportunity to produce snapshot images of a motionless heart. The implementation of electrocardiographic gating remains one of the most significant advances to facilitating imaging in this respect. This has been further optimized by the addition of k-space segmentation (Fig. 14-1).

In electrocardiographic triggering, data acquisition is synchronized to the cardiac cycle. The R wave is used as a starting point from which a defined trigger delay can be timed to acquire a portion of k-space. The trigger delay is typically set at mid-diastole, where minimal motion occurs.[1] This partitioning allows each package of data to be acquired in a short time interval, ideally less than 50 ms, and therefore without motion degradation. In k-space segmentation, the full complement of k-space data is compiled by imaging over several successive cardiac cycles, each of which contributes its respective portion of information. Electrocardiographic triggering can be implemented in a prospective fashion, where the R wave is an actual trigger for data acquisition. More often, however, retrospective triggering is used, in which the R wave is a marker for sorting information already acquired through the entire R-R interval. The latter allows complete diastolic phase imaging, which is important in accurate functional assessment for which end-systolic and end-diastolic views of the cine sequence are required.

Electrocardiographic gating may be impaired in patients with large thoracic cavities, such as in emphysema, or when large pericardial effusions decrease the electrical signal. Another artifact, the magnetohydrodynamic effect, occurs when ions contained within blood pass through the magnetic field, inducing a voltage that distorts the electrocardiographic tracing. This particular limitation can be minimized with an optimized version of gating available through vector electrocardiography, which is

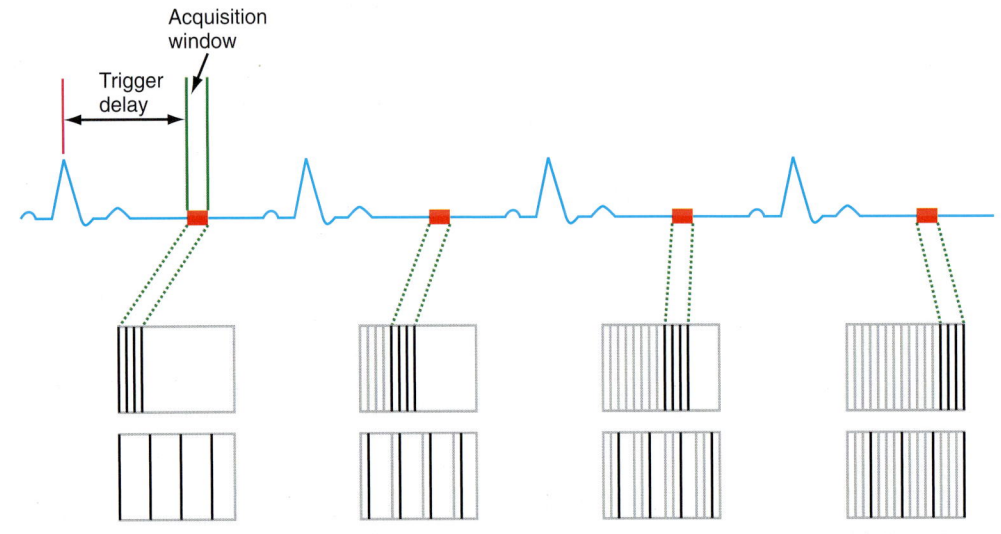

■ **FIGURE 14-1** Electrocardiographic triggering and k-space segmentation. Data collection occurs during a restricted acquisition window at a fixed trigger delay following each R wave on the electrocardiogram (ECG). Different segments of the data matrix required for image generation are acquired during different cardiac cycles and the pieces are combined to yield a full data set. Two possible strategies for the order of data collection are shown in the two rows below the ECG tracing. In both cases, *vertical black lines* represent data acquired during the current cardiac cycle, whereas *gray lines* represent data from previous cycles. (Adapted from Manning WJ, Pennell DJ. Cardiovascular Magnetic Resonance Imaging. Philadelphia, Churchill-Livingstone, 2002.)

less prone to distortion of the cardiac tracing by the magnetohydrodynamic effect.[2]

The second significant motion hurdle to overcome has been the elimination of respiratory artifacts. This has been addressed in abdominal imaging by using breath-holding during image acquisition, when possible, and has been adapted to MRI as well. Although this produces excellent image quality with fast imaging techniques such as turbo field echo and echo-planar imaging, there remain limitations. Breath-hold reproducibility can be low, resulting in potential slice misregistration in multislice acquisitions. This is particularly problematic in left ventricular function assessment on short-axis cine imaging. Instructing patients to breath-hold at end-expiration has been shown to provide the most consistent data and to minimize variability in position.[3] Breath-hold imaging is also limited by the amount of time that can be spent on other aspects of the image quality, such as the signal-to-noise ratio (SNR) and spatial and temporal resolution. This limitation is in part offset by parallel imaging techniques that can speed up imaging and provide magnetic resonance (MR) currency of time, which can be used for optimization of other imaging parameters.

Certain patients have difficulty with breath-holding, particularly those with cardiac and/or respiratory diseases, and then other compensation techniques must be considered. Free-breathing techniques include compensation by respiratory bellows gating. In this approach, an air-filled bellow within a belt placed around the abdomen converts information about respiration into a pressure tracing that can be used to infer cardiac position (from diaphragm position, which in turn is inferred by chest wall position).

Multiple signal averages can be used to minimize motion artifacts in free-breathing techniques. This can be used alone or combined with the techniques described. In this scenario, patients are allowed to free-breathe with repeated imaging to increase the SNR and minimize any individual motion artifact by averaging out any occasional motion.

More recently, an alternate method for respiratory compensation has been developed in the form of the navigator echo technique (Fig. 14-2). First described by Ehman and Felmlee,[4] this technique uses an interleaved column of excitation perpendicular to the direction of motion for assessment of tissue displacement. The navigator echo is typically prescribed at interfaces with high tissue contrast; such as the right hemidiaphragm, where signal is compared to a reference echo for displacement. Information on displacement can then be used to select echoes for image reconstruction that reflect nonmotion. The scan efficiency depends on operator-dependent factors such as stringency of gating criteria, with windows of 3 to 5 mm being typical for acceptance or rejection of echo information. The larger the acceptance window, the higher the efficiency and shorter overall acquisition time, but with consequent increase in motion blurring. Other factors that can be manipulated in the navigator technique include prospective versus retrospective acquisition and the number of navigator echoes acquired, with a resulting balance between image quality and time efficiency. By avoiding breath-holding in this technique, patient comfort and compliance are improved. One of the primary advantages of the navigator technique is the ability to spend time currency to improve SNR and spatial resolution.

Limitations to navigator techniques include respiratory drift of the diaphragm beyond the acceptance window, which occurs in patients who fall asleep or are anxious during the early part of an examination but later settle into a different rhythm.[5] Careful monitoring of patients' breathing patterns and keeping them alert during the scan acquisition can minimize respiratory drift. Further improvements

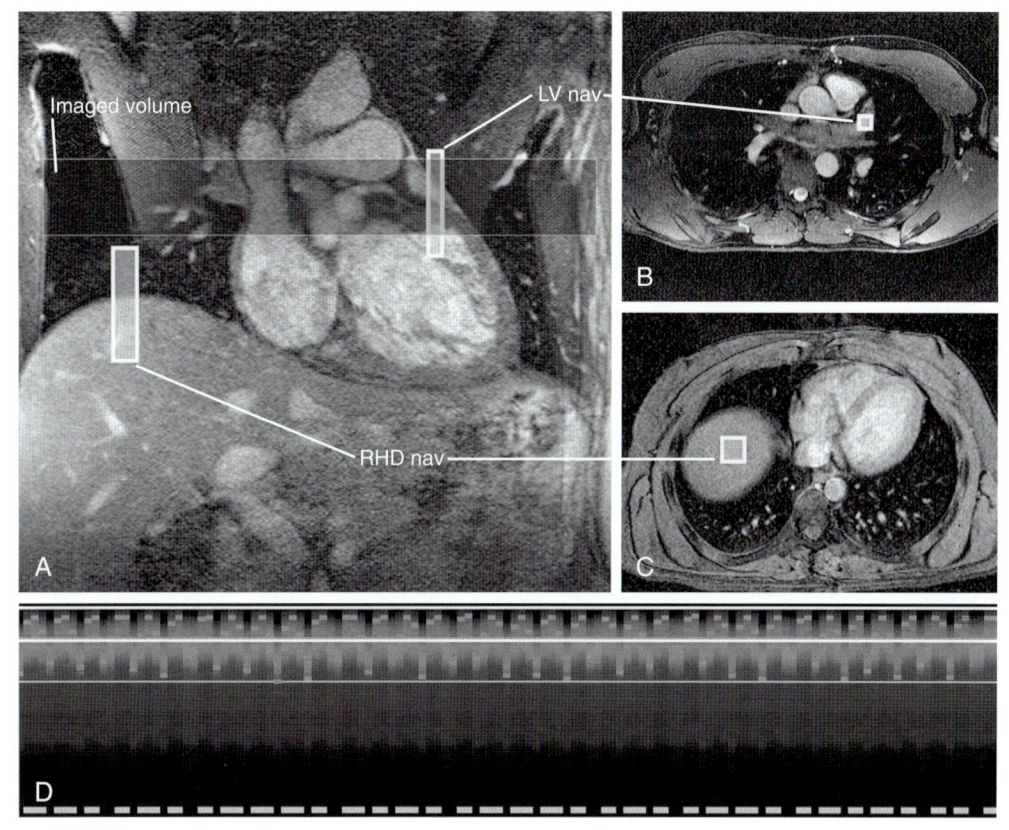

FIGURE 14-2 Navigator echo gating. One or more columns of magnetization traversing a tissue interface are excited using a tailored excitation sequence, and the displacements of the interface are calculated and used as a measure of respiratory motion. **A**, Coronal scout image showing two possible placements of the navigator echo excitation, one through the right hemidiaphragm (RHD NAV), and one through the left ventricular free wall (LV NAV). The navigator excitation may or may not overlap the imaged volume. **B**, Transverse scout image showing the LV NAV in cross section. **C**, Transverse scout image in a more caudal plane showing the RHD NAV in cross section. **D**, Sample navigator echo tracing, with navigator signal on the vertical axis shown as a function of time on the horizontal axis. Respiration results in a cyclic motion of the tissue interface. *Gray dots* superimposed on the tracing represent automatically detected interface positions in successive cardiac cycles. *Thick white lines* indicate the gating acceptance window. In a prospective gating strategy, only cardiac cycles in which the interface position falls within this range (indicated also by *gray bars* at the bottom of the tracing) are used for data acquisition. *Thin white lines* on either side of the acceptance window indicate a range or kernel used by the automatic interface detection algorithm. *(From Manning WJ, Pennell DJ. Cardiovascular Magnetic Resonance Imaging. Philadelphia, Churchill-Livingstone, 2002.)*

have been made to the navigator technique specifically for coronary MR angiography (MRA) by phase ordering.

Development continues in the area of real-time cardiac imaging, in which cine imaging is acquired throughout respiration. This allows for assessment of additional aspects of physiologic changes in cardiac function related to phases of respiration not obtained by conventional breath-hold cine techniques. However, real-time imaging of the heart remains beyond routine clinical practice at this time.

TECHNIQUES

Anatomic Overview

Indications

Cardiac examinations generally begin with a morphologic overview of the heart, pericardium, mediastinum, and great vessels. T1-weighted images provide an excellent overview of this anatomy and thus remain standard in most MRI protocols. Tissue characterization can also be performed on T1-weighted images, looking for fat in entities such as arrhythmogenic right ventricular dysplasia or cardiac mass lesions. T2-weighted images, which can further characterize focal masses, are now demonstrating increased usefulness for several clinical diseases, often reflecting edema in the myocardium. This can be especially helpful in ischemic heart disease, in which differentiation of acute from chronic infarcts, which can look similar on viability sequences (see later), can be made by the presence of a bright T2 signal in the acute scar.[6] Similarly, T2 edema can be identified in areas of disease involvement in acute myocarditis[7] and nonischemic cardiomyopathy.[8]

MRI has also been demonstrated to be useful in the noninvasive assessment of cardiac iron overload. Patients with thalassemia, for example, may have transfusion-related iron overload. The presence of iron has prognostic implications for these patients with an increased risk of heart failure. Iron deposition in the heart is also an important cause for mortality in this patient population compared with other organs. Early detection can be difficult by serum ferritin measurements, which are not necessarily reflective of myocardial content, and routine biopsy of the myocardium is not feasible. T2*-weighted imaging can provide noninvasive measures of iron deposition in the myocardium, with correlation to deterioration in ventricular function.[9]

Technique Description

Turbo spin-echo (TSE) sequences are most commonly used for routine morphologic assessment. In contrast to other anatomic locations, the TSE sequence in cardiac imaging is modified by the implementation of a dual inversion preparatory pulse that produces black blood (BB) images. The absence of signal in the blood pool is achieved by using a selective and nonselective 180-degree inversion pulse, which is followed by a long inversion time chosen to null blood magnetization (Fig. 14-3). These preparatory pulses are followed by a gated TSE readout with k-space segmentation. This can be performed with either breath-holding or free-breathing.

The black blood pulse produces good myocardium–blood pool differentiation. These static images are of high SNR, with good tissue contrast (Fig. 14-4). Furthermore, image parameters are easily manipulated to allow for T1- or T2-weighted tissue characterization. If fat saturation is required, an additional selective 180-degree inversion pulse can be added with a short inversion time to null fat, also known as STIR (short tau inversion recovery).

Single-shot TSE or half-Fourier acquisition single-shot turbo spin-echo (HASTE) imaging can provide significant reduction in imaging time and shorten breath-holding. The rapid acquisition is achieved by long echo train lengths and half-Fourier reconstruction but results in a tradeoff in SNR. This type of sequence may be useful for patients who cannot breath-hold and for whom respiratory gating techniques have failed. Manual triggering during end-expiration with these subsecond single images can yield diagnostic scans.

When evaluating iron content in myocardium, one can assess the degree of deposition by the shortening in relaxation times on T2* sequences. Myocardial T2* sequences are obtained at varying TE times to calculate the degree of signal loss relative to normal muscle. Decay curves derived from these images can provide information on the presence and severity of myocardial iron content.

Pitfalls and Solutions

Signal loss in the myocardium can occur when the BB pulse is too thick and oversaturation of tissue occurs within the slice of interest. Decreasing the thickness of the BB pulse can prevent this artifactual oversaturation of normal tissue. In contrast, poor blood pool nulling may occur as a result of an inadequate BB pulse above or below the slice of interest.

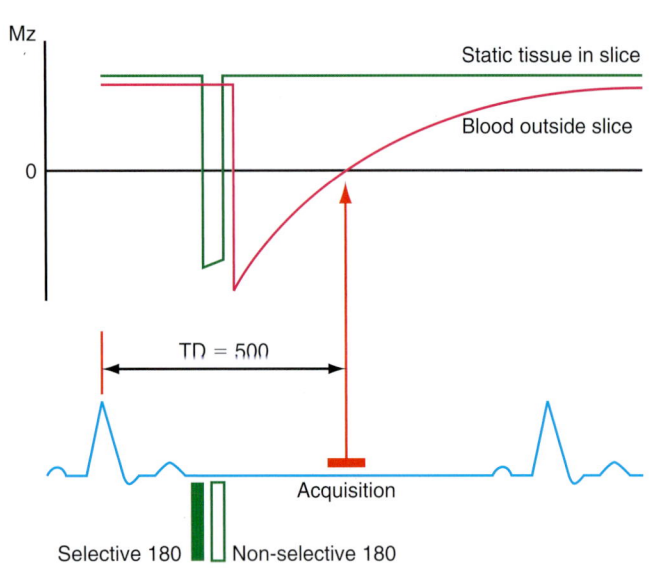

FIGURE 14-3 Schematic diagram of black blood pulse sequence.

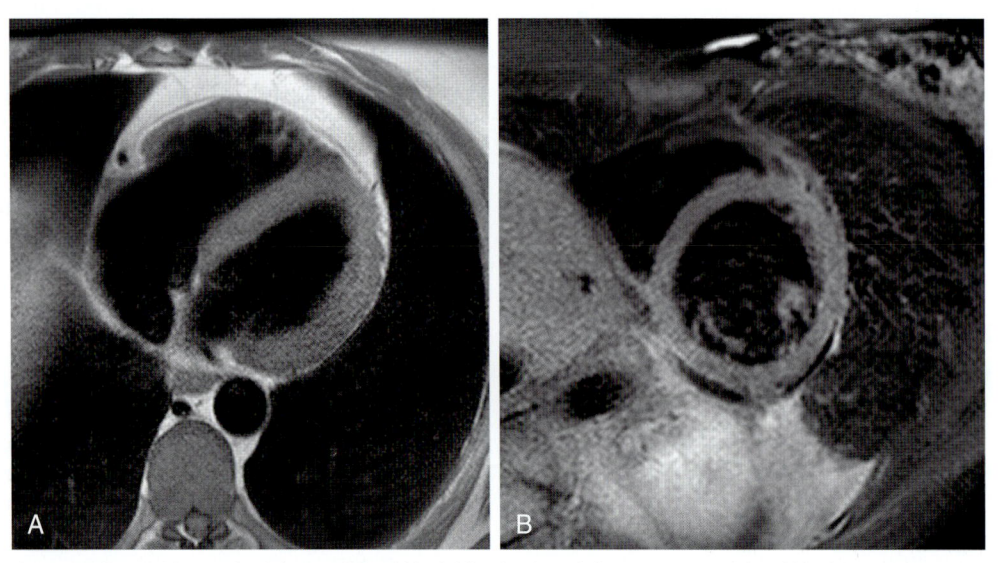

FIGURE 14-4 Electrocardiographic gated axial T1-weighted black blood (A) and short-axis T2-weighted black blood fat-saturated (B) images of the heart. Normal intermediate signal myocardium is identified with similar signal intensity to chest wall muscle. T2-weighted image also demonstrates intermediate signal intensity myocardium.

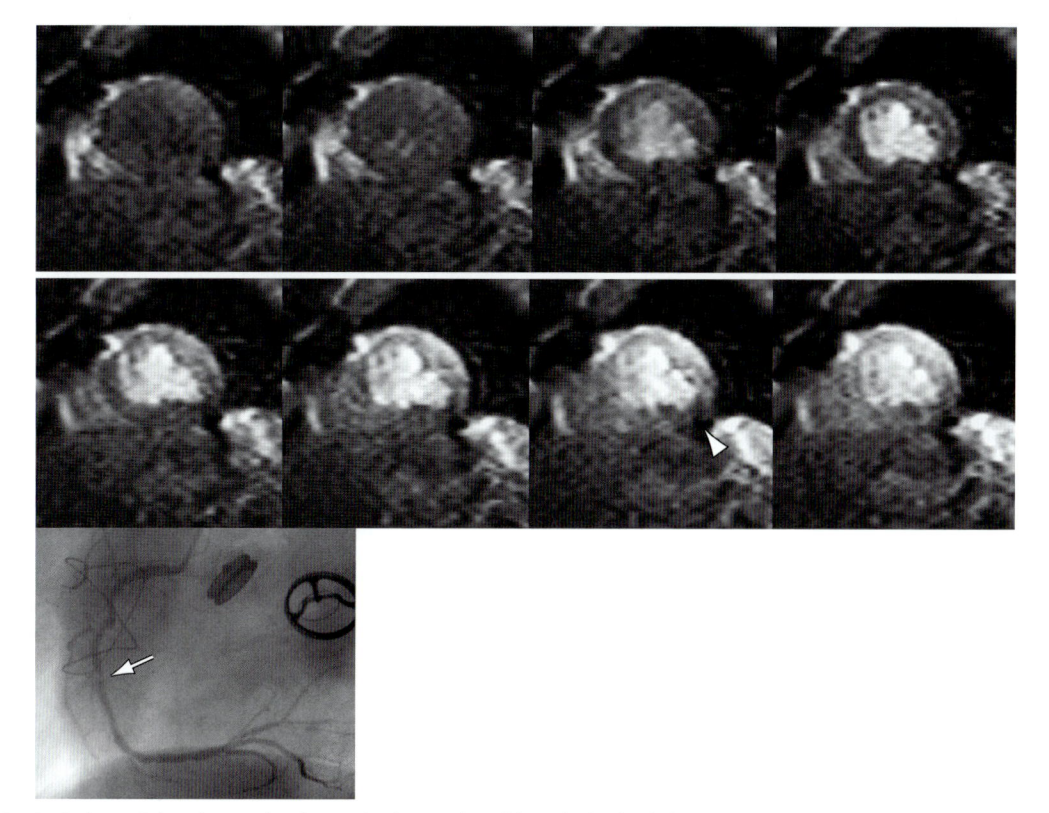

■ **FIGURE 14-5** Perfusion MR imaging study. Short-axis view at the midventricular level shows a perfusion defect in the posterior wall (*arrowhead*) corresponding to a stenosis of the right coronary artery (*arrow*). (From Pujadas S, Reddy GP, Lee JJ, Higgins CB. Magnetic resonance imaging in ischemic heart disease. Semin Roentgenol 2003; 38:320-329.)

Slow-flowing blood can result in poor blood suppression, producing an endocardial border of hyperintensity on T2-weighted images. When a thin layer of pseudo-T2 involvement is isolated to the endocardium, correlation should be made to other imaging sequences to help determine the true anatomic location of signal changes. If the changes are determined to be adjacent to the endocardium, then they are likely artefactual. This artefact is particularly notable in regions adjacent to wall motion abnormality, at the ventricular apex, or the interstices of trabeculae.[11]

Perfusion

Indications

Myocardial perfusion is important in determining the hemodynamic significance of coronary artery stenoses identified at angiography. Nuclear cardiology currently fulfills the role of perfusion assessment by single photon emission computed tomography (SPECT)[12] and positron emission tomography (PET) imaging.[13] However, both techniques share the relative limitation of spatial resolution and radiation exposure. SPECT imaging also suffers from soft tissue attenuation, whereas access to PET imaging, despite its usefulness, is limited at this time.

Cardiac MR strengths include good tissue contrast, spatial resolution, and temporal resolution, which make it a natural candidate for perfusion imaging. First-pass perfusion MRI with gadolinium-based contrast agents is an accepted tool in the evaluation of coronary artery disease (Fig. 14-5).[14] When perfusion MRI is compared with current scintigraphic techniques, it performs well.[15] Overall, numerous studies evaluating the performance of MR perfusion in detecting obstructive coronary artery disease produce sensitivity and specificity of 83% and 82%, respectively.[16]

Contraindications

Perfusion imaging is not performed if the patient cannot receive the stress agent. Table 14-1 lists contraindications to pharmacologic stress agents. General contraindications to MR examination and to gadolinium-based contrast agents, including nephrogenic systemic fibrosis are also reasons that preclude cardiac MR perfusion examinations.

Technique Description

Perfusion imaging methods are less standardized with several sequences currently in use, depending on MRI vendor and site preference. Generally, a T1-weighted sequence during administration of gadolinium permits visualization of normally enhancing (brightening) myocardium to be differentiated from hypoenhancing (dark) ischemic tissue. Careful pulse sequence implementation is necessary to balance several factors,

TABLE 14-1 Contraindications to Pharmacologic Stress Agents

Agents	Contraindications
Dobutamine	Known hypersensitivity to agent
	Unstable angina pectoris
	Severe arterial hypertension (≥220/120 mm Hg)
	Hemodynamically significant aortic stenosis
	Complex cardiac arrhythmias
	Hypertrophic obstructive cardiomyopathy
	Myocarditis, pericarditis, or endocarditis
	Other major diseases
Adenosine, dipyridamole	Known hypersensitivity to agent
	Unstable angina pectoris
	Severe arterial hypertension (≥220/120 mm Hg)
	Systolic blood pressure < 90 mm Hg
	Asthma, severe obstructive pulmonary disease
	Atrioventricular block ≥ IIa
	Carotid artery stenosis
	Sick sinus syndrome
	Atrial fibrillation, flutter
	QT prolongation
	Decompensated heart failure
	Severe valvular stenosis

including spatial and temporal resolution, acquisition time, and SNR.

Currently a T1-GRE, hybrid gradient-echo–echoplanar imaging (GRE-EPI), or balanced steady-state free precession (SSFP) sequence can be used for perfusion imaging. The T1-GRE sequence is limited by lower spatial and/or temporal resolution so the other two techniques are now favored. Both the hybrid GRE-EPI and balanced SSFP techniques have been validated recently.[14] T1 weighting using a saturation recovery preparatory pulse has replaced inversion recovery as the current method of contrast preparation. Generally, short-axis views with at least three slice locations should be acquired—ideally each heartbeat, but every other one is acceptable. The in-plane resolution should be less than 3 mm with a temporal resolution of approximately 150 ms or less. Imaging duration should be long enough for the contrast to pass through the LV myocardium. As in many other areas, parallel imaging may be used to shorten the acquisition time. This is particularly useful in perfusion imaging to reduce motion artifacts and increase spatial or temporal resolution but it is limited by the tradeoff in SNR.

Stress and resultant hyperemia can be induced by the administration of pharmacologic agents such as adenosine or dipyrimadole because it is impractical to have patients exercise within the magnet environment. Normal coronary arteries will respond to the stress agent by hyperemic vasodilation, with a resultant increase in myocardial perfusion. However, arteries with significant stenoses are already maximally dilated at rest to compensate for the existing luminal compromise, and are thus unable to produce a response to the stress agent. The difference in response of each region produces an imbalance, with a delayed arrival of contrast and lower contrast agent concentration in the ischemic myocardium compared with the normal myocardium. Many centers prefer the use of adenosine because of its extremely short half-life, which allows more control with respect to side effects from pharmacologic administration. The recommended dose for adenosine is at a rate of 0.14 mg/kg/min by intravenous infusion generally for 3 to 6 minutes for a total dose of 0.42 to 0.84 mg/kg to achieve maximal vasodilation. To minimize the risk of heart block, adenosine and the contrast agent should be administered by separate IV setups to avoid a large bolus of drug delivery. Side effects associated with adenosine include flushing, chest pain, palpitations, and breathlessness. More severe side effects include transient heart block, hypotension, sinus tachycardia, and bronchospasm. Dipyridamole is administered for a total dose of 0.56 mg/kg over 4 minutes. The effects of dipyridamole are longer lasting; which is not desirable when considering side effects but advantageous for the extended imaging window. Xanthine inhibitors (caffeine, theophylline) will counteract the vasodilatory effects of both agents and should be avoided for 24 hours prior to examination. Aminophylline, however, should be available to counteract the effects of adenosine, if necessary, by slow IV infusion of 250 mg.

Contrast media used in perfusion imaging are typically gadolinium-based extracellular agents. The dosing range is between 0.025 to 0.15 mmol/kg body weight. MR-IMPACT, a multicenter, multivendor trial assessing the diagnostic performance of MRI perfusion with coronary angiography and SPECT, evaluated different contrast agent dosing regimens. Patients were randomized to receive 0.01, 0.025, 0.05, 0.075, or 0.10 mmol/kg per stress and rest injection, with the 0.10-mmol/kg dose resulting in the best performance of MRI perfusion.[17] Nonetheless, variability still exists between imaging protocols and dosing regimens at different institutions, reflecting the lack of uniform agreement on the optimal imaging protocol. In routine clinical practice with qualitative visual analysis, the upper limit of dosing is preferable. In distinction, when performing semiquantitative analysis, a lower concentration dose regimen (e.g., 0.025 mmol/kg) is optimal for ensuring the relative linear relationship between gadolinium concentration and myocardial signal intensity.

Injection rates should be 3 to 5 mL/sec followed by saline flush of at least 30 mL. Injection speed should not be less than 3 mL/sec to avoid limitations in myocardial enhancement.

Different imaging protocols can be implemented when performing MR perfusion, which may vary depending on the information desired. Most protocols will include stress perfusion and delayed hyperenhancement, but rest perfusion imaging is less consistently included. Traditionally, stress-rest SPECT imaging involves administering a radioactive tracer to assess perfusion and hence the presence of ischemia. This is followed by rest injection, which evaluates the redistribution of radioactive tracer into viable tissue, reflecting scar in areas of absent activity. The analogous MRI approach would be a stress perfusion and delayed hyperenhancement protocol for similar ischemia-viability assessment. In contrast, PET imaging allows assessment of perfusion reserve that reflects hemodynamically significant coronary artery stenoses, which is accomplished on MR perfusion with a combined stress-rest protocol.

Combined stress-rest protocols with delayed hyperenhancement afford the added value of distinguishing true perfusion defects from artifacts (see later). In adenosine stress studies, the stress component is typically determined first, with a short interval delay followed by rest perfusion. The longer lasting effects of dipyrimadole make it preferable to perform a rest study first because a stress-first study might lead to an excessive time interval before being able to perform rest perfusion imaging.

Pitfalls and Solutions

The most prominent and troublesome artifact encountered in perfusion imaging is the dark rim artifact (DRA). Although not completely understood, one theory about its presence is that this represents a Gibbs artifact that produces dark bands at high-contrast interfaces, such as between the bright contrast-containing left ventricular cavity and dark myocardium. Increasing resolution, which can be challenging within the existing MR perfusion constraints, may minimize DRA. Parallel imaging and 3-T magnets may provide the flexibility for achieving this result.

Recognizing DRA is important because it may occur despite technique optimization. DRA is suspected if the subendocardial rim of hypointense signal is noted to be most prominent at peak left ventricular (LV) cavity enhancement with subsequent lessening. The transient nature reflects the temporal relationship of this artifact to the balance between blood and myocardial contrast. When a subendocardial rim of hypointense signal is identified that persists longer than the contrast agent's first pass through the LV cavity, a true hypoperfusion defect is suspected. In protocols with dual perfusion studies (rest and stress) and DE imaging, if a perfusion abnormality is demonstrated on both components of the perfusion study without corresponding delayed hyperenhancement, this should be interpreted as DRA.

Excessively high concentration doses of gadolinium contrast may result in dominant T2* effects, with potential decreases in signal intensity within blood pool and the myocardium. Either could lead to difficult or inappropriate assessment of perfusion changes. Maintaining concentration doses less than 0.15 mmol/kg body weight will minimize the possibility of this confounding factor. Furthermore, maintaining perfusion parameters at minimal "echo times" will also limit the susceptibility to T2* effects.

Reporting

Qualitative interpretation remains the primary method of clinical reporting of perfusion MR imaging at this time. Full examination review, which requires interpretation of the delayed hyperenhancement (DHE) images in conjunction with stress perfusion images, is ideal in clinical practice.[18]

Delayed Hyperenhancement Normal, Stress Perfusion Normal

If the myocardium demonstrates no scar and perfusion demonstrates uniform enhancement, then the patient does not have ischemia and does have viable tissue.

Delayed Hyperenhancement Normal, Stress Perfusion Abnormal, Rest Perfusion Normal

If the myocardium demonstrates no scar and stress perfusion demonstrates a defect that normalizes at rest perfusion, then the patient has ischemia with viable tissue.

Delayed Hyperenhancement Abnormal, Concordant Stress Perfusion Abnormal

If the myocardium demonstrates delayed gadolinium enhancement of scar and perfusion demonstrates a corresponding defect on stress imaging, then the patient has scar without ischemia.

Delayed Hyperenhancement Abnormal, Discordant Stress Perfusion Abnormal

If the myocardium demonstrates delayed gadolinium enhancement of scar and perfusion demonstrates a defect on stress imaging that involves a larger region than the nonviable tissue on DHE, then the patient has peri-infarct ischemia adjacent to scar. This can assist in determining the benefit of revascularization.

Quantitative interpretation involves placing region of interest (ROI) measurements within the wall to assess signal intensity changes. One can then determine parameters that are perfusion-linked or absolute tissue perfusion.

Delayed Hyperenhancement

Indications

LV function is an important factor in the long-term survival of patients with ischemic heart disease (IHD) for whom severe LV dysfunction is associated with a poor prognosis. However, LV function can improve after revascularization procedures, including both percutaneous transluminal coronary angioplasty (PTCA) and stent placement or coronary artery bypass grafting (CABG).[19] Thus, the determination of tissue viability becomes paramount.

Identifying and differentiating viable from nonviable myocardium is currently performed by PET scanning, thallium or technetium SPECT scintigraphy, and dobutamine stress echocardiography (DSE). However, each technique has certain drawbacks or limitations. PET availability remains limited and is relatively high in cost, whereas SPECT has poor spatial resolution and signal attenuation artifacts. Furthermore, the nuclear techniques expose patients to radiation, which is particularly concerning if repeated studies are required. Dobutamine stress echocardiography also suffers from poor spatial resolution and has greater operator dependence and examination failure rates (up to 15%).

The concept of infarct-related hyperenhancement in MRI has long existed but has rapidly gained acceptance as a standard investigative tool with newer imaging techniques and their ability to detect and size infarcted tissue in vivo.[20] The mechanism of delayed hyperenhancement in acute infarcts, although still incompletely understood, is thought to occur because of the increased volume of

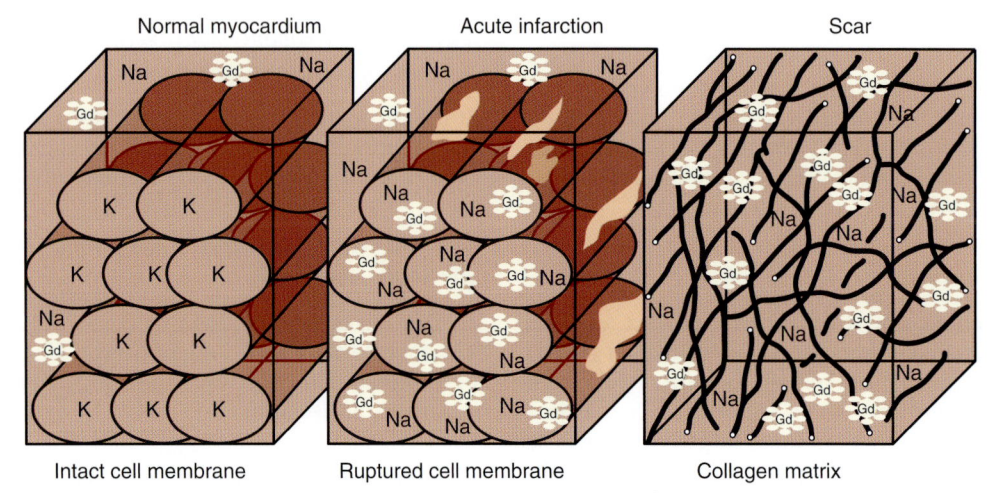

■ **FIGURE 14-6** Potential mechanisms of delayed hyperenhancement in acute and chronic infarctions. See text for details. *(From Weinsaft J, Klem I, Judd RM. MRI for the assessment of myocardial viability. In Kim RJ [ed]. Cardiovascular MR Imaging. Philadelphia, WB Saunders, 2007, p 509.)*

distribution of contrast agent resulting from myocardial interstitial edema and myocyte membrane disruption (Fig. 14-6).[21] Similarly, in chronic infarcts, delayed hyperenhancement can be seen because the dense collagen of scar tissue may contain greater interstitial space than that between myocytes of viable myocardium, which also results in greater accumulation of contrast agent.

MRI thus represents a new tool to assess viability. Advantages to MRI include the lack of ionizing radiation and provision of simultaneous functional assessment. One particular advantage of DHE-MRI is the improvement in spatial resolution compared with existing techniques. The superior resolution of DHE-MRI provides a distinct advantage for imaging nontransmural infarction.[22] Numerous studies have since compared DHE-MRI with current imaging modalities and confirmed this advantage. When Klein and colleagues[23] compared PET and DHE-MRI in study patients, both performed well in the assessment of nonviable tissue but more infarcts were detected by DHE-MRI. Furthermore, when evaluating subendocardial infarcts (nontransmural), approximately one half (55%) were identified by DHE-MRI but classified as normal by PET. Similar differences have been shown in comparisons of DHE-MRI with SPECT imaging, where subendocardial infarcts (<50% wall thickness by histopathology) were identified in 92% (MRI) and 28% (SPECT) of patients, respectively.[24]

The superior spatial resolution of DHE-MRI is important to consider in conjunction with the ability to identify the viable component of myocardium adjacent to infarct (Fig. 14-7). When considering the transmural extent of infarction, DHE-MRI is ideally suited for quantifying the viable nonenhancing myocardium versus nonviable delayed enhancing scar. The percentage of wall thickness involvement is a direct measurement compared with the entire wall thickness at that level. In contrast, other techniques, such as dobutamine stress echocardiography, infer viability by response to exogenous drug administration. Nuclear techniques visualize viable tissue but do not directly see the nonviable tissue; they compare it with a remote normal zone. This degree of visualization may have implications for management and prognostic stratification.

DHE imaging has been shown to be particularly useful in the setting of IHD with reversible myocardial dysfunction of stunned and hibernating myocardium. In the acute period, after an episode of ischemia during which infarction does not occur and reperfusion is established, reversible dysfunction can occur; this is known as stunning. Myocyte death has not occurred but contractile dysfunction persists, and DHE can predict the extent of salvageable myocardium by demonstrating the absence of scar in the region of contractile dysfunction. The presence of viability is important because patients with LV dysfunction from stunning versus myocardial necrosis have a better prognosis. In hibernating myocardium, there is downregulation of function related to the chronic decrease in blood flow to the region of interest. The underlying myocardium is viable and will regain function if there is restoration of regional blood flow; thus, DHE-MRI is ideally suited to detecting hibernating myocardium as well.

In large areas of acute infarctions, one may observe microvascular obstruction (MO) with capillary occlusion and accumulation of debris. This phenomenon is thought to occur from damage and obstruction at the microcirculatory level, with reduced perfusion resulting in limited penetration of gadolinium contrast agent to the infarct core.[25] The presence of MO can be identified on DHE-MRI as an area of no-reflow and has important implications for patients because they are at increased risk of recurrent chest pain, heart failure, and infarction (Fig. 14-8).[26] The presence of MO was better demonstrated by DHE-MRI compared with contrast echo in one study, also confirming the importance of this finding as a prognostic factor in immediate postinfarct complications.[27] Thus, there is extensive literature supporting the usefulness of DHE-MRI as a first-line test for imaging viability.

However, not all DHE is related to infarcted scar tissue. DHE-MRI imaging can be used to assess nonischemic origin cardiac disease as well. Patients with acute myocarditis can present with acute coronary syndrome but if a comprehensive cardiac work-up is performed, they show no evidence of coronary artery disease (CAD). The differential diagnosis of acute coronary syndrome includes acute myocarditis, which is often challenging to assess

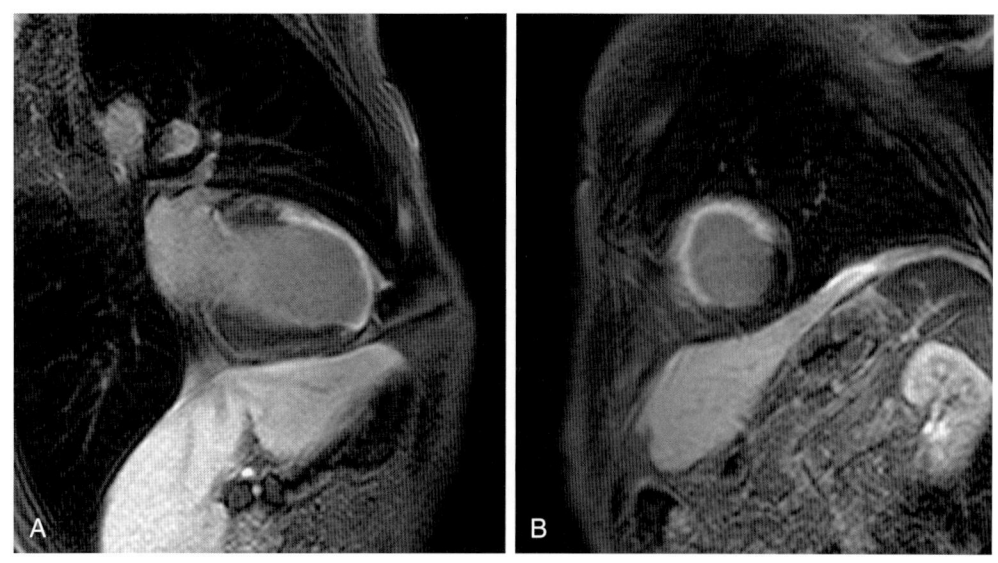

■ **FIGURE 14-7** Vertical long-axis (**A**) and short-axis (**B**) DHE views of the heart demonstrate transmural hyperenhancement with wall thinning of the anterior wall involving the apex (**A**). Extension is also seen toward the anteroseptum (**B**). The distribution of DHE is typical for left anterior descending artery vascular territory.

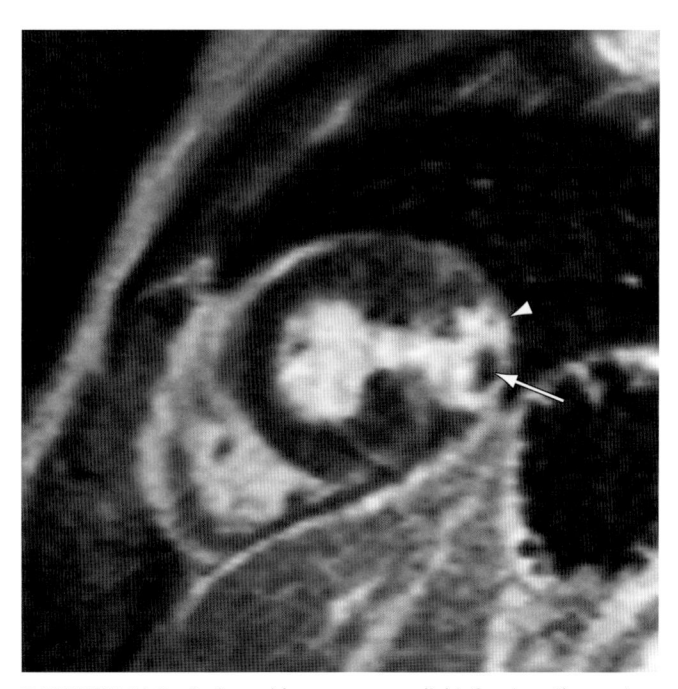

■ **FIGURE 14-8** Patient with acute myocardial infarction. Short-axis view at midventricular level shows transmural hyperenhancement (*arrowhead*) of the posterolateral wall, with a dark area (*arrow*) in the core corresponding to a no-reflow area. (*From Pujadas S, Reddy GP, Lee JJ, Higgins CB. Magnetic resonance imaging in ischemic heart disease. Semin Roentgenol 2003; 38:320-329.*)

clinically and is a diagnosis of exclusion. In these patients, MRI can be helpful in the initial diagnosis and follow-up of the disease, with DHE-MRI reflecting inflammation in the acute phase. The presence of DHE may be the most common finding at diagnosis and can have a unique nonischemic distribution. Furthermore, the DHE on follow-up MRI may have prognostic implications with respect to long-term outcome in patients with myocarditis.[28]

DHE can also be seen in hypertrophic cardiomyopathy (CMO), with distinct nonischemic patterns involving the midwall, subepicardium, or right ventricular free wall. The presence and degree of enhancement may be related to risk factors for sudden death in this population.[29]

Similarly, cardiac involvement in sarcoidosis can be demonstrated by DHE-MRI with a predilection for the subepicardium of the anteroseptal and inferolateral walls (Fig. 14-9). In one small study, the degree of enhancement was inversely related to treatment with steroids, which suggests that DHE could be used as a surrogate marker for response to therapy.[30] In a study of 81 patients by Patel and associates,[31] a relatively high prevalence of delayed hyperenhancement was demonstrated, which was twice as sensitive for the detection of cardiac involvement compared with the current consensus criteria. More importantly, this study showed DHE-MRI to be the only independent predictor of adverse clinical events including cardiac death.

Cardiac involvement in amyloid remains a difficult diagnosis to make, even with endomyocardial biopsy, and carries a poor prognosis, with a decrease in median survival. Not only has DHE-MRI been shown to be able to image patients with characteristic subendocardial enhancement positively,[32] but it also demonstrates prognostic value with decreased median survival and increased rate of death or heart transplantation.[33]

DHE-MRI has demonstrated similar usefulness in Anderson-Fabry and Chagas disease. Much interest has also been generated in cardiac noncompaction, iron overload CMO, endomyocardial fibroelastosis, and uremic CMO, although the role of DHE-MRI is still unclear at this time.

Finally, DHE-MRI has also been shown to be helpful in evaluating certain complications of IHD. False aneurysms may develop postinfarction when there is disruption of the complete wall thickness but integrity is maintained by overlying pericardium. Differentiating true from false aneurysms in the heart is crucial because the latter are at

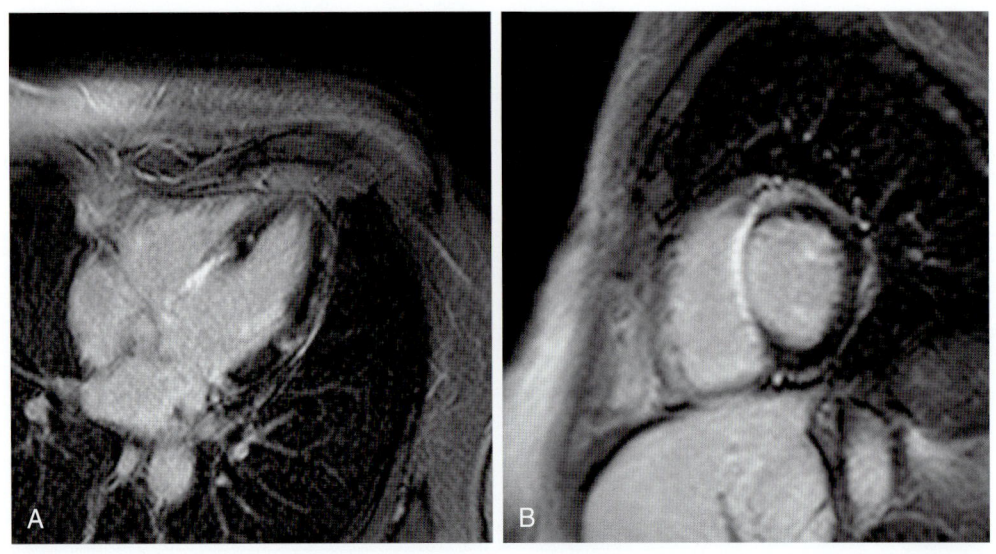

■ **FIGURE 14-9** Horizontal long-axis (HLA; **A**) and short-axis (SA; **B**) DHE views of the heart in cardiac sarcoidosis. The HLA view demonstrates DHE at the base of the septum, with midmyocardial distribution. The SA view demonstrates septal involvement extending toward the RV side of the myocardium with sparing of the endocardium (**B**). Patchy mid to outer wall enhancement in the mid-septum and lateral wall is also present (**A**).

greater risk for rupture and surgical treatment is considered first-line therapy. Although classic imaging features exist for differentiating the two types of aneurysms, DHE may play an additional role in distinguishing these entities. In a small study of 22 patients, Konen and coworkers[34] have demonstrated a pericardial DHE pattern, with false aneurysms being more commonly identified than true aneurysms.

Patients with intracardiac thrombi are at risk of distal embolization and are currently imaged by echocardiography. Correct identification is important for the initiation of medical therapy to prevent cerebrovascular events. Echocardiography, however, has mixed results in identifying thrombi and is subject to interobserver variability. In one study by Srichai and colleagues,[35] MRI was more sensitive to the detection of thrombi (88%) compared with transthoracic (23%) and transesophageal echocardiography (40%). Typically, MRI imaging with cine sequences is used to identify thrombus but the routine addition of DHE may have incremental value, as suggested in a recent study by Weinsaft and associates.[36] In their study of 784 patients with systolic dysfunction, DHE-MRI demonstrated a significant increase in the number of thrombi detected (55 patients) compared with cine MRI (37 patients) alone (Fig. 14-10).

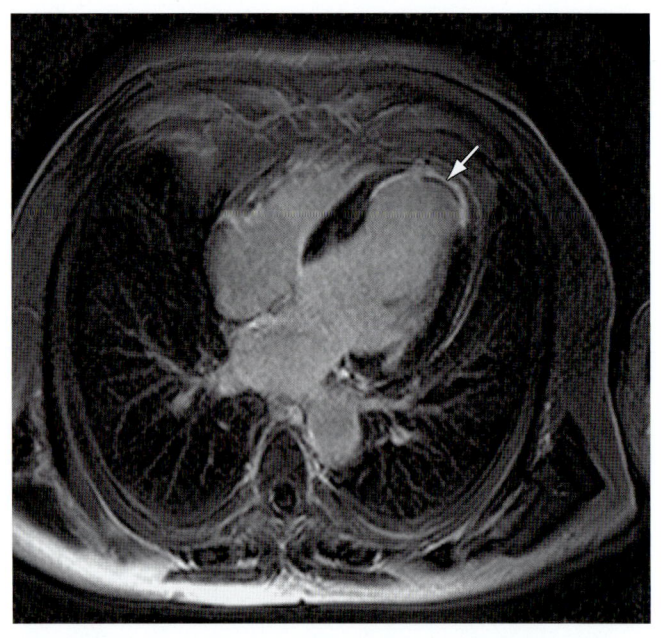

■ **FIGURE 14-10** Horizontal long-axis DHE view of the heart. The infarction is identified in the LV apex, which is aneurysmal, and demonstrates transmural involvement. The enhancement is nontransmural toward the edge of infarction. A thin curvilinear hypointense structure underlies the apical infarct and represents a thrombus (*arrow*).

Contraindications

No specific contraindications exist aside from those related to contrast administration.

Technique Description

Imaging can be performed at any time between 5 and 30 minutes but typically at 15 minutes to balance contrast delivery and washout. Total administered dose for DHE is approximately 1.5 to 2 times the standard dose by weight using standard gadolinium agents. Alternate agents such as gadobenate dimeglumine (MultiHance, Bracco, Milan, Italy) or gadobutrol (Gadovist, Bayer Healthcare, Leverkusen, Germany) may allow for a reduction in dose because of differences in their respective molecules.

Although many techniques have been described for imaging delayed hyperenhancement, currently a segmented k-space turbo field echo sequence with a trigger delay for diastole to minimize cardiac motion and an inversion pulse set to null normal myocardium is most commonly used (Fig. 14-11).[37] The inversion pulse maximizes the contrast between abnormal myocardium with gadolinium accumulation (delayed hyperenhancement) and normal myocardium, which will appear dark.

Inversion time (TI) is determined by running a trial of pre-DHE images at varying TI times and selecting the most appropriate time for nulling normal myocardium (Fig. 14-12). Vendor-specialized software is available, such as Look-Locker (Philips Medical Systems, Best, The Netherlands) or TI Surf (Siemens Medical Solutions, Erlangen, Germany), which simplifies this process by acquiring a range of TI sample images in a single breath-hold for comparison.

Newer techniques for DHE may obviate the need for a Look-Locker and the time required to determine the optimal inversion time. Whereas classic inversion recovery–turbo field echo (IR-TFE) sequences are magnitude based, with image quality and infarct depiction significantly dependent on IR time selection, the phase-sensitive inversion recovery sequence produces a spectrum of DHE-MRI images that maintain DHE to normal myocardium differentiation across a spectrum of IR times.[38]

Despite the success of the IR-TFE sequence for delayed hyperenhancement, there are limitations of two-dimensional imaging. Slice gap misregistration and time-consuming breath-holds may lead to loss of patient cooperation, fatigue, or inadequate image quality. To overcome some of these issues, three-dimensional techniques are now being used with potential benefits in contrast-to-noise ratio, SNR, and time savings.[39]

However, if patients are still unable to breath-hold, then navigator-facilitated methods can produce diagnostic images, which may be shorter in overall acquisition time. The patients can breathe freely and comfortably while the scanner acquires the imaging volume so that patients are not subjected to repetitive exhaustive breath-holding. However, many patients undergoing investigation for cardiac DHE are poor breath-holders and have irregular cardiac rhythms, which may render all motion compensation techniques useless. In this subset of patients, newer subsecond DHE sequences are superior to the segmented IR technique.[40]

Future advances include a combined cine DHE sequence, which will allow for improved correlation of wall motion changes to tissue viability.

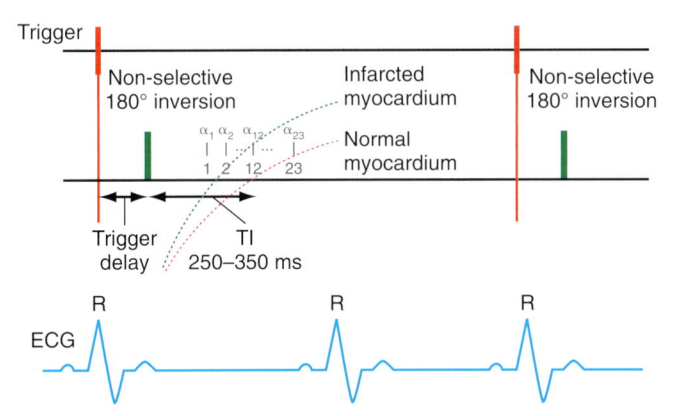

■ FIGURE 14-11 Schematic representation of inversion recovery sequence for nulling of the myocardium.

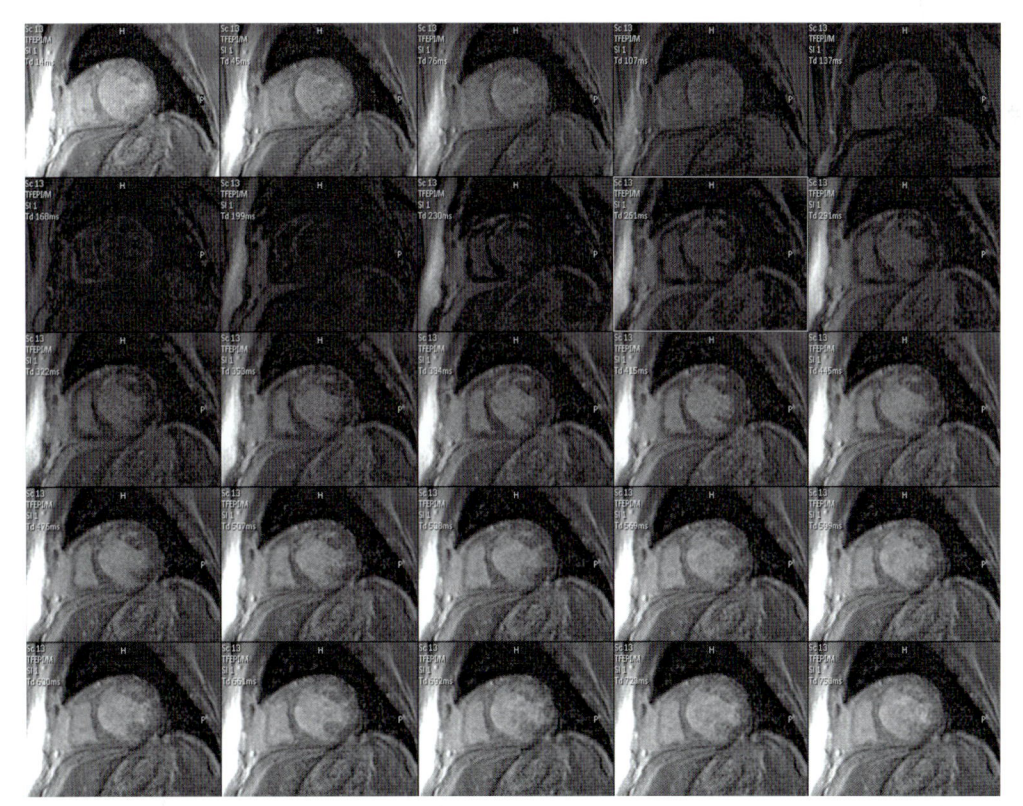

■ FIGURE 14-12 Look-Locker series of images for determination of DHE sequence IR time. Sequential images with varying inversion times are taken in the mid-LV chamber in short axis to compare the signal intensities of myocardium. The image demonstrating the optimal saturation of normal myocardium is selected as the ideal IR time for the subsequent DHE sequence to optimize infarct visualization.

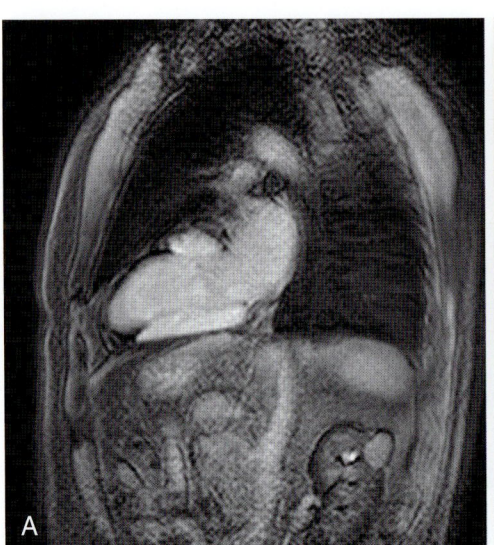

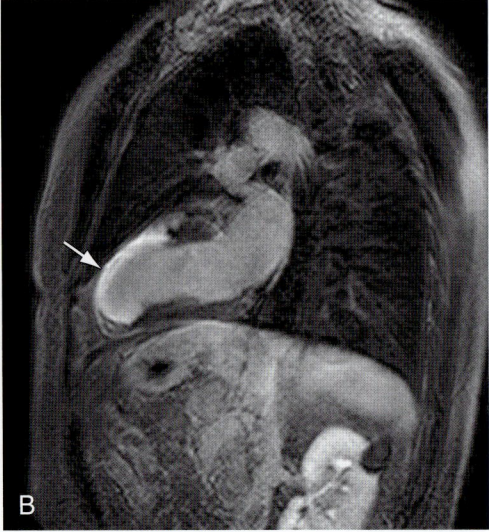

FIGURE 14-13 Selection of inversion time. **A,** Image with improper inversion time. Note the poor differentiation of scar tissue from normal myocardium. **B,** Image with appropriate inversion time, with maximal differentiation of delayed hyperenhancing infarct (*arrow*) from the viable myocardium.

Pitfalls and Solutions

Appropriate selection of inversion time is crucial to the image quality and subsequent scar visualization on DHE-MRI. The optimal time relies on a subjective assessment of optimal suppression; the MR technologist or radiologist must decide, based on pre-DHE images, which portion of myocardium is normal to determine the IR time that will produce suppressed (dark) viable myocardium. Optimal suppression leads to maximal differentiation of delayed enhancing infarct from the viable myocardium. Improper IR time selection will lead to poor differentiation of scar tissue from normal myocardium or accidental reversal of signal intensities, with a dark infarct and bright normal myocardium (Fig. 14-13). Careful assessment of Look-Locker or TI Surf scouts and correlation to cine imaging can help identify normal myocardium and assist in optimizing the differentiation of scar from normal myocardium.

Infarct sizing is important in assessing response to therapy, particularly in research trials. Improper timing of DHE-MRI outside of the 15- to 20-minute window can lead to improper assessment of scar tissue extent (up to 28% discrepancy). Imaging earlier may overestimate enhancement, whereas late imaging may result in underestimation.[41] The simple recognition of infarct evolution over time on DHE-MRI is sufficient to maintain constant imaging within the optimal imaging range of 15 minutes.

The presence of no-reflow is generally diagnosed when a large region of DHE is identified in acute infarction with the presence of a hypoenhanced region at its core. This should not be mistaken as a region of infarct sparing because the wavefront phenomenon of infarction occurs from inside, at the endocardial border, to outside, at the epicardial border. No-reflow regions can be differentiated from viable myocardium by their location because they will be completely surrounded by DHE or may be at the endocardial border adjacent to the LV cavity but otherwise surrounded by DHE in three dimensions. The area of no-reflow has a significantly depressed but not absent flow, so repeat imaging at later delay times will eventually demonstrate hyperenhancement, unlike viable myocardium.

Reporting

When considering ischemic heart disease, DHE-MRI images are usually interpreted in conjunction with cine imaging in three main combinations (Fig. 14-14).

Delayed Hyperenhancement Normal, Wall Motion Normal

If the myocardium demonstrates no scar and cine imaging demonstrates normal wall motion, then the patient has viable tissue.

Delayed Hyperenhancement Normal, Wall Motion Abnormal

If the myocardium demonstrates no scar and stress perfusion demonstrates a defect, which normalizes at rest perfusion, then the patient has ischemia with viable tissue. This may represent stunned or hibernating myocardium.

Delayed Hyperenhancement Abnormal, Wall Motion Abnormal

If the myocardium demonstrates scar and cine imaging demonstrates corresponding wall motion abnormalities, then the patient has nonviable tissue.

When the presence of DHE is demonstrated in a patient without CAD, in a noncoronary artery distribution or in a nonwavefront distribution, then nonischemic causes of cardiac disease must be considered. The segment of wall involvement and the inner, mid-wall, or outer wall pattern of involvement can assist in determining a specific cause.

Hyperenhancement patterns

Ischemic

A. Subendocardial infarct

B. Transmural infarct

Nonischemic

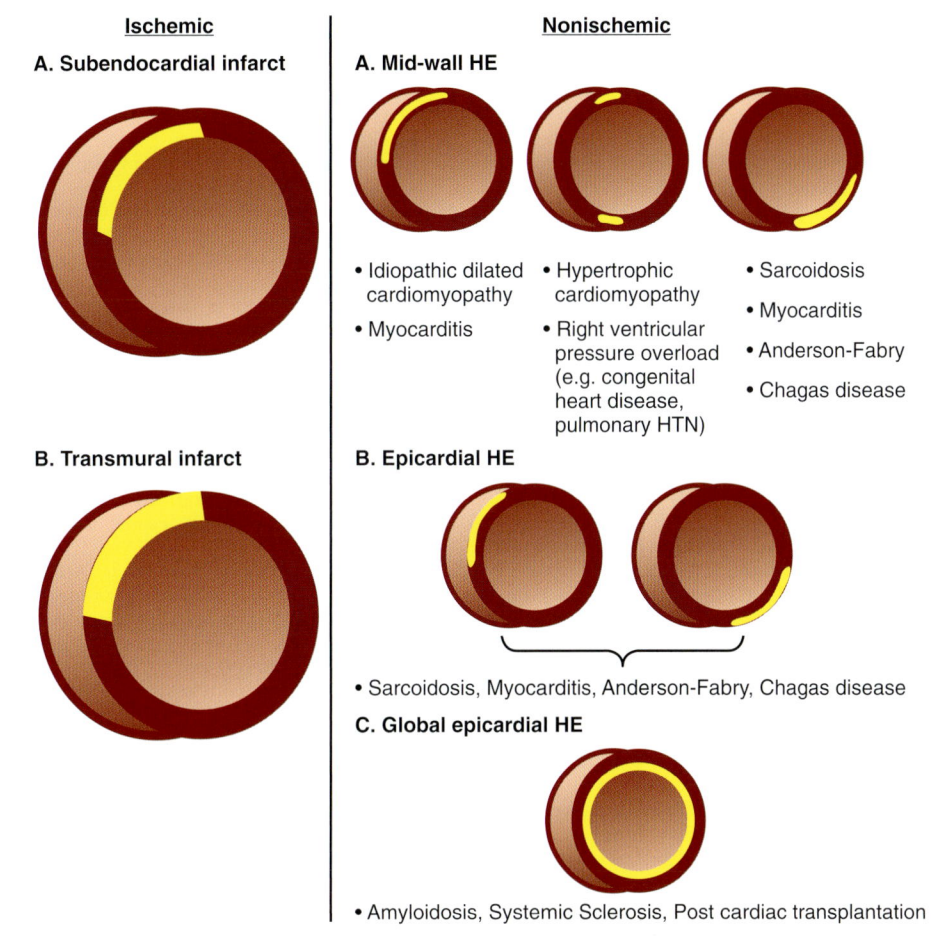

A. Mid-wall HE

- Idiopathic dilated cardiomyopathy
- Myocarditis

- Hypertrophic cardiomyopathy
- Right ventricular pressure overload (e.g. congenital heart disease, pulmonary HTN)

- Sarcoidosis
- Myocarditis
- Anderson-Fabry
- Chagas disease

B. Epicardial HE

- Sarcoidosis, Myocarditis, Anderson-Fabry, Chagas disease

C. Global epicardial HE

- Amyloidosis, Systemic Sclerosis, Post cardiac transplantation

■ **FIGURE 14-14** Schematic diagrams illustrating the patterns of enhancement in ischemic and nonischemic disease. Infarction occurs from the endocardium inside to the epicardium on the outer side of the ventricle, according to the wavefront phenomenon. In contrast, when enhancement occurs in a mid-wall, epicardial, or patchy noncoronary artery territory of supply, nonischemic causes should be considered. *(From Weinsaft J, Klem I, Judd RM. MRI for the assessment of myocardial viability. In Kim RJ [ed]. Cardiovascular MR Imaging. Philadelphia, WB Saunders, 2007, p 519.)*

KEY POINTS

- Turbo spin echo black blood images are frequently used for morphologic assessment of the heart.
- MR myocardial perfusion imaging is performed with the use of a hybrid gradient echoplanar or a steady-state free precession sequence during the first pass of contrast agent.
- The delayed hyperenhancement technique is used for MR viability imaging of the myocardium.

SUGGESTED READINGS

Abdel-Aty H, Simonetti O, Friedrich MG: T2-weighted cardiovascular magnetic resonance imaging. J Magn Reson Imaging 2007; 26:452-459.

Kramer CM, Barkhausen J, Flamm SD, et al: Standardized cardiovascular magnetic resonance imaging (CMR) protocols. Society for Cardiovascular Magnetic Resonance: board of trustees task force on standardized protocols. J Cardiovasc Magn Reson 2008; 10:35.

Sakuma H: Magnetic resonance imaging for ischemic heart disease. J Magn Reson Imaging 2007; 26:3-13.

Vogel-Claussen J, Rochitte CE, Wu KC, et al: Delayed enhancement MR imaging: utility in myocardial assessment. RadioGraphics 2006; 26:795-810.

REFERENCES

1. Hofman MBM, Wickline SA, Lorenz CH. Quantification of in-plane motion of the coronary arteries during the cardiac cycle: implications for acquisition window duration for MR flow quantification. J Magn Reson Imaging 1998; 8:568-576.
2. Fischer SE, Wickline SA, Lorenz CH. Novel real-time R-wave detection algorithm based on the vectorcardiogram for accurate gated magnetic resonance acquisitions. Magn Reson Med 1999; 42:361-370.
3. Palthow C, Ley S, Zaporozhan J, et al. Assessment of reproducibility and stability of different breath-hold manoeuvres by dynamic MRI: comparison between healthy adults and patients with pulmonary hypertension. Eur Radiol 2006; 16:173-179.
4. Ehman R, Felmlee JP. Adaptive technique for high-definition MR imaging of moving structures. Radiology 1989; 173:255-263.
5. Taylor AM, Jhooti P, Weismann F, et al. MR navigator-echo monitoring of temporal changes in diaphragm position: implications for MR coronary angiography. J Magn Reson Imaging 1997; 7:629-636.
6. Abdel-Aty H, Zagrosek A, Schulz-Menger J, et al. Delayed enhancement and T2-weighted cardiovascular magnetic resonance imaging differentiate acute from chronic myocardial infarction. Circulation 2004; 109:2411-2416.
7. Abdel-Aty H, Boye P, Zagrosek A, et al. Diagnostic performance of cardiovascular magnetic resonance imaging in patients with suspected acute myocarditis: comparison of different approaches. J Am Coll Cardiol 2005; 45:1815-1822.
8. Sharkey SW, Lesser JR, Zenovich AG, et al. Acute and reversible cardiomyopathy provoked by stress in women from the United Sates. Circulation 2005; 111:472-479.
9. Anderson LJ, Holden S, Davis B, et al. Cardiovascular T2-star (T2*) magnetic resonance for the early diagnosis of myocardial iron overload. Eur Heart J 2001; 22:2171-2179.
10. Reference deleted in proofs.
11. Abdel-Aty H, Simonetti O, Friedrich M. T2-weighted cardiovascular magnetic resonance imaging. J Magn Reson Imaging 2007; 26:452-459.
12. Maddahi J, Van Train K, Prigent F, et al. Quantitative single photon emission computed thallium-201 tomography for detection and localization of coronary artery disease: optimization and prospective validation of a new technique. J Am Coll Cardiol 1989; 14:1689-1699.
13. Muzik O, Duvernoy C, Beanlands RS, et al. Assessment of diagnostic performance of quantitative flow measurements in normal subjects and patients with angiographically documented coronary artery disease by means of nitrogen-13 ammonia and positron emission tomography. J Am Coll Cardiol 1998; 31:534-540.
14. Giang TH, Nanz D, Coulden R, et al. Detection of coronary artery disease by magnetic resonance myocardial perfusion imaging with various contrast medium doses: first European multi-centre experience. Eur Heart J 2004; 25:1657-1665.
15. Schwitter J, Nanz D, Kneifel S, et al. Assessment of myocardial perfusion in coronary artery disease by magnetic resonance: a comparison with positron emission tomography and coronary angiography. Circulation 2001; 103:2230-2235.
16. Kim HWJ, Klem I, Kim RJ. Detection of myocardial ischemia by stress perfusion cardiovascular magnetic resonance. In Kim RJ (ed). Cardiovascular MR Imaging. Philadelphia, WB Saunders, 2007, pp 527-540.
17. Schwitter J, Wacker CM, van Rossum AC, et al. MR-IMPACT: comparison of perfusion-cardiac magnetic resonance with single-photon emission computed tomography for the detection of coronary artery disease in a multicentre, multivendor, randomized trial. Eur Heart J 2008; 29:480-489.
18. Klem I, Heitner JF, Shah DJ, et al. Improved detection of coronary artery disease by stress perfusion cardiovascular magnetic resonance with the use of delayed enhancement infarction imaging. J Am Coll Cardiol 2006; 47:1630-1638.
19. Elefteriades JA, Tolis G, Levi E, et al. Coronary artery bypass grafting in severe left ventricular dysfunction: excellent survival with improved ejection fraction and functional state. J Am Coll Cardiol 1993; 22:1411-1417.
20. Kim RJ, Fieno JS, Parrish TB, et al. Relationship of MRI delayed contrast enhancement to irreversible injury, infarct age, and contractile function. Circulation 1999; 100:1992-2002.
21. Saeed M, Wendland MF, Masui T, Higgins CB. Reperfused myocardial infarctions on T1- and susceptibility-enhanced MRI: evidence for loss of compartmentalization of contrast media. Magn Reson Med 1994; 31:31-39.
22. Kim RJ, Wu E, Rafael A, et al. The use of contrast-enhanced magnetic resonance imaging to identify reversible myocardial dysfunction. N Engl J Med 2000; 343:1445-1453.
23. Klein C, Nekolla SG, Bengel FM, et al. Assessment of myocardial viability with contrast-enhanced magnetic resonance imaging: comparison with positron emission tomography. Circulation 2002; 105:162-167.
24. Wagner A, Mahrholdt H, Holly TA, et al. Contrast-enhanced MRI and routine single photon emission computed tomography (SPECT) perfusion imaging for detection of the subendocardial myocardial infarcts: an imaging study. Lancet 2003; 361:374-379.
25. Rochitte CE, Lima JA, Bluemke DA, et al. Magnitude and time course of microvascular obstruction and tissue injury after acute myocardial infarction. Circulation 1998; 98:1006-1014.
26. Wu KC, Zerhouni EA, Judd RM, et al. Prognostic significance of microvascular obstruction by magnetic resonance imaging in patients with acute myocardial infarction. Circulation 1998; 97:765-772.
27. Wu KC, Kim RJ, Bluemke DA, et al. Quantification and time course of microvascular obstruction by contrast-enhanced echocardiography and magnetic resonance imaging following acute myocardial infarction and reperfusion. J Am Coll Cardiol 1998; 32:1756-1764.
28. Wagner A, Schultz-Menger J, Deitz R, Friedrich MG. Long-term follow-up of patients with acute myocarditis by magnetic resonance imaging. MAGMA 2003; 16:17-20
29. Moon JCC, McKenna WJ, McCrohon JA, et al. Toward clinical risk assessment in hypertrophic cardiomyopathy with gadolinium cardiovascular magnetic resonance imaging. J Am Coll Cardiol 2003; 41:1561-1567.
30. Vignaux O, Dhote D, Duboc D, et al. Cardiac magnetic resonance imaging findings in sarcoidosis. J Cardiovasc Magn Reson 2003; 5:15-16.
31. Patel M, Cawley P, Heitner JE, et al. Detection of myocardial damage in patients with sarcoidosis. Circulation 2009; 120:1969-1977.
32. Kwong RY, Falk RH. Cardiovascular magnetic resonance in cardiac amyloidosis. Circulation 2005; 111:122-124.
33. White J, Patel M, Shah DJ, et al. Prognostic utility of delayed enhancement cardiac magnetic resonance imaging in patients with systemic amyloidosis and suspected cardiac involvement. Circulation 2006; 114:679.
34. Konen E, Merchant N, Gutierrez C, et al. True versus false aneurysm: differentiation with MR imaging—initial experience. Radiol 2005; 236:65-70.
35. Srichai MB, Junor C, Rodriguez LL, et al. Clinical, imaging, and pathologic characteristics of left ventricular thrombus: a comparison of contrast enhanced magnetic resonance imaging, transthoracic echocardiography and transesophageal echocardiography with surgical or pathologic validation. Am Heart J 2006; 152:75-84.
36. Weinsaft JW, Kim HW, Shah DJ, et al. Detection of left ventricular thrombus by delayed enhancement cardiovascular magnetic resonance. J Am Coll Cardiol 2008; 52:148-157.
37. Simonetti OP, Kim RJ, Fieno DS, et al. An improved MR imaging technique for the visualization of myocardial infarction. Radiology 2001; 218:215-223.
38. Huber AM, Schoenberg S, Hayes C, et al. Phase-sensitive inversion-recovery MR imaging in the detection of myocardial infarction. Radiology 2005; 237:854-860.
39. Tatli S, Zou K, Fruitman M, et al. Three-dimensional magnetic resonance imaging for myocardial-delayed hyperenhancement: a comparison with the two-dimensional technique. J Magn Reson Imaging 2004; 20:378-382.
40. Burkhard S, Rehwald WG, Albert TSE, et al. Respiratory motion and cardiac arrhythmia effects on diagnostics accuracy of myocardial delayed-enhancement MR imaging in canines. Radiology 2008; 247:106-114.
41. Oshinski JN, Yang Z, Jones JR, et al. Imaging time after Gd-DTPA injection is critical in using delayed enhancement to determine infarct size accurately with magnetic resonance imaging. Circulation 2001; 104:2838-2842.

CHAPTER 15

Clinical Techniques of Cardiac Magnetic Resonance Imaging: Function

Rahul Kumar and W. Gregory Hundley

The assessment of cardiac function provides valuable diagnostic and prognostic information when managing patients with cardiovascular disease. Advancements in magnetic resonance imaging (MRI) technology have allowed for routine noninvasive assessment of left and right ventricular regional and global systolic and diastolic function.[1] With the image acquisition methods described in Chapter 13, MRI is well suited to measure these crucial parameters, as evidenced by results produced from studies of phantoms, cadavers, animals, and human clinical trials.

In addition to resting measures of left ventricular (LV) performance, MRI may also be used to assess dynamic indices, such as the response to exercise and inotropic agents, and load-independent measures, such as myocardial stress and strain. In addition, regional LV or right ventricular (RV) abnormalities may be present, despite somewhat preserved global function that may be indicative of an underlying cardiomyopathy. This chapter will review the use of MRI in the assessment of cardiac systolic function.

Technical Requirements

Technical requirements for evaluating resting cardiac function require an MRI scanner with capabilities and protocols described in Chapter 13. Evaluating for dynamic measures of ventricular function, such as with dobutamine or exercise, necessitates further equipment (see later).

DETERMINING GLOBAL MEASURES OF CARDIAC FUNCTION

Indications and Clinical Utility

An accurate assessment of LV function is important for determining prognosis and appropriate therapy. MRI determinations of LV volumes using Simpson's rule have been rigorously validated with cadaver studies. An early study showed excellent correlation ($r = 0.997$) between MRI-derived volume measurements of latex casts of excised human ventricles and the actual volume measurements from the casts themselves.[2] Data derived from multiple autopsy series have shown a similarly high degree of correlation,[3] as have animal studies using canine, porcine, rat, and mouse models.[4,5,6]

Several studies have demonstrated high reproducibility of MRI in the assessment of ejection fraction (EF) via Simpson's rule methods. In one such investigation, intraobserver, interobserver, and interexamination variability were analyzed rigorously and measurements of LV volumes using MRI were more consistent compared with those obtained by other imaging modalities in prior studies.[7] Another study found a 5% interobserver and interstudy variability in EF with cardiac MRI,[8] superior to the 10% that has been reported for echocardiography.[9] Notably, such consistency has been demonstrated in normal and morphologically abnormal (dilated and hypertrophied) left ventricles,[10] for which other methods are vulnerable to inaccuracy.

Direct comparisons between MRI and other imaging techniques in the evaluation of EF have further bolstered the value of MRI in clinical practice. One of the first such studies compared MRI with ventricular angiography in calculating EF using the area-length method and found excellent correlation between the two ($r = 0.88$).[11] More recently, MRI assessment of EF using Simpson's rule has proved more reproducible (less interstudy, intraobserver, and interobserver variability) than two-dimensional echocardiography, currently the most widely available imaging modality to assess cardiac function.[12,13] Also of note, direct comparisons among MRI, echocardiography, and radionuclide ventriculography revealed considerable differences in calculated EF, suggesting that MRI is the more accurate and preferred method to assess cardiac function, especially in dilated ventricles.[14] Because of its consistent performance in clinical evaluations, MRI assessment of LV volumes using Simpson's rule is now widely accepted as the most accurate and precise noninvasive estimation of EF.[15]

These benefits of MRI have research and clinical implications. Better reproducibility has resulted in the need for smaller sample sizes (sometimes by a factor of 80% to 90%) in studies using MRI measures of ventricular volumes than in those using other imaging modalities.[3] Furthermore, MRI is now routinely used as the gold standard when evaluating other imaging techniques, such as three-dimensional echocardiography.[16,17] MRI may be particularly important in evaluating patients for prophylactic implantable cardioverter-defibrillator placement,[18] in which an EF of 35% is commonly used to guide the implantation of a device. MRI may also be useful in serial evaluations to detect changes in EF that are smaller than the limits of sensitivity of echocardiography. This can be especially relevant in identifying the subclinical cardiotoxic effects of chemotherapy.[19]

Contraindications

Because no stimulant or contrast agent is required to assess resting EF, the contraindications for this technique coincide with those pertaining to any MRI scan, such as the presence of certain metal implants or devices (see Chapter 19) or severe claustrophobia.

Technique Description

Determination of resting EF by MRI requires no intravenous contrast agent or stimulant. The protocols that are most commonly used include steady-state free precession (SSFP) and gradient echo sequences, which are discussed in detail in Chapter 13.

Pitfalls and Solutions

Although generally very useful in accurately determining global EF, MRI does occasionally present obstacles that need to be overcome. The most frequent pitfall in MRI is inferior quality images because of respiratory motion artifact. One often-used remedy is a free-breathing protocol that uses respiratory gating or the use of real-time imaging rather than postacquisition reconstruction. Either of these techniques can improve image quality by reducing artifacts introduced by suboptimal breath-holding.

Image Interpretation

Once acquired, the global EF is determined by calculating volumes at end-diastole and end-systole. Most frequently, postprocessing involves using Simpson's rule to determine ventricular chamber volumes. The function is then reported as a percentage (calculated by dividing the stroke volume by the end-diastolic volume and multiplying by 100), with 50% to 70% considered to be the normal range.

RESTING REGIONAL WALL MOTION ABNORMALITIES

Indications and Clinical Utility

Although ventricular EF provides a global assessment of cardiac function, it is still a relatively insensitive index of myocardial pathology. A patient with an EF of 50% may have regional wall motion abnormalities indicative of underlying coronary disease. Because of its excellent spatial resolution, cine MR images of the left ventricle allow a qualitative assessment of regional cardiac function without the acoustic limitations inherent in echocardiography.[20] In addition, because the quality and resolution of white blood MR images is not closely related to body habitus or cardiac orientation, images can be acquired in almost any tomographic plane, allowing for a more comprehensive evaluation of regional function.[3]

Quantitation of regional myocardial function can be accomplished with MRI using a variety of techniques (see Chapter 14). Local wall thickening can be assessed and has been shown to correlate well with the size and extent of myocardial infarction, as measured by enzymatic release.[21] Myocardial tagging can also be used to calculate regional strain, an appealing concept because the dynamics of ventricular systole are complex and consist not only of thickening but also of contraction, expansion, twisting, and through-plane motion.[20] Strain calculation can potentially detect more subtle wall motion abnormalities than visual qualitative assessment and may provide valuable functional information in patients who have infarctions, hypertension, and nonischemic cardiomyopathies.[22-24] It is again worth noting that many of these patients may have a preserved global EF, despite having abnormal segmental myocardial mechanics. Although myocardial tagging and quantification of regional wall function is currently not a routine part of the cardiac MRI examination at most centers, considerable data suggest that it may have significant clinical utility in the future.

Contraindications

As for global EF, because no stimulants or contrast agents are required, contraindications for this technique coincide with those pertaining to any MRI scan.

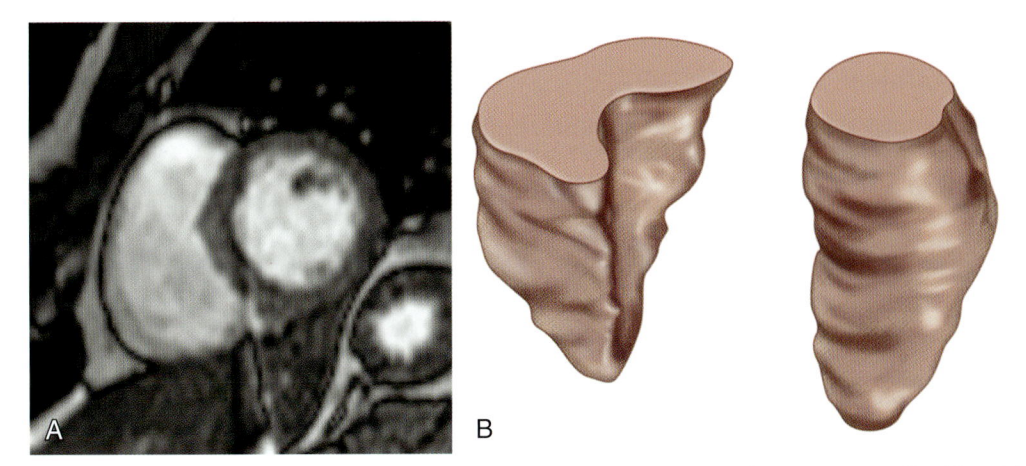

FIGURE 15-1 Short-axis MRI image of the right and left ventricles in end-diastolic phase (**A**) and representation of healthy adult ventricles (with the right ventricle on the left side of the picture) as geometrically reconstructed from MRI images (**B**). The bulging of the septum to the right side creates an irregular meniscus-shaped right ventricle that is not always amenable to certain imaging modalities.

Description

Also as for the assessment of global EF, evaluation of regional wall motion abnormalities usually involves SSFP or gradient echo sequences. Although qualitative visual assessment of wall motion is most often used and is often feasible, given the formidable spatial resolution of MRI, quantitation of wall thickening using myocardial tagging may have a more significant clinical role in the future (see earlier, "Indications and Clinical Utility"). Myocardial tagging techniques are discussed in detail in Chapter 13.

Pitfalls and Solutions

The challenges pertaining to the determination of global cardiac function also apply to the assessment of regional wall motion abnormalities—namely the need to acquire good-quality images, free of artifact. Evaluating for regional wall motion abnormalities can also be particularly daunting to those who are inexperienced because it is sometimes difficult to discern true wall thickening from simple translation. It is thus important to have interpreters who are well versed in assessing regional cardiac function.

Image Interpretation

The interpretation of wall motion is often done in a qualitative manner, as noted. Reporting wall motion entails the use of a bull's-eye diagram, with the left ventricle divided into 17 segments from the base to the apex, and assigning a score to each segment, ranging from normal to aneurysmal.

RIGHT VENTRICULAR FUNCTION

Indications and Clinical Utility

Just as for the left ventricle, RV function has important clinical and therapeutic implications. A depressed RV function predisposes patients to hypotension and confers a poor prognosis for patients with acute myocardial infarctions and chronic LV dysfunction.[25] In addition, RV function is a focus of attention in those with congenital heart disease. Because of its geometry and location beneath the sternum, the right ventricle is particularly difficult to assess with echocardiography and radionuclide ventriculography (Fig. 15-1). MRI is not bound by these constraints and thus allows for an accurate assessment of this cardiac chamber.

MRI-derived volumes and mass of the right ventricle have shown robust correlations with in vitro casts and with clinical standards, such as invasive dilution techniques and radionuclide ventriculography.[26,27] Studies have also shown high reproducibility, with low intraobserver, interobserver, and interstudy variability in normal volunteers[28] and low interstudy variability in a diverse patient population.[29] The accuracy and precision of MRI allow for rigorous clinical evaluation of the right ventricle while obviating the risk of invasive procedures and radiation exposure.

Contraindications

Contraindications to the assessment of RV function by MRI are the same for any MR scanning procedure not requiring contrast, inotropic, or vasoactive agents.

Pitfalls and Solutions

Challenges associated with the assessment of RV function by MRI are the same as those presented by left ventricular evaluation.

Image Interpretation

Unless otherwise requested, RV function is usually not quantified but is graded subjectively as normal or mildly, moderately, or severely depressed. When a more precise assessment is warranted, RV volumes can be measured using short-axis slices and an EF can thus be calculated. An EF ranging from 47% to 80% is considered normal for the right ventricle.

DIASTOLIC FUNCTION

Indications and Clinical Utility

Although echocardiography is currently the established technique for diastolic assessment, there are inherent limitations to ultrasound that may be overcome with MRI, which can be used to evaluate the ventricle in three dimensions, taking into account the untwisting, longitudinal, and radial movement that occurs in diastole. Using myocardial tagging, strain assessment in these different orientations can be determined, thereby yielding a potentially more comprehensive evaluation of ventricular diastole than that offered by echocardiography. Transmitral flow velocities can also be determined, as in echocardiography, to ascertain the LV filling pattern and degree of diastolic dysfunction.

Contraindications

Contraindications to assessment of diastolic function are the same as for any MRI scan not requiring contrast, inotropic, or vasoactive agents.

Pitfalls and Solutions

Given the rapidity of diastolic flow propagation, the limited temporal resolution of MRI can be a hindrance in accurately assessing diastolic function. This can be overcome by adjusting the views per segment, compromising some degree of spatial resolution, and/or using a free-breathing as opposed to a breath-hold protocol, so a longer time of acquisition can be used. Generally, a temporal resolution of at least 35 ms is warranted for diastolic evaluation.

Image Interpretation

In addition to evaluating the motion and strain of the myocardial tissue, which is currently not widely used clinically for diastole, MRI can also determine LV flow velocities and propagation during diastole. Using phase contrast imaging (see Chapter 17), the transmitral flow pattern can be determined much like it is with echocardiography. It is important to note, however, that some aspects of the transmitral E signal, such as acceleration and deceleration time, have not been validated with phase contrast MRI. Further characterization of diastolic LV flow can be achieved using a combination of phase contrast imaging and color vector mapping (Fig. 15-2). This is an experimental technique at present and is not yet widely used in clinical practice, but it does represent the potential of phase contrast imaging for assessing flow propagation in LV diastole. There is currently no standardized method of reporting diastolic function assessed by MRI.

DYNAMIC LEFT VENTRICULAR FUNCTION USING DOBUTAMINE

Indications and Clinical Utility

Like resting cardiac function, LV response to chronotropic and inotropic stimulation provides considerable clinical information, both physiologic and prognostic. Advances in software and hardware, specifically the development of phased-array surface coils, faster scanning, and advanced gating have increased the practicality and clinical utility of cardiac MRI wall motion stress testing.[3] The focus of this subject will be the use of dobutamine and exercise stress testing in clinical practice. See Chapter 53 for a discussion of myocardial contrast perfusion imaging.

Physiology and Safety Profile of Dobutamine

Dobutamine is a synthetic catecholamine with mild β_1 receptor selectivity.[30,31] It is a positive inotrope and, because of its peripheral vasodilatory effects, it induces a reflex tachycardia.[32] At doses of up to 10 μg/kg/min, dobutamine augments myocardial contractility and promotes coronary vasodilation; doses of 20 to 40 μg/kg/min increase heart rate and myocardial oxygen demand[33] and, in the setting of significant epicardial coronary artery stenoses, can induce wall motion abnormalities by way of a supply-demand mismatch (Fig. 15-3).[34,35] Several large-scale investigations have evaluated the safety of dobutamine as a stress agent and have found a low incidence (often less than 1%) of major complications.[36,37]

Dobutamine Magnetic Resonance Imaging and Myocardial Ischemia

Perhaps the most common use of dobutamine stress imaging is to identify those patients who have physiologically significant coronary stenoses. The first clinical trials investigating the use of MRI in dobutamine studies were relatively small but showed excellent agreement between wall motion abnormalities seen on MRI at peak dobutamine levels and areas of abnormal myocardial perfusion as assessed by dobutamine thallium perfusion.[38,39] The sensitivity of dobutamine MRI compared favorably with that of dipyridamole MRI in detecting coronary stenoses in another study consisting exclusively of patients with high-grade (70% or more) lesions of at least one major coronary vessel.[40] In this series, the sensitivity of dobutamine MRI in detecting this degree of coronary stenosis was higher than 80% and increased with multivessel involvement. These early studies implied the safety and effectiveness of dobutamine as a pharmacologic stress agent and the utility of cardiac MRI in assessing for wall motion abnormalities.

A larger, more recent study compared dobutamine MRI with dobutamine stress echocardiography (DSE),[41] a routinely used method of detecting inducible ischemia. In this study, 208 consecutive patients underwent DSE, dobutamine MRI, and biplane coronary angiography within a 14-day period. Dobutamine MRI demonstrated better sensitivity (86% vs. 74%) and specificity (86% vs. 70%) than DSE in detecting coronary artery disease (defined as more than 50% luminal narrowing) seen on angiography. Examinations were feasible in approximately 90% of patients with both DSE and dobutamine MRI, although the reasons for exclusion differed for the two techniques. Insufficient image quality was the major reason for exclusion from DSE and claustrophobia for dobutamine MRI. On the basis of these results, it was concluded that dobutamine MRI

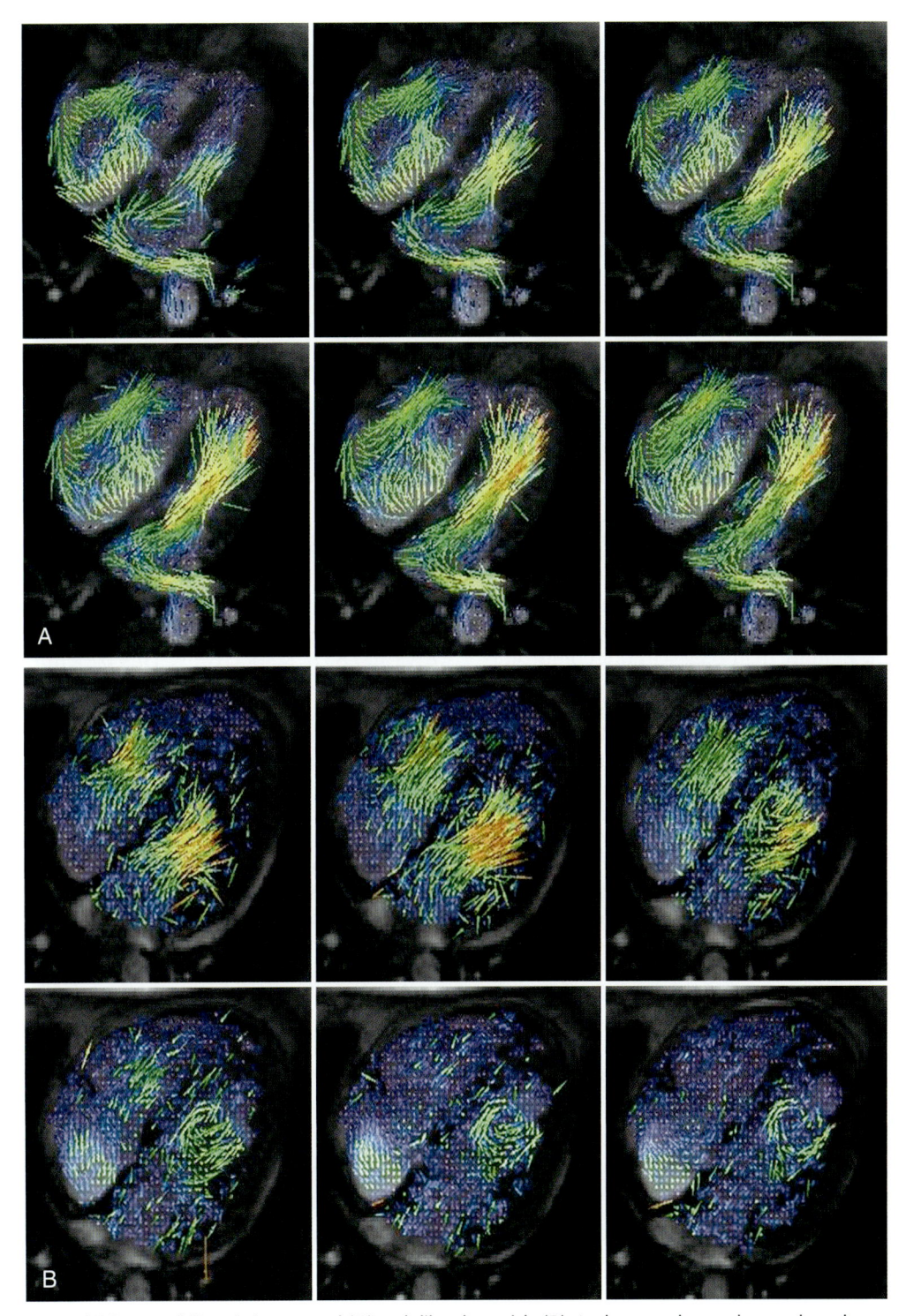

FIGURE 15-2 Sequential frames of diastole in a normal (**A**) and dilated ventricle (**B**). In the normal example, note how the streamlines extend all the way to the apex. By contrast, flow propagation is markedly less and degenerates into a vortex in the middle of the dilated left ventricle.

can detect wall motion abnormalities with significantly higher diagnostic accuracy than DSE because of improved image quality.

In keeping with this hypothesis, another large-scale, single-center trial evaluated 163 patients referred for DSE who did not have adequate imaging windows, despite the use of second harmonic imaging and contrast agents.[42] These patients underwent dobutamine MRI instead and the vast majority (more than 80%) were able to complete their study without complications. Of patients who underwent coronary angiography, dobutamine MRI had a sensitivity and specificity higher than 80% in the detection of coronary arterial luminal narrowing of at least 50%, similar to the results of the study detailed earlier. Of note, this study included patients who had resting wall motion abnormalities, whereas the study by Nagel and colleagues[41] specifically excluded patients with previous myocardial infarction and reduced resting EF. The authors concluded

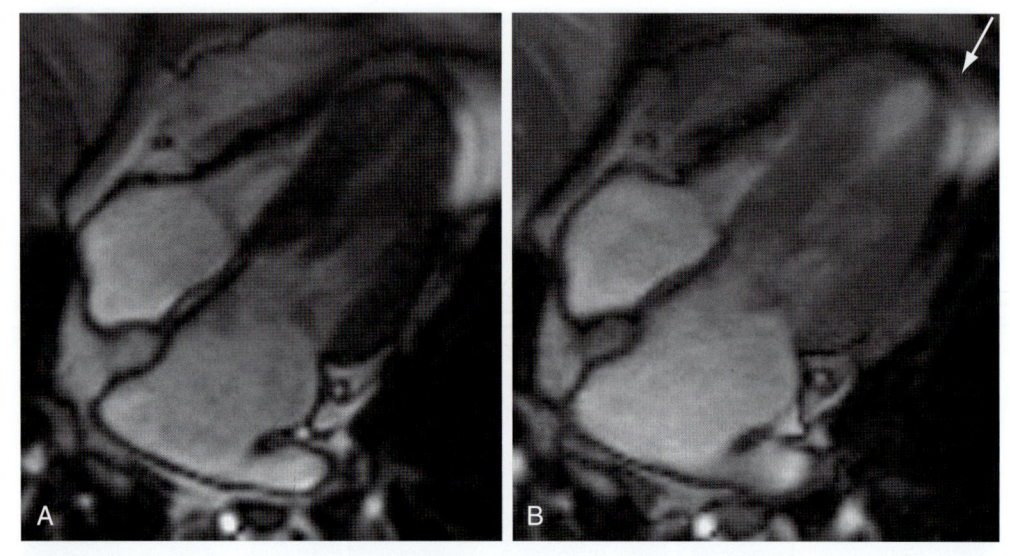

FIGURE 15-3 Wall motion abnormality during dobutamine infusion. **A,** At baseline, the end-systolic frame shows all segments contracting normally. **B,** The apex (*arrow*) becomes akinetic at peak dobutamine infusion, however.

that dobutamine MRI could be performed safely using fast imaging techniques and that dobutamine MRI had potentially greater clinical utility than DSE, without compromising sensitivity or specificity.

Further studies have increasingly substantiated the clinical utility of dobutamine MRI. In a small series consisting exclusively of patients with known epicardial coronary disease, low-dose dobutamine MRI was effective in differentiating normal, ischemic, hibernating, and nonviable myocardium.[43] There was also robust correlation seen with stress perfusion in these patients. In another study, which looked exclusively at patients with known coronary disease, Wahl and associates[44] performed high-dose dobutamine MRI prior to coronary angiography on 160 consecutive patients who had undergone prior coronary revascularization and had resting wall motion abnormalities. The sensitivity and specificity of dobutamine MRI in detecting coronary luminal narrowing of at least 50% was 89% and 84%, respectively. This patient population (with underlying wall motion abnormalities and low EF) is especially difficult to evaluate with DSE because of frequently poor acoustic windows. The fact that the diagnostic accuracy of dobutamine MRI is maintained in this group further broadens its clinical utility (Table 15-1).

In these studies and in current routine clinical practice, wall motion abnormalities are identified and graded in a qualitative manner. The heightened image clarity of MRI, however, is well suited for quantitative analysis; this may attenuate the subjectivity involved in dobutamine stress assessment. Dobutamine MRI was performed in 39 consecutive patients referred for coronary angiography and in 10 normal volunteers; wall thickening was quantified

TABLE 15-1 Summary of Studies Validating the Clinical Utility of Dobutamine Magnetic Resonance Imaging in Detecting Significant Coronary Disease

Study	Subjects and Imaging	Methods	Results and Conclusions
Baer et al[40]	61 patients with significant coronary artery disease and normal EF underwent dobutamine and dipyridamole MRI.	Wall motion abnormalities were assessed on each study to determine safety and sensitivity for both tests.	Overall sensitivity for both tests in the detection of coronary disease exceeded 80%, with no serious side effects reported.
Nagel et al[41]	208 patients underwent dobutamine MRI, DSE, and coronary angiography within a 14-day period.	Sensitivity and specificity in detecting coronary stenoses of >50% were determined for both modalities.	Dobutamine MRI demonstrated higher sensitivity (86% vs. 74%) and specificity (86% vs. 70%) than DSE.
Hundley et al[42]	153 consecutive patients with poor echocardiographic windows underwent dobutamine MRI.	The safety of performing dobutamine MRI in patients who could not undergo DSE because of poor acoustic windows was assessed.	No serious events occurred in any patients undergoing dobutamine MRI. In 41 patients who underwent coronary angiography, the sensitivity and specificity of dobutamine MRI in detecting significant coronary lesions exceeded 80%.
Wahl et al[44]	160 consecutive patients who had undergone prior revascularization procedures and had resting wall motion abnormalities underwent dobutamine MRI followed by coronary angiography.	The sensitivity and specificity of dobutamine MRI in detecting significant coronary disease in abnormal left ventricles was assessed.	Sensitivity and specificity of dobutamine MRI in detecting coronary stenoses of >50% were 89% and 84%, respectively.

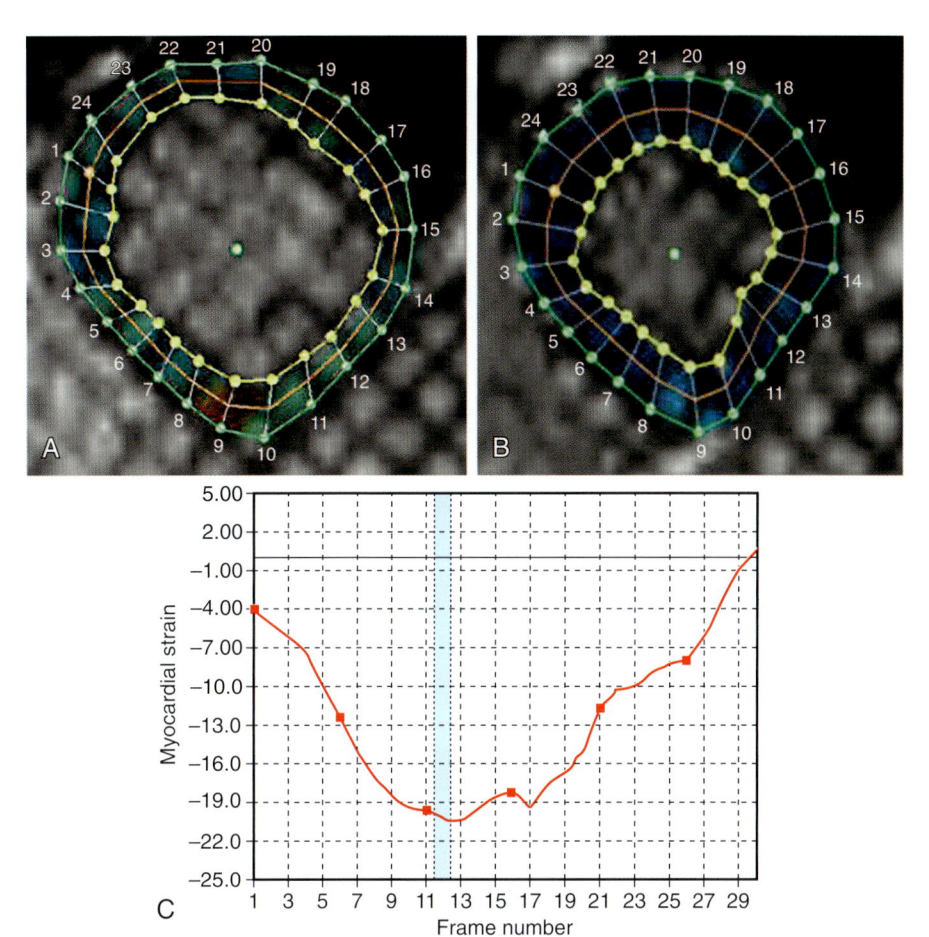

FIGURE 15-4 Strain assessment by way of myocardial tagging. Tagged end-diastolic (**A**) and end-systolic (**B**) images are seen, along with the quantitative assessment of strain (**C**).

using the modified center line technique.[45] This technique yielded a sensitivity of 91% and specificity of 80% in the detection of significant coronary artery disease. Myocardial tagging has also been applied to dobutamine MRI studies and yields significantly different strain and strain rates in ischemic and infarcted myocardium than in remote normal segments.[46] Comparing tagged and nontagged images in dobutamine MRI studies, Kuijpers and coworkers[47] found that tagged images detected inducible wall motion abnormalities in 10 patients who were judged to have normal nontagged studies. All these patients were found to have coronary disease on subsequent coronary angiography. Of note, this trial did not use quantitative methods to determine strain via the tagged images. Further studies are required to determine whether myocardial tagging and quantitative techniques are truly superior to visual assessment of wall motion and whether they should become a standard part of clinical practice (Fig. 15-4).

Dobutamine Magnetic Resonance Imaging and Myocardial Viability

Following an ischemic event, differentiating between viable and nonviable myocardial tissue is an important clinical distinction that can help determine the utility of revascularization. Early studies evaluating the use of cardiac MRI for this found that wall thinning and shortened T2 relaxation time at rest could identify regions of chronic infarction (i.e., nonviable myocardium).[48] Corroborating the importance of wall thickness in assessing for myocardial viability was a study by Baer and colleagues,[49] which correlated a diastolic wall thickness more than 2.5 standard deviations below the normal mean value and systolic akinesis to markedly reduced technetium uptake.

Another study by this group sought to determine which markers could predict contractile recovery of dysfunctional myocardium following revascularization, a functional definition of myocardial viability.[50] In this series, 43 patients who suffered a remote myocardial infarction underwent resting and low-dose dobutamine cardiac MRI as well as a follow-up resting MRI after a revascularization procedure (either bypass grafting or angioplasty). A resting diastolic wall thickness of 5.5 mm or more was 92% sensitive but only 56% specific in predicting contractile recovery on postrevascularization MRI. Dobutamine-induced systolic wall thickening of 2 mm or more was highly sensitive (89%) but also very specific (94%) in predicting functional recovery. The authors concluded that low-dose dobutamine cardiac MRI provided more information on myocardial viability than resting MRI alone. Other studies evaluating the use of low-dose dobutamine MRI in assessing for contractile recovery in patients with a recent myocardial infarction have also yielded favorable results, with diagnostic accuracy exceeding 80%.[51,52]

Just as for the detection of coronary stenoses, DSE is also widely used to identify myocardial viability. An early study comparing dobutamine MRI with DSE found a

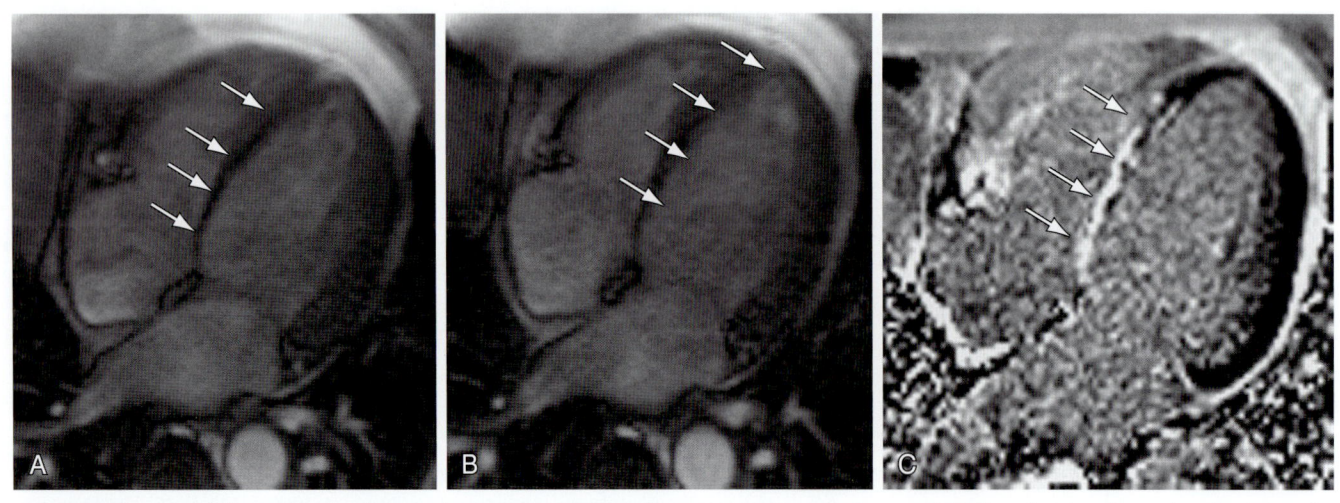

FIGURE 15-5 Viability study using dobutamine to evaluate contractile reserve. End-systolic frames of the four-chamber view at baseline (A) and with low-dose dobutamine (B) show persistent akinesis of the inferior septum (arrows). There is extensive transmural delayed enhancement of this area with gadolinium (C), confirming the lack of viability.

high degree of concordance in the diagnosis of viability.[53] Baer and associates[54] compared dobutamine transesophageal echocardiography (TEE) with dobutamine MRI using positron emission tomography (PET) scanning as the reference standard for viability. Both modalities yielded similar results but MRI was slightly more sensitive and specific than echocardiography. In a follow-up study, a similar head-to-head comparison was performed, this time using contractile recovery following revascularization as the end point. The investigators determined that there was no significant difference between dobutamine TEE and dobutamine MRI in the assessment of viability.[55] These studies indicated that dobutamine MRI compared favorably with an already accepted technique in the assessment of myocardial viability.

Dobutamine MRI has also been compared with contrast MRI imaging for the assessment of viability (Fig. 15-5). Delayed hyperenhancement techniques using gadolinium contrast are widely used in determining the extent of viable and scarred myocardium, discussed in detail in Chapter 57. Partial wall thickness enhancement (less than 75%) represents an area of uncertainty in predicting contractile recovery, which may be clarified with low-dose dobutamine testing. Kaandorp and colleagues sought to investigate the relevance of intermediate degrees of enhancement[56] and found that regions with only subendocardial enhancement (encompassing 1% to 50% of total ventricular wall thickness) often exhibited contractile reserve with low-dose dobutamine, whereas areas with transmural involvement (enhancement extending to 76% to 100% of wall thickness) did not improve with dobutamine. Segments with 51% to 75% enhancement varied in their response, with 61% of these segments improving with dobutamine and 39% demonstrating no contractile reserve. The authors concluded that in cases of intermediate hyperenhancement, assessment of contractile reserve with dobutamine may allow optimal identification of segments that are likely to improve with revascularization.

In keeping with this hypothesis, two studies have compared dobutamine MRI with delayed contrast-enhanced MRI in predicting functional improvement after a revascularization procedure in patients with coronary artery disease.[57,58] Dobutamine MRI exhibited a greater diagnostic accuracy than contrast enhancement; this advantage was largest in segments with intermediate degrees of enhancement (51% to 75%). Low-dose dobutamine MRI compares favorably with echocardiography and delayed hyperenhancement, which is a reflection of its clinical accuracy and utility in evaluating for myocardial viability.

Dobutamine Magnetic Resonance Imaging and Patient Prognosis

Aside from providing physiologic information, the results of a clinically relevant cardiac study should have prognostic implications and risk stratification value. To this end, Hundley and colleagues[59] followed 279 patients over an average of 20 months after the completion of full-dose dobutamine MRI. Evidence of inducible ischemia or a resting EF lower than 40% was associated with myocardial infarction and cardiac death independently of the presence of coronary risk factors (Fig. 15-6). Of note, these patients had previous transthoracic echocardiography that was not adequate for wall motion analysis and so the authors concluded that in patients with poor echocardiograms, the results of dobutamine MRI stress tests can be used to forecast myocardial infarction or cardiac death.

The results of another investigation by Kuijpers and associates[60] further suggested the clinical utility of dobutamine MRI in patient risk stratification. Consecutive patients (299) suspected of myocardial ischemia but with indeterminate resting and bicycle exercise electrocardiograms underwent resting and full-dose dobutamine MRI. Patients who had resting wall motion abnormalities were at higher risk for major adverse cardiac events at 2-year follow-up than patients with normal resting wall motion (18% vs. 0.56%; $P < .001$). Furthermore, the results of dobutamine MRI could classify patients with unknown or

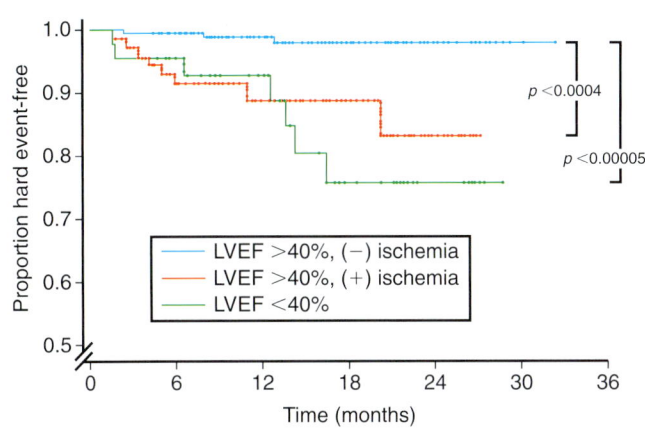

FIGURE 15-6 Kaplan-Meier event-free survival curves in patients with an LVEF < 40% or ≥ 40%, with or without inducible ischemia. Compared with patients with an LVEF ≥ 40% and no evidence of inducible ischemia, event-free survival was significantly lower in patients with inducible ischemia ($P < .0004$) or an LVEF < 40% ($P < .00005$). (Adapted from Hundley WG, Morgan TM, Neagle CM, et al. Magnetic resonance imaging determination of cardiac prognosis. Circulation 2002; 106:2328-2333.)

intermediate risk (e.g., patients in this study with no prior history of coronary disease, indeterminate resting electrocardiograms, and no resting wall motion abnormalities) more definitively into a high or low coronary risk group. It was concluded that dobutamine MRI may be a valuable tool in risk-stratifying patients, especially those with unclear cardiac risk.

Dobutamine MRI has also been used in the assessment of preoperative cardiovascular risk in patients undergoing noncardiac surgery.[61] In 102 consecutive patients unable to undergo stress echocardiography because of inadequate acoustic windows, 6 patients suffered a perioperative cardiac event and 5 of them had inducible ischemia on their dobutamine MRI. Just as in the earlier study, the investigators though that dobutamine MRI was a significant predictor of cardiac events and could be especially useful for clarifying risk in patients who have intermediate clinical predictors of perioperative cardiac events.

Contraindications

In addition to having the usual contraindications to any MR scan, dobutamine MRI also presents the added risk of an intravenous inotrope. Patients with ongoing ischemia, tachyarrhythmias, intracardiac thrombi, and severe baseline hypertension may not be suitable candidates for dobutamine infusion.

Pitfalls and Solutions

Image quality with dobutamine can be problematic because the tachycardia may decrease temporal and spatial resolution. Using different protocols, including those involving free-breathing sequences, may be a viable option. In cases in which the patient does not reach target heart rate (usually 85% of maximum predicted in tests for ischemia), administering atropine to decrease vagal tone may be required. On the other hand, if the patient develops persistent tachycardia or hypertension with dobutamine infusion, intravenous β blockade may be warranted.

Image Interpretation

In clinical practice, wall motion is assessed visually at rest and at peak stress. The left ventricle is divided into 17 segments and each is given a score ranging from normal to aneurysmal. If wall motion abnormalities are inducible with dobutamine, the location of coronary stenosis that corresponds to the wall motion territory in question is reported.

DYNAMIC LEFT VENTRICULAR FUNCTION USING EXERCISE

Indications and Clinical Utility

In patients who are capable of physical exertion, it may be possible to perform exercise rather than pharmacologic stress MRI. Both bicycle and treadmill exercise have been evaluated as stress agents (Fig. 15-7) and have

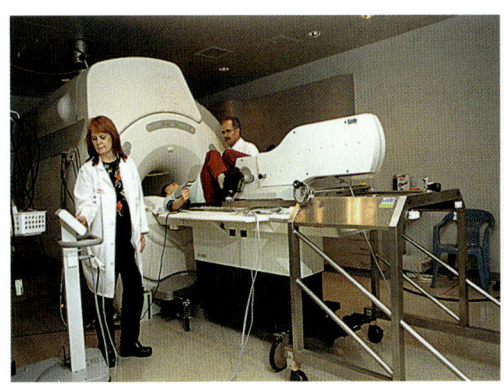

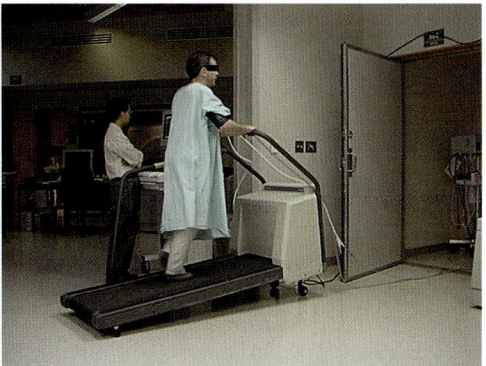

Exercise bike attached to the scanner | Treadmill positioned outside the scan room

FIGURE 15-7 Exercise cardiovascular magnetic resonance. Shown is a diagrammatic representation of an exercise bike used for MRI stress studies made from nonferromagnetic materials (*left panel*). In the *right panel*, a treadmill is positioned outside the magnetic resonance scanner. With this treadmill approach, heightened diagnostic accuracy is achieved when images are collected within 1 minute of exercise cessation. (Adapted from Walsh TF, Hundley G. Assessment of ventricular function with cardiovascular magnetic resonance. Cardiol Clin 2007; 25:15-33.)

shown favorable preliminary results. In one study, 16 healthy patients successfully completed supine bicycle stress tests and underwent MR imaging using an ultrafast sequence.[62] Both the right and left ventricles demonstrated physiologic changes with exercise, such as increased stroke volume and EF and decreased end-systolic volumes, all of which were consistent with previous exercise physiology data. Because of the difficulty in imaging the right ventricle with conventional modalities, this is one of the few reports detailing the response of the right ventricle to exercise. In another trial, which used treadmill exercise, 27 patients with exertional chest pain completed an exercise protocol and subsequent MRI imaging.[63] The sequence was 79% sensitive and 85% specific for detecting more than 70% coronary artery stenoses on coronary angiography. These values are similar to those obtained by stress echocardiography and nuclear studies. The authors noted that one of the major limitations of performing treadmill MRI tests is the inability to acquire images within 60 to 90 seconds of cessation of exercise. This report suggests that treadmill MRI testing is at least feasible and further studies are needed to determine the clinical utility of exercise stress MRI in the evaluation of ischemic heart disease.

Contraindications

Any patient who is unable to exercise, has unstable angina, or has any exercise-limiting condition such as chronic lung disease or peripheral arterial disease would not be a suitable candidate for exercise MRI.

Pitfalls and Solutions

The major challenge in exercise MRI is acquiring images at peak heart rate. After cessation of exercise, the heart rate often drops rapidly and significantly, necessitating a very prompt transfer from exercise equipment to the scanner. Delays in this transition can produce a suboptimal stress test. Optimal placement of exercise equipment and coordination among MRI staff are essential in performing exercise MRI.

Image Interpretation

Exercise MRI studies are interpreted and reported much the same way as those involving dobutamine—namely, an assessment of wall motion at rest and at peak heart rate and the coronary territory that corresponds to any inducible wall motion abnormalities.

SUMMARY AND CONCLUSION

Much data have been accumulated with respect to the MRI assessment of ventricular function. Because of its excellent spatial resolution, MRI is now the gold standard for measuring resting cardiac chamber volumes and has shown greater accuracy and precision than other imaging modalities in this regard. The same holds true for evaluation of segmental wall motion abnormalities. Further studies are needed to determine whether myocardial tagging and strain quantification should be a standard part of the clinical examination.

There is also a growing body of data suggesting the clinical utility of stress MRI in several areas, both physiologic and prognostic. Larger scale trials and longer term follow-up are warranted to confirm the clinical power of pharmacologic and exercise stress MRI. In addition, research is underway to address the shortcomings of stress MRI, including long scan times, limited access to patients during stress, and distortion of electrocardiogram tracings by the magnetic field. As a whole, however, clinical trials suggest that MRI is a clinically useful means of assessing many aspects of cardiac function.

KEY POINTS

- The assessment of cardiac function can be done at rest and with stress.
- MRI is generally a safe, effective, and clinically effective tool for determining resting and dynamic left ventricular function, as well as right ventricular function.
- There are relatively few contraindications to the determination of resting left ventricular function by MRI.
- Future directions include strain assessment and diastolic evaluation.

SUGGESTED READING

Walsh TF, Hundley G. Assessment of ventricular function with cardiovascular magnetic resonance. Cardiol Clin 2007; 25:15-33.

REFERENCES

1. Ganz W, Donoso R, Marcus HS, et al: A new technique for measurement of cardiac output by thermodilution in man. Am J Cardiol 1971; 27:392-396.
2. Rehr RB, Malloy CR, Filipchuk NG, et al. Left ventricular volumes measured by MR imaging. Radiology 1985; 156:717-719.
3. Walsh TF, Hundley G. Assessment of ventricular function with cardiovascular magnetic resonance. Cardiol Clin 2007; 25:15-33.
4. Nahrendorf M, Hiller KH, Hu K, et al. Cardiac magnetic resonance imaging in small animal models of human heart failure. Med Image Anal 2003; 7:369-375.

5. Koch JA, Poll LW, Godehardt E, et al. Right and left ventricular volume measurements in an animal heart model in vitro: first experiences with cardiac MRI at 1.0 T. Eur Radiol 2000; 10:455-458.
6. Caputo GR, Tscholakoff DT, Sechtem U, Higgins CB. Measurement of canine left ventricular mass by using MR imaging. Am J Roentgenol 1987; 148:33-38.
7. Pattynama PMT, Lamb HJ, van der Velde EA, et al. Left ventricular measurements with cine and spin-echo MR imaging: a study of reproducibility with variance component analysis. Radiology 1993; 187:261-268.
8. Semelka RC, Tomei E, Wagner S, et al. Normal left ventricular dimensions and function: interstudy reproducibility of measurements with cine MR imaging. Radiology 1990; 174:763-768.
9. Gordon EP, Schnittger I, Fitzgerald PJ, et al. Reproducibility of left ventricular volumes by two-dimensional echocardiography. J Am Coll Cardiol 1983; 2:506-513.
10. Semelka RC, Tomei E, Wagner S, et al. Interstudy reproducibility of dimensional and functional measurements between cine magnetic resonance studies in the morphologically abnormal left ventricle. Am Heart J 1990; 119:1367-1373.
11. Stratemeier EJ, Thompson R, Brady TJ, et al. Ejection fraction determination by MR imaging: comparison with left ventricular angiography. Radiology 1986; 158:775-777.
12. Grothues F, Smith GC, Moon JCC, et al. Comparison of interstudy reproducibility of cardiovascular magnetic resonance with two-dimensional echocardiography in normal subjects and in patients with heart failure or left ventricular hypertrophy. Am J Cardiol 2002; 90:29-34.
13. Bellenger NG, Marcus NJ, Davies C, et al. Left ventricular function and mass after orthotopic heart transplantation: a comparison of cardiovascular magnetic resonance with echocardiography. J Heart Lung Transplant 2000; 19:444-452.
14. Bellenger NG, Burgess MI, Ray SG, et al. Comparison of left ventricular ejection fraction and volumes in heart failure by echocardiography, radionuclide ventriculography and cardiovascular magnetic resonance. Are they interchangeable? Eur Heart J 2000; 21:1387-1396.
15. Rumberger JA, Behrenbeck T, Bell MR, et al. Determination of ventricular ejection fraction: a comparison of available imaging methods. Mayo Clin Proc 1997; 72:360-370.
16. Ioannidis JPA, Trikalinos TA, Danias PG. Electrocardiogram-gated single-photon emission computed tomography versus cardiac magnetic resonance imaging for the assessment of left ventricular volumes and ejection fraction: a meta-analysis. J Am Coll Cardiol 2002; 39:2059-2068.
17. Chuang MI, Hibberd MG, Salton CJ, et al. Importance of imaging method over imaging modality in noninvasive determination of left ventricular volumes and ejection fraction: assessment by two- and three-dimensional echocardiography and magnetic resonance imaging. J Am Coll Cardiol 2000; 35:477-484.
18. Zimetbaum PJ. A 59-year-old man considering implantation of a cardiac defibrillator. JAMA 2007; 297:1909-1916.
19. Oberholzer K, Kunz RP, Dittrich M, Thelen M. Anthracycline-induced cardiotoxicity: cardiac MRI after treatment for childhood cancer. Fortschr Roentgenstr 2004; 176:1245-1250.
20. Bellenger NG, Grothues F, Smith GC, Pennell DJ. Quantification of right and left ventricular function by cardiovascular magnetic resonance. Herz 2000; 25:392-399.
21. Holman E, van Jonbergen HPW, van Dijkman PRM, et al. Comparison of magnetic resonance imaging studies with enzymatic indexes of myocardial necrosis for quantification of myocardial infarct size. Am J Cardiol 1993; 71:1036-1040.
22. Kramer CM, Rogers WJ, Theobald TM, et al. Remote noninfarcted region dysfunction soon after first anterior myocardial infarction. A magnetic resonance tagging study. Circulation 1996; 94:660-666.
23. Palmon LC, Reichek N, Yeon SB, et al. Intramural myocardial shortening in hypertensive left ventricular hypertrophy with normal pump function. Circulation 1994; 89:122-131.
24. MacGowan GA, Shapiro EP, Azhari H, et al. Noninvasive measurement of shortening in the fiber and cross-fiber directions in the normal human left ventricle and in idiopathic dilated cardiomyopathy. Circulation 1997; 96:535-541.
25. Zehender M, Kasper W, Kauder E, et al. Right ventricular infarction as an independent predictor of prognosis after acute inferior myocardial infarction. N Engl J Med 1993; 328:981-988.
26. Longmore DB, Underwood SR, Hounsfield GN, et al. Dimensional accuracy of magnetic resonance in studies of the heart. Lancet 1985; 1:1360-1362.
27. Culham JA, Vince DJ. Cardiac output by MR imaging: an experimental study comparing right ventricle and left ventricle with thermodilution. Can Assoc Radiol J 1988; 39:247-249.
28. Lorenz CH, Walker ES, Morgan VL, et al. Normal human right and left ventricular mass, systolic function, and gender differences by cine magnetic resonance imaging. J Cardiovasc Magn Reson 1999; 1:7-21.
29. Grothues F, Moon JC, Bellenger NG, et al. Interstudy reproducibility of right ventricular volumes, function, and mass with cardiovascular magnetic resonance. Am Heart J 2004; 147:218-223.
30. Vallet B, Dupuis B, Chopin C. Dobutamine: mechanisms of action and use in acute cardiovascular pathology. Ann Cardiol Angiol (Paris) 1991; 40:397-402.
31. Ruffolo RR Jr. The pharmacology of dobutamine. Am J Med Sci 1987; 294:244-248.
32. Baig MW. Pharmacologic perfusion imaging. Who needs it and why? Postgrad Med J 1992; 91:185-187.
33. Iskandrian AS, Verani MS, Heo J. Pharmacologic stress testing: mechanism of action, hemodynamic responses, and results in detection of coronary artery disease. J Nucl Cardiol 1994; 1:94-111.
34. Kugiyama K, Inobe Y, Ohgushi M, et al. Comparison of coronary hemodynamics during infusions of dobutamine and adenosine in patients with angina pectoris. Jpn Circ J 1998; 62:1-6.
35. Warltier DC, Zyvoloski M, Gross GJ, et al. Redistribution of myocardial blood flow distal to a dynamic coronary arterial stenosis by sympathomimetic amines: comparison of dopamine, dobutamine and isoproterenol. Am J Cardiol 1981; 48:269-279.
36. Kuijpers D, Janssen CH, van Dijkman PR, et al. Dobutamine stress MRI. Part I: safety and feasibility of dobutamine cardiovascular magnetic resonance in patients suspected of myocardial ischemia. Eur Radiol 2004; 14:1823-1828.
37. Hamilton CA, Link KM, Salido TB, et al. Is imaging at intermediate doses necessary during dobutamine stress magnetic resonance imaging? J Cardiovasc Magn Reson 2001; 3:297-302.
38. Pennell DJ, Underwood SR. The cardiovascular effects of dobutamine assessed by magnetic resonance imaging. Postgrad Med J 1991; 67(Suppl 1):S1-S8.
39. Pennell DJ, Underwood SR, Manzara CC, et al. Magnetic resonance imaging during dobutamine stress in coronary artery disease. Am J Cardiol 1992; 70:34-40.
40. Baer FM, Theissen P, Smolarz K, et al. Dobutamine versus dipyridamole magnetic resonance tomography: safety and sensitivity in the detection of coronary stenoses. Z Kardiol. 1993; 82:494-503.
41. Nagel E, Lehmkuhl HB, Bocksch W, et al. Noninvasive diagnosis of ischemia-induced wall motion abnormalities with the use of high-dose dobutamine stress MRI: comparison with dobutamine stress echocardiography. Circulation 1999; 99:763-770.
42. Hundley WG, Hamilton CA, Thomas MS, et al. Utility of fast cine magnetic resonance imaging and display for the detection of myocardial ischemia in patients not well suited for second harmonic stress echocardiography. Circulation 1999; 100:1697-1702.
43. Sensky PR, Jivan A, Hudson NM, et al. Coronary artery disease: combined stress MR imaging protocol—one-stop evaluation of myocardial perfusion and function. Radiology 2000; 215:608-614.
44. Wahl A, Paetsch I, Roethemeyer S, et al. High-dose dobutamine-atropine stress cardiovascular MR imaging after coronary revascularization in patients with wall motion abnormalities at rest. Radiology 2004; 233:210-216.
45. Van Rugge FP, van der Wall EEE, Spanjersberg SJ, et al. Magnetic resonance imaging during dobutamine stress for detection and localization of coronary artery disease. Circulation 1994; 90:127-138.
46. Edvardsen T, Gerber BL, Garot J, et al. Quantitative assessment of intrinsic regional myocardial deformation by Doppler strain rate echocardiography in humans: validation against three-dimensional tagged magnetic resonance imaging. Circulation 2002; 106:50-56.
47. Kuijpers D, Ho KY, van Dijkman PR, et al. Dobutamine cardiovascular magnetic resonance for the detection of myocardial ischemia with the use of myocardial tagging. Circulation 2003; 107:1592-1597.
48. McNamara MT, Higgins CB. Magnetic resonance imaging of chronic myocardial infarcts in man. AJR Am J Roentgenol 1986; 146:315-320.

49. Baer FM, Smolarz K, Theissen P, et al. Regional 99mTc-methoxyiso-butyl-isonitrile-uptake at rest in patients with myocardial infarcts: comparison with morphological and functional parameters obtained from gradient-echo magnetic resonance imaging. Eur Heart J 1994; 15:97-107.
50. Baer FM, Theissen P, Schneider CA, et al. Dobutamine magnetic resonance imaging predicts contractile recovery of chronically dysfunctional myocardium after successful revascularization. J Am Coll Cardiol 1998; 31:1040-1048.
51. Dendale P, Franken PR, Holman E, et al. Validation of low-dose dobutamine magnetic resonance imaging for assessment of myocardial viability after infarction by serial imaging. Am J Cardiol 1998; 82:375-377.
52. Sandstede JJW, Bertsch G, Beer M, et al. Detection of myocardial viability by low-dose dobutamine cine MR imaging. Magn Reson Imaging 1999; 17:1437-1443.
53. Dendale PA, Franken PR, Waldman G-J, et al. Low-dosage dobutamine magnetic resonance imaging as an alternative to echocardiography in the detection of viable myocardium after acute infarction. Am Heart J 1995; 130:134-140.
54. Baer FM, Voth E, LaRosee K, et al. Comparison of dobutamine transesophageal echocardiography and dobutamine magnetic resonance imaging for detection of residual myocardial viability. Am J Cardiol 1996; 78:415-419.
55. Baer FM, Theissen P, Crnac J, et al. Head to head comparison of dobutamine–transoesophageal echocardiography and dobutamine–magnetic resonance imaging for the prediction of left ventricular functional recovery in patients with chronic coronary artery disease. Eur Heart J 2000; 21:981-991.
56. Kaandorp TAM, Bax JJ, Schuijf JD, et al. Head-to-head comparison between contrast-enhanced magnetic resonance imaging and dobutamine magnetic resonance imaging in men with ischemic cardiomyopathy. Am J Cardiol 2004; 93:1461-1464.
57. Motoyasu M, Sakuma H, Ichikawa Y, et al. Prediction of regional functional recovery after acute myocardial infarction with low dose dobutamine stress cine MR imaging and contrast enhanced MR imaging. Cardiovasc Magn Reson 2003; 5:563-564.
58. Wellnhofer E, Olariu A, Klein C, et al. Magnetic resonance low-dose dobutamine test is superior to scar quantification for the prediction of functional recovery. Circulation 2004; 109:2172-2174.
59. Hundley WG, Morgan TM, Neagle CM, et al. Magnetic resonance imaging determination of cardiac prognosis. Circulation 2002; 106:2328-2333.
60. Kuijpers D, van Dijkman PRM, Janssen CHC, et al. Dobutamine stress MRI. Part II. Risk stratification with dobutamine cardiovascular magnetic resonance in patients suspected of myocardial ischemia. Eur Radiol 2004; 14:2046-2052.
61. Rerkpattanapipat P, Morgan TM, Neagle CM, et al. Assessment of preoperative cardiac risk with magnetic resonance imaging. Am J Cardiol 2002; 90:416-419.
62. Roest AAW, Kunz P, Lamb HJ, et al. Biventricular response to supine physical exercise in young adults assessed with ultrafast magnetic resonance imaging. Am J Cardiol 2001; 87:601-605.
63. Rerkpattanapipat P, Gandhi SK, Darty SN, et al. Feasibility to detect severe coronary artery stenoses with upright treadmill exercise magnetic resonance imaging. Am J Cardiol 2003; 92:603-606.

CHAPTER 16

Clinical Techniques of Cardiac Magnetic Resonance Imaging: Functional Interpretation and Image Processing

Chirapa Puntawangkoon and W. Gregory Hundley

Accurate assessments of global and regional left and right ventricular (LV and RV) function are important when managing patients with cardiovascular disease. Magnetic resonance imaging (MRI) has been developed to characterize cardiac function, yielding high-quality images in patients, regardless of body habitus. Using fast imaging protocols with high temporal resolution, MRI allows one to identify resting and stress-induced changes in LV wall motion to predict the contractile reserve in patients with ischemic heart disease, detect improvement in regional LV performance after coronary artery revascularization[1] or transmyocardial placement of stem cells,[2] and visualize evidence of ethanol ablation of the myocardium in patients with hypertrophic obstructive cardiomyopathy.[3] With MRI, RV function can be defined in those with congenital heart disease,[4] arrhythmogenic right ventricular dysplasia (ARVD), and primary pulmonary hypertension.[5] The purpose of this chapter is to describe the various MRI techniques used to assess LV and RV function.

IMAGE ACQUISITION TECHNIQUES

"White blood" imaging with fast field gradient-echo, or steady-state free precession (SSFP), sequences provides the basis whereby cine images of LV and RV mass, volume, and ejection fraction (EF) are determined with MRI.[6] By grouping the phase encodes and coordinating image acquisition with the rhythmic contraction of the heart, crisp, clear images of cardiac contraction can be obtained in 2 to 4 seconds.

Spoiled Gradient Echo

Indication

This method, also known as a fast low-angle shot (FLASH), or fast-field echo (FFE), is the most extensively studied for assessing ventricular wall motion, volumes, mass, and EF. It is particularly useful for visualizing turbulent flow associated with valvular stenosis and regurgitation.

Limitation

In patients with severe ventricular dysfunction, slow blood flow along the endocardial surface reduces one's ability to visualize low contrast in the LV myocardium.

Description

Using spoiled gradient-echo techniques, the movement of blood through the LV cavity provides bright contrast against the gray appearance of the myocardium.

TABLE 16-1 Imaging Techniques

Technique	Advantage	Disadvantage	Diastole	Systole
FLASH	Identifies turbulent flow associated with intracardiac shunts or valvular heart disease	Flow artifact in patients with severe ventricular dysfunction Longer acquisition times (10 seconds)	TA = 16.26 seconds	
SSFP	High SNR and CNR between the blood pool and myocardial interface Shorter scan times with high temporal resolution Accurate LV volume and mass measurements	Difficult to visualize small turbulent flow jets associated with suspected ASD, VSD, or valvular heart disease	TA = 12.57 seconds	
EPI	Shorter imaging times Decreased motion-related artifact	Low SNR (compared with FLASH) Chemical shift artifact Reduced temporal resolution; thus, difficult to obtain precise LV volume measurement	Real-time + retrospective gating TA = 3.37 seconds	Real-time + retrospective gating
SENSE	Shorter scan times with high temporal resolution for both cardiac breath-hold and real-time cine imaging Increases data sampling rate in real-time imaging	Decreased SNR	(SSFP + SENSE) TA = 6.79 seconds	(SSFP + SENSE)

ASD, atrial septal defect; CNR, contrast-to-noise ratio; LV, left ventricle; SNR, signal-to-noise ratio; TA, acquisition time; VSD, ventricular septal defect.

Steady-State Free Precession

Indication

This method, also known as true fast imaging with steady-state precession (TrueFISP), is also used for assessing ventricular wall motion, volumes, mass, and EF.

Limitation

This technique underestimates turbulent flow associated with intracardiac shunts or valvular heart disease (Table 16-1).

Description

SSFP imaging exhibits high signal-to-noise ratio (SNR) and high contrast-to-noise ratio (CNR) with the blood-myocardial interface. With SSFP, cine MR images depict the endocardial surface, regardless of blood flow velocity.[7,8] This technique can be used with brief repetition times repetition times (TR) (<3 ms), leading to short scan times with high temporal resolution. Studies comparing FLASH and SSFP imaging have demonstrated significant improvements with SSFP in the blood-myocardial interface in patients with decreased LV ejection fraction.[9] With short echo times of less than 1.5 ms, the blood pool within the cavity appears more uniform and image quality is not hampered by turbulent flow.

Echo-Planar Imaging

Indication

Echo-planar imaging (EPI) is useful for obtaining a qualitative assessments of LV wall motion in patients unable to perform breath-holding.

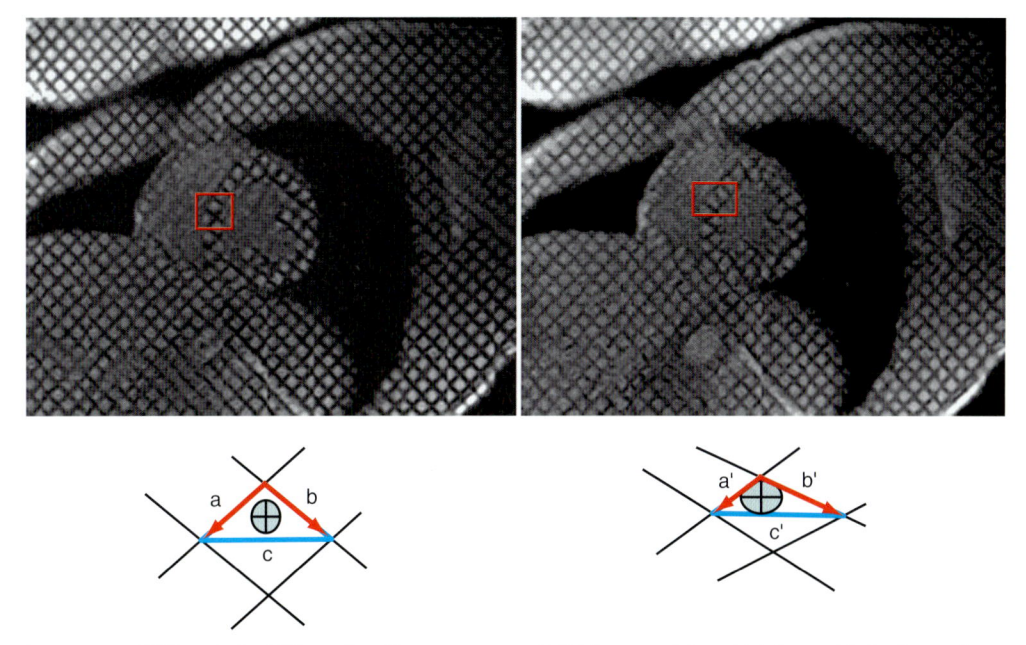

FIGURE 16-1 Assessment of LV strain by MRI tagging. Shown are tagged MRI images of the mid–left ventricle in short axis at end-diastole (*left*) and end-systole (*right*). The deformation of the grid can be seen visually and can be used to determine the quantitative circumferential strain. For two-dimensional analysis, motion of the heart wall that transformed a hypothetical unit circle during diastole into an ellipse during systole corresponds to the directions of the eigenvectors of the transformation. Their lengths are the eigenvalues shown in the diagram below the images. The radial thickening or displacement is the difference between c' length and c length.

Limitation

Because of low spatial and temporal resolution, this technique is not well suited for precise determination of volumes and EF.[10]

Description

Ultrafast EPI is a fast imaging sequence in which multiple echoes are acquired following each excitation that are then used to perform single-shot imaging. "Snapshots" of LV wall motion acquired during relatively short imaging times (e.g., 30-40 ms/slice) are produced with this technique by using advanced hardware to switch the gradients rapidly during scanning. This fast gradient-echo technique exhibits a relatively low SNR and more chemical shift artifacts compared with conventional gradient-echo methods.

Sensitivity Encoding Parallel Imaging

Indication

The sensitivity-encoding (SENSE) technique obtains images during short periods of breath-holding.

Limitation

There is a loss of SNR in some images.

Description

This technique uses sensitivity information from multiple coil elements to correct for k-space undersampling in the post-Fourier domain. Each coil has a different sensitivity profile so that undersampled acquisitions may be unfolded that result in decreased scan time. Images produced with the SENSE technique exhibit consistent contrast, with preserved spatial resolution (see Table 16-1).

TECHNIQUE FOR ASSESSING QUANTITATIVE ANALYSIS OF MYOCARDIAL MOTION

Tagged Imaging

Indication

This is highly accurate for assessing LV midwall myocardial function.

Limitation

With this technique, it is difficult to measure LV function along the LV epicardial and endocardial surfaces.[11]

Description

Myocardial motion can be tracked in one, two, or three dimensions using tissue tagging.[12,13] With tagging, dark saturation bands, or "markers," are placed across the myocardium for the purpose of quantifying LV function. These markers are induced by prepulse sequences applied immediately after the R wave, usually in planes perpendicular to the imaging plane. Quantification of intramyocardial deformations can be accomplished by tracking the intersection points of the tagging lines to demonstrate myocardial rotation, contraction, relaxation, and strain (Fig. 16-1). The SPAMM (**spa**tial **m**odulation of **m**agnetization)

TABLE 16-2 Technique for Assessing Quantitative Analysis of Myocardial Motion

Technique	Advantage	Limitations
Tagged imaging	Provides the data suited for strain assessment.	Difficulty resolving subendocardial and subepicardial differences. Requires high temporal resolution to avoid motion blurring. Uses cine gradient-echo techniques
Phase contrast imaging	Provides comparable data with TDI for assessment of diastolic function and LV dyssynchrony. Can be used with retrospective gating to view the entire complete cardiac cycle.	Difficult to calculate myocardial strain. Requires high temporal and spatial resolution Susceptibility to motion artifact (such as blood related artifact and beat to beat variation) Cannot used to measure large movements
DENSE	Provides regional LV myocardial function assessments across the endocardium, mid wall, and epicardium. Provides data needed for tissue tracking for strain assessments.	Requires experienced center and specialized software

DENSE, displacement encoding with stimulated echoes technique; LV = left ventricle; TDI, tissue Doppler imaging.

technique,[14] uses two perpendicular sets of parallel lines that form a rectangular grid on the image that can be tracked throughout the cardiac cycle. These tagging lines move with the myocardium during the contraction and relaxation phases of the cardiac cycle (see Fig. 16-1).

Another tagging technique, complementary SPAMM (C-SPAMM), results in myocardial tag persistence throughout the entire cardiac cycle by using a negative tagging signal during the diastolic phases of image acquisition. The C-SPAMM technique allows for the study of both systolic and diastolic myocardial deformation resulting from improved tag contrast relative to the background myocardium. A disadvantage of C-SPAMM involves a longer image acquisition time. However, this technique is useful for patients with diastolic dysfunction or elevated heart rates (e.g., during dobutamine stress).

As soon as the images are acquired, there are three methods for extraction of motion data from tagged images: (1) tracking the dark tag lines as intensity minima; (2) eusing optical flow analysis; or (3) applying harmonic phase (HARP) determinates. All three of the tracking methods (Table 16-2) are highly accurate for assessing midwall myocardial function but exhibit some difficulty for discriminating tag intersection points near the epicardial and endocardial surfaces.[11]

Phase-Contrast Velocity Mapping

Indication

This method, also known as tissue phase mapping (TPM), measures intramyocardial motion velocity during the cardiac cycle.

Limitation

With this method, it is difficult to calculate myocardial strain.

Description

The change in the phase of the net magnetization inside each pixel is proportional to the velocity of the tissue during systole and diastole. Studies by Markl, Kvitting, and colleagues[15,16] have demonstrated the utility of this technique for tracking LV displacement in a manner similar to that performed with tissue Doppler imaging (TDI) during transthoracic echocardiography. Paelinck and associates[17] have compared TDI with phase contrast MRI when studying diastolic function in patients with hypertensive heart disease and found a good agreement between MRI and TDI. Westenberg and coworkers[18] compared TDI with phase contrast MRI in patients with conduction delay and idiopathic dilated cardiomyopathy and found that MRI was able to classify them as having minimal, intermediate, or extensive disease.

Displacement Encoding with Stimulated Echoes

Indication

Displacement encoding with stimulated echoes (DENSE) is useful for quantifying myocardial motion.

Limitation

This technique needs specialized software and expertise.

Description

The DENSE technique was developed in an attempt to combine the advantages of the tagging and cine phase contrast velocity imaging techniques. The DENSE technique provides three-dimensional displacement vectors of each pixel at one point in time and then tracks tissue displacement throughout the cardiac cycle.[19] With DENSE, regional LV myocardial function data across the entire LV myocardium, endocardium, midwall, and epicardium can be obtained (see Table 16-2).

IMAGE INTERPRETATION

Left Ventricular Volume and Function

Global Left Ventricular Function

The two most common methods used to measure LV volume and EF are the area-length technique and the multislice Simpson's rule technique.

Area-Length Method

The area-length technique is based on formulas that assume that the left ventricle exhibits the shape of a simple prolate ellipsoid.[20] LV end-diastolic and end-systolic volumes are calculated from the corresponding tracings at both these points of the cardiac cycle. The single-plane ellipsoid method uses the length (L) and two-dimensional area (A) in a single apical long-axis view (usually apical four-chamber view).[21]

$$\text{Volume} = 0.85A^2/L$$
$$\text{LVEF} = (\text{LV EDV} - \text{LV ESV})/(\text{LV EDV}) \times 100\%$$

(where EDV is the end-diastolic volume and ESV is the end-systolic volume)

This technique may be imprecise when patients exhibit distorted LV geometry caused by LV dilation or resting regional wall motion abnormalities.[22]

Multislice Simpson's Rule Method

Quantification of global function using multiple cine MRI provides measurements of volumes, EF, and mass that do not depend on assumed LV geometry. Using Simpson's rule, stacked disks are assessed and the end-diastolic and end-systolic volumes are calculated by summing the volume of the blood pool in each slice. This method is highly accurate and reproducible, and has been validated in ex vivo and in vivo models. Figure 16-2 illustrates the method for obtaining standard views and Figure 16-3 shows some standard multislice and LV volume and mass calculations.

Comparison of Left Ventricular Volume Measurements Between SSFP and FLASH

Previous studies at 1.5 T compared FLASH and SSFP techniques for the quantitation of ventricular volumes, mass, and EF. Consistently, SSFP imaging provides larger volume and smaller LV mass determinations with a negligible effect on LVEF. The reason for these volume and mass discrepancies relates to the higher blood-myocardial contrast and higher myocardial SNR in SSFP images. During SSFP imaging, this results in improved definition of the endocardial border without flow artifacts from the LV cavity (see Table 16-1). Of note, these differences at

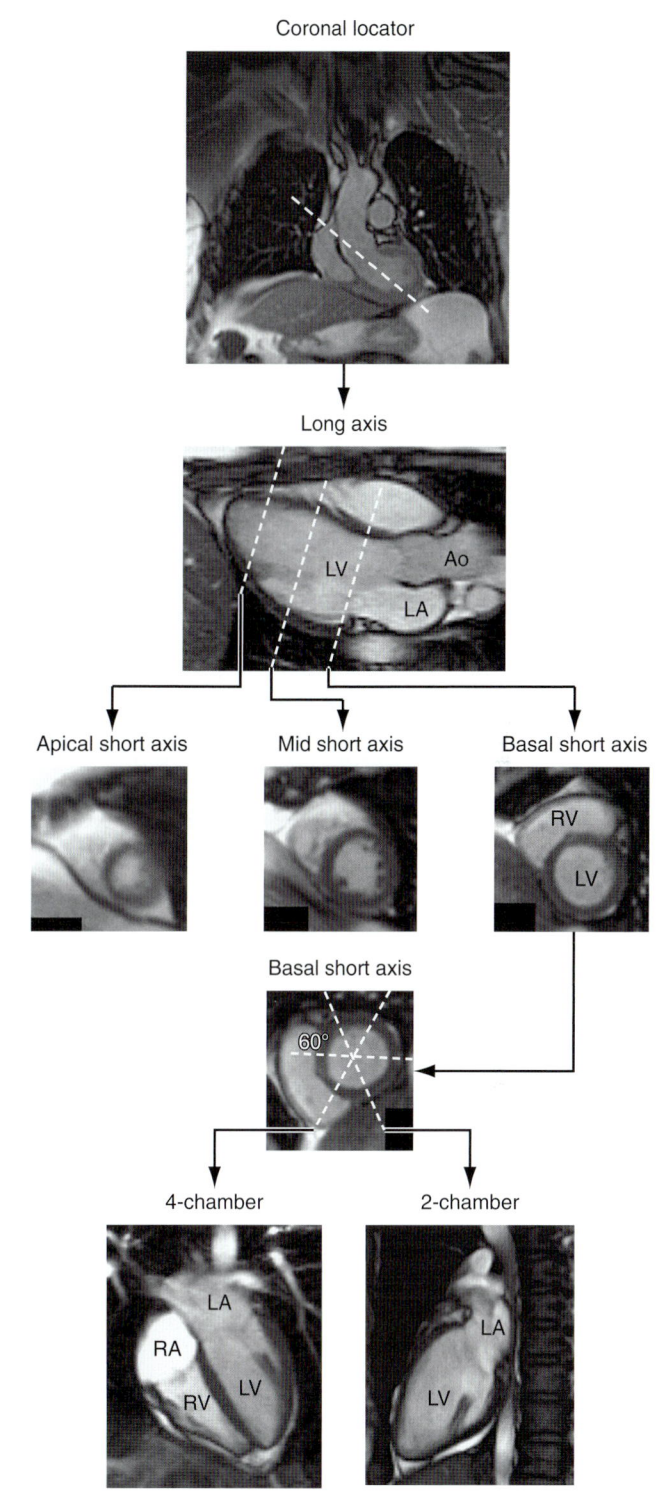

■ **FIGURE 16-2** Method for obtained standard views, obtaining three short-axis (basal, mid, and apical) and three apical long axis views (long-axis, four-chamber, and two-chamber views). In all images, the myocardium is gray and the blood pool is white. The *white dashed lines* indicate the slice positions for obtaining the subsequent views demarcated by the *arrows*. Ao, aorta; LA, left atrium; LV, left ventricle; RA, right atrium; RV, right ventricle.

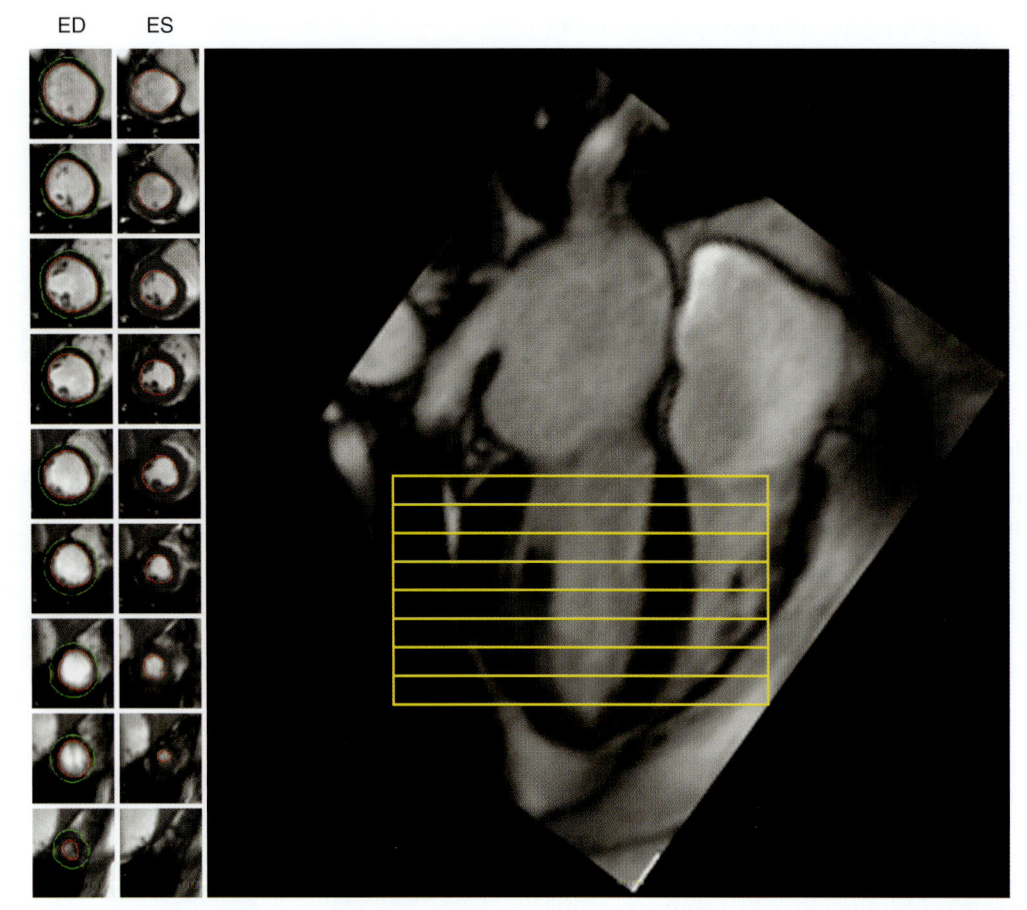

FIGURE 16-3 Method for obtaining standard multislice short-axis views from the four-chamber plane. The horizontal *yellow lines* indicate the slice positions for obtaining the short-axis view. **Left,** Each short axis slice is shown with the endocardial (*red*) and epicardial (*green*) borders used for the calculation of LV volume and LV mass.

$$\text{LV volume} = \sum_{i=0}^{n}[\text{area in endocardial contour on each slide} \times (\text{slice thickness} + \text{gap in between slice})]$$

$$\text{LV mass} = 1.05 \times \sum_{i=0}^{n}[\text{myocardial area} \times (\text{slice thickness} + \text{gap in between slice})]$$

(myocardial area = the difference in area between the endocardial and epicardial contour in the end-diastole, n = number of total slices. The specific gravity of the myocardial tissue = 1.05 g/dL.)

$$\text{LVEF} = (\text{LV EDV} - \text{LV ESV})/(\text{LV EDV}) \times 100\%$$

(EF = ejection fraction, EDV = end-diastolic volume, ESV = end-systolic volume.)

1.5 T may be present when individuals are scanned at 3.0 T.[23]

Left Ventricular Mass

Typically, LV mass is measured at end-diastole from multiple short-axis images. The epicardial and endocardial borders are traced in each slice, and papillary muscles and endocardial trabeculae may or may not be included in the LV mass calculation. Left ventricular mass is reported in grams and is calculated by multiplying the volume of the LV myocardium by the specific gravity of the myocardial tissue, 1.05 g/dL. The accuracy of LV mass has been established in autopsy studies of the heart and from studies in live human and animal subjects (see Fig. 16-3).

Regional Left Ventricular Function

Systolic Left Ventricular Function

Qualitative (Wall Motion)

With MRI, regional LV contractile function can be assessed qualitatively by visual inspection. Normally, LV free wall thickness increases more than 40% during systole. Regional hypokinesia is defined as systolic wall thickening less than 30%, akinesia is defined as systolic wall thickening less than 10%, and dyskinesia is defined as systolic outward movement or diastolic bulging of the ventricular wall.[24]

Left ventricular wall motion is also visualized in orthogonal planes oriented parallel to the long axis of the heart. A combination of three short-axis cines spanning from the base to the apex are routinely acquired (Table 16-3) and

TABLE 16-3 Normal Values of Left Ventricular Function from Short-Axis View in Healthy Persons*

	1.5-T Studies											3-T Studies			
	Lorenz et al. (1999)[1] (SPGR)		Sandstede et al. (2000)[2] (SPGR)		Salton et al. (2002)[3] (SPGR)		Natori et al. (MESA,† 2006)[4] (SPGR)				Hudsmith et al. (2006)[5] (SPGR)	Alfakih et al. (2006)[6] (b-SSFP)		Hudsmith et al. (2005)[7] (b-SSFP)	Hudsmith et al. (2006)[5] (SPGR)	Hudsmith et al. (2006)[7] (b-SSFP)
Parameter	Age 8-57 yr		Age 45-74 yr		Age 36-78 yr		Age 45-84 yr (400 cases)				Age 28 ± 5 yr			Age 28 ± 5 yr	Age 28 ± 5 yr	Age 28 ± 5 yr
	Male	Female	Male	Female	Male	Female	White	Asian	Male	Female		Male	Female			
LVEDV (mL)	136	96	103	91	115	84	148 ± 30.5	116.5 ± 18.4	142.2 ± 34	109.2 ± 22.5	128 ± 30	168	135	157 ± 37	133 ± 31	149 ± 37
LVESV (mL)	45	32	34	26	36	25	50.1 ± 14.7	36.5 ± 7	47.4 ± 19.4	30.9 ± 9.5	44 ± 12	61	49	57 ± 18	51 ± 21	59 ± 16
LVSV (mL)	92	65	68	72	79	69	97.9 ± 21.4	80 ± 14.9	94.8 ± 21.3	78.2 ± 17	85 ± 24	108	86	100 ± 32	82 ± 24	91 ± 28
LVEF (%)	67	67	68	72	69	70	66.3 ± 6.4	68.5 ± 4.4	67.2 ± 7.2	71.8 ± 5.6	66 ± 8	64	64	63 ± 9	62 ± 12	60 ± 8
LV mass (g)	178	125	152	111	155	103	170 ± 32.1	129.1 ± 20	163.8 ± 35.8	113.6 ± 24.2	128 ± 31	133	90	108 ± 29	142 ± 37	109 ± 30
CO (L/min)	5.8	4.3	5.1	5.1			5.7 ± 1.4	4.8 ± 1	5.6 ± 1.2	4.9 ± 1.1						
LVEDVI (mL/m²)	69	61	52	53	58	50	74.5 ± 14	68.3 ± 7.4	73.9 ± 14.7	64.5 ± 10.8		82	78			
LVESVI (mL/m²)			17	15	18	15	25.2 ± 7.1	21.4 ± 3.4	24.5 ± 8.8	18.2 ± 5.1						
LVSVI (mL/m²)	47	41			40	35	49.3 ± 10.1	46.9 ± 6.7	49.4 ± 9.9	46.3 ± 8.4						
LVMI (g/m²)	91	79	77	66	78	61	85.6 ± 14.7	75.7 ± 8.2	85.1 ± 15.2	66.9 ± 10.9		65	52			
CI (L/min/m²)	3	2.8	2.6	3			2.9 ± 0.6	2.8 ± 0.5	2.9 ± 0.6	2.9 ± 0.6						

*Mean or mean ± standard deviation.
†In the MESA study, the papillary muscles were included in the LV end-diastolic volume and LV end-systolic volume and excluded from the LV mass.
b-SSFP, balance steady-state free precession; CI, cardiac index; CO, cardiac output; EDV, end-diastolic volume; EDVI, end-diastolic volume index; EF, ejection fraction; ESV, end-systolic volume; ESVI, end-diastolic volume index; MESA, Multi-Ethnic Study of Atherosclerosis; MI, mass index; RV, right ventricle; SPGR, fast spoiled gradient-echo; SV, stroke volume; SVI, stroke volume index.

[1] Lorenz CH, Walker ES, Morgan VL, et al. Normal human right and left ventricular mass, systolic function, and gender differences by cine magnetic resonance imaging. J Cardiovasc Magn Reson 1999; 1:7-21.
[2] Sandstede J, Lipke C, Beer M, et al. Age- and gender-specific differences in left and right ventricular cardiac function and mass determined by cine magnetic resonance imaging. Eur Radiol 2000; 10:438-442.
[3] Salton CJ, Chuang ML, O'Donnell CJ, et al. Gender differences and normal left ventricular anatomy in an adult population free of hypertension. A cardiovascular magnetic resonance study of the Framingham Heart Study Offspring cohort. J Am Coll Cardiol 2002; 39:1055-1060.
[4] Natori S, Lai S, Finn JP, et al. Cardiovascular function in multiethnic study of atherosclerosis (MESA): normal values by age, sex, and ethnicity. AJR Am J Roentgenol 2006; 186:S357-S365.
[5] Hudsmith LE, Petersen SE, Tyler DJ, et al. Determination of cardiac volumes and mass with FLASH and SSFP cine sequences at 1.5 vs 3 Tesla: A validation study. J Magn Reson Imaging 2006; 24:312-318.
[6] Alfakih K, Reid S, Hall A, Sivananthan MU. The assessment of left ventricular hypertrophy in hypertension. J Hypertens 2006; 24:1223-1230.
[7] Hudsmith LE, Petersen SE, Francis JM, Robson MD, Neubauer S. Normal human left and right ventricular and left atrial dimensions using steady state free precession magnetic resonance imaging. J Cardiovasc Magn Reson 2005; 7:775-782.

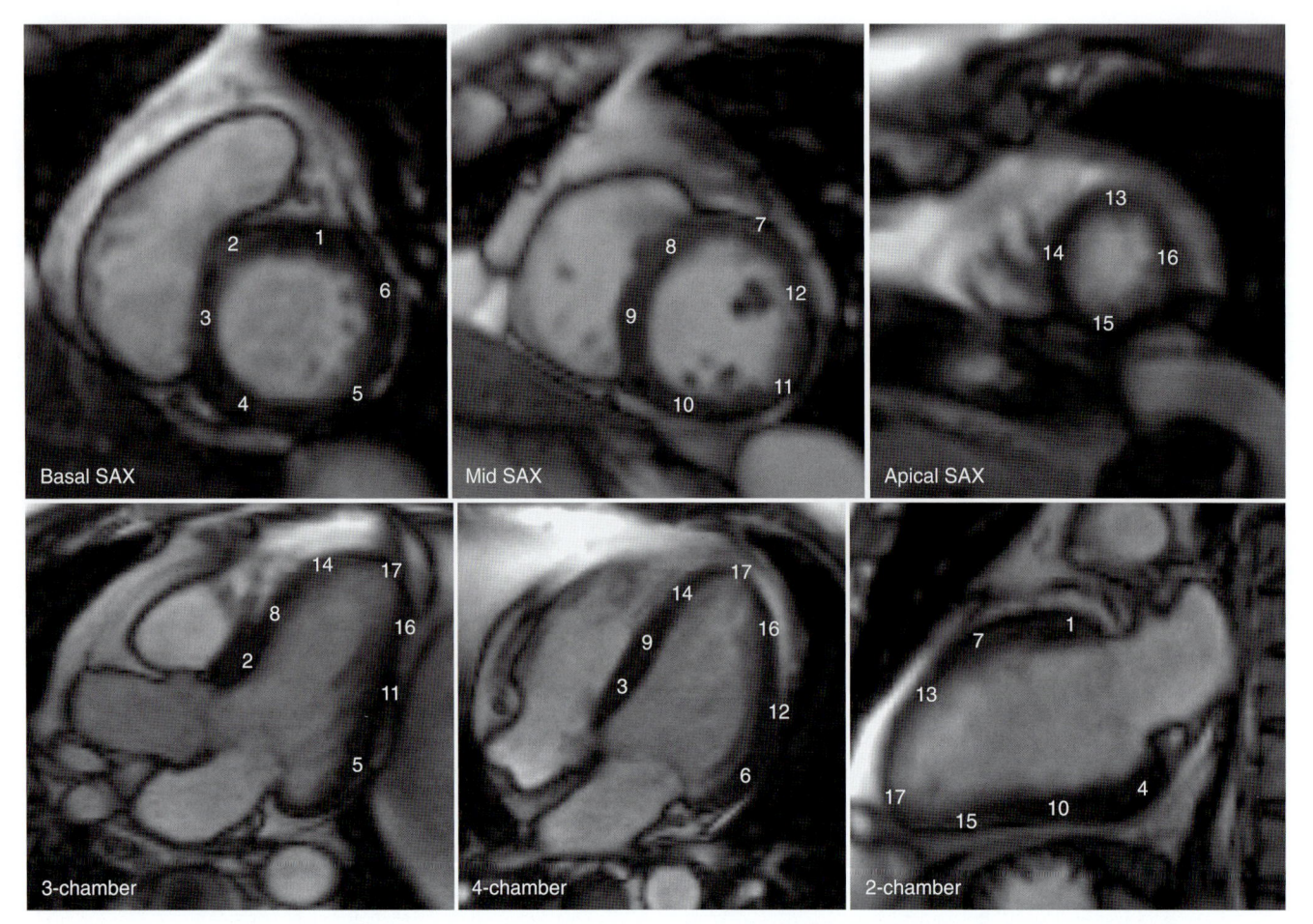

FIGURE 16-4 Cine MR images of the left ventricle are displayed in three short-axis (*upper row*) and three long-axis (*lower row*) views. Myocardial regions are divided into 17 segments, as identified: 1, basal anterior; 2, basal anteroseptum; 3, basal inferoseptum; 4, basal inferior; 5, basal inferolateral; 6, basal anterolateral; 7, mid-anterior; 8, mid-anteroseptum; 9, mid-inferoseptum; 10, mid-inferior; 11, mid-inferolateral; 12, mid-anterolateral; 13, apical anterior; 14, apical septum; 15, apical inferior; 16, apical lateral; and 17, apical cap. SAX, short axis.

apical planes are also acquired. These include the vertical long-axis (VLA) view, or four-chamber view, the horizontal long-axis (HLA) view, or two-chamber view, and the long axis or three-chamber view (Fig. 16-4; also see Fig. 16-2).[24]

Quantitative (Wall Thickening)

1. Modified center line method. Radial wall thickness is quantified by creating a radian emanating from the center of the left ventricle that courses perpendicularly across the endocardium and epicardium. The length between the endocardial and epicardial surface evenly spaced transmyocardial lines or chords identifies the local LV wall thickness. The difference between end-diastolic and end-systolic chord lengths represents local end-systolic wall thickening. This technique can overestimate wall thickness if the MRI slice is not acquired in a true short-axis plane.
2. Thickening or thinning assessed with tagging. Most tagged MRI data consist of two or three sets of two-dimensional images (see earlier). Tag deformation associated with ventricular motion and deformation provides information regarding circumferential and longitudinal shortening and lengthening, and radial

thickening and thinning. Assessment of radial deformation can be compared within different myocardial segments to characterize regional wall motion (see Fig. 16-1).

Left Ventricular Strain

Left ventricular strain measurements reflect the direction and spatial variation of LV myocardial displacement without dependence on LV preload.[25,26] The LV myocardium has a complex architecture—subepicardial and subendocardial fibers are longitudinal, whereas mid-wall fibers are circumferential in direction. LV deformation is therefore composed of radial thickening, circumferential shortening and torsion, and longitudinal shortening. There are two coordinate systems in three orthogonal directions that are used to determine principle strains; radial strain is the myocardial deformation in the radial direction (R), longitudinal strain (L) is myocardial shortening from base to apex (negative value), and circumferential strain is the intramural circumferential shortening (C).[27] Shear strains represent the changes in angles between coordinate axes (Fig. 16-5).[28]

The circumferential-longitudinal shear angle describes the twisting motion of the heart and is closely related to

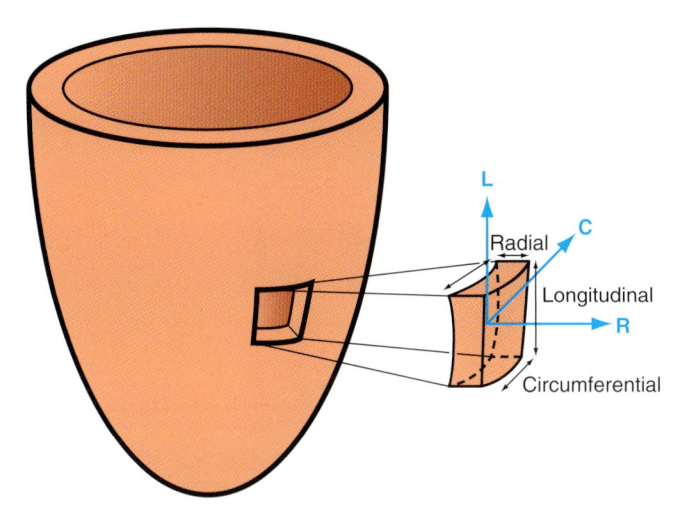

FIGURE 16-5 Diagram showing the LV coordinate system includes radial (R), circumferential (C), and longitudinal (L) directions.

Diastolic Left Ventricular Function and Regional Relaxation

Parameters of diastolic function are determined from rates of inflow into the left ventricle or from the outward relaxation of the myocardium. Phase contrast velocity mapping can be used to quantify ventricular inflow in real time. This information is useful for evaluating the impact of respiratory motion on ventricular filling to demonstrate constrictive physiology (e.g., in constrictive pericarditis). Using the transmitral velocity to measure the mitral inflow pattern can also demonstrate LV filling patterns similar to these obtained with Doppler echocardiographic techniques (Fig. 16-6).

The assessment of outward movement of the LV myocardium can be acquired with tissue tagging techniques. By using myocardial tagging to evaluate the diastolic parameters, reverse myocardial strain and shear strain can be assessed at rest or during high-dose dobutamine stress to identify patients with flow-limiting epicardial coronary artery luminal narrowings.[31]

torsion of the left ventricle. The twisting motion of the left ventricle stores potential elastic energy by straining the extracellular matrix, which is released during early diastole, and therefore contributes to early diastolic suction.[29] The contraction and relaxation of the spiraling myofibers cause the LV torsion and untwisting. Torsion is defined as the circumferential-longitudinal shear on the epicardial surface between two short-axis slices. The net ventricular torsion is the result of the subepicardial contraction and subendocardial counterbalancing contraction.[29] Both tagged imaging and DENSE techniques are well suited for tissue tracking for strain assessment. Several studies have reported the use of myocardial strain assessments to evaluate regional systolic and diastolic LV function in patients with myocardial ischemia, infarction, and postinfarction remodeling.[29,30]

Right Ventricular Volume and Function

Global Right Ventricular Function

Cardiac MRI demonstrates high interstudy reproducibility for determining RV function (volumes and EF) in healthy subjects, patients with heart failure, and patients with hypertrophy.[32] The intraobserver, interobserver, and interstudy variability was demonstrated to be 5% to 6% in normal volunteers.[33] Cardiac MRI has been used to follow patients with repaired tetralogy of Fallot. Davlouros and colleagues[34] have demonstrated pulmonary regurgitation and RV outflow tract aneurysm associated with RV dilation and a decrement in RV ejection fraction in patients after tetralogy of Fallot repair. Similar to the left ventricle, Simpson's rule method is used to calculate RV volume and EF. Table 16-4 summarizes normal measures of RV function from various studies.

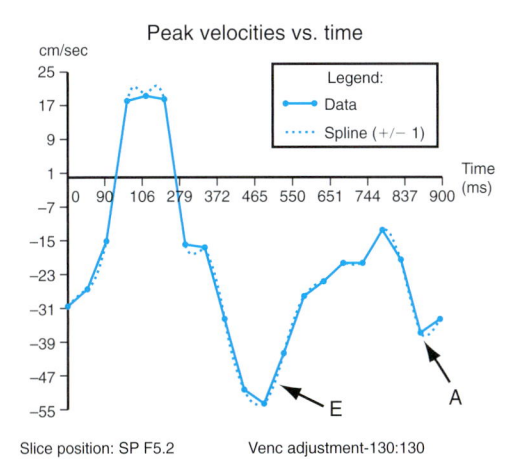

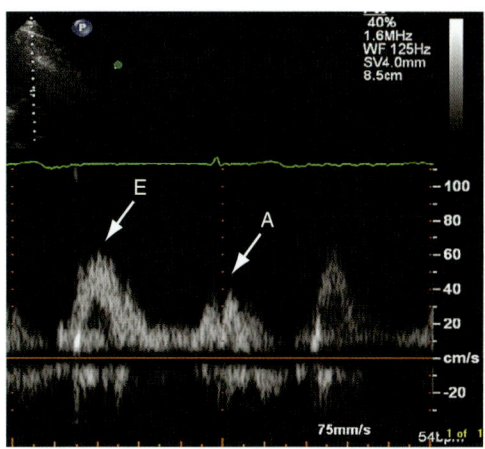

FIGURE 16-6 Mitral inflow velocities as seen by MRI phase contrast (*left*) and echo Doppler (*right*). Close agreement between the peak E and A velocities (about 55 and 35 cm/second, respectively) can be seen in both modalities

TABLE 16-4 Normal Values of Right Ventricular Function in Healthy Persons*

	1.5-T Studies							3-T Studies			
	Lorenz et al. (1999)[1] (SPGR)		Sandstede et al. (2000)[2] (SPGR)		Grothues et al. (2004)[3] (SPGR)	Tandri et al. (2007)[4] Natori et al. (2006)[5] (SPGR)		Hudsmith et al. (2006)[6] (SPGR)	Alfakih et al. (2006)[7] (b-SSFP)		Hudsmith et al. (2005)[8] (b-SSFP)	Hudsmith et al. (2006)[6] (SPGR)	Hudsmith et al. (2005)[8] (b-SSFP)
	Age 8-57 yr		Age 45-74 yr		Age 26-57 yr	Age 45-84 yr (394 cases)		Age 28 ± 5 yr			Age 28 ± 5 yr	Age 28 ± 5 yr	Age 28 ± 5 yr
Parameter	Male	Female	Male	Female		Male	Female		Male	Female			
RVEDV (mL)	157	106	119	91	153 ± 34	142.4 ± 31.1	110.2 ± 24	159 ± 41	176	131	171 ± 42	171 ± 41	167 ± 40
RVESV (mL)	63	40	50	26	58 ± 20	54.3 ± 16.9	55.1 ± 12.5	55 ± 16	79	52	61 ± 15	59 ± 15	63 ± 16
RVSV (mL)	95	66	60	72	95 ± 16	88.3 ± 21.6	75 ± 17.9	104 ± 27	98	78	110 ± 29	111 ± 29	104 ± 27
RVEF (%)	60	63	54	39	63 ± 7	62 ± 10	69 ± 10	66 ± 3	55	60	64 ± 4	65 ± 4	62 ± 4
RV mass (g)	50	40	5.1	5.1	60 ± 14			33 ± 6			35 ± 8	35 ± 5	34 ± 7
CO (L/min)			5.1										
RVEDVI (mL/m²)	80	67	59	53		82 ± 16.2	68.6 ± 14						
RVESVI (mL/m²)			24	15		31.2 ± 9.2	21.7 ± 7.5						
RVMI (g/m²)	48	42	27	23		50.7 ± 11	46.8 ± 9.9						
CI (L/min/m²)	26	25	2.6	3									

*Mean or mean ± standard deviation.
†In the MESA study, the moderator band was included as part of the RV volume.

b-SSFP, balance steady-state free precession; CI, cardiac index; CO, cardiac output; EDV, end-diastolic volume; EDVI, end-diastolic volume index; EF, ejection fraction; ESV, end-systolic volume; ESVI, end-diastolic volume index; MESA, Multi-Ethnic Study of Atherosclerosis; MI, mass index; RV, right ventricle; SPGR, fast spoiled gradient-echo; SV, stroke volume; SVI, stroke volume index.

[1] Lorenz CH, Walker ES, Morgan VL, et al. Normal human right and left ventricular mass, systolic function, and gender differences by cine magnetic resonance imaging. J Cardiovasc Magn Reson 1999; 1:7-21.
[2] Sandstede J, Lipke C, Beer M, et al. Age- and gender-specific differences in left and right ventricular cardiac function and mass determined by cine magnetic resonance imaging. Eur Radiol 2000; 10:438-442.
[3] Grothues F, Moon JC, Bellenger NG, et al. Interstudy reproducibility of right ventricular volumes, function, and mass with cardiovascular magnetic resonance. Am Heart J 2004; 147:218-223.
[4] Tandri H, Taya SK, Nasir K, et al. Normal reference values for the adult right ventricle by magnetic resonance imaging. Am J Cardiol 2006; 98:1660-1664.
[5] Natori S, Lai S, Finn JP, et al. Cardiovascular function in multiethnic study of atherosclerosis (MESA): normal value by age, sex and ethnicity. AJR AM J Roentgenol 2006; 186:S357-S365.
[6] Hudsmith LE, Petersen SE, Tyler DJ, et al. Determination of cardiac volumes and mass with FLASH and SSFP cine sequences at 1.5 vs 3 Tesla: A validation study. J Magn Reson Imaging 2006; 24:312-318.
[7] Alfakih K, Reid S, Hall A, Sivananthan MU. The assessment of left ventricular hypertrophy in hypertension. J Hypertens 2006; 24:1223-1230.
[8] Hudsmith LE, Petersen SE, Francis JM, et al. Normal human left and right ventricular and left atrial dimensions using steady state free precession magnetic resonance imaging. J Cardiovasc Magn Reson 2005; 7:775-782.

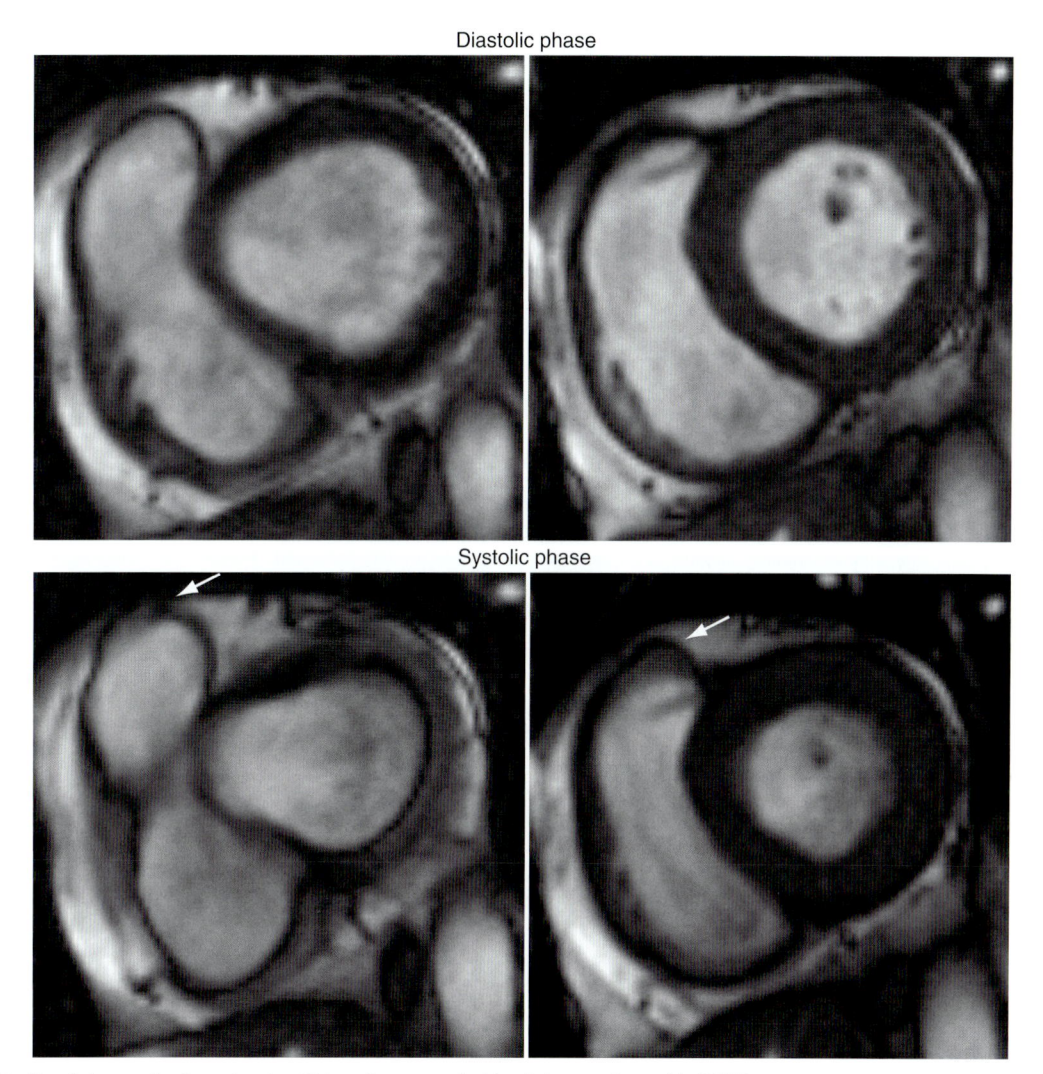

FIGURE 16-7 Basal short-axis slices showing RV outflow tract dyskinesis in a patient with ARVC.

Regional Right Ventricular Function

There is no standard convention for segmenting the RV myocardium to determine regional RV function. In short-axis views, the RV free wall can be divided into four regions—the inflow tract, outflow tract, midventricular region, and apex. Arrhythmogenic right ventricular cardiomyopathy (ARVC) is a clinically important syndrome with regional RV motion abnormalities (akinesis or dyskinesis) on cine MRI that correspond to areas of adipose tissue replacement.[35] As shown in Figure 16-7, MRI is useful for identifying this condition.

Although most myocardial tagging studies have been performed on the left ventricle, tagging of the right ventricle can be used to study RV myocardial deformation in patients with congenital heart diseases such as postoperative atrial switch procedures for transposition of the great arteries.[35] Complex RV geometry and the presence of a thin RV wall (normal < 6 mm) result in muscle tagging analyses being technically more demanding relative to the thicker walled left ventricle.

Right Ventricular Diastolic Function

Tricuspid transvalvular flow profiles may be used to assess RV diastolic filling patterns (E and A waves). Diastolic dysfunction within the walls of the right ventricle have been demonstrated using phase contrast velocity mapping in patients with hypertrophic cardiomyopathy.[25]

> **KEY POINTS**
> - Cardiac MRI yields fast, accurate, reproducible assessments of global and regional systolic and diastolic LV and RV function.
> - Multislice Simpson's rule methods with cine white blood imaging techniques can be used to provide accurate measures of ventricular volume, mass, and ejection fraction.
> - A variety of quantitative analysis techniques incorporating tagging, phase contrast MRI, or displacement encoding with stimulated echoes (DENSE) can be used to provide precise measures of right or left ventricular systolic and diastolic function.

SUGGESTED READINGS

Petitjean C, Rougon N, Cluzel P. Assessment of myocardial function: a review of quantification methods and results using tagged MRI. J Cardiovasc Magn Reson 2004; 7:501-516.

Walsh TF, Hundley WG: Assessment of ventricular function with cardiovascular magnetic resonanace. Cardiol Clin 2007; 25:15-33.

REFERENCES

1. Gerber BL, Garot J, Bluemke DA, et al. Accuracy of contrast-enhanced magnetic resonance imaging in predicting improvement of regional myocardial function in patients after acute myocardial infarction. Circulation 2002; 106:1083-1089.
2. Mathur A, Martin JF. Stem cells and repair of the heart. Lancet 2004; 364:183-192.
3. Sigwart U. Non-surgical myocardial reduction for hypertrophic obstructive cardiomyopathy. Lancet 1995; 346:211-214.
4. Reddy GP, Higgins CB. Magnetic resonance imaging of congenital heart disease: evaluation of morphology and function. Semin Roentgenol 2003; 38:342-351.
5. Van Wolferen SA, Marcus JT, Boonstra A, et al. Prognostic value of right ventricular mass, volume, and function in idiopathic pulmonary arterial hypertension. Eur Heart J 2007; 28:1250-1257.
6. Grothues F, Smith GC, Moon JC, et al. Comparison of interstudy reproducibility of cardiovascular magnetic resonance with two-dimension echocardiography in normal subjects and in patients with heart failure or left ventricular hypertrophy. Am J Cardiol 2002; 90:29-34.
7. Moon JC, Lorenz CH, Francis JM, et al. Breath-hold FLASH and FISP cardiovascular MR imaging: left ventricular volume differences and reproducibility. Radiology 2002; 223:789-797.
8. Ichikawa Y, Sakuma H, Kitagawa K, et al: Evaluation of left ventricular volumes and ejection fraction using fast steady-state cine MR imaging: comparison with left ventricular angiography. J Cardiovasc Magn Reson 2003; 5:333-342.
9. Shors SM, Cotts WG, Pavlovic-Surjancev, et al: Non-invasive cardiac evaluation in heart failure patients using magnetic resonance imaging: a feasibility study. Heart Fail Rev 2005; 10:265-273.
10. Poustchi-Amin M, Mirowitz SA, Brown JJ, et al: Principles and application of echo-planar imaging: a review for the general radiologist. Radiographics 2001; 21:767-779.
11. Axel L, Montillo A, Kim D. Tagged magnetic resonance imaging of the heart: a survey. Med Image Anal 2005; 9:376-393.
12. Young AA, Axel L. Three-dimensional motion and deformation of the heart wall: estimation with spatial modulation of magnetization—a model-based approach. Radiology 1992; 185:241-247.
13. Ryf S, Spiegel MA, Gerber M, Boesiger P. Myocardial tagging with 3D-CSPAMM. J Magn Reson Imaging 2002; 16:320-325.
14. Axel L, Dougherty L. MR imaging of motion with spatial modulation of magnetization. Radiology 1989; 171:841-845.
15. Markl M, Schneider B, Hennig J, et al. Cardiac phase contrast gradient echo MRI: measurement of myocardial wall motion in healthy volunteers and patients. Int J Cardiol Imaging 1999; 15:441-452.
16. Kvitting JP, Ebbers T, Engvall J, et al. Three-directional myocardial motion assessed using 3D phase contrast MRI. J Cardiovasc Magn Reson 2004; 6:627-636.
17. Paelinck BP, de Roos A, Bax JJ, et al. Feasibility of tissue magnetic resonance imaging: a pilot study in comparison with tissue Doppler imaging and invasive measurement. J Am Coll Cardiol 2005; 45:1109-1116.
18. Westenberg JJ, Lamb HJ, van der Geest RJ, et al. Assessment of left ventricular dyssynchrony in patients with conduction delay and idiopathic dilated cardiomyopathy: head-to-head comparison between tissue Doppler imaging and velocity-encoded magnetic resonance imaging. J Am Coll Cardiol 2006; 47:2042-2048.
19. Rademakers FE, Rogers WJ, Guier WH, et al. Relation of regional cross-fiber shortening to wall thickening in the intact heart. Three-dimensional strain analysis by NMR tagging. Circulation 1994; 89:1174-1182.
20. Van Rossum AC, Visser FC, Sprenger M, et al. Evaluation of magnetic resonance imaging for determination of left ventricular ejection fraction and comparison with angiography. Am J Cardiol 1988; 62:628-633.
21. Cranney GB, Lotan CS, Dean L, et al. Left ventricular volume measurement using cardiac axis nuclear magnetic resonance imaging. Validation by calibrated ventricular angiography. Circulation 1990; 82:154-163.
22. Martin ET, Fuisz AR, Pohost GM. Imaging cardiac structure and pump function. Cardiol Clin 1998; 16:135-160.
23. Hudsmith LE, Petersen SE, Tyler DJ, et al. Determination of cardiac volumes and mass with FLASH and SSFP cine sequences at 1.5 vs 3 Tesla: A validation study. J Magn Reson Imaging 2006; 24:312-318.
24. Cerqueira MD, Weissman NJ, Dilsizian V, et al; American Heart Association Writing Group on Myocardial Segmentation and Registration for Cardiac Imaging. Standardized myocardial segmentation and nomenclature for tomographic imaging of the heart: a statement for healthcare professionals from the Cardiac Imaging Committee of the Council on Clinical Cardiology of the American Heart Association. Circulation 2002; 105:539-542.
25. Dong SJ., Hees PS, Huang WM, et al. Independent effects of preload, afterload, and contractility on left ventricular torsion. Am J Physiol 1999; 277:H1053-H1060.
26. Dong SJ, Hees PS, Siu CO, et al. MRI assessment of LV relaxation by untwisting rate: a new isovolumetric phase measure of t. Am J Physiol 2001; 281:H2002-H2009.
27. Göttte Marco JW, Germans T, et al. Myocardial strain and torsion quantified by cardiovascular magnetic resonance tissue tagging: studies in normal and impaired left ventricular function. J Am coll Cardiol 2006; 48:2002-2011.
28. Reichek N. MRI myocardial tagging. J Magn Reson Imaging 1999; 10:609-616.
29. Bogaert J, Bosmans H, Maes A, et al. Remote myocardial dysfunction after anterior myocardial infarction: impact on left ventricular shape on regional function: a magnetic resonance myocardial tagging study. J Am Coll Cardiol 2000; 35:1525-1534.
30. Marcus JT, Gotte MJ, Van Rossum AC, et al. Myocardial function in infracted and remote regions early after infarction in man assessment by magnetic resonance tagging and strain analysis. J Magn Reson Imaging 1997; 38:803-810.
31. Paetsch I, Foll D, Kaluza A et al. Magnetic resonance stress tagging in ischemic heart disease. Am Physiol Heart Circ Physiol 2005; 288:H2708-H2714.
32. Grothues F, Moon JC, Bellenger NG, et al: Interstudy reproducibility of right ventricular volumes, function, and mass with cardiovascular magnetic resonance. Am Heart J 2004; 147:218-223.
33. Lorenz CH, Walker ES, Morgan VL, et al. Normal human right and left ventricular mass, systolic function, and gender differences by cine magnetic resonance imaging. J Cardiovasc Magn Reson 1999; 1:7-21.
34. Davlouros PA, Kilner PJ, Hornung TS, et al. Right ventricular function in adults with repaired tetralogy of Fallot assessed with cardiovascular magnetic resonance imaging: determental role of right ventricular outflow aneurysm or akinesia and adverse right to left ventricular interaction. J Am Coll Cardiol 2002; 40:2044-2052.
35. Pettersen E, Helle-Valle T, Edvardsen T, et al. Contraction pattern of the systemic right ventricle shift from longitudinal to circumferential shortening and absent global ventricular torsion. J Am Coll Cardiol 2007; 49:2450-2456, 2007.

CHAPTER 17

Magnetic Resonance Evaluation of Blood Flow

Michael D. Hope, Karen G. Ordovas, Thomas A. Hope, Alison Knauth Meadows, Charles B. Higgins, and Gautham P. Reddy

Magnetic resonance imaging (MRI) is highly motion sensitive and can noninvasively offer accurate and reproducible quantification of blood velocity and flow. There are a variety of flow-sensitive MRI sequences, including phase contrast, time of flight, and arterial spin labeling, that allow visualization and varying degrees of quantification of blood flow. In this chapter, we focus on phase contrast MRI (also referred to as velocity-encoded cine MRI), which is routinely used in clinical practice for quantitative assessment of cardiovascular physiology and flow dynamics.

DESCRIPTION OF TECHNICAL REQUIREMENTS

Phase Contrast Magnetic Resonance Imaging

Velocity-encoded cine phase contrast MRI employs a bipolar gradient pulse to encode the velocity of moving protons. The two lobes of the bipolar gradient pulse are equal in strength but opposite in orientation, one positive, the other negative. A stationary proton will experience equal and opposite gradients that cancel one another and will have no resulting phase shift. However, a moving proton will not experience an equal but opposite second lobe of the gradient pulse and consequently will acquire a phase shift (Fig. 17-1). The angle of acquired phase shift is proportional to the velocity of the moving proton. An MRI sequence with this type of bipolar gradient is thus flow sensitive.

To calculate the angle of acquired phase shift of a moving proton to determine its velocity, the flow-sensitive sequence is subtracted from a flow-insensitive sequence (i.e., a gradient sequence without a bipolar pulse). Stationary protons are subtracted out, leaving behind only the motion-induced phase shifts of moving protons. This subtraction gives rise to phase images, in which signal intensity is proportional to blood flow velocity. The unsubtracted combination of signal from the flow-sensitive and flow-insensitive sequences gives rise to magnitude images.

Multiple phase contrast acquisitions can be obtained over the cardiac cycle. With appropriate cardiac gating, these data can be segmented into time-resolved images of dynamic blood flow, which is referred to as velocity-encoded cine MRI. Compared with echocardiography, which also offers real-time evaluation of blood flow, velocity-encoded cine MRI is operator independent and consequently more reproducible.

Flow-Encoding Axes

Flow sensitivity occurs in the orientation of the applied bipolar gradient. For example, if the bipolar gradient pulses are applied in the z-axis, the resulting motion-induced phase shifts are induced along that axis, and the velocity of blood moving from the head to the feet is encoded. Bipolar gradients can be applied in all three dimensions, allowing flow encoding in any direction. However, increasing the number of flow-encoding axes also increases scan time.

Flow quantification is performed by prescribing an imaging plane orthogonal to the direction of flow within a vessel. During postprocessing, the borders of the vessel are delineated with a flexible region of interest for each segment of the cardiac cycle. This creates a cross-sectional area for each time point and defines the pixels that contain velocities representing intravascular flow. The spatial mean velocity is then calculated from these pixels and multiplied by the cross-sectional area for each time point in the cardiac cycle (Fig. 17-2). The result is blood flow calculated in milliliters per heartbeat.[1]

Pressure gradients can be estimated with the modified Bernoulli equation, $\Delta P = 4v^2$, where ΔP is the peak

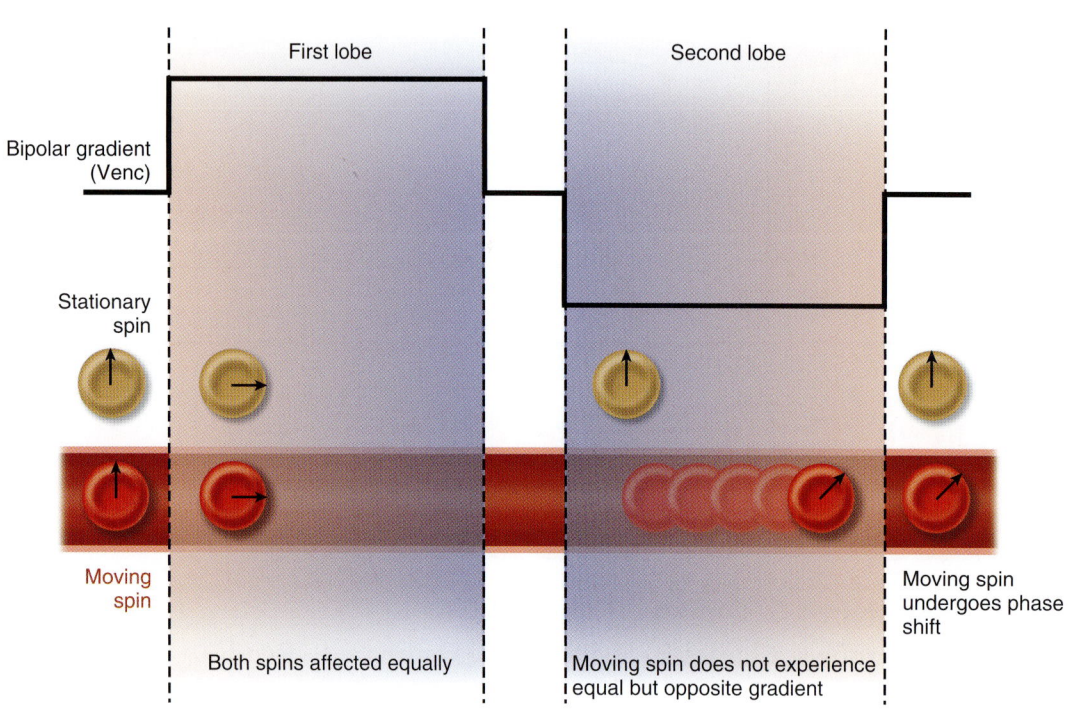

FIGURE 17-1 Diagram of the effect of bipolar gradients on stationary and moving spins. Venc, velocity encoding value. *(Modified from Westbrook C, Roth CK, Talbot J. MRI in Practice, 3rd ed. Oxford, Wiley-Blackwell, 2005.)*

pressure gradient in millimeters of mercury and v is the peak blood flow velocity in meters per second. Unlike flow quantification, phase contrast imaging planes may be prescribed in a parallel or perpendicular orientation with respect to the direction of blood flow to capture the point of peak velocity of flow downstream from a stenosis (Fig. 17-3). It is important to select a relatively high velocity encoding (Venc) value because peak velocities associated with stenotic valves can exceed 5 m/sec.[2]

Velocity Encoding

Phase contrast MRI can be optimized for different velocities of blood flow. The encoding velocity of a given sequence, or Venc, is selected on the basis of the maximum anticipated velocity of the blood flow of interest. The scanner will use this value to adjust the amplitude and duration of the phase contrast bipolar gradients so that a proton moving at the selected Venc value will give rise to a phase shift of 180 degrees. For example, for a Venc value of 100 cm/sec, the range of phase shifts will be adjusted to encode velocities from −100 cm/sec to +100 cm/sec (Fig. 17-4). The lower the Venc value selected, the greater the sensitivity to slower flow but also the stronger the required gradients and the longer the repetition time (TR) of the sequence. An ideal Venc value is slightly greater than the maximum expected velocity.

Imaging Limitations and Pitfalls

There are some pitfalls to be aware of in employing phase contrast MRI for blood flow quantification. Signal aliasing will occur if the peak velocity of blood flow surpasses the Venc value at any point in the cardiac cycle. This phenomenon takes place because positive velocities that surpass the Venc value will give rise to phase shifts that are interpreted as negative velocities (e.g., a phase shift of 185 degrees will be interpreted as −175 degrees). On phase images, areas of aliasing are easily identifiable: the sudden loss of signal in regions of maximum signal brightness (Figs. 17-5 and 17-6).

Underestimation of velocity and flow can occur if a vessel is not evaluated in a plane orthogonal to the direction of flow or if partial volume averaging occurs. In addition, peak flow velocity downstream of a stenosis, and thus the associated pressure gradient, can be underestimated for two reasons: (1) as the accuracy of peak velocity measurement is dependent on temporal resolution, the value may be underestimated by MRI compared with echocardiography, which has a higher temporal resolution; and (2) the precise, three-dimensional location of the peak velocity downstream from a stenosis may not be included in the two-dimensional phase contrast evaluation.[3,4]

TECHNIQUES
Indications

Two-dimensional phase contrast MRI is currently the most common flow-sensitive cardiac sequence used in clinical practice. A two-dimensional plane is prescribed in the appropriate orientation for evaluation of the vascular area of interest, and time-resolved phase contrast data are acquired in a single direction during a breath-hold. The technique allows quantification of cardiac output, pulmonary-to-systemic flow ratio (shunt), valvular regurgitation, differential lung perfusion, coronary flow reserve, and severity of vascular and valvular stenosis. We focus our discussion here on valvular disease, aortic coarctation, shunt, and pulmonary blood flow evaluation.

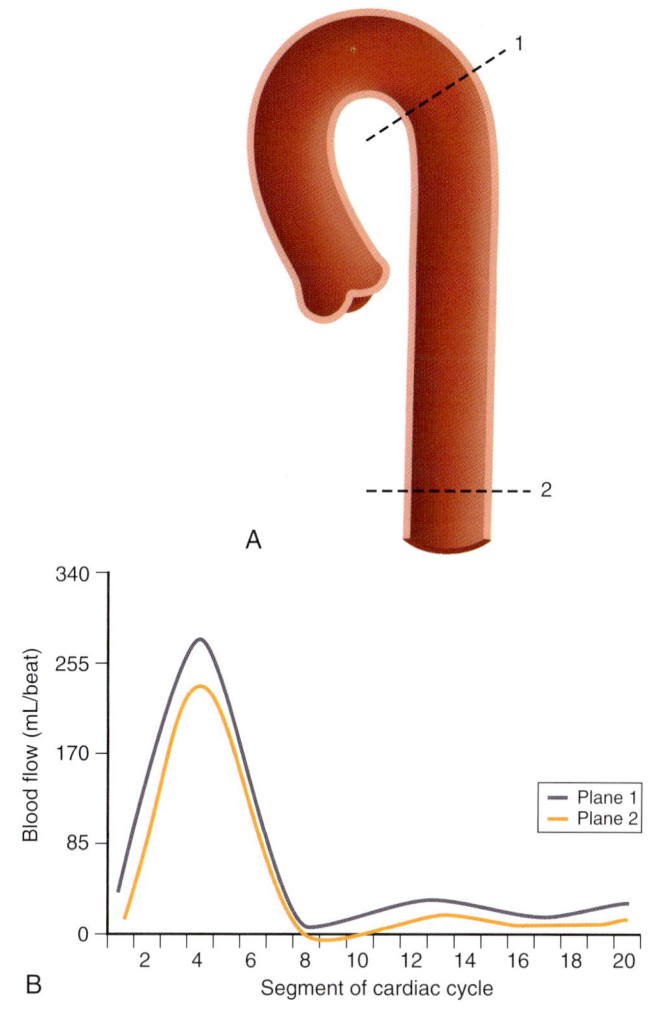

FIGURE 17-2 **A,** Two-dimensional velocity-encoded cine phase contrast scan planes in the proximal (plane 1) and distal (plane 2) descending thoracic aorta. **B,** Typical aortic blood flow with two-dimensional velocity-encoded cine phase contrast MR imaging.

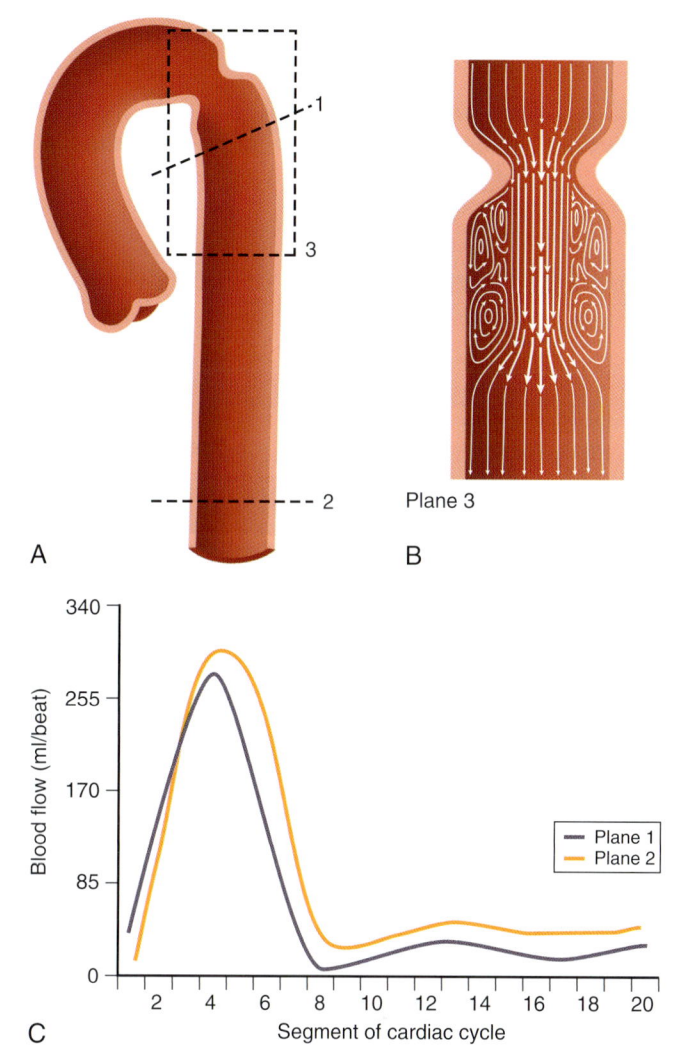

FIGURE 17-3 **A** and **B,** Two-dimensional velocity-encoded cine phase contrast scan planes in the proximal (plane 1) and distal (plane 2) descending thoracic aorta for quantification of collateral blood flow in coarctation of the aorta. Plane 3 is prescribed in the direction of flow to measure peak velocity, which is used to derive the pressure gradient across the stenosis used in the modified Bernoulli equation.[11] **C,** Typical aortic blood flow with two-dimensional velocity-encoded phase contrast MR imaging. Note that the distal blood flow (plane 2) is higher than the proximal flow (plane 1). The area between the curves represents collateral flow.

Contraindications

None.

Technique Description

Valvular Disease

Although echocardiography is the initial imaging modality of choice for assessment of cardiac valves because it is significantly cheaper and faster than MRI, cardiac MRI does play an important role in evaluation of valvular heart disease. MRI can augment the echocardiographic assessment with (1) reproducible and accurate calculation of ventricular size, function, and mass with steady-state free precession sequences and (2) quantitative evaluation of the severity of valvular stenosis and regurgitation with phase contrast sequences.

Precise quantification of aortic, pulmonary, and mitral regurgitation has been demonstrated with phase contrast MRI.[5-7] Aortic and pulmonary regurgitant volume can be quantified directly, resulting in more accurate and reproducible data than with echocardiography, by which blood flow is estimated on the basis of the apparent size of flow jets, which can be significantly affected by imaging parameters and orientation. The imaging plane is prescribed perpendicular to the direction of blood flow at approximately 1 to 2 cm above the level of the semilunar valve in question (Fig. 17-7). Valvular regurgitant fraction is the ratio of retrograde to antegrade flow across a valve.

Mitral regurgitation can also be assessed directly, but through-plane movement of the valve during systole may introduce significant error.[8] Another approach for estimation of mitral regurgitation is subtraction of the flow in the aorta during systole (left ventricular outflow) from flow across the mitral valve during diastole (left ventricular inflow); the base of the heart is less prone to movement during diastole, so by prescribing a two-dimensional plane

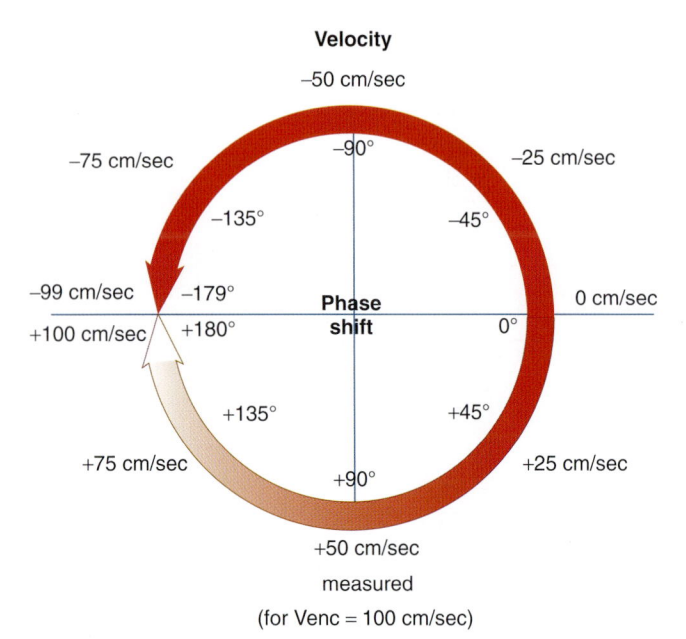

FIGURE 17-4 Diagram of phase shifts and velocity for a given velocity encoding value (Venc). (Modified from Lee VS. Cardiovascular MR Imaging: Physical Principles to Practical Protocols. Philadelphia, Lippincott Williams & Wilkins, 2005.)

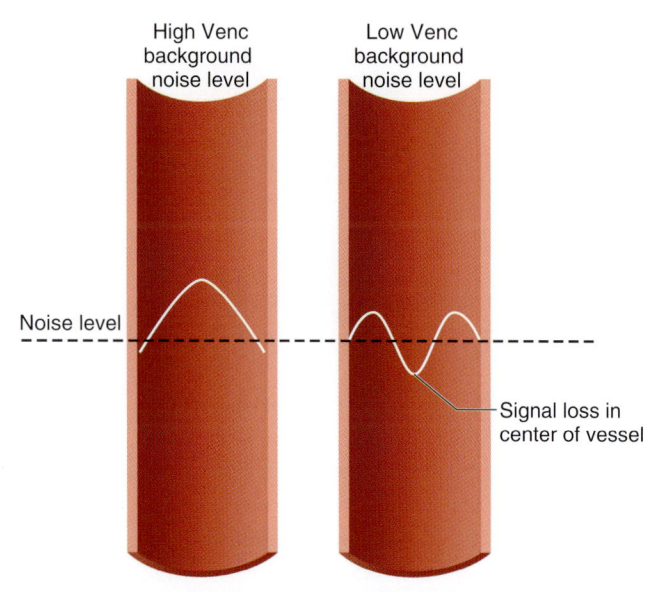

FIGURE 17-5 Diagram of aliasing with low but not with high velocity encoding value (Venc). (Modified from Westbrook C, Roth CK, Talbot J. MRI in Practice, 3rd ed. Oxford, Wiley-Blackwell, 2005.)

across the mitral valve during end-diastole, diastolic flow can be reliably calculated. Assuming normal aortic valve function, any difference between the outflow and inflow measurements can be attributed to mitral regurgitation.[5] Tricuspid regurgitation can be estimated in a similar fashion from measurements of pulmonic outflow and right ventricular inflow.

The degree of valvular stenosis is estimated by use of the modified Bernoulli equation, $\Delta P = 4v^2$ (discussed earlier in the section on flow-encoding axes), which is also used routinely for Doppler echocardiography. The technique has demonstrated good accuracy compared with Doppler echocardiography for both mitral and aortic stenosis.[9,10]

Aortic Coarctation

Aortic coarctation is narrowing of the aortic arch that restricts forward flow at or near the junction with the descending aorta. MRI can lend to the evaluation and management of coarctation by providing both anatomic and functional data on the location and degree of stenosis. Specifically, phase contrast MRI allows quantification of the functional significance of coarctation in two ways: (1) estimation of the pressure gradient across the lesion by using the maximum associated flow velocity in conjunction with the modified Bernoulli equation as discussed elsewhere[11] and (2) quantification of collateral flow.

Collateral flow arises in coarctation as blood must find an alternate path to the descending thoracic aorta and below. It indicates a hemodynamically significant lesion that may require intervention. Evaluation of collateral flow

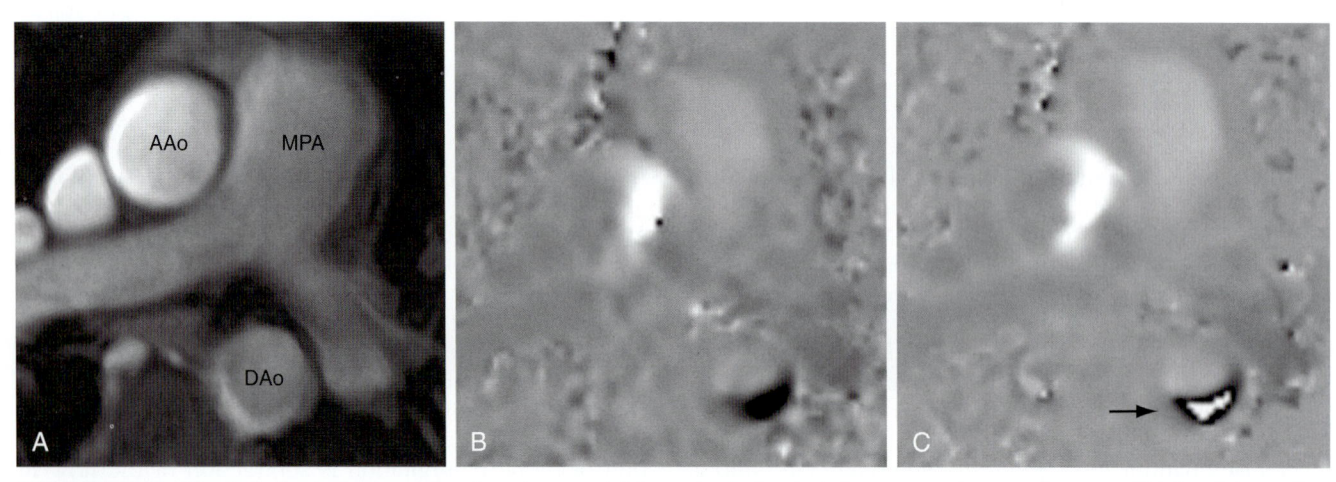

FIGURE 17-6 Signal aliasing in the descending thoracic aorta. Axial magnitude data in **A** demonstrate the ascending aorta (*AAo*) and descending aorta (*DAo*) in cross section and the bifurcation of the main pulmonary artery (*MPA*) into the right and left pulmonary arteries. Corresponding phase images demonstrate flow toward the head in the ascending aorta (*white area*) and toward the feet in the descending aorta (*black area*) during systole depicted in **B**, with aliasing of signal in the descending aorta at a slightly later systolic time point in **C**. The abrupt loss of signal within the fast flow channel in the descending aorta (*arrow*) is characteristic for aliasing.

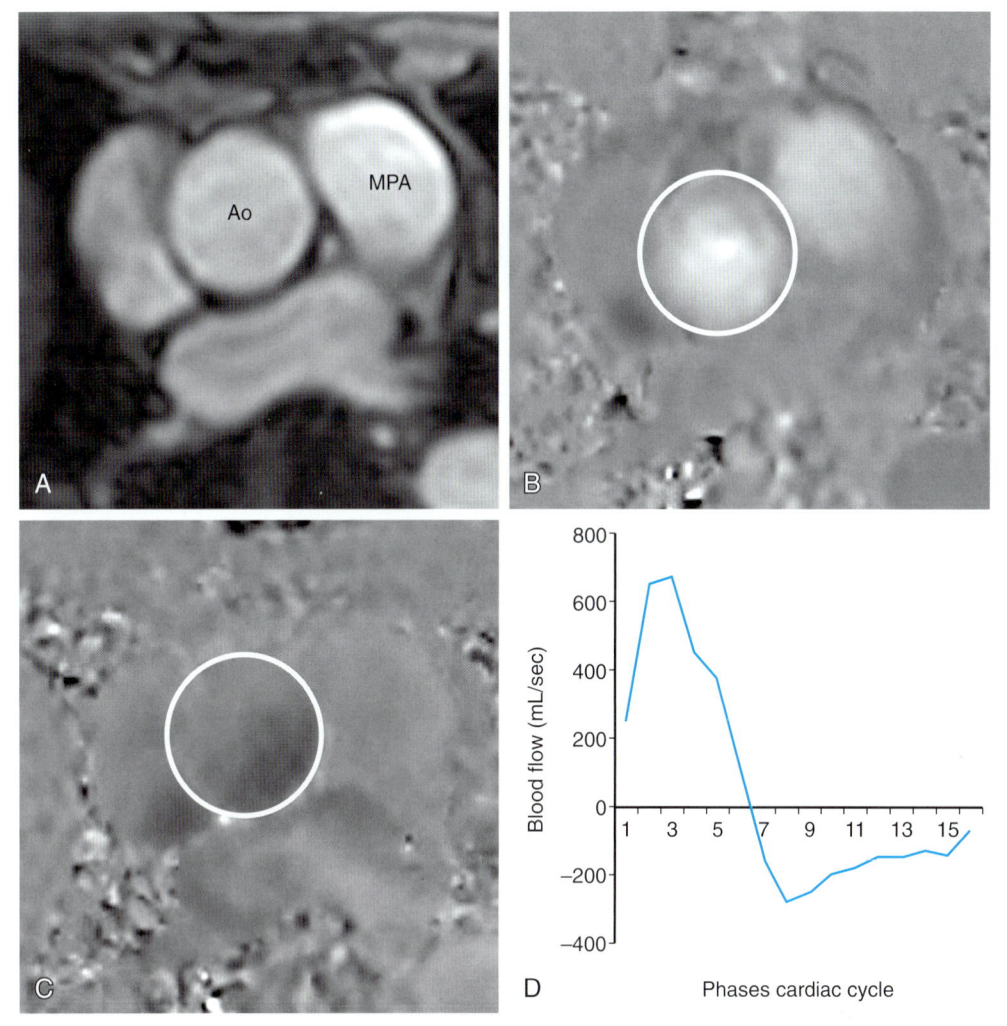

FIGURE 17-7 Quantification of aortic regurgitation. Axial magnitude data in **A** demonstrate the aorta (Ao) and main pulmonary artery (MPA). Corresponding phase images demonstrate flow toward the head in the aorta (white) during systole in **B** but flow toward the feet (black) in diastole in **C**, consistent with aortic regurgitation. The degree of aortic regurgitation is demonstrated graphically over the cardiac cycle in **D**.

is achieved by prescribing imaging planes orthogonal to aortic blood flow just distal to the coarctation and at the level of the diaphragm (Figs. 17-3 and 17-8). In healthy individuals, blood flow will decrease by approximately 7% over this interval spanning the descending aorta.[12] In hemodynamically significant coarctation, however, blood flow will increase rather than decrease over this interval as blood bypassing the coarctation will be delivered to the distal descending aorta through collaterals; the percentage increase in blood flow gives a quantitative measure of the degree of collateralization.[12-14] Study of surgically created coarctation in a porcine model confirms that phase contrast MRI is an accurate method of measuring collateral flow and that these collaterals develop within weeks.[15]

For an accurate assessment of collateral flow, phase images must be reviewed carefully for aliasing. If aliasing is present in the imaging plane just downstream of the coarctation, blood flow in the proximal descending aorta will be underestimated, and consequently, there may be an apparent but erroneous increase in flow in the distal descending aorta. Correction of this artifact can be achieved by increasing the Venc value in subsequent acquisitions.

Shunts

Quantification of shunt severity is performed clinically to determine if a patient may need surgery or to assess postsurgical outcomes. Intracardiac shunt quantification is achieved with phase contrast MRI by determining the ratio of flow in the pulmonary artery to that in the aorta, referred to as the Qp:Qs ratio, where Qp is the net flow in the main pulmonary artery and Qs is the net flow in the ascending aorta. This type of analysis can be used for both left-to-right and right-to-left shunts; the shunted volume is the difference between the pulmonary and aortic blood flow in either case. Phase contrast MRI has been deemed a first-line clinical study for quantification of shunt volume.[16]

Measurement of the Qp:Qs ratio is performed with two separate phase contrast acquisitions orthogonal to the direction of blood flow in the main pulmonary artery and ascending aorta, both at approximately 1 cm above the respective semilunar valves (Fig. 17-9). As the placement of this plane will be distal to the coronary ostia in the aorta, aortic flow will be approximately 3% to 5% less than pulmonic flow because of coronary runoff. A normal

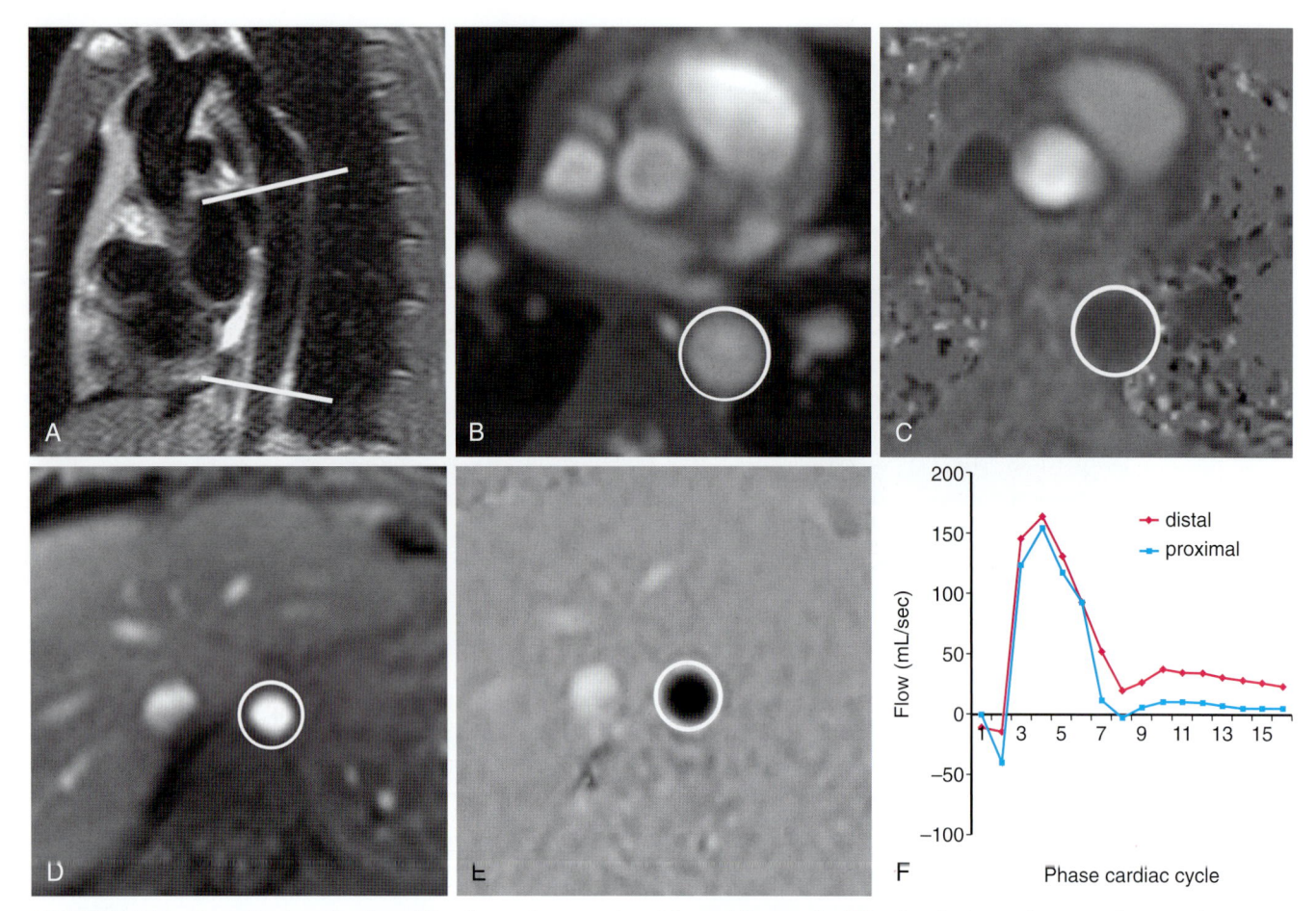

FIGURE 17-8 Quantification of collateral flow for aortic coarctation. **A** is an oblique sagittal T1 spin-echo image demonstrating a moderate juxtaductal coarctation. Two planes are depicted for quantification of collateral flow. Magnitude and phase images from the more superior plane just downstream of the coarctation in the proximal descending aorta are shown in **B** and **C**, respectively, and from the more inferior plane in the distal descending aorta at the level of the diaphragm in **D** and **E**, respectively. Relative flow at these planes is graphically demonstrated in **F** and reveals collateral flow of 35%, consistent with a hemodynamically significant aortic coarctation.

Qp:Qs ratio, therefore, should be slightly greater than 1. MRI-based measurement of Qp:Qs ratio in this fashion has been extensively validated.[17-20]

Pulmonary Flow Evaluation

Phase contrast MRI can be used to assess differential flow in the right and left pulmonary arteries and relative flow within the pulmonary veins. Branch pulmonary artery stenosis, which can be seen after arterial switch repair performed for transposition of the great vessels, may go undetected with other imaging modalities.[21] Direct quantification of blood flow to both lungs is crucial for determination of the hemodynamic significance of such a stenosis. Measurement of differential pulmonary flow is achieved with two phase contrast acquisitions orthogonal to the direction of blood flow in the proximal right and left pulmonary arteries (Fig. 17-10). The normal blood flow distribution is 55% to the right lung and 45% to the left lung.

MR blood flow evaluation has also been used clinically to assess pulmonary venous obstruction[22] and to characterize the complex postsurgical pulmonary inflow in patients after total cavopulmonary connection, with quantification of the relative contributions of the superior and inferior caval veins to the right and left lungs.[23] In addition, some investigators have proposed use of the time-resolved velocity data that underlie MR flow evaluations to noninvasively estimate the degree of pulmonary artery hypertension.[24]

Time-Resolved, Three-Dimensional Phase Contrast MRI

Acquisition of three-dimensional phase contrast data in a time-resolved fashion over the cardiac cycle for an imaging volume that contains the heart and great vessels is an attractive approach to cardiac MRI flow evaluation, but one that has been limited in its clinical application by long scan time. Work in the early 1990s with two-dimensional planes stacked to achieve three-dimensional data sets showed the utility of this type of imaging for uncovering of complex, secondary aortic blood flow characteristics such as helices and vortices, which are not easily appreciated by two-dimensional imaging.[25] More recently, true three-dimensional phase contrast acquisitions have been validated, and time-saving measures such as parallel imaging and other approaches to k-space subsampling have been implemented to make this type of comprehensive MR flow evaluation a more viable clinical tool.[26-28] The technique has been termed flow-sensitive four-dimensional MRI or simply four-dimensional flow, where the fourth dimension refers to time, and seven-

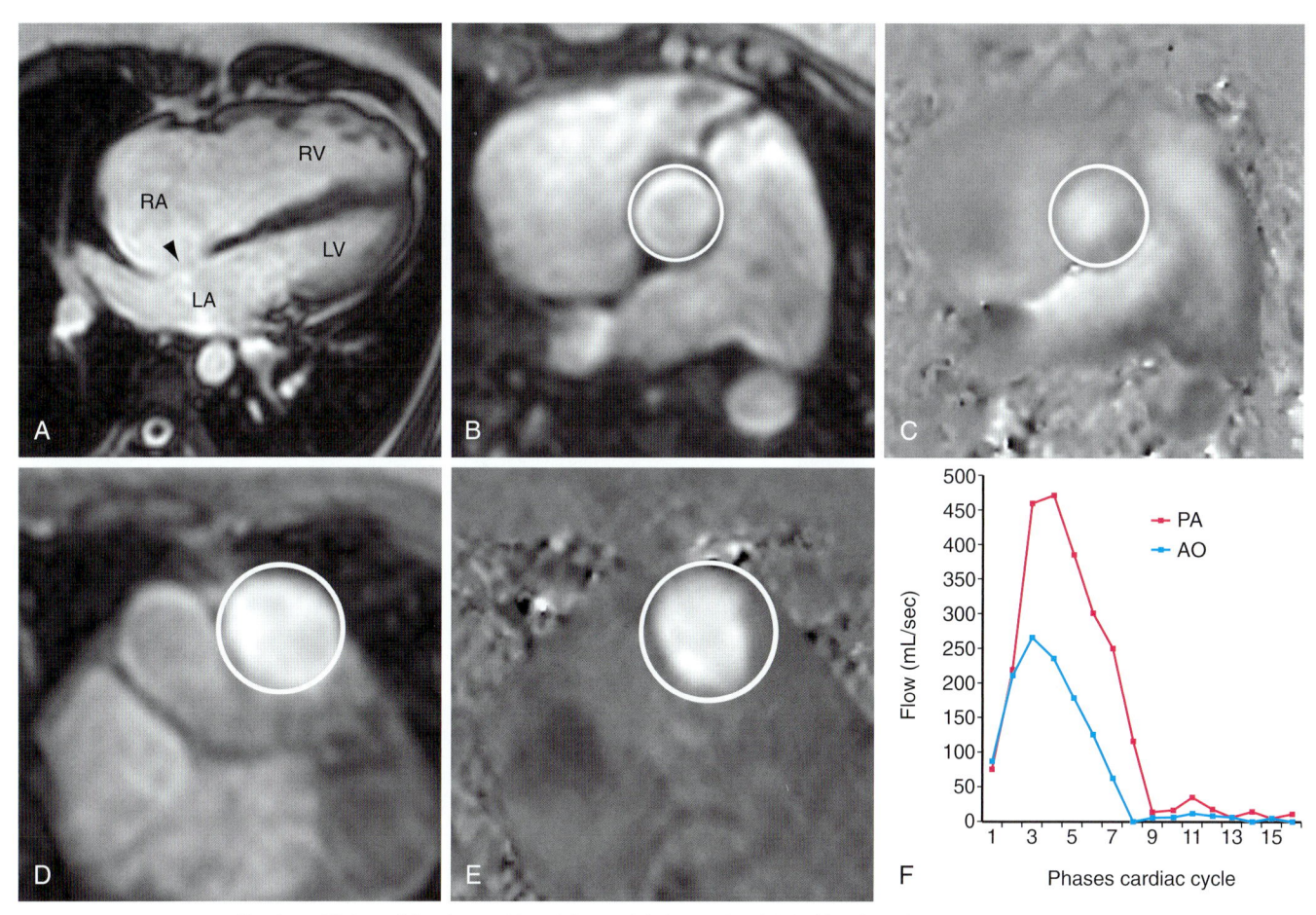

■ **FIGURE 17-9** Quantification of left-to-right shunt with atrial septal defect. **A** is a bright blood gradient echo image in a four-chamber orientation demonstrating an atrial septal defect (*arrowhead*). To quantify the degree of shunting across the atrial septum, relative flow in the aorta and main pulmonary artery is measured. Magnitude and phase images from the aorta are shown in **B** and **C**, respectively, and from the main pulmonary artery in **D** and **E**, respectively. Relative flow is graphically demonstrated in **F**, revealing a ratio of pulmonary to aortic blood flow (Qp:Qs) of 2 to 1, consistent with a significant left-to-right shunt.

dimensional flow, referring to the seven data components that are encoded for each voxel that composes a data set.

Advantages of this technique include complete temporal and spatial coverage of the vascular area of interest, continuous breathing, no requirement for prospective placement of two-dimensional planes for phase contrast acquisition, and a variety of unique visualization and quantification options for velocity data that are not available by conventional two-dimensional phase contrast imaging. Rich and extensive data analysis is possible in the postprocessing stage with appropriate software. Interactive navigation throughout these volumetric data sets allows evaluation of blood velocity and flow in user-defined regions of interest at any phase of the cardiac cycle (Fig. 17-11). Three-dimensional visualization tools such as streamlines and particle traces allow four-dimensional visual presentation of secondary blood flow features that may not otherwise be evident (Figs. 17-12 and 17-13).

Secondary Parameters

The three-dimensional velocity vector fields that are generated by this technique can be used for applications beyond the mapping and quantification of blood velocity and flow. These data are starting to be used clinically to estimate important secondary vascular parameters including vascular wall shear stress, relative blood pressure, and pulse wave velocity.

Wall shear stress refers to the force per unit area exerted on the vascular wall by fluid in motion in a tangential plane. Abnormal shear values have been strongly implicated in atherogenesis.[29] Recently, this parameter has been estimated by use of near wall velocity gradients generated by three-dimensional phase contrast MRI and reported for the carotid arteries as well as for thoracic and intracranial aneurysms.[30-33] Confirmation of these reported shear stress values with an accepted standard such as computational fluid dynamics is forthcoming.

Relative pressure mapping has been demonstrated and validated in vivo by use of multidirectional velocity data and the Navier-Stokes equations.[34,35] Pulse wave velocity, which reflects the degree of vascular stiffness, is another secondary parameter that can be estimated with time-resolved velocity data, although a much higher temporal resolution than that typically provided by the three-dimensional phase contrast sequence is required for accurate calculation.[36]

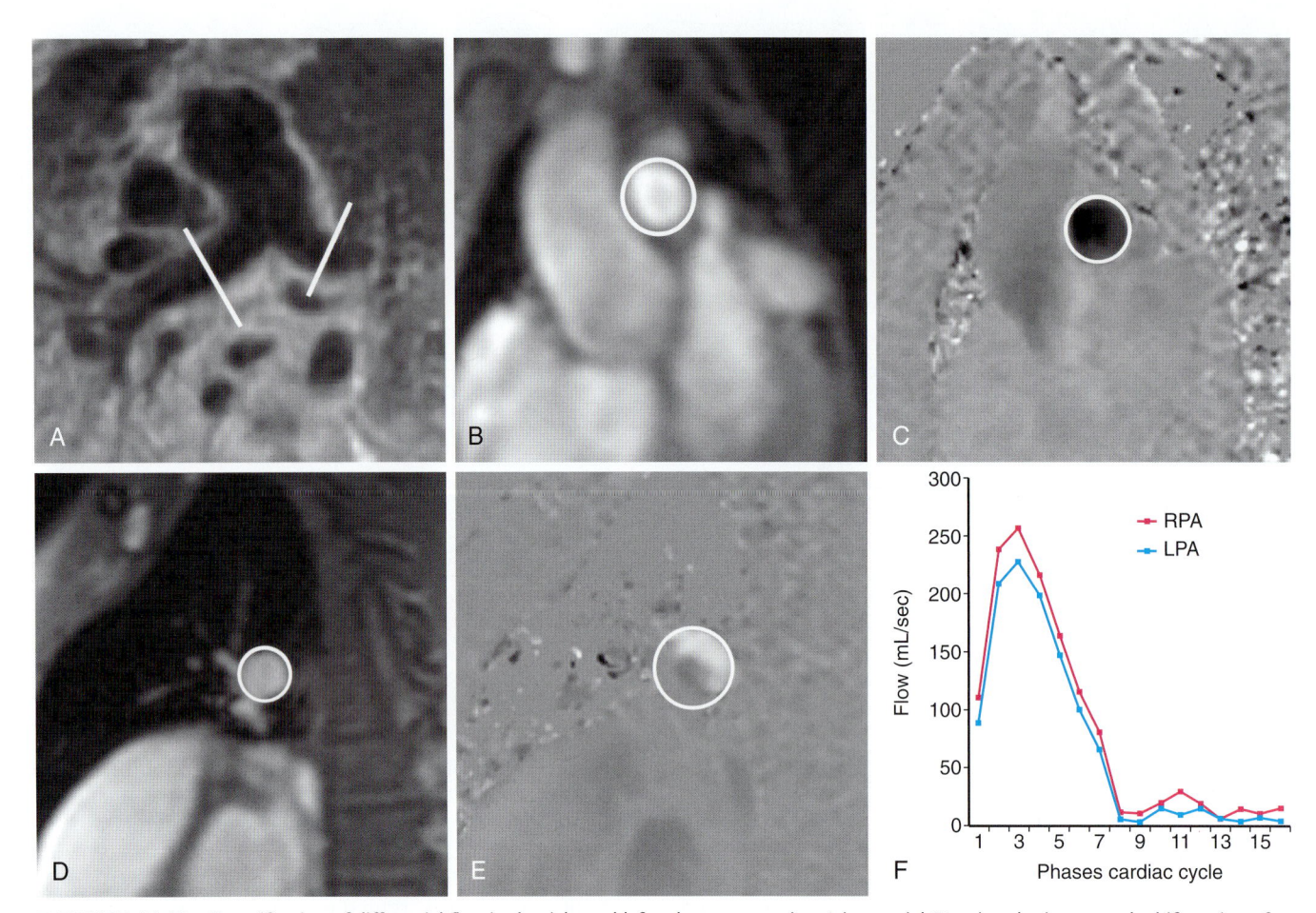

FIGURE 17-10 Quantification of differential flow in the right and left pulmonary arteries. **A** is an axial T1 spin-echo image at the bifurcation of the main pulmonary artery with two planes depicted for quantification of flow into the right and left pulmonary arteries. Magnitude and phase images from the right pulmonary artery are shown in **B** and **C**, respectively, and from the left pulmonary artery in **D** and **E**, respectively. Relative flow at these planes is graphically demonstrated in **F** and reveals that 55% of pulmonary flow is directed toward the right lung and 45% to the left, which is a normal distribution.

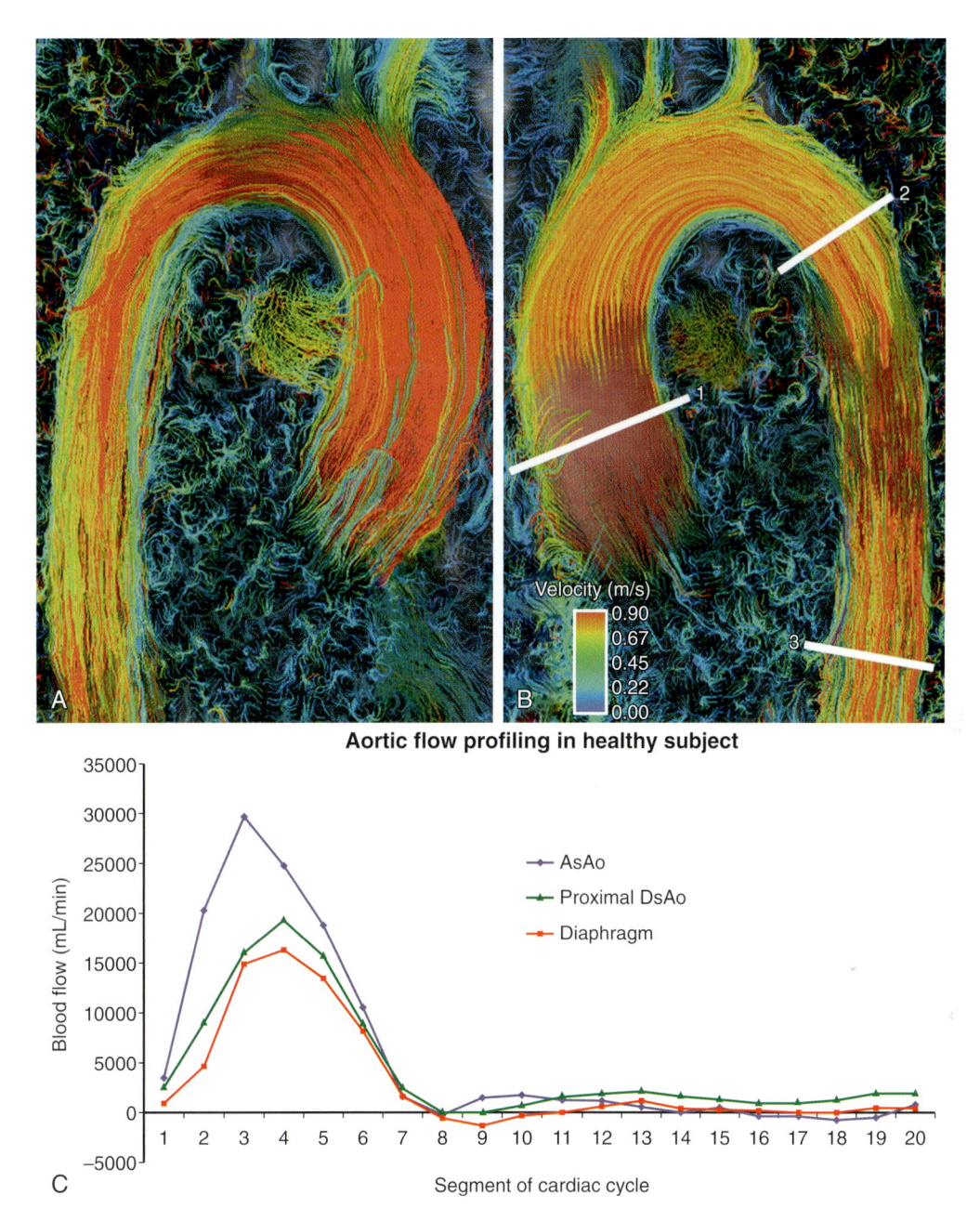

CHAPTER 17 ● *Magnetic Resonance Evaluation of Blood Flow* 247

■ **FIGURE 17-11** Visualization of three-dimensional phase contrast data from a healthy subject in oblique sagittal orientation from the right (**A**) and left (**B**) sides of the aortic arch with streamlines during mid-systole. Streamlines are imaginary lines aligned with local vector fields and represent the flow field at a given moment in the cardiac cycle. They are color coded for velocity. Note the smooth trajectory of streamlines and absence of significant secondary flow features throughout the thoracic aorta. Flow quantification was performed for the three planes depicted in **B**: orthogonal to aortic blood flow in the proximal ascending aorta (plane 1), in the proximal descending aorta (plane 2), and at the level of the diaphragm (plane 3). **C** is a graph of blood flow over the cardiac cycle at these three planes.

248 PART TWO • *Cardiac Imaging Techniques*

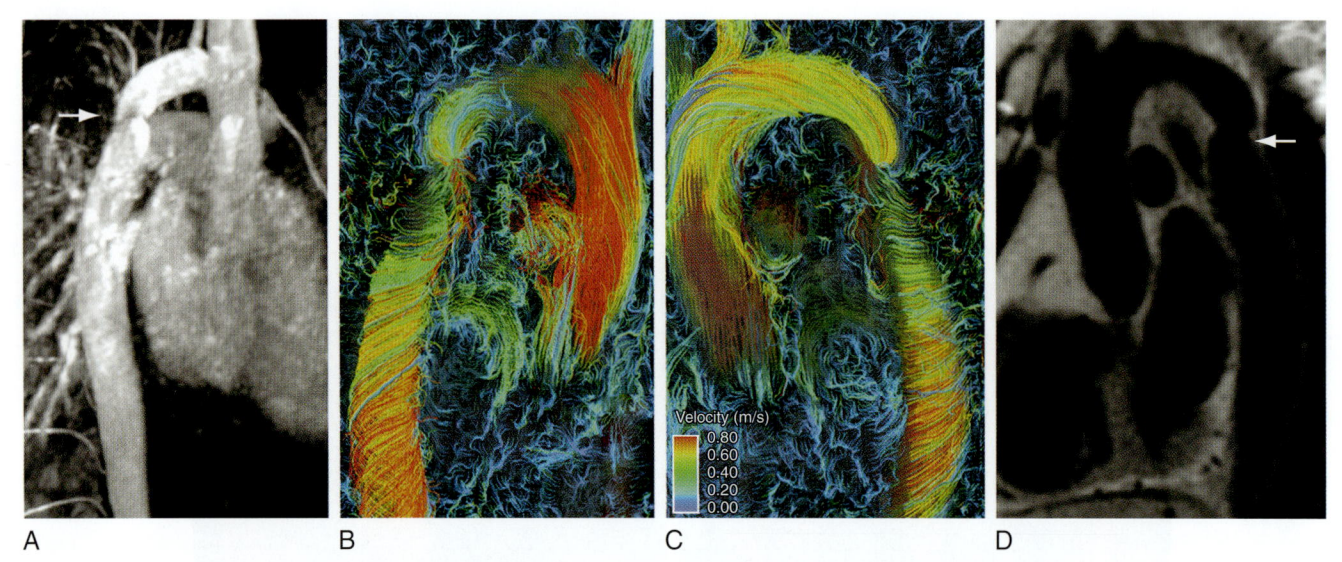

■ **FIGURE 17-12** Abnormal helical flow in a patient with aortic coarctation. **A,** Three-dimensional contrast-enhanced MR angiography demonstrates a focal juxtaductal coarctation (*arrow*). **B** and **C,** Views of the right and left aspect of the aortic arch, respectively, with streamlines to visualize three-dimensional phase contrast data in mid-systole. Marked flow disturbance is seen at and distal to the coarctation, with abnormal right-handed helical flow in the descending thoracic aorta. **D,** Oblique sagittal T1 spin-echo image in the same orientation as **C** demonstrating the coarctation (*arrow*).

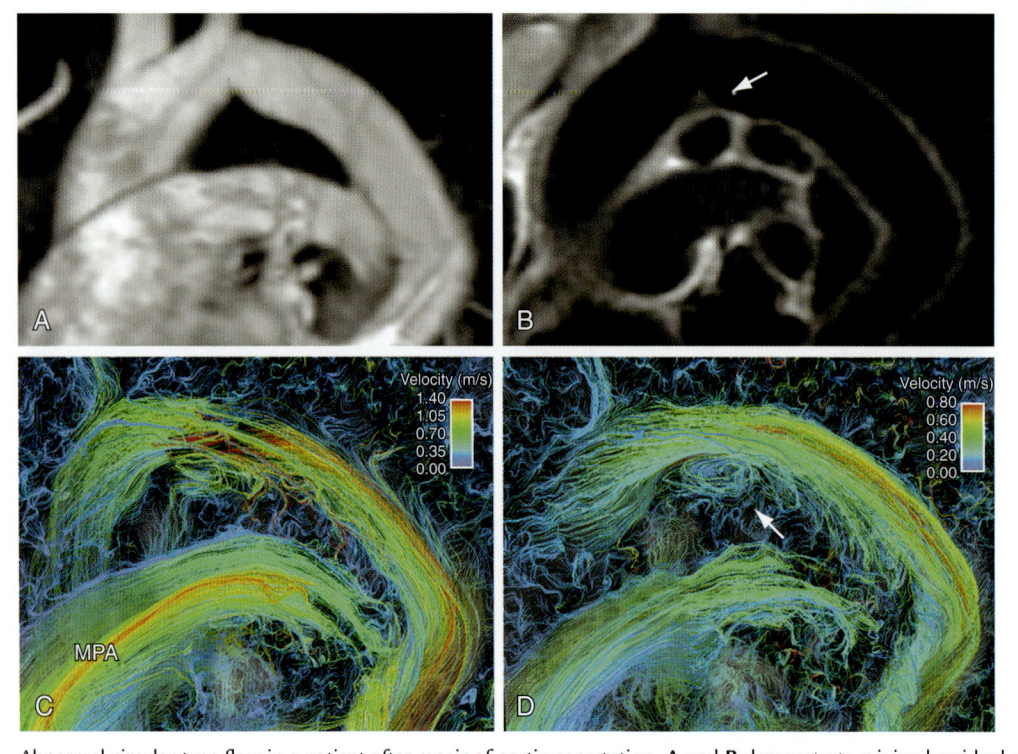

■ **FIGURE 17-13** Abnormal circular-type flow in a patient after repair of aortic coarctation. **A** and **B** demonstrate minimal residual narrowing (*arrow*) of the mid-aortic arch with three-dimensional contrast-enhanced MR angiography and oblique sagittal T1 spin-echo imaging, respectively. **C** and **D** represent streamline evaluation of the aortic arch at mid and late systole, respectively. Disturbed flow is revealed, with acceleration and signal dropout secondary to aliasing as well as circular-type flow (*arrow*) downstream of the focal region of mild aortic narrowing.

KEY POINTS

- Velocity-encoded cine phase contrast MRI can be used to evaluate velocity, flow, and pressure gradients.
- Phase contrast MRI can be applied for quantitative assessment of regurgitant volume and fraction in valvular regurgitation; pressure gradient in valvular stenosis; collateral flow and pressure gradient in coarctation of the aorta; differential pulmonary blood flow in the presence of pulmonary artery stenosis; and pulmonary-to-systemic flow ratio in the setting of a cardiac shunt.

SUGGESTED READINGS

Glockner JF, Johnston DL, McGee KP. Evaluation of cardiac valvular disease with MR imaging: qualitative and quantitative techniques. Radiographics 2003; 23:e9.

Higgins CB, Sakuma H. Heart disease: functional evaluation with MR imaging. Radiology 1996; 199:307-315.

Malek AM, Alper SL, Izumo S. Hemodynamic shear stress and its role in atherosclerosis. JAMA 1999; 282:2035-2042.

Markl M, Chan FP, Alley MT, et al. Time-resolved three-dimensional phase-contrast MRI. J Magn Reson Imaging 2003; 17:499-506.

Pennell DJ, Sechtem UP, Higgins CB, et al. Clinical indications for cardiovascular magnetic resonance (CMR): Consensus Panel report. Eur Heart J 2004; 25:1940-1965.

Varaprasathan GA, Araoz PA, Higgins CB, Reddy GP. Quantification of flow dynamics in congenital heart disease: applications of velocity-encoded cine MR imaging. Radiographics 2002; 22:895-905.

REFERENCES

1. Varaprasathan GA, Araoz PA, Higgins CB, Reddy GP. Quantification of flow dynamics in congenital heart disease: applications of velocity-encoded cine MR imaging. Radiographics 2002; 22:895-905.
2. Glockner JF, Johnston DL, McGee KP. Evaluation of cardiac valvular disease with MR imaging: qualitative and quantitative techniques. Radiographics 2003; 23:e9.
3. Higgins CB, Sakuma H. Heart disease: functional evaluation with MR imaging. Radiology 1996; 199:307-315.
4. Tang C, Blatter DD, Parker DL. Accuracy of phase-contrast flow measurements in the presence of partial-volume effects. J Magn Reson Imaging 1993; 3:377-385.
5. Dulce MC, Mostbeck GH, O'Sullivan M, et al. Severity of aortic regurgitation: interstudy reproducibility of measurements with velocity-encoded cine MR imaging. Radiology 1992; 185:235-240.
6. Rebergen SA, Chin JG, Ottenkamp J, et al. Pulmonary regurgitation in the late postoperative follow-up of tetralogy of Fallot. Volumetric quantitation by nuclear magnetic resonance velocity mapping. Circulation 1993; 88:2257-2266.
7. Fujita N, Chazouilleres AF, Hartiala JJ, et al. Quantification of mitral regurgitation by velocity-encoded cine nuclear magnetic resonance imaging. J Am Coll Cardiol 1994; 23:951-958.
8. Hundley WG, Li HF, Willard JE, et al. Magnetic resonance imaging assessment of the severity of mitral regurgitation. Comparison with invasive techniques. Circulation 1995; 92:1151-1158.
9. Kilner PJ, Manzara CC, Mohiaddin RH, et al. Magnetic resonance jet velocity mapping in mitral and aortic valve stenosis. Circulation 1993; 87:1239-1248.
10. Heidenreich PA, Steffens J, Fujita N, et al. Evaluation of mitral stenosis with velocity-encoded cine-magnetic resonance imaging. Am J Cardiol 1995; 75:365-369.
11. Kilner PJ, Firmin DN, Rees RS, et al. Valve and great vessel stenosis: assessment with MR jet velocity mapping. Radiology 1991; 178:229-235.
12. Steffens JC, Bourne MW, Sakuma H, et al. Quantification of collateral blood flow in coarctation of the aorta by velocity encoded cine magnetic resonance imaging. Circulation 1994; 90:937-943.
13. Holmqvist C, Ståhlberg F, Hanséus K, et al. Collateral flow in coarctation of the aorta with magnetic resonance velocity mapping: correlation to morphological imaging of collateral vessels. J Magn Reson Imaging 2002; 15:39-46.
14. Araoz PA, Reddy GP, Tarnoff H, et al. MR findings of collateral circulation are more accurate measures of hemodynamic significance than arm-leg blood pressure gradient after repair of coarctation of the aorta. J Magn Reson Imaging 2003; 17:177-183.
15. Chernoff DM, Derugin N, Rajasinghe HA, et al. Measurement of collateral blood flow in a porcine model of aortic coarctation by velocity-encoded cine MRI. J Magn Reson Imaging 1997; 7:557-563.
16. Pennell DJ, Sechtem UP, Higgins CB, et al. Clinical indications for cardiovascular magnetic resonance (CMR): Consensus Panel report. Eur Heart J 2004; 25:1940-1965.
17. Arheden H, Holmqvist C, Thilen U, et al. Left-to-right cardiac shunts: comparison of measurements obtained with MR velocity mapping and with radionuclide angiography. Radiology 1999; 211:453-458.
18. Powell AJ, Maier SE, Chung T, Geva T. Phase-velocity cine magnetic resonance imaging measurement of pulsatile blood flow in children and young adults: in vitro and in vivo validation. Pediatr Cardiol 2000; 21:104-110.
19. Sieverding L, Jung WI, Klose U, Apitz J. Noninvasive blood flow measurement and quantification of shunt volume by cine magnetic resonance in congenital heart disease. Preliminary results. Pediatr Radiol 1992; 22:48-54.
20. Brenner LD, Caputo GR, Mostbeck G, et al. Quantification of left to right atrial shunts with velocity-encoded cine nuclear magnetic resonance imaging. J Am Coll Cardiol 1992; 20:1246-1250.
21. Gutberlet M, Boeckel T, Hosten N, et al. Arterial switch procedure for D-transposition of the great arteries: quantitative midterm evaluation of hemodynamic changes with cine MR imaging and phase-shift velocity mapping—initial experience. Radiology 2000; 214:467-475.
22. Videlefsky N, Parks WJ, Oshinski J, et al. Magnetic resonance phase-shift velocity mapping in pediatric patients with pulmonary venous obstruction. J Am Coll Cardiol 2001; 38:262-267.
23. Houlind K, Stenbøg EV, Sørensen KE, et al. Pulmonary and caval flow dynamics after total cavopulmonary connection. Heart 1999; 81:67-72.
24. Laffon E, Vallet C, Bernard V, et al. A computed method for noninvasive MRI assessment of pulmonary arterial hypertension. J Appl Physiol 2004; 96:463-468.
25. Kilner PJ, Yang GZ, Mohiaddin RH, et al. Helical and retrograde secondary flow patterns in the aortic arch studied by three-directional magnetic resonance velocity mapping. Circulation 1993; 88(pt 1):2235-2247.
26. Markl M, Chan FP, Alley MT, et al. Time-resolved three-dimensional phase-contrast MRI. J Magn Reson Imaging 2003; 17:499-506.
27. Wentland AL, Korosec FR, Vigen KK, et al. Cine flow measurements using phase contrast with undersampled projections: in vitro validation and preliminary results in vivo. J Magn Reson Imaging 2006; 24:945-951.

28. Bammer R, Hope TA, Aksoy M, Alley MT. Time-resolved 3D quantitative flow MRI of the major intracranial vessels: initial experience and comparative evaluation at 1.5T and 3.0T in combination with parallel imaging. Magn Reson Med 2007; 57:127-140.
29. Malek AM, Alper SL, Izumo S. Hemodynamic shear stress and its role in atherosclerosis. JAMA 1999; 282:2035-2042.
30. Katritsis D, Kaiktsis L, Chaniotis A, et al. Wall shear stress: theoretical considerations and methods of measurement. Prog Cardiovasc Dis 2007; 49:307-329.
31. Sui B, Gao P, Lin Y, et al. Assessment of wall shear stress in the common carotid artery of healthy subjects using 3.0-tesla magnetic resonance. Acta Radiol 2008; 49:442-449.
32. Meckel S, Stalder AF, Santini F, et al. In vivo visualization and analysis of 3-D hemodynamics in cerebral aneurysms with flow-sensitized 4-D MR imaging at 3T. Neuroradiology 2008; 50:473-484.
33. Frydrychowicz A, Berger A, Russe MF, et al. Time-resolved magnetic resonance angiography and flow-sensitive 4-dimensional magnetic resonance imaging at 3 Tesla for blood flow and wall shear stress analysis. J Thorac Cardiovasc Surg 2008; 136:400-407.
34. Thompson RB, McVeigh ER. Fast measurement of intracardiac pressure differences with 2D breath-hold phase-contrast MRI. Magn Reson Med 2003; 49:1056-1066.
35. Moftakhar R, Aagaard-Kienitz B, Johnson K, et al. Noninvasive measurement of intra-aneurysmal pressure and flow pattern using phase contrast with vastly undersampled isotropic projection imaging. AJNR Am J Neuroradiol 2007; 28:1710-1714.
36. Groenink M, de Roos A, Mulder BJ, et al. Changes in aortic distensibility and pulse wave velocity assessed with magnetic resonance imaging following beta-blocker therapy in the Marfan syndrome. Am J Cardiol 1998; 82:203-208.

CHAPTER 18

Contrast Agents in Magnetic Resonance Imaging

Michael V. Knopp

INTRODUCTION

Intravenous contrast agents have become integral to the clinical practice of cardiovascular magnetic resonance (MR) imaging. Myocardial perfusion and myocardial delayed enhancement MR are important contrast-enhanced techniques for the clinical evaluation for myocardial disease. Contrast-enhanced magnetic resonance angiography (CE MRA) has become the preferred method for fast and accurate assessment of common arterial structures such as the thoracic aorta, abdominal aorta, carotid arteries, renal arteries, and peripheral arteries. These applications were facilitated by innovations in MRI instrumentation that improved acquisition speed and in optimization of cardiovascular imaging protocols.[1] This chapter will focus solely on those MR contrast agents that have, or promise to have, value for cardiovascular applications.

The value of a contrast agent depends on its ability to generate image contrast for a given imaging modality. Radiographic contrast agents lead to an attenuation of the transmitted x-rays; MR agents rely on a completely different biophysical principle. MR contrast agents generate image contrast by locally changing the relaxivity of the recipient tissue. For example, all contrast agents for x-ray computer tomography (CT) use iodine as their central ion, whereas MR contrast agents depend on the magnetic moment of the central atom. For cardiovascular MR imaging, we classify today's available agents into paramagnetic (mostly gadolinium-based) and super-paramagnetic (mostly iron oxide-based).[2] We also experience a substantial variability in country specific availability of MR contrast agents for cardiovascular imaging as well as regulatory approvals, which is especially evident for cardiovascular imaging. Therefore, we will initially discuss the development and safety of MR contrast agents before we will review some of their type-specific characteristics for cardiovascular MR and MRA.

Development of MR Contrast Agents

Before a discussion of the different characteristics of contrast agents, it should be recognized that contrast agents are medications or drugs and as such they require a stringent safety evaluation as well as an assessment of suitable clinical indications for their use. MR contrast agents are, therefore, clinically developed similarly to any other therapeutic medication. After completion of preclinical evaluations and extensive toxicology, contrast agents undergo a typical phase I (feasibility), phase II (dose-ranging) and multiple phase (III) (efficacy and safety) assessments prior to submission for regulatory approval to market and distribute a contrast agent. Similar to therapeutic drugs, such a full clinical development program is more than a 10-year process that typically includes more than 500 patient examinations and costs in the range between tens to hundreds of millions of U.S. dollars.

Regulatory Label of MR Contrast Agents

The regulatory approval by an agency such as the Food and Drug Administration (FDA) in the United States defines the *indicated use* frequently—also referred to as the *labeled use*—as well as how to use it appropriately, any warnings and contraindications. For healthcare providers, the package insert and the prescribing information is the locally appropriate and always updated contrast agent specific information source. Although our scientific community is global and the contrast agents we use are virtually available worldwide, the regulatory environment remains a national responsibility with considerable differences among jurisdictions reflected in the availability and approved label. Reading information product labels (package inserts) is not only essential to the good practice of healthcare, it is mandatory! Having stressed this labeling and its importance, we must recognize that health care technologic and methodologic advances are frequently much faster than regulatory solutions.

Using a medication or drug, which requires a physician order or prescription, outside its regulatory defined *approved, labeled* use is considered to be at least *off-label*; however it could also be *against-label* if such a use is defined as a contraindication or a defined warning applies. The vast majority of contrast-enhanced MRI examinations of the cardiovascular system performed globally to date has been done "off-label".[3] In 2010, none of the marketed MR contrast agents in the United States has an FDA-approved indication for use in cardiac MRI despite a huge number of clinical trials and clinical experience; and only one, gadofosveset trisodium (Ablavor, Lantheus Medical Imaging, North Billerica, MA) has an FDA-approved MRA indication and only "to evaluate aortoiliac occlusive disease (AIOD) in adults with known or suspected peripheral vascular disease."

Our imaging community is frequently perplexed with this situation and asks, "What is the difference if I use a contrast agent to do a brain MRI compared to the same dose injected in the same way for a cardiac MRI or vascular MRA?" The most important aspect here is that a regulatory approval requires proof of both efficacy and safety in an indication-specific population. Our community frequently does not appreciate that both are imperative. Furthermore, a population studied for evaluation of the brain does have a substantially different safety profile than one for a cardiovascular question. This is an important aspect and has led to issues that have changed how we appropriately use contrast agents today and in the future. Before we discuss the safety in more detail, let us complete the review on labeling. Labels of contrast agents (i.e., the official drug prescribing information that is contained on drug package inserts) are regulated, regularly updated, do change, and require that the health care provider has a process in place that ensures timely updates. Phase IV studies are also called postmarketing studies and are frequently requested from regulatory agencies to "review" the safety and efficacy in clinical practice populations, which can be different from the time of the original clinical trials or population studied. Magnetic resonance imaging has undergone a tremendous growth in the last two decades—not only in the number and performance of MR systems available, but also in the patient population being served. In particular, more frail patients are being studied more frequently and the overall outstanding safety of MR has led to some complacency that is not warranted and requires a review of appropriate training and standard operating procedures for the whole healthcare team involved in MRI. In this regard, the *label* or *regulatory approved use* becomes important because substantially more diligence must be expected for *off-label use* where safety considerations and contraindications might not yet have been fully established.

An off-label use has its foundation in the declaration of Helsinki and is basically founded in the physician's prerogative to provide the most appropriate care to patients. Off-label use is a common and essential part of today's practice of medicine, but it also requires appropriate diligence in its use. First of all, off-label use and clinical research are quite different. An investigational use (i.e., research use) requires a formal protocol approved by the Institutional Review Board (IRB) or an equivalent ethics board and typically informed consent; whereas off-label use requires only peer reviewed evidence. Why peer reviewed evidence? The regulatory agencies and legal interpretations expect objectivity without bias or conflict of interest. It is well recognized that regulatory agencies are appropriately very sensitive on the propagation of off-label use of drugs and therefore disallow drug vendors to advertise, market, or otherwise incentivize such off-label use as can be seen by a $2.3 billion[4] fine recently enforced for off-label propagation of a therapeutic drug and numerous warning letters being posted by FDA.[5] A key distinction of off-label use versus an investigational use is that off-label use pertains only to applications for patient care (i.e., clinical practice) and not for a research aim or objective.

Use of a drug or contrast agent for a listed contraindication or excluded use cannot be considered to be off-label; they are against label however they might still be necessary and patient-specific appropriate if used with the proper diligence. A new situation arose when the FDA decided to put a *black box warning label* on all gadolinium-based contrast agents in 2007 as a response to the occurrence of cases with NSF (nephrogenic systemic fibrosis).[6] Before we review the current status of this severe adverse reaction to gadolinium-containing MR contrast agents, let us finish with the labeling aspects. What is the intent of such a warning and what does it mean from a practical point of view? First, it is the strongest warning mechanism that the regulatory agencies have to ensure the user/health care professional is aware of a change in a label and product or class-associated warning, and second, gives regulatory guidance on the appropriate use. The FDA black box label means, for example, that any contrast dosage outside the contrast agent-specific label cannot be considered off-label anymore but will have to be considered against the label. In summary, the country-specific label of an MR contrast agent must be known and appropriately considered in the clinical practice of cardiovascular MR/MRA and will continue to change.

Safety of MR Contrast Agents

Although any contrast agent that received marketing approval needed to previously prove safety and identify use and warnings labels, cardiovascular MR imaging had its share of specific issues in the recent past that are highlighted to raise proper awareness and understanding in managing patients with cardiovascular disease.

The nonimaging community was warned in a 2003 letter to the editor of the *New England Journal of Medicine* that severe pseudohypocalcemia was observed after gadolinium-enhanced MRA.[7] The authors noted lower calcium values in blood samples obtained in patients immediately after they had an MRA performed with gadodiamide (Omniscan, GE Healthcare Medical Diagnostics) as MR contrast agent. The interaction of excess chelate in the gadodiamide with colorimetric calcium tests was recognized by experts but was neither included in the product label nor commonly known and caused multiple issues, especially in patients who had undergone CE

MRA.[8,9] A subsequent letter and editorial revealed that these drug laboratory test interactions are not specific to MRA, but to two contrast agent formulations, gadodiamide and gadoversetamide (Optimark, Mallinckrodt) that interact to lead to false lower calcium levels in colorimetric but not in ionic calcium tests.[10] These observations and subsequent public discussion can be credited with increasing awareness about MR contrast agent safety, which was perceived as entirely safe with considerable complacency evolving.

One of the most essential safety aspects of a contrast agent is that it needs to be completely eliminated after injection into the patient. Although this sounds trivial, imaging agents did have some dark clouds in their history when thorium dioxide (Thorotrast, Heyden) was discovered and subsequently used as a capable x-ray contrast agent, however, its retention in the body and radioactivity (alpha-particle) was not readily recognized in the early part of the last century.[11] Most MR imaging agents including gadolinium chelates are eliminated via renal clearance; iron oxides, with the liver and reticuloendothelial system (RES). It is important to understand the specific characteristics and elimination pathway of an agent as well as what happens if elimination is impaired. Therefore, it should not be a surprise that a drug that depends on renal elimination has the potential to change its biologic behavior if the pathway is impaired, consequently making agents with multiple or other elimination pathways highly desirable for patient populations with renal impairment. Contrast agents should always be given at the lowest effective dose to enable diagnostic-appropriate visualization of the target organ system, here the cardiovascular system; however, at this juncture, is also the pitfall. For a time some in our community suggested that "more is better" which frequently did improve the image quality obtainable by still evolving MR methodologies, however, the safety profile does change with changing populations and dosages. Similar to the speed rating of a tire, safety of medications can and does vary when we use it beyond recommended usage. From a safety perspective, the rapid elimination from the body, no or limited drug to drug interactions and no or limited toxicity are the key desirable safety aspects of a contrast agent.

Pharmacovigilance of MR Contrast Agents

Pharmacovigilance is the analysis of observed adverse events of an available drug, in this case MR contrast agent, and is the methodology employed to monitor the safety when a drug is broadly available. It is still a growing science as we continue to learn more about how to assess, manage, and predict the safety of drugs in large, diverse patient populations and with considerable changes in the way we practice medicine. Aside from post-marketing, phase IV studies, the information source is solely based on adverse event reporting. A healthcare provider is encouraged and sometimes mandated by country-specific laws to report any adverse event observed during the clinical use of medications/drugs—either directly to the vendor or to a regulatory body sponsored website such as MedWatch by the FDA.[12] Although this spontaneous adverse event reporting has its shortcomings, it is the best and only broad-based mechanism currently available. Unfortunately, drug manufacturers and, as such, also the vendors of MR contrast agents do not commonly voluntarily release their adverse event reporting database which they are required to compile on a global basis. The manufacturer does know how many doses of a drug are sold and those sales data are then related to the adverse event reporting rates. In an adverse event report, the reporter documents the observations, some patient characteristics, severity of the adverse event, and assesses the relationship to the contrast agent. Depending on the severity and expectancy of the adverse event, the regulatory agency and/or manufacturer may further investigate such a report. As part of country-specific marketing approvals, a manufacturer may have to report the noted observations, however these are typically not publically available documents. The largest released reporting of pharmacovigilance data on an MR contrast agent is available on the use of Gd-DTPA (Magnevist, Bayer HealthCare Pharmaceutical) and has been voluntarily reported. These data indicate for specific event categories, such as cardiovascular reactions rates, of 4 to 8 events per 100,000 doses administered.[13] Renal impairment was identified in adverse event reports from 0.1 to 0.8 events per 100,000 doses and was with angioedema, the only major category that showed an increasing trend in the recent years of adverse event reporting. Further analysis of those reports indicating renal impairment revealed that patients most commonly had preexisting renal conditions due to nephrotoxic medications and were receiving higher than labeled contrast agent doses. Unfortunately, these data are not publically available for the other commonly used MR contrast agents. The current annual global use of MR contrast agents is estimated to be around 12 million patient doses. Although no broad-based data are currently available on the cardiovascular MRA examinations being performed, estimates suggest an annual rate of about 2 to 3 million procedures. In order to further put adverse event reporting in perspective, it must be highlighted that those for the Gd-DTPA MR contrast agent are two to three times lower than those reported for nonionic monomeric iodinated contrast agents used in x-ray, and allergic reactions are reported about eight times more frequently for nonionic iodinated contrast media used in x-ray than for the Gd-DTPA, an MR contrast agent.[14] Anaphylactoid reactions have been seen in Gd-DTPA at a reporting rate of 3 to 4 per million, whereas urticaria has been reported at a rate of 29 to 79 per million.

NEPHROGENIC SYSTEMIC FIBROSIS (NSF)

Nephrogenic systemic fibrosis (NSF) initially also referred to as nephrogenic fibrosing dermopathy (NFD) is a condition that, to date, has occurred only in people with kidney disease. NSF is a systemic disorder with its most prominent and visible effects in the skin, hence its original designation as a dermopathy.[15] Our current knowledge recognizes that kidney disease seems to be a prerequisite for developing NSF and, therefore, it has been accepted as the terminology most reflective of the reality of the disorder. Although the pathophysiology of this disease mechanism is not yet fully understood and is still evolving, it is simultaneously subject to intense litigation, such as those consolidated by a judicial panel to the U.S. District court in Cleveland, Ohio.

As the knowledge continues to evolve, it is important for the reader to review current literature to ensure being aware of recent observations. The following paragraph summarizes the current and broadly accepted knowledge.

Neither the duration of kidney disease nor its underlying cause appears to be related to the development of NSF. No specific form of dialysis has been linked to NSF, although most patients with NSF do undergo dialysis procedures which are coinciding with severe renal impairment. Some patients who have never been dialyzed have developed NSF. NSF affects males and females in approximately equal numbers. NSF has been confirmed in all age groups but tends to affect the middle-aged population most commonly. It has been identified in patients from a variety of ethnic backgrounds from North and South America, Europe, Asia and Australia with the majority of reported cases occurring in the United States.

The current concepts on the underlying causative factors are the combination of two factors: severe renal impairment and exposure to gadolinium. Gadolinium (Gd), an element of the lanthanide series (atomic number 64), is used in nearly all currently marketed MRI contrast agents. It is always used in a chelated form because it is toxic in its free form. All standard, nonprotein interacting Gd-chelates are virtually entirely excreted via the kidneys; therefore any impairment leads to increased in vivo retention and circulation times. If there is no residual urine output, the only way such agents can exit the body is through dialysis. In patients with normal kidney function, the Gd-chelates are considered safe because the bond between the toxic Gd atom and its ligand molecule is very strong; however, differences between agents are established. There is a small risk that Gd atoms can unbind from their carrier ligands and the unbound "free" Gd reacts like calcium ions, most likely binding to readily-available phosphates and forming insoluble molecules. In patients who receive large doses of Gd-chelates and who do not undergo rapid and effective dialysis, there is a risk that larger amounts of these gadolinium compounds could develop and remain in the body in a form that is not readily removable. Although several Gd-chelate formulations exist as detailed subsequently, only some appear to be more frequently associated with NSF, and only one, gadodiamide, has been associated with the vast majority of cases of NSF. Some clinicians have suggested that because this agent is slightly more likely to dissociate chemically, Gd dissociation (de-chelation) might be the trigger of NSF at the cellular level; however, this aspect is currently not only in scientific but also in legal discovery discussion. Another relevant drug to drug interaction might be caused by the co-administration of erythropoietin (EPO) and intravenous iron. Erythropoietin has the potential to affect the growth of other cells in the bone marrow and curiously, the cell responsible for producing much of the collagen deposition seen in NSF develops in the bone marrow. Initial preclinical experiments indicate that EPO could facilitate the development of NSF in some cases by increasing the number of circulating fibrocytes.

Besides kidney disease, medical conditions that may be associated with NSF include hypercoagulation abnormalities and deep venous thrombosis, recent surgery (particularly vascular surgery), recent failure of a transplanted kidney, and sudden onset kidney disease with severe swelling of the extremities. It is very common for the NSF patient to have undergone a vascular surgical procedure (such as revision of an arteriovenous fistula, or angioplasty of a blood vessel) or to have experienced a thrombotic episode (thrombotic loss of a transplant or deep venous thrombosis) approximately 2 weeks before the onset of the skin changes.

The underlying clinical question as identified in the cases above frequently justifies the use of gadolinium-enhanced MRI or MRA studies. Whether there is an independent risk associated with endothelial damage or hypercoagulation remains an open question, although circulating fibrocyte migration from the blood is facilitated in both scenarios. In summary, the pathophysiological trigger and disease mechanism is still under investigation and our knowledge continues to evolve.

The current status with a focus on cardiovascular imaging in regard to the NSF risk of Gd-containing MR contrast agents (GBCA) can be outlined in the following way. First, we need to confirm prior to any administration of GBCA that the patient does not have a severe renal impairment. Our community has and is evolving guidance on how to most appropriately manage this risk assessment. The wide availability of point-of-care testing for serum creatine levels and the estimated glomerular filtration rate (eGFR), enables a just-in-time risk assessment. It appears prudent at the current time that in outpatients, a recent (less than 3 months old) blood lab readout of serum creatine (and eGFR) should be available. However, in patients being imaged for a cardiovascular question, a concomitant renal ailment might be rapidly evolving, the patient might have recently received medications or undergone other diagnostic studies such as contrast-enhanced CT or diagnostic angiogram using iodinated contrast agents and the patient could have experienced a new renal impairment. In such situations, as well as in instances in which a patient has undergone multiple imaging examinations, a very recent eGFR is strongly recommended. As highlighted in the FDA warning, a GFR below 30 mL/min/1.73 m^2, which means patients with chronic kidney disease (CKD) of 4 or 5 or patients who have had or are waiting for a liver transplantation, have an elevated risk for this severe adverse event. Some investigators see patients with CKD 3 or a GFR between 30 to 60 mL/min/1.73 m^2 as a potential or lower risk group.

The issue of multiple imaging studies in short time periods is evolving as a safety concern in that potential cumulative effects are difficult to study and are frequently superimposed on other underlying medical ailments. Therefore, it is also highly advisable to have a current eGFR available in such patients.

How to most appropriately handle the medical indications to use Gd-chelates in patients with renal impairment requires a patient-specific assessment and continues to rapidly evolve. As with all procedures that have elevated

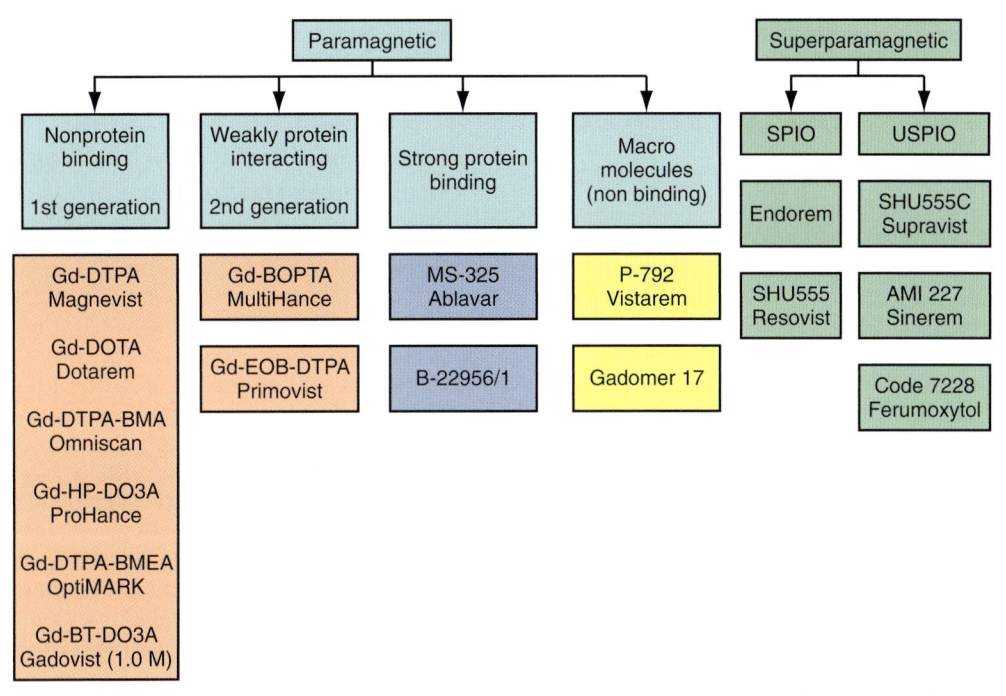

FIGURE 18-1 Classification scheme for MR contrast agents that are potentially applicable to cardiovascular imaging. The paramagnetic gadolinium chelates can be classified according to their degree of protein interaction. The ultra-small iron oxide particles are "blood pool agents" that demonstrate long intravascular enhancement.

risks, a patient-specific risk-benefit analysis must be done by the physician prescribing the MR contrast agent and current literature should be consulted. In addition to the already identified medical conditions, special considerations need to include a review of frequency of imaging studies and potential drug to drug interactions, patient compliance, and appropriate follow-up capabilities. There are alternate MR contrast agents on the horizon that are iron oxide-based and do not use the renal elimination pathway that appear promising for use in the patients with severe renal impairment. Although non–contrast-enhanced MR angiography is frequently not as capable as CE MRA, it still might be the most appropriate alternative if ultrasound-based imaging cannot clarify the medical question to be resolved. In summary, the awareness of the potential for NSF has substantially changed our practice with the unambiguous need to be able to identify patients with renal impairment prior to dosing with Gd-chelates, the need to follow the labeled use and indications as well as being more aware of cumulative effects of multiple imaging studies and/or drug to drug interaction.

Cost

The cost of MR contrast agents varies regionally and is strongly dependent on the degree of discounting. All MR contrast agents have weight-based dosing in the label and most pharmaceutical companies manufacture contrast agent vials in different sizes. Multi-vial dosing combined with patient-specific dosing can be accommodated if appropriately approved injection/infusion systems are being used. It can be further anticipated that upcoming contrast agents will use alternate elimination pathways or will be capable of use at substantially lower concentrations, albeit at a cost premium to existing contrast agent options.

First Pass versus Steady State Imaging

The time window of increased vascular signal enhancement is a critical component for MRA. Although this time window is influenced by the injection/infusion protocol used, the dosage, and cardiac output, it is most importantly dependent on the kind of contrast agent used—a first pass agent or a blood-pool agent. The vast majority of MRA development and clinical use has been done as first pass imaging. The availability and market introduction of gadofosveset trisodium has for the first time enabled a combined clinical first pass and steady-state imaging of the vasculature. The challenges and opportunities of steady-state imaging will be discussed in other chapters of this book. The next sections will focus on the specific characteristics of the different MR contrast agents and are approached by classifying the agents into appropriate groupings.

CLASSIFICATION OF MR CONTRAST AGENTS FOR CARDIOVASCULAR IMAGING

MR contrast agents currently fall into two broad categories; those based on gadolinium, which are predominately paramagnetic in nature, and those based on iron oxide particles of different coating and size that are superparamagnetic (Fig. 18-1). The broadest use for cardiovascular imaging is based on gadolinium chelates which can be subclassified into agents revealing no interaction with proteins, those that have weak temporary interaction with proteins leading to increased relaxivity and/or having an additional extrarenal elimination pathway, and those that have strong protein binding. Table 18-1 summarizes the contrast agents that are currently available or have been in clinical trials at varying stages relevant for cardiovascular MR imaging.[16]

Currently, nine GBCAs are approved in one or more countries. Seven of those have been developed as multipurpose imaging contrast agents and all have at least neuroimaging as a labeled indication. Two gadolinium chelates are approved with targeted indications, gadoxetate disodium (Eovist, Bayer Healthcare) as a liver-specific imaging "to detect and characterize lesions in adults with known or suspected focal liver disease and gadofosveset trisodium (Ablavor, Lantheus) as an MRA agent "to evaluate aortoiliac occlusive disease (AIOD) in adults with known or suspected periperipheral vascular disease."

Nonprotein Interacting Standard Gadolinium Chelates

This group of "conventional" gadolinium chelate agents was introduced more than 20 years ago with nearly simultaneous approval of gadopentetate dimeglumine (Gd-DTPA, Magnevist, Bayer Healthcare) in all three key markets: European Union, United States, and Japan. Five of these agents are available as 0.5 molar formulations and one, gadobutrol (Gd-BT-DO3A, Gadovist, Bayer Healthcare) is being marketed at a 1.0 molar formulation. Although differences exist between these agents in terms of the molecular structure and chemical and physical properties (Tables 18-1 and 18-2), all agents are nonspecific and are eliminated unchanged via the renal pathway by glomerular filtration. The T1 relaxation rates of these agents are comparable and fall in the range between 4.3 and 5.6 L/mmol · s^{-1}. These similarities lead to equivalent imaging characteristics at the same dose and injection rate.

From the molecular structure, the agents can be subclassified into ionic or nonionic, linear, or macrocyclic. The concept of the nonionic agents was that they would have an even better safety profile with fewer adverse events comparable to the impact of reducing ionicity in iodinated contrast agents. This idea could not be realized with the agents and the stability of the binding of the gadolinium central atom has become much more critical. From this perspective, the nonionic linear molecules are the least stable and the ionic macrocyclic agents are the most stable. Therefore, the binding strength of the gadolinium by its surrounding chelating complex has become a differentiating factor. The two agents, gadodiamide (Gd-DTPA-BMA, Omniscan, GE-Healthcare) and gadoversetamide (Gd-DTPA-BMEA) have substantially lower binding and, therefore, include excess chelate in the formulation to trap any dissociated gadolinium ion in the vial which has also been the causative factor for the interference with colorimetric calcium tests and the spurious hypocalcemia.[10]

Gadobutrol (Gadovist, Bayer Healthcare) is the only agent that is available at 1.0 molar formulation that enables twice the concentration of gadolinium to be delivered into the vasculature per unit volume, thereby enabling a stronger vasculature signal for perfusion and vasculature imaging, which has led to the initial preferred use of this type of agent for susceptibility weighted perfusion imaging of the brain.

Gadolinium Chelates with Weak Protein Interaction

This class represents a second generation of gadolinium chelates that possess a higher T1 relaxivity in blood such as for gadobenate (Gd-BOPTA, Multihance, Bracco) (9.7 L/mmol · s^{-1}) due to the weak transient interaction between the agent and serum proteins, particularly albumin and a T1 relaxivity of 8.2 L/mmol · s^{-1} in human plasma for gadotexetate disodium (Eovist, Bayer Healthcare). Both agents are ionic, linear chelates and have a dual elimination pathway with partially hepatobiliary elimination, gadobenate is weaker than gadoxetate. The higher T1 relaxivity manifests as a significantly greater intravascular signal intensity enhancement compared to that achieved with conventional gadolinium chelates at equivalent doses with the benefits of a more pronounced effect in smaller vessels as well as in the margins of the tumors. To objectively assess if differences in intravascular image contrast exist between the first group of standard gadolinium chelates and the new group, an intraindividual cross-over study was performed that revealed that gadobenate dimeglumine presented a significantly more intense contrast enhancement with a higher, longer peak duration and larger area under the vascular contrast enhancement curve.[17] This finding was confirmed in subsequent larger MRA studies for the run-off vasculature,[18] pelvic and carotid vasculature. The practical impact is that for the same dose and administration approach, a more intense and longer duration intravascular signal intensity benefit was noted. The clinical advantages of the increased relaxivity also have been demonstrated for many vascular territories that range from the carotid vasculature[16] to the distal run-off vessels.[16] Like the conventional nonprotein interacting GBCAs, gadobenate dimeglumine has an excellent safety profile with a very low incidence of adverse events noted for the clinical development program as a whole,[16] however the potential risk to cause NSF cannot be excluded and the same level of diligence also applies to this group. The fact that more signal/enhancement can be obtained for the same dosing more readily enables full diagnostic quality at lower doses, thereby reducing dose and accumulation-dependent potential effects.

Gadoxetate disodium has only recently been developed and is being marketed in many countries for liver imaging and is packaged in a 0.25 mol/L concentration, one half that of the standard GBCAs. This agent is not currently being used nor has it been clinically evaluated for cardiovascular imaging; however, it can certainly be used for MR angiography associated with liver imaging.

Gadolinium Chelates with Strong Protein Interaction

The contrast agents in this category exhibit strong affinity for serum proteins which increase the relaxivity and also have extended intravascular half-life making them by

TABLE 18-1 Physicochemical Characteristics of Clinically Developed Gadolinium-Based MR Contrast Agents

Characteristics	Gd-DTPA Gadopentate Dimeglumine Magnevist (0.5 mol/L)	Gd-BOPTA Gadobenate Dimeglumine MultiHance (0.5 mol/L)	Gd-EOB-DTPA Gadoxetate Disodium Eovist (0.25 mol/L)	Gadofosveset Trisodium Ablavar (0.25 mol/L)	Gd-DTPA-BMA Gadodiamide Omniscan (0.5 mol/L)	Gd-DTPA-BMEA Gadoversetamide OptiMARK (0.5 mol/L)	Gd-DOTA Gadoterate Meglumine Dotarem (0.5 mol/L)	Gd-HP-DO3A Gadoteridol ProHance (0.5 mol/L)	Gd-BT-DO3A Gadobutrol Gadovist (1.0 mol/L)
Molecular structure	Linear ionic	Linear ionic	Linear ionic	Linear ionic	Linear nonionic	Linear nonionic	Cyclic ionic	Cyclic nonionic	Cyclic nonionic
Thermodynamic stability constant (log K_{eq})	22.1	22.6	23.5	22.1	16.9	16.6	25.8	23.8	21.8
Osmolality (Osm/kg)	1.96	1.97	0.69	0.83	0.65	1.11	1.35	0.63	1.60
Viscosity (mPa · s at 37° C)	2.9	5.3	1.2	1.8	1.4	2.0	2.0	1.3	4.96
T1 relaxivity (L/mmol · s^{-1}), plasma	4.9	9.7	8.7	Variable	4.8	N/A	4.3	4.6	5.6

N/A, not available.

Table 18-2 Physicochemical Characteristics of Small and Ultra-Small Particles of Iron Oxides Developed as MR Contrast Agents

Characteristics	AMI 25 Ferumoxide (Feridex)	SHU555 Ferucarbotran (Resovist)	NC100150 Feruglose (Clariscan)	SHU555C Ferucarbotran (Supravist)	AMI 227 Ferumoxtran (Combidex)	Code 7228 Ferumoxytol (Feraheme)
Particle/coating	SPIO dextran	SPIO	USPIO	USPIO	USPIO	USPIO Polyglucose
Osmolality (Osm/kg)	0.34	0.33				0.27-0.33
Concentration	11.2 mg Fe/mL		29.8 mg Fe/ML			
Imaging approach	T2	T2, T1	T2		T1, T2	
Market status	Discontinued	Available	Discontinued	Clinical development	Clinical development	Therapeutic

design cardiovascular imaging agents. Gadofosveset trisodium, developed under the identifier MS-325 (then under the proposed product name of Vasovist and now under the new product name of Ablavar) has gone through full clinical development and is approved in several countries, including the United States, for specific MRA indications. This agent is available in a 0.25 mol/L concentration, has been reported to be 88% to 96% noncovalently bound to albumin in human plasma and to exhibit a relaxivity at 0.5T that is 6 to 10 times that of gadopentetate dimeglumine. The agent has a recommended dosing of 0.03 mmol/kg body weight[19] and achieves its desired intravascular contrast at a substantially lower dose because of its higher relaxivity. The elimination pathway is primarily renal but it also has some hepatobiliary elimination. This agent can be used for first pass contrast-enhanced MRA and for steady-state imaging in a number of vascular territories. Although this agent has been investigated in trials in many vascular territories, its 2008 FDA approval and label states the indication as "MRA to evaluate aortoiliac occlusive disease (AIOD) in adults with known or suspected peripheral vascular disease". The European Medicines Agency (EMA) had already approved the agent in 2005 with the labeled indication "for contrast-enhanced magnetic resonance angiography for visualization of abdominal or limb vessels in patients with suspected or known vascular disease", which is a much broader indication. The agent also exhibits an extravasation in the case of blood brain-barrier breakdown and is currently the only approved agent that will allow first pass and steady-state imaging.

The second agent with strong affinity for serum proteins and increased relaxivity is gadocoletic acid (B22956, Bracco). This agent has undergone phase II trials for enhanced coronary MRA and has been shown to have even stronger affinity for serum albumin than gadofosveset (approximately 94% bound noncovalently) with a similarly long intravascular residence time.[20]

There are two principal types of paramagnetic "blood pool" contrast agents: those whose intravascular residence time is prolonged due to a capacity of the gadolinium chelate for strong interaction with serum proteins, and those that have a macromolecular structure whose large size limits the extent of extravasation compared to the first pass gadolinium agents. Another important factor to characterize blood pool agents is in their capability and efficacy to be used in first pass as well as for steady-state vascular imaging.

Gadolinium Contrast Agents with Macromolecular Structures

Examples of gadolinium-based blood pool agents with macromolecular structures are P792 (Vistarem, Guebert) and Gadomer-17 (Bayer Healthcare).[16] These agents differ from the currently available low molecular weight gadolinium agents in possessing large molecular structures that prevent extravasation of the molecules from the intravascular space following injection, but do have slow, reduced leakage in case of blood-brain barrier breakdown. The molecular weights of P792 and gadomer-17 are 6.5 kDa and 35 kDa, respectively, which compare with weights of between approximately 0.56 kDa and 1.0 kDa for the purely first pass gadolinium agents. Whereas the structure of P792 is based on that of gadoterate substituted with four large hydrophilic spacer arms, gadomer-17 is a much larger polymer of 24 gadolinium cascades. In addition to differences in molecular weight and structure, these two agents appear to differ in terms of their rates of vascular clearance, with P792 considered a rapid clearance blood pool agent. Despite these differences, both agents have cardiovascular imaging capabilities and have been evaluated for these indications in clinical trials. Currently, it is not clear if and when any of these agents will receive regulatory approval or would be marketed.

Superparamagnetic Iron Oxide Agents

The second major category of potential contrast agents for cardiovascular imaging consists of the superparamagnetic group, which is based on particles of iron oxide (PIO) that are differentiated by the size and by its coating and are frequently also referred to as nanoparticles. Those with a diameter larger than 50 nanometer are referred to as small (SPIO) and those smaller as ultra-small (USPIO). Iron oxide particles have either a starch, dextran, or carbohydrate coating and its biologic characteristics are predominately dependent on its coating, whereas its imaging characteristics as either beneficial for T1-weighted or T2*-weighted imaging, is based on its size.

The first approved and marketed iron oxide-based contrast agent was AMI 25, also known as ferumoxide and marketed as Endorem (Guebert) or Feridex (Bayer Healthcare), with an indication for T2*-weighted liver imaging. This SPIO has also been used for cell-tracking and has a demonstrated potential for molecular-based cardiovascular imaging applications.[21] Although there were no regulatory issues, the sole manufacturer of this agent, AMAG Pharmaceuticals, decided in November 2008 to cease its manufacture.

The second available iron oxide was developed under the code name of SHU555, also known as Ferrixan or Ferucarbotran, and subsequently marketed as a liver imaging agent under the brand name of Resovist (Bayer). These superparamagnetic iron oxide particles are coated with carboydextran and are accumulated by phagocytosis in cells of the reticuloendothelial system (RES) of the liver. The product formulation had a distribution of particle sizes that predominately led to the RES uptake. However, a filtered subfraction of this agent SHU555 C consists only of USPIOs and has been developed as a cardiovascular imaging agent for first pass and steady-state MR angiography. Another USPIO with starch coating was developed for MRA known as Feruglose, NC100150 or Clariscan, however development was discontinued after substantial longer term liver retention was observed.

All iron oxides have been used as carrier molecules for targeted imaging and it remains a highly exciting research area with great potential for molecular targeted cardiovascular imaging. AMI 227 (Ferumoxtran), also known as Combidex or Sinerem, is another USPIO that has been specifically evaluated for lymphatic MR imaging[22,23] but has not yet received final regulatory approval. The fifth iron oxide agent that has been evaluated for MRA imaging is ferumoxytol, formerly known as Code 7228 and now as Feraheme (AMAG). Although its initial development goal envisioned it to be an imaging agent, it was subsequently developed as an iron replacement therapeutic drug indicated for the treatment of iron deficiency anemia in adult patients with chronic kidney disease (CKD), the very same population at higher risk for NSF from Gd chelate imaging agents. This agent received its therapeutic FDA approval in 2009 and is being marketed with its labeled therapeutic indications. The potential for cardiovascular applications of this agent are high because it has a first pass and steady-state imaging ability and a well established safety profile at even higher doses than needed for imaging in a high-risk population for Gd chelates. Overall, it can be speculated that iron oxides, especially the USPIOs, will have an important place in cardiovascular MRA in the future, not only for intravascular contrast but also as a molecular targeted MR contrast agent. The contrast agent field will continue to evolve and the efforts over the last decade are leading to exciting new, safe, and robust imaging approaches, further increasing the clinical importance of safe, effective, and noninvasive MR cardiovascular imaging.

Although contrast agents for both CT and MR did not reveal distinctively different imaging characteristics in the past, now new agents provide truly distinctive characteristics that advance the capabilities in noninvasive disease detection and characterization. The advent of molecular targeted agents is on the horizon for cardiovascular cross-sectional imaging that will enable us to further improve imaging capabilities.

> **KEY POINTS**
> - Most commonly, gadolinium-chelate contrast agents are used off-label for cardiac MRI and contrast-enhanced MRA in clinical practice. Off-label use requires peer-review evidence. New contrast agents and cardiovascular indications are evolving and vigilance by practitioners is recommended to ensure that they have the most current information.
> - Contrast agents can be classified as paramagnetic (e.g., nonprotein binding, weakly protein binding, strong protein binding, macromolecules [nonbinding]) or super-paramagnetic (e.g., iron oxide agents).
> - Nephrogenic systemic fibrosis (NSF) is a serious, potentially fatal condition associated with use of gadolinium-chelate contrast agents in patients with severe renal impairment, notably patients with a glomerular filtration rate (GFR) of less than 30 mL/min/1.73 m^2.

SUGGESTED READINGS

Bleicher AG, Kanal E: Assessment of adverse reaction rates to a newly approved MRI contrast agent: review of 23,553 administrations of gadobenate dimeglumine. AJR Am J Roentgenol 2008; 191: W307-W311.

Knoff MV, Balzer T, Esser M, Kashanian FK, et al: Assessment of utilization and pharmacovigilance based on spontaneous adverse event reporting of gadopentetate dimeglumine as a magnetic resonance contrast agent after 45 million administrations and 15 years of clinical use. Invest Radiol 2006; 41:491-499.

Neuwelt EA, Hamilton BE, Varallyay CG, et al: Ultrasmall superparamagnetic iron oxides (USPIOs): a future alternative magnetic resonance (MR) contrast agent for patients at risk for nephrogenic systemic fibrosis (NSF)? Kidney Int 2009; 75:465-474.

Prompona M, Cyran C, Nikolaou K, Bauner K, et al: Contrast-enhanced whole-heart MR coronary angiography at 3.0 T using the intravascular contrast agent gadofosveset. Invest Radiol 2009; 44:369-374.

REFERENCES

1. Runge VM, Kirsch JE, Lee C. Contrast-enhanced MR angiography. J Magn Reson Imaging 1993; 3(1): 233-239.
2. Knopp MV, von Tengg-Kobligk H, Floemer F, Schoenberg SO. Contrast agents for MRA: future directions. J Magn Reson Imaging 1999; 10(3):314-316.
3. Knopp MV, Runge VM. Off-label use and reimbursement of contrast media in MR. J Magn Reson Imaging 1999; 10(3):48-95.
4. http://www.businessweek.com/bwdaily/dnflash/content/sep2009/db2009092_913433.htm
5. www.fda.gov/downloads/ICECI/EnforcementActions/WarningLetters/2000/UCM068176.pdf
6. www.fda.gov/bbs/topics/NEWS/2007/NEW01638.html
7. Doorenbos CJ, Ozyilmaz A, van Wijnen M. Severe pseudohypocalcemia after gadolinium-enhanced magnetic resonance angiography. N Engl J Med 2004; 350(1):87-88; author reply 87-88.
8. Choyke P, Knopp M. Pseudohypocalcemia with MR imaging contrast agents: a cautionary tale. Radiology 2003;227:627-628.
9. Prince M, Erel H, Lent R, Blumenfeld J, et al. Gadodiamide administration causes spurious hypocalcemia. Radiology 2003; 227:639-646.
10. Prince MR, Choyke PL, Knopp MV. More on pseudohypocalcemia and gadolinium-enhanced MRI. N Engl J Med 2004; 350(1):87-88; author reply 87-88.
11. Becker N, Liebermann D, Wesch H, Van Kaick G. Mortality among Thorotrast-exposed patients and an unexposed comparison group in the German Thorotrast study. Eur J Cancer 2008; 44(9):1259-1268.
12. www.fda.gov/safety/MedWatch/default.htm
13. Knopp M, Balzer T, Esser M, et al. Assessment of utilization and pharmacovigilance based on spontaneous adverse event reporting of gadopentetate dimeglumine as a magnetic resonance contrast agent after 45 million administrations and 15 years of clinical use. Invest Radiol 2006; 41:491-499.
14. Niendorf HP, Haustein J, Corenlius I, et al. Safety of gadolinium-DTPA: extended clinical experience. Magn Reson Med 1991; 22(2):222-228.
15. Marckmann P, Skov L, Rossen K, et al. Nephrogenic systemic fibrosis: suspected causative role of gadodiamide used for contrast-enhanced magnetic resonance imaging. J Am Soc Nephrol 2006; 17:2359-2362.
16. Knopp M, Kirchin M. Contrast agents for magnetic resonance angiography: current status and future perspectives. In Arlart I, Bongartz G, Marchal G (eds). Magnetic Resonance Angiography, 2nd rev ed. Berlin: Springer, 2005.
17. Knopp MV, Schoenberg SO, Rehm C, et al. Assessment of gadobenate dimeglumine for magnetic resonance angiography: phase I studies. Invest Radiol 2002; 37(12):706-715.
18. Knopp MV, Giesel FL, von Tengg-Kobligk H, et al. Contrast-enhanced MR angiography of the run-off vasculature: intraindividual comparison of gadobenate dimeglumine with gadopentetate dimeglumine. J Magn Reson Imaging 2003; 17(6):694-702.
19. Hartman M, Wiethoff A, Hentrich H, Rohrer M. Initial imaging recommendations for vasovist angiography. Eur Radiol [Suppl 2] 2006; B15-BB23.
20. de Haën C, Anelli PL, Lorusso V, et al. Gadocoletic acid trisodium salt (b22956/1): a new blood pool magnetic resonance contrast agent with application in coronary angiography. Invest Radiol 2006; 41(3):279-291.
21. Anderson S, Glod J, Arbab A. Noninvasive MR imaging of magnetically labeled stem cells to identify neovasculature in a glioma model. Blood 2005; 105:420-425.
22. Bellin M, Roy C, Kinkel K, Thoumas D, et al. Lymph node metastases: safety and effectiveness of mr imaging with ultrasmall superparamagnetic iron oxide particles—initial clinical experience. Radiology 1998; 207:799-808.
23. Harisinghani M, Barentsz J, Hahn P, et al. Noninvasive detection of clinically occult lymph-node metastases in prostate cancer. N Engl J Med 2003; 348:2491-2499.

CHAPTER 19

Magnetic Resonance Imaging Safety

Maureen N. Hood*

Safety of MRI is essential for any patient evaluation, and is especially critical for cardiovascular MRI, where high-risk patients, procedures, and implanted devices are common. Safety of patients is a priority for the American Medical Association and The Joint Commission. Safety in MRI has been a source of controversy, however, among health care providers and patients. Growth in medical technology has resulted in more patients receiving implanted devices, many of which were not specifically designed to be safe for MRI. Many devices lack definitive evidence to support their MRI safety.

In 2008, MRI safety came under scrutiny by The Joint Commission when a sentinel event alert was issued in the United States because of widespread adverse events. The alert was based on 398 adverse events reported to the U.S. Food and Drug Administration's (FDA) Manufacturer and User Facility Device Experience Database (MAUDE) over a 10-year period, 9 of which were deaths.[1] Burns from significant heating of wires and leads were the most common problem reported at more than 70% of the MRI-related incidents. Adverse events and accidents in the MRI environment happen because of failures in adherence to proper MRI safety procedures, inappropriate use of equipment, outdated safety information, lack of training for individuals working in the MRI environment, and lack of appropriate supervision of the MRI suite.[1,2] The safety problems in MRI cannot be taken lightly because the safety issues surrounding MRI are complicated and often unpredictable. The Joint Commission's recommendations for reducing accidents and injuries in MRI follow the "ACR Guidance Document for Safe MR Practices,"[3] and can be found at http://www.jointcommission.org/Sentinel Events/SentinelEventAlert/sea_38.htm or http://www.acr.org/SecondaryMainMenuCategories/quality_safety/MRSafety/safe_mr07.aspx.

This chapter provides an overview of MRI safety as it pertains to patients with cardiovascular disease, with suggestions of supplemental information and references. MRI safety is an enormous topic that is constantly changing, and a host of Web-based resources are available. Questions of MRI safety need to be evaluated with the most up-to-date information possible, which is why providers need to research the specific devices and scanning circumstances carefully. Box 19-1 lists useful websites for the reader's reference. MRI safety guidelines are updated on a regular basis. Failure to follow current safety guidelines puts patients at increased risk for injury and, in some instances, results in unnecessary avoidance of clinically necessary MRI examinations.

GENERAL CONCERNS

Hazards

MRI is based mainly on magnetism and radio waves. These properties sound safe compared with the ionizing radiation from x-rays, radioisotopes, or external-beam radiation. MRI is not without its hazards, however. The main sources of problems with MRI are as follows:

1. Static magnetic field
2. Gradient fields (transient)
3. Radiofrequency (RF)
4. Cryogens (superconducting scanners)
5. Ignorant or inadequately trained individuals

Not only do magnetism and radio waves have potential to cause harm, but also MRI is a sophisticated technology that has a variety of possible combinations of magnetic fields, RF fields, and electronics. The complexity of MRI combined with the variability of patients and growth of imaging procedures makes MRI safety increasingly challenging and unpredictable.

Individuals who are not educated and trained for safety in the MRI environment cause an added level of danger

---

*The opinions or assertions contained herein are the private views of the author and are not to be construed as official or reflecting the views of the Department of Defense or the Uniformed Services University of the Health Sciences.

BOX 19-1 Recommended Websites

ACR Practice Guideline for Adult Sedation/Analgesia—
http://www.acr.org/SecondaryMainMenuCategories/quality_safety/guidelines/iv/adult_sedation.aspx

ACR Practice Guideline for Pediatric Sedation/Analgesia—
http://www.acr.org/SecondaryMainMenuCategories/quality_safety/guidelines/iv/pediatric_sedation.aspx

International Society for Magnetic Resonance in Medicine—
http://www.ismrm.org/

Institute for Magnetic Resonance Safety, Education, and Research—http://www.imrser.org/

Magnetic Resonance Safety Testing—http://www.magneticresonancesafetytesting.com/

MRI Safety—http://www.mrisafety.com

North American Society of Cardiovascular Imaging—
http://www.nasci.org/

Section for Magnetic Resonance Technologists—http://www.ismrm.org/smrt/

United States Food and Drug Administration—http://www.fda.gov/MedicalDevices/Safety/AlertsandNotices/ucm135362.htm

Society of Cardiac Magnetic Resonance—http://www.scmr.org/

University of Nottingham: Magnetic Resonance Group, Safety Information—http://www.magres.nottingham.ac.uk/safety/

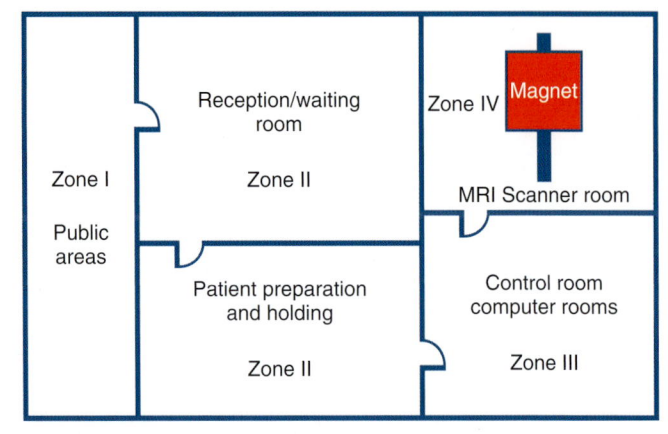

FIGURE 19-1 The four zones (I, II, III, and IV) of an MRI suite. (From Kanal E, Barkovich AJ, Bell C, et al; ACR Blue Ribbon Panel on MR Safety. ACR guidance document for safe MR practices: 2007. AJR Am J Roentgenol 2007; 188:1447-1474.)

because they are unfamiliar with the dangers and safety precautions needed to ensure safe operation of equipment in the MRI scanner area. Many accidents are a result of noncompliance with safety guidelines, or of adherence to outdated guidelines. The ECRI Institute, a nonprofit health services research organization, recommends that MRI clinics appoint a safety officer to oversee the establishment, implementation, and maintenance of MRI safety policies and procedures, something The Joint Commission and American College of Radiology (ACR) also recommend as a prudent preventive measure.[1,3,4]

Magnetic Resonance Imaging Clinic

The physical facilities of an MRI facility play a direct role in safety. Site planning for an MRI system should be done to limit access of non-MRI personnel to the actual MRI scanner room. Only properly screened patients and personnel should be allowed into the MRI scan room, and they should be allowed in the scan room only with the direct supervision of qualified MRI professionals. The ACR has recommended a clinic design safety template that includes control of site access restriction.[3] An MRI facility should be considered to be made up of four zones as outlined by the "ACR Guidance Document for Safe MR Practices" (Fig. 19-1).[3] Zone I is the area outside the actual MRI facility, and it is open to the general public. This is the area where the general public, patients, health care workers, and MRI center employees enter the MRI facility.

Zone II is accessible by the general public, but has controlled access to zones III and IV. Zone II is typically where reception and general waiting are located. Initial MRI screening, medical histories, and insurance issues are attended to in zone II. Safety guidelines recommend that the patient preparation and holding be included in zone II to protect the patients and other individuals. The design of the facility must also take into consideration the need to have the patient holding area well thought out to ensure that patients can still be monitored as needed by health care personnel.

Zone III is the area in which all non-MRI personnel should be escorted and supervised at all times. All individuals and equipment entering zone III should be screened. A physical restriction such as a locking mechanism needs to be in place for zone III to prevent entrance by non-MRI personnel. Key locks, pass card systems, or other types of security locks are recommended. Combination locks are not recommended because lock codes are easy to disseminate. Only MRI personnel who have been properly trained in MRI safety should have free access to zone III.

Zone IV is the MRI system room, which is inside zone III. This room has the highest restrictions and should be clearly marked as being hazardous. Only MRI personnel, screened patients, and MRI approved equipment may enter zone IV. Zone IV needs to be locked and to have otherwise controlled access. MRI system operators need to have direct visual control (direct sight or camera) over zone IV. In the event of a patient emergency, such as a "Code Blue," a plan must be in place to remove the patient from zone IV and into a safe area in zone II or III for emergency personnel to manage the patient safely.

No patient should undergo an MRI examination without proper identification of an implanted device and the potential risk to the patient ascertained relative to the intended MRI conditions. The potential hazards associated with MRI procedures are affected by, but are not limited to, the static magnetic field, gradient switching, transmit RF coil, imaging sequences, RF energy heating and induction, device specifications, body part to be imaged, and patient. The safety of the patient and the device must be considered with all potential hazards in mind. Many devices have been tested by scientists and manufacturers so that the risk/benefit ratios can be more confidently evaluated. Not all devices have been tested under all

MRI scanning conditions, however, plus new devices are constantly being introduced into clinical care. MRI scanners and procedures have also evolved over time and are very complex, making MRI safety a particular challenge.

Cardiovascular MRI has extra considerations beyond the general MRI safety requirements and recommendations because cardiovascular imaging often includes advanced imaging techniques, such as ECG gating, cardiac stress imaging with pharmacologic stress agents, and interventional procedures. Advanced vascular work may include an MRI "runoff" or "bolus chase" angiogram, in which a dynamic injection of contrast agent is administered while moving the table and patient through the MRI system to visualize the vessels in the chest, abdomen, pelvis, legs, and feet. Many of these techniques require extra care of the patient, availability of specialized personnel for advanced cardiac care, and specialized equipment to maintain safety and image quality. More patients with implanted devices are being requested to be scanned with MRI. Improving MRI facilities and safety training is imperative for imaging suites and procedures that are based on the latest information to prevent negative outcomes, while providing the best possible health care.

Physics of Electricity and Magnetism

Maxwell's equations are the building blocks of our understanding of electricity and magnetism. The four equations known as Gauss' law for electricity, Gauss' law for magnetism, Faraday's law, and Ampere-Maxwell law help in understanding many of the important elements of MRI safety.[5] The mathematical predictions for safety cannot be calculated easily. Ensuring the safety of a device in a patient undergoing an MRI examination requires knowledge of the device, the specific MRI system, the type of RF coils used, the sequences employed for imaging, the way the patient loads the scanner and transmit RF coil, and whether or not monitoring or gating equipment is also being used. It is nearly impossible to predict all of the possible ways for heat deposition or current induction that may occur with a given implant in a patient—hence the safety dilemma.

Static Magnetic Field Strength

Currently, most clinical scanners for cardiac use are operating at a static magnetic field of 1.5 T or 3 T. Table 19-1 outlines the FDA significant risk recommendations. Magnetic fields have the potential for translational and rotational (or torque) effects. Basically, magnetic field interactions increase as the static magnetic field strength increases. If a device is considered to pose a potential safety concern, it is prudent to consider carefully the potential options for such scanning at the lowest field strength appropriate for the imaging needs (e.g., coil selection, imaging pulse sequence selection). Imaging time is also important because the increase in scan time may prolong the requirements for monitoring a child or a sedated claustrophobic patient. Discussion with the patient on what to expect and the need for the patient to communicate any unusual sensations immediately is imperative. Devices and scanners vary considerably, so many factors must be considered. Substances that are attracted to the magnetic field are often referred to as having ferromagnetic properties. Devices that are ferromagnetic have the potential to interact with the magnetic field in a translational or rotational manner (or both), possibly causing great harm to the patient or equipment or both. The plethora of MRI accident pictures that are available via the Internet provide some idea of the danger of the static magnetic field of the MRI scanner. Many pictures of objects flying into scanners can be found at sites such as Simply Physics (http://www.simplyphysics.com/flying_objects.html).

Gradient Magnetic Fields

MRI scanners use time-varying magnetic fields called gradients to encode for field of view, slice thickness, and other imaging parameters, and in certain aspects of pulse sequence image contrast. Stronger and faster gradients and more powerful RF transmission coils are being used in MRI scanners.[6] The current FDA limit for gradient magnetic field rates of change (dB/dt) varies depending on operating conditions. Significant risk for dB/dt is classified as when painful nerve stimulation or severe discomfort is produced.[7] Gradient fields are magnetic fields that are much weaker than the main magnetic field, but they are switched on and off very quickly and, according to Maxwell's equations, can induce time-varying electrical currents.[8] Gradients can induce currents in conductive materials[9] and potentiate peripheral nerve stimulation, but are typically not painful on current FDA-approved MRI systems.[10] This is a safety concern because these gradient currents have the potential also to induce currents in certain cardiac devices, which could induce arrhythmias.[9] Tandri and coworkers[8] reported that gradient currents may be strong enough under certain conditions to distort pacing pulses, which is significant enough to interfere with myocardial capture or loss of capture when patients with pacemakers are scanned in MRI. This finding reinforces the need for prudent screening and risk/benefit considerations with patients with any kind of implanted cardiac device.

Radiofrequency Fields

The transmit RF coils of the MRI scanner emit RF energy that is specifically tuned to the tissue of interest at a given

TABLE 19-1 Static Main Magnetic Field Limit Recommendations by the U.S. Food and Drug Administration*

Population	Main Static Magnetic Field Greater than (tesla)
Adults, children, and infants >1 month old	8
Neonates (<1 month old)	4

*The FDA considers an MRI scanner to be of significant risk when it is operating above the levels listed.
From United States Food and Drug Administration, Center for Devices and Radiological Health. Guidance for Industry. Criteria for significant risk investigations of magnetic resonance diagnostic devices. Available at: http://www.fda.gov/cdrh/ode/guidance/793.pdf. Accessed June 5, 2008.

static magnetic field strength. RF energy is absorbed by the tissue and released, producing signals that receiver coils can detect. RF energy may cause heating of biologic tissues, however, when the tissues are exposed to excessive RF energy levels. To ensure patient safety, levels of RF energy used for MRI procedures indicated in the units of specific absorption rate (SAR), are recommended by the FDA. Generally, MRI scanners calculate or estimate SAR based on the patient's weight and report values in W/kg. In 2003, the FDA relaxed the SAR limits as follows: 4 W/kg—whole body for 15 minutes, 3 W/kg—head for 10 minutes, 8 W/kg—peak 1 g of tissue (head or torso) for 15 minutes, 12 W/kg—peak 1 g of tissue (extremities) for 15 minutes.[7]

SAR increases with increasing static magnetic field strength, flip angle, duty cycle of the equipment, and patient size.[11] The SAR experienced at 3 T is approximately four times the absorption rate as 1.5 T,[12] making some of the cardiac imaging at 3 T potentially challenging. The SAR can be reduced, however, by modifying parameters such as flip angle, repetition time, slice thickness, imaging matrix, and echo train length, depending on the pulse sequence and the desired image contrast. Parallel imaging schemes have been a successful strategy for SAR reduction at 3 T.

TABLE 19-2 Terminology for the Labeling of Items for MRI Purposes*

Old Terminology	Definition
MRI safe†	This term indicates that the device, when used in the MRI environment, has been shown to present no additional risk to the patient, but may affect the quality of the diagnostic information.
MRI compatible†	This term indicates that the device, when used in the MRI environment, is MRI safe, and has been shown neither to affect significantly the quality of the diagnostic information nor to have its operations affected by the MRI device.

*The older terminology from the FDA's Center for Devices and Radiological Health of 1997 is still in use because the updated, new terminology has not been applied retrospectively.
†The use of the terms *MRI compatible* and *MRI safe* without specification of the MRI environment to which the device was tested should be avoided because interpretation of these claims may vary, and they are difficult to substantiate rigorously. Statements such as "intended for use in the MRI environment" or similar claims *along with* appropriate qualifying information are preferred (i.e., test conditions should be specifically stated).
From United States Food and Drug Administration, Center for Devices and Radiological Health. A primer on medical device interactions with magnetic resonance imaging systems, 1997. Available at: http://www.fda.gov/cdrh/ode/primerf6.html. Accessed June 5, 2008.

Cryogens

Cryogens are used to create superconducting MRI scanners. Liquid helium is the most common cryogen used in MRI scanners today, but liquid nitrogen is also used in some systems. Generally, only service engineers come in contact with the cryogens; however, if the cryogen system malfunctions, a quench can occur. A quench is the rapid release of the cryogen liquid (in the form of gas) from the MRI scanner that brings the magnetic field strength of the MRI scanner down very quickly. A quench can be problematic if the MRI scan room is built with the door opening inward, and there is not a pressure release mechanism.[3] This situation can set up the potential for a pressure lock to occur because helium expands at 754:1 as it turns to gas. Helium is also very cold (liquid helium is <−268° C). Ruptured eardrums, frostbite, and asphyxiation are potential adverse consequences to individuals in the scan room if a quench occurs whereby the helium gas escapes into the scan room instead of through the ventilation system.

CARDIAC DEVICES AND MAGNETIC RESONANCE IMAGING INFORMATION

An increasing number of implantable cardiovascular devices are being made available for patients with cardiovascular disease. Each device has a different composition, mass, geometry, potential for heating and functionality that affects the possible risks associated with MRI procedures. Devices such as cardiac pacemakers, pacing leads, and implantable cardioverter-defibrillators (ICDs) are controversial devices in patients today. Because of the variety and complexity of devices, the safety of implanted devices should never be assumed.[3] Patients entering zones III and IV need to have the safety of their implanted devices documented in writing and other external devices carefully tested.

Terminology Issues

The FDA originally adopted the terms *MRI safe* and *MRI compatible* in 1997 (Table 19-2). More recently, to try to minimize confusion from the older *MRI compatible* term, the FDA has adopted new terminology (*MRI safe, MRI conditional*, and *MRI unsafe*), developed by the American Society of Testing and Materials, which is based on specified MRI conditions and device interactions (Table 19-3).[2,3,14] The overall goal remains the same: to test devices, document the specific findings, and categorize the device for guidance concerning the scanning of patients. Because of the complexity of MRI scanners, RF coils, and devices, it is imperative that the detailed safety information be adequately reviewed by the responsible physicians overseeing the MRI procedure to be as safe as possible with the vast amount of devices implanted in patients today.

Cardiac Pacemakers, Implantable Cardioverter-Defibrillators, and Other Devices

Cardiac pacemakers, ICDs, and other electronic devices pose several potential problems to patients relative to the MRI environment. The devices can harm the patients through possible movement of the device, potential to heat or burn the patient, potential to cause arrhythmias, and potential of malfunction or damage occurring to the device.[8,15] These problems can lead to harm and even fatalities. Patients with these devices are generally

TABLE 19-3 Terminology for MRI Implants, Devices, and Labeling from the American Society of Testing and Materials

New Terminology	Definition
MRI safe	An item that poses no known hazards in all MRI environments
MRI conditional	An item that has been shown to pose no known hazards in a specified MRI environment with specified conditions of use. Field conditions that define the specified MRI environment include static magnetic field strength, spatial gradient, dB/dt (time varying magnetic fields), radiofrequency fields, and specific absorption rate. Additional conditions, including specific configurations of the item, may be required
MRI unsafe	An item that is known to pose hazards in all MRI environments

From American Society for Testing and Materials (ASTM) International, Designation: F2503-05. Standard Practice for Marking Medical Devices and Other Items for Safety in the Magnetic Resonance Environment. West Conshohocken, PA, ASTM International, 2005.

restricted from the MRI environment, but this policy is starting to change.

In January 2008, the FDA granted approval to begin the first clinical trials on a pacemaker system designed for safe use within an MRI scanner.[16] The pacemaker system (EnRhythm MRI SureScan; Medtronic, Minneapolis, MN) has gone through extensive design steps to improve the safety and efficacy of the cardiac pacemaker. Many physicians have been insisting for many years that pacemakers made with the newer technologies in recent years are safe; however, no manufacturer currently claims MRI safety. It has been reported that patients with pacemakers can safely undergo MRI scanning under certain highly specific and controlled conditions.[17] There are many potential problems associated with pacemakers that relate to such issues as the reed switches, lead lengths, circuitry, batteries, capacitors, types of functions, and types of patient therapies that must be considered. According to the recommendations from the American Heart Association Scientific Statement of 2007, only sites with expertise in cardiac MRI and electrophysiology should be attempting to scan patients with pacemakers and ICDs.[9] The risk/benefit ratio must clearly show the clinical benefit to the patient.

Pacemaker leads are also problematic, even when the pulse generator is detached. The problem is that long lengths of any wire can potentially cause heating, which may be excessive, and cardiac excitation.[9,18] Leads are often wound up with the tip of the lead still embedded in the myocardium. The amount of heating varies according to the size, shape, and composition of the metal; the location in the body; the location of the implant with respect to the RF coil; and the amount of SAR deposition.[18] Leads that are fractured pose a higher risk for excessive heating. The American Heart Association Scientific Statement in 2007 recommends that retained leads follow the same guidelines as pacemakers and ICDs.[9] Clinical studies are unavailable on fractured leads; MRI scanning in patients with damaged or fractured transvenous leads is discouraged.

Insertable Loop Recorders

Insertable loop recorders (ILR), also known as event monitors, are subcutaneously implanted devices used to monitor patients with unexplained syncope continuously. One ILR (Reveal; Medtronic, Minneapolis, MN) has been tested and has not shown adverse effects to the patient, but data retrieved from the recorder after scanning showed artifacts on the recorded ECG data retrieved from the ILR device.[19] There is also a theoretical risk of the electromagnetic fields from the MRI scanner compromising the data on the ILR.[9] Data on the ILR should be retrieved before the MRI examination. The ILR is considered to be MRI conditional.

Prosthetic Heart Valves

Prosthetic heart valves are made from various metals and biomaterials, and come in a wide variety of designs. Some valves may not contain any metal, and some may be made only of metal. Many heart valves have been tested at 1.5 T and 3 T. Many of the tested heart valves have been found to have measurable magnetic field interactions at 1.5 T.[2] The blood flow and beating of the heart exerted on the valve in vivo have been found to be greater, however, than the forces of the magnetic field at 1.5 T.[20] In a study of excised heart valves, it was measured that the forces necessary to dislodge sutures in a heart valve were greater than those found at 4.7 T.[21] Similarly, the forces necessary to cause valve dehiscence were found to be clinically insignificant at exposures of 4.7 T.

The Lenz effect theorizes significant electromotive force when metal heart valves interact in the MRI environment. The heart valves can theoretically create, in themselves, a little magnetic field that could oppose the static magnetic field of the MRI scanner, and possibly inhibit the opening and closing of the heart valve.[22] The potential for the hazards with heart valves are at this point theoretical only because serious adverse events have not been reported with heart valves at 1.5 T.[22] The Lenz effect increases linearly with field strength, so the potential for adverse interactions increases with field strength. In any case, patients with metallic heart valves should be monitored more closely because of the potential for heart valves to have magnetic field interactions at any field strength.

Stents

Many types of stents are available for cardiovascular and other applications. Most of these stents are made of 316L stainless steel or nitinol, but other materials, such as tantalum, MP35N, titanium, platinum, Elgiloy, and cobalt chromium, are also used.[2] Most of these stents are non-ferromagnetic or weakly ferromagnetic. If the stent is nonferromagnetic, an MRI procedure may be performed immediately after implantation.[9] There may be a potential problem with stents that are overlapped as two or more devices. Overlapped stents or long length stents may be

TABLE 19-4 Four Levels of Depth of Sedation According to the American Society of Anesthesiologists*

	Responsiveness	Airway	Spontaneous Ventilation	Cardiovascular Function
1. Minimal sedation (anxiolysis)	Normal response to verbal stimulation	Unaffected	Unaffected	Unaffected
2. Moderate sedation/analgesia ("conscious sedation")	Purposeful response to verbal or tactile stimulation	No intervention required	Adequate	Usually maintained
3. Deep sedation/analgesia	Purposeful response after repeated or painful stimulation	Intervention may be required	May be inadequate	Usually maintained
4. General anesthesia	Unarousable even with painful stimulus	Intervention often required	Frequently inadequate	May be impaired

*Sedation is considered a continuum, and qualified personnel need to be present for monitoring and care of the sedated patient. It is not always possible to predict how each patient will respond to sedation, and practitioners providing the sedation for each level must be able to rescue the patient if he or she is more deeply sedated than intended. Qualified practitioners proficient at airway management and advanced life support must be available for sedation.
From American Society of Anesthesiologists. Standards, guidelines and statements: guidelines for ambulatory anesthesia and surgery. 2004. Available at: http://www.asahq.org/publicationsAndServices/standards/04.pdf. Accessed August 22, 2008.

able to heat up substantially in the MRI environment because of current induction from RF power deposition, but this is a theoretical hazard. One key concept to remember is that new stents are being developed on a regular basis, and that not all stents are made in the United States under rigorous FDA guidelines. With the increase in globalization of health care and medical tourism, a growing number of patients in the United States are getting devices that may be available only in other countries. Obtaining specific stent information before performing an MRI examination on a patient is necessary to optimize patient safety.

MAGNETIC RESONANCE IMAGING CONTRAST AGENTS

Gadolinium (Gd)-chelate contrast agents are the primary contrast agents used in cardiovascular MRI and are cleared by the kidney. For individuals with normal renal function, Gd contrast agents are considered non-nephrotoxic when given intravenously at FDA-approved doses.[23] In 2000, findings of nephrogenic systemic fibrosis were reported, however, in patients who had received Gd-chelate contrast agents. Nephrogenic systemic fibrosis is found almost exclusively in patients with severe renal impairment and acidosis.[24] At this time, the FDA and the ACR recommend that patients with glomerular filtration rate less than 30 mL/min/1.73 m² should not receive Gd-chelate contrast agents. Currently, the FDA recommends that patients on dialysis be dialyzed immediately after receiving Gd-chelate contrast agents because they are dialyzable. More detailed recommendations are discussed in Chapter 18; see also the FDA and ACR websites (http://www.fda.gov/cder/drug/infopage/gcca/qa_200705.htm and http://www.acr.org/SecondaryMainMenuCategories/quality_safety/MRSafety/recommendations_gadolinium-based.aspx).

SEDATION

Generally, it is preferable to avoid sedation for cardiovascular patients, especially when the assessment includes the heart. Cardiac MRI works best when the patient can cooperate with breath-holding and other instructions. In addition, when patients fall asleep, their breathing pattern may become erratic, making image acquisition more difficult. Some patients are unable to tolerate an MRI examination, however, because of anxiety, pain, or other discomfort without some sort of assistance. Medications are often given to these patients. Free-breathing cardiac MRI techniques can often provide diagnostic quality images, albeit with motion blurring artifacts.

The Joint Commission requires that institutions have a plan of care for all sedation/anesthesia performed for procedures. The ACR follows the recommendations of The Joint Commission for their practice guidelines for adult sedation/analgesia, which can be found at http://www.acr.org/SecondaryMainMenuCategories/quality_safety/guidelines/iv/adult_sedation.aspx. The guidelines for sedation/anesthesia are designed to assist in the safe administration of sedation/analgesia and monitoring in the radiology department. Regardless of the sedation/anesthesia state, qualified personnel must be available, and patients must be monitored throughout the MRI examination. Sedation is considered to be a continuous spectrum; the health care provider must always be qualified to be able to reverse a patient if the patient unexpectedly slips into a deeper level of sedation than that intended.[25] Patient management procedures before and after the MRI examination must also be taken into consideration.

There are four generally accepted levels of sedation/analgesia according to the American Society of Anesthesiologists and The Joint Commission, ranging from light sedation to general anesthesia (Table 19-4).[1,26] Each level requires increasing level of qualifications for the personnel administering and monitoring the patients. The ACR recommends that patients should not be discharged until level of consciousness, vital signs, and motor function return to acceptable levels as assessed by health care personnel, and that written discharge instructions be given to the patient and family.[27] Discharge instructions should include possible adverse effects of the medication, a physician contact number, and warning not to drive for at least 12 hours.[27]

Pediatric patients represent a special challenge in cardiovascular MRI. Similar to adult patients, it is best if the pediatric patient is not sedated for cardiac studies. It is unreasonable, however, to expect a young child to hold still for a long MRI study. MRI sites that perform pediatric MRI must carefully develop a detailed protocol for the sedation of the pediatric patient. The American Academy of Pediatrics and the American Academy of Pediatric Dentistry have emphasized that children are different when it comes to sedation.[28] A child's respiratory system is vulnerable to sedative medications, and a child can easily slip from a state of sedation to anesthesia during a procedure.[29-31] Children are at risk for complications during sedation, such as apnea, hypoventilation, laryngospasm, and cardiopulmonary impairment, even under carefully monitored conditions.[31,32] Experienced teams that are able to rescue pediatric patients when they slip into unintended levels of sedation must be available. The American Academy of Pediatrics, American Academy of Pediatric Dentistry, and ACR all agree that the specific guidelines established by the American Society of Anesthesiologists for the personnel and delivery of sedation/analgesia should be followed.[3,27,28]

ACOUSTIC NOISE AND HEARING PROTECTION

MRI scanners are noisy. Patients complain often about the banging noises the MRI systems make. The noise may be very loud, may interfere with patient-operator communication, may increase patient anxiety, may interfere with functional MRI responses to stimuli, and may be annoying to patients and health care workers.[33,34] The loud noises made by the MRI scanners have the potential for temporary hearing loss, and patients need to be given hearing protection. In clinical tests performed at 0.35 T, the noise generated by the coils of the scanner were loud enough to cause a temporary hearing loss of more than 15 dB in 5 of 14 patients who were scanned in the scanner without hearing protection.[33]

Noise is measured as the sound pressure level. The FDA rates an MRI scanner as having significant risk if it generates peak unweighted sound pressure levels greater than 140 dB. Hearing loss is multifaceted, but generally the FDA recommends hearing protection for dB levels greater than 85 for more than 15 minutes of exposure. Many MRI systems operate at dB levels greater than 100. Passively reducing the acoustic noise through the use of earplugs or earmuffs can reduce the noise level by 25 to 29 dB (earplugs) and 31 to 38 dB (earmuffs),[35] reducing the impact on hearing. Some patients may be much more sensitive to acoustic noise than others, so attention to the patient's needs (e.g., using earplugs and earmuffs) may help, or trying to minimize total scan time may be considered. Because sound travels through the body, totally eliminating the sound to the patient is impossible. Educating the patient as to what to expect during the study is helpful for compliance and patient satisfaction.

STRESS TESTING AND SAFETY IN MAGNETIC RESONANCE IMAGING

Cardiac pharmacologic stress is becoming a more common procedure in the MRI setting. Monitoring for stress MRI requires the same level of precautions and emergency equipment as required for any other type of stress testing. The patient must be screened and prepared at least 24 to 72 hours before the study to allow for specific preprocedural instructions, depending on the pharmacologic stress agent selected for use. Qualified personnel must be present in the MRI suite for stress testing. At a minimum, an advanced cardiac life support (ACLS)–certified physician must be present. ACLS-qualified nurses with MRI safety training are also highly recommended for overall patient monitoring during the procedure. MRI-acceptable monitoring equipment is necessary to monitor the patient adequately during the stress procedure. A "crash cart" must be located in a safe place near the MRI system room. The crash cart should *never* go into the MRI system room because some equipment on it may be unsafe. The powerful static magnetic field of an MRI system may cause the defibrillator to function improperly.

Emergency procedures for rapid evacuation need to be practiced in the MRI suite. Codes cannot be performed inside the MRI system room because of the emergency equipment, and non-MRI personnel entering from outside the MRI department and typically carrying unsafe devices (e.g., scissors, stethoscopes). Patients must be removed from the scanner room for emergency personnel to attend the patient safely and conduct the code. Detachable MRI beds are preferred to minimize the time it takes to evacuate a patient. Otherwise, an MRI safe or MRI conditional stretcher for rapid patient transport must be in the room during pharmacologic stress testing.

Stress testing requires two intravenous access sites for the MRI procedure because two drugs (the stress agent and the Gd-chelate contrast agent) are being infused. Two venous access lines give an extra measure of safety in case the patient has an adverse reaction to any of the medications being given during stress testing. Typically, an MRI conditional power injector is used for the contrast agent infusion, and a separate MRI conditional medication infusion pump is used for the pharmacologic stress agent administration.

The most commonly used medications for cardiac MRI stress are adenosine and dobutamine. Adenosine is a vasodilator that is used for myocardial perfusion studies.[36,37] Adenosine is well tolerated and has a half-life of only 10 seconds. For this reason, adenosine is considered a safer drug of choice for perfusion stress testing in MRI. Another vasodilator that has been used for perfusion is dipyridamole.[38] Although inexpensive, dipyridamole has a longer half-life than adenosine, requiring a longer monitoring period. Dipyridamole is also much more likely to require theophylline to be used to normalize the patient's response. Caution must be used because theophylline is a shorter acting drug than dipyridamole, so the patient must be counseled and monitored about having recurrence of the vasodilator symptoms.

Dobutamine is a positive inotrope that is used for the wall motion studies.[39] Stress perfusion can also be achieved in dobutamine patients if atropine is added to the medication protocol. Dobutamine is a much riskier drug to use for stress than adenosine. A 12-lead ECG must be performed before and after the procedure to monitor for arrhythmias. The effects of the dobutamine start quickly, with the patient often needing an increased dose during the scanning. Caution must be used because dobutamine's half-life is 2 minutes with the effects lasting in some cases for 20 or 30 minutes. Dobutamine may precipitate or exacerbate ventricular ectopy. Severe hypotension and ventricular tachycardia can occur with dobutamine, so the crash cart and fluid expanders must be readily available in the MRI suite during these procedures. To help the patient recover from dobutamine stress faster, β-blockers may be given. In all stress procedures, the patient must be assessed by a physician or nurse practitioner before discharge. For additional information on cardiac stress imaging, see Chapter 26.

FUTURE ISSUES

Intraoperative MRI and combination x-ray and MRI suites are already in existence. The growth of invasive procedures in cardiovascular MRI brings a higher level of MRI safety considerations. These interventional MRI suites need to have extra areas where personnel can prepare for the MRI procedures at the level required for surgical asepsis or interventional/cardiac catheterization suite asepsis. All equipment entering these areas must be carefully screened for MRI safety issues. A system to ensure sterility and MRI safety needs to be in place that follows standard of care. Some facilities provide pocket-less scrubs and laboratory coats to help reduce the chance for projectile accidents.

CONCLUSION

As MRI technology advances, we must continue to update our knowledge and risk assessments for MRI safety. MRI systems have potential risks related to the static magnetic field strength, the gradient magnetic fields, the RF fields, and the cryogens that supercool the superconducting scanners. In addition, medical devices that are implanted into patients and other equipment that may go into an MRI suite come with various potential safety issues, such as material composition; mass of the device; shape of the device; and position of the device within, on, or around the patient. The safety of devices and equipment must be carefully considered in the MRI environment for optimal outcomes.

Medications used for cardiovascular MRI are generally related to the need for contrast agents, patient sedation, or cardiac stress testing. These medications require properly trained and licensed and certified personnel to administer the medications and monitor the patients. The ultimate goal is the welfare of the patient. Well-trained staff, well-designed facilities, diligence to adhere to recommended safety standards, and open communication lead to the safest possible MRI examinations.

KEY POINTS

- MRI scanners should be considered to be always on and dangerous at all times.
- No patient should be scanned without adequate screening.
- No patient should be scanned without proper identification of an implanted device.
- Properly trained and licensed personnel for imaging, sedation, stress testing, and other procedures are required for MRI safety.
- Communication among health care personnel and with the patient is of paramount importance for the safety and well-being of the patient being scanned.

ACKNOWLEDGMENT

The author acknowledges the insight and editing support of Frank G. Shellock, PhD, in this chapter. Dr. Shellock is a world-renowned expert on MRI safety. He is the founder of the Institute for Magnetic Resonance Safety, Education, and Research and is a fellow of the International Society for Magnetic Resonance in Medicine. The author thanks Dr. Shellock for his assistance with this chapter, and acknowledges his invaluable support for MRI education and safety worldwide.

SUGGESTED READINGS

American Academy of Pediatrics; American Academy of Pediatric Dentistry, Coté CJ, Wilson S; Work Group on Sedation. Guidelines for monitoring and management of pediatric patients during and after sedation for diagnostic and therapeutic procedures: an update. Pediatrics 2006; 118:2587-2602.

Faris OP, Shein M. Food and Drug Administration perspective: magnetic resonance imaging of pacemaker and implantable cardioverter-defibrillator patients. Circulation 2006; 114:1232-1233.

Kanal E, Barkovich AJ, Bell C, et al. ACR Blue Ribbon Panel on MR Safety. ACR guidance document for safe MR practices: 2007. AJR Am J Roentgenol 2007; 188:1447-1474.

Lee VS, Hecht EM, Taouli B, et al. Body and cardiovascular MR imaging at 3.0 T. Radiology 2007; 244:692-705.

Levine GN, Gomes AS, Arai AE, et al. Safety of magnetic resonance imaging in patients with cardiovascular devices: an American Heart Association scientific statement from the Committee on Diagnostic and Interventional Cardiac Catheterization. Circulation 2007; 116: 2878-2891.

Roguin A, Schwitter J, Vahlhaus C, et al. Magnetic resonance imaging in individuals with cardiovascular implantable electronic devices. Europace 2008; 10:336-346.

Shellock FG. Reference Manual for Magnetic Resonance Safety, Implants, and Devices: 2008 Edition. Los Angeles, Biomedical Research Publishing Group, 2008.

Shellock FG, Spinazzi A. MRI safety update 2008—parts 1 and 2. AJR Am J Roentgenol 2008; 191:1129-1139, 1140-1149.

Shinbane JS, Colletti PM, Shellock FG. MR in patients with pacemakers and ICDs: defining the issues. J Cardiovasc Magn Reson 2007; 9:5-13.

Zhuo J, Gullapalli RP. AAPM/RSNA physics tutorial for residents: MR artifacts, safety, and quality control. RadioGraphics 2006; 26:275-297.

REFERENCES

1. The Joint Commission. Preventing accidents and injuries in the MRI suite. Issue 38, February 14, 2008. Available at: http://www.jointcommission.org/SentinelEvents/SentinelEventAlert/sea_38.htm. Accessed June 5, 2008.
2. Shellock FG. Reference Manual for Magnetic Resonance Safety, Implants, and Devices: 2008 Edition. Los Angeles, Biomedical Research Publishing Group, 2008.
3. Kanal E, Barkovich AJ, Bell C, et al. ACR Blue Ribbon Panel on MR Safety. ACR guidance document for safe MR practices: 2007. AJR Am J Roentgenol 2007; 188:1447-1474.
4. ECRI. Hazard report: patient death illustrates the importance of adhering to safety precautions in magnetic resonance environments. Health Devices 2001; 30.
5. Maxwell JC. A Treatise on Electricity and Magnetism, Vol 1, 2nd ed. Oxford, Clarendon Press, 1881.
6. Shellock FG, Crues JV. MR procedures: biological effects, safety, and patient care. Radiology 2004; 232:635-652.
7. United States Food and Drug Administration, Center for Devices and Radiological Health. Guidance for Industry. Criteria for significant risk investigations of magnetic resonance diagnostic devices. Available at: http://www.fda.gov/cdrh/ode/guidance/793.pdf. Accessed June 5, 2008.
8. Tandri H, Zviman MM, Wedan SR, et al. Determinants of gradient field-induced current in a pacemaker lead system in a magnetic resonance imaging environment. Heart Rhythm 2008; 5:462-468.
9. Levine GN, Gomes AS, Arai AE, et al. Safety of magnetic resonance imaging in patients with cardiovascular devices: an American Heart Association scientific statement from the Committee on Diagnostic and Interventional Cardiac Catheterization. Circulation 2007; 116:2878-2891.
10. Schaefer DJ. Bioeffects of MRI and patient safety. In Bronskill MJ, Sprawls P (eds). The Physics of MRI: 1992 AAPM Summer School Proceedings. Woodbury, NY, American Association of Physics in Medicine, 1993.
11. Zhuo J, Gullapalli RP. AAPM/RSNA physics tutorial for residents: MR artifacts, safety, and quality control. RadioGraphics 2006; 26:275-297.
12. Lee VS, Hecht EM, Taouli B, et al. Body and cardiovascular MR imaging at 3.0 T. Radiology 2007; 244:692-705.
13. United States Food and Drug Administration, Center for Devices and Radiological Health. A primer on medical device interactions with magnetic resonance imaging systems, 1997. Available at: http://www.fda.gov/cdrh/ode/primerf6.html. Accessed June 5, 2008.
14. American Society for Testing and Materials (ASTM) International, Designation: F2503-05. Standard Practice for Marking Medical Devices and Other Items for Safety in the Magnetic Resonance Environment. West Conshohocken, PA, ASTM International, 2005.
15. Shinbane JS, Colletti PM, Shellock FG. MR in patients with pacemakers and ICDs: defining the issues. J Cardiovasc Magn Reson 2007; 9:5-13.
16. Medtronic. FDA grants Medtronic approval to begin clinical trial of first pacemaker system designed for safe use in MRI machines: innovations in pacing technology advance access to non-invasive diagnostics. Available at: http://wwwp.medtronic.com/Newsroom/NewsReleaseDetails.do?itemId=1201527823548&lang=en_US. Accessed June 5, 2008.
17. Sommer T, Naehle CP, Yang A, et al. Strategy for safe performance of extrathoracic magnetic resonance imaging at 1.5 tesla in the presence of cardiac pacemakers in non-pacemaker-dependent patients: a prospective study with 115 examinations. Circulation 2006; 114:1285-1292.
18. Bassen H, Kainz W, Mendoza G, et al. MRI-induced heating of selected thin wire metallic implants—laboratory and computational studies—findings and new questions raised. Minim Invasive Ther Allied Technol 2006; 15:76-84.
19. Gimbel JR, Zarghami J, Machado C, et al. Safe scanning, but frequent artifacts mimicking bradycardia and tachycardia during magnetic resonance imaging (MRI) in patients with an implantable loop recorder (ILR). Ann Noninvasive Electrocardiol 2005; 10:404-408.
20. Soulen RL, Budinger TF, Higgins CB. Magnetic resonance imaging of prosthetic heart valves. Radiology 1985; 154:705-707.
21. Edwards MB, Ordidge RJ, Hand JW, et al. Assessment of magnetic field (4.7 T) induced forces on prosthetic heart valves and annuloplasty rings. J Magn Reson Imaging 2005; 22:311-317.
22. Condon B, Hadley DM. Potential MR hazard to patients with metallic heart valves: the Lenz effect. J Magn Reson Imaging 2000; 12:171-176.
23. Prince MR, Arnoldus C, Frisoli JK. Nephrotoxicity of high-dose gadolinium compared with iodinated contrast. J Magn Reson Imaging 1996; 6:162-166.
24. United States Food and Drug Administration, Center for Devices and Radiological Health. Information on gadolinium-containing contrast agents. Available at: http://www.fda.gov/Cder/Drug/infopage/gcca/default.htm. Accessed June 10, 2008.
25. American Society of Anesthesiologists. Standards, guidelines and statements: guidelines for ambulatory anesthesia and surgery. 2004. Available at: http://www.asahq.org/publicationsAndServices/standards/04.pdf. Accessed August 22, 2008.
26. American Society of Anesthesiologists. Standards, guidelines and statements: continuum of depth of sedation: definition of general anesthesia and levels of sedation/analgesia. Available at: http://www.asahq.org/publicationsAndServices/standards/20.pdf. Accessed June 5, 2008.
27. American College of Radiology. ACR practice guideline for adult sedation/analgesia. 2005. Available at: http://www.acr.org/SecondaryMainMenuCategories/quality_safety/guidelines/iv/adult_sedation.aspx. Accessed June 5, 2008.
28. American Academy of Pediatrics; American Academy of Pediatric Dentistry, Coté CJ, Wilson S; Work Group on Sedation. Guidelines for monitoring and management of pediatric patients during and after sedation for diagnostic and therapeutic procedures: an update. Pediatrics 2006; 118:2587-2602.
29. Dial S, Silver P, Bock K, Sagy M. Pediatric sedation for procedures titrated to a desired degree of immobility results in unpredictable depth of sedation. Pediatr Emerg Care 2001; 17:414-420.
30. Motas D, McDermott NB, VanSickle T, et al. Depth of consciousness and deep sedation attained in children as administered by nonanaesthesiologists in a children's hospital. Paediatr Anaesth 2004; 14:256-260.
31. American Academy of Pediatrics Committee on Drugs. Guidelines for monitoring and management of pediatric patients during and after sedation for diagnostic and therapeutic procedures: addendum. Pediatrics 2002; 110:836-838.
32. Coté CJ, Notterman DA, Karl HW, et al. Adverse sedation events in pediatrics: a critical incident analysis of contributing factors. Pediatrics 2000; 105(4 Pt 1):805-814.
33. Brummett RE, Talbot JM, Charuhas P. Potential hearing loss resulting from MR imaging. Radiology 1988; 169:539-540.
34. Bandettini PA, Jesmanowicz A, Van Kylen J, et al. Functional MRI of brain activation induced by scanner acoustic noise. Magn Reson Med 1998; 39:410-416.
35. Ravicz ME, Melcher JR, Kiang NY. Acoustic noise during functional magnetic resonance imaging. J Acoust Soc Am 2000; 108:1683-1696.
36. Nagel E, Klein C, Paetsch I, et al. Magnetic resonance perfusion measurements for the noninvasive detection of coronary artery disease. Circulation 2003; 108:432-437.
37. Gudmundsson P, Winter R, Kitlinski M, et al. Real-time perfusion adenosine stress echocardiography versus myocardial perfusion adenosine scintigraphy for the detection of myocardial ischemia in patients with stable coronary artery disease. Clin Physiol Funct Imaging 2006; 25:32-38.
38. Picano E, Sicari R, Varga A. Dipyridamole stress echocardiography. Cardiol Clin 1999; 17:481-499.
39. Nagel E, Lehmkuhl HB, Bocksch W, et al. Noninvasive diagnosis of ischemia-induced wall motion abnormalities with the use of high-dose dobutamine stress MRI: comparison with dobutamine stress echocardiography. Circulation 1999; 99:763-770.

CHAPTER 20

Physics and Instrumentation of Cardiac Single Photon Emission Computed Tomography

Edward J. Miller and Raymond R. Russell*

Successful performance and interpretation of cardiac single photon emission computed tomography (SPECT) studies relies on a basic understanding of the physics and instrumentation that allows for the generation of the images. The first practical system for the in vivo imaging of radionuclides was developed in the late 1950s by Anger and became commercially available in 1962.[1] Despite more than 45 years of use and technical advances, the basic physics and design principles used today for cardiac SPECT imaging are remarkably similar to Anger's initial concept.

This chapter provides the reader with a basic understanding of the physical principles underlying cardiac SPECT imaging, with a particular focus on how basic physics impacts image acquisition and the problems of imaging artifacts. We also focus on the basic aspects of SPECT imaging camera design and briefly highlight advances in new solid-state detector systems.

PHYSICS AND SPECT IMAGING

Basic Atomic Structure

The classically described structure of an atom is known as the *Bohr atom*. It depicts a set of electrons orbiting the nucleus in stable electron shells (K, L, M, N) (Fig. 20-1). Each of the shells represents an energy state, with the innermost shell (K) associated with the greatest potential energy. Each electron's energy state is defined further by a discrete set of four quantum numbers per electron. The Pauli exclusion principle states that no two electrons in the same atom can have an identical set of quantum numbers. By definition, a stable atom exists in its lowest possible energy state. When the energy state of an electron is increased (i.e., moved to a higher energy orbital shell or via absorption of external energy), the electron emits energy spontaneously as it returns to its lower, more stable energy state. This emission of energy by unstable electrons provides one mechanism for radionuclide imaging and is described in detail in the next section.

Electrons orbit a nucleus composed of a dense conglomerate of protons and neutrons that are bound together by a network of so-called strong nuclear forces. A proton contains a charge of 1.6×10^{-19} coulombs, which is the exact opposite charge of an electron. Neutrons are particles of slightly greater mass than protons, but are uncharged. The number of protons present in its nucleus, or Z number, defines each element, whereas the mass number, or A, represents the number of protons plus the number of neutrons. Specific nomenclature defines the relationship between the number of protons and neutrons in a nucleus (Table 20-1). The ratio of protons to neutrons defines the stability of a particular nucleus (Fig. 20-2); the transformation of an unstable nucleus to a more stable state is responsible for many of the radioactive emissions used in nuclear imaging.

Radioactivity: Electron Transition, Unstable Nuclei, and Radioactive Decay

Radiation refers to the transfer of energy across distance, and can be in the form of kinetic energy transfer through the interaction of charged particles or through electromagnetic energy transfer in the form of photons. Our discussion focuses primarily on the physics of electromagnetic/photon radiation because this is the most relevant to cardiac nuclear imaging. A photon is a massless, chargeless carrier of energy that behaves much like a wave, traveling at the speed of light. Photons generated from

---

*The views expressed in this chapter are those of the authors and do not reflect the official policy or position of the Department of the Navy, Department of Defense, or U.S. Government.

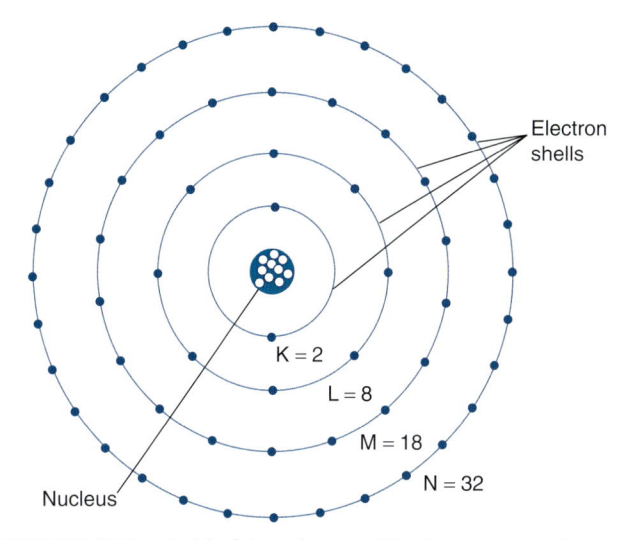

FIGURE 20-1 Model of the Bohr atom. The Bohr atom predicts an atomic model where the nucleus is surrounded by electron shells.

TABLE 20-1 Nuclear Nomenclature

Name	Symbol	Description
Z number	$_ZX$	Number of protons
A number	^AX	Mass number; number of neutrons + protons
N number	N	Number of neutrons
Nuclide		Common elementary characteristics
Isomer	m	Equal protons and neutrons, different energy state (e.g., Tc 99m)
Isotope		Same number of protons; $Z_1 = Z_2$
Isotone		Same number of neutrons; $N_1 = N_2$
Isobar		Same mass number; $A_1 = A_2$

energy transitions occurring in the electron cloud are termed *x-rays*, and photons emitted from nuclear transitions are termed *gamma rays*.

The energy (*E*) transmitted by a photon is proportional to its wavelength (λ, in nm). Because photons travel at the speed of light (*c*), the energy carried by a photon (in keV) is governed by the equation:

$$E = 1.24(\lambda)$$

Photons released from different radionuclides have different wavelengths and different energies. The characteristic energy (or energies) of photons released from different radionuclides plays a crucial role in image generation (photopeak generation) and in the creation of imaging artifacts (e.g., attenuation, scatter).

Radiation can involve energy contained either in electrons or in the nucleus. An electron of a particular element exists in a characteristic energy state defined by its unique quantum number. This energy is a combination of the kinetic energy of motion of the electron and potential energy between the electron and the charges contained within the nucleus. The strength of this potential energy is proportional to the number of protons in the nucleus, and is inversely proportional to the distance of the electron from the nucleus. A heavy element (i.e., large Z number) with many protons exerts more force on an orbital electron and has more potential energy, and an inner shell electron has greater potential energy than an outer shell electron. This potential energy is commonly referred to as the *binding energy* for that electron and represents the energy required to separate that electron from the atom. With the introduction of energy equal to its binding energy, an electron can be removed from an atom with a resulting orbital electron vacancy. This process is called *ionization*. In contrast to ionization, if the energy transmitted to the orbital electron is insufficient to remove it from its shell, the transferred energy is dissipated as heat in a process known as *excitation*.

Two types of ionization electron transition can occur. In heavy elements (elements with a high number of protons, or Z number), a *characteristic x-ray* is produced when an electron from an outer shell fills an inner shell vacancy (Fig. 20-3). The energy difference between two electron shells is characteristic of the element, given the different Z number and nuclear charge that define that element. The energy released as the characteristic x-ray represents the difference in potential energy between the outer shell electron and its new quantum state in the inner shell. The movement of an electron from an outer shell to an inner shell produces an x-ray with a characteristic energy, which can be described as a K, L, M, or N x-ray, and the energy of a characteristic x-ray from a particular element can be predicted based on the subatomic structure of the element. An example of a characteristic x-ray emission is the 68- to 70-keV mercury characteristic x-ray that is emitted from thallium 201.

Another mechanism of electron transition that leads to energy emission occurs when an outer shell electron fills an inner shell vacancy, but transfers the energy difference to an outer shell orbital electron (rather than emitting a characteristic x-ray), leading to the emission of an *Auger electron* (see Fig. 20-3). Because the release of an Auger electron leads to an orbital vacancy, a cascade of subsequent characteristic x-rays or further Auger electrons can

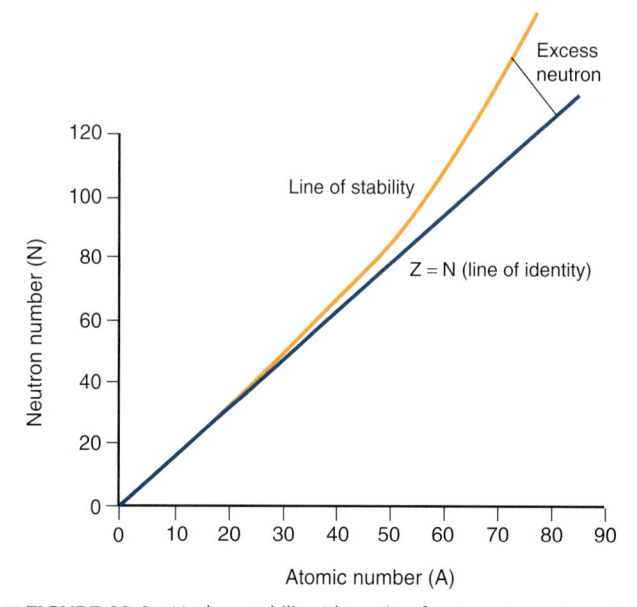

FIGURE 20-2 Nuclear stability. The ratio of protons to neutrons in a nucleus defines its stability and potential for radioactive decay. The line of stability diverges from the line of identity (equal proton/neutron ratio) at higher N numbers.

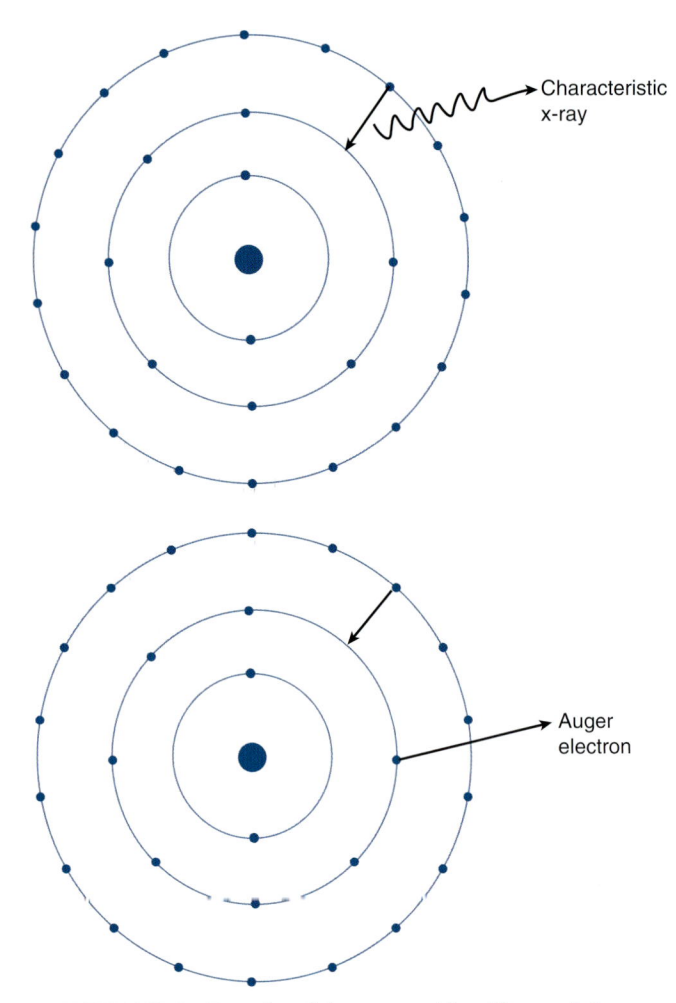

FIGURE 20-3 Examples of electron transition. Characteristic x-rays (*top*) and Auger electrons (*bottom*) can be emitted during electron transition.

TABLE 20-2   Types of Radioactive Decay

Name	Symbol	Schema	Type
Alpha decay	α	$^AX_Z \rightarrow {}^{A-4}Y_{Z-2} + \alpha$	
Beta decay	β⁻	$^AX_Z \rightarrow {}^AY_{Z+1} + \beta^- + \bar{\upsilon}$ (antineutrino)	Isobaric
Positron emission	β⁺	$^AX_Z \rightarrow {}^AY_{Z-1} + \beta^+ + \upsilon$ (neutrino)	Isobaric
Electron capture		$^AX_Z \rightarrow {}^AY_{Z-1} + \upsilon$ (neutrino) + x-ray	Isobaric
Gamma emission	γ	$^AX_Z \rightarrow {}^AX_Z + \gamma$	Isomeric
Internal conversion		$^AX_Z \rightarrow {}^AX_Z + \gamma$	Isomeric

occur after the initial emission. Auger electrons are usually produced when orbital electron vacancies are filled in elements of low Z number.

Besides energy transfer involving electrons, energy can also be released from the nucleus. Unstable nuclei can release energy in an attempt to reach a more stable energy state through the process of radioactive decay. This process is also called *nuclear transformation*. Radioactive decay of a particular unstable nucleus can occur in a series of decay steps, involving one or more of the types of radioactive decay described subsequently. Molybdenum-99 decays by β⁻ emission (discussed in detail later) to Tc 99m. Tc 99m undergoes subsequent gamma emission by isomeric transition producing the stable daughter Tc 99m. The "m" notation refers to a metastable excited nucleus with a measurable life span before its decay (approximately 10^{-12} seconds), which is an intermediate between the "excited" and "stable" states.

Radioactive decay can involve particulate and nonparticulate emissions. Different types of radioactive decay are described in Table 20-2 and include alpha particle emission, beta particle emission, positron emission, electron capture, gamma ray emission, and internal conversion.

Alpha particles are equivalent to a He nucleus (two protons, two neutrons). Alpha particles are massive in size compared with other particulate emissions, and because of their large size cannot travel far in matter before an interaction occurs, and their energy is released. Because alpha particles cannot travel significant distances, their use in imaging is limited. The much higher linear energy transfer of alpha particles compared with beta particles or gamma photons results in significantly greater effective doses of absorbed radiation.

Beta particle emission occurs when a nucleus is unstable because of an elevated neutron/proton ratio (Fig. 20-4). When this occurs, a neutron is converted to a proton with the emission of an electron (β⁻) and an antineutrino ($\bar{\upsilon}$). Because of the ejection of the electron and antineutrino from the nucleus, the daughter has an atomic number that is one greater than the parent. This decreases the instability generated by the elevated number of neutrons.

In contrast to beta particle (β⁻) emission, when a nucleus is unstable because of an increased number of protons, radioactive decay can occur through *positron emission* (β⁺) or *electron capture* (see Fig. 20-4). A positron, which is effectively an electron with a positive charge, is emitted during times of proton excess with the simultaneous generation of a neutron. When a positron is emitted from the nucleus, it quickly encounters an electron in the environment, leading to the annihilation of both particles. This annihilation event converts all of the mass of the two particles into energy, with the subsequent generation of two photons of equal energy that travel at 180 degrees to each other. Because the total energy generated by the annihilation reaction is 1.02 MeV, each of the photons emitted from the reaction carries an energy of 511 keV. The high energy of these photons and their simultaneous generation allowing for coincidence detection underlie the mechanisms for positron emission tomography (PET).

A separate process by which a proton-rich nucleus can obtain nuclear stability is through *electron capture* (see Fig. 20-4). In electron capture, an inner shell electron combines with a nuclear proton to form a neutron, creating a more stable nucleus. An outer shell electron fills the vacant inner shell with the subsequent generation of characteristic x-rays or Auger electrons. Positron emission and electron capture are competitive processes, with β⁺ emission occurring more frequently in "lighter" elements, and electron capture occurring in "heavier" elements. The

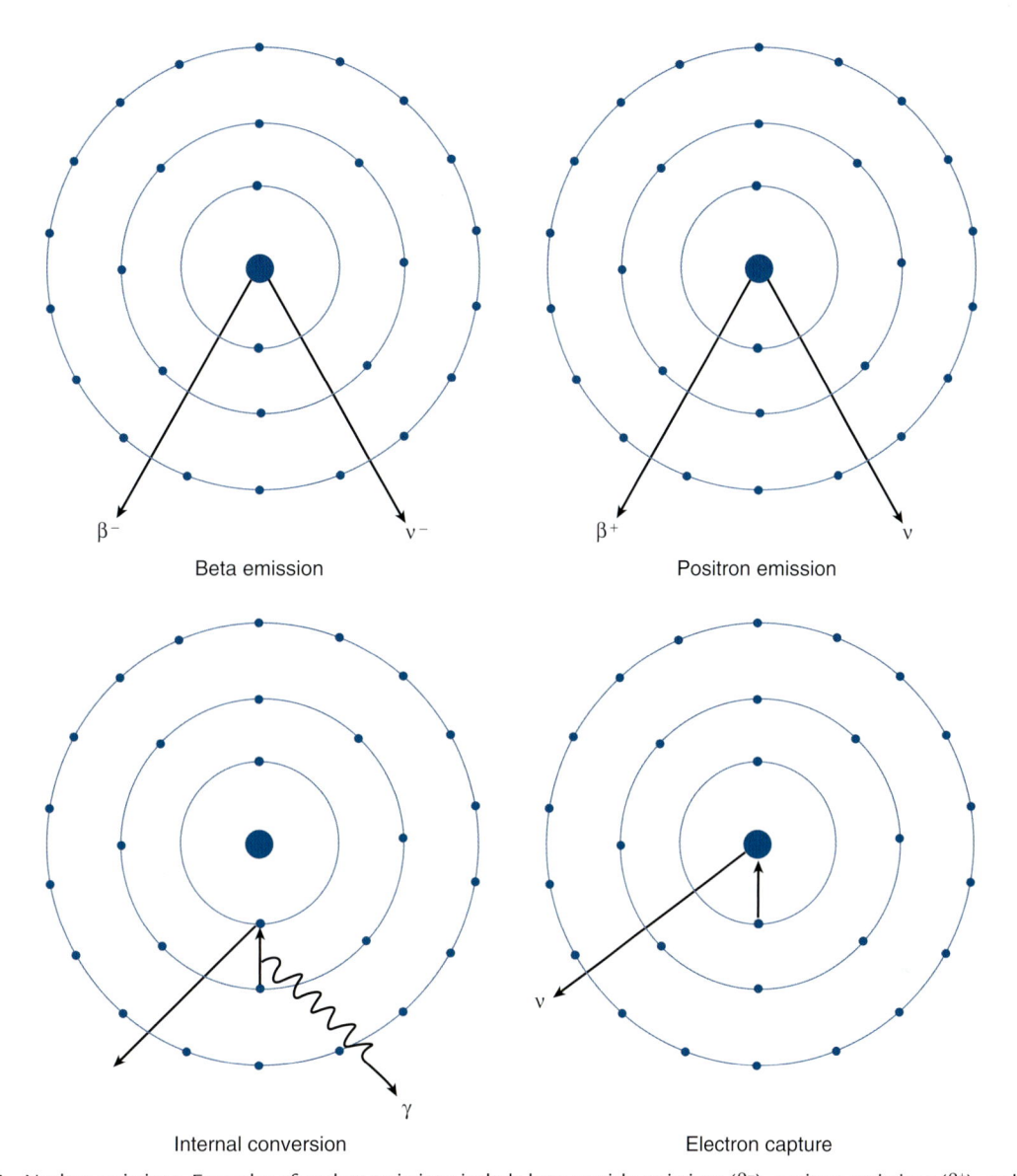

FIGURE 20-4 Nuclear emissions. Examples of nuclear emissions include beta particle emissions (β⁻), positron emissions (β⁺), and electron capture. υ, neutrino, υ⁻, antineutrino.

characteristic x-rays that are produced during thallium 201 decay (described previously) are produced through electron capture.

Gamma ray emission occurs during nuclear transformation when the process of radioactive decay does not completely dissipate the energy required for the atom to reach its most stable state. Gamma rays are a form of electromagnetic radiation with variable energy without mass or charge (i.e., a photon). Gamma rays carry off the excess nuclear energy through the process of *isomeric transition*. Isomeric transition occurs when a metastable nucleus is present from a prior radioactive decay. This can commonly occur after β⁻ decay, but can also occur as a consequence of *internal conversion* (see Fig. 20-4), where an unstable nucleus transfers its energy to an inner shell (K or L) electron, leading to its expulsion as a conversion electron. An outer shell electron, releasing energy via a characteristic x-ray or Auger electron, fills the subsequent electron vacancy. The ability of gamma rays to penetrate tissue (and be used as an imaging tool) depends on their energy. An example of isomeric transition is the gamma photon emitted from the decay of the metastable Tc 99m nucleus.

Radioactive Decay

Radioactive decay is a spontaneous process that can be described by mathematical modeling of the probability of decay. Although it is impossible to predict the exact moment of decay for a particular unstable nucleus, it is possible to predict how many unstable nuclei of an element will decay over time. This time is commonly referred to as the *half-life* ($t_{1/2}$) of the element, or the time it takes for a spontaneously decaying radionuclide to decrease its activity by 50%. The $t_{1/2}$ of a radionuclide is a function of its exponential rate of decay (dN/dt) or activity (A), and this rate of decay is specific for an element and related to the *decay constant* (λ) by:

$$dN/dt = -\lambda N$$

or

$$A = \lambda N$$

To describe the number of radioactive nuclei present (N_t) at a given time (t) compared with the number present initially (N_0), one can solve the previous differential equation, yielding:

$$N_t = N_0 e^{-\lambda t}$$

If we solve this equation for the time at which one half of the original quantity of nuclei are present ($t_{1/2}$), or:

$$N_t/N_0 = \frac{1}{2} = e^{-\lambda t}$$

then

$$t_{\frac{1}{2}} = \ln 2 / \lambda = 0.693 / \lambda$$

This exponential decay relationship and the concept of the decay constant are clinically useful. Because the decay constants for clinically relevant radionuclides are known, if the activity at a particular time (i.e., arrival of a radiopharmaceutical shipment) is known, one can calculate the activity present at a point of time in the future when it is to be used. The Système International unit of activity of radioactivity is the becquerel (Bq; 1 Bq = 1 decay/second), although the curie (Ci; 1 Ci = 3.7×10^{10} decay/second) is commonly used in clinical settings: 1 Bq = 27 $\times 10^{-12}$ Ci. When a radionuclide is mixed with a nonradioactive carrier, the *specific activity* of the nuclide is expressed as activity per gram (Bq/g).

Manufacture of Radionuclides

Medical radionuclides can be produced in a nuclear reactor, cyclotron, or a generator on site. This section describes the production of three commonly employed radionuclides in nuclear cardiology: thallium 201, Tc 99m, and rubidium 82.

Thallium 201 is usually produced in a cyclotron from the proton-bombardment of nonradioactive thallium 203, lead, or bismuth. Additionally, thallium 201 can be produced from lead 201 ($t_{1/2}$ 9.3 hours) by a generator-based method. Most cyclotron-produced radionuclides have an elevated proton/neutron ratio, and decay by electron capture or positron emission. Because of its long $t_{1/2}$ (74 hours), thallium 201 can be transported from the cyclotron to the end-user.

In contrast to thallium 201, Tc 99m can be produced on-site using a commercially available generator (Fig. 20-5) from nuclear reactor–produced molybdenum 99. Molybdenum 99 is a fission reaction product of ^{235}U. As molybdenum 99 slowly undergoes β^- decay with a $t_{1/2}$ of 66 hours, 87.5% of the decay product is Tc 99m, with the remaining 12.5% being the stable isomer Tc 99. When the generator is prepared at the radiopharmaceutical manufacturer, molybdenum 99 is tightly bound to a supporting alumina (Al_2O_3) column. Molybdenum 99 is more negatively charged than Tc 99m, and Tc 99m can be eluted ("milked") from the column with normal saline into a collection vial as Tc 99m-pertechnetate.

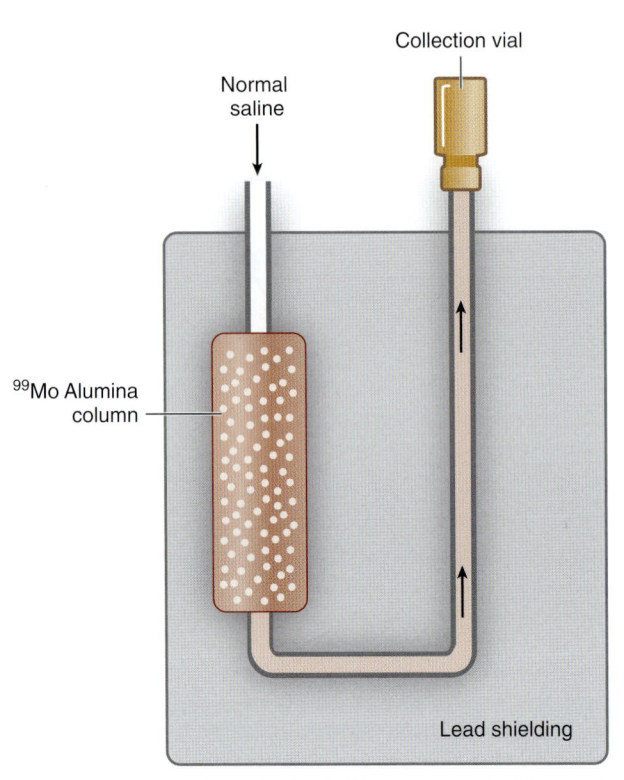

■ **FIGURE 20-5** Schematic of a Tc 99m generator. Tc 99m can be eluted from a generator as it is produced from the spontaneous decay of molybdenum 99 (^{99}Mo), which is adsorbed to an alumina column. Normal saline is used to elute the Tc 99m, which is collected in a sterile vial.

Rubidium 82 is the most commonly used PET tracer for evaluating myocardial perfusion. Rubidium 82 is produced from the electron capture decay of cyclotron-produced strontium 82 ($t_{1/2}$ 25.3 days). Similar to a Tc 99m generator, strontium 82 is adsorbed on a shielded column (stannic oxide), and rubidium 82 is eluted from the generator with normal saline. Because the $t_{1/2}$ of rubidium 82 is short (75 seconds), the generator elution occurs directly into the patient's intravenous line. In addition to rubidium 82, other PET tracers may be used for assessment of cardiac perfusion, metabolism, and viability, including [2-^{18}F]-2-fluoro-2-deoxyglucose (^{18}FDG), [^{13}N]-ammonia, [1-^{11}C]-glucose, and [1-^{11}C]-palmitate. These tracers are generated by a cyclotron, however, and because of their short half-lives, generally must be produced by an on-site cyclotron. The exception is ^{18}FDG, which has a $t_{1/2}$ of 110 minutes and can be produced by a cyclotron in a radiopharmaceutical network for regional distribution.

Interactions with Matter

The interactions of radiation with matter depend on the type of radiation and the composition of the interacting matter. Generally, the interactions of charged particles with matter (alpha particles, beta particles, and electrons) can lead to ionization and excitation as described earlier. In addition, another charged particle interaction is called *bremsstrahlung*, which involves the interaction of charged particles (electrons) with the strong forces in the nucleus, leading to photon emission. Because most medical imaging involves photon (gamma and x-ray) detection, our discussion focuses on the three primary ways photons interact with matter: photoelectric effect, Compton scatter, and pair production (Fig. 20-6).

The *photoelectric effect* is the photon-matter interaction responsible for the production of a photoelectron in scintillation crystals (used in gamma camera detectors—see later). In the photoelectric effect, a photon interacts with an orbital electron; if the photon's energy is greater than the binding energy of the electron, the electron is ejected from its orbital shell with an energy equal to the energy of the incident photon minus the binding energy of the electron. The net effect is a 100% conversion of the photon's electromechanical energy. Three main ancillary radiations can occur as a consequence of the photoelectric effect. The first two involve the production of secondary electrons, the high-energy photoelectron from the initial photon interaction and an Auger electron as the orbital electron's position is filled. The other radiation occurs with the production of a characteristic x-ray during the initial photon-orbital electron interaction.

Compton scatter occurs when a photon interacts with a loosely bound electron. The photon releases part of its energy to the interacting electron, proportional to the incident angle of interaction (0 to 90 degrees) between the photon and electron. In contrast to the photoelectric effect, the photon in Compton scatter is not destroyed. The two types of radiation products during a Compton scatter interaction include the scattered photon and the interacting electron, termed the *recoil electron*. The subsequent path of travel of the scattered photon and recoil electron are altered during this interaction, producing "scatter" of the photon from its original path. The angle of the photon after Compton scatter depends on the energy of the incident photon, with lower energy incident photons more likely to have a greater angle of deflection after this interaction. This scatter of photons from their original angle of travel provides a significant difficulty for defining from where these photons originated during an imaging procedure.

The final type of interaction between a photon and matter is called *pair production*. When a high-energy photon (>1.02 MeV) interacts with a nucleus, the photon's energy can be converted to mass with the production of a positive (β^+) and a negative (β^-) electron. The amount of energy required to create the mass of an electron is 0.51 MeV; pair production does not occur with photons less than 1.02 MeV and does not occur during normal cardiac imaging procedures.

The probability of a particular type of interaction between a photon and matter depends on the energy of the photon and the Z number of the material (Fig. 20-7). In elements with a high Z number, an interaction with a low-energy (<1 MeV) photon has a high likelihood of interacting via the photoelectric effect, whereas high-energy photons predominantly interact via pair produc-

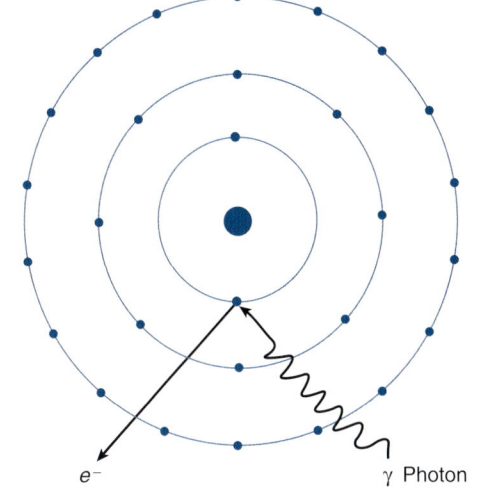

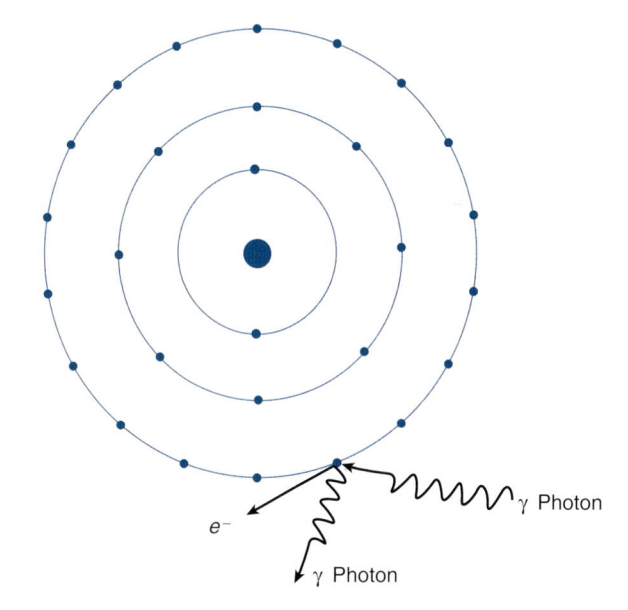

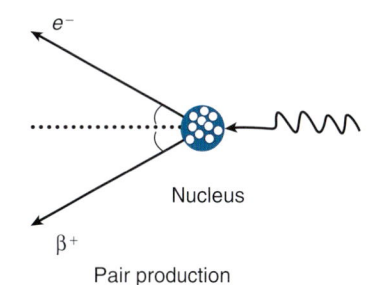

■ **FIGURE 20-6** Types of photon interactions with matter. Gamma photons (γ) can interact with matter by the photoelectric effect (*top*), Compton scatter (*middle*), or pair production (*bottom*). β^+, positron; e^-, electron.

tion. Compton scatter occurs when photons carrying an energy in the range associated with radionuclides that are used in medical imaging (60 to 500 keV) interact with matter with a high density of loosely bound electrons (i.e., high physical density tissues such as bone) and is for the

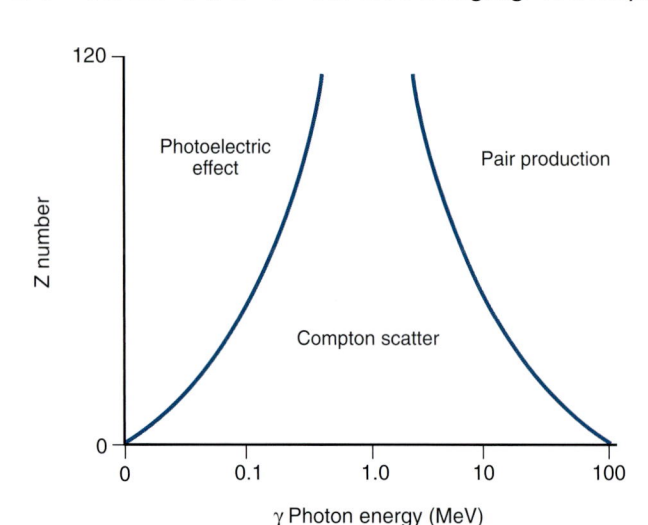

FIGURE 20-7 Photon and matter interaction probability. The energy of the interacting photon and the Z number of the interacting element determine the probability of a particular type of photon-matter interaction.

most part independent of the Z number of the absorbing material. The most likely effect of an imaging photon interaction within the human body before its arrival at the detection camera is one of Compton scatter.

The final concept in the interactions with photons with matter is called *attenuation* and refers to the percentage of photons that interact with a given thickness of matter. Photons that interact with matter by one of the aforementioned processes do not pass through the matter directly, or are "attenuated." The amount of attenuation occurring in a given material depends on the energy of the photon beam and the thickness of the material (x) and the Z number. The Z number defines the *linear attenuation coefficient* (μ) for the particular material, with higher Z number elements increasing the probability of photon attenuation. The mathematical equation that describes the number of photons for a given energy that pass through a material (I_x) compared with the number of incident photons (I_0) is:

$$I_x = I_0 e^{-\mu x}$$

Because photon beams occur with variable energy, it is useful to express the amount of thickness of a particular material that leads to the attenuation of one half of a particular photon energy beam. This is termed the *half value thickness* (HVT) of a material, and is defined by the linear attenuation coefficient (μ) for that material by the equation:

$$HVT = \ln 2/\mu = 0.693/\mu$$

INSTRUMENTATION AND SPECT IMAGING

SPECT imaging uses the photons arising from radioactive decay to generate an image of the coronary perfusion of the heart. This technique requires a method of detecting photons, defining the spatial origination of these photons, determining their energy characteristics and number, and

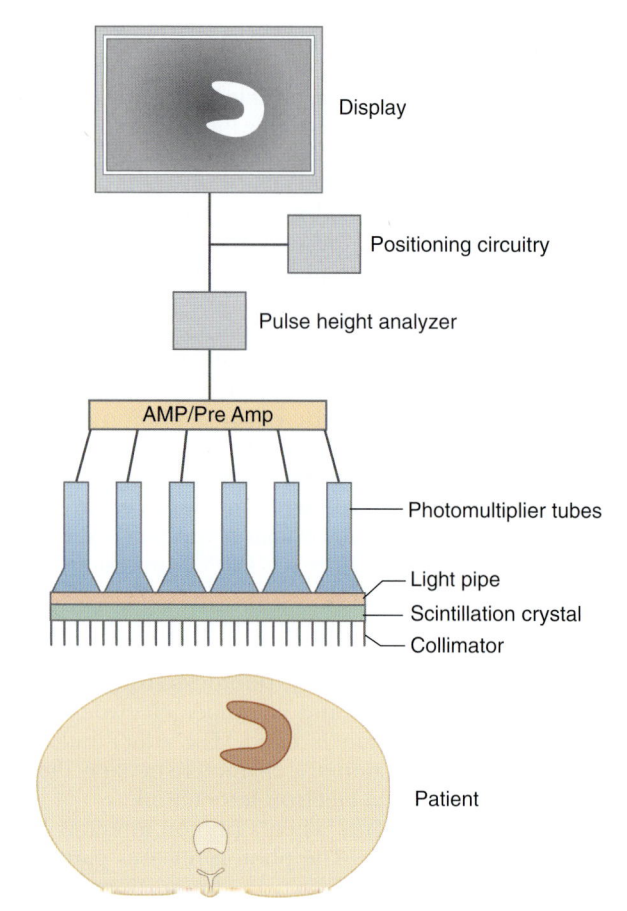

FIGURE 20-8 Components of a gamma camera.

displaying an interpretable image of these data. This section details the basic instrumentation that makes up gamma (Anger) cameras and highlights some more recent innovations in this technology.

The prototypic gamma detector is composed of the following elements (Fig. 20-8): collimator, scintillation crystal, light pipe, photomultiplier tubes, preamplifiers/amplifiers, pulse-height analyzer, positioning circuitry, analog-to-digital converter, and display device. A photon emitted from a patient must travel along a path that allows it to pass through the collimator holes where it encounters the scintillation crystal. In the scintillation crystal, the photon's energy is converted to light. The photomultiplier tubes detect this light and generate an electrical signal relative to the intensity of the detected light. These electrical signals are individually detected and allow for determination of the originating location of the photon by the use of computerized electronics and algorithms, and are amplified and converted to a digital image. The details of each component of the gamma detector are discussed in sequence.

Collimators

A *collimator* is a device that restricts the passage of photons into the scintillation crystal to select for photons traveling along particular paths. Because radionuclides emit photons in all directions, a collimator ensures that only photons traveling along the desired path from the patient are available for detection. Collimators are typically made of lead and are composed of multiple holes of defined diameter and depth, separated by intervening septa. To reach the scintillation crystal, photons must pass through one of these holes, traveling parallel to the long axis of the hole. Otherwise, the photons are absorbed by the septa. The most commonly used collimator type in SPECT imaging is a parallel-hole collimator (Fig. 20-9). Other types of collimators include slant-hole, converging, diverging, and pin-hole.

The choice of a particular collimator depends on the object being imaged, the energy of the imaging photon, and the desired relationship between image sensitivity and resolution, with sensitivity defined as the percentage of emitted photons from a given source that are able to pass through the collimator and interact with the crystal. As part of the ability to restrict or permit photon transmission, collimators also affect the spatial resolution of the camera. The spatial resolution is usually measured by imaging a point source of radioactivity, and is measured as the width of a plot of image intensity (peak photon counts) versus distance and is expressed at one half of the maximum intensity (Fig. 20-10). This measurement of resolution is termed the *full width half maximum* (FWHM), with small FWHM values indicating that a camera can resolve two distinct points that are more closely spaced. For two different collimators with identical hole lengths, those with smaller diameter holes have lower sensitivity, but are able to resolve photon sources that are closely opposed. Similarly, thicker septa can also decrease sensitivity, but increase resolution. Most gamma camera systems used clinically today have a FWHM of approximately 9 mm for 140 keV Tc 99m gamma photons emitted 10 cm from the detector head. The most common collimator used in SPECT imaging is a parallel hole design, termed the *low-energy all purpose collimator*.

Scintillation Crystals

When a photon passes through a collimator, it interacts with the *scintillation crystal*. This crystal is made up of a material that converts the photon's energy to a flash of light, also known as a "scintillation event." The most common material used for scintillation crystals in gamma cameras is sodium iodide (NaI) doped with small amounts of thallium that enable the crystal to scintillate when struck with a photon. NaI crystals have a high probability of photoelectric interactions between photons with energies commonly used in imaging and produce light in proportion to the exciting photon's energy. The excited electrons return to their stable quantum state with the release of energy as light, and the amount of light produced is proportional to the energy of the exciting photon. In the case of Tc 99m photons, the scintillation event produces a flash of 410-nm light. The crystal scintillates via excitation of the crystal's electrons by Compton scatter or, most prominently, by the photoelectric effect. The potential disadvantages of NaI scintillation crystals are that they are hydroscopic (absorb moisture) and must be sealed and are very fragile. Other materials can also be used for scintillation crystals (Table 20-3).

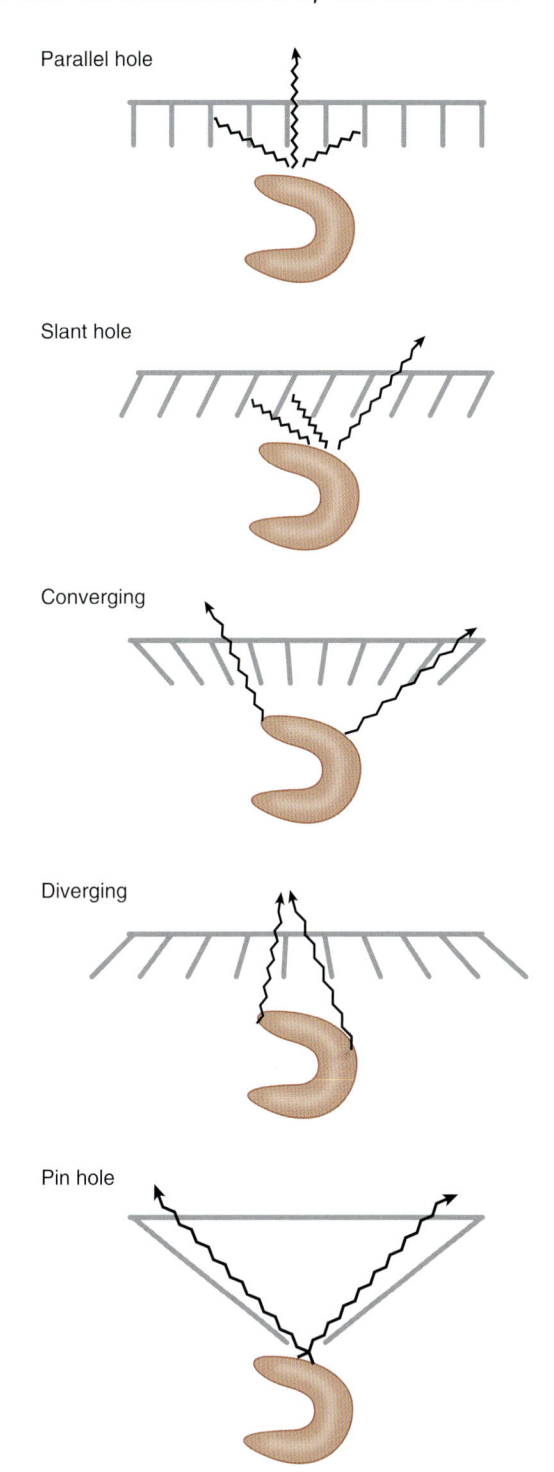

■ **FIGURE 20-9** Types of collimators used in SPECT imaging. Collimator type affects spatial resolution and magnification. The particular type of collimator employed depends on the particular imaging agents and requirements.

Photomultiplier Tubes

The flashes of light produced by the scintillation crystal are detected and converted to an electrical signal by a type of photodetector called a *photomultiplier tube*. This device is a cathode-tipped vacuum tube, which produces an electron every time it is struck by a light photon. This electron signal is "multiplied" within the tube every time

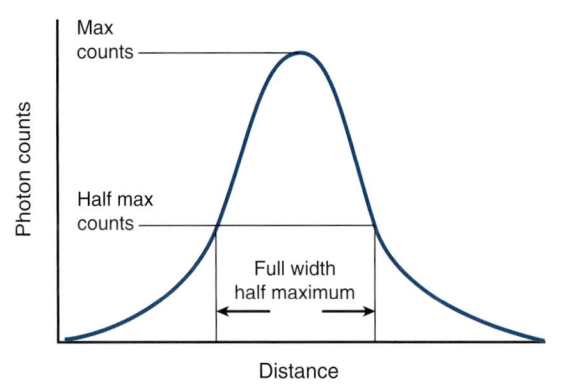

FIGURE 20-10 Example of full width half maximum plot.

an electron strikes one of the tube's dynodes to produce a measurable signal for each light emission from the scintillation crystal. The number of photons produced by the scintillation crystal is proportional to the number of photons that interact with the crystal. For each approximately 10 photons that enter a photomultiplier tube, only 1 to 3 electrons would be produced without amplification. The photomultiplier tube increases the electron output to approximately 10^5 to 10^8 electrons, however, allowing a measurable electrical signal to be available for image generation. This electronic signal that exits the photomultiplier tube is increased further using preamplifiers and amplifiers.

Multiple photomultiplier tubes are arranged in an array on top of the scintillation crystal, coupled to the scintillation crystal by an optical glass–transparent gel interface that has the same refractive index as the scintillation crystal. This glass-gel coupling is termed the *light pipe* raising the photomultiplier tubes above the surface of the scintillation crystal. This height allows for multiple tubes to visualize a scintillation event, allowing the camera array to localize the scintillation event within the X, Y plane. Event localization is one of the hallmarks of the gamma camera and allows for generation of a SPECT image (Fig. 20-11).

Event Localization

A gamma camera uses the concept of proportional energy generation from scintillation events to ascribe arithmetically each event to a particular location within the crystal. This process was initially described by Anger,[1] and is summarized as follows: Each scintillation event is simultaneously detected at multiple photomultiplier tubes, and the photomultiplier tube overlying the event receives the largest proportion of light generated from that event. Other photomultiplier tubes near to, but not directly overlying, the scintillation event receive proportionally less light from the event. The thickness of the light pipe enables simultaneous visualization of scintillation events by multiple photomultiplier tubes by elevating them a critical distance above the crystal. By integrating all of the signals from all of the photomultiplier tubes from each scintillation event using positioning circuitry, the X, Y coordinates of each scintillation event can be obtained. The "intrinsic resolution" of a particular gamma camera refers to the accuracy of the positioning circuitry and computer algorithms to determine the location of a scintillation event. "Extrinsic resolution" refers to the combination of the resolution of the collimator along with intrinsic resolution.

Energy Discrimination

In addition to being able to determine the physical location of a scintillation event, a photomultiplier array can discriminate the energy of the exciting photon. This permits the use of acquisition protocols that specifically detect scintillation events from photons from a particular radionuclide, and can allow for simultaneous acquisition of images using two radionuclides of different energies. In simplistic terms, a photomultiplier array visualizes all of the light produced by a given scintillation event, although each individual photomultiplier tube visualizes only a portion of the light. By summing all of the signals from all of the photomultiplier tubes in an array, it is possible to know the total amount of light for a given scintillation event. Because the light produced by a given scintillation event is proportional to the energy of the exciting photon, the summed signal from the photomultiplier tubes is proportional to the exciting photon's energy and is known as the "photopeak," which approximates a gaussian distribution for a given radionuclide photon emission.

In actuality, not all photons interact in a linear fashion with respect to energy and light generation because of the combined effects of Compton scatter and instrumental uncertainty. The gamma camera can be set up to acquire only events that meet certain energy criteria, or fall within an "energy window" around the photopeak. This energy window is generated by a pulse-height analyzer, which rejects the photon signals that do not fall within a predetermined range surrounding the photopeak.

TABLE 20-3 Materials Used for Scintillation Crystals

Material	Symbol	Hydroscopic	Photons per keV	Scintillation Decay Time (ns)	Use
Sodium iodide	NaI	Yes	40	230	SPECT/general nuclear imaging
Bismuth germanium oxide	BGO	No	4.8	300	PET
Cesium fluoride	CsF_2	Yes	2.5	2.5	PET
Barium fluoride	BaF_2	Minimal	6.5	0.8	PET
Lutetium orthosilicate	LSO	No	25	47	Hybrid SPECT/PET
Gadolinium orthosilicate	GSO	No	6.4	60	PET>SPECT
Plastic		No	Variable	Variable	Multiple

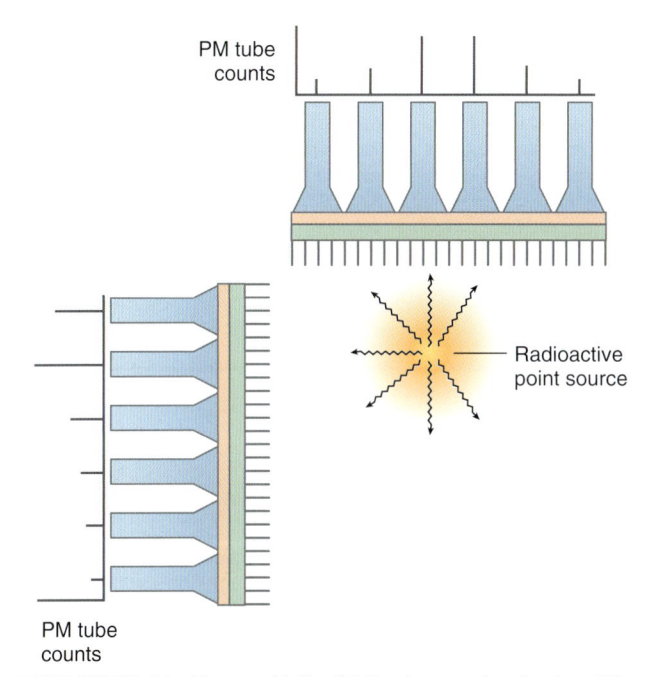

FIGURE 20-11 Photomultiplier (PM) tube event localization. When analyzing the emissions from a point source of radioactivity, the photomultiplier tubes directly overlying the point source in either the X or the Y planes detect the most scintillation events (greatest number of "counts"). Position logic circuitry is used to place this particular photon emission in a given set of X, Y coordinates.

Image Generation

When a scintillation event has been localized and falls within the required energy window for detection, the generation of an image can occur. First, the analog signal obtained from the energy peak needs to be converted to a digital signal using an analog-to-digital converter. This digital signal can be transformed from a spatial domain to a frequency domain by way of the Fourier transformation.

When the event localized digital information is in the frequency domain, it can be used for the construction of an image. Classically, SPECT images have been constructed by "back projecting" sequentially acquired planar images obtained by rotating the camera around the patient onto an imaginary center point to create the three-dimensional SPECT image. This method requires the raw projection data to be passed through a so-called ramp filter to omit certain frequencies (filter "cutoff") and enhance other frequencies ("power") to optimize image quality. This method of SPECT reconstruction is termed *filtered back projection*. Filters function to remove inherent reconstruction artifacts (particularly the "star" artifact inherent in back projection), optimize the signal-to-noise ratio in image reconstruction, and provide image enhancement. This method allows for rapid image reconstruction, but loss of image information occurs because of filtering.

Newer reconstruction algorithms have sought to reconstruct SPECT images using a mathematical computational method called *iterative reconstruction*. Iterative methods use mathematical equations to model the particular imaging physics and geometry of the acquisition and to reconstruct the image after discriminating the image into pixels. Each of these pixels represents an unknown value at the beginning of the reconstruction, which after passing the projection data through multiple "iterations" of the mathematical equations, approaches a recognizable image. This method allows for image generation in the setting of low counts, scatter, and noise. This method of image reconstruction also permits the image to be reconstructed using information acquired from an attenuation map, correcting for nonuniform attenuation. After reconstruction by filtered back projection or iterative reconstruction, a tomographic image can be displayed and statistically quantified and interpreted.

Quality Control

The performance and acquisition of reproducible and interpretable SPECT images using a gamma camera requires strict attention to quality control. Procedures are required to ensure that energy peaking, uniformity, linearity, resolution, and sensitivity fall within standard norms. The American Society of Nuclear Cardiology (www.asnc.org) has published guidelines on instrumentation quality assurance and performance,[2] which detail these quality assurance issues.

Advances in SPECT Instrumentation

Despite the validated utility over the past 40 years of the traditional gamma (Anger) camera, advances in SPECT instrumentation technology in the coming years may dramatically alter how SPECT images are acquired and processed. These advances include multidetector imaging systems that allow for a smaller size imaging system, allowing imaging rooms to use less floor space. In addition, most SPECT imaging vendors are developing improved iterative reconstruction algorithms that allow for faster (two to four times) acquisition. Last, fundamental advances in photon detector technology have the potential to change fundamentally how SPECT images are obtained. Solid-state, semiconductor-based detectors, such as cadmium zinc telluride, have the potential to improve energy and spatial resolution, decrease scan times, reduce radiation exposure, and allow for simultaneous dual-isotope imaging in small footprint imaging systems. American Society of Nuclear Cardiology guidelines (available at www.asnc.org) on the incorporation of new imaging technology will help to define when and how these new technologies should be incorporated into standard clinical practice.

CONCLUSION

Successful acquisition and interpretation of SPECT myocardial perfusion images requires knowledge and understanding of the basic physics governing radioactive decay and the interactions of radiation with matter. An understanding of these principles helps the clinician select the appropriate and safest imaging study for the patient and recognize potential sources of imaging error and artifacts. Similarly, a working knowledge of the basics of SPECT imaging instrumentation is crucial to acquiring good quality images and providing an accurate interpretation of the imaging data.

KEY POINTS

- Radiation is the transfer of energy across distance; photons carry energy at the speed of light.
- Radioactive decay can produce alpha particles, beta particles, positrons, and gamma photons.
- Photons interact with matter via the photoelectric effect, Compton scatter, and pair production.
- Attenuation occurs when photons interact with matter, proportional to the attenuation coefficient for the interacting matter.
- Gamma cameras are composed of a collimator, a scintillation crystal, a light pipe, photomultiplier tubes, a pulse-height analyzer, position circuitry, an analog-to-digital converter, and a display device.
- Future SPECT imaging systems will use advanced reconstruction methods and possibly solid-state semiconductor detectors.

SUGGESTED READINGS

Chandra R. Nuclear Medicine Physics: The Basics, 6th ed. Baltimore, Lippincott Williams & Wilkins, 2004.

Cherry SR, Sorensen JA, Phelps MC. Physics in Nuclear Medicine, 3rd ed. Philadelphia, Saunders, 2003.

Hendee WR, Ritenour ER. Medical Imaging Physics, 4th ed. New York, Wiley-Liss, 2002.

Iskandrian AE, Verani MS. Nuclear Cardiac Imaging: Principles and Applications, 3rd ed. New York, Oxford University Press, 2003.

Stefaan T, Getkin A, Grinyov B, et al. Radiation Detectors for Medical Applications, Vol 1. Dordrecht, The Netherlands, Springer, 2006.

REFERENCES

1. Anger HO. Scintillation camera. Rev Sci Instrum 1958; 29:27-33.
2. Nichols KJ, Bacharach SL, Bergmann SR, et al; Quality Assurance Committee of the American Society of Nuclear Cardiology. Instrumentation quality assurance and performance. J Nucl Cardiol 2006; 13:e25-e41.

CHAPTER 21

Clinical Single Photon Emission Computed Tomography Cardiac Protocols

Miguel Hernandez-Pampaloni

Nuclear medicine has become a remarkable diagnostic tool to identify and to stratify patients with suspected coronary artery disease (CAD) with pivotal prognostic implications. Myocardial perfusion imaging (MPI) provides an accurate measurement of coronary narrowing leading to inducible perfusion abnormalities with prognostic implications (Fig. 21-1). The relationship between the degree of coronary stenosis and the maximal hyperemic response was first reported more than 30 years ago.[1] Myocardial regions with relatively decreased post-stress radiotracer uptake and resting normalization indicate a misbalance between oxygen supply and myocardial demands, characteristic of ischemia. Nonreversible myocardial perfusion defects normally relate to necrosis or infarction. Current imaging protocols allow the accurate assessment of relative regional perfusion and myocardial function at rest and stress based on regional blood flow heterogeneity. Gated single photon emission computed tomography (SPECT) represents nearly 95% of all procedures performed today in cardiac nuclear medicine. This chapter reviews the different imaging SPECT acquisition protocols that are currently in use as well as the principal indications.

TECHNICAL REQUIREMENTS
^{201}Tl Imaging Protocols

During the last two decades, thallium 201 (^{201}Tl) has been used as a myocardial perfusion tracer. After an intravenous injection, the initial myocyte uptake is mainly determined by regional myocardial perfusion, whereas the integrity of the cell membrane is predominantly important for delayed imaging of tracer retention (potassium ion total distribution). Regional thallium activity on delayed images acquired early (3 to 4 hours) or late (8 to 72 hours) after stress has been used to demonstrate the presence and extent of viable myocardium based on the phenomenon termed *thallium redistribution*.[2] Intracellular thallium uptake through the sarcolemmal membrane is maintained during long periods if regional myocardial blood flow is sufficiently preserved to be able to deliver the isotope to the myocytes. Redistribution is thought to represent areas of ischemic but viable myocardium, whereas fixed, non-redistributing defects are thought to represent nonviable, fibrotic scar.

When ^{201}Tl alone is used, a variety of different acquisition protocols of stress imaging have been employed, including redistribution and reinjection imaging. Although different ^{201}Tl imaging protocols have been employed, stress-redistribution-reinjection and rest-redistribution SPECT imaging protocols are the most currently used to assess myocardial viability.[3] Reinjection of 1 mCi of ^{201}Tl after 3 to 4 hours of redistribution imaging detects viable tissue in 35% to 49% of segments with fixed irreversible ^{201}Tl defects with conventional stress-redistribution protocols.[4] An inverse relationship has been reported between regional thallium activity in irreversible defects and the amount of myocardial fibrosis.[5] Perrone-Filardi and colleagues[6] demonstrated the nearly linear relation between thallium activity and the likelihood of recovery of regional function after revascularization. Overall sensitivity of several stress-redistribution-reinjection studies averaged 85% with a lower specificity (averaging 47%), suggesting that this protocol tends to overestimate the potential for contractile function recovery.[2]

Rest-redistribution ^{201}Tl imaging is a valid alternative to discriminate viable from nonviable myocardium when the clinical question is to identify viability and not inducible ischemia.[7,8] Studies have reported that 24-hour imaging

Evaluation of CAD: A prognostic approach

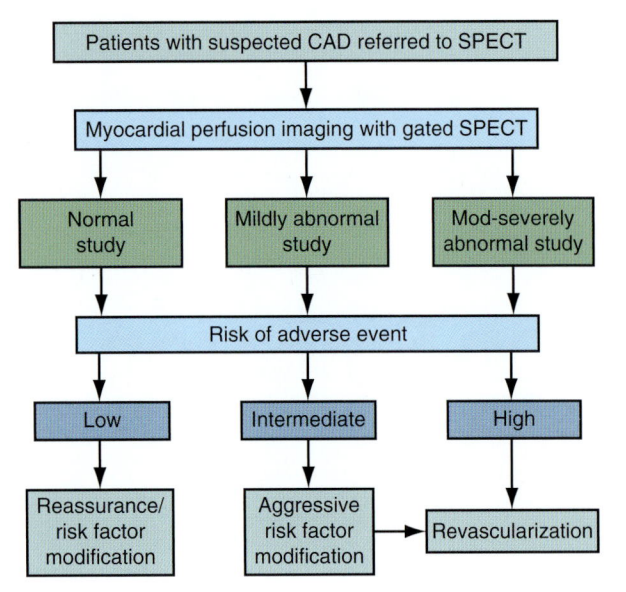

■ FIGURE 21-1 Evaluation of CAD: a prognostic approach.

after rest injection detects additional areas of viable myocardium compared with 4-hour imaging alone, possibly related to higher resting blood flow levels.[9]

Tc 99m Labeled Imaging Protocols

A technetium Tc 99m labeled compound, either sestamibi or tetrofosmin, is a synthetic lipophilic cationic perfusion agent that distributes passively across sarcolemmal and mitochondrial membranes remaining fixed to the mitochondria. A negative mitochondrial gradient charge is essential for its accumulation and retention within the myocyte. Unlike ^{201}Tl, it does not redistribute over time. This lack of significant redistribution means that separate rest and stress injections are standard with ^{99m}Tc-labeled compounds. Different acquisition protocols can be used with these agents, including 2-day stress/rest, same-day rest/stress, same-day stress/rest, and dual-isotope protocols.

Two-Day Protocol

From a technical point of view, to optimize imaging quality, the 2-day stress/rest is one of the most preferred acquisition protocols. The main advantage is the use of two high doses of Tc 99m labeled compounds, which enables high-quality images to be obtained because of the elevated high count rate. The stress study should be performed first because the rest study can be omitted if the stress study is normal. Obviously, the major disadvantage is the delay in reporting of the final analysis.

One-Day Protocol

This is probably the most commonly employed protocol with low-dose rest/high-dose stress; its major drawback is the risk of reducing the stress image's contrast; up to 15% of the radiotracer uptake observed at the time of stress imaging comes from the preexisting resting myocardial distribution. The order sequence for this protocol should be related to the main indication. If the study is performed for the diagnosis of myocardial ischemia, the stress portion should be done first because that will avoid the reduction of contrast that a previously resting injection would have on a stress-induced defect. If detection of viable myocardium or assessment of the reversibility of a perfusion defect is the indication, performance of the resting study first may be preferable.

As with all Tc 99m labeled compounds, imaging should begin between 60 and 90 minutes after injection to allow hepatobiliary clearance and to minimize subdiaphragmatic activity if vasodilators were administered. To enhance the washout of gastrointestinal activity from liver and gallbladder, fluids or a fatty meal can be suggested.

Regarding viability assessment, earlier studies using primarily planar scintigraphy and visual interpretation suggested that Tc 99m sestamibi underestimates myocardial viability in chronic CAD and left ventricular dysfunction. Dilsizian and colleagues[10] described the utility of quantitative Tc 99m sestamibi imaging when the severity of decrease in Tc 99m sestamibi uptake within irreversible defects was considered or when an additional redistribution image was acquired after the rest injection for detection of dysfunctional but viable myocardium. A significant inverse linear relationship has been described between Tc 99m sestamibi uptake and myocardial fibrosis in biopsy specimens.[11] Several approaches have been introduced to increase the diagnostic performance of Tc 99m sestamibi for the identification of viable myocardium, such as functional evaluation of the left ventricle by first-pass radionuclide ventriculography, gated SPECT acquisition perfusion images,[12] and intravenous administration of nitrates to reduce resting hypoperfusion and to increase the correspondence of the resting images with myocardial viability.[13]

Fatty acid analogues marked with iodine isotopes (^{123}I, ^{131}I) have been employed to study myocardial metabolism on the basis of the principle that in a viable but ischemic myocardium, fatty acids are mainly esterified and incorporated into the triglyceride and phospholipid blood pool and are slowly metabolized, with subsequent clearance rate reduction.[14] Early data suggested that this method may provide data comparable to ^{201}Tl protocols in patients with left ventricular dysfunction or after an acute myocardial infarction. These tracers may prove to be of more value in the near future, considering the key role that oxidative metabolism plays in preservation of myocardial function.

Dual-Isotope Protocols

Dual-isotope imaging protocols using Tc 99m labeled compounds and ^{201}Tl are based on the ability of the Anger camera to collect data from the two different energy windows representing each radiotracer. Simultaneous and separate dual-isotope imaging protocols have been described.[15,16] Two of the major advantages of these protocols are the possibility of shortening the duration of a complete stress or rest redistribution protocol and the superior capability of ^{201}Tl to assess myocardial viability. Separate acquisition times can reduce the necessity of downscatter correction that can diminish ^{201}Tl contrast images, leading to an overestimation of defect reversibility; this can be achieved by acquiring ^{201}Tl data sets before the administration of Tc 99m because of the very limited (2.2%) contribution of ^{201}Tl into the Tc 99m energy window.

Gated SPECT

Most of the current imaging protocols perform a simultaneous ECG gating during at least the stress data set acquisition.[17] Gated SPECT can be performed with ^{201}Tl or Tc 99m compounds. One of the major advantages is the possibility of measuring contractile function and the left ventricular ejection fraction.

STRESS PROTOCOLS

The primary aim of stress MPI is to detect CAD and to risk stratify those patients with known CAD. To achieve this goal, SPECT MPI is based on the assessment of the relative regional blood flow perfusion to myocardial regions supplied by stenotic vessels and its comparison with myocardial territories supplied by normal vessels. The principal difference between stress methods relates to the mechanisms used to disclose regional myocardial blood flow abnormalities as an indication of coronary stenosis. It is critical to select the most appropriate test by the indication on a patient by patient basis. When the goal is to evaluate exercise tolerance, the duration of the exercise, symptoms developed, and hemodynamic changes are the primary factors to consider. On the other hand, if the aim is to detect CAD or to risk stratify the patient, the factors that determine myocardial oxygen demand are the most important to take into account.

Exercise Testing

This is the most common form of stress during MPI. Exercise testing is performed on the treadmill according to the Bruce protocols and allows the assessment of different hemodynamic variables, such as exercise capacity, blood pressure, and heart rate responses. It is imperative that the intravenous injection of the radiotracer be performed at maximal stress and that exercise continue for at least an additional 60 seconds to ensure optimal myocardial concentration. The traditional goal of the test as an acceptable level of cardiac workload has been the achievement of at least 85% of the maximum predicted heart rate (220 − age). Prognostic information from the exercise test should be integrated with MPI because the patients with mild to moderate perfusion defects who achieved a heart rate higher than 80% had a very low risk for major cardiac events and cardiac death.[18] At the same time, patients with a reported normal MPI study but abnormal heart rate reserve were at the same risk for suffering a major cardiac event as those with normal heart rate reserve achieved and abnormal MPI studies (Tables 21-1 and 21-2). A maximal stress test may satisfy diagnostic purposes if it goes beyond the hemodynamic threshold of triggering the ischemic symptoms. However, it may not reveal the full amount of jeopardized myocardium and may be inadequate for the evaluation of cardiac risk in a patient scheduled to have major noncardiac surgery. A submaximal exercise test (not achieving 85% of the targeted heart rate) may still be a valid alternative for evaluation of ischemic risks after cardiac events. To achieve the most adequate level of cardiac stress and to avoid suboptimal stress testing, patients should discontinue antianginal medications (β blockers and calcium blockers for 36 to 48 hours and long-acting nitrates for 12 hours).[19] Furthermore, all patients should be studied in the fasting state, having been in a nothing-by-mouth status for at least 4 hours before the study, regardless of the stress method to be employed. All caffeine, including beverages and chocolate, especially before pharmacologic stress testing, should be avoided for at least 24 to 48 hours to avoid block of the endothelial receptors and their dilatory effect.

Pharmacologic Stress Protocols

These tests are generally performed in those patients who cannot achieve an adequate level of exercise. The two types of drugs used for pharmacologic stress are vasodilators and inotropics such as dobutamine. Coronary local autoregulatory mechanisms maintain adequate regional blood flow at rest, even when a significant coronary stenosis is present. For this reason, patients may be asymptomatic at rest, having normal myocardial perfusion studies. The hyperemic pharmacologic stress response is based on the ability of the coronary vessel to preserve its vasodilatory response. When this autoregulation fails, the vessel is unable to augment the supply required for an increased demand, producing therefore a related image defect. This is a manifestation of a decreased coronary flow reserve when it is considered as the ratio between the peak myocardial blood flow achieved at stress and its counterpart at rest. Thus, a hemodynamically significant

TABLE 21-1 Exercise Protocols

Bicycle or treadmill
Maximal exercise and at least 85% of age-predicted maximum heart rate
Monitor ECG continuously (9 or 12 leads)
Blood pressure recorded every 2 to 3 minutes
Tracer injection at peak exercise; keep exercising for at least 1 additional minute
Assess electrical changes or symptoms

TABLE 21-2 Exercise Stress Contraindications

Acute aortic dissection
Symptomatic aortic stenosis
Uncontrolled cardiac arrhythmias
Severe pulmonary hypertension
Acute myocardial infarction within the last 5 days
Uncontrolled, severe hypertension (blood pressure > 200/110 mm Hg)
Decompensated congestive heart failure
Uncontrolled unstable angina

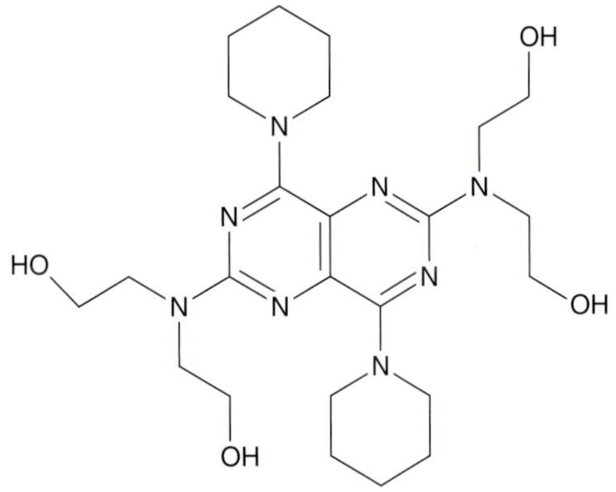

FIGURE 21-2 Structure of dipyridamole.

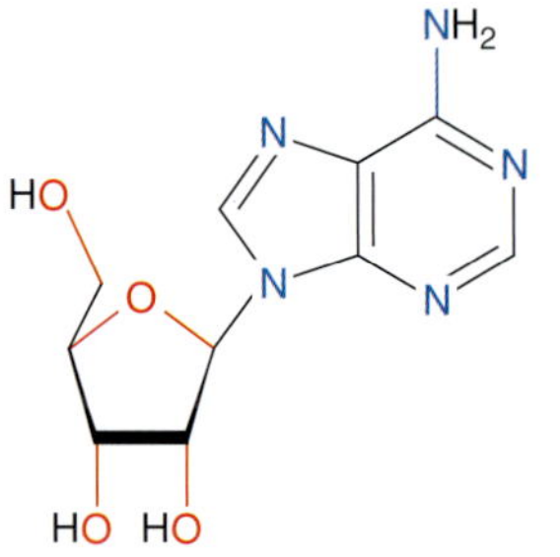

FIGURE 21-3 Structure of adenosine.

coronary narrowing could be defined by a blunted coronary flow reserve in the presence of hyperemic stress; the greater the stress and the related increase in flow in normal vessels, the greater the possibility of identifying those regions with different degrees of coronary stenosis. Normal vessels increase their blood flow four to five times after adequate stress. Current SPECT instruments allow the detection of regional perfusion distribution when there is a 30% change in radiotracer concentration.

Vasodilators

Dipyridamole and adenosine are the most commonly used coronary vasodilators (Figs. 21-2 and 21-3). Briefly, dipyridamole is a pyrimidopyrimidine that has been widely used since 1987. Its blocks the cellular reuptake of adenosine, increasing its extracellular concentration, which produces vasodilation. Dipyridamole denies the extracellular access to the activity of red cell membrane–bound adenosine deaminase. The coronary dilating effect is related to the A_2 receptor binding and activation mediated by G proteins, which ultimately result in vascular smooth muscle relaxation and vasodilation. The stimulation of the A_1 receptor in the sinus and atrioventricular nodes reduces the sinus rate and the atrioventricular conduction that may cause heart block during stress testing.

Individuals with normal coronary arteries increase their blood flow up to four times of the resting levels. In patients with CAD, there is heterogeneity of perfusion without ischemia that may be observed in cases of severe CAD, often in association with a coronary steal.[20] It has been reported that diagnostic accuracy for the detection of CAD with pharmacologic stress MPI is similar to that with exercise MPI, despite the fact that coronary flow may be increased to a greater degree than during exercise. Symptomatic myocardial ischemia is less commonly produced with vasodilators, possibly owing to the lower oxygen demands as opposed to exercise.[21] Unlike with exercise, patients are instructed to withhold the use of methylxanthines, such as theophylline and caffeine, for at least 24 hours before the study to minimize interference with vasodilators due to the competition for the adenosine receptors. As with exercise, it appears preferable to withhold antianginal medications and calcium blockers for at least 24 hours before imaging; some studies have suggested that they may diminish the extent of myocardial perfusion defects.[22] On the other hand, patients with known CAD should be imaged without withholding of medications, similar to exercise testing, to evaluate the effect of medical therapy.

A mild increase in the incidence of ischemia has been described by the addition of low-level exercise to the pharmacologic stress, which may add more diagnostic sensitivity to the test. The low-level exercise reduces the splanchnic blood flow and therefore the liver uptake of the radiopharmaceuticals.[23]

Dipyridamole is infused intravenously at rest, in the supine position, at a rate of 0.142 mg/kg/min for 4 minutes for a total dose of 0.57 mg/kg. The maximal vasodilator effect is achieved 3 minutes after completion of the infusion, the time of injection of the radiopharmaceutical. It persists at this level for 30 to 60 minutes. Injection of the radiotracer can be done earlier than 7 to 8 minutes if severe hemodynamic effects develop or clear symptoms are noted or there are acute ischemic ECG changes that can jeopardize the safety of the test. A wide range of side effects occur in up to 30% to 40% of all patients. They are mostly mild and nonspecific and should be accepted as an indicator of the drug effect. They include symptoms such as chest discomfort, dizziness, shortness of breath, and headache.[24] Side effects are commonly reversed with a single intravenous dose of aminophylline (75 to 125 mg), although the dose may have to be repeated on some occasions, or rarely nitroglycerin is used. Aminophylline occupies endothelial adenosine binding sites and ends dipyridamole-induced vasodilation. Aminophylline is administered 3 to 4 minutes after administration of the radionuclide to allow adequate time for radiotracer extraction, and then the dipyridamole test is ended. It should be given slowly, however, to avoid some of its own side effects, including nausea, tachycardia, and hypotension. Unlike with adenosine, whose hemodynamic effects occur during the drug infusion, a fall in blood pressure and an increase in heart rate occur when the dipyridamole infusion is completed. There is generally no significant change in the double product and myocardial oxygen demand.

Adenosine is a heterocyclic compound with a purine base and ribose, synthesized intracellularly through the breakdown of adenosine triphosphate (ATP) through the S-adenosylhomocysteine pathways. During myocardial ischemia, there is ATP breakdown; the generated adenosine binds the endothelial A_2 receptors, dilates the coronary arteries, and restores flow. Adenosine has a partial A_1

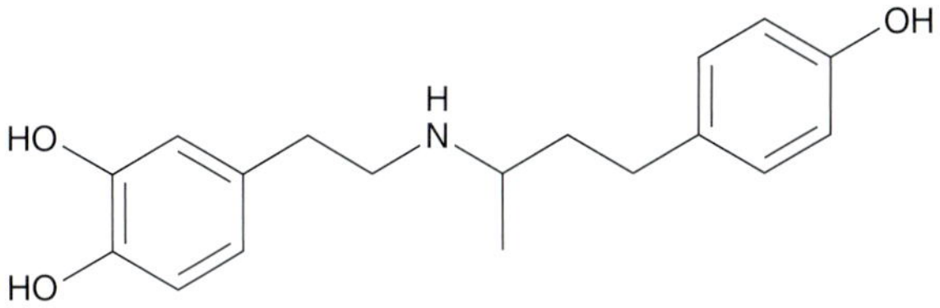

FIGURE 21-4 Structure of dobutamine.

receptor effect and can decrease the heart rate and attenuate the effects of β-adrenergic agonists, causing bronchospasm. However, even patients with a history of bronchospasm may be studied safely if symptoms are controlled with sympathomimetic inhalers or steroids.

Adenosine is infused intravenously at a standard dose of 140 μg/kg/min during 4 to 6 minutes, with administration of the radiopharmaceutical at 2 minutes with a 4-minute infusion or at 3 minutes with the 6-minute infusion protocol. Because of the very limited (several seconds) half-life of adenosine, the number of side effects are generally time limited. The only major side effect is an increased risk of heart block; thus, adenosine is considered to be contraindicated in patients with second-degree atrioventricular block and sick sinus syndrome. Common episodes of atrioventricular block are normally overridden by the vagolytic effect of the drug, and they do not produce severe symptoms or cerebral hypoperfusion. ST segment depression has been reported in approximately 15% of those patients with adenosine-induced chest pain, which occurs in a third of the patients tested with this drug. Because of the potency of adenosine, it must be administered through a pump infusion. Like dipyridamole, it may be irritative for the skin and should be infused through a large proximal vein.

Inotropic Agents

Dobutamine, an adrenergic agonist, is generally used in patients with severe chronic obstructive pulmonary disease or asthma (Fig. 21-4). Dobutamine stimulates α_1 receptors and β_1 receptors, increasing myocardial contractility, and β_2 receptors, which may cause hypotension due to peripheral vasodilation. As a consequence, there is an increase in heart rate, systolic blood pressure, cardiac output, and stroke volume. The cardiac effect varies, depending on the infused dose. At doses up to 10 μg/kg/min, dobutamine preferentially stimulates α_1 and β_1 receptors to increase contractility, making it a good tool for assessment of myocardial viability. Increased chronotropic effects occur at higher doses, with a subsequent increase in contractility and thickening that may be useful for identification of hibernating myocardium. When it is performed with echocardiography, the infusion is stopped when wall motion abnormalities develop. Dobutamine infusion should be maintained while the radiotracer is distributed. In recent years, different protocols have been recommended.[25]

Dobutamine is infused in a stepwise increased titration at 3-minute intervals, from low (5 to 10 μg/kg/min) to high (40 μg/kg/min) doses, with increments that are based on the patient's symptoms to produce ischemia. The endpoint of the dobutamine test is a true ischemic response.

The main side effect is nonsustained tachycardia; however, because of its ischemic mechanism, it has increased risks for development of serious events in patients with known severe proximal CAD or dynamic coronary syndromes. Because of its peripheral vasodilatory effect, dobutamine has been described to produce hypotension at higher doses in 20% of the patients.[26] β Blockers are the antidote to dobutamine side effects. Esmolol drip should also be available in serious situations because of the short half-life of dobutamine (2.4 minutes). Dobutamine has been reported to have a diagnostic sensitivity of 91% and specificity of 86% in patients with suspected CAD.[27] Dobutamine stress SPECT is more sensitive than dobutamine echocardiography, and it is generally used as an alternative to dipyridamole or adenosine in the presence of their contraindications. Dobutamine is the only pharmacologic stress for use with echocardiography.

BASIC IMAGE INTERPRETATION

Location, size, and intensity of the perfusion defect are determined by the conventional correlation of image findings with anatomic relationships, generally the 17-segment model of the left ventricle standardized by the American Society of Nuclear Cardiology. Determination of the degree of reversibility is made by visual or semiquantitative comparison between the post-stress images and the resting data sets.

Transient, stress-induced cavitary dilation has been demonstrated in planar and SPECT studies, being related to either true enlargement or induced subendocardial ischemia. It has been related to a higher likelihood of major cardiac events and death.

As a general rule, use of a computer monitor and a linear color scale is recommended to interpret the results, even though the gray scale has been largely used as well. It is critical to follow a systematic approach to the images and to properly align stress and rest images, displayed on the three standard image sets—short axis, vertical long axis, and horizontal long axis (Figs. 21-5 to 21-16). Review of the projection (raw) data is crucial to provide evidence for motion of the patient that would create artifacts and reduce diagnostic accuracy. Projection data also provide information on the cardiac size and other potential areas of thoracic radiotracer uptake, such as lung uptake. Lung uptake in the presence of reversible perfusion defects is another sign of more severe disease. Although it is sometimes difficult to fully appreciate lung uptake in SPECT images, additional projection images should help accurately identify this finding.[28] Extracardiac radiopharmaceutical activity may reflect a variety of neoplastic lesions, either primary or metastatic, that may involve the lung, breast, thyroid, parathyroid glands, mediastinum, or liver. In addition, intense subdiaphragmatic activity from the gastrointestinal tract or from the liver may confound the interpretation of the inferior wall by creating virtual perfusion defects, or it may obscure the presence of a true perfusion abnormality. When substantial activity is noted in the gastrointestinal tract, the image acquisition should be repeated. Soft tissue attenuation, such as breast activity, may reduce the specificity for the detection of CAD.

Text continued on p. 296

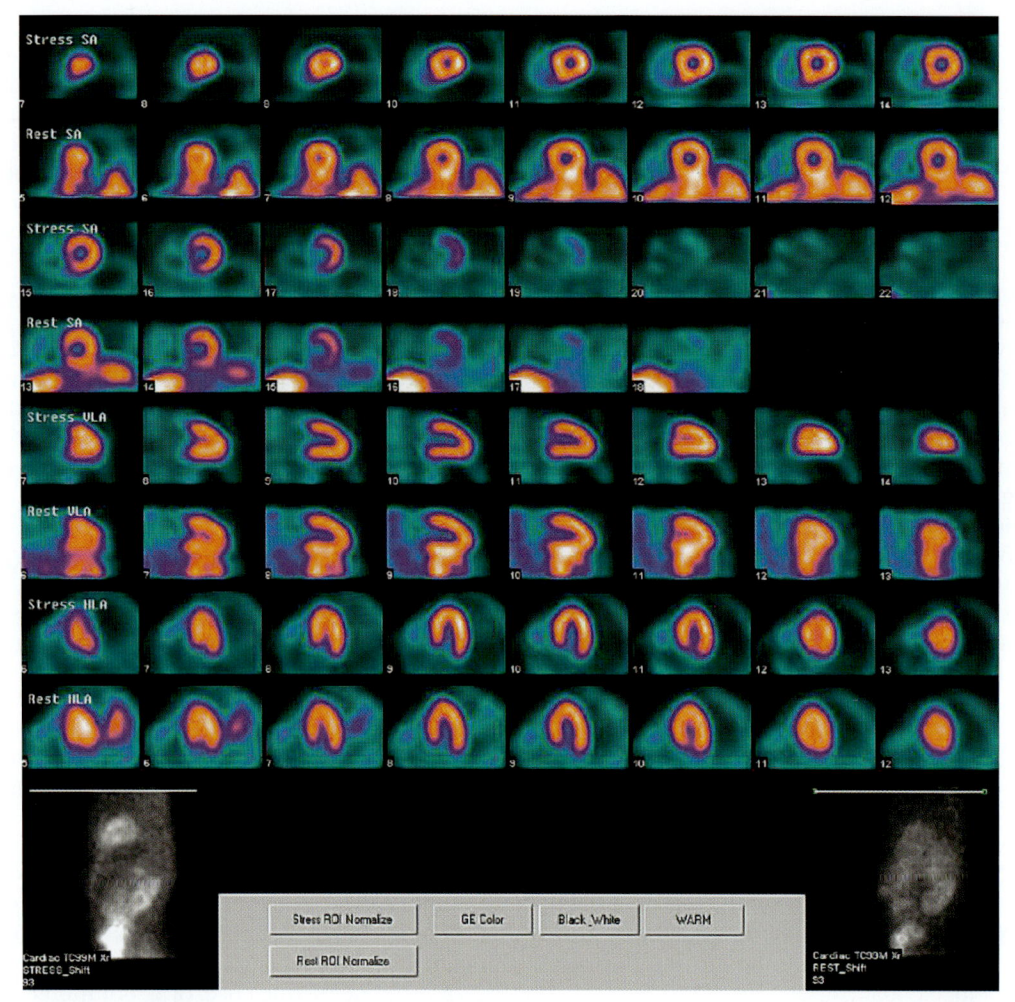

FIGURE 21-5 Stress/rest Tc 99m sestamibi short-axis, vertical long-axis, and horizontal long-axis left ventricular images showing a homogeneous tracer distribution along the entire left ventricle.

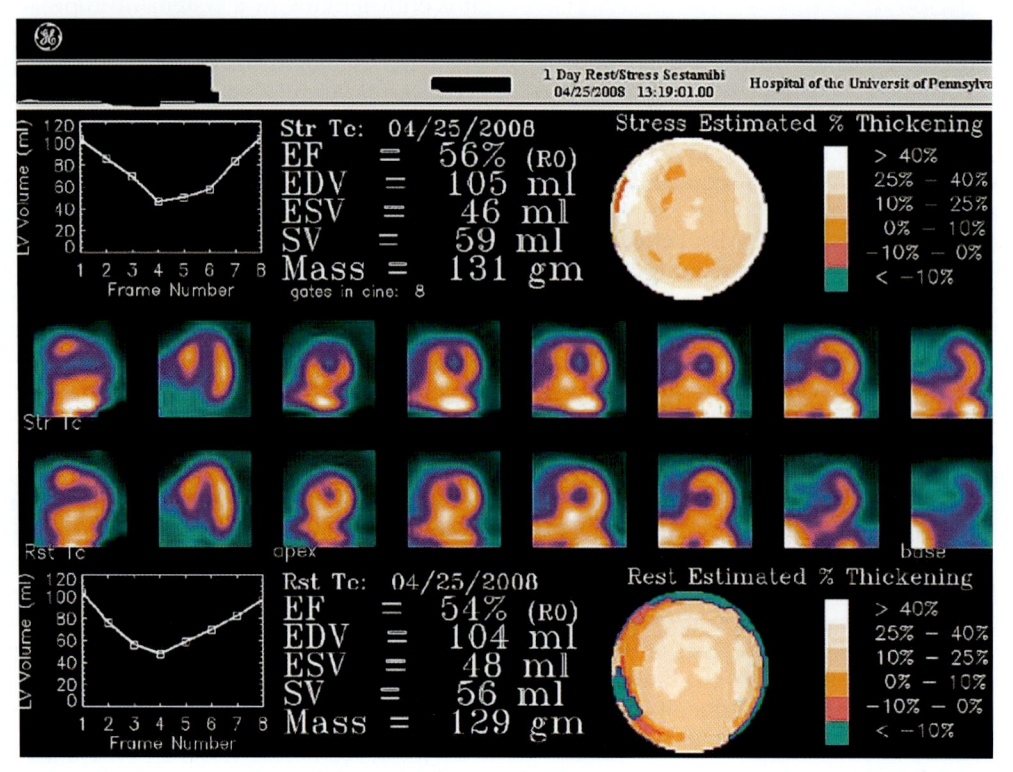

FIGURE 21-6 Stress/rest Tc 99m sestamibi gated short-axis left ventricular images showing normal left ventricular ejection fraction and volumes.

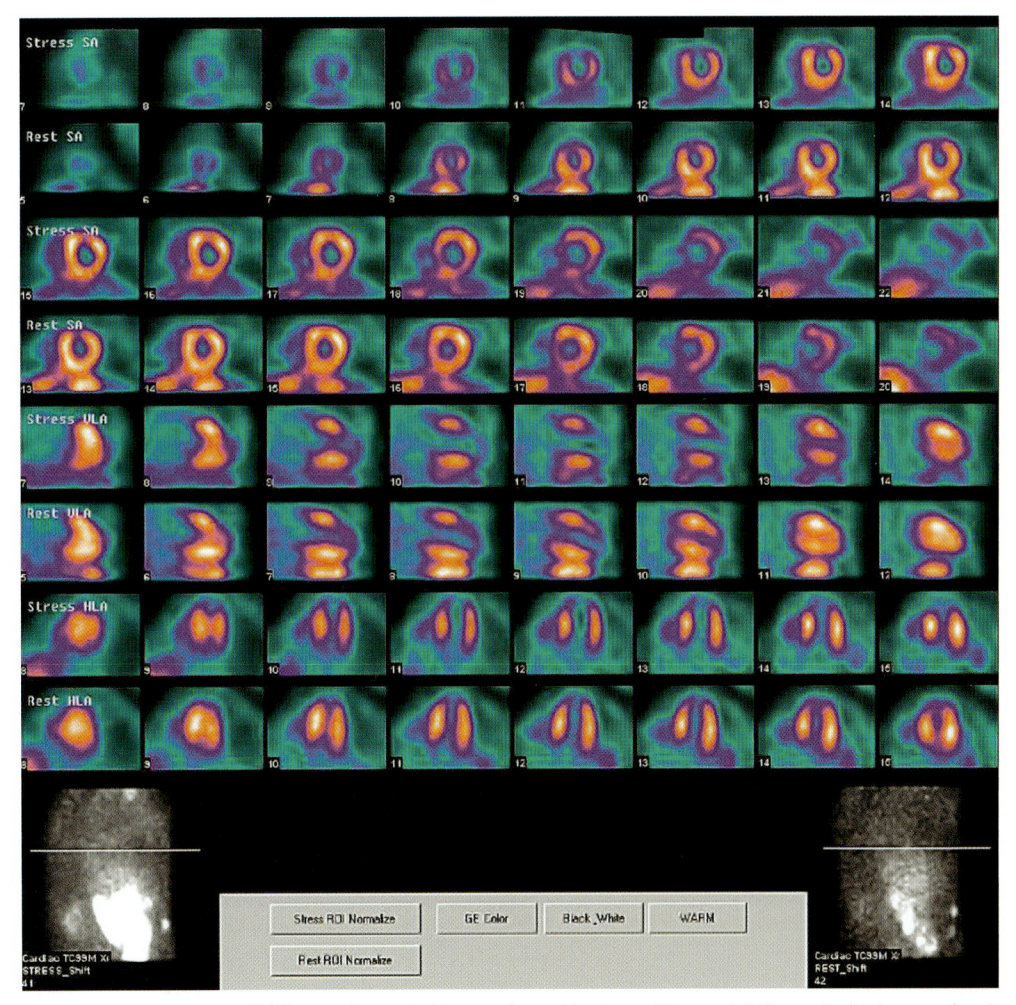

■ **FIGURE 21-7** Stress/rest Tc 99m sestamibi short-axis, vertical long-axis, and horizontal long-axis left ventricular images showing a moderate, predominantly fixed myocardial perfusion defect, representing infarct or scar, with mild reversible ischemia, in the mid to distal anterior wall and the apex, likely corresponding to a stenosis in the territory of the left anterior descending coronary artery.

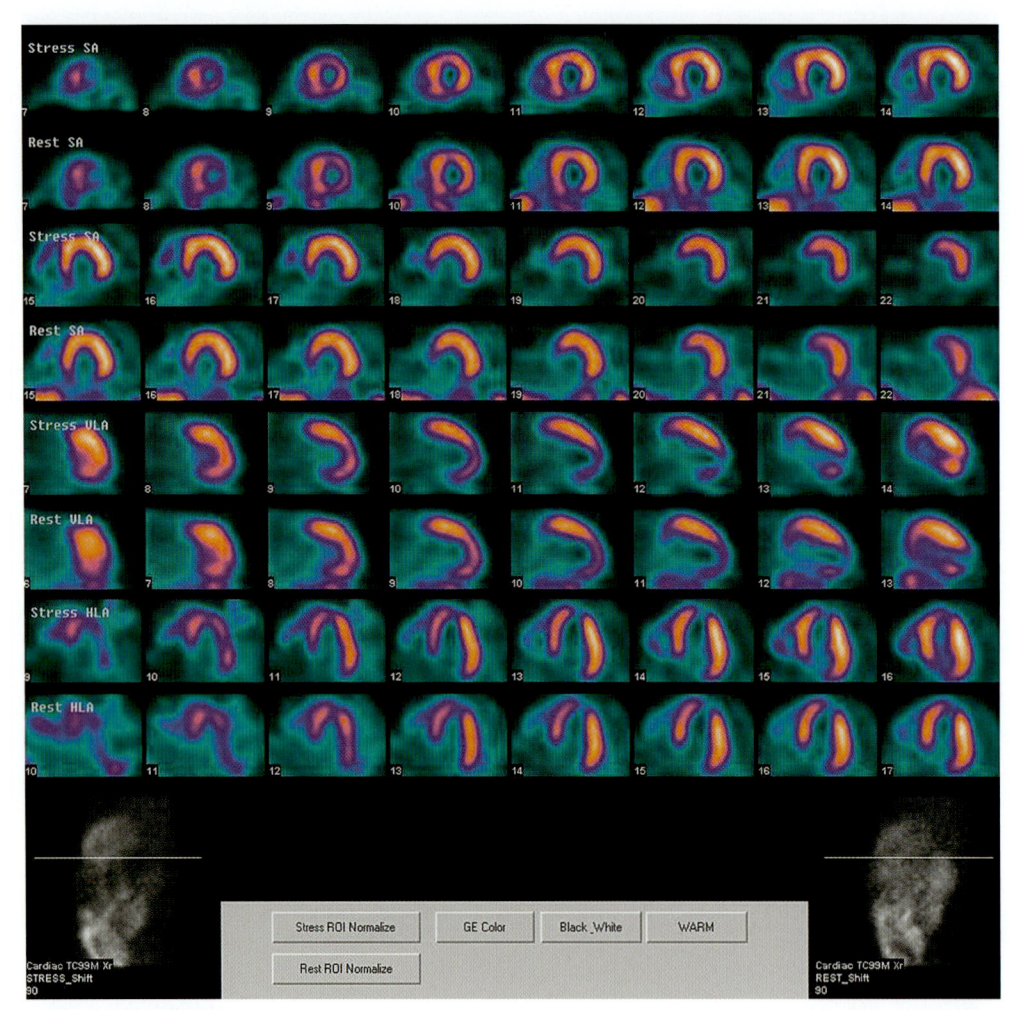

■ **FIGURE 21-8** Stress/rest Tc 99m sestamibi short-axis, vertical long-axis, and horizontal long-axis left ventricular images showing a severe, fixed myocardial perfusion defect in the inferior wall, consistent with previous infarct or myocardial necrosis.

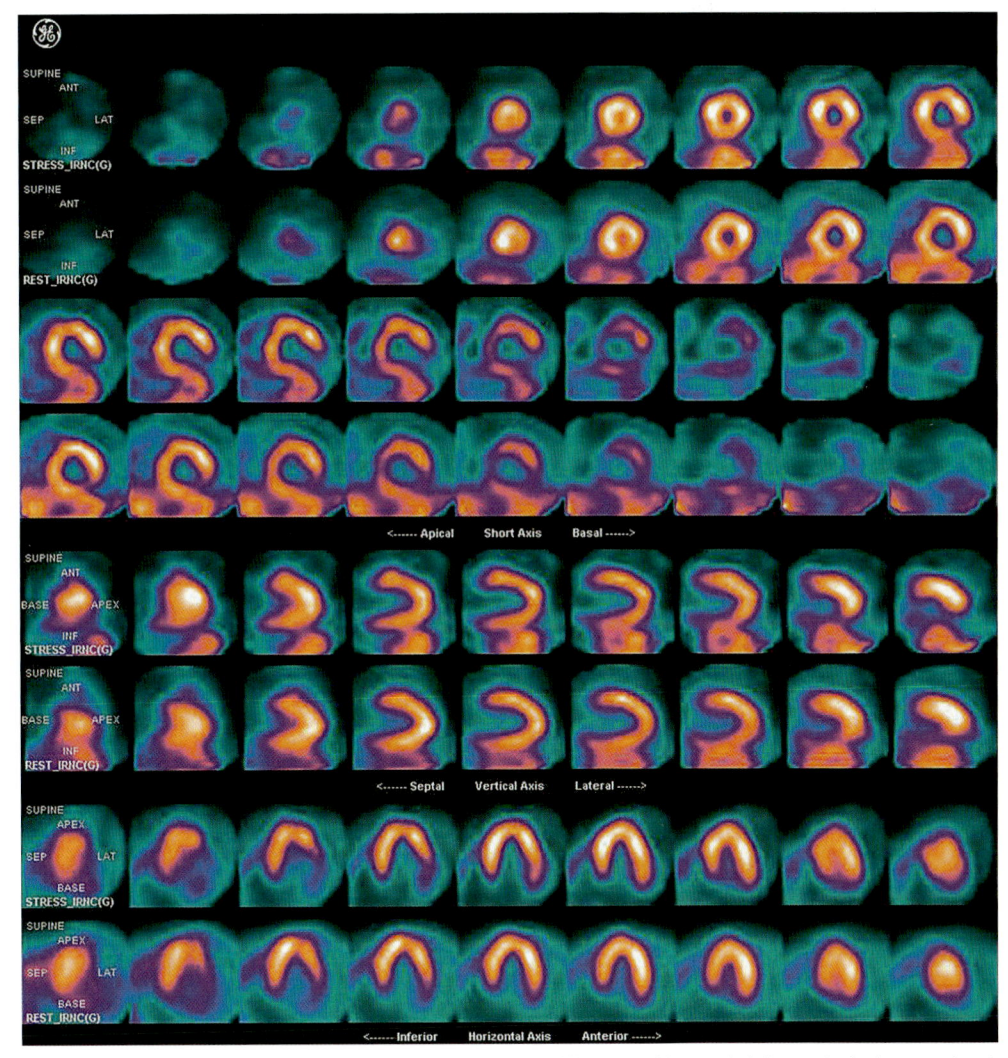

■ **FIGURE 21-9** Stress/rest Tc 99m sestamibi short-axis, vertical long-axis, and horizontal long-axis left ventricular images showing a severe, fixed myocardial perfusion defect in the inferolateral wall from the base to the mid ventricular wall, with no reversibility, consistent with a previous infarct or myocardial necrosis.

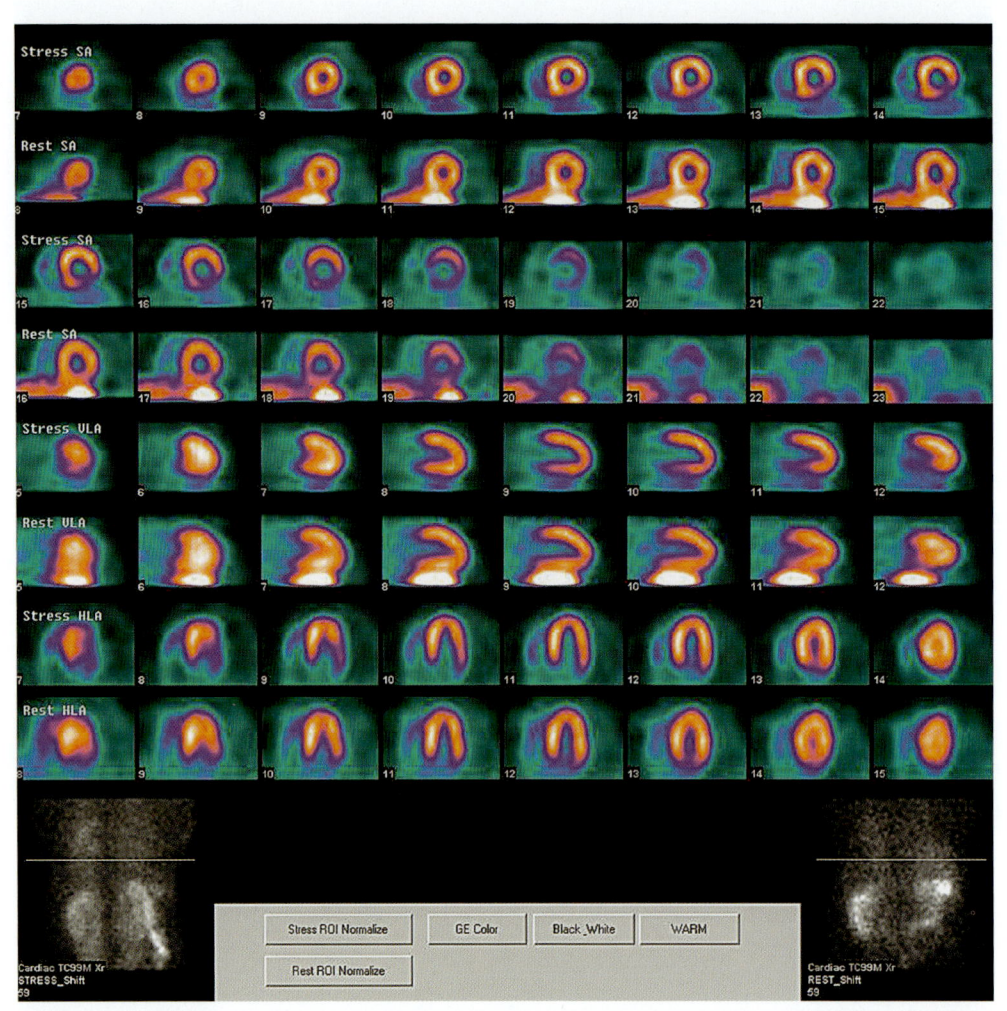

■ **FIGURE 21-10** Stress/rest Tc 99m sestamibi short-axis, vertical long-axis, and horizontal long-axis left ventricular images showing a myocardial perfusion defect in the inferior wall at stress, moderate in size and intensity, with complete reversibility at rest, consistent with myocardial ischemia in the territory of the right coronary artery.

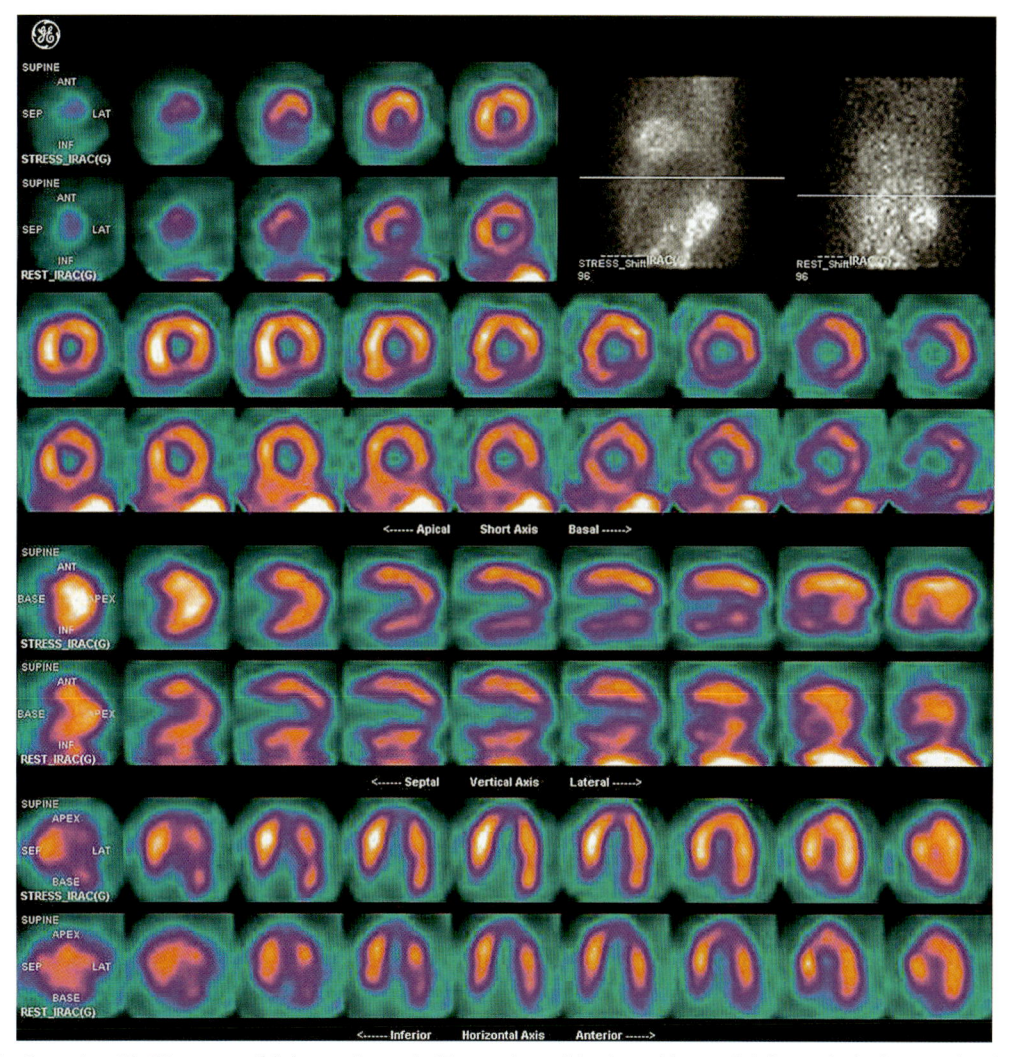

FIGURE 21-11 Stress/rest Tc 99m sestamibi short-axis, vertical long-axis, and horizontal long-axis left ventricular images showing a fixed myocardial perfusion defect in the distal inferior wall and the apex, moderate in intensity and mild in size, consistent with prior infarct or myocardial necrosis.

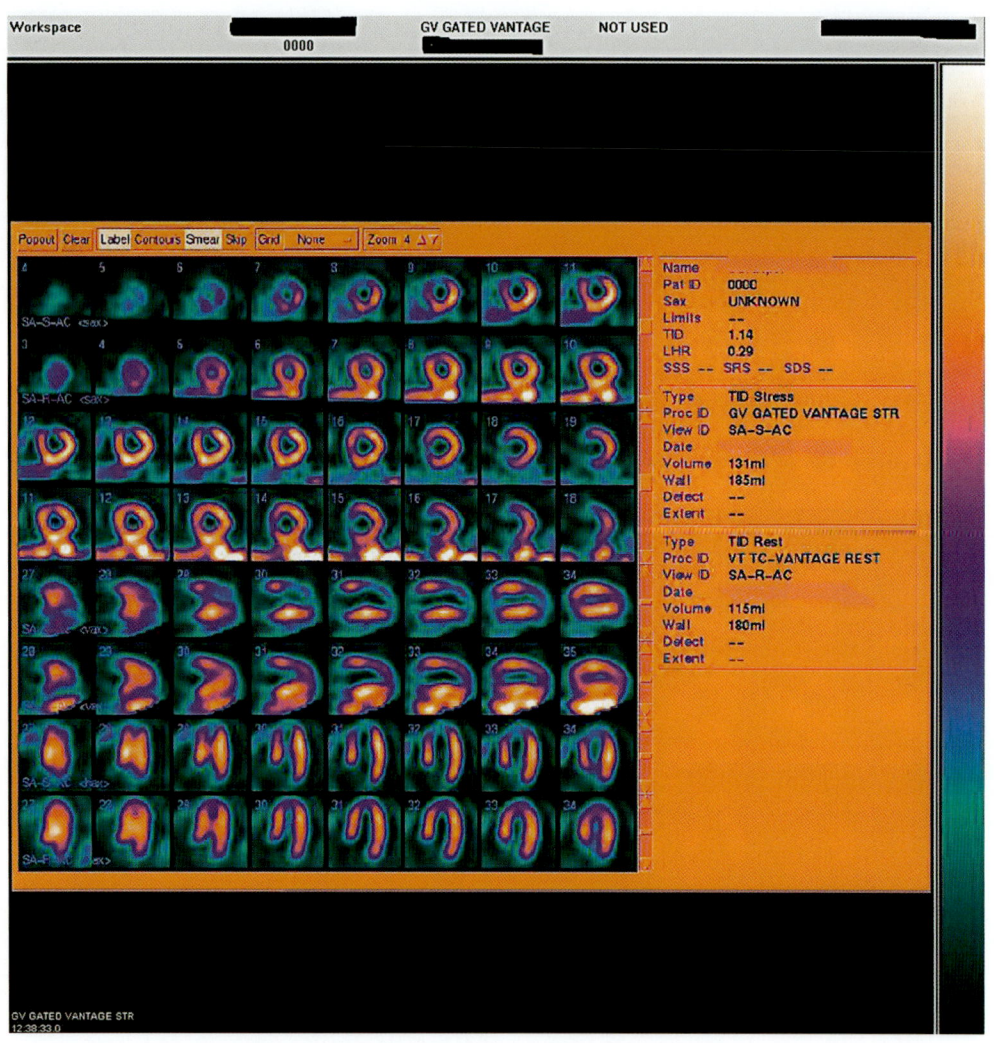

■ **FIGURE 21-12** Stress/rest Tc 99m sestamibi short-axis, vertical long-axis, and horizontal long-axis left ventricular images showing a stress-induced myocardial perfusion defect in the mid to distal anterior wall, severe in intensity and moderate in size, with partial perfusion reversibility at rest, consistent with myocardial ischemia in the territory of the left anterior descending coronary artery.

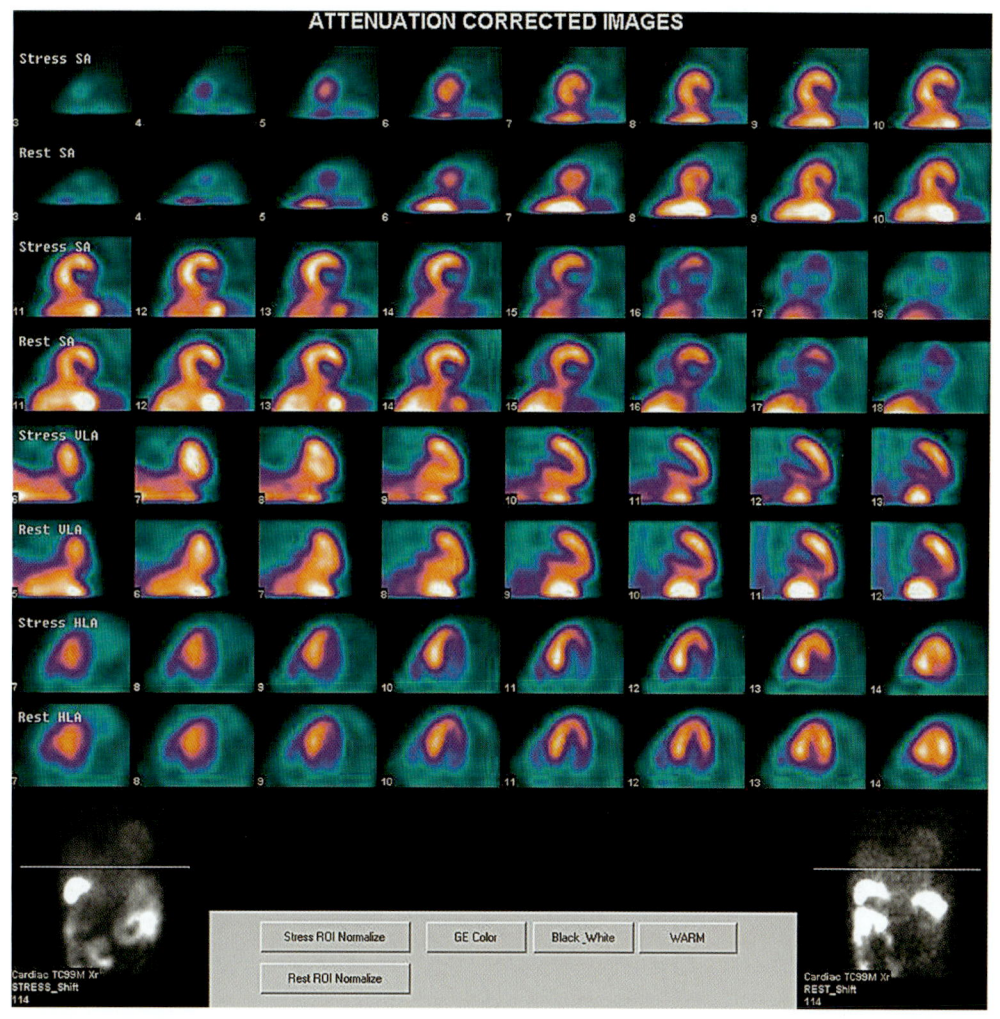

CHAPTER 21 ● *Clinical Single Photon Emission Computed Tomography Cardiac Protocols* 293

■ **FIGURE 21-13** Stress/rest Tc 99m sestamibi short-axis, vertical long-axis, and horizontal long-axis left ventricular images showing a stress-induced myocardial perfusion defect in the upper lateral wall, moderate in size and intensity, with partial to complete reversibility at rest, consistent with myocardial ischemia in the territory of the circumflex coronary artery.

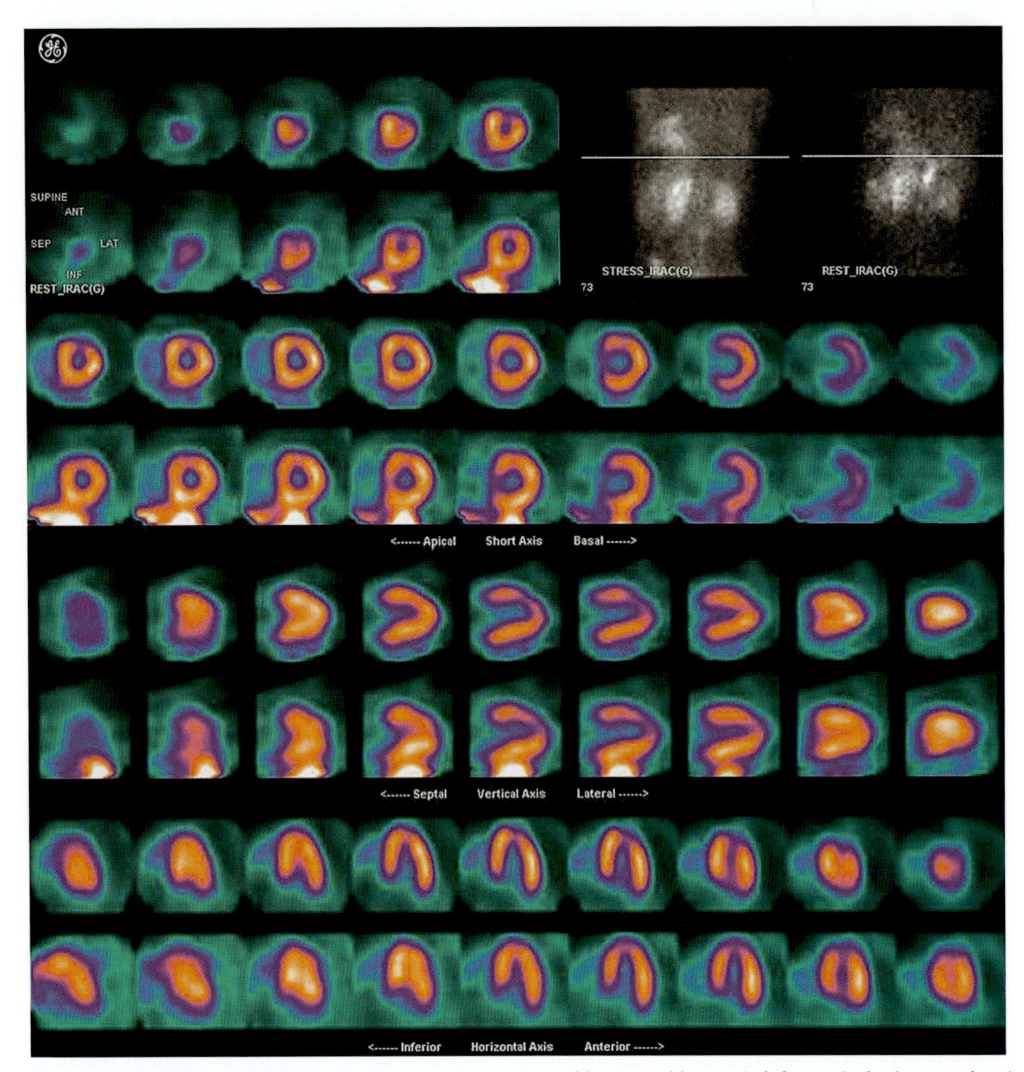

■ **FIGURE 21-14** Stress/rest Tc 99m sestamibi short-axis, vertical long-axis, and horizontal long-axis left ventricular images showing a small distal anterior wall, stress-induced myocardial perfusion defect, with total reversibility at rest, suggestive of myocardial ischemia in the territory of the left descending coronary artery.

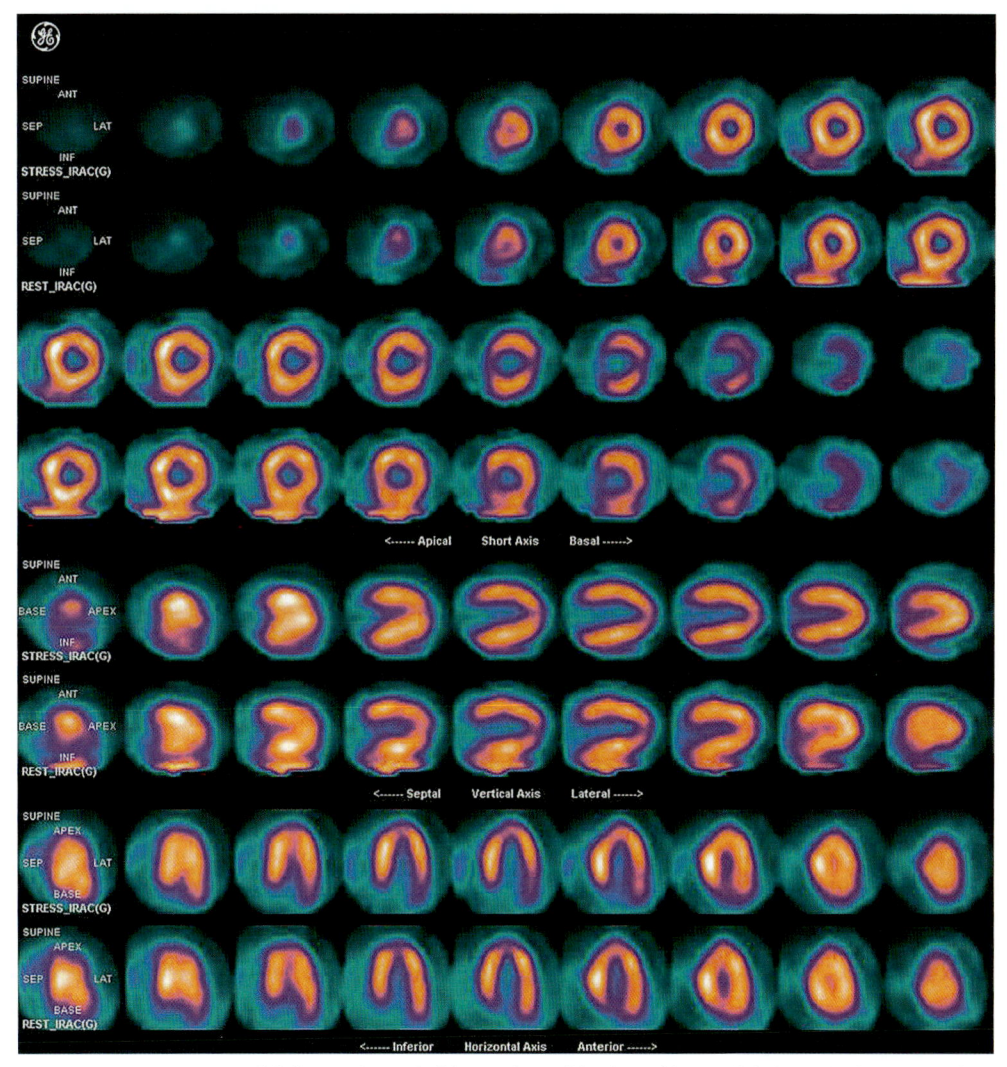

CHAPTER 21 • Clinical Single Photon Emission Computed Tomography Cardiac Protocols 295

■ **FIGURE 21-15** Stress/rest Tc 99m sestamibi short-axis, vertical long-axis, and horizontal long-axis left ventricular images showing a small, mild stress–induced myocardial perfusion defect in the mid lateral wall, with complete reversibility, suggestive of myocardial ischemia in the territory of the circumflex coronary artery.

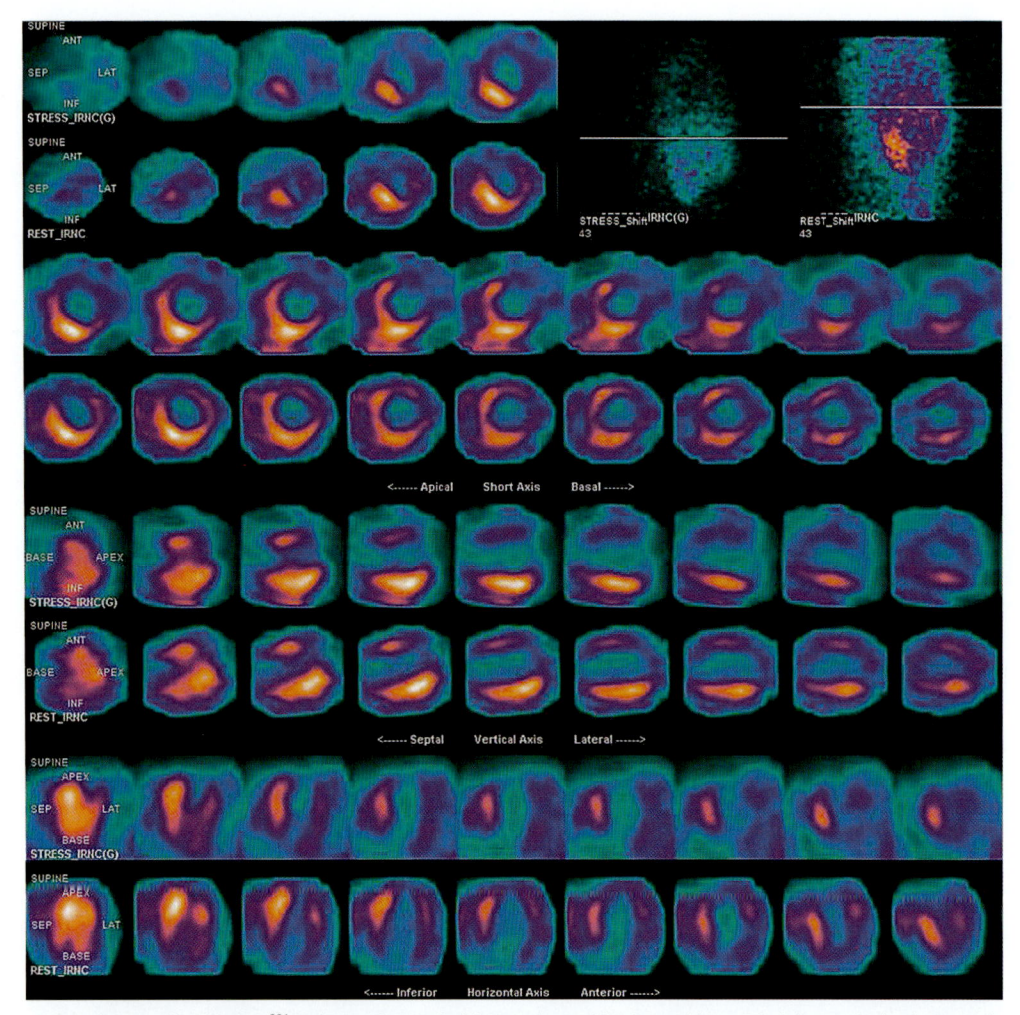

FIGURE 21-16 Rest/4-hour redistribution ^{201}Tl short-axis, vertical long-axis, and horizontal long-axis left ventricular images showing a severe, large fixed myocardial perfusion defect in the anterior and lateral walls with no redistribution, consistent with infarct or myocardial necrosis in those territories.

Rotating SPECT images will clarify this point and help in the correct image interpretation.

The degree of the perfusion defects is described in a qualitative fashion as mild, moderate, or severe. The extent of the perfusion defects may be reported as small, medium, or large. Different scoring systems have been developed to describe the severity of the perfusion defects, normally using the standard 17-segment model of the left ventricle, on a scale of 0 to 4; 0 is absent perfusion equal to the background, and 4 corresponds to normal perfusion. A perfusion defect in at least two consecutive image sets and in two projection image reconstruction displays is considered significant. A fixed perfusion defect with no significant change between the rest and post-stress images is often reported as myocardial scar or necrosis. The presence of severe myocardial ischemia cannot be completely excluded in some studies. A perfusion defect noted in the post-stress images that partially or completely normalizes at rest is termed partial or full reversibility, and it indicates myocardial ischemia. Further, perfusion abnormalities should be identified by location and presumptive coronary vascular distribution. During the last two decades, several quantitative software-based package programs have been developed and are commercially available. These programs are based on the comparison of a patient's individual regional myocardial uptake with a database of normal controls. The most common way to present these data is by use of a circumferential profile of the left ventricle, known popularly as a bull's-eye. However, quantitative analysis should not be considered a substitute for a visual interpretation, but it should be used as an adjunct.

KEY POINTS

- Imaging protocols allow the accurate assessment of relative regional perfusion and myocardial function at rest and stress.
- Stress-redistribution-reinjection and rest-redistribution ^{201}Tl SPECT imaging can be used to assess myocardial viability.
- The one-day protocol using Tc 99m labeled compounds is commonly employed with low-dose rest and high-dose stress imaging.

SUGGESTED READING

Henzlova MJ, Cerqueira MD, Hanson CL, et al. ASNC Imaging Guidelines for Nuclear Cardiology Procedures: Stress protocols and tracers. J Nucl Cardiol 2009; in press. Available at: www.ASNC.org.

REFERENCES

1. Gould KL, Lipscomb K, Hamilton GW. Physiologic basis for assessing critical coronary stenosis. Instantaneous flow response and regional distribution during coronary hyperemia as measures of coronary flow reserve. Am J Cardiol 1974; 33:87-94.
2. Pohost GM, Zir LM, McKusick KA, et al. Differentiation of transiently ischemic from infarcted myocardium by serial imaging after a single dose of thallium-201. Circulation 1977; 55:294-302.
3. Dilsizian V, Bonow R. Current diagnostic techniques of assessing myocardial viability in patients with hibernating and stunned myocardium. Circulation 1993; 87:1-20.
4. Dilsizian V, Rocco TP, Freedman NMT, et al. Enhanced detection of ischemic but viable myocardium by the reinjection of thallium after stress-redistribution imaging. N Engl J Med 1990; 323:141-146.
5. Zimmerman R, Mall G, Rauch B, et al. ^{201}Tl activity in irreversible defects as a marker of myocardial viability: clinicopathological study. Circulation 1995; 91:1016-1021.
6. Perrone-Filardi P, Pace L, Prastaro M, et al. Assessment of myocardial viability in patients with chronic coronary artery disease: rest–4-hour–24-hour ^{201}Tl tomography versus dobutamine echocardiography. Circulation 1996; 94:2712-2719.
7. Galassi AR, Centamore G, Fiscella A, et al. Comparison of rest-redistribution thallium-201 imaging and reinjection after stress-redistribution for the assessment of myocardial viability in patients with left ventricular dysfunction secondary to coronary artery disease. Am J Cardiol 1995; 75:436-442.
8. Qureshi U, Nagueh SF, Afridi I, et al. Dobutamine echocardiography and quantitative rest-redistribution ^{201}Tl tomography in myocardial hibernation: relation of contractile reserve to ^{201}Tl uptake and comparative prediction of recovery of function. Circulation 1997; 95:626-635.
9. Wagdy HM, Christian TF, Miller TD, Gibbons RJ. The value of 24-hour images after rest thallium injection. Nucl Med Commun 2002;23:629-637.
10. Dilsizian V, Arrighi JA, Diodati JG, et al. Myocardial viability in patients with chronic coronary artery disease. Comparison of ^{99m}Tc-sestamibi with thallium reinjection and ^{18}F-fluorodeoxyglucose. Circulation 1994; 89:578-587.
11. Maes AF, Borgers M, Flameng W, et al. Assessment of myocardial viability in chronic coronary artery disease using technetium-99m sestamibi SPECT. Correlation with histologic and positron emission tomography studies and functional follow-up. J Am Coll Cardiol 1997; 29:62-68.
12. Levine MG, McGill CC, Ahlberg AW, et al. Functional assessment with electrocardiographic gated single-photon emission computed tomography improves the ability of technetium-99m sestamibi myocardial perfusion imaging to predict myocardial viability in patients undergoing revascularization. Am J Cardiol 1999; 83:1-5.
13. Rambaldi R, Poldermans D, Bax JJ, et al. Dobutamine stress echocardiography and technetium-99m-tetrofosmin/fluorine 18-fluorodeoxyglucose single-photon emission computed tomography and influence of resting ejection fraction to assess myocardial viability in patients with severe left ventricular dysfunction and healed myocardial infarction. Am J Cardiol 1999; 84:130-134.
14. Vanzetto G, Janier M, Fagret D, et al. Metabolic myocardial viability assessment with iodine 123–16-iodo-3-methylhexadecanoic acid in recent myocardial infarction: comparison with thallium-201 and fluorine-18 fluorodeoxyglucose. Eur J Nucl Med 1997; 24:170-178.
15. Berman DS, Kiat HS, Van Train KF, et al. Myocardial perfusion imaging with technetium-99m-sestamibi: comparative analysis of available imaging protocols. J Nucl Med 1994; 35:681-688.
16. Kiat H, Germano G, Friedman J, et al. Comparative feasibility of separate or simultaneous rest thallium-201/stress technetium-99m-sestamibi dual-isotope myocardial perfusion SPECT. J Nucl Med 1994; 35:542-548.
17. Bateman TM, Berman DS, Heller GV, et al. American Society of Nuclear Cardiology position statement on electrocardiographic gating of myocardial perfusion SPECT scintigrams. J Nucl Cardiol 1999; 470-471.
18. Azarbal B, Hayes SW, Lewin HC, et al. The incremental prognostic value of percentage of heart rate reserve achieved over myocardial perfusion single-photon emission computed tomography in the prediction of cardiac death and all-cause mortality: superiority over 85% of maximal age-predicted heart rate. J Am Coll Cardiol 2004; 44:423-430.
19. Klocke FJ, Bairb MG, Lorell BH, et al. ACC/AHA/ASNC guidelines for the clinical use of cardiac radionuclide imaging—executive summary. J Am Coll Cardiol 2003; 42:1318-1333.
20. Takeishi Y, Chiba J, Abe S, et al. Adenosine-induced heterogeneous perfusion accompanies myocardial ischemia in the presence of advanced coronary artery disease. Am Heart J 1994; 127:1262-1268.
21. Iskandrian A. State of the art for pharmacologic stress imaging. In Zaret BL, Beller G (eds). Nuclear Cardiology: State of the Art and Future Directions, 2nd ed. St. Louis, Mosby, 1998, pp 312-330.
22. Sharir T, Rabinowitz B, Livschitz S, et al. Underestimation of extent and severity of coronary artery disease by dipyridamole stress thallium-201 single-photon emission computed tomographic myocardial perfusion imaging in patients taking antianginal drugs. J Am Coll Cardiol 1998; 31:1540-1546.
23. Pennell DJ, Mavrogeni SI, Forbat SM, et al. Adenosine combined with dynamic exercise for myocardial perfusion imaging. J Am Coll Cardiol 1995; 25:1300-1309.
24. Lette J, Tatum JL, Fraser S, et al. Safety of dipyridamole testing in 73,806 patients: the Multicenter Dipyridamole Safety Study. J Nucl Cardiol 1995; 2:3-17.
25. Secknus MA, Marwick TH. Evolution of dobutamine echocardiography protocols and indications: safety and side effects in 3011 studies over 5 years. J Am Coll Cardiol 1997; 29:1234-1240.
26. Marcovitz PA, Bach DS, Mathias W, et al. Paradoxic hypotension during dobutamine stress echocardiography: clinical and diagnostic implications. J Am Coll Cardiol 1993; 21:1080-1086.
27. Bonow RO. Diagnosis and risk stratification in coronary artery disease: nuclear cardiology versus stress echocardiography. J Nucl Cardiol 1997; 4:S172-S178.
28. Veilleux M, Lette J, Mansur A, et al. Prognostic implications of transient left ventricular cavity dilation during exercise and dipyridamole-thallium imaging. Can J Cardiol 1994; 10:259-266.

CHAPTER 22

Radiopharmaceutical Single Photon Emission Computed Tomography Imaging Agents

Alexander Bustamante and Gautam Nayak*

Myocardial perfusion imaging agents have become critical to diagnosis, prognosis, and clinical decision-making in the setting of coronary artery disease. Radiopharmaceuticals have been used to determine regional perfusion since the 1950s, although the imaging techniques have been refined and improved over time. In general, myocardial perfusion radiotracers share many of the following common characteristics:

1. Tracer uptake within the myocardium must be proportional to the regional myocardial blood flow over a relatively wide range of blood flow.
2. Myocardial uptake of tracers should be high enough to allow the detection of regional heterogeneity by external gamma scintigraphy.
3. Myocardial radiotracer distribution at the time of injection must remain stable during the acquisition time of the images.
4. The effect of blood flow on the myocardial transport of radiotracers must be greater than the effect of metabolic cellular alterations.
5. Agents should be labeled to a radionuclide having adequate physical characteristics to provide high photon flux and optimal counting statistics.

With these principles in mind, the advent of radiopharmaceuticals has followed a diverse course and continues to expand.

*The views expressed in this chapter are those of the author and do not necessarily reflect the official policy or position of the Department of the Navy, Army, Department of Defense, or the U.S. government.

We certify that all individuals who qualify as authors have been listed; each has participated in the conception and design of this work, the analysis of data (when applicable), the writing of the document, and the approval of the submission of this version; that the document represents valid work; that if we used information derived from another source, we obtained all necessary approvals to use it and made appropriate acknowledgments in the document; and that each takes public responsibility for it.

DESCRIPTION OF TECHNICAL REQUIREMENTS

Thallium 201

The Saperstein principle states that a given type of radiopharmaceutical will be distributed in proportion to regional perfusion if its extraction by the organ of interest is high and if its clearance from the blood is rapid.[1] This principle led to the development of the potassium analogues, one of the first radiopharmaceuticals used to image myocardial perfusion. These agents are monovalent cations of potassium, cesium, rubidium, and thallium. They enter the myocardium by active channels through the Na^+, K^+-ATPase pump. Thallium 201 (^{201}Tl) has many of the best physical and biologic characteristics for imaging in humans, making it one of the most popular myocardial perfusion agents used since the 1970s.[1] Thallium continues to find significant utility in the diagnosis of coronary artery disease and in the evaluation of prognosis and revascularization in those with ischemic heart disease.

Physical Properties

Thallium, a metallic element in group IIIA of the periodic table, has a crystal radius (1.44 Å) between that of potassium and rubidium. It is a cyclotron-produced monovalent cation with a physical half-life of 73.1 hours. As thallium decays by electron capture to mercury 201, it produces low-energy gamma rays with principal photopeaks at 135.3 keV (2.7% abundance) and 167.4 keV (10% abundance) and x-rays emitted from the mercury daughter at 68 to 80.3 keV (95% abundance). These photopeaks of 68 to 80 keV are the primary photon energies used in gamma ray imaging with thallium. Unlike technetium-based agents, thallium requires no in-house preparation.

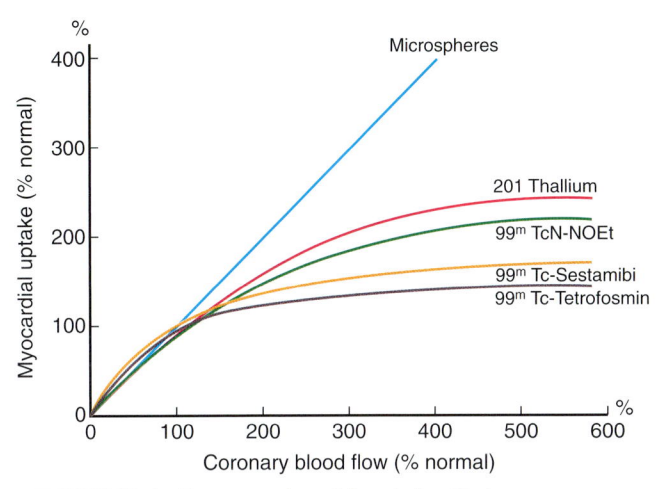

FIGURE 22-1 Representation of the relationship between coronary blood flow and myocardial uptake of various perfusion imaging radiotracers.

Extraction and Biodistribution

The flow dependence of myocardial tracer uptake limits the sensitivity of a given tracer for the detection of coronary artery disease. In Figure 22-1, the curves of tracer myocardial uptake versus myocardial blood flow flatten as coronary blood flow increases. This implies that at a given level of coronary blood flow, the tracer imaging defect will be much less than the actual coronary blood flow disparity. In Figure 22-1, there is a linear relation of uptake over a wide range of coronary blood flow using a standard of radiolabeled microspheres. At high flow rates (~2.5 mL/min/g), there is a diffusion limitation and a fall in tracer extraction with increased cellular tracer washout, leading to a plateau of myocardial uptake. This phenomenon leads to an underestimation of coronary blood flow at high flow rates and overestimation at very low flow rates when there is increased myocardial extraction relative to blood flow.

In general, ^{201}Tl has an extraction fraction of 87% at normal flow rates. Only viable myocardial cells that maintain a transmembrane potassium gradient will retain ^{201}Tl. In general, a maximum of 4% of the injected dose is taken up in the myocardium (occurring within 10 to 15 minutes of injection), with high concentrations also found in the liver and kidney. ^{201}Tl disappearance from the blood compartment is rapid; more than 90% of blood activity clears with a half-life of 5 minutes, resulting in a decreased blood pool background.[2]

Redistribution

Myocardial redistribution is one of the most clinically important characteristics of ^{201}Tl. On a practical level, redistribution is manifested as a "filling in" of a myocardial perfusion defect occurring 3 to 5 hours after the injection of ^{201}Tl at peak stress. The myocardial uptake of thallium is not static over time, and redistribution is related to the rate of influx of ^{201}Tl into the myocardium from the blood pool and the rate of clearance or washout of thallium from the myocardium. As described in the previous section, no more than 3% to 5% of tracer is delivered to the myocardium. The amount of washout from the myocardium depends not only on the amount of tracer leaving through blood flow but also on how much is being continuously accumulated by exchange from other compartments.[3] Figure 22-2 further illustrates this concept for various levels of myocardial blood flow. All the curves show some level of rapid early myocardial uptake, roughly proportional to myocardial perfusion. Blood levels of tracer fall rapidly as tracer is extracted by the heart and other systemic compartments. After this initial extraction, tracer molecules are slowly released back into the blood from body compartments, maintaining a constant low-level blood concentration of tracer. There is a subsequent exchange of tracer between the blood and myocardial cells until an equilibrium point is reached. This exchange equilibrium is not dependent on blood flow but only on the relative concentration of intravascular and extravascular tracer molecules and the subsequent concentration gradient supported by the membrane potentials or by active membrane transport.[4] All tracers must redistribute to some extent, although thallium displays this property to a greater extent because of the ease with which its molecules are transported in and out of the myocardium through active channels. With thallium, a reversible myocardial perfusion defect related to ischemic heart disease will show normalization of ^{201}Tl uptake at 3 to 4 hours after injection at stress because of delayed accumulation into the ischemic segment and a more rapid washout from normal myocardial segments than from hypoperfused segments.[1]

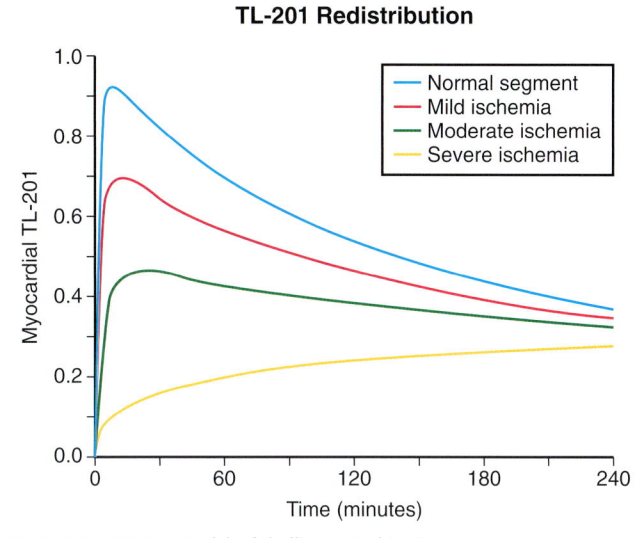

FIGURE 22-2 Model of thallium 201 kinetics incorporating extraction, redistribution, and systemic excretion. Myocardial thallium uptake is shown for normal flow and transiently reduced flows of various degrees. *(From Zaret BL, Beller GA [eds]. Clinical Nuclear Cardiology: State of the Art and Future Directions, 3rd ed. Philadelphia, Mosby, 2005, p 7.)*

Clinical Considerations

Viability

In many clinical scenarios, patients with known coronary artery disease and history of myocardial infarction are considered for revascularization. However, exposure of patients to the risks of possible complex percutaneous or surgical revascularization options in the absence of true long-term benefit, either from a mortality or on a symp-

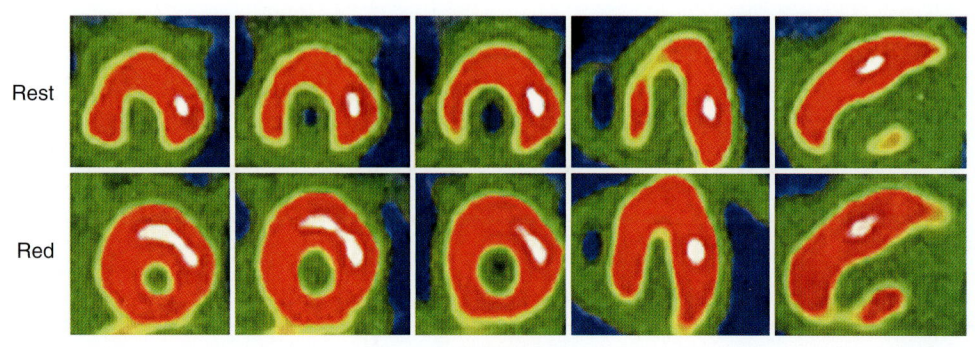

FIGURE 22-3 Rest and redistribution imaging of thallium 201 showing viable myocardium in the inferior and septal walls. *(From Iskandrian AE, Verani MS [eds]. Nuclear Cardiac Imaging: Principles and Applications, 3rd ed. New York, Oxford University Press, 2002.)*

TABLE 22-1 Radiopharmaceutical SPECT Imaging Agents

	²⁰¹Tl	Sestamibi	Teboroxime	Tetrofosmin
Uptake	Active	Passive	Passive	Passive
Preparation	Cyclotron	Kit	Kit	Kit
Chemical $t_{1/2}$	72 hr	6 hr	6 hr	6 hr
Myocardial clearance	6 hr	5 hr	10 min	3 hr
Redistribution	Yes	Minimal	Yes	Minimal
SPECT studies	Yes	Yes	Possible	Yes
Gated SPECT	No	Yes	No	Yes
Effective dose equivalent	16 mSV/2 mCi	11 mSv/30 mCi	18 mSv/30 mCi	8 mSV/30 mCi
Clearance	Renal	Hepatic	Hepatic	Hepatic

tomatic basis, may preclude a more aggressive approach. Truly infarcted myocardium will not improve in contractile function regardless of coronary blood flow to the region of interest. Myocardium that is chronically ischemic or hibernating but not truly infarcted can achieve significant benefit from revascularization. These myocardial cells have downregulated their metabolic processes as a protective mechanism to counteract a lack of blood flow until future oxygen delivery capabilities return. Optimization of blood flow to hibernating myocardium indeed does improve long-term outcomes and can improve symptoms in carefully selected patients.[5] This concept has led to an enormous growth in the use of nuclear perfusion imaging to assess for viability to guide clinical decision-making with regard to revascularization.

Thallium has proved to be a useful agent in the assessment of viability. Its redistribution properties lend themselves to a sensitive physiologic assessment of tissue integrity, even in the absence of adequate blood flow to a region of myocardium.[6] In general, cationic tracers that are retained by membrane potentials will be "viability" agents. Significant tracer uptake into the myocardium requires delivery, implying perfusion, and retention, implying enough cellular integrity to generate membrane potentials to fuel active transport channels. Even in the absence of a delivery mechanism, thallium can redistribute over time to myocardial cells that have intact cell membranes. Practically, this would be manifested as a lack of perfusion (or counts) on rest imaging with a "filling in" of any defects with delayed imaging. Infarcted tissue would not display similar count statistics owing to an inability of thallium tracer molecules to enter dead myocardial cells (Fig. 22-3). As a result, patients with symptoms of ischemic heart disease but history of prior infarction (and, often, systolic left ventricular dysfunction) may benefit from revascularization in the setting of viability in the region subtended by obstructive epicardial coronary lesions. In general, redistribution imaging is performed at least 4 to 6 hours after rest imaging to allow maximal thallium uptake into hibernating but viable myocardium. Some studies have shown that 24-hour late thallium imaging enhances the detection of myocardial viability after myocardial infarction.[7] From a practical perspective, 24-hour thallium redistribution imaging is often preferred to early (4- to 6-hour) redistribution studies for the assessment of viability.

Radiation Exposure

In the 21st century, the medical use of radiation is the largest man-made source of radiation. More than 5 billion imaging examinations are performed worldwide each year, with a majority employing ionizing radiation with radiology or nuclear medicine.[8] In modern medicine, attributable cancer risk increases significantly with increasing lifetime radiation exposure. Cardiac studies account for 57% of all nuclear medicine examinations and 85% of the effective dose.[9] Radiologic dose estimates can be expressed as multiples of a single posterior-anterior chest radiograph (equivalent to 0.02 mSv). As can be seen in Table 22-1, a stress technetium sestamibi study is the radiation dose equivalent of 600 chest radiographs, and a similar thallium study is the equivalent of 1500 chest radiographs. For thallium, this corresponds to an extra lifetime cancer risk of about 1 in 1000 patients (Fig. 22-4). Indeed, as our technology improves and the demand grows for noninvasive cardiac studies, radiation exposure will continue to be a strong consideration in choosing the most

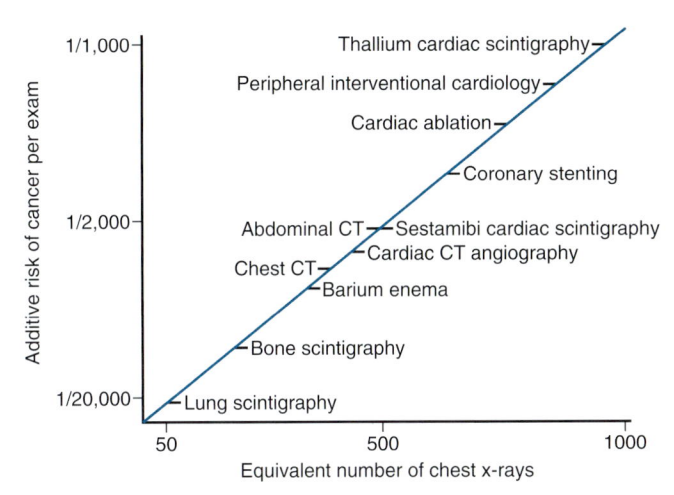

FIGURE 22-4 Additive risk of cancer with various radiologic studies with respect to equivalent number of chest radiographs.

appropriate imaging modality with consideration of balancing lifetime cancer risk with the optimal, cost-efficient diagnostic approach.

Dose and Image Quality

The major driving force behind the increased radiation exposure risk for thallium is its long half-life, especially compared with technetium. As a result, dosing is limited to 2 to 4 mCi, a fraction of that feasible for technetium-based agents (25 to 30 mCi), for a typical myocardial perfusion study. Count statistics for thallium therefore prove to be less robust, often making imaging artifacts more prominent and actual scan interpretation more of a problem. Studies have consistently shown that image quality is better and interobserver reader variability is lower with technetium-based agents compared with thallium.[10] In addition, the ability to inject much higher doses of technetium and the improved counts therein allow ECG-based gating of technetium images, adding left ventricular wall motion to the perfusion data, which can improve image interpretation sensitivity and specificity.

Technetium Tc 99m Labeled Myocardial Perfusion Agents

Despite the clinical value of ^{201}Tl as a myocardial perfusion agent, its physical characteristics are suboptimal for gamma camera imaging. Since its introduction to clinical use in the 1970s, intense research subsequently led to the discovery of other cardiac nuclear tracers, particularly technetium Tc 99m labeled agents. These agents have many physical properties that are superior to ^{201}Tl as listed in Table 22-1, but the two of most interest are its ideal photon energy peak (140 keV) and short half-life (6 hours) that allows a 10-fold dose increase in comparison with ^{201}Tl. These two attributes result in image quality superior to that of ^{201}Tl-based cardiac imaging, particularly in obese patients.[10,11,12] The two Tc 99m labeled perfusion agents of most clinical use today are sestamibi and tetrofosmin. Two other tracers that have been developed are N-NOET and teboroxime.

As opposed to ^{201}Tl, which is cyclotron produced and thus must be obtained from commercial suppliers, Tc 99m is eluted from a small molybdenum 99 (^{99}Mo) generator, allowing possible 24-hour use. Tc 99m is produced in the form of Tc 99m pertechnetate, which can be eluted from the generator with sterile normal saline. After an elution of the ^{99}Mo generator, maximal activity is achieved after 24 hours, but clinical doses of Tc 99m are available as soon as 3 to 6 hours later. The free Tc 99m pertechnetate can then be reconstituted with the aforementioned perfusion agents to be used for myocardial perfusion imaging.[13]

Tc 99m Sestamibi

Physical Properties

Tc 99m sestamibi was the first Tc 99m labeled myocardial perfusion agent developed in the class of cationic technetium compounds, the hexakis alkylisonitrile technetium(I) complexes. Tc 99m sestamibi is a lipophilic complex of six isonitriles that is taken up predominantly by passive diffusion across the cellular membrane. Sequestration in the cell is related to the transmembrane potential particularly across the mitochondria, where it is preferentially localized.

Extraction and Biodistribution

Tc 99m sestamibi has an in vivo first-pass myocardial extraction of 55% to 68%, which is significantly less than that of ^{201}Tl. Related to a reduced extraction rate is a non-linear cellular uptake particularly above coronary flow rates of 2 to 2.5 mL/min/g, which theoretically reduces its sensitivity to detect less critical stenosis. Cellular uptake of Tc 99m sestamibi, like that of ^{201}Tl, is more linear at basal flow rates and actually increases relative to absolute blood flow at lower rates. Approximately 1% of the dose is taken up by the myocardium and remains in the blood pool 1 hour after injection.[14]

Redistribution and Viability

Tc 99m sestamibi clearance from the myocardium is slow and redistribution is minimal. Unlike ^{201}Tl, technetium-based agents are more firmly trapped within the myocardium and as a result decay before they exchange with the blood pool, making redistribution insignificant. Uptake of Tc 99m sestamibi remains significant at low-flow ischemic states, and the agent is not taken up by necrotic or infarcted tissue. Thus, the ability to assess for viability is implied by the differential retention of the tracer between ischemic and infarcted myocardium. Also as a result of minimal redistribution, images may be acquired at a time remote from injection, permitting the potential use in patients with acute coronary syndromes.

Tc 99m Tetrofosmin

Physical Properties

Tc 99m tetrofosmin is a lipophilic cationic complex that demonstrates myocardial retention, uptake, and clearance kinetics similar to those of Tc 99m sestamibi. Sequestration of the tracer is similarly related to the transmembrane potential of the myocardial mitochondrial membrane.

Extraction and Biodistribution

The first-pass myocardial extraction rate for Tc 99m tetrofosmin is 54%, which is somewhat lower than that of Tc 99m sestamibi, with a slow rate of myocardial clearance and redistribution. As a result of the lower extraction rate, uptake of the tracer plateaus at higher coronary flow rates, particularly above 2 mL/min/g, potentially underestimates more modest coronary stenosis.[14]

Redistribution and Viability

Tc 99m tetrofosmin demonstrates essentially no redistribution, and uptake, such as that of Tc 99m sestamibi, is related to the presence of an intact cellular membrane. Ischemic myocardium retains the ability to transfer Tc 99m tetrofosmin across the cell membrane, but no uptake is measurable in necrotic tissue.

Tc 99m Teboroxime

Physical Properties

Tc 99m teboroxime is a neutral lipophilic tracer and a member of the boronic acid adducts of technetium complexes. This compound is smaller than Tc 99m sestamibi and larger than ^{201}Tl and chemically distinct. Partitioning of the tracer in the lipid phase of the cell membrane appears to result in a conformational change, with a reduced ability for cellular reuptake.

Extraction and Biodistribution

The neutral lipophilic characteristics of Tc 99m teboroxime result in an extraction rate that exceeds 90%. Tc 99m teboroxime approximates a freely diffusible radiotracer with a concomitant rapid myocardial washout that is independent of metabolic activity. Myocardial uptake is linear with coronary blood flow even at high flow rates and thus does not experience a "roll-off" phenomenon as does Tc 99m sestamibi or even ^{201}Tl. However, as a result of the rapid myocardial washout of Tc 99m teboroxime, subsequent gamma imaging needs to occur rapidly to avoid underestimation of a potential defect. In animal models, defect normalization can occur as rapidly as 8 minutes by use of adenosine stress in dogs with and without coronary occlusions. This has led to the limited use of this agent for clinical applications.[10]

Redistribution and Viability

Tc 99m teboroxime demonstrates a rapid myocardial washout and redistribution that appears to be related to differential clearance without particular reuptake of the tracer. This is likely a result of a conformational change in the tracer on sequestration in the plasma lipid layer, impeding further reuptake. This has led to little clinical application of this perfusion tracer for viability assessment.

Tc 99m N-NOET

Physical Properties

Tc 99m N-NOET is a member of the Tc 99m nitrido dithiocarbamates and the newest of the Tc 99m labeled agents for use in myocardial perfusion imaging. Sequestration of the tracer appears to be localized to hydrophobic components of myocardial cells, particularly the cell membrane, with no specific association to mitochondria. Tc 99m N-NOET uptake appears in part to be mediated through an interaction with L-type calcium channels as verapamil and diltiazem reduced its uptake, and furthermore, BayK 8644, a calcium channel activator, increased its uptake in cultured myocardial cells.

Extraction and Biodistribution

The myocardial extraction fraction of Tc 99m N-NOET is similar to that of ^{201}Tl at 82% to 87%, with an initial cardiac retention higher than that of ^{201}Tl. This linear uptake with flow in the hyperemic range has the potential to increase sensitivity for detection of subtle ischemic changes in relation to the other Tc 99m based tracers. Cardiac transport of Tc 99m N-NOET appears to be less sensitive than ^{201}Tl to ischemic injury. Myocardial washout of Tc 99m N-NOET is rapid, resulting in reductions in defect contrast soon after injection, which is related to the rapid redistribution of the tracer. This is similar to Tc 99m teboroxime, but to a lesser extent with Tc 99m N-NOET.[10]

Redistribution and Viability

Myocardial redistribution of Tc 99m N-NOET appears to have an imaging pattern similar to that of ^{201}Tl, although this pattern is a result of differential clearance between ischemic and normally perfused myocardium rather than a true redistribution as in the case of ^{201}Tl. Hence, Tc 99m N-NOET demonstrates an apparent myocardial redistribution mechanistically different from that of ^{201}Tl and not truly a function of cellular integrity. The ability of Tc 99m N-NOET to truly detect viable myocardium is as yet unproven. Because Tc 99m N-NOET uptake is related more to myocardial blood flow, it has unique clinical utility in the setting of recent infarction with revascularization. Tc 99m N-NOET proves to be a better marker of reperfused myocardium acutely than is ^{201}Tl, which is a better marker of viability.

KEY POINTS

- Thallium 201 is a potassium analogue with usefulness is stress imaging and viability assessment.
- Technetium permits improved image quality in stress imaging with lower overall radiation exposure.
- As new myocardial tracers are being developed, image quality will need to be balanced with radiation exposure.

SUGGESTED READING

Henzlova MJ, Cerqueira MD, Henson CL, et al. ASNC Imaging Guidelines for Nuclear Cardiology Procedures: stress protocols and tracers. J Nucl Cardiol 2009; in press. Available at: www.ASNC.org.

REFERENCES

1. Taillefer R. Kinetics of myocardial perfusion imaging radiotracers. In Iskandrian AE, Verani MS (eds). Nuclear Cardiac Imaging: Principles and Applications, 3rd ed. New York, Oxford University Press, 2003, p 51.
2. Krahwinkel W, Herzog H, Feinendegen LE. Pharmacokinetics of thallium-201 in normal individuals after routine myocardial scintigraphy. J Nucl Med 1988; 29:1582-1587.
3. Grunwald AM, Watson DD, Hoszgrete HH, et al. Thallium-201 kinetics in normal and ischemic myocardium. Circulation 1981; 64:610-618.
4. Watson D, Glover D. Overview of Kinetics and Modeling. In Zaret BL, Beller GA (eds). Clinical Nuclear Cardiology: State of the Art and Future Directions, 3rd ed. Philadelphia, Mosby, 2005, pp 6-7.
5. Sansoy V, Glover DK, Watson DD, et al. Comparison of thallium-201 resting redistribution with technetium-99m–sestamibi uptake and functional response to dobutamine for assessment of myocardial viability. Circulation 1995; 92:994-1004.
6. Dilsizian V, Rocco TP, Nanette MD, et al. Enhanced detection of ischemic but viable myocardium by the reinjection of thallium after stress-redistribution imaging. N Engl J Med 1990; 323:141-146.
7. Allman KC, Shaw LJ, Hachamovitch R, Udelson JE. Myocardial viability testing and impact of revascularization on prognosis in patients with coronary artery disease and left ventricular dysfunction. J Am Coll Cardiol 2002; 39:1151-1158.
8. Picano E, Vano E, Semelka R, Regulla D. The American College of Radiology white paper on radiation dose in medicine: deep impact on the practice of cardiovascular imaging. Cardiovasc Ultrasound 2007; 5:37-43.
9. Thompson R, Cullon S. Issues regarding radiation dosage of cardiac nuclear and radiography procedures. J Nucl Cardiol 2006; 13: 19-23.
10. Beller GA, Bergmann SR. Myocardial perfusion imaging agents: SPECT and PET. J Nucl Cardiol 2004;11:71-86.
11. Kailasnath P, Sinusas AJ. Technetium-99m–labeled myocardial perfusion agents: are they better than thallium-201? Cardiol Rev 2001; 9:160-172.
12. Kailasnath P, Sinusas AJ. Comparison of Tl-201 with Tc-99m-labeled myocardial perfusion agents: technical, physiologic, and clinical issues. J Nucl Cardiol 2001; 8:482-498.
13. Baggish AL, Boucher CA. Radiopharmaceutical agents for myocardial perfusion imaging. Circulation 2008; 118:1668-1674.
14. Hendel R, Parker M, Zaret B, et al. Reduced variability of interpretation and improved image quality with a technetium 99m myocardial perfusion agent: comparison of thallium-201 and technetium 99m–labeled tetrofosmin. J Nucl Cardiol 1994; 509-514.

CHAPTER 23

Physics and Instrumentation of Cardiac Positron Emission Tomography/Computed Tomography

John R. Votaw and Jonathan A. Nye

This chapter concerns the physics of cardiac PET/CT and the difference between scanning the heart and scanning other parts of the body. Because of the desire to image a beating organ and because stress can cause the diaphragm and heart to move within the thoracic cavity, pitfalls can be part of cardiac imaging that are less important for whole-body imaging. These include obtaining a proper attenuation correction, imaging at the correct time relative to injection, and determining whether there has been motion of the patient during the study. Before these issues can be addressed, some background into the data acquisition is necessary.

SCANNER PHYSICS

Positron emission tomography (PET) takes advantage of the unique characteristics of positron decay. A proton-rich nucleus, such as ^{82}Rb or ^{18}F, can eliminate its excess charge by emitting a positron, which is the antiparticle of the electron. The positron will scatter around in the body (within a millimeter or so of where the decay took place) until it meets an electron, and then they are annihilated. The annihilation converts the mass of the positron and electron into energy, in this case two 511-keV photons that travel in nearly opposite directions (Fig. 23-1). If both of these photons can be detected, then it is known that there is activity somewhere along the line between the two responding detectors. After enough of these events have been recorded, the information can be combined to form an image.

At the heart of a PET camera are scintillation detectors. A scintillation detector is a crystal that gives off many low-energy photons when a high-energy photon interacts with its molecules. The low-energy photons are collected by photomultiplier tubes, which convert them into an electronic signal. The precise time of arrival of the event and the energy of the event are recorded. This is diagrammed in Figure 23-2. The timing is critical because it is used to decide if two photons came from the same annihilation. If two photons are detected within a very short time (called the time window, typically 3 to 12 ns, depending on the type of detector used in the scanner), it is assumed that they were created from a single positron-electron annihilation that occurred somewhere on the line that connects the two recording detectors. This is called a *coincident event*, and the line is termed a *line of response*. If the time between detecting two photons is greater than the time window, the two detected events must have originated from two separate annihilations because light travels at approximately 0.3 m/ns and the scanner is only about 1 m in diameter. The primary data set from the scanner is the number of coincident events that are recorded for each line of response.

Recording the energy of the event is important to determine first if the photon came from a positron annihilation and then if it scattered off tissue in the body on its way to the detector. If the photon arrives with 511 keV of energy, it is overwhelmingly likely that it originated in a positron-electron annihilation. This is useful for preventing background events of different energy from entering the data stream. The detectors are not perfect, and there are some physical effects that cause the energy to vary, so scanner electronics are generally set to accept events with a range of energies, typically 430 to 650 keV. One of the

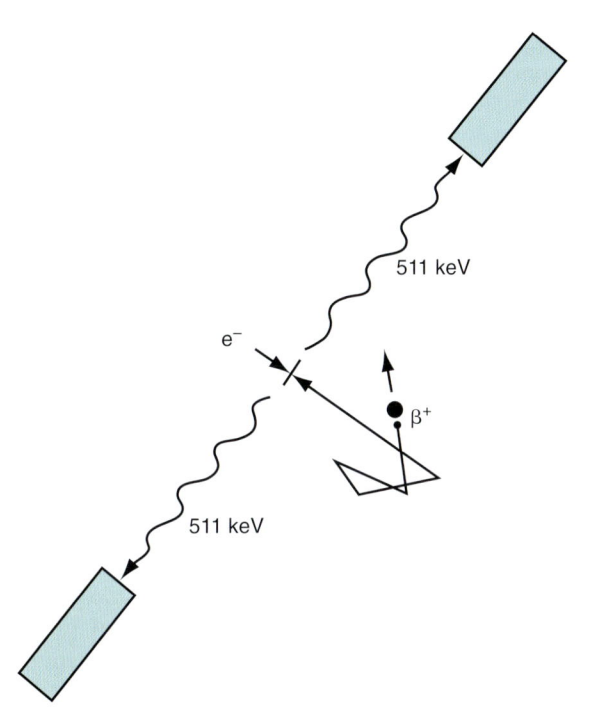

FIGURE 23-1 Depiction of coincidence detection and the basic physics involved in PET imaging. The nuclide decays, giving off a positron that eventually meets an electron and annihilates into two 511-keV photons. These two photons are detected, giving the information that a decay took place between the two detectors. Events that happen this way, as is desired, are called true events.

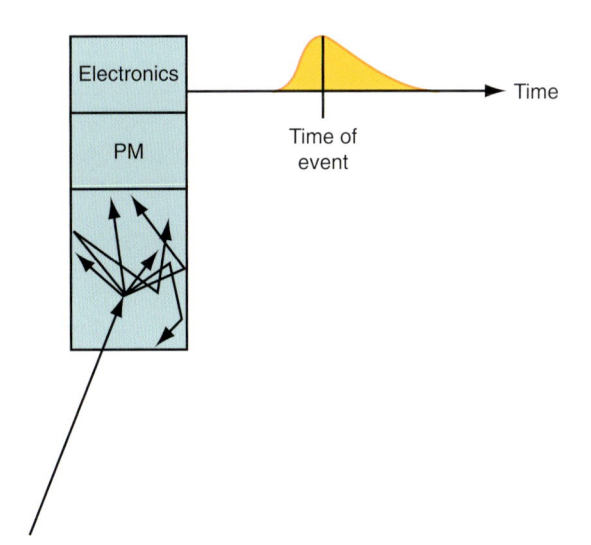

FIGURE 23-2 Schematic of a scintillation detector typical of those used in PET scanners. The high-energy (511 keV) photon interacts in the detector crystal, which then glows in a shower of low-energy (visible) photons. These visible photons are collected by the photomultiplier (PM), which converts the light into an electronic signal. The electronics identify the time of the event and the area of the pulse, which is proportional to energy.

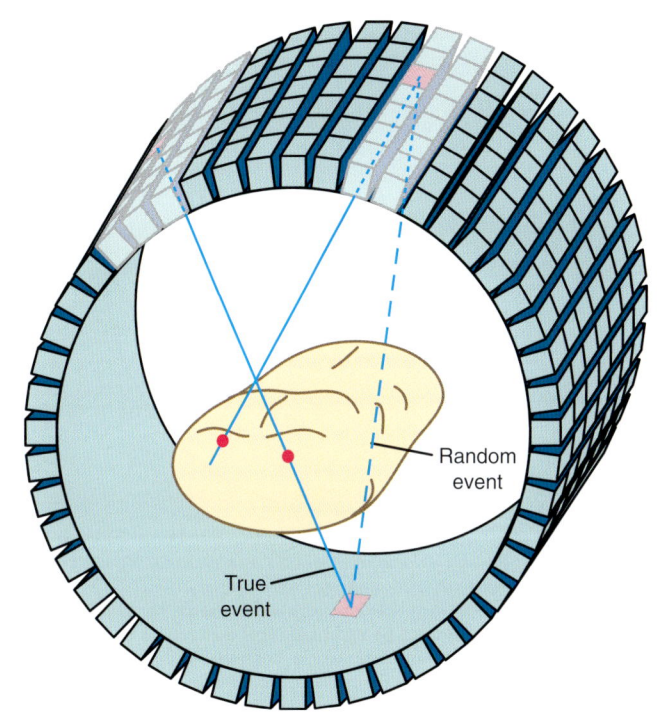

FIGURE 23-3 Depiction of the geometry in a typical PET scanner and the nature of a random event. The scanner is made of many small individual detectors arranged in a cylinder. The scanner electronics can record events between any pair of these detectors. Note that the photons need not be "in the plane" of a particular detector ring. A true event and a random event are depicted. In the random event, two separate decays have led to photons that are detected by the scanner. Unfortunately, neither of the decays takes place on the line connecting the two responding detectors. These types of events must be removed from the data set before an accurate image can be reconstructed.

are continually monitoring for photons. The main advantage of PET imaging over SPECT is the vastly increased count rate capability. All detectors in the PET ring are continuously monitoring for events versus a gamma camera, which uses a lead collimator to detect only events along certain projections at any given time.

There are several types of events that can be recorded in a PET scanner. The example shown in Figure 23-1 is called a *true event*. "True" comes from a positron-electron annihilation generating two photons that travel in opposite directions and are both recorded. This is the raw data that we desire to accurately reconstruct an image. Unfortunately, collecting data as described also results in recording of other types of events. It is possible for photons from two different positron annihilations that by random chance happen to decay within a few nanoseconds of each other to be detected in separate detectors within the time window. This situation is depicted in Figure 23-3. When this happens, there is the potential for incorrectly assuming that radioactivity is present between the two responding detectors. This type of event is called a *random event* because the two detectors that are involved and the time between detection of the two photons are both completely random. Random events add a uniform background to the primary data set.

The randomness in time between the two detections can be exploited to estimate the number of random events that are confounding the primary data set. The number of

physical effects is scatter. When a photon scatters, it loses some energy to the scatterer. Hence, with better energy resolution, the number of contaminating background and scattered events accepted into the primary data set can be reduced.

A PET camera is made by arranging detectors in a cylindrical geometry as depicted in Figure 23-3. All detectors

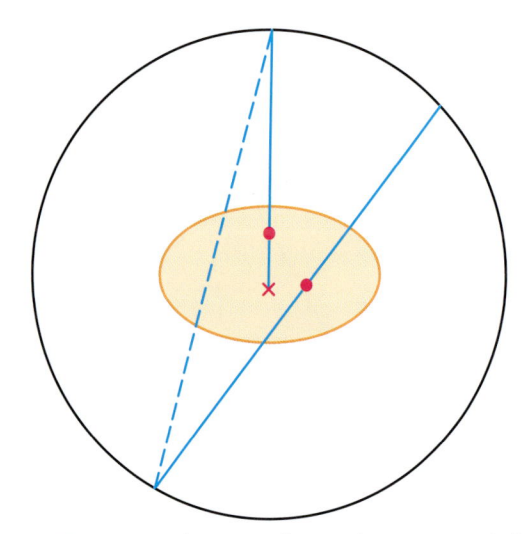

FIGURE 23-4 Two other types of events that can occur during a PET acquisition. The *straight line* represents a true event as depicted in Figure 23-1. The line with the *x* indicates an attenuation event. One of the photons heading toward the detectors is attenuated by the body, so a coincidence event could not be recorded. This leads to an underestimate of the amount of activity in the body. This is fixed by the attenuation correction derived from the collected CT scan. If these two events happen to occur at the same time, the event is termed a *multiple*. In this case, it is not clear from the collected data if there is activity along the *dotted* or *solid* line. The data set is corrected for multiple events during the correction for random events.

random events is estimated by one of two methods. The first method is the "delayed window" method. In this technique, a second data set is simultaneously acquired that includes only random events.[1] The second method probabilistically calculates the number of expected random events based on the count rates in each of the detectors. In either case, the estimate is subtracted from the primary data set to produce a random corrected data set.

A *multiple event* is a combination of a true event and a random event as shown in Figure 23-4. By random chance, a third photon falls within the time window of a true event. When this occurs, it is unknown which pair of detectors represents the true event and which pair represents the random event. In all cases, one of the potential lines of response can be eliminated because it does not go through the imaged field of view. This leaves two lines of response, one true and one random. Both of the events are recorded. On average, the random events are corrected in the process described earlier. Recording both events and later correcting for the random yields additional information that can be used to reconstruct the image. This is as opposed to the archaic practice of ignoring multiple events because it cannot be known which two detectors recorded the true event.

Photon attenuation by the patient's body leads to potential underestimation of the amount of activity in the patient. This is also depicted in Figure 23-4. Keep in mind that unless both photons are detected, no event can be recorded. It is the total amount of tissue that both photons must traverse that determines the probability of attenuation. Note that the probability of an event's being attenuated is greater if the line of response traverses the center of the patient. On the other hand, some of the events originating at the edge of the body can reach the detectors after traversing only a small amount of tissue. Because of this, more events that originate at the center of the body are attenuated compared with the edge of the body. If this is not taken into account when images are reconstructed, the center parts of the image will be depressed (Fig. 23-5).

A scatter event is when one of the photons scatters in the patient so that the line of response between the two responding detectors does not include the location of the event (Fig. 23-6). Essentially all scattering of importance to PET is photons scattering off free electrons, called *Compton scattering*. When a photon scatters, it transfers some of its energy to the electron. The greater the scattering angle, the greater the energy transfer. A 511-keV photon that scatters by 30 degrees is reduced in energy to 450 keV, approximately the lower level threshold used in setting up PET detectors. Hence, if one or both of the annihilation photons scatter by less than 30 degrees, they can be recorded by the PET system. With this much scattering, a recorded event with a line of response that passes near the center of the scanner could be off by up to 10 cm. Scattering by small angles is more probable than by larger angles, so scatter affects PET images by reducing resolution and contrast.

The final type of event that needs to be considered for cardiac imaging is called a prompt gamma and is shown in Figure 23-7. This is a property of ^{82}Rb decay that is not present with ^{18}F. When a rubidium nucleus decays, it converts to a krypton nucleus by giving off its charge in the form of a positron. A significant fraction of the time, the krypton is in an excited state and almost immediately gives off another gamma ray. This is a situation that looks very much like the multiple event depicted in Figure 23-4, but there is a significant difference. The prompt gamma event is not random. The annihilation photons and the prompt gamma all are generated from a single decay process. In this case, the true and random events are correlated in time, that is, they happen at the same time. (Actually, the prompt gamma can be delayed by a few picoseconds, but this extremely small time is insignificant compared with the duration of the time window.) Compared with a multiple event, the random is equally likely to occur at any time.

PET Detectors

All of the different types of events need to be accounted for in image reconstruction. The first defense against the confounding types of events is the detector itself. There are several different types of detector materials (Table 23-1). The three main characteristics for the detector material in PET are the stopping power, energy resolution, and time resolution. The greater the stopping power, the less detector material is needed to stop one of the annihilation photons. This is important for economic and image quality reasons. The detector material is the dominating cost of a scanner, so it pays to have higher stopping power material. It can also lead to better images. If a photon is detected in a smaller detector, the line of response is better defined, which leads to better images. Finally, for detectors of equal size, the one with the higher stopping power is more likely to record the event, leading to a higher sensitivity scanner and, again, better images.

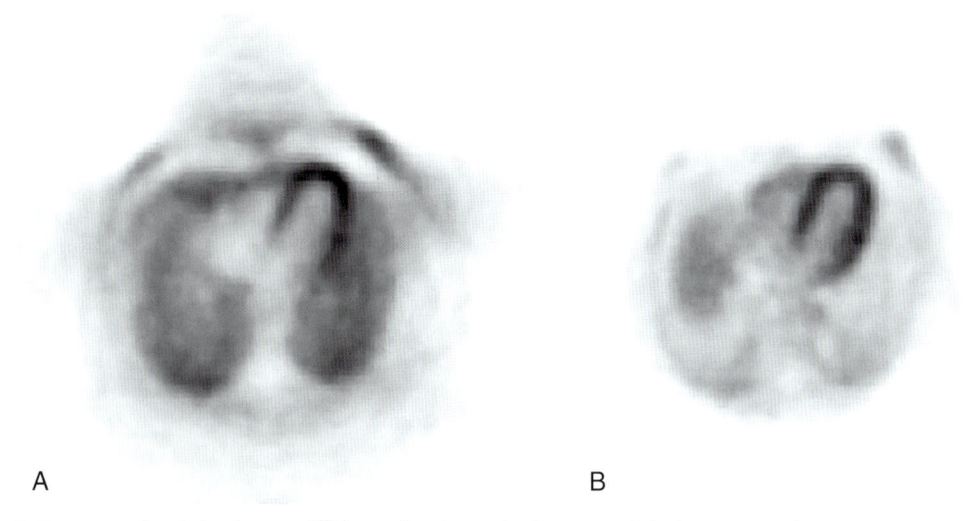

CHAPTER 23 • Physics and Instrumentation of Cardiac PET/CT

A   B

FIGURE 23-5 **A,** Uncorrected emission image of ^{82}Rb uptake. Counts in the center of the image are underestimated because of photon attenuation by the patient's body. This is most noticeable in the myocardial septum. **B,** A random event, scatter, and attenuation-corrected emission image of ^{82}Rb uptake. The depressed uptake in the myocardial septum and basal lateral wall has been recovered after attenuation correction is applied to the uncorrected image.

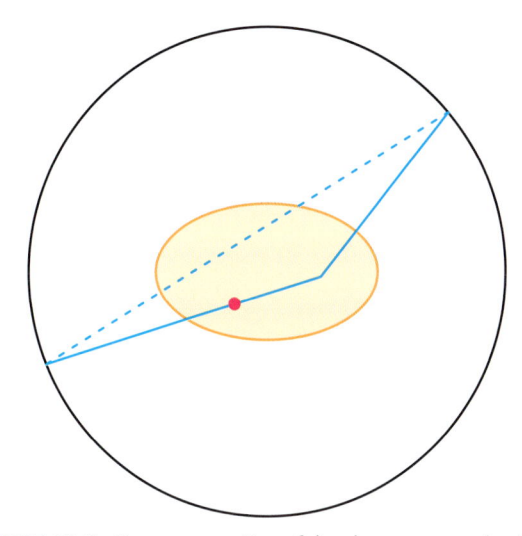

FIGURE 23-6 Scatter event. One of the photons emanating from the positron-electron annihilation has scattered off of an electron in the body and so is detected by an inappropriate detector. If it is not removed from the data set, activity will be assumed to be present along the dotted line in error.

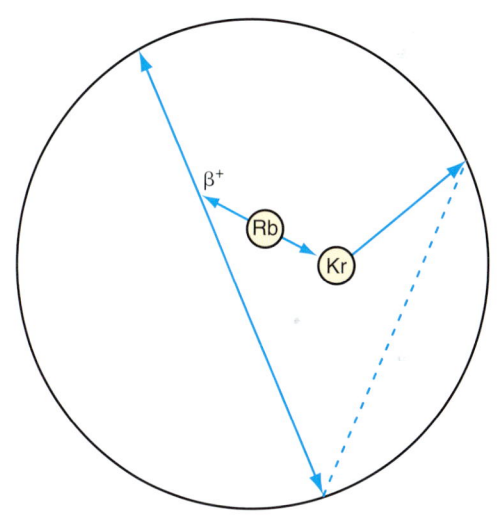

FIGURE 23-7 Prompt gamma event. This type of event can occur in scanning with rubidium (Rb). Rubidium decays to an excited state of krypton (Kr), which gives off its excess energy in the form of a photon. If all three of these photons are detected, the event has the appearance of a multiple event (see Fig. 23-4). The difference is that one event precipitated all three photons as opposed to the two decays that just happened to occur at the same time in Figure 23-4. Hence, there is no randomness in the timing between these photons, so a conventional correction for random events will not remove them from the data set. A separate prompt gamma contamination estimate must be performed to account for these events before an image is reconstructed.

Energy resolution is important for determining whether an event is scattered or not as discussed earlier. Because no detector is perfect, some number of scattered photons will always be recorded. However, with better energy resolution, the lower level energy threshold can be increased, which reduces the maximal angle through which a photon can be scattered and still be recorded. There is a subtle point worth mentioning here. As more scattered photons are rejected, the number of recorded events decreases. Because almost all photons are scattered to some degree, a perfect scatter rejection would result in very few events being recorded, which would result in very poor images. The scattered events do carry information as to the location of the source of activity. Hence, it is beneficial always to accept some level of scatter. As computer power and the scatter estimation and image reconstruction routines improve, more scatter events should be included in the data set.

Finally, the time resolution of the detector is important because it affects the number of random events that are recorded. The better the time resolution, the smaller the time window, and the fewer random events will enter the data set. Random events truly are random and therefore are equally likely to occur at any time. Therefore, a detector that permits a time window half as large

TABLE 23-1 PET Detector Material Properties

Property	LSO	BGO	Na(Tl)
Density (g/cm^3)	7.4	7.1	3.7
Stopping power (1/cm)	.87	.96	.34
Decay time (ns)	40	300	230
Energy resolution (%)	13	23	6.6

will result in a data set that has half the number of random events.

The choice of detector materials involves a tradeoff. Generally speaking, more detected events leads to better images. The number of detected events is greatly increased if the scanner is operated in three-dimensional mode. Unfortunately, the number of confounding events (randoms and scatter) is increased as well as the number of good events (true). At some point, the detriment of dealing with the bad events outweighs the benefit of collecting more good events. This tradeoff will be discussed later after a short discussion of three-dimensional imaging, which greatly increases the counts in PET imaging.

In many of the preceding diagrams, it appears as if the PET scanner is a ring of detectors within a single plane. Historically, this was the case. A volumetric PET scanner was built by stacking a set of independent detector rings to make a scanner. At some point, it was realized that if the detected events are limited to those occurring only within a plane, the number of detected events will be many times less than it could be. On the other hand, it takes much more computer memory and processing power to reconstruct images when nonplanar events are also included. The computing threshold was passed around 1999, and in modern scanners, the acceptance of events is opened up so that any pair of detectors can record an event. This is depicted in Figure 23-3.

Opening up the scanner has advantages and disadvantages. The advantage is collecting many more counts. When you collect more counts, you have better statistics, and the images look much better. On the other hand, many more random, scatter, and prompt gamma events are also recorded. Consider a scatter event. It might stay within a plane of detectors or it might scatter outside the plane. Because the plane is very thin, the overwhelming probability is that it will scatter out of the plane. If you have only a two-dimensional scanner, these scatter events will not become part of the data. However, if the scanner is operating in three-dimensional mode, scatter into neighboring planes will be recorded. Because of this, the fraction of recorded events that are scattered in a three-dimensional scanner can approach 50%. Hence, a robust and accurate scatter correction must be performed. The same consideration can be applied to the detection of random events. If there is a possibility of detecting events between any pair of detectors anywhere within the scanner, it is much more likely that a random event will be recorded. In many imaging situations, when the time window can be reduced to approximately 6 ns or less, the advantage of collecting more events outweighs the disadvantages. For this reason, scanners that are made with the faster, better time resolution detectors are those that principally operate in three dimensions. The quantitative technique for calculating how these unwanted events affect image quality is called *noise equivalent counting*.

Attenuation Correction

A requisite for recovering absolute activity concentrations and artifact-free images is proper estimation of the attenuating structures in the thorax. Coincidence detection requires both collinear photons to reach the detector pairs within a timing window. Attenuation correction in PET takes advantage of the fact that the total path-length traveled by the photon pair is the same, irrespective of the position along the line where the annihilation took place. The total attenuation can then be measured directly by placing a source of activity at the edge of the field of view and acquiring counts with the patient in the scanner and comparing to counts acquired with nothing in the scanner. Before the introduction of combined PET and CT systems, attenuation was measured with external radionuclide sources. This technique required several minutes of data collection to achieve good statistics and closely represents the average position of the dynamically changing the thorax contents observed during the emission study. Now, collection of attenuation data with CT takes a few seconds or less to capture an instance of the thoracic contents. The temporal mismatch between CT for attenuation correction and PET for the emission study can lead to artifacts in the reconstructed images that confound interpretation and quantitation. The use of CT for attenuation correction and protocols to minimize temporal mismatch are discussed later.

Conversion of CT Images to PET Attenuation Maps

Photon transmission through a dense body can be expressed in terms of the linear attenuation coefficient, μ [1/cm]; μ is a function of the photon energy and electron density of the material traversed. Photon attenuation at CT diagnostic energies is dominated by the photoelectric effect and Compton scattering. Measured linear attenuation coefficients in CT imaging are determined with a continuous photon spectrum composed of bremsstrahlung and characteristic x-rays ranging from approximately 10 keV to the peak x-ray tube potential. Reconstructed CT attenuation values are expressed relative to water and termed *Hounsfield units* [HU = 1000 $(\mu - \mu_{water})/\mu_{water}$]. PET imaging occurs at 511 keV, where photon attenuation is dominated by Compton scattering. Therefore, CT data cannot be used directly to correct for attenuation of PET emission data. Instead, CT data are converted to 511-keV linear attenuation coefficients by segmentation or direct scaling.

Segmentation takes advantage of there being only a few primary tissue types in the field of view, such as bone, tissue, and lung. CT numbers (Hounsfield units) that fall within one of these groups are replaced with the appropriate linear attenuation coefficient at 511 keV. The advantage of this technique is that it reduces variation and noise in the image. The disadvantage is that it does not permit interindividual or intraindividual variation in the coefficients. It also forces all tissues into one of the segmented types. This method is now rarely used.

Direct scaling assumes a linear relationship between CT and PET attenuation. This is a good assumption in low-density tissues such as lung and soft tissue. Bone is an exception because its CT attenuation is dominated primarily by photoelectric contributions. Therefore, the linear relationship depends on the effective energy of the CT scan. So, an appropriate calibration curve needs to be a combination of two or more linear curves that cover the range of attenuation commonly found in the body. A bilinear relationship is a common conversion technique used in PET/CT scanners (Fig. 23-8).

CT data are collected at higher resolution (typically 1- × 1- × 1-mm voxels) than are PET data (typically 6- × 6- × 6-mm voxels), requiring the converted CT image to be down-sampled to the PET image matrix size and smoothed with an appropriate kernel to match the PET resolution (Fig. 23-9). The attenuation map data are then used to correct the emission data.

Attenuation Mismatch

Artifacts can arise from improper registration between the transmission and emission scans. The cause of such artifacts can be placed in three primary groups: (1) motion of the patient, such as large rigid body movements, which may occur during or between scans; (2) breathing motion, resulting from the mismatch in temporal resolution between the CT attenuation correction (acquired in <1 breath cycle) and the emission (acquired over many breath cycles) scans; and (3) drift of the contents of thoracic cavity drift, such as that induced by the administration of pharmacologic stressing agents and other factors leading to a shift in the heart's position within the thoracic cavity. Each of these sources is discussed.

Motion of the Patient

Voluntary motion of the patient commonly occurs in response to discomfort experienced during long imaging scans. A motion event may occur between the CT and PET acquisition or, more commonly, during the PET study. Intra-scan motion is evident by mismatched boundaries and uptake in regions not normally associated with perfusion or increased metabolism (Fig. 23-10). Motion during a scan appears as blurred edges and loss of anatomic detail (Fig. 23-11).

Respiratory and Contractile Cardiac Motion

In dedicated PET systems, the long transmission time required for rotating radionuclide transmission sources around the body provides good respiratory and cardiac temporal averaging as is present in the emission scan. With the introduction of CT for attenuation correction, respiratory and contractile cardiac motion has consider-

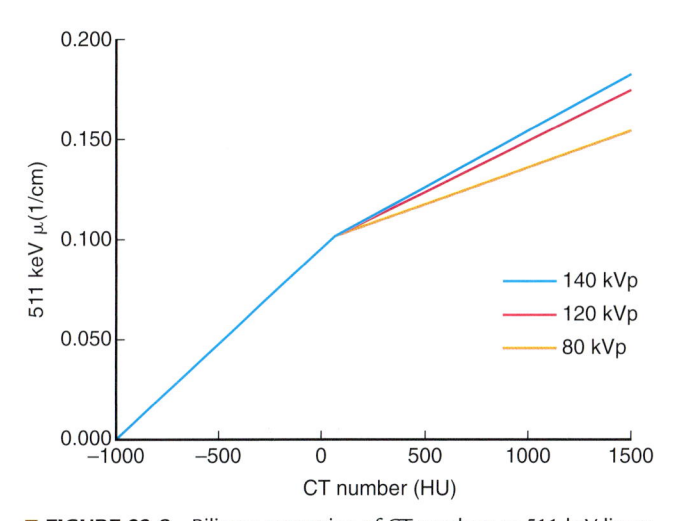

■ **FIGURE 23-8** Bilinear conversion of CT numbers to 511-keV linear attenuation coefficients. The change in slope occurs at 0 HU (water) and is a function of the different attenuation properties of soft tissue and bone and the voltage on the x-ray tube.

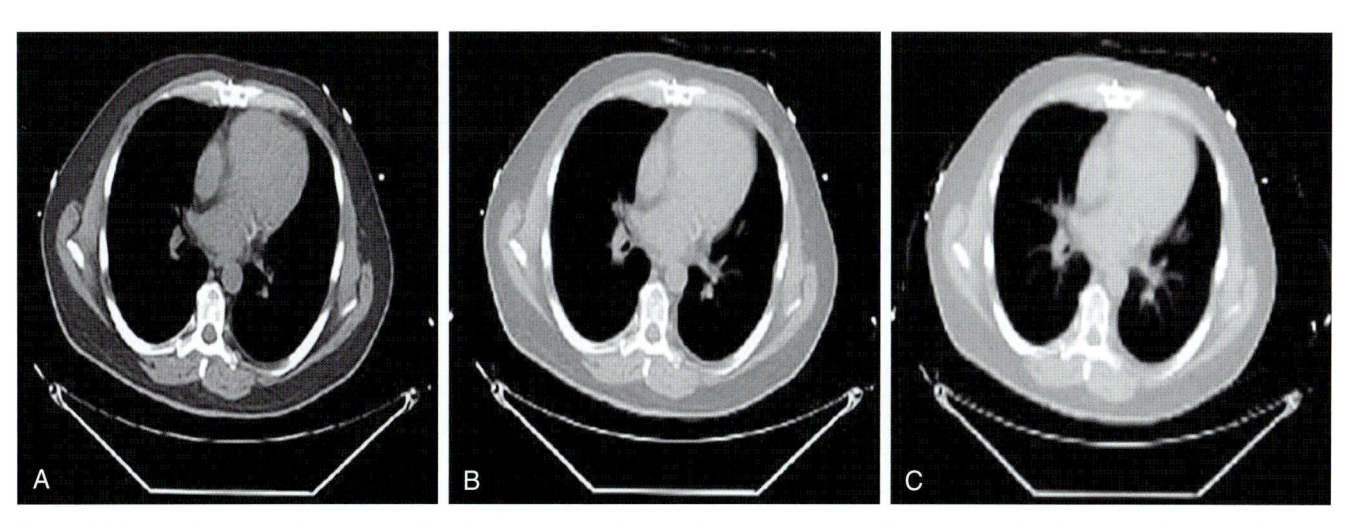

■ **FIGURE 23-9** CT image collected at 120 kVp (**A**), converted to 511 keV linear attenuation coefficients using the bilinear curve in Figure 23-8 (**B**), and down-sampled to the PET matrix size and smoothed with a 6-mm gaussian filter (**C**). The image in C is used to correct PET data for attenuation.

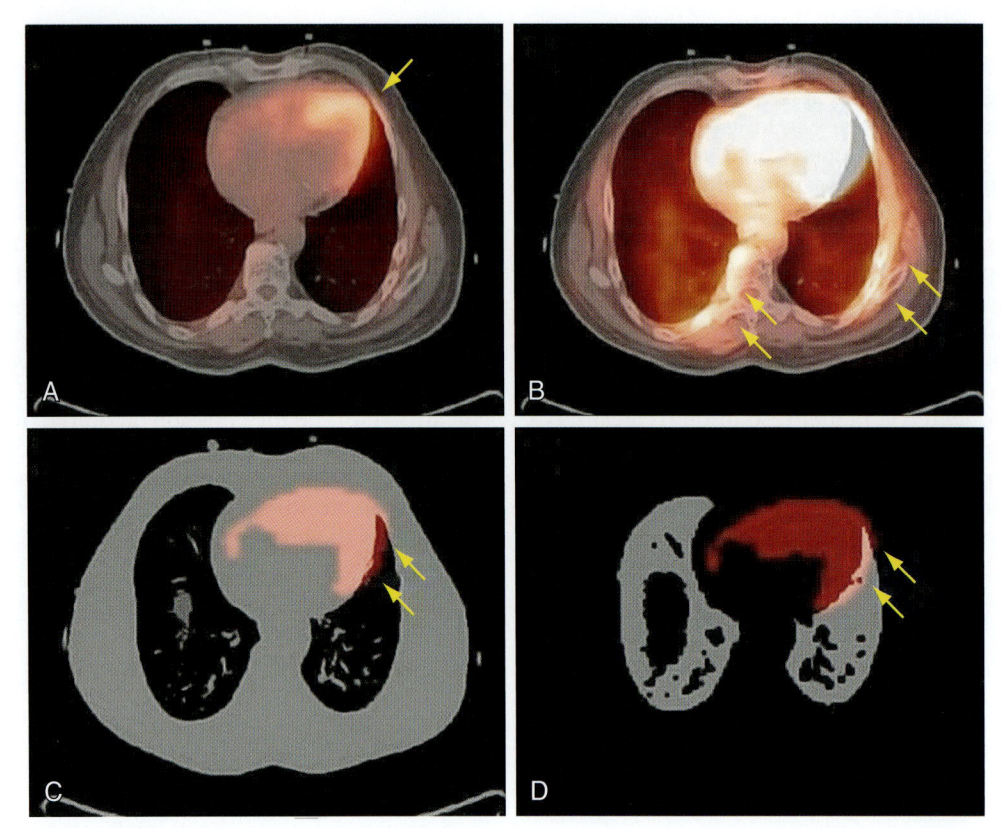

FIGURE 23-10 **A,** Patient scanned with ^{82}Rb identified as having intra-scan motion evident from the apex of the myocardium positioned in the left chest wall. **B,** Lowering of the upper level display threshold of the PET scan makes the mismatch more apparent and reveals streak artifacts along the boundaries of the lungs, which is another sign of movement. **C,** A binary representation of myocardial uptake and attenuating tissue shows uptake overlying the left lung of the CT image. Overlying tissue is a strong indicator of misregistration. **D,** A binary myocardial uptake image overlaid on a segmented lung image again shows the myocardial uptake overlying the CT lung field.

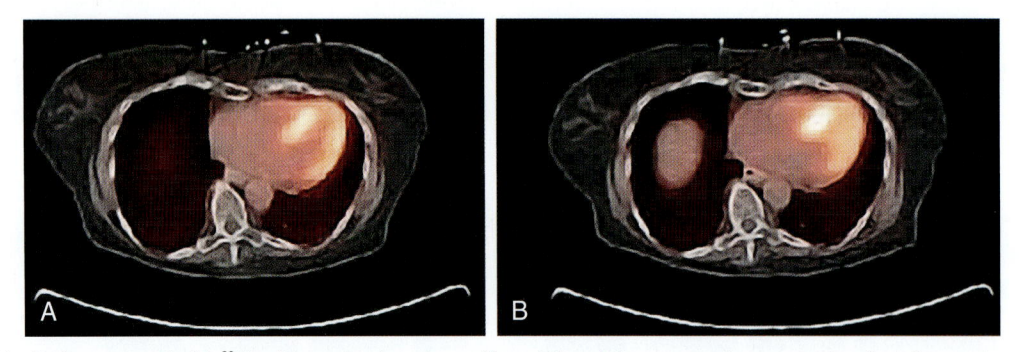

FIGURE 23-11 Patient scanned with ^{82}Rb with no visual motion artifacts (**A**) and the same patient scanned earlier after moving during the emission study (**B**). Note the decreased blood pool to myocardium contrast and apparent loss of resolution.

ably greater potential to unduly influence the attenuation correction because a fast helical CT scan fails to account for the time averaging observed in the emission acquisition (Fig. 23-12). As a result, the reported frequency of registration errors between the transmission and emission sequences has increased dramatically from dedicated PET systems[2] to PET/CT hybrid systems.[3]

Drift of Thoracic Contents

Drift of the thoracic contents, such as slow continuous movement of the heart, occurs in response to changes in the patient's state, such as changes in lung volume as a result of the introduction of a pharmacologic stressing agent.[2] Misregistration caused by this mechanism is commonly observed as cardiac uptake overlying the CT lung field (Fig. 23-13). Furthermore, even in the presence of

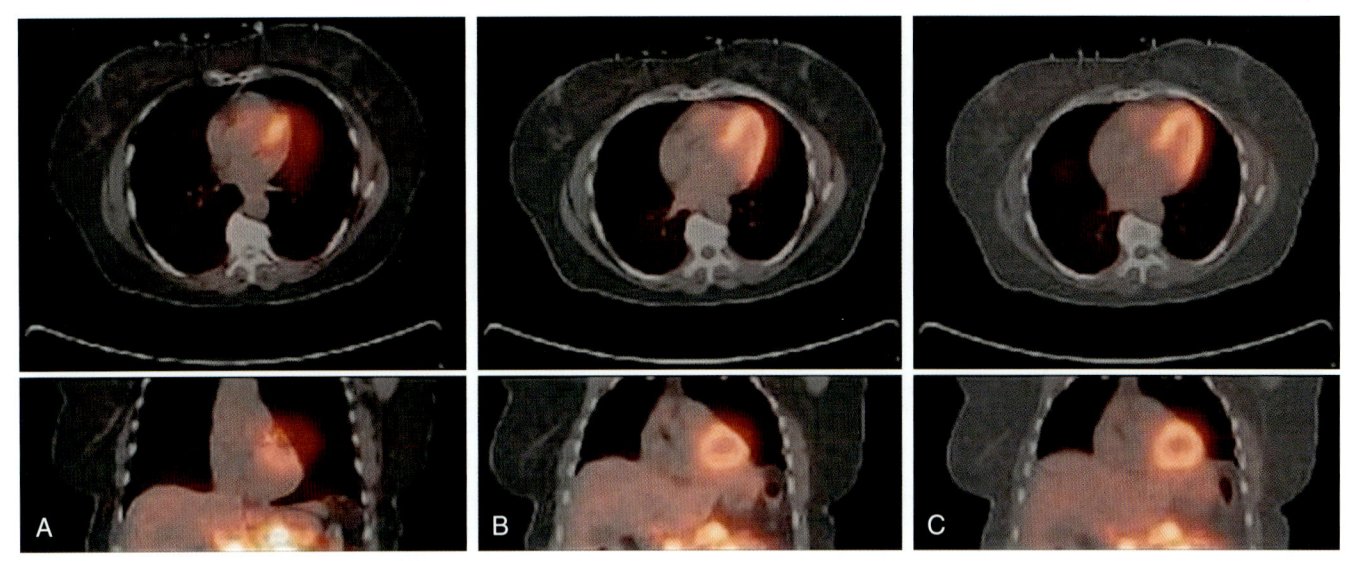

FIGURE 23-12 An example of three different CT protocols for attenuation correction. **A,** Breath-hold CT at inspiration. This is unsuitable for attenuation correction. **B,** Free-breathing low-pitch CT. **C,** Free-breathing time-averaged cine CT. In **B** and **C,** note the superior alignment between the PET and CT images compared with the breath-hold CT.

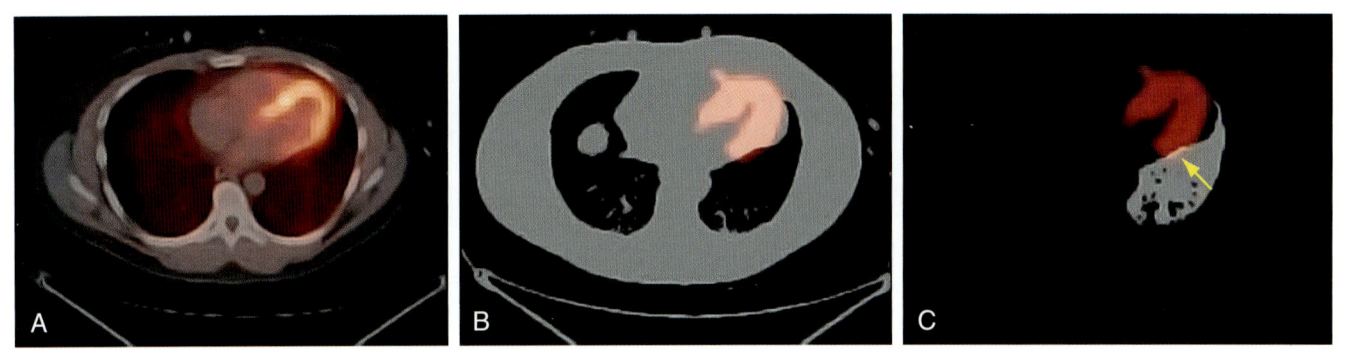

FIGURE 23-13 An example of misalignment between the emission and transmission examinations caused by drift of the heart. Notice that the myocardium in the PET image appears to have rotated relative to that in the CT image. **A,** Fused ^{82}Rb adenosine stress image. **B,** Segmented image of ^{82}Rb uptake overlaid on CT image. **C,** Segmented image of ^{82}Rb uptake overlaid on left lung of the CT volume.

good respiratory averaged transmission data, drift of thoracic contents is still prevalent and is a main factor along with motion of the patient leading to registration errors in approximately one quarter of clinical perfusion studies. Given the nature of its mechanism, motion of the patient often cannot be accounted for by altering the transmission protocol and therefore requires that a post-reconstruction image registration method be available.

Attenuation Correction Protocols

Correction schemes to address the motion problem in the thorax have concentrated on gating techniques in the PET/CT acquisition and blurring or averaging of the transmission data.[4] The first method uses either prospective (sinogram mode) or retrospective (list mode) gating of the respiratory and cardiac cycles. The respiratory cycle is normally monitored by use of a bellows, chest band, or infrared tracking system, of which the sinusoidal phase is then divided into a predetermined number of bins, commonly 10. Monitoring of the cardiac cycle is performed with an electrocardiograph; the phase is similarly divided into a preset number of bins between successive R-R waves, commonly eight bins. The data can then be binned into a two-dimensional histogram and reconstructed into separate image volumes of any cardiac-respiratory phase combination that matches the CT phase collected. The disadvantage of this technique is that the collected prompt events are distributed into many separate images (~80), and reconstruction of a single image results in poor quality because of the low number of counts. Therefore, multiple gates are often added together to improve image quality at the sacrifice of motion-free image information. These multiple gating techniques are achievable on PET/CT systems, but there are limited software resources capable of efficiently processing these events.

A second approach to matching PET emission and CT transmission data is blurring or averaging of the CT data to match the averaged nature of the PET study. This approach is referred to as *time-averaged CT* and has been explored more extensively because the protocols employed are used routinely in stand-alone cardiac CT units. Time-averaged CT protocols have been proposed in place of a breath-hold because they permit the patient to be scanned under free-breathing conditions (see Fig. 23-12B&C). The motivation is that the free-breathing state provides a more accurate representation of attenuating structures present in the emission examination. One method for obtaining a time-averaged CT scan is use of a low-pitch helical protocol whereby data are collected at a pitch of 0.5 or lower. This approach increases the axial sampling, which suppresses motion artifacts and results in blurring when linear interpolation algorithms are used in the reconstruction. In this case, the cardiac and respiratory phases are spread along the axial direction (see Fig. 23-12B).[5] A second method is collecting an average CT by successive cine mode acquisitions (also referred to as sequential), whereby multiple images are collected over one or more breath cycles at a single bed position. The table is then stepped to the next position, and acquisition resumes. This sequence is repeated until the entire chest cavity is covered. The multiple image data are then averaged at each bed position and interpolated to the PET slice thickness for attenuation correction (see Fig. 23-12C).[6]

Placement of the CT Attenuation Correction in the Imaging Protocol

Ideally, it is desirable to collect a CT attenuation correction (CTAC) in the rest and stress states by placing the CT protocol before rest perfusion and after stress perfusion. The latter condition can be logistically difficult in centers performing cardiac perfusion examinations by using adenosine to stress the patient. This is because the recovery from adenosine is too fast to permit a post–CT image to capture the thoracic contents in the peak stress state. Studies performed with dipyridamole or regadenoson (Lexiscan), which have a longer duration of effect, permit a second CTAC to be placed at the end of the stress emission study.

PET and CT Coregistration

Drift of the thoracic contents and motion of the patient cannot be fully corrected by altering the CTAC protocol and thus require a post-imaging correction method to align the transmission and emission data. Registration packages are becoming standard on PET/CT cardiac systems and employ a six-parameter (three translations, three rotations) rigid-body transformation of the CTAC image to match the emission data. The process of coregistration has not yet been automated; therefore, it remains a source of variability introduced by individual user preferences in subjectively assessing alignment quality.

It is recommended that the emission study be reconstructed without corrections to reduce the likelihood of mistaking a low-count region for an anatomic edge. Variability in the coregistration can further be reduced by implementing a quality control procedure. A straightforward method is to count the number of myocardial uptake pixels that overlie the left lung of the CTAC image. Then, as the CT myocardium is altered to match the myocardium uptake in the emission images, the number of emission myocardial pixels in the CT left lung field can be monitored (see Fig. 23-13).[7]

A disadvantage of the rigid-body transformation method is the concomitant relocation of highly attenuating structures. In the case of drift of the thoracic contents, bony structures such as the spine are repositioned to an area that does not correspond to spine in the emission study. This leads to streaking artifacts discussed in the section on quality control. Therefore, an alternative to the rigid-body registration method is needed. One proposed technique is an emission-driven approach wherein pixels in the left CT lung field that overlap with myocardial uptake in the emission image are reassigned values corresponding to soft tissue.[3]

Scatter Correction

The presence of scatter in the data set leads to images with reduced resolution and contrast. Scattered events add to the background, but because small-angle scattering is more probable, scatter adds more events to the lines of response that pass through the central areas of the body. For example, an image that contains scatter would have greater apparent activity at the center. On the other hand, if the scatter correction is overzealous, there will be a decrease in apparent activity near the center. This situation happens if prompt gammas are not properly handled as described later. The fraction of scattered events in three-dimensional scanners can approach 50%. Hence, scatter correction is a substantial modification to the primary data set. If an image contains photopenic regions that do not correspond to expected anatomy, it is wise to investigate the scatter correction. A comparison of images with and without the correction is valuable for determining if there is a problem in the original reconstruction.

Scatter correction is a difficult problem because to calculate the amount of scatter, you must know the location of both the radioactivity and the scattering material. The distribution of scatterers is derived from the CT scan, but the location of the radioactivity is unknown. After all, it is the purpose for performing the scan. Hence, scatter correction is necessarily an iterative procedure.

Photons can scatter off any electron in the body, but considering every possibility is unwieldy. The calculation becomes much easier if all of the scattering is considered to occur from a single scattering source. The most common simplification is to assume that the scatter always takes place at the midpoint of the particular line of response[8]; with this assumption, it is straightforward to calculate the number of scatter events that would be detected in neighboring lines of response, and an iterative process can be used to reduce the effect of scatter in the final images.

There is a fundamental difficulty with this algorithm for scatter correction. Some of the scattering takes place outside the field of view, where there is no information about the scatter sources. Hence, the calculation, even in principle, cannot be done without simplifying assumptions. Scatter events that originate outside of the field of view tend to contribute a uniform or very slowly varying background throughout the field of view. The following algorithm is often used to account for scatter from unknown sources. The scatter calculation is performed as described before for the known scatterers. This sets the shape of the scatter background. The calculated distribution is then linearly scaled so that it matches the number of events detected outside of the patient. This assumes that after random events correction, the only events outside of the patient are from scatter. The critical point here is that practical scatter correction is a two-step process: the first step estimates the shape of the scatter distribution, and the second scales it to match the data outside the patient.

A difficulty is encountered when scanning ^{82}Rb. Recall that ^{82}Rb often emits a prompt gamma that looks like a random event when it is detected. Further, the standard randoms correction using the delayed window will not correct for this type of event because it never occurs in the delayed window. This is important in thinking about the scatter correction. With other PET nuclides, after the randoms correction, the only type of event that is seen outside the body is scatter, which is why the scaling step is valid. However, in the ^{82}Rb case, there are also apparent random events outside the body. Therefore, if the scatter distribution is scaled to match the background, it will be made artificially high. This leads to overestimation of the amount of scatter in the body. Subtracting this supposed large contribution leaves behind photopenic areas. Often, these photopenic areas overlap the heart and could be read as a defect, leading to a false-positive study result. See the later section on quality control for figures showing this effect.

Scatter correction remains an area of active investigation. As computer power continues to increase, more and more sophisticated algorithms can be used to estimate and to correct for scatter. On first consideration, most people consider scattered photons to be contaminants that should be discarded from the data set. However, the scattered photons carry information about the location of activity. This is because scatter by small angles is more likely than by large angles. So, the line of response from a scattered event is likely to pass near the actual source of activity. An algorithm that makes use of this fact could potentially produce better images. Currently, state-of-the-art reconstructions model the scatter and subtract it from the primary data set. Rather than discarding the information in these events, it is likely that reconstruction algorithms in the future will take advantage of the information to produce images with better resolution and contrast.

Image Reconstruction

There are two broad approaches to reconstruction of images from PET data. One is a direct calculation of the image from the data, and the other is an iterative approach that calculates successive approximations that lead to the final image. The direct approach is called filtered backprojection (FBP). Historically, FBP has been used because it requires fewer computing resources and the algorithm is fast. On the other hand, several assumptions must be made about the data for the calculation to be performed. The implications of these are discussed later. The most common iterative approach is called ordered subsets expectation maximization or OSEM. Iterative methods have the advantage of being able to more appropriately incorporate the physics of the decay and detecting device. There are two main disadvantages: it takes longer, and because it is a series of successive approximations, each getting closer to the "true" image, it is very difficult to know when to stop the iterations.

FBP requires that the recorded data will be equivalent (except for a simple shift in position) no matter where the activity is placed in the scanner. In general, this is not the case. Photons from the center of the field of view enter the detectors perpendicular to the front surface. On the other hand, photons from the edge can impinge on the detectors with a high angle of incidence and so have high probability of passing through one detector and interacting with its neighbor. (This is generally called the depth of interaction problem in PET.) More detectors are involved when activity is at the edge of the field of view, so the assumption required by FBP is not fully justified. FBP has other assumptions that are not fully justified. FBP is built on equations derived mathematically after assuming a perfect set of data. It does not consider the statistical nature of radioactive decay. The actual number of detected events varies from scan to scan because of inherent randomness. Also implied in assuming a perfect data set is that it consists of only true events. This means that randoms, scatter, and attenuation must all be corrected (perfectly) before reconstruction. Finally, the perfect data set implies that there are no gaps in the data. All practical scanners have gaps between separate detectors. Often, there are gaps between individual detectors that are assembled into detector modules. These modules are assembled into the scanner ring, leaving different-sized gaps at their edges. The greater these assumptions are violated, the greater will be the negative impact on the final image.

The most visible breakdown of the assumptions in FBP is streaks in the images. These are primarily caused because the data are not perfect. Some lines of response will have an excess number of recorded events, and some neighbors will have too few just by the random nature of radioactive decay. Because of this, certain lines of response will project too much activity and other lines too little. There are two situations in which this is particularly apparent. Outside the image, the process can produce both positive and negative streaks. Most often, negative pixel values are simply ignored. The other situation is in the vicinity of very hot structures that are next to somewhat cool structures. The bladder is such a case in normal fluorodeoxyglucose (FDG) imaging. The lines of response that pass through the bladder generally have many times more recorded events than do neighboring lines of response. Any error in the detected number of events in the large lines of response will have a large effect on the neighboring lines. Because of the random nature of the decay process, the calculated number of events to project will never be exactly correct. In this situation, the errors appear as streaks and are readily apparent in nearby structures that contain little radioactivity.

Iterative reconstruction methods do not have the FBP difficulties resulting from violated assumptions necessary for the mathematics. However, they do have some drawbacks of their own that will be discussed after an introduction to the technique is presented. The start of an iterative routine is a guess of the image. Assuming that the image represents the activity distribution in the field of view, the

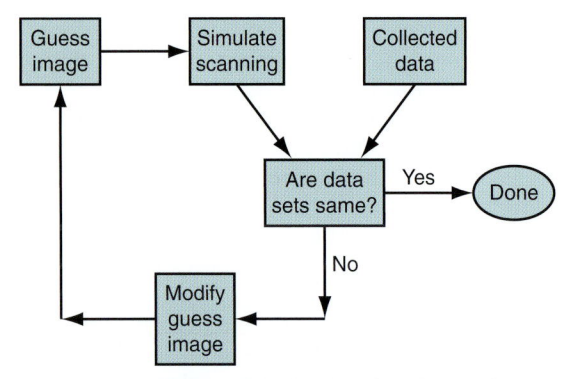

FIGURE 23-14 Diagram of the iterative algorithm used to reconstruct images. Initially, a guess is made for the image. On the basis of assuming that the activity is at the locations in the guessed image, scanning is simulated to produce a simulated data set. The simulated and measured data sets are compared, and if they are significantly different, the guess image is modified and the process is repeated. The quality of this routine is in the "simulate scanning" box. This box can include very sophisticated physics to provide the best images, or it can contain many approximations to make the computations easier and faster.

scanning process is simulated to produce a simulated data set. The simulated data set is compared with the actual data set, and differences are noted. Where the simulated data are too large, the corresponding pixels in the guess image are reduced, and vice versa, to produce the next estimate of the true image (Fig. 23-14). The process is repeated many times until the simulated and measured data sets are the same or as close as possible. In the literature, there is considerable discussion about how many iterations should be performed. Because the statistics of radioactive decay are well known to be Poisson distributions, the simulated data set can be compared with the actual data set in a probabilistic sense. Hence, the probability that that particular data set could have arisen from the guess image distribution is calculated. Iterations can be continued as long as this probability continues to increase. After each of the first few iterations, the probability increases rapidly; but after many iterations, the incremental increase is much less. Hence, from a practical point of view, images are generally reconstructed with a fixed number of iterations.

The advantage of the iterative reconstruction procedure is that the physics of scanning is more realistically built into the algorithm. This includes the scattering process, any gaps in detector spacing within the scanner, variation in resolution across the field of view, and the noise inherent with radioactive decay. These processes are all part of the "simulate scanning" box in Figure 23-14. The disadvantage is the time required to reconstruct the image. As a matter of practical implementation, the physics built into the reconstruction algorithm is not the best available. As discussed before, the scatter correction estimation involves assuming that scattering takes place at the center of the scanner. Another problem area is the geometry of the lines of response. Photons in different lines of response interact differently with the detectors, depending on whether the line of response is normally incident or incident at an angle with respect to the detectors. To make the calculation faster, it is usually assumed that all lines of response have the same interaction with the detector. These are examples of problems with the practical implementation. In principle, the iterative reconstruction can be much more accurate. As computing power has increased over the years, the physics built into the reconstruction algorithm has become more sophisticated. For example, including the difference in detection response as a function of the geometry of the detectors and line of response is becoming more common.

As computing power continues to improve, the algorithms will incorporate even more of the physics of the scanning process, and there is little doubt that iterative reconstruction will dominate all image reconstruction. Currently, iterative reconstruction is superior in low-count studies. In these studies, the noise is proportionately higher and the perfect data assumption of FBP is more violated. Iterative reconstruction with its proper handling of the noise in radioactive decay is superior in these imaging situations. This is why nearly all whole-body FDG imaging is reconstructed with the iterative routine. Cardiac imaging is generally not in this regimen; the count rate is much higher. For this reason, the reconstruction method used at different centers is divided between FBP and iterative reconstruction. When there are sufficient counts, as there is in both ^{82}Rb and FDG cardiac imaging, the assumption of perfect data is much more reliable for the FBP reconstruction algorithm. When this is the case, it may be that the indecision in knowing how many iterations to perform is a dominant factor in choosing the algorithm. From a practical point of view, it is very difficult to determine any difference between the two reconstruction methods for cardiac imaging. Because of this, almost all centers decide on the method they use for historical reasons or some other preconceived bias. There is little question that in the future, iterative reconstruction will be the method of choice.

TRACER KINETICS

In this section, the properties of rubidium for measuring flow and of FDG for measuring glucose metabolism are discussed. Both of these tracers have unique properties that influence how they interact with the tissue and permit specific physiologic parameters to be determined.

Rubidium 82

Rubidium is a microsphere-like tracer. Microspheres are radiolabeled molecules or physical spheres that will flow through arteries but are trapped in capillaries. In a microsphere experiment, the microspheres are injected into the left atrium or ventricle, and they are distributed throughout the body by the circulatory system. Areas that get more blood flow get more microspheres. Because they are trapped in the capillaries, subsequent determination of the number of microspheres in a volume of tissue is a measure of the amount of blood that flows into that tissue. Hence, if one could measure the number of microspheres per volume and make a relative image, it would depict a distribution proportional to the amount of blood flowing into the tissue at each pixel location.

Rubidium acts like a microsphere because after it crosses the capillary membrane, it becomes charged.

Once it has a positive ionic charge, it will not re-cross the capillary membrane to return to the blood supply. A fixed amount of rubidium is generally injected into an arm vein. It circulates through the heart, to the lung, back to the heart, and then to the rest of the body including the coronary arteries. Rubidium that enters the coronary arteries eventually passes to capillaries, where it can cross the membrane into the tissue, change charge state, and become trapped. The amount that crosses the membrane depends on the amount that is delivered, which is by definition blood flow. So, an image of the rubidium distribution is very highly correlated with the amount of blood flowing into each gram of tissue.

Unfortunately, rubidium is not a perfect microsphere analogue. Some of the rubidium will stay in the capillary and pass directly through the tissue. Also, the change in charge state is not instantaneous after it crosses the capillary membrane. In the time before it becomes charged, some rubidium will re-cross the capillary membrane, re-enter the blood supply to leave, and never be seen again. Because of this, the amount of rubidium trapped is less than one would expect if it behaved truly as a microsphere. The situation is worse at high flow; when blood is traveling faster, the tracer spends less time in the capillary and therefore has less chance to cross the capillary membrane. That is, the greater the flow, the greater the underestimate of that flow as measured by rubidium. Search the Internet for "^{82}Rb flow-dependent extraction" for more details.

Many investigators have taken this behavior into account when using rubidium to measure myocardial blood flow for the purpose of research studies.[9-11] In general, in these types of studies, a group of patients with a particular disease or in a particular flow state are scanned and then averaged together. These patients are then compared with another group of patients to determine if there is a difference in flow. With this technique, researchers have found that there are flow-dependent effects caused by different drugs and different lifestyles. See, for example, references 12 to 15.

An area of current research is to determine whether this technique is valid and clinically useful in individual patients. Because of the difficulties mentioned, the calculation of absolute blood flow has a fairly large error associated with it. If absolute blood flow can be reliably determined in individual patients, it could have a large impact in the assessment of coronary artery disease. It would make identification of triple-vessel disease apparent, and it would permit quantitative longitudinal studies of individual patients. In this way, the effectiveness of either a medical or invasive treatment could be better monitored.

Fluorodeoxyglucose

FDG is used to measure carbohydrate metabolism in myocardial tissue. This is only one of the energetic pathways used by the heart (fatty acid metabolism is another), so depending on the state of the heart, FDG may not measure the total energy budget. For information on estimating fatty acid metabolism with PET, search the Internet for "myocardial fatty acid PET." FDG has several unique properties that make it ideally suited to measurement of carbohydrate metabolism. The critical ones are that (1) the extraction across the capillary membranes during a single pass is relatively small; (2) the clearance of FDG from the body through the kidneys is relatively slow; (3) when FDG enters the metabolic pathway, it is trapped in cardiac tissue (nearly) irreversibly; and (4) FDG that does not enter the metabolic pathway re-enters the circulatory system and is eventually cleared from the body by the kidneys. In some sense, FDG acts like a microsphere because it is irreversibly trapped, but the trapping is due to a metabolic process rather than a flow process.

The four properties of FDG are important for the following reasons. The first two lead to the uptake of FDG being flow independent. The extraction is low; typically only 10% of the FDG crosses the capillary membrane during a single pass. If the extraction were high, similar to rubidium, the amount of FDG trapped in the tissue would be more a function of how much is delivered than of how much is metabolized. Regions of high flow would get more FDG regardless of their metabolic rate. Because the extraction is relatively small, the FDG needs to remain in the body for a suitable length of time for all tissues to have equal access to FDG. The kidneys clear FDG from the body relatively slowly, permitting FDG to make many circulations through the body before it is removed. This permits all tissues to have equal access to FDG regardless of the amount of blood flow to them. On the other hand, the clearance from the body cannot be so slow that activity remains in the blood throughout the study, leading to high background. The clearance of FDG by the kidneys happens to be nicely situated between too fast to allow equal uptake and too slow to permit high-contrast images.

In a typical FDG experiment, activity is injected and becomes trapped in tissue proportionally to glucose metabolic rate during approximately 15 minutes. The remainder of the activity is cleared by the kidneys during the next 15 to 25 minutes. Hence, by approximately 45 minutes after the injection, there is very good contrast between activity in the myocardial tissue and low activity in the blood, and the uptake is very highly correlated with the glucose metabolic rate.

PROTOCOLS

Prescreening, instruction and consent, preparation, and comfort are important components to a successful imaging examination that provides high medical value to the patient. The patient's history should be reviewed before the examination to determine if specific instructions are required or if specific demographic information is missing. Information required for a successful PET/CT cardiac examination includes the patient's height and weight, medications, dietary state, diabetic state, recent medical history pertaining to chest discomfort, and previous interventions or procedures. The following information represents the adopted protocols of the authors' institution and reflects the specific situations and demographics of the surrounding population of patients.

Dietary Restrictions

Perfusion Imaging

One to two days before the scheduled examination, the patient should be instructed to fast (except for water) 6 hours before the examination and to abstain from caffeine-containing foods (e.g., chocolate) and beverages (e.g., soda) for a minimum of 24 hours before the examination. This creates a more consistent background state that enables a higher sensitivity study. The patient should also be instructed to discontinue use of theophylline- or aminophylline-containing medications because they are antagonistic to pharmacologic stressing agents (e.g., adenosine). In addition, β blockers and calcium channel blockers should be held up to 24 hours prior.

Viability Imaging

Recommended dietary restrictions for assessment of myocardial viability are similar to those detailed for perfusion imaging. Insulin-dependent patients require more rigorous monitoring to stabilize blood glucose levels. It is desirable for the myocardium to preferentially use glucose during the uptake of FDG. This is accomplished by fasting followed by a glucose loading protocol.

Glucose Loading

Viability imaging employs FDG as the marker for glucose metabolism. FDG enters cells by the same transport mechanism as glucose does and is trapped in the myocardium after undergoing phosphorylation to FDG-6-phosphate. In a glucose-deprived state, such as that after fasting, the myocardium derives the majority of its energy from free fatty acids, so the uptake of FDG will be heterogeneous and variable across patients. The myocardium's preference for glucose can be invoked by a glucose load given either orally or intravenously.

The general principle of glucose loading is to mobilize glucose transporters on the cell membrane by shifting the myocardium from the fasting state to the preferential fed state. A subsequent decline in glucose, by insulin injection, then promotes the transport of FDG into the myocardial cells. Monitoring of the glucose blood levels is complicated in patients with a history of diabetes mellitus, who may not present sufficiently low blood glucose levels after the fasting and dietary requirements. In this situation, a blood glucose analyzer is critical in managing plasma glucose levels and may exclude the patient if levels cannot be stabilized during the uptake and scanning period. The reader is referred to the step-by-step guidelines for FDG viability imaging published by the American Society of Nuclear Cardiology.[16]

Preparation and Positioning of the Patient

On the patient's arrival, the dietary requirements are reviewed and then the patient is asked to change into a hospital gown. The patient is prepared with a peripheral intravenous line placed in an antecubital vein large enough to permit the simultaneous injection of the pharmacologic stress agent and the radiopharmaceutical. Additional monitoring devices to measure baseline vital signs, such as electrocardiographic leads, blood pressure cuff, and oxygen pulse oximeter, can also be fixed to the patient.

Ensuring the patient's comfort on the scanner bed is essential to minimize artifacts associated with motion of the patient. This care is especially relevant during administration of the pharmacologic stress agent because a second injection of the pharmacologic stress agent is typically not advisable. The patient's arms should be placed overhead and supported by a cradle or pillows to prevent muscle fatigue. Sometimes overhead is not possible, so strict instructions about stillness should be emphasized. Once the patient is resting comfortably on the table and the monitoring devices are hooked up, protocol instruction is given including breathing instructions for the attenuation correction, timing of injections, administration of pharmacologic stress, and frequency of monitoring. If movement of the patient is detected early in the study, the resting acquisition can be repeated, whereas the stress portion of the study is less flexible when pharmacologic stress agents are employed.

Pharmacologic Stress

It is very difficult logistically to treadmill stress then transport the patient to an imaging camera for PET perfusion imaging because of the short half-lives of the radiopharmaceuticals (^{82}Rb, 75 seconds; ^{13}N, 10 minutes). Therefore, pharmacologic agents are preferred for the stressing portion of perfusion studies and provide some benefits, including reduction in radiation exposure to the imaging staff. Also, some patients may require pharmacologic stress because of an inability to reach a desired level of exercise, and it potentially provides a more consistent level of stress simulation in patient groups that present physical handicaps or myocardial infarction. However, protocols involving drug infusion are generally more complex, requiring calculation of dosage, infusion equipment, timing, additional personnel, and continuous monitoring for adverse effects.

The two most common pharmacologic stress agents are adenosine, a direct vasodilator, and dipyridamole, which inhibits facilitated reuptake of adenosine to indirectly increase the endogenous plasma level of adenosine.[17] The primary adverse effects associated with adenosine are flushing, dizziness, chest pain, and bronchoconstriction, which can be relieved by termination of the infusion or intravenous aminophylline. Dipyridamole has similar adverse effects, but the side effects are prolonged, and reversal often requires drug intervention.[18] The peak onset is induced within 3 to 7 minutes after infusion with a half-life of approximately 30 to 45 minutes. The choice between adenosine and dipyridamole is generally given to adenosine because of rapid onset of action and short half-life, lower cost per dose, and easier monitoring after study completion.[19] Peak vasodilatory effects with adenosine occur after 2 minutes of infusion and return to baseline within 2 minutes after termination.[20] The stress perfusion protocols discussed in this section involve the use of adenosine.

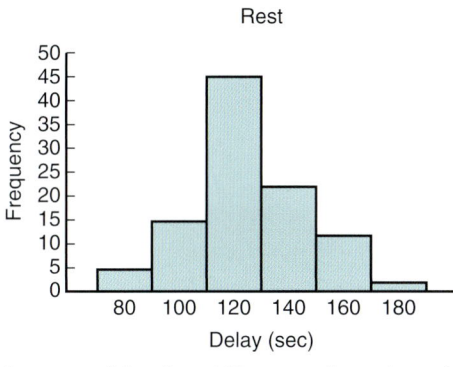

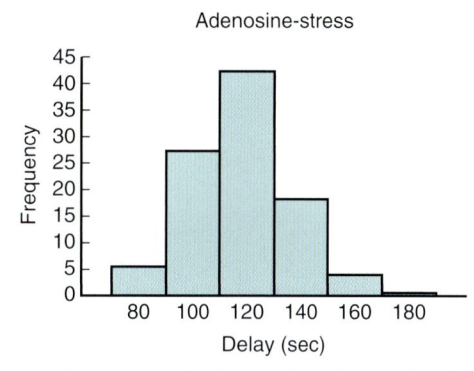

FIGURE 23-15 Histogram of data from 100 consecutive patients showing the time required for the blood pool to reach half of the myocardial tissue concentration after injection of ^{82}Rb. This time is referred to as the postinjection delay. Image data after this delay time are summed to create images for clinical interpretation.

An alternative coronary vasodilator is regadenoson, a selective A_{2A} adenosine agonist, recently approved by the Food and Drug Administration for myocardial perfusion imaging.[21] Adverse effects are similar to those of adenosine but less severe in some cases because of the weak affinity for the A_1, A_{2B}, and A_3 subtypes. The agent is packaged as a single dose and administered in a slow bolus (<10 seconds) at fixed concentration irrespective of the patient's weight. Peak onset is rapid, resulting in an increase in coronary blood flow up to twice resting rate 10 to 20 seconds after injection and decreasing to resting rate within 10 minutes. The slightly longer duration at peak coronary output for this agent compared with adenosine allows a second CTAC after stress.

FIGURE 23-16 An example of an acquisition protocol for perfusion imaging by list mode acquisition. The rest and stress scan durations are 7.5 minutes beginning at the injection of the radiopharmaceutical. The electrocardiographic signal is recorded in the list mode file.

Rest-Stress Protocols

A number of rest-stress protocols are in use in perfusion imaging. These protocols incorporate several features primarily focused on reducing the total scan time; others are tailored to extract more specific information, such as cardiac function and blood flow. Uptake of perfusion tracers is relatively rapid; the myocardial–blood pool ratio reaches 2:1 as soon as 80 seconds after infusion and sometimes as late as 180 seconds (Fig. 23-15). The data acquisition is often delayed after injection to wait for the blood pool to clear and thereby to obtain high-contrast images. The American Society of Nuclear Cardiology guidelines recommend a minimum delay of 90 seconds.[22] This technique streamlines the imaging protocol, allowing more consistent throughput. However, this practice can lead to loss of useful counts in patients with fast blood pool clearance or loss of image quality in patients with poor myocardial function or perfusion. In addition, the clearance time between rest and stress studies may vary. Thus, allowing a flexible delay permits more accurate comparison between the two image sets.

PET scanners are moving toward "list mode" acquisition. In this mode, the responding detectors and time of every event are stored in a very large data file. This is another advance made possible by increased computing power and it permits a retrospective decision as to which counts should be combined to form an image. The data collection can begin at the time of injection and later parsed to create optimal images. This is an added processing step compared with traditional data collection. However, its flexibility results in more consistent high-quality imaging at the cost of adding two steps in the image processing protocol. Therefore, the greatest flexibility in the study is achieved with a list mode acquisition, followed by initial fast reconstruction of images at predefined times, then analysis and a second reconstruction with optional timing.

Common perfusion protocols consist of the following components: (1) CT-based transmission scan at rest, (2) rest perfusion examination, (3) pharmacologic stress perfusion examination, and (4) CT-based transmission scan at stress. Two workflows are given for list mode (Fig. 23-16) and sinogram mode (Fig. 23-17) acquisition. The primary difference between the two sequences is that in sinogram mode acquisition, a second resting injection is required with electrocardiographic trigger if gated information is desired. The list mode acquisition stores the electrocardiographic triggers in the event list, which can then be binned retrospectively. This acquisition feature reduces scan time and saves radiation dose to the patient. The CTAC scan protocol is collected under free-breathing conditions to incorporate contractile and respiratory averaging (see the section on CT protocol). The extended

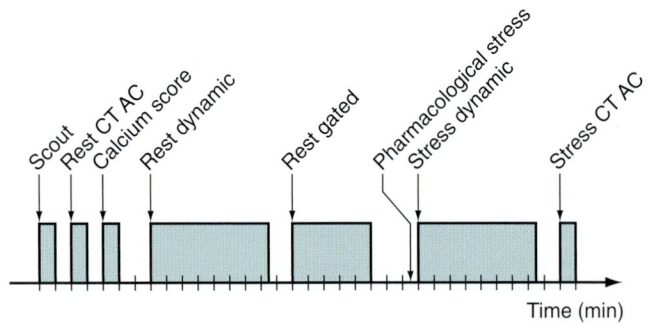

FIGURE 23-17 An example of an acquisition protocol for perfusion imaging by sinogram mode acquisition. The rest and stress scan durations are 7.5 minutes beginning at the injection of the radiopharmaceutical. Note that an extra injection is needed to collect gated data compared with the list mode protocol.

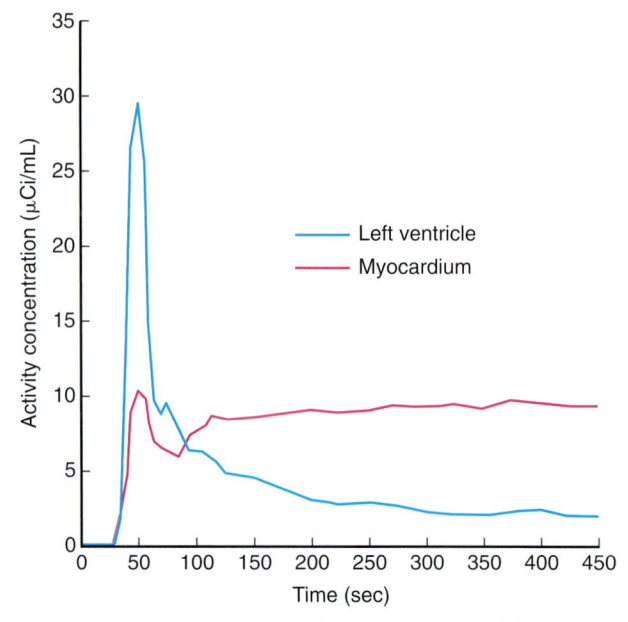

FIGURE 23-18 Representative time-activity curves of the left ventricle and myocardial tissue from an ^{82}Rb perfusion study. High-contrast images can be obtained by waiting for the blood pool to reach half of the myocardium activity concentration.

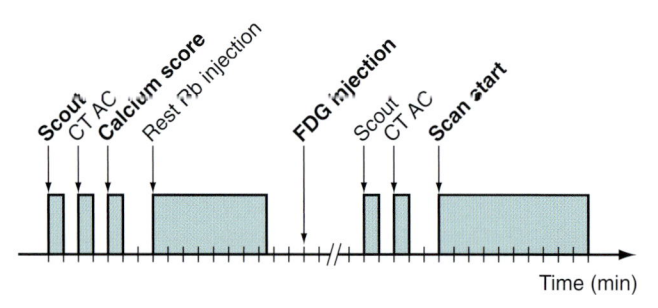

FIGURE 23-19 An example of a viability acquisition protocol. The rest acquisition duration is 7.5 minutes starting at infusion. The FDG scan is 10 minutes, which is sufficient to produce high-contrast, low-noise images.

duration of certain pharmacologic stress agents, such as regadenoson, permits the collection of an additional CTAC scan after the stress portion of the examination. Last, an optional diastolic gated CT can be incorporated to assess calcium burden by Agatston scoring. This is increasingly common for PET/CT systems sold with 64-slice or more CT scanners.

After the CTAC and Ca scoring examination, the patient table is moved to the PET position and the infusion lines are prepared. The Rb injection should be administered as a slow bolus (10 to 30 seconds). Prolonged infusion times will not allow the blood to clear sufficiently and will degrade image quality. Two infusions are performed with electrocardiographic monitoring, a 7.5-minute rest acquisition started at the time of infusion followed by a 7.5-minute pharmacologic stress acquisition. For example, pharmacologic stress with use of regadenoson is delivered in a 10-second bolus before the stress radiotracer infusion. The data are histogrammed into a specified number of frames, and regions are drawn over the left myocardium and ventricular cavity. These regions are applied identically to all frames and plotted over time to construct a time-activity curve (Fig. 23-18). The time that the blood pool concentration drops to one-half the myocardial concentration is identified and set as the scan delay. The list mode data are then rehistogrammed by starting at the delay point to reconstruct static and gated images. This is the "optimal timing" advantage made possible by list mode data collection.

Before the final reconstruction, PET images can be overlaid on the CTAC to check for proper registration. Registration with the CTAC is performed by using the techniques described before for both the rest and stress data sets. The newly registered CTAC images are saved and used to correct the rehistogrammed data in the final reconstructions.

Viability Protocols

Viability of recovering or dysfunctional myocardium requires both sufficient blood flow and metabolic activity. Therefore, this protocol consists of a resting perfusion study followed by a glucose metabolism study with electrocardiographic monitoring (Fig. 23-19). As previously mentioned, the mobilization of glucose transporters is promoted by shifting the myocardium from using fatty acids to glucose by administration of a glucose load. Plasma glucose levels must be continuously monitored to keep the myocardium in the preferential glucose state (<140 mg/dL). Patients with diabetes mellitus present a particular challenge because of their inability to reliably produce endogenous insulin and their reduced cell response to exogenous insulin stimulation. This may lead to troubles in stabilizing blood glucose levels during uptake after infusion and during imaging. The reader is referred to the American Society of Nuclear Cardiology and Society of Nuclear Medicine guidelines on FDG viability imaging.[22]

Data Reconstruction and Display

The final data are corrected for randoms, scatter, and attenuation and reconstructed by FBP or ordered subset expectation maximization (OSEM). The transaxial data are then reoriented along the short axis and imported into the user-desirable display software for interpretation.

DOSIMETRY

The radiation burden to the whole body from PET radiopharmaceuticals is low compared with general nuclear medicine cardiac procedures because of their short half-lives. Added doses in PET/CT perfusion and viability protocols are primarily attributed to exposure from added diagnostic CT procedures. The effective dose from a CT examination depends on the acquisition parameters. In general, a CTAC with good spatial resolution can be acquired with a total radiation burden of 1 mSv or less.

For a 370-MBq injection of FDG, the total whole-body effective dose is 7 mSv.[23] For a rest-stress ^{82}Rb injection (2 × 1850 MBq), the total effective radiation dose is 2.4 mSv.[24] With the addition of a scout for localization, CTAC, and two perfusion injections, a typical total effective whole-body dose for a rest-stress ^{82}Rb study is 0.5 mSv + 2 mSv + 2.4 mSv = 5 mSv.

QUALITY CONTROL

A well-designed quality control program involves monitoring of different aspects of the imaging instrumentation on daily, weekly, and monthly intervals. The procedures outlined are essential to maintaining high diagnostic accuracy and anticipating potential equipment failures before they compromise image quality. Scanners can vary considerably in construction geometry and materials. The quality control program should be adapted to the specific characteristics of the system and take into consideration individual manufacturer recommendations. However, the data collection, storage, and reconstruction are more standardized across manufacturers, and a thorough quality control program can be developed that is independent of the hardware configuration. Quality control procedures outlined by task groups (i.e., American Society of Nuclear Cardiology)[26] and accreditation agencies (i.e., American College of Radiology, Intersocietal Commission for the Accreditation of Nuclear Medicine Laboratories)[27,28] are general and applicable across several configurations. These procedures should be considered in developing a program for your institution.

A thorough PET/CT instrumentation quality control program cannot anticipate all image quality problems. The patient is potentially a large source of visually complex image artifacts that may be indistinguishable from true myocardial defects. Artifacts are often associated with multiple mechanisms, including motion of the patient, poor count statistics, poor blood pool clearance, CT image artifacts, and improper scatter correction. The largest contributor of poor image quality is motion of the patient that results in erroneous attenuation correction. These events lead to areas of artificially high and low uptake in the image.

The following section provides details of common instrumentation quality control procedures and examples of image quality problems observed in scanning of patients.

PET/CT Quality Control

From a software standpoint, the operation of a PET/CT scanner is completely integrated, giving the sense of a common unified gantry. From a hardware point of view, the PET and CT systems are completely autonomous. Thus, it is crucial that a quality control program includes an independent evaluation of the individual PET and CT systems and an evaluation of their combined use. Because of the construction of the scanner, the CT and PET portions of a study cannot be acquired simultaneously. The following quality control procedures are standard for several manufacturers and found in several guidelines, such as those of the American Society of Nuclear Cardiology.[26] Daily procedures are best performed in the morning before clinical scanning to anticipate potential problems with scanning of patients.

PET Quality Control

A baseline performance evaluation of the scanner following the National Electronic Manufacturers Association (NEMA) procedures is recommended.[29,30] These measurements should be performed by the installation engineers and hospital staff physicist. The NEMA performance evaluation includes standards for measurements of count rate, resolution, and contrast that provide objective criteria for comparing the scanner with published manufacturer specifications. It will also establish the baseline performance of the camera, from which the user can document changes that occur over time. The NEMA performance measurements should be conducted after installation of a new scanner and after major hardware upgrades. Good practice should involve a yearly NEMA performance evaluation to be compared with the baseline performance evaluation.

Daily Procedures

Changes in PET system performance are typically slow in evolving, and a rigorous daily quality control routine should be sensitive enough to track trends in system sensitivity. Changes in sensitivity may be associated with hardware and software malfunction and include changes in gantry temperature, amplifier drift, and high-voltage drift. Many of these changes can be detected visually by reviewing the raw PET data or tabulated individual detector or block count performance. The most efficient way to collect this information is by scanning a uniform phantom.

Most software systems come with the capability to view the sinogram data. In this view, differences in individual detector blocks can be detected visually that may otherwise be masked in the reconstructed images. A quantitative approach may be available that will report the singles count rate in each detector block or series of detectors. For a uniform phantom centered in the field of view, the detector singles rates should be similar. These values should be recorded by the user for comparison to the baseline.

Monthly

Small variations in detector response due to drift in photomultiplier tube gain are expected during routine use of the scanner and can be corrected by collecting a normalization scan. This scan is usually acquired with a low-activity rotating rod source that uniformly irradiates all detectors. Multiplicative factors for each line of response are calculated by comparing the counts received in individual lines of response with the average across all detector pairs. Several hours of counting are required to achieve good statistical accuracy, and therefore the scan is best collected overnight.

CT Quality Control

Quality control for CT pertains to both its performance as a stand-alone procedure and its use to correct PET data for attenuation. Errors in the CT number (Hounsfield unit) may misrepresent structure densities in the images used for anatomic localization and can propagate to inaccurate attenuation correction in the PET image.

Daily Procedures

Accurate CT numbers are a critical component and should be checked by performing a calibration test. Absolute calibration is performed by the service engineers at installation or after a major hardware upgrade. The calibration should be checked daily by scanning a uniform water-filled cylinder. A common threshold of action is ±5 CT units. By definition, the CT value of water is zero.

Other phantoms may be provided by the manufacturer that allow more rigorous testing of the CT number calibration and uniformity. Incorporation of these phantoms into a daily quality control routine will provide additional measures of image quality and performance and be helpful to the service engineers if a problem is detected.

Combined PET and CT Quality Control

Errors present in the individual PET and CT quality control procedures propagate to the final attenuation-corrected PET data. Aside from the procedures before, the sequential acquisition of the CT and PET examinations presents additional challenges associated with registration. If the individual PET and CT daily quality controls yield acceptable results, misregistration may still occur from sources of misalignment after bed motion and deflection of the cantilevered scanner bed. The latter source can be difficult to anticipate as the deflection of a cantilevered scanning bed will be dependent on the patient's weight. These differences lead to errors in localization on fused image sets.

Mechanical alignment of the CT and PET gantries is difficult to perform within the precision of PET/CT spatial measurements. It is much easier to make small changes to align the CT and PET reference frames in software by rigidly transforming one matrix to match the other. For this reason, manufacturers often provide a phantom and automated routine to check the alignment and to calculate an offset that would be applied to one of the image reference frames during the reconstruction. If no phantom exists, it is recommended that at least four point sources be placed in air in different planes. To make these point sources opaque to the CT, they can be loaded with diluted CT contrast media. In performing these measurements, it is recommended that a weight be placed on the edge of the table closest to the scanner to simulate any possible bed deflection. Once the phantom is arranged on the bed, acquire a CT image and static PET image. Load them into a fused workstation and visually check the alignment.

Accuracy of the attenuation correction requires correct transformation of CT number to 511 keV attenuation coefficients, where 0 HU is set to 0.096/cm. Potential errors in attenuation correction are best assessed by reconstructing the daily PET quality control image with the accompanying CT image used to check uniformity. The reconstruction parameters should be the same as those used for clinical scans. On any slice in the phantom field of view, the activity profile across the diameter should be flat. Concave or convex profiles are a sign of inaccurate attenuation correction.

^{82}Rb Generator

Daily Procedures

Calibration of the ^{82}Rb generator activity and breakthrough of the ^{82}Sr parent should be checked on a daily basis. This procedure is conducted in the morning before scanning of patients. First, elute the generator and discard the eluent to waste. Allow the generator to recover (~10 minutes), perform a second elution into a vial, and record the elution time. Place the vial in the dose calibrator and record the reading 75 seconds after the completed elution. Multiply this reading by two and compare with the calibrated printout from the generator. If the value and reading deviate by more than 10%, the generator calibration should be adjusted. Repeat the procedure to check the new calibration.

^{82}Sr breakthrough can be checked with the same eluent used in the calibration check. After approximately 20 minutes, the dose calibrator reading should be less than 0.02 µCi per millicurie of ^{82}Rb eluted. If not, it implies that there is ^{82}Sr in the eluent. Replace the line filters on the generator and repeat the measurement.

Image Quality Control

Motion of the patient is a potentially large source of image degradation requiring careful inspection of the image data. The effects on the image of motion by the patient are blurred contours and mismatch between the emission and transmission image data. This situation can often be remedied by collecting a second emission scan, which is feasible for perfusion imaging agents and FDG for viability. Overall, proper instruction to the patient, ensuring the patient's comfort during the imaging course, and attention to motion of the patient during the rest-stress acquisitions can make the relative occurrence of this quality problem very small. Nonetheless, the position of the patient should be monitored throughout the study by the laser alignment system supplied with the scanner.

FIGURE 23-20 Overcorrection of the lateral wall after rigid-body translation of the CT image. Streaks are observed extending from the spine to the lateral wall caused by concomitant relocation of the spine in the CT and PET images.

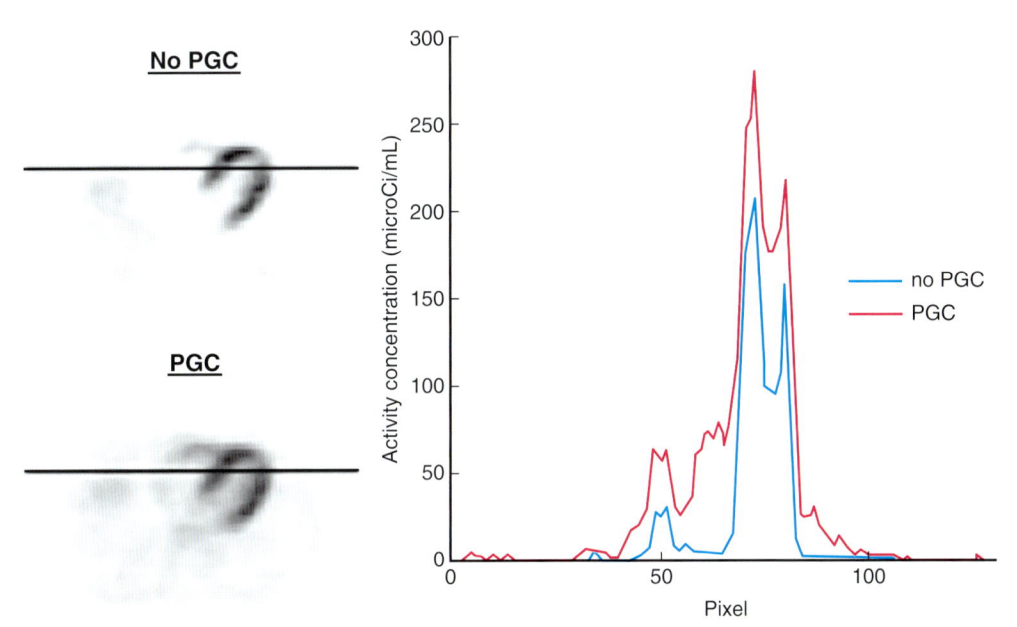

FIGURE 23-21 ^{82}Rb perfusion images reconstructed with and without prompt gamma correction (PGC). Line profiles show severe count reduction in the background regions outside the myocardium in the no PGC data.

Streaking and Lateral Wall Overcorrection

Registration of the PET and CT data can be difficult to judge because of the blurred boundaries of the heart in the emission and lack of other anatomic references due to poor uptake in the surrounding body tissues. As a result, it is possible to shift the CT image to a location where bony structures such as the ribs and spine do not correspond to their same location in the PET data. Shifting of these highly attenuating structures will cause erroneous attenuation correction that affects the entire image, but is most visible in areas along the left ventricular wall and spinal column. The concomitant relocation of the spine causes artificially increased uptake in the left ventricle wall and along the left lung boundary and distortion of the lateral wall contour (Fig. 23-20).

Prompt Gamma

Isotopes with gamma transitions in addition to positron decay represent a significant problem in three-dimensional scanning because of the wide acceptance angle for prompt events. Failure to properly correct prompt gamma events causes overcorrection of the scatter fraction, leaving photopenic areas in the image as previously described. These artificially low-count regions are most apparent in the center of the image field of view where the scatter correction is the largest. In cardiac PET imaging, this region includes the septa and apical portion of the myocardium (Fig. 23-21). In addition, sharp edges are often observed at the left ventricle–left lung interface and near the chest wall.

Metal Implants

Implanted metallic components associated with implantable cardioverter-defibrillators and pacemaker leads pose a potential problem when they are located near the myocardium.[31] Devices such as these have high mass attenuation coefficients due to their strong photoelectric absorption at x-ray photon energies, resulting in high CT values (>200 HU). However, the interaction of 511-keV gammas with metallic implants occurs primarily through Compton scattering; therefore, the attenuation varies little

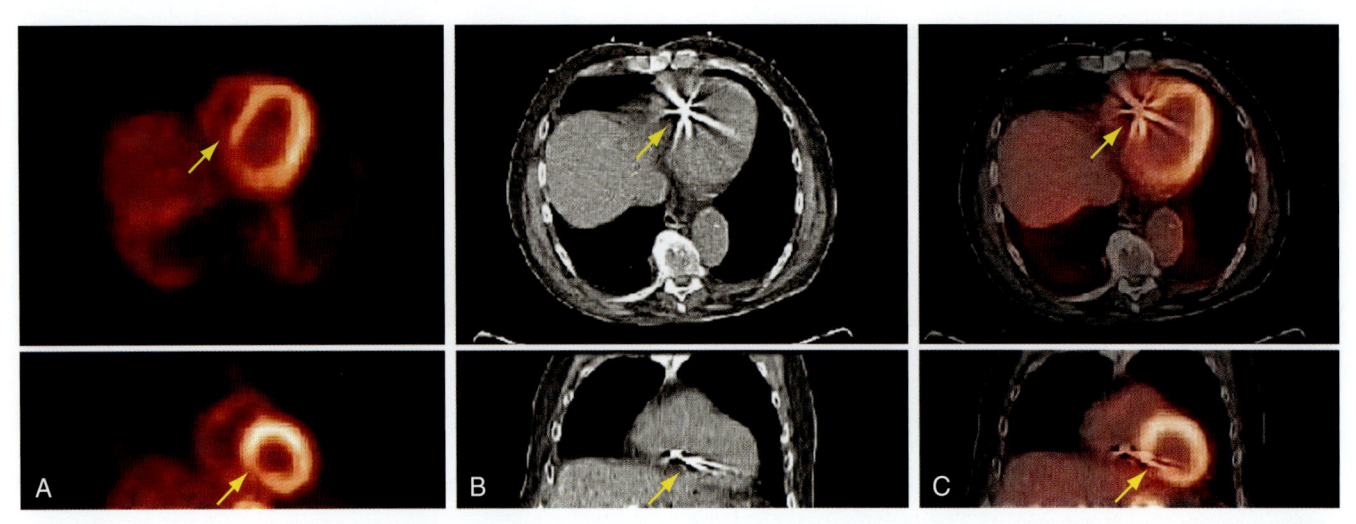

■ **FIGURE 23-22** A small artifact in the septal wall (**A**) is present from erroneous attenuation correction caused by the presence of an implantable cardioverter-defibrillator (**B**). The fused image (**C**) shows the location of the implantable cardioverter-defibrillator in relation to the PET image artifact.

with that of water. Employing bilinear conversion schemes overestimates the attenuation coefficients of metallic implants at 511 keV, which then propagate to the PET image (Fig. 23-22). Several metal artifact algorithms have been introduced to compensate for the misclassification of metal implants in the creation of PET attenuation maps.[32-34]

Truncation

The acquisition fields of view in PET and CT scanners are typically not matched. The CT gantry field of view is often 10 to 20 cm less in diameter than that of the PET gantry. Therefore, the reconstructed CT data may be missing portions of tissue at the outer boundaries of the patient (Fig. 23-23). This typically occurs when the arms are down or in patients with large torsos. The truncation of the attenuation data to the CT field of view leaves portions of the PET data with no corresponding attenuation correction factors. As a result, data at the outer rim of the PET image are underestimated. Truncation is less pronounced in perfusion imaging because of low uptake in the extremities.

Elevated Activity in Inferior Wall at Stress

At stress, the increase in lung volume causes dilation of the diaphragm and a downward shift of the heart. Therefore, when a rest CTAC is used to correct the stress study, a large portion of the diaphragm is present in the transaxial slices of the inferior portion of the myocardium. This results in an overcorrection of the attenuation in those planes and an artificially high activity concentration in the emission study. Most often, the data are scaled for display to the hottest regions, which can lead to the lateral or superior regions appearing decreased (Fig. 23-24).

> ### KEY POINTS
> - Cardiac PET/CT imaging presents more challenges than whole-body PET/CT because of the beating heart, respiratory cycle, and need to stress the patient.
> - Mismatch between the positions of organs during the CT and PET data acquisitions is the main source of image artifacts.
> - Mismatch can be minimized by protocol selection but in the end requires software alignment for optimal imaging.
> - Rubidium acts like a microsphere for monitoring of myocardial blood flow.
> - Rubidium emits a prompt gamma that will lead to false-positive study results if it is not properly handled in three-dimensional PET image reconstruction.
> - Myocardial viability can be assessed with FDG.

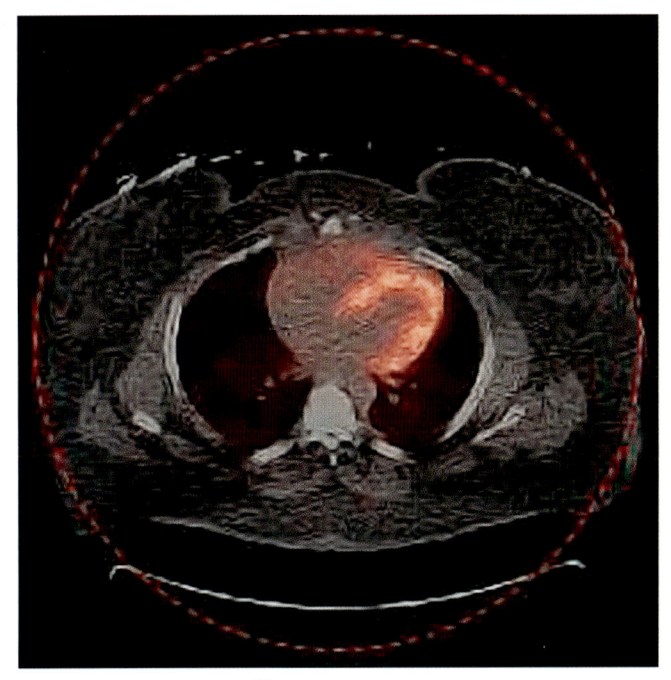

■ **FIGURE 23-23** Fused ^{82}Rb and CT study showing truncation of the CT image indicated by the reconstruction field of view outlined in red. When a CT image is truncated, the resulting attenuation map is inaccurate along lines that traverse the truncated regions. Erroneous attenuation correction at the edges of the image field of view produce the most usually apparent artifacts. The low perfusion of cardiac tracers in the extremities makes these artifacts difficult to visualize.

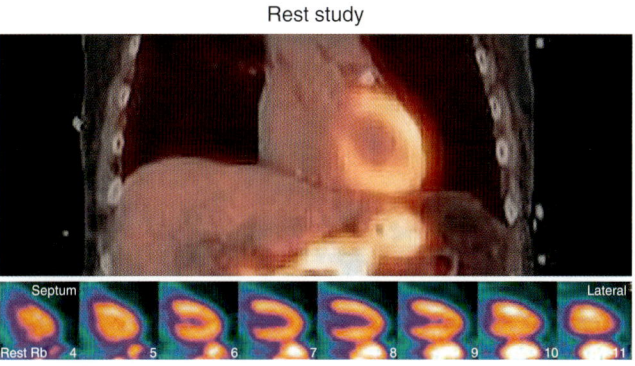

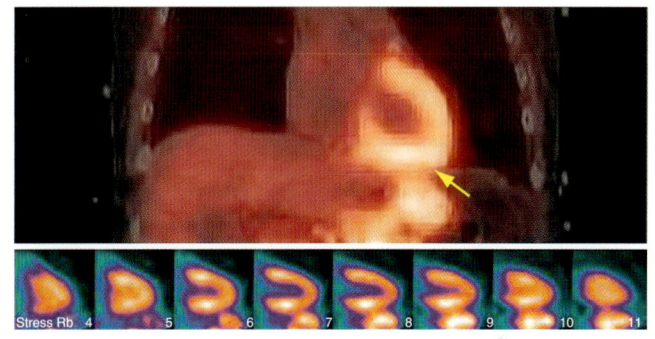

■ **FIGURE 23-24** An ^{82}Rb rest and adenosine stress perfusion study using a resting CT image for attenuation correction. The short biologic half-time of adenosine does not permit collection of a second CT image at peak stress. There is potential for an image artifact in this case because the lung volume in the stress state is typically larger than at rest. The result is a lower diaphragm position in the stress emission compared with that in the rest CT image, causing overcorrection in the inferior wall of the myocardium.

SUGGESTED READINGS

Bendriem B, Townsend DW (eds). The Theory and Practice of 3D PET. Dordrecht, The Netherlands, Kluwer Academic, 1998.
Bushberg JT, Seibert JA, Leidholdt EM Jr, Boone JM. The Essential Physics of Medical Imaging, 2nd ed. Philadelphia, Lippincott Williams & Wilkins, 2002.
Cherry S, Sorenson J, Phelps M. Physics in Nuclear Medicine. Philadelphia, WB Saunders, 2003.
Johns HE, Cunningham JR. Physics of Radiology, 4th ed. Springfield, Ill, Charles C Thomas, 1983.
Kalender WA. Computed Tomography: Fundamentals, System Technology, Image Quality, Applications. New York, Wiley, 2006.
Phelps ME. PET: Physics, Instrumentation, and Scanners. New York, Springer, 2006.

REFERENCES

1. Knoll GF. Radiation Detection and Measurement. New York, John Wiley & Sons, 1979, p 694.
2. Loghin C, Sdringola S, Gould KL. Common artifacts in PET myocardial perfusion images due to attenuation-emission misregistration: clinical significance, causes, and solutions. J Nucl Med 2004; 45: 1029-1039.
3. Martinez-Möller A, Souvatzoglou M, Navab N, et al. Artifacts from misaligned CT in cardiac perfusion PET/CT studies: frequency, effects, and potential solutions. J Nucl Med 2007; 48:188-193.
4. Martinez-Möller A, Zikic D, Botnar RM, et al. Dual cardiac-respiratory gated PET: implementation and results from a feasibility study. Eur J Nucl Med Mol Imaging 2007; 34:1447-1454.
5. Nye JA, Esteves F, Votaw JR. Minimizing artifacts resulting from respiratory and cardiac motion by optimization of the transmission scan in cardiac PET/CT. Med Phys 2007; 34:1901-1906.
6. Pan T, Mawlawi O, Luo D, et al. Attenuation correction of PET cardiac data with low-dose average CT in PET/CT. Med Phys 2006; 33:3931-3938.
7. Schuster DM, Halkar RK, Esteves FP, et al. Investigation of emission-transmission misalignment artifacts on rubidium-82 cardiac PET with adenosine pharmacologic stress. Mol Imaging Biol 2008; 10:201-208.
8. Watson CC, Newport D, Casey ME. A single scatter simulation technique for scatter correction in 3D PET. In Grangeat P, Amans JL (eds). 1995 International Meeting on Fully Three-dimensional Image Reconstruction in Radiology and Nuclear Medicine. Dordrecht, The Netherlands, Kluwer Academic, 1996.
9. Hutchins GD, Schwaiger M, Rosenspire KC, et al. Noninvasive quantification of regional blood flow in the human heart using N-13 ammonia and dynamic positron emission tomographic imaging. J Am Coll Cardiol 1990; 15:1032-1042.
10. Hutchins GD. What is the best approach to quantify myocardial blood flow with PET? J Nucl Med 2001; 42:1183-1184.
11. Krivokapich J, Smith GT, Huang SC, et al. ^{13}N ammonia myocardial imaging at rest and with exercise in normal volunteers. Quantification of absolute myocardial perfusion with dynamic positron emission tomography. Circulation 1989; 80:1328-1337.

12. Campisi R, Nathan L, Pampaloni MH, et al. Noninvasive assessment of coronary microcirculatory function in postmenopausal women and effects of short-term and long-term estrogen administration. Circulation 2002; 105:425-430.
13. Czernin J, Barnard RJ, Sun KT, et al. Effect of short-term cardiovascular conditioning and low-fat diet on myocardial blood flow and flow reserve. Circulation 1995; 92:197-204.
14. Laine H, Nuutila P, Luotolahti M, et al. Insulin-induced increment of coronary flow reserve is not abolished by dexamethasone in healthy young men. J Clin Endocrinol Metab 2000; 85:1868-1873.
15. Mellwig KP, Baller D, Gleichmann U, et al. Improvement of coronary vasodilatation capacity through single LDL apheresis. Atherosclerosis 1998; 139:173-178.
16. Bacharach SL, Bax JJ, Case J, et al. PET myocardial glucose metabolism and perfusion imaging: Part 1—Guidelines for data acquisition and patient preparation. J Nucl Cardiol 2003; 10:543-556.
17. Iskandrian AS, Verani MS, Heo J. Pharmacologic stress testing: mechanism of action, hemodynamic responses, and results in detection of coronary artery disease. J Nucl Cardiol 1994; 1:94-111.
18. Leppo JA. Comparison of pharmacologic stress agents. J Nucl Cardiol 1996; 3(pt 2):S22-S26.
19. Holmberg MJ, Mohiuddin SM, Hilleman DE, et al. Outcomes and costs of positron emission tomography: comparison of intravenous adenosine and intravenous dipyridamole. Clin Ther 1997; 19:570-581; discussion 538-539.
20. Wilson RF, Wyche K, Christensen BV, et al. Effects of adenosine on human coronary arterial circulation. Circulation 1990; 82:1595-1606.
21. Thompson CA. FDA approves pharmacologic stress agent. Am J Health Syst Pharm 2008; 65:890.
22. Schelbert HR, Beanlands R, Bengel F, et al. PET myocardial perfusion and glucose metabolism imaging: Part 2—Guidelines for interpretation and reporting. J Nucl Cardiol 2003; 10:557-571.
23. Radiation dose to patients from radiopharmaceuticals. Ann ICRP 1987; 18:1-29.
24. deKemp R, Beanlands R. A revised effective dose estimate for the PET perfusion tracer Rb-82. J Nucl Med Meeting Abstracts 2008; 49(MeetingAbstracts_1):183P-b-.
25. Radiation Dose to Patients from Radiopharmaceuticals, vol 18/1-4. ICRP, 1988. Publication 53.
26. Nichols KJ, Bacharach SL, Bergmann SR, et al. Instrumentation quality assurance and performance. J Nucl Cardiol 2006; 13:e25-e41.
27. PET Phantom Instructions for Evaluation of PET Image Quality/ACR Nuclear Medicine Accreditation Program. Reston, VA, American College of Radiology, 2009.
28. EC Standard 61675-1. Radionuclide Imaging Devices—Characteristics and Test Conditions. Part 1. Positron Emission Tomographs. Geneva. International Electrotechnical Commission, 1998.
29. Daube-Witherspoon ME, Karp JS, Casey ME, et al. PET performance measurements using the NEMA NU 2-2001 standard. J Nucl Med 2002; 43:1398-1409.
30. Watson CC, Casey ME, Eriksson L, et al. NEMA NU 2 performance tests for scanners with intrinsic radioactivity. J Nucl Med 2004; 45:822-826.
31. DiFilippo FP, Brunken RC. Do implanted pacemaker leads and ICD leads cause metal-related artifact in cardiac PET/CT? J Nucl Med 2005; 46:436-443.
32. Yu H, Zeng K, Bharkhada DK, et al. A segmentation-based method for metal artifact reduction. Acad Radiol 2007; 14:495-504.
33. Kennedy JA, Israel O, Frenkel A, et al. The reduction of artifacts due to metal hip implants in CT-attenuation corrected PET images from hybrid PET/CT scanners. Med Biol Eng Comput 2007; 45:553-562.
34. Hamill JJ, Brunken RC, Bybel B, et al. A knowledge-based method for reducing attenuation artefacts caused by cardiac appliances in myocardial PET/CT. Phys Med Biol 2006; 51:2901-2918.

CHAPTER 24

Clinical Techniques of Positron Emission Tomography and PET/CT

Marcelo F. Di Carli and Mouaz H. Al-Mallah

Positron emission tomography (PET) is a powerful tool that provides high-quality assessment of myocardial diseases. Although PET has been used for more than 25 years as a powerful investigative tool to understand physiologic processes such as myocardial perfusion and metabolism, neuronal and receptor function, and, more recently, molecularly targeted imaging, it is increasingly being accepted in routine clinical practice as a noninvasive tool to evaluate patients with known or suspected coronary artery disease (CAD). The reasons for this increased acceptance are likely multifactorial and related to the exponential growth in the number of PET/CT systems, attributable primarily to the widely accepted role of the technology in clinical oncology, which has led to increased availability; approval by the U.S. Food and Drug Administration of PET radiopharmaceuticals for cardiac imaging; changes in reimbursement; and the increasing documentation of clinical efficacy of PET/CT. All of these factors have contributed to help advance the clinical role of PET/CT in clinical cardiovascular medicine. This chapter reviews the current clinical uses of cardiac PET/CT imaging with a focus on the diagnosis of CAD and assessment of myocardial viability.

RADIOPHARMACEUTICALS

Although several tracers have been used for evaluating myocardial perfusion with PET, the most widely used in clinical practice are rubidium 82 and ammonia N 13. In addition, [18]FDG is the radiotracer of choice for the evaluation of myocardial viability.[1]

Rubidium 82

Rubidium 82 is the most widely used radiotracer for clinical PET myocardial perfusion imaging (MPI). It is a potassium analogue that is a generator-product and does not require a cyclotron on site. It has a physical half-life of 76 seconds. This physical characteristic allows the generator to be eluted with greater than 90% yield every 10 minutes. In addition, the rapid reconstitution of the generator allows for fast sequential perfusion imaging and laboratory throughput, maximizing clinical efficiency. The generator is replaced every 28 days (reflecting the physical half-life of its parent radionuclide, strontium 82).

After infusion, rubidium 82 rapidly crosses the capillary membrane and is actively transported to the cell via the sodium/potassium ATP transporter, which depends on coronary blood flow.[2] Compared with fluorine 18 or nitrogen 13, the positron range and the spatial uncertainty in the location of the decaying nucleus of rubidium 82 (2.6 mm FWHM [full width at half maximum]) is greater than for fluorine 18 (0.2 mm FWHM) or nitrogen 13 (0.7 mm FWHM), mitigating the improved spatial resolution of PET.

Ammonia N 13

Being a cyclotron product, ammonia N 13 use in routine clinical practice is limited to institutions that have a cyclotron on site. It has a physical half-life of 9.96 minutes and has a shorter positron range compared with rubidium 82, resulting in higher signal-to-noise ratio. After injection, ammonia N 13 rapidly disappears from the circulation, permitting the acquisition of images of excellent quality. Although the sequestration of ammonia N 13 in the lungs is usually minimal, it may be increased in patients with depressed left ventricular systolic function or chronic pulmonary disease and, occasionally, in smokers; this may adversely affect the quality of the images. In these cases, it may be necessary to increase the time between injection and image acquisition to optimize the contrast between myocardial and background activity. When inside the myocyte, ammonia N 13 is incorporated into the glutamine pool and becomes metabolically trapped. Only a small fraction diffuses back into the intravascular space.[3]

Myocardial retention of ammonia N 13 is heterogeneous, with retention in the lateral left ventricular wall being about 10% lower than that of other segments, even in normal subjects. This heterogeneous retention could result in an apparent perfusion defect in the inferolateral wall, limiting its evaluation. Ammonia N 13 allows the acquisition of ungated and gated images of excellent quality. These studies take full advantage of the superior resolution of PET relative to single photon emission computed tomography (SPECT) because the half-life of ammonia N 13 is sufficiently long, and its average positron range is very short. Gated ammonia N 13 imaging can provide accurate assessments of regional and global cardiac function.[4] This imaging agent is not well suited for peak stress gated imaging, however, because of the 3- to 4-minute time interval between radiotracer injection and start of imaging, and the relatively long (20 minutes) acquisition time.

^{18}FDG

^{18}FDG is an imaging agent that is used to assess myocardial metabolic activity. Fluorine 18 has a physical half-life of 109 minutes, allowing regional distribution to clinical sites from local cyclotrons. Although normal myocardium preferentially uses free fatty acids, ischemic myocardium switches to preferential glucose metabolism. Because ^{18}FDG is a glucose analogue, it provides a unique opportunity to image ischemic but viable myocardium. ^{18}FDG traces the initial transport of glucose across the myocyte membrane and its subsequent hexokinase-mediated phosphorylation to FDG-6-phosphate. Because the latter is a poor substrate for further metabolism and is impermeable to the cell membrane, it becomes virtually trapped in the myocardium, allowing the imaging of viable cells.

ASSESSMENT OF MYOCARDIAL PERFUSION

Imaging Protocols

Figure 24-1 illustrates common protocols used for imaging myocardial perfusion with PET/CT, where the low-dose CT scan is used for attenuation correction.[1] This scan is also called a *CT-based attenuation correction scan* (CTAC).

Computed Tomography Scans

After obtaining the topogram, a low-dose CT scan covering the heart region is obtained. The parameters of this low-dose, non–ECG gated CT scan include a slow gantry rotation combined with a high pitch (e.g., 0.5:1 to 0.6:1), a high tube potential (e.g., 140 kVp), and a low tube current (10 to 20 mA). The scan is obtained during tidal expiration breath-hold or shallow breathing. The rest and stress emission images should each be corrected with its own dedicated transmission scan because of known changes in cardiac and pulmonary volumes during pharmacologic stress. Whether one attenuation scan (e.g., one CTAC) is sufficient to correct the stress and rest transmission scans is yet to be determined.

Emission Scans

For rubidium 82, approximately the same dose (40 to 60 mCi) is injected for the rest and stress myocardial perfusion studies because of the short physical half-life of rubidium 82 (76 seconds). For ammonia N 13, the general trend is to use a lower dose for the rest images (10 mCi) and a higher dose for the stress images (30 mCi), analogous to 1-day SPECT imaging protocols. The low-dose/high-dose protocol is faster than same-dose protocols for rest and stress because it does not require waiting for decay of ammonia N 13 to background levels before a second dose can be administered. Large patients may require large doses for the rest and stress studies. Some laboratories perform stress imaging first because a normal scan may avoid the need for rest imaging. This approach limits the ability to assess rest myocardial blood flow and coronary vasodilator reserve, however, limiting the ability to identify patients with extensive CAD and "balanced" ischemia, as discussed subsequently.

Different protocols can be used to acquire emission scans (see Fig. 24-1), as follows:

1. *ECG gated imaging*. This is the most common clinical approach. Imaging begins 90 to 120 seconds after rubidium 82 injection, or 3 to 5 minutes after ammonia N 13 injection, to allow for clearance of radioactivity from the lungs and blood pool; the scan duration is approximately 5 minutes for rubidium 82 or 20 minutes for ammonia 13 N (see Fig. 24-1B).

2. *Multiframe or dynamic imaging*. Imaging begins with the bolus (short infusion) of rubidium 82 or ammonia 13 N and continues for 7 to 8 minutes or 20 minutes (see Fig. 24-1C). The advantage of this approach is that it allows quantification of myocardial blood flow (in mL/min/g) by fitting regional tissue and blood time-activity curves to a suitable kinetic model. Its main disadvantage is that one needs to perform a separate radionuclide injection to obtain ECG gated images from which to assess cardiac function, especially when using rubidium 82. Using ammonia 13 N, one can acquire a short multiframe or dynamic scan (4 minutes) that can be followed with a separate, approximately 15-minute ECG gated scan to assess myocardial perfusion and left ventricular ejection fraction (LVEF), without the need of an additional radionuclide injection owing to its longer physical half-life (approximately 10 minutes) (see Fig. 24-1D). To measure the left ventricular blood time-activity curves noninvasively, one must acquire many dynamic PET image

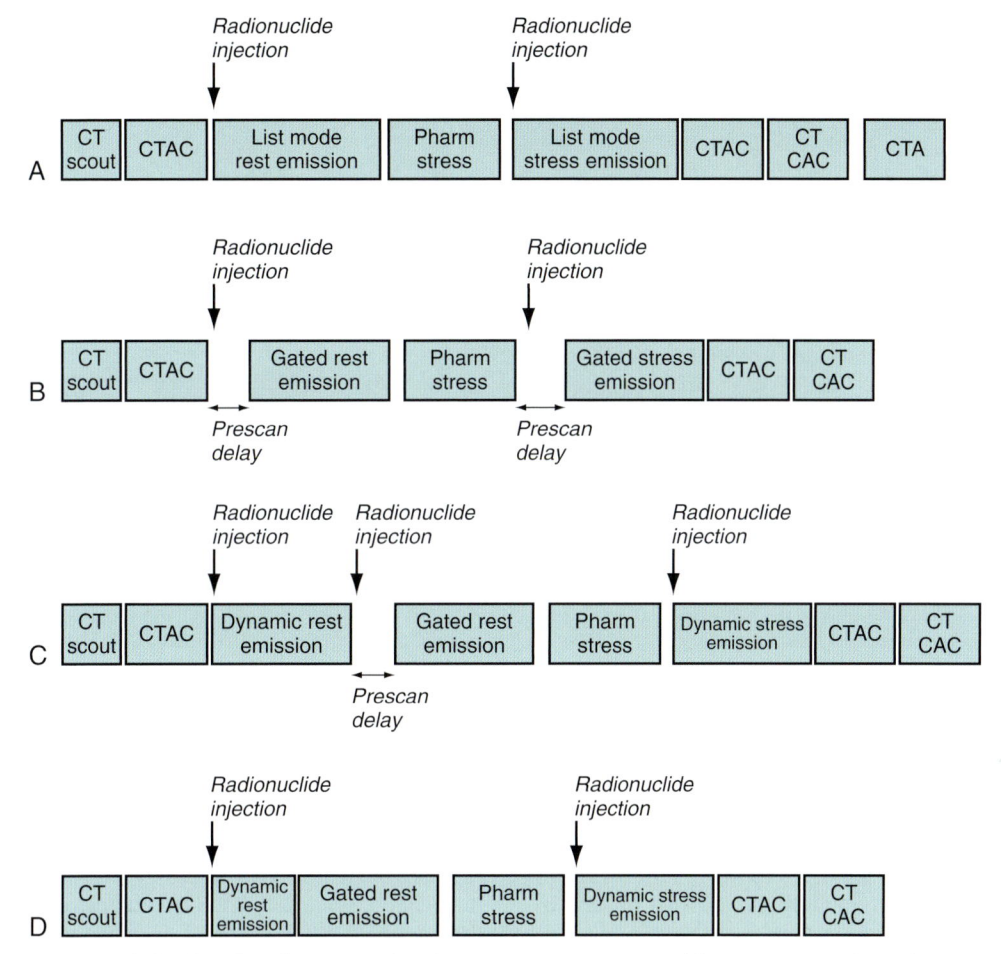

■ **FIGURE 24-1** A-D, Protocols for clinical cardiac PET/CT imaging. CAC, coronary artery calcium; CTA, CT angiography; CTAC, CT-based attenuation scan. *(From Di Carli MF, Dorbala S, Meserve J, et al. Clinical myocardial perfusion PET/CT. J Nucl Med 2007; 48:783-793.)*

frames while the tracer bolus passes through the right ventricle, the lungs, and the left ventricle. During this interval, it is common for a large amount of activity (approximately 20 to 30 mCi) to be located entirely within the PET scanner's axial field of view. Because of possible count-rate limitations under such conditions, particularly in three-dimensional scan mode, great care must be taken to ensure the accuracy of the PET system's corrections for random and scatter coincidences and dead time.

3. *List mode imaging.* This is the ideal approach because a single injection and data acquisition allows multiple image reconstructions (i.e., summed, ECG gated, and multiframe or dynamic) for a comprehensive physiologic examination of the heart. With this approach, image acquisition begins with the bolus injection of the radionuclide and continues for 7 to 8 minutes for rubidium 82 or 20 minutes for ammonia N 13 (see Fig. 24-1A). List mode imaging requires significant computer power to perform the multiple reconstructions, especially for the three-dimensional image acquisition mode.

Stress testing is most commonly performed using adenosine, dipyridamole, or dobutamine. Protocols using exercise stress testing with PET/CT have been described.[5] The use of exercise PET in clinical practice is very limited, however, especially with shorter half-life agents such as rubidium 82 (half-life 76 seconds).

Quality Assurance for Cardiac PET/CT

Hybrid imaging using PET/CT is prone to significant artifacts if not performed correctly. Quality control measures, including routine inspection of the transmission and emission data and the transmission-emission alignment, should always be enforced to obtain high-quality studies. These quality control measures include the following:

1. *Count density.* The level of statistical noise in the emission and transmission images should be checked to see if enough counts have been acquired; this is crucial with rubidium 82 imaging because of the short half-life of the isotope. Although the image quality of CT transmission images may be suboptimal in heavy patients, this does not seem to compromise the quality of the attenuation correction because the attenuation map is integrated along the PET lines of response to obtain attenuation-correction factors. The most common sources of count-poor emission studies include large patient size, inadequate radionuclide dose or delivery (e.g., problems with intravenous access), and inadequate scan duration.

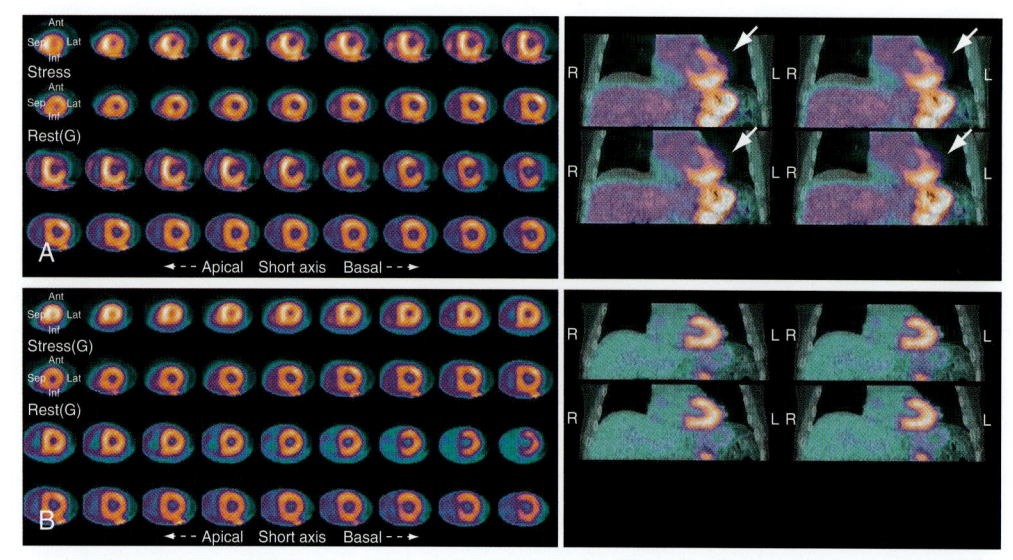

■ **FIGURE 24-2** Transmission-emission misalignment. **A,** The misaligned CT transmission and rubidium 82 images (*right*), and the resulting anterolateral perfusion defect on stress-rest rubidium 82 PET (*left*). The perfusion defect results from applying incorrect attenuation coefficients during tomographic reconstruction to the area of the left ventricular myocardium overlaying on the lung field on the CT transmission scan (*arrows*). **B,** The correction of the emission-transmission misalignment (*right*), and the resulting normal perfusion study. *(From Di Carli MF, Dorbala S, Meserve J, et al. Clinical myocardial perfusion PET/CT. J Nucl Med 2007; 48:783-793.)*

2. *Heart-to-blood pool count ratio.* Acquisition of emission images before complete clearance of radiotracer from the blood pool may potentially degrade image quality. The optimal prescan delay for acquisition of ammonia 13 N images is about 3 minutes and for rubidium 82 images is approximately 90 seconds in healthy subjects. The most common factors that prolong circulation time of the radionuclide include severe left ventricular systolic dysfunction (LVEF <30%, either chronic or acute secondary to severe ischemia during stress), right ventricular systolic dysfunction, and primary lung disease. In these clinical settings, increased prescan delay is usually required to improve image quality.[1,6] The use of the list mode imaging protocols is very helpful because assumptions regarding prescan delay are not required.

3. *Transmission-emission misalignment.* Misregistration of transmission and emission images can result from respiratory or patient motion, and can lead to inaccurate clinical results (Fig. 24-2). Because transmission and emission imaging are sequential, patient or respiratory (e.g., deep inspiration) motion during the emission images is most likely to lead to transmission-emission misalignment and potential attenuation-correction artifacts (see Fig. 24-2). The extent and direction of this misalignment determine whether artifacts are apparent in the attenuation-corrected images. Most commercial PET/CT systems now include software tools to correct for transmission-emission misalignments.

Diagnostic Accuracy

Table 24-1 summarizes the published studies documenting the diagnostic accuracy of myocardial perfusion PET imaging for detecting obstructive CAD.[7] The average weighted sensitivity for detecting at least one coronary artery with greater than 50% stenosis is 90% (range 83% to 100%), and the average specificity is 89% (range 73% to 100%). The corresponding average positive and negative predictive values are 94% (range 80% to 100%) and 73% (range 36% to 100%), and the overall diagnostic accuracy is 90% (range 84% to 98%). Most of the available data have been obtained with dedicated PET cameras, rather than with PET/CT systems. In a more recent study using PET/CT (where the CT was used only for attenuation correction), Sampson and colleagues[8] reported a sensitivity of 93%, a specificity of 83%, and a normalcy rate of 100%. In this study of patients without known prior CAD, the positive and negative predictive values of PET/CT were 80% and 94%, with an overall accuracy of 87%. All patients with a low likelihood for CAD showed normal scans, for a normalcy rate of 100%. The sensitivity for detecting CAD in patients with single vessel and multivessel (two or more vessels) disease was 92% and 95%. These results were applicable to men and women and to obese and nonobese individuals.

Comparative Studies of Positron Emission Tomography versus Single Photon Emission Computed Tomography

Two studies have performed a direct comparison of the diagnostic accuracy of rubidium 82 myocardial perfusion PET and thallium 201 imaging in the same patient populations. Go and colleagues[9] compared PET and SPECT in 202 patients and showed higher sensitivity with PET than with SPECT (93% vs. 76%), without significant changes in specificity (78% vs. 80%). Stewart and coworkers[10] compared PET and SPECT in 81 patients and observed a higher specificity with PET than with SPECT (83% vs. 53%), without significant differences in sensitivity (86% vs. 84%). The differences between these two studies are likely to be attributable to patient selection resulting in differences in prescan likelihood of CAD.

TABLE 24-1 Summary of Published Literature Regarding Diagnostic Accuracy of PET

First Author	Patients	Women	Prior CAD	PET Radiotracer	Sensitivity	Specificity	PPV	NPV	Accuracy
Sampson[8]*	102	0.42	0	^{82}Rb	0.93	0.83	0.80	0.94	0.87
Bateman[33]	112	0.46	0.25	^{82}Rb	0.87	0.93	0.95	0.81	0.89
Marwick[34]	74	0.19	0.49	^{82}Rb	0.90	1	1	0.36	0.91
Grover-McKay[35]	31	0.01	0.13	^{82}Rb	1	0.73	0.80	1	0.87
Stewart[10]	81	0.36	0.42	^{82}Rb	0.83	0.86	0.94	0.64	0.84
Go[9]	202	NR	0.47	^{82}Rb	0.93	78	0.93	0.80	0.90
Demer[36]	193	0.26	0.34	^{82}Rb/^{13}NH$_3$	83	0.95	0.98	0.60	0.85
Tamaki[37]	51	NR	0.75	^{13}NH$_3$	0.98	1	1	0.75	0.98
Gould[38]	31	NR	NR	^{82}Rb/^{13}NH$_3$	0.95	1	1	0.90	0.97
Weighted summary	877	0.29	0.35		0.90	0.89	0.94	0.73	0.90

*Study using PET/CT (where CT is used for attenuation correction only).
NPV, negative predictive value; NR, not reported; PPV, positive predictive value.
From Di Carli MF, Hachamovitch R. New technology for noninvasive evaluation of coronary artery disease. Circulation 2007; 115:1464-1480.

More recently, Bateman and associates[11] compared rubidium 82 PET and Tc 99m sestamibi SPECT in two matched patient cohorts undergoing clinically indicated pharmacologic stress perfusion imaging using contemporary technology for SPECT and PET. Overall diagnostic accuracy was higher for PET than for SPECT (87% vs. 71% with a 50% angiographic threshold, and 89% vs. 79% with a 70% angiographic threshold). Differences in diagnostic accuracy reflected primarily the increased specificity (with a marginal advantage in sensitivity) of PET versus SPECT, and applied to men and women and to obese and nonobese individuals.

Evaluation of Multivessel Coronary Artery Disease

The diagnosis of multivessel or left main CAD with diffuse balanced ischemia using MPI remains a challenge. PET (similar to SPECT) often uncovers only the coronary territory supplied by the most severe stenosis. The use of ancillary high-risk markers often helps in ascertaining the presence of multivessel CAD. ECG gating provides a unique opportunity to assess left ventricular function at rest and during *peak stress* (as opposed to *poststress* with gated SPECT). More recent data suggest that in normal subjects, LVEF increases during peak vasodilator stress.[12] In the presence of CAD, changes in LVEF (from baseline to peak stress) are inversely related to the magnitude of perfusion abnormalities during stress (reflecting myocardium at risk) (Fig. 24-3) and the extent of angiographic CAD (Fig. 24-4). In patients with three-vessel or left main CAD, LVEF during peak stress decreases even in the absence of apparent perfusion abnormalities (Fig. 24-5). In contrast, patients without significant CAD or with one-vessel disease show a normal increase in LVEF. Consequently, the negative predictive value of an increase in LVEF (from rest to peak stress) of 5% or greater to exclude the presence of three-vessel or left main CAD or both is 97%.[12]

PET measurements of myocardial blood flow (in mL/min/g of myocardium) and coronary vasodilator reserve may also help overcome the limitations of relative perfusion assessments with PET to uncover the presence of multivessel CAD. Because myocardial blood flow (in mL/min/g of tissue) and coronary vasodilator reserve (the ratio between peak and rest myocardial blood flow) are inversely and nonlinearly related to stenosis severity, quantitative estimates of coronary hemodynamics by PET allow better definition of the extent of obstructive CAD. PET quantification of myocardial blood flow is well validated using ammonia 13 N.[13,14] Quantitative approaches with rubidium 82 have also been developed.[15,16] Validation studies in animals and humans are currently under way.

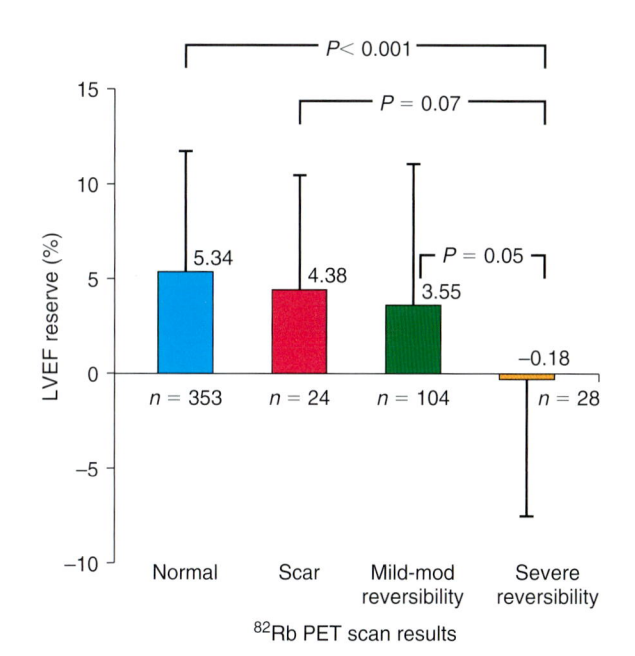

■ FIGURE 24-3 Bar graph showing the relationship between the magnitude of stress-induced perfusion abnormalities and the delta change in left ventricular ejection fraction (LVEF) (from baseline to peak stress). *(From Dorbala S, Vangala D, Sampson U, et al. Value of vasodilator left ventricular ejection fraction reserve in evaluating the magnitude of myocardium at risk and the extent of angiographic coronary artery disease: a 82Rb PET/CT study. J Nucl Med 2007; 48:349-358.)*

Risk Stratification

Studies documenting the incremental prognostic value of PET perfusion imaging in predicting patient outcomes are beginning to emerge. Yoshinaga and coworkers[17] studied

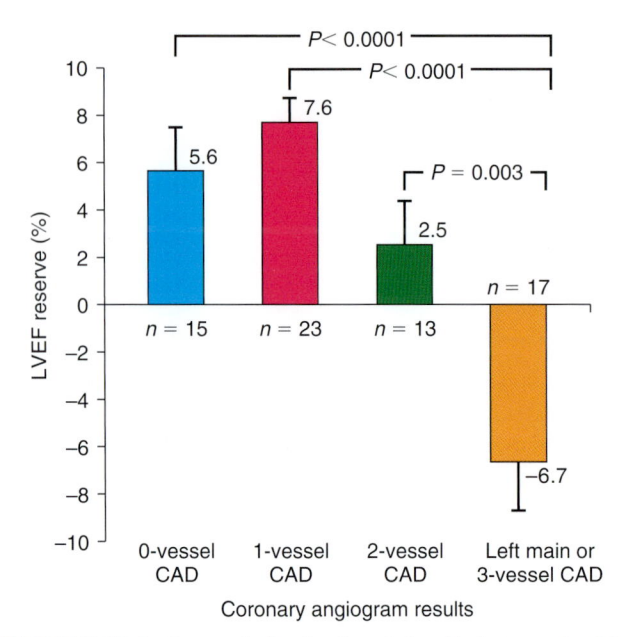

FIGURE 24-4 Bar graph showing the relationship between the delta change in left ventricular ejection fraction (LVEF) and the extent of angiographic coronary artery disease (CAD) (>70% stenosis). *(From Dorbala S, Vangala D, Sampson U, et al. Value of vasodilator left ventricular ejection fraction reserve in evaluating the magnitude of myocardium at risk and the extent of angiographic coronary artery disease: a 82Rb PET/CT study. J Nucl Med 2007; 48:349-358.)*

the prognostic value of dipyridamole stress rubidium 82 PET in 367 patients who were followed for 3.1 ± 0.9 years. The extent and severity of perfusion defects with stress PET were associated with increasing frequency of adverse events. The negative predictive value of a normal scan to predict hard events (i.e., myocardial infarction or cardiac death) was very high; patients with normal stress PET had an event rate of 0.4%/year. This study, the largest published PET prognosis study to date, was limited, however, by the occurrence of only 17 hard events.

Preliminary data from our laboratory in 1602 consecutive patients undergoing rest-stress rubidium 82 myocardial perfusion PET/CT imaging also suggest that this technique provides incremental value to clinical variables in predicting overall survival.[18] In contrast to previous studies, this study was adequately powered by the occurrence of 113 deaths (7% of the study cohort) during a median follow-up period of 511 days. In keeping with previous studies, increases in the extent and severity of stress perfusion defects translated into proportional increases in predicted mortality. In addition, preliminary data from our laboratory in 1274 consecutive patients also confirm the incremental prognostic value of LVEF over stress perfusion imaging.[19] As expected, this analysis showed that mortality hazard was inversely related to LVEF. MPI added incremental value to LVEF (at any LVEF, a higher summed stress score had greater risk), and LVEF added incremental value to MPI (i.e., at any summed stress score, a lower LVEF had greater risk).

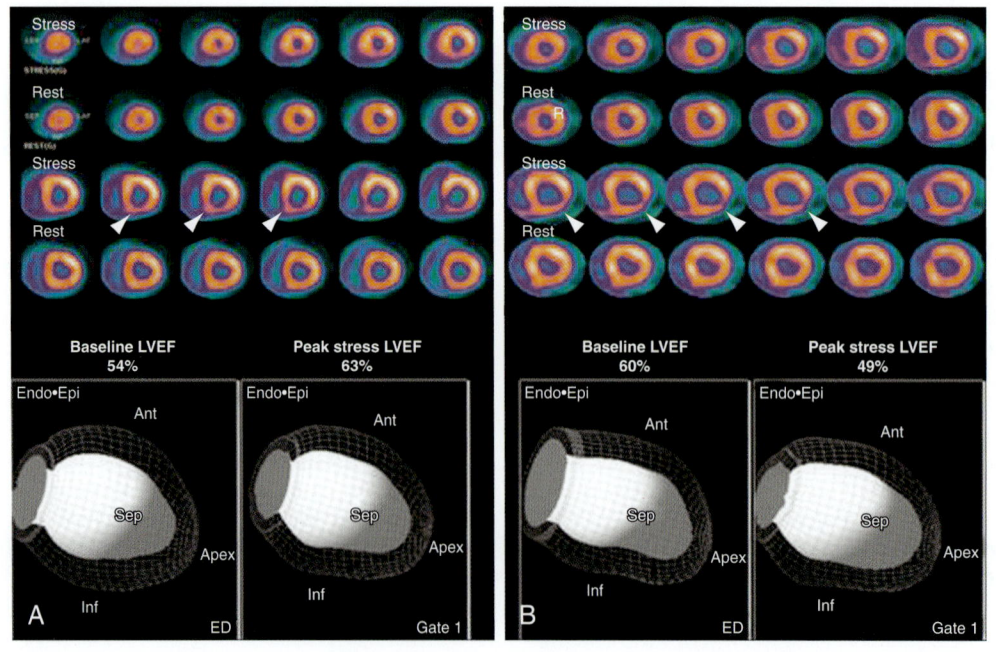

FIGURE 24-5 Gated rest-stress rubidium 82 myocardial perfusion PET images illustrating the added value of left ventricular function over the perfusion information. **A,** Normal increase in left ventricular ejection fraction (LVEF) from rest to peak stress (*bottom*) in a patient with angiographic single vessel coronary artery disease, showing a single perfusion defect in the inferior wall on the PET images (*arrows*). **B,** Abnormal decrease in LVEF from rest to peak stress in a patient with angiographic multivessel vessel coronary artery disease, also showing a single perfusion defect in the inferolateral wall on the PET images (*arrows*). *(From Di Carli MF, Hachamovitch R. New technology for noninvasive evaluation of coronary artery disease. Circulation 2007; 115:1464-1480.)*

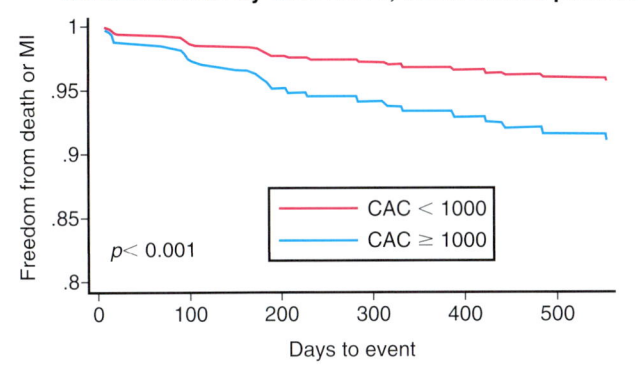

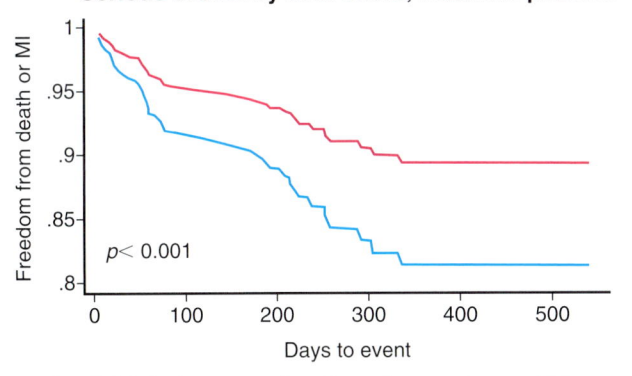

FIGURE 24-6 Cox proportional hazards regression model for freedom from death or myocardial infarction (MI) adjusted for age, sex, symptoms, and conventional coronary artery disease risk factors in patients without ischemia (*top panel*) and with ischemia (*lower panel*). CAC, coronary artery calcium. *(From Schenker MP, Dorbala S, Hong ECT, et al. Relationship between coronary calcification, myocardial ischemia, and outcomes in patients with intermediate likelihood of coronary artery disease: a combined positron emission tomography/computed tomography study. Circulation 2008; 117:1693-1700.)*

The potential to acquire and quantify rest and stress myocardial perfusion and CT information from a single dual-modality study opens the door to expand the prognostic potential of stress nuclear imaging. More recent data from our laboratory suggest that quantification of coronary artery calcium (CAC) scores at the time of stress nuclear imaging using a hybrid approach with PET/CT can enhance risk predictions in patients with suspected CAD.[20] In a consecutive series of 621 patients undergoing stress PET imaging and CAC scoring in the same clinical setting, risk-adjusted analysis showed a stepwise increase in adverse events (death and myocardial infarction) with increasing levels of CAC score for any level of perfusion abnormality. This finding was observed in patients with and without evidence of ischemia on PET MPI.

The annualized event rate in patients with normal PET MPI and no CAC was substantially lower than in patients with normal PET MPI and a CAC score of 1000 or greater (Fig. 24-6). Likewise, the annualized event rate in patients with ischemia on PET MPI and no CAC was lower than in patients with ischemia and a CAC score of 1000 or greater. These findings suggest incremental risk stratification by incorporating information regarding the anatomic extent of atherosclerosis in conventional models using nuclear imaging alone, a finding that may serve as a more rational basis for personalizing the intensity and goals of medical therapy in a more cost-effective manner. Although CT angiography as an adjunct to perfusion imaging could expand the opportunities to identify patients with noncalcified plaques at greater risk of adverse cardiovascular events, it is unclear how much added prognostic information there is in the contrast-enhanced coronary CT angiography scan over the simple noncontrast CT scan for CAC determination.[21]

ASSESSMENT OF MYOCARDIAL VIABILITY

In addition to assessment of myocardial perfusion, PET/CT plays an important role in the evaluation of viability in patients with ischemic cardiomyopathy. This evaluation is of utmost clinical importance because high-risk surgical revascularization seems to afford a long-term survival benefit based on small series.[22] Data from large-scale randomized clinical trials are still pending, however, and the selection of patients with severe left ventricular dysfunction for high-risk revascularization is controversial. It is very important to differentiate left ventricular dysfunction caused by scarring from that arising from viable but dysfunctional myocardium. PET/CT plays an important role in the evaluation of these patients and makes this distinction possible.

Hibernation versus Stunning

In patients with CAD and left ventricular dysfunction, the cause of the decrease in the left ventricular contractile function could be secondary to scarring, stunning, or hibernation. The differentiation between these three different pathophysiologic mechanisms is of utmost importance to developing a treatment strategy.

Myocardial scarring results from myocardial infarction or other inflammatory or infiltrative diseases that involve the myocardium. *Myocardial stunning* is a reversible state of regional contractile dysfunction that can occur after restoration of coronary blood flow following a brief episode of ischemia despite the absence of necrosis.[23] Although commonly regarded as an acute phenomenon, stunned myocardium may also occur in patients with chronic coronary stenosis who experience recurrent episodes of ischemia (symptomatic or asymptomatic) in the same territory. This mechanism is probably the most common form of stunning in patients with chronic left ventricular dysfunction secondary to CAD. *Myocardial hibernation* refers to a state of persistent left ventricular dysfunction associated with chronically reduced blood flow but preserved viability.[24] This chronic downregulation in contractile function at rest is thought to represent a protective mechanism whereby the heart reduces its oxygen requirements to ensure myocyte survival. This protective mechanism can result in a considerable amount of myocardium that is rendered hypocontractile, however, and it may contribute to overall left ventricular dysfunction. Different metabolic patterns are seen in these three states with PET metabolic imaging using ^{18}FDG, which provides the basis for PET/CT ^{18}FDG imaging.

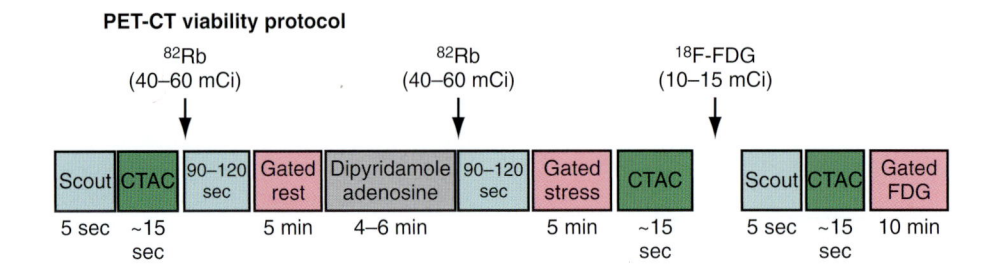

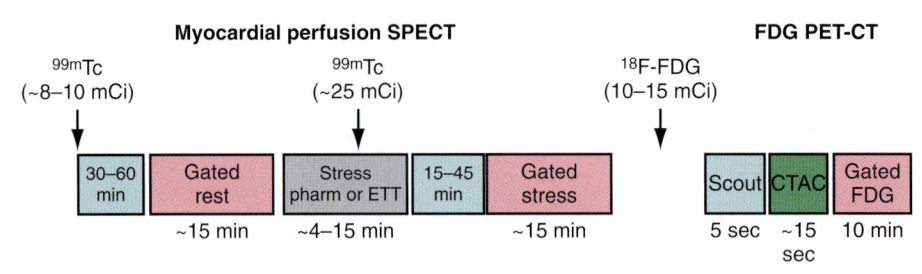

FIGURE 24-7 Myocardial viability PET/CT protocols. CTAC, CT-based attenuation scan; ETT, exercise treadmill testing. *(From Di Carli MF. Myocardial viability assessment with PET and PET/CT. In Di Carli MF, Lipton MJ [eds]. Cardiac PET and PET/CT Imaging. New York, 2007, Springer, pp 250-269.)*

Normal myocardium uses different energy-producing substrates to fulfill its energy requirements.[25] In the fasting state, free fatty acids (FFA) are mobilized in large quantities from triglycerides stored in adipose tissue. The increased availability of FFA in plasma makes them the preferred energy-producing fuel in the myocardium. In the fed state, however, the increase in plasma glucose and the subsequent increase in insulin levels significantly reduce FFA release from adipose tissue and, consequently, its availability in plasma. In addition, the increased insulin levels mobilize glucose transporters onto the cell membrane, resulting in increased transport and use of exogenous glucose by the myocardium.

Under ischemic conditions, there is a shift to preferential glucose uptake by the myocardium. Noninvasive approaches that can assess the magnitude of exogenous glucose use play an important role in the evaluation of tissue viability in ischemic cardiomyopathy. In addition, prolonged severe reduction of myocardial blood flow rapidly precipitates depletion of high-energy phosphate, cell membrane disruption, and cellular death. Assessment of regional blood flow also provides important information regarding the presence of tissue viability within dysfunctional myocardial regions.

PET/CT Viability Imaging Protocols

Because dysfunctional myocardium that improves functionally after revascularization must retain sufficient blood flow and metabolic activity to sustain myocyte viability, the combined assessment of regional blood flow and glucose metabolism seems most attractive for delineating myocardial viability. With this approach, regional myocardial perfusion is first evaluated after the administration of ammonia 13 N or rubidium 82. Because data regarding the magnitude of stress-induced ischemia and resting viability are important for management decisions, the ideal approach should include rest and stress perfusion imaging (Fig. 24-7). Regional glucose uptake is assessed with ^{18}FDG, as described subsequently.

Patient Preparation for ^{18}FDG Imaging

A detailed step-by-step description of the available methods for ^{18}FDG imaging is provided by the "Guidelines for PET Imaging" published by the American Society of Nuclear Cardiology and the Society of Nuclear Medicine.[6] The most commonly used approaches for ^{18}FDG imaging include the following (Fig. 24-8):

1. *Glucose loading.* This is the most commonly used approach to ^{18}FDG imaging. The goal of glucose loading is to stimulate the release of endogenous insulin to decrease the plasma levels of FFA and to facilitate the transport and use of ^{18}FDG. Patients are usually fasted for at least 6 hours and then receive an oral or intravenous glucose load. Most patients require the administration of intravenous insulin to maximize myocardial ^{18}FDG uptake. With this approach, image quality is generally of diagnostic quality, and the reported diagnostic accuracy is very good.

2. *Hyperinsulinemic-euglycemic clamp.* This approach is technically demanding and time-consuming. It provides the highest and most consistent image quality, however. Based on the reported predictive accuracies, the high image quality does not translate into improved predictions of functional outcome. Because the

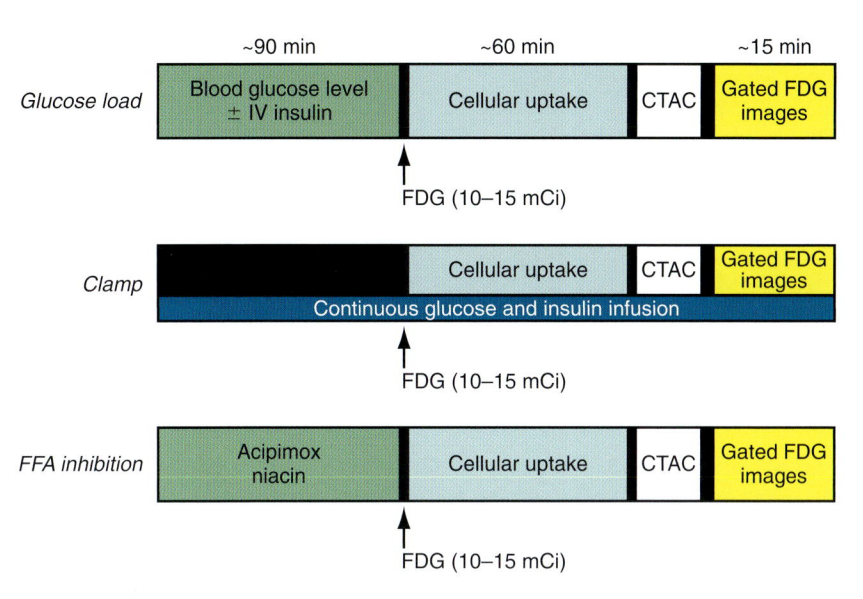

FIGURE 24-8 Timeline of protocols for patient preparation before ^{18}FDG imaging. FFA, free fatty acids; IV, intravenous. *(From Di Carli MF. Myocardial viability assessment with PET and PET/CT. In Di Carli MF, Lipton MJ [eds]. Cardiac PET and PET/CT Imaging. New York, 2007, Springer, pp 250-269.)*

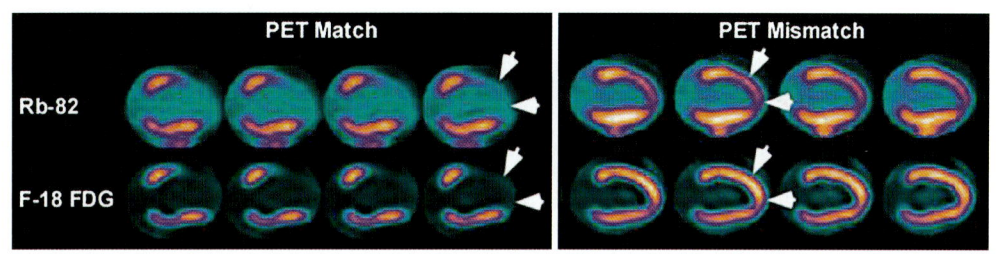

FIGURE 24-9 PET patterns of myocardial viability. *Left panel,* Concordant reductions in myocardial perfusion (rubidium 82) and glucose metabolism (^{18}FDG), reflecting myocardial infarction. *Right panel,* Preserved glucose metabolism (^{18}FDG) in a territory with decreased myocardial perfusion (rubidium 82), reflecting complete tissue viability. *(From Di Carli MF, Hachamovitch R. New technology for noninvasive evaluation of coronary artery disease. Circulation 2007; 115:1464-1480.)*

hyperinsulinemic-euglycemic clamp is technically demanding, most laboratories reserve this approach for challenging conditions (e.g., diabetes and severe congestive heart failure).

3. *Acipimox.* This is a nicotinic acid derivative that inhibits peripheral lipolysis, reducing plasma FFA levels and, indirectly, forcing a switch to preferential myocardial glucose use. The drug is usually given in combination with a glucose load 60 minutes before ^{18}FDG administration. The approach is practical and provides consistent image quality. Acipimox is not available for clinical use in the United States, however.

Although several methods have been proposed, only the glucose-loading approach has undergone extensive validation worldwide, and it remains the most commonly used in clinical practice. This approach can be technically challenging, especially in patients with diabetes and congestive heart failure, and aggressive patient preparation is mandatory to optimize diagnostic accuracy. The available evidence suggests that this approach can provide accurate predictions of functional, symptomatic, and prognostic improvement after revascularization, and improve management decisions in patients with poor cardiac function.

Myocardial Perfusion and Glucose-Loaded ^{18}FDG Patterns

Using the sequential-perfusion ^{18}FDG approach, four distinct perfusion-metabolism patterns can be observed in dysfunctional myocardium, as follows:

1. Normal perfusion associated with normal ^{18}FDG uptake
2. Reduced perfusion associated with preserved or enhanced ^{18}FDG uptake (so-called perfusion-metabolism mismatch), reflecting myocardial viability (Fig. 24-9)
3. Proportional reduction in perfusion and ^{18}FDG uptake (so-called perfusion-metabolism match), reflecting nonviable myocardium (see Fig. 24-9)
4. Normal or near-normal perfusion with reduced ^{18}FDG uptake (so-called reversed perfusion-metabolism mismatch) (Fig. 24-10)[26]

The patterns of normal perfusion and metabolism or of a PET mismatch identify potentially reversible myocardial dysfunction, whereas the PET match pattern identifies irreversible myocardial dysfunction. The reversed perfusion-metabolism mismatch has been described in the context of repetitive myocardial stunning,[26] and in patients with left bundle branch block.[27] Quantitation of regional

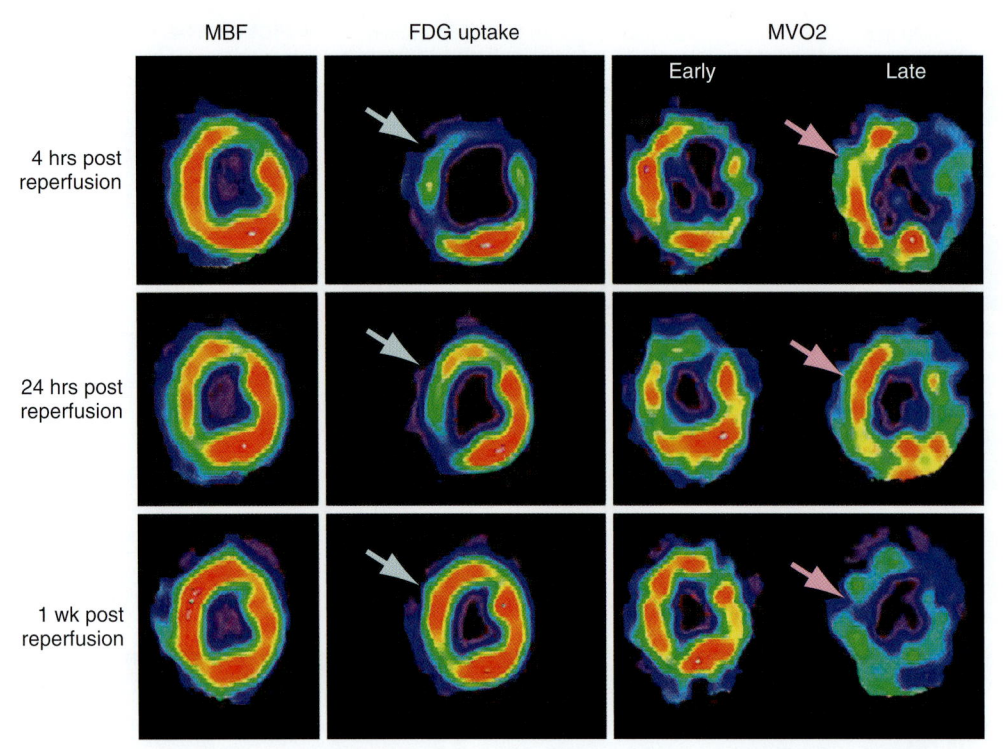

FIGURE 24-10 PET images of a dog heart in short-axis views obtained at corresponding mid-ventricular levels obtained after reperfusion following four 5-minute left anterior descending coronary artery occlusions, each followed by 5 minutes of reperfusion. Images of blood flow (*left column*) were obtained with ammonia 13 N and images of glucose metabolism (*middle column*) were obtained with ^{18}FDG. Images of oxidative metabolism (reflecting regional myocardial oxygen consumption [MV_{O_2}]) (*right column*) were obtained with acetate 11 C; the *early* phase denotes delivery of the tracer to the myocardium, whereas the *late* phase represents regional washout of the tracer through the tricarboxylic acid cycle (myocardial oxidation). *Top panel,* Corresponding mid-ventricular short-axis sections of regional blood flow, glucose, and MV_{O_2} 4 hours after reperfusion. The flow images (*left*) show near-normal perfusion in the stunned regions (i.e., anterior and anterior septum). Stunned regions showed reduced ^{18}FDG use (*arrow*), however, and slow clearance of acetate 11 C (impaired oxidation) relative to normal myocardium (lateral wall). *Middle panel,* One day after reperfusion. Myocardial perfusion in stunned myocardium is near-normal, glucose uptake (*arrow*) remains depressed, and the MV_{O_2} is still lower (*arrow*) than in normal myocardium. *Bottom panel,* One week after reperfusion. Blood flow, glucose uptake, and MV_{O_2} are largely homogeneous. Wall motion and metabolism showed a parallel recovery with time. MBF, myocardial blood flow. *(From Di Carli MF, Prcevski P, Singh TP, et al. Myocardial blood flow, function, and metabolism in repetitive stunning. J Nucl Med 2000; 41:1227-1234.)*

myocardial perfusion and ^{18}FDG tracer uptake and their difference can be helpful to assess objectively the magnitude of viability. In addition, gated ^{18}FDG-PET/CT images can be used to assess global left ventricular function.

Accuracy of PET/CT to Predict Functional Recovery

Myocardial Perfusion

Using only regional myocardial perfusion information, contractile dysfunction was predicted to be reversible after revascularization when regional blood flow was only mildly or moderately reduced (>50% of normal), and irreversible when regional blood flow was severely reduced (<50% of normal). Using these criteria, the average positive predictive accuracy of blood flow estimates for predicting functional recovery after revascularization is 63% (range 45% to 78%), whereas the average negative predictive accuracy is 63% (range 45% to 100%). ^{18}FDG imaging adds significant independent information for distinguishing reversible from irreversible myocardial dysfunction and improving the diagnostic accuracy of PET/CT in predicting functional recovery.[28]

Combined Myocardial Perfusion and ^{18}FDG

The experience with the combined blood flow/^{18}FDG approach using PET or the PET/SPECT hybrid technique (SPECT perfusion with ^{18}FDG-PET imaging) has been extensively documented in 17 studies including 462 patients (Table 24-2).[28] Contractile dysfunction was predicted to be reversible after revascularization in regions with increased ^{18}FDG uptake or a perfusion-metabolism mismatch, and irreversible in regions with reduced ^{18}FDG uptake or a perfusion-metabolism match pattern. Using these criteria, the average positive predictive accuracy for predicting improved segmental function after revascularization is 76% (range 52% to 100%), whereas the average negative predictive accuracy is 82% (range 67% to 100%).

Several studies using different PET approaches have shown that the gain in global left ventricular systolic function after revascularization is related to the magnitude of viable myocardium assessed preoperatively (Table 24-3).[28] These data show that clinically meaningful changes in global left ventricular function can be expected after revascularization only in patients with large areas of hibernating or stunned myocardium (≥17% of the left ventricular mass). Patients with large areas of PET mismatch (≥18%

TABLE 24-2 Predictive Values for Segmental Functional Recovery after Revascularization Using Combined Estimates of Myocardial Perfusion and ^{18}FDG Metabolism with PET

First Author	N	LVEF %	Criteria for Viability	PPV % (Segments)	NPV % (Segments)	Diagnostic Accuracy
Tillisch[39]	17	32 ± 14	Mismatch	85 (35/41)	92 (24/26)	88 (59/67)
Tamaki[40]	22	NR	Mismatch	78 (18/23)	78 (18/23)	78 (36/46)
Tamaki[41]	11	NR	Mismatch	80 (40/50)	100 (0/6)	82 (46/56)
Carrel[42]	23	34	Mismatch	84 (16/19)	75 (3/4)	83 (19/23)
Lucignani[43]	14	38 ± 5	Mismatch	95 (37/39)	80 (12/15)	91 (49/54)
Gropler[44]	16	NR	Mismatch	79 (19/24)	83 (24/29)	81 (43/53)
Marwick[45]	16	NR	^{18}FDG >2 SD	67 (25/37)	79 (38/48)	74 (63/85)
Gropler[46]	34	NR	^{18}FDG >2 SD	52 (38/73)	81 (35/43)	63 (73/116)
Vanoverschelde[47]	12	55 ± 7	Mismatch	100 (12/12)	—	100 (12/12)
vom Dahl[48]	37	34 ± 10	Mismatch	53 (29/55)	86 (90/105)	74 (119/160)
Knuuti[49]	48	53 ± 11	^{18}FDG >85%	70 (23/33)	93 (53/57)	84 (76/90)
Maes[50]	20	48 ± 9	Mismatch	75 (9/12)	75 (6/8)	75 (15/20)
Grandin[51]	25	49 ± 11	Mismatch	79 (15/19)	67 (4/6)	76 (19/25)
Tamaki[52]	43	41	FDG UI	76 (45/59)	91 (65/71)	85 (110/130)
Baer[53]	42	40 ± 13	FDG >50%	72 (167/232)	91 (126/139)	79 (293/371)
vom Dahl[54]	52	47 ± 10	Mismatch	68 (19/28)	96 (25/26)	81 (44/54)
Wolpers[55]	30	42 ± 11	FDG >50%	78	85	-
Mean ± SD	462			76 ± 12	82 ± 14	79 ± 10

LVEF, left ventricular ejection fraction; NPV, negative predictive value; NR, not reported; PPV, positive predictive value.
From Di Carli MF. Myocardial viability assessment with PET and PET/CT. In Di Carli MF, Lipton MJ (eds). Cardiac PET and PET/CT Imaging. New York, 2007, Springer, pp 250-269.

TABLE 24-3 Relationship between the Extent of Viability and the Change in Left Ventricular Ejection Fraction after Revascularization Using Combined Estimates of Myocardial Perfusion and ^{18}FDG Metabolism with PET

First Author	N	Criteria for Viability	Pre LVEF (%)	Post LVEF (%)
Tillisch[39]	17	Mismatch ≥25% LV	30 ± 11	45 ± 14
Carrel[42]	23	Mismatch ≥17% LV	34 ± 14	52 ± 11
Vanoverschelde[47]	12	Anterior wall mismatch	55 ± 7	65 ± 8
Maes[50]	20	Anterior wall mismatch	51 ± 11	60 ± 10
Grandin[51]	25	Mismatch ≥20% LV	51 ± 12	63 ± 18
Schwarz[56]	24	Anterior wall mismatch	44 ± 12	54 ± 9
Wolpers[55]	30	Anterior wall mismatch	39 ± 10	49 ± 17
vom Dahl[57]	82	Mismatch ≥1 CAT	46 ± 9	54 ± 11

CAT, coronary artery territory; LV, left ventricle; LVEF, left ventricular ejection fraction.
From Di Carli MF. Myocardial viability assessment with PET and PET/CT. In Di Carli MF, Lipton MJ (eds). Cardiac PET and PET/CT Imaging. New York, 2007, Springer, pp 250-269.

of the left ventricle), in particular areas located in the territory served by the left anterior descending coronary artery, had the greatest clinical benefit.

Data evaluating the improvement in the global left ventricular function are limited. Most of the published studies included patients with normal or mild left ventricular dysfunction. The direct extrapolation of the excellent results obtained in patients with regional or mild to moderate left ventricular dysfunction to patients with very low LVEF is problematic. In addition to the degree of viability by ^{18}FDG-PET/CT, many other factors affect functional outcome after revascularization, including the presence and magnitude of stress-induced ischemia, the stage of cellular degeneration within viable myocytes, the degree of left ventricular remodeling, the timing and success of revascularization procedures, the adequacy of the target coronary vessels, and the timing of left ventricular functional assessment after revascularization.

Impact of Viability Assessment on Patient Outcomes

The goal of viability assessment by PET in the setting of severe ischemic cardiomyopathy is to identify patients in whom revascularization can potentially improve left ventricular function, symptoms, and survival. Multiple studies have addressed this question and are summarized in Table 24-4. The studies included a total of 288 patients with CAD and moderate or severe left ventricular dysfunction. Most of these patients had a history of myocardial infarction and multivessel CAD. Patients with viable myocardium had a consistently higher event rate than patients without viability suggesting an increased risk of a cardiac event for patients with viable myocardium treated medically.

These data suggest that the presence of ischemic but viable myocardium as assessed by ^{18}FDG-PET seems to identify consistently patients with left ventricular

TABLE 24-4 Risk of Cardiac Events for Patients with Moderate to Severe Left Ventricular Dysfunction and Hibernating Myocardium Compared with Patients without Hibernating Myocardium

First Author	Year	Viability Assessment	Patients	LVEF (%)	Follow-up (mo)*	OR	Lower 95% CI	Upper 95% CI
Eitzman[58]	1992	PET	42	34 ± 13	12	7.00	1.53	32.08
Di Carli[59]	1994	PET	50	24 ± 7	13	7.00	1.51	32.33
Lee[60]	1994	PET	61	38 ± 16	17	7.66	2.31	25.44
vom Dahl[57]	1997	MIBI/^{18}FDG	77	≤50	29	1.21	0.22	6.51
Rohatgi[61]	2001	PET	58	22 ± 6	25	1.27	0.44	3.66

*Reflects reported average.
CI, confidence interval; OR, odds ratio.

dysfunction who are at high risk for cardiac events when treated with medical therapy alone. In addition, Allman and colleagues[29] reported a meta-analysis of 24 studies that documented long-term patient outcomes after viability imaging by SPECT, PET, or dobutamine echocardiography in 3088 patients (2228 men, 860 women) with a mean LVEF 32% ± 8% and follow-up for 25 ± 10 months. There was no apparent benefit for revascularization over medical therapy in the absence of demonstrated viability. Meta-regression of the pooled study data in patients with viable myocardium showed an inverse relationship between LVEF and the prognostic benefit associated with revascularization.

The multicenter randomized PARR-2 study did not show a significant reduction in cardiac events in patients with left ventricular dysfunction and suspected coronary disease for ^{18}FDG-PET–assisted management versus standard care.[30] The study included 440 patients with severe left ventricular dysfunction and coronary disease being considered for revascularization, heart failure, or transplantation. Patients were randomly assigned to management assisted by ^{18}FDG-PET or standard care. The primary outcome, a composite of cardiac death, MI, or hospitalization within 1 year, was not different between the two groups (30% for the PET arm vs. 36% for the standard arm; relative risk 0.82, P = .16); however, 25% of the patients with PET-indicated revascularization did not have it done. In patients who adhered to PET recommendations and in patients without recent angiography, significant benefits were observed (hazard ratio 0.4, P = .035).

Another target for revascularization in these patients is the control of symptoms and hospital admissions for congestive heart failure. We showed a significant linear correlation between the global extent of a preoperative perfusion-metabolism PET mismatch (reflecting hibernating myocardium) and the percent improvement in functional capacity after coronary artery bypass graft surgery in 36 patients with ischemic cardiomyopathy (LVEF 28% ± 6%) (Fig. 24-11).[31] In this study, a perfusion-metabolic PET mismatch involving 18% or greater of the left ventricle on quantitative analysis was associated with a sensitivity of 76% and a specificity of 78% for predicting a significant improvement in heart failure class after bypass surgery.

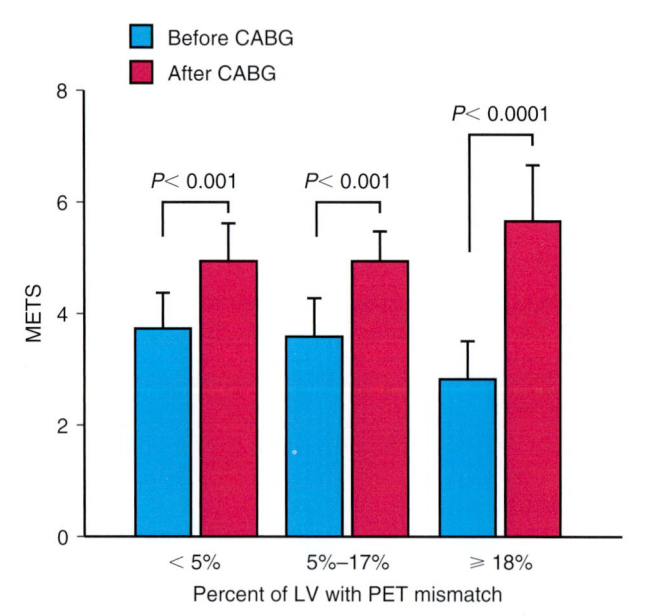

■ **FIGURE 24-11** Relationship between the anatomic extent of the perfusion–^{18}FDG-PET mismatch (% of the left ventricle [LV]) and the change in functional capacity (metabolic equivalents of oxygen consumption [METS]) after coronary artery bypass graft (CABG) surgery in patients with severe left ventricular dysfunction. (Based on data from Di Carli MF, Asgarzadie F, Schelbert HR, et al. Quantitative relation between myocardial viability and improvement in heart failure symptoms after revascularization in patients with ischemic cardiomyopathy. Circulation 1995; 92:3436-3444.)

CONCLUSIONS AND FUTURE DIRECTIONS

The clinical evidence presented in this chapter indicates that PET and PET/CT are accurate and reproducible techniques for the evaluation of CAD. For PET perfusion imaging, future studies should focus on important patient subgroups that had relatively limited representation—women, obese patients, and diabetics. These subgroups are relevant because they constitute large segments of patients referred for testing for known or suspected CAD. In addition, more information is needed to identify where PET/CT would fit in a clinical strategy as an alternative to SPECT. Many of these questions may be addressed by SPARC (Study of Perfusion versus Anatomy's Role in CAD), a prospective, multicenter registry comparing stress SPECT, stress PET, and CT angiography alone with respect to outcomes and resource use.[32] This study, designed to enroll approximately 3000 patients in 35 to 40 sites, is expected to shed light on the relative value of these newer modalities (PET, CT angiography, hybrid PET/CT) compared with standard approaches (SPECT). In particular, insights may be gained into questions such as which test or combination of tests, sequentially or in combination, in which patients should be used.

PET provides important clinical and prognostic data that aids in the management of patients with ischemic cardiomyopathy. Results from multiple studies imply that despite an increasing clinical risk of revascularization with worsening left ventricular dysfunction, noninvasive imaging evidence of preserved viability may provide information on clinical benefit to balance against that risk, informing clinical decision making. There appears to be a significant reduction, however, in the accuracy of viability testing, including PET, for predicting functional recovery in patients with severely depressed left ventricular function (LVEF <30%). The ongoing STICH (Surgical Treatment for Ischemic Heart Failure) trial is expected to shed light on the utility of viability testing in patients with CAD and decreased LVEF. Until then, PET/CT perfusion and viability testing will continue to be the cornerstone in the evaluation of these patients.

REFERENCES

1. Di Carli MF, Dorbala S, Meserve J, et al. Clinical myocardial perfusion PET/CT. J Nucl Med 2007; 48:783-793.
2. Selwyn AP, Allan RM, L'Abbate A, et al. Relation between regional myocardial uptake of rubidium-82 and perfusion: absolute reduction of cation uptake in ischemia. Am J Cardiol 1982; 50:112-121.
3. Schelbert HR, Phelps ME, Huang SC, et al. N-13 ammonia as an indicator of myocardial blood flow. Circulation 1981; 63:1259-1272.
4. Hickey KT, Sciacca RR, Bokhari S, et al. Assessment of cardiac wall motion and ejection fraction with gated PET using N-13 ammonia. Clin Nucl Med 2004; 29:243-248.
5. Chow BJ, Beanlands RS, Lee A, et al. Treadmill exercise produces larger perfusion defects than dipyridamole stress N-13 ammonia positron emission tomography. J Am Coll Cardiol 2006; 47:411-416.
6. Bacharach SL, Bax JJ, Case J, et al. PET myocardial glucose metabolism and perfusion imaging. Part 1: guidelines for data acquisition and patient preparation. J Nucl Cardiol 2003; 10:543-556.
7. Di Carli MF, Hachamovitch R. New technology for noninvasive evaluation of coronary artery disease. Circulation 2007; 115:1464-1480.
8. Sampson UK, Dorbala S, Limaye A, et al. Diagnostic accuracy of rubidium-82 myocardial perfusion imaging with hybrid positron emission tomography/computed tomography in the detection of coronary artery disease. J Am Coll Cardiol 2007; 49:1052-1058.
9. Go RT, Marwick TH, MacIntyre WJ, et al. A prospective comparison of rubidium-82 PET and thallium-201 SPECT myocardial perfusion imaging utilizing a single dipyridamole stress in the diagnosis of coronary artery disease. J Nucl Med 1990; 31:1899-1905.
10. Stewart RE, Schwaiger M, Molina E, et al. Comparison of rubidium-82 positron emission tomography and thallium-201 SPECT imaging for detection of coronary artery disease. Am J Cardiol 1991; 67:1303-1310.
11. Bateman TM, Heller GV, McGhie AI, et al. Diagnostic accuracy of rest/stress ECG-gated Rb-82 myocardial perfusion PET: comparison with ECG-gated Tc-99m sestamibi SPECT. J Nucl Cardiol 2006; 13:24-33.
12. Dorbala S, Vangala D, Sampson U, et al. Value of vasodilator left ventricular ejection fraction reserve in evaluating the magnitude of myocardium at risk and the extent of angiographic coronary artery disease: a 82Rb PET/CT study. J Nucl Med 2007; 48:349-358.
13. Kuhle WG, Porenta G, Huang SC, et al. Quantification of regional myocardial blood flow using 13N-ammonia and reoriented dynamic positron emission tomographic imaging. Circulation 1992; 86:1004-1017.
14. Muzik O, Beanlands RS, Hutchins GD, et al. Validation of nitrogen-13-ammonia tracer kinetic model for quantification of myocardial blood flow using PET. J Nucl Med 1993; 34:83-91.
15. El Fakhri G, Sitek A, Guerin B, et al. Quantitative dynamic cardiac 82Rb PET using generalized factor and compartment analyses. J Nucl Med 2005; 46:1264-1271.
16. Lin JW, Sciacca RR, Chou RL, et al. Quantification of myocardial perfusion in human subjects using 82Rb and wavelet-based noise reduction. J Nucl Med 2001; 42:201-208.
17. Yoshinaga K, Chow BJ, Williams K, et al. What is the prognostic value of myocardial perfusion imaging using rubidium-82 positron emission tomography? J Am Coll Cardiol 2006; 48:1029-1039.
18. Dorbala S, Hachamovitch R, Kwong R, et al. Incremental prognostic value of rubidium-82 myocardial perfusion PET-CT imaging in patients with known or suspected CAD. J Am Coll Cardiol 2007; 49:109A.
19. Dorbala S, Hachamovitch R, Kwong R, et al. Incremental prognostic value of left ventricular ejection fraction assessment over myocardial perfusion imaging: a rubidium-82 PET/CT study. J Am Coll Cardiol 2007; 49:109A.
20. Schenker MP, Dorbala S, Hong ECT, et al. Relationship between coronary calcification, myocardial ischemia, and outcomes in patients with intermediate likelihood of coronary artery disease: a combined positron emission tomography/computed tomography study. Circulation 2008; 117:1693-1700.
21. Mahmarian JJ. Computed tomography coronary angiography as an anatomic basis for risk stratification: deja vu or something new? J Am Coll Cardiol 2007; 50:1171-1173.
22. Baker DW, Wright RF. Management of heart failure, IV: anticoagulation for patients with heart failure due to left ventricular systolic dysfunction. JAMA 1994; 272:1614-1618.
23. Braunwald E, Kloner RA. The stunned myocardium: prolonged, postischemic ventricular dysfunction. Circulation 1982; 66:1146-1149.
24. Rahimtoola SH. The hibernating myocardium. Am Heart J 1989; 117:211-221.
25. Opie LH. The Heart: Physiology and Metabolism, 2nd ed. New York, Raven Press, 1991.
26. Di Carli MF, Prcevski P, Singh TP, et al. Myocardial blood flow, function, and metabolism in repetitive stunning. J Nucl Med 2000; 41:1227-1234.
27. Nowak B, Sinha AM, Schaefer WM, et al. Cardiac resynchronization therapy homogenizes myocardial glucose metabolism and perfusion in dilated cardiomyopathy and left bundle branch block. J Am Coll Cardiol 2003; 41:1523-1528.
28. Di Carli MF. Predicting improved function after myocardial revascularization. Curr Opin Cardiol 1998; 13:415-424.
29. Allman KC, Shaw LJ, Hachamovitch R, et al. Myocardial viability testing and impact of revascularization on prognosis in patients with coronary artery disease and left ventricular dysfunction: a meta-analysis. J Am Coll Cardiol 2002; 39:1151-1158.
30. Beanlands RS, Nichol G, Huszti E, et al. F-18-fluorodeoxyglucose positron emission tomography imaging-assisted management of patients with severe left ventricular dysfunction and suspected coronary disease: a randomized, controlled trial (PARR-2). J Am Coll Cardiol 2007; 50:2002-2012.

31. Di Carli MF, Asgarzadie F, Schelbert HR, et al. Quantitative relation between myocardial viability and improvement in heart failure symptoms after revascularization in patients with ischemic cardiomyopathy. Circulation 1995; 92:3436-3444.
32. The Study of Myocardial Perfusion and Coronary Anatomy Imaging Roles in CAD (SPARC). Available at: www.sparctrial.org. Accessed July 15, 2010.
33. Bateman TM, Heller GV, McGhie AI, et al. Diagnostic accuracy of rest/stress ECG-gated Rb-82 myocardial perfusion PET: comparison with ECG-gated Tc-99m sestamibi SPECT. J Nucl Cardiol 2006; 13:24-33.
34. Marwick TH, Nemec JJ, Stewart WJ, et al. Diagnosis of coronary artery disease using exercise echocardiography and positron emission tomography: comparison and analysis of discrepant results. J Am Soc Echocardiogr 1992; 5:231-238.
35. Grover-McKay M, Ratib O, Schwaiger M, et al. Detection of coronary artery disease with positron emission tomography and rubidium 82. Am Heart J 1992; 123:646-652.
36. Demer LL, Gould KL, Goldstein RA, et al. Assessment of coronary artery disease severity by positron emission tomography: comparison with quantitative arteriography in 193 patients. Circulation 1989; 79:825-835.
37. Tamaki N, Yonekura Y, Senda M, et al. Value and limitation of stress thallium-201 single photon emission computed tomography: comparison with nitrogen-13 ammonia positron tomography. J Nucl Med 1988; 29:1181-1188.
38. Gould KL, Goldstein RA, Mullani NA, et al. Noninvasive assessment of coronary stenoses by myocardial perfusion imaging during pharmacologic coronary vasodilation. VIII. Clinical feasibility of positron cardiac imaging without a cyclotron using generator-produced rubidium-82. J Am Coll Cardiol 1986; 7:775-789.
39. Tillisch J, Brunken R, Marshall R, et al. Reversibility of cardiac wall-motion abnormalities predicted by positron tomography. N Engl J Med 1986; 314:884-888.
40. Tamaki N, Yonekura Y, Yamashita K, et al. Positron emission tomography using fluorine-18 deoxyglucose in evaluation of coronary artery bypass grafting. Am J Cardiol 1989; 64:860-865.
41. Tamaki N, Yonekura Y, Yamashita K, et al. Prediction of reversible ischemia after coronary artery bypass grafting by positron emission tomography. J Cardiol 1991; 21:193-201.
42. Carrel T, Jenni R, Haubold-Reuter S, et al. Improvement in severely reduced left ventricular function after surgical revascularization in patients with preoperative myocardial infarction. Eur J Cardiothorac Surg 1992; 6:479-484.
43. Lucignani G, Paolini G, Landoni C, et al. Presurgical identification of hibernating myocardium by combined use of technetium-99m hexakis 2-methoxyisobutylisonitrile single photon emission tomography and fluorine-18 fluoro-2-deoxy-D-glucose positron emission tomography in patients with coronary artery disease. Eur J Nucl Med 1992; 19:874-881.
44. Gropler RJ, Geltman EM, Sampathkumaran K, et al. Functional recovery after coronary revascularization for chronic coronary artery disease is dependent on maintenance of oxidative metabolism. J Am Coll Cardiol 1992; 20:569-577.
45. Marwick TH, MacIntyre WJ, Lafont A, et al. Metabolic responses of hibernating and infarcted myocardium to revascularization: a follow-up study of regional perfusion, function, and metabolism. Circulation 1992; 85:1347-1353.
46. Gropler RJ, Geltman EM, Sampathkumaran K, et al. Comparison of carbon-11-acetate with fluorine-18-fluorodeoxyglucose for delineating viable myocardium by positron emission tomography. J Am Coll Cardiol 1993; 22:1587-1597.
47. Vanoverschelde JL, Wijns W, Depre C, et al. Mechanisms of chronic regional postischemic dysfunction in humans: new insights from the study of noninfarcted collateral-dependent myocardium. Circulation 1993; 87:1513-1523.
48. vom Dahl J, Eitzman DT, al-Aouar ZR, et al. Relation of regional function, perfusion, and metabolism in patients with advanced coronary artery disease undergoing surgical revascularization. Circulation 1994; 90:2356-2366.
49. Knuuti MJ, Saraste M, Nuutila P, et al. Myocardial viability: fluorine-18-deoxyglucose positron emission tomography in prediction of wall motion recovery after revascularization. Am Heart J 1994; 127(4 Pt 1):785-796.
50. Maes AF, Borgers M, Flameng W, et al. Assessment of myocardial viability in chronic coronary artery disease using technetium-99m sestamibi SPECT: correlation with histologic and positron emission tomographic studies and functional follow-up. J Am Coll Cardiol 1997; 29:62-68.
51. Grandin C, Wijns W, Melin JA, et al. Delineation of myocardial viability with PET. J Nucl Med 1995; 36:1543-1552.
52. Tamaki N, Kawamoto M, Tadamura E, et al. Prediction of reversible ischemia after revascularization: perfusion and metabolic studies with positron emission tomography. Circulation 1995; 91:1697-1705.
53. Baer FM, Voth E, Deutsch HJ, et al. Predictive value of low dose dobutamine transesophageal echocardiography and fluorine-18 fluorodeoxyglucose positron emission tomography for recovery of regional left ventricular function after successful revascularization. J Am Coll Cardiol 1996; 28:60-69.
54. vom Dahl J, Altehoefer C, Sheehan FH, et al. Recovery of regional left ventricular dysfunction after coronary revascularization: impact of myocardial viability assessed by nuclear imaging and vessel patency at follow-up angiography. J Am Coll Cardiol 1996; 28:948-958.
55. Wolpers HG, Burchert W, van den Hoff J, et al. Assessment of myocardial viability by use of 11C-acetate and positron emission tomography: threshold criteria of reversible dysfunction. Circulation 1997; 95:1417-1424.
56. Schwarz ER, Schaper J, vom Dahl J, et al. Myocyte degeneration and cell death in hibernating human myocardium. J Am Coll Cardiol 1996; 27:1577-1585.
57. vom Dahl J, Altehoefer C, Sheehan FH, et al. Effect of myocardial viability assessed by technetium-99m-sestamibi SPECT and fluorine-18-FDG PET on clinical outcome in coronary artery disease. J Nucl Med 1997; 38:742-748.
58. Eitzman D, al-Aouar Z, Kanter HL, et al. Clinical outcome of patients with advanced coronary artery disease after viability studies with positron emission tomography. J Am Coll Cardiol 1992; 20:559-565.
59. Di Carli M, Davidson M, Little R, et al. Value of metabolic imaging with positron emission tomography for evaluating prognosis in patients with coronary artery disease and left ventricular dysfunction. Am J Cardiol 1994; 73:527-533.
60. Lee KS, Marwick TH, Cook SA, et al. Prognosis of patients with left ventricular dysfunction, with and without viable myocardium after myocardial infarction: relative efficacy of medical therapy and revascularization. Circulation 1994; 90:2687-2694.
61. Rohatgi R, Epstein S, Henriquez J, et al. Utility of positron emission tomography in predicting cardiac events and survival in patients with coronary artery disease and severe left ventricular dysfunction. Am J Cardiol 2001; 87:1096-1099.

CHAPTER 25

Radiopharmaceuticals and Radiation Dose Considerations in Cardiac Positron Emission Tomography and PET/CT

Gaby Weissman and Albert J. Sinusas

The application of positron emission tomography (PET) for evaluation of cardiovascular disease is rapidly growing with the increased availability of hybrid PET and computed tomography (CT) scanners and new radiopharmaceuticals. Traditionally, PET imaging was employed as a unique research tool for the in vivo quantitative monitoring of myocardial perfusion, metabolism, and receptor binding. However, PET is emerging as a routine clinical approach, primarily for assessment of myocardial perfusion in patients with nondiagnostic single photon emission computed tomography (SPECT) imaging. The flexibility of radiolabeled probes for PET imaging facilitates early pilot or developmental studies. It has become increasingly clear that the molecular or physiologic information provided by PET could be substantially enhanced with the addition of anatomic information, leading to the development of hybrid PET/CT imaging systems. These hybrid systems not only improve the quantification of PET radiotracers but also allow the simultaneous evaluation of coronary physiology and coronary anatomy as derived from computed tomographic angiography (CTA).

The flexibility and power provided by radiolabeled PET probes and PET/CT come at some cost. PET tracers undergo positron decay, yielding high-energy photons (511 keV) that are more difficult to shield, and lead to a potentially increased risk of occupational exposures. In addition, most PET tracers are cyclotron produced and have a relatively short half-life ranging from minutes to hours, necessitating the availability of a cyclotron and local radiochemistry expertise as well as expensive equipment for radiation handling. However, the commercial availability of rubidium 82 (^{82}Rb) generators has improved access to PET imaging for evaluation of myocardial perfusion. Last, the addition of high-resolution multidetector CT scanners requires expertise not only in PET but also in cardiac CT physics. The merging of two imaging technologies that both deliver ionizing radiation to the patient also presents an important problem regarding radiation safety management. In this chapter, we review currently available PET radiotracers for cardiovascular application as well as the radiation issues associated with PET and PET/CT.

PET RADIOPHARMACEUTICALS

Perfusion Agents

There are currently three PET perfusion agents that are approved for clinical use (^{13}N-ammonia, ^{15}O-water, and ^{82}Rb), although several other PET perfusion agents are under preclinical and clinical evaluation. We focus on the clinically available agents (Table 25-1).

^{13}N-Ammonia

^{13}N-Ammonia is a cyclotron produced PET perfusion agent with a physical half-life of 10 minutes requiring an on-site cyclotron and radiochemistry synthesis capability. In the blood, ^{13}N-ammonia exists in equilibrium between two states, neutral ammonia (NH_3) and charged ammonium (NH_4^+). The neutral ammonia rapidly crosses cell membranes. Once it is inside the cell, glutamine synthase takes

TABLE 25-1 PET Perfusion Tracers and Their Characteristics

PET Tracer	Tracer Type	Half-life	Production
^{13}N-Ammonia	Extracted	10 minutes	Cyclotron
^{15}O-Water	Diffusible	2 minutes	Cyclotron
^{82}Rb	Extracted	75 seconds	Strontium 82 generator

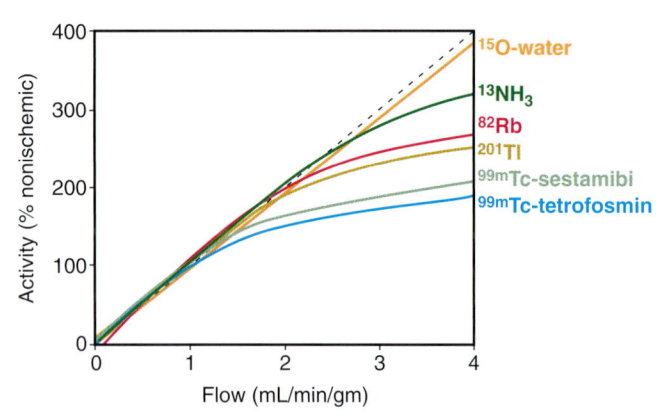

Note that ^{13}N-ammonia and ^{82}Rb are extracted tracers and demonstrate roll-off at higher flows. ^{82}Rb is generator produced, allowing production at centers that do not possess an on-site cyclotron.

FIGURE 25-1 True myocardial blood flow as measured by microspheres (x-axis) is plotted versus radiotracer uptake. At lower (physiologic) flows, there is a linear relationship between the two. However, at higher flow rates, tracer uptake "rolls off." This is not true of ^{15}O-water, which is a freely diffusible tracer and can track flows across a wide range of rates. (From Glover DK, Gropler RJ. Journey to find the ideal PET flow tracer for clinical use: are we there yet? J Nucl Cardiol 2007; 14:765-768.)

glutamate, ammonia, and ATP and produces glutamine, which remains intracellular, thereby fixing the ^{13}N within the cell with very little diffusion back into the blood pool. ^{13}N-Ammonia has a high extraction rate, with a significant percentage of the agent entering the myocyte.[1] Animal models demonstrate, however, a nonlinear extraction of ^{13}N-ammonia compared with the gold standard of microsphere flow measurements. At flows in the normal resting physiologic range of about 50 to 150 mL/min/100 g, ^{13}N-ammonia uptake is nearly linear. However, at higher flows of more than 200 mL/min/100 g, such as those produced with vasodilator stress, there is a plateau effect, and higher flow rates are not associated with a further linear increase of ^{13}N-ammonia uptake and retention.[2] The nonlinear uptake at higher flow rates does not reflect a limitation of the diffusion of ^{13}N-ammonia; rather, it is a limitation of metabolic trapping through the glutamine synthase pathway. This roll-off phenomenon may lead to underestimation of the true myocardial perfusion at higher flows, a statement true for all extracted radiotracers (Fig. 25-1). ^{13}N-Ammonia image quality is generally excellent, with rapid clearance of the tracer from the blood pool and lung, although lung uptake can be an issue in patients with chronic lung disease or depressed left ventricular function.[3]

Imaging with ^{13}N-ammonia is typically initiated either simultaneously with or shortly after a 10- to 20-mCi radiotracer infusion. For estimation of absolute blood flow, a dynamic image acquisition must be initiated with the infusion to determine the arterial input function and myocardial uptake and clearance kinetics for application of compartmental analysis. When ECG-gated PET imaging is performed only for the determination of relative perfusion and function, the acquisition begins 90 seconds to 3 minutes after infusion, which allows clearance of tracer activity from the blood pool. Image acquisition lasts 5 to 15 minutes, and attenuation correction is used in image generation. ^{13}N-Ammonia perfusion information is used as part of a rest-stress protocol, defining myocardial ischemia, or it is used in conjunction with 2-fluorodeoxyglucose (FDG) to delineate the classic mismatch between myocardial perfusion and metabolic activity in the evaluation of myocardial viability.

^{15}O-Water

^{15}O-Water is also a cyclotron-produced agent with an ultrashort half-life of 2 minutes. Unlike ^{13}N-ammonia and ^{82}Rb, ^{15}O-water is a diffusible agent that is not extracted by or trapped within the myocytes but rather freely diffuses across membranes. The kinetics of ^{15}O-water are dependent only on myocardial perfusion and are not affected by the metabolic rate-limiting steps that affect extracted tracers, eliminating the issues with tracer roll-off. However, PET ^{15}O-water imaging generally is performed only as a dynamic study to determine uptake kinetics. Application of a single-compartment model to the dynamic image data allows a highly accurate estimation of absolute myocardial flow across a wide range of blood flow rates (0.29 to 5.04 mL/min/g).[4] ^{15}O-water can be administered as an intravenous bolus, as a slow infusion, or by inhalation of ^{15}O-CO_2, which is converted to ^{15}O-water in the lungs by carbonic anhydrase.

The advantage of ^{15}O-water as an "ideal" flow tracer is counterbalanced by the complex acquisition protocols and analyses required for use in clinical practice. Because the ^{15}O-water is not extracted from the blood pool, the images are contaminated by the high level of residual activity within the blood pool, which must be subtracted from the final image to properly evaluate myocardial perfusion. Two techniques are used to accomplish this goal. The blood pool can be labeled with ^{15}O-carbon monoxide (CO). Inhalation of ^{15}O-CO leads to irreversible binding of the CO to hemoglobin, thereby labeling the red blood cells and the blood pool. Blood pool data obtained during this acquisition can be subtracted from the ^{15}O-water perfusion, eliminating the contribution of the blood pool from the final ^{15}O-water data set. Alternatively, very early acquisitions (20 to 40 seconds after tracer infusion) provide an image of the blood pool before tracer flow has reached the myocardium; these are then used to remove background blood pool signal from the myocardium.[5] The difficulties in image processing as well as the increased radiation exposure to the lung with use of the inhaled ^{15}O-CO technique limit the clinical application of ^{15}O-water.

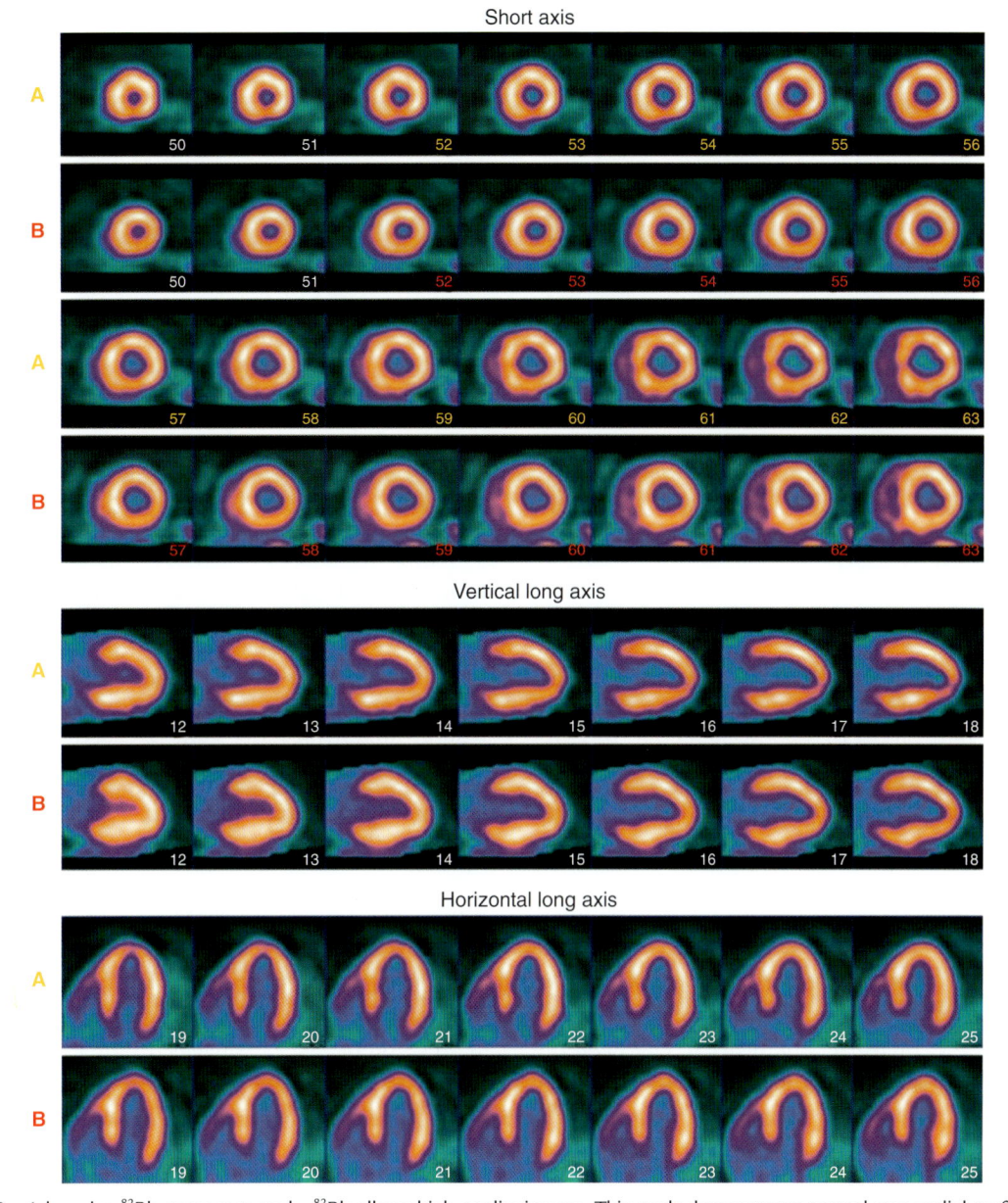

■ **FIGURE 25-2** Adenosine ^{82}Rb stress-rest study. ^{82}Rb allows high-quality images. This study demonstrates normal myocardial perfusion at stress and rest with homogeneous uptake throughout.

Rubidium 82

^{82}Rb is a radioactive monovalent cationic potassium analogue. Unlike the other perfusion agents used in cardiac PET, ^{82}Rb is produced in a commercially available generator, alleviating the need for an on-site cyclotron, which makes it a more practical perfusion tracer for widespread clinical application. ^{82}Rb is obtained by elution of 25 to 50 mL of normal saline with use of a computerized pump through a strontium 82 (^{82}Sr) generator. The generator is rapidly replenished, with 90% of the maximal activity available after 5 minutes, and full replenishment occurs by 10 minutes. ^{82}Rb has an ultrashort half-life of 75 seconds, which allows rapid acquisition of sequential stress and rest images (Fig. 25-2). The half-life of ^{82}Sr is 25.5 days, and therefore the generator needs to be replaced every 4 weeks.

^{82}Rb is extracted from the blood pool by the Na$^+$,K$^+$-ATPase pump. Extraction of ^{82}Rb is similar to that of thallium 201 (^{201}Tl), another potassium analogue,[6] but it is less than that of ^{13}N-ammonia[7]; therefore, the issues associated with roll-off may be present in ^{82}Rb as they are in all other extractable tracers. Extraction of ^{82}Rb is affected by myocardial perfusion as well as by the metabolic milieu. Severe acidosis and hypoxemia can affect ^{82}Rb extraction.[6] In addition, ^{82}Rb is a less ideal imaging agent because the ^{82}Rb positron has a high kinetic energy, which allows the positron to travel a relatively long distance before an annihilation event occurs. The increased positron range of the parent molecule results in a reduced spatial resolution of ^{82}Rb imaging compared with that possible with other PET agents. Despite these issues, ^{82}Rb has become one of the most commonly used PET

TABLE 25-2 Diagnostic Accuracy of Myocardial PET Perfusion Imaging for Detection of Coronary Artery Disease				
Sensitivity (%)	Specificity (%)	N	Agent	Author
95	100	50	NH_3, ^{82}Rb	Gould
94	95	193	^{82}Rb	Demer
93	78	202	^{82}Rb	Go
97	100	45	NH_3	Schelbert
93	100	49	NH_3	Yonekura
98	93	146	^{82}Rb	Williams
84	88	81	^{82}Rb	Stewart
95	95	25	NH_3	Tamaki
93	92	791		Average

Overall, PET perfusion studies have an excellent sensitivity and specificity for the detection of coronary artery disease.
Modified from Machac J. Cardiac positron emission tomography imaging. Semin Nucl Med 2005; 35:17-36.

perfusion agents because of the availability, ease of use, and acceptable image quality.

Summary of PET Perfusion Imaging

PET perfusion has become a routine tool in the management of cardiac patients. Multiple studies have evaluated the accuracy of perfusion PET for the detection of coronary artery disease. PET has consistently been found to have a high sensitivity and specificity for the detection of coronary artery disease. The accuracy of this technique makes the use of PET perfusion an attractive option in patients with chest pain or suspected coronary artery disease despite the increased cost and relative technical complexity (Table 25-2).[8-15]

Metabolic Agents

The flexibility of PET pharmacochemistry has allowed the development of tracers to track multiple metabolic processes within the heart. Glucose metabolism has been the primary target of clinical cardiac PET. Other processes, including fatty acid metabolism and neurohormonal innervation, have been studied as well.

^{18}F-Fluorodeoxyglucose (^{18}F-FDG)

Fluorodeoxyglucose (2-fluoro-2-deoxy-D-glucose, FDG) is a glucose analogue that enters the cell through facilitated diffusion. Once inside cells, it is phosphorylated by hexokinase into FDG 6-phosphate, which is metabolically inert and is trapped within the myocyte. Therefore, retention of FDG is an energy-requiring process and is dependent on intact metabolic pathways (Fig. 25-3). FDG can be labeled with fluorine18 (^{18}F), which decays by positron emission with a half-life of 110 minutes. The prolonged half-life of ^{18}F allows local distribution of the agent from a central cyclotron site to regional imaging centers. Whereas it is the most commonly used agent in oncologic PET imaging, ^{18}F-FDG is used primarily for the evaluation of myocardial viability in cardiac imaging.

Myocytes generally favor fatty acids derived from adipose tissue stores as their primary source of energy. However, after a glucose load, glucose becomes the primary metabolic energy substrate as systemic release of insulin limits free fatty acid release and increases transmembrane transport of glucose. In the setting of myocardial ischemia, free fatty acid metabolism decreases while glucose metabolism increases, resulting in increased uptake of ^{18}F-FDG in the ischemic tissue. As the phosphorylation of ^{18}F-FDG is an energy-requiring process, uptake of ^{18}F-FDG can occur only in metabolically active (viable) myocytes. Therefore, in the clinical setting, ^{18}F-FDG is used to determine viability in chronically ischemic myocardium.

Preparation of the patient is important in the proper acquisition of ^{18}F-FDG images. In the fasting state, glucose uptake is low and inhomogeneous. To maximize glucose

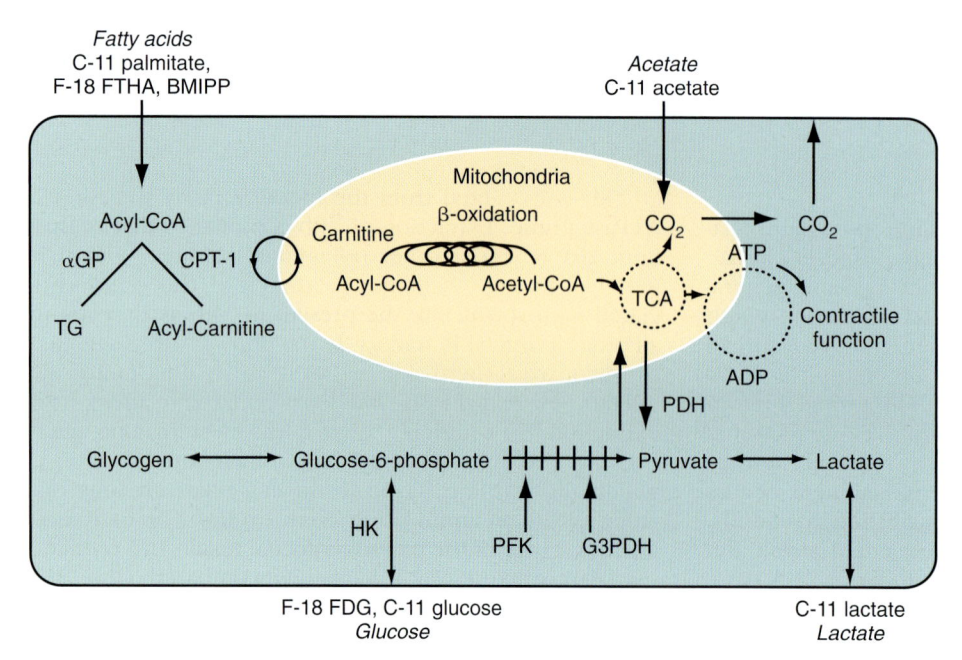

■ FIGURE 25-3 Glucose and fatty acid pathways in the myocytes. FDG enters as glucose and after phosphorylation becomes trapped intracellularly. Free fatty acids such as acetate and palmitate enter the cell and participate in the beta-oxidation pathway. (From Herrero P, Gropler RJ. Imaging of myocardial metabolism. J Nucl Cardiol 2005; 12:345-358.)

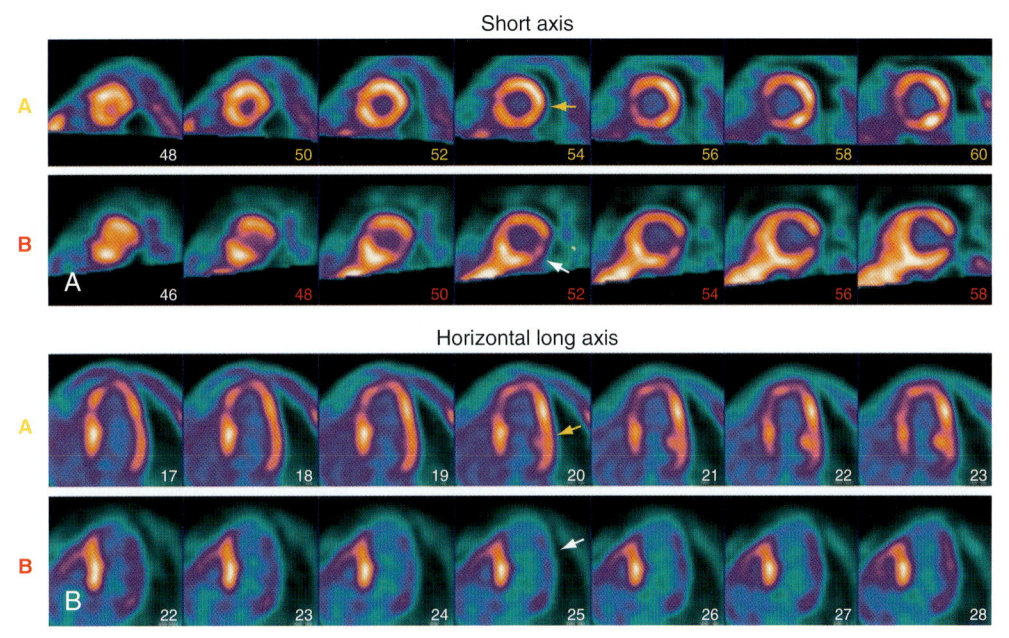

FIGURE 25-4 Cardiac viability study. Top rows (**A**) represent FDG study; bottom rows (**B**) represent ^{82}Rb perfusion examination. Short-axis images demonstrate a large perfusion defect in the lateral segments (*white arrow*). There is uptake of FDG in these segments (*yellow arrow*), indicating viable myocardium. Horizontal long-axis images demonstrate that the perfusion defect involves the apex as well as the lateral wall; all segments are viable as indicated by FDG uptake.

use by the myocardium, the patient is asked to fast for 6 to 12 hours. An oral glucose load (25 to 100 g) or an intravenous glucose load is administered and followed by insulin as needed before imaging. In diabetic patients, a more rigorous methodology is necessary to produce high-quality scans, and a euglycemic hyperinsulinemic clamp is often used. A dose of 5 to 15 mCi is injected, and imaging begins at least 45 minutes after tracer infusion. Viability studies with ^{18}F-FDG are performed in conjunction with a perfusion study. Perfusion can be acquired with PET perfusion agents as described before or with SPECT perfusion agents such as ^{201}Tl or technetium Tc 99m. Preserved FDG uptake in the setting of reduced perfusion suggests the presence of viable myocardium. These segments are likely to have improved function after revascularization. Segments that have both diminished perfusion and diminished FDG uptake are unlikely to recover function with revascularization and consist mostly of infarcted tissue (Fig. 25-4).

^{11}C-Palmitate and ^{11}C-Acetate

As noted previously, free fatty acids are the primary source of energy in normal myocardium, accounting for 60% to 80% of ATP produced in nonischemic myocytes. Free fatty acids are activated as acyl coenzyme A. Acyl coenzyme A enters the mitochondria through the acyl carnitine transport system and becomes part of the beta-oxidation pathway. Whereas this pathway is a rich source of ATP, it is highly oxygen dependent. During periods of ischemia, there is a rapid shift away from fatty acid metabolism to increased glucose use (see Fig. 25-3). Free fatty acids account for the preponderance of myocardial energy formation, and these pathways are dramatically altered by ischemia. Therefore, free fatty acid imaging is an attractive target for noninvasive imaging of ischemia and the associated alterations in oxidative metabolism. PET imaging of fatty acid metabolism generally involves imaging with carbon 11 (^{11}C)–labeled medium-sized straight-chain fatty acids like palmitate, which undergo beta-oxidation. ^{11}C has also been used to label acetate as an alternative approach for imaging of oxidative metabolism. ^{11}C is cyclotron produced and has a relatively short half-life of 20.4 minutes. Initially produced in 1934 and first studied in humans in 1945, it has the advantage of being an organic molecule and therefore can potentially be used to target a wide variety of metabolic processes.[16] Unfortunately, ^{11}C-labeled metabolic agents are more difficult to employ in clinical practice and have been primarily used for research purposes. However, both ^{11}C-palmitate and ^{11}C-acetate have been effectively employed for the evaluation of myocardial oxidative metabolism.

Several studies have evaluated fatty acid metabolism in normal volunteers and patients. Walsh and colleagues[17] demonstrated decreased mitochondrial metabolism in infarcted myocardium. In addition, ^{11}C-palmitate infusion during dobutamine stress testing demonstrated the expected rise in fatty acid metabolism in the normal myocardial segments, whereas areas supplied by stenosed vessels did not show a rise in fatty acid use.[18] Last, free fatty acid metabolism imaging has been used to demonstrate differences in myocardial metabolism in the elderly[19] as well as in inherited nonischemic cardiomyopathies.[20] In both cases, fatty acid metabolism was decreased compared with normal controls. Although the clinical application of some of these findings is not fully elucidated, free fatty acid PET offers a powerful method for the in vivo evaluation of myocardial metabolism and therefore provides an important tool for gaining insight into disease processes associated with altered myocardial metabolism.

Neurohormonal Cardiac PET

The heart is innervated by both the sympathetic and parasympathetic nervous systems. Sympathetic activation leads to increased cardiac activation, an increase in contractility, and an increase in heart rate. The parasympathetic system acts in opposition, slowing heart rate and decreasing contractility. Neurohormonal activation plays an important role in several disease processes. Neurohormonal activation is altered in heart failure, in diabetes, after myocardial infarction, and after cardiac transplantation. In addition, cardiac arrhythmias have been associated with abnormalities of the autonomic nervous system. Therefore, a compelling case can be made for imaging of the cardiac autonomic activation.

Multiple tracers have been developed for the evaluation of both the sympathetic and parasympathetic pathways (Table 25-3). One PET agent that has been extensively used in the evaluation of neurohormonal activation in heart failure and other cardiac disease states is m-hydroxyephedrine (HED). HED, a derivative of the amine metaraminol, is an analogue of norepinephrine that is resistant to metabolism through the typical monoamine oxidase pathway. Therefore, sympathetic activation of the heart can be effectively evaluated with ^{11}C-labeled HED ([^{11}C]HED) PET imaging. This radiopharmaceutical has been studied in multiple conditions including cardiac transplantation, cardiomyopathies, diabetes, and myocardial infarction. Evaluation of neuroactivation can infer disease outcome; for example, lower levels of [^{11}C]HED are associated with a poor prognosis in heart failure.[21] Whereas neurohormonal PET imaging remains in an early stage of development, many potential future avenues of investigation are present, including the prediction of sudden cardiac death.

TABLE 25-3 Nuclear Medicine Tracers for Sympathetic Neurons

Tracer	PET/SPECT Tracer	Type
^{11}C-m-hydroxyephedrine (^{11}C-HED)	PET	Analogue
^{123}I-MIBG (metaiodobenzylguanidine)	SPECT	Analogue
^{18}F-6-fluorodopamine	PET	Catecholamine
^{11}C-epinephrine	PET	Catecholamine
^{18}F-6-fluoronorepinephrine	PET	Catecholamine
^{11}C-phenylephrine	PET	Analogue
^{18}F-fluorometaraminol	PET	Analogue
^{18}F-p-fluorobenzylguanidine	PET	Analogue
^{18}F-fluoroiodobenzylguanidine	PET	Analogue
^{18}F-6-fluorometaraminol	PET	Analogue

^{123}I-MIBG has been the most studied SPECT agent. The PET agents are divided into those that are radiolabeled catecholamines and those that are catecholamine analogues.
Modified from Langer O, Halldin C. PET and SPECT tracers for mapping the cardiac nervous system. Eur J Nucl Med Mol Imaging 2002; 29:416-434.

IONIZING RADIATION IN PET/CT

Medical PET and CT imaging involves the use of ionizing radiation. Particles emitted by CT x-ray tubes or from the decay of radiopharmaceuticals used in nuclear medicine contain sufficient energy to detach electrons from atoms and are therefore labeled ionizing. Ionizing radiation poses several potential negative effects on biologic tissues. These effects are broadly divided into two groups: deterministic and stochastic effects. Deterministic effects have a threshold level below which there are no adverse events. When the threshold for biologic effect is reached, the severity of the effect is proportional to the final dose delivered, with increasing doses causing increasingly severe effects. Conditions in which an acute exposure to a high level of radiation leads to cell death are deterministic and include skin toxicity, bone marrow toxicity, gastrointestinal effects, and central nervous system syndrome. These effects are usually seen at doses above those experienced in diagnostic medical procedures. Stochastic effects, on the other hand, are related to DNA damage and are probabilistic in nature. There is no threshold level below which exposure is completely safe, and increasing exposure increases the probability of an adverse effect but not necessarily the severity. The risk of future malignant disease is an important stochastic effect of ionizing radiation and is the focus of concern in diagnostic radiology procedures.

There has been an increasing focus on the effects of medical radiation, especially in the realm of cardiac imaging, and consideration must be given to maximizing the patient's safety when tests with ionizing radiation are performed. The concept of ALARA (as low as reasonably achievable) is the primary dictate in performing diagnostic studies involving ionizing radiation. Absorbed dose refers to the amount of energy deposited in tissue by the radiation passing through it. The absorbed radiation dose is measured in grays (Gy); 1 Gy corresponds to the amount of radiation required to deposit 1 joule of energy in 1 kilogram of matter. The equivalent dose, expressed in sieverts (Sv), corrects for the different effects that different types of radiation have on tissues, with alpha particles depositing more energy than beta or gamma radiation. X-rays and gamma rays have a correction factor of 1. This measurement does not take into account the sensitivity of different tissues to radiation. The effective dose, also expressed in sieverts, is the sum of the tissue-weighted equivalent doses to all the exposed organs. This measurement is most useful in comparing the risk posed by a nonuniform radiation exposure to the patient through exposure to a diagnostic test or to nuclear medicine staff through occupational exposure. Because tissues such as lung and breast tissue are more sensitive to the effects of ionizing radiation than are other organs such as skin, radiation to those organs is of greater concern. Diagnostic procedures vary significantly in the dose delivered to the patient. CT and nuclear medicine examinations tend to be relatively high dose diagnostic examinations, with the effective dose potentially reaching 30 mSv, although it is generally in the range of 3 to 15 mSv. By way of comparison, the average annual background radiation at sea level is about 2.5 mSv, and the

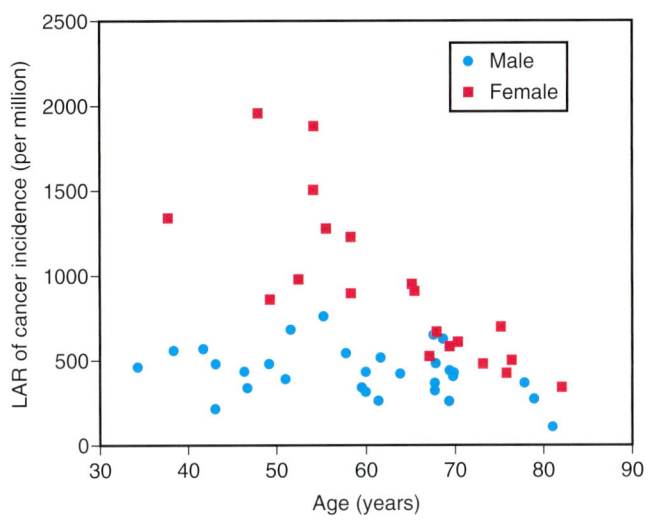

FIGURE 25-5 Estimated lifetime attributable risk (LAR) of malignant disease estimated with models developed in the National Academies' Biological Effects of Ionizing Radiation VII (BEIR VII) report. Note that with decreasing age and female sex, the risk of malignant transformation increases. *(From Einstein AJ Sanz J, Dellegrottaglie S, et al. Radiation dose and cancer risk estimates in 16-detector computed tomography coronary angiography. J Nucl Cardiol 2008; 15:232-240.)*

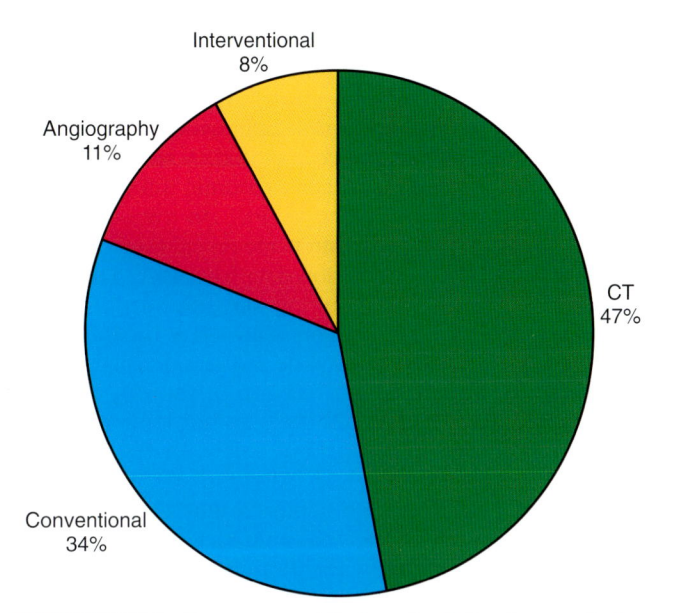

FIGURE 25-6 Percentage contribution of radiation from medical imaging, 2001-2002, in the United Kingdom. Note that a significant portion of the dose is from CT examinations. *(From Hart D, Wall BF. UK population dose from medical X-ray examinations. Eur J Radiol 2004; 50:285-291.)*

dose associated with a chest x-ray is very low at about 0.01 mSv.

The true risk to the patient from exposure to diagnostic medical radiation is difficult to estimate. The relatively low dose of radiation delivered with each exposure and the long latency time before the development of adverse events make it difficult to establish a causal link as large studies with long follow-up times are necessary to evaluate such effects. Therefore, much of the data available is derived from the study of nuclear plant workers involving occupational or accidental exposures or from the atom bomb experience at Hiroshima and Nagasaki. There are increased rates of leukemia and breast, thyroid, colorectal, and lung cancer in the exposed population.[22] Excessive radiation exposure also has an adverse effect on mortality.[23] Radiation exposure to young people carries a greater risk than to the elderly as the longer time horizon allows the clinical appearance of malignant change. In addition, the variable sensitivity of different tissues places women at higher risk from exposure to the thorax as breast tissue is sensitive to the effects of radiation (Fig. 25-5). Einstein and colleagues[24] estimated a lifetime risk of 1 in 143 for a 20-year-old woman exposed to a single coronary CT study as opposed to a lifetime risk of 1 in 3261 for an 80-year-old man. It is therefore reasonable to exercise greater caution in scanning younger patients, especially a pediatric population.

In 2006, nuclear medicine scans and CT scans accounted for 22% of all radiologic studies, excluding dental studies. These procedures accounted for 75% of the effective dose administered with diagnostic procedures, with CT making up 46% and nuclear medicine accounting for 26% of the total exposure. The number of CT scans has increased by 10% annually since 1993, with an estimated 67 million CT scans being performed in the United States in 2006. In 2005, it was estimated that 19.7 million nuclear medicine procedures were performed in the United States. Nuclear cardiology accounted for 57% of all nuclear studies; most of these studies were myocardial perfusion scans.[25] Therefore, it is important to take into account the radiation issues associated with PET/CT. PET/CT poses a unique challenge in diagnostic imaging as two separate systems with significant associated radiation exposure are employed (Fig. 25-6 and Table 25-4).

PET/CT

CT may serve several purposes in the context of PET imaging. One important function is that of attenuation correction of the PET scans. As photons from the positron

TABLE 25-4 Growth in Radiology Procedures Involving Ionizing Radiation in the United Kingdom from 1997 to 2002

Study	1997-1998	1998-1999	1999-2000	2000-2001	2001-2002
Radiographs	19,474,590	19,876,933	19,967,296	19,913,022	19,806,876
CT	1,172,656	1,254,474	1,359,852	1,488,752	1,625,304
Fluoroscopy	1,179,979	1,244,632	1,256,965	1,253,847	1,222,296
Radioisotopes	722,096	699,654	727,255	539,141	537,653

CT volume grew by 39%, radiography remained stable, and radioisotope use declined during the same time period.
Modified from Hart D, Wall BF. UK population dose from medical X-ray examinations. Eur J Radiol 2004; 50:285-291.

annihilation event pass through tissues, they are variably attenuated before they reach the PET camera, which can lead to artifacts in the final image. An attenuation map allows the scanner to take particle attenuation into account when the final PET image is composed. A second role of CT in PET/CT imaging is to add anatomic information to the physiologic data provided by PET. In the context of cardiac imaging, this most often means adding coronary anatomy from CTA to perfusion data from PET. There are several techniques for acquiring the attenuation scan. Almost all current PET scanners sold today include a CT scanner, which is used to provide a tissue density attenuation map for attenuation correction of the PET images. This attenuation CT scan can be acquired with very low radiation exposure to the patient solely for the purpose of creating an attenuation map. Alternatively, a high-dose diagnostic CT scan can be acquired and used for both attenuation correction and anatomic localization.

An alternative technique for attenuation correction that was employed routinely in the previous generation PET scanners involves the use of a rotating external radionuclide source, such as germanium 68 (^{68}Ge), for creation of a transmission attenuation scan. The effective radiation dose from the ^{68}Ge transmission scan is negligible compared with a CT scan. This represents a significant advantage over PET/CT.[26] Whereas an external source may be adequate for attenuation correction, CT provides important anatomic data that can be used to localize and to quantify radiotracer activity as well as to provide complementary diagnostic information. Even a low-dose nongated CT scan, which is inadequate for quantification of coronary calcifications, or coronary CTA provides diagnostic anatomic information of the thorax and heart that is unavailable with an external radionuclide dose.

The combination of CTA and PET perfusion imaging provides complementary information about coronary physiology and detailed coronary anatomy. The hybrid procedures also permit the assessment of other functional or physiologic information (i.e., myocardial viability, sympathetic function) along with structural abnormalities (i.e., pericardial effusion, myocardial hypertrophy). This additional information, of course, comes at a cost of additional radiation exposure; therefore, understanding of the mechanisms of dose reduction becomes important in the proper administration of these tests. The rest of this chapter focuses on the issues related to the radiation exposure associated with PET/CT imaging.

Radiation Exposure Associated with CT

The radiation associated with CT is related to several sources of exposure: the primary x-ray beam, leakage of radiation from the x-ray tube housing, and scatter of photons due to the interaction of x-rays and tissues as the beam passes through the patient. The total radiation to which the patient is exposed is determined by the tube current, the voltage applied across the tube, the length of the field scanned, the rotation time, the speed of the table through the scanner, and the x-ray beam width. As exposure increases, the signal-to-noise ratio increases, improving image quality. The operator can manipulate these parameters to achieve the best balance of image quality

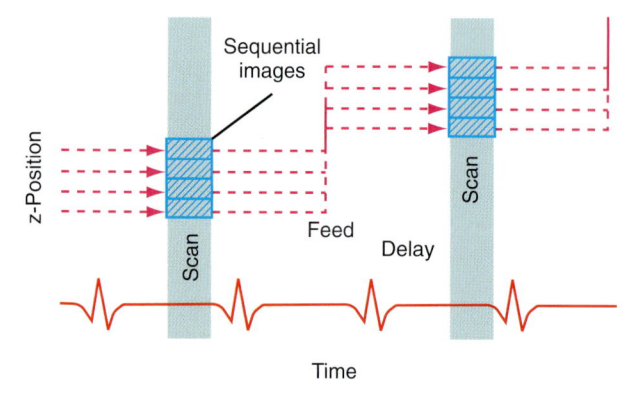

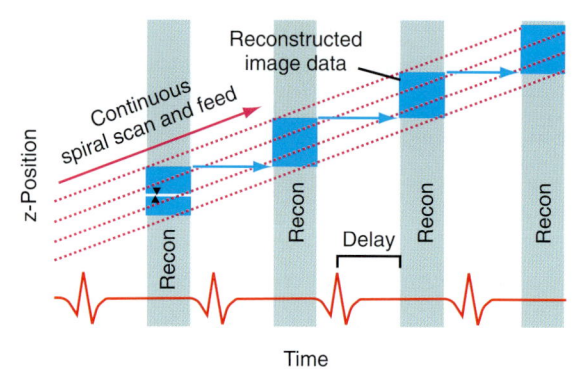

■ **FIGURE 25-7** Prospective versus retrospective ECG gating. **A,** In prospective gating, the patient is scanned only during the short time window effective for coronary imaging. **B,** In retrospective scans, there is continuous exposure and reconstruction after acquisition eliminates data acquired at times outside of the effective window. This difference allows lower exposure with prospective scans. *(From Wintersperger BJ, Nikolaou K. Basics of cardiac MDCT: techniques and contrast application. Eur Radiol 2005; 15[Suppl 2]:B2-B9. Reproduced with permission of Springer Science and Business Media.)*

and the lowest dose achievable (the principle of ALARA). Cardiac CT can deliver relatively high radiation doses compared with noncardiac chest CT because of the need for ECG gating to optimize visualization of the coronary arteries at selected phases of the cardiac cycle and for evaluation of cardiac function over the entire cardiac cycle. Toward this end, images are acquired continuously throughout the cardiac cycle with an ECG trigger reference to acquire a series of images in multiple phases of the cardiac cycle. This requires relatively slow table speed in relation to the rotation of the x-ray tube (pitch), leading to increased exposure when helical scanning techniques are used. In addition, the small size of the coronary arteries requires a high spatial resolution, demanding increased radiation energy and exposure times to maximize the signal-to-noise ratio and to improve image quality.

One of two principal scanning methods can be used in cardiac CTA (Fig. 25-7). Traditional CTA uses a retrospective ECG gating technique. In this scan, a helical acquisition necessitates continuous radiation exposure throughout the cardiac cycle, increasing the overall ionizing radiation exposure. Several acquisition strategies can be employed to reduce exposure during retrospective ECG-gated cardiac CT. One strategy involves dose modulation, which allows lowering of the tube current during preselected portions of the cardiac cycle that are unlikely to provide diagnostic information. The coronary arteries move relatively rapidly through the imaging field during the cardiac cycle, while the temporal resolution of cardiac CT is relatively low. Therefore, data obtained during much of the cardiac cycle are unnecessary for the evaluation of the coronary arteries because the coronaries are in motion and cannot be imaged optimally secondary to through-plane motion. The coronaries are relatively still during end-systole and diastasis, and therefore only information acquired during those two selected phases of the cardiac cycle is generally clinically useful in the evaluation of epicardial coronary arteries. By maximizing the x-ray tube output during those two phases and, importantly, lowering tube output during the rest of the cardiac cycle, dose savings of 30% to 40% can be achieved.

The second CTA technique, which is increasingly used, is prospective ECG-gated image acquisition. This technique allows greater dose savings than those available with helical techniques. This scan uses an axial acquisition as opposed to the helical acquisition in the retrospective technique. The CT scanner is turned on only during the phase of the cardiac cycle in which coronary motion is minimized, avoiding radiation exposure at other portions of the cardiac cycle. This scanning approach requires longer scan times and therefore longer breath-hold times as well as a stable cardiac rhythm. However, as the number of CT detector rows has increased from 4 to 64 and beyond, breath-hold times are sufficiently short, making this technique more clinically viable in practice. Whereas the main advantage of prospective gating is decreased radiation dose, the primary disadvantage is the loss of functional information as the heart is imaged for only a short period of the entire cardiac cycle. In the context of PET/CT imaging, this limitation is partially overcome as ECG-gated PET scans can provide information about regional and global left ventricular function. Therefore, in the context of PET/CT imaging, prospective CTA is an especially appealing technologic advancement. Exposure from cardiac CT ranges from 7 to 21.4 mSv with use of 64–detector row scanners employing the retrospective acquisition techniques[27]; however, the newer prospective CT acquisition techniques offer much lower effective doses, potentially less than 3 mSv.[28] This represents a substantial radiation dose savings to the patient.

In addition to the choice between helical and axial scanning, there are other CT parameters that can be used to minimize exposure. Tube current and tube voltage can and should be adjusted to the lowest levels that produce diagnostic-quality images. These adjustments are especially applicable in smaller and thinner patients because less x-ray attenuation occurs in these patients. Last, the width of the scan field in the z direction should be minimized to include only the heart and coronary arteries to avoid unnecessary radiation to adjacent structures (Table 25-5).

TABLE 25-5 Dose Reduction Strategies for the CT Portion of the PET/CT Examination

CT Dose Reduction Strategy	Disadvantages
Low-dose transmission scan	Nondiagnostic-quality CT Useful for attenuation correction only
Prospective ECG gating	Lack of functional information Data limited to a single phase of the cardiac cycle
Dose modulation with retrospective ECG gating	Diagnostic data limited to a single phase of the cardiac cycle
Decrease tube current	Decreased signal-to-noise ratio
Decrease scan length in the z plane	Limited by size of the heart

Radiation Exposure Associated with PET

Radiation exposure associated with PET imaging is also related to several factors. Positrons deposit their energy locally, which accounts for much of the radiation exposure to the patient. The high-energy photons released in the annihilation events are penetrating particles and often cause radiation exposure to bystanders and PET facility staff as opposed to the patient. The relatively short half-life of the most commonly used PET imaging agents (seconds to minutes) and the limitation of total dose that is imposed by the response time of the often uncollimated or minimally collimated PET detectors result in relatively low radiation exposure to the patient compared with SPECT imaging. The use of three-dimensional cardiac PET scanning without collimation will improve system sensitivity and necessitate use of lower doses, which will offer potential advantages in reducing radiation exposure.

Radiation dosimetry of nuclear radiopharmaceuticals is calculated by a mathematical biokinetic model that incorporates the tissue biodistribution of the agent as well as biologic and physical decay. Different PET agents have different target organs, dictating which tissues receive the maximal radiation exposure. The bladder is the organ of maximal dose for ^{13}N-ammonia and ^{18}F-FDG. The heart is the target organ for ^{15}O-water, and the lungs are the target organ for inhaled ^{15}O-CO gas. Total effective dose is then calculated from the sum of the organ doses. Effective radiation dose to the patient associated with PET imaging varies with the type of agent used, from 2.4 mSv for ^{13}N-ammonia perfusion studies to 13.5 mSv for ^{82}Rb perfusion studies (Fig. 25-8). Note that these radiation doses compare favorably with standard SPECT agents, for which doses can range from 6.6 mSv for stress-only ^{99m}Tc-tetrofosmin studies to 29.2 mSv for dual-isotope stress-rest studies using Tc 99m and ^{201}Tl because those agents have significantly longer half-lives.[27]

Last, in addition to consideration of the radiation exposure to the patient, occupational exposure related to PET radiopharmaceuticals is also important. As positron annihilation events produce high-energy photons, these photons can travel long distances and affect bystanders. This is of particular importance to the staff of a PET facility. Technologists working with PET agents tend to have higher exposure to radiation compared with those

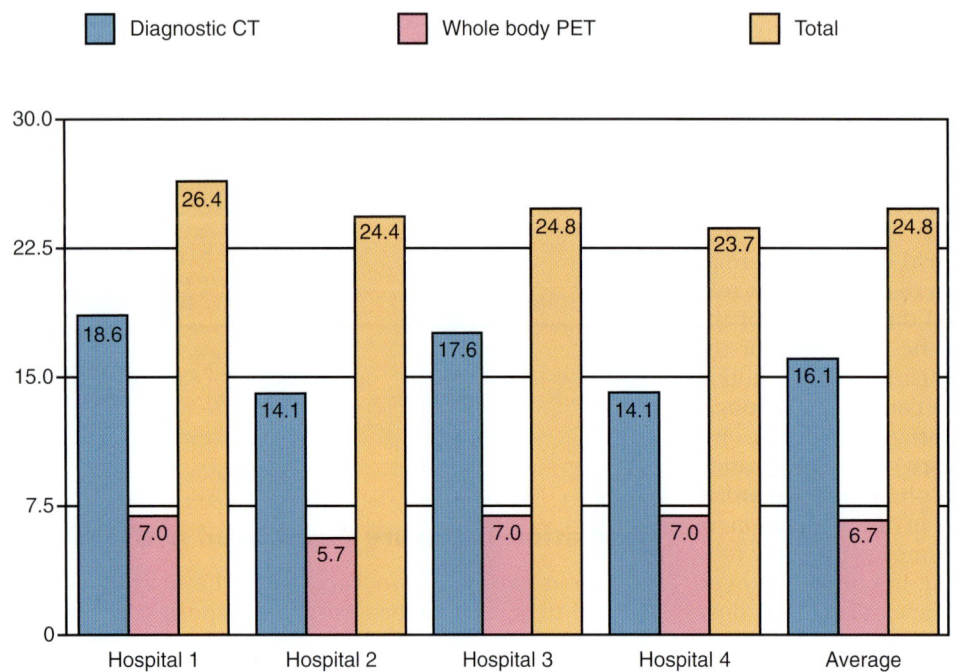

FIGURE 25-8 Radiation exposure (mSv) from whole-body FDG-PET/CT in four hospitals. Much of the total radiation dose is attributable to the diagnostic CT examination of the PET/CT; the PET scan and the transmission images account for a minority of the radiation. *(Modified from Brix G, Lechel U, Glatting G, et al. Radiation exposure of patients undergoing whole-body dual-modality ^{18}F-FDG PET/CT examinations. J Nucl Med 2005; 46:608-613. Reproduced with permission of the Society of Nuclear Medicine.)*

working with SPECT agents.[29] Mitigation strategies for occupational exposure center on the three principles of radiation safety, maximizing distance and shielding while minimizing exposure time. Proper shielding of syringes and vials reduces hand doses. Maintaining an appropriate distance from a recently injected patient reduces occupational exposure. Finally, proper setup of the patient before injection of the tracer and an efficient system of removal of intravenous lines and equipment and handling after the procedure can reduce the time of exposure for the PET laboratory staff. Used in concert, these techniques reduce radiation exposure and increase safety for PET personnel.

Dose Reduction in Cardiac PET/CT

Because PET/CT may potentially involve significant radiation exposure to the patient, care must be taken to maximize safety of the patient while maintaining image quality. Each technique should be optimized individually, allowing the best results in each portion of the study. Several considerations are taken into account in reducing radiation exposure from PET/CT studies. The first consideration is whether additional information is gained from combining both modalities. In some cases, a normal or abnormal test result from one of the two imaging techniques may be sufficient to make the diagnosis and to define future management of the patient. In such cases, the second study may be avoided entirely, saving the patient unnecessary cost and exposure. If just the PET study is necessary, an attenuation map can be constructed from either an external radionuclide transmission scan or a low-dose transmission CT scan for attenuation correction, minimizing the radiation exposure. Conversely, a normal coronary CTA study may obviate the need for perfusion imaging, avoiding the additional radiation associated with PET imaging. Considering which population of patients will benefit most from the combination of physiologic and anatomic information allows the greatest dose savings overall (Figs. 25-9 and 25-10).

When both studies are performed, efforts should be made to reduce exposure with each modality. The appropriate radionuclide dose should be selected according to the patient's size. Exposure to radiation with ^{18}F-FDG can be mitigated by encouraging hydration and frequent bladder emptying after the scan; radioisotope in the bladder is a major source of radiation exposure to the bladder and abdominal organs.[30]

A large proportion of the effective radiation dose in PET/CT is related directly to the CT scan. In a study involving four centers using diagnostic-quality contrast-enhanced CT as part of a whole-body ^{18}F-FDG-PET/CT protocol (Fig. 25-11), an average of 16.1 mSv of the total 24.8 mSv for the entire procedure was accounted for by the diagnostic-quality CT (65%).[30] By comparison, low-dose (not "diagnostic quality") CT has an effective dose of 4.5 mSv. The logical conclusion is that low-dose CT for attenuation correction alone should be preferentially performed in instances in which a high-dose diagnostic CT examination is unnecessary.

When diagnostic-quality CTA is needed, strategies such as those discussed previously can minimize exposure of patients to ionizing radiation. Exposure of the patient can be further lowered by limiting the CT scan length (i.e., cranial-caudal coverage in the z dimension) to the patient's heart. Tube current should be set at the lowest level that will produce images of diagnostic quality. During retrospective ECG-gated acquisition, tube current dose modulation can be used to minimize radiation during the portions of the cardiac cycle that are unlikely to produce diagnostic images. Last, when possible, prospective ECG-gated CT scan protocols should be favored because they lead to the greatest dose reduction.

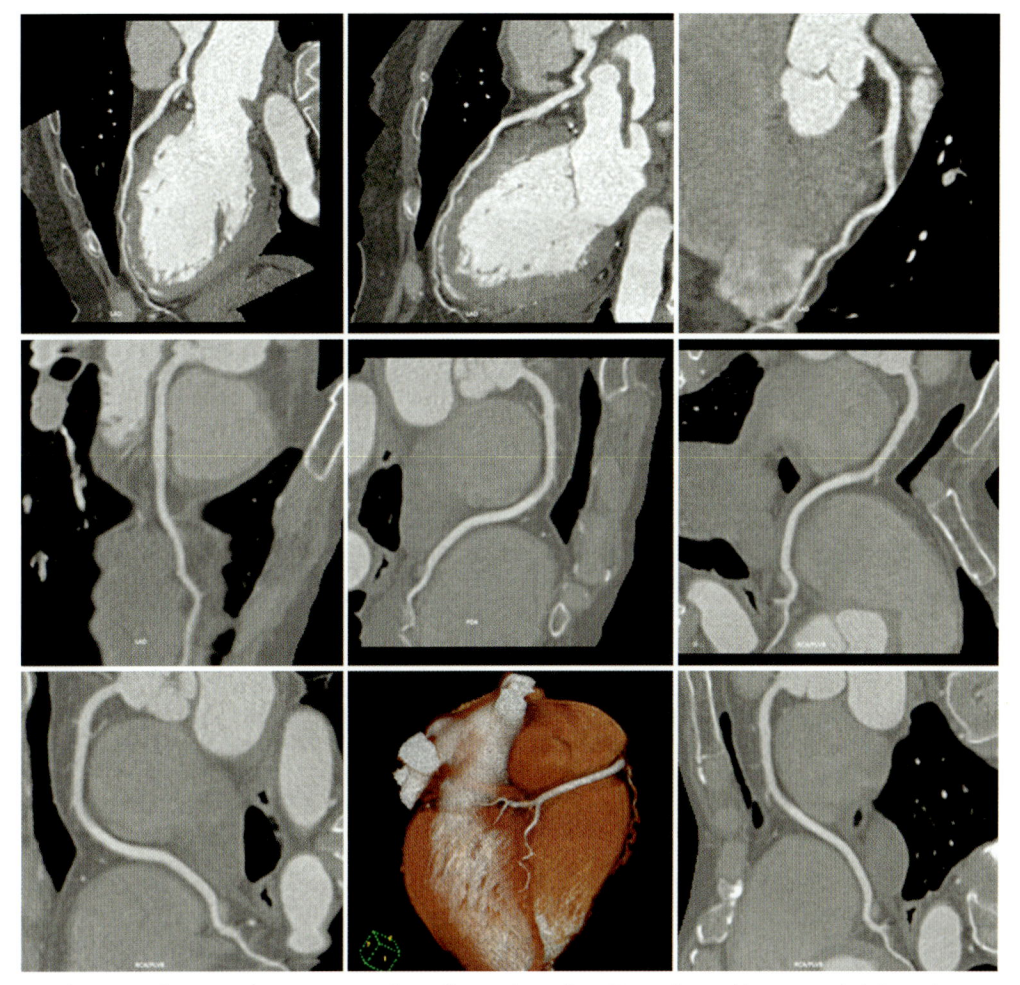

CHAPTER 25 • *Radiopharmaceuticals and Radiation Dose Considerations in Cardiac PET* 349

■ **FIGURE 25-9** CTA demonstrating normal coronary vessels. A diagnostic-quality CTA study provides anatomic information to supplement the physiologic data obtained from PET in addition to serving as an attenuation map.

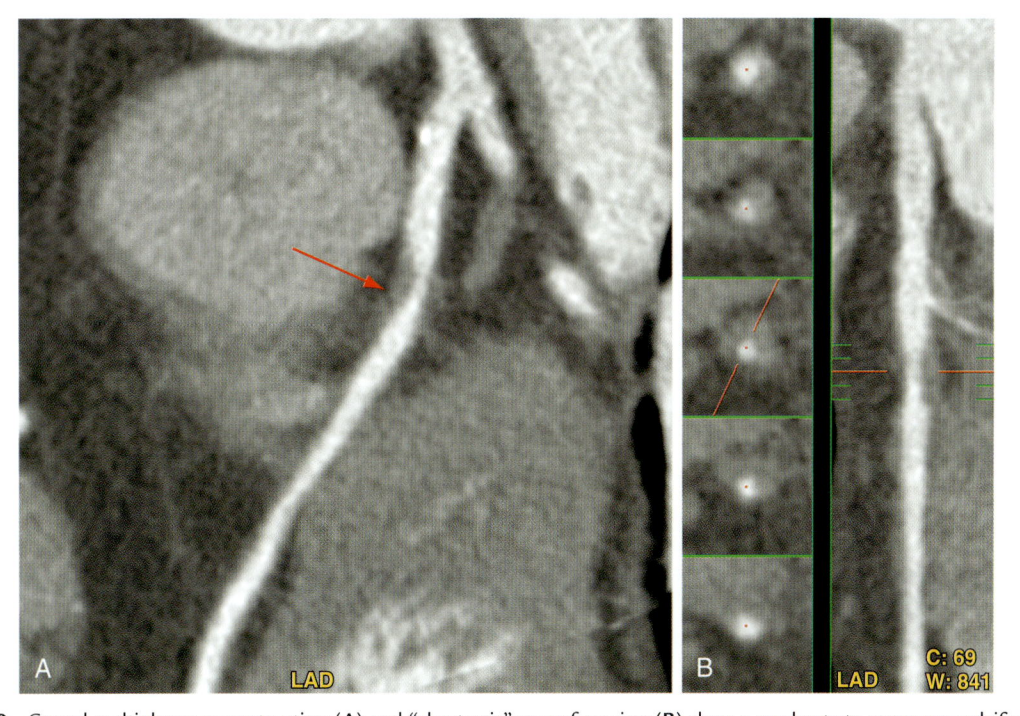

■ **FIGURE 25-10** Curved multiplanar reconstruction (**A**) and "short-axis" or en face view (**B**) show a moderate to severe noncalcified plaque (*arrow*) in the mid left anterior descending artery (LAD). It is in these cases that functional information provided by a PET perfusion scan can be most valuable.

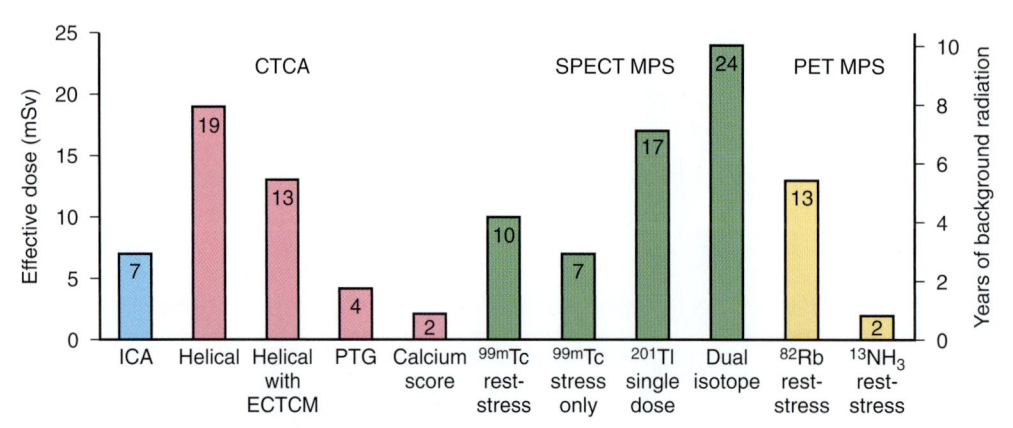

■ **FIGURE 25-11** Radiation exposure (mSv) from cardiac procedures. On the left is the effective dose. On the right is the equivalent in years of background radiation, assuming 2.4 mSv annual background radiation. CTCA, computed tomographic coronary angiography; ICA, invasive coronary angiography; ECTCM, electrocardiographically controlled tube current modulation; PTG, prospective triggered gating; ^{99m}Tc, technetium Tc 99m; MPS, myocardial perfusion scintigraphy. *(From Einstein AJ. Radiation risk from coronary artery disease imaging: how do different diagnostic tests compare? Heart 2008; 94:1519-1521. Reproduced with permission from BMJ Publishing Group, Ltd.)*

KEY POINTS

- Increasing prevalence of hybrid PET/CT imaging systems permits the evaluation of anatomy and physiology in a single test.
- PET tracers are most commonly produced in a cyclotron, with ^{82}Rb a notable exception.
- PET perfusion agents are divided into extractable agents (^{13}N-ammonia and ^{82}Rb) and diffusible agents (^{15}O-water).
- ^{82}Rb provides high-quality myocardial perfusion images and has become more widely used since the isotope can be produced by a small, on-site, fully shielded, portable generator and infusion system.
- Myocytes use fatty acids as their main energy source. However, in ischemia, the heart quickly switches to glucose metabolism. PET tracers can be used to image these metabolic processes.
- ^{18}F-FDG, a cyclotron-produced tracer with a relatively long half-life, identifies viable tissues by identifying intact glucose metabolism within myocytes.
- CT and nuclear medicine individually account for a substantial proportion of medical radiation exposure in the population.
- Radiation exposure in PET/CT is related to exposure from both scans. Careful attention to each technique as well as technologic advances such as prospective acquisition in cardiac CT can minimize exposure.
- A significant proportion of PET/CT exposure comes from the CT portion of the examination. Hence, emphasis on prospective CTA allows a significant dose reduction.

SUGGESTED READINGS

Beller GA, Bergmann SR. Myocardial perfusion imaging agents: SPECT and PET. J Nucl Cardiol 2004; 11:71-86.
Bergmann SR. Imaging of myocardial fatty acid metabolism with PET. J Nucl Cardiol 2007; 14:S118-S124.
Brix G, Beyer T. PET/CT: dose-escalated image fusion? Nuklearmedizin 2005; 44(Suppl 1):S51-S57.
Di Carli MF. Advances in positron emission tomography. J Nucl Cardiol 2004; 11:719-732.
Einstein AJ, Moser KW, Thompson RC, et al. Radiation dose to patients from cardiac diagnostic imaging. Circulation 2007; 116:1290-1305.
Hall EJ, Brenner DJ. Cancer risks from diagnostic radiology. Br J Radiol 2008; 81:362-378.
Machac J. Cardiac positron emission tomography imaging. Semin Nucl Med 2005; 35:17-36.
Townsend DW. Combined positron emission tomography–computed tomography: the historical perspective. Semin Ultrasound CT MR 2008; 29:232-235.
Townsend DW. Positron emission tomography/computed tomography. Semin Nucl Med 2008; 38:152-166.

REFERENCES

1. Schelbert HR, Phelps ME, Huang SC, et al. N-13 ammonia as an indicator of myocardial blood flow. Circulation 1981; 63:1259-1272.
2. Shah A, Schelbert HR, Schwaiger M, et al. Measurement of regional myocardial blood flow with N-13 ammonia and positron-emission tomography in intact dogs. J Am Coll Cardiol 1985; 5:92-100.
3. Wahl RL, Buchanan JW. Principles and Practice of Positron Emission Tomography. Philadelphia, Lippincott Williams & Wilkins, 2002.
4. Bergmann SR, Herrero P, Markham J, et al. Noninvasive quantitation of myocardial blood flow in human subjects with oxygen-15–labeled water and positron emission tomography. J Am Coll Cardiol 1989; 14:639-652.
5. Beller GA, Bergmann SR. Myocardial perfusion imaging agents: SPECT and PET. J Nucl Cardiol 2004; 11:71-86.
6. Goldstein RA, Mullani NA, Marani SK, et al. Myocardial perfusion with rubidium-82. II. Effects of metabolic and pharmacologic interventions. J Nucl Med 1983; 24:907-915.

7. Becker L, Ferreira R, Thomas M. Comparison of Rb-86 and microsphere estimates of left ventricular blood flow distribution. J Nucl Med 1977; 15:969-973.
8. Gould KL, Goldstein RA, Mullani NA, et al. Noninvasive assessment of coronary stenoses by myocardial perfusion imaging during pharmacologic coronary vasodilation. VIII. Clinical feasibility of positron cardiac imaging without a cyclotron using generator-produced rubidium-82. J Am Coll Cardiol 1986; 7:775-789.
9. Demer LL, Gould KL, Goldstein RA, et al. Assessment of coronary artery disease severity by positron emission tomography. Comparison with quantitative arteriography in 193 patients. Circulation 1989; 79:825-835.
10. Go RT, Marwick TH, MacIntyre WJ, et al. A prospective comparison of rubidium-82 PET and thallium-201 SPECT myocardial perfusion imaging utilizing a single dipyridamole stress in the diagnosis of coronary artery disease. J Nucl Med 1990; 31:1899-1905.
11. Schelbert HR, Wisenberg G, Phelps ME, et al. Noninvasive assessment of coronary stenoses by myocardial imaging during pharmacologic coronary vasodilation. VI. Detection of coronary artery disease in human beings with intravenous N-13 ammonia and positron computed tomography. Am J Cardiol 1982; 49:1197-1207.
12. Yonekura Y, Tamaki N, Senda M, et al. Detection of coronary artery disease with ^{13}N-ammonia and high-resolution positron-emission computed tomography. Am Heart J 1987; 113:645-654.
13. Williams BR, Jansen DE, Wong LF, et al. Positron emission tomography for the diagnosis of coronary artery disease: a non-university experience and correlation with coronary angiography. J Nucl Med 1989; 30:845.
14. Stewart RE, Schwaiger M, Molina E, et al. Comparison of rubidium-82 positron emission tomography and thallium-201 SPECT imaging for detection of coronary artery disease. Am J Cardiol 1991; 67:1303-1310.
15. Tamaki N, Yonekura Y, Senda M, et al. Value and limitation of stress thallium-201 single photon emission computed tomography: comparison with nitrogen-13 ammonia positron tomography. J Nucl Med 1988; 29:1181-1188.
16. Allard M, Fouquet E, James D, Szlosek-Pinaud M. State of art in ^{11}C labelled radiotracers synthesis. Curr Med Chem 2008; 15:235-277.
17. Walsh MN, Geltman EM, Brown MA, et al. Noninvasive estimation of regional myocardial oxygen consumption by positron emission tomography with carbon-11 acetate in patients with myocardial infarction. J Nucl Med 1989; 30:1798-1808.
18. Tamaki N, Kawamoto M, Takahashi N, et al. Assessment of myocardial fatty acid metabolism with positron emission tomography at rest and during dobutamine infusion in patients with coronary artery disease. Am Heart J 1993; 125:702-710.
19. Kates AM, Herrero P, Dence C, et al. Impact of aging on substrate metabolism by the human heart. J Am Coll Cardiol 2003; 41:293-299.
20. Davila-Roman VG, Vedala G, Herrero P, et al. Altered myocardial fatty acid and glucose metabolism in idiopathic dilated cardiomyopathy. J Am Coll Cardiol 2002; 40:271-277.
21. Pietila M, Malminiemi K, Ukkonen H, et al. Reduced myocardial carbon-11 hydroxyephedrine retention is associated with poor prognosis in chronic heart failure. Eur J Nucl Med 2001; 28:373-376.
22. Pierce DA, Shimizu Y, Preston DL, et al. Studies of the mortality of atomic bomb survivors. Report 12, Part I. Cancer: 1950-1990. Radiat Res 1996; 146:1-27.
23. Cologne JB, Preston DL. Longevity of atomic-bomb survivors. Lancet 2000; 356:303-307.
24. Einstein AJ, Henzlova MJ, Rajagopalan S. Estimating risk of cancer associated with radiation exposure from 64-slice computed tomography coronary angiography. JAMA 2007; 298:317-323.
25. Mettler FAJ, Thomadsen BR, Bhargavan M, et al. Medical radiation exposure in the U.S. in 2006: preliminary results. Health Phys 2008; 95:502-507.
26. Wu TH, Huang YH, Lee JJ, et al. Radiation exposure during transmission measurements: comparison between CT- and germanium-based techniques with a current PET scanner. Eur J Nucl Med Mol Imaging 2004; 31:38-43.
27. Einstein AJ, Moser KW, Thompson RC, et al. Radiation dose to patients from cardiac diagnostic imaging. Circulation 2007; 116:1290-1305.
28. Abada HT, Larchez C, Daoud B, et al. MDCT of the coronary arteries: feasibility of low-dose CT with ECG-pulsed tube current modulation to reduce radiation dose. AJR Am J Roentgenol 2006; 186:S387-S390.
29. Chiesa C, De Sanctis V, Crippa F, et al. Radiation dose to technicians per nuclear medicine procedure: comparison between technetium-99m, gallium-67, and iodine-131 radiotracers and fluorine-18 fluorodeoxyglucose. Eur J Nucl Med 1997; 24:1380-1389.
30. Brix G, Lechel U, Glatting G, et al. Radiation exposure of patients undergoing whole-body dual-modality ^{18}F-FDG PET/CT examinations. J Nucl Med 2005, 46:608-613.

CHAPTER 26

Pharmacologic Stress Agents

Alexander Bustamante and Gautam Nayak*

As imaging modalities for the detection of heart disease continue to evolve and the elderly patient population expands, alternatives to traditional exercise stress testing are becoming more important in clinical practice. Increasingly, patients with conditions precluding exercise treadmill testing are being referred for diagnostic evaluations for possible coronary artery disease using pharmacologic stress tests. Exercise stress imaging provides significant diagnostic and prognostic information and is ideal for otherwise able patients. Not all patients can tolerate the rigorous activity inherent in an exercise treadmill test, however. In these patients, including patients with degenerative joint disease, pulmonary conditions, peripheral vascular disease, congestive heart failure, and other systemic processes that prevent the attainment of adequate exercise stress levels, pharmacologic agents have become pivotal.

Two major categories of pharmacologic agents are most frequently used: vasodilators and inotropes. Although both types of agents can be used in either stress perfusion imaging or stress echocardiography, vasodilators have found their niche in nuclear perfusion studies, and inotropes have become more common in stress echocardiography. More recently, vasodilators and inotropes have been used for stress MRI, and vasodilators have been used for stress CT perfusion. This chapter explores both types of pharmacologic stress agents from their physiologic basis to their diagnostic and prognostic value. The clinical implications of each modality and their inherent advantages and disadvantages are specifically emphasized.

---

*The views expressed in this chapter are those of the author and do not necessarily reflect the official policy or position of the Department of the Navy, Army, Department of Defense, or the U.S. government.

We certify that all individuals who qualify as authors have been listed; each has participated in the conception and design of this work, the analysis of data (when applicable), the writing of the document, and the approval of the submission of this version; that the document represents valid work; that if we used information derived from another source, we obtained all necessary approvals to use it and made appropriate acknowledgments in the document; and that each takes public responsibility for it.

VASODILATOR AGENTS

Vasodilators are primarily used in single photon emission computed tomography (SPECT) myocardial perfusion imaging with radiotracers such as thallium 201 and Tc 99m. As positron emission tomography (PET) and MRI perfusion studies become more ubiquitous, these agents are expected to have an expanding role. The two agents most extensively studied and in current clinical use are adenosine and dipyridamole. The use of these vasodilators was spurred by insight into the pathophysiology of coronary blood flow (CBF). Their utility continues to grow based on a wealth of clinical evidence and expanding indications and imaging modalities.

Coronary Blood Flow

As heart muscle contracts during systole, the myocardium impedes its own blood supply because most CBF occurs during diastole. This pulsatile flow is conducted through a highly curved, branching vascular system composed of larger epicardial vessels and smaller intramural vessels. While epicardial coronary arteries serve as conductance vessels, intramural arteries distribute and regulate blood flow. This adaptation, termed *autoregulation,* occurs rapidly in response to changes in myocardial oxygen demands, primarily through functional hyperemia.[1] This ability of the coronary tree to alter its resistance and increase CBF in response to myocardial metabolic demands is maintained by a balance between vasoconstrictors, such as endothelin, and vasodilators, such as nitric oxide. Acting in smaller arteries and arterioles, these vasoactive factors are integral in allowing rapid, sustained adaptation of CBF based on the requirements of the myocardium.

Coronary Flow Reserve

As atherosclerosis develops in epicardial coronary arteries, the resulting stenosis produces resistance to blood flow. The physiologic effect of a coronary stenosis depends on

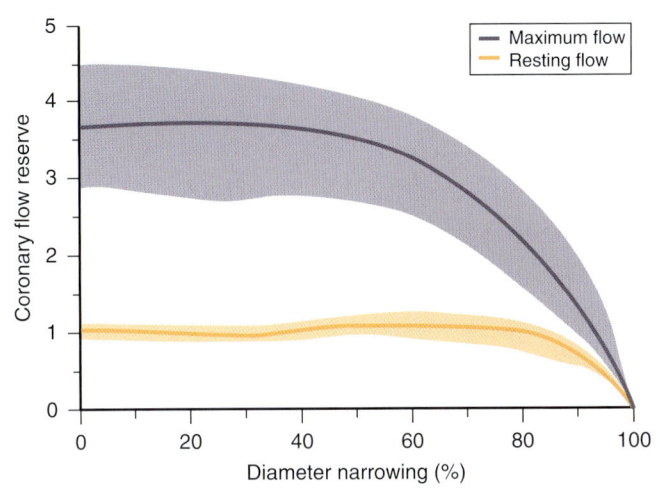

FIGURE 26-1 Coronary flow reserve as a function of coronary artery diameter narrowing. Maximum (i.e., hyperemic) coronary blood flow and normal resting coronary artery flow are depicted. With progressive narrowing, resting flow is not affected until 80% to 90% stenosis, whereas hyperemic flow is impaired at 50% narrowing. *(From Gould KL, Lipscomb K, Hamilton GW. Physiologic basis for assessing critical coronary stenosis: instantaneous flow response and regional distribution during coronary hyperemia as measures of coronary flow reserve. Am J Cardiol 1974; 33:87-94.)*

the degree to which the resistance to flow can be compensated by dilation of the microcirculation distal to the stenosis. This mechanism, regulated by vasoactive factors, maintains resting CBF at a constant level despite the presence of a growing burden of atherosclerosis. When an epicardial coronary constriction exceeds 80% to 90% of the normal segment diameter, the distal vasodilatory mechanisms are unable to compensate, and resting CBF cannot provide adequate oxygen to meet the resting needs of the myocardium.[1,2] When a stenotic vessel is exposed to a vasodilator (e.g., adenosine or dipyridamole) intended to induce hyperemic (or maximal) flow, the relative increase in flow decreases proportionately when a stenosis exceeds 50%, and is generally abolished at a 90% occlusion (Fig. 26-1).

This concept of coronary flow reserve is integral to understanding the physiologic effects of chronic atherosclerosis within the lumen of the coronary tree. The response of coronary arteries to vasodilators depends on the degree of stenosis and the chronic effects of coronary flow reserve at the time of vasodilator administration.

Coronary Blood Flow and Radiotracer Uptake

Vasodilators can increase CBF five times normal levels. This large increase in CBF occurs in myocardium supplied by normal coronary arteries, in contrast to the lack of an increase to myocardium supplied by stenosed arteries as discussed previously; this forms the basis for vasodilator perfusion imaging (Fig. 26-2). If the myocardial uptake of radiotracers such as thallium 201 and Tc 99m were purely linear and based on CBF, a high level of image contrast would theoretically exist between myocardium supplied by normal arteries (i.e., without stenosis) and arteries with hemodynamically significant stenoses. In reality, the extraction fraction of most tracers decreases when CBF increases beyond 2.5 times baseline values. The practical effect of this "roll-off" in the uptake-flow relationship is a physiologic constraint in detecting mild-to-moderate stenoses. The flow increase in response to vasodilators in vessels with a mild-to-moderate stenosis may still be two to three times normal because of coronary flow reserve. This prevents differentiation with a normal coronary artery owing to radiotracer roll-off at a fixed level of hyperemic flow because the normal and mildly stenotic arteries would have identical tracer uptake. Generally with the more common radiotracers, it is difficult to identify noninvasively stenoses that are less than 50% because of the preservation of CBF in the resting and hyperemic states through natural vascular response mechanisms.

Adenosine

Adenosine is a small heterocyclic compound that is endogenously produced in variable amounts as part of a normal cellular metabolism and during ischemia. Through adenosine receptors, it serves as a potent coronary vasodilator (adenosine A_2 receptors) and inhibitor of the sinoatrial and atrioventricular (AV) nodes (adenosine A_1 receptors).[3] Adenosine is produced intracellularly, but interacts on the adenosine receptors on the outer cell membrane (Fig. 26-3). Theophylline and caffeine act at these receptors as competitive blockers, reducing the effects of adenosine.

Clinically, adenosine is infused intravenously and has a very short half-life of less than 2 seconds. As a result, the time-to-peak effect occurs in the first minute of infusion. Adenosine is given typically as a continuous infusion of 140 µg/kg/min for 4 to 6 minutes, with radiotracer injection halfway into the infusion. To avoid an unintended rapid bolus of residual adenosine, radionuclide dose injection and flushing and adenosine infusion should be done through separate intravenous lines or through the use of a dual port.[3] Hemodynamically, adenosine causes a modest decrease in systolic blood pressure and increase in heart rate, in total leading to an increase in cardiac output and mild increase in pulmonary capillary wedge pressure.

Side effects are common with adenosine infusion, occurring in more than 75% of patients (Table 26-1). These side effects are transient, usually resolving within 1 to 2 minutes of stopping the infusion, and rarely require reversal with aminophylline. Most side effects are related to stimulation of the adenosine A_1 and A_3 receptors. Chest pain is common, although it is not specific for the presence of coronary artery disease, occurring in patients with no coronary artery disease at the same frequency as in patients with documented coronary artery disease. Although stimulation of the adenosine A_3 receptors can theoretically lead to bronchospasm, most dyspnea occurring with adenosine infusion is likely related to hyperventilation. Caution should be used in patients with a history of asthma, severe chronic obstructive pulmonary disease (COPD), or active wheezing because of the potential for bronchospasm. Changes in AV conduction usually result in transient first-degree or second-degree AV block. Most bradyarrhythmias are transient and resolve despite continued adenosine infusion.

Dipyridamole

Dipyridamole is a pyrimidine base that induces vasodilation by elevating blood and interstitial levels of adenosine.

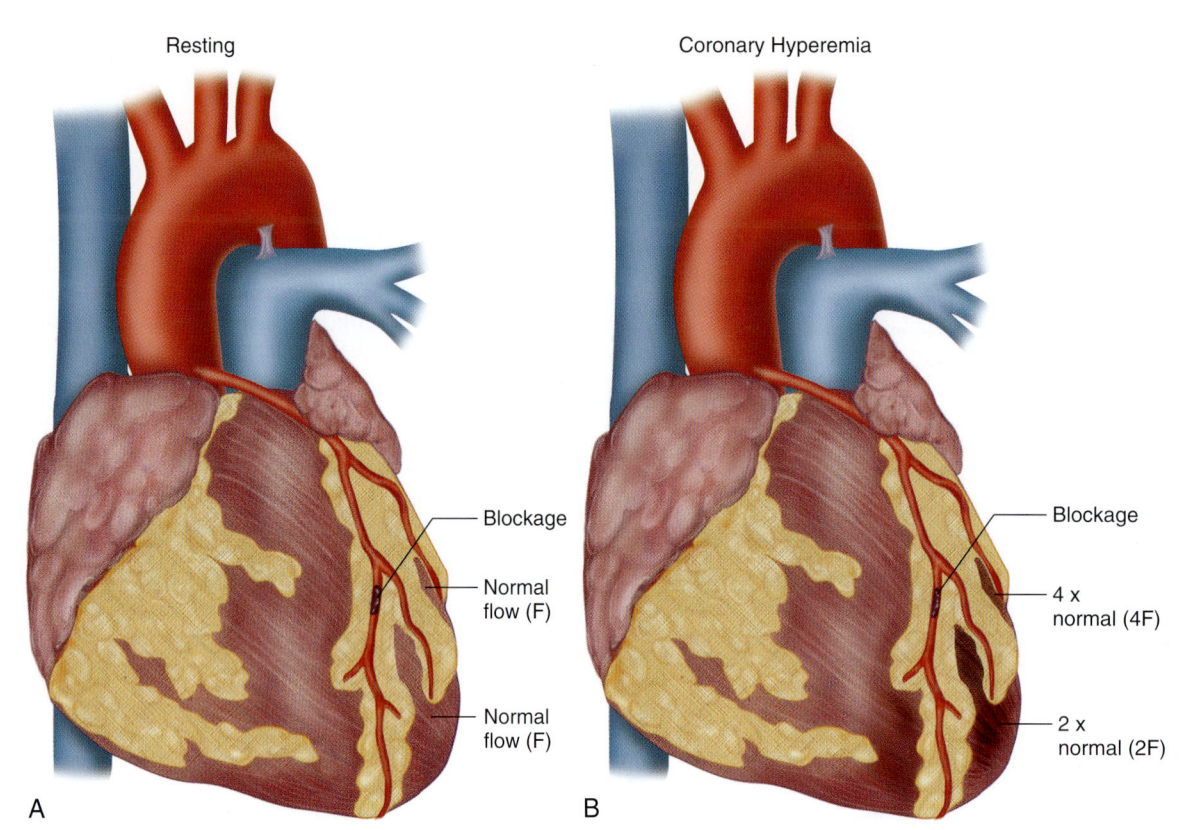

FIGURE 26-2 Comparison of coronary flow at rest versus hyperemia. **A,** Myocardial flow proximal and distal to a stenosis are equal at rest. **B,** Myocardial flow with hyperemia increases four times above resting flow in the arteries with no coronary artery disease. In the territory supplied by the stenotic artery, hyperemic flow increases only twofold. As a result, radiotracer uptake is relatively decreased in the territory supplied by the stenotic vessel, resulting in a perfusion defect. *(Adapted from Iskandrian AE, Verani MS. Nuclear Cardiac Imaging: Principles and Applications. New York, Oxford University Press, 2003.)*

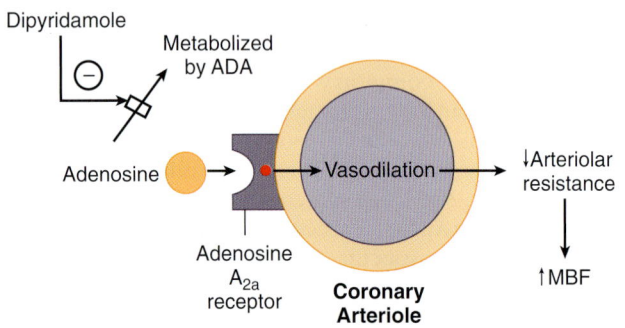

FIGURE 26-3 Schematic of the mechanism of action of dipyridamole and adenosine. Exogenously administered adenosine acts directly on its receptor to result in coronary arteriolar vasodilation, and an increase in myocardial blood flow (MBF) as resistance is minimized. The adenosine A_{2a} receptor mediates coronary arteriolar vasodilation, which is the basis for pharmacologic stress testing. Dipyridamole blocks the intracellular retransport of adenosine and inhibits adenosine deaminase (ADA), resulting in increased intracellular and interstitial concentrations of adenosine, which then interacts with its receptor. *(Adapted from Follansbee WP. Alternatives to leg exercise in the evaluation of patients with coronary artery disease: functional and pharmacological stress modalities. In Gerson MC [ed]. Cardiac Nuclear Medicine. New York, McGraw-Hill, 1997.)*

TABLE 26-1 Side Effects of Pharmacologic Stress Agents

Signs/Symptoms (%)	Adenosine	Dipyridamole	Dobutamine
Chest pain	35	20	39
Flushing	37	3	<1
Dyspnea	35	3	6
Dizziness	9	3	4
Gastrointestinal discomfort	15	1	1
Headache	14	12	7
Arrhythmia	3	5	45
Atrioventricular block	8	0	0
ST segment changes	6	8	20-31
Any adverse effect	81	50	50-75
Major Event			
Death	0	2	0
Myocardial infarction	1	2	0
Bronchospasm	12	6	0

Adapted from Zaret BL, Beller GA. Clinical Nuclear Cardiology: State of the Art and Future Directions, 3rd ed. Philadelphia, Mosby, 2005.

By blocking reuptake of adenosine into cells, dipyridamole increases extracellular levels of adenosine, allowing interaction with adenosine A₂ receptors on the outer cell membrane. Activation of the adenosine A₂ receptor leads to a complex series of events mediated by G proteins and leading to a decrease in intracellular calcium uptake, culminating in coronary vasodilation (see Fig. 26-3). Dipyridamole also exhibits antiplatelet activity, likely related to phosphodiesterase inhibition, increased adenosine triphosphate (ATP) levels, potentiation of aspirin effects, and increased adenosine.[3]

Clinically, dipyridamole is infused intravenously and has a biologic half-life of 88 to 136 minutes. It is given as a continuous infusion of 0.57 mg/kg over 4 minutes, with radiotracer injection 3 to 4 minutes *after* the dipyridamole infusion is completed. This is distinct from adenosine, where tracer injection is during vasodilator infusion (Fig. 26-4). The standard intravenous dose of dipyridamole results in a slight increase in heart rate, a decrease in systolic blood pressure, a modest increase in cardiac output, and a slight increase in pulmonary capillary wedge pressure.

Side effects occur in about 50% of patients and include chest pain, nausea, dizziness, and headache (see Table 26-1). As with adenosine, chest pain is mostly nonanginal and does not correlate with the presence of coronary artery disease. Bronchospasm is rare, but can be precipitated in patients with asthma or severe COPD. Arrhythmias, including AV block, are highly uncommon. Dipyridamole has generally been extensively studied and has an excellent safety record. Most significant side effects can be reversed with slow intravenous administration of theophylline (100 to 300 mg), which is a competitive blocker of adenosine receptors.

INOTROPIC AGENTS

Mechanism of Action

Synthetic inotropic agents act similarly to endogenous catecholamines, such as epinephrine and norepinephrine. Normal exercise results in the release of norepinephrine from sympathetic nerve endings that are abundant on the cardiac ventricles, atria, and conduction system. Norepinephrine stimulates β₁ receptors located on the cardiac cell membrane resulting in a complex protein signaling cascade that results in the enhancement of calcium entry into the cell. Calcium potentiates the action between actin and myosin increasing myofibril contraction (Fig. 26-5). The cardiac conduction system also contains β₁ receptors allowing for increased AV conduction and increases in

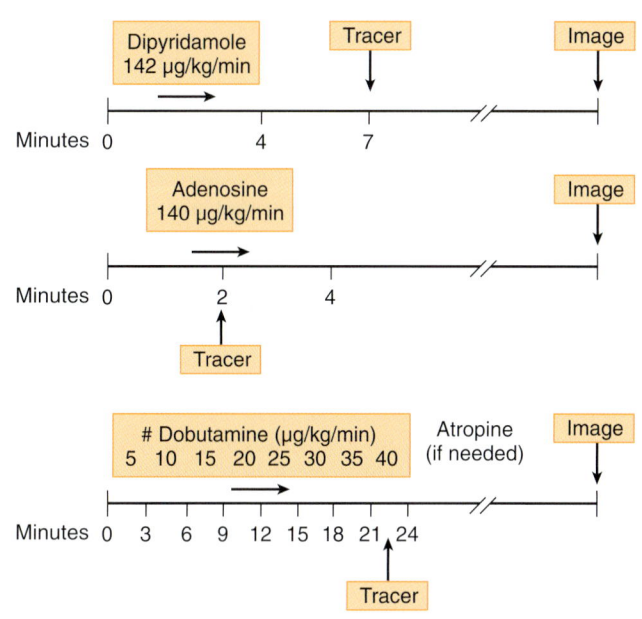

■ **FIGURE 26-4** Pharmacologic stress protocols based on nuclear perfusion imaging. Dobutamine is incrementally increased to a maximum dose of 40 μg/kg/min. If target heart rate has not been reached, the addition of 0.5 to 1 mg of atropine is typically needed. Echocardiographic images are typically obtained at the beginning of the dobutamine infusion, and at prespecified intervals to include peak heart rate and recovery phases. Tracer can be injected for perfusion imaging after target heart rate is reached. (Adapted from Zaret BL, Beller GA. *Clinical Nuclear Cardiology: State of the Art and Future Directions*, 3rd ed. Philadelphia, Mosby, 2005.)

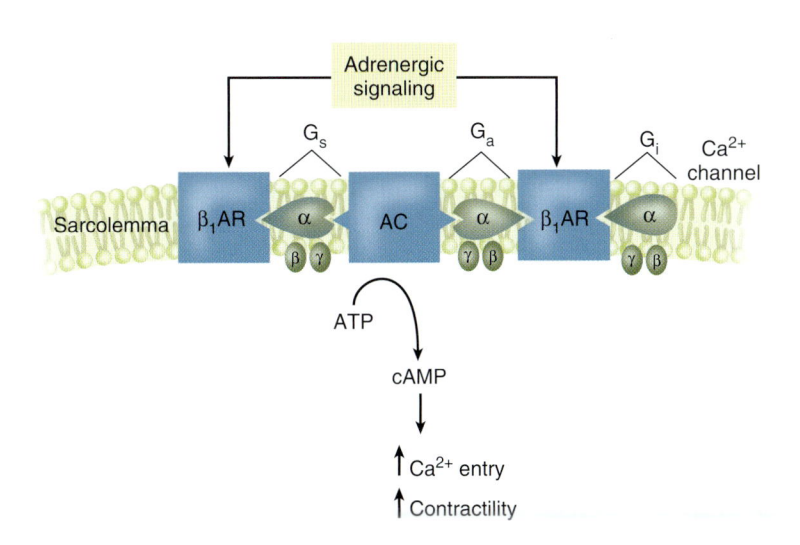

■ **FIGURE 26-5** Schematic representation of selected components of the cardiac myocyte β₁-adrenergic and β₂-adrenergic receptor pathways. The β₁-adrenergic receptor is illustrated with direct coupling through G_s to voltage-sensitive Ca²⁺ channels. (Modified from Bristow MR, Linas S, Port JD. Drugs in the treatment of heart failure. In Zipes DP, Lippy P, Bonow RO, et al [eds]. *Braunwald's Heart Disease*, 7th ed. Philadelphia, Saunders, 2005.)

heart rate. The actions of specific inotropes depend on the balance of β and α activity, which predominantly mediates peripheral vasoconstriction. Other catecholamines stimulate $β_2$ receptors located in vascular smooth muscle and result in vasodilation.[4]

Dobutamine

Dobutamine is a synthetic catecholamine with potent inotropic activity mediated by $β_1$ receptor stimulation. At low doses (2.5 to 10 μg/kg/min), dobutamine can be used therapeutically to increase cardiac output and decrease left ventricular filling pressures with only a modest increase in heart rate. As a result, this agent has been used extensively in patients with decompensated heart failure without profound hypotension. The additional $β_2$ properties may result in aggravating preexisting hypotension, and may require the need for concomitant $α_1$ stimulating vasoconstrictors to improve peripheral arterial resistance. At higher doses of dobutamine, heart rate is incrementally increased via $α_1$ stimulation. The combination of inotropic and chronotropic effects results in an increase in myocardial oxygen demand with secondary coronary vasodilation making for an effective stress agent.

Dobutamine has a short half-life and is given typically as a continuous infusion at a starting dose of 5 μg/kg/min, increasing by 5 to 10 μg/kg/min doses up to 40 μg/kg/min at 3-minute intervals. The patient is instructed to discontinue β blockers before the imaging study at a minimum of 24 to 48 hours to mitigate its negative inotropic and chronotropic effects. Atropine at 0.5- to 1-mg doses can be added in patients who are not reaching target heart rate with higher doses of dobutamine (see Fig. 26-4). Continuous heart rate monitoring and periodic ECG and blood pressure recordings are required. Criteria for termination of the infusion include severe hypotension or hypertension, malignant arrhythmia, severe chest pain, ST segment elevation greater than 1 mm or ST segment depression 2 mm or greater, or intractable noncardiac symptoms.

Coronary hyperemia induced by higher doses of dobutamine depends on increasing myocardial oxygen demand in response to increases in cardiac contractility and heart rate. This effect is less than that of vasodilators such as adenosine, and the latter agent is preferred if nuclear myocardial perfusion imaging is the modality of choice unless contraindicated. Near-equivalent coronary vasodilation can be achieved with the combination of dobutamine and atropine as with dipyridamole in younger patients.[5]

Despite the advantages of vasodilators over inotropic agents such as dobutamine, there are clinical situations in which they are contraindicated. Patients with active reversible airway disease, such as asthma, and some patients with COPD may experience an exacerbation of their symptoms with vasodilators. Dobutamine infusion is a safe alternative in these patients without the risk of airway compromise.

Side effects with dobutamine are varied, but usually well tolerated (see Table 26-1). Chest pain, palpitations, and nausea are common during prolonged infusions. Ventricular and supraventricular arrhythmias can be seen, but they often resolve on cessation of the infusion or treatment with low-dose intravenous β blockers. Hypotension can occur in some patients, but because of the short half-life of dobutamine, this generally resolves on discontinuation of the infusion.[3]

UTILITY IN CORONARY ARTERY DISEASE

Commonly used imaging modalities for detection of myocardial ischemia include myocardial perfusion studies and stress echocardiography. As discussed earlier, vasodilators are used primarily in nuclear perfusion studies, whereas dobutamine plays an integral part in detecting physiologically significant coronary artery disease in both. With myocardial perfusion imaging, flow heterogeneity develops when myocardial oxygen demand is increased in the setting of a fixed coronary stenosis with normal coronary vessels compensating by dilating and essentially "stealing" flow from the diseased vessel (see Fig. 26-2); this results in decreased nuclear tracer uptake in the territory of the obstructed vessel relative to the distribution of the disease-free vessels, manifesting as a perfusion defect. With stress echocardiography, ischemia develops in a territory supplied by a coronary vessel with a high-grade stenosis when demand outstrips the ability of the coronary vessel to dilate and is typically reflected in regional wall motion abnormalities. In the ischemia cascade, perfusion abnormalities precede that of wall motion dysfunction, making myocardial perfusion imaging typically more sensitive than stress echocardiography for detection of ischemic heart disease. Stress echocardiography has a relatively higher specificity, however.

Diagnosis and Prognosis in Coronary Artery Disease

The primary utility of pharmacologic stress agents is in the diagnosis of coronary artery disease. In patients with and without known coronary artery disease, pharmacologic myocardial perfusion studies help to localize ischemia and quantify the burden of disease. The prognostic information gained is additive to clinical and historical data. After a normal myocardial perfusion examination, most clinical trials looking at risk have reported cardiac event rates of less than 1%[6]; this is generally independent of imaging type, radiopharmaceutical, or patient clinical characteristics. In patients undergoing pharmacologic stress, reported cardiac event rates are higher, ranging from 1.3% to 2.7% per year.[6] This higher rate is probably secondary to the generally higher clinical risk in patients referred for pharmacologic stress testing (vs. exercise stress), who typically have an inherently higher cardiac event risk rate secondary to their underlying debilitating disease, such as peripheral occlusive arterial disease or diabetes. Numerous studies have confirmed that simply having vasodilator stress testing is associated with the same long-term cardiac event risk as having known coronary artery disease.

In patients with abnormal pharmacologic stress perfusion studies, there is a close relationship between the extent and severity of the perfusion abnormalities and the risk of adverse outcomes. The risk of major cardiac events progressively increases as a function of the myocardial

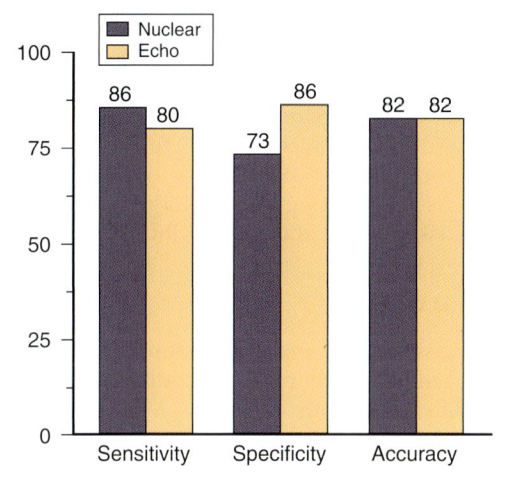

■ **FIGURE 26-6** Comparison of accuracy of dobutamine stress myocardial perfusion imaging and simultaneous echocardiography for diagnosis of coronary artery disease. Results represent pooled data from 12 studies in 593 patients. *(Adapted from Elhendy A, Bax JJ, Poldermans D. Dobutamine stress myocardial perfusion imaging in coronary artery disease. J Nucl Med 2002; 43:1634-1646.)*

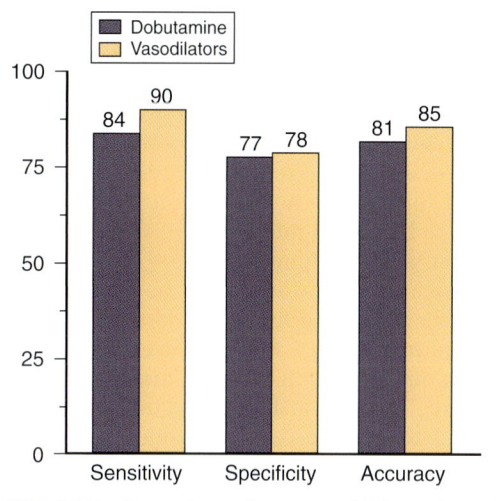

■ **FIGURE 26-7** Comparison of accuracy of dobutamine and vasodilator stress myocardial perfusion imaging for the diagnosis of coronary artery disease. Results represent pooled data from two studies in 157 patients. *(Adapted from Elhendy A, Bax JJ, Poldermans D. Dobutamine stress myocardial perfusion imaging in coronary artery disease. J Nucl Med 2002; 43:1634-1646.)*

perfusion imaging results, with large defects associated with an incrementally higher risk than small defects; this is true for adenosine and dipyridamole stress testing. With dipyridamole, testing with thallium 201 SPECT imaging yields an average sensitivity of 89% and specificity of 75%.[7] For adenosine thallium 201 SPECT myocardial perfusion imaging, the average sensitivity is 88%, and specificity is 85%.[7]

Walking Adenosine Protocols

For patients able to walk, it is advantageous to combine low-level exercise with adenosine myocardial perfusion imaging. In addition to mitigating the side effects of adenosine, there is generally less hepatic uptake of radiotracer and a higher heart/background ratio, which improves overall imaging quality. In limited studies, this improved imaging quality has translated into improved sensitivity and additional prognostic implications, with an inability to walk associated with greater adverse risk.[8]

DOBUTAMINE: SPECT IMAGING VERSUS ECHOCARDIOGRAPHY

Dobutamine stress myocardial perfusion imaging generally has a higher sensitivity and lower specificity for detecting significant coronary artery disease compared with dobutamine stress echocardiography (Fig. 26-6). In two clinical trials that directly compared dobutamine stress myocardial perfusion imaging with stress echocardiography, the sensitivities were 86% and 80%, and specificities were 73% and 86%.[9,10] This difference reflects the earlier detection of ischemia with perfusion stress testing based on its earlier occurrence in the myocardial ischemic cascade. The sensitivity of detecting coronary artery disease increases incrementally with the extent of disease involvement. Dobutamine stress myocardial perfusion imaging has a sensitivity of 80%, 92%, and 97% for one-vessel, two-vessel, and three-vessel disease, respectively. Compared with vasodilator stress myocardial perfusion imaging, dobutamine has a slightly lower sensitivity with similar specificity for the diagnosis of coronary artery disease (Fig. 26-7).[10]

Pharmacologic Agents and Medications

For patients on anti-ischemic medications, such as β blockers, calcium channel blockers, and nitrates, the sensitivity of exercise perfusion studies in the diagnosis of coronary artery disease is lower when patients test while taking these medications compared with testing after being removed from these medications (i.e., after a suitable period to ensure "washout" of the medications). This issue is less clear with vasodilator testing, although limited studies have shown a significant decrease in individual vessel sensitivity with no change in specificity in patients on anti-ischemic medications at the time of testing. For dobutamine testing, β blockers may blunt the capacity of the agent to achieve adequate stress heart rates for imaging, although this is usually overcome with atropine and isometric supine exercise. Generally, this blunting caused by β blockers translates into no significant loss of sensitivity or specificity in patients on these medications, although most protocols advise patients to hold β blockers before dobutamine stress imaging.

Post-infarct Myocardial Imaging

In the United States, most patients presenting with myocardial infarction undergo early definitive risk stratification with coronary angiography. There is still a role, however, in low-risk myocardial infarction patients for predischarge noninvasive risk stratification in lieu of an early invasive strategy. Pharmacologic stress imaging has numerous advantages over exercise stress testing. Patients do not need to exercise, which has inherent safety advantages after myocardial infarction, where most guidelines advocate a delay in submaximal stress testing of at least 7 days after an event and waiting 3 to 4 weeks after myocardial infarction for full exercise protocols. Dobutamine and vasodilator use early after a myocardial infarction have the potential for adverse hemodynamic events, but have been shown to be safe in multiple cardiac imaging studies 2 days after an acute ischemic event.[7,11,12]

Because pharmacologic stress can be performed safely 48 hours after a myocardial infarction, it can provide equivalent information to full exercise protocols at an earlier time point. If pharmacologic imaging shows a significant degree of ischemia or infarction in the infarct zone, referral to cardiac catheterization would be indicated. Pharmacologic imaging in the post–myocardial infarction period provides significantly better prognostic information compared with submaximal exercise stress testing because pharmacologic stress imaging identifies the infarct and ischemic territories.

Viability Assessment with Dobutamine

Patients with ischemic heart disease may have large territories of dysfunctional myocardium that may recover function on revascularization. The detection of this myocardial viability is uniquely suited to dobutamine as a stress agent. Examinations using a protocol of low dose followed by higher doses of dobutamine infusion with the aid of echocardiography may unmask areas of viability. These myocardial segments would show a biphasic response to dobutamine. At low doses, the ventricular myocardium would show an improvement in contractility compared with the resting state, but at higher doses, owing to increasing oxygen demand, would show a decrement in function. Many small studies have shown a survival advantage and an improvement in global left ventricular function in patients with viability who underwent surgical revascularization compared with medical therapy alone. Similar to the detection of coronary artery disease, dobutamine stress myocardial perfusion imaging shows a higher sensitivity and lower specificity for the identification of myocardial viability than echocardiography.[13]

EXERCISE VERSUS PHARMACOLOGIC STRESS

Generally, exercise stress imaging provides a wealth of information from a physiologic, functional, and prognostic perspective. Exercise stress imaging is the preferred stress modality in patients who can exercise and achieve an adequate workload. When patients are able to complete only a submaximal (<85% target heart rate) exercise protocol, stress imaging becomes less sensitive and can underestimate the degree and extent of ischemia. It has been estimated that at least 25% of outpatients and 50% of hospitalized patients cannot perform adequate exercise to achieve a maximum workload.[7] Pharmacologic stress imaging has become the optimal modality of testing in these patients for diagnosis of coronary artery disease, quantification of ischemic burden, and important prognostic determination. As with all types of stress testing, patient selection is crucial, and certain underlying conditions may make pharmacologic stress testing better than exercise testing, even in patients with normal functional capacity. In addition, similar to exercise testing, the physiologic, ECG, and imaging parameters obtained during pharmacologic stress testing have unique implications that can often assist in accurate image interpretation.

Patient Selection

Beyond patients who are unable to exercise, pharmacologic stress imaging, whether with vasodilators or inotropic agents, is often the study of choice. A prime example in which vasodilator stress perfusion imaging is most accurate is in the setting of patients with underlying left bundle branch block (LBBB). Myocardial perfusion imaging in patients with LBBB may show reversible anteroseptal defects with exercise or dobutamine stress in the absence of obstructive coronary artery disease. These defects are a result of asynchronous and delayed systolic septal contraction secondary to the conduction system delay in septal depolarization associated with LBBB. Fifty percent of patients with LBBB undergoing exercise SPECT and 84% to 100% of patients with LBBB undergoing dobutamine SPECT show falsely reversible anteroseptal defects.[14] Patients with ventricular paced rhythms show similar false-positive stress perfusion results owing to asynchronous septal depolarization (and a "pseudo"-LBBB), although this is generally less of an issue with exercise testing—unless patients are pacemaker-dependent.[15] The best way to avoid this scenario is to use vasodilator stress with either adenosine or dipyridamole in patients with LBBB or in patients who are pacemaker-dependent.[16]

Another patient characteristic that may influence stress modality is underlying severe reactive airways disease. In patients with active wheezing or a propensity for bronchospasm, it is preferable to avoid adenosine and dipyridamole, both of which have cross-reactivity with the adenosine A_3 receptor, which can induce bronchoconstriction. Multiple studies have shown that vasodilators are generally safe in patients with COPD, unless there is a significant reactive airway component or there is an acute exacerbation of the underlying condition. Prophylactic bronchodilator use before vasodilator infusion is also an option, although limited data are available to support routine use with standard protocols. Table 26-2 reviews many of these conditions, most of which have been described in this chapter.

Electrocardiographic Changes

Monitoring of the ECG during exercise or pharmacologic stress imaging is crucial to accurate test assessment, and often provides important additional information to help with image interpretation. During exercise, ST segment depression has been associated with higher clinical risk. With pharmacologic stressors, ST segment changes have also been correlated with future adverse outcomes. With vasodilator stress perfusion imaging, ST segment depression is infrequent because of minimal change in heart rate and blood pressure. When it occurs, ST segment

TABLE 26-2 Selection of Stress Test

Condition	Test of Choice
If patient can achieve an adequate level of exercise	Use exercise
If patient has exercise limitations	Use adenosine, dipyridamole, or dobutamine
If patient has bronchospasm	Use dobutamine
If patient has LBBB/pacemaker	Use adenosine, dipyridamole, or dobutamine
If patient is <72 hr after acute MI	Use adenosine or dipyridamole
If patient is <24 hr after PCI	Use adenosine or dipyridamole

LBBB, left bundle branch block; MI, myocardial infarction; PCI, percutaneous coronary intervention.
Adapted from Zaret BL, Beller GA. Clinical Nuclear Cardiology: State of the Art and Future Directions, 3rd ed. Philadelphia, Mosby, 2005.

depression during vasodilator infusion has been shown to be a significant predictor of adverse outcomes and is independent of and incremental to the subsequent perfusion data.[17,18] There has been a significant association with severe, multivessel coronary artery disease and higher cardiac event rates in patients with vasodilator-induced ST segment depression even in the setting of normal SPECT images.

With dobutamine, ST segment changes have also been shown to be additive to imaging information, although to a lesser extent. Patients undergoing dobutamine stress imaging show improved positive predictive value for significant coronary artery disease with a positive stress ECG in addition to the stress images.[19] Generally, ECG abnormalities with vasodilator or inotropic stress are additive to the stress images obtained. They often provide information independent of SPECT or echocardiographic data to assist in better risk stratification.[20,21]

Other Perfusion Imaging Indices

The ability to incorporate ECG data and SPECT images is pivotal in the interpretation of myocardial perfusion studies. Beyond stress/rest mismatch, nuclear stress imaging uses other indices to delineate higher risk studies. Transient ischemic dilation (TID) occurs as a result of subendocardial ischemia during stress, resulting in the appearance of cavity dilation in the stress images compared with rest. TID is a very specific indicator of high cardiac risk, often occurring in the setting of severe, multivessel coronary artery disease. Multiple studies have shown the same diagnostic and prognostic implications of TID with exercise compared with pharmacologic stress, although the threshold ratio of stress to rest cavity size is larger with vasodilators and inotropes.[3]

Similarly, increased lung uptake of thallium in SPECT studies is also an indicator of elevated pulmonary capillary wedge pressure (or left atrial pressure), delineating a higher risk of subsequent cardiac events and severe coronary artery disease. As with TID, the diagnostic and prognostic information gained from increased lung uptake of thallium is similar when using exercise or pharmacologic stress.[3] With myocardial perfusion imaging, TID and increased thallium lung uptake with pharmacologic stress provide incremental diagnostic and prognostic indices comparable to exercise studies.

CONCLUSION

Pharmacologic stress testing with SPECT myocardial perfusion imaging and echocardiography has become a key modality in the evaluation of coronary artery disease. As imaging expands into newer modalities such as contrast echocardiography, PET, and MRI, these agents will have expanding roles. Vasodilators such as adenosine and dipyridamole are primarily used in SPECT nuclear perfusion imaging, whereas dobutamine is mainly used in stress echocardiography with additional use in SPECT imaging. The safety record and side-effect profile of all pharmacologic agents are highly favorable for inpatient and outpatient care in a broad range of patients and disease states.

The sensitivity and specificity of adenosine, dipyridamole, and dobutamine rival that of exercise stress imaging. Under certain clinical conditions, these agents are superior in improving test accuracy and minimizing false-positive results. The diagnostic and prognostic information achieved through pharmacologic stress imaging is excellent and incremental to the other clinical parameters measured during the course of stress testing. The cardiovascular evaluation of patients unable to exercise because of underlying comorbidities, such as degenerative joint disease, vascular disease, lung disease, and other conditions, has been enhanced through pharmacologic stress testing. Pharmacologic stress imaging with vasodilators and inotropes provides key clinical insights into the mechanisms of ischemic heart disease, and is instrumental in the diagnosis and associated prognosis of coronary artery disease.

KEY POINTS

- Pharmacologic stress imaging is an effective method to evaluate coronary artery disease in patients with comorbid conditions that preclude exercise.
- Vasodilators such as adenosine and dipyridamole and inotropes such as dobutamine are safe and tolerated in most clinical conditions.
- In the evaluation of coronary artery disease, pharmacologic stress imaging provides excellent diagnostic and prognostic information, similar to that achieved with exercise.
- As imaging modalities for the detection of heart disease continue to evolve from SPECT and echocardiography to PET and MRI, pharmacologic stress agents will increasingly become vital for accurate evaluation of coronary artery disease.

SUGGESTED READINGS

Hendel RC, Jamil T, Glover DK. Pharmacologic stress testing: new methods and new agents. J Nucl Cardiol 2003; 10:197-204.

Iskandrian AE, Verani MS. Nuclear Cardiac Imaging: Principles and Applications. New York, Oxford University Press, 2003.

Klocke FJ, Baird MG, Lorell BH, et al. ACC/AHA/ASNC guidelines for the clinical use of cardiac radionuclide imaging—executive summary: a report of the American College of Cardiology/American Heart Association Task Force on Practice Guidelines (ACC/AHA/ASNC Committee to Revise the 1995 Guidelines for the Clinical Use of Cardiac Radionuclide Imaging). J Am Coll Cardiol 2003; 42:1318-1333.

Libby P, Bonow RO, Zipes DP, et al (eds). Braunwald's Heart Disease, 8th ed. Philadelphia, Saunders, 2008.

Miyamoto MI, Vernotico SL, Majmundar H, et al. Pharmacologic stress myocardial perfusion imaging: a practical approach. J Nucl Cardiol 2007; 14:250-255.

Orlandi C. Pharmacology of coronary vasodilation: a brief review. J Nucl Cardiol 1996; 3:S27-S30.

Zaret B, Beller G. Clinical Nuclear Cardiology: State of the Art and Future Directions, 3rd ed. Philadelphia, Mosby, 2005.

REFERENCES

1. Lim M, Kern M. Coronary pathophysiology in the cardiac catheterization laboratory. Curr Prob Cardiol 2006; 31:497-504.
2. Zipes DP, Lippy P, Bonow RO, et al (eds). Braunwald's Heart Disease. A Textbook of Cardiovascular Medicine, 7th ed, Vol 2. Philadelphia, Saunders, 2005.
3. Zaret B, Beller G. Clinical Nuclear Cardiology: State of the Art and Future Directions, 3rd ed. Philadelphia, Mosby, 2005.
4. Frishman WH, Sonnenblick EH. Cardiovascular Pharmacotherapeutics. New York, McGraw-Hill, 1997.
5. Tadamura E, Iida H, Matsumoto K, et al. Comparison of myocardial blood flow during dobutamine-atropine infusion with that after dipyridamole administration in normal men. J Am Coll Cardiol 2001; 37:130-136
6. Heller GV, Herman SD, Travin MI, et al. Independent prognostic value of intravenous dipyridamole with technetium-99m sestamibi tomographic imaging in predicting cardiac events and cardiac-related hospital admissions. J Am Coll Cardiol 1995; 26.1202-1208.
7. Klocke FJ, Baird MG, Lorell BH, et al. ACC/AHA/ASNC guidelines for the clinical use of cardiac radionuclide imaging—executive summary: A report of the American College of Cardiology/American Heart Association Task Force on Practice Guidelines (ACC/AHA/ASNC Committee to Revise the 1995 Guidelines for the Clinical Use of Cardiac Radionuclide Imaging). J Am Coll Cardiol 2003; 42:1318-1333.
8. Thomas GS, Prill NV, Majmundar H, et al. Treadmill exercise during adenosine infusion is safe, results in fewer adverse reactions, and improves myocardial perfusion image quality. J Nucl Cardiol 2000; 7:439-446.
9. Calnon DA, McGrath PD, Doss AL, et al. Prognostic value of dobutamine stress technetium-99m sestamibi single-photon emission computed tomography myocardial perfusion imaging: stratification of a high-risk population. J Am Coll Cardiol 2001; 38:1511-1517.
10. Elhendy A, Bax JJ, Poldermans D. Dobutamine stress myocardial perfusion imaging in coronary artery disease. J Nucl Med 2002; 43:1634-1636.
11. Smart SC, Knickelbine T, Stoiber TR, et al. Safety and accuracy of dobutamine-atropine stress echocardiography for the detection of residual stenosis of the infarct-related artery and multivessel disease during the first week after acute myocardial infarction. Circulation 1997; 95:1394-1401.
12. Carlos ME, Smart SC, Wynsen JC, et al. Dobutamine stress echocardiography for risk stratification after myocardial infarction. Circulation 1997; 95:1402-1410.
13. Camici PG, Prasad SK, Rimoldi OE. Stunning, hibernation, and assessment of myocardial viability. Circulation 2008; 117:103-114.
14. O'Keefe JH Jr, Bateman TM, Barnhart CS. Adenosine thallium-201 is superior to exercise thallium-201 for detecting coronary artery disease in patients with left bundle branch block. J Am Coll Cardiol 1993; 21:1332-1338.
15. Tse HF, Yu C, Wong KK, et al. Functional abnormalities in patients with permanent right ventricular pacing: the effect of the sites of electrical stimulation. J Am Coll Cardiol 2002; 40:1451-1458.
16. Skalidis EI, Kochiadakis GE, Koukaraki SI, et al. Myocardial perfusion in patients with permanent ventricular pacing and normal coronary arteries. J Am Coll Cardiol 2001; 37:124-129.
17. Hachamovitch R, Berman DS, Kiat H, et al. Value of stress myocardial perfusion single photon emission computed tomography in patients with normal resting electrocardiograms: an evaluation of incremental prognostic value and cost-effectiveness. Circulation 2002; 105:823-829.
18. Klodas E, Miller TD, Christian TF, et al. Prognostic significance of ischemic electrocardiographic changes during vasodilator stress testing in patients with normal SPECT images. J Nucl Cardiol 2003; 10:4-8.
19. Shaheen LJ, Klutstein MW, Rosenmann D, et al. Diganostic value of 12 lead electrocardiogram during dobutamine echocardiographic studies. Am Heart J 1998; 136:1061-1064.
20. Kim C, Kwok YS, Heagerty P, et al. Pharmacologic stress testing for coronary artery disease diagnosis: a meta-analysis. Am Heart J 2001; 142:934-944.
21. Levine MG, Ahlberg AW, Mann A, et al: Comparison of exercise, dipyridamole, adenosine and dobutamine stress with the use of Tc-99m tetrofosmin tomographic imaging. J Nucl Cardiol 1999; 6:389-396.

PART THREE

Cardiac Interventions

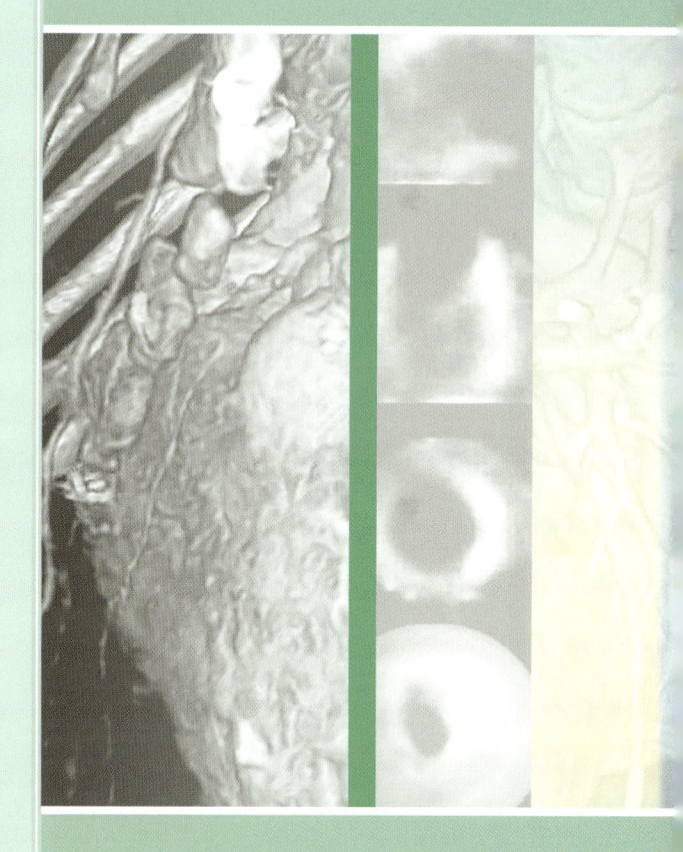

CHAPTER 27

Congenital Percutaneous Interventions

Phillip Moore

Imaging has always played a key diagnostic role in the management of children with congenital heart disease. During the last 20 years, two major developments in the field have transformed the use of imaging in clinical management: (1) with the development of interventional catheter-based treatment strategies, the majority of common congenital heart diseases are now treated in the catheterization laboratory instead of in the operating suite; and (2) because of the successful treatment of children with congenital heart disease, there are now as many adults living with congenital heart disease as there are children. These changes have led to the evolution and use of imaging techniques to guide procedural treatments applicable to infants, children, and adults. This chapter reviews the common percutaneous interventional procedures for the treatment of congenital heart disease and illustrates the key role that imaging plays in their success.

ATRIAL SEPTAL DEFECT

Description and Special Anatomic Considerations

Secundum atrial septal defect (ASD), one of the more common congenital heart defects, represents 6% to 10% of all congenital anomalies, occurring in 1 in 1500 live births.[1] Secundum ASDs are due to absence, perforation, or deficiency of the septum primum. This defect typically occurs sporadically but has been linked to genetic abnormalities such as Holt-Oram syndrome and mutations on chromosome 5p.

Device closure of an ASD was first performed in 1974 by King and Mills[2] with a 24-gauge surgically placed femoral sheath and a double-sided disk device. Technology and technique have been modified and refined over the years; however, the procedure remains conceptually identical. A collapsible double-sided disk device with a metal frame and fabric patches is positioned antegrade through a long femoral sheath (6F to 10F) across the secundum ASD. On extrusion from the sheath, the device expands, creating a patch on both sides of the septum, clamping the rim of tissue surrounding the ASD. The endocardium grows in to cover the device to create a permanent seal. Because of the need for surrounding rim tissue, device closure is limited to secundum-type defects and is not applicable to either primum (no inferior posterior rim) or venosus (no superior rim) ASDs. With recent technologic advances, device closure has rapidly become the treatment of choice for secundum ASDs.

Indications

Device closure is indicated for any size secundum ASD with evidence on echocardiography of right ventricular volume overload. ASD should also be closed in patients with symptoms of exercise intolerance or history of cryptogenic stroke. There is mounting evidence that ASD closure, even in the elderly, can improve maximal oxygen consumption.[3] ASDs have been closed by device in small children, including infants; however, the most common timing for elective closure appears to be between 2 and 4 years of age.

Contraindications

There are no absolute contraindications to device ASD closure except for patients with active thrombus in the left atrium and those with a known allergy to the device implant materials, particularly the nickel in the device frames, although this is an extremely rare condition. Patients who are hypercoagulable, particularly those with disorders that predispose to arterial clots, should be considered very carefully as the post-placement risk of clot formation during the endocardialization process may be significantly increased. Patients with significant left ventricular dysfunction also must be monitored closely after

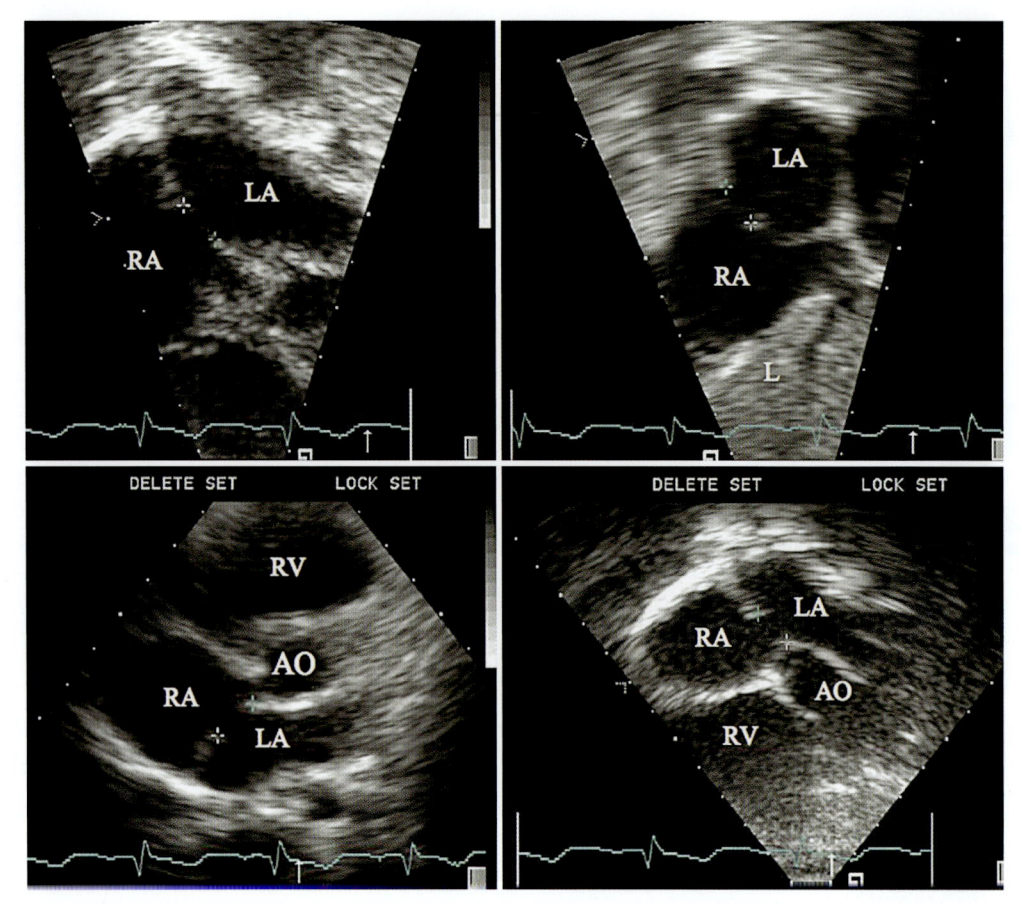

FIGURE 27-1 Transthoracic echocardiograms in various planes evaluating size of ASD and presence of surrounding rim tissue. AO, aortic valve; L, liver; LA, left atrium; RA, right atrium; RV, right ventricle.

the procedure because of the potential for the development of acute left atrial hypertension and resultant pulmonary edema. Diuretics immediately after closure may be helpful in this subgroup of patients. Patients with pulmonary hypertension must be considered carefully but may benefit as long as there is a left-to-right shunt at rest.

Outcomes and Complications

Concurrent controlled trials comparing surgical closure with device closure have shown efficacy rates of more than 96% with significantly lower complication rates and hospital stay.[4] Most patients can be discharged on the day of the procedure, with return to full activity within 48 to 72 hours, significantly reducing costs and medical resources.[5] Early complications have been minor and occur in fewer than 9% of patients; they consist primarily of transient arrhythmias, vascular injury, and asymptomatic device embolization. Serious complications have been rare but include thrombus formation on the device, heart block requiring pacing, and cardiac perforation.[6]

Imaging Findings

Preoperative Planning

When an ASD has been diagnosed, complete transthoracic echocardiography should be performed to evaluate the suitability for device closure. This includes specific attention to the pulmonary vein drainage as well as to the size and location of the defect, including tissue rims to the atrioventricular valves, inferior vena cava, right pulmonary veins, aortic valve, and roof of the atrium. If the transthoracic study is inadequate to delineate these structures, OmniPlane transesophageal echocardiography should be performed. Documentation of an adequate atrial septal rim circumferentially (>3 mm, especially at the posterior inferior inlet portion; Fig. 27-1) and evaluation for additional defects, tissue strands, or septal aneurysms with perforations are essential (Fig. 27-2). Identification of all pulmonary veins, particularly the right upper, is essential because of the association of partial anomalous pulmonary venous return with sinus venosus ASD.

There is current interest in the use of three-dimensional echocardiography as well as MRI for the preprocedure evaluation of ASD. Certainly, these modalities improve detection of an anomalous pulmonary vein and give a more complete understanding of the shape of the defect. This may permit more accurate measurement of the long-axis dimension of the defect, which is helpful for choosing the appropriate type and size of device. Although these modalities give additional information, their clinical advantage in typical ASDs is not proved, and they do add to cost and medical service use. In patients with unusual anatomy, they are invaluable (Fig. 27-3).

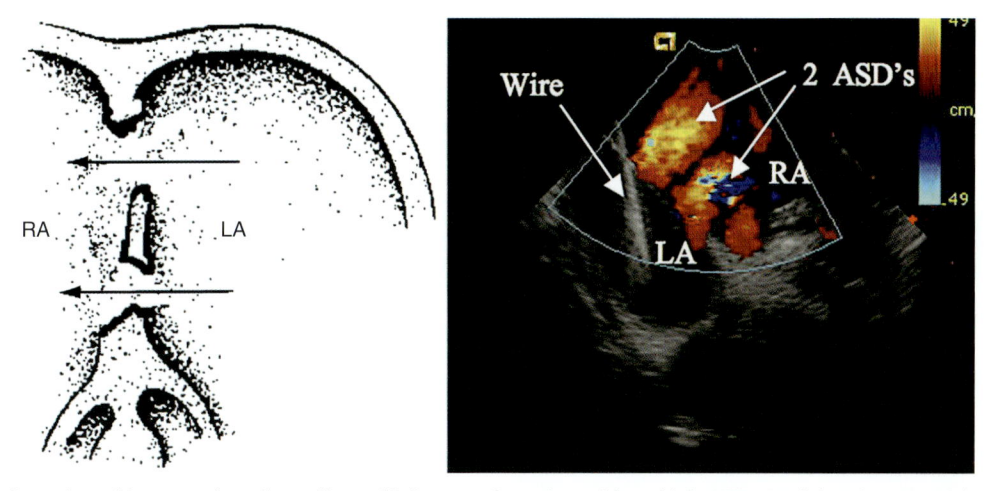

FIGURE 27-2 Schematic and intravascular echocardiographic images of a patient with multiple ASDs. LA, left atrium; RA, right atrium.

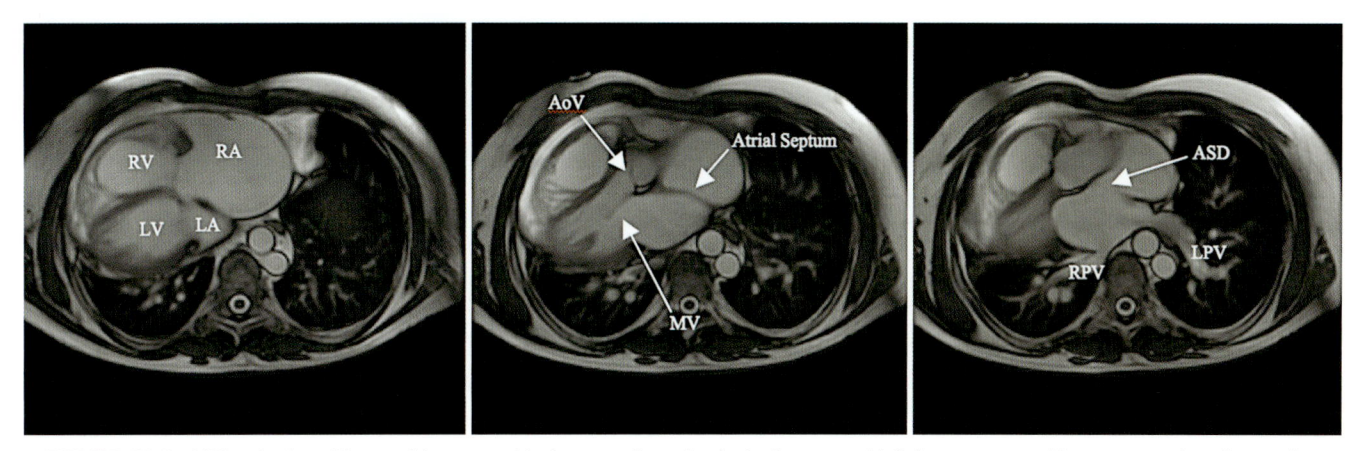

FIGURE 27-3 MRI series in a 50-year-old person with dextrocardia, polysplenia, interrupted inferior vena cava with azygos continuation, and large ASD. AoV, aortic valve; LA, left atrium; LPV, left pulmonary vein; LV, left ventricle; MV, mitral valve; RA, right atrium; RPV, right pulmonary vein; RV, right ventricle.

Procedural imaging for device implantation is a combination of echocardiography and biplane fluoroscopy. In my practice, I use surface echocardiography for implantation in children younger than 6 years (Fig. 27-4) and intracardiac echocardiography for older patients (Fig. 27-5). Transesophageal echocardiography is used in older patients in some institutions; however, it necessitates general anesthesia for the procedure. Balloon sizing of the defect is often done and can be useful to detect multiple defects (Fig. 27-6). There has been experimental animal work with active MRI for device implantation (Fig. 27-7), although there has been no human clinical application to date.

Postoperative Surveillance

The cornerstone of surveillance after implantation remains transthoracic echocardiography. Patients are seen 1, 6, and 12 months after implantation to ensure appropriate device position, to rule out thrombus formation, and to assess right ventricular size and function. In most patients

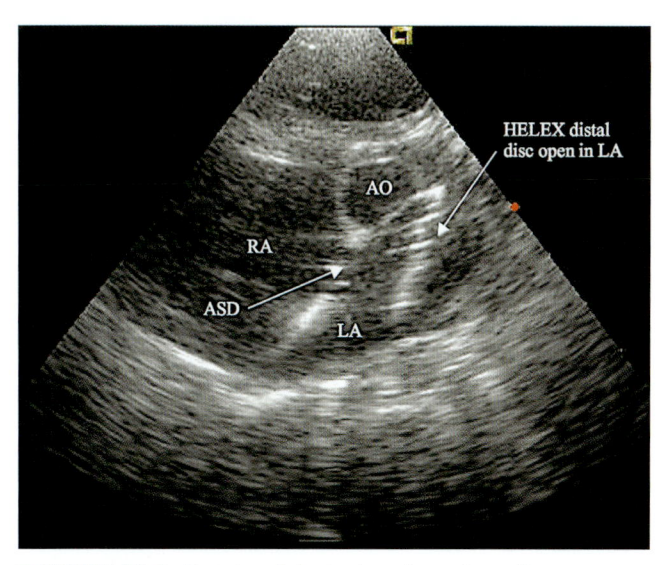

FIGURE 27-4 Parasternal short-axis surface echocardiogram guiding delivery of a HELEX device for ASD closure in a 3-year-old child. AO, aorta; LA, left atrium; RA, right atrium.

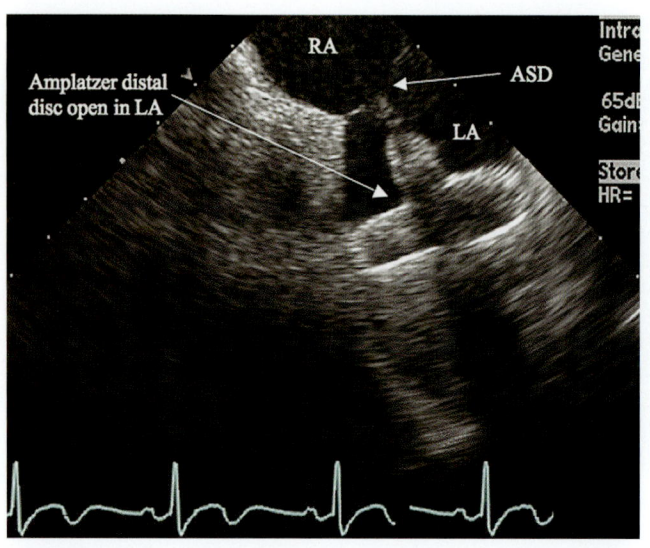

FIGURE 27-5 Intracardiac echocardiogram guiding delivery of an Amplatzer device for ASD closure in a 16-year-old. LA, left atrium; RA, right atrium.

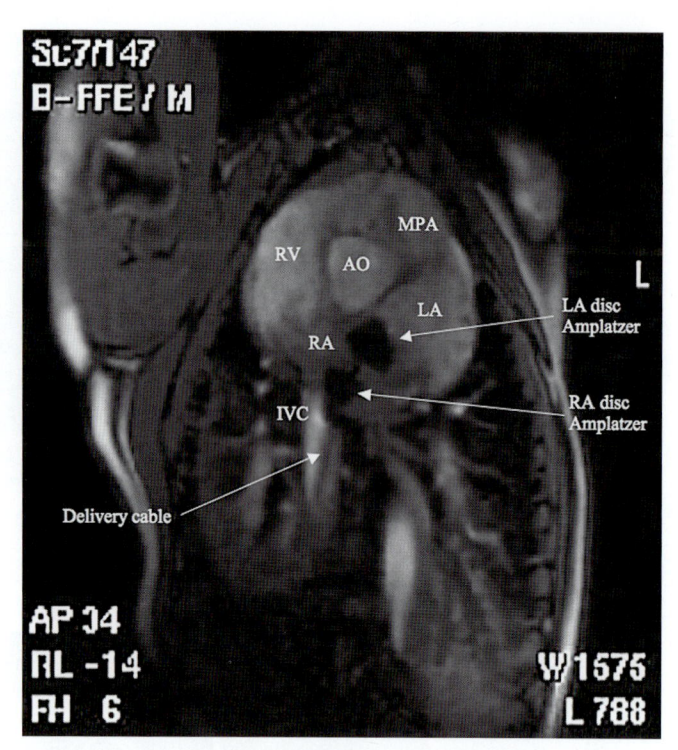

FIGURE 27-7 MRI-guided Amplatzer ASD closure in a swine model. AO, aorta; IVC, inferior vena cava; LA, left atrium; MPA, main pulmonary artery; RV, right ventricle; RA, right atrium.

with right ventricular dilation, ventricular size returns to normal by 12 months after implantation. Commonly used devices have different imaging properties by echocardiography and radiography (Fig. 27-8). There have been frame fractures after implantation in certain devices (STARFlex and HELEX); therefore, chest radiography or, if necessary, fluoroscopy is needed at 6 to 12 months of follow-up (Fig. 27-9). MRI (Fig. 27-10) and CT can be used to image septal devices after implantation but have not shown additional clinical utility to date.

PATENT FORAMEN OVALE

Description and Special Anatomic Considerations

Device closure of patent foramen ovale (PFO) was first described in 1987[7] for the prevention of recurrent stroke associated with paradoxical embolus.[8] It has also been used to prevent right-to-left shunting causing desaturation in patients with orthodeoxia-platypnea syndrome.[9] The foramen ovale is a flap valve in the atrial septum created by overlap of the superior anterior septum secundum on the inferior posterior septum primum (Fig. 27-11). It is present in all fetuses during development to direct oxygenated venous return from the placenta through the inferior vena cava across the atrial septum, bypassing the right ventricle and unexpanded lungs, to fill the left ventricle, allowing optimal cerebral perfusion. After birth, with redistribution of flow due to lung expansion resulting in an increased left atrial pressure, the PFO closes and seals permanently in 65% to 80% of people, age dependent.[10] However, in 20% to 35% of the normal population, the foramen ovale does not fibrose closed and remains patent, allowing unidirectional flow from right to left if right atrial pressure exceeds left atrial pressure. This is physiologically insignificant for most people unless the amount of right-to-left shunting is significant, causing orthodeoxia-platypnea syndrome, or an embolus crosses right to left, resulting in a cryptogenic transient ischemic attack or stroke. Approximately 55% of patients who have had a stroke have a PFO,[11] suggesting that it plays an important role in some of these patients.

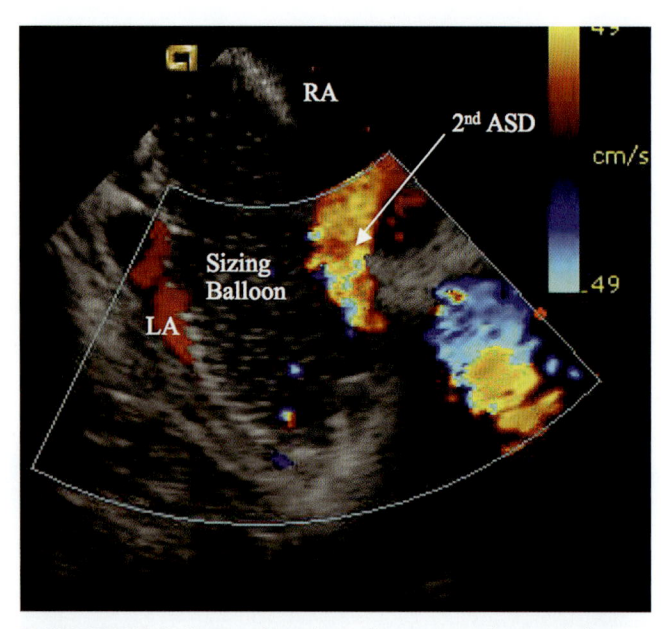

FIGURE 27-6 Intracardiac echocardiogram assessing test balloon occlusion diameter showing a second ASD. LA, left atrium; RA, right atrium.

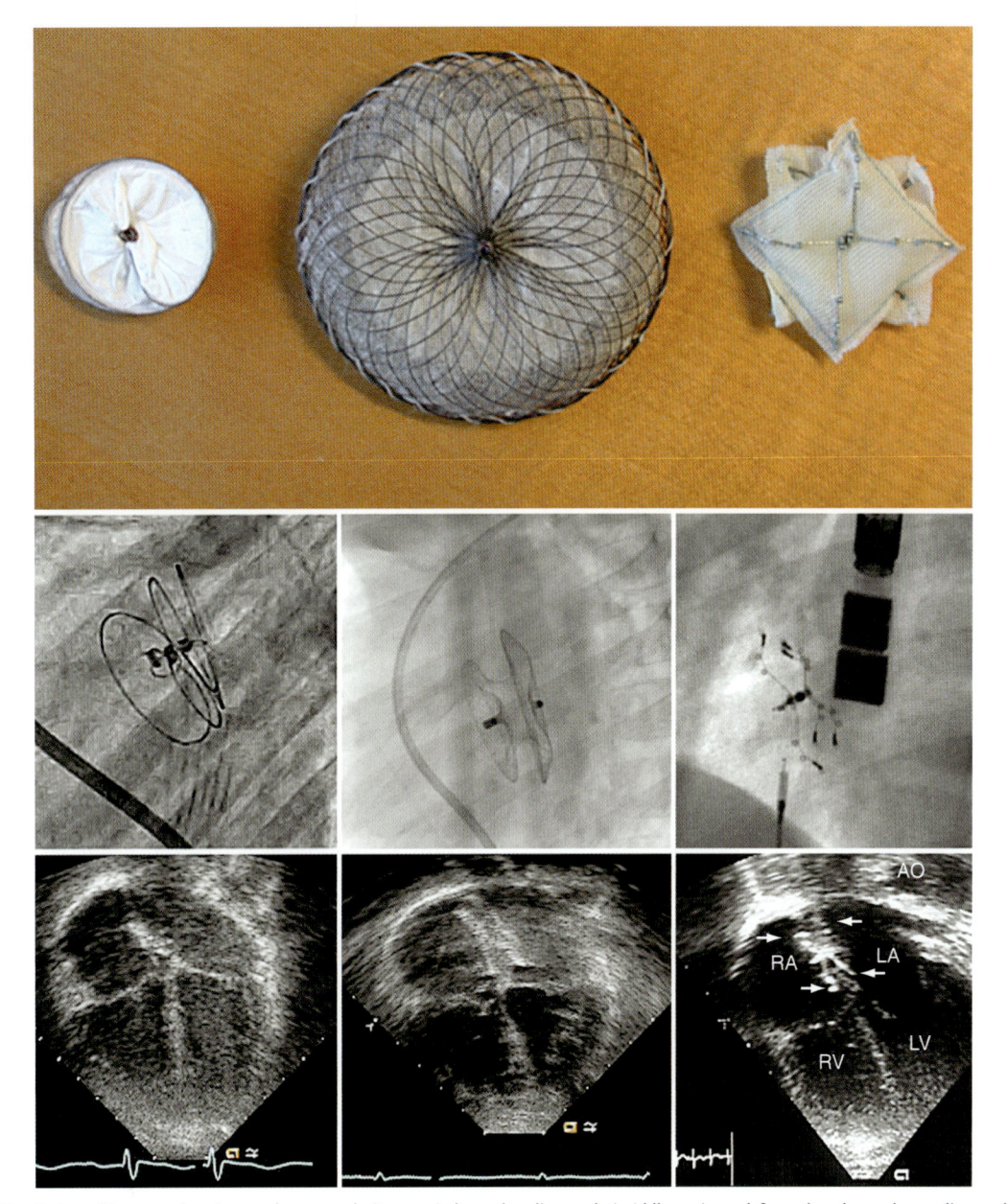

■ **FIGURE 27-8** Series of images showing a photograph (*top row*), lateral radiograph (*middle row*), and four-chamber echocardiographic image (*bottom row*) of the three most common devices currently available for ASD closure: HELEX (*left column*), Amplatzer ASO (*middle column*), and STARFlex (*right column*).

During the last 14 years, interventional device closure of PFO has become an attractive alternative therapeutic strategy to surgical PFO closure or lifelong anticoagulation for stroke prevention. No controlled comparative studies with these other treatment strategies exist for PFO closure, although several active multicenter protocols in stroke patients are currently comparing device closure with medical therapy for prevention of recurrent stroke. Good comparative data from the ASD literature suggest that the efficacy of device closure of ASD is similar to that of surgical closure, with a significant reduction in complications, hospital stay, recovery time, and medical resource use.[4]

Indications

Potential indications for PFO device closure include any patient who has had or has substantial risk for a cryptogenic stroke in the setting of a PFO. Absolute indications for PFO device closure remain controversial because there are limited controlled data comparing different treatment strategies and evaluating long-term follow-up. However, several clinical situations clearly warrant device closure, including patients with active venous thrombosis in the setting of a cryptogenic stroke, patients with recurrent cryptogenic stroke while they are receiving anticoagulation, patients with recurrent cryptogenic stroke and

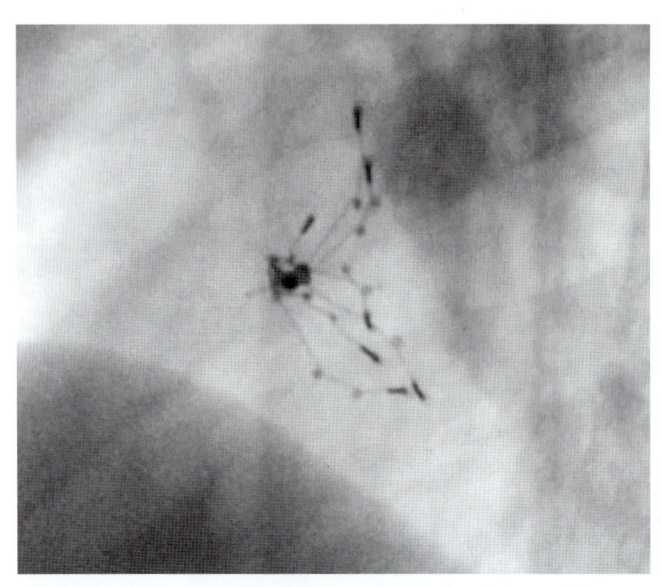

■ **FIGURE 27-9** Lateral chest radiograph showing fracture of the two superior arms of the right atrial disk in a STARFlex device 6 months after implantation.

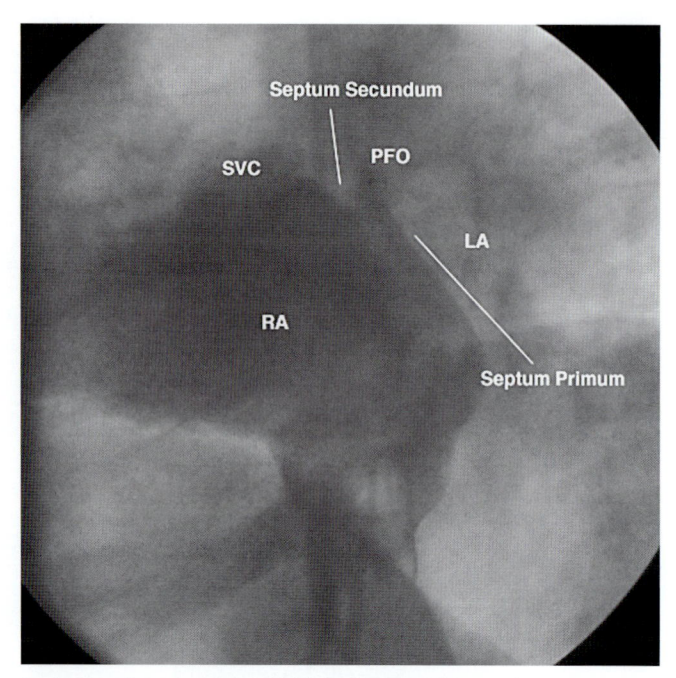

■ **FIGURE 27-11** Right atrial left anterior oblique and caudal angiogram showing the most common PFO anatomy. LA, left atrium; RA, right atrium; SVC, superior vena cava.

contraindications to anticoagulation, and scuba divers who have had significant decompression sickness but insist on continuing to dive. On the basis of current data, PFO device closure may be a reasonable therapeutic alternative for patients with an initial cryptogenic stroke and no additional risk factors.

Contraindications

There are no absolute contraindications to device PFO closure except for patients with active thrombus in the left atrium and those with a known allergy to the device implant materials, particularly the nickel in the frame, although this is extremely rare. Patients who are hypercoagulable, particularly those with disorders that predispose to arterial clots, should be considered very carefully as the post-placement risk of clot formation on the device during the endocardialization process may be significantly increased. However, those patients who are predisposed to venous clots may be the very patients who benefit the most in the long term, albeit with a potentially increased thrombus risk during the first 6 months after implantation. Patients who require anticoagulation long term for other issues may obtain limited benefit from device closure.

Outcomes and Complications

Procedural success with PFO device closure is 98% to 100%, with complete closure rates of 51% to 96% at 6 months on evaluation by saline contrast transesophageal echocardiography.[12,13] Recurrent neurologic event risk after PFO device closure is 1% to 2% annually, with a 96% 1-year and a 90% to 94% 5-year event-free rate.[12,13] These results are significantly influenced by selection of patients because some patients who undergo device closure may have recurrent strokes unrelated to either the PFO or the device. More definitive information about recurrent stroke risk will be available from controlled randomized trials now under way comparing device closure with medical therapy. Procedural complications are uncommon, occurring in fewer than 2% of patients; they include stroke, transient ischemic attack, transient myocardial ischemia (these three due to air or clot embolism with the large delivery sheaths in the left atrium), device malposition or embolization, cardiac perforation with tamponade, and local femoral vein injury.[12] Late complications include atrial arrhythmias in 4% of patients, although most are mild and require no treatment,[14] and thrombus formation on the device.

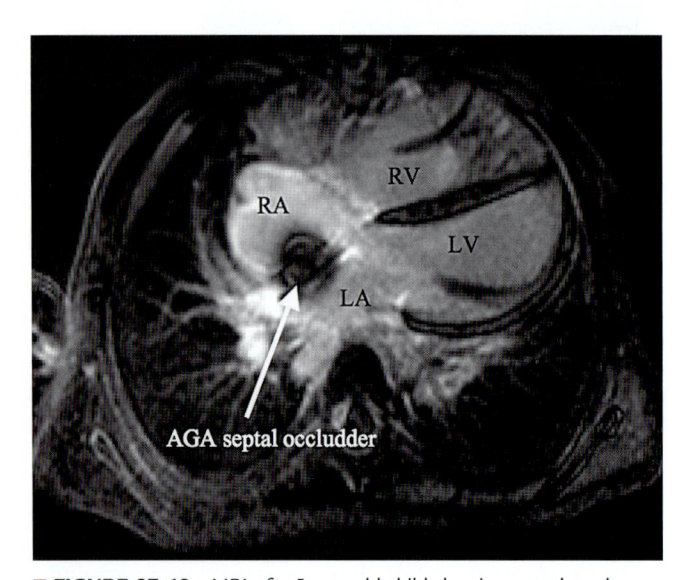

■ **FIGURE 27-10** MRI of a 5-year-old child showing complete closure of a large ASD with an Amplatzer septal occluder device. LA, left atrium; LV, left ventricle; RA, right atrium; RV, right ventricle.

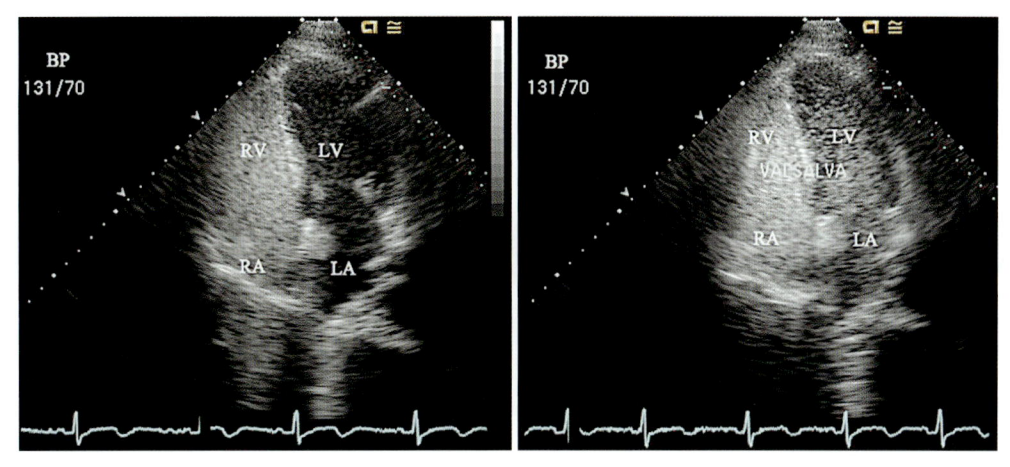

■ **FIGURE 27-12** Four-chamber transthoracic echocardiogram with saline contrast injection. *Left,* No right-to-left shunting at rest. *Right,* Repeated saline injection with Valsalva maneuver demonstrates large right-to-left shunt through the PFO. LA, left atrium; LV, left ventricle; RA, right atrium; RV, right ventricle.

Imaging Findings

Preoperative Planning

Because most patients undergo PFO device closure for prevention of stroke recurrence, it is essential to evaluate the patient's prior neurologic events and to ensure that they were cryptogenic and likely related to the PFO. Stroke associated with paradoxical embolism is a diagnosis of exclusion, so it is imperative to rule out other potential causes of stroke including cerebral aneurysm, carotid or vertebral vessel abnormalities, atrial arrhythmias, left atrial appendage thrombus, cardiomyopathy, and a hypercoagulable state. Standard pre–device closure evaluation includes head and neck MRI or MRA; carotid ultrasonography; saline contrast transesophageal echocardiography with Valsalva maneuver (Fig. 27-12); and hypercoagulable screen, including proteins C and S, antithrombin III, factor V Leiden, prothrombin 20210, methylenetetrahydrofolate reductase (MTHFR), anticardiolipin antibody, and homocysteine. This work-up is essential to help guide decisions about the appropriateness of implanting a device and the optimal medical strategy during the endocardialization process. If there is controversy about the presence or size of the PFO, a saline contrast transcranial Doppler study of the middle cerebral artery with Valsalva maneuver is sensitive,[15] allowing quantification of the amount of right-to-left shunting. The test is not specific to a PFO; pulmonary arteriovenous malformations will also result in a positive test result. Because of a small incidence of atrial arrhythmias after device placement, a baseline electrocardiogram should also be obtained.

Procedural imaging includes fluoroscopy with or without echocardiography, most commonly intracardiac imaging. Unlike for an ASD, the angiogram must be performed in the right atrium to demonstrate the right-to-left shunting, best shown on profile in the lateral plane (75 degrees left anterior oblique and 5 degrees caudal; see Fig. 27-11).

Postoperative Surveillance

Surveillance after implantation relies primarily on transthoracic echocardiography with saline contrast. Patients are seen 1, 6, and 12 months after implantation to ensure appropriate device position, to rule out thrombus formation, and to assess residual right-to-left shunt. Transesophageal echocardiography with saline contrast should be performed at 6 months if there is an abnormal or questionable thoracic echocardiographic study. Quantification of a residual shunt by transcranial Doppler examination is useful to determine the need for repeated intervention.

PATENT DUCTUS ARTERIOSUS

Description and Special Anatomic Considerations

Patent ductus arteriosus (PDA) is the persistence of a normal fetal connection between the proximal descending aorta and the proximal left pulmonary artery that allows the right ventricle to bypass the lungs and pump deoxygenated blood through the descending aorta to the placenta for oxygenation. Normal ductal closure occurs within the first 12 hours after birth by contraction and cellular migration of the medial smooth muscle in the wall of the ductus, resulting in protrusion of the thickened intima into the lumen, causing functional closure. Final closure with creation of the ligamentum arteriosum is completed by 3 weeks of age; permanent sealing of the duct by infolding of the endothelium, disruption of the internal elastic lamina, and hemorrhage and necrosis in the subintimal region lead to replacement of muscle fibers with fibrosis. This process of closure is incomplete in 1 in 2000 live births and accounts for up to 10% of all congenital heart disease.[16]

PDA was one of the first congenital heart lesions treated by interventional techniques, first reported by Porstmann in 1967.[17] There have been substantial refinements in devices and techniques during the last 35 years, but for the last 15 years, interventional catheter treatment has been the preferred therapy in most large centers worldwide. It is a particularly attractive technique in adults, in whom surgical ligation and division can be a problem because of calcified ductal tissue and increased surgical risks. The technique is simple, consisting of placement of a device or vascular occlusion coil in the PDA either antegrade from the femoral vein or retrograde from the femoral artery. Once it is implanted, the device physically occludes ductal flow, and during the first 6 to 8 weeks after implantation, endothelial overgrowth covers the device or coil from both the pulmonary artery and aorta, sealing the PDA permanently closed.

Several different closure devices are currently used because of the significant variability of ductal anatomy. The most common anatomic shape is conical with a large aortic ampulla that narrows at the pulmonary artery end; however, other distinct anatomic forms exist, including "tubular" without a narrowing at the pulmonary artery end, "complex" with narrowing at both the aortic and pulmonary ends, and a short "window" that is an anatomy commonly found in adults.[18] Different closure tools and techniques may be needed to effectively address these less common PDA anatomic subtypes. The most commonly used technique for closure of PDAs less than 2.5 mm is retrograde placement of embolization coils. For large ducts, antegrade placement of an Amplatzer duct occluder device is the preferred method.

Indications

PDA closure is indicated in all patients with left atrial or left ventricular enlargement due to left-to-right shunting or pulmonary artery pressure elevation. Small PDAs that do not result in hemodynamic effects are still at risk for the development of endocarditis. Controlled trials comparing antibiotic prophylaxis with device closure for the prevention of endocarditis have not and will not be performed because of the limited number of patients and the low incidence of endocarditis. There have been no late reports of endocarditis after interventional closure of the ductus, although procedural infections have occurred rarely. Current clinical recommendations are for device or coil closure in small PDAs if they are audible on physical examination.

Contraindications

Patients with systemic pulmonary hypertension and right-to-left ductal shunting should not have the PDA closed. If pulmonary hypertension is noted during catheterization, an accurate assessment of the degree of hypertension and the reactivity of the pulmonary bed must be made during temporary occlusion of the ductus. A second venous sheath should be placed so that simultaneous pulmonary artery pressure measurement and pulmonary vascular resistance calculations can be made while balloon occlusion of the PDA is performed. If there is a baseline left-to-right shunt and a decrease in pulmonary artery pressures with balloon occlusion, ductal closure is indicated.

Outcomes and Complications

Transcatheter ductal closure procedural success has been extremely high, with rates of complete closure above 96%.[19,20] The procedure takes approximately 2 hours, with discharge within 6 hours. Full activity may resume within 48 hours of the procedure. No anticoagulation or antiplatelet therapy is recommended after the coil closure procedure, although most centers recommend daily aspirin for 4 to 6 months after Amplatzer duct occluder or device closure. Procedural complications are uncommon, occurring in fewer than 5%.[19,20] Hemolysis causing anemia may occur if a residual shunt is present after closure with either coils or a device and requires repeated catheterization with placement of additional embolization coils. The major complication associated with coil closure of the PDA is coil embolization to the lungs; however, this is a technical issue that occurs at or immediately after implantation, and the incidence significantly decreases with the operator's experience. It is related to either undersizing of the coil or malposition on placement. In all but a very few patients, the coils can be snared from their embolized position in the pulmonary artery and removed from the body without sequela. Device embolization, thrombus, and ductal aneurysm have been reported in fewer than 1%.

Imaging Findings

Preoperative Planning

A complete physical examination and thoracic echocardiography are necessary to make the diagnosis before intervention. Transthoracic echocardiography will show an abnormal systolic left-to-right color flow jet into the main pulmonary artery or proximal left pulmonary artery directed inferiorly and anteriorly. The central pulmonary arteries will be dilated, as will the left atrium and left ventricle if the shunt is significant. The ductus itself can be imaged from the left parasternal area. Pulmonary artery pressure estimate can be obtained with the PDA Doppler flow velocity. The hemodynamic significance of the PDA can be assessed by measurement of retrograde flow in the descending aorta (Fig. 27-13). In the adult, in whom echocardiography imaging may be poor, MRI should be performed to demonstrate the PDA anatomy clearly. Unusual variations of the ductus arteriosus include origin from the inferior aspect of the transverse arch and from the proximal innominate or subclavian artery (Fig. 27-14). These are usually associated with more complex forms of congenital heart disease. The anatomy of the ductus can vary significantly; the most common is conical, with the narrowing at the pulmonary artery end (Fig. 27-15). The ductus in the adult tends to be short or window-like (Fig. 27-16) and may have significant calcification. These various ductal anatomies can all be closed interventionally but require a variety of closure devices (Fig. 27-17).

Postoperative Surveillance

The majority of patients can be discharged on the same day or the next morning after the procedure. Predischarge evaluation should include a physical examination to assess for recurrence of ductal murmur (it will have disappeared with successful closure) and sheath insertion site. If a murmur is present or there is concern of device or coil positioning at the time of closure, imaging of the ductal device is necessary, either chest radiography or echocardiography. Uncommon but significant complications associated with ductal closure include proximal left pulmonary

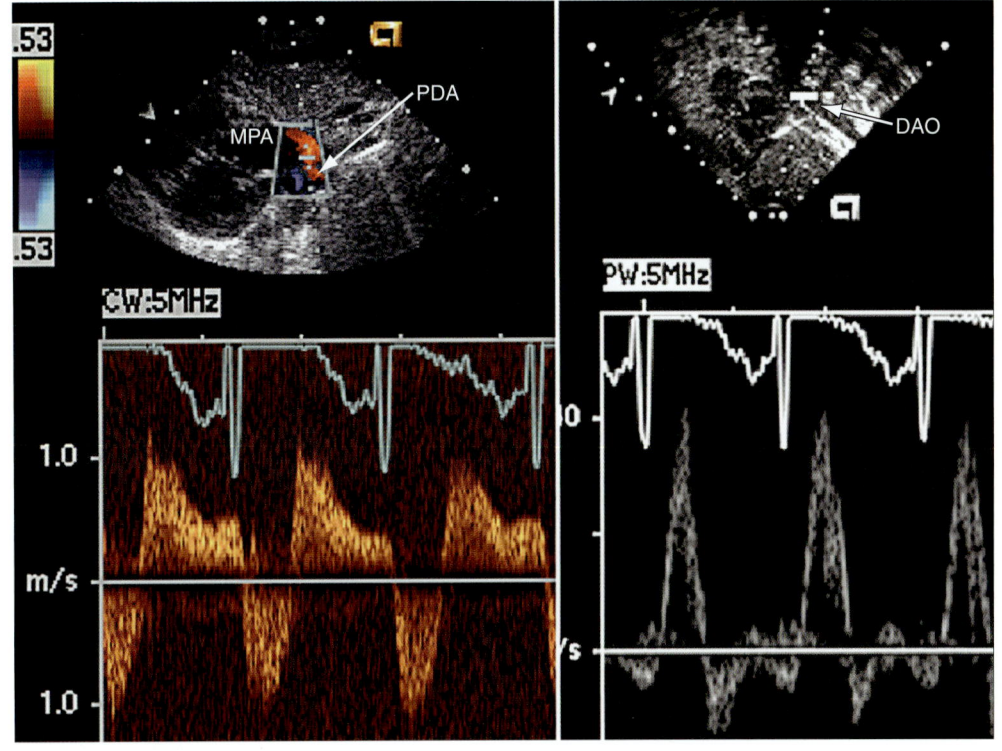

FIGURE 27-13 *Left,* Parasternal echocardiographic image of a PDA with Doppler assessment of diastolic left-to-right flow into the main pulmonary artery (MPA). *Right,* Doppler assessment of the descending aorta (DAO) with significant retrograde flow.

artery stenosis and mild coarctation related to device protrusion, both of which can and should be evaluated by echocardiography. If left pulmonary artery stenosis is confirmed on echocardiography, a nuclear medicine pulmonary flow scan should be obtained to evaluate the physiologic significance of the obstruction. After device placement, endothelialization occurs during the first 6 to 12 weeks. Although it is uncommon, development of a small leak next to the coil (Fig. 27-18) or device can occur (<1%), so follow-up echocardiography at 4 to 6 months after closure is critical to ensure complete closure.

COARCTATION OF THE AORTA

Description and Special Anatomic Considerations

Balloon dilation and more recently stent repair are becoming the treatments of choice for coarctation of the aorta in many centers in older children and adults. Coarctation is most often a discrete narrowing of the proximal descending thoracic aorta just distal to the origin of the left subclavian artery at the site of the ductus ligamentum. It represents 7% of all patients with congenital heart disease and results in upper extremity hypertension, left ventricular hypertrophy, and eventually ventricular failure if it is left untreated. Hypoplasia of the distal transverse arch occurs in up to 10% of patients. Although it is much less common, coarctation of the distal thoracic aorta or abdominal aorta does occur, often in association with vasculitis or genetic syndromes such as Williams syndrome. It should be considered during the initial evaluation of systemic hypertension and can easily be diagnosed on physical examination by decreased femoral pulses with a delay compared with radial pulses and blood pressure differential between the arms and legs. A 2/6 systolic

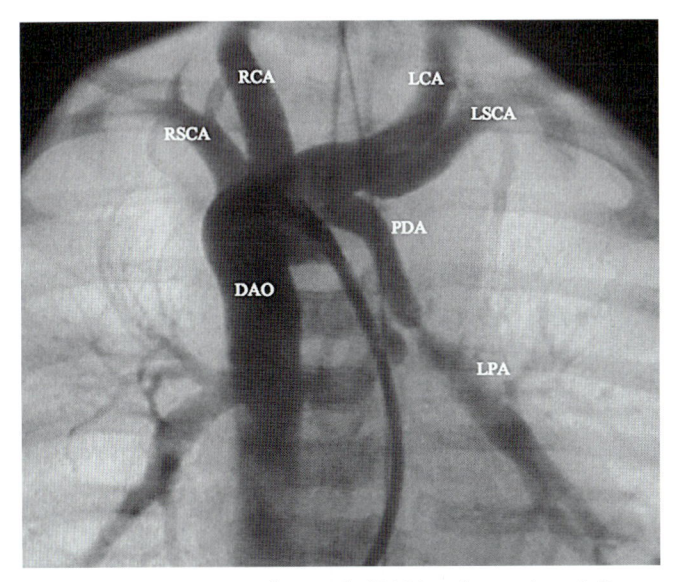

FIGURE 27-14 Descending aortic (DAO) angiogram in an infant with right aortic arch and PDA arising from the left innominate artery supplying the left pulmonary artery (LPA). LCA, left carotid artery; LSCA, left subclavian artery; RCA, right carotid artery; RSCA, right subclavian artery.

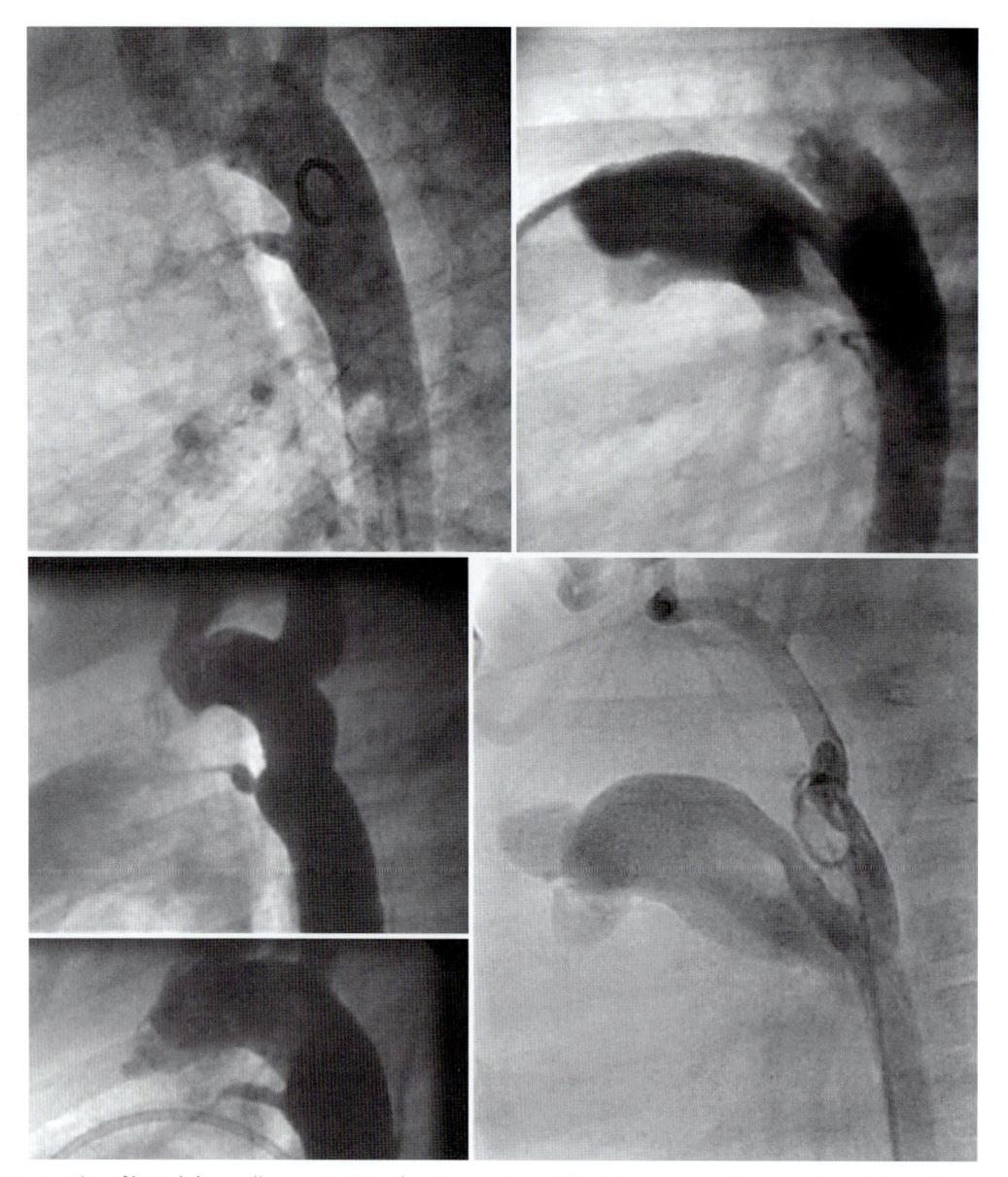

FIGURE 27-15 A series of lateral descending aortograms showing a variety of ductal anatomies, all amenable to interventional closure.

ejection murmur can often be heard at the left upper sternal border and over the left side of the back. The narrowing is due to thick intimal and medial ridges that protrude posteriorly and laterally into the aortic lumen.[21] Intimal proliferation and elastic lamina disruption occur distal to the ridges because of the high-velocity jet impact on the distal aortic wall. Cystic medial necrosis with disarray and loss of medial elastic tissue occurs commonly in the adjacent aorta and may extend to the ascending aorta as well. It is this abnormality that may lead to late aneurysm formation. The body's compensatory response to coarctation is the development of vessels that bypass the obstruction, collateral vessels from the innominate, carotid, and subclavian arteries that connect to the thoracic aorta below the level of the coarctation, often connecting through the intercostal arteries. Enlargement of the intercostal arteries due to this collateral flow is the mechanism for rib notching seen on chest radiography in older patients with severe native coarctation.

Indications

Any coarctation with a gradient of more than 10 mm Hg and significant upper body hypertension or left ventricular hypertrophy without additional cause should be treated. For mild coarctation, it is imperative to use stent implantation to ensure complete resolution of the mild obstruction. Mild coarctations with a gradient of less than 20 mm Hg without hypertension or left ventricular hypertrophy should be considered for stent repair if collaterals are present or the patient has an abnormal blood pressure response to exercise. Patients with coarctation gradients of more than 20 mm Hg at rest even without upper body

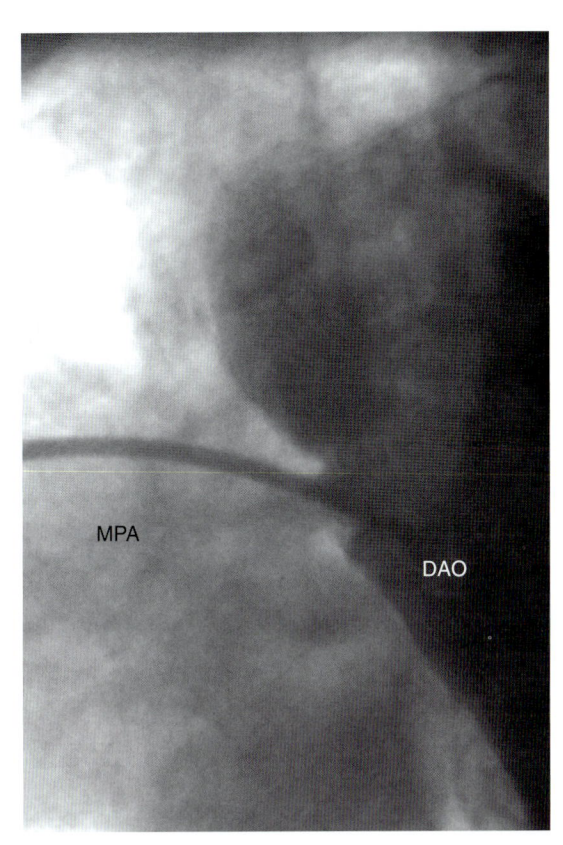

FIGURE 27-16 Lateral angiogram in a 65-year-old patient showing a short window-like ductus arteriosus, commonly seen in adults. DAO, descending aorta; MPA, main pulmonary artery.

Outcomes and Complications

Balloon dilation for treatment of coarctation was first performed in the early 1980s in children with good success in both native and postoperative recoarctation.[23] Its efficacy in adults was found to be similar to that in children[24]; however, there remained a small but significant failure rate with residual gradient of more than 20 mm Hg in approximately 15% of patients treated. Stent implantation for repair of coarctation was performed sporadically in the early 1990s in children; it was first reported in adults in 1995 with very promising results.[25] Since that time, stent repair has become the treatment of choice for coarctation in many centers because of the improved success rate and low restenosis rate, although controlled trials are not available. Procedural success has been reported in more than 95% of patients, with residual obstruction of less than 20 mm Hg. Recurrent stenosis has been extremely rare, occurring in fewer than 5%, usually in younger patients, and is generally mild. Complications have been reported in up to 20% and include aneurysm, perforation, stroke, and death in fewer than 3%.[26] In addition, femoral artery complications including arteriovenous fistula and pseudoaneurysm have been reported in association with the larger arterial sheaths required for the procedure.

Imaging Findings

Preoperative Planning

Echocardiography is useful to confirm the diagnosis and to evaluate location and severity of the obstruction. However, spatial resolution is limited, particularly in older adolescents and adults, so to determine exact anatomic dimensions, either thoracic CT or MRI (Fig. 27-19) is needed. MRI gives the added benefit of assessment of the severity of obstruction as well as the significance of collateral flow (Fig. 27-20). Special attention should be paid to the surrounding aortic diameter, including the distal transverse arch, the coarctation diameter, and the location relative to the carotid and left subclavian arteries, as well as to the presence of existing aneurysm, poststenotic dilation, and calcification. Final assessment of the coarctation is performed during the procedure with biplane angiography, including during and after balloon dilation or stent implantation (Fig. 27-21).

Postoperative Surveillance

Most patients are discharged on the day after the implantation or dilation, and chest radiography should be performed before discharge to ensure stable stent placement. Because late aneurysms may occur in up to 7% as late as 10 years, ongoing imaging surveillance is required. Current recommendations are for CT or MRI scan 6 to 12 months after implantation (Fig. 27-22). If an aneurysm is detected, annual evaluations are required. If no aneurysm is detected, repeated imaging every 4 to 5 years is recommended.

hypertension should be repaired. Patients with mild coarctation (<20 mm Hg) without upper body hypertension should have blood pressure checks every 6 to 12 months with ongoing surveillance for the development of left ventricular hypertrophy.

Contraindications

Patients with coarctation gradients of less than 20 mm Hg with no evidence of collateral flow, hypertension, left ventricular hypertrophy, or abnormal blood pressure response to exercise do not need treatment. Patients with significant hypoplasia and obstruction of the transverse aortic arch in the area of the origin of the carotids should be excluded. Stent repair with jailing of the carotids may be appropriate in the rare patient at extremely high surgical risk; however, for the majority of patients with this lesion, surgical repair should be performed. Any patient with an existing aneurysm should also be cautiously considered. Covered thoracic stents may have a role in this setting, although there are limited data at present. Aortic wall dissection, aneurysm, and rupture associated with stent implantation are uncommon but increase in frequency with the age of the patient and the degree of aortic calcification associated with the coarctation.[22] These patients must be considered carefully, and covered stent implantation versus surgery should be considered.

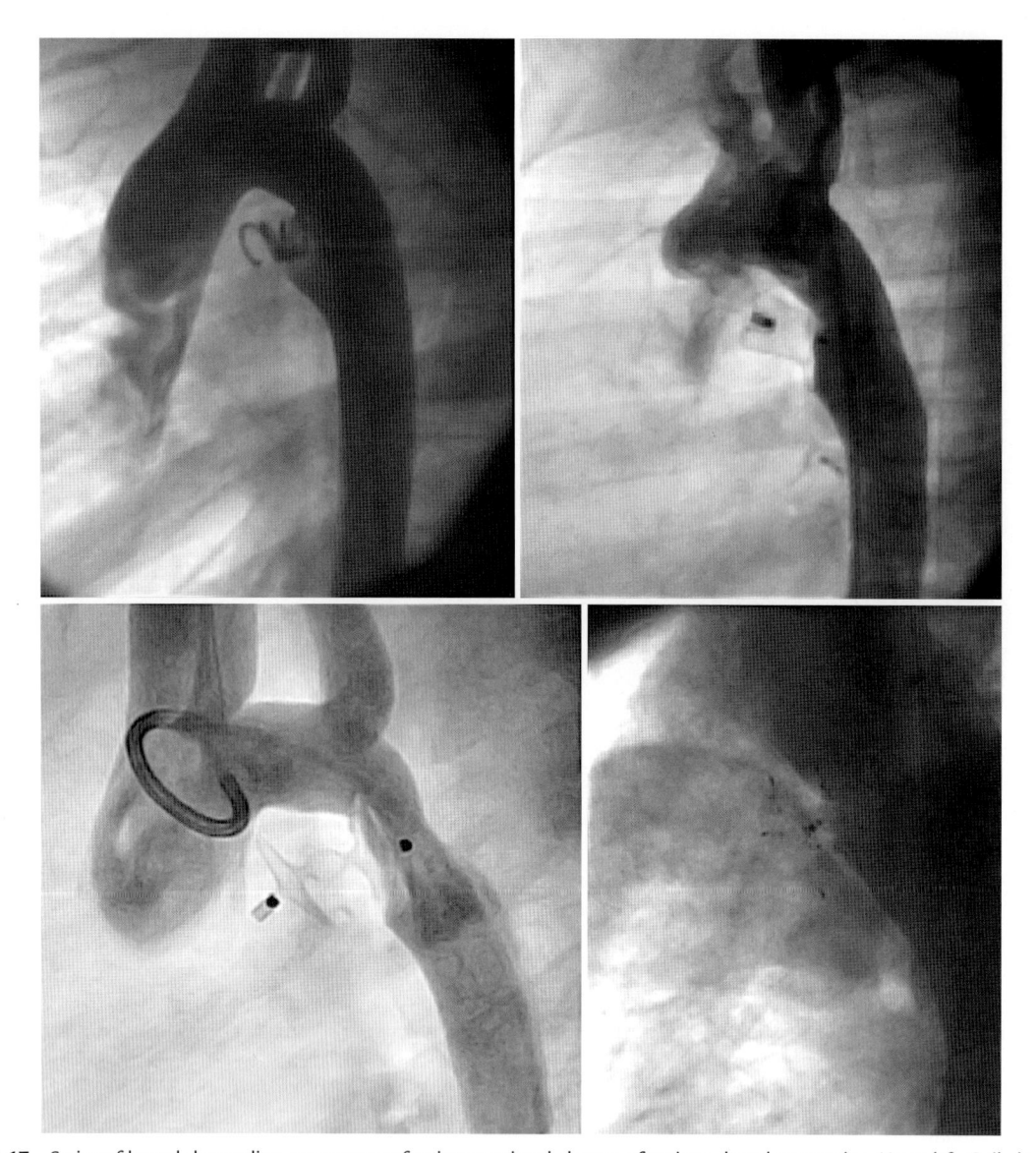

■ **FIGURE 27-17** Series of lateral descending aortograms after interventional closure of various ductal anatomies. *Upper left,* Coil closure. *Upper right,* Amplatzer duct occluder I. *Lower left,* Amplatzer duct occluder II. *Lower right,* STARFlex device.

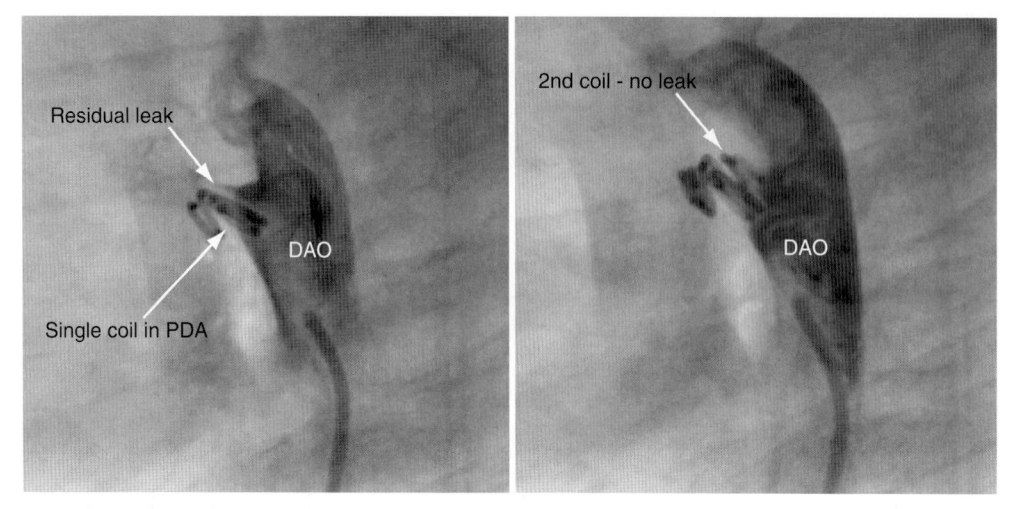

■ **FIGURE 27-18** Lateral angiogram of a 2-year-old child after single coil closure of a moderately sized PDA. *Left,* Residual leak through the ductus over the superior edge of existing coil. *Right,* Complete closure after placement of a second coil. DAO, descending thoracic aorta.

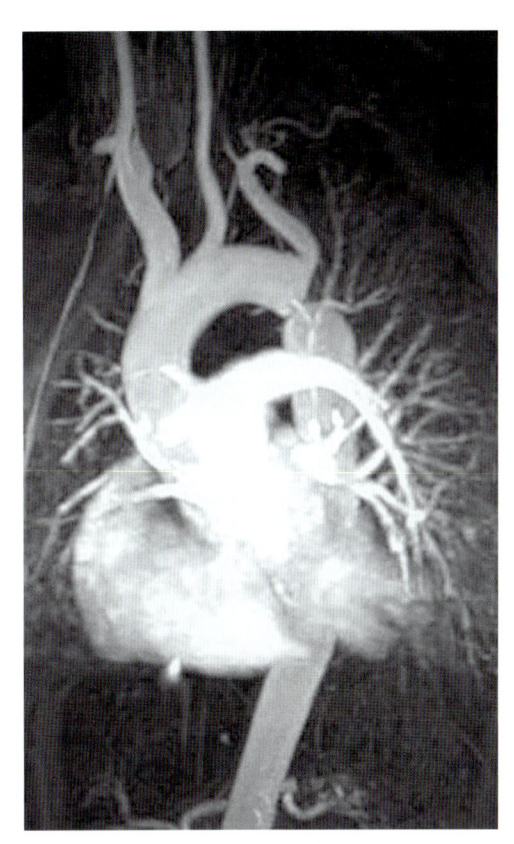

FIGURE 27-19 Three-dimensional reconstruction of MR angiogram in a patient with severe discrete native coarctation of the aorta.

PULMONARY ARTERY STENOSIS

Description and Special Anatomic Considerations

Balloon dilation of segmental pulmonary artery stenosis with stent repair of more proximal lesions has become the standard of care because of limited and challenging surgical success. Branch pulmonary artery stenosis is a rare congenital lesion in isolation but is often associated with complex congenital heart lesions after surgical repair, especially tetralogy of Fallot. Other associated lesions include truncus arteriosus or pulmonary atresia with ventricular septal defect after right ventricle-to-pulmonary artery conduit placement, transposition of the great arteries after arterial switch repair, and pulmonary artery sling after reimplantation. Branch pulmonary artery stenosis decreases perfusion to the affected lung and, if severe, causes hypertension in the nonaffected lung and right ventricle. Distal pulmonary artery stenosis promotes pulmonary insufficiency, which compounds the decrease in cardiac output and increased workload on the right ventricle seen in these patients. Patients can be asymptomatic with right ventricular hypertension but often present with exercise intolerance.

Indications

The systolic gradient across branch pulmonary artery stenosis is, in isolation, a poor determinant of the need for treatment and can be interpreted only by also considering quantitative pulmonary flow data. Normal distribution of pulmonary flow is 55% to the right lung and 45% to the left lung. Patients with a reduction of more than 15% of flow or an absolute flow of less than 1 L/min/m² in the affected lung should be considered for stent repair. Patients with any degree of contralateral pulmonary artery hypertension, right ventricular hypertension, or right ventricular hypertrophy should be aggressively treated to prevent progression, as should patients with significant pulmonary insufficiency associated with the branch pulmonary artery stenosis.

Contraindications

Adult patients after repair of complex congenital heart disease such as tetralogy of Fallot or truncus arteriosus are complex, often with multiple anatomic, hemodynamic, and arrhythmia issues in addition to their branch pulmonary artery stenosis. It is critical that these patients are evaluated completely and that a comprehensive plan is made in coordination with a cardiologist familiar with congenital heart disease and involving an electrophysiologist, cardiothoracic surgeon, and interventionalist. If surgical revision of the underlying repair is required, a surgical approach to the branch pulmonary artery stenosis may be preferable.

Outcomes and Complications

Balloon dilation of branch pulmonary artery stenosis was initially described in 1983 by Lock and colleagues[27]; however, only 50% of lesions responded, with a significant restenosis rate. With the availability of larger peripheral stents in the early 1990s and their application to pulmonary artery branch stenosis,[28] stent placement has rapidly become the treatment of choice in school-age children and adults because of improved success and low restenosis rates. Shaffer and coworkers[29] reported results in more than 130 children and adults with postoperative branch pulmonary artery stenosis; in more than 65%, stent implantation increased lesion diameter by more than 100%, with a median gradient reduction from 46 to 10 mm Hg and right ventricle–to–systemic pressure ratio reduction from 60% to 40%. Long-term results have been excellent, with restenosis rates below 5%. Complications are rare, occurring in fewer than 4% of cases overall, and include hemoptysis, aneurysm, perforation, refractory ventilation-perfusion mismatch, and death. Technical issues, such as device malposition and embolization, have been reported in less than 2% and are quite rare with recent improvements in balloon and stent technology. Recent use of cutting balloons has further improved results to more than 90% success for segmental pulmonary artery stenosis resistant to standard dilation and stenting techniques.[30]

Imaging Findings

Preoperative Planning

Echocardiography allows accurate assessment of tricuspid regurgitation, right ventricular hypertrophy and dilation,

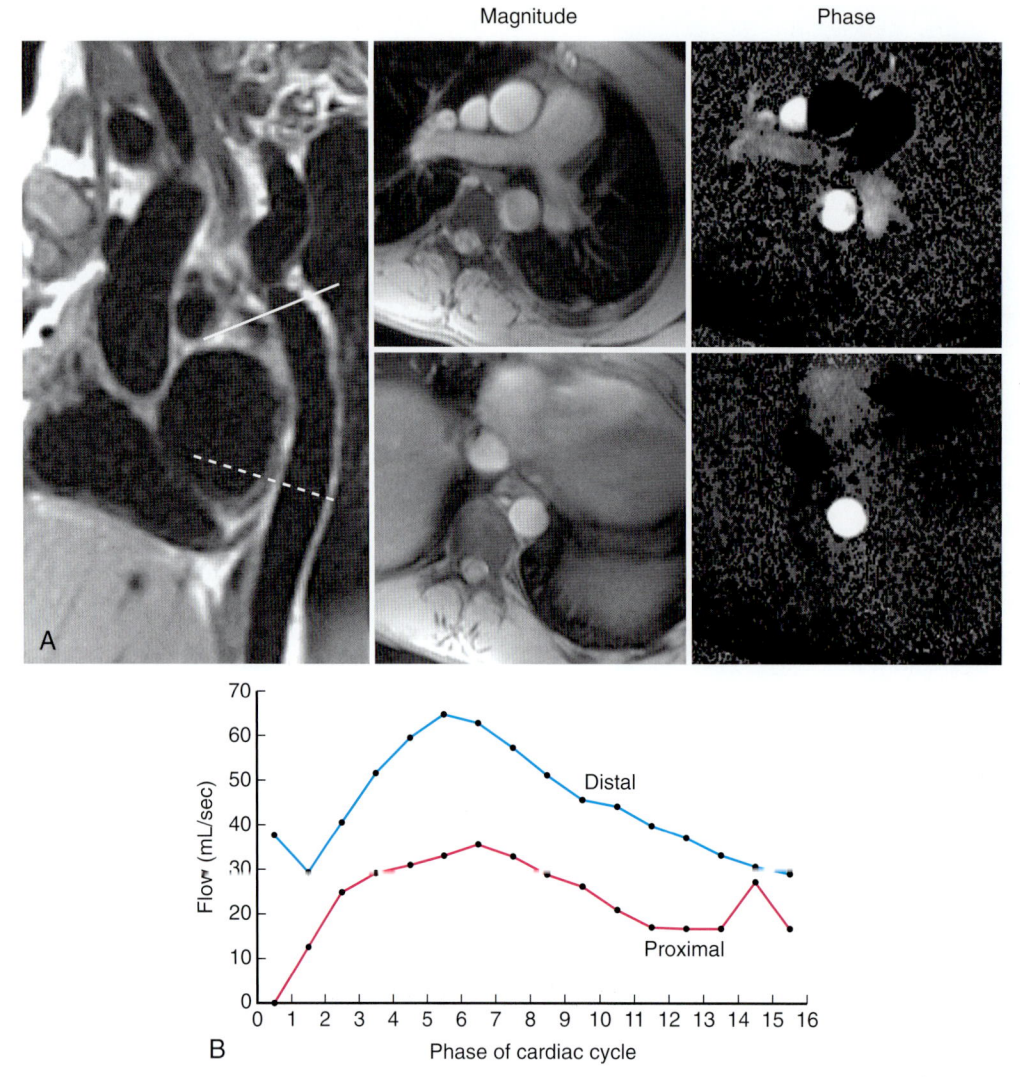

■ **FIGURE 27-20** **A,** MRI series in a teenager with coarctation assessing proximal and distal vessel magnitude and phase to calculate flow. **B,** Flow data from images in **A** indicate significant collateral flow bypassing the area of coarctation, with greater flow seen in the distal thoracic aorta than immediately after the site of coarctation.

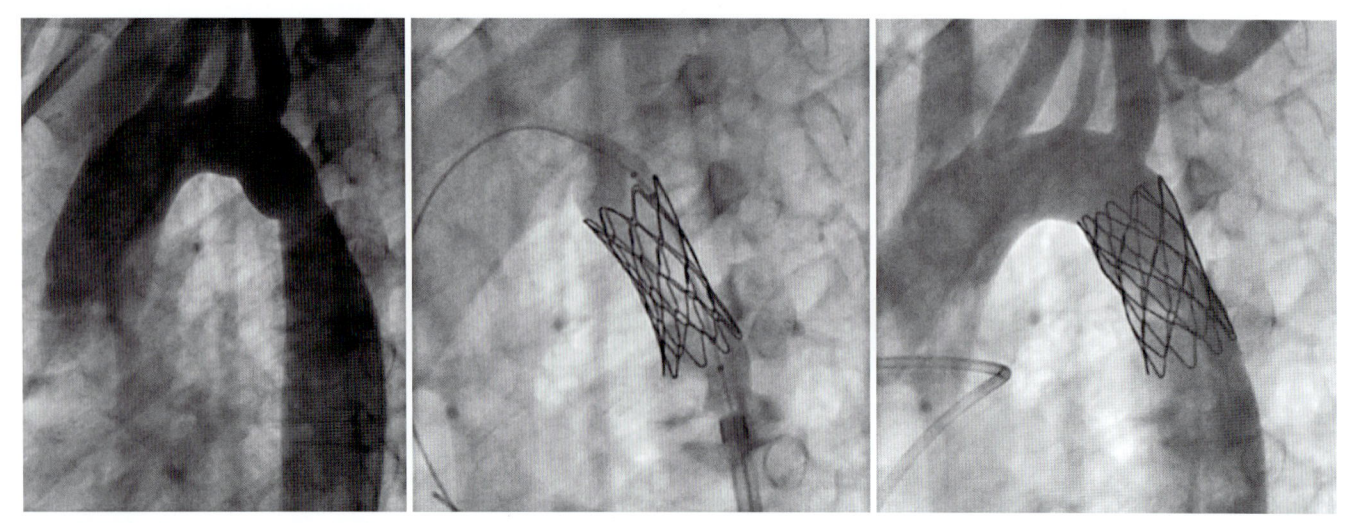

■ **FIGURE 27-21** Serial lateral ascending aortic angiograms in a 16-year-old with coarctation: *left,* discrete coarctation; *middle,* platinum bare-metal stent implant; and *right,* resolution of obstruction after implantation.

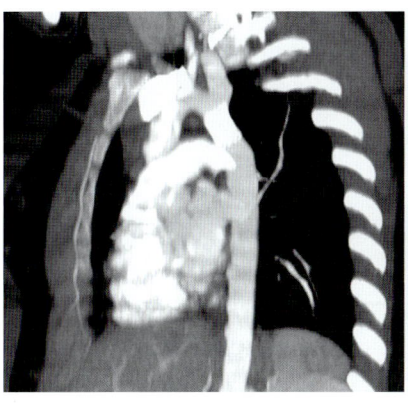

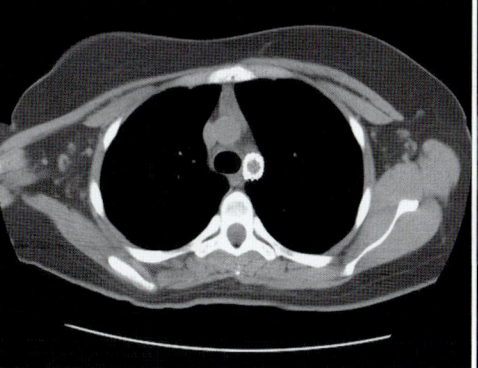

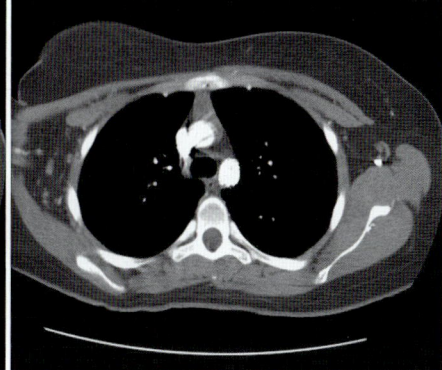

FIGURE 27-22 Cardiac CT in 16-year-old girl several years after stent repair of native coarctation.

and pulmonary insufficiency before the procedure. It is limited in the evaluation of proximal pulmonary artery stenosis and poor in the evaluation of segmental branch stenosis. MRI, CT, and angiography (Fig. 27-23) remain the best imaging for anatomic stenosis information in the pulmonary arteries. In addition to anatomic information, physiologic information of relative flow to pulmonary segments is crucial before the procedure for interventional decision-making. This should be assessed with either nuclear medicine pulmonary flow scan (Fig. 27-24) or MRA. These flow data are critical and must be coupled with anatomic and pressure data at the procedure to optimize clinical decision-making.

Postoperative Surveillance

Postoperative type and frequency depend on the type and location of treatment (angioplasty alone versus stent implantation) as well as on the presence of vessel injury or aneurysm after treatment. For proximal pulmonary artery lesions treated with balloon angioplasty alone, echocardiography coupled with pulmonary flow scan evaluation at 4 months, then yearly thereafter, is adequate. For more distal stenosis with stent implantation, CT angiography is optimal for imaging, although cardiac MRI (Fig. 27-25) can be used (artifact will depend on stent type—currently both stainless steel and nitinol stents are commonly being used). Nuclear medicine pulmonary flow scan evaluation yearly is needed if flow data cannot be accurately obtained by MRI. If an acute aneurysm develops with the procedure early (Fig. 27-26), more frequent CT or MRI is required during the first year to ensure no progression.

PULMONARY INSUFFICIENCY

Description and Special Anatomic Considerations

Pulmonary valve implantation for pulmonary insufficiency is an active area of development in percutaneous treatment of congenital heart disease. Pulmonary insufficiency with associated right-sided heart dilation and dysfunction is a common occurrence late after repair of tetralogy of Fallot and truncus arteriosus. Although it is tolerated well in childhood, recent information shows that chronic pulmonary insufficiency limits right ventricular function and shortens life span. Surgical repair requires tissue valve implantation, either a homograft or stented autograft. Although quite effective, these valves last only 15 to 20 years, necessitating multiple repeated operations over a lifetime. In 2000, Bonhoeffer and colleagues[31] reported the first percutaneous pulmonary valve implantation using a bovine jugular valve sewn inside a balloon-expandable platinum stent. Since that time, more than 450 patients have been treated. Commercial valves are now available in Europe and are currently under investigation in the United States.

Anatomic considerations before percutaneous pulmonary valve implantation include degree of pulmonary insufficiency and stenosis, degree of right ventricular dilation and dysfunction, size and anatomy of the right ventricular outflow tract (RVOT) and main pulmonary artery, and presence of branch pulmonary artery stenosis.

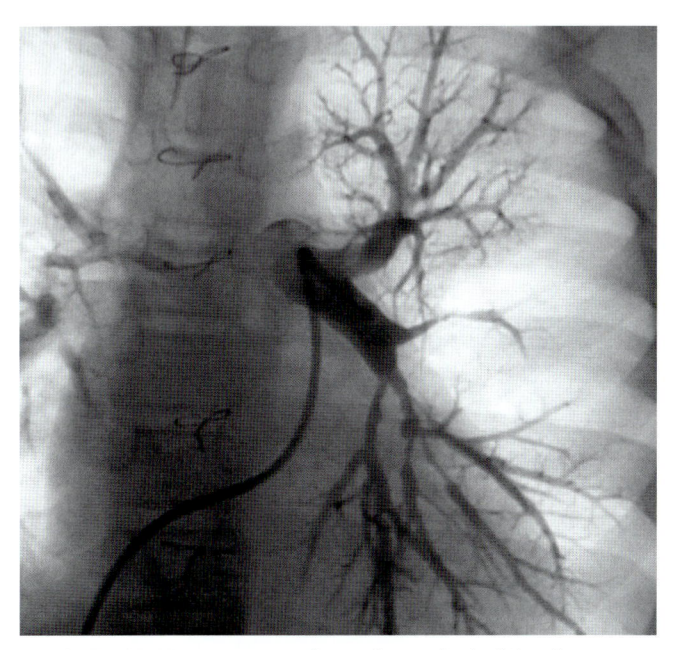

FIGURE 27-23 Anteroposterior angiogram in the left pulmonary artery of an 8-year-old girl with severe subpulmonary artery segmental stenosis due to a chronic thrombotic disorder.

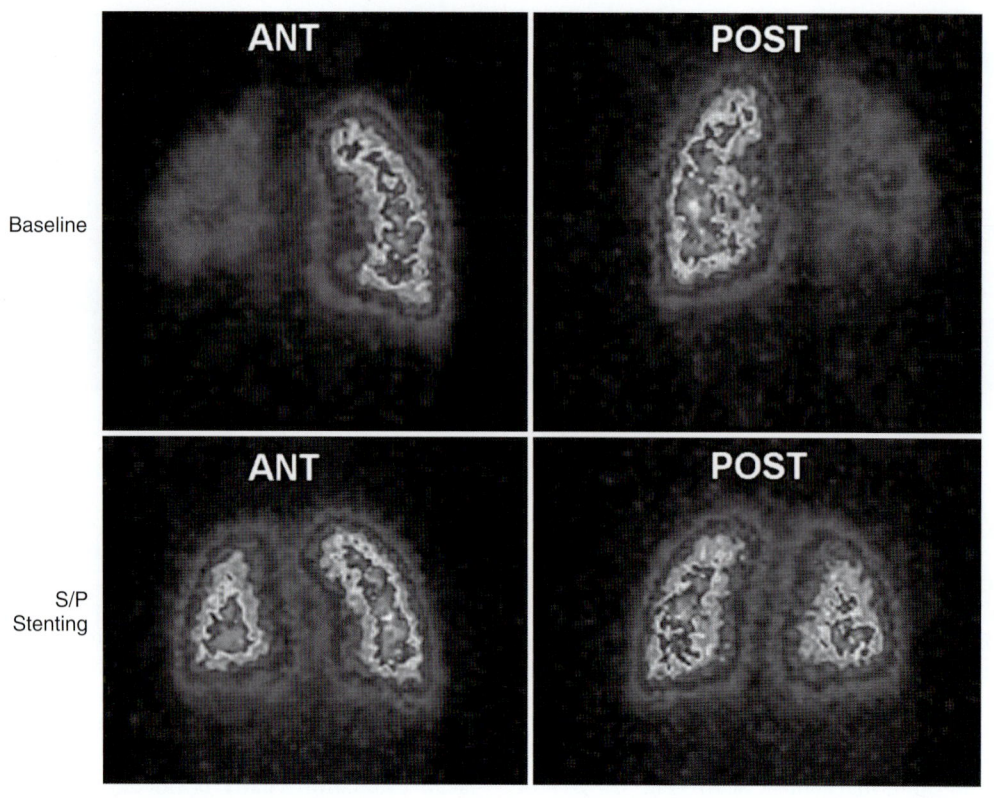

FIGURE 27-24 Nuclear pulmonary flow scan in a child with severe proximal right pulmonary artery stenosis before and after stent repair showing a marked increase in flow to the right lung.

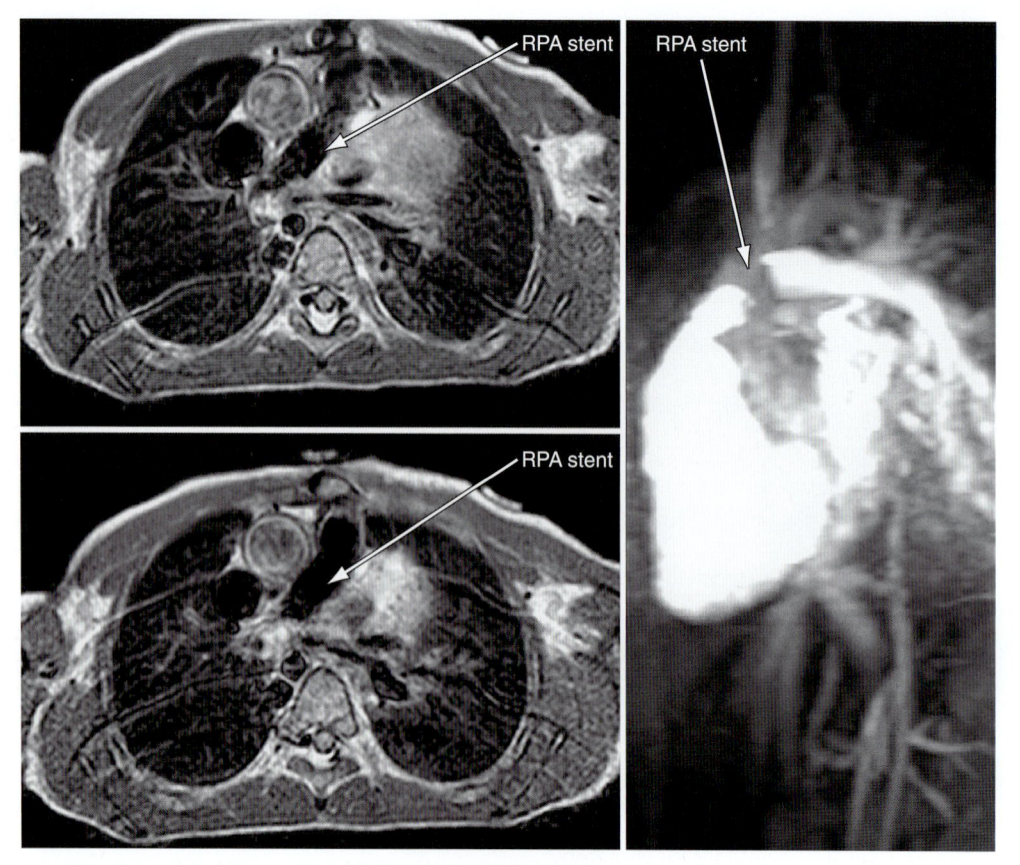

FIGURE 27-25 *Left,* Axial black blood MRI images of a 5-year-old child 1 year after right pulmonary artery (RPA) stainless steel stent repair. *Right,* MRA reconstruction. Note the stent artifact in the proximal right pulmonary artery.

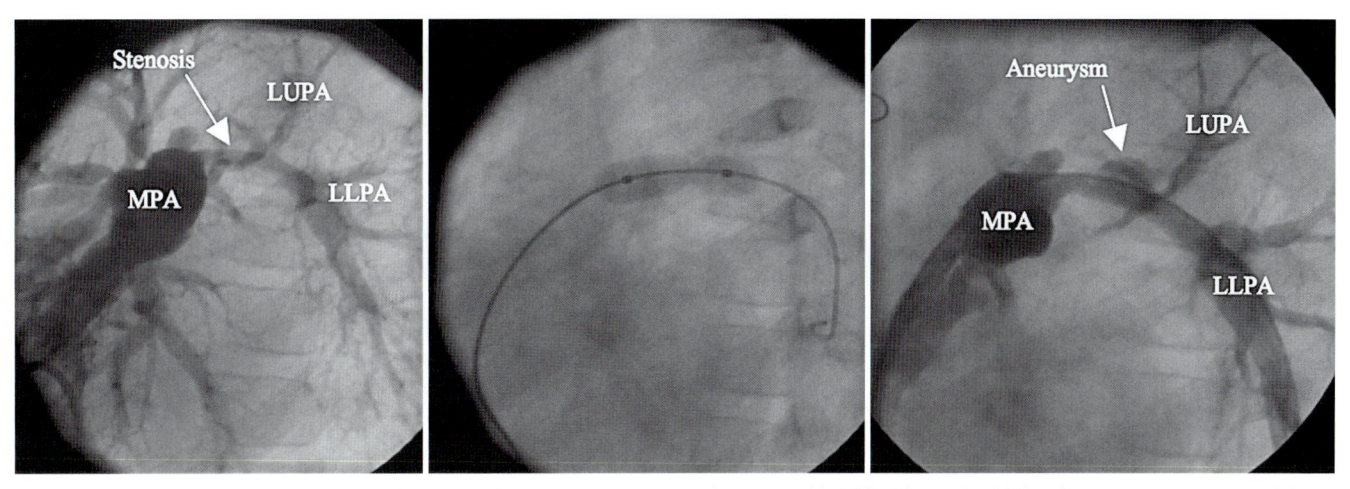

FIGURE 27-26 Lateral angiograms in the main pulmonary artery (MPA) of a 3-year-old child with proximal left pulmonary artery stenosis: *left,* angiogram before dilation; *middle,* balloon dilation; and *right,* after dilation, showing a significant aneurysm extending to the origin of the left upper lobe segment (LUPA). LLPA, left lower lobe segmental branch.

Indications

Indications for treatment of pulmonary insufficiency include right ventricular dilation (>140 mL/m^2), regurgitant fraction above 20%, worsening tricuspid regurgitation, and symptoms of exercise intolerance. Pulmonary stenosis with insufficiency should be treated if there is significant right ventricular hypertrophy, right ventricular pressures above 3/4 systemic, worsening tricuspid regurgitation, or symptoms of exercise intolerance (peak $\dot{V}_{O_2}$ < 65% predicted).

Contraindications

Current limitations to percutaneous pulmonary valve implantation are due to both the large sheath size required for the implant and the stented valve maximum diameter (Fig. 27-27). The procedure currently requires a sheath larger than 20F; therefore, most operators restrict use to patients weighing 25 kg or more. Commercially available implants are limited to a maximum diameter of 24 mm, limiting their use in the RVOT or main pulmonary artery to lesions no larger than 22 mm in diameter. This limitation will be relaxed as newer devices are developed to expand to larger diameters. The RVOT must be more than 14 mm in diameter to ensure proper functioning of the valve with expansion. In addition, the location of the coronary arteries relative to the RVOT and main pulmonary artery area is crucial for determination of eligibility. Although uncommon, there are patients after surgical repair of tetralogy of Fallot or truncus arteriosus whose left or right coronary artery courses directly behind the obstructive RVOT. Placement of a stent in these patients will result in coronary compromise and myocardial infarction and can cause death.

Outcomes and Complications

The procedure is successful in 95% of implantations, with significant reduction in right ventricular systolic pressures (63 mm Hg to 45 mm Hg) and of RVOT gradients (37 mm Hg to 17 mm Hg).[32] Pulmonary insufficiency, severe in all patients before implantation, was absent in more than 60% and trivial or mild in 38% after 18 months of follow-up. Procedural complications included acute surgery for RVOT and existing homograft dissection in 5%, with no associated mortality. Late complications included endocarditis and reobstruction due to sternal compression or stent fracture. Repeated stent dilation or stent implantation inside the existing stent is needed in up to 12% because of late stenosis or fracture. Freedom from reoperation is 84% at 5 years. Percutaneous valve implantation results in resolution of right ventricular dilation (142 to 91 mL/m^2) and improved submaximal exercise tolerance at 1 year.[33]

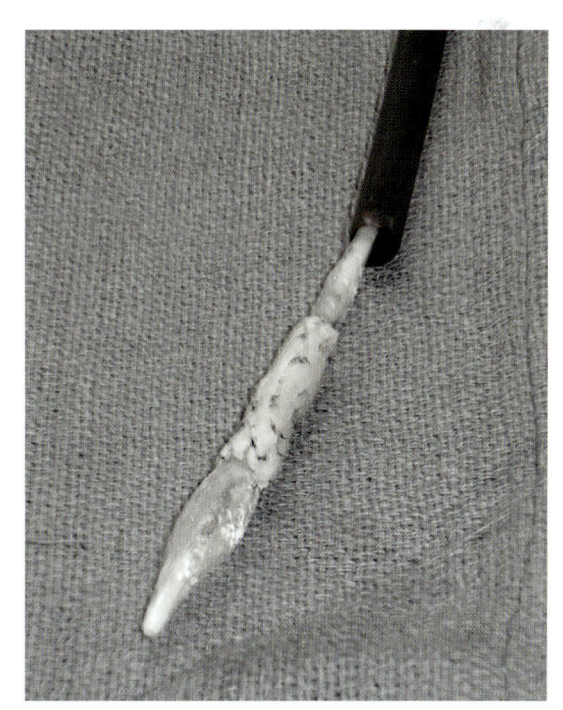

FIGURE 27-27 Bovine jugular venous valve sewn onto a stainless steel stent mounted on an 18-mm balloon. Note compressed size relative to the 22F sheath.

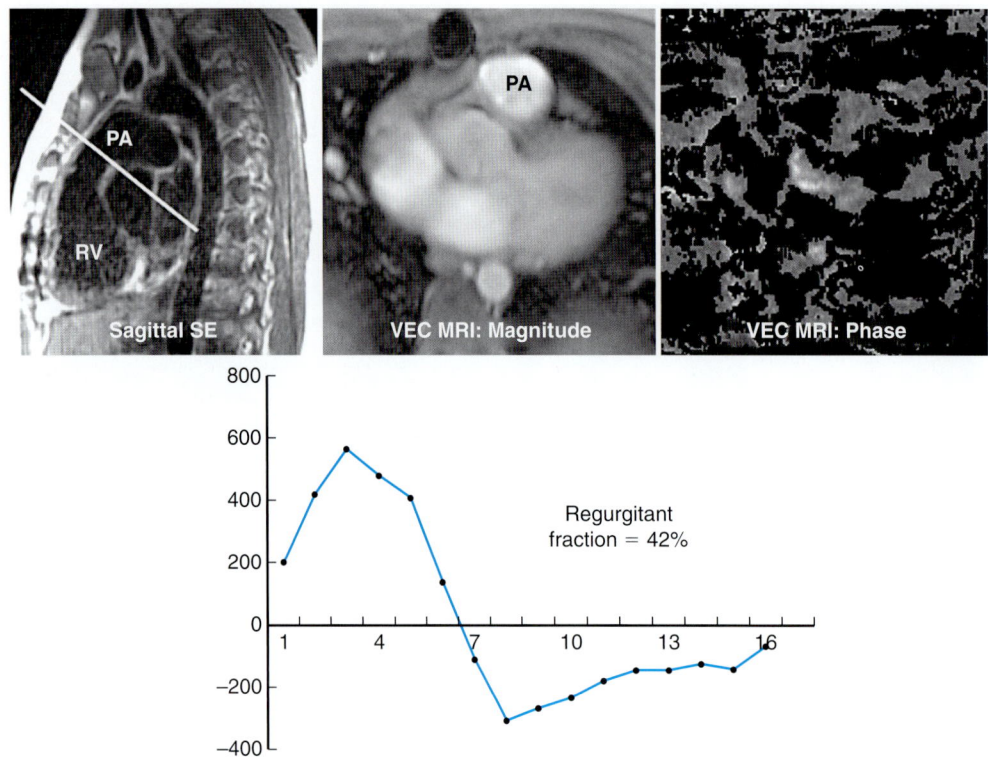

■ **FIGURE 27-28** *Left,* Black blood cardiac MRI of 14-year-old patient after repair of tetralogy of Fallot with right ventricular dilation due to pulmonary regurgitation. *Middle and right,* The velocity-encoded cine MRI for magnitude and phase in the main pulmonary artery (PA). *Lower image,* The data graphed, demonstrating pulmonary flow with a 42% regurgitant fraction.

Imaging Findings

Preoperative Planning

Preoperative imaging is crucial to determination of eligibility for this procedure as well as for planning. CT or MRI is required to adequately assess the right ventricle, RVOT, main pulmonary artery, and branch pulmonary artery anatomy to determine dimensions. MRI gives the added benefit of pulmonary regurgitant fraction assessment (Fig. 27-28) as well as relative branch pulmonary flows. Specific attention to coronary artery anatomy in the area of the RVOT to assess for large coronary branches immediately posterior to the RVOT is crucial. If coronary artery anatomy is not clear from CT or MRI or there are significant concerns, selective coronary angiography with simultaneous test RVOT balloon expansion is required during the procedure (Fig. 27-29). Angiography in the main pulmonary artery is performed after implantation to assess valve

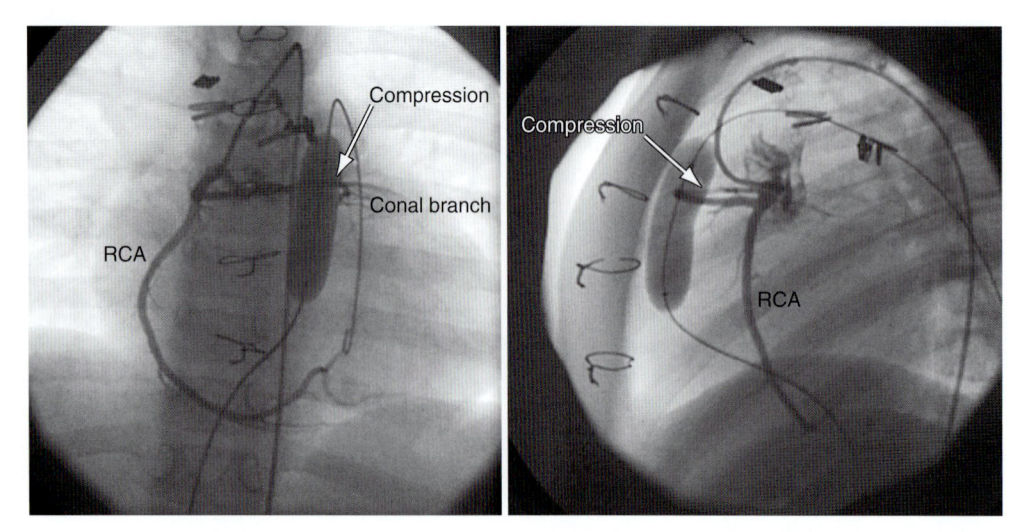

■ **FIGURE 27-29** *Left,* Anteroposterior selective right coronary artery (RCA) angiogram during balloon dilation of stenotic right ventricle-to-pulmonary artery homograft. Notice the large conal branch of the right coronary artery crossing just posterior to the homograft with significant compression from the inflated balloon. *Right,* The corresponding lateral image.

and stent integrity. Repeated echocardiographic evaluation (Fig. 27-31) is appropriate every 6 months with CT or MRI evaluation annually to assess right ventricle size, in-stent restenosis, stent integrity, and pulmonary regurgitant fraction. If the patient is stable with a competent valve, these assessments can be lengthened to every 2 to 3 years.

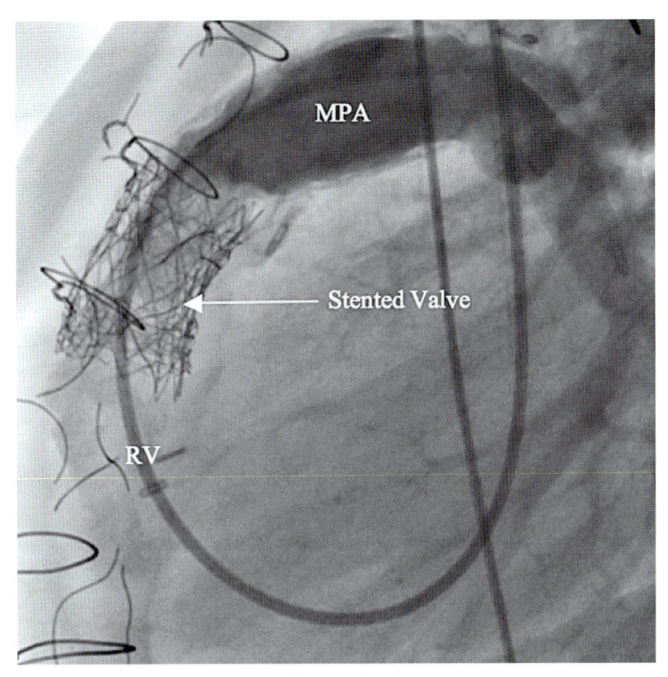

FIGURE 27-30 Lateral angiogram in the main pulmonary artery (MPA) of a 6-year-old child after valved stent implantation. Notice the trivial degrees of regurgitation into the right ventricle (RV).

positioning and function (Fig. 27-30). Procedural echocardiography, either transesophageal echocardiography or intracardiac, is useful as well for assessing residual stenosis and insufficiency immediately after implantation to determine the need for additional dilation or stenting.

Postoperative Surveillance

Before discharge, echocardiography and chest radiography are repeated to assess residual stenosis, insufficiency,

KEY POINTS

- A majority of common congenital heart defects are now repaired in the catheterization laboratory with transcatheter techniques.
- Device closure is now the treatment of choice for secundum atrial septal defect and patent foramen ovale.
- Coil or device closure is currently the treatment of choice for patent ductus arteriosus.
- Stent repair is an effective option for treatment of both native and recurrent coarctation for school-age children, adolescents, and adults.
- Pulmonary insufficiency can now be treated with transcatheter stented valve implantation in adolescents and adults.
- Imaging modalities including echocardiography, angiography, CT, and MRI are crucial for pretreatment evaluation, implantation guidance, and surveillance after repair in patients with congenital heart disease treated with interventional catheterization.

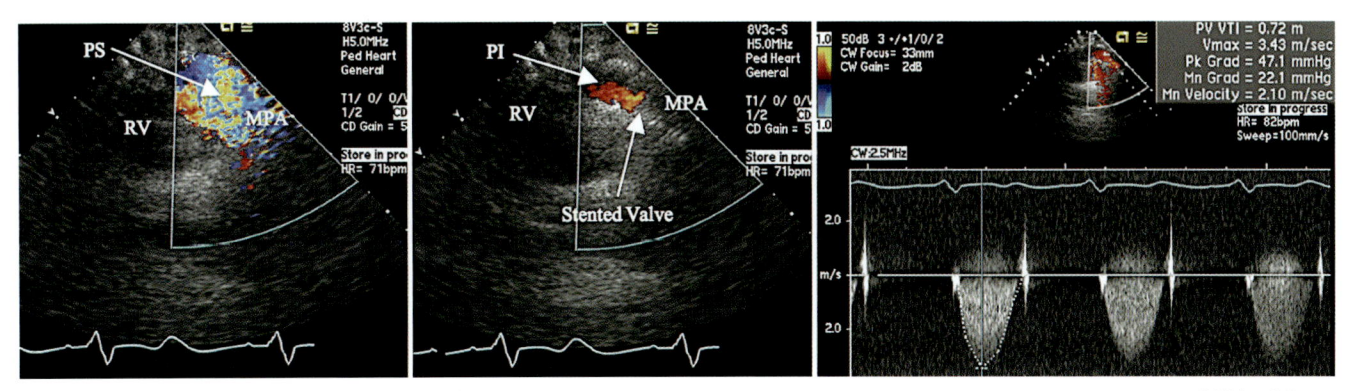

FIGURE 27-31 Echocardiogram 6 months after stent pulmonary valve implantation in a 6-year-old. *Left*, Systolic frame showing mild blood flow acceleration across the stent valve, indicating mild residual stenosis. *Middle*, Diastolic frame showing trivial regurgitant flow. *Right*, Doppler image quantifying mild stenosis with no significant regurgitation, indicating that the implanted valve is functioning well. MPA, main pulmonary artery; PI, pulmonary insufficiency; PS, pulmonary stenosis; RV, right ventricle.

SUGGESTED READINGS

Del Rosario M, Arora N, Gupta V. Role of percutaneous interventions in adult congenital heart disease. J Invasive Cardiol 2008; 20:671-679.

Hijazi ZM, Awad SM. Pediatric cardiac interventions. J Am Coll Cardiol Cardiovasc Interv 2008; 1:603-611.

REFERENCES

1. Samánek M. Children with congenital heart disease: probability of natural survival. Pediatr Cardiol 1992; 13:152-158.
2. King TD, Mills NL. Nonoperative closure of atrial septal defects. Surgery 1974; 75:383-388.
3. Suchoń E, Podolec P, Tomkiewicz-Pajak L, et al. Cardiopulmonary exercise capacity in adults with atrial septal defect. Acta Cardiol 2002; 57:75-76.
4. Du ZD, Hijazi ZM, Kleinman CS, et al. Comparison between transcatheter and surgical closure of secundum atrial septal defect in children and adults: results of a multicenter nonrandomized trial. J Am Coll Cardiol 2002; 39:1836-1844.
5. Hughes ML, Maskell G, Goh TH, Wilkinson JL. Prospective comparison of costs and short term health outcomes of surgical versus device closure of atrial septal defect in children. Heart 2002; 88:67-70.
6. Chessa M, Carminati M, Butera G, et al. Early and late complications associated with transcatheter occlusion of secundum atrial septal defect. J Am Coll Cardiol 2002; 39:1061-1065.
7. Lock JE, Cockerham JT, Keane JF, et al. Transcatheter umbrella closure of congenital heart defects. Circulation 1987; 75:593-599.
8. Bridges ND, Hellenbrand W, Latson L, et al. Transcatheter closure of patent foramen ovale after presumed paradoxical embolism. Circulation 1992; 86:1902-1908.
9. Landzberg MJ, Sloss LJ, Faherty CE, et al. Orthodeoxia-platypnea due to intracardiac shunting—relief with transcatheter double umbrella closure. Cathet Cardiovasc Diagn 1995; 36:247-250.
10. Hagen PT, Scholz DG, Edwards WD. Incidence and size of patent foramen ovale during the first 10 decades of life: an autopsy study of 965 normal hearts. Mayo Clin Proc 1984; 59:17-20.
11. Lechat P, Mas JL, Lascault G, et al. Prevalence of patent foramen ovale in patients with stroke. N Engl J Med 1988; 318:1148-1152.
12. Martín F, Sánchez PL, Doherty E, et al. Percutaneous transcatheter closure of patent foramen ovale in patients with paradoxical embolism. Circulation 2002; 106:1121-1126.
13. Sievert H, Horvath K, Zadan E, et al. Patent foramen ovale closure in patients with transient ischemia attack/stroke. J Interv Cardiol 2001; 14:261-266.
14. Beitzke A, Schuchlenz H, Gamillscheg A, et al. Catheter closure of the persistent foramen ovale: mid-term results in 162 patients. J Interv Cardiol 2001; 14:223-229.
15. Telman G, Yalonetsky S, Kouperberg E, et al. Size of PFO and amount of microembolic signals in patients with ischaemic stroke or TIA. Eur J Neurol 2008; 15:969-972.
16. Mitchell SC, Korones SB, Berendes HW. Congenital heart disease in 56,109 births: incidence and natural history. Circulation 1971; 43:323-332.
17. Portsmann W, Wierny L, Warnke H. Closure of persistent ductus arteriosus without thoracotomy. Ger Med Mon 1967; 12:259-261.
18. Krichenko A, Benson LN, Burrows P, et al. Angiographic classification of the isolated, persistently patent ductus arteriosus and implications for percutaneous catheter occlusion. Am J Cardiol 1989; 63:877-880.
19. Wang JK, Liau CS, Huang JJ, et al. Transcatheter closure of patent ductus arteriosus using Gianturco coils in adolescents and adults. Catheter Cardiovasc Interv 2002; 55:513-518.
20. Bilkis AA, Alwi M, Hasri S, et al. The Amplatzer duct occluder: experience in 209 patients. J Am Coll Cardiol 2001; 37:258-261.
21. Edwards JE, Christensen NA, Clagett OT, et al. Pathologic considerations in coarctation of the aorta. Mayo Clin Proc 1948; 23:324-332.
22. Forbes TJ, Garekar S, Amin Z, et al. Procedural results and acute complications in stenting native and recurrent coarctation of the aorta in patients over 4 years of age: a multi-institutional study. Catheter Cardiovasc Interv 2007; 70:276-285.
23. Lock JE, Bass JC, Amplatz K, et al. Balloon dilation angioplasty of aortic coarctations in infants and children. Circulation 1983; 68:109-116.
24. Tynan M, Finley JP, Fontes V, et al. Balloon angioplasty for the treatment of native coarctation: results of Valvuloplasty and Angioplasty of Congenital Anomalies Registry. Am J Cardiol 1990; 65:790-792.
25. Diethrich EB, Heuser RR, Cardenas JR, et al. Endovascular techniques in adult aortic coarctation: the use of stents for native and recurrent coarctation repair. J Endovasc Surg 1995; 2:183-188.
26. Marshall AC, Perry SB, Keane JF, Lock JE. Early results and medium-term follow-up of stent implantation for mild residual or recurrent aortic coarctation. Am Heart J 2000; 139:1054-1060.
27. Lock JE, Castaneda-Zuniga WR, Fuhrman BP, Bass JL. Balloon dilation angioplasty of hypoplastic and stenotic pulmonary arteries. Circulation 1983; 67:962-967.
28. O'Laughlin MP, Perry SB, Lock JE, Mullins CE. Use of endovascular stents in congenital heart disease. Circulation 1991; 83:1923-1939.
29. Shaffer KM, Mullins CE, Grifka RG, et al. Intravascular stents in congenital heart disease: short- and long-term results from a large single-center experience. J Am Coll Cardiol 1998; 31:661-667.
30. Bergersen LJ, Perry SB, Lock JE. Effect of cutting balloon angioplasty on resistant pulmonary artery stenosis. Am J Cardiol 2003; 91:185-189.
31. Bonhoeffer P, Boudjemline Y, Saliba Z, et al. Percutaneous replacement of pulmonary valve in a right-ventricle to pulmonary-artery prosthetic conduit with valve dysfunction. Lancet 2000; 356:1403-1405.
32. Lurz P, Coats L, Khambadkone S, et al. Percutaneous pulmonary valve implantation: impact of evolving technology and learning curve on clinical outcome. Circulation 2008; 117:1964-1972.
33. Frigiola A, Tsang V, Bull C, et al. Biventricular response after pulmonary valve replacement for right ventricular outflow tract dysfunction: is age a predictor of outcome? Circulation 2008; 118(Suppl):S182-S190.

CHAPTER 28

Congenital Cardiac Surgery

Frederick K. Emge and Christian L. Gilbert

Pediatric cardiology as a specific discipline can track its beginnings to the first ligation of a patent ductus arteriosus by Gross in 1938.[1] Much anatomic research had been done up to that time, but surgical treatment was now an option (Table 28-1). In 1945, Crafoord and Nylin[2] reported the first surgical repair of coarctation of the aorta, and in the same year, surgical palliation of tetralogy of Fallot with an aortopulmonary shunt was described by Taussig and Blalock.

For the repair of intracardiac defects, cardiopulmonary bypass was needed, and in 1955, Lillehei[3] reported successful repair of ventricular septal defect, atrioventricular septal defect, and tetralogy of Fallot with use of this human cross-circulating technique. Kirklin[4] demonstrated the successful use of mechanical cardiopulmonary bypass, reporting eight cases in 1955.

The development of prostaglandins has had an impact on pediatric cardiology and cardiac surgery most significantly. The introduction of prostaglandin E_1 in routine clinical use in the mid-1970s[5] has allowed proper diagnosis in a timely fashion of a child with congenital heart disease while permitting further clinical stabilization and refinement of the medical management and surgical intervention.

With imaging, cardiac catheterization was a necessary advance for the diagnosis and treatment of congenital cardiac defects, and by the 1950s,[6] many centers were routinely studying children with heart defects and planning surgical interventions on the basis of these studies. However, the development of two-dimensional echocardiography and color flow Doppler imaging by the 1980s significantly changed the ability to diagnose infants and children with heart disease and refined the ability of surgeons to perform more complex procedures in infants and young children. Three- and four-dimensional multiplanar echocardiography is a developing imaging modality that is affecting how we visualize intracardiac anatomy and great vessel disease, and it is rapidly becoming an expectation of the surgeon as surgical intervention is planned.

The more intriguing aspect of congenital heart disease is the fact that within the next few years, there will be more adults with congenital heart disease than children with congenital heart disease (Table 28-2).[7] Survival to adulthood with a diagnosis of congenital heart disease is now an expectation.

This chapter serves as a general overview of congenital heart disease, surgical considerations, and imaging strategies. More detailed aspects of these defects (Table 28-3) are addressed in subsequent chapters.

SURGERY FOR ACYANOTIC CONGENITAL HEART LESIONS WITH A SHUNT

Description and Special Anatomic Considerations

Acyanotic congenital heart disease (Table 28-4) is characterized by a lack of cyanosis. In further defining these disorders, they are often classified on the basis of the presence or absence of left-to-right shunt.

Ventricular septal defect (VSD), the most common form of congenital heart disease, represents approximately one third of all major congenital cardiac defects. VSDs are generally classified into one of four groups, depending on their location in the interventricular septum (Fig. 28-1). These may be associated with other cardiac defects, such as atrioventricular valve defects, coarctation of the aorta, and other left-to-right shunts. The ventricular septum anatomy is complex, and many associated anatomic structures are key in the consideration of the repair, such as location of the conduction system of the heart.

Atrial septal defects, which usually cause volume overload of the right ventricle and increased pulmonary blood flow, are also categorized on the basis of their location within the atrial septum. These defects can go undiagnosed for decades and can be associated with other defects, such as partial anomalous pulmonary venous return. Unfortunately, when they are undiagnosed for several decades, fixed pulmonary vascular changes may develop that prohibit surgical correction.

TABLE 28-1	Chronology of Selected Milestones in Pediatric Cardiology
1936	Maude Abbott publishes landmark atlas with historical data on patients with congenital heart disease.
1939	Gross and Hubbard publish case reports of a 7½-year-old patient with successful ligation of a patent ductus.
1945	Crafoord and Nylin publish report of successful coarctation repair in two patients.
1945	Blalock and Taussig publish report of successful shunts in three tetralogy patients.
1949	Janeway invites Nadas to develop pediatric cardiology at Boston Children's Hospital.
1955	Kirklin and associates report open heart surgery in eight patients with congenital heart disease.
1964	Mustard reports atrial repair of transposition of the great vessels in a 23-month-old.
1966	Raskind and Miller report balloon atrial septostomy in three infants.
1966	Ross and Somerville report homograft repair of pulmonary atresia in an 8-year-old.
1968	McGoon and associates report repair of truncus in an 8-year-old.
1971	Fontan and Baudet report successful repair of tricuspid atresia in two of three patients aged 12, 23, and 35 years.
1975	Jatene and associates report arterial switch for transposition of the great arteries.
1975	Norwood and associates report successful palliatives of hypoplastic left heart syndrome in two of three patients. Early 1970s M-mode echocardiography begins widespread use.
1975	Elliot and associates report ductal dilation with prostaglandin E in two patients.
1976	Bargeron and associates describe axial cineangiography; late 1970s, echocardiography is introduced.
1982	Kan and associates report percutaneous valvuloplasty for valvular pulmonary stenosis.
1980s-1990s	Doppler studies, color flow, fetal studies, and transesophageal echocardiography become vital part of pediatric cardiology.
1980s	Explosion of studies show possibility and success of percutaneous treatment of pulmonary artery stenosis, coarctation, and aortic stenosis.
1990s	Interventional catheterization therapy for patent ductus arteriosus, pulmonary and aortic stenosis, pulmonary artery stenosis, and many atrial septal defects becomes standard part of management.

From Graham TP Jr. Minimizing the morbidity of pediatric cardiovascular disease—historical perspective; pediatric cardiology. Prog Pediatr Cardiol 2005; 20:1-6.

TABLE 28-2 Extrapolated Prevalence of Adult Congenital Heart Disease in the General Population and Extrapolated Numbers to the United States and Canada

Country	Group	Country Population (year 2000)	Prevalence per 1000 Population		Total Population Living with CHD (year 2000)		
			Severe	Other	Severe	Other	Total
United States	Children	72,293,812	1.45	10.44	104,826	754,747	859,573
	Adults	209,128,094	0.38	3.71	79,469	775,865	855,334
Canada	Children	7,137,778	1.45	10.44	10,350	74,518	84,868
	Adults	23,551,257	0.38	3.71	8,949	87,375	96,324

CHD, congenital heart disease.
Data from Marelli AJ, Mackie AS, Ionescu-Ittu R, et al. Congenital heart disease in the general population: changing prevalence and age distribution. Circulation 2007; 115:163-172.

TABLE 28-3 Relative Frequency of Major Congenital Heart Lesions*

Lesion	Percentage of all Lesions
Ventricular septal defect	35-30
Atrial septal defect (secundum)	6-8
Patent ductus arteriosus	6-8
Coarctation of aorta	5-7
Tetralogy of Fallot	5-7
Pulmonary valve stenosis	5-7
Aortic valve stenosis	4-7
D-Transposition of great arteries	3-5
Hypoplastic left ventricle	1-3
Hypoplastic right ventricle	1-3
Truncus arteriosus	1-2
Total anomalous pulmonary venous return	1-2
Tricuspid atresia	1-2
Single ventricle	1-2
Double-outlet right ventricle	1-2
Others	5-10

*Excluding patent ductus arteriosus in preterm neonates, bicuspid aortic valve, physiologic peripheral pulmonic stenosis, and mitral valve prolapse.

Aortopulmonary-level shunts, such as a patent ductus arteriosus, are less common as isolated defects because they typically close spontaneously in the newborn period. However, they are often seen in conjunction with other complex congenital heart disease. If they are undiagnosed during the course of many years, there is some risk for bacterial endocarditis (rare), and if the connection is large, Eisenmenger syndrome or fixed irreversible pulmonary vascular changes may develop. Aortopulmonary windows, which are direct communications between the great vessels, are much more uncommon and can be challenging to diagnose if one is not attentive to subtle echocardiographic findings.

Aortic root–to–right heart shunts, such as a ruptured sinus of Valsalva aneurysm, coronary artery fistula, or anomalous origin of the left coronary artery from the pulmonary artery, are uncommon. However, a high index of suspicion must be present when one evaluates a newborn or older infant with a diagnosis of dilated cardiomyopathy because anomalous origin of the left coronary artery from the pulmonary artery may be difficult to exclude as a source of the dysfunction.

TABLE 28-4 Acyanotic Congenital Heart Disease with a Left-to-Right Shunt

Atrial-Level Shunt
Atrial septal defect: causes diastolic overload of the right ventricle and increased pulmonary blood flow
  Ostium secundum, the most common defect, involves fossa ovalis in midseptal location.
    Ostium primum anomalies, a form of atrioventricular septal defect, occur immediately adjacent to atrioventricular valves, either of which may be deformed and incompetent.
Sinus venosus type occurs high in the atrial septum, near entry of the superior vena cava.
Partial anomalous pulmonary venous connection
Atrial septal defect with mitral stenosis (Lutembacher syndrome)

Ventricular-Level Shunt
Ventricular septal defects: either isolated defects or one component of a combination of anomalies
  Usually one opening situated in the septum membrane
  Functional disturbance depends on size and pulmonary vascular bed status rather than on defect location.
Ventricular septal defect with aortic regurgitation
Ventricular septal defect with left ventricular-to-right atrial shunt

Aortic Root–to–Right Heart Shunt
Ruptured sinus of Valsalva aneurysm with fistula
Coronary arteriovenous fistula (unusual)
  Consists of communication between a coronary artery and another coronary chamber, usually the coronary sinus, right atrium, or right ventricle
Anomalous origin of left coronary artery from pulmonary trunk

Aortopulmonary-Level Shunt
Patent ductus arteriosus
  Failure of the ductus arteriosus to close after birth
Aortopulmonary window

Multiple-Level Shunts
Complete common atrioventricular canal (endocardial cushion defect with atrial and ventricular septal defect)
Ventricular septal defect with atrial septal defect (unassociated with endocardial cushion defect)
Ventricular septal defect with patent ductus arteriosus

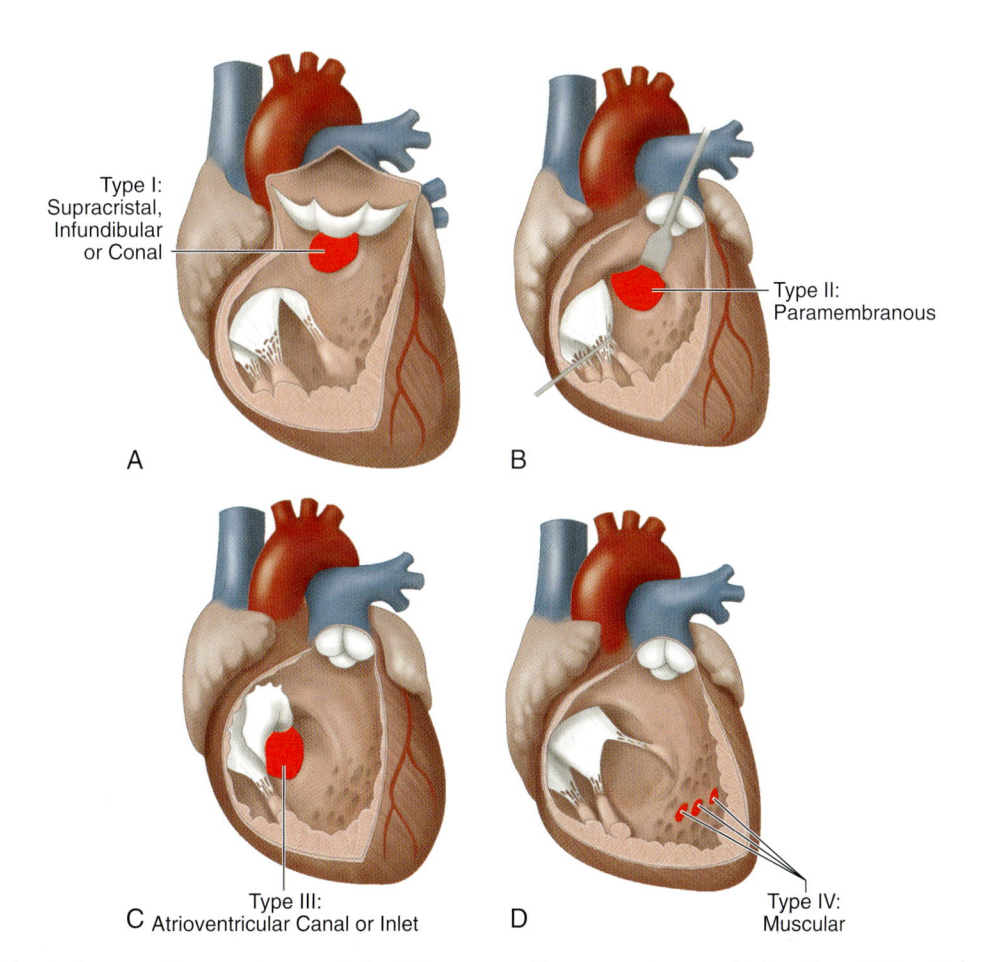

■ **FIGURE 28-1** The classic anatomic nomenclature assigning VSDs to one of four anatomic types. *(Redrawn from Wells WJ, Lindesmith GG. Ventricular septal defect. In Arciniegas E [ed]. Pediatric Cardiac Surgery. Chicago, Year Book Medical, 1985.)*

Multiple-level shunts are typified by the complete atrioventricular septal defect (AVSD, previously known as endocardial cushion defect) with a common atrial- and ventricular-level shunt. A variety of any or all of these defects can combine to present with multiple-level shunts. The most challenging aspect for the surgeon in addressing AVSD is often the common valve function and anatomy.

Indications

Surgical intervention for acyanotic heart defects with left-to-right shunt is almost always primarily driven by clinical symptoms and secondarily by risks of not intervening in a timely fashion. Many lesions can be corrected in infancy but do not need to be addressed until the child is older (or larger) to allow better surgical field access or more optimal tissue "durability." For example, atrioventricular valve tissue is very thin and friable and may be better manipulated at some point later than 1 month of age, if surgery can be safely delayed without resulting in any negative clinical outcomes.

In this broad category of defects, the usual driving indication for early surgical intervention is congestive heart failure and how difficult it is to control with medical management. This is balanced against the surgical risks for the various procedures and the possible comorbidities that may exist as a part of a clinical syndrome or initial clinical presentation. An infant's weight and gestational age also may play a role in the surgical timing for many of these defects. A typical scenario for surgical intervention based on prematurity and significant lung disease as a result of left-to-right shunt is a patent ductus arteriosus. The advent of indomethacin[8] as medical management for closure of these defects has significantly reduced the need for surgical intervention.[9] However, in extreme prematurity, renal disease, and severe diastolic "runoff" through a large patent ductus arteriosus, surgery may be a relative emergency.

For example, surgical timing for closure of a hemodynamically significant VSD may be indicated at a few weeks or as late as a few years. The later closure may be indicated for a late-identified supracristal VSD or a perimembranous VSD with a coexistent subaortic membrane or prolapse of the aortic valve leaflets. Both of these defects have been implicated in progressive aortic valve damage,[10,11] even though they may be quite small and have no risks for long-term pulmonary vascular disease or congestive heart failure.

The diagnosis of anomalous left coronary artery is typically an emergent one; acute surgical intervention is indicated to reestablish appropriate coronary blood flow and to avert continued or permanent myocardial damage or infarction. Less commonly, these anomalies may present after a referral for a murmur in an otherwise normal infant or child. Although they are rare presentations, surgical intervention may be delayed for a few days to allow further diagnostic evaluation, if indicated, or when other medical considerations exist.

With the diagnosis of AVSD, there can be tremendous variability of the surgical timing based on the level of shunting (i.e., atrial vs. ventricular), the complexity of the associated common atrioventricular valve disease, and the associated clinical status (Fig. 28-2).

Finally, the surgical timing and types of surgery that may be employed to correct these defects are biased against the surgical experience of the performing center. This bias will be derived from a variety of issues—a surgeon's level of expertise, perfusion and anesthesia support, and, in some cases, the presence of advanced support in the postoperative period, such as extracorporeal membrane oxygenation programs.

Contraindications

As discussed, there are many relative contraindications to surgical intervention that are usually related to weight, gestational age, coexistent disease, and surgical center bias. However, there are a few absolute contraindications to surgical interventions for acyanotic cardiac defects with left-to-right shunt. The primary contraindication to cardiac surgery for complete repair of these defects is the presence of fixed pulmonary hypertension. A pulmonary-to-systemic vascular resistance ratio greater than 0.9:1 or pulmonary arteriolar resistance greater than 12 Wood units is regarded as an absolute contraindication to surgery. A pulmonary arteriolar resistance of more than 8 Wood units obtained during cardiac catheterization with pulmonary vasodilation is also a contraindication to surgery.

A reactive pulmonary vascular bed noted during provocative testing in the catheterization laboratory may be a relative contraindication and merits further discussion. Small atrial septal defects with systemic-to-pulmonary shunts of less than 0.7 may be a relative contraindication to surgical or device closure, depending on other pathologic processes.

Outcomes and Complications

Overall surgical results for this diverse spectrum of diseases are very good, with disease-specific mortality much less than 5% for the majority of these lesions and morbidity generally in the same range. Surgical center bias and preexistent morbidity or complicating factors will dramatically affect these predicted results.

Imaging Findings

Preoperative Planning

Echocardiography is the typical diagnostic modality that is used to plan for surgical intervention, but on occasion, cardiac catheterization is still needed to help define questions surrounding physiology or other defects. Intraoperative transesophageal echocardiography is routine and helpful in the immediate preoperative surgical decision process and in defining postoperative residual anatomic defects, such as persistent or residual VSD or peri-patch "leak" with left-to-right shunt.

The role of cardiac catheterization is to answer highly specific questions related to physiology that cannot be deduced from other noninvasive imaging modalities, such as Doppler echocardiography or phase contrast velocity cardiac MR sequences. Other risk factors (e.g., mechanical

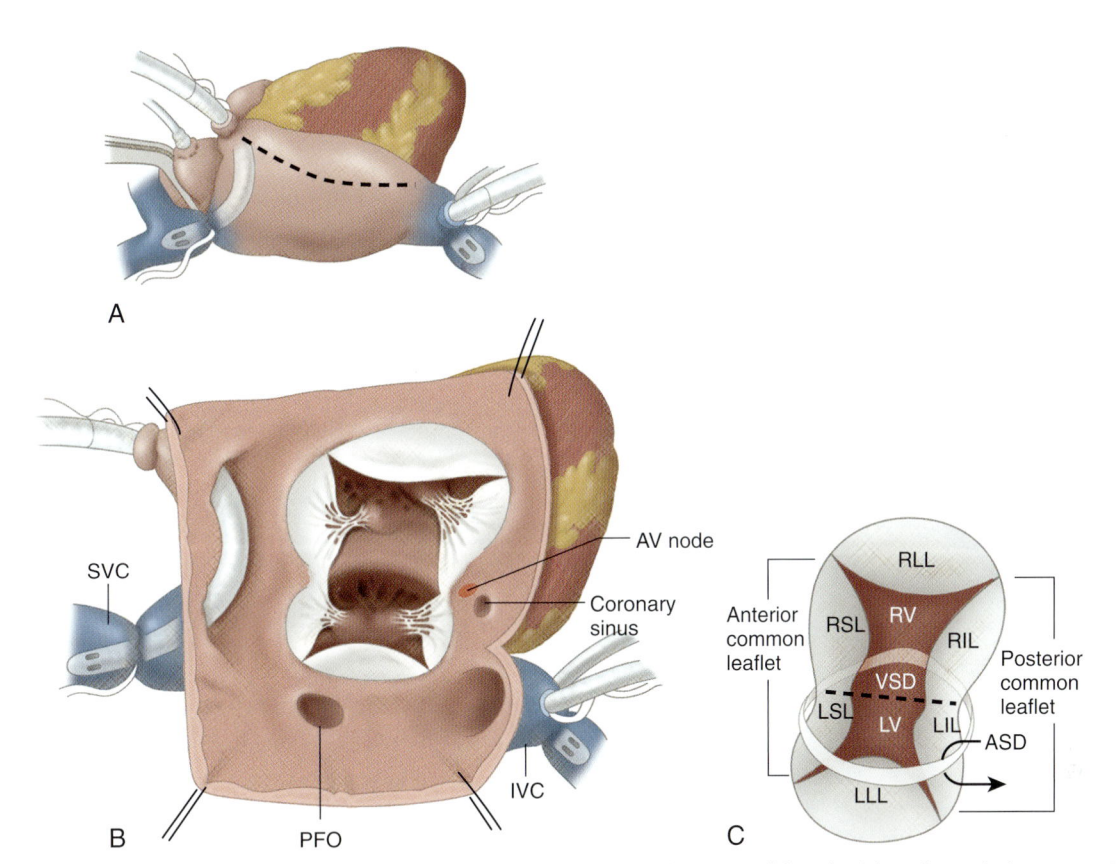

FIGURE 28-2 Exposure and assessment of anatomy. **A,** The atrial incision (*broken line*) is parallel to the right atrioventricular groove. **B,** The right atrium has been opened after administration of cardioplegia. Note the coronary sinus and the location of the atrioventricular (AV) node. **C,** Relationship of ventricular septal defect (VSD), atrial septal defect (ASD), and common atrioventricular valve. The valve leaflets are identified as follows: LIL, left inferior leaflet; LLL, left lateral leaflet; LSL, left superior leaflet; RIL, right inferior leaflet; RLL, right lateral leaflet; and RSL, right superior leaflet. IVC, inferior vena cava; LV, left ventricle; PFO, patent foramen ovale; RV, right ventricle; SVC, superior vena cava. *(Redrawn from Backer CL, Mavroudis C, Alboliras ET, Zales VR. Repair of complete atrioventricular canal defects: results with the two-patch technique. Ann Thorac Surg 1995; 60:530-537.)*

ventilation, extreme prematurity, or marked hemodynamic instability) may preclude cardiac MR because of the extended time and limited access to the patient and may influence the decision to perform a diagnostic cardiac catheterization or CT as well.

The role of MRI is in diagnosis of anomalous pulmonary venous drainage in complex defects and particularly in the sinus venosus atrial septal defects, in which the incidence of partial anomalous pulmonary venous return may be as high as 85%.[12] Their location within the mediastinum may make reliable echocardiographic diagnosis impossible, particularly in the operating room at the time of operative intervention.

Postoperative Surveillance

Because of the echocardiogram's portability, time to complete a study, and relative cost and safety, it remains the standard of care for routine postoperative surveillance of the majority of pediatric cardiac surgical interventions. However, cardiac MRI and, to a lesser extent, cardiac and thoracic CT angiography have an increasingly important role in long-term assessment of selected defects.

Consideration is given to these modalities when there is concern about the patency of repaired anomalous pulmonary veins or for periodic evaluation of regurgitant volumes and absolute chamber size in persistent or progressive aortic or mitral insufficiency after surgery.

SURGERY FOR ACYANOTIC CONGENITAL HEART LESIONS WITHOUT A SHUNT

Description and Special Anatomic Considerations

Acyanotic heart defects without a shunt generally have normal oxygen saturations at rest, unless they suffer from an A-a gradient secondary to pulmonary vascular congestion from their cardiac defect. These defects[5] include left-sided and right-sided heart obstructive lesions and regurgitant valve disease (Table 28-5).

Mitral valve disease is a rare entity in children as a primary defect although it is a common sequela in postoperative AVSD patients. As in aortic valve disease, in the younger children and infants with mitral valve disease, there is much effort made to delay surgical interventions for these disease entities. Surgical palliation with surgical repairs of the valves has been the preferred choice because homograft replacements have limited durability. Both repair and homograft replacement may provide early hemodynamic success but often require early reoperation

TABLE 28-5 Acyanotic Congenital Heart Disease without a Shunt

Left-Sided Heart Malformations
Congenital obstruction to left atrial inflow
    Cor triatriatum
    Pulmonary vein stenosis
    Mitral stenosis
Mitral regurgitation
    Atrioventricular septal (endocardial cushion defect)
    Congenitally corrected transposition of the great arteries
    Anomalous origin of the left coronary artery from the pulmonary trunk
    Miscellaneous (e.g., double-orifice mitral valve, congenital perforations, accessory commissures with anomalous chordal insertion, congenitally short or absent chordae, cleft posterior leaflet, parachute mitral valve)
Primary dilated endocardial fibroelastosis
Aortic stenosis
    Valvular stenosis
    Subaortic stenosis
Idiopathic hypertrophic subaortic stenosis is most common; also called hypertrophic cardiomyopathy
Discrete subvalvular: resembles valvular aortic stenosis
    Supravalvular stenosis: localized or diffuse narrowing of the ascending aorta originating just above coronary arteries at the superior margin of the sinuses of Valsalva
Aortic valve regurgitation
Coarctation of the aorta
    Narrowing or constriction of the aorta lumen may occur anywhere along the length but most commonly distal to origin of left subclavian artery near insertion of the ligamentum arteriosum.
Hypoplastic left heart syndrome

Right-Sided Heart Malformations
Acyanotic Ebstein anomaly of the tricuspid valve
Pulmonic stenosis
    Valvular pulmonic stenosis: the most common form of isolated right ventricular obstruction
    Infundibular
    Subinfundibular
    Supravalvular (stenosis of pulmonary artery and its branches)
Congenital pulmonary valve regurgitation
Idiopathic dilation of the pulmonary trunk

and ultimate mechanical valve replacement. Although it is a durable solution for many decades, the size of the patient often limits the size of the mechanical valve that can be used. Furthermore, the need for long-term anticoagulation can be of significant medical risk for the complications of bleeding in these children while having a negative impact on their quality of life.

Coarctation of the aorta may occur as an isolated defect or in association with various other lesions, most commonly bicuspid aortic valve and VSD.[13] Surgical repair of coarctation of the aorta has been one of the oldest surgical procedures available. Early limitations revolved around the size or weight of the infant, but these considerations have virtually disappeared. The controversy that continues to smolder is the role of balloon dilation or stent for the native coarctation of the aorta. Additional intracardiac defects, such as a posterior malaligned VSD, may complicate the surgery and the surgical approach. Complete repair has become the generally accepted approach to these complex defects because the prior approach of repair of the coarctation of the aorta and pulmonary artery banding has resulted in complications such as double-outlet obstruction early postoperatively and a more complicated medical and surgical management approach long term.

The extreme forms of obstructive left-sided heart lesions include hypoplastic left heart syndrome and its many variants.[14] These patients can have varying degrees of hypoplasia or atresia of the left ventricle, aorta, and mitral or aortic valves, usually in some combination thereof. They all have coarctation of the aorta. Because these are duct-dependent lesions, they tend to be manifested in the first few days of life, although they may on occasion present late at several weeks of age. It is a lethal condition. Norwood first presented his approach to palliation of this entity in 1979. It essentially created a hemodynamically stable single ventricle, which could proceed down the single ventricle pathway of palliation with a bidirectional caval anastomosis and a subsequent Fontan procedure.

Acyanotic right-sided heart lesions are few in number but tend to be more approachable through interventional cardiac catheterization procedures of balloon pulmonary valvuloplasty, angioplasty, or pulmonary artery stent placement.

Anomalies of the tricuspid valve, such as Ebstein anomaly,[15] tend to be manifested with cyanosis in the newborn period, and the infants can be quite ill. If acyanotic, they are typically diagnosed after an echocardiogram is obtained as part of evaluation of a murmur. The diagnosis of Ebstein anomaly may be a coincident finding made as part of a work-up for Wolff-Parkinson-White syndrome–mediated supraventricular tachycardia. The mean age at diagnosis of the acyanotic forms of this disease is the middle teenage years. These anomalies are almost uniformly associated with atrial septal defects.

Indications and Contraindications

Surgical interventions for both aortic and mitral valve disease share similar indications and contraindications.

The primary indications for early intervention in the neonate or young infant are primarily clinically driven. As previously discussed, there are limited options in the smaller patient for operative intervention because mechanical valve replacement is fraught with an extraordinary number of risks and the need for early and repeated surgeries to essentially "up-size" these valves as the patient grows.

Catheter-based intervention for severe aortic valve stenosis in the newborn[16] is typically the preferred option. However, often less than perfect reduction in the stenosis gradient is tolerated such that one minimizes the risks for significant aortic insufficiency.

Aortic insufficiency is a much more difficult disease to treat in infants and children. A variety of clinical parameters have been used to prompt surgical intervention.[17] Decreasing clinical activity level, decreasing left ventricular performance (as measured by echocardiography or MRI), and progressive left ventricular dilation and secondary mitral insufficiency or left atrial hypertension have been considered useful in formulating surgical intervention plans.

The Ross procedure has been an effective surgical procedure to provide good relief of aortic valve disease in children while avoiding many of the long-term medical management concerns of a mechanical aortic valve replacement. However, this has some significant controversy associated with it.[18] More recent surgical approaches have aimed at "reconstruction" of the valve leaflets, although this is controversial as well and appears to be dependent on the surgical center's abilities.

Mitral valve repair continues to be the optimal goal of most surgeons when possible, secondary to the issues revolving around mitral valve replacement at an early age. Somatic growth and the issues of chronic anticoagulation in the younger and more active patients empower surgeons to continue to develop surgical repair procedures for the mitral valve.

The Norwood procedure for the hypoplastic left heart constellation of defects has significantly altered the approach to these formerly uniformly fatal lesions. Modifications of this procedure have resulted in the Sano shunt and a move toward even more creative attempts at palliation, such as the hybrid procedure, or patent ductus arteriosus stent and bilateral pulmonary artery banding.

Pulmonary valve stenosis has long been a disease that lends itself to interventional catheterization procedures.[19] More recent use of radiofrequency catheters to perforate pulmonary atresia, as a method to pass a wire and then a balloon catheter across such an obstruction to achieve some degree of palliation, is an exciting advancement in the hands of the skilled interventionalist. Surgical open pulmonary valvotomy is still an option, but it is often reserved for unique circumstances at this time.

Postoperative Surveillance

As is repeatedly emphasized in the diagnosis and surveillance of children with cardiac defects, the consideration of noninvasive and radiation-free imaging modalities is mandatory. The role of echocardiography as a standard follow-up imaging modality is typical. Exercise treadmill testing and periodic rhythm monitoring are also common for children and adults with congenital heart disease.

What is important is the growing role of cardiac MR for both functional and routine anatomic surveillance. In combination with newer technologies such as three-dimensional echocardiography to evaluate valve morphology, much can be done to mitigate complications of surgery or the natural history of these defects.

Cardiac CT is an added modality, although it does carry with it some risk of radiation exposure.

SURGERY FOR CYANOTIC CONGENITAL HEART LESIONS WITH INCREASED PULMONARY BLOOD FLOW

Description and Special Anatomic Considerations

These congenital cardiac lesions are characterized by cyanosis or bluish coloration of the skin due to arterial oxygen desaturation resulting from the shunting of systemic venous blood to the arterial circulation. To help understand the basic physiology involved in these lesions, they are typically classified by degree of pulmonary blood flow (Table 28-6).

Complete transposition of the great arteries is the most common cyanotic congenital heart lesion that presents in neonates.[20] This entity was first described more than 200 years ago. However, until the development of the surgical atrial septectomy in the 1950s and the balloon atrial septostomy in the 1960s, early death was expected. These palliative interventions allowed the development of physiologic palliative procedures, such as the atrial switch operation (Mustard and Senning),[21] and later the anatomic correction with the arterial switch procedure. Although survival rates for the arterial switch procedure approach 95%, significant anatomic variations influence the outcome. These include associated cardiac anomalies, relationship of the great arteries to each other, and coronary artery anatomy variants.[22] Echocardiography is the mainstay of this diagnosis, which is one that often may be made in utero by fetal echocardiography.

Single-ventricle defects are rare defects and can present with either increased or decreased pulmonary blood flow.

TABLE 28-6 Cyanotic Congenital Heart Disease with Increased Pulmonary Blood Flow

Complete Transposition of the Great Arteries
Aorta arises rightward anteriorly from the right ventricle.
Pulmonary artery emerges leftward and posteriorly from the left ventricle.
Two separate and parallel circulations result.
Communication between the two circulations must exist after birth to sustain life.
  Two thirds of patients have patent ductus arteriosus.
  One third have associated ventricular septal defect.

Single Ventricle
A family of complex lesions with both atrioventricular valves or a common atrioventricular valve opening into a single ventricular chamber

To strictly fit this diagnosis, the single ventricle is missing the nontrabeculated inflow region of either ventricle. This differentiates these defects from tricuspid atresia patients, who typically have a smooth inlet of the remaining ventricle. These cardiac defects invariably have other associated cardiac defects, such as complex outflow tract obstruction or interrupted aortic arch. They also may have significant noncardiac congenital defects.[23] Two-dimensional echocardiography is diagnostic for single ventricle and usually provides most detail of the associated cardiac defects.

Indications

The surgical intervention in these defects depends on the age at presentation, the size and weight of the patient, and the presence of associated congenital cardiac and extracardiac defects.

Complete repair of the patient with transposition of the great arteries with the arterial switch operation is the goal of the experienced cardiothoracic surgeon. The age at which to attempt complete repair is generally within the first 1 to 2 weeks of life because the left ventricular function and mass change as pulmonary vascular resistance changes with age. However, many variables have an impact on these decisions.[24]

There is still the occasional patient for whom the atrial switch or a Rastelli procedure may be the optimal intervention. The surgical approach to the patient with single ventricle remains one in which the preoperative medical management and the skill of the congenital cardiac surgeon dictate much of the operative timing and decision-making.

The single-ventricle pathway,[25] as it has become known, requires careful medical and surgical management of pulmonary vascular resistance and single-ventricle systolic function, with an attempt to preserve single-ventricle diastolic function. The staged approach to ultimate palliation with a Fontan variant repair of these defects is now common. These palliative procedures may include pulmonary artery banding, pulmonary artery transection and creation of systemic-to-pulmonary artery shunt, and the Damus-Kaye-Stansel approach for selected defects. Caval anastomoses, hemi-Fontan, and the Fontan variant are the typical considerations for subsequent surgery for these patients. However, when this palliation fails or the poor hemodynamics of the patient preclude consideration of a Fontan intervention, cardiac transplantation remains a viable option.

Contraindications

Pulmonary vascular resistance has a common role for this category of defects, although for different reasons. The ability to perform the arterial switch operation for transposition of the great arteries is influenced by "deconditioning," changes that occur within the left ventricular myocardium as a result of decreasing pulmonary artery resistance, which typically occurs within the first several days after birth. Although it is not an absolute contraindication to the arterial switch operation, alternative approaches may be needed to "recondition" the left ventricle; extracorporeal membrane oxygenation or left ventricular support may be employed, or in certain cases, the atrial switch operation may be considered. Abnormal coronary artery patterns, an early contraindication, are no longer considered a contraindication to this operation.

Palliative operations for the single ventricle are dependent on preservation of good ventricular systolic and diastolic function as well as a low-resistance pulmonary vascular bed to allow passive return of blood from the pulmonary vascular bed to the receiving atrium of the single ventricle. Problems with either, and often both, may limit the ability to fully palliate these patients.

Outcomes and Complications

Surgical results of the arterial switch operation are influenced by a large number of factors. However, the simple arterial switch procedure in a patient with an intact ventricular septum has survival results that are above 95%. It is the associated congenital cardiac defects that often increase the potential morbidity and increase the need for a diverse approach to monitoring of these patients postoperatively. Clinical follow-up, complemented by echocardiography and cardiac MRI, has become common in the long-term assessment of these patients.

The single-ventricle patients have more issues involving close follow-up of the passive cavopulmonary circuits, which are necessary to provide adequate cardiac output and oxygenation of blood.[26] The role of MRI and, for selected patients, CT has become common as a regular method to serially observe them longitudinally and to plan for any necessary interventions.

SURGERY FOR CYANOTIC CONGENITAL HEART LESIONS WITH DECREASED PULMONARY BLOOD FLOW

Description and Special Anatomic Considerations

The typical congenital cardiac lesions considered in this category of defects include tetralogy of Fallot, tricuspid atresia, and Ebstein anomaly (Table 28-7). Acyanotic patients can also present these defects, as noted before, and their manifestations are influenced by the degree of pulmonary blood flow.

Tetralogy of Fallot represents approximately 7% to 10% of cases of congenital heart disease and is the most common cause of cyanotic congenital heart disease in all ages. This defect is composed of four abnormalities: VSD with anterior malalignment, over-riding aorta, right ventricular outflow tract hypertrophy, and valvular pulmonary stenosis. The degree of valvular pulmonary stenosis and right ventricular hypertrophy or outflow tract obstruction dictates the time of presentation because these patients may be acyanotic at birth and infancy if this is not significant. However, the natural history of this lesion is progression of the cyanosis as the hypertrophy and pulmonary stenosis worsen with age.

TABLE 28-7 Cyanotic Congenital Heart Disease with Decreased Pulmonary Blood Flow

Tricuspid Atresia
Tricuspid valve atresia
Interatrial communication
Hypoplasia of right ventricle and pulmonary artery frequently occurs.

Ebstein Anomaly
Downward displacement of tricuspid valve into the right ventricle
 Caused by anomalous attachment of tricuspid leaflets
 Valve tissue is dysplastic and results in tricuspid regurgitation.
Right ventricle is often hypoplastic.
Abnormally situated tricuspid orifice produces "atrialized" portion of the right ventricle between the atrioventricular ring and valve origin, continuous with the right atrium chamber.

Tetralogy of Fallot
Obstruction to right ventricular outflow, usually infundibular (subpulmonary valvular) stenosis
Malaligned ventricular septal defect
Aortic override of the ventricular septal defect
Right ventricular hypertrophy

Tricuspid atresia is the third most common cyanotic congenital defect. Again, these patients can present with varying amounts of pulmonary blood flow and a variety of associated congenital cardiac defects. Pulmonary obstruction is usually associated with normally related great vessels. This is a cyanotic defect for which electrocardiography can be quite helpful in the diagnosis because right-sided electrical forces are typically diminished or absent.

Ebstein anomaly can be manifested in the neonatal period with intense cyanosis. This presentation is often associated with right ventricular outflow obstruction from the inferiorly displaced septal leaflet of the tricuspid valve, right ventricular hypoplasia, and elevated pulmonary vascular resistance. These are perhaps some of the sickest infants with congenital heart disease because of the associated defects and complicating physiology.

Indications

Definitive surgical repair for the patients with tetralogy of Fallot has become the goal of the pediatric cardiologist and cardiothoracic surgeon.[27] However, palliation is still needed for a variety of complicating cardiac and extracardiac issues.

Some adult patients may have undergone initial palliation with either a Potts shunt (descending aorta to pulmonary artery) or a Waterston shunt (ascending aorta to pulmonary artery) as a method to improve pulmonary blood flow. These carried significant risks for pulmonary artery hypertension and distorted pulmonary artery anatomy. For this reason, these procedures have been abandoned and replaced with the modified Blalock-Taussig shunt (typically Gore-Tex) as a palliative procedure to augment pulmonary blood flow. This procedure often provides several months to years of time to allow other medical issues to be addressed as well as adequate growth to permit corrective surgery.

Definitive surgery involves closure of the VSD, resection of the right ventricular outflow tract muscle obstruction, and elimination of the valvular pulmonary stenosis. Because of the long-term chronic right ventricular volume overload from the common pulmonary insufficiency seen after resection of the right ventricular outflow tract or pulmonary stenosis, there have been recent attempts to preserve some pulmonary valve tissue and to tolerate some degree of pulmonary stenosis. The belief is that this may limit the degree of insufficiency and protect the right ventricle from the damage of chronic volume overload and ventricular dilation.

Tricuspid atresia patients are almost always confined to a single-ventricle palliation pathway. This may involve a Blalock-Taussig shunt to augment pulmonary blood flow but limit damage to the pulmonary vascular bed for chronic pressure or volume overload of the pulmonary arteries.[28]

Contraindications

The contraindications to definitive surgery for correction of tetralogy of Fallot are related to the native pulmonary artery architecture. In more extreme forms of the lesion, the pulmonary arteries may be very small, noncontinuous, or almost exclusively supplied by systemic collaterals. On rare occasion, there may not be a corrective or palliative option. Much work has been done to try to improve pulmonary blood flow through unifocalization procedures with systemic-to-pulmonary artery shunts. However, these patients have varied native pulmonary architecture, so no absolute surgical options may be available.

Patients with tricuspid atresia have contraindications to single-ventricle palliation options similar to those of other single-ventricle patients. Pulmonary vascular resistance and ventricular performance dictate whether these are viable options or if cardiac transplantation is the only endpoint.

Outcomes and Complications

Surgical outcomes for patients with tetralogy of Fallot are very much dependent on the native pulmonary artery anatomy. With proper anatomic substrate, surgical survival for definitive repair approaches 95%. Palliative shunts can be associated with pulmonary artery distortion and stenosis at the anastomosis site between the shunt and pulmonary artery. Although uncommon, acute thrombosis of the shunt can precipitate a life-threatening event from a lack of pulmonary blood flow and severe cyanosis.

Tricuspid atresia patients tend to do quite well with the single-ventricle pathway for palliation. Because these patients have a normally functioning left ventricle, they tend to be the ideal patients for excellent long-term survival after the Fontan procedure, with a good quality of life. Three patients with tricuspid atresia were the first to undergo the Fontan operation, which he published in 1971. It is not uncommon for these patients who have done well to be able to successfully carry a pregnancy to term with little adverse hemodynamic effect. However, this does require close pre-conception planning and cardiac surveillance during the pregnancy.[29]

KEY POINTS

- Repair of left-to-right shunts is primarily driven by clinical symptoms, and many lesions can be corrected in later childhood rather than in infancy.
- Coarctation of the aorta is amenable to early surgery. There is some controversy related to the role of angioplasty and stent placement as a primary treatment.
- Admixture lesions, such as transposition of the great arteries, are usually treated with a complete repair.
- In tetralogy of Fallot, definitive repair is the usual treatment. To reduce the risk of postoperative pulmonary regurgitation that can lead to right ventricular volume overload, some surgeons have recently tolerated a degree of postoperative pulmonary stenosis.
- For congenital heart disease, echocardiography is the mainstay of preoperative planning and postoperative monitoring. The role of MRI and CT has grown to replace catheterization in many instances for anatomic and functional information.

SUGGESTED READINGS

Keane JF, Fyler DC, Lock JE. Nadas' Pediatric Cardiology. 2nd ed. Philadelphia, Saunders, 2006.

Lai W, Mertens L, Cohen M, et al, eds. Echocardiography in Pediatric and Congenital Heart Disease: From Fetus to Adult. Hoboken, NJ, Wiley-Blackwell, 2009.

Nichols DG, Cameron DE (eds). Critical Heart Disease in Infants and Children. 2nd ed. St Louis, Mosby, 2006.

REFERENCES

1. Gross RE, Hubbard JP. Surgical ligation of a patent ductus arteriosus. Report of first successful case. JAMA 1939; 112:729-731.
2. Crafoord C, Nylin G. Congenital coarctation of the aorta and its surgical treatment. J Thorac Surg 1945; 14:347-361.
3. Lillehei CW, Cohen M, Warn HE, Varco RL. The direct vision intracardiac correction of congenital anomalies by controlled cross circulation. Surgery 1955; 38:11-29.
4. Kirklin JW, DuShane JW, Patrick RT, et al. Intracardiac surgery with the aid of a mechanical pump oxygenator system (Gibbon type): report of 8 cases. Proc Staff Meet Mayo Clin 1955; 30:201-206.
5. Olley PM, Coceani F, Bodach E. E-type prostaglandin—a new emergency therapy for certain congenital cardiac malformations. Circulation 1976; 53:728-731.
6. Bargeron LM, Elliott LP, Soto B, et al. Axial cineangiography in congenital heart disease. Circulation 1977; 56:1075-1083.
7. Marelli AJ, Mackie AS, Ionescu-Ittu R, et al. Congenital heart disease in the general population: changing prevalence and age distribution. Circulation 2007; 115:163-172.
8. Douidar SM, Richardson J, Snodgrass WR. Role of indomethacin in ductus closure: an update evaluation. Dev Pharmacol Ther 1988; 11:196-212.
9. Malviya M, Ohlsson A, Shah S. Surgical versus medical treatment with cyclooxygenase inhibitors for symptomatic patent ductus arteriosus in preterm infants. Cochrane Database Syst Rev 2008; 1:CD003951.
10. Mori K, Matsuoka S, Tatara K, et al. Echocardiographic evaluation of the development of aortic valve prolapse in supracristal ventricular septal defect. Eur J Pediatr 1995; 154:176-181.
11. Tweddell JS, Pelech AN, Frommelt PC. Ventricular septal defect and aortic valve regurgitation: pathophysiology and indications for surgery. Semin Thorac Cardiovasc Surg Pediatr Card Surg Annu 2006:147-152.
12. Dellegrottaglie S, Pedrotti P, Pedretti S, et al. Atrial septal defect combined with partial anomalous pulmonary venous return: complete anatomic and functional characterization by cardiac magnetic resonance. J Cardiovasc Med (Hagerstown) 2008; 9:1184-1186.
13. Syamasundar P, Rao MD. Coarctation of the aorta. Available at: http://emedicine.medscape.com/article/895502-overview.
14. Wernovsky G, Ghanayem N, Ohye RG, et al. Hypoplastic left heart syndrome: consensus and controversies in 2007. Cardiol Young 2007; 17(Suppl 2):75-86.
15. Paranon S, Acar P. Ebstein's anomaly of the tricuspid valve: from fetus to adult: congenital heart disease. Heart 2008; 94:237-243.
16. Zain Z, Zadinello M, Menahem S, Brizard C. Neonatal isolated critical aortic valve stenosis: balloon valvuloplasty or surgical valvotomy. Heart Lung Circ 2006; 15:18-23. Epub 2005 Jul 25.
17. Backer CL. Techniques for repairing the aortic and truncal valves. Cardiol Young 2005; 15(Suppl 1):125-131.
18. Luciani GB, Mazzucco A. Aortic root disease after the Ross procedure. Curr Opin Cardiol 2006; 21:555-560.
19. Kutty S, Zahn EM. Interventional therapy for neonates with critical congenital heart disease. Catheter Cardiovasc Interv 2008; 72: 663-674.
20. Skinner J, Hornung T, Rumball E. Transposition of the great arteries: from fetus to adult. Heart 2008; 94:1227-1235.
21. Mustard WT. Successful two-stage correction of transposition of the great vessels. Surgery 1964; 55:469-472.
22. Angelini P, de la Cruz MV, Valencia AM, et al. Coronary arteries in transposition of the great arteries. Am J Cardiol 1994; 74: 1037-1041.
23. Cohen MS, Anderson RH, Cohen MI, et al. Controversies, genetics, diagnostic assessment, and outcomes relating to the heterotaxy syndrome. Cardiol Young 2007; 17(Suppl 2):29-43.
24. Warnes CA. Transposition of the great arteries (review). Circulation 2006; 114:2699-2709.
25. Rodefeld MD, Ruzmetov M, Schamberger MS, et al. Staged surgical repair of functional single ventricle in infants with unobstructed pulmonary blood flow. Eur J Cardiothorac Surg 2005; 27:949-955.
26. Driscoll DJ. Long-term results of the Fontan operation. Pediatr Cardiol 2007; 28:438-442.
27. van Doorn C. The unnatural history of tetralogy of Fallot: surgical repair is not as definitive as previously thought. Heart 2002; 88: 447-448.
28. Warnes CA. Tricuspid atresia and univentricular heart after the Fontan procedure. Cardiol Clin 1993; 11:665-673.
29. Drenthen W, Pieper PG, Roos-Hesselink JW, et al. Pregnancy and delivery in women after Fontan palliation. Heart 2006; 92:1290-1294. Epub 2006 Jan 31.

CHAPTER 29

Percutaneous Catheter-Based Treatment of Coronary and Valvular Heart Disease

Mark Sheldon and Warren Laskey

Although catheter-based therapy for the management of obstructive vascular disease in humans began with the pioneering work of Dotter and Judkins,[1] the extension and application of catheter-based therapy to the management of obstructive coronary artery disease (CAD) is properly credited to Gruntzig, working in Switzerland, and Myler, working in the United States. The mid-to-late 1970s were a period of intense efforts toward the miniaturization of catheter design along with feasibility studies beginning with a canine model and extending to the operating room setting and, finally, the cardiac catheterization laboratory.[2,3] With Gruntzig's move from Zurich, Switzerland, to Atlanta, Georgia, in 1980, the technique and technology of what was then termed *percutaneous transluminal coronary angioplasty (PTCA)* developed rapidly.

First-generation angioplasty balloon catheters were crude (and hazardous) by today's standards—generally 2 mm in diameter and "guided" into the target vessel by large-bore (9F to 10F) stiff guide catheters. The range of these early PTCA catheters was severely limited by the lack of optimal directional control and the large profile of the balloon catheter itself. Consequently, over the next several decades, the promise of this noninvasive approach to the management of patients with symptomatic coronary heart disease was realized with an explosion in the technology of catheter materials and manufacturing. Without such advances, the indications for this procedure would remain limited to clinically stable patients who are suitable for coronary artery bypass graft (CABG) surgery, and in whom a discrete, proximal, concentric, noncalcified, nonangulated stenosis in a large epicardial vessel was identified as the cause of disease (Fig. 29-1A).[4]

The early double-lumen design allowed for distal coronary artery pressure monitoring (Fig. 29-1B through D), enabling immediate assessment of the hemodynamic result of PTCA, and the large-bore guide catheter allowed for the injection of contrast material to assess the result fluoroscopically (Fig. 29-1E). As the popularity of PTCA grew, and the clinical and anatomic spectrum of disease encountered in diagnostic angiography laboratories expanded, it became clear, however, that (1) "lower profile" PTCA catheters would be necessary to treat many stenoses, and (2) improved "manipulability" and "directionality" were mandatory. PTCA catheter systems were modified with quantum leaps in technology—elimination of the double-lumen design (with consequent loss of ability to monitor distal pressure) and the creation of a (re)movable PTCA guidewire (in contrast to the fixed balloon–short wire design of prototypic catheters). These two fundamental changes, along with continued modifications in catheter and guidewire design, allowed for the explosive growth in PTCA procedures over the last 30 years. The development of "niche" devices,[5,6] each designed for a specific anatomic situation, allowed for broader application in a wider spectrum of lesions and patients. During this explosive growth period in primarily nonballoon catheter technology, the procedure assumed a new name—percutaneous coronary intervention (PCI).

This chapter primarily reviews percutaneous catheter-based treatments of CAD in adults. The emerging application of percutaneous catheter-based management of valvular heart disease is briefly discussed at the end of the chapter.

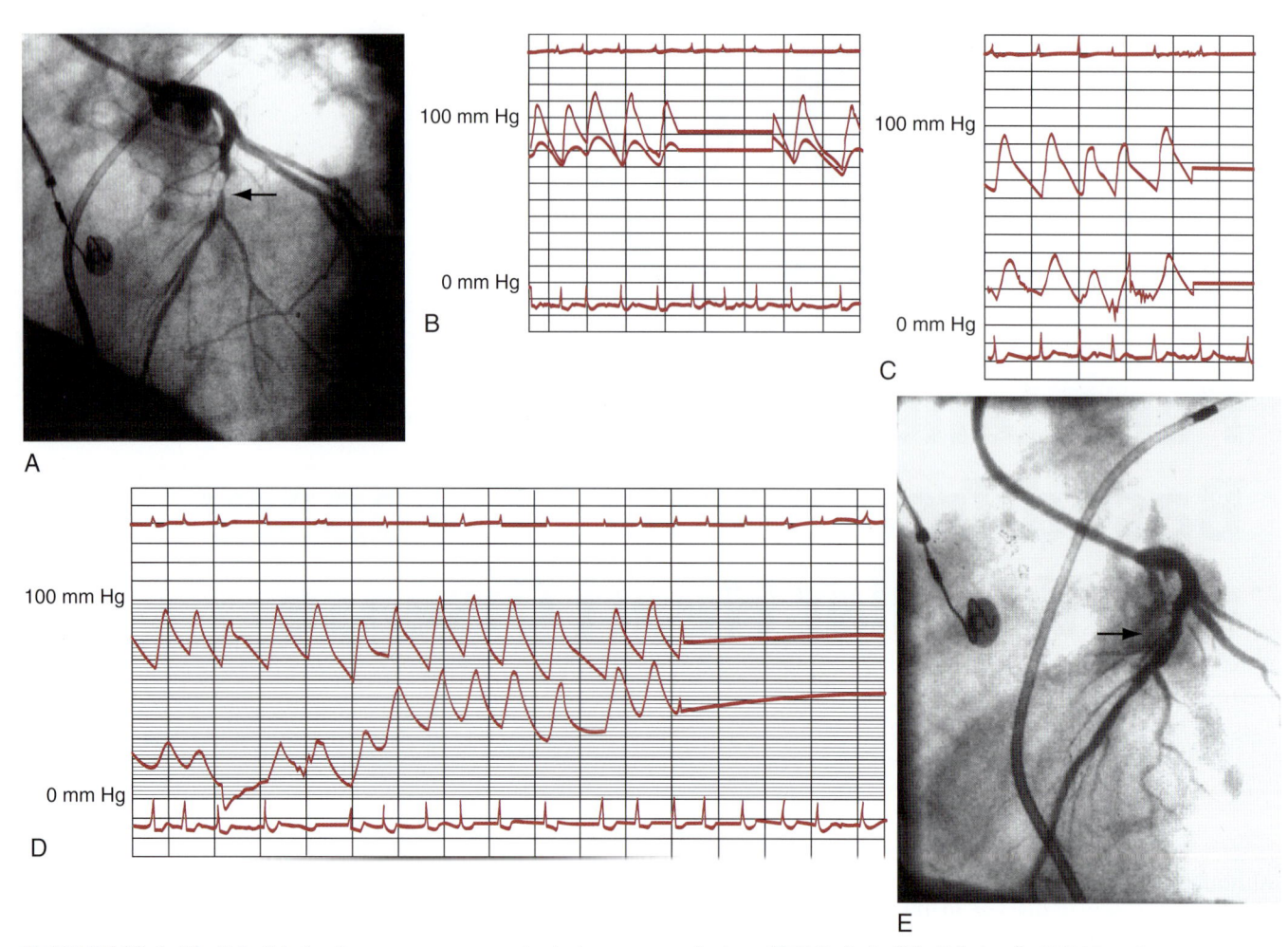

FIGURE 29-1 The "ideal" lesion for percutaneous transluminal coronary angioplasty (PTCA). **A,** An "ideal" lesion for PTCA is a discrete, concentric, noncalcified stenosis in the proximal portion of the left anterior descending coronary artery (*arrow*). **B,** Arterial pressure recordings from the guiding catheter (*upper tracing*) and distal lumen of the PTCA catheter (*lower tracing*) in a nonstenotic arterial segment. **C,** Translesional pressure gradient recording with PTCA catheter distal to stenosis. The gradient represents the hemodynamic severity of the stenosis. **D,** On balloon deflation, translesional pressure gradient begins to decrease (*left-hand side*) to control levels noted in **B**; this indicates improvement in the hemodynamic severity of the stenosis. **E,** Confirming the hemodynamic results in **A**, coronary angiogram shows virtual elimination of stenosis (*arrow*).

PROCEDURE

Description and Special Anatomic Considerations

Birfurcation-Type Lesions

When plaque is present at, around, or within the ostium of a significant side-branch (i.e., bifurcation [Fig. 29-2]), the chances of short-term and long-term ischemic complications are increased. There is much debate on the best way to approach these lesions. When the side-branch is small (<1.5 mm in diameter or subtending a small vascular territory), simply stenting over that side-branch is sufficient. In this situation, the chances of possible ischemic complications of displacing plaque into the side-branch, causing acute occlusion, are relatively small, and do not warrant increased procedural complexity and duration. When the side-branch approaches the diameter of the main branch or has a large vascular territory that it supplies, the ischemic complications of such plaque shift become significant. Myriad approaches to catheter-based management of bifurcation lesions have been described,[7,8] which reflect the anatomic diversity of this category. Despite the use of stents and potent anticoagulant and antiplatelet regimens, however, clinical outcomes in patients with such anatomy remain suboptimal.[9]

Saphenous Vein Bypass Grafts

With the half-life of saphenous vein bypass grafts generally around 8 to 10 years, the number of post-CABG patients needing intervention continues to grow. Lesions in such older grafts (Fig. 29-3) present difficult issues: The veins themselves are characterized by diffuse fibrointimal hyperplasia even when nonobstructive—the vascular disease process continues to varying degrees, and a complex plaque consisting of platelets, thrombin, fibrin, inflammatory cells, and cholesterol crystals adheres to the endoluminal surface. Debris from large, bulky atherosclerotic plaque during PCI is frequently "liberated" downstream[10]; this often results in a "no-flow" phenomenon wherein such embolization results in occlusion of the distal vasculature with dramatic clinical consequences. Subsequently, it was found that the risk of peri-procedural ischemic

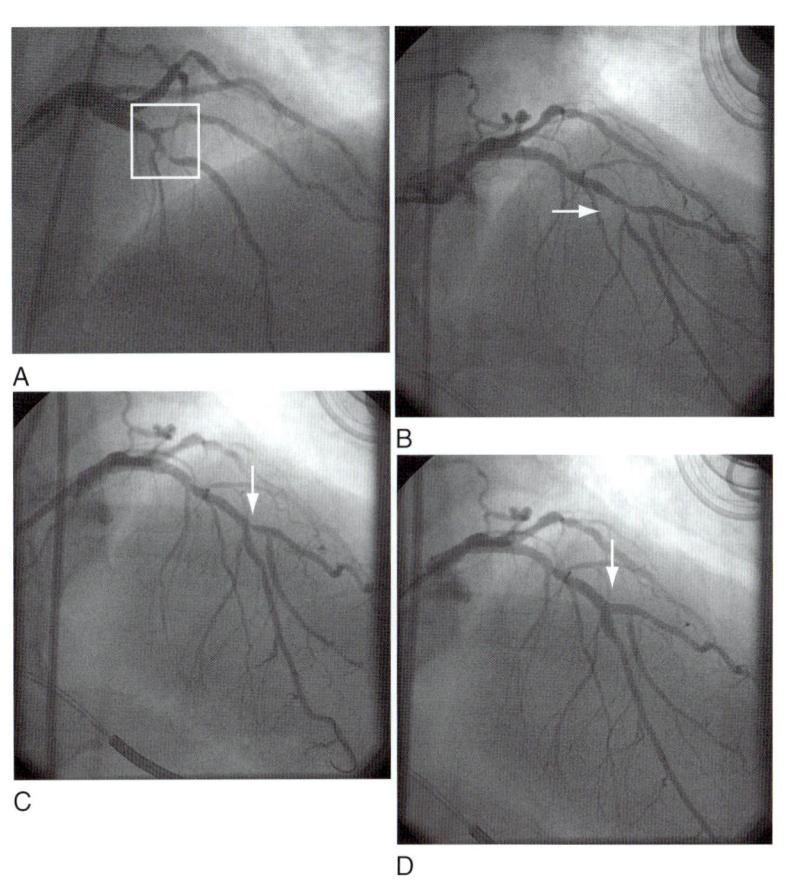

FIGURE 29-2 Bifurcation coronary artery lesions. **A,** Complex bifurcation lesion at the origin of a large diagonal artery. Note disease of native left anterior descending (LAD) artery, disease of diagonal artery, and disease of LAD artery distal to bifurcation (*outlined by box*). **B,** Bifurcation lesion in a different patient from **A,** in whom target lesion is in mid-LAD artery (*arrow*) after the origin of a diagonal artery. **C,** After percutaneous transluminal coronary angioplasty of LAD artery, there is plaque shift from the target area into the origin of the aforementioned diagonal artery (*arrow*). **D,** Because of occlusive behavior in diagonal artery (*arrow*), the latter is "treated" as well.

complications during saphenous vein graft PCI can be reduced by up to 50% with the use of distal protection devices (Fig. 29-4).[11]

Complex Lesions, Angulated Lesions, and Lesions Distal to Proximal Vessel Tortuosity

Complex lesions, angulated lesions, and lesions distal to proximal vessel tortuosity (Figs. 29-5 through 29-7) also characterize "high-risk" anatomic subsets. Although especially true in the PTCA era, negotiation of severe tortuosity and proximal curvatures is still a challenge for even the most "low-profile" devices. Similarly, complex lesions, generally encountered in the setting of acute coronary syndromes, remain unpredictable in their response to PCI.

A key to working in tortuous arteries is having proper guide catheter support (i.e., adequate support to enable the PCI instrument to reach, and cross, the distal or post-curvature target lesion). The hazard here is dissection of the proximal vessel by the tensile forces exerted by the guide and, in some instances, propagation of the proximal vessel with complete occlusion. Advances in guidewire technology have vastly improved the ability to deliver various devices into or through excessively angulated arteries. The additional support provided by stiffer wires or wires specifically designed to decrease friction (by moving the balloon catheter or stent away from the arterial wall) has been a major advance in these difficult situations. Perhaps the most important improvements in these situations have been in stent design. Over the past decade, coronary stents have gone from very stiff and bulky catheter designs to designs that provide more flexibility and, consequently, deliverability. Not only are stents easier to pass to the lesion distal to a tortuous segment, but they are now also able to conform to angulated lesions with a minimal loss of radial force (Fig. 29-8).

Chronic Total Occlusions

Chronic total occlusion (Fig. 29-9), one of the last frontiers of interventional cardiology, refers to a native coronary artery (or vein graft) that has been occluded for at least 2

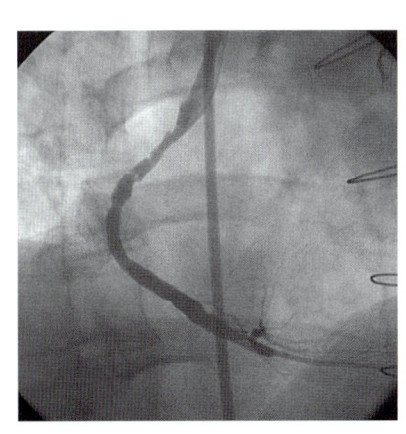

FIGURE 29-3 An 8-year-old aorto–right coronary artery saphenous vein bypass graft. Note irregular borders consistent with endoluminal deposits of atherosclerotic debris and fibrointimal hyperplasia.

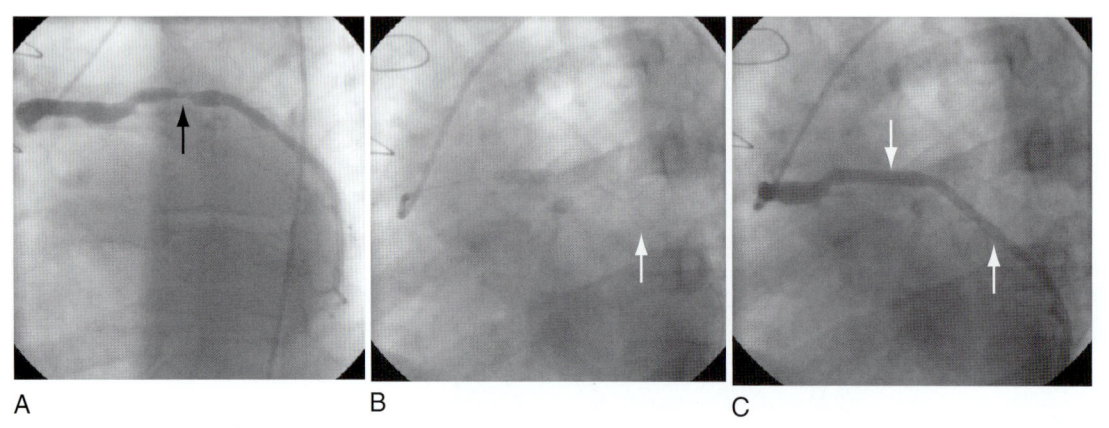

FIGURE 29-4 Saphenous vein bypass graft. **A,** Use of distal protection device during intervention on a saphenous vein bypass graft stenosis (*arrow*). **B,** *Arrow* indicates collection system distal to balloon segment of percutaneous transluminal coronary angioplasty catheter. **C,** *Up arrow* indicates distal collecting portion of the catheter (see **B**), whereas *down arrow* indicates lesion appearance after percutaneous coronary intervention with stent placement.

weeks. Such totally occluded vessels are commonly found during diagnostic catheterization. Although they may or may not be associated with a discernible myocardial infarct in the subtended territory, such anatomy still may predispose to symptoms of coronary insufficiency that medical therapy cannot treat adequately. In this setting, an attempt at recanalization is often contemplated.

Historically, successful recanalization of a chronic total occlusion was achieved in only 50% to 70% of attempts even with very experienced operators. The difficulty arises from the nature of the lesion itself. The usual process of passing a soft, flexible guidewire distal to the target lesion (to pass balloons and stents) becomes considerably more troublesome with no patent lumen to follow. Until a wire can be passed beyond the obstruction, no other devices can be used to treat the lesion. Often a fibrotic and calcified cap forms on the occluded end of the vessel, which can be very difficult to penetrate. Even when penetration is successful, entry into the distal lumen can be problematic, and dissection of the distal vessel is common. This inability to traverse the occlusion with a guidewire is still the most common mode of failure when treating a chronic total occlusion. The advent of newer "coated," stiffer, and tapered-tip wires and the use of techniques such as simultaneous bilateral coronary angiography have increased success rates modestly. Other, more innovative (and aggressive) techniques under study are a subject requiring more in-depth discussion.

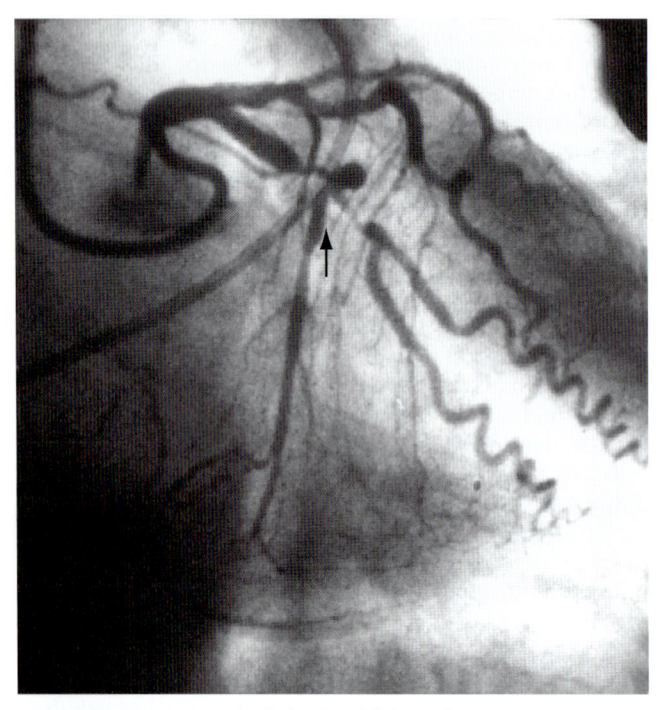

FIGURE 29-5 Complex lesion in mid-circumflex coronary artery extending proximal and distal to tortuous segment of circumflex artery proper (*arrow*).

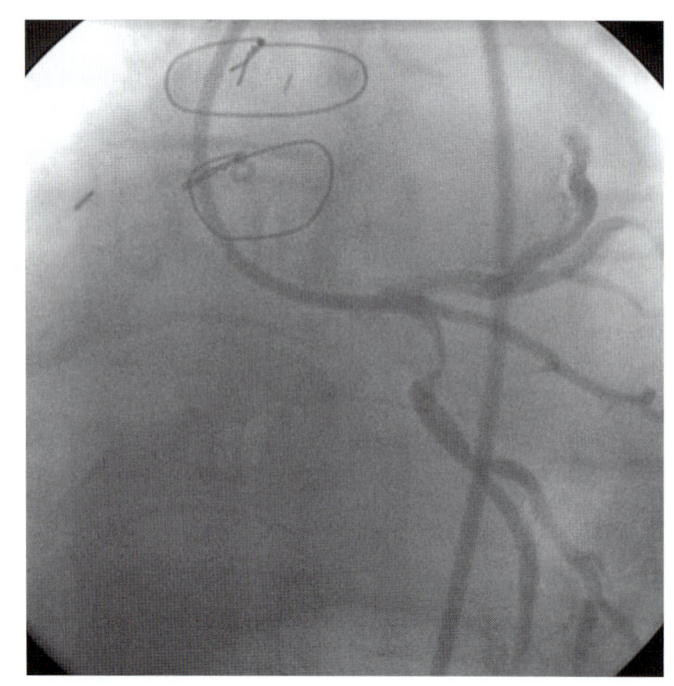

FIGURE 29-6 Complex "lesion on a bend" involving proximal left circumflex artery.

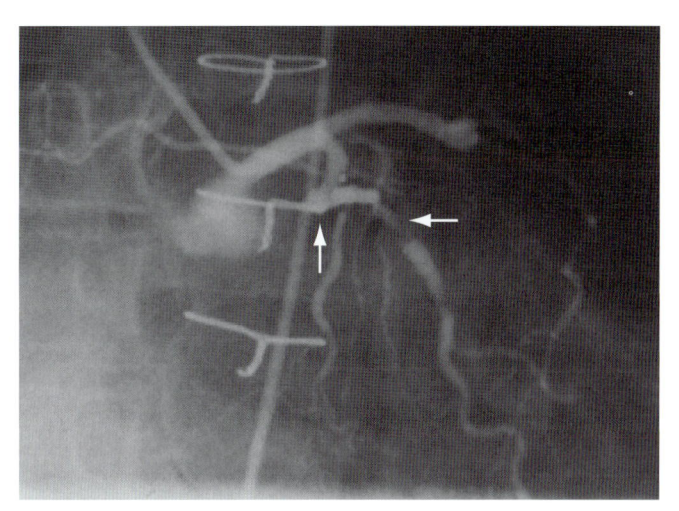

FIGURE 29-7 Complex lesion in circumflex marginal artery (*horizontal arrow*) distal to a sharp bend in artery (*up arrow*).

When a wire is across the occluded segment, there can still be difficulty in getting the catheter into position. Even with immediate procedural success, chronic total occlusions are characterized by higher rates of restenosis compared with similar procedures in initially patent arteries. Currently, the presence of a chronic total occlusion is often the deciding factor in the decision to refer a patient to surgery rather than attempt a PCI, particularly when complete revascularization is desired in the setting of multivessel disease.[12]

Long Lesions and Diffuse Disease

The presence of diffuse disease (i.e., >20 mm in length [Fig. 29-10]) within a vessel was always one of the biggest dilemmas for PCI, and remains one of the largest contributing factors for restenosis. Restenosis rates after PTCA in long lesions can be 80%. Although stenting these lesions was often necessary for more angiographically acceptable immediate results, persistent rates of (in-stent) restenosis of 40% temper enthusiasm for this subset of lesions. The advent of drug-eluting stents has enabled these lesions to be successfully treated with dramatically reduced restenosis rates. These stents have successfully reduced restenosis rates and the need for repeat revascularization in patients with diffuse disease to the 9% to 20% range.[13]

Left Main Coronary Artery Disease

Traditionally, significant disease of the left main coronary artery (Figs. 29-11 and 29-12) has been one of the firmest indications for CABG surgery.[14] When "protected" by a previous bypass graft to either the left anterior descending artery or the circumflex artery, these procedures can be done with a minimum of risk and high likelihood of success. In the unprotected state, however, the complexity of anatomy (typically a bifurcation or trifurcation) and the amount of myocardium at risk make these procedures high risk for the short-term and mid-term. In the United States, Canada, and most of Europe, left main coronary artery PCI remains a procedure used only for patients who

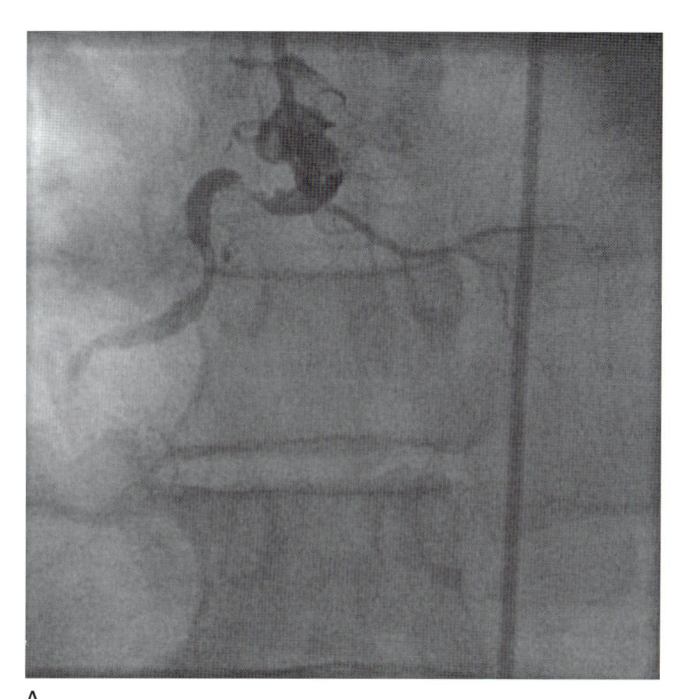

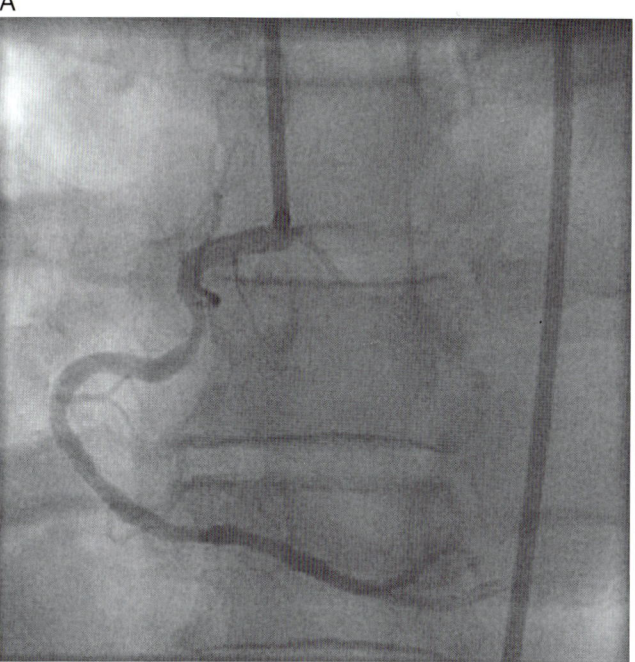

FIGURE 29-8 Complex coronary artery lesion. **A,** "Lesion on a bend" in proximal portion of right coronary artery. **B,** Apparent "straightening" of arterial segment after stent placement.

have a prohibitive risk for CABG surgery. In parts of Asia and certain other countries in Eastern Europe and South America, these procedures have continued to be used on a wider basis.[15] The main issues that have continued to limit wider acceptance of this procedure are the ramifications of the complications of in-stent restenosis and stent thrombosis (see later). When ongoing procedural and technologic modifications (e.g., designs to "fit" a bifurcation specifically) are established, PCI extended to this previously contraindicated group may become more frequent.[16]

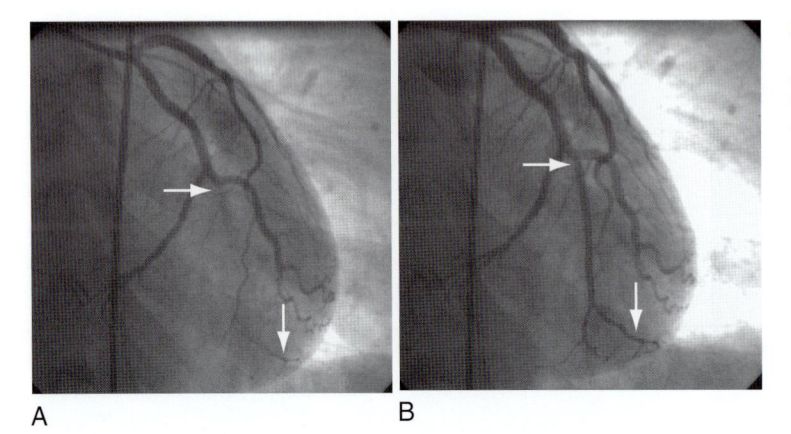

FIGURE 29-9 Chronic total occlusion of distal circumflex marginal artery. **A,** Arterial occlusion begins at the *horizontal arrow*. *Down arrow* indicates branch filling of the distal vessel via intracoronary collaterals. **B,** Recanalization of total occlusion in **A** with stent placement. *Arrows* indicate same areas as defined in **A**.

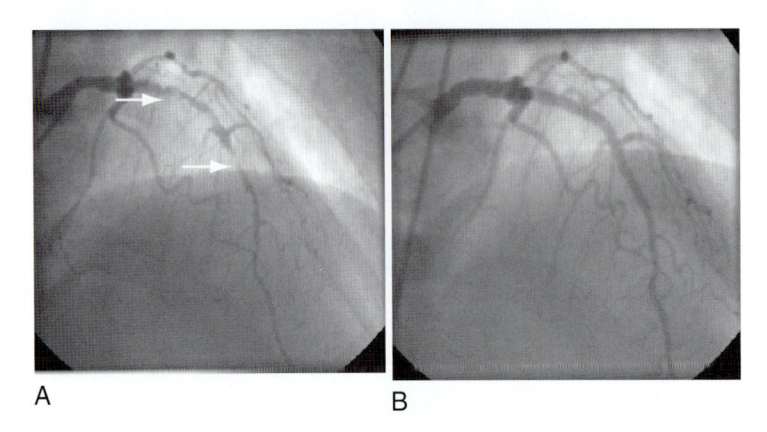

FIGURE 29-10 Long segment (diffuse) coronary artery disease. **A,** Long, diffusely diseased segment of the left anterior descending artery beginning at *top arrow* and terminating at *bottom arrow*. **B,** Same region of artery as in **A** after placement of multiple stents.

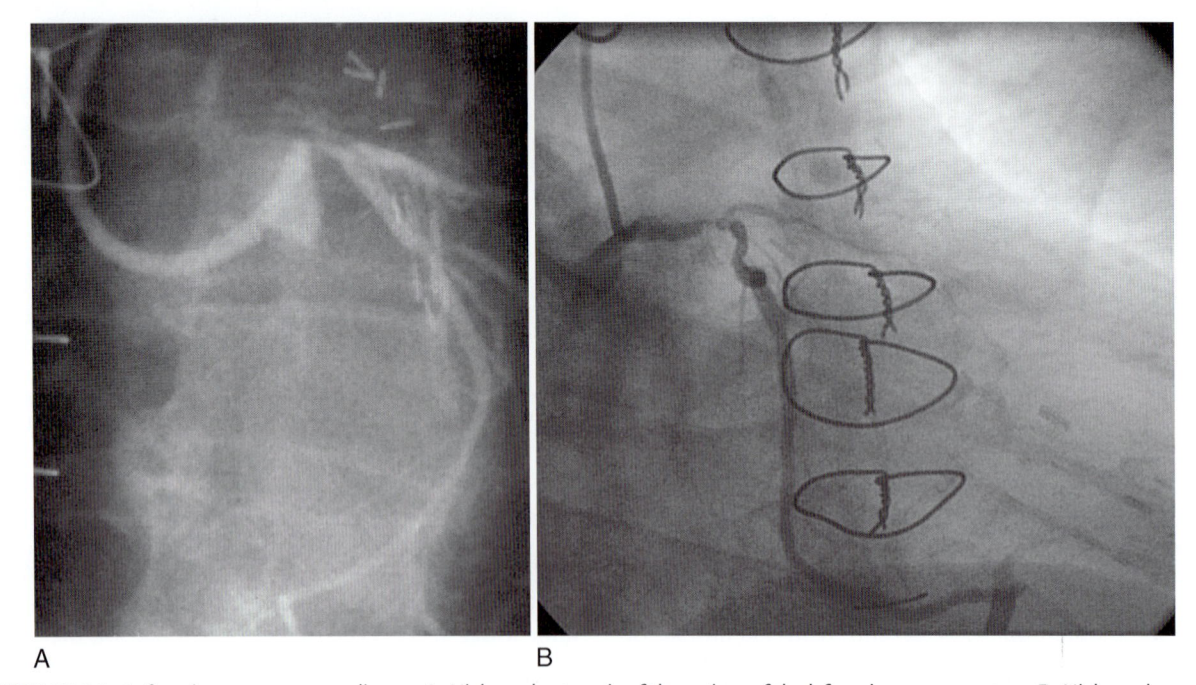

FIGURE 29-11 Left main coronary artery disease. **A,** High-grade stenosis of the ostium of the left main coronary artery. **B,** High-grade stenosis of the distal portion of the left main coronary artery.

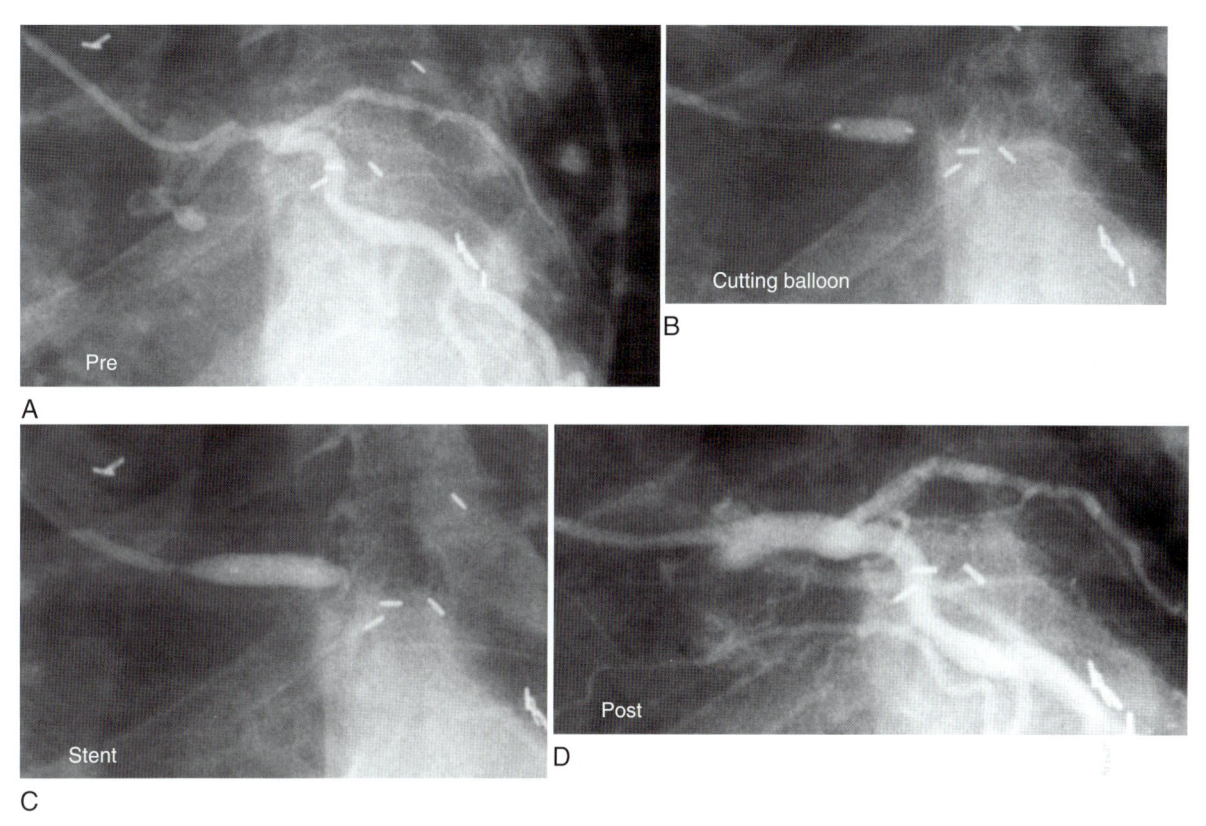

FIGURE 29-12 Left main coronary artery disease. **A,** Percutaneous coronary intervention for a stenosis in the body of the left main coronary artery (before intervention). **B,** A cutting balloon is used to "prepare" the fibrotic lesion for stent placement. **C,** A bare-metal stent is successfully deployed at the target lesion. **D,** Satisfactory final angiographic result. *(Courtesy of Raoul Bonan, MD.)*

ST Segment Elevation Myocardial Infarction

The most dramatic clinical presentation for a patient with CAD is ST segment elevation myocardial infarction (STEMI). Prompt triage, diagnosis, medical stabilization, and reperfusion are the mainstays of treatment. Considerable effort has been expended in developing and optimizing the care that these patients receive. The goal for successful reperfusion ("door-to-balloon" time) is as quickly as possible, but at least no more than 90 minutes. In settings where a cardiac catheterization laboratory is not immediately available, the choice is clear—prompt thrombolytic therapy should be initiated in patients who are eligible within 30 minutes. These patients should be transferred to a PCI-capable facility for further care, especially if there is evidence of ongoing ischemia, heart failure, significant arrhythmias, or lack of clinical reperfusion.

"Primary" PCI is considered the gold standard for treatment and has been compared with thrombolytic therapy multiple times.[17] Traditionally, the preferred procedural method has been to perform an initial balloon angioplasty followed by stent placement for definitive recanalization. Only when a large thrombus burden was obvious was thrombectomy with either an aspiration or rheolytic device considered necessary (Fig. 29-13). Poor myocardial tissue level perfusion despite the apparently "normal flow" in the epicardial vessel has continued to be a significant problem, however, which has been linked to distal embolization of thrombus, plaque, or both. This problem has led to a resurgence in the use of aspiration or rheolytic thrombectomy devices (Fig. 29-14) as a means of initial reperfusion followed by stenting for definitive recanalization.[18]

Stent Thrombosis

Stent thrombosis (Fig. 29-15) is a dramatic event that can occur immediately, acutely (within 24 hours), subacutely (within 30 days), late (within 1 year), or very late (after 1 year). Stent thrombosis can be a devastating event, which frequently manifests with STEMI. Risk factors for early, acute, and subacute stent thrombosis include inadequate (or resistance to) antithrombotic or antiplatelet therapy, untreated dissection at the site of implant, prothrombotic substrate, and premature cessation of dual antiplatelet therapy. The treatment is emergent recatheterization, removal of thrombus with aspiration thrombectomy, or balloon angioplasty. It is also generally recommended to perform intravascular ultrasound to ensure that no mechanical complications, such as undetected dissection, undersized or underdeployed stents, or residual obstructive plaque proximal or distal to the stent, are present. These complications must be dealt with appropriately by ensuring proper expansion, using further stenting, maximizing medical therapy, and ensuring compliance. With the present armamentarium of devices, medications, and adjunctive procedures, stent thrombosis is a rare event (overall risk by 1 year approximately 1%).

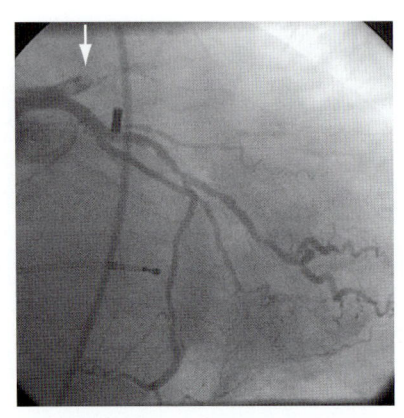

FIGURE 29-13 Total occlusion of the proximal portion of the left anterior descending artery is found in this patient presenting with an acute ST segment elevation myocardial infarction. Notice the presence of thrombus in the segment of artery immediately proximal to the occlusion (*arrow*).

Catheter Modification for Specific Lesion Subsets

As alluded to earlier, specific balloon catheter modifications were required for unique anatomic situations in which conventional technology frequently failed. These situations included lesions that were heavily calcified or characterized by extensive fibrosis. In either situation, the response to balloon expansion was either inadequate or excessively disruptive. The concept of "lesion modification" was introduced along with a technique called *percutaneous transluminal coronary rotational atherectomy*.[19] Employing a high-speed rotating (160,000 to 180,000 rpm) diamond-studded "burr" mounted on a traditional balloon catheter, "pretreatment" of such lesions frequently enabled definitive lesion treatment with excellent immediate results (Fig. 29-16).

Persistently unacceptable rates of restenosis,[20] the complexity (and risk) of the procedure, and further refinements in traditional catheter technology have reduced the use of percutaneous transluminal coronary rotational atherectomy from a significant minority of all PCI to a niche indication at present. The development of the less cumbersome "cutting balloon" (see Fig. 29-12) with the similar philosophy of plaque/lesion "modification" as percutaneous transluminal coronary rotational atherectomy has led to more widespread acceptance at present in these situations.[21]

Another limitation of traditional balloon angioplasty was the inability to treat eccentric lesions or lesions characterized by substantial plaque mass. An innovative catheter design, directional coronary atherectomy, allowed for more precise directional control, allowing for more specific lesion targeting and physical removal of the plaque (Fig. 29-17).[22] Despite the intellectual attractiveness of this concept, and the often pristine angiographic appearance of the result, the technology was bulky and cumbersome. In addition, an excess hazard of directional coronary atherectomy was identified in one of the early randomized trials of device evaluation,[23] further limiting the application of this truly innovative technique.

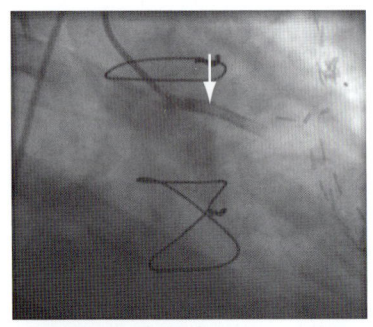

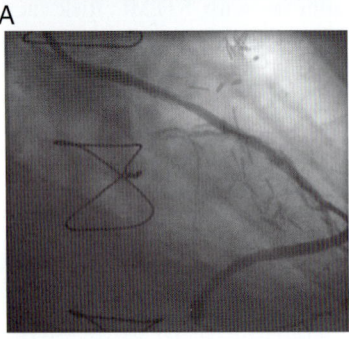

FIGURE 29-14 Thrombotic occlusion. **A,** Total (thrombotic) occlusion in the proximal portion of a saphenous vein bypass graft. Notice the abrupt disappearance of the column of contrast material within the proximal portion of the vessel (*arrow*). **B,** Immediately after extraction thrombectomy, prompt restitution of flow is noted in the large vascular bed supplied by this bypass graft.

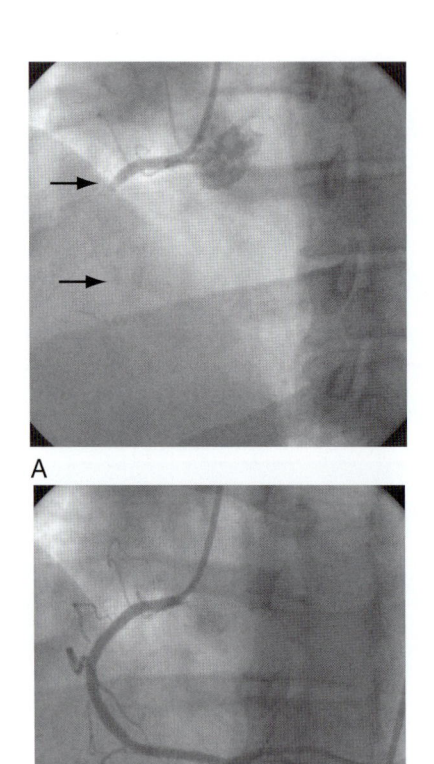

FIGURE 29-15 Stent thrombosis. **A,** Late stent thrombosis within a bare-metal stent. *Arrows* demarcate proximal and distal ends of stent. **B,** Successful recanalization of totally occluded stent.

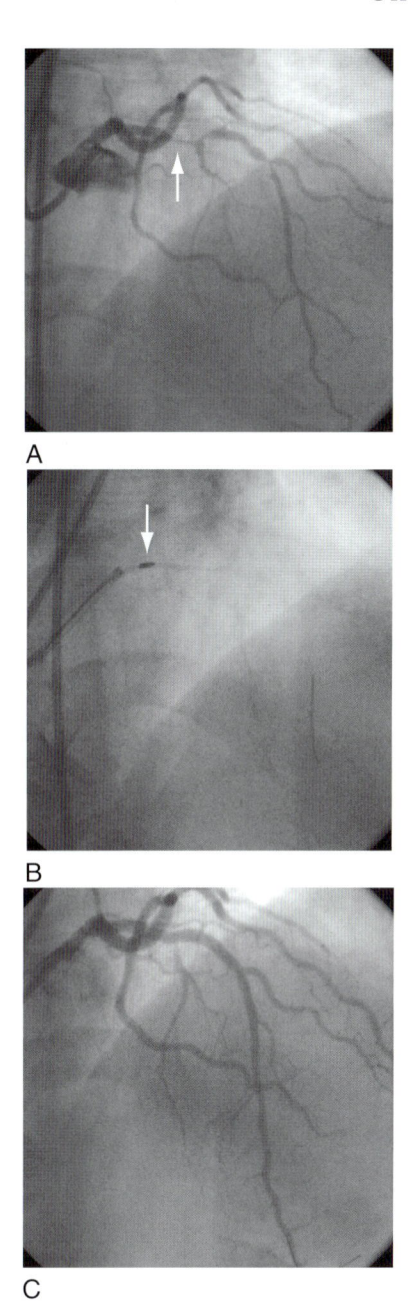

FIGURE 29-16 Percutaneous transluminal coronary rotational atherectomy. **A,** A long, diffusely calcified lesion involving the proximal portion (*arrow*) of the left anterior descending artery. **B,** The burr of the rotational atherectomy catheter (*arrow*) is advanced to the target and activated at 180,000 rpm. **C,** After lesion "preparation" by percutaneous transluminal coronary rotational atherectomy, a stent is deployed with an excellent final angiographic result.

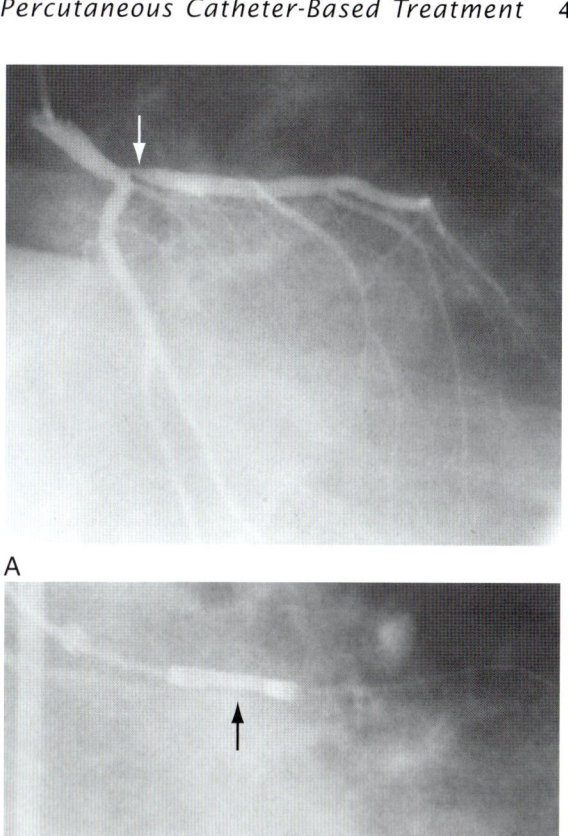

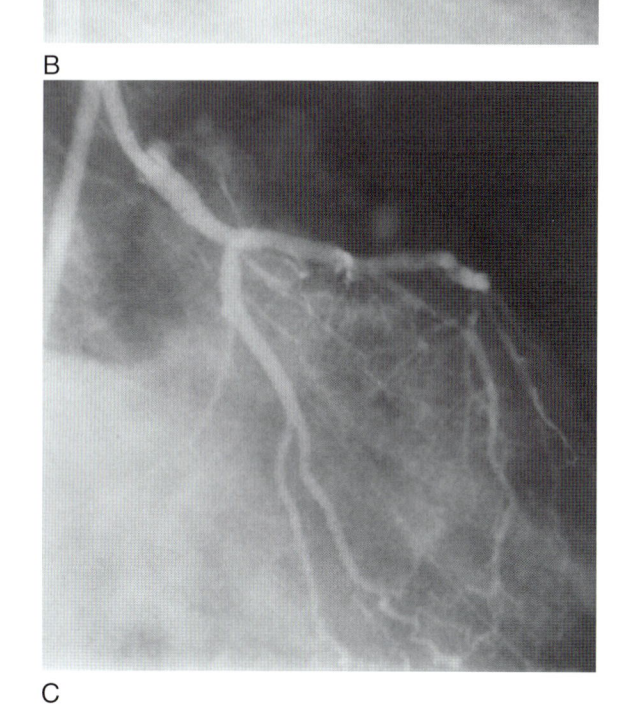

FIGURE 29-17 Directional coronary atherectomy. **A,** High-grade stenosis of the proximal (ostial) portion of the left anterior descending artery (*arrow*). **B,** Collecting chamber of the directional atherectomy catheter is rotated toward the plaque (*arrow*), and excision is performed. **C,** An excellent angiographic result is achieved without evidence of disruption of the left main or circumflex arteries.

Indications

The indications for coronary revascularization procedures have been generally accepted through a consensus of opinion from the various academic societies and organizations that give direction to and advise the cardiology profession. The strongest and most agreed on indications (class I and IIa) are summarized from the American College of Cardiology/American Heart Association Clinical Guidelines on PCI from 2005 and the update from 2007.[24,25]

Stable Coronary Disease

1. PCI is reasonable for asymptomatic patients or patients with mild to moderate angina (Canadian Cardiovascular Society [CCS] class I to II) and one-vessel or two-vessel disease including lesions with a good chance of success, low risk of morbidity, and subtending a moderate or large area of myocardium or causing a moderate or large area of ischemia on noninvasive testing.
2. PCI is reasonable for PCI-related restenosis causing significant ischemia in asymptomatic patients or in patients with mild to moderate angina.
3. PCI is reasonable for asymptomatic patients or patients with mild to moderate angina and a left main artery stenosis of 50% or greater who are ineligible for surgical revascularization.
4. PCI is reasonable in patients with severe angina (CCS class III) and single-vessel or multivessel CAD who are undergoing medical therapy, and who have one or more significant lesions in one or more coronary arteries suitable for PCI with a high likelihood of success and a low risk of morbidity or mortality.
5. PCI is reasonable in patients with severe angina (CCS class III) and single-vessel or multivessel CAD who are undergoing medical therapy with focal saphenous vein graft lesions or multiple stenoses who are poor candidates for reoperative surgery.
6. PCI is reasonable in patients with severe angina (CCS class III) with significant left main CAD (>50% diameter stenosis) who are candidates for revascularization, but are ineligible for CABG surgery.

Acute Coronary Syndromes

1. An early invasive PCI strategy is indicated for patients with unstable angina/non–ST segment elevation myocardial infarction (NSTEMI) who have no serious comorbid conditions, and who have coronary lesions amenable to PCI and who have characteristics for invasive therapy.
2. PCI (or CABG surgery) is recommended for patients with unstable angina/NSTEMI with one-vessel or two-vessel CAD with or without significant proximal left anterior descending CAD, but with a large area of viable myocardium and high-risk criteria on noninvasive testing.
3. PCI (or CABG surgery) is recommended for patients with unstable angina/NSTEMI with multivessel coronary disease with suitable coronary anatomy, with normal left ventricular function, and without diabetes mellitus.
4. An intravenous platelet glycoprotein IIb/IIIa inhibitor is useful in patients with unstable angina/NSTEMI undergoing PCI.
5. An early invasive strategy (i.e., diagnostic angiography with intent to perform revascularization) is indicated in patients with unstable angina/NSTEMI who have refractory angina or hemodynamic or electrical instability (without serious comorbid conditions or contraindications to such procedures).
6. PCI is reasonable for focal saphenous vein graft lesions or multiple stenoses in patients with unstable angina/NSTEMI who are undergoing medical therapy, and who are poor candidates for reoperative surgery.
7. PCI (or CABG surgery) is reasonable for patients with unstable angina/NSTEMI with one-vessel or two-vessel CAD with or without significant proximal left anterior descending CAD, but with a moderate area of viable myocardium and ischemia on noninvasive testing.
8. PCI (or CABG surgery) can be beneficial compared with medical therapy for patients with unstable angina/NSTEMI with one-vessel disease with significant proximal left anterior descending CAD.
9. Use of PCI is reasonable in patients with unstable angina/NSTEMI with significant left main CAD (>50% diameter stenosis) who are candidates for revascularization, but are ineligible for CABG surgery, or who require emergency intervention at angiography for hemodynamic instability.

ST Elevation Myocardial Infarction

1. If immediately available, primary PCI should be performed in patients with STEMI (including true posterior myocardial infarction) or myocardial infarction with new or presumably new left bundle branch block who can undergo PCI of the infarct artery within 12 hours of symptom onset, if performed in a timely fashion (balloon inflation goal within 90 minutes of presentation) by clinicians skilled in the procedure. Primary PCI should be performed as quickly as possible, with a goal of a medical contact-to-balloon or door-to-balloon time within 90 minutes.

Contraindications

Contraindications to performing catheterization with an expectation of proceeding on to PCI are relative with few, if any, that would be considered absolute. Generally, the lack of one of the above-listed indications or the presence of significant comorbid conditions, such as recent stroke, acute renal failure, active bleeding, or a life expectancy for another reason that is severely limited, would be a contraindication for PCI.

Outcomes and Complications

Largely as a result of the foresight of Gruntzig, Myler, and others, the assessment of procedural outcomes (short-term and long-term) was considered to be an inherent aspect of PTCA. The National Heart, Lung and Blood Institute Registry was established in 1979 and served as a rich source of clinical and procedural data.[26] Detailed clinical and anatomic information provided the basis for the estimation of procedural risk.[27] Although less applicable in the current "stent" era, the prediction of risk for adverse procedural outcomes could be linked to lesion morphology.[28] Anatomic subsets that are associated with an increased risk for procedural failure, complication, or restenosis are bifurcation lesions, vein graft lesions, complex lesions, chronic total occlusions, and left main coronary artery disease. Examples of each of these anatomic subsets and the nontraditional catheter technology developed for such situations are discussed next.

The major adverse cardiac events after PCI are death, myocardial infarction, and emergent CABG surgery. Although the rates of these events, individually and in composite, decreased consistently throughout the PCI era, it was not until the advent of coronary stents and advances in adjunctive pharmacotherapy that procedural major adverse cardiac event rates overall declined to current levels of approximately 5%.[29,30] Generally, the risk of adverse procedural outcomes can be assessed using a few easily identifiable preprocedural clinical variables.[31,32] Important clinical subsets that are associated with an increased risk for procedural failure, complication, or restenosis are diabetes, left ventricular dysfunction, chronic kidney disease, and acute myocardial infarction. Additionally, the compounding and confounding effects of age must always be taken into account because there are biologic and statistical interactions between advanced age and each of the latter subsets.[33]

Diabetes

Diabetes mellitus not only increases the risk for coronary atherosclerosis, but also, when diagnosed, increases the risk for poor outcomes. Dyslipidemia is more prevalent and often more severe, renal disease is more frequent, and the atherosclerotic plaque burden is often more extensive and more diffuse than in nondiabetics. In addition, increased inflammatory markers, widespread endothelial dysfunction, and a prothrombotic state are linked to the diabetic condition. These factors conspire not only to make the acute outcomes of PCI less successful, but also contribute to the inferior long-term outcomes compared with nondiabetic patients.[34] These inferior outcomes are particularly significant in patients who are receiving insulin therapy.

Diabetic patients clearly do better with revascularization, however. PCI and CABG surgery can provide important benefits, including symptomatic relief and, in many patients, improved survival. To date, randomized trials suggest that diabetics with multivessel disease fare better with CABG surgery than with PTCA with respect to survival and the need for repeat revascularization procedures.[34] Ongoing trials comparing multivessel PCI (stent) with CABG surgery should help in defining which procedure offers greater benefit, and in which populations a specific strategy can be defined as the procedure of choice.

Long-term outcomes in diabetic patients are further compromised by increased risk of restenosis. The introduction of drug-eluting stents has had a great impact on the treatment of CAD in all patients, but more so in diabetic patients.[35] The findings of lower restenosis and major adverse cardiac event rates when using drug-eluting stents compared with bare-metal stents[36] have led to more diabetic patients being treated with PCI.

Left Ventricular Dysfunction

Left ventricular dysfunction is frequently found in patients with, and is often a result of, CAD. With proper medical treatment and, in many cases, revascularization therapy, left ventricular function may significantly improve. Although poor left ventricular function is often one of the indications for recommending a revascularization procedure, it also increases the risk for PCI and CABG surgery. The lack of cardiac reserve and the possibility of causing a decrease or loss of blood flow in arteries subtending large areas of myocardium or in collaterals supporting these areas are some of the purported mechanisms that increase the risk with left ventricular dysfunction.[31,37,38] Various strategies have been employed to lessen procedural risk in very-high-risk patients with advanced left ventricular dysfunction,[39-41] but data are uncontrolled and inconsistent in supporting the need for such extreme measures.

Chronic Kidney Disease

The presence of preexisting renal disease in patients undergoing any revascularization procedure is one of the strongest predictors of poor outcome.[42-44] Temporary or permanent worsening of renal function is frequently seen in patients with chronic kidney disease and portends poor short-term and long-term outcomes. Despite the use of low osmolar nonionic contrast agents, an increased risk of in-hospital death or myocardial infarction and repeat revascularization procedures is significant after PCI.[42,45]

Perhaps the most disheartening long-term adverse outcome is the development of restenosis at the PTCA site. Although a detailed discussion of the biology of restenosis and the many pharmacologic trials designed to decrease the incidence of restenosis are beyond the scope of this chapter, to understand better the importance and timing of the "stent era," a brief review of the restenosis process is in order. Histopathologic studies in the early years of PTCA suggested a "response to injury" as a mechanism for the benefit of the procedure and the risk of restenosis.[46-48] Developments in molecular and cell biology provided further insight into the complex cellular, autocrine, and paracrine responses to vascular disruption.[49,50] Although some degree of intimal hyperplasia and lumen compromise is noted in all patients after PTCA,[51,52] the final common pathway for patients with restenosis is the development of excessive neointimal hyperplasia. The time course for this process in humans is similar to wound healing. With the incidence of restenosis after conventional PTCA ranging from 30% to 50%, and the failure of specific devices or pharmacologic therapies to reduce the risk of restenosis, the stage was set for the stent era.

STENT ERA

As with balloon angioplasty, much of the seminal work in coronary stent design and materials technology was done in collaboration with vascular and interventional radiologists. Although the first coronary stent technology applied in humans was designed to treat occlusive dissections (Fig. 29-18) after PTCA,[53,54] it was not until the pivotal STRESS[55] and BENESTENT[56] randomized controlled trials showed a reduction in the incidence of restenosis compared with PTCA that the use of coronary stents exponentially increased. Although the risk of restenosis was reduced with stents, the main driver for the rapid acceptance of this technology was the predictable final

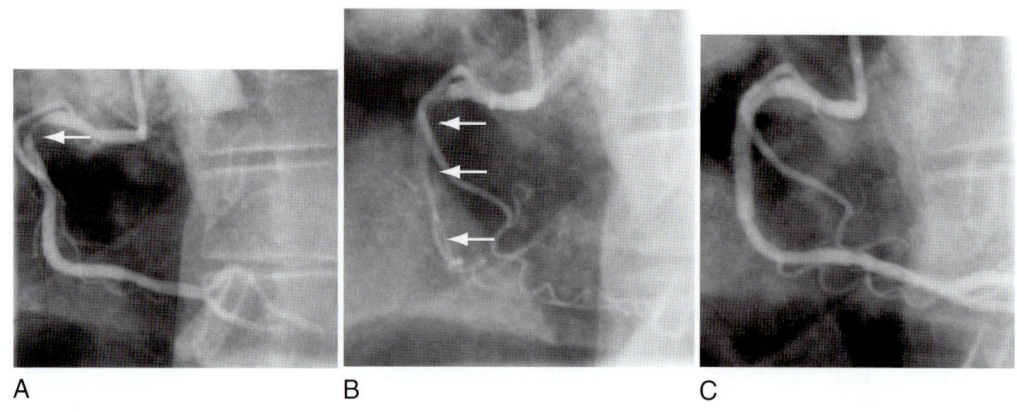

FIGURE 29-18 Stenting of coronary artery dissection. **A,** High-grade stenosis in the proximal portion of a large dominant right coronary artery. Notice the location of the lesion within the angulated segment of the artery (*arrow*). **B,** After percutaneous transluminal coronary angioplasty, an extensive dissection, initiated at the target site, propagates distally with near-total cessation of blood flow (*arrows*). **C,** Immediate stent deployment with full coverage of dissection results in restitution of antegrade blood flow and avoidance of the need for emergent coronary artery bypass surgery.

angiographic result (Fig. 29-19) and the diminished risk of abrupt vessel closure. As with all new technologies, however, important limitations to this addition to the interventional cardiologists' armamentarium rapidly became apparent. The first limitation, relating to the complex and prolonged in-hospital anticoagulation and antithrombotic regimen required after the placement of a coronary stent, was ultimately addressed with the use of high-pressure deployment techniques to optimize stent expansion and apposition to the vessel wall and thienopyridine derivatives for platelet antagonism.[57-59]

The second limitation to the use of metallic stents was not only the persistence of the restenosis problem, albeit of lessened absolute magnitude though still of clinical consequence, but also the high rate of failure of conventional means of treating in-stent restenosis (Fig. 29-20). Another rapid period of innovative catheter-based technologies ensued, each with its own limitations and, importantly, each characterized by persistently unacceptable rates of recurrent in-stent restenosis. In the mid-1990s, the introduction of vascular brachytherapy for the treatment of in-stent restenosis offered some promise,[60,61] although the technique was logistically complex and labor intensive.

Coincident with the declining enthusiasm for vascular brachytherapy for the treatment of patients with in-stent restenosis was the introduction of drug-eluting stents. Early reports from small series of selected patients documenting essentially zero restenosis after implantation of a sirolimus-eluting stent were met with considerable relief and enthusiasm.[62] In short order, the pivotal randomized trials with sirolimus-eluting stents[63] and paclitaxel-eluting stents[64] showed short-term safety and efficacy with virtually single-digit restenosis rates. The rapid acceptance of this revolutionary technology led to the increasing realization, however, that the inhibition of the normal vascular healing process might increase the risk of inadequate re-endothelialization with an increased risk of stent thrombosis.[65,66] Results from numerous nonrandomized studies and uncontrolled case series suggested an increased risk compared with bare-metal stents, although the magnitude of this risk was believed to be small and the time course delayed.[67] These same studies failed to identify an increased risk of death and myocardial infarction, which generally accompany stent thrombosis. Larger and longer term studies continue to note a slightly increased risk of late (>1 year) stent thrombosis without an increased risk of death or myocardial infarction.

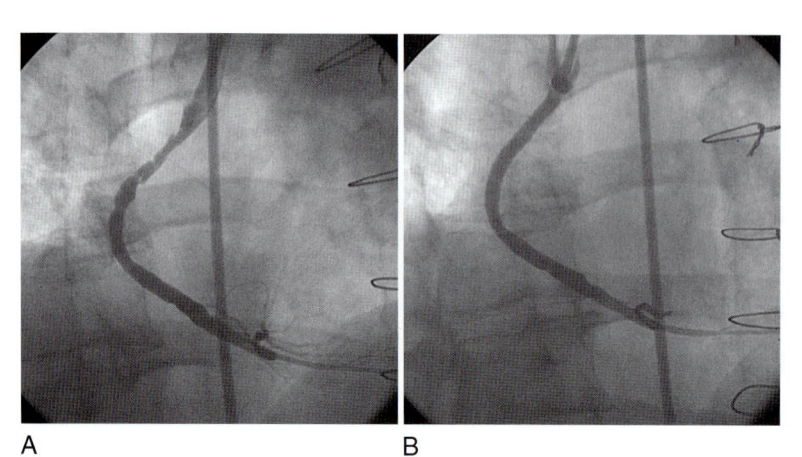

FIGURE 29-19 Coronary artery stent placement. **A,** Baseline angiogram of severely diseased saphenous vein bypass graft. **B,** After successful stent placement, the final angiographic result is visually pleasing.

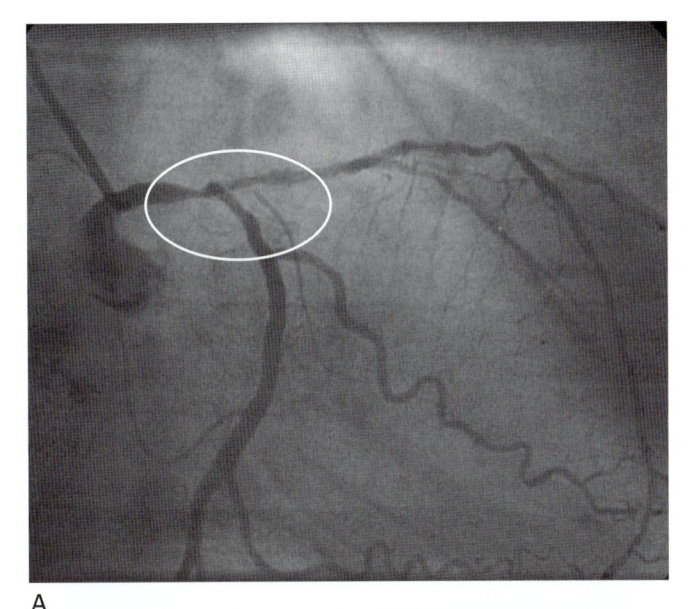

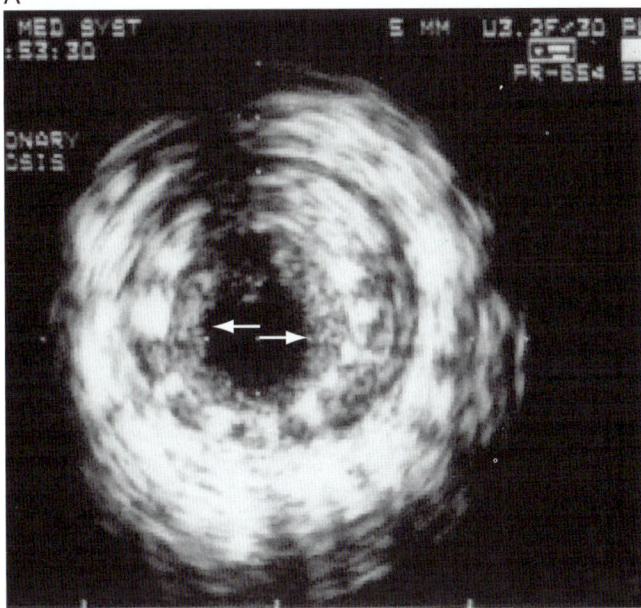

■ FIGURE 29-20 In-stent restenosis. **A,** Long segment of in-stent restenosis (*oval*). **B,** Intravascular ultrasound scan confirms extensive obstructing material within the stent (*arrows*).

Current recommendations for postprocedural management call for extended dual antiplatelet therapy (thienopyridine plus aspirin) for 1 year after implantation of a drug-eluting stent[68] and, of equal importance, careful consideration of the relative merits of a drug-eluting stent compared with a bare-metal stent in each individual case.[69]

Major adverse periprocedural events, most of which are associated with adverse clinical events and some of which are interrelated, are significant coronary dissection, coronary perforation, thromboembolization, and abrupt vessel closure. Examples of each are shown in Figures 29-21 through 29-23. In the present era of very low profile balloon catheters, potent antithrombotic agents, near-universal use of stents, and increased operator experience, the incidences of these undesirable events have decreased individually to less than 1%.

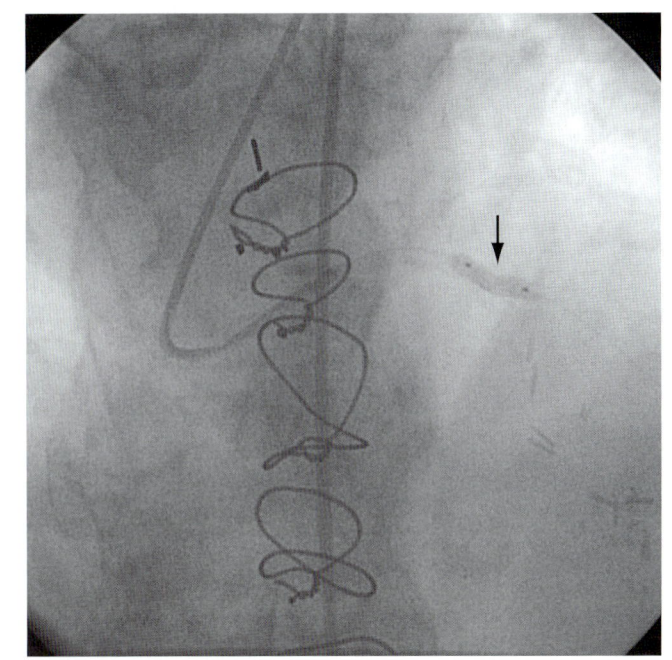

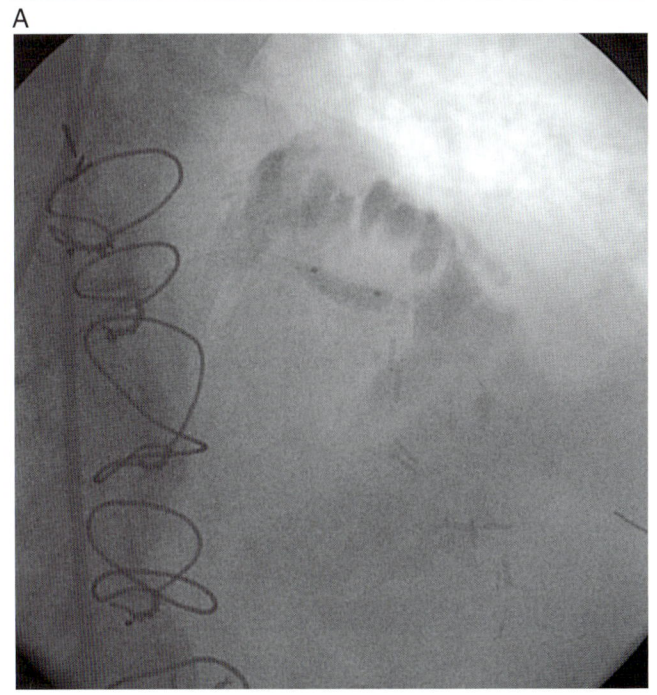

■ FIGURE 29-21 Percutaneous transluminal coronary angioplasty–related coronary artery perforation. **A,** Expansion of percutaneous transluminal coronary angioplasty balloon to 20 atm in a rigid, calcified stenosis. Notice persistent indentation of balloon indicating incomplete dilation of stenosis (*arrow*). **B,** Rupture of artery with extravasation of contrast media (from the balloon) is noted in the extravascular and pericardial space.

CATHETER-BASED MANAGEMENT OF VALVULAR HEART DISEASE

Beginning with the dramatic hemodynamic and clinical improvement in patients with congenital pulmonic valve stenosis,[70] the era of nonsurgical management of congenital and acquired valvular heart disease began. Because the

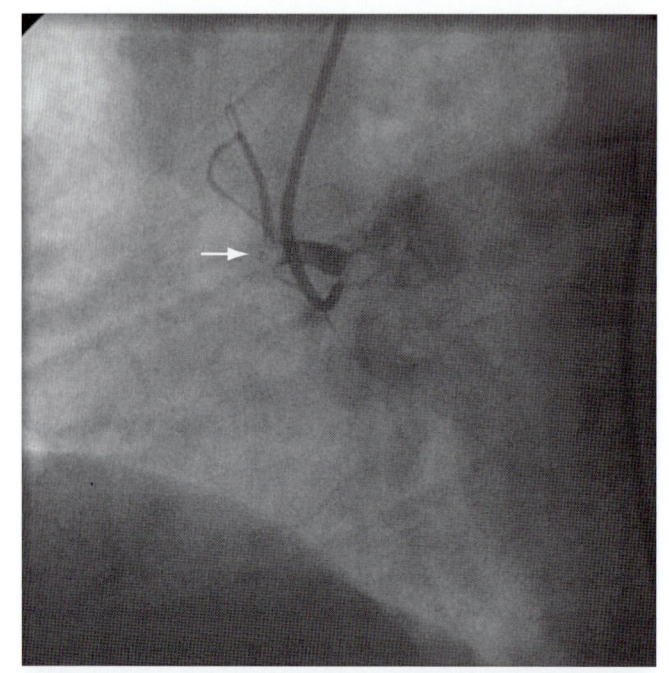

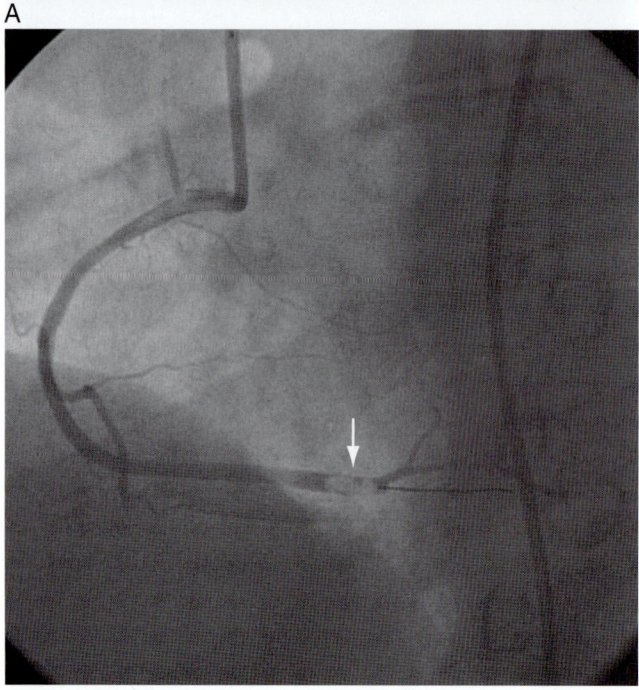

■ **FIGURE 29-22** Distal thromboembolization after percutaneous coronary intervention. **A,** Intervention performed on a total occlusion (*arrow*) of the proximal right coronary artery. **B,** Despite successful recanalization of this totally occluded vessel, with an excellent angiographic result at the target site, distal embolization of thrombus is noted (*arrow*). The patient sustained a large postprocedural myocardial infarction.

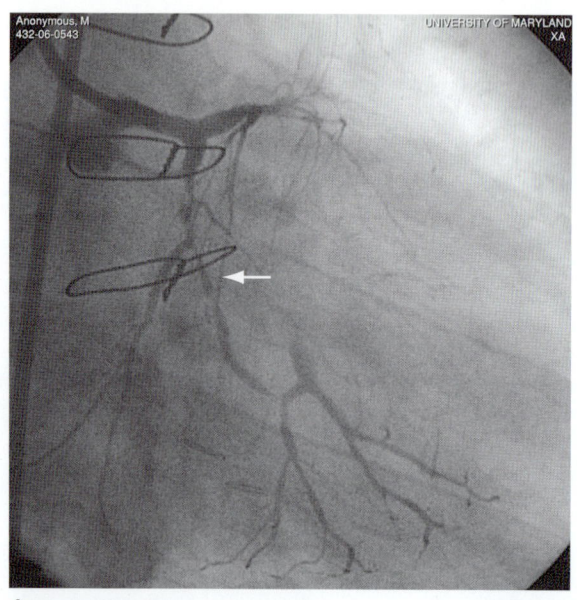

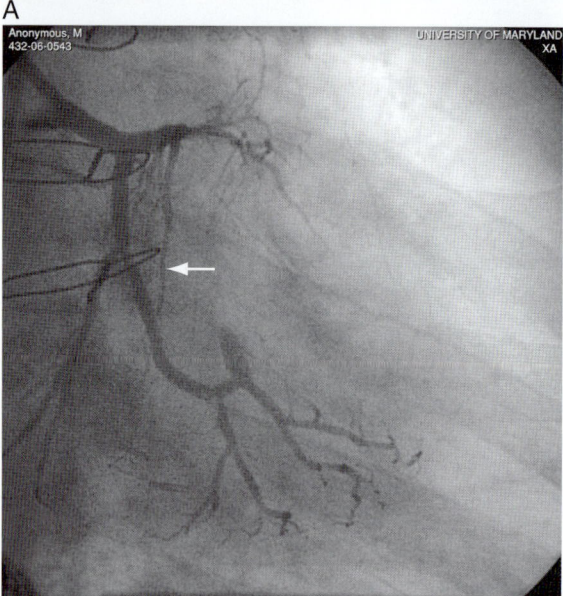

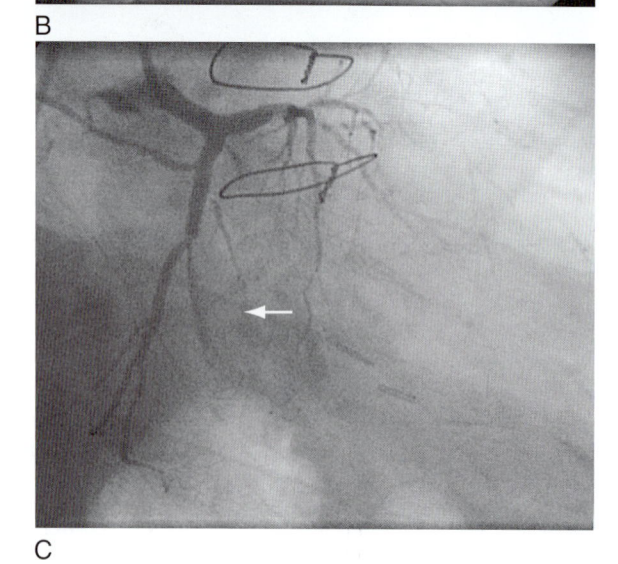

■ **FIGURE 29-23** Abrupt arterial closure after percutaneous transluminal coronary angioplasty. **A,** Long, high-grade stenosis in the circumflex marginal artery (*arrow*). **B,** Excellent angiographic result immediately after percutaneous transluminal coronary angioplasty. **C,** Abrupt vessel closure at the target site (*arrow*) 10 minutes after the angiogram in **B**.

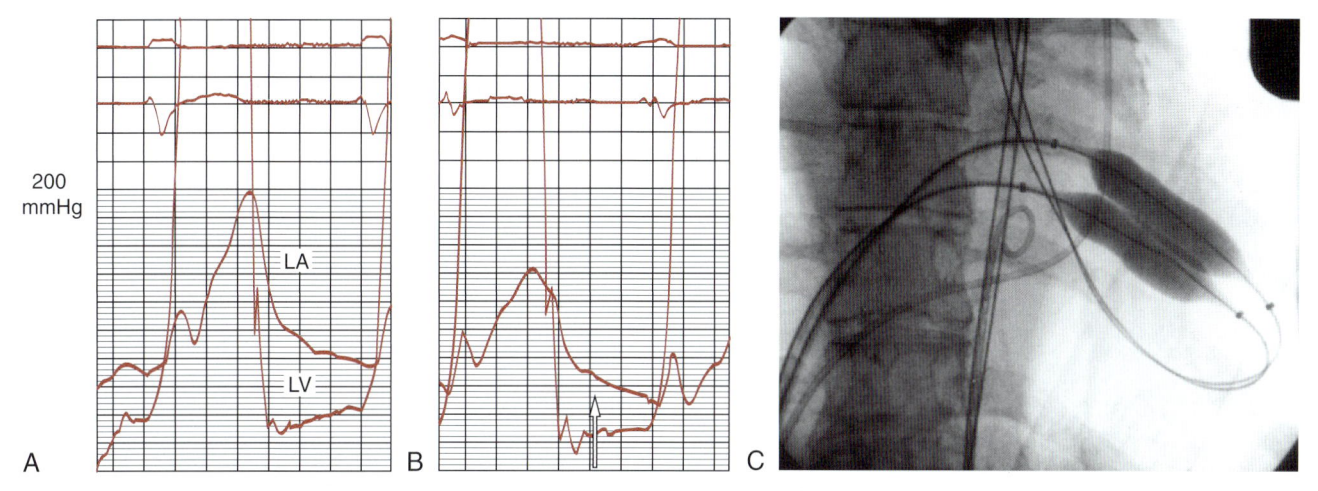

FIGURE 29-24 Mitral balloon valvotomy. **A,** Left atrial (LA) and left ventricular (LV) pressure recordings in a patient with mitral stenosis (baseline). **B,** After balloon valvotomy, the gradient during diastole (*arrow*) is significantly reduced. **C,** Two balloons expanded within the mitral orifice during balloon valvotomy.

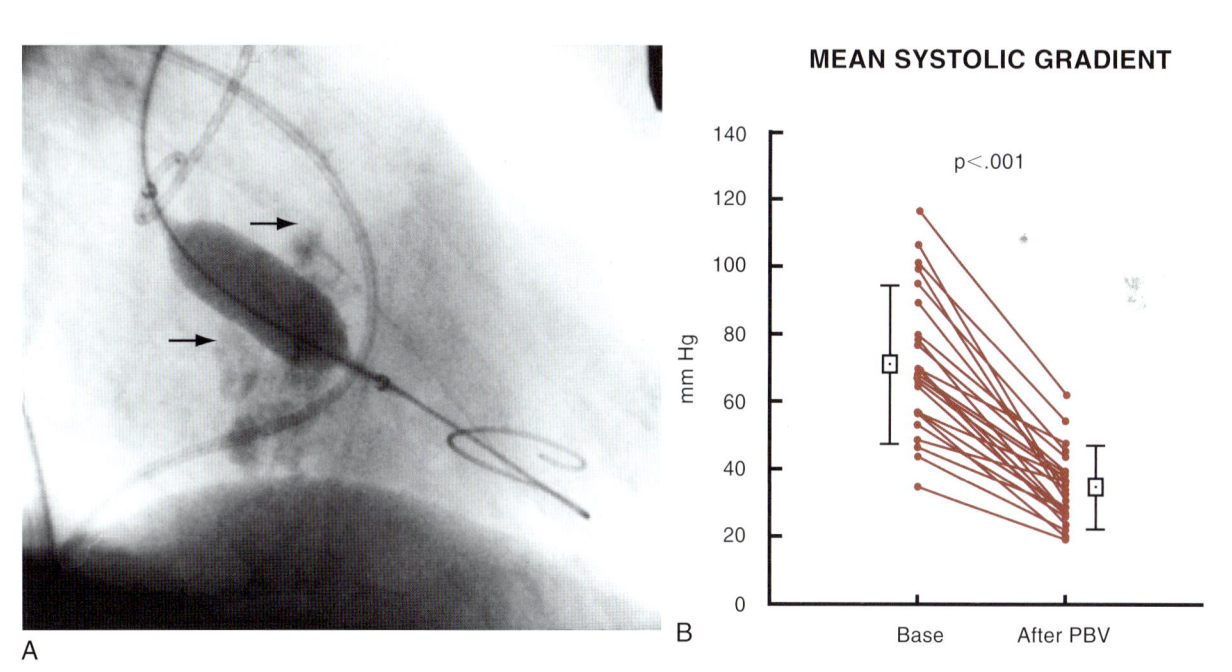

FIGURE 29-25 Aortic balloon valvotomy. **A,** Balloon valvotomy of stenotic, calcified (*arrows*) aortic valve in a 92-year-old patient. **B,** Immediate hemodynamic improvement after aortic balloon valvotomy (author's personal series). PBV, percutaneous balloon valvotomy.

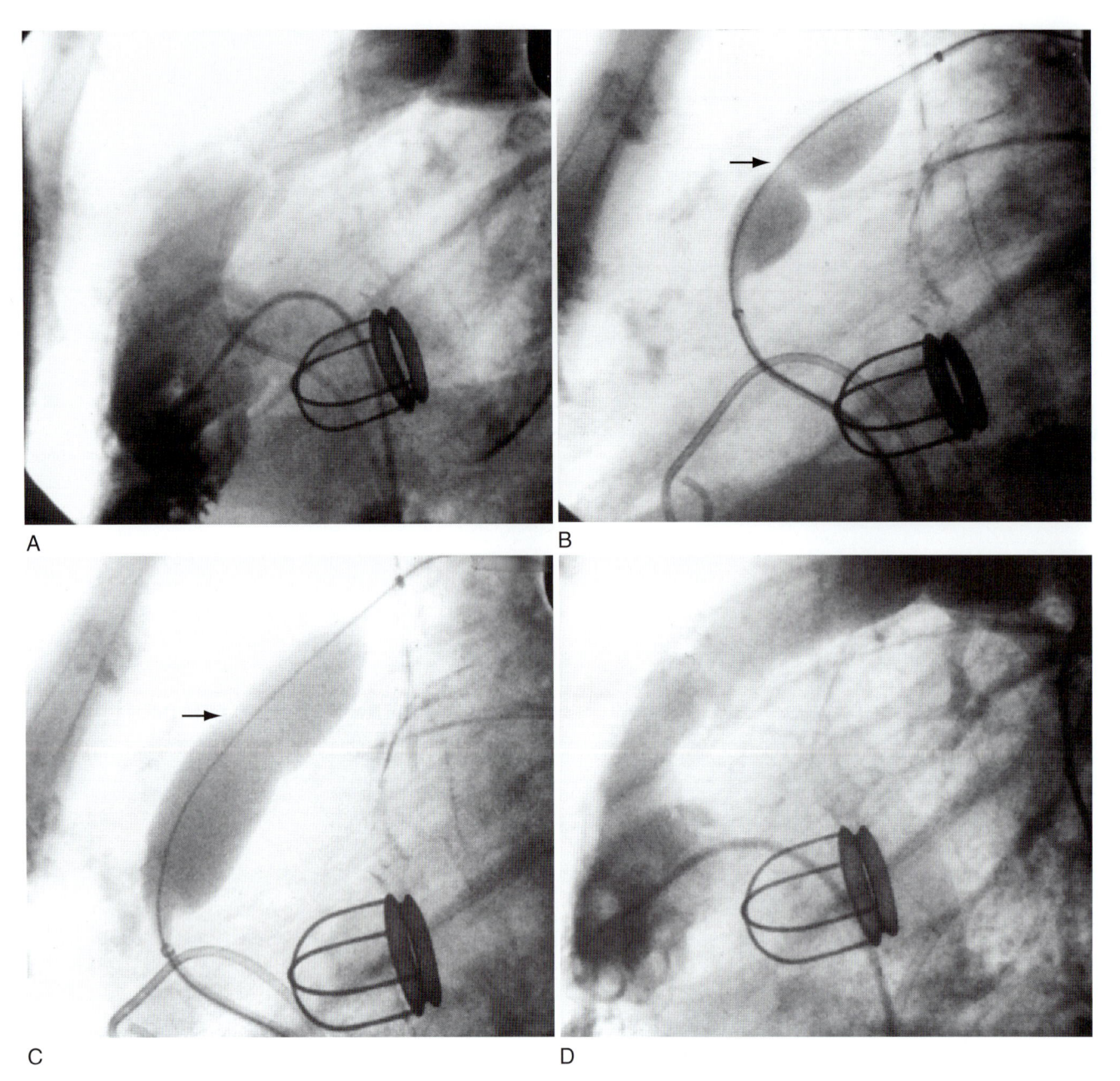

■ **FIGURE 29-26** Pulmonary balloon valvotomy. **A,** Right ventriculogram showing a domed, thickened pulmonic valve. The peak transvalvular gradient was 70 mm Hg. **B,** Balloon expansion at low pressure within the stenotic valve showing indentation indicative of incomplete dilation (*arrow*). **C,** Balloon expansion at higher pressure showing full expansion indicative of complete dilation (*arrow*). **D,** Right ventriculogram showing improved valve mobility. The postdilation transvalvular gradient was reduced to 20 mm Hg. (*Courtesy of J.P. Kleaveland, MD.*)

management of patients with congenital heart disease is discussed elsewhere, the current discussion focuses on catheter-based management of adults with acquired valvular heart disease.

Balloon catheter valvotomy was first applied to patients with rheumatic heart disease—most commonly mitral stenosis[71]—and has now become the preferred treatment for such patients in the absence of specific contraindications.[72] In properly selected patients and with experienced operators, the results are generally highly predictable (Fig. 29-24) with low complication rates.

Balloon catheter valvotomy in adult patients with calcific aortic valve stenosis was first reported in 1985 by the group from Rouen.[73] An immediate reduction in gradient and an increase in aortic valve area (Fig. 29-25) were thought to connote procedural success and, it was hoped, longer term overall clinical improvement. Mid-term to long-term follow-up indicated a high incidence of "restenosis," however, and a persistently elevated increased risk of death.[74] The current role of aortic valvuloplasty in the management of elderly patients or patients at high risk for surgical aortic valve replacement is unclear because there are no randomized trials to assess comparative outcomes. Nevertheless, aortic valvuloplasty represents a reasonable palliative option for "end-stage" patients at increased surgical risk or increased risk from progressive heart failure. In such patients, the procedure may be viewed as a "bridge" to surgical valve replacement, or as a compassionate procedure with clearly prespecified expectations. The emerging era of percutaneous catheter-based valve replacement (see next) may have a significant impact on treatment options for such patients.

In adults, balloon pulmonic valvotomy is generally performed in patients who are symptomatic or in patients who have progressed through adolescence and early adulthood without signs or symptoms of hemodynamic deterioration, but in whom critical values for right ventricular pressure and transvalvular gradient are documented.[72] Rarely, the procedure may be successfully performed on a noncongenitally stenosed pulmonic valve as well (Fig. 29-26). Data in the literature on longer term outcomes after native pulmonic valvuloplasty in adults are scarce.[75]

Finally, rapid developments in stent and catheter technology now allow for "hybrid devices" (balloon/stent/ ancillary device) to be used in the management of stenotic or insufficient valves. Beginning with the nonsurgical replacement of malfunctioning pulmonic valves,[76] the concept of stent-mounted valves has attracted great interest. Although this field is in its infancy,[77] early reports from ongoing clinical trials for mitral valve repair and aortic valve replacement are encouraging.[78]

KEY POINTS

- Percutaneous coronary intervention has become a highly successful and safe procedure to treat chronic CAD and its many acute presentations.
- Many adjunctive procedures and medical therapies have proven effectiveness in specific patient populations or lesion types.
- Percutaneous valve replacement is an investigational procedure that has promise to extend the present surgical treatments.

SUGGESTED READINGS

Babaliaros V, Block P. State of the art percutaneous intervention for the treatment of valvular heart disease: a review of the current technologies and ongoing research in the field of percutaneous valve replacement and repair. Cardiology 2007; 107:87-96.

Bravata DM, Gienger AL, McDonald KM, et al. Systematic review: the comparative effectiveness of percutaneous coronary interventions and coronary artery bypass graft surgery. Ann Intern Med 2007; 147:703-716.

Gunn J, Crossman D, Grech ED, et al. New developments in percutaneous coronary intervention. BMJ 2003; 327:150-153.

Holmes DR Jr, Kereiakes DJ, Laskey WK, et al. Thrombosis and drug-eluting stents: an objective appraisal. J Am Coll Cardiol 2007; 50:109-118.

Kereiakes DJ. Effects of GP IIb/IIIa inhibitors on vascular inflammation, coronary microcirculation, and platelet function. Rev Cardiovasc Med 2006; 7(Suppl 4):S3-S11.

Nallamothu BK, Bradley EH, Krumholz HM. Time to treatment in primary percutaneous coronary intervention. N Engl J Med 2007; 357: 1631-1638.

Rajagopal V, Kapadia SR, Tuzcu EM. Advances in the percutaneous treatment of aortic and mitral valve disease. Min Cardioangiol 2007; 55:83-94.

Routledge HC, Lefevre T, Morice MC, et al. Percutaneous aortic valve replacement: new hope for inoperable and high-risk patients. J Invasive Cardiol 2007; 19:478-483.

Sarkar K, Sharma SK, Sachdeva R, et al. Coronary artery restenosis: vascular biology and emerging therapeutic strategies. Expert Rev Cardiovasc Ther 2006; 4:543-556.

Soon KH, Selvanayagam JB, Cox N, et al. Percutaneous revascularization of chronic total occlusions: review of the role of invasive and non-invasive imaging modalities. Int J Cardiol 2007; 116:1-6.

REFERENCES

1. Dotter CT, Judkins MP. Transluminal treatment of arteriosclerotic obstruction: description of a new technique and preliminary report of its application. Circulation 1964; 30:654.
2. Gruentzig AR, Senning A, Siegenthaler WE. Non-operative dilatation of coronary artery stenosis: percutaneous transluminal coronary angioplasty. N Engl J Med. 1979; 301:61.
3. Stertzer SH, Myler RK, Bruno MS, et al. Transluminal coronary artery dilation. Pract Cardiol 1979; 5:25.
4. Myler RK, Gruentzig AR, Stertzer SH. Coronary angioplasty. In Rapaport E (ed). Cardiology Update. New York, Elsevier Biomedical, 1983, pp 1-66.
5. King SB, Yeh W, Holubkov R, et al. Balloon angioplasty versus new device intervention: clinical outcomes. A comparison of the NHLBI PTCA and NACI Registries. J Am Coll Cardiol 1998; 31:558-566.
6. Waller BF. "Crackers, breakers, stretchers, drillers, scrapers, shavers, burners, welders and melters"—the future treatment of atherosclerotic coronary artery disease? A clinico-morphologic assessment. J Am Coll Cardiol 1989; 13:969.
7. Iakovou I, Ge L, Colombo A. Contemporary stent treatment of coronary bifurcations. J Am Coll Cardiol 2005; 46:1446-1555.
8. Assali AR, Assa HV, Ben-Dor I, et al. Drug-eluting stents in bifurcation lesions: to stent one branch or both? Catheter Cardiovasc Interv 2006; 68:891-896.
9. Al Suwadi J, Yeh W, Cohen HA, et al. Immediate and one year outcome in patients with coronary bifurcation lesions in the modern era. Am J Cardiol 2001; 87:1139-1144.
10. Topol EJ, Yadav JS. Recognition of the importance of embolization in atherosclerotic vascular disease. Circulation 2000; 101:570-580.
11. Baim DS, Wahr D, George B, et al; on behalf of the SAFER trial investigators. Randomized trial of a distal embolic protection device during percutaneous intervention of saphenous vein aorto-coronary bypass grafts. Circulation 2002; 105:1285-1290.
12. Aziz S, Ramsdale DR. Chronic total occlusions—a stiff challenge requiring a major breakthrough: is there light at the end of the tunnel? Heart 2005; 91(Suppl 3):iii-42-iii-48.

13. Stone GW, Ellis SG, Cannon L, et al; TAXUS V investigators. Comparison of a polymer-based paclitaxel-eluting stent with a bare metal stent in patients with complex coronary artery disease: a randomized controlled trial. JAMA 2005; 294:1215-1223.
14. Smith SC, Feldman TE, Hirshfeld JW Jr, et al. ACC/AHA/SCAI 2005 guideline update for percutaneous coronary intervention—summary article: a report of the American College of Cardiology/American Heart Association Task Force on Practice Guidelines (ACC/AHA/SCAI Writing Committee to Update the 2001 Guidelines for Percutaneous Coronary Intervention). Circulation 2006; 113:156-175.
15. Seung KB, Park D-W, Kim Y-H, et al. Stents versus coronary artery bypass grafting for left main coronary artery disease. N Engl J Med 2008; 358:1781-1792.
16. Buszman PE, Kiesz SR, Bochenek A. Acute and late outcomes of unprotected left main stenting in comparison with surgical revascularization. J Am Coll Cardiol 2008; 51:538-545.
17. Keeley EC, Boura JA, Grines CL. Primary angioplasty versus intravenous thrombolytic therapy for acute myocardial infarction: a quantitative review of 23 randomised trials. Lancet 2003; 361:13-20.
18. Svilaas T, Vlaar PJ, van der Horst IC, et al. Thrombus aspiration during primary percutaneous coronary intervention. N Engl J Med 2008; 358:557-567.
19. Bertrand ME, Van Belle E. Rotational atherectomy. In Topol EJ (ed). Textbook of Interventional Cardiology. Philadelphia, Saunders, 2003, pp 549-557.
20. Reifart N, Vandormael M, Krajcar M, et al. Randomized comparison of angioplasty of complex coronary lesions at a single center. Excimer Laser, Rotational Atherectomy, Balloon Angioplasty Comparison (ERBAC) study. Circulation 1997; 96:91-98.
21. Popma JJ, Lansky AJ, Purkayastha DD, et al. Angiographic and clinical outcome after cutting balloon angioplasty. J Interv Cardiol 1996; 8(Suppl):12A-19A.
22. Safian RD. Coronary atherectomy: directional and extraction techniques. In Topol EJ (ed). Textbook of Interventional Cardiology. Philadelphia, Saunders, 2003, pp 523-548.
23. Topol E, Leya F, Pinkerton C, et al. A comparison of directional atherectomy with coronary angioplasty in patients with coronary artery disease. N Engl J Med 1993; 321:221-227.
24. King SB 3rd, Smith SC Jr, Hirshfeld JW Jr, et al. 2007 focused update of the ACC/AHA/SCAI 2005 guideline update for percutaneous coronary intervention: a report of the American College of Cardiology/American Heart Association Task Force on Practice guidelines. J Am Coll Cardiol 2008; 51:172-209.
25. Smith SC Jr, Feldman TE, Hirshfeld JW Jr, et al; American College of Cardiology/American Heart Association Task Force on Practice Guidelines; ACC/AHA/SCAI Writing Committee to Update 2001 Guidelines for Percutaneous Coronary Intervention. ACC/AHA/SCAI 2005 guideline update for percutaneous coronary intervention: a report of the American College of Cardiology/American Heart Association Task Force on Practice Guidelines. Circulation 2006; 113:e166-e286.
26. Detre K, Holubkov R, Kelsey S, et al. Percutaneous transluminal coronary angioplasty in 1985-1986 and 1977-1981. N Engl J Med 1988; 318:265.
27. Ryan T, Faxon DP, Gunnar RP, et al. Guidelines for percutaneous transluminal coronary angioplasty. Circulation 1988; 78:486.
28. Ellis SG, Guetta V, Miller D, et al. Relation between lesion characteristics and risk with percutaneous intervention in the stent and glycoprotein IIb/IIIa era: an analysis of results from 10,907 lesions and proposal for new classification scheme. Circulation 1999; 100:1971-1976.
29. Williams DO, Holubkov R, Yeh, W, et al. Percutaneous coronary intervention in the current era compared with 1985-1986: the National Heart, Lung and Blood Institute registries. Circulation 2000; 102:2945-2951.
30. Kimmel SE, Localio AR, Krone RJ, et al. The effects of contemporary use of coronary stents on in-hospital mortality. Registry Committee of the Society for Cardiac Angiography and Interventions. J Am Coll Cardiol 2001; 37:499-504.
31. Kimmel SE, Berlin JA, Strom BL, et al; for the Registry Committee of the Society for Cardiac Angiography and Interventions. Development and validation of a simplified predictive index for major complications in contemporary percutaneous transluminal coronary angioplasty practice. J Am Coll Cardiol 1995; 26:931-938.
32. Block PB, Peterson EC, Krone R, et al. Identification of variables needed to risk adjust outcomes of coronary interventions: evidence-based guidelines for efficient data collection. J Am Coll Cardiol 1998; 32:275-282.
33. Wennberg DE, Makenka DJ, Sengupta A, et al. Percutaneous transluminal coronary angioplasty in the elderly: epidemiology, clinical risk factors, and in-hospital outcomes. The Northern New England Cardiovascular Disease Study Group. Am Heart J 1999; 137:639-645.
34. The BARI Investigators. Influence of diabetes on 5-year mortality and morbidity in a randomized trial comparing CABG and PTCA in patients with multivessel disease: the Bypass Angioplasty Revascularization Investigation. Circulation 1997; 96:1761-1769.
35. Marroquin OC, Selzer F, Mulukutla SR, et al. A comparison of bare-metal and drug-eluting stents for off-label indications. N Engl J Med 2008; 358:342-353.
36. Babapulle MN, Joseph L, Belisle P, et al. A hierarchical Bayesian meta-analysis of randomised clinical trials of drug-eluting stents. Lancet 2004; 364:583-591.
37. Singh M, Lennon RJ, Holmes DR Jr, et al. Correlates of procedural complications and a simple integer risk score for percutaneous coronary intervention. J Am Coll Cardiol 2002; 40:387-393.
38. Keelan PC, Johnston JM, Koru-Sengul T, et al. Comparison of in-hospital and one-year outcomes in patients with left ventricular ejection fractions ≤40-49% and ≥50% having percutaneous coronary revascularization. Am J Cardiol 2003; 91:1168-1172.
39. Aragon J, Lee MS, Kar S, et al. Percutaneous left ventricular assist device: "TandemHeart" for high-risk coronary intervention. Catheter Cardiovasc Interv 2005; 65:346-352.
40. Henriques JP, Remmelink M, Baan J Jr, et al. Safety and feasibility of elective high-risk percutaneous coronary intervention procedures with left ventricular support of the Impella Recover LP 2.5. Am J Cardiol 2006; 97:990-992.
41. Vogel RA, Shawl F, Tommaso C, et al. Initial report of the National Registry of Elective Cardiopulmonary Bypass Supported Coronary Angioplasty. J Am Coll Cardiol 1990; 15:23-29.
42. Best PJ, Lennon R, Ting HH, et al. The impact of renal insufficiency on clinical outcomes in patients undergoing percutaneous coronary interventions. J Am Coll Cardiol 2002; 39:1113-1119.
43. Naidu SS, Selzer F, Jacobs A, et al. Renal insufficiency is an independent predictor of mortality after percutaneous coronary intervention. Am J Cardiol 2003; 92:1160-1164.
44. Sadeghi HM, Stone GW, Grines CL, et al. Impact of renal insufficiency in patients undergoing primary angioplasty for acute myocardial infarction. Circulation 2003; 108:2769-2775.
45. Rihal CS, Textor SC, Grill DE, et al. Incidence and prognostic importance of acute renal failure after percutaneous coronary intervention. Circulation 2000; 105:2259-2264.
46. Block PC, Myler RK, Stertzer S, et al. Morphology after transluminal angioplasty in human beings. N Engl J Med 1981; 305:382-385.
47. Block PC. Mechanism of transluminal angioplasty. Am J Cardiol 1984; 53:69C-71C.
48. Schwartz RS. Animal models of human coronary restenosis. In Topol EJ (ed). Textbook of Interventional Cardiology. Philadelphia, Saunders, 2003, pp 391-414.
49. Forrester JS, Fishbein M, Helfant R, et al. A paradigm for restenosis based on cell biology: clues for the development of new preventive therapies. J Am Coll Cardiol 1991; 17:758.
50. Libby P, Simon DI, Rogers C. Inflammation and arterial injury. In Topol EJ (ed). Textbook of Interventional Cardiology. Philadelphia, Saunders, 2003, pp 381-389.
51. Nobuyoshi M, Kimura T, Nosaka H, et al. Restenosis after successful percutaneous coronary transluminal coronary angioplasty: serial angiographic follow-up of 229 patients. J Am Coll Cardiol 1988; 12:616.
52. Kuntz RE, Gibson M, Nobuyoshi M, et al. Generalized model of restenosis after conventional balloon angioplasty, stenting and directional atherectomy. J Am Coll Cardiol 1993; 21:15.
53. Sigwart U, Puel J, Mirkovitch V, et al. Intravascular stents to prevent occlusion and restenosis after transluminal angioplasty. N Engl J Med 1987; 316:701-706.
54. Roubin GS, Cannon AD, Agarwal SK, et al. Intracoronary stenting for acute and threatened closure complicating percutaneous transluminal angioplasty. Circulation 1992; 85:916-927.

55. Fischman DL, Leon MB, Baim DS, et al. A randomized comparison of coronary stent placement and balloon angioplasty in the treatment of coronary disease. N Engl J Med 1994; 331:496-501.
56. Serruys PW, de Jaegere P, Kiemeneij F, et al. A comparison of balloon-expandable stent implantation with balloon angioplasty in patients with coronary artery disease. N Engl J Med 1994; 331:489-495.
57. Colombo A, Hall P, Nakamura S, et al. Intracoronary stenting without anticoagulation accomplished with intravascular ultrasound guidance. Circulation 1995; 91:1676-1688.
58. Schomig A, Neumann FJ, Kastrati A, et al. A randomized comparison of antiplatelet and anticoagulant therapy after the placement of coronary-artery stents. N Engl J Med 1996; 334:1084-1089.
59. Leon MB, Baim DS, Popma JJ, et al. A clinical trial comparing three antithrombotic drug regimens after coronary artery stenting. N Engl J Med 1998; 339:1665-1671.
60. Teirstein PS, Massullo V, Jani S, et al. Catheter-based radiotherapy to inhibit restenosis after coronary stenting. N Engl J Med 1997; 336:1697-1703.
61. Popma JJ, Suntharalingham M, Lansky AJ, et al; for the Stents and Radiation Therapy (START) investigators. Randomized trial of 90Sr/90Y(beta) radiation versus placebo control for treatment of in-stent restenosis. Circulation 2002; 106:1090-1096.
62. Morice MC, Serruys PW, Sousa JE, et al. Randomized study with the sirolimus-coated Bx velocity balloon-expandable stent in the treatment of patients with de novo native coronary artery lesions: a randomized comparison of a sirolimus-eluting stent with a standard stent for coronary revascularization. N Engl J Med 2002; 346:1773-1780.
63. Moses JW, Leon MB, Popma JJ, et al. Sirolimus-eluting stents vs. standard stents in patients with stenosis in a native coronary artery. N Engl J Med 2003; 349:1315-1323.
64. Stone GW, Ellis SG, Cox DA, et al. A polymer-based, paclitaxel-eluting stent in patients with coronary artery disease. N Engl J Med 2004; 350:221-231.
65. Holmes DR Jr, Kereiakes DJ, Laskey WK, et al. Thrombosis and drug-eluting stents: an objective appraisal. J Am Coll Cardiol 2007; 50:109-118.
66. Maisel WH. Unanswered questions—drug-eluting stents and the risk of late thrombosis. N Engl J Med 2007; 356:981-984.
67. Laskey WK, Yancy CW, Maisel WH. Thrombosis in coronary drug-eluting stents: report from the meeting of the Circulatory System Medical Devices Advisory Panel of the Food and Drug Administration Center for Devices and Radiologic Health, December 7-8, 2006. Circulation 2007; 115:2352-2357.
68. Grines C, Bonow R, Casey D Jr, et al. Prevention of premature discontinuation of dual antiplatelet therapy in patients with coronary artery stents. A science advisory from the American Heart Association, American College of Cardiology, Society for Cardiovascular Angiography and Interventions, American College of Surgeons and American Dental Association, with representation from the American College of Physicians. J Am Coll Cardiol 2007; 49:734-739.
69. Hodgson JMcB, Bottner RK, Klein LW, et al; Drug-Eluting Stent Task Force. Final report and recommendations of the working committees on cost effectiveness/economics, access to care and medico-legal issues. Cathet Cardiovasc Interv 2004; 62:1-17.
70. Kan JS, White RI, Mitchell SE, et al. Percutaneous balloon valvuloplasty: a new method for treatment of congenital pulmonary valve stenosis. N Engl J Med 1982; 307:540.
71. Inoue K, Owaki T, Nakamura T, et al. Clinical application of transvenous mitral commissurotomy by a new balloon catheter. J Thorac Cardiovasc Surg 1984; 87:394-402.
72. Bonow RO, Carabello BA, Chatterjee K, et al. ACC/AHA 2006 guidelines for the management of patients with valvular heart disease: a report of the American College of Cardiology/American Heart Association Task Force on Practice Guidelines. Circulation 2006; 114:e84-e231.
73. Cribier A, Savin T, Saoudi N, et al. Percutaneous transluminal valvuloplasty of acquired aortic stenosis in elderly patients: an alternative to valve replacement? Lancet 1986; 1:63-67.
74. O'Neill WW; Mansfield Scientific Aortic Valvuloplasty Registry Investigators. Predictors of long-term survival after percutaneous aortic valvuloplasty: report of the Mansfield Scientific Aortic Valvuloplasty Registry. J Am Coll Cardiol 1991; 17:909-913.
75. Chen CR, Cheng TO, Huang T, et al. Percutaneous balloon valvuloplasty for pulmonic stenosis in adolescents and adults. N Engl J Med 1966; 335:21-25.
76. Bonhoeffer P, Boudjemline Y, Saliba Z, et al. Percutaneous replacement of pulmonary valve in a right ventricle to pulmonary artery prosthetic conduit with valve dysfunction. Lancet 2000; 356:1403-1405.
77. Vassiliades TA, Block PC, Cohn LH, et al. The clinical development of percutaneous heart valve technology. A position statement of the Society for Thoracic Surgeons, the American Association for Thoracic Surgery and the Society for Cardiovascular Angiography and Interventions. J Thorac Cardiovasc Surg 2005; 129:970-976.
78. Rosengart TK, Feldman T, Borger MA, et al. Percutaneous and minimally-invasive valve procedures: a scientific statement from the American Heart Association Council on Cardiovascular Surgery and Anesthesia, Council on Clinical Cardiology, Functional Genomics and Translational Biology Interdisciplinary Working Group and Quality of Care and Outcomes Research Interdisciplinary Working Group. Circulation 2008; 117:1750-1767.

CHAPTER 30

Surgery for Acquired Cardiac Disease

John S. Thurber* and Subrato J. Deb

The history of cardiac surgery dates back to the late 19th century, with the repair of pericardial and cardiac trauma by Williams of Chicago in 1893. The modern era of cardiac surgery began in earnest with the development of the cardiopulmonary bypass machine by Gibbon of Boston in 1953. The modern concepts and techniques of extracorporeal circulation were refined further by Lillehei and Kirklin in the early 1950s. Extracorporeal circulation, along with improved techniques of myocardial protection, has allowed surgeons to perform the most complex procedures in the current realm of cardiothoracic surgical practice. The most commonly performed procedure since its inception in the 1960s is coronary artery bypass graft (CABG) surgery.

The development of coronary cine angiography in the early 1960s enabled the identification of stenoses of the coronary arteries in living patients (Fig. 30-1). This identification made it possible for the directed treatment of ischemic heart disease through CABG surgery and percutaneous interventions of obstructed arteries. The treatment for coronary artery disease was revolutionized, dramatically improving the therapeutic options for patients with this commonly occurring condition.

---

*The views expressed in this chapter are those of the author and do not necessarily reflect the official policy or position of the Department of the Navy, Army, Department of Defense, or the U.S. government.

We certify that all individuals who qualify as authors have been listed; each has participated in the conception and design of this work, the analysis of data (when applicable), the writing of the document, and the approval of the submission of this version; that the document represents valid work; that if we used information derived from another source, we obtained all necessary approvals to use it and made appropriate acknowledgments in the document; and that each takes public responsibility for it.

SURGERY FOR CORONARY ARTERY DISEASE

Description and Special Anatomic Considerations

Myocardial blood flow is provided by the left and right coronary arteries, originating from the aortic root. The left main coronary artery bifurcates into the left anterior descending (LAD) and the left circumflex arteries. The left circumflex artery further branches into the obtuse marginal arteries, which together with the LAD artery provide most blood flow to the left ventricle. The right coronary artery provides blood flow to the right ventricle and terminates as the posterior descending artery, providing blood flow to the inferior wall of the left ventricle (Fig. 30-2).

The basic goal of CABG surgery is to provide new blood flow beyond significantly stenotic epicardial vessels. Stenosis is considered hemodynamically significant when the diameter is reduced by greater than 50%, which equates to a reduction in the cross-sectional area of 75% (Fig. 30-3). The technique of CABG surgery involves four stages: (1) conduit harvest, (2) institution of extracorporeal circulation, (3) construction of vascular anastomoses, and (4) separation from cardiopulmonary bypass. Most commonly used conduits for bypass grafts include the left internal mammary artery and greater saphenous vein. Other possible conduits include the right internal mammary artery, the radial artery, the right gastroepiploic artery, and the lesser saphenous vein. Generally, arterial conduits have better long-term patency than venous grafts.

CABG surgery is performed with the use of cardiopulmonary bypass, which provides circulatory support and gas exchange during the operation. Anticoagulation with heparin is typically used during the period of cardiopulmonary bypass. To establish a still and bloodless field on

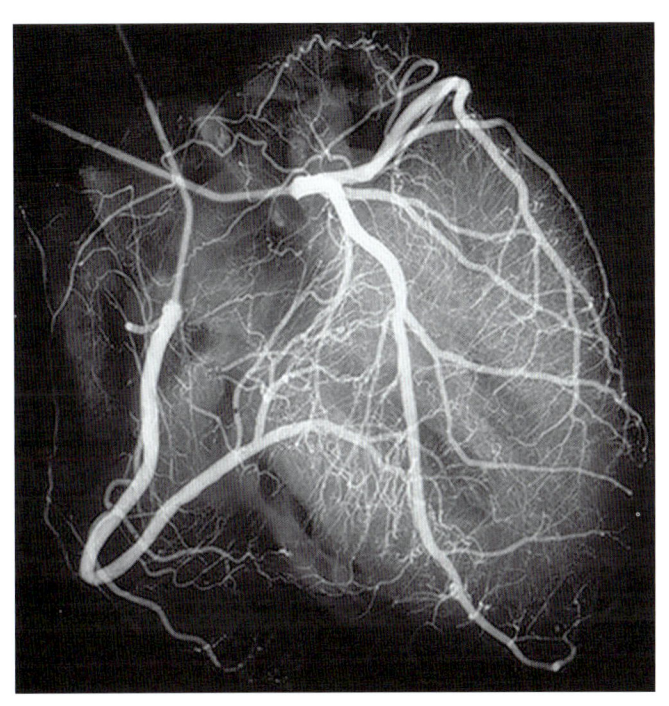

FIGURE 30-1 Coronary angiogram of right and left coronary artery systems. *(From Mayo Clinic Cardiothoracic Grand Rounds, picture used in slide presentation, 2002.)*

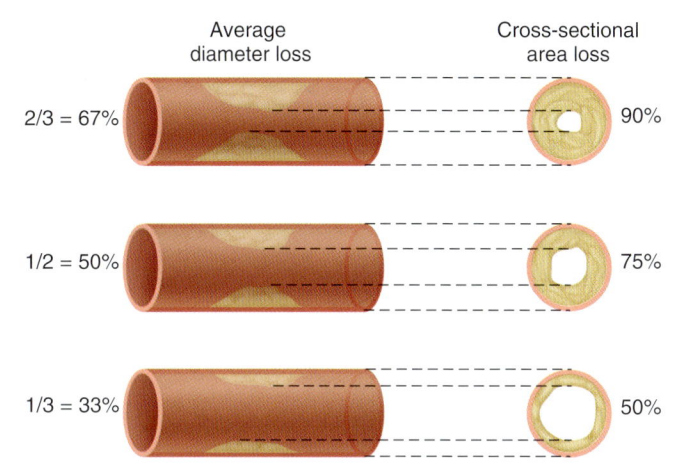

FIGURE 30-3 Relationship of coronary artery stenosis in diameter and cross-sectional area. *(From Brandt PW, Partridge JB, Wattie WJ. Coronary arteriography: a method of presentation of the arteriogram report and a scoring system. Clin Radiol 1977; 28:361.)*

which to sew the anastomoses, the heart is arrested using hyperkalemic cardioplegia solution. The basic cardiopulmonary bypass circuit is shown in Figure 30-4. When the heart is arrested, and epicardial arteries are exposed (Fig. 30-5), the vascular anastomoses may be constructed.

The microvascular anastomoses are constructed using fine suture material, under loupe magnification, as shown in Figure 30-6. The left internal mammary artery is most commonly placed to the LAD artery as an in-situ graft (Fig. 30-7), whereas the greater saphenous vein is placed as a reversed graft from the ascending aorta to the coronary artery (Fig. 30-8).

The final stage of the operation involves separation of the patient from cardiopulmonary bypass and obtaining hemostasis. Protamine is typically administered to reverse heparin anticoagulation.

Indications

Over the years, accepted indications for CABG surgery have changed slightly, primarily as a result of the advent of catheter-based revascularization techniques, especially coronary artery stenting. The American Heart Association (AHA) has published comprehensive guidelines regarding the indications for CABG.[1] These recommendations generally are classified into one of eight subsets of patients as shown in Table 30-1. Class I or II indications for surgery include patients with stable or unstable angina and three-vessel disease (including the main branches of the right coronary artery, LAD artery, and left circumflex artery), patients with two-vessel disease with proximal LAD artery stenosis, or asymptomatic patients with significant left main stenosis. CABG surgery after acute myocardial infarction is indicated in these same conditions and is usually delayed for 1 week, if possible, to allow myocardial recovery before surgery. Emergent CABG surgery may be indicated for cardiogenic shock secondary to acute myocardial infarction in patients younger than 75 years (which can salvage 50% of patients) or for post–percutaneous intervention complications.

Contraindications

The only contraindications to a patient undergoing CABG surgery are the absence of adequate target vessels, as seen on cardiac catheterization, or a lack of a suitable conduit.

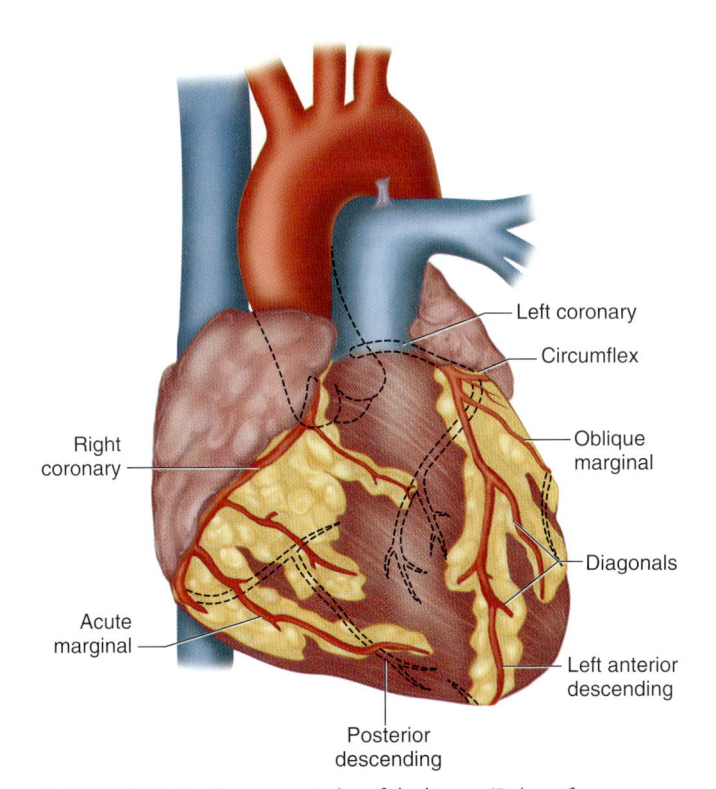

FIGURE 30-2 Coronary arteries of the heart. *(Redrawn from University of Utah Health Sciences Center. 2002. Available at: http://healthcare.utah.edu/healthinfo/adult/cardiac/arteries.htm.)*

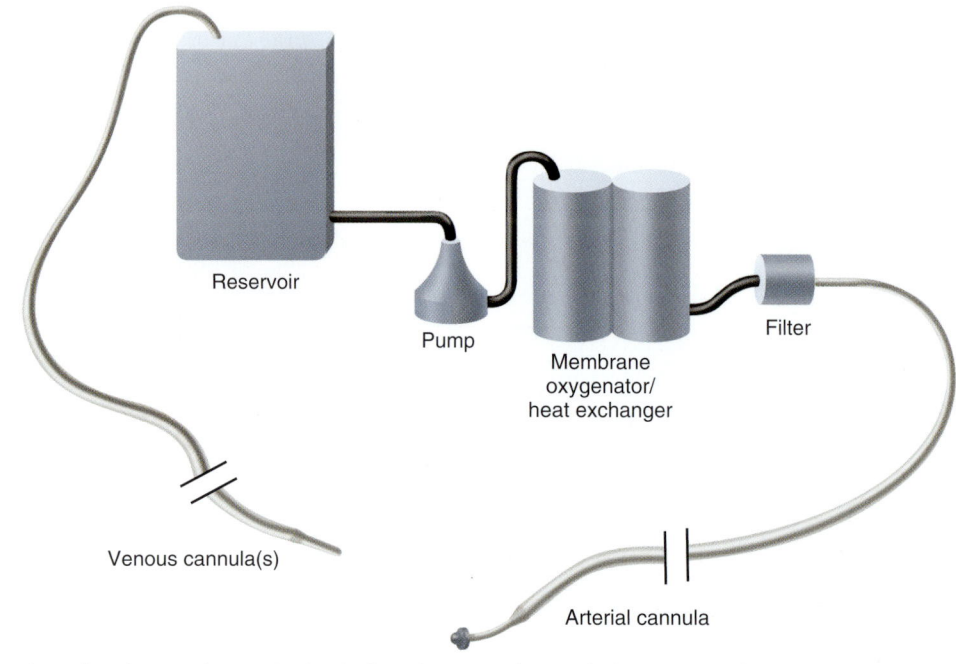

FIGURE 30-4 Basic cardiopulmonary bypass circuit. *(Redrawn from Mayo Clinic Cardiothoracic Grand Rounds, picture used in slide presentation, 2002.)*

Patients in this category with refractory angina may be considered for alternative forms of therapy, such as transmyocardial revascularization, stem cell therapy, and coronary endarterectomy.

All patients are risk-stratified to predict the probability of operative morbidity and mortality. Factors that increase risk for surgery are presented in Table 30-2. The most important predictor of operative mortality is the preoperative left ventricular ejection fraction. There are several acceptable methods to calculate perioperative risk in cardiac surgery. The Society of Thoracic Surgeons (STS) Risk Calculator and the EUROSCORE are two of the most commonly used methods. When the calculated risks of surgery outweigh the potential benefits of the operation, surgery should not be performed.

Outcomes and Complications

Overall hospital mortality after CABG surgery has declined over the past 20 years and presently is 2% to 3%, according to the STS surgical database. Most in-hospital deaths after CABG surgery are due to cardiac failure. Overall 5-year survival is greater than 90%, and overall 10-year survival is 70% to 80%. The frequent use of the left internal mammary artery

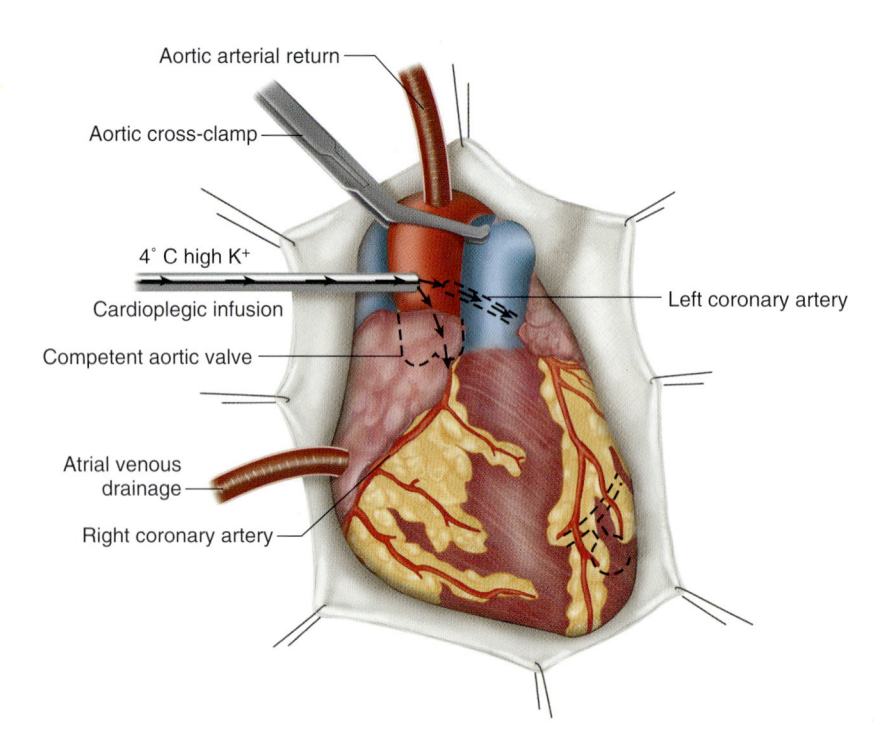

FIGURE 30-5 Common cannulation and myocardial protection techniques used for cardiopulmonary bypass. *(Redrawn from Roberts AJ. Efficacy of intraoperative myocardial protection in adult cardiac surgery. In Roberts AJ [ed]. Difficult Problems in Adult Cardiac Surgery. Chicago, Year Book Medical Publishers, 1985, p 386.)*

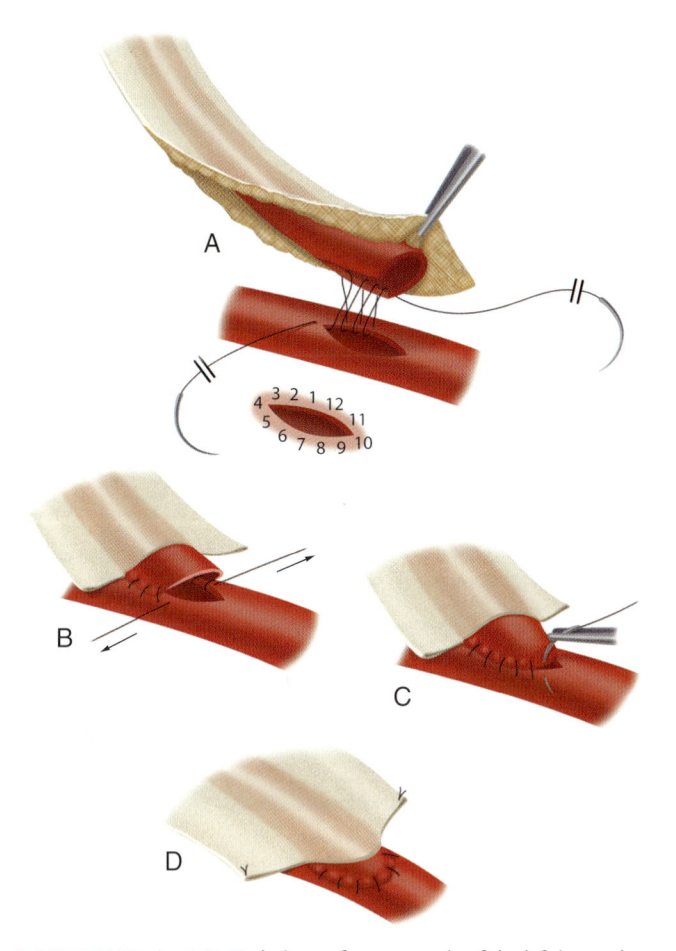

■ **FIGURE 30-6** A-D, Technique of anastomosis of the left internal mammary artery to the left anterior descending coronary artery. (Redrawn from Rankin JS, Morris JJ. Utilization of autologous arterial grafts for coronary artery bypass. In Sabiston D, Spencer F [eds]. Surgery of the Chest, 6th ed. Philadelphia, Saunders, 1996, p 1913.)

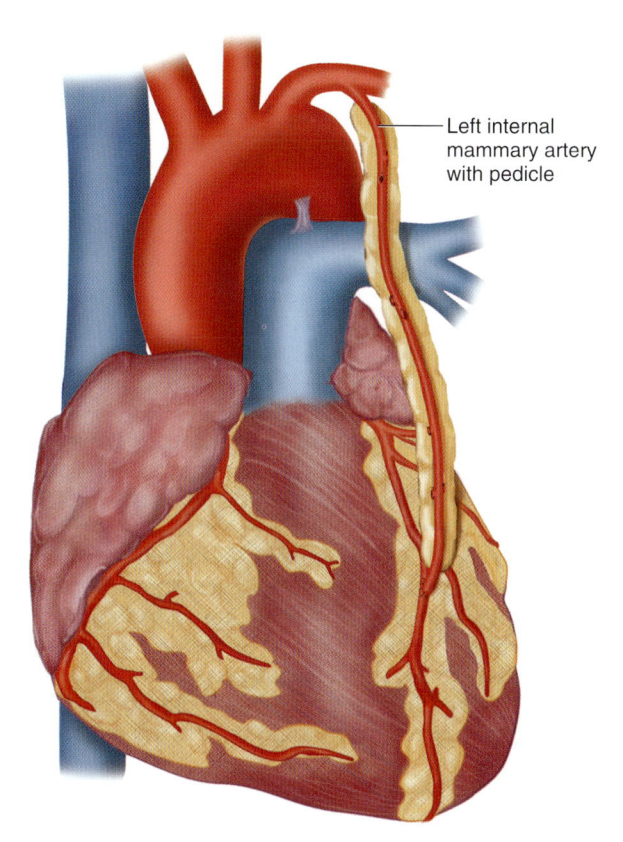

■ **FIGURE 30-7** In-situ left internal mammary artery graft to left anterior descending coronary artery. (Redrawn from Rhead J, Sundt TM. What is coronary artery bypass grafting? Society of Thoracic Surgeons, 2008. Available at: www.sts.org/sections/patientinformation/adultcardiacsurgery/cabg.)

has favorably affected short-term and long-term survival. For patients with preoperative angina, resolution of symptoms is approximately 60% at 10 years. Recurrent angina is typically due to progression of atherosclerotic disease of the native coronary arteries or vein grafts. The aggressive use of statin therapy and β blockers can delay the progression of coronary artery or vein graft disease after CABG surgery.[2]

The results of three randomized prospective studies comparing CABG surgery with medical management conclusively showed survival advantages with CABG surgery, particularly among patients with three-vessel disease, left main disease, and decreased left ventricular ejection fraction (35% to 50%).[3-5] In diabetic patients with multivessel disease, CABG surgery has been shown to be superior to percutaneous coronary interventions. In the current era of drug-eluting stents, CABG surgery has been shown to have a reduced rate of reintervention, particularly in the setting of multivessel disease.

Potential early postoperative complications after CABG surgery include cardiac failure/low cardiac output syndrome, stroke, bleeding, renal failure requiring hemodialysis, pneumonia, mediastinitis/wound infection, pericardial tamponade, and atrial fibrillation. Atrial fibrillation is the most frequent complication after cardiac surgery, seen in 15% to 30% of patients. The incidence of this arrhythmia has decreased with the use of perioperative prophylaxis with agents such as amiodarone or β blockers. Possible late complications (>2 weeks postoperatively) include delayed pericardial or pleural effusion, late saphenous vein graft failure, and wound infection (sternal or saphenectomy site).

Imaging Findings

Preoperative Planning

With the advent of selective coronary angiography by Mason Sones in 1967, and the CASS study,[4] the gold standard for assessment of coronary artery anatomy and disease was established. Several projections obtained using fluoroscopic guidance allow the surgeon to obtain a three-dimensional assessment of the coronary arteries (Table 30-3). Figure 30-9 shows several commonly used projections of coronary artery catheterization. Additionally, by injecting contrast material with the catheter positioned in the left ventricle, an image of the left ventricle throughout the cardiac cycle may be obtained to assess left ventricular function.

The high-resolution, 64-detector CT scanner has emerged as a tool for performing coronary angiography quickly and less invasively.[6] Data quality is high, and has improved with increasingly sophisticated technology.

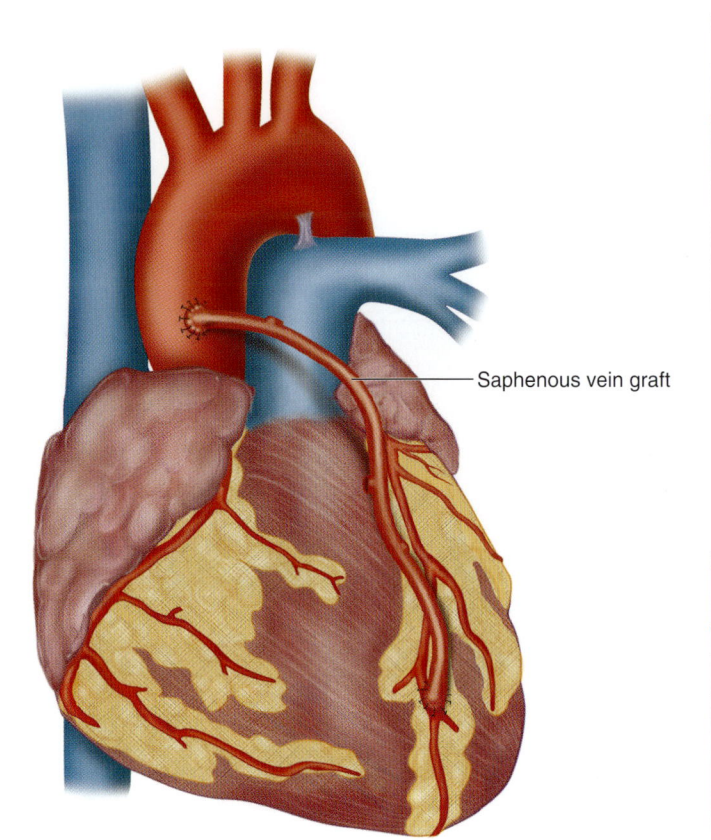

FIGURE 30-8 Reversed aorto–saphenous vein graft to left anterior descending coronary artery. *(Redrawn from Rhead J, Sundt TM. What is coronary artery bypass grafting? Society of Thoracic Surgeons, 2008. Available at: www.sts.org/sections/patientinformation/adultcardiacsurgery/cabg.)*

Saphenous vein graft

TABLE 30-1	American Heart Association Recommended Indications for Coronary Artery Bypass Graft (CABG) Surgery: Clinical Subsets of Patients
Asymptomatic or mild angina	
Stable angina	
Unstable angina/non–ST segment elevation myocardial infarction	
ST segment elevation myocardial infarction	
Poor left ventricular function	
Life-threatening ventricular arrhythmias	
CABG surgery after failed previous percutaneous intervention	
Previous CABG surgery	

From Eagle KA, Guyton RA, Davidoff R, et al. ACC/AHA 2004 guideline update for coronary artery bypass surgery: a report of the American College of Cardiology/American Heart Association Task Force on Practice Guidelines (Committee to Update the 1999 Guidelines for Coronary Artery Bypass Graft Surgery. Circulation 2004; 110:e340-e437.

TABLE 30-2	Preoperative Risk Factors for Coronary Artery Bypass Graft Surgery
Decreased left ventricular ejection fraction	
Pulmonary disease	
Renal insufficiency	
Peripheral vascular disease, including ascending aorta	
Prior sternotomy	
Advanced age	
Obesity	

Sensitivity and specificity of CT angiography have been shown to be comparable to conventional coronary angiography in detecting stenoses in symptomatic patients.[7] Positive and negative predicted values also are comparable. Current limitations of CT angiography that reduce the reliability for image interpretation include heavy vessel wall calcifications, persistent irregular heart rhythm (and

TABLE 30-3	Standard Projectional Views for Cardiac Catheterization
Anteroposterior	
Right anterior oblique (RAO)	
RAO caudal	
RAO cranial	
Left anterior oblique (LAO)	
LAO caudal	
LAO cranial	
Lateral	

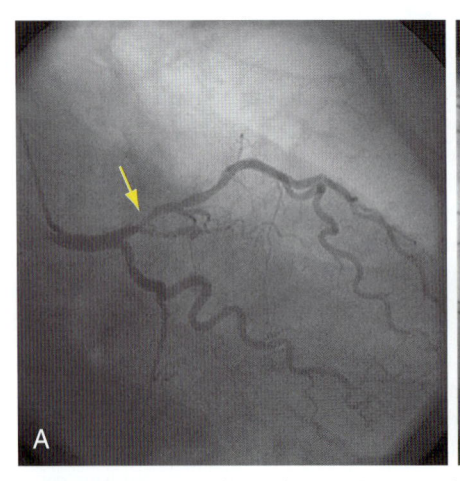

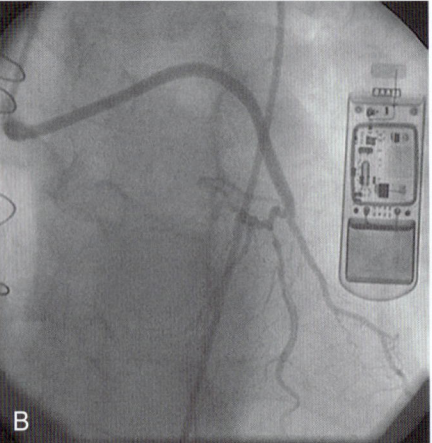

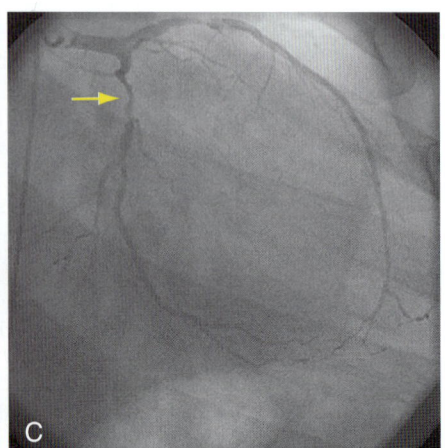

FIGURE 30-9 Cardiac catheterization views showing coronary artery lesions. **A,** Right anterior oblique (cranial) projection showing proximal left anterior descending coronary artery lesion (*arrow*). **B,** Left anterior oblique (cranial) projection showing patent vein graft to obtuse marginal artery. **C,** Right anterior oblique (caudal) projection showing left anterior descending coronary artery and left circumflex coronary artery disease (*arrow*).

the need for heart rates <70 beats/min), and existing coronary stents.[8] The estimated radiation dose used for CT angiography is also higher than the dose used for conventional angiography. MR angiography is another modality used to assess coronary artery anatomy, particularly in patients with coronary anomalies.

Preoperative echocardiogram is recommended to evaluate valvular competency and ventricular function. For patients with peripheral vascular disease who are at risk for perioperative stroke, a non–contrast-enhanced CT scan of the chest to rule out aortic atheroma and a carotid duplex image to rule out significant carotid artery stenosis are useful.

Postoperative Surveillance

Routine (scheduled) postoperative radiographic surveillance is typically not performed unless the patient has new findings consistent with cardiac ischemia, such as angina, shortness of breath symptoms, a positive exercise stress test, or a change in myocardial contractility on echocardiogram. A myocardial perfusion scan can be obtained if persistent or recurrent ischemia is suspected after CABG surgery. Currently, the most sensitive and specific method to assess bypass graft patency is cardiac catheterization. Coronary CT angiography may become more commonly used in the near future for graft surveillance in patients with equivocal findings.

SURGERY FOR AORTIC VALVULAR DISEASE

Description and Special Anatomic Considerations

Although the number of coronary artery bypass procedures has gradually declined in current cardiovascular surgical practice in the United States, the number of valve procedures has steadily increased over the last 10 years. In the executive summary of the STS Spring 2007 Report, the number of isolated aortic valve replacements (AVRs) and tricuspid valve procedures showed the greatest increase since 1997.[9]

Aortic Valve Anatomy

Situated centrally at the base of the heart, the aortic valve resides in a unique position because of its proximity to all chambers of the heart and the three other cardiac valves (Fig. 30-10). The aortic valve is trileaflet, consisting of three semilunar cusps and the fibrous aortic annulus to which the cusps are attached. Sinuses of Valsalva are areas of aortic dilation adjacent to the aortic valve cusps, and are identified by the respective coronary artery origination as left, right, and noncoronary (Fig. 30-11). The commissures are structures where adjacent aortic cusps abut each other and have special anatomic significance during surgery. The commissure between the noncoronary and right coronary cusps is directly cephalad to the penetration of the atrioventricular bundle and membranous septum (see Fig. 30-11). The commissure between the noncoronary and left coronary cusps bisects the aortic-mitral curtain and the anterior leaflet of the mitral valve (see Fig. 30-11). This area is of particular significance during aortic root enlargement and in cases of aortic valve endocarditis as an avenue of spread for infection to the mitral valve. The last commissure between the left and right cusps defines the adjacent pulmonary valve and right ventricular outflow tract (see Figs. 30-10 and 30-11).

The aortic valve operates via a passive mechanism of valve opening and closing that is driven by small differences in pressure between the ascending aorta and left ventricle. This mechanism is quite different from the mitral valve discussed later in this section.

Pathophysiology of Aortic Stenosis and Regurgitation

Acquired calcific aortic valvular stenosis is most commonly due to degeneration and calcification of the aortic valve leaflets; this disease primarily affects elderly patients. In contrast, significant aortic stenosis in younger patients is most commonly due to premature calcification and degeneration of a bicuspid aortic valve, and typically occurs in the fourth or fifth decade of life. In calcific aortic stenosis, the calcification and thickening of the aortic

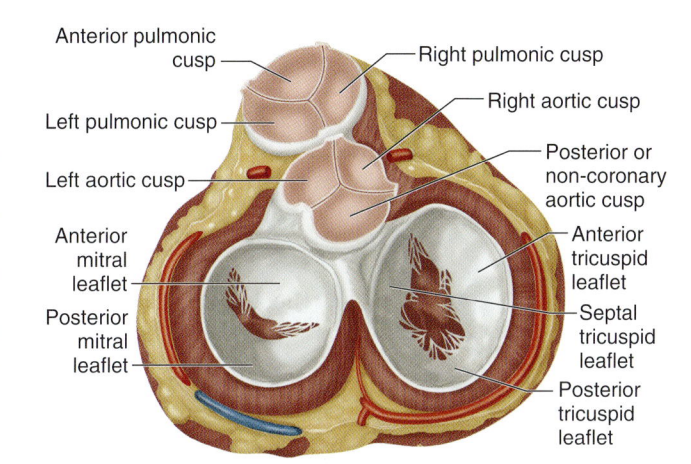

■ FIGURE 30-10 Aortic valve position in base of the heart. (Redrawn from Miljevic T, Sayeed MR, Stamou SC, et al. Pathophysiology of aortic valve disease. In Cohn LH [ed]. Cardiac Surgery in the Adult. New York, McGraw-Hill, 2008, pp 825-840.)

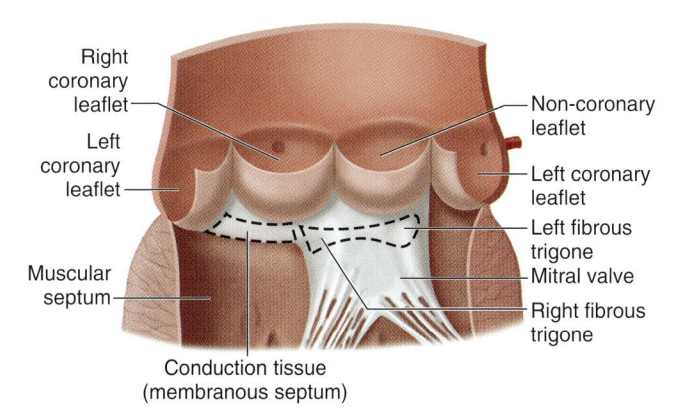

■ FIGURE 30-11 Aortic annulus. (Redrawn from Miljevic T, Sayeed MR, Stamou SC, et al. Pathophysiology of aortic valve disease. In Cohn LH [ed]. Cardiac Surgery in the Adult. New York, McGraw-Hill, 2008, pp 825-840.)

valve leaflets occurs through an active inflammatory process, partially related to hypercholesterolemia, similar to the process of coronary atherosclerosis.[10-13] As the leaflets calcify and fuse together, the functional area of the valve decreases to cause a measurable obstruction to outflow. The progressive pressure overload to the left ventricle results in maladaptive left ventricular hypertrophy, and eventually results in clinically significant obstruction.

In contrast to aortic stenosis, the causes of aortic valvular regurgitation are numerous and include pathology of the aortic annulus, aortic valve, ascending aorta, or a combination. Common causes of aortic regurgitation include ascending aortic aneurysm or dissection; annuloaortic ectasia; and abnormalities of the aortic valve, such as bicuspid aortic valve, calcific degeneration, rheumatic disease, infectious endocarditis, and myxomatous degeneration. In contrast to aortic stenosis, in which there is a pressure overload, aortic regurgitation is characterized by pressure and volume overload to the left ventricle. Maladaptive compensatory mechanisms include eccentric and concentric left ventricular hypertrophy to maintain forward flow.

Over time, changes include an increase in chamber compliance to accommodate the increased volume state, with an increase in left ventricular end-diastolic and end-systolic dimensions. Eventually, left ventricular systolic dysfunction develops with progressive chamber enlargement as the left ventricular chamber conforms to a more spherical geometry from the normal ellipsoid shape. This change results in a decrease in left ventricular myocardial contractility and correlates with the onset of symptoms of heart failure.[13] This process is gradual and can take many years until the development of clinically relevant aortic regurgitation. In contrast to chronic aortic regurgitation, acute severe aortic regurgitation is less well tolerated. The sudden volume overload to the ventricle creates marked hemodynamic changes frequently resulting in pulmonary edema and cardiogenic shock unless the volume overload is corrected. Infective endocarditis of the aortic valve and ascending aortic dissection are two common causes of acute severe aortic regurgitation.

Aortic Valve Replacement

The technique of AVR is similar for aortic stenosis and aortic regurgitation. Implementations of cardiopulmonary bypass and cardioplegic arrest of the heart are important steps in the successful conduct of the operation. Because of the location of the aortic valve, it is crucial to avoid injury to related structures (see Figs. 30-10 and 30-11). In all AVRs, the concept of adequate myocardial protection must be ensured. This is particularly true in operations on the aortic valve because the ventricle is hypertrophic and susceptible to injury during surgery. Delivery of cardioplegia should include antegrade cardioplegia either into the aortic root (aortic stenosis) or directly into the coronary ostia in cases of aortic regurgitation and retrograde cardioplegia into the coronary sinus for balanced myocardial protection.

The ascending aorta is opened, and the aortic valve is inspected and excised carefully (Fig. 30-12). In cases of aortic stenosis, the annulus requires débridement of calcium to seat the prosthesis and prevent paravalvular regurgitation. The aortic annulus is sized for an appropriate-sized valve. Sutures (supported with pledgets on either the ventricular or aortic side) are placed around the aortic annulus and then passed through the sewing cuff of the prosthetic valve, which is then seated (Figs. 30-13 and 30-14). After seating the prosthesis, the aortotomy is closed, the heart is deaired, and the cross-clamp is released.

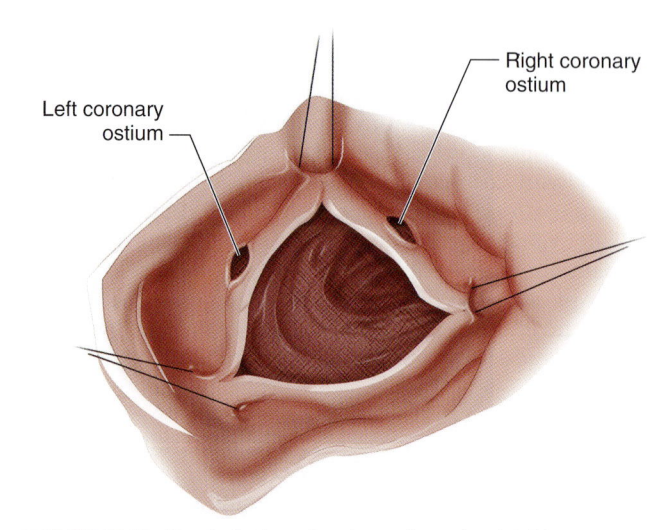

■ **FIGURE 30-12** Excised aortic valve and annular débridement. *(Redrawn from Desai ND, Christakis GT. Bioprosthetic aortic valve replacement: stented pericardial and porcine valves. In Cohn LH [ed]. Cardiac Surgery in the Adult. New York, McGraw-Hill, 2008, pp 857-894.)*

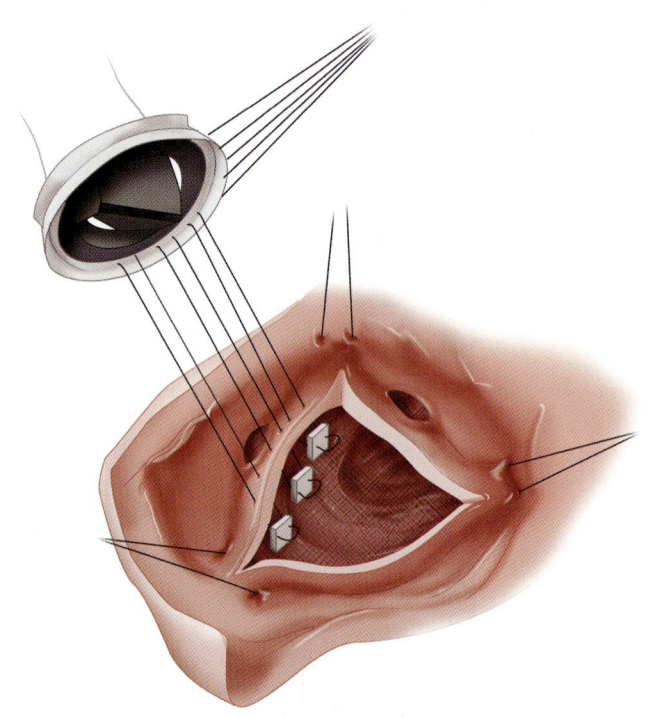

■ **FIGURE 30-13** Suture placement for seating prosthesis. *(Redrawn from Desai ND, Christakis GT. Bioprosthetic aortic valve replacement: stented pericardial and porcine valves. In Cohn LH [ed]. Cardiac Surgery in the Adult. New York, McGraw-Hill, 2008, pp 857-894.)*

CHAPTER 30 ● *Surgery for Acquired Cardiac Disease* 419

TABLE 30-5 Indications for Aortic Valve Replacement for Aortic Stenosis (AS)

Indication	Class of Evidence*
Symptomatic	
Severe AS that is symptomatic	I
Asymptomatic	
Severe AS and undergoing coronary artery bypass graft surgery	I
Severe AS and undergoing surgery of the aorta	I
Severe AS and undergoing surgery for other heart valves	I
Severe AS and left ventricular systolic dysfunction (ejection fraction <50%)	I
Moderate AS and undergoing other heart surgery	IIa

*Class I refers to conditions for which there is evidence or general agreement (or both) that the procedure or treatment is beneficial, useful, and effective. Class IIa refers to conditions for which there is conflicting evidence or a divergence of opinion (or both). Weight of evidence/opinion is in favor of usefulness or efficacy or both.

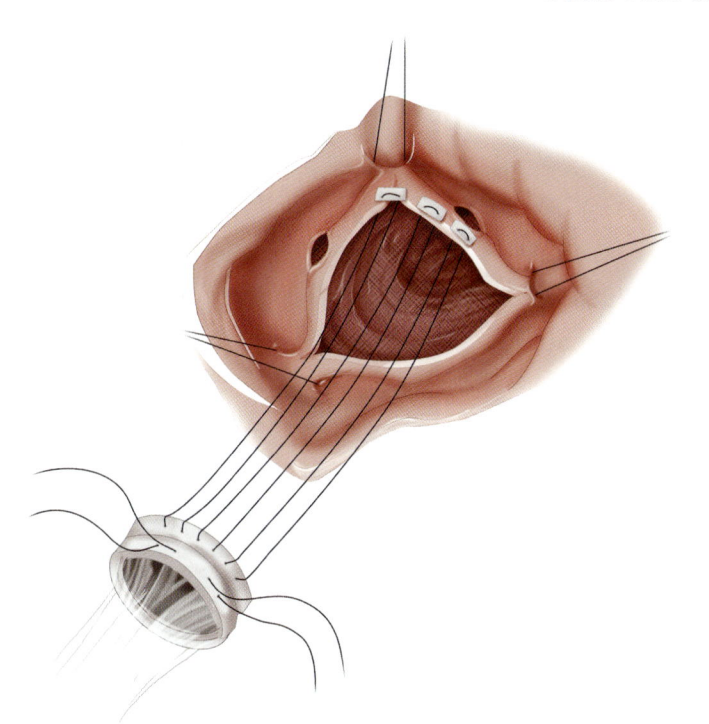

■ **FIGURE 30-14** Seating prosthesis. *(Redrawn from Desai ND, Christakis GT. Bioprosthetic aortic valve replacement: stented pericardial and porcine valves. In Cohn LH [ed]. Cardiac Surgery in the Adult. New York, McGraw-Hill, 2008, pp 857-894.)*

After confirmation of satisfactory hemodynamics and adequate prosthesis function by intraoperative transesophageal echocardiography (TEE), the patient is separated from extracorporeal circulation, and anticoagulation is reversed.

Indications

The evaluation and degree of severity of aortic stenosis can be estimated using echocardiography with Doppler measurements and cardiac catheterization, and can be graded based on several parameters (Table 30-4).[13] Hemodynamically, but not clinically significant obstruction occurs when the valve area decreases from the normal 3 to 4 cm² to less than 1.5 to 2 cm². The classic symptoms of aortic stenosis are angina; syncope; and symptoms of congestive heart failure, such as dyspnea. When symptoms occur, survival is dismal, unless the valve is replaced. About 75% of patients with symptomatic aortic stenosis die within 3 years after the onset of symptoms unless the aortic valve is replaced.[10,11] Current indications for AVR as defined by the American College of Cardiology (ACC) and AHA are listed in Table 30-5.[13] Asymptomatic patients with severe aortic stenosis can be observed until symptoms develop.

The severity of aortic regurgitation can be quantified by echocardiography or MRI as defined by Table 30-6. Operative therapy for chronic aortic regurgitation is controversial in asymptomatic patients. Because the natural history of severe asymptomatic aortic regurgitation is a gradual decline in ventricular function, patients require close follow-up to detect the onset of clinically evident heart failure. The rate of progression and the predictors of outcome are debatable and not well defined based on randomized trials. Observational data support surgery in asymptomatic patients with evidence of ventricular enlargement or decrease in ejection fraction. Extreme left ventricular dilation (left ventricular end-diastolic dimension >80 mm) may be a risk factor for sudden death.[14] The use of vasodilators in delaying the rate of progression of aortic regurgitation is controversial. Afterload-reducing agents such as calcium channel blockers and angiotensin-converting enzyme inhibitors have been examined, and the results are equivocal.[15] Similarly, the regulation of

TABLE 30-4 Classification of Severity of Aortic Valve Stenosis

Indicator	Mild	Moderate	Severe
Jet velocity (m/s)	<3	3-4	>4
Mean gradient (mm Hg)*	<25	25-40	>40
Valve area (cm²)	>1.5	1-1.5	<1

*Mean gradient is flow dependent and should be evaluated with knowledge of cardiac output.
Adapted from Bonow RO, Carabello BA, Chatterjee K, et al. ACC/AHA 2006 guidelines for the management of patients with valvular heart disease: a report of the American College of Cardiology/American Heart Association Task Force on Practice Guidelines (writing committee to revise the 1998 Guidelines for the Management of Patients with Valvular Heart Disease): developed in collaboration with the Society of Cardiovascular Anesthesiologists: endorsed by the Society for Cardiovascular Angiography and Interventions and the Society of Thoracic Surgeons. Circulation 2006; 114:e84-e231.

TABLE 30-6 Classification of Severity of Aortic Valve Insufficiency

Indicator	Mild	Moderate	Severe
Regurgitation volume (mL/beat)	<30	30-59	>60
Regurgitation fraction (%)	<30	30-49	>50
Regurgitation orifice area (cm²)	<0.1	0.1-0.29	>0.3

TABLE 30-7 Indications for Aortic Valve Replacement in Severe Aortic Regurgitation (AR)

Indication	Class of Evidence*
Symptomatic	
Severe AR with NYHA class III-IV	I
Asymptomatic	
Severe AR and evidence of LV dysfunction (EF <50%)	I
Severe AR and undergoing coronary bypass graft surgery	I
Severe AR and undergoing other valve or aortic surgery	I
Severe AR and normal EF and evidence of LV dilation (LVEDD >75 mm or LVESD >55 mm)	IIa

*Class I refers to conditions for which there is evidence or general agreement (or both) that the procedure or treatment is beneficial, useful, and effective. Class IIa refers to conditions for which there is conflicting evidence or a divergence of opinion (or both). Weight of evidence/opinion is in favor of usefulness or efficacy or both.
EF, ejection fraction; LV, left ventricular; LVEDD, left ventricular end-diastolic dimension; LVESD, left ventricular end-systolic dimension; NYHA, New York Heart Association.

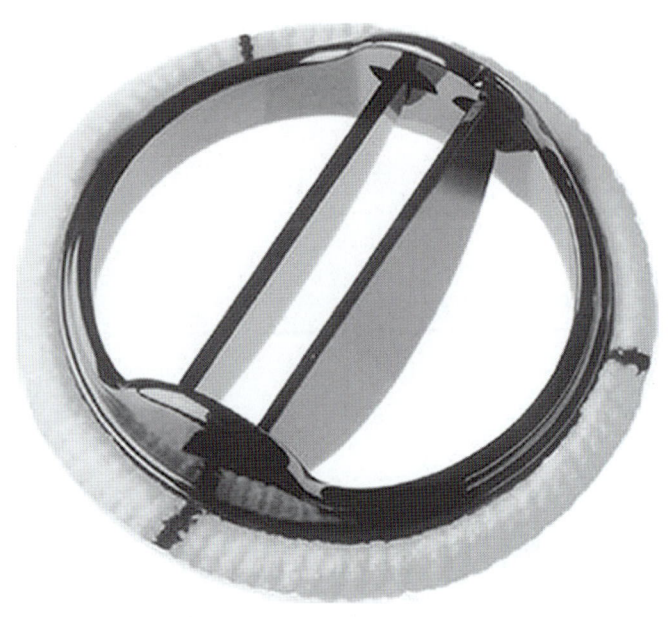

FIGURE 30-15 Mechanical bileaflet prosthetic aortic valve. (St. Jude Regent valve courtesy of St. Jude Medical, Minneapolis, MN.)

serum lipid levels to delay the progression of aortic stenosis has been studied with mixed results.[16]

Patients with aortic regurgitation and the presence of severe symptoms, categorized as New York Heart Association class III-IV, should have aortic valve surgery. The indications of AVR for aortic regurgitation are summarized in Table 30-7.[13]

Contraindications

There is no effective medical therapy for severe aortic stenosis, and given the fatality of symptomatic aortic stenosis, there are no absolute contraindications for AVR. Three situations warrant special discussion when considering the risks of AVR. (1) AVR has been shown to be lifesaving in octogenarians or older individuals in the absence of major coexisting illnesses.[17] Age by itself is not a contraindication. (2) Among patients with left ventricular dysfunction and substantial transvalvular gradients (mean >40 mm Hg), the result of surgery is excellent.[13] Patients with a reduced ejection fraction and a low transvalvular gradient (mean <30 mm Hg) have high operative risk and reduced survival after surgery.[18] Even these high-risk patients benefit from surgery, however, and such patients should be considered for operative therapy unless prohibitive risks are encountered. (3) Asymptomatic patients with severe aortic stenosis have an excellent prognosis without valve replacement; however, there is a risk of sudden death in 1% to 2% of asymptomatic patients. In addition, the onset of symptoms can be insidious and not clinically apparent. Exercise testing and echocardiography may help identify asymptomatic patients who may benefit from early valve surgery.

Otto and colleagues[12] found patients whose transvalvular velocity exceeded 4 m/s had a 70% risk of becoming symptomatic and requiring AVR in 2 years. In patients with prohibitive risk of AVR, aortic balloon valvotomy has been used as a bridge to surgery in hemodynamically unstable adults with severe left ventricular dysfunction. The acute complication rate is greater than 10%, and restenosis is rapid in most patients. This form of therapy should be limited to centers with extensive experience in this procedure.[13]

There are no absolute contraindications for AVR in patients with aortic regurgitation. Among patients with prohibitive risk of death because of serious comorbid conditions, vasodilator therapy may be indicated.

Outcomes and Complications

To discuss the outcomes of AVR, we first briefly discuss the various types of prostheses because the prosthesis is one of the most important determinants of long-term results. Prosthetic aortic valves are divided into two major types: tissue and mechanical. A mechanical prosthesis requires lifelong anticoagulation to prevent thromboembolic complications and is associated with long-term bleeding risk, particularly in elderly patients. Structural valve degeneration does not occur with mechanical valves, and they can last the lifetime of the patient. The evolution of mechanical valves has progressed from the "ball in cage" valve (e.g., Starr-Edwards valve) through the tilting disk valve (e.g., Björk-Shiley valve) to the current design of a bileaflet valve (e.g., St. Jude valve) (Fig. 30-15). Bileaflet anatomy of the valve provides the best flow dynamics and the least trauma to red blood cells.

In contrast to mechanical valves, a tissue prosthesis provides the surgeon a variety of choices. Tissue valves can be separated into three major classes based on tissue origin: autograft, allograft, and xenograft. Xenograft tissue prosthesis (bovine or porcine) can be divided further into stent supported (Fig. 30-16A) and unsupported (see Fig. 30-16B). Nonstented valves are supported by the native aortic root and provide better hemodynamics than stented valves.

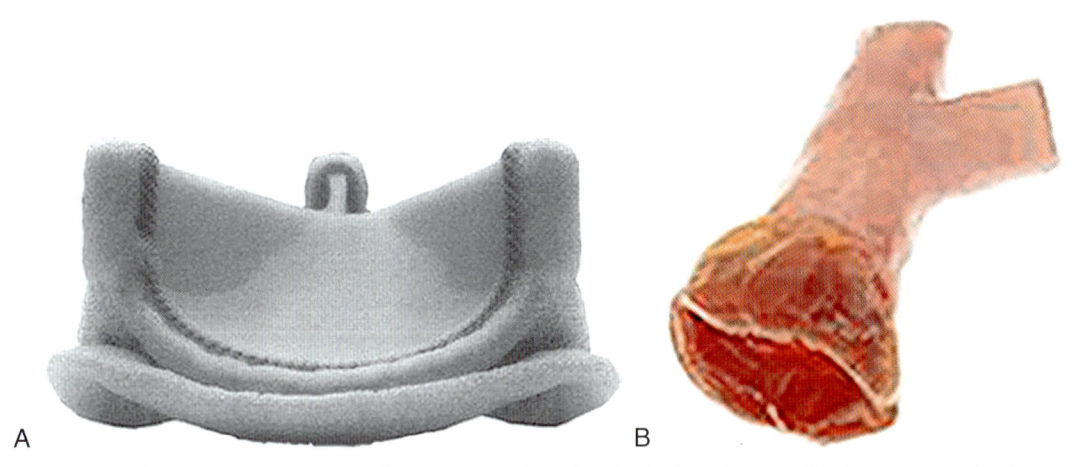

FIGURE 30-16 **A,** Stented tissue prosthetic aortic valve. **B,** Unstented aortic valve (cadaver homograft). *(A, Carpentier-Edwards Perimount Magna valve courtesy of Edwards Lifesciences, Irvine, CA.)*

The major advantage of a tissue prosthesis is that long-term anticoagulation is not required, decreasing the risk of bleeding complications and lifestyle modifications necessary for mechanical valves. Limitations of tissue valves include structural valve degeneration that may require replacement during the lifetime of the patient. The risk of replacement is greatest in patients younger than 60 years and patients with hypercalcemic conditions, such as renal dysfunction or hyperparathyroidism. Although there is no conclusive evidence that unstented prostheses offer a survival advantage to stented valves, there are clinical situations where an unstented valve provides advantages. In cases of aortic valve endocarditis complicated by an aortic root abscess, an unstented cadaver allograft (homograft) provides native tissue to reconstruct the aortic annulus and decreases the risk of reinfection of the prosthesis compared with other types of valves. A second situation includes a small aortic root, often seen in calcific aortic stenosis among elderly women. In this situation, an unstented valve may provide a larger orifice and superior flow dynamics than a stented valve. Last, the autograft aortic valve includes the transposition of the pulmonary valve to the aortic position and reconstruction of the pulmonary valve with an unstented valve (also known as Ross procedure).

A second important consideration to AVR outcome is the concept of patient-prosthesis mismatch as described in detail by Pibarot and Dumesnil.[19] Patient-prosthesis mismatch is due to the inherent limitations in effective orifice area (EOA) obligatory in all stented tissue prostheses. To overcome this problem, much technology has been invested in designing stented tissue valves with larger EOA. Although it is unclear if a particular type of stented tissue valve offers an advantage compared with another, it is important to index the EOA to the patient's body surface area (EOA index). Generally, a minimum EOA index greater than 0.75 is necessary, and an EOA index greater than 0.85 is optimal to prevent patient-prosthesis mismatch.[19] Unless an adequate-sized valve is replaced at the aortic position, continued obstruction of left ventricular outflow can result in decreased functional improvement and progression of left ventricular hypertrophy with increased short-term and long-term mortality.[19] To prevent the problems related to patient-prosthesis mismatch, two options are available: aortic root enlargement or placing an unstented tissue prosthesis. Aortic root enlargement usually allows the seating of a prosthesis one size larger and is required in 10% of patients undergoing AVR.[17]

The results of surgery for aortic stenosis are excellent compared with medical therapy (Fig. 30-17) with improvement in long-term survival. In the executive summary of the STS Spring 2007 Report, the unadjusted aortic valve operative mortality was 3% to 4% for the last 10 years.[13] If CABG surgery is required in addition to AVR, the mortality is increased to 5% to 7%. If concomitant mitral valve surgery is required, the risk of death increases further to 7% to 11%.[13]

Specific postoperative complications of AVR can be categorized as patient-related and valve-related. All patients are at risk of perioperative stroke, with the individual rates varying according to existing medical conditions and age. Increased risk is seen in patients with advanced age, diabetes, and peripheral vascular disease. Risks of injury to adjacent structures include myocardial infarction, ventricular septal defect, pulmonary and mitral valve injury, heart block with the need for a permanent pacemaker, and aortic disruption or dissection. Valve-related complications, which are similar between mechanical and tissue prostheses, include endocarditis, paravalvular leak, and hemolysis. Long-term issues include problems related to anticoagulation, patient-prosthesis mismatch, and structural valve degeneration if a tissue prosthesis was implanted.

Imaging Findings

Preoperative Planning

All patients older than 40 years should undergo selective left heart catheterization to exclude concomitant coronary artery disease that may require bypass grafting. Among patients with severe aortic stenosis and angina, the prevalence of coronary artery disease is 40% to 50%.[13] In cases where noninvasive testing is equivocal to the severity of aortic stenosis, left heart catheterization can measure

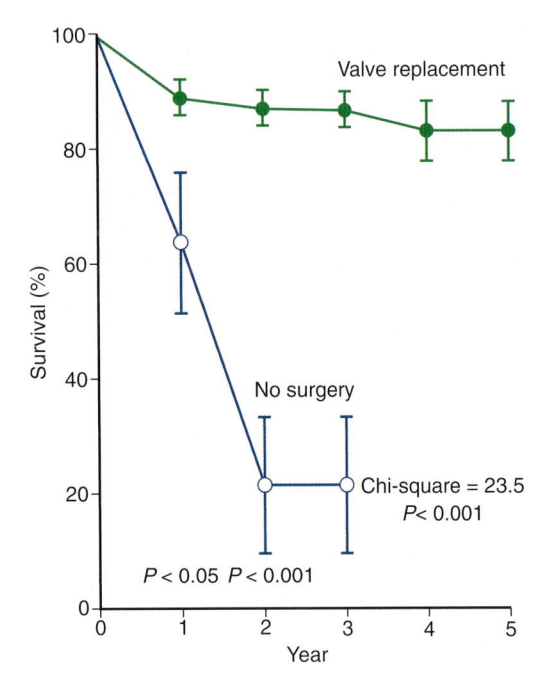

FIGURE 30-17 Survival comparison between surgical and medical therapy for symptomatic aortic stenosis. (From Emery RW, Emery AM, Knutsen AI, et al. Aortic valve replacement with a mechanical cardiac valve prosthesis. In Cohn LH [ed]. Cardiac Surgery in the Adult. New York, McGraw Hill, 2008, pp 841 856.)

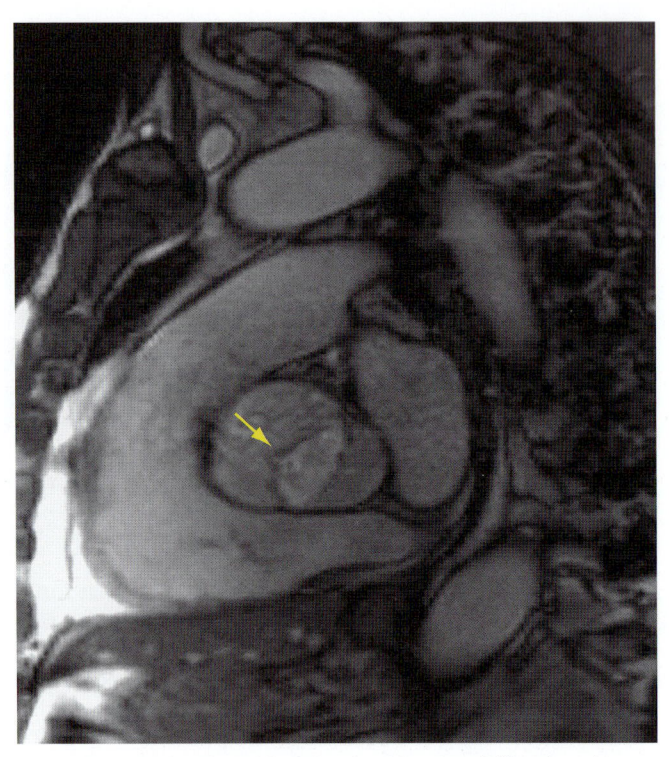

FIGURE 30-18 Bicuspid aortic valve (*arrow*) and dilated aortic root as seen on a double oblique steady-state free precession MR image obtained en face to the aortic valve.

transvalvular pressure gradient and calculate the aortic valve area.

MRI may be used to characterize further left ventricular volume, function, and mass in aortic stenosis and aortic regurgitation. MRI can be used to determine the severity of valvular disease and to characterize specific valvular anatomy, such as a bicuspid valve (Fig. 30-18). MRI can quantify the severity of aortic stenosis by determining the valve area by direct planimetry, negating the need for TEE. Cardiac CT has the ability to detect and quantify aortic valve calcification, which may have prognostic significance or allow the monitoring of progression of aortic stenosis (Fig. 30-19). Imaging of the thoracic aorta with either CT or MRI should be obtained in patients at risk of aortic root or ascending aortic aneurysm (Figs. 30-20 and 30-21).

Postoperative Surveillance

The ACC/AHA guidelines provide some guidance regarding the follow-up of patients who have undergone valve replacement.[13] For patients with prosthetic heart valves, a history and physical examination and Doppler transthoracic echocardiography (TTE) is obtained at 2 to 4 weeks. Routine follow-up should be conducted annually with earlier evaluation if there is a change in the clinical status. Education for patients who are to take oral warfarin (Coumadin) anticoagulation and antibiotic prophylaxis is essential for excellent long-term results.

SURGERY FOR MITRAL VALVULAR DISEASE

Description and Special Anatomic Considerations

Situated between the left atrium and left ventricle, the integrity of the mitral valve is paramount to the normal

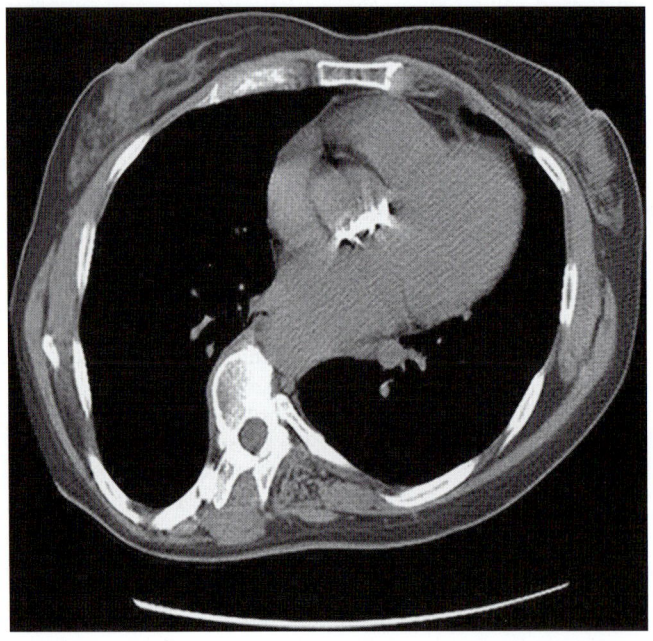

FIGURE 30-19 CT image showing severe calcification of the aortic valve.

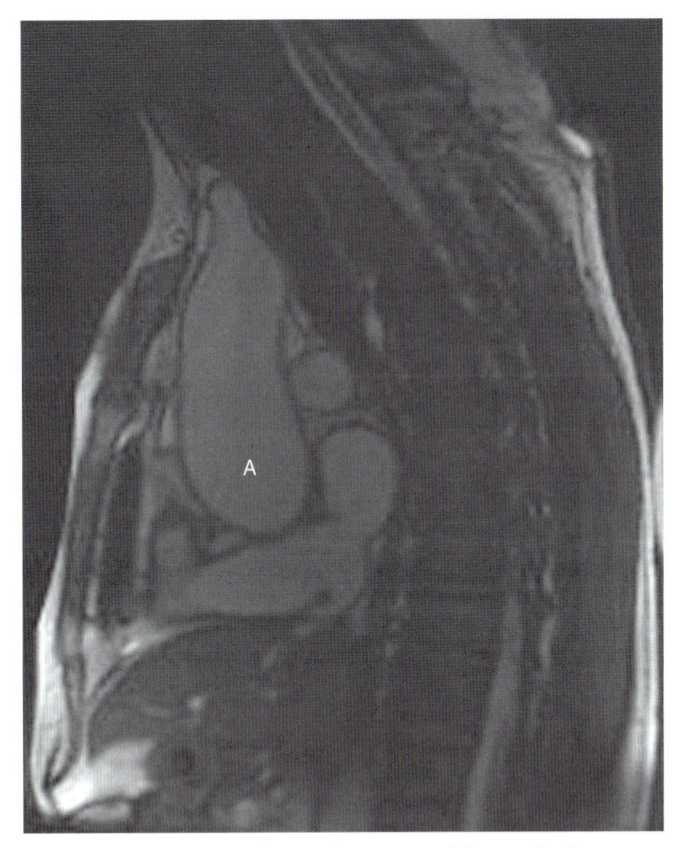

■ **FIGURE 30-20** Ascending aortic aneurysm (A) on sagittal steady-state free precession MR image.

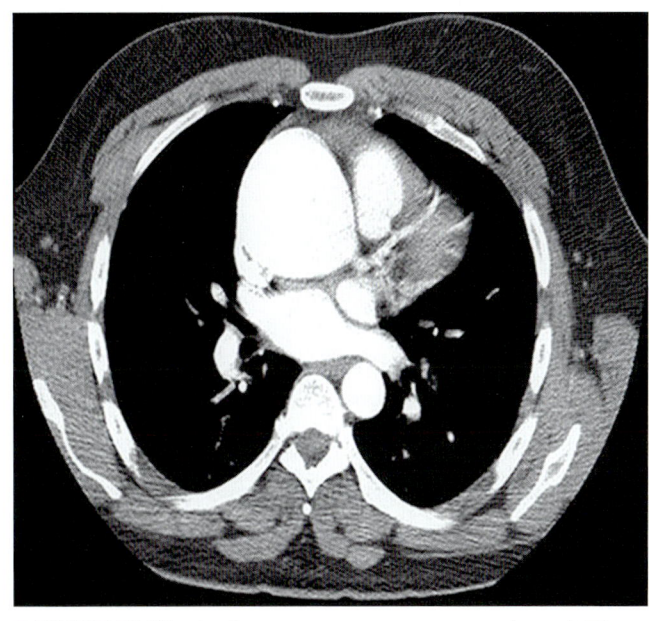

■ **FIGURE 30-21** Aortic root aneurysm on contrast-enhanced CT image.

function of the heart. Mitral valve anatomy can be viewed as valvular and subvalvular components. The valvular components include the anterior and posterior leaflets, the leaflet scallops, the anterior and posterior commissures, and the left and right trigones (Fig. 30-22A). Subvalvular components include the chordal attachments to the free edges of the anterior and posterior leaflets, the antero- lateral and posteromedial papillary muscles, and the left ventricle (see Fig. 30-22B). The mitral valve annulus is a ring of fibroconnective tissue on which each leaflet is attached and is a dynamic structure that varies with each cardiac cycle. Valve coaptation is enhanced by the fact that the annulus reduces the effective mitral valve orifice by 25% to 40% during systole.[13]

The surface area of the valve together with the annulus comprises the total cross-sectional area, which ranges from 5 to 12 cm^2. The mobile anterior leaflet accounts for two thirds of the valve area and one third of the anterior circumference, whereas the posterior leaflet accounts for one third of the area and two thirds of the circumference. The two leaflets are separated by commissures, which must be differentiated from the trigones during valve

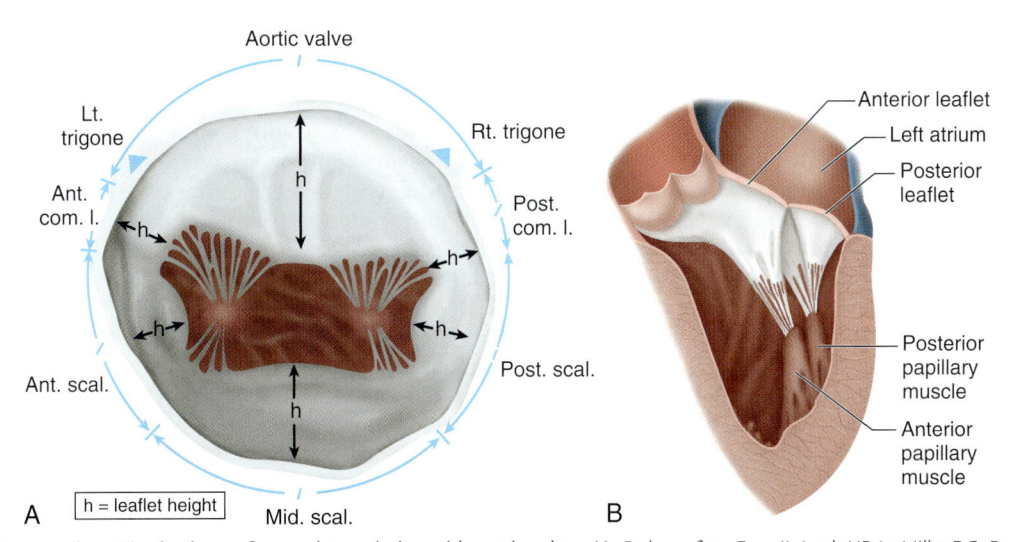

■ **FIGURE 30-22** A and B, Mitral valve en face and association with aortic valve. (A, Redrawn from Fann JI, Ingels NB Jr, Miller DC. Pathophysiology of mitral valve disease. In Cohn LH [ed]. Cardiac Surgery in the Adult. New York, McGraw-Hill, 2008, pp 973-1012.)

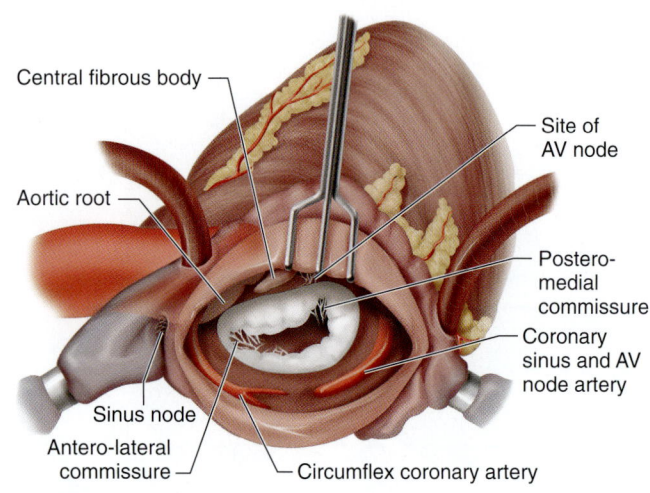

FIGURE 30-23 Surgical view of mitral valve and proximity of crucial structures. AV, aortic valve.

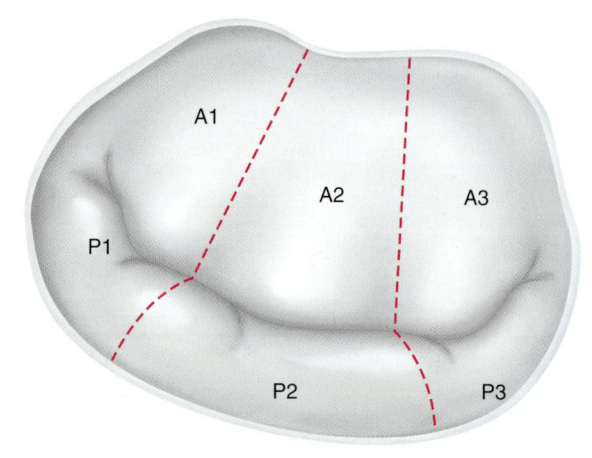

FIGURE 30-24 Mitral valve scallops. (Redrawn from Chen FY, Cohn LH. Mitral valve repair. In Cohn LH [ed]. Cardiac Surgery in the Adult. New York, McGraw-Hill, 2008, pp 1013-1030.)

surgery (see Fig. 30-22A). The trigones are relatively fixed structures that are part of the fibrous skeleton of the heart.

Similar to the aortic valve, the mitral valve sits in proximity to several important cardiac structures (Fig. 30-23). Each leaflet is divided by three roughly equal scallops: left, middle, and right corresponding to the proximity with the left and right trigones. The left scallop closest to the left trigone of the posterior leaflet is designated as P1; the middle, as P2; and the right, as P3. The anterior leaflet is similarly designated as A1 to A3 (Fig. 30-24).

The papillary muscles constitute approximately 30% of the left ventricular mass,[13] and are integral to normal mitral valve function. Ischemic injury to the either papillary muscle can result in significant mitral valve regurgitation.

Mitral Regurgitation

Mitral valve regurgitation is usually due to myxomatous degeneration. Other causes include collagen vascular and rheumatic heart disease, certain drugs, and infective endocarditis. Ischemic mitral regurgitation is differentiated from organic mitral regurgitation by the presence of coronary artery disease and ischemic injury to the left ventricle and papillary muscles. Severe chronic mitral regurgitation results from the inability of proper leaflet coaptation and can be due to valvular and subvalvular pathology. Carpentier identified three basic pathoanatomic lesions resulting in mitral regurgitation (Fig. 30-25). Type II lesions are most common and are due to myxomatous disease of the mitral valve with either elongated or ruptured chordae. Type I and III lesions are typically seen in ischemic mitral regurgitation. The severity of mitral regurgitation can be quantified using Doppler echocardiographic measurements. Severe mitral regurgitation is classified as a regurgitation volume greater than 60 mL or an effective regurgitant orifice greater than 40 mm.

Severe mitral regurgitation is characterized initially by eccentric ventricular hypertrophy with increases in ventricular dimensions to maintain forward flow. This compensated phase is accompanied by increases in left atrial size. Eventually, the mitral regurgitation results in increased left ventricular dimensions indicating contractile dysfunction. As the left ventricle dilates, the annulus enlarges along the unsupported posterior circumference (Fig. 30-26). This annular dilation results in further worsening of mitral regurgitation.

Acute severe mitral regurgitation is poorly tolerated and results in death unless urgently treated. Acute volume overload on the unprepared left atrium and ventricle results in cardiogenic shock. These situations are seen in infective endocarditis and papillary muscle rupture from myocardial infarction.

Mitral Stenosis

Mitral stenosis is an obstruction to left ventricular inflow and is the result of a structural abnormality of the mitral valve. The most common cause of mitral stenosis is rheumatic heart disease. Other causes include congenital malformations, endocarditis, left atrial myxoma, mitral annular calcification, and various inflammatory causes. When the mitral valve area decreases to less than 2.5 cm^2, clinical symptoms develop. As the valve area decreases further to less than 1.5 cm^2, symptoms at rest can occur because of the development of secondary pulmonary hypertension and left ventricular dysfunction. Common complications of mitral stenosis include atrial fibrillation, embolism, hemoptysis owing to bronchial vascular congestion, and heart failure. Classification of the severity of mitral stenosis can be based on the decrement of the valve area, the increase in the diastolic gradient across the mitral valve, and the degree of pulmonary hypertension.

The treatment of mitral stenosis is based on a continuum and includes medical therapy, percutaneous balloon valvuloplasty, and surgery. Medical therapy is primarily focused on prevention of systemic embolization and includes anticoagulation and the treatment of atrial fibrillation. Three different operations are used to treat mitral valve disorders: (1) mitral valve repair, (2) mitral valve replacement with chordal preservation, and (3) mitral valve replacement without chordal preservation. Valve

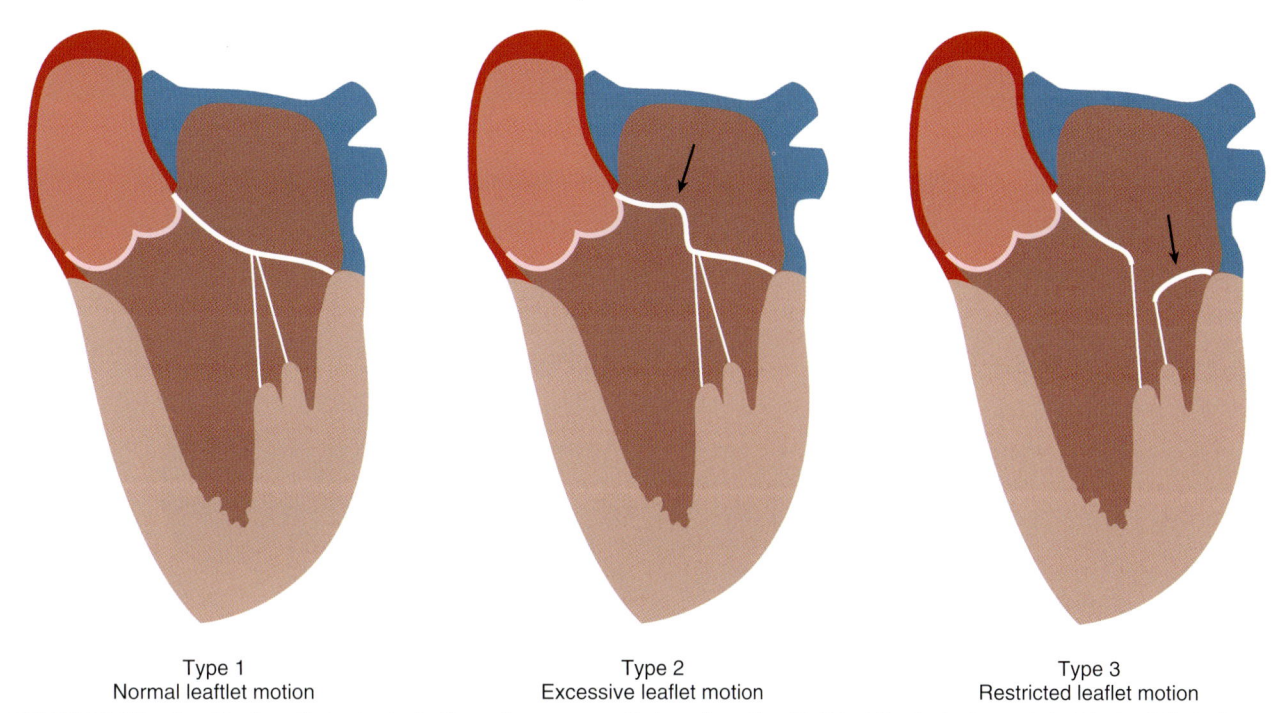

Carpentier classification

Type 1
Normal leaflet motion

Type 2
Excessive leaflet motion

Type 3
Restricted leaflet motion

■ **FIGURE 30-25** Classification of mitral valve leaflet pathoanatomy. *(Redrawn from Chen FY, Cohn LH. Mitral valve repair. In Cohn LH [ed]. Cardiac Surgery in the Adult. New York, McGraw-Hill, 2008, pp 1013-1030.)*

repair is superior to valve replacement. If the valve is replaced, chordal preservation is preferred for better postoperative left ventricular function and survival.

Detailed description of mitral valve repair techniques is beyond the scope of this chapter. The basic operative steps are presented. Mitral valve procedures can be performed via sternotomy, left or right thoracotomy, and minimally invasive approaches.

The patient is placed on cardiopulmonary bypass, and the heart is arrested using cold cardioplegia. The left atrium is opened anterior to the right pulmonary veins longitudinally (Fig. 30-27). The mitral apparatus is brought into view being cognizant of surrounding important structures (Fig. 30-28A). If the patient has atrial fibrillation, the left atrial appendage may be sutured closed to reduce stroke risk. Valve competency is evaluated with cold saline injection into the left ventricular cavity, and a determination of either valve repair or valve replacement is made (see Fig. 30-28B). For replacement, excision of variable amounts of anterior leaflet and posterior leaflet is performed with the goal of preserving the papillary muscles and chordal attachments of the subvalvular apparatus (Fig. 30-29). After the proper sizing of the mitral valve orifice, pledget-supported sutures are placed around

Annular Dilation

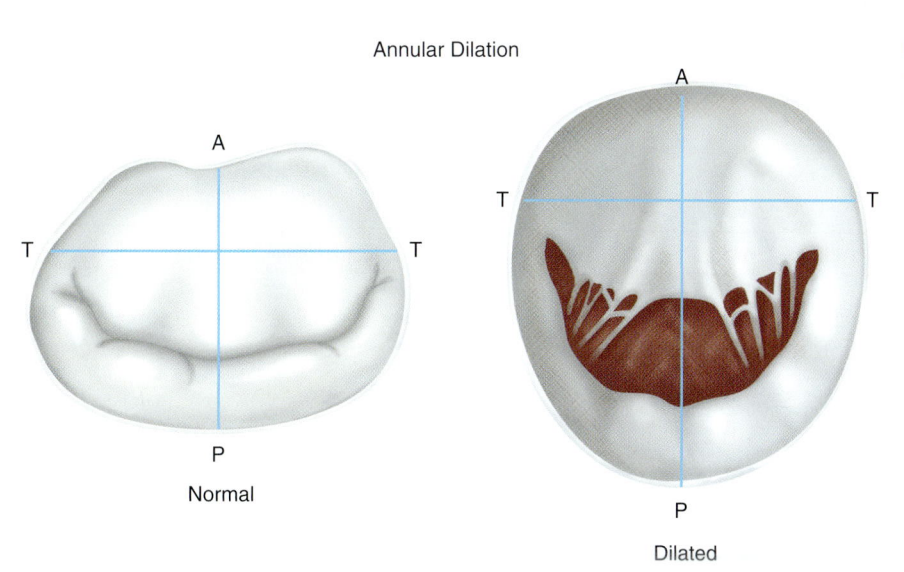

Normal

Dilated

■ **FIGURE 30-26** Posterior enlargement of the annulus. *(Redrawn from Chen FY, Cohn LH. Mitral valve repair. In Cohn LH [ed]. Cardiac Surgery in the Adult. New York, McGraw-Hill, 2008, pp 1013-1030.)*

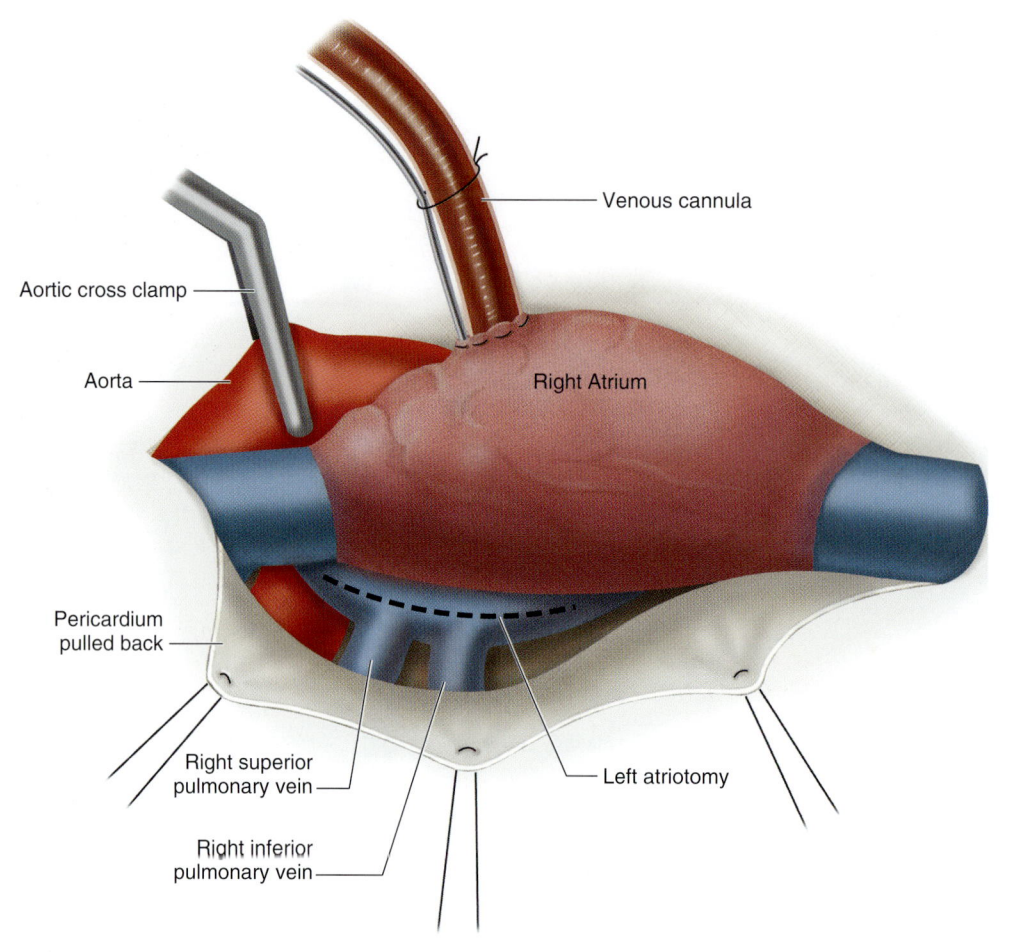

■ **FIGURE 30-27** Left atriotomy to view the mitral valve. *(Redrawn from Mayo Clinic Cardiothoracic Grand Rounds, picture used in slide presentation, 2002.)*

the mitral valve annulus and the sewing cuff of the prosthesis (Fig. 30-30). After seating the prosthesis, the left atriotomy is closed, the heart is deaired, and the patient is separated from cardiopulmonary bypass. Intraoperative TEE is essential, particularly in cases where valve repair is entertained.

Indications

The indications for mitral valve replacement for mitral regurgitation were defined by the ACC/AHA guidelines in 2006 (Table 30-8). In addition to these indications, some authors have recommended early mitral valve surgery if

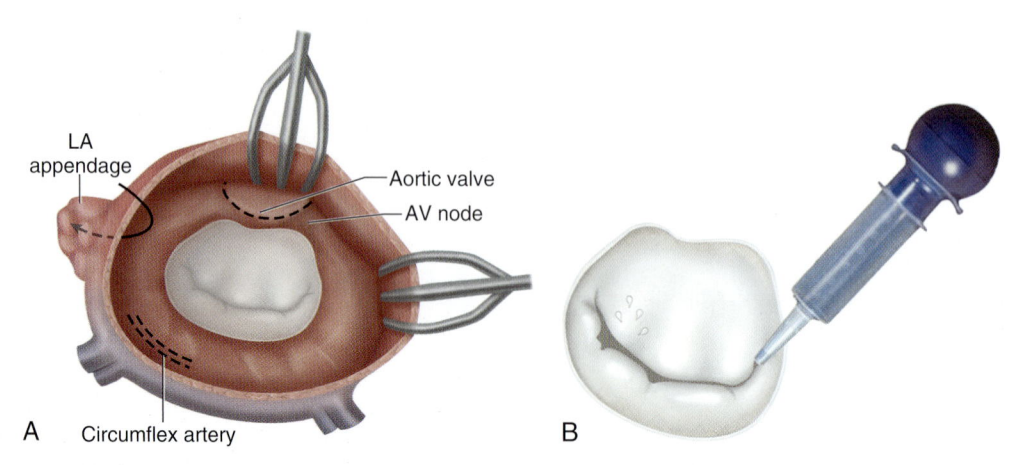

■ **FIGURE 30-28** **A,** Critical structures at risk and ideal surgical view of mitral valve leaflets. AV, aortic valve; LA, left atrial. **B,** Testing the mitral valve with cold saline. *(**A,** Redrawn from Gudbjartsson T, Absi T, Aranki S. Mitral valve replacement. In Cohn LH [ed]. Cardiac Surgery in the Adult. New York, McGraw-Hill, 2008, pp 1031-1068; **B,** redrawn from Mayo Clinic Cardiothoracic Grand Rounds, picture used in slide presentation, 2002.)*

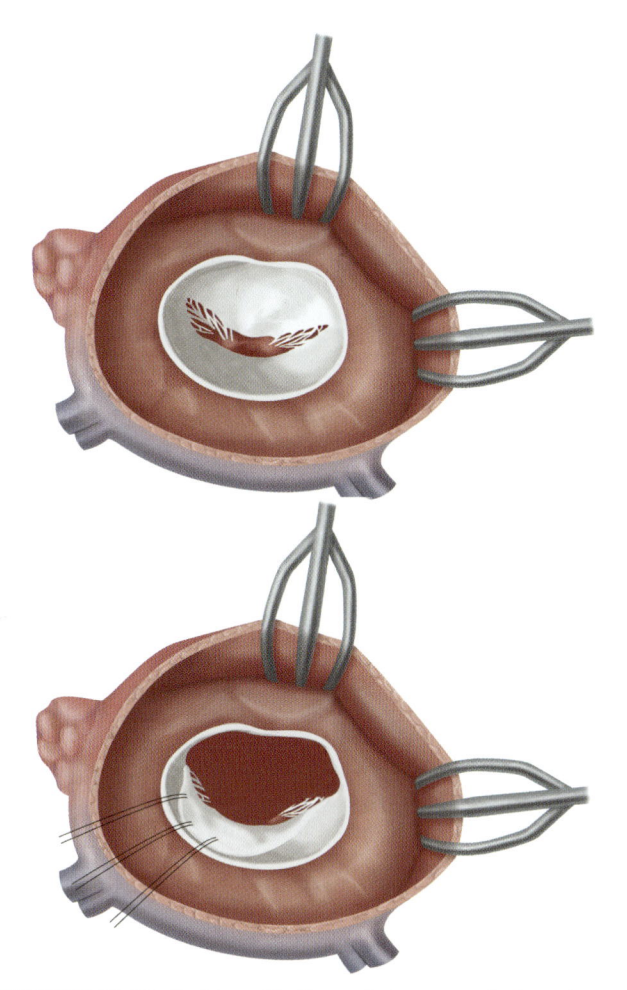

FIGURE 30-29 Excision of leaflets and placement of valve sutures. *(Redrawn from Gudbjartsson T, Absi T, Aranki S. Mitral valve replacement. In Cohn LH [ed]. Cardiac Surgery in the Adult. New York, McGraw-Hill, 2008, pp 1031-1068.)*

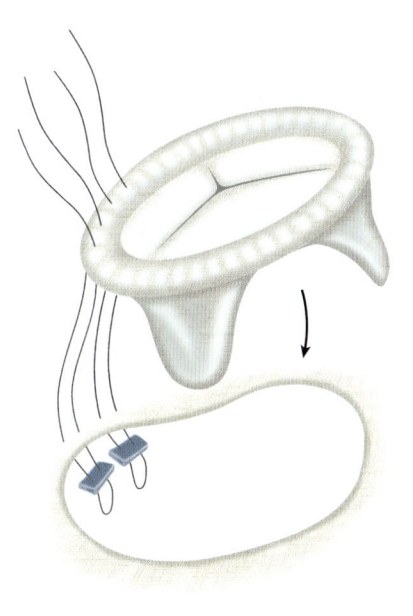

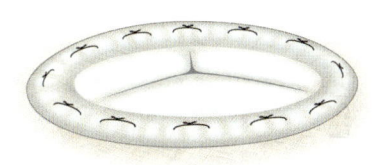

FIGURE 30-30 Seating of mitral prosthesis. *(Redrawn from Gudbjartsson T, Absi T, Aranki S. Mitral valve replacement. In Cohn LH [ed]. Cardiac Surgery in the Adult. New York, McGraw-Hill, 2008, pp 1031-1068.)*

the effective regurgitant orifice is greater than 40 mm, and there is a high probability of mitral valve repair.

Interventions for mitral stenosis are more complex because percutaneous balloon valvuloplasty and surgery have similar outcomes. Indications for percutaneous balloon valvuloplasty have been defined by the ACC/AHA (Table 30-9). Key determinants of successful percutaneous balloon valvuloplasty are based on valve leaflet mobility, leaflet and subvalvular thickening, and the degree of leaflet calcification. These parameters can be determined by echocardiography. Favorable anatomy includes little valvular calcification, minimal valvular and subvalvular fibrosis, and nominal thickening of the valve. Mitral valve replacement is indicated when percutaneous balloon valvuloplasty is impossible and in cases where percutaneous balloon valvuloplasty has failed or is contraindicated. Surgical indications for repair of mitral stenosis are listed in Table 30-10.

Contraindications

Contraindications include isolated mitral valve surgery in patients with mild or moderate mitral regurgitation and in patients in whom valve repair is impossible. Surgery is also contraindicated in asymptomatic patients with mitral

TABLE 30-8 Indications for Mitral Valve Surgery in Patients with Mitral Regurgitation (MR)

Indication	Class of Evidence*
Symptomatic	
Severe MR and symptoms	I
Severe MR and NYHA class II-IV	I
Asymptomatic	
Severe MR and decreased EF (normal >60%) and LVESD >40 mm	I
Severe MR and preserved EF and LVESD <40 mm†	IIa
Severe MR and new-onset atrial fibrillation	IIa
Severe MR and pulmonary hypertension‡	IIa
Severe MR and NYHA class II-IV and severe LV dysfunction in which valve repair is likely	IIa

*Class I refers to conditions for which there is evidence or general agreement (or both) that the procedure or treatment is beneficial, useful, and effective. Class IIa refers to conditions for which there is conflicting evidence or a divergence of opinion (or both). Weight of evidence/opinion is in favor of usefulness or efficacy or both.
†Only if valve repair is likely.
‡Pulmonary artery systolic pressure at rest >50 mm Hg and >60 mm Hg with exercise.
EF, ejection fraction; LV, left ventricular; LVESD, left ventricular end-systolic dimension; NYHA, New York Heart Association.

TABLE 30-9 Indications for Percutaneous Mitral Balloon Valvotomy in Moderate to Severe Mitral Stenosis

Indication	Class of Evidence*
NYHA class II-IV failure	I
Asymptomatic with pulmonary hypertension†	I
NYHA class II-IV failure and not surgical candidate	IIa
Asymptomatic with new-onset atrial fibrillation	IIb
NYHA class II-IV and mitral valve area >1.5 cm² and pulmonary hypertension	IIb
Alternative to surgery	IIb

*Class I refers to conditions for which there is evidence or general agreement (or both) that the procedure or treatment is beneficial, useful, and effective. Class IIa refers to conditions for which there is conflicting evidence or a divergence of opinion (or both). Weight of evidence/opinion is in favor of usefulness or efficacy or both. Class IIb refers to conditions for which usefulness/efficacy is less well established by evidence or opinion.
†Pulmonary artery systolic pressure >50 mm Hg at rest or >60 mm Hg with exercise.
NYHA, New York Heart Association.

TABLE 30-10 Indications for Surgery for Mitral Stenosis (MS)

Indication	Class of Evidence*
Symptomatic NYHA class III-IV failure and PMBV is unavailable, contraindicated, or not favorable owing to valve morphology	I
Symptomatic with moderate to severe MS and moderate to severe MR	I
Severe pulmonary hypertension, NYHA class I-II, and not candidate for PMBV	IIa
Asymptomatic with moderate to severe MS and recurrent emboli while on anticoagulation if valve morphology is favorable to valve repair	IIb

*Class I refers to conditions for which there is evidence or general agreement (or both) that the procedure or treatment is beneficial, useful, and effective. Class IIa refers to conditions for which there is conflicting evidence or a divergence of opinion (or both). Weight of evidence/opinion is in favor of usefulness or efficacy or both. Class IIb refers to conditions for which usefulness/efficacy is less well established by evidence or opinion.
MR, mitral regurgitation; NYHA, New York Heart Association; PMBV, percutaneous mitral balloon valvotomy.

regurgitation and preserved left ventricular function (left ventricular ejection fraction >60%) and no evidence of dilation (left ventricular end-systolic dimension <40 mm).

Special caution should be exercised in elderly patients with mitral regurgitation, in particular patients 75 years old or older who require valve replacement. Operative mortality in this subgroup can be particularly high, exceeding 20% in low-volume centers.[13] Among patients with asymptomatic or mildly symptomatic mitral regurgitation, medical therapy should be implemented in lieu of surgery. In cases of moderate to severe mitral regurgitation and mitral stenosis or in the presence of a left atrial thrombus, percutaneous balloon valvuloplasty is contraindicated, and surgery should be pursued.

Outcomes and Complications

When treated medically, severe mitral regurgitation secondary to myxomatous disease is associated with excess mortality and high morbidity. Survival rates ranging from 27% to 97% at 5 years have been reported. Surgery is almost unavoidable within 10 years of diagnosis and is associated with improved prognosis.[20]

The durability of mitral valve repair is excellent. The Mayo Clinic published the results of 917 patients who underwent isolated mitral valve procedures over a 15-year period.[21] In this study, the authors found survival was superior after repair compared with replacement. The reoperation rate was higher after repair of the anterior leaflet compared with the posterior leaflet, and reoperation was similar after repair or replacement of the valve. A reoperation rate of 28% was noted at 15 years for anterior leaflet repair and 11% for posterior leaflet repair. The authors also noted that the reoperation rate decreased for both leaflets in patients treated more recently with a decrease to 5% for posterior leaflet repairs and 10% for anterior leaflet repairs at 10 years. In another study of 170 consecutive patients over a 14-year period who underwent mitral valve repair owing to nonrheumatic causes, the authors found the 20-year Kaplan-Meier survival rate was similar to the survival rate for a normal population with the same age.[22] The primary determinant of operative mortality in mitral valve procedures is left ventricular function.[20-23]

Overall, the 10-year survival for untreated symptomatic mitral stenosis is 50% to 60%, whereas asymptomatic patients have a greater than 80% 10-year survival.[13] When patients with symptomatic mitral stenosis undergo valve intervention (percutaneous balloon valvuloplasty or mitral valve replacement), survival is improved to near survivals of asymptomatic patients. Key determinants of long-term outcome in mitral stenosis include the degree of pulmonary hypertension, the presence of atrial fibrillation, and left ventricular function.[12]

The unadjusted mortality for mitral valve repair as noted in the STS Spring 2007 Report is 2% or less.[9] Operative mortality for mitral valve replacement is higher at 5% and 6%. Combined procedures have a higher mortality as noted with AVR. Concomitant coronary artery surgery increases the risk of surgery, as do procedures involving multiple valves. Mitral valve replacement and CABG surgery has one of the highest unadjusted mortality rates (>10%). This high mortality is due to the fact that these patients have significant left ventricular impairment and ischemic mitral regurgitation.

Structures at risk for injury during mitral valve surgery are shown in Figures 30-23 and 30-27. These structures include the atrioventricular node or nodal artery; circumflex coronary artery, particularly in cases of left-sided dominance; aortic valve; and coronary sinus. Similar to AVR, there are patient-related and valve-related complications.

Imaging Findings

Preoperative Planning

Patients older than 40 years should have coronary angiography before surgery. Because of the possibility of pulmonary hypertension, particularly among patients with mitral stenosis, preoperative right heart catheterization should be done. All patients undergoing mitral valve surgery should have preoperative TEE, particularly if valve repair is considered. It is important to rule out associated functional tricuspid valve disease, particularly among patients with elevated pulmonary pressures. Although concomitant tricuspid valve repair increases the risks of surgery, the long-term outcomes are better if the tricuspid valve is made competent at the time of initial mitral valve surgery. If the patient has atrial fibrillation, an ablative procedure should be considered. The role of CT or MRI in mitral valve disease is not well defined. Both modalities can be used to determine chamber dimensions and to evaluate annular calcification similar to aortic valve disease.

Postoperative Surveillance

Early close follow-up is important because most valve repairs fail early, typically within the first year of surgery. Annual echocardiographic evaluation and physical examination are recommended in the ACC/AHA guidelines.[13] Endocarditis prophylaxis is important to implement regardless of repair or replacement. Long-term anticoagulation is unnecessary with tissue prosthesis unless associated atrial fibrillation is present.

INFECTIVE ENDOCARDITIS

Description and Special Anatomic Considerations

Endocarditis is a microbial infection of the endocardial surface of the heart. Such infections include most commonly the cardiac valves, but also the chambers of the heart and the great vessels. Preexisting valve lesions and indwelling cardiac devices, such as pacemakers, predispose patients to these infections. Endocardial vegetation is the characteristic lesion defining infective endocarditis and is a complex of fibrin, microbial organisms, and inflammatory cells. Native valve endocarditis is typically due to mitral valve prolapse, the most common cardiovascular diagnosis predisposing patients to endocarditis in North America. Prosthetic valve endocarditis is a serious infection typically involving the sewing cuff of the prosthesis, and has an equal frequency between mechanical and tissue prostheses in the aortic and mitral positions. Mechanical prostheses have a slightly higher incidence of endocarditis in the initial 3 months after surgery. Microbiologic features in most series include staphylococci and viridans streptococci as the most common pathogens. *Streptococcus bovis* is prevalent in elderly patients and is associated with colonic neoplasms.[24]

Clinical manifestations of infective endocarditis can be due to cardiac and extracardiac consequences of the infection. Destruction of the cardiac valve or fistulization between heart chambers results in poorly tolerated congestive heart failure. Acute mitral or aortic regurgitation is less well tolerated than right-sided valvular failure and requires urgent surgical intervention. Additional cardiac findings include heart block owing to injury of the conduction system, often associated with aortic root abscess and coronary ischemia secondary to emboli. Extracardiac

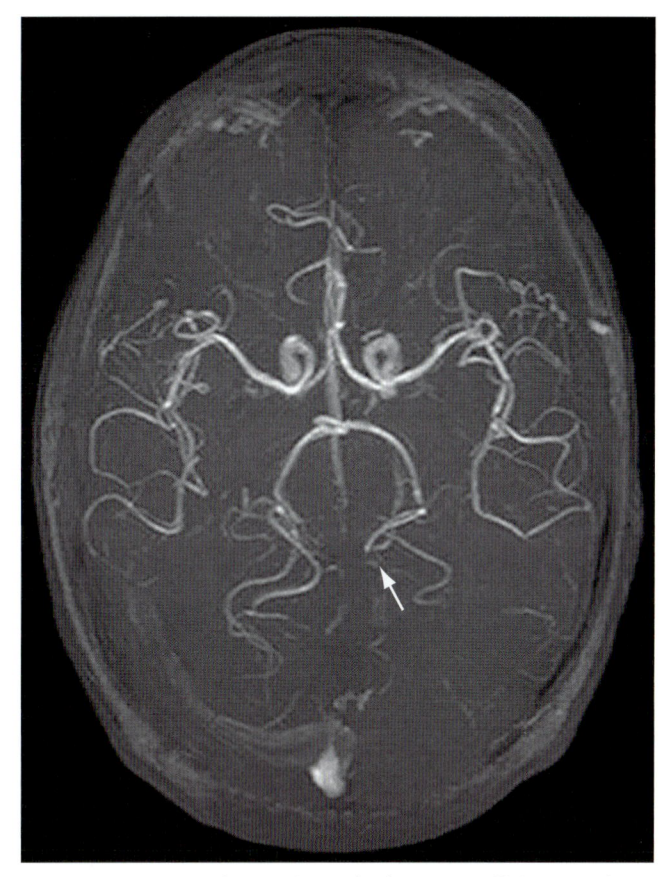

■ **FIGURE 30-31** Left posterior cerebral artery cutoff sign secondary to embolic occlusion from mitral valve vegetation in infective endocarditis.

manifestations are primarily due to septic microembolism and the intense immunologic response to the infection. Common peripheral manifestations include splinter hemorrhages, which are small areas of bleeding found underneath the fingernails or toenails and conjunctival petechiae. Painful tender nodules in the subcutaneous pads of the fingers and hand are known as Osler nodes and are due to neutrophilic vasculitis, whereas painless Janeway lesions are erythematous or hemorrhagic lesions noted on the palms or soles and caused by septic embolism.

One of the most devastating manifestations of infective endocarditis is embolic injury to the brain (Fig. 30-31). More than 65% of embolic events in infective endocarditis involve the central nervous system, and neurologic complications develop in 20% to 40% of all patients with infective endocarditis.[24] Different diagnostic criteria exist for the diagnosis of infective endocarditis with differing levels of sensitivity. The von Reyn and Duke criteria are less useful than the modified Duke criteria, which have a sensitivity near 90% (Table 30-11).[25] Echocardiography is the most important initial diagnostic evaluation, and TTE is highly cost-effective. In cases of prosthetic valve endocarditis, TEE may provide better detail than TTE. Death from infective endocarditis is usually due to CNS complications or due to congestive heart failure, and the overall mortality rate is 20% to 25% for native valve endocarditis and prosthetic valve endocarditis. Right-sided endocarditis (tricuspid valve) has a lower mortality.[24]

TABLE 30-11 Modified Dukes Criteria for Infective Endocarditis

Major Criteria
A. Positive blood culture for infective endocarditis (1 of the following 3)
  1. Typical microorganism consistent with infective endocarditis from 2 separate blood cultures
     a. Viridans streptococci, *Streptococcus bovis*, or HACEK* group, *or*
     b. Community-acquired *Staphylococcus aureus* or enterococci, in the absence of a primary focus
  2. Microorganisms consistent with infective endocarditis from persistently positive blood cultures defined as
     a. 2 positive cultures of blood samples drawn >12 hr apart, *or*
     b. All of 3 or most of 4 separate cultures of blood (with first and last sample drawn 1 hr apart)
  3. Single positive blood culture for *Coxiella burnetii* or phase I antibody titer >1:800.
B. Evidence of endocardial involvement
  1. Positive echocardiogram for infective endocarditis defined as
     a. Oscillating intracardiac mass on valve or supporting structures, in the path of regurgitant jets, or on implanted material in the absence of an alternative anatomic explanation, *or*
     b. Abscess, *or*
     c. New partial dehiscence of prosthetic valve
  or
  2. New valvular regurgitation (worsening or changing of preexisting murmur not sufficient)

Minor Criteria
Predisposition: predisposing heart condition or intravenous drug use
Fever: temperature >38° C (>100.4° F)
Vascular phenomena: major arterial emboli, septic pulmonary infarcts, mycotic aneurysm, intracranial hemorrhage, conjunctival hemorrhages, and Janeway lesions
Immunologic phenomena: glomerulonephritis, Osler nodes, Roth spots, and rheumatoid factor
Microbiologic evidence: positive blood culture, but does not meet a major criterion, or serologic evidence of active infection with organism consistent with infective endocarditis
Echocardiographic findings: consistent with infective endocarditis, but do not meet a major criterion

Clinical Criteria for Infective Endocarditis Requires:
2 major criteria, *or*
1 major and 2 minor criteria, *or*
5 minor criteria

*HACEK group—*Haemophilus* spp., *Actinobacillus actinomycetemcomitans*, *Cardiobacterium hominis*, *Eikenella* spp., and *Kingella kingae*.
From Li JS, Sexton DJ, Mick N, et al. Proposed modifications to the Duke criteria for the diagnosis of infective endocarditis. Clin Infect Dis 2000; 30:633-638.

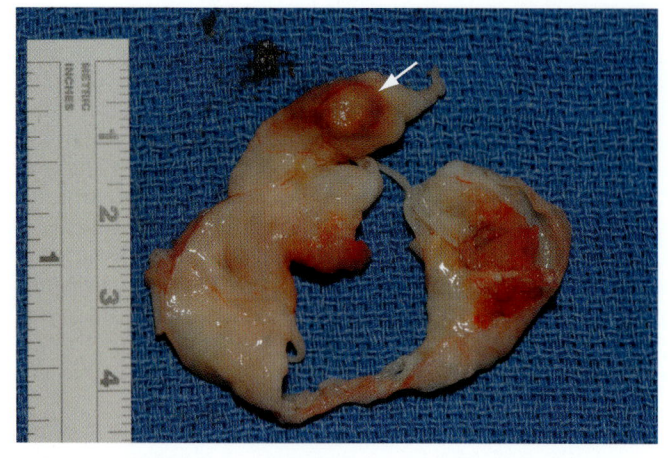

FIGURE 30-32 Excised mitral valve with bileaflet vegetations with posterior intraleaflet abscess (*arrow*) at P1 (see Fig. 30-24).

ditis. In situations where only the posterior leaflet is involved, repair may be more feasible than situations where the anterior or both leaflets are involved (Fig. 30-32). If the annulus is destroyed by infection, repair is unlikely.

Indications

Indications for surgery in infective endocarditis as recommended by the ACC/AHA are detailed in Tables 30-12 and 30-13. The most important indication for surgery is the development of congestive heart failure.

Contraindications

Recent neurologic complications of infective endocarditis are considered a relative contraindication to surgery in infective endocarditis. Owing to the numerous patients

Specific surgical techniques are similar to the techniques described in earlier discussions of the aortic and mitral valves. Goals of surgical therapy are to reverse the process of heart failure and remove the source of sepsis and systemic embolization. The degree of valve destruction and extravalvular extension dictates if valve repair is possible in this situation. Infective endocarditis of the aortic valve often results in extensive paravalvular destruction with aortic root abscess, which negates valve repair. Aortic root reconstruction with a cryopreserved allograft offers the patient the best chance of survival and decreases the risk of reinfection. If isolated leaflet perforation is found, a pericardial patch repair may be possible as may be seen in cases of mitral or healed aortic valve endocar-

TABLE 30-12 Indications for Surgery in Native Valve Infective Endocarditis

Indication	Class of Evidence*
Congestive heart failure	I
Elevated left ventricular end-diastolic pressure	I
Elevated left atrial pressure†	I
Endocarditis caused by highly resistant organism‡	I
Complications of extravalvular extension§	I
Recurrent emboli or persistent vegetations	IIa
Mobile vegetations >10 mm	IIb

*Class I refers to conditions for which there is evidence or general agreement (or both) that the procedure or treatment is beneficial, useful, and effective. Class IIa refers to conditions for which there is conflicting evidence or a divergence of opinion (or both). Weight of evidence/opinion is in favor of usefulness or efficacy or both. Class IIb refers to conditions for which usefulness/efficacy is less well established by evidence or opinion.
†Evidence of premature closure of mitral valve with aortic regurgitation, rapid decelerating mitral regurgitation signal by continuous-wave Doppler, or moderate to severe pulmonary hypertension.
‡Fungal, gram-negative bacilli (*Pseudomonas*); *Staphylococcus* spp. in some cases.
§Evidence of heart block, annular abscess, or destructive penetrating lesions resulting in intracardiac or extracardiac fistulas or, in the case of atrioventricular endocarditis, mitral valve leaflet perforation.

TABLE 30-13 Indications for Surgery in Prosthetic Valve Endocarditis

Indication	Class of Evidence*
Congestive heart failure	I
Evidence of prosthesis dehiscence†	I
Evidence of increasing obstruction or regurgitation	I
Extravalvular complications such as abscess	I
Evidence of persistent bacteremia despite antibiotics	IIa
Evidence of recurrent emboli despite antibiotics	IIa
Relapsing infection after initial therapy	IIa

*Class I refers to conditions for which there is evidence or general agreement (or both) that the procedure or treatment is beneficial, useful, and effective. Class IIa refers to conditions for which there is conflicting evidence or a divergence of opinion (or both). Weight of evidence/opinion is in favor of usefulness or efficacy or both.
†Cine fluoroscopic examination showing "rocking" prosthesis.

who have cerebral emboli from infective endocarditis, the timing of operative therapy becomes critical because anticoagulation necessary for cardiopulmonary bypass can result in injury expansion. Although standardized recommendations are lacking, the longer the patient is allowed to recover from a recent cerebral injury, the better the outcome. Hemorrhagic infarcts portend a worse prognosis than purely ischemic injury. Hemodynamically unstable patients with multiorgan failure, particularly renal failure, are a subgroup with very high mortality. In such a situation, a multidisciplinary discussion involving the patient and family should be undertaken before embarking on operative therapy. It is always preferable to allow the initiation of antimicrobiologic therapy, even if only for a few days before surgery. Valve replacement in a patient with positive blood cultures increases the risk of relapse up to 10% to 15% and is highest if the offending organism is *Staphylococcus,* and should be avoided if the hemodynamic status of the patient is stable.[13]

Outcomes and Complications

A systematic review of the literature showed mitral valve repair to be superior to mitral valve replacement in infective endocarditis with lower in-hospital mortality, long-term mortality, recurrent endocarditis, and early and late cerebrovascular events.[26] The choice of a tissue versus a mechanical prosthesis is debatable; prosthetic mechanical valves have a slightly higher rate of infection early after surgery.

The mortality rate for infective endocarditis varies depending on the causative organism and coexisting conditions at the time of operation. Staphylococci, gram-negative bacilli, and fungi have the highest reported rates (up to 50%). Patients with congestive heart failure treated with antibiotics alone have mortality rates greater than 56% to 86%, whereas patients treated with surgery and antibiotics have mortality rates of 11% to 35%.[24] Shock, ventricular dysfunction, and concomitant coronary artery disease are predictors of poor outcome. The hemodynamic status of the patient is the principal determinant of operative mortality, and early intervention before the onset of ventricular dysfunction is preferred.

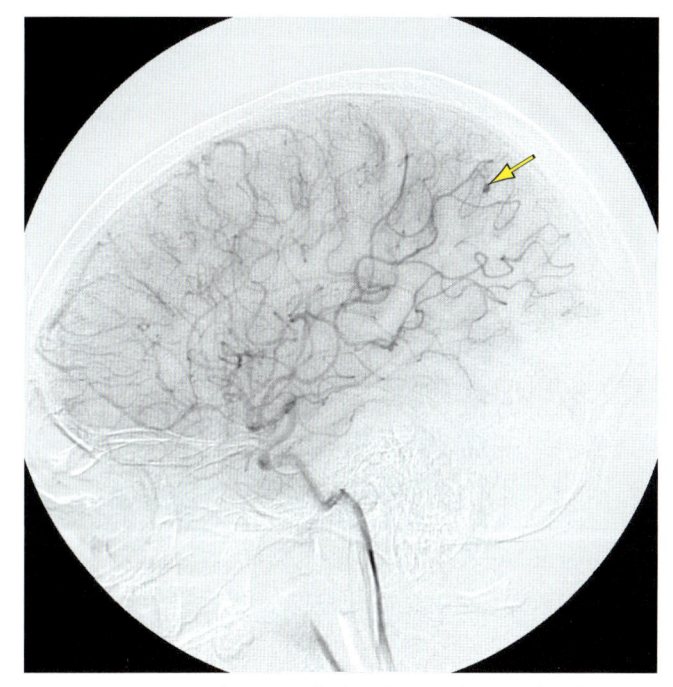

■ FIGURE 30-33 Selective cerebral angiogram showing distal occipital/parietal middle cerebral artery mycotic aneurysm (*arrow*).

Imaging Findings

Preoperative Planning

In situations where a mechanical prosthesis is being considered, and concern for mycotic aneurysm exists, selec-

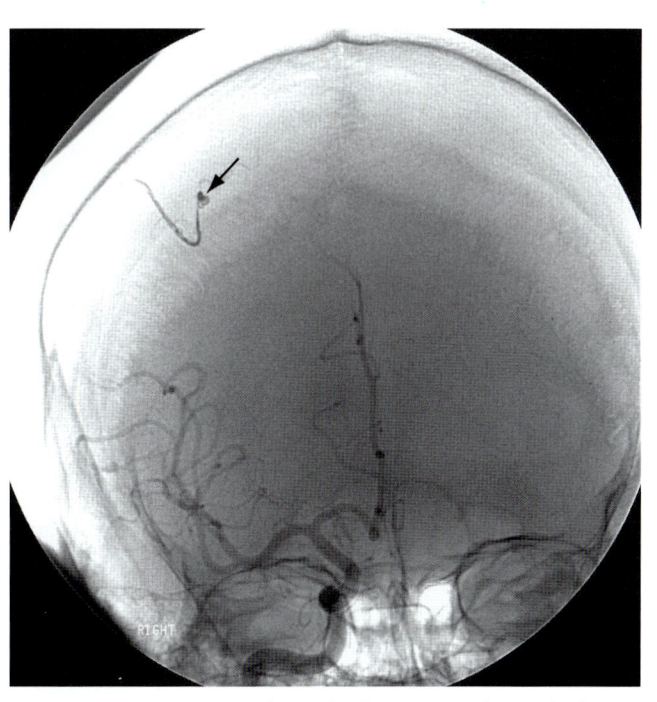

■ FIGURE 30-34 Same patient as in Figure 30-33 after cerebral artery embolization (*arrow*).

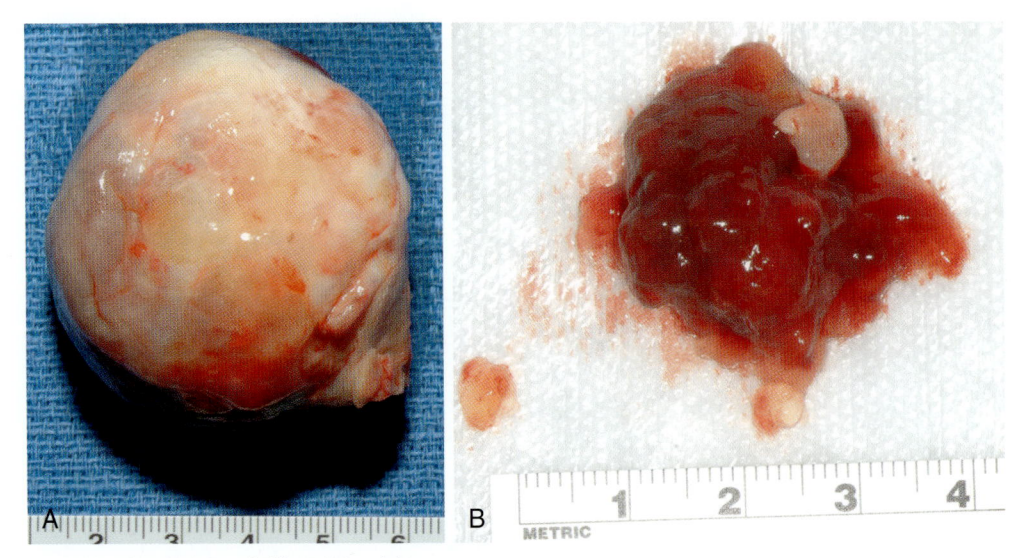

FIGURE 30-35 Excised polypoid (**A**) and villous (**B**) atrial myxomas.

tive cerebral angiography may be indicated to rule out mycotic aneurysm (Fig. 30-33). Catheter-based selective cerebral artery embolization offers a less invasive form of therapy (Fig. 30-34).

Postoperative Surveillance

The risk of prosthetic valve endocarditis is greatest the first 4 to 6 weeks after surgery. Patients should be followed closely, and there should be a low threshold for echocardiographic examination in cases where recurrent endocarditis is suspected.

For patients with prosthetic heart valves, a history, physical examination, and appropriate testing should be performed on the first outpatient visit after surgery, typically 2 to 4 weeks after hospital discharge. Doppler TTE should be obtained at this visit to establish a new baseline echocardiogram. Thereafter, annual examinations should be performed. Although some authors recommend against echocardiography during the first 5 years after bioprosthetic valve replacement, we believe that annual examinations can identify early valve failure, particularly in cases of valve repair.

SURGERY FOR CARDIAC MYXOMA

Description and Special Anatomic Considerations

Primary tumors of the heart are mostly benign and constitute more than 75% of such neoplasms. Cardiac myxoma is the most common primary tumor of the heart; it constitutes more than 50% of all benign cardiac tumors.[27] Other benign neoplasms include lipomas, papillary fibroelastomas, and rhabdomyomas. Cardiac myxomas occur in all age groups, but are particularly common among women 30 to 60 years old. Myxomas typically originate from the endocardium of the interatrial septum and are found most commonly in the left atrium. The right atrium and very rarely the ventricular cavity are other sites.

Two distinct morphologic types of myxomas are identified: polypoid and pedunculated round tumors with a gelatinous consistency (Fig. 30-35A) and the less common, villous myxoma, which is characterized by multiple, fine villous extensions and has a propensity for embolism owing to fragility (Fig. 30-35B). Clinical presentation includes the triad of congestive heart failure owing to either inflow or outflow obstruction from tumor bulk; embolism; and constitutional symptoms such as fever, myalgia, and anorexia. Cardiac obstruction manifests with findings similar to either mitral or tricuspid valve stenosis. Embolism is found in 30% to 40% of patients and typically occurs to the central nervous system. Diagnosis is made by echocardiography and the findings of an intracavitary mass.

The treatment for myxoma and other benign tumors of the heart is surgical resection and is curative. For malignant neoplasms, a multidisciplinary approach is recommended. Specific anatomic considerations for the resection of cardiac tumors depend on the location of the tumor and its attachment.

For left atrial myxomas, the approach is similar to that of a mitral valve procedure. After the implementation of cardiopulmonary bypass, a left atriotomy is made, and the left atrial cavity is examined thoroughly. The myxoma is removed with full thickness of the atrial septum to ensure negative margins. Occasionally, a parallel incision is required in the right atrium to remove large myxomas in the left atrium. The resulting atrial septal defect can be closed primarily or with a patch of autologous pericardium. It is important to exclude synchronous tumor in the ventricular cavity.

For right atrial tumors, special consideration is required before implementation of cardiopulmonary bypass because of the risk of tumor fragmentation during cannulation of the right atrium. In situations with large bulky tumors in the right atrium, femoral cannulation is preferred. If the tumor is sitting near the orifice of the tricuspid valve, the potential for injury to the atrioventricular node exists, and in this situation, a subendocardial resection "shaving" the tumor is necessary in this area.

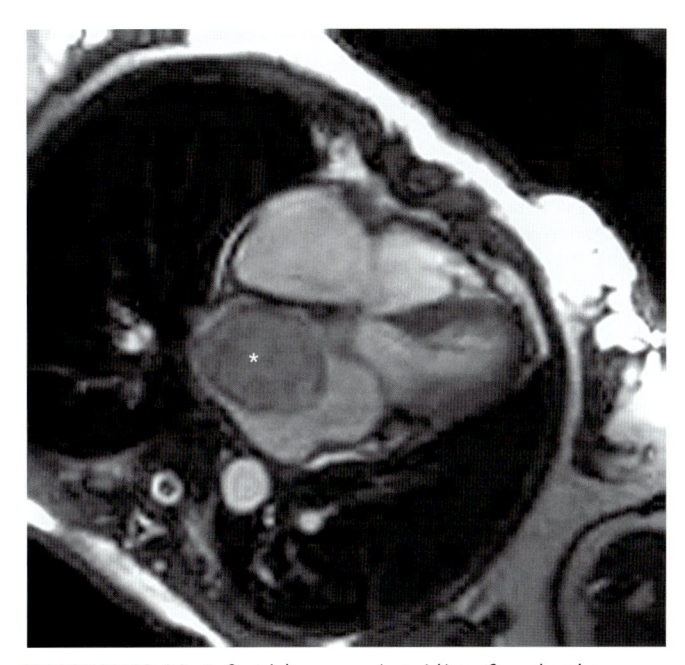

■ FIGURE 30-36 Left atrial myxoma (*asterisk*) on four-chamber steady-state free precession MR image.

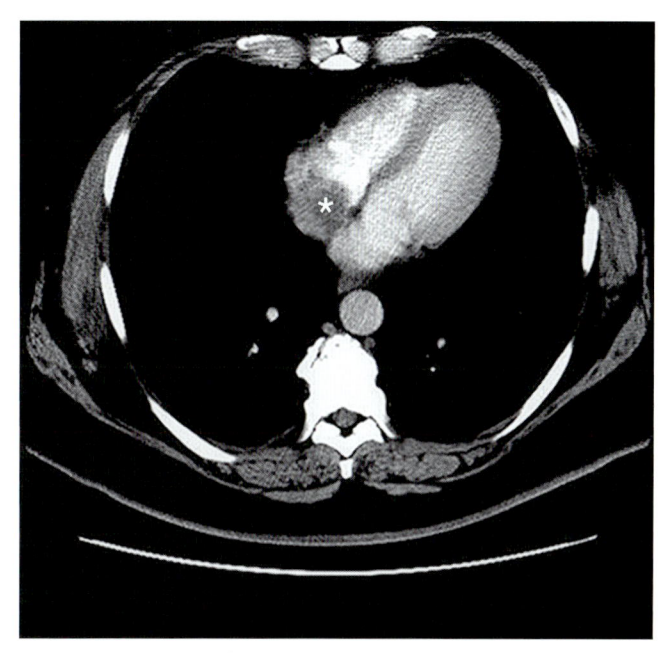

■ FIGURE 30-37 Right atrial myxoma (*asterisk*) on contrast-enhanced CT image.

Indications

Resection of a benign intracardiac tumor is indicated in all situations because there is no effective alternative therapy. When an atrial myxoma is identified, surgery should not be delayed because there is a risk of embolization and death while awaiting surgery.[27]

Contraindications

There are no contraindications to removal of a benign cardiac tumor.

Outcomes and Complications

The results are excellent in most cases. In most patients, myxomas are sporadic, and recurrence is rare. Risk of recurrence is higher in patients with familial or complex myxomas with rates of 12% to 22%, whereas patients with sporadic myxomas have a rate of recurrence of 1% to 3%.[27] Specific complications related to resection depend on the location of the tumor. Surgical risks include conduction abnormalities, valve injury, atrial septal defect, and embolization.

Imaging Findings

Preoperative Planning

Imaging with either CT or MRI can differentiate tissue composition making it possible to identify solid, liquid, and fatty space-occupying tumors within the heart (Figs. 30-36 and 30-37). In situations of a right atrial myxoma, CT angiography to image the pulmonary vasculature is important to rule out synchronous tumor deposits.

Postoperative Surveillance

There is no consensus follow-up. Semiannual echocardiographic surveillance is recommended for the first 2 years after surgery and annually thereafter for the ensuing 3 years. These recommendations are based on surveillance programs applied to other tumors of the thorax.

SURGERY FOR THE ASCENDING THORACIC AORTA

Pathologic conditions of the ascending thoracic aorta requiring surgical repair include aneurysmal dilation and acute aortic syndromes. Acute aortic syndromes include aortic dissection, penetrating ulcer of the aorta, and intramural hematoma. In cases of acute aortic dissection and in some cases of intramural hematoma, repair is done emergently. Ascending aneurysms may be electively repaired, unless the patient is symptomatic or has threatened or realized rupture.

Aortic Dissection

Aortic dissection occurs when blood enters between the medial layers of the aortic wall through an intimal tear. The blood propagates and creates a false lumen, which may eventually communicate across the dissection flap with the true lumen through another downstream intimal tear (Fig. 30-38). Causes of dissection are listed in Table 30-14, and include iatrogenic causes (as during cannulation for cardiopulmonary bypass or during catheterization) and numerous pathologic conditions, including hypertension, Marfan syndrome, or bicuspid aortic valve. Of patients with acute aortic dissection, 40% die before reaching a hospital, and 50% die within the initial 48 hours from presentation.[28] Causes of death from ascending aortic

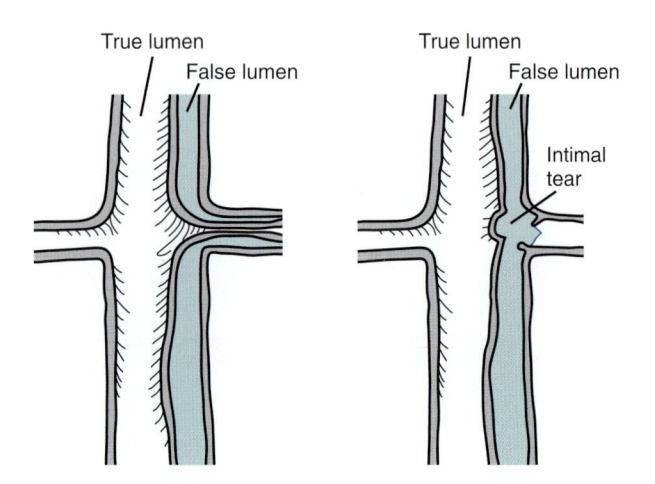

■ FIGURE 30-38 Aortic dissection. Intimal tear allows blood to enter the vessel wall, creating an intimal flap and false lumen, which can compress and obstruct flow into a branch vessel. (Redrawn from Reece TB, Green GR, Kron IL. Aortic dissection. In Cohn LH [ed]. Cardiac Surgery in the Adult. New York, McGraw-Hill, 2008, pp 1195-1222.)

TABLE 30-14 Risk Factors for Type A and B Thoracic Aortic Dissection

Hypertension
Connective tissue disorders
   Ehlers-Danlos syndrome
   Marfan disease
   Turner syndrome
Iatrogenic
Bicuspid aortic valve
Trauma
Atherosclerosis
Thoracic aortic aneurysm
Coarctation of the aorta
Cystic medial disease of aorta
Pharmacologic effects
Polycystic kidney disease
Pheochromocytoma

dissection include rupture into the pericardial sac causing tamponade, severe acute aortic incompetence, occlusion of coronary arteries or branch vessels causing myocardial infarction or stroke, and free rupture into the pleural space with exsanguination.

Two classification systems are used to characterize aortic dissection (Fig. 30-39). The Stanford classification is the simplest and most closely correlated with the clinical implications. Type A dissections are treated surgically and constitute a cardiovascular emergency. Type B dissections are treated medically and only rarely require surgery.

Aortic Aneurysm

Ascending aortic aneurysms are associated with many conditions, including degenerative conditions such as cystic medial degeneration and atherosclerosis, connective tissue disorders such as Marfan and Ehlers-Danlos syndrome, bicuspid aortic valve, infectious aortitis (mycotic), chronic dissection, coarctation, and trauma. The natural history of this entity has been studied extensively, and the indications for elective repair have become clearer over the past decade.[29,30] The goal is to perform elective repair before potential complications of rupture (spontaneous or traumatic), or dissection may occur.

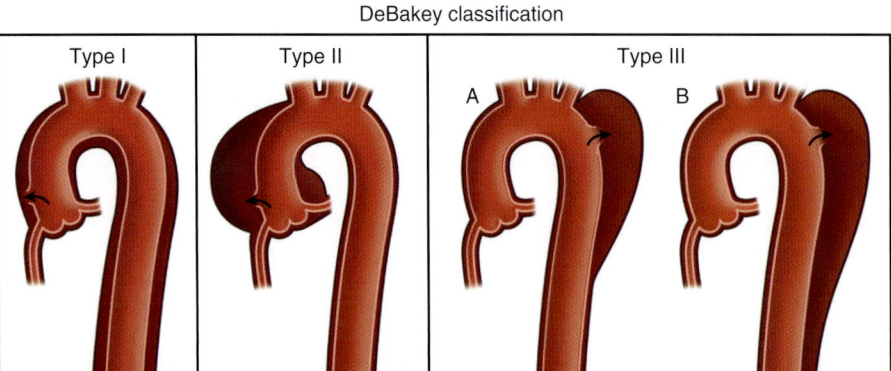

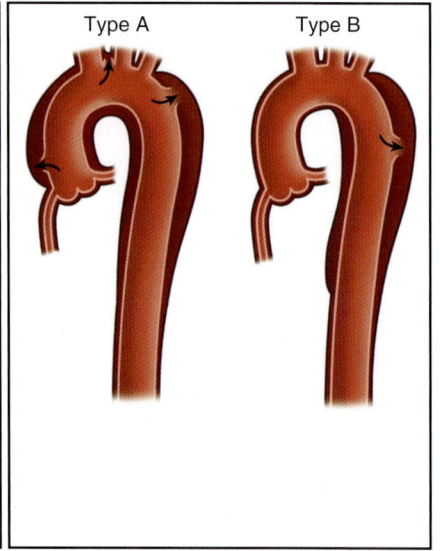

■ FIGURE 30-39 Classification system for thoracic aortic dissection. (Redrawn from Kouchokos NT, Dougenis D. Surgery of the thoracic aorta. N Engl J Med 1997; 336:1878.)

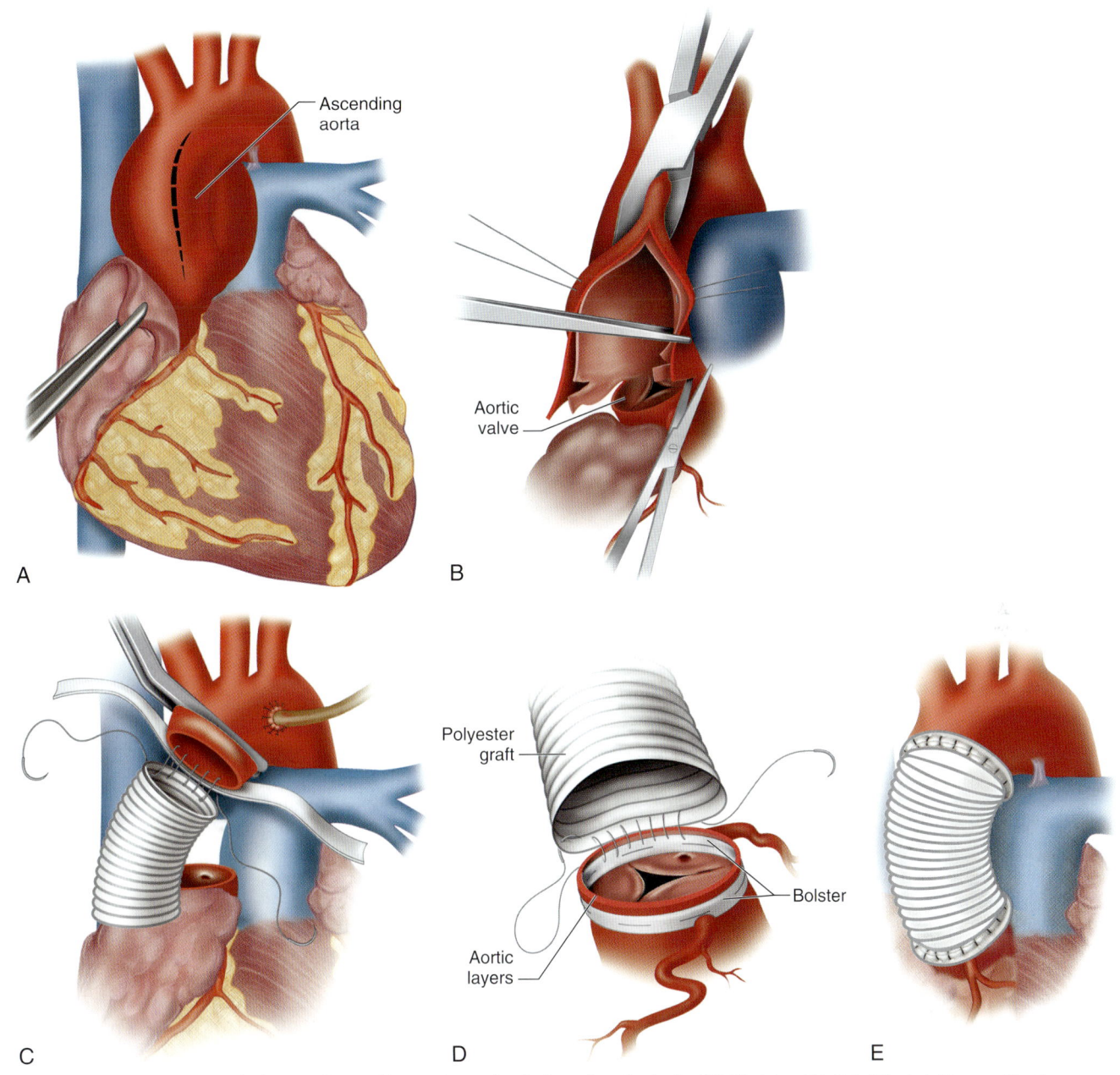

CHAPTER 30 • Surgery for Acquired Cardiac Disease   435

FIGURE 30-40 A-E, Surgical steps of ascending aortic repair. *(Redrawn from Kouchoukos NT, Blackstone EH, Doty DB, et al. Diseases of the thoracic arteries and veins. In Kirklin J, Barrett-Boyes B [eds]. Cardiac Surgery, 3rd ed. Philadelphia, PA, Churchill Livingstone, 2003, pp 1828-1830, 1864.)*

Description and Special Anatomic Considerations

Regardless of the pathology (dissection or aneurysm), the basic steps of repair of the ascending thoracic aorta are the same. Occasionally, pathology dictates that repair of the aortic arch be included. All repairs require the use of cardiopulmonary bypass. Arterial cannulation may be required in a location other than the ascending aorta, such as the femoral artery or axillary artery, depending on the anatomy of the aneurysm. The ascending dissection or aneurysm is excised beginning proximally 2 to 3 cm above the aortic valve commissures, to a point distally where the aorta becomes normal in diameter. It is replaced with an interposition textile graft. Hypothermic circulatory arrest may be required if the aneurysm or dissection involves the aortic arch, using an open anastomosis without cross-clamp.

Concomitant aortic valve repair or replacement along with CABG surgery may be performed as needed (Fig. 30-40). The complexity of the graft repair is determined by the extent of aorta that must be excised. The repair may involve anastomosis to or reconstruction of the branch vessels, or may require excision and replacement of the aortic root, with composite valve-conduit graft and reimplantation of the coronary arteries onto the graft. The goal of surgery is to excise and replace the entire pathologic area of the ascending aorta.

Indications

Emergent surgical repair is indicated in all cases of Stanford type A dissection, acute aortic syndrome, and spontaneous or traumatic aortic rupture. Elective surgical repair of thoracic aortic aneurysm is generally indicated if the ascending aorta diameter reaches 5 to 5.5 cm, the descending aorta reaches 6 cm, or the rate of growth is 1 cm/yr or greater (see Fig. 30-39). These criteria are based on extensive analysis of the natural history of thoracic aortic aneurysms by Coady and associates,[29] which showed a fourfold increase in risk of rupture or dissection after the ascending aorta reaches a diameter of 6 cm. In patients with Marfan syndrome or other familial aneurysms, earlier intervention is recommended. Bicuspid or unicuspid aortic valve has been associated with an abnormality of elastin formation in the aortic wall, and earlier intervention is indicated in these patients. Finally, patients undergoing valve or CABG surgery as the primary indication for surgery may also have a moderately dilated ascending aorta. Based on several studies, including one by Prenger and colleagues,[30] it is recommended that an aorta with a diameter of 4 to 5 cm be repaired concomitantly because of a 27% risk of future dissection without repair.

Contraindications

Contraindications for surgical repair of the aorta include comorbid conditions that would make the mortality risk of the surgery outweigh the risk of nonoperative management. There are few conditions that would make patients' surgical risk higher than that involving medical management of an acute ascending aortic dissection. Relative contraindications include patients older than 80 years and patients presenting with stroke with dense neurologic deficit. For elective aneurysm repair, patients with recent significant stroke or recent myocardial infarction with reduced ejection fraction may be at inordinate risk not to survive the operation, and may not be considered reasonable surgical candidates. Patients who do not undergo surgical repair because of comorbid conditions but who may be considered for surgery at a later date should be followed with serial CT scans (with contrast material), with the interval determined by the individual's clinical situation.

Outcomes and Complications

Operative mortality for elective repair of thoracic aortic aneurysm is very low, in most series 2% to 4%. The overall hospital mortality for repair of acute aortic dissection is higher, approximately 10% to 20%. Mortality is increased for patients presenting with hemodynamic instability, and is higher for patients requiring repair of the aortic arch, as shown in several series. Published 5-year survival for patients undergoing repair of acute type A aortic dissection is roughly 80%, and 60% at 10 years, whereas 5-year and 10-year postoperative survival for type B dissections is lower, 50% and 30%, respectively.[28]

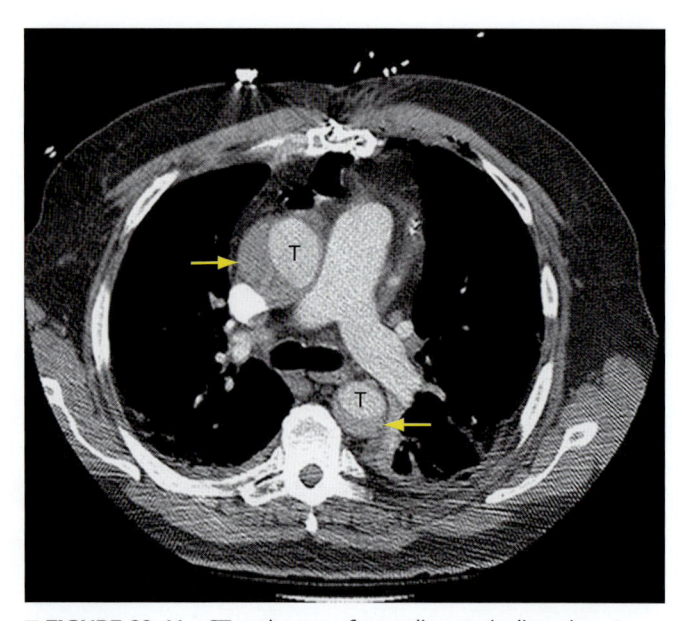

■ FIGURE 30-41 CT angiogram of ascending aortic dissection. *Arrows* shows false lumens. T, true lumen.

Imaging Findings

Preoperative Planning

For evaluation of thoracic aortic aneurysm and acute aortic syndrome, the most common method of assessment is CT, or more specifically CT angiography. CT scanning provides a quick identification of size, location, and extent of dissection, ulcer, or intramural hematoma and calcification (Fig. 30-41). Three-dimensional reconstruction provides increased accuracy regarding the size of the aneurysm in patients whose aorta is tortuous. Serial CT scanning provides valuable information in documenting the rate of growth of ascending aneurysms, to determine timing of surgery for asymptomatic patients.

Over the past decade, MRI has become a more commonly used modality in the assessment of thoracic aortic diseases because it can provide information on myocardial and aortic valve function, with the added advantages of enhanced three-dimensional imaging and avoidance of need for iodinated contrast agent. In dissections, MRI can depict sites of intimal tear with blood entry into the false channel. MRI can merge the information similar to that obtained from CT, echocardiogram, and angiography into one study, and in many centers is now the study of choice for imaging the thoracic aorta. Disadvantages are that MRI is generally more time-consuming and more costly than CT.

Conventional x-ray aortography is another modality used to evaluate suspected aortic dissection or traumatic transection. This study can accurately show the anatomy of the tear, including intimal flap and true lumen/false channel; depict the relationship of the arch vessels; and assess the aortic valve for incompetence. For patients undergoing elective repair of ascending aneurysm, this study provides accurate information regarding the size, location, and relationship to the branch vessels of the aorta and can depict the presence of aortic valve regurgita-

TABLE 30-15 Surveillance Studies after Repair of Acute Ascending Aortic Dissection

Timing of Study	Study	Indication
Before hospital discharge	MRI or CT	All patients
	TTE	Valve procedure
	Arteriography	Suspected malperfusion
After hospital discharge		
3 mo	MRI or CT	Dilated aorta or residual dissection
	TTE	Valve procedure
9 mo	MRI or CT	Dilated aorta or residual dissection
	TTE	Valve procedure
Subsequent examinations		
Every 6 mo	MRI or CT	Progression of aortic disease, Marfan syndrome
	TTE	Aortic incompetence
Every 12 mo	MRI or CT	Aortic diameter ≥5 cm
Every 24 mo	MRI or CT	Aortic diameter <5 cm

From Borst HG, Heinemann MK, Stone CD. Surgical Treatment of Aortic Dissection. New York, Churchill Livingstone, 1996, p 343.

tion. If the patient is older than 40 years, coronary angiography may be performed concomitantly. A significant contrast bolus is required for this study, which may be problematic in patients with preexisting renal insufficiency.

Finally, TEE with color Doppler imaging may be performed to rule out aortic dissection or transection and assess aortic valvular function. This is also an important tool for intraoperative assessment during operations on the ascending aorta, providing information on atherosclerotic disease, and cardiac valvular and ventricular function. Advantages are that this study may be done quickly at the bedside, and it requires no intravenous contrast agent.

Postoperative Surveillance

All patients who have had surgery of the thoracic aorta should undergo periodic, long-term surveillance. Aortic tissue remaining after aneurysm repair is often abnormal, and patients should undergo periodic CT or MRI because of their risk of aneurysm, dissection, or pseudoaneurysm formation. This risk is elevated in patients who have undergone surgical repair of aortic dissection, and they should have a more vigilant follow-up program. Table 30-15 shows an acceptable surveillance schedule as reported by Borst and associates.[31] Before hospital discharge, CT or MRI should be performed as a baseline postoperative evaluation, then repeated at the appropriate interval, depending on whether the patient has residual dissection, dilated aorta, or normal diameter. If valve reconstruction was performed, TTE should be performed before hospital discharge, then serially examined in follow-up. Patients with suspected malperfusion at any time should undergo aortography.

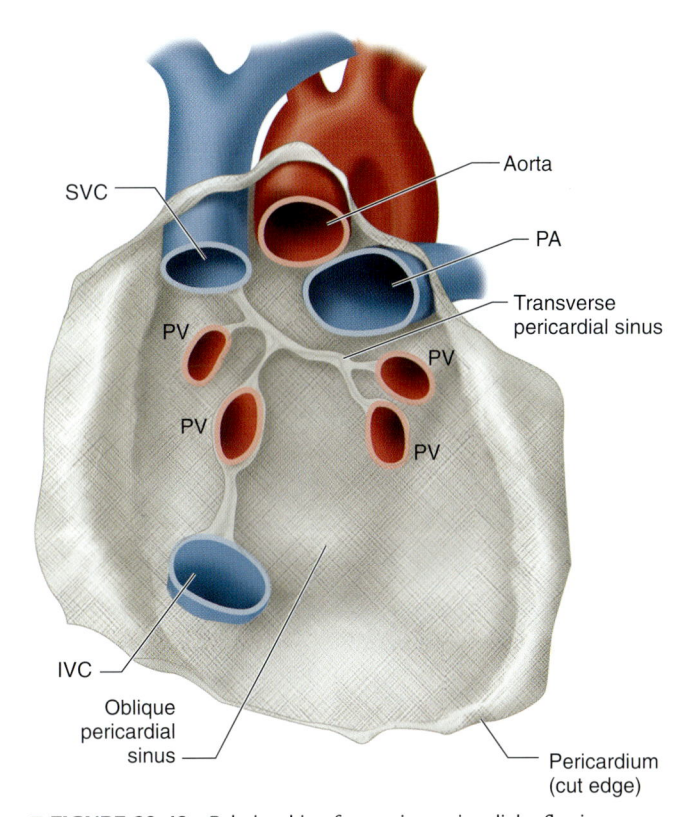

■ **FIGURE 30-42** Relationship of posterior pericardial reflections to anatomic structures. IVC, inferior vena cava; PA, pulmonary artery; PV, pulmonary vein; SVC, superior vena cava. (Redrawn from Mangi AA, Torchiana DF. Pericardial disease. In Cohn LH [ed]. Cardiac Surgery in the Adult. New York, McGraw-Hill, 2008, pp 1465-1478.)

DISORDERS OF THE PERICARDIUM

The pericardium is composed of a serous component and a fibrous, semicompliant membranous component that envelops the heart like a cocoon. The serous portion is bordered by the visceral pericardium (a layer on the epicardium) and parietal pericardium. The fibrous component is a membrane in continuity with the parietal pericardium. The function of the pericardium is to maintain the heart's position in the mediastinum and preserve cardiac performance by preventing myocardial distention when volume overload occurs. The serous pericardium contains fluid that provides lubrication during cardiac motion, reducing friction with the pericardial sac. Two natural recesses called sinuses provide a pathway around the heart within the pericardium (Fig. 30-42). Common disorders of the pericardium include conditions of excessive fluid accumulation within the serous pericardium and involvement of the pericardium with disease (pericarditis). The end result of inflammatory pericarditis is constrictive pericarditis. These derangements cause hemodynamic effects that can be fatal. Table 30-16 lists conditions associated with these pericardial disorders.

Constrictive Pericarditis

Constrictive pericarditis can occur with any condition that causes inflammation of the pericardium with subsequent fibrosis. Causes of constrictive pericarditis are listed in

TABLE 30-16 Disorders Associated with Pericardial Disease
Chronic constrictive pericarditis
Previous cardiac surgery, trauma
Post-mediastinal radiation
Tuberculosis
Chronic idiopathic
Acute or recurrent effusive pericarditis
Idiopathic
Infectious—viral, bacterial, tuberculous
Acute myocardial infarction
Uremia
Malignancy
Post-mediastinal radiation
Systemic autoimmune diseases (rheumatoid arthritis, systemic lupus erythematosus, sarcoidosis, vasculitides)
Post–cardiac injury syndrome (trauma, cardiac surgery)
From Little WC, Freeman GL. Pericardial disease. Circulation 2006; 113:1622-1632.

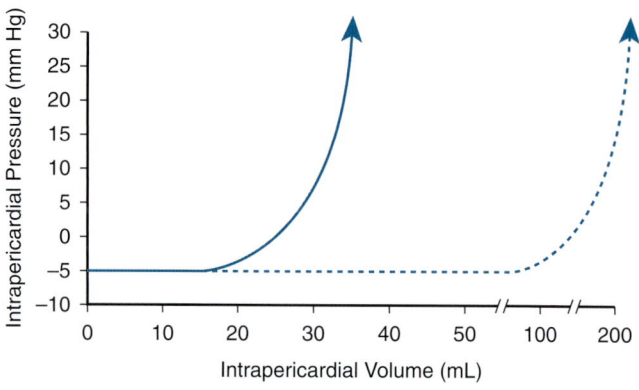

FIGURE 30-43 Relationship of volume of pericardial fluid to intrapericardial pressure. *(Redrawn from Mangi AA, Torchiana DF. Pericardial disease. In Cohn LH [ed]. Cardiac Surgery in the Adult. New York, McGraw-Hill, 2008, pp 1465-1478.)*

Table 30-16. Constrictive pericarditis is seen in 4% to 5% of patients who have undergone previous cardiac surgery.[32] This insidious condition can manifest in a widely variable postoperative time interval (days to years after surgery). Patients may present with worsening symptoms of congestive heart failure with a normal left ventricular ejection fraction and in the absence of other cardiac pathology. Constrictive pericarditis can also be caused by radiation therapy to the mediastinum, malignancy, and infection. Tuberculous pericarditis is less common today than in the early 20th century.

The basic physiologic derangement in constrictive pericarditis is the inability of the heart to fill normally because the constricting membrane prevents chamber distention. The diagnosis of constrictive pericarditis is made using hemodynamic measurements as listed in Table 30-17. The most specific of these findings, ventricular interdependence, is seen as a decrease in left ventricular systolic pressure with an increase in right ventricular systolic pressure during inspiration, measured in the cardiac catheterization laboratory.

Effusive Pericarditis

Acute and chronic effusive pericarditis with pericardial effusion may manifest with acute pericardial tamponade. Tamponade occurs as the semicompliant fibrous pericardium accommodates an increase in volume up to a point at which the compliance is exceeded, and intrapericardial pressure acutely increases. Figure 30-43 illustrates the hemodynamic derangement that only a small increase in the amount of pericardial fluid can result in a dramatic increase in intrapericardial pressure. A common finding on physical examination is pulsus paradoxus, which is a dissociation of cardiac and intrathoracic pressures, causing a decrease in systolic pressure of greater than 10 mm Hg with inspiration.

Chronic effusive pericarditis is related to numerous diseases, including renal disease, hemodialysis, malignancy, medications, and (rarely) infection, and is more common in young women. Acute pericarditis with effusion may be seen after cardiac surgery and after myocardial infarction (Dressler syndrome). This condition may be seen in any post–cardiac surgery patient, and commonly occurs in patients who have undergone valve replacement with mechanical prosthesis, who are on warfarin anticoagulation, and who may present days to weeks after surgery.

Description and Special Anatomic Considerations

The surgical treatment for constrictive pericarditis is complete pericardiectomy (Fig. 30-44). This may be performed through a median sternotomy or a left thoracotomy, and requires meticulous dissection of the visceral (off the epicardium) and parietal layers of the pericardium. The use of cardiopulmonary bypass may be necessary to complete the operation. The pericardiectomy includes removal of all encasing pericardial tissue (visceral, parietal, and fibrous). The extent of removal is limited laterally by the phrenic nerves, inferiorly by the diaphragm, and superiorly by the great vessels. The goal of the surgery is to free the left and right ventricles sufficiently to allow normal filling in diastole. Technically, this can be extremely challenging and bloody because of the dense pericardial adhesions and calcification that may be encountered.

For acute or chronic pericarditis with tamponade, the indicated surgery is urgent/emergent pericardial drainage. This surgery may be performed via an open "pericardial window" with a subxyphoid approach, or by using a minimally invasive approach with video-assisted thoracic surgery. If the effusion is chronic or due to malignancy, a

TABLE 30-17 Hemodynamic Findings with Constrictive Pericarditis
Equal, elevated end-diastolic pressures in all four cardiac chambers
Ventricular interdependence
Pulmonary artery systolic pressure <50 mm Hg
LV end-diastolic pressure/RV end-diastolic pressure <5 mm Hg
RV diastolic pressure/RV systolic pressure > one third
LV, left ventricular; RV, right ventricular.

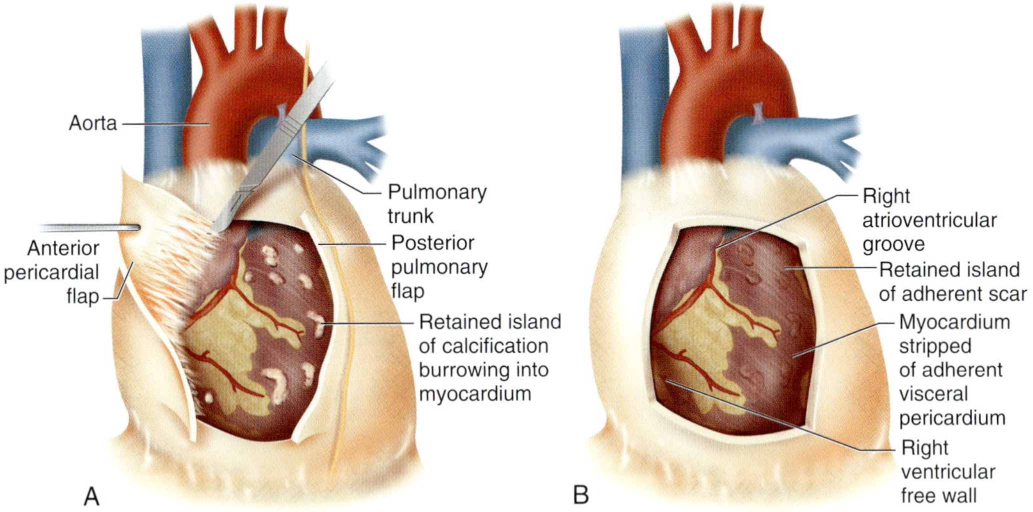

FIGURE 30-44 A and B, Technique of pericardiectomy. *(Redrawn from Kouchoukos NT, Blackstone EH, Doty DB, et al. Pericardial disease. In Kirklin J, Barrett-Boyes B [eds]. Cardiac Surgery, 3rd ed. Philadelphia, PA, Churchill Livingstone, 2003, p 1786.)*

portion of the pericardium should be excised to ensure definitive drainage. The pericardium may be sent for pathologic analysis to determine the cause of the condition, if unclear.

Indications

The mere existence of a pericardial effusion or thickened pericardium is not an indication for surgical intervention. Surgery is considered only when a patient is experiencing signs and symptoms of tamponade or of constriction with hemodynamic findings by catheterization or echocardiogram. In cases of acute pericardial tamponade, prompt intervention is lifesaving. With chronic effusive pericarditis, patients should undergo drainage when symptoms develop (usually shortness of breath) or after failing intensive medical therapy.

Contraindications

For constrictive pericarditis, the only contraindication for surgery is the patient's inability to tolerate the procedure because of comorbid conditions. No contraindications exist for open pericardial drainage for tamponade because this is a potentially lifesaving intervention.

Outcomes and Complications

The results of surgical procedures for pericardial disease vary with the etiology and severity of the disease. Total pericardiectomy for constrictive pericarditis has an operative mortality risk of 10% to 20%,[33] depending on the degree of preoperative congestive heart failure, elevated right atrial pressure, and other significant comorbid conditions. Operative morbidity includes bleeding owing to the difficulty dissecting dense epicardial adhesions, injury to the phrenic nerve, and injury to epicardial vessels and bypass grafts. Patients usually respond well to surgery with a decrease in heart failure symptoms, and generally shed much of the accumulated preoperative water weight. Long-term survival is diminished, however, in patients with previous cardiac surgery, reduced preoperative ejection fraction, or radiation-induced disease. Results after postpericardiotomy open pericardial drainage are very good, with immediate improvement in hemodynamics and alleviation of symptoms, with low morbidity and mortality.[34]

Imaging Findings

Preoperative Planning

Chest radiograph and echocardiography often provide sufficient information in the diagnosis of acute pericardial tamponade. Figure 30-45 shows a typical chest radiograph of a patient with a large pericardial effusion and tamponade.

In patients with constrictive pericarditis, echocardiography, CT, or MRI may show a thickened pericardium (Fig. 30-46); however, echocardiography provides much more useful information with the ability to assess hemodynamics. Echocardiography may reveal a respiratory variation in early mitral filling, along with increased diastolic flow reversal in the hepatic veins during expiration. Right and left cardiac catheterization provide the most accurate assessment of hemodynamic criteria to diagnose constrictive pericarditis, as stated previously.

Postoperative Surveillance

TTE is the most common modality used to evaluate patients after surgical treatment of pericardial disease. Important findings include the recurrence of effusion, along with persistent derangements in hemodynamics with impaired chamber filling in diastole. Patients typically undergo at least one postoperative echocardiogram before discharge from the hospital. Depending on the clinical situation, one or more studies are performed as an outpatient as appropriate.

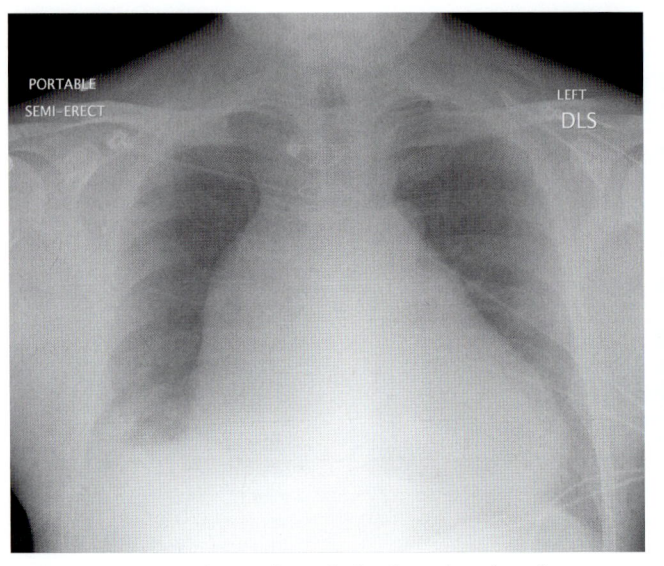

■ **FIGURE 30-45** Chest radiograph showing enlarged cardiac silhouette in a patient with a large pericardial effusion.

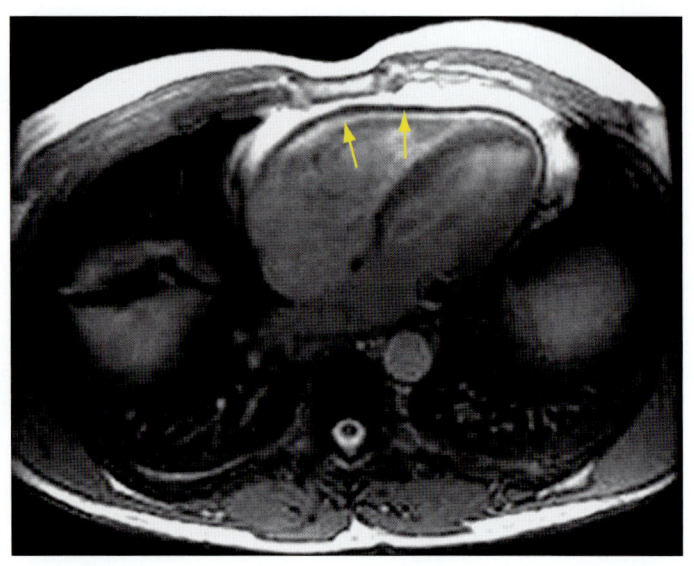

■ **FIGURE 30-46** Gradient-echo image of a patient with a thickened pericardium (*arrows*) that is hypointense in signal.

KEY POINTS

- Revascularization using CABG can be performed with very low morbidity and mortality.
- Catheter coronary angiography remains the gold standard to assess for coronary disease, but coronary CT angiography has emerged as a promising technique for screening of patients with suspected coronary disease or surveillance of patients with known coronary disease.
- Patients with symptomatic aortic stenosis have increased risk for mortality (75% die by 3 years) and require AVR. Patients with severe aortic regurgitation are at risk for progressive heart failure and benefit from AVR.
- Surgical options for mitral valve surgery include valve replacement, valve repair, and percutaneous balloon valvuloplasty.
- Infective endocarditis can occur especially in patients with mitral valve prolapse or in patients who have undergone prosthetic valve replacement.
- Cardiac myxomas are the most common primary cardiac tumor. Surgical resection is curative.
- Ascending aortic surgery is most commonly performed for repair of a type A aortic dissection and aortic aneurysm. In patients with concomitant aortic valve disease, replacement of the aortic valve is often considered at the time of ascending aortic surgery.
- The diagnosis of constrictive pericarditis is typically made based on hemodynamic criteria.
- Pericardiectomy is the surgical treatment of choice for constrictive pericarditis.

SUGGESTED READING

Kouchoukos NT, Dougenis D. Surgery of the thoracic aorta. N Engl J Med 1997; 336:1876-1888.

REFERENCES

1. Eagle KA, Guyton RA, Davidoff R, et al. ACC/AHA 2004 guideline update for coronary artery bypass surgery: a report of the American College of Cardiology/American Heart Association Task Force on Practice Guidelines (Committee to Update the 1999 Guidelines for Coronary Artery Bypass Graft Surgery). Circulation 2004; 110:e340-e437.
2. Post Coronary Artery Bypass Graft Trial Investigators. The effect of aggressive lowering of low-density lipoprotein cholesterol levels and low-dose anticoagulation on obstructive changes in saphenous vein coronary artery bypass grafts. N Engl J Med 1997; 336:153-162.
3. Veterans Administration Coronary Artery Bypass Surgery Cooperative Study Group. Eleven-year survival in the Veterans Administration randomized trial of coronary bypass surgery for stable angina. N Engl J Med 1984; 311:1333-1339.
4. Coronary Artery Surgery Study (CASS). A randomized trial of coronary artery bypass surgery: quality of life in patients randomly assigned to treatment groups. Circulation 1983; 68:951-960.
5. Varnauskas E. Twelve-year follow-up of survival in the randomized European Coronary Surgery Study. N Engl J Med 1988; 319:332-337.

6. Simon AR, Baraki H, Weidemann J, et al. High-resolution 64-slice helical-computer-assisted-tomographical-angiography as a diagnostic tool before CABG surgery: the dawn of a new era? Eur J Cardiothorac Surg 2007; 32:896-901.
7. Mollett NR, Cademartiri F, van Meighem CA, et al. High-resolution spiral computed tomography coronary angiography in patients referred for diagnostic conventional coronary angiography. Circulation 2005; 112:2318-2323.
8. Plass A, Grunenfelder J, Leschka S, et al. Coronary artery imaging with 64-slice computed tomography from cardiac surgical perspective. Eur J Cardiothorac Surg 2006; 30:109-116.
9. Society of Thoracic Surgeons Executive Summary, STS Sprint 2007 Report. Duke Clinical Research Institute. Available at: www.sts.org/documents/pdf/ndb/Fall_2007_Executive_Summary.pdf—2007-01-01 (accessed August 1, 2007).
10. Carabello BA. Aortic stenosis. N Engl J Med 2002; 346:677-682.
11. Carabello BA, Crawford FA. Valvular heart disease. N Engl J Med 1997; 337:32-41.
12. Otto CM, Burwash IG, Leggert ME, et al. Prospective study of asymptomatic valvular aortic stenosis: clinical, echocardiographic and exercise predictors of outcome. Circulation 1997; 95:2262-2270.
13. Bonow RO, Carabello BA, Chatterjee K, et al. ACC/AHA 2006 guidelines for the management of patients with valvular heart disease: a report of the American College of Cardiology/American Heart Association Task Force on Practice Guidelines (writing committee to revise the 1998 Guidelines for the Management of Patients with Valvular Heart Disease): developed in collaboration with the Society of Cardiovascular Anesthesiologists: endorsed by the Society for Cardiovascular Angiography and Interventions and the Society of Thoracic Surgeons. Circulation 2006; 114:e84-e231.
14. Enriquez-Sarano M, Tajik AJ. Aortic regurgitation. N Engl J Med 2004; 351:1539-1546.
15. Carabello BA. Vasodilators in aortic regurgitation—where is the evidence of their effectiveness? N Engl J Med 2005; 353:1400-1402.
16. Cowell SJ, Newby DE, Prescott RJ, et al. A randomized trial of intensive lipid-lowering therapy in calcific aortic stenosis. N Engl J Med 2005; 352:2389-2397.
17. Mullany CJ. Aortic valve surgery in the elderly. Cardiol Rev 2000; 8:333-339.
18. Connolly HM, Oh JK, Schaff HV, et al. Severe aortic stenosis with low transvalvular gradient and severe left ventricular dysfunction: result of aortic valve replacement in 52 patients. Circulation 2000; 101:1940-1946.
19. Pibarot P, Dumesnil JG. Prosthesis-patient mismatch: definition, clinical impact and prevention. Heart 2006; 92:1022-1029.
20. Ling LH, Enriquez-Sarano M, Seward JB, et al. Clinical outcome of mitral valve regurgitation due to flail leaflet. N Engl J Med 1996; 335:1417-1423.
21. Mothy D, Orszulak TA, Schaff HV, et al. Very long-term survival and durability of mitral valve repair for mitral valve prolapse. Circulation 2001; 104:11-17.
22. Braunberger E, Deloche A, Berrebi A, et al. Very long-term results (more than 20 years) of valve repair with Carpentier's techniques in nonrheumatic mitral valve insufficiency. Circulation 2001; 104:8-11.
23. Enriquez-Sarano M, Avierinos JF, Messika-Zeitoun D, et al. Quantitative determinants of the outcome of asymptomatic mitral regurgitation. N Engl J Med 2005; 352:875-883.
24. Mylonakis E, Calderwood SB. Infective endocarditis in adults. N Engl J Med 2001; 345:1318-1330.
25. Li JS, Sexton DJ, Mick N, et al. Proposed modifications to the Duke criteria for the diagnosis of infective endocarditis. Clin Infect Dis 2000; 30:633-638.
26. Feringa HH, Shaw LJ, Poldermans D, et al. Mitral valve repair and replacement in endocarditis: a systematic review of the literature. Ann Thorac Surg 2007; 83:564-570.
27. Reynen K. Cardiac myxomas. N Engl J Med 1995; 333:1610-1617.
28. Reece TB, Green GR, Kron IL. Aortic dissection. In Cohn LH (ed): Cardiac Surgery in the Adult. New York, McGraw-Hill, 2008, pp 1195-1222.
29. Coady MA, Rizzo JA, Elefteriades JA. Developing surgical intervention criteria for thoracic aortic aneurysms. Cardiol Clin 1999; 17:827.
30. Prenger K, Pieters F, Cheriex E. Aortic dissection after aortic valve replacement: incidence and consequences for strategy. J Card Surg 1994; 9:495.
31. Borst HG, Heinemann MK, Stone CD. Surgical Treatment of Aortic Dissection. New York, Churchill Livingstone, 1996.
32. Ling LH, Oh JK, Schaff HV, et al. Constrictive pericarditis in the modern era: evolving clinical spectrum and impact on outcome after pericardiectomy. Circulation 1999; 100:1380.
33. McCaughan BC, Schaff HV, Piehier JM, et al. Early and late results of pericardiectomy for constrictive pericarditis. J Thorac Cardiovasc Surg 1985; 89:340.
34. Aksöyek A, Tütün U, Ulus T, et al. Surgical drainage of late cardiac tamponade following open heart surgery. Thorac Cardiovasc Surg 2005; 53:285-290.

CHAPTER 31

Imaging of Atrial Fibrillation Intervention

Cristopher A. Meyer and Mehran Attari

There has been great deal of interest in left atrial anatomy and function, and particularly pulmonary veins owing to the increase in popularity of ablative procedures for atrial fibrillation (AF). This chapter reviews the clinical data relevant to AF, the treatment options, and the complementary role of imaging in treatment planning.

DEFINITION

AF, a supraventricular tachyarrhythmia, is the most common cardiac arrhythmia with an overall prevalence of 0.4% to 1%.[1] AF manifests clinically with an "irregularly irregular" heart rate, lack of P waves on ECG, and heart rates of up to 200 beats/min. To guide treatment options, the American College of Cardiology/American Heart Association/European Society of Cardiology (ACC/AHA/ESC) has issued guidelines classifying AF into paroxysmal, persistent, and permanent.[2] Paroxysmal AF is defined as AF lasting less than 7 days and terminating spontaneously. Persistent AF lasts longer than 7 days and requires cardioversion to achieve normal sinus rhythm. Permanent AF lasts longer than 1 year. When AF occurs in individuals younger than 60 years and without underlying risk factors, it is termed *lone AF*.

PREVALENCE AND EPIDEMIOLOGY

AF affects approximately 2.3 million people in the United States and more than 6 million people in Europe.[3] Its prevalence increases with age. Although AF is rare in children, in adults, the incidence and prevalence double every 10 years after age 50. The lifetime risk of developing AF is one in four after age 40.

Epidemiologic studies have linked AF to underlying structural heart disease, particularly mitral valvular disease, hypertension, and coronary artery disease.[4] Age, diabetes, smoking, obesity, male sex, and white race are also independently associated with increased risk of AF.[1,2] The epidemics of obesity and chronic heart failure are expected to contribute to an increased incidence of AF. The total annual cost for treatment of AF is estimated at $6.65 billion.[5] AF results in approximately 350,000 hospitalizations, 5 million office visits, and 276,000 emergency department visits annually in the United States.

PATHOPHYSIOLOGY OF ATRIAL FIBRILLATION AND PULMONARY VEINS

The pathophysiology of AF is complex and not fully understood. AF is initiated by rapid firing of ectopic foci or reentrant wavelets most often (94%) originating from the pulmonary veins.[6] Other sources of ectopic foci have been identified in superior vena cava, coronary sinus, ligament of Marshal, crista terminalis, body of left atrium and right atrium, and more distal pulmonary veins.[7-9] Pathologic studies have shown the extension of myocardial sleeves into pulmonary veins.[10] A sleeve of myocardium surrounds the proximal aspect of the pulmonary vein and when measured from the venoatrial junction extends 0.2 to 1.7 cm out of the pulmonary veins with the longest sleeves associated with the superior pulmonary veins. The longest extensions occur in the following order: left superior pulmonary vein, right superior pulmonary vein, left inferior pulmonary vein, and right inferior pulmonary vein.[11] Haissaguerre and colleagues[6] showed a similar rank order when identifying ectopic foci for ablation. More than 90% of these ectopic beats arise from pulmonary veins; 50% arise from the left superior pulmonary vein alone. The posterior left atrium and pulmonary veins have become the focus of attention in treatment efforts of AF. When initiated, an abnormal atrial substrate maintains AF in susceptible individuals. Current AF treatments strive to isolate electrically the originating foci in the pulmonary veins from the atrial substrate and to modify the substrate.

MANIFESTATIONS OF DISEASE

Clinical Presentation

AF prevents ventricular preload and is associated with increased cardiovascular morbidity or mortality.[12] It is an independent risk factor for stroke, increasing the risk by threefold to fivefold.[4,13] It is also associated with increased risk of systemic embolism. The source of the embolism is left atrial appendage (LAA) in most patients.[14] AF is associated with an increase in overall mortality in multiple studies.[15,16]

Clinically Relevant Anatomy

The left atrium can be divided into four components: the septum, the vestibule, the appendage, and the venous portion. The walls of the left atrium are described as superior, posterior, left lateral, septal, and anterior.[17] The anterior wall behind the transverse pericardial sinus posterior to the aorta is very thin, averaging 2 mm in thickness.[18] The thickest portion of the left atrium is the superior wall, averaging 4.5 ± 0.6 mm in thickness.[18]

The interatrial septum comprises the foramen ovale. The foramen ovale is a flap valve that typically fuses by early adulthood. The prevalence of patent foramen ovale is reported to be 25%.[19] The foramen ovale is the only portion of the septum that can be traversed without risk of injury to the sinoatrial nodal artery or exiting the heart.[18]

The vestibular component is smooth and is the thinnest portion of the left atrium surrounding the orifice of the mitral valve. The great cardiac vein runs just external to this thin structure in the atrioventricular groove. Posteriorly, the vestibule abuts the wall of the coronary sinus.

Most of the left atrium is smooth-walled. The exception is the LAA, which is derived from the primitive atrium and contains multiple pectinate muscles and a trabeculated surface. The LAA is a common source of atrial thrombi because of relative stasis of blood flow in this region in AF and the narrow neck of the appendage. Accessory atrial appendages (also termed *roof pouch*) have been reported in 0.06% of patients; these are of unclear clinical significance, but they may result in discontinuity of a roof ablation line if unrecognized (Fig. 31-1).[20,21]

The venous component comprises most of the left atrium. Classic left atrial anatomy consists of bilateral superior and inferior pulmonary veins and is present about two thirds of the time (Fig. 31-2).[22,23] Accessory pulmonary veins are named for the lobes or segments they drain. Common anatomic variants include a conjoined left pulmonary trunk, which bifurcates to form the left superior pulmonary vein and left inferior pulmonary vein (under incorporation) and has been reported as a consistent source of arrhythmogenic atrial ectopy (Fig. 31-3).[24,25] An accessory right middle pulmonary vein is the most common variant, occurring 20% to 30% of the time; it originates from the intervenous saddle and is typically 1 cm or less in diameter (Fig. 31-4).[26] The next most common accessory vein drains the superior segment of the right lower lobe independently. One of the most striking accessory veins is the "top vein" (3%), which can drain the posterior segment right upper lobe or superior segment right lower lobe, and is particularly important to describe for patients being considered for the Wolf mini-Maze procedure; this unusual location is blind to the thoracoscopist (Fig. 31-5).[27,28] Overincorporation of the right inferior pulmonary vein commonly results in multiple orificial branches and has been reported in 66% to 99% of

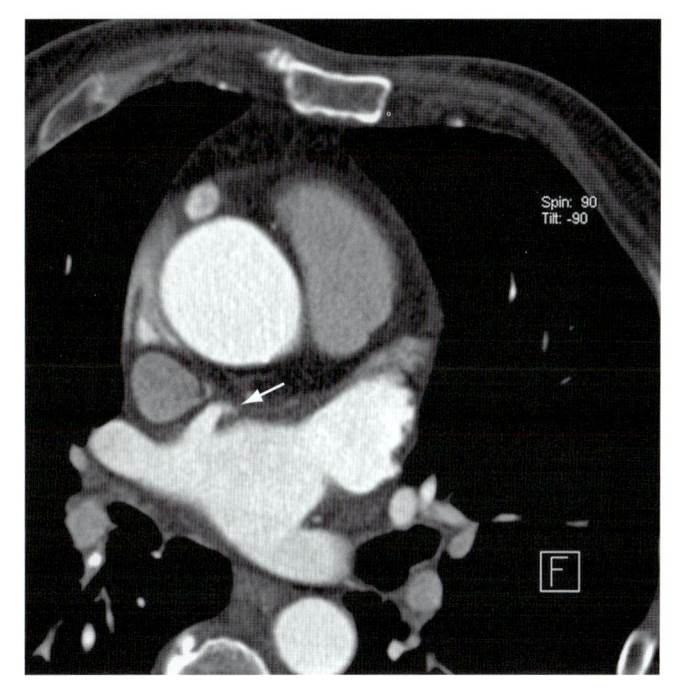

■ FIGURE 31-1 Accessory LAA. A focal outpouching (*arrow*) is seen anterior to the right superior pulmonary vein.

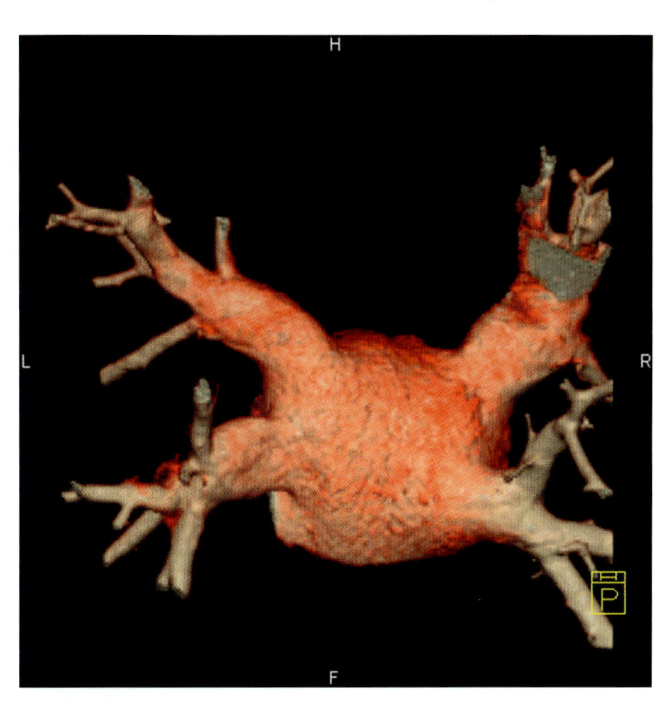

■ FIGURE 31-2 Classic view of the left atrium in this volume rendered image of the dorsal left atrium showing four pulmonary veins.

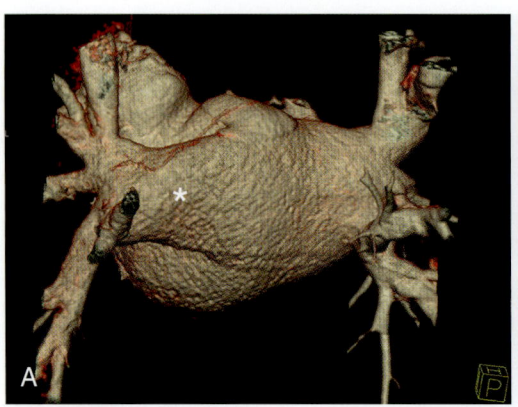

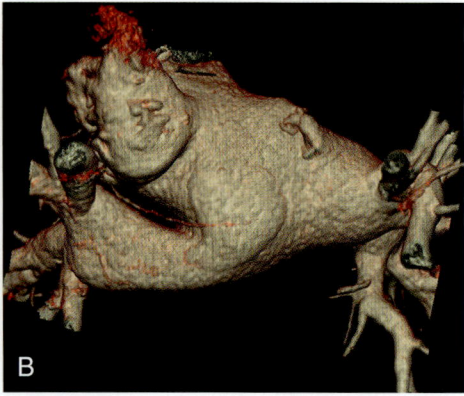

FIGURE 31-3 A and B, A common left pulmonary vein (*asterisk*) is illustrated in dorsal (**A**) and roof (**B**) volume rendered images of the left atrium. This variant anatomy is a consistent source of arrhythmogenic atrial ectopy.

cases (Fig. 31-6).[29] Rarely, the inferior pulmonary veins can be conjoined resulting in an inferior truncus (Fig. 31-7).[30]

The sinoatrial node is found along the course of the sinoatrial artery in the subepicardium. This subepicardial location makes the node more vulnerable to select cardiac surgery and pericardial disease.[31] The node artery arises from the right coronary artery in 66% of cases, arises from the left circumflex artery in 27%, and has a dual supply in 6%.[32] Most arise from the proximal right coronary artery and course along the anterior interatrial groove toward the cavoatrial junction (Figs. 31-8 and 31-9).

CLINICAL TREATMENT OF ATRIAL FIBRILLATION

Traditionally, treatment of AF has included electrical or chemical cardioversion followed by long-term antiarrhythmic therapy. This strategy is unsatisfactory in maintenance

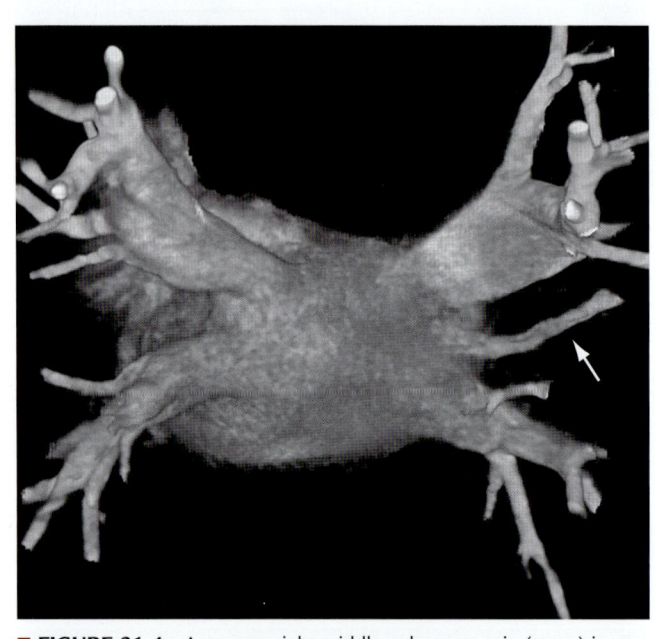

FIGURE 31-4 Accessory right middle pulmonary vein (*arrow*) is seen arising from the intervenous saddle of the superior and inferior pulmonary veins on this volume rendered dorsal image of the left atrium.

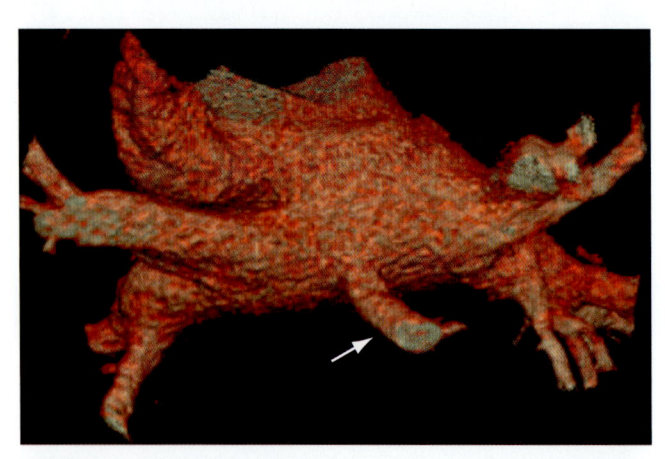

FIGURE 31-5 Volume rendered image of the roof of the left atrium shows an unusual venous variant, the "top vein" (*arrow*). Because of its unusual location, the top vein is prone to misadventure at catheter ablation or thoracoscopy unless identified prospectively.

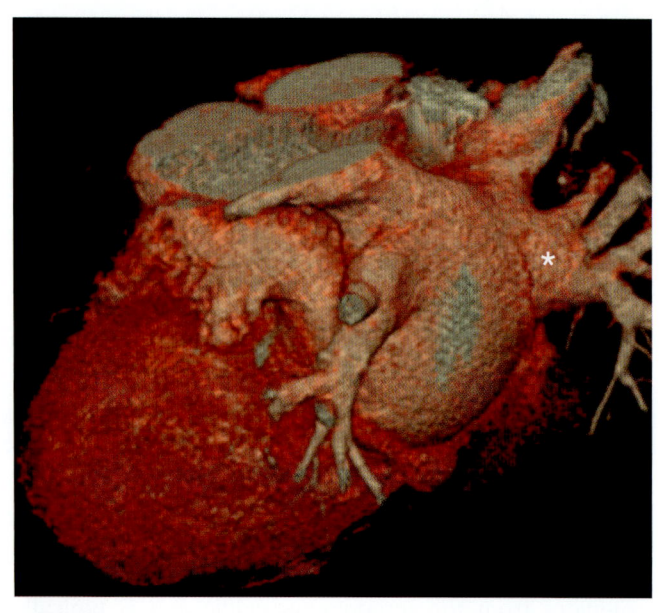

FIGURE 31-6 Posterior oblique volume rendered image of the right inferior pulmonary vein reveals multiple branches (*asterisk*) within 5 mm of the venoatrial junction consistent with overincorporation.

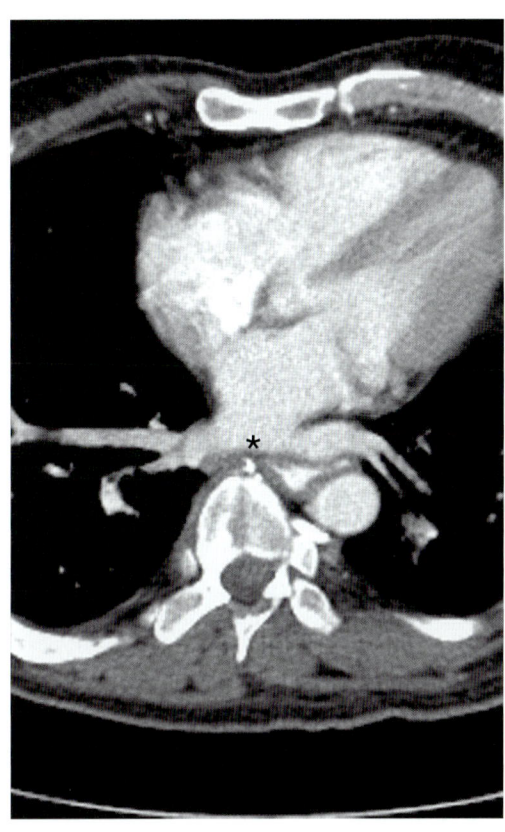

FIGURE 31-7 Curved multiplanar reconstruction showing a rare variant: conjoined right and left inferior pulmonary veins. Note the common trunk (*asterisk*) of the inferior pulmonary veins draining to the left atrium.

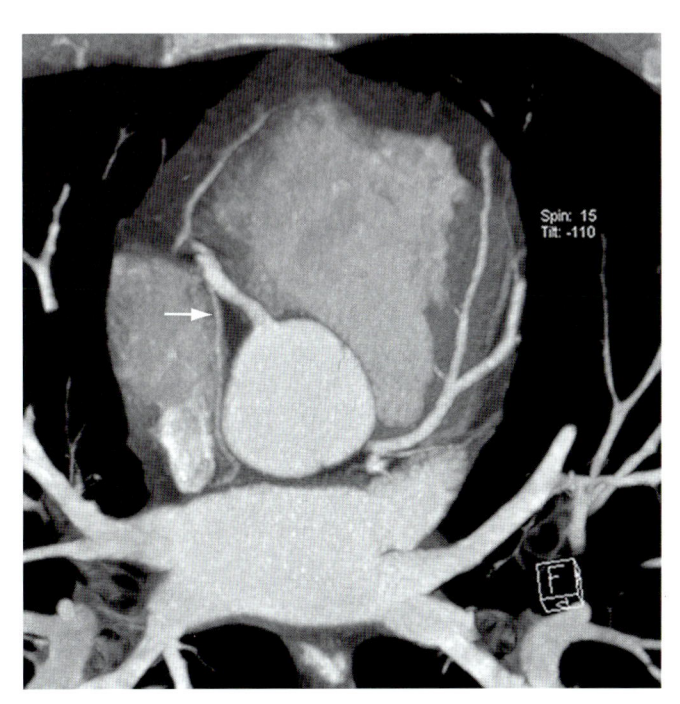

FIGURE 31-8 The sinoatrial node artery (*arrow*) typically arises from the right coronary artery approximately two thirds of the time.

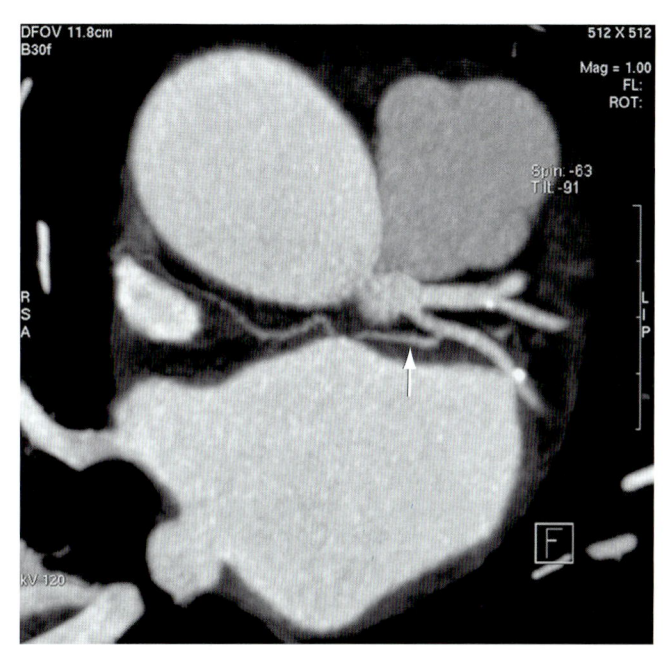

FIGURE 31-9 In some patients, the sinoatrial node artery (*arrow*) arises from the proximal or middle circumflex coronary artery.

of sinus rhythm, with less than 50% of patients being in sinus rhythm after 1 to 2 years.[33] It also has the accompanying disadvantage of requiring lifelong anticoagulation. Maintenance of sinus rhythm is important in younger active individuals to decrease the incidence of stroke, and in older patients with heart failure, the loss of the "atrial kick" affects overall cardiac output.

In an effort to improve treatment efficacy, a surgical procedure called the Cox Maze procedure was developed; this procedure results in isolation of the pulmonary veins and compartmentalization of the atria.[34] Multiple incisions in both atria result in scar tissue that reduces the amount of atrial tissue between scars to below the critical re-entry circuit size, preventing AF. A thoracoscopic variant of this procedure, the Wolf mini-Maze, was developed in an effort to prevent the more morbid median sternotomy necessitated by the Cox-Maze procedure.[35] It is a bilateral video-assisted thoracoscopic off-pump procedure. A curved bipolar radiofrequency (RF) ablation device is used to create bilateral, transmural, linear lesions around an atrial cuff of the right and left pulmonary veins achieving electrical isolation (Fig. 31-10). In addition, a staple excision of the LAA is performed. Relevant to the Wolf mini-Maze procedure, the surgeon is "blind" to the anatomy of the posterior wall of the left atrium. Accessory veins in this region are particularly vulnerable to surgical mishap.[28]

Catheter-based procedures have been developed that aim at treating the triggers and the substrate for the AF. Ablation involves the purposeful devitalization of arrhythmogenic myocardial tissue to treat arrhythmias. This devitalization may be accomplished using cryotherapy or, more commonly, RF current to induce a thermal injury. RF lesions are typically 3 to 6 mm in diameter and 3 mm deep.[36] More recently, use of externally irrigated catheters has increased in an effort to improve lesion delivery and reduce char formation at the catheter tip, which decreases

FIGURE 31-10 Illustration of the Wolf mini-Maze procedure approach to the right pulmonary vein showing incision of the pericardium and a curved bipolar RF ablation device at the venoatrial junction.

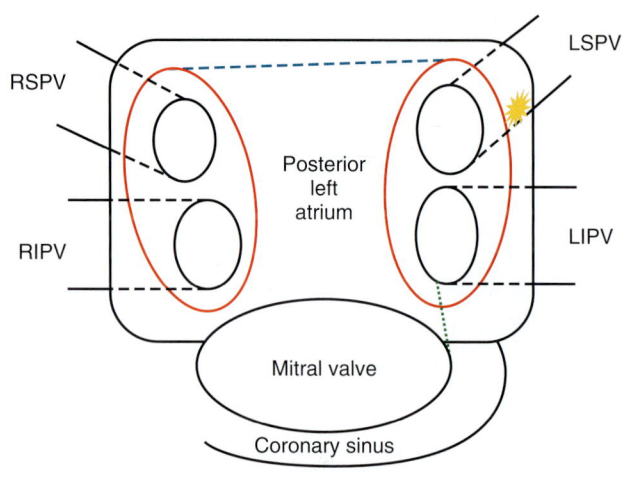

FIGURE 31-11 Line diagram showing commonly employed ablation techniques. A point ablation is illustrated in the left superior pulmonary vein (LSPV) (*irregular yellow area*). This technique resulted in an unacceptably high incidence of stenosis and has been abandoned. Common sites for ablation in the left atrium include the circumferential extraostial ablation (*solid red ovals*), the left atrium roof line (*blue dashed squares*) and the mitral isthmus line (*green dotted line*). LIPV, left inferior pulmonary vein; RIPV, right inferior pulmonary vein; RSPV, right superior pulmonary vein.

thermal efficiency.[37] The choice of catheter and energy delivery varies among different centers with an emphasis on smaller, lower energy systems. The most recent ACC/AHA/ESC guideline recommends ablation of AF in symptomatic patients who have not responded to medical therapy.[2,38] Currently, ablation is performed in a wider array of patients, however, particularly in patients with congestive heart failure, in whom ablation of AF has been shown to improve ventricular systolic function.[39]

The first contemporary approach to AF ablation was performed by Haissaguerre and colleagues[6] in 1994 by point ablation of distal pulmonary vein foci. This procedure was moderately successful, although it was complicated by a high percentage of pulmonary vein stenosis. Since then, multiple approaches have been developed, including segmental isolation of pulmonary veins and circumferential ablation, a stepwise approach that requires additional ablation lines in the roof of the left atrium, mitral annulus and isthmus, and coronary sinus and isolation of the superior vena cava (Fig. 31-11). Ablation of continuous atrial fractionated signals and autonomic ganglia around the pulmonary veins has also been tried.[38,40-43] The most common technique includes isolation of pulmonary veins using a circumferential extraostial ablation 1 to 2 cm on the atrial side of the pulmonary veins and isolation of the posterior left atrium.[38,44,45] Additional ablation lines may be created in the posterior left atrium, termed the *roof ablation line*, and at the mitral isthmus.

Although advanced volumetric imaging has already been shown to shorten the procedure, it remains a lengthy procedure requiring deep sedation or general anesthesia. Before converting the patient to normal sinus rhythm, a transesophageal or intracardiac echocardiogram is performed to exclude LAA thrombus, which is an absolute contraindication to the procedure. A catheter is advanced on the venous side of the circulation into the right atrium. The left atrium is accessed from the right atrium via a patent foramen ovale or using a transseptal puncture of the intact septum. Circumferential contiguous lesions are created around the pulmonary veins. A circular mapping catheter may be used to guide the ablation and confirm the electrical isolation of the pulmonary veins.

Left atrium function is partially preserved with the surgical Maze procedure.[46,47] With catheter ablation techniques targeting the posterior left atrium, the pulmonary vein orifices, and the mitral isthmus line, 30% to 40% of left atrial surface area may be ablated.[48] Multidetector CT evaluation of left atrial transport after circumferential RF ablation of paroxysmal AF found a decrease in left atrium function, although it is unclear whether this impairment is severe enough to predispose to thrombus formation.[49] More recently, Takahashi and coworkers[45] reported recovery of left atrium function with stepwise catheter ablation for chronic AF. Patient selection may also be important because pulmonary vein electrical isolation has been shown to be more effective in paroxysmal than in persistent AF.[50]

Imaging Techniques

The anatomy of the pulmonary veins can be delineated during the procedure by retrograde contrast venography in conjunction with intracardiac ultrasonography.[51] More often, a CT or MRI examination of the left atrium is performed before the procedure.[52]

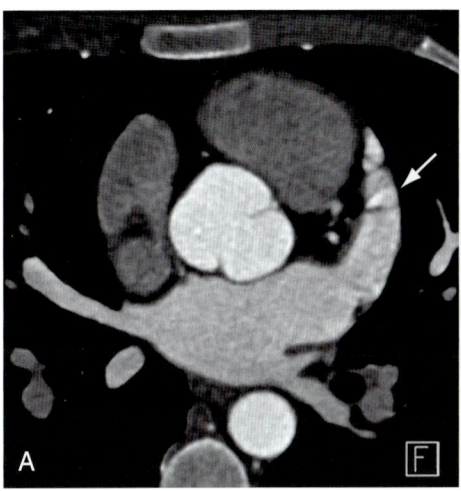

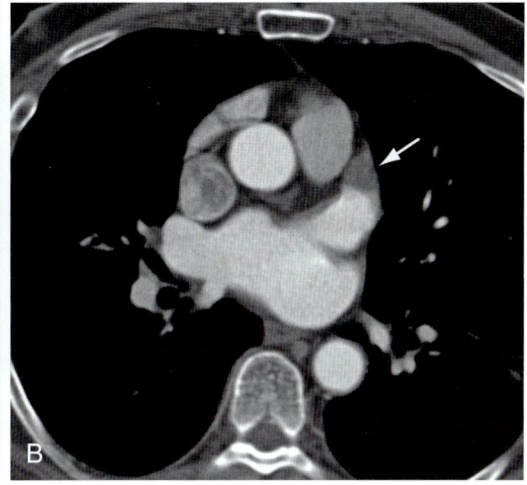

FIGURE 31-12 A, Normal triangular LAA (*arrow*) with contrast material filling the entire lumen. Hypodense lines perpendicular to the wall are the normal pectinate muscles. B, Filling defect (*arrow*) in the tip of the LAA in another patient is consistent with thrombus.

Multidetector Computed Tomography

All patients are prepared for multidetector CT as for cardiac CT angiography. They are instructed to avoid stimulants such as caffeine or pseudoephedrine 24 hours before the study. They are also prescribed an oral dose of β blockers to be taken the night before and 1 hour before the time of the study. Most patients are in paroxysmal AF, and imaging is done with the patient in normal sinus rhythm, if possible. The choice of gated or nongated CT for pulmonary vein mapping depends on the institution; adequate images can be obtained for pulmonary vein measurements and defining pulmonary venous anatomy without cardiac gating at lower radiation dose. ECG gated cardiac CT provides a more precise definition of the pulmonary vein orifice measurements in atrial diastole, better image quality for advanced three-dimensional postprocessing and catheter guidance systems, and the ability to detect unsuspected coronary artery pathology.

The examinations are performed on a multidetector CT scanner using retrospective ECG gating. The study is typically performed with a gantry rotation time of 330 ms and 0.6 mm detector collimation. Contrast material is administered based on the scan length times; the injection rate is typically 5 to 6 mL/s. Dose modulation is often employed; however, the tube current is maximized from end-systole to end-diastole. Esophageal contrast material can be administered orally before the scan so that three-dimensional volumetric reconstructions fully define the relationship of the esophagus to the left atrium. Reconstructions can be performed at 10% increments throughout the cardiac cycle in addition to three fixed temporal delay reconstructions in end-systole at 150 ms, 200 ms, and 250 ms. Images are generally processed on a three-dimensional workstation and are reviewed in axial, multiplanar reformats, maximum intensity projection, and volume rendered formats.

These examinations are reviewed as comprehensive cardiac CT angiography. The pulmonary veins are reported based on standard nomenclature, and two-dimensional diameter orifice measurements are defined at the venoatrial junction. Many authors report the distance to the first bifurcation (trunk length), although in our experience, this is less important now that electrophysiologists are performing circumferential extraostial ablations. We report all orificial pulmonary veins, defined as branches that occur within 5 mm of the venoatrial junction. It has been shown that ablation within 5 mm of the ostium of a pulmonary vein or first bifurcation increases risk of stenosis after the procedure.[50,53] All accessory veins must be identified and reported; these veins are frequently less than 1 cm in diameter, increasing the risk of stenosis if they are unrecognized before ablation. In addition, the left atrium is fully described, including a left atrial diameter measurement defined in transesophageal echocardiographic terms as the distance from the posterior wall of the left atrium abutting the esophagus to the anterior wall of the left atrium.

An evaluation for LAA thrombus must be performed because LAA thrombus is an absolute contraindication to cardioversion and RF ablation. Although transesophageal echocardiography has been the gold standard in the detection of LAA thrombus, 64-row multidetector CT reliably excludes LAA thrombus (Fig. 31-12).[54] Using a ratio threshold density of the LAA to the ascending aorta of greater than 0.75 had 100% negative predictive value in excluding LAA thrombus.[55] Occasionally, the equivalent of spontaneous echocardiographic contrast is identified as failure to opacify the LAA on first pass of contrast material.[54] Sluggish flow through the narrow neck of the LAA and loss of atrial contractility can result in poor mixing of blood that may mimic a clot in the LAA. Delayed images can be performed if this is recognized at the time of the scan to show diffusion of contrast material into the tip of the LAA (Fig. 31-13).[56]

Patent foramen ovale can be identified as a fine linear hypodensity paralleling the foramen (Fig. 31-14).[57] Atrial septal aneurysms are defined as a bulge of the interatrial septum of greater than 15 mm into either atrium. This defect has been associated with strokes and migraine headaches.[58]

The course of the esophagus should be defined relative to the pulmonary veins and is crucial information that assists the electrophysiologist when performing circumferential RF ablation. Although the course of the esophagus varies, it often lies close to, or parallels, the ostia of

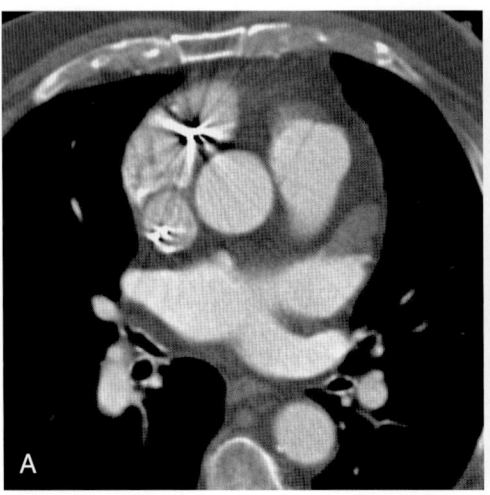

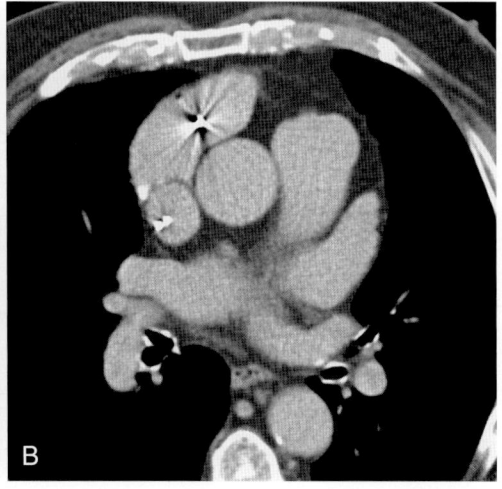

■ FIGURE 31-13 A, Immediate contrast-enhanced CT image of the LAA shows a filling defect in the tip of the LAA that simulates thrombus. B, On 1 minute delayed CT image through the same region, contrast medium has diffused into the tip, filling the LAA, confirming the absence of thrombus. The appearance in A was secondary to sluggish flow within the LAA.

the left pulmonary veins. The walls of the left atrium and esophagus are thin (often <5 mm in thickness), and the left inferior pulmonary vein can often course immediately adjacent to the esophagus, making thermal injury to the esophagus a possible complication of RF ablation (Fig. 31-15).[59] Esophageal mobility of greater than or equal to 2 cm has been reported in most patients under conscious sedation, so real-time imaging of the esophagus is not replaced by cross-sectional imaging.[60] The electrophysiology cardiologist typically passes an esophageal stethoscope as a marker of esophageal location at fluoroscopy throughout the RF ablation.

Certain anatomic variants are important to identify before the procedure, including persistent left superior vena cava and partial anomalous pulmonary venous return. In persistent left superior vena cava, the anomalous vein drains to the coronary sinus with a course along the left lateral wall running along the ligament of Marshall. This is in the expected location for a typical pulmonary vein ablation line. A fistula at this level would create a right-to-left shunt (Fig. 31-16). Partial anomalous pulmonary venous return must be identified to avoid confusion at fluoroscopy (Fig. 31-17). In addition, based on the anomalous draining vein, associated defects may be present. Right upper lobe partial anomalous pulmonary venous

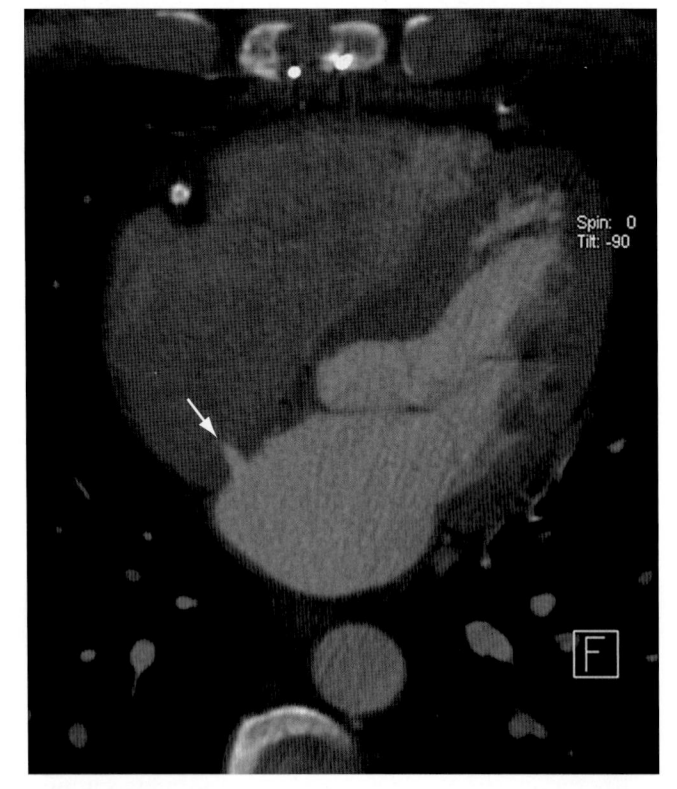

■ FIGURE 31-14 A jet of contrast material (*arrow*) is seen extending from the left atrium to the less opacified right atrium consistent with an atrial septal defect. (*Case courtesy of Dr. William Strub, Cincinnati, OH.*)

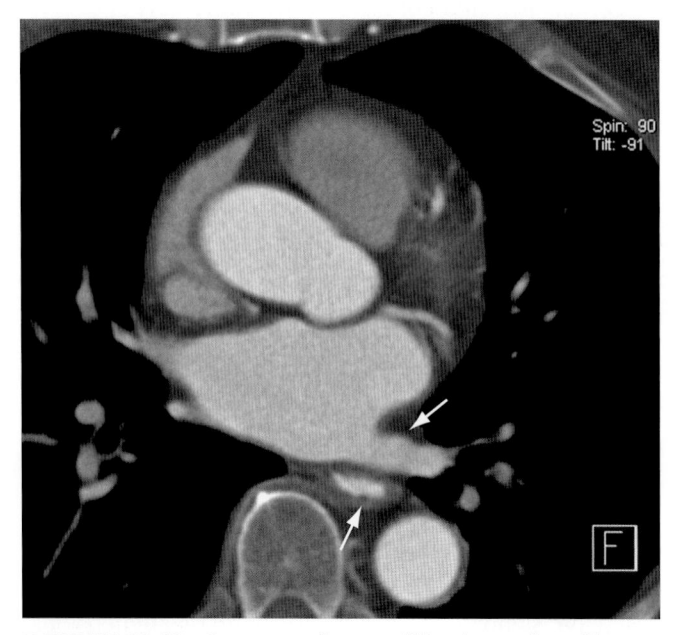

■ FIGURE 31-15 Contrast medium opacifying the esophageal lumen (*anterior white arrow*) shows the close approximation of the esophagus to the left atrium, in this case, the venoatrial junction of the left inferior pulmonary vein (*posterior white arrow*).

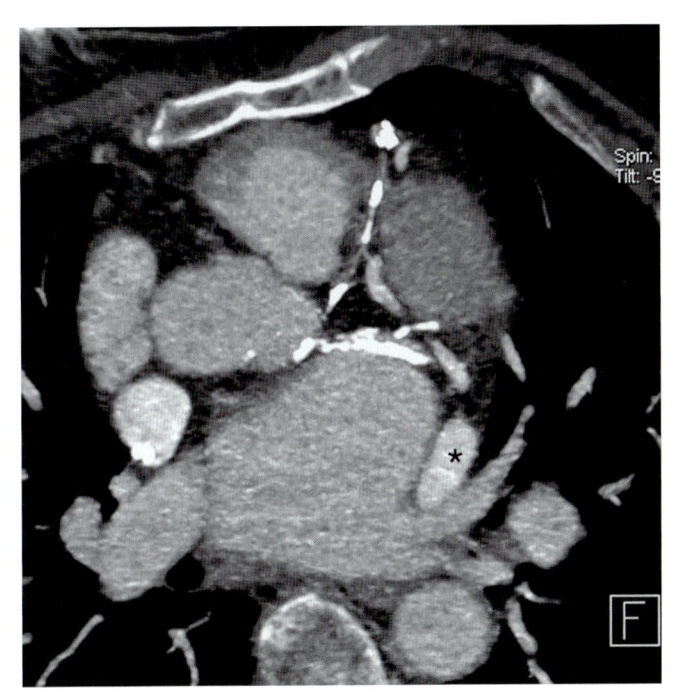

■ **FIGURE 31-16** Persistent left superior vena cava (*asterisk*) is seen anterior to the left inferior pulmonary vein in the expected location of the ligament of Marshall.

end-systole.[61,62] More recent advances with the improved temporal resolution of dual source imaging may result in reliable evaluation of the coronary arteries in AF patients.[63,64]

Magnetic Resonance Imaging

As an alternative to CT, MRI evaluation of the left atrium and pulmonary veins may be performed.[65] This examination characteristically is divided into several sequences: an ECG gated fat-suppressed two-dimensional fast spin-echo sequence for morphology, an ECG gated single-slice cine mode single breath-hold sequence such as steady-state free precession (SSFP) to show cyclical blood flow, and a three-dimensional gadolinium-enhanced MR angiography sequence such as a breath-hold three-dimensional fast spoiled gradient-recalled-echo imaging sequence (Fig. 31-18).[66] It has been shown more recently that a three-dimensional noncontrast free breathing MR angiography examination using SSFP can adequately evaluate pulmonary veins in patients unable to suspend respiration or at high risk for contrast complications.[67] Lickfett and associates[68] reported a 32.5% change in pulmonary vein ostial diameters during the cardiac cycle with the largest diameter in late diastole and the minimum diameter occurring in early systole. One potential limitation of pulmonary vein imaging with MRI is the contraindication to imaging patients with pacemakers and defibrillators.

return is frequently associated with sinus venosus atrial septal defect.

It is crucial to evaluate these examinations similar to other cardiac CT angiography examinations for unsuspected ancillary findings. In a review of patients before Wolf mini-Maze procedure, Meyer and colleagues[28] reported a high incidence of ancillary findings, including mitral stenosis, coronary artery disease, pulmonary nodules, and pleural abnormalities. Pleural abnormalities are particularly important to identify before thoracoscopic procedures because unfettered access to the pleural space may be an issue. Evaluation of the coronary arteries in AF patients is challenging, but not impossible with 64-row (or more) multidetector CT if the patients are evaluated in

Image Fusion

Using these volumetric data sets, a three-dimensional model of the left atrium can be reconstructed. This model can be referenced in the electrophysiology laboratory for catheter manipulation. More recent innovations have merged three-dimensional electroanatomic mapping systems with the three-dimensional cardiac model to permit tracking of catheter movement and more precise anatomic localization of ablation points. Three mapping technologies are in common use. The first uses electromagnetic positioning established by means of a locator pad consisting of three ultra-low emitting coil magnets

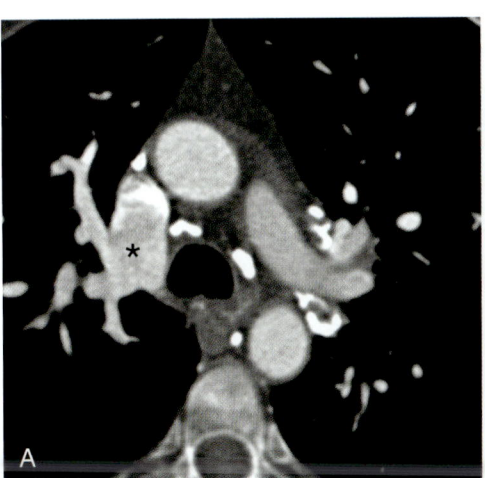

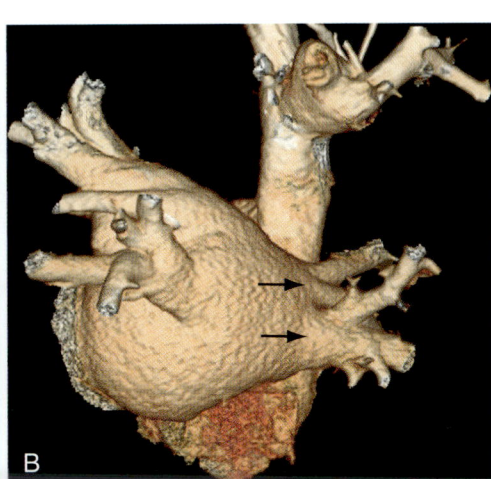

■ **FIGURE 31-17** **A,** Axial CT image reveals the right upper lobe superior pulmonary vein draining to an enlarged azygos vein (*asterisk*). **B,** Medial posterior view from a volume rendered reconstruction shows the partial anomalous pulmonary venous return draining to the azygos vein. The right middle pulmonary vein and right inferior pulmonary vein drain normally to the left atrium (*arrows*).

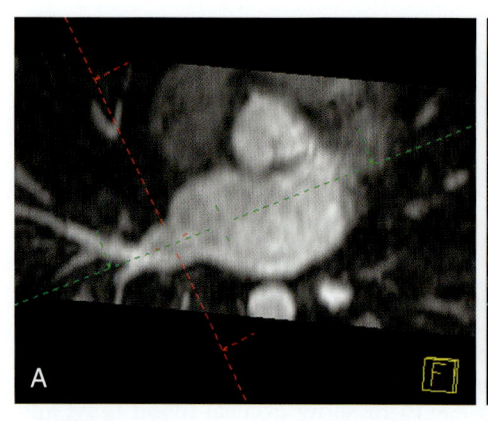

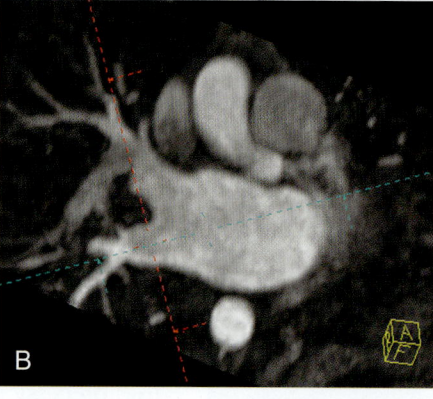

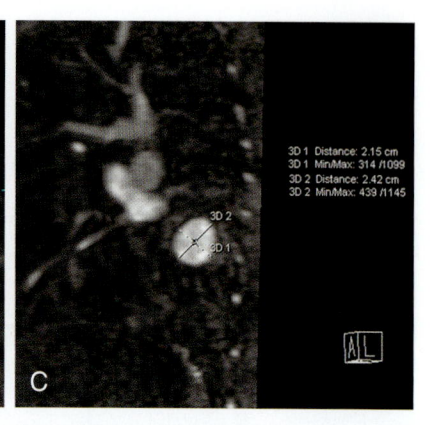

FIGURE 31-18 A-C, Multiplanar reconstruction of a gadolinium-enhanced three-dimensional MR angiography acquisition data set shows the right inferior pulmonary vein in axial oblique long-axis (**A**), coronal oblique long-axis (**B**), and sagittal oblique short-axis (en face) (**C**) views for measuring the pulmonary vein orifice at the venoatrial junction.

placed below the patient, a reference external catheter usually positioned posterior to the patient, and the mapping catheter with a magnetic field sensor. The location of the sensor is determined from the intersection of the theoretical spheres whose radii are the distances measured by the sensor.[69] A second system uses cutaneous pads to generate electrical fields that track the catheter.[70] Finally, a third approach involves the use of a multielectrode balloon to track catheter position.[71]

With all these systems, an anatomic shell is created by moving the catheter along the walls of the cardiac chamber and recording multiple catheter positions. Electrograms and points of interest (e.g., anatomic markers, ablation points) can be represented on the shell. Image fusion is usually achieved with a point registration algorithm using fiducial points gathered during mapping at fixed anatomic locations, such as pulmonary vein–left atrium junctions; this is later refined by the process of surface registration minimizing the distance between the two surfaces.[72,73] The integrated image provides a map of RF ablation points and real-time catheter localization (Fig. 31-19). Multiple studies have evaluated these registration methods and shown clinically acceptable accuracy.[74-83]

The major obstacles to optimal registration seem to be inherent inaccuracies of mapping systems, effect of respiration and heart rate, the effect of indentation caused by the mapping catheter on the real-time map, limitation of rigid registration algorithms, lack of accurate anatomic landmarks, and differences in chamber size and alignment between the time of image acquisition and mapping.[73,83,84] Lickfett and associates[68] showed a mean phasic change in ostial position of 7.2 mm. In a nonrandomized study, decreased fluoroscopy times were reported along with improved clinical outcomes when AF ablations were performed with image integration software.[85]

Postprocedure Imaging

In a survey of 9000 procedures, Cappato and colleagues[86] found an overall rate of major complications of 6% associated with AF catheter ablation procedures. Complications include death, stroke, cardiac tamponade, venous stenosis, and atrioesophageal fistula.

Pulmonary Venous Stenosis

Pulmonary venous stenosis is reported in 1.5% to 42.4% of patients after RF ablation for AF.[86] This complication was considerably more common when point ablations were performed within the pulmonary veins. Current

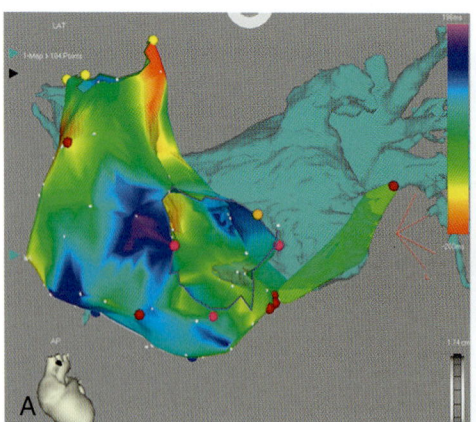

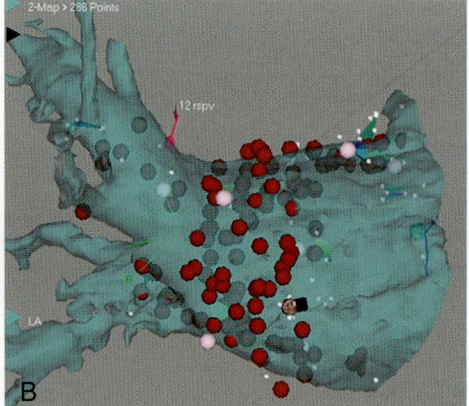

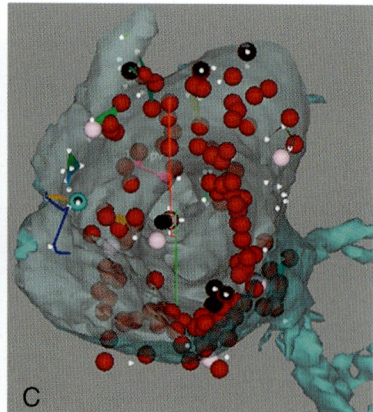

FIGURE 31-19 **A,** Three-dimensional volume rendered shell of the left atrium (*turquoise*) is extracted from a cardiac-gated multidetector CT data set and fused with electroanatomic mapping points in the right atrium and coronary sinus. **B** and **C,** Surface (**B**) and endoscopic (**C**) maps of the left atrium record the site of ablation points (*red dots*) and the location of the catheter tip (*central black dot with white crosshairs*).

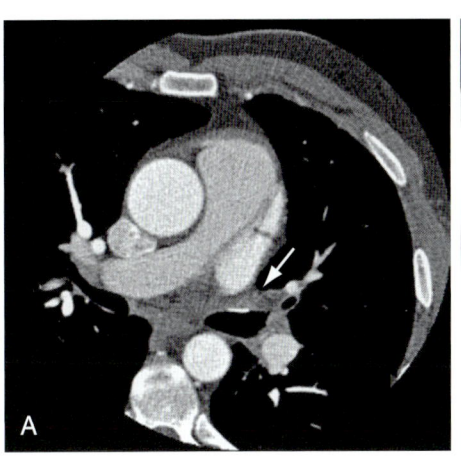

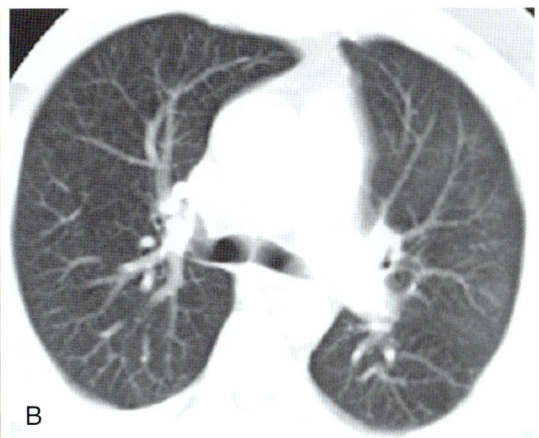

■ FIGURE 31-20 A, Axial image at the level of the LAA. There is no enhancement of the left superior pulmonary vein (*arrow*) in the expected location anterior to the left upper lobe bronchus. B, Lung windows reveal ground-glass opacity in the left upper lobe consistent with lobar edema owing to venous obstruction.

extraostial techniques combined with lower energy delivery, decreased ablation temperatures, and intracardiac echocardiography result in an incidence of moderate to severe stenosis of less than 1.4% at centers experienced in these techniques.[87] Nevertheless, pulmonary vein stenosis (Fig. 31-20) may result in focal edema, veno-occlusive disease, parenchymal hemorrhage, venous thrombosis, and venous infarcts. Pulmonary vein balloon angioplasty and stenting can be used for symptomatic severe stenosis.

Atrioesophageal Fistula

Atrioesophageal fistula is a rare but potentially devastating complication of left atrium RF ablation procedures with a reported 50% mortality. The increased prevalence of this complication of RF ablation for AF and its increased frequency are thought to be due to the increased use of circumferential pulmonary vein ablation and posterior left atrium ablation instead of point ablations.[87,88] In a prospective study using endoscopic analysis of the esophagus after pulmonary vein ablation, 53% of patients had erythema 24 hours after pulmonary vein ablation, and 18% had focal necrosis/ulceration.[89] Transesophageal echocardiography and esophagoscopy are contraindicated if this diagnosis is suspected because of air insufflation. CT is the study of choice, and shows infiltration of the mediastinal fat and subtle fluid collections between the posterior wall of the left atrium and the esophagus (Fig. 31-21).[90]

Recurrent Atrial Fibrillation

The left atrial isthmus has been implicated in recurrent AF. The left atrial isthmus is the region between the left inferior pulmonary vein orifice and the posteroinferior mitral annulus, and is typically longer in AF patients.[91] The precise anatomic relationships of the adjacent coronary sinus and left circumflex artery should be determined. Injury to the circumflex coronary artery has been reported with atrial isthmus line ablation.[92] Circumferential pulmonary vein ablation effectively eliminates AF, but may result in organized atrial tachycardias, of which 90% are re-entrant and related to gaps in the ablation lines.[93] Early studies suggest that myocardial delayed enhancement MRI may be an effective noninvasive tool for identifying ablation-related atrial scarring.[94,95]

REPORTING: INFORMATION FOR REFERRING PHYSICIANS

1. Left atrial anatomy—pulmonary vein location and number, variants, and orificial veins
2. Left atrial anatomy and size and presence of thrombus (especially LAA thrombus)
3. Atrial septal abnormalities
4. Presence of major anomalies, such as partial anomalous pulmonary venous return
5. Ancillary findings, such as coronary artery disease and pulmonary disease

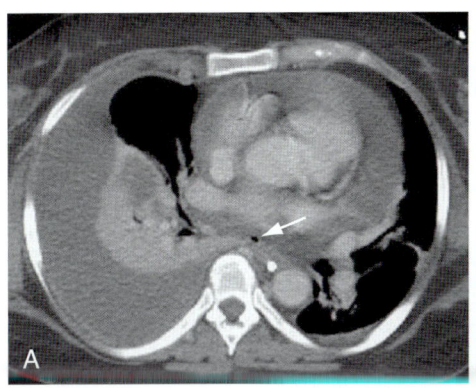

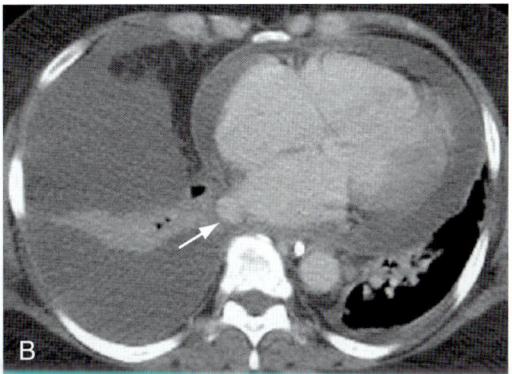

■ FIGURE 31-21 A, A focus of gas (*arrow*) is seen in the mediastinum posterior to the left atrium consistent with an atrioesophageal fistula. B, A pseudoaneurysm of the left atrium (*arrow*) is identified as an oval contrast collection protruding beneath the right inferior pulmonary vein. (*Case courtesy of Dr. Diane Strollo.*)

> **KEY POINTS**
>
> - AF is the most common cardiac arrhythmia, initiated by rapid firing of ectopic foci or re-entrant wavelets most often originating from the pulmonary veins.
> - RF ablation of AF involves isolation of the pulmonary veins and the posterior left atrium.
> - Pulmonary vein anatomy can be delineated with CT or MRI.
> - Common pulmonary vein anatomic variants include a conjoined left pulmonary trunk and an accessory right middle lobe pulmonary vein.
> - Image fusion can be used to track catheter movement and to obtain precise anatomic localization of ablation points.
> - Postprocedure imaging can identify complications such as pulmonary vein stenosis or atrioesophageal fistula.

ACKNOWLEDGMENT

The authors thank Ms. Rhonda Strunk, RT, R(CT), for her assistance in the preparation of images for this chapter.

SUGGESTED READINGS

Cappato R, Calkins H, Chen SA, et al. Worldwide survey on the methods, efficacy and safety of catheter ablation for human atrial fibrillation. Circulation 2005; 111:1100-1105.

Cronin P, Sneider MB, Kazerooni EA, et al. MDCT of the left atrium and pulmonary veins in planning radiofrequency ablation for atrial fibrillation: a how-to guide. AJR Am J Roentgenol 2004; 183:767-778.

Fuster V, Rydén LE, Cannom DS, et al. ACC/AHA/ESC 2006 guidelines for the management of patients with atrial fibrillation—executive summary: a report of the American College of Cardiology/American Heart Association Task Force on Practice Guidelines and the European Society of Cardiology Committee for Practice Guidelines (Writing Committee to Revise the 2001 Guidelines for the Management of Patients With Atrial Fibrillation). J Am Coll Cardiol 2006; 48:854-906.

Lacomis JM, Wigginton W, Fuhrman C, et al. Multi-detector row CT of the left atrium and pulmonary veins before radiofrequency ablation for atrial fibrillation. RadioGraphics 2003; 23:S35-S48.

Saremi F, Krishnan S. Cardiac conduction system: anatomic landmarks relevant to interventional electrophysiologic techniques demonstrated with 64-detector CT. RadioGraphics 2007; 27:1539-1567.

REFERENCES

1. Feinberg WM, Blackshear JL, Laupacis A, et al. Prevalence, age distribution, and gender of patients with atrial fibrillation: analysis and implications. Arch Intern Med 1995; 155:469-473.
2. Fuster V, Rydén LE, Cannom DS, et al. ACC/AHA/ESC 2006 guidelines for the management of patients with atrial fibrillation—executive summary: a report of the American College of Cardiology/American Heart Association Task Force on Practice Guidelines and the European Society of Cardiology Committee for Practice Guidelines (Writing Committee to Revise the 2001 Guidelines for the Management of Patients With Atrial Fibrillation). J Am Coll Cardiol 2006; 48:854-906.
3. Heeringa J, van der Kuip DA, Hofman A, et al. Prevalence, incidence and lifetime risk of atrial fibrillation: the Rotterdam study. Eur Heart J 2006; 27:949-953.
4. Ryder KM, Benjamin EJ. Epidemiology and significance of atrial fibrillation. Am J Cardiol 1999; 84:131R-138R.
5. Coyne KS, Paramore C, Grandy S, et al. Assessing the direct costs of treating nonvalvular atrial fibrillation in the United States. Value Health 2006; 9:348-356.
6. Haissaguerre M, Jais P, Shah DC, et al. Spontaneous initiation of atrial fibrillation by ectopic beats originating in the pulmonary veins. N Engl J Med 1998; 339:659-666.
7. Yamada T, McElderry HT, Doppalupadi H, et al. Catheter ablation of focal triggers and drivers of atrial fibrillation. J Electrocardiol 2008; 41:138-143.
8. Saksena S, Skadsberg ND, Rao HB, et al. Biatrial and three-dimensional mapping of spontaneous atrial arrhythmias in patients with refractory atrial fibrillation. J Cardiovasc Electrophysiol 2005; 16:494-504.
9. Li J, Wang L. Catheter ablation of atrial fibrillation originating from superior vena cava. Arch Med Res 2006; 37:415-418.
10. Saito T, Waki K, Becker AE. Left atrial myocardial extension onto pulmonary veins in humans: anatomic observations relevant for atrial arrhythmias. J Cardiovasc Electrophysiol 2000; 11:888-894.
11. Nathan H, Eliakin M. The junction between the left atrium and the pulmonary veins. Circulation 1966; 34:412-422.
12. Lloyd-Jones DM, Wang TJ, Leip EP, et al. Lifetime risk for development of atrial fibrillation: the Framingham Heart Study. Circulation 2004; 110:1042-1046.
13. Wolf PA, Abbott RD, Kannel WB. Atrial fibrillation as an independent risk factor for stroke: the Framingham Study. Stroke 1991; 22:983-988.
14. Aschenberg W, Schluter M, Kremer P, et al. Transesophageal two-dimensional echocardiography for the detection of left atrial appendage thrombus. J Am Coll Cardiol 1986; 7:163-166.
15. Stewart S, Hart CL, Hole DJ, et al. A population-based study of the long term risks associated with atrial fibrillation: 20-year follow-up of the Renfrow/Paisley study. Am J Med 2002; 113:359-364.
16. Dries DL, Exner DV, Gersh BJ, et al. Atrial fibrillation is associated with an increased risk for mortality and heart failure progression in patients with asymptomatic and symptomatic left ventricular systolic dysfunction: a retrospective analysis of the SOLVD trials. Studies of Left Ventricular Dysfunction. J Am Coll Cardiol 1998; 32:695-703.
17. McAlpine WA. Heart and Coronary Arteries. Springer-Verlag, Berlin, 1975, pp 58-59.
18. Ho SY, Sanchez-Quintana D, Cabrera JA, et al. Anatomy of the left atrium: implications for radiofrequency ablation of atrial fibrillation. J Cardiovasc Electrophysiol 1999; 10:1525-1533.
19. Anderson RH, Brown NA, Webb S. Development and structure of the atrial septum. Heart 2002; 88:104-110.

20. Vanovermeire OM, Duerinckx AJ. Accessory appendages if the left atrium as seen during 64-slice coronary CT angiography. Presented at the Scientific Sessions at the Syllabus Society of Thoracic Radiology, March 13, 2006; Orlando, FL.
21. Wongcharoen W, Tsao HM, Wu MH, et al. Morphologic characteristics of the left atrial appendage, roof, and septum: implications for the ablation of atrial fibrillation. J Cardiovasc Electrophysiol 2006; 17:951-956.
22. Lacomis J, Schwartzman D, Wigginton W, et al. 3D-multidetector CT and variations in pulmonary venous and left atrial anatomy: implications in atrial fibrillation patients undergoing ablative therapy. Radiology 2002; S225:631.
23. Marom EM, Herndon JE, Kim YH, et al. Variations in pulmonary venous drainage to the left atrium: implications for radiofrequency ablation. Radiology 2004; 230:824-829.
24. Mansour M, Holmvang G, Sosnovik D, et al. Assessment of pulmonary vein anatomic variability by magnetic resonance imaging: implications for catheter ablation techniques for atrial fibrillation. J Cardiovasc Electrophysiol 2004; 15:387-393.
25. Schwartzman D, Bazaz R, Nosbisch J. Common left pulmonary vein: a consistent source of arrhythmogenic atrial ectopy. J Cardiovasc Electrophysiol 2004; 15:560-566.
26. Tsao HM, Wu MH, Yu WC, et al. Role of right middle pulmonary vein in patients with paroxysmal atrial fibrillation. J Cardiovasc Electrophysiol 2001; 12:1353-1357.
27. Lickfett L, Kato R, Tandri H, et al. Characterization of a new pulmonary vein variant using magnetic resonance angiography: incidence, imaging and interventional implications of the "right top pulmonary vein." J Cardiovasc Electrophysiol 2004; 15:538-543.
28. Meyer CA, Hall JE, Mehall JR, et al. Impact of preoperative 64-slice CT scanning on mini-Maze atrial fibrillation surgery. Innovations 2007; 2:169-175.
29. Perez-Lugones A, Schwartzman PR, Schweikert R, et al. Three-dimensional reconstruction of pulmonary veins in patients with atrial fibrillation and controls: morphological characteristics of different veins. Pacing Clin Electrophysiol 2003; 26:8-15.
30. Sra J, Malloy A, Shah H, et al. Common ostium of the inferior pulmonary veins in a patient undergoing left atrial ablation for atrial fibrillation. J Interv Card Electrophysiol 2006; 15:203.
31. James TN. The sinus node. Am J Cardiol 1977; 40:965-986.
32. Saremi F, Abolhoda A, Ashikyan O, et al. Arterial supply to sinuatrial and atrioventricular nodes: imaging with multidetector CT. Radiology 2008; 246:99-109.
33. van Gelder IC, Hagens VE, Bosker HA, et al. A comparison of rate control and rhythm control in patients with recurrent persistent atrial fibrillation. N Engl J Med 2002; 347:1834-1840.
34. Cox JL, Ad N, Palazzo T, et al. Current status of the maze procedure for the treatment of atrial fibrillation. Semin Thorac Cardiovasc Surg 2000; 12:15-19.
35. Wolf RK, Schneeberger EW, Osterday R, et al. Video-assisted bilateral pulmonary vein isolation and left atrial appendage exclusion for atrial fibrillation. J Thorac Cardiovasc Surg 2005; 130:797-802.
36. Saremi F, Krishnan S. Cardiac conduction system: anatomic landmarks relevant to interventional electrophysiologic techniques demonstrated with 64-detector CT. RadioGraphics 2007; 27:1539-1567.
37. Macle L, Jais P, Weerasooriya R, et al. Irrigated-tip catheter ablation of pulmonary veins for treatment of atrial fibrillation. J Cardiovasc Electrophysiol 2002; 13:1067-1073.
38. Calkins H, Brugada J, Packer DL, et al. HRS/EHRA/ECAS expert consensus statement on catheter and surgical ablation of atrial fibrillation: recommendations for personnel, policy, procedures and follow-up. A report of the Heart Rhythm Society (HRS) Task Force on catheter and surgical ablation of atrial fibrillation. Heart Rhythm 2007; 4:816-861.
39. Hsu LF, Jais P, Sanders P, et al. Catheter ablation for atrial fibrillation in congestive heart failure. N Engl J Med 2004; 351:2373-2383.
40. Wright M, Haissaguerre M, Knecht S, et al. State of the art: catheter ablation for atrial fibrillation. J Cardiovasc Electrophysiol 2008; 9:583-592.
41. O'Neill MD, Jais P, Hocini M, et al. Catheter ablation for atrial fibrillation. Circulation 2007; 116:1515-1523.
42. Nademanee K, Schwab M, Porath J, et al. How to perform electrogram-guided atrial fibrillation ablation. Heart Rhythm 2006; 3:981-984.
43. Pappone C, Rosanio S, Oreto G, et al. Circumferential radiofrequency ablation of pulmonary vein ostia: a new anatomic approach for curing atrial fibrillation. Circulation 2000; 102:2619-2628.
44. Sanders P, Hocini M, Jais P, et al. Complete isolation of the pulmonary veins and posterior left atrium in chronic atrial fibrillation: long-term clinical outcome. Eur Heart J 2007; 28:1862-1871.
45. Takahashi Y, O'Neill MD, Hocini M, et al. Effects of stepwise ablation of chronic atrial fibrillation on atrial electrical and mechanical properties. J Am Coll Cardiol 2007; 49:1306-1314.
46. Lonnerholm S, Blomstrom P, Nilsson L, et al. Atrial size and transport function after Maze III procedure for paroxysmal atrial fibrillation. Ann Thorac Surg 2002; 73:107-111.
47. Albirini A, Scalia GM, Murray RD, et al. Left and right atrial transport function after the Maze procedure for atrial fibrillation: an echocardiographic Doppler follow-up study. J Am Soc Echocardiogr 1997; 10:937-945.
48. Pappone C, Manguso F, Vicedomini G, et al. Prevention of iatrogenic atrial tachycardia after ablation of atrial fibrillation: a prospective randomized study comparing circumferential pulmonary vein ablation with a modified approach. Circulation 2004; 110:3036-3042.
49. Lemola K, Desjardins B, Sneider M, et al. Effect of left atrial circumferential ablation for atrial fibrillation on left atrial transport function. Heart Rhythm 2005; 2:923-928.
50. Oral H, Knight BP, Tada H, et al. Pulmonary vein isolation for paroxysmal and persistent atrial fibrillation. Circulation 2002; 105:1077-1081.
51. Callans DJ, Wood MA. How to use intracardiac echocardiography for atrial fibrillation ablation procedures. Heart Rhythm 2007; 4:242-245.
52. Lacomis JM, Pealer K, Fuhrman CR, et al. Direct comparison of computed tomography and magnetic resonance imaging for characterization of posterior left atrial morphology. J Interv Card Electrophysiol 2006; 16:7-13.
53. Scharf C, Sneider M, Case I, et al. Anatomy of the pulmonary veins in patients with atrial fibrillation and effects of segmental ostial ablation analyzed by computed tomography. J Cardiovasc Electrophysiol 2003; 14:150-155.
54. Kim YY, Klein AL, Halliburton SS, et al. Left atrial appendage filling defects identified by multidetector computed tomography in patients undergoing radiofrequency pulmonary vein antral isolation: a comparison with transesophageal echocardiography. Am Heart J 2007; 154:1199-1205.
55. Patel A, Au E, Donegan K, et al. Multidetector row computed tomography for identification of left atrial appendage filling defects in patients undergoing pulmonary vein isolation for treatment of atrial fibrillation: comparison with transesophageal echocardiography. Heart Rhythm 2008; 5:253-260.
56. Saremi F, Channual S, Gurudevan SV, et al. Prevalence of left atrial appendage pseudothrombus filling defects in patients with atrial fibrillation undergoing coronary computed tomography angiography. J Cardiovasc CT 2008; 2:164-171.
57. Saremi F, Attai SF, Narula J. 64 multidetector CT in patent foramen ovale. Heart 2007; 93:505.
58. Mugge A, Daniel WG, Angermann C, et al. Atrial septal aneurysm in adult patients: a multi-center study using transthoracic and transesophageal echocardiography. Circulation 1995; 91:2785-2792.
59. Lemola K, Sneider M, Desjardins B, et al. Computed tomographic analysis of the anatomy of the left atrium and esophagus: implications for left atrial catheter ablation. Circulation 2004; 110:3655-3660.
60. Good E, Oral H, Lemola K, et al. Movement of the esophagus during left atrial catheter ablation for atrial fibrillation. J Am Coll Cardiol 2005; 46:2107-2110.
61. Sato T, Anno H, Kondo T, et al. Applicability of ECG-gated multislice helical CT to patients with atrial fibrillation. Circulation J 2005; 69:1068-1073.
62. Strub WM, Vagal A, Meyer C. Optimizing coronary artery imaging in patients with atrial fibrillation with ECG-gated 64 MDCT. AJR Am J Roentgenol 2007; 189:W50-W51.
63. Oncel D, Oncel G, Tastan A. Effectiveness of dual-source CT coronary angiography for the evaluation of coronary artery disease in patients with atrial fibrillation: initial experience. Radiology 2007; 245:703-711.
64. Wolak A, Gutstein A, Cheng VY, et al. Dual-source coronary computed tomography angiography in patients with atrial fibrillation: initial experience. J Cardiovasc CT 2008; 2:172-180.

65. Lacomis J, Schwarzman D, Fuhrman C, et al. Ablation imaging of left atrial and pulmonary venous anatomy in atrial fibrillation patients: comparison of 3D multidetector CT and magnetic resonance angiography. Radiology 2002; S225:626.
66. Ghaye B, Szapiro D, Dacher JN, et al. Percutaneous ablation for atrial fibrillation: the role of cross-sectional imaging. RadioGraphics 2003; 23:S19-S33.
67. Singhal A, Tomasian A, Sassani A, et al. 3D noncontrast free breathing MR angiography (MRA) of pulmonary veins by steady state free precession (SSFP) technique. Annual Meeting of the American Roentgen Ray Society Meeting, Washington, DC, April 15, 2008.
68. Lickfett L, Dickfeld T, Kato R, et al. Changes of pulmonary vein orifice size and location throughout the cardiac cycle: dynamic analysis using magnetic resonance cine imaging. J Cardiovasc Electrophysiol 1999; 10:136-144.
69. Gepstein L, Hayam G, Ben-Haim SA. A novel method for nonfluoroscopic catheter-based electroanatomical mapping of the heart: in vitro and in vivo accuracy results. Circulation 1997; 95:1611-1622.
70. Takahashi Y, Rotter M, Sanders P, et al. Left atrial linear ablation to modify the substrate of atrial fibrillation using a new nonfluoroscopic imaging system. Pacing Clin Electrophysiol 2005; 28(Suppl 1):S90-S93.
71. Schilling RJ, Peters NS, Davies DW. Feasibility of a noncontact catheter for endocardial mapping of human ventricular tachycardia. Circulation 1999; 99:2543-2552.
72. Dong J, Calkins H, Solomon SB, et al. Integrated electroanatomic mapping with three-dimensional computed tomographic images for real-time guided ablations. Circulation 2006; 113:186-194.
73. Sra J, Ratnakumar S. Cardiac image registration of the left atrium and pulmonary veins. Heart Rhythm 2008; 5:609-617.
74. Bertaglia E, Bransolino G, Zoppo F, et al. Integration of three-dimensional left atrial magnetic resonance images into a real-time electroanatomic mapping system: validation of a registration method. Pacing Clin Electrophysiol 2008; 31:273-282.
75. Dong J, Dalal D, Scherr D, et al. Impact of heart rhythm status on registration accuracy of the left atrium for catheter ablation of atrial fibrillation. J Cardiovasc Electrophysiol 2007; 18:1269-1276.
76. Richmond L, Rajappan K, Voth E, et al. Validation of computed tomography image integration into the EnSite NavX mapping system to perform catheter ablation of atrial fibrillation. J Cardiovasc Electrophysiol 2008; 19:821-827.
77. Zhong H, Lacomis JM, Schwartzman D. On the accuracy of CartoMerge for guiding posterior left atrial ablation in man. Heart Rhythm 2007; 4:595-602.
78. Dong J, Dickfeld T, Dalal D, et al. Initial experience in the use of integrated electroanatomic mapping with three-dimensional MR/CT images to guide catheter ablation of atrial fibrillation. J Cardiovasc Electrophysiol 2006; 17:459-466.
79. Ector J, De Buck S, Adams J, et al. Cardiac three-dimensional magnetic resonance imaging and fluoroscopy merging: a new approach for electroanatomic mapping to assist catheter ablation. Circulation 2005; 112:3769-3776.
80. Fahmy TS, Mlcochova H, Wazni OM, et al. Intracardiac echo-guided image integration: optimizing strategies for registration. J Cardiovasc Electrophysiol 2007; 18:276-282.
81. Kistler PM, Earley MJ, Harris S, et al. Validation of three-dimensional cardiac image integration: use of integrated CT image into electroanatomic mapping system to perform catheter ablation of atrial fibrillation. J Cardiovasc Electrophysiol 2006; 17:341-348.
82. Sra J, Krum D, Hare J, et al. Feasibility and validation of registration of three-dimensional left atrial models derived from computed tomography with a noncontact cardiac mapping system. Heart Rhythm 2005; 2:55-63.
83. Sra J, Krum D, Malloy A, et al. Registration of three-dimensional left atrial computed tomographic images with projection images obtained using fluoroscopy. Circulation 2005; 112:3763-3768.
84. Noseworthy PA, Malchano ZJ, Ahmed J, et al. The impact of respiration on left atrial and pulmonary venous anatomy: implications for image-guided intervention. Heart Rhythm 2005; 2:1173-1178.
85. Kistler PM, Rajappan K, Jahngir M, et al. The impact of CT images integration into an electroanatomic mapping system on clinical outcomes of catheter ablation of atrial fibrillation. J Cardiovasc Electrophysiol 2006; 17:1093-1101.
86. Cappato R, Calkins H, Chen SA, et al. Worldwide survey on the methods, efficacy and safety of catheter ablation for human atrial fibrillation. Circulation 2005; 111:1100-1105.
87. Lacomis JM, Goitein O, Deible C, et al. CT of the pulmonary veins. J Thorac Imaging 2007; 22:63-76.
88. Pappone C, Oral J, Santinelli V, et al. Atrioesophageal fistula as a complication of percutaneous transcatheter ablation of atrial fibrillation. Circulation 2004; 109:2724-2726.
89. Schmidt M, Nolker G, Marschang H, et al. Incidence of oesophageal wall injury post-pulmonary vein antrum isolation for treatment of patients with atrial fibrillation. Europace 2008; 10:205-209.
90. Schley P, Gulker H, Horlitz M. Atrio-esophageal fistula following circumferential pulmonary vein ablation: verification of diagnosis with multislice computed tomography. Europace 2006; 8:189-190.
91. Chiang SJ, Tsao HM, Wu MH, et al. Anatomic characteristics of the left atrial isthmus in patients with atrial fibrillation: lessons from computed tomographic images. J Cardiovasc Electrophysiol 2006; 17:1274-1278.
92. Takahashi Y, Jais P, Hocini M, et al. Acute occlusion of the left circumflex coronary artery during mitral isthmus linear ablation. J Cardiovasc Electrophysiol 2005; 16:1104-1107.
93. Chae S, Oral H, Good E, et al. Atrial tachycardia after circumferential pulmonary vein ablation of atrial fibrillation: mechanistic insights, results of catheter ablation, and risk factors for recurrence. J Am Coll Cardiol 2007; 50:1781-1787.
94. Reddy VY, Schmidt EJ, Holmvang G, et al. Arrhythmia recurrence after atrial fibrillation ablation: can magnetic resonance imaging identify gaps in atrial ablation lines? J Cardiovasc Electrophysiol 2008; 19:434-437.
95. Peters DC, Wylie JV, Hauser TH, et al. Detection of pulmonary vein and left atrial scar after catheter ablation with three-dimensional navigator gated delayed enhancement MR imaging: initial experience. Radiology 2007; 243:690-695.

PART FOUR

Coronary Artery Imaging

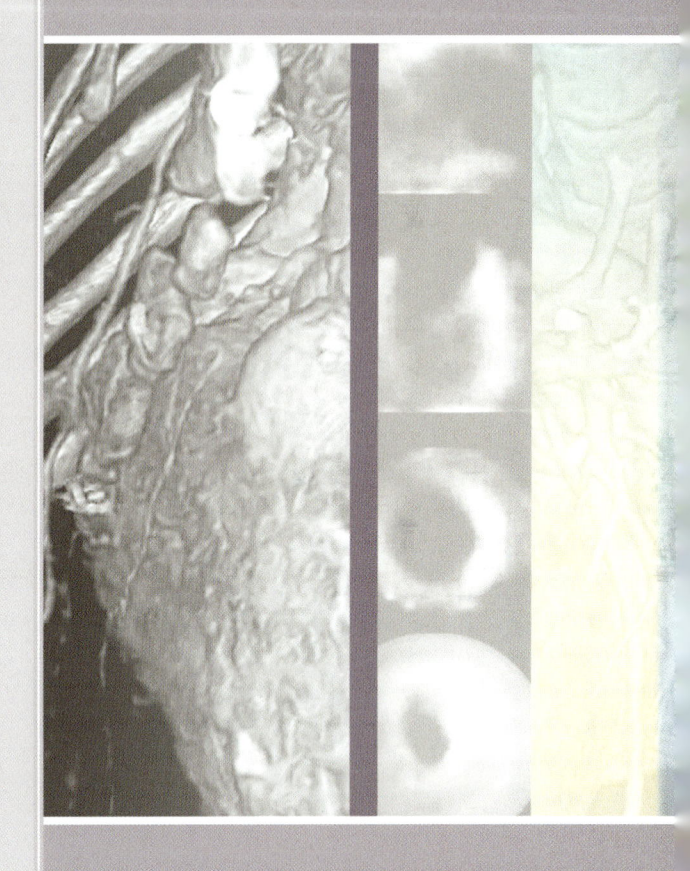

CHAPTER 32

Coronary Calcium Assessment

William Stanford

Coronary artery calcification (CAC) has long been recognized as an indicator of atherosclerosis. Numerous clinical and pathologic studies have shown strong associations between calcium and atherosclerotic plaque formation. Initially, the calcium plaque was identified using fluoroscopy, plain films, and conventional CT. These imaging studies required relatively large deposits of calcium for visualization, however. The potential for CT to detect early coronary artery disease (CAD) was not realized until the development of the electron-beam CT scanner in the 1980s. The introduction of this technology with its excellent temporal and spatial resolution allowed the visualization of small calcium deposits, and the ability to identify early coronary atherosclerotic plaque took a giant leap forward.

This chapter reviews the impact of CAD and briefly reviews the pathophysiology involved in the development of calcified plaque. We discuss the ability of CT to identify stenotic lesions and the potential of calcium in identifying individuals at risk for cardiac events. Last, we briefly discuss the role of calcium in different ethnic populations, how the identification of coronary calcium is being used in specific population groups, and how calcium is being used clinically in the diagnosis and the treatment of coronary heart disease.

IMPORTANCE OF CALCIUM IN IDENTIFYING CORONARY HEART DISEASE

In 2004, more than 15.8 million individuals in the United States developed CAD, and more than 450,000 died.[1] Of the estimated 700,000 Americans who are expected to experience an acute coronary event this year, only 50% will have a prior history of CAD. About 17% of individuals who die of an acute coronary event are younger than 65 years. The estimated economic loss from coronary heart disease in 2007 was estimated to be greater than $151.6 billion, making CAD the largest single component of U.S. health care expenditures.

Traditional risk factors predict only approximately 60% of patients who eventually die of heart disease, and one third of these individuals possess no identifiable Framingham risk indices that would predict a future "hard" coronary event. Although traditional risk factors, such as age, smoking, hypertension, hyperlipidemia, diabetes, and family history, are associated with an increasing risk for developing coronary heart disease, the assessment of such risk factors often underestimates an individual's overall risk for sudden cardiac death.

The association of calcium with atherosclerosis coupled with the ability of current scanner technologies to identify small coronary calcium deposits allows the identification of atherosclerotic plaque early in its development, often before the plaque has produced myocardial damage or has progressed to critical stenosis. The early identification of calcium has the potential of significantly reducing the impact of CAD.

PATHOPHYSIOLOGY

Atherosclerotic Plaque Development

Coronary atherosclerotic plaque development begins early in life and is characterized by the accumulation of lipid-laden macrophages within the intima of arterial walls.[2] With increasing accumulations, the lesions often progress to Stary type IV and type V atheroma, which are well-developed plaques characterized by intramural collections of cholesterol and phospholipids. These lipid collections are often covered by a thin, fibrous cap (fibroatheroma). Because of remodeling, the lesions initially have little significant luminal narrowing and are often undetected by angiography. Two thirds of individuals with acute myocardial infarctions or unstable angina have only minimal angiographic narrowing at the culprit site of occlusion. Myocardial perfusion studies that attempt to identify the hemodynamic effects of coronary stenoses may be normal and often underestimate an individual's risk for a cardiac event.

Because these plaques are predisposed to spontaneous rupture, the lesions are often referred to as "vulnerable plaques." Why plaques rupture is unclear, but the process is likely multifactorial and related to biomechanical stresses and localized plaque inflammation. The histologic composition of these plaques may predict eventual outcomes from CAD; screening examinations that can identify plaque morphology may provide the best assessment of risk for coronary heart disease.

When a fibrous cap ruptures, the lipid core is exposed to circulating blood, and an acute thrombogenic reaction may ensue. Advanced lesions that produce stenoses have a greater prevalence in patients with chronic or stable angina, and they are more frequently detected by traditional diagnostic techniques that either identify the stenosis or screen for their hemodynamic effects.

A strong correlation has been found between the quantitative measurements of coronary artery calcium and pathologic measurements of plaque area and volume. Rumberger and colleagues[3] showed that calcium is identifiable by CT when plaque area measures 5 to 10 mm^2 per 3-mm-thick voxel. It has been established that as calcium increases, so does the likelihood of hemodynamically significant stenoses. Heavy concentrations of calcium suggest a greater atherosclerotic burden and a greater likelihood of hemodynamically significant stenoses. Supporting this concept is an article by Kragel and associates,[4] who reported that atherosclerotic plaques associated with significant stenosis often contain more calcium than nonobstructive plaques.

Autopsy studies have shown that large CAC burdens correlate with greater likelihoods of significant arterial luminal narrowing, especially when distributed over multiple vessels. One such study was by Mautner and coworkers,[5] who examined 1298 segments from 50 heart specimens and observed that 93% of arteries with stenoses greater than 75% had CAC. Conversely, only 14% of arteries with stenoses less than 25% were associated with calcification. Many other studies have shown that heavier CAC burdens were strongly associated with significant stenoses on angiography and with overall poorer patient outcomes. Calcium measurements derived from CT cannot predict site-specific stenoses. CAC measurements cannot be used to predict the site or the severity of the stenoses.[6]

Coronary calcium is a frequent constituent of vulnerable and hard plaques, and the presence and quantity of CAC correlate well with the overall severity of the atherosclerotic process, and make these lesions potentially identifiable by traditional noninvasive methods, such as fluoroscopy and CT. There are no diagnostic tests that can identify a priori vulnerable plaques that are susceptible to rupture. Postmortem analysis of coronary arteries of adults with sudden cardiac death have shown that histologically determined calcium scores for stable and ruptured plaques were similar (4.5 vs. 5.2).[7] Despite this, plaque calcification is frequently present in most patients who have acute plaque disruption and sudden death. In addition, intravascular ultrasound examinations performed on patients with acute cardiac events (infarct or unstable angina) have shown that vulnerable plaques tend to be associated with less calcification than plaques found in patients with stable angina, and that moderate levels of coronary calcium portend a greater number of vulnerable plaques and a subsequent higher risk for sudden death. Complicating this issue further is evidence suggesting that small to moderate amounts of calcium within plaque may be associated with a more unstable plaque configuration, which may facilitate their eventual rupture, and may make plaques less tolerable to shear stresses and promote endothelial lining disruption.

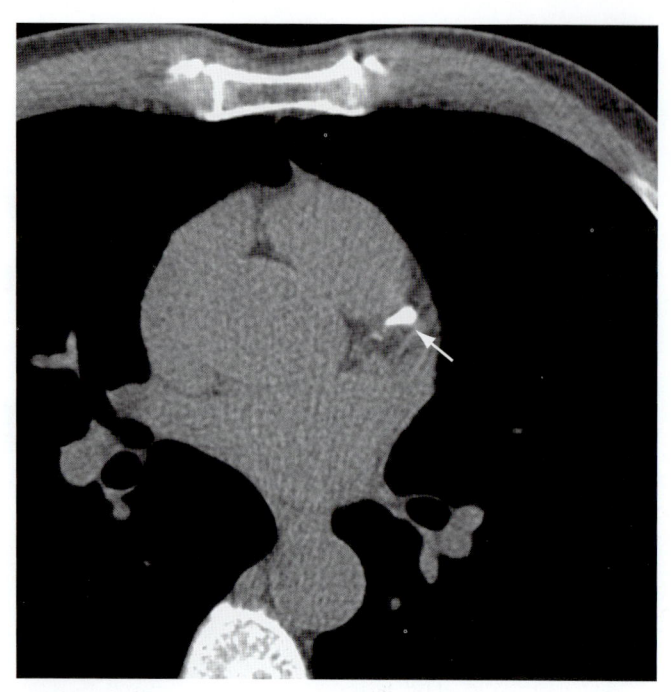

FIGURE 32-1 A 64-row multidetector CT image of a calcification (*arrow*) in the left anterior descending coronary artery.

IMAGING OF CORONARY ARTERY CALCIUM

CT imaging of small deposits of coronary calcium became available in the 1980s with the development of the electron-beam CT scanner. The electron-beam CT scanner has now been superseded by multidetector CT scanners, and few electron-beam CT scanners continue in operation. Multidetector CT scanners initially had a single detector ring technology, but now have progressed to dual source and 64-detector to 256-detector ring technology. Much of today's coronary calcium imaging is being done on dual source and 64-detector CT scanners (Fig. 32-1).

Electron-Beam Computed Tomography

The electron-beam CT scanner was introduced in 1980. It generated images by having electrons sweep tungsten target rings located beneath the patient to produce x-rays that traversed the patient to be collected by solid-state detectors in the gantry above the patient. This technology, with its absence of moving parts, allowed temporal resolutions of 50 to 100 ms, which for the first time could essentially "freeze" cardiac motion.

Older electron-beam CT scanners operated at 130 kV, 625 mA to produce 50-ms to 100-ms 1.5-mm, 3-mm, and

6-mm slice thickness images at resolutions of 9.5 1 p/cm. Later model electron-beam CT scanners operated at 140 kV, 1000 mA, and were able to generate dual 1.5-mm, 3-mm, and 8-mm slices at 50-ms temporal resolution. The spatial resolution was 10 1 p/cm. This updated version provided a 100-ms mode for higher spatial resolution and a 33-ms mode for higher temporal resolution.

Multidetector Computed Tomography

Electron-beam CT scanners have now been replaced by multidetector CT scanners, which have detectors capable of generating 256 detector images of varying thicknesses with each gantry rotation. Gantry rotation times have been reduced from 1000 ms to 330 ms, and with segmented reconstruction and dual source imaging, times approximating 83 ms are possible. An added advantage with most scanners is that the information generated is as a volumetric data set, and this permits reformations at different slice thicknesses. Multidetector CT images are commonly ECG gated, and this further decreases motion unsharpness by allowing image acquisitions during the quieter phase of the cardiac cycle. The latter is particularly important in coronary calcification and CT angiography imaging.

Current multidetector CT scanners can generate images by *prospective gating,* wherein the scanner is activated only during the time needed to acquire an image; this is roughly at one half the gantry rotation time. The time of data collection is initiated from the R wave of the ECG, and the operator can select the desired delay. This mode is frequently used in CAC imaging because patient radiation dose can be kept to a minimum. Rapid or irregular heartbeats can affect image quality and reproducibility, however. Previous 4-detector ring scanners rotating at 0.5 seconds and programmed to provide 2.5-mm slice thicknesses could acquire data in about a 20-second breath-hold; however, current 64-detector scanners are able to reduce scanning times to 8 to 12 seconds.

Retrospective gating is the more commonly used operating mode. In this sequence, there is helical scanning of the entire heart while recording the patient's ECG. On completion of the scan, the images are reconstructed at a preselected phase of the cardiac cycle. To avoid anatomic gaps in the data set, the pitch is set very low; the patient radiation exposure is higher. Nevertheless, the ability to reconstruct images during multiple phases of the cardiac cycle from the same high-resolution data set provides important information. Submillimeter slices 0.6 mm thick can be obtained to achieve high spatial resolution. The patient's heart rate can be a major factor influencing image quality, however, and if the heart rate exceeds 65 to 70 beats/min, β blockers are commonly administered to allow data collection during a single heartbeat.

Calcium Score Reporting

Calcium scores are reported using the Agatston score, volume score, and mass score.[8] The Agatston score was the initial reporting score and is used in much of the older literature. It used electron-beam CT technology to identify lesions with a threshold of +130 Hounsfield units (HU) and 2 to 3 contiguous pixels located over the course of the coronary artery. To calculate the score, a region of interest is placed around each lesion, and the area of the lesion is multiplied by a weighted factor of 1 to 4 based on the peak signal anywhere in the lesion. A weighted factor of 1 is used for a peak calcification of 130 to 199 HU; 2, for a peak calcification of 200 to 299 HU; 3, for a peak calcification of 300 to 399 HU; and 4, for a peak calcification of greater than 400 HU.

The volume score linearly interpolates the data for isotropic volumes and represents the volume (in mm^3) of each lesion above the 130 HU threshold. Lesions with similar area but differing amounts of calcium may have different volume scores.[8]

The mass score uses a calibration factor derived from scanning a phantom containing a known amount of calcium. The phantom is placed in the scanning field, and a calibration factor is determined. From it, the calibration factor times the number of voxels containing threshold calcium times the volume of one voxel times the mean CT number for each lesion equates to the mass score (in mg). The total score is the sum of all individual scores.

Rumberger and Kaufman[8] reviewed the Agatston, volume, and mass scores, and found equivalence of the three CAC scoring methods for stratification of their cohort of 11,490 individuals who had undergone electron-beam CT. Likewise, comparable agreement was found among the three CAC scoring methods over successive electron-beam CT scans. Based on phantom experiments, however, these investigators reported nonlinearity of the Agatston and volume scores with the volume score overestimating lesion volume. Using the same phantoms, mass scores were found to be linear with a few exceptions.

Standardization of Computed Tomography Scanners

To ensure that calcium scores are meaningful, it is important that CT scanners and protocols are standardized so that scores from one scanner can be compared with another. Toward that end, the Physics Task Group of the International Consortium on Standardization in Cardiac CT was formed.[9] Using a phantom with inserts of calcium and water density material embedded in an epoxy anthropomorphic body torso, scanning algorithms for all five commercially available scanners were developed (Fig. 32-2). The manufacturers included were Toshiba, Imatron, General Electric, Phillips, and Siemens.

Multidetector CT scanners were calibrated against the phantom for temporal and spatial resolution and noise. Minimum requirements included not less than 4 slices per rotation, rotation times less than 0.5 second, and an ability to reference an ECG signal. The target noise baseline was set at ± 20 HU for the water insert of the phantom. To accommodate different patent sizes, external circumferential rings can be added. Using consortium-developed scanner algorithms, variations of 4% for Agatston scores, 7.9% for volume scores, and 4.9% for mass scores were achieved. The calculated calcium score was within ± 5 mg of the actual calcium mass of the phantom. For the calibrations, a fixed density of 100 mg/mL of calcium hydroxyapatite was used. Subsequently, all manufacturers have now implemented these recommendations into their clinical protocols. To determine the approximate phantom size, the lateral skin-to-skin mea-

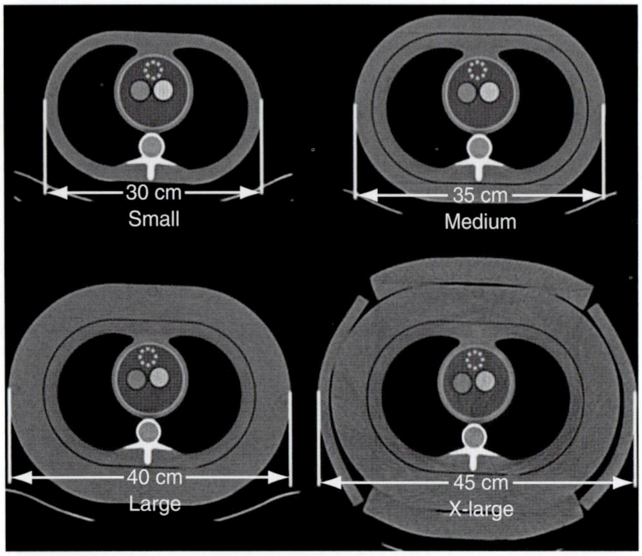

FIGURE 32-2 A semi-anthropomorphic thoracic phantom and three additional attenuation layers were used to represent small, medium, large, and extra-large adults. Two syringes were placed in the water-filled cardiac regions of the phantoms. The *dotted circle* on each phantom represents the ROI where the background noise level was measured. (From Yu L, Primak AN, Liu X, McCollough CH: Image quality optimization and evaluation of linearly-mixed images in dual-source, dual-energy CT. Med Phys 2009; 36:1019-1024.)

surement width at mid-liver measured from an anteroposterior radiograph is used. A multidetector CT database registry is currently under development.

RADIATION DOSAGE

The effective radiation dosage is a measure of the total radiation exposure to the patient. This is reported in millisieverts (mSv) and is frequently equated to months of background radiation exposure. For an electron-beam CT calcium study, the effective dose approximates 1 mSv in men and 1.3 mSv in women (4 and 5.2 months of background radiation).

For a multidetector CT prospectively triggered CAC study, the effective dose approximates 1.5 mSv in men and 1.8 mSv in women (6 months and 7.2 months of background radiation). If the multidetector CT CAC study were retrospectively gated, the radiation exposure would increase to approximately 3 mSv in men and 3.6 mSv in women, which would equate to 12 months and 14.4 months of background radiation. More recent developments in modulation techniques can now ramp down the power during noncritical imaging times, and this can decrease radiation exposure by 80%.[10]

Comparison of Multidetector Computed Tomography and Electron-Beam Computed Tomography in Coronary Artery Calcium Score Determinations

Numerous articles have compared multidetector CT and electron-beam CT in CAC score determinations. Knez and colleagues[11] scanned 99 symptomatic men (mean age 60 years) with 4-detector multidetector CT and electron-beam CT (prospective triggering at 80% R–R interval) and found a correlation coefficient of $r = 0.99$ for volume and $r = 0.98$ for mass scoring. These investigators found a mean overall variability of 17%, but no significant differences for scores 1 to 100, 101 to 400, 401 to 1000, and greater than 1000. Knez and colleagues[11] concluded that multidetector CT was equivalent to electron-beam CT for CAC scoring.

Becker and associates[12] also compared 4-detector multidetector CT with electron-beam CT (prospective triggering) in 100 patients. They calculated Agatston, volume, and mass scores, and concluded that the variability was highest for the Agatston score (32%), and that the correlation between multidetector CT and electron-beam CT was excellent for volume and mass scores.

Horiguchi and colleagues[13] compared electron-beam CT and 16-multidetector CT with retrospective gating in 100 patients and reported a high correlation between these scanners for the Agatston score ($r^2 = 0.95$), volume score ($r^2 = 0.95$), and mass score ($r^2 = 0.97$). Last, Daniell and coworkers[14] compared the results of electron-beam CT and 4-detector multidetector CT in 68 patients. Electron-beam CT and multidetector CT scores correlated well ($r = 0.98$-0.99). The variability between electron-beam CT and multidetector CT Agatston score was 25%, and for the volume score the variability was 16%. The electron-beam CT scores were higher than multidetector CT scores in approximately 50% of the cases. Numerous investigators have documented high correlation coefficients for multidetector CT versus electron-beam CT in coronary calcium scoring.

Interscan Reproducibility

A major consideration in the use of calcium scores is the variability of changes in CAC between serial CT scans on repeat imaging. Although interscan variability is predominantly affected by motion and table position, it is influenced further by the extent of CAC burden, scanner type, scan protocol starting position, and image artifacts. With optimal ECG triggering, variability can be reduced to less than 15% for electron-beam CT. The correlation coefficients of Agatston score, volume score, and mass score are excellent ($r = 0.96$).[15] The conclusion was that the electron-beam CT and multidetector CT scanners have equivalent reproducibility.

Differences between scanner types have been reported in many studies. In the Multi-Ethnic Study of Atherosclerosis (MESA) trial of 6814 multiethnic individuals scanned on three electron-beam CT and three multidetector CT scanners, the differences were 20.1% for the Agatston score, and 18.3% for the interpolated volume score ($P < .01$).[16] Other authors[17] reported a multidetector CT variation of 12% for Agatston scores, 7.5% for volume scores, and 7.5% for mass scores. Overall, reported variabilities on 16-detector to 64-detector multidetector CT scanners seem to be in the range of 8% to 18% for the Agatston, volume, and mass scores.

TABLE 32-1 Results from Knez et al: Presence of Significant Stenosis (>50% Stenosis)			
Calcium Score	Sensitivity (%)	Specificity (%)	Predictive Accuracy (%)
>0	99	28	70
>10	94	70	84
>100	87	79	83
75th percentile	85	80	82

TABLE 32-2 Results from Budoff et al: Presence of Significant Stenosis (>50% Stenosis)		
Calcium Score	Sensitivity (%)	Specificity (%)
>20	90	58
>80	79	72
>100	76	75
Overall	95	60

CLINICAL IMPORTANCE OF CORONARY CALCIUM IMAGING

Current indications include determining the overall atherosclerotic burden, evaluating risk assessment, and following progression of calcification after dietary or drug therapy. Other indications include evaluating patients before coronary CT angiography with regard to excluding individuals with excessively high calcium scores and evaluating individuals entering emergency departments with acute chest pain in whom the absence of calcium may be helpful in excluding a cardiac etiology for the chest pain.

Coronary Artery Calcification as an Indicator of Coronary Stenosis

Many electron-beam CT studies have addressed the issue of CAC as an indicator of coronary stenosis. Haberl and coworkers[18] looked at electron-beam CT calcium scores as an indicator of coronary luminal stenoses. They studied 1764 patients undergoing conventional coronary angiography and found that electron-beam CT CAC scores were a highly sensitive but only moderately specific determinant of stenosis. Knez and colleagues[19] reviewed 16 electron-beam CT trials (N = 2115 patients) comparing electron-beam CT–derived Agatston scores with volume scores. The reference standard was conventional coronary angiography. Knez and colleagues[19] found that electron-beam CT–derived CAC scores were an accurate predictor of the presence of greater than 50% luminal stenosis. Their results are shown in Table 32-1.

In another study, Budoff and colleagues[20] analyzed electron-beam CT volume scores as a predictor of luminal stenoses in 1851 patients undergoing conventional coronary angiography. Their results are shown in Table 32-2. From these studies, the investigators concluded that electron-beam CT volume scores provided incremental value in predicting the severity and extent of angiographically significant coronary artery stenosis. Last, the American College of Cardiology/American Heart Association Expert Consensus Document on Electron-Beam CT for the Diagnosis and Prognosis of Coronary Artery Disease[21] evaluated these and many additional studies, and reported a pooled sensitivity of 91.8% and specificity of 55% for detection of greater than 50% coronary artery stenoses.

Value of Zero Calcium Score

More important than the total score may be the implications of a 0 calcium score. Several investigators have addressed this issue. Becker and associates[22] studied 1347 symptomatic subjects with suspected CAD, and found an overall sensitivity of any calcium score to predict stenosis was 99%, with a specificity of 32%. An absolute score greater than or equal to 100 and an age-specific and gender-specific score greater than the 75th percentile were identified as the cutoff levels that provide the highest sensitivities (86% to 89%) and lowest false-positive rates (20% to 22%). Becker and associates[22] also concluded that absence of coronary calcium was highly accurate for exclusion of CAD.

Several other studies have addressed this issue. Cheng and coworkers[23] assessed the presence and severity of noncalcified coronary plaques on 64-detector multidetector CT versus coronary angiography in 554 symptomatic patients with low to intermediate pretest likelihood for CAD, and concluded that the absence of CAC is associated with a very low presence of significantly occlusive CAD.

Coronary Artery Calcium as a Predictor of Cardiac Events

In an American College of Cardiology/American Heart Association Consensus Document on Coronary Artery Calcium Scoring, it was concluded that CAC scores added incremental prognostic value in the evaluation of patients at intermediate risk for a coronary event. A study by Raggi and coworkers[24] supported this conclusion. These investigators screened 632 patients with electron-beam CT for hard cardiac events (myocardial infarction and death), and found in 32-month follow-up that most events occurred in individuals with high calcium scores (>75th percentile) compared with age-matched and gender-matched controls. Arad and colleagues[25] used electron-beam CT to screen 1172 asymptomatic patients. They followed patients for a mean of 3.6 years to determine the incidence of cardiovascular end points (myocardial infarction, death, and need for revascularization) and concluded that in asymptomatic adults electron-beam CT calcium scores were highly predictive of events.

Pletcher and associates[26] reported a meta-analysis of studies between 1980 to 2003. In an analysis of 13,000 asymptomatic patients screened with electron-beam CT and followed for 3.6 years, they found the odds ratios for Agatston CAC scores less than 100, 100 to 400, and greater than 400 were 2.1, 4.2, and 7.2, and concluded that the electron-beam CT–derived Agatston calcium scores were independent predictors for hard coronary events in asymptomatic subjects. Several additional studies were reported in the American College of Cardiology Foundation/American Heart Association consensus document on CAC scoring, and all reported similar or better odds ratios for electron-beam CT as a predictor of a cardiac event.[27]

In patients experiencing acute hard cardiac events, coronary calcium is almost always present in amounts exceeding those found in asymptomatic individuals. Although acute cardiac events do occur in individuals who have little or no demonstrable calcium, the absence of detectable CAC does portend a low likelihood of a major cardiac event within the next 2 to 5 years (5% to 10% overall risk).[21]

IMPORTANCE OF CORONARY CALCIUM IN SPECIALIZED POPULATIONS

Risk Assessment in Asymptomatic Individuals

Traditional risk assessment algorithms such as the Framingham Risk Score have been the standard used in assessing an individual's 10-year risk. Current definitions of risk are as follows:

- Low risk = 1% per year or 10% in 10 years
- Intermediate risk = 1% to 2% per year or 10% to 20% in 10 years
- High risk = greater than 2% per year or greater than 20% in 10 years

Present recommendations are that individuals at high risk are more likely to benefit from intensive risk modification and that individuals at low risk should adhere to a healthy lifestyle. In individuals at intermediate risk, the situation is uncertain, and further tests are often indicated. Calcium scoring has been advocated in the assessment of risk over measured conventional risk factors[28,29] in intermediate-risk patients. Many authors believe it is reasonable to use CAC measurement as a treatment modifier in this group of patients.

Patients Presenting to Emergency Departments with Chest Pain

In patients presenting to emergency departments with chest pain, functional tests such as treadmill, nuclear stress tests, or stress-echocardiography are frequently used, especially when cardiac enzymes and the admitting ECG do not show evidence of acute coronary syndrome. In these patients, the absence of calcium has a high correlation with the absence of a coronary etiology for the pain.

Laudon and colleagues[30] performed CAC scoring in the emergency department in 104 patients, and reported a negative predictive value of 100% for a CAC score of 0. In another study, McLaughlin and associates[31] reported a negative predictive value of 98% in 134 patients in a similar emergency department setting.[31] Additionally, Georgiou and coworkers[32] followed 198 patients presenting to the emergency department with chest pain and normal ECG and cardiac enzymes. They found that patients without CAC may safely be discharged from the emergency department because of the extremely low rate of future events (approximately 0.1%/yr). Numerous studies indicated the high negative predictive value of a 0 CAC score ($r > 90\%$). The positive predictive value is lower, however, which results in CAC screening being a highly sensitive, but poorly specific modality for assessing patients with acute coronary syndrome.

More recently, Rubinshtein and coworkers[33] assessed the severity of CAD using 64-multidetector CT in patients undergoing investigation for acute coronary syndrome. In 668 consecutive patients, 231 had a low (<100) or 0 CAC score, and of these patients, obstructive CAD was present in 9 of 125 (7%) with a 0 score, and in 18 of 106 (17%) with a low score (1 to 100). Rubinshtein and coworkers[33] concluded a 0 CAC score seemed to be a good predictor for the exclusion of significant CAD in patients with intermediate to high pretest likelihood of obstructive CAD. Low CAC scores remain controversial, however, because many studies have shown that the presence of noncalcified and potentially obstructive lesions is higher in patients with low calcium scores compared with patients with a score of 0.

Relationship Between Race and Calcium Score

Many studies have shown differences in scores between men and women and between subjects of different ethnicities. Bild and colleagues,[34] evaluating data from the MESA study, found that the prevalence of CAC (score >0) was highest in whites followed by Chinese, Hispanics, and blacks. Also from the MESA study of 6722 multiethnic individuals, Detrano and coworkers[35] reported that CAC is a strong predictor of cardiovascular death, nonfatal myocardial infarction, angina, and need for revascularization. They concluded that CAC adds incremental prognostic value beyond traditional risk factors for the prediction of events. It seems appropriate to consider CAC as an indicator of increased risk in all races.

Elderly Populations

The assessment of CAC in elderly individuals is of interest because a small reduction in risk results in a significant reduction in event rates. Because the Framingham Risk Score has age thresholds that limit its applicability, one may miscalculate the true risk of CAD, and this may lead to inaccurate selection, especially in elderly patients for aggressive risk factor modification.

Currently, only a few studies have focused on the predictive value of CAC in elderly individuals. One of these was the Rotterdam Coronary Calcification Study, which evaluated older individuals with a mean age of 71 years. This study found that during a mean follow-up period of 3.3 years, 50 of the 1795 initially asymptomatic subjects had a coronary event.[29] From these data, the researchers reported that increasing calcium scores showed relative risks for CAD up to 8.2 for a calcium score greater than 1000 compared with absent or low calcium score (0 to 100). Increasing calcium scores seem to be strongly associated with an increasing incidence of events, and low calcium scores seem to be important even in elderly individuals. Supporting these findings is a study by LaMonte and associates,[36] in which CAD event rates were adjusted for gender. These investigators showed that in subjects older than 65 years there was a graded increase in event rates for calcium scores of 100 and 400 (7.1 and 8.2 per 1000 person-years). Conversely, the absence of coronary calcium was associated with a very low event rate (0.9 per 1000 person-years). There is support that CAC screening is valuable in all age groups.

Diabetes Mellitus and Coronary Artery Calcium Screening

It is well known that diabetes mellitus is associated with a high prevalence of CAD. Limited outcome data exist for diabetic patients, however. Anand and colleagues[37] performed sequential CAC and myocardial perfusion imaging in 180 patients with type 2 diabetes. The incidence of myocardial ischemia was found to be proportional to the CAC score. For patients with type 2 diabetes with a CAC score of 0, 11 to 100, 101 to 400, 401 to 1000, and greater than 1000, the incidence of myocardial ischemia on stress perfusion imaging was 0%, 18%, 23%, 48%, and 71%. Anand and colleagues[37] concluded that patients with a CAC score greater than 100 have an increased frequency of ischemia on myocardial perfusion imaging.

Raggi and coworkers[38] evaluated 903 diabetic patients from a database of 10,377 asymptomatic individuals followed for an average of 5 years after CAC screening. The end point of the study was all-cause mortality. The authors showed that all-cause mortality was higher in diabetic patients than nondiabetic patients for any degree of CAC, and the risk increased as the score increased. They also found the absence of CAC predicted a low short-term risk of death (approximately 1% at 5 years) for diabetic patients and nondiabetic subjects. It seems that the presence and the absence of CAC are important modifiers of risk even in the presence of established risk factors.

Renal Failure and Coronary Artery Calcium

It is also well known that the prevalence of CAC increases with declining renal function. Russo and colleagues[39] reported the prevalence of CAC to be 40% in 85 predialysis patients compared with 13% with normal renal function. In this prospective study of 313 high-risk hypertensive patients, a reduced glomerular filtration rate was shown to be the major determinant of the rate of progression of CAC. Consistent with these findings, Sigrist and associates[40] reported prevalence of CAC to be 46% in 46 predialysis patients compared with 70% and 73% in 60 hemodialysis patients and 28 peritoneal dialysis patients ($P = .02$).

In another study of patients undergoing hemodialysis followed for almost 5 years, Block and colleagues[41] reported a low mortality rate for patients with a negative calcium score (3.9%/yr). This is a remarkable finding in view of the extremely high mortality and cardiovascular event rate in these patients (approximately 25%/yr to 30%/yr). CAC seems to be predictive of an adverse outcome in renal dialysis patients; however, its absence is associated with a low event rate.

Comparison of Coronary Calcium Screening with Treadmill and Nuclear Stress Imaging

Exercise stress testing is frequently used in patients with suspected CAD. There are often numerous false-negative results, however. Lamont and colleagues[42] studied 153 patients who underwent electron-beam CT and coronary angiography because of a positive treadmill stress test. In patients with a CAC score of 0, the negative predictive value was 93%. The authors concluded that the absence of CAC reliably identified patients with a false-positive treadmill stress test result. Raggi and coworkers[43] also evaluated treadmill stress test and showed that in patients with low to intermediate pretest probabilities of disease, CAC scoring as the initial test provided a substantial cost benefit over exercise stress testing, and that a CAC score of 0 can reliably exclude CAD.

Berman and associates[44] also reported a positive relationship between stress-induced myocardial ischemia as seen on single-photon emission computed tomography (SPECT) myocardial perfusion studies and electron-beam CT CAC. They studied 1195 patients without known coronary disease and found the frequency for ischemic SPECT was less than 2% with CAC scores less than 100 and increased progressively with CAC greater than 100 ($P \leq .0001$). Symptomatic patients with CAC scores equal to or greater than 400 had a higher likelihood of myocardial ischemic changes versus asymptomatic patients ($P < .025$). Berman and associates[44] concluded that ischemic SPECT was associated with a high likelihood of subclinical atherosclerosis, but is rarely seen in CAC scores less than 100, and that most low CAC scores would obviate the need for subsequent noninvasive testing.

CALCIUM SCORE PROGRESSION

Serial changes in CAC score have important implications for monitoring responses to therapy and in identifying patients with aggressive disease who are at higher risk for CAD. Progression of CAC is generally calculated as a percent or absolute change from the baseline score. Raggi and colleagues[45] defined a change of greater than 15% as true progression. Annual CAC progression rates typically are 20% to 24% per year using either the Agatston or the volume score. Factors modifying the rate of change include the patient's CAC score, gender, age, family history of premature CAD, ethnicity, diabetes, body mass index, hypertension, and renal insufficiency. Most patients exhibit a positive change in CAC scores over time. A few (29% to 34%) may exhibit no change, however, especially if they have a low Framingham Risk Score, are women, or are individuals with a 0 score.

EFFECT OF STATIN THERAPY ON CORONARY ARTERY CALCIUM PROGRESSION

Numerous studies have evaluated changes in CAC scores after treatment with statins. In observational studies, untreated patients had an average CAC progression of

36%, whereas patients receiving statin therapy had changes averaging 13%.[46] Randomized trials have sometimes failed to confirm these findings, however, and comparisons of intensive versus moderate statin therapy have shown no differences in CAC progression. This lack of effect suggests that a longer observational period may be needed, and that statins may reduce cardiac events independent of any effect on calcified plaque. Despite this suggestion, several reports have noted that rapid increases in the CAC score are associated with worsening of clinical outcomes, including myocardial infarction.

> **KEY POINTS**
> - CAC is a predictor of cardiac events and adds incremental value to risk factors in intermediate-risk populations.
> - Absence of CAC is associated with very low cardiac event rates.
> - Rapid CAC progression is associated with higher risk of cardiac events.
> - CAC may be a good predictor for cardiac events in elderly patients, diabetic patients, and patients of different ethnic backgrounds.
> - CAC scores can be used to predict the presence of obstructive CAD. Despite a high sensitivity, however, CAC has a low specificity; the main use of CAC should be assessment of risk of cardiac events, rather than the detection of obstructive CAD.

SUGGESTED READING

Greenland P, Bonow RO, Brundage BH, et al. ACCF/AHA 2007 clinical expert consensus document on coronary artery calcium scoring by computed tomography in global cardiovascular risk assessment and in evaluation of patients with chest pain: a report of the American College of Cardiology Foundation Clinical Expert Consensus Task Force (ACCF/AHA Writing Committee to Update the 2000 Expert Consensus Document on Electron Beam Computed Tomography). Circulation 2007; 115:402-426.

REFERENCES

1. American Heart Association. Heart Disease and Stroke Statistics: 2007 update. Dallas, TX, American Heart Association, 2007.
2. Stary HC, Chandler AB, Glagov S, et al. A definition of initial, fatty streak, and intermediate lesions of atherosclerosis. Circulation 1994; 89:2462-2478.
3. Rumberger, JA, Simons DB, Fitzpatrick LA, et al. Coronary artery calcium area by electron-beam computed tomography and coronary atherosclerotic plaque area: a histopathologic correlative study. Circulation 1995; 92:2157-2162.
4. Kragel AH, Reddy SG, Wittes JT, et al. Morphometric analysis of the composition of the atherosclerotic plaques in the four major epicardial coronary arteries in acute myocardial infarction and in sudden coronary death. Circulation 1989; 80:1747-1756.
5. Mautner GC, Mautner SL, Froehlich J, et al. Coronary artery calcification: Assessment with electron beam CT and histomorphometric correlation. Radiology 1994; 192:619-623.
6. Bormann JL, Stanford W, Stenberg RG, et al. Ultrafast tomographic detection of coronary artery calcification as an indicator of stenosis. Am J Card Imaging 1992; 6:191-196.
7. Taylor AJ, Burke AP, O'Malley PG, et al. A comparison of the Framingham Risk Index, coronary artery calcification, and culprit plaque morphology in sudden cardiac death. Circulation 2000; 101: 1243-1248.
8. Rumberger JA, Kaufman L. A Rosetta stone for coronary calcium risk stratification: Agatston, volume, and mass scores in 11,490 individuals. AJR Am J Roentgenol 2003; 181:743-748.
9. McCollough CH, Ulzheimer S, Halliburton SS, et al. Coronary artery calcium: a multi-institutional, multimanufacturer international standard for quantification at cardiac CT. Radiology 2007; 243:527-538.
10. Hunold P, Vogt FM, Schmermund A, et al. Radiation exposure during cardiac CT: effective doses at multi-detector row CT and electron-beam CT. Radiology 2003; 226:145-152.
11. Knez A, Becker C, Becker A, et al. Determination of coronary calcium with multi-slice spiral computed tomography: a comparative study with electron-beam CT. Int J Cardiovasc Imaging 2002; 18:295-303.
12. Becker CR, Kleffel T, Crispin A, et al. Coronary artery calcium measurement: agreement of multirow detector and electron beam CT. AJR Am J Roentgenol 2001; 176:1295-1298.
13. Horiguchi J, Yamamoto H, Akiyama Y, et al. Coronary artery calcium scoring using 16-MDCT and a retrospective ECG-gating reconstruction algorithm. AJR Am J Roentgenol 2004; 183:103-108.
14. Daniell AL, Wong ND, Friedman JD, et al. Concordance of coronary artery calcium estimates between MDCT and electron beam tomography. AJR Am J Roentgenol 2005; 185:1542-1545.
15. Hoffman U, Siebert U, Bull-Stewart A, et al. Evidence for lower variability of coronary artery calcium mineral mass measurements by multidetector computed tomography in a community-based cohort—consequences for progression studies. Eur J Radiol 2006; 57:396-402.
16. Detrano RC, Anderson M, Nelson J, et al. Coronary calcium measurements: effect of CT scanner type and calcium measure on rescan reproducibility-MESA study. Radiology 2005; 236:477-484.
17. Ohnesorge B, Flohr T, Fischback R, et al. Reproduction of coronary calcium quantification in repeat examinations with retrospective ECG-gated multisection spiral CT. Eur Radiol 2002; 12:1532-1540.
18. Haberl R, Becker A, Leber A, et al. Correlation of coronary calcification and angiographically documented stenoses in patients with suspected coronary artery disease: results of 1,764 patients. J Am Coll Cardiol 2001; 37:451-457.
19. Knez A, Becker A, Leber A, et al. Relation of coronary calcium scores by electron beam tomography to obstructive disease in 2,115 symptomatic patients. Am J Cardiol 2004; 93:1150-1152.
20. Budoff MJ, Diamond GA, Raggi P, et al. Continuous probabilistic prediction of angiographically significant coronary artery disease using electron beam tomography. Circulation 2002; 105:1791-1796.
21. O'Rourke RA, Brundage BH, Froelicher VF, et al. American College of Cardiology/American Heart Association Expert Consensus document on electron-beam computed tomography for the diagnosis and prognosis of coronary artery disease. Circulation 2000; 102: 126-140.
22. Becker A, Leber A, White CW, et al. Multislice computed tomography for determination of coronary artery disease in a symptomatic patient population. Int J Cardiovasc Imaging 2007; 23:361-367.
23. Cheng VY, Lepor NE, Madyoon H, et al. Presence and severity of noncalcified coronary plaque on 64-slice computed tomographic coronary angiography in patients with zero and low coronary artery calcium. Am J Cardiol 2007; 99:1183-1186.

24. Raggi P, Callister TQ, Cooil B, et al. Identification of patients at increased risk of first unheralded acute myocardial infarction by electron-beam computed tomography. Circulation 2000; 101:850-855.
25. Arad Y, Spadaro LA, Goodman K, et al. Prediction of coronary events with electron beam computed tomography. J Am Coll Cardiol 2000; 36:1253-1260.
26. Pletcher MJ, Tice JA, Pignone M, et al. Using the coronary artery calcium score to predict coronary heart disease events: a systematic review and meta-analysis. Arch Intern Med 2004; 164:1285-1292.
27. Greenland P, Bonow RO, Brundage BH, et al. ACCF/AHA 2007 clinical expert consensus document on coronary artery calcium scoring by computed tomography in global cardiovascular risk assessment and in evaluation of patients with chest pain: a report of the American College of Cardiology Foundation Clinical Expert Consensus Task Force (ACCF/AHA Writing Committee to Update the 2000 Expert Consensus Document on Electron Beam Computed Tomography). Circulation 2007; 115:402-426.
28. Greenland P, LaBree L, Azen SP, et al. Coronary artery calcium score combined with Framingham score for risk prediction in asymptomatic individuals. JAMA 2004; 291:210-215.
29. Vliegenthart R, Oudkerk M, Hofman A, et al. Coronary calcification improves cardiovascular risk prediction in the elderly. Circulation 2005; 112:572-577.
30. Laudon DA, Vukov LF, Breen FJ, et al. Use of electron-beam computed tomography in the evaluation of chest pain patients in the emergency department. Ann Emerg Med 1999; 33:15-21.
31. McLaughlin VV, Balogh T, Rich S. Utility of electron beam computed tomography to stratify patients presenting to the emergency room with chest pain. Am J Cardiol 1999; 84:327-328, A328.
32. Georgiou D, Budoff MJ, Kaufer E, et al. Screening patients with chest pain in the emergency department using electron beam tomography: a follow-up study. J Am Coll Cardiol 2001; 38:105-110.
33. Rubinshtein R, Gaspar T, Halon DA, et al. Prevalence and extent of obstructive coronary artery disease in patients with zero or low calcium score undergoing 64-slice cardiac multidetector computed tomography for evaluation of a chest pain syndrome. Am J Cardiol 2007; 99:472-475.
34. Bild DE, Detrano R, Peterson D, et al. Ethnic differences in coronary calcification: the Multi-Ethnic Study of Atherosclerosis (MESA). Circulation 2005; 111:1313-1320.
35. Detrano R, Guerci AD, Carr JJ, et al. Coronary calcium as a predictor of coronary events in four racial or ethnic groups. N Engl J Med 2008; 358:1336-1345.
36. LaMonte MJ, FitzGerald SJ, Church TS, et al. Coronary artery calcium score and coronary heart disease events in a large cohort of asymptomatic men and women. Am J Epidemiol 2005; 162:421-429.
37. Anand DV, Lim E, Hopkins D, et al. Risk stratification in uncomplicated type 2 diabetes: prospective evaluation of the combined use of coronary artery calcium imaging and selective myocardial perfusion scintigraphy. Eur Heart J 2006; 27:713-721.
38. Raggi P, Shaw LJ, Berman DS, et al. Prognostic value of coronary artery calcium screening in subjects with and without diabetes. J Am Coll Cardiol 2004; 43:1663-1669.
39. Russo D, Palmiero G, De Blasio AP, et al. Coronary artery calcification in patients with CRF not undergoing dialysis. Am J Kidney Dis 2004; 44:1024-1030.
40. Sigrist M, Bungay P, Taal MW, et al. Vascular calcification and cardiovascular function in chronic kidney disease. Nephrol Dial Transplant 2006; 21:707-714.
41. Block GA, Spiegel OM, Erlich J, et al. Effects of sevelamer and calcium on coronary artery calcification in patients new to hemodialysis. Clin Exp Nephrol 2004; 8:54-58.
42. Lamont DH, Budoff MJ, Shavelle R, et al. Coronary calcium scanning adds incremental value to patients with positive stress tests. Am Heart J 2002; 143:861-867.
43. Raggi P, Callister TQ, Cooil B, et al. Evaluation of chest pain in patients with low to intermediate pretest probability of coronary artery disease by electron beam computed tomography. Am J Cardiol 2000; 85:283-288.
44. Berman DS, Wong ND, Gransar H, et al. Relationship between stress-induced myocardial ischemia and atherosclerosis measured by coronary calcium tomography. J Am Coll Cardiol 2004; 44:923-930.
45. Raggi P, Cooil B, Ratti C, et al. Progression of coronary artery calcium and occurrence of myocardial infarction in patients with and without diabetes mellitus. Hypertension 2005; 46:238-243.
46. Callister TQ, Raggi P, Cooil B, et al. Effect of HMG-CoA reductase inhibitors on coronary artery disease as assessed by electron-beam computed tomography. N Engl J Med 1998; 339:1972-1978.

CHAPTER 33

Congenital Coronary Anomalies

James P. Earls

Anomalies of the coronary arteries are uncommon, but sometimes can be clinically significant. Most coronary artery anomalies are benign and clinically insignificant; however, some may lead to compromise to coronary flow causing ischemia, heart failure, and death. Clinical presentation depends on the specific anomaly.

Noninvasive imaging has emerged as the preferred way to image coronary anomalies. Electron-beam CT and MR angiography are valuable for the diagnosis of anomalous coronary arteries. More recently, multidetector CT also has been shown to be very useful in the detection and characterization of anomalous coronary arteries. This chapter reviews the appearance of the most commonly encountered coronary anomalies on noninvasive imaging using CT and MRI.

DEFINITION

Anomalous coronary arteries can be grouped into three general categories. Angelini and colleagues[1] have written one of the most complete works on this subject, and this text can serve as an excellent reference for additional study. Anomalies generally can be divided into three general classifications: (1) anomalies of origin and course (ectopic ostium within proper sinus, ostium outside normal sinus, and absent vessel); (2) anomalies of intrinsic coronary arterial anatomy (congenital stenosis of ostium, congenital aneurysms, and myocardial bridging); and (3) anomalies of coronary termination (fistulas) (Table 33-1).

One of the most commonly encountered anomalies of origin and course is that of a retroaortic circumflex coronary artery that arises from the right sinus of Valsalva. This has an anomalous ectopic ostium (right sinus of Valsalva) and course (retroaortic), but terminates in the usual location (left atrioventricular groove). Myocardial bridging is a commonly encountered anomaly of intrinsic coronary anatomy. Although the artery, which is almost always the left anterior descending (LAD) artery, arises from the usual sinus and travels in the usual course (anterior interventricular groove), but it takes an unusual temporary dip into the myocardium of the anterior wall before re-emerging in the epicardial fat.

Finally, anomalies of coronary termination include coronary artery fistulas. These are coronary arteries that arise from the proper sinus, but eventually terminate in an unusual location. The coronary artery blood flow does not supply the myocardium, but may flow into the pulmonary artery, coronary sinus, cardiac chamber, or superior vena cava. Small fistulas are incidental findings; however, large fistulas may have serious hemodynamic and clinical consequences.

PREVALENCE AND EPIDEMIOLOGY

Congenital anomalies of the coronary arteries affect about 1.3% (range 0.2% to 5.6%) of individuals.[2-10] Approximately 80% of anomalies are considered benign without significant clinical sequelae; the remaining 20% can potentially cause symptoms, and may be responsible for significant disease.[3]

We have found a slightly higher prevalence of coronary anomalies than was previously reported. A review of 2087 coronary CT examinations (JP Earls, unpublished data) found an overall prevalence of coronary anomalies of 3.83%. Of those, 54% (or 2.1% of the total) were not previously suspected, whereas 46% (or 1.8% of the total) were either previously known or suspected based on prior imaging studies. One might expect to see anomalies in a larger percentage of clinical cases than one would believe based on epidemiologic studies.

ETIOLOGY AND PATHOPHYSIOLOGY

Coronary anomalies are congenital in origin. In many cases, blood flow to the myocardium remains intact, even in periods of high myocardial oxygen demand, and when

TABLE 33-1 Classification of Coronary Anomalies
Anomalies of origin and course
Anomalous coronary artery from the opposite sinus of Valsalva
LCA, LAD artery, or left circumflex artery from the right coronary sinus
Interarterial course
Intraseptal course
Anterior wall course
Posterior (retroaortic) course
RCA from the left coronary sinus
Interarterial course
Intraseptal course
Anterior wall course
Posterior (retroaortic) course
Anomalous RCA, LCA, LAD artery, or left circumflex artery arising from the pulmonary artery
Anomalous LCA arising from the noncoronary sinus of Valsalva
High origin of the LCA or RCA from the ascending aorta
Absent left main (separate origins of LAD artery and left circumflex artery)
Arterial duplication
Single coronary artery arising from the right or left sinus of Valsalva
Anomalies of Intrinsic Coronary Arterial Anatomy
Congenital ostial stenosis
Congenital coronary aneurysms
Myocardial bridging
Anomalies of Termination
Coronary artery fistula

no clinical consequences are present. In other cases, the abnormal origin or course leads to compromised blood flow either during exercise or at rest, and symptoms may develop.

The terminology used to describe coronary anomalies is not standardized and sometimes can be confusing. In addition, the actual number of different coronary anomalies is large. The most common anomalies involve variations in the origin or course of the coronary arteries themselves; examples include an artery that arises from the incorrect coronary sinus, which must travel back to its anatomically correct location before terminating in the anatomically correct region of myocardium. In most cases, anomalies are sporadic isolated findings. They may also be associated with other cardiac pathology, however, including valvular lesions, such as a bicuspid aortic valve, or congenital heart disease, such as tetralogy of Fallot or transposition of the great vessels.

MANIFESTATIONS OF DISEASE
Clinical Presentation

Presentation depends greatly on the specific anomaly. Most coronary artery anomalies are benign and never have any clinical symptoms. These are usually detected as incidental findings. Other anomalies are potentially significant and are sometimes ominously termed *malignant* or *potentially lethal*; these increase the risk of myocardial ischemia and sudden death because their position or orientation may lead to coronary flow compromise.[11-15] Although anomalies are uncommon, they can have a substantial impact on premature cardiac morbidity and mortality among young adults. Eckart and associates[16] found coronary anomalies present in more than 30% of sudden nontraumatic deaths in young individuals.

Imaging Indications and Algorithm

Noninvasive imaging has emerged as the preferred way to diagnose and evaluate coronary anomalies. Echocardiography can often detect anomalous origins and even some anomalous courses or, as in the case of larger fistulas, anomalous terminations. Electron-beam CT and MR angiography are useful for the comprehensive diagnosis of anomalous coronary arteries.[17-22] More recently, multidetector CT has proved to be useful in the detection and characterization of anomalous coronary arteries.[23-28]

IMAGING TECHNIQUE AND FINDINGS
Computed Tomography

Cardiac multidetector CT using contrast-enhanced technique is capable of detecting and characterizing coronary artery anomalies. Most anomalies are incidental findings and are frequently detected when the coronary arteries are being evaluated for atherosclerotic stenoses. The same CT angiographic technique is used when imaging coronary anomalies and atherosclerotic coronary artery disease. This technique is discussed in depth in Chapter 9.

With the exception of anomalous coronary arteries arising from the pulmonary artery, anomalous arteries fill with contrast material at the same time as anatomically normal arteries. Timing of contrast administration and data acquisition for the examination should not be altered. If anomalous origin from the pulmonary artery is suspected, a longer contrast infusion may be appropriate. In situations where the anomalies are seen in conjunction with other cardiac conditions, such as transposition of the great vessels, the amount of imaged anatomy in the z-axis may be increased from the standard heart and aortic root only selection.

Magnetic Resonance Imaging

MRI has been used for a long time to image potential coronary anomalies. It has the advantage of not using ionizing radiation, and has many different pulse sequences to help identify and evaluate the anomalous artery. MRI has been especially used in children and young adults to minimize radiation dose because this population is more susceptible to radiation-induced malignancies owing to their young age. Techniques vary widely and include bright blood and dark blood sequences, contrast-enhanced and non–contrast-enhanced sequences, and breath-hold and non–breath-hold sequences. No single technique has yet emerged as the dominant coronary MRI technique for coronary analysis. MRI sometimes can be less reliable, however, than its newer competitor, multidetector CT. MRI does not expose patients to the higher risks of ionizing radiation and of iodinated contrast agents. The relatively small amount of radiation exposure and of need for an intravenous catheter are particular advantages for imaging children.

Interarterial course   Septal course   Anterior course   Retroaortic course

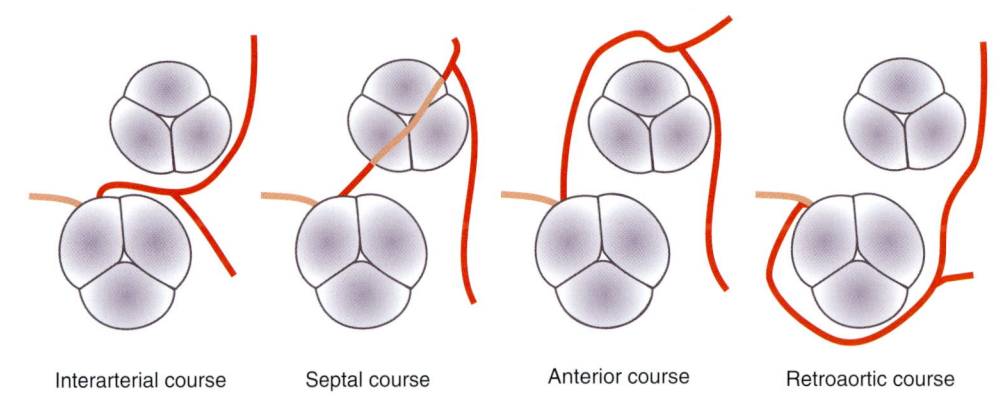

■ **FIGURE 33-1** There are four possible pathways for the anomalous LCA: (1) an interarterial course between the aortic root and the pulmonary artery, (2) a septal course through the myocardium below the pulmonary artery, (3) an anterior or prepulmonic course anterior to the right ventricular outflow tract, and (4) a retroaortic or posterior course behind the aortic root.

DIFFERENTIAL DIAGNOSIS

Anomalies of Origin and Course

Anomalous Origin of a Coronary Artery from the Opposite Sinus of Valsalva

One of the most commonly encountered potentially serious anomalies involves the anomalous origination of a coronary artery from the opposite sinus of Valsalva. Either the right coronary artery (RCA) or the left coronary artery (LCA) can arise from the opposite sinus, and then traverse across the heart to resume a normal position. Alternatively, a single branch of the LCA, the LAD artery, or the left circumflex artery can arise from the opposite sinus, whereas the remainder of the LCA may arise from the correct sinus.

There are several potential courses for an anomalous LCA arising from the right sinus of Valsalva or the RCA (Fig. 33-1). Diagnosis of the exact course is important because it determines if intervention is necessary. There are four possible pathways for the anomalous LCA: (1) between the aortic root and the pulmonary artery (interarterial course), (2) a transseptal (intraseptal or subpulmonic) course, (3) anterior to the right ventricular outflow tract (anterior or prepulmonic course), and (4) posterior to the aortic root (retroaortic course). Although the anterior, posterior, and septal (subpulmonic) courses are benign, an interarterial course carries a high risk for sudden cardiac death.[29,30]

Axial reconstructions from a multidetector CT coronary angiogram can depict the anatomic course. The exact position and course of the anomalous artery can be viewed in relation to the aortic root and pulmonary artery (Fig. 33-2). The LCA arises from the right sinus of Valsalva or directly from the RCA in 0.10% of patients, and an interarterial course is present in approximately 75% of these patients.[31]

Three-dimensional volume rendered multidetector CT images of the coronary arteries and aortic root can also be helpful in depicting the course and anatomic relationships. An anomalous coronary artery originating from the opposite sinus of Valsalva can cause syncope, myocardial infarction, and sudden death in the absence of critical, fixed stenosis. Patients with an anomalous LCA that takes an interarterial course have a high risk for sudden cardiac death because of the acute angle of the ostium, the stretch of the intramural segment of the anomalous artery, or the compression between the commissures of the right and left coronary cusps.[1,31] This anomalous LCA may narrow the origin or proximal aspect of the vessel and limit flow. An anomalous interarterial coronary artery is frequently an underlying cause for sudden death in young athletes. Often, MRI can also show an anomalous coronary artery with an interarterial course (Fig. 33-3).

The other three types of anomalous coronary artery originating from the opposite sinus of Valsalva have predominantly benign clinical outcomes. Anomalous coronary arteries originating from the opposite sinus of Valsalva can have an intraseptal (intramyocardial) course (Fig. 33-4). In this anomaly, the proximal portion of the anomalous coronary artery is completely surrounded by the gray

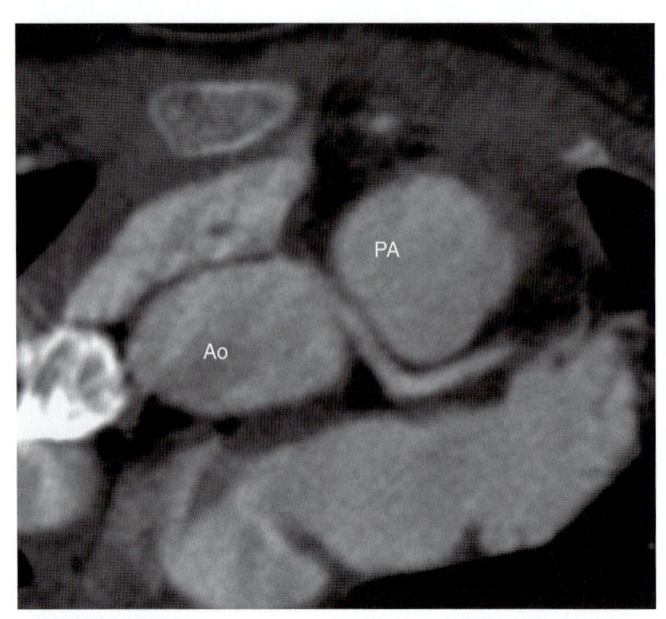

■ **FIGURE 33-2** Axial reconstruction from a multidetector CT coronary angiogram confirms that the anomalous LCA arises with the RCA from the right sinus of Valsalva and has an interarterial course, passing between the aorta (Ao) and pulmonary artery (PA).

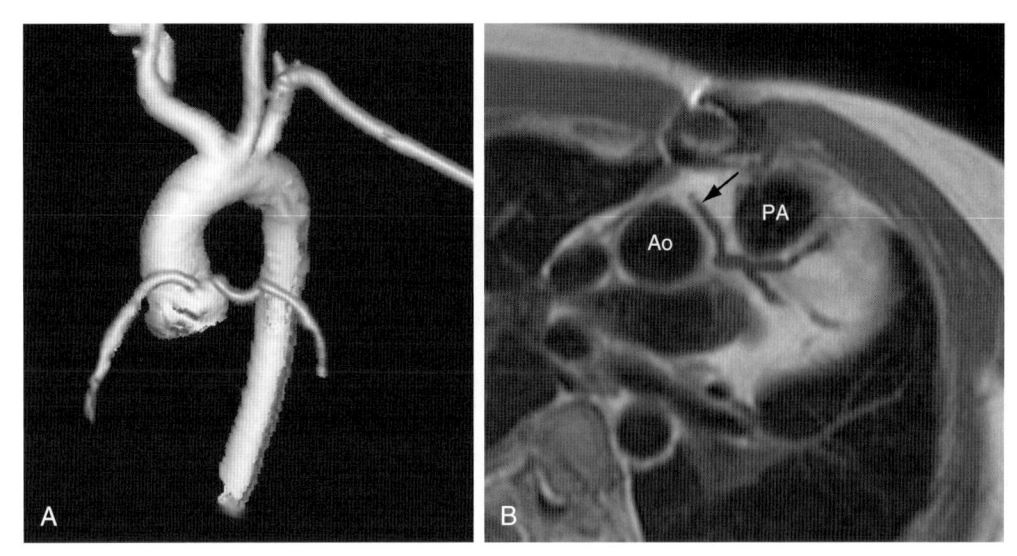

■ **FIGURE 33-3** MRI of an anomalous RCA that takes an interarterial course. **A,** Volume rendered view of a gadolinium-enhanced three-dimensional MR angiogram depicts the anomalous RCA arising from a near common origin with the LCA from the left sinus of Valsalva. **B,** Double inversion recovery fast spin-echo black blood image depicts the anomalous interarterial RCA (*arrow*) as a low signal intensity structure passing between the aorta (Ao) and pulmonary artery (PA).

myocardium of the interventricular septum, and is believed to be "protected" from possible compression as seen more typically with the interarterial course. Care must be taken, however, because a portion of the anomalous coronary, especially the initial proximal segment, may be extracardiac, in which case it assumes the same risks noted for the anomalous interarterial course. The intraseptal pathway is mostly located within the upper, anterior interventricular septum. Frequently, septal branches can be seen to arise from the anomalous vessel, a distinction that may help differentiate an interarterial course from an intraseptal course on conventional angiography.

In cases with an anomalous LCA or LAD artery with an anterior course, the anomalous LCA or LAD artery arises from the proximal RCA and takes a course anterior to the pulmonary artery (Fig. 33-5). Because the anomalous vessel is long and is associated primarily with the low-pressure pulmonary outflow tract, it does not get compressed or stretched as does the interarterial course of an anomalous artery arising from the opposite coronary sinus. It is considered a benign anomaly without significant clinical sequelae. This particular anomaly is commonly seen in patients with tetralogy of Fallot. An anterior course may also be seen with an anomalous RCA that arises from the LCA or LAD artery.

The fourth variant of anomalous coronary artery originating from the opposite sinus of Valsalva involves a course posterior to the aorta (i.e., retroaortic course) (Fig. 33-6). In this case, an anomalous circumflex coronary artery arises with the RCA from the right sinus of Valsalva. The retroaortic course is the most common pathway for an anomalous origin of a coronary artery from the opposite sinus of Valsalva. The retroaortic left circumflex artery is seen in 0.1% to 0.9% of the population.[1]

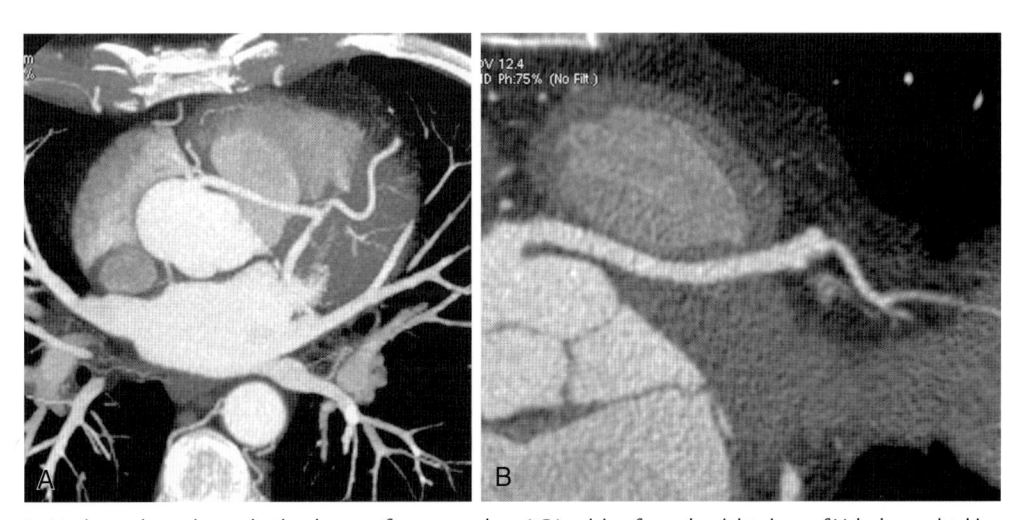

■ **FIGURE 33-4** **A,** Maximum intensity projection image of an anomalous LCA arising from the right sinus of Valsalva and taking an intraseptal course. **B,** On a curved multiplanar reconstruction image, the proximal portion of the LCA is completely surrounded by the gray myocardium of the interventricular septum. This anomalous pathway is mostly located within the upper, anterior interventricular septum.

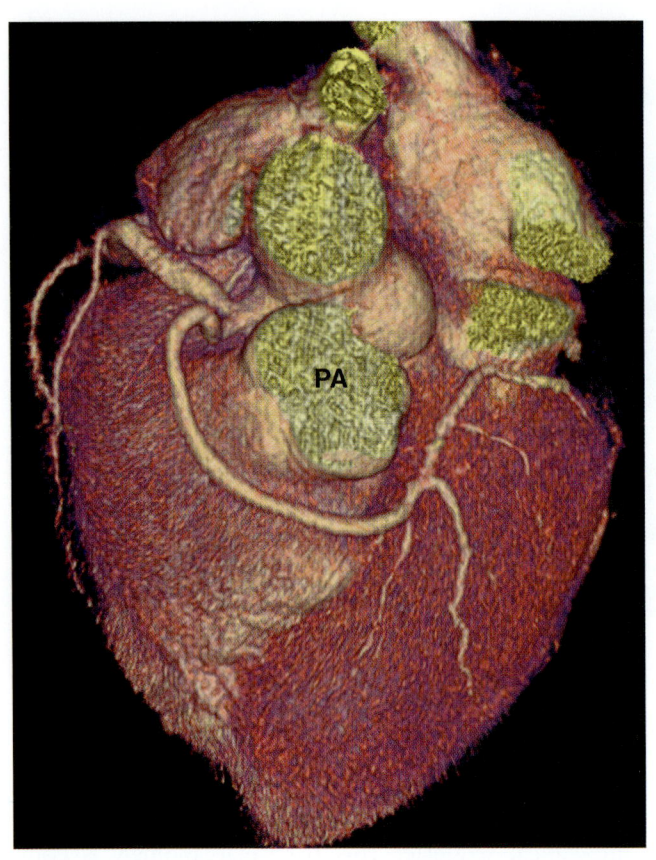

FIGURE 33-5 An anomalous LCA arises from the proximal RCA and takes a course anterior to the pulmonary artery (PA).

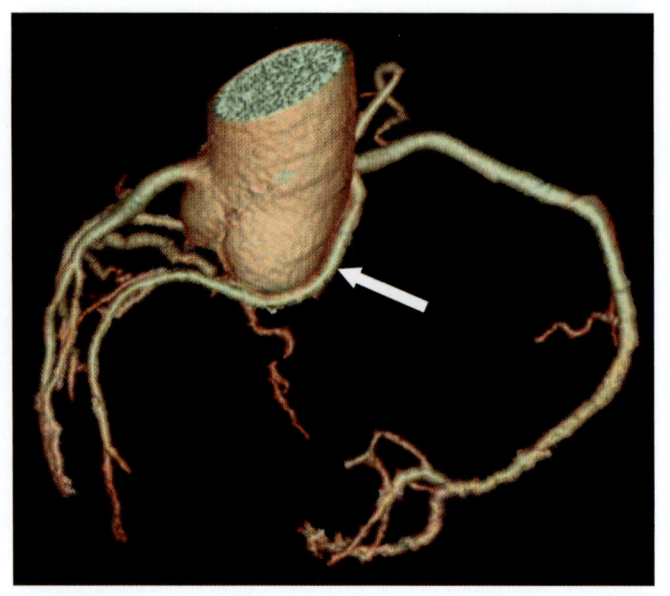

FIGURE 33-6 Volume rendered view depicts an anomalous circumflex coronary artery (*arrow*) arising from the RCA and passing posterior to the aortic root. The retroaortic course is the most common pathway for an anomalous origin of a coronary artery from the opposite sinus of Valsalva.

Anomalous Origin of a Coronary Artery from the Pulmonary Artery

Anomalous origin of the left coronary artery from the pulmonary artery (ALCAPA) is a very serious anomaly, reported in 1 of every 300,000 live births.[32] Most patients become symptomatic in infancy and early childhood. Ninety percent of untreated infants die before 1 year of age, and only a few patients survive to adulthood.[33] In ALCAPA, the LCA arises from the pulmonary artery (Fig. 33-7), and the RCA arises normally from the aorta; this is also known as Bland-White-Garland syndrome.[1] ALCAPA is usually an isolated anomaly, but rarely it has been described with patent ductus arteriosus, ventricular septal defect, tetralogy of Fallot, and coarctation of the aorta.

In patients with ALCAPA, initially myocardial ischemia is transient; however, increases in myocardial oxygen consumption lead to infarction, dysfunction, and mitral insufficiency. Collateral circulations between the right and left coronary systems develop, and LCA flow eventually reverses and enters the pulmonic trunk because of the low pulmonary vascular resistance (coronary steal phenomenon). Eventually, the combination of left ventricular dys-

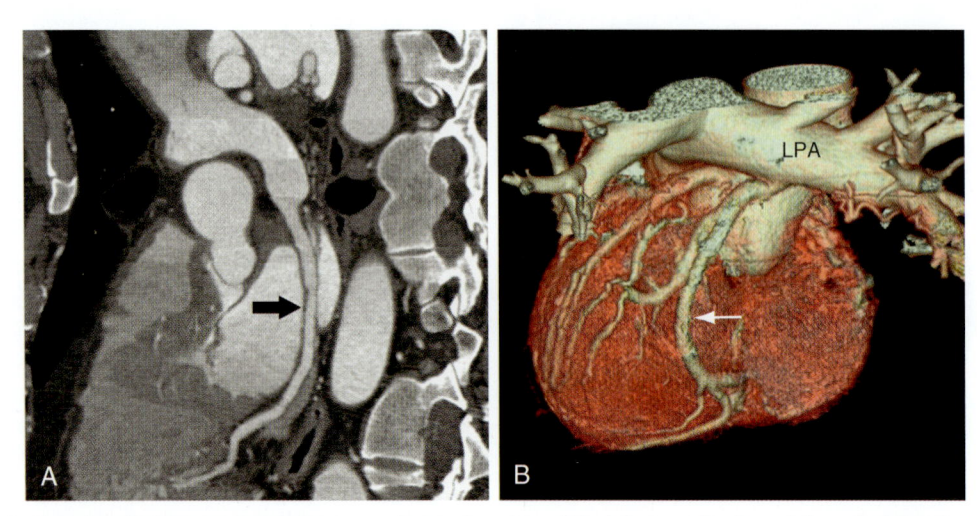

FIGURE 33-7 **A,** Curved multiplanar reconstruction image depicts the origin of the left circumflex (*arrow*) from the left pulmonary artery (LPA). **B,** Posterior view of a three-dimensional volume rendered multidetector CT coronary angiogram provides a better three-dimensional view of the anomalous dominant left circumflex (*arrow*) and LPA.

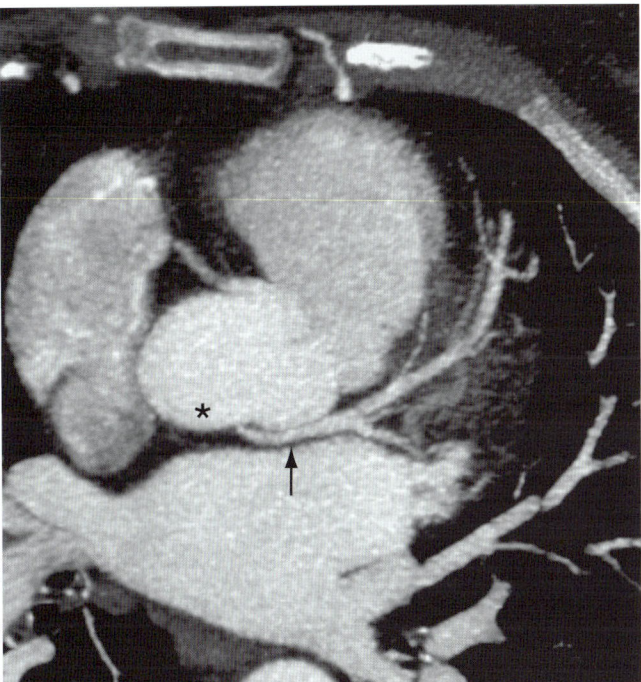

FIGURE 33-8 Multidetector CT depicts an anomalous LCA (*arrow*) arising from the noncoronary sinus of Valsalva (*asterisk*).

FIGURE 33-9 Volume rendered view from a multidetector CT scan depicts high origins of the RCA and LCA; both arise from the ascending aorta above the right and left sinuses of Valsalva.

function and significant mitral valve insufficiency leads to congestive heart failure.

Current surgical treatment for ALCAPA is directed at establishing revascularization by recreating a two–coronary artery system. This is done via a number of methods: a left subclavian artery–coronary artery anastomosis, a saphenous vein bypass graft, Takeuchi procedure (creation of an intrapulmonary tunnel), or direct reimplantation. After surgery, most patients experience normalization of left ventricular function, improving long-term survival.[32] An anomalous origin of the RCA from the pulmonary artery may also occur, but with ischemic complications affecting the RCA versus LCA vascular distribution.

Anomalous Coronary Artery Arising from the Noncoronary Sinus

Either the RCA or the LCA may arise from the noncoronary sinus of Valsalva (Fig. 33-8). Both of these anomalies are rare, and in an otherwise normal heart, they usually have no clinical relevance. These anomalies may also be seen with transposition of the great vessels.[34] Although of minimal clinical importance, documentation of the anomaly would be useful before conventional coronary angiography or intervention. As patients age, the aortic root can rotate clockwise, causing the normal LCA origin to turn more posterior than usual. One needs to be careful not to misdiagnose anomalous LCA arising from a non-coronary sinus in this situation.

High Origin of a Coronary Artery

A high origin of a coronary artery refers to origin outside of the coronary sinus (Fig. 33-9), above the junctional zone between its sinus and the tubular part of the ascending aorta. High coronary ostia, located above the sinotubular junction, have been reported in 6% of adult hearts.[35] A high origin of a coronary artery is generally not related to hemodynamic or clinical problems; however, it may lead to difficulty in cannulating the artery during conventional coronary arteriography. Intra-arterial cannulation of an RCA with a high origin, especially when it is above the right sinus of Valsalva, can be particularly difficult.

Multiple Ostia

Another commonly encountered benign anomaly is absence of the left main coronary artery resulting in separate origins of the LAD artery and left circumflex artery (Fig. 33-10). Separate origins of the LCA and left circumflex artery are reported in a few (0.41%) patients and are unrelated to other anomalies or cardiac disease.[36] The clinical relevance of separate origins of the LAD artery and left circumflex artery is limited because there are no known adverse hemodynamic effects. This anomaly may present difficulty for the angiographer because multiple ostia need to be recognized and require separate cannulation during selective diagnostic catheterization studies. Separate origins may have some protective effects because this configuration allows for alternative collateral sources in patients with proximal coronary stenoses.[34]

Arterial Duplication

Arterial duplication is another form of coronary anomaly and often involves the LAD artery (Fig. 33-11). Clinically this anomaly had been termed *duplication of the LAD artery*, and it is seen in 0.13% to 1% of the general population.[37] This anomaly consists of a short LAD artery, which courses and terminates in the anterior interventricular

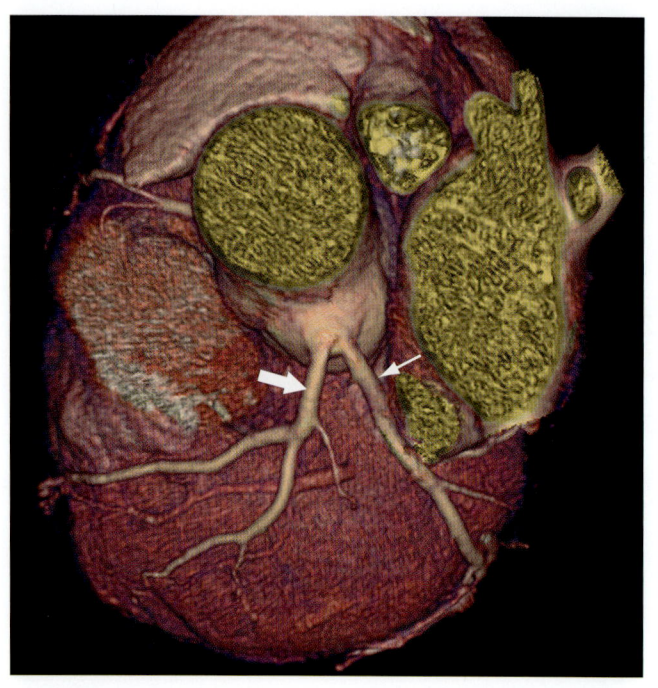

■ **FIGURE 33-10** Three-dimensional volume rendered multidetector CT coronary angiogram depicts absence of the left main coronary artery and separate origins of the LAD artery (*thick arrow*) and left circumflex (*thin arrow*) arteries. This anomaly may present difficulty for the angiographer because multiple ostia need to be recognized and require separate cannulation during diagnostic catheterization examinations.

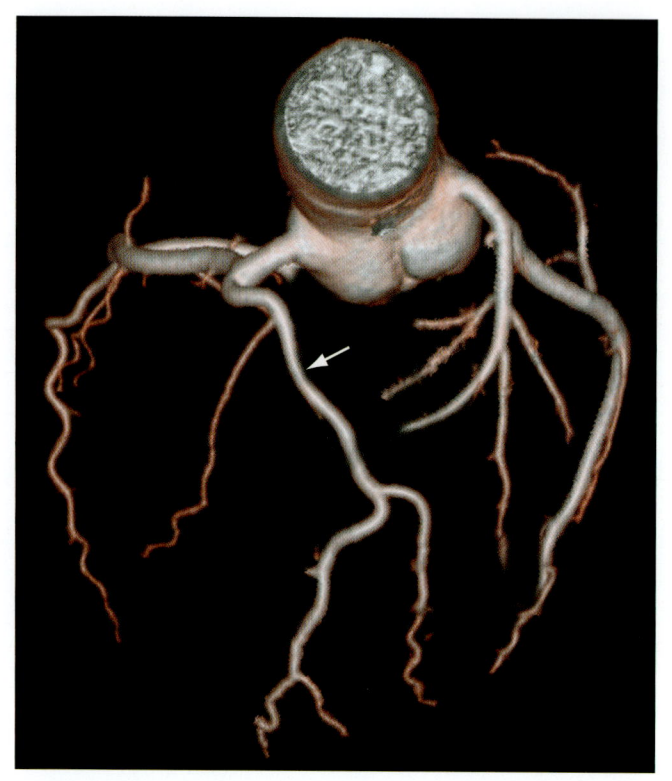

■ **FIGURE 33-11** Multidetector CT coronary angiogram shows that the LAD artery has a dual origin. The proximal portion arises normally from the left main coronary artery. The mid to distal portion of the LAD artery arises from the RCA via a branch (*arrow*) that traverses anterior to the pulmonary outflow tract.

sulcus, and a long LAD artery, which originates from either the LAD artery or the RCA and enters the distal interventricular sulcus and courses to the apex.[37] Because the LAD artery is frequently bypassed surgically, it is important to recognize this anomaly before surgical revascularization so that the surgical arteriotomy is correctly placed.[37]

Single Coronary Artery

A single coronary artery (Fig. 33-12) is a rare anomaly in which only one coronary artery arises from the aortic trunk by a single ostium. The artery supplies the blood to the entire heart. The presence of a single coronary artery is rare, reported in approximately 0.024% to 0.066% of the population.[1,38] A single coronary artery has many different patterns of distribution. It may follow the pattern of a normal artery, divide into two branches with distributions of the RCA and the LCA, or have a distribution different from that of the normal coronary arterial tree.[39] Single coronary artery is a very heterogeneous group of anomalies in which the single artery can arise from the right, left, or noncoronary sinus of Valsalva, and the pathways of the branches can vary greatly, taking retrocardiac, retroaortic, interarterial, intraseptal, and anterior courses.

Anomalies of Intrinsic Coronary Arterial Anatomy

Congenital Ostial Stenosis

Coronary arteries may have an ostial stenosis that is not due to atherosclerosis or other type of acquired disease. Congenital ostial stenoses are due to a membrane or fibrotic ridge.[1] This membrane or ridge is sometimes found with anomalous coronary arteries, and is believed to be due to the tangential orientation of the anomalous artery as it passes through the aortic wall. Ostial stenoses may be present in some cases where the RCA arises ectopically from the left sinus of Valsalva and runs in an interarterial path (Fig. 33-13).

Congenital Coronary Aneurysms

Ectasia, or aneurysm formation, may be localized to a single coronary segment or can involve the coronaries diffusely. Patients with either focal or diffuse coronary ectasia, not related to atherosclerosis, have abnormal arterial walls, with medial degeneration, intimal thickening, and eventual ulceration and mural thrombus formation.[40] Congenital coronary aneurysms are often associated with Kawasaki disease (Fig. 33-14).

Myocardial Bridging

Normal coronary arteries traverse the epicardial fat before entering the myocardium. In complete myocardial bridging, a short segment of the artery, known as a tunneled segment, passes into and through the myocardium for a short segment before re-entering the epicardial fat. It then branches normally and terminates within the myocardium (Figs. 33-15 and 33-16). Complete myocardial bridging is seen in 20% of asymptomatic patients and is

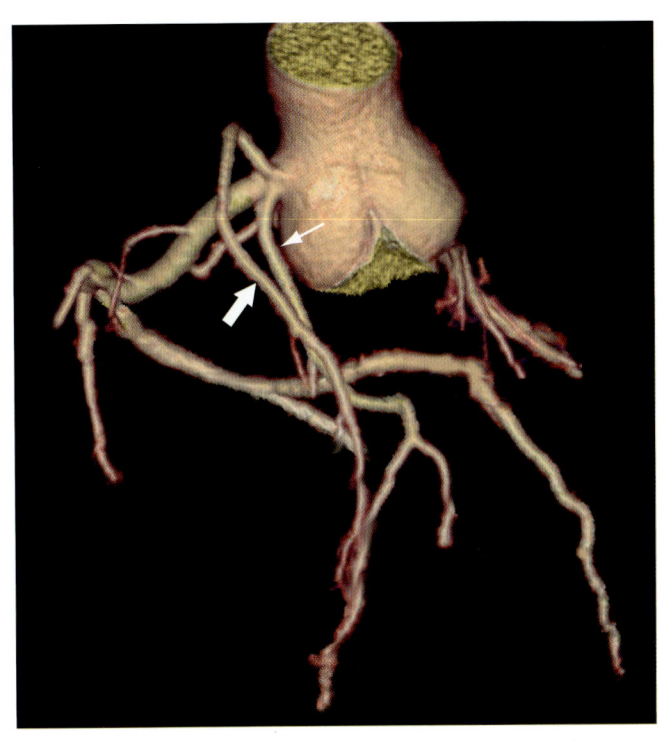

FIGURE 33-12 A single coronary artery arises from the right sinus of Valsalva, with associated retroaortic circumflex artery, and interarterial (*thin arrow*) and anterior (*thick arrow*) courses of a duplicated LAD artery.

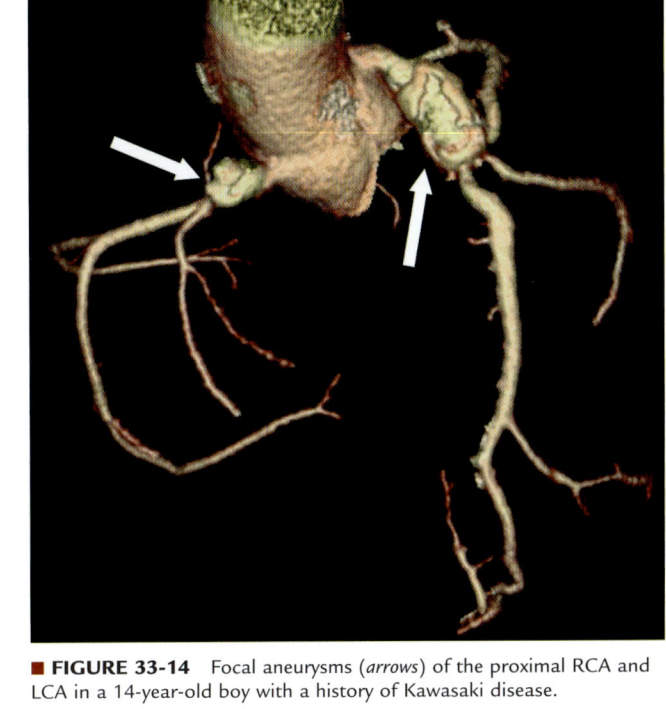

FIGURE 33-14 Focal aneurysms (*arrows*) of the proximal RCA and LCA in a 14-year-old boy with a history of Kawasaki disease.

a very rare cause of ischemia secondary to spasm. In incomplete myocardial bridging, the involved artery extends down to and touches the myocardium, but does not completely enter before extending back up into the myocardium.

FIGURE 33-13 Curved multiplanar reconstruction of an anomalous RCA, arising from the left sinus of Valsalva and taking an interarterial course. The proximal portion of the RCA is significantly narrowed consistent with congenital ostial stenosis. PA, pulmonary artery.

Myocardial bridging typically involves the middle portion of the LAD artery, but the circumflex artery, diagonal arteries, and RCA are occasionally involved.[41] The prevalence of myocardial bridging varies greatly in reported series, ranging from 0.5% to 2.5% on angiography examinations to 15% to 85% at pathologic analysis.[41] Multidetector CT coronary angiography depicts the intramyocardial path of the involved coronary arterial segment. Although most patients with myocardial bridging are asymptomatic, in rare cases myocardial bridging is responsible for angina pectoris, myocardial infarction, life-threatening arrhythmias, or death.[41]

Anomalies of Termination: Coronary Artery Fistula

A coronary fistula is an abnormal connection between a coronary artery and the pulmonary artery (Fig. 33-17), coronary sinus, cardiac chamber, or superior vena cava. Fistulas are present in approximately 0.1% to 0.2% of patients at coronary angiography.[42] Small fistulas are often incidental findings; however, large fistulas have serious hemodynamic and clinical consequences. Fistulas represent a left-to-right or a left-to-left shunt, depending on where they communicate, and they result in dilation of the coronary artery to varying degrees, depending on the shunt volume. Myocardial ischemia may develop in the portion of the myocardium supplied by the abnormally connecting coronary artery. The right ventricle is the most common site of drainage (45% of cases), followed by the right atrium (25%) and the pulmonary artery (15%).[43]

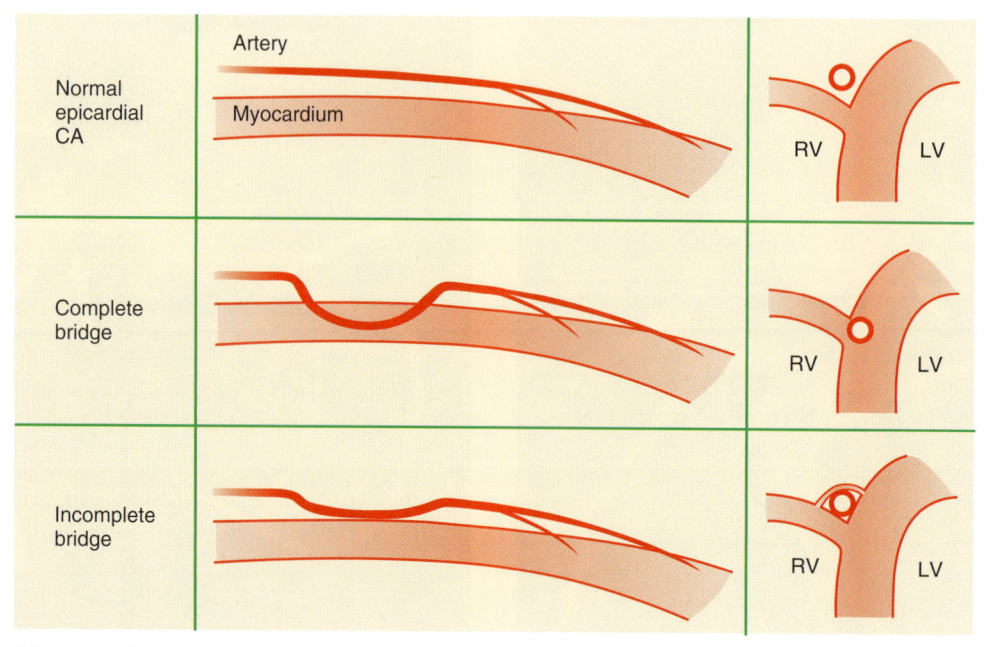

FIGURE 33-15 Diagram depicts a normal coronary artery (CA) and complete and incomplete myocardial bridging. Normal coronary arteries traverse the epicardial fat before entering the myocardium. In complete myocardial bridging, a short segment of the artery, known as a tunneled segment, passes into and through the myocardium for a short segment before re-entering the epicardial fat. It then branches normally and terminates within the myocardium. LV, left ventricle; RV, right ventricle. *(Redrawn from Earls JP. Coronary artery anomalies. In Narula J, Budoff MJ, Achenbach SS [eds]. Atlas of Cardiovascular Computed Tomography. New York, Springer, 2007.)*

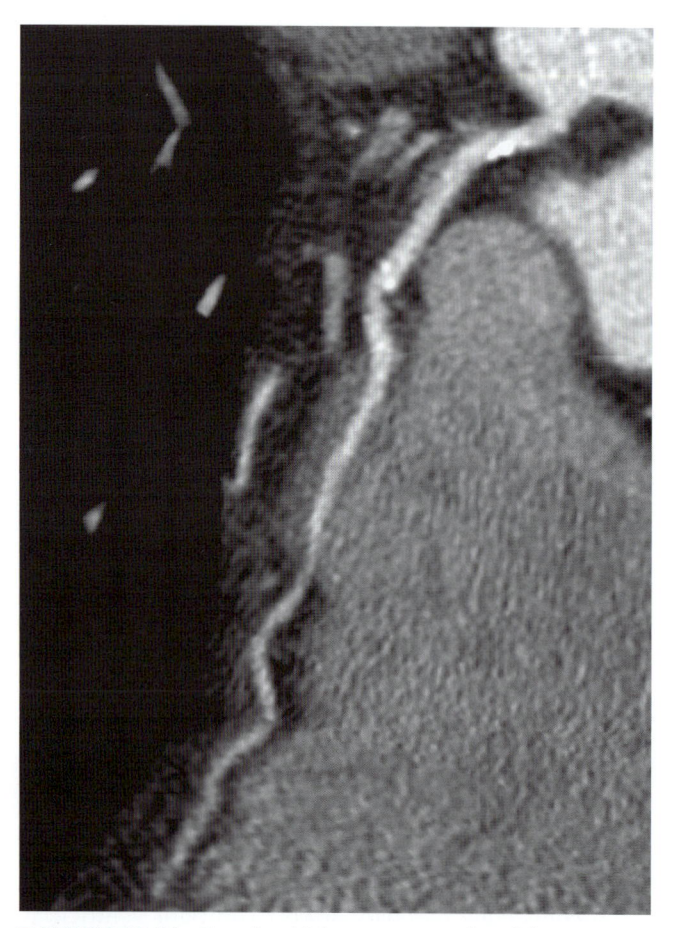

FIGURE 33-16 Curved multiplanar reconstruction of the LAD artery in a patient with complete myocardial bridging shows that the artery enters the myocardium for a short segment then re-enters the epicardial fat.

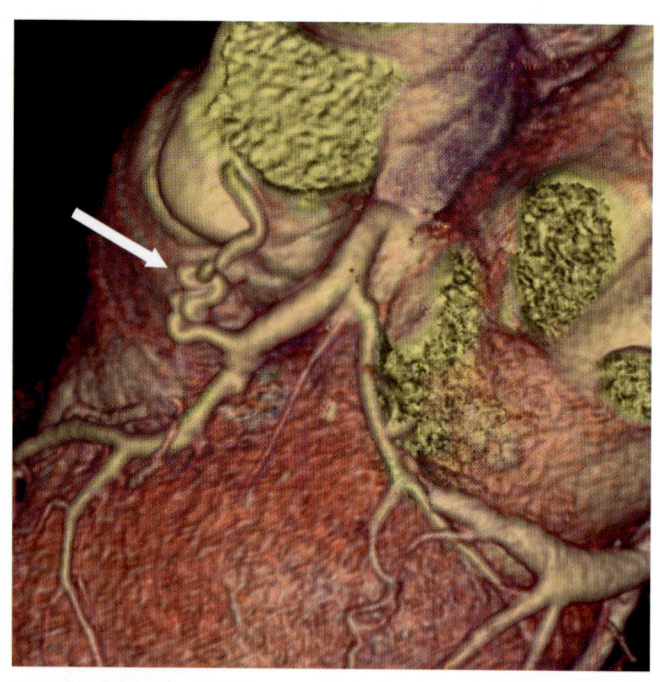

FIGURE 33-17 Multidetector CT depicts a small fistula (*arrow*) with communication between the LAD artery and pulmonary artery.

CONCLUSION

This chapter has reviewed the appearance of the most commonly encountered coronary anomalies. Coronary artery anomalies are uncommon, but they can be clinically significant. Approximately 80% of anomalies are considered benign without significant clinical sequelae; the remaining 20% can potentially cause symptoms and may be responsible for significant disease. Physicians interpreting coronary CT and MR angiography need to be aware of the appearance, prevalence, and clinical significance of coronary artery anomalies. MRI and multidetector CT are very useful in the detection and characterization of anomalous coronary arteries.

> **KEY POINTS**
>
> - Coronary anomalies are encountered in approximately 2% of patients.
> - CT and MRI can accurately depict the origin and course of coronary anomalies.
> - Potentially serious coronary anomalies are anomalous interarterial coronary arteries that pass between the aorta and pulmonary artery, single coronary arteries, arteries arising from the pulmonary arteries, and coronary fistulas.

SUGGESTED READINGS

Angelini P, Flamm SD. Newer concepts for imaging anomalous aortic origin of the coronary arteries in adults. Catheter Cardiovasc Interv 2007; 69:942-954.

Cademartiri F, Runza G, Luccichenti G, et al. Coronary artery anomalies: incidence, pathophysiology, clinical relevance and role of diagnostic imaging. Radiol Med (Torino) 2006; 111:376-391.

Dodd JD, Ferencik M, Liberthson RR, et al. Congenital anomalies of coronary artery origin in adults: 64-MDCT appearance. AJR Am J Roentgenol 2007; 188:W138-W146.

Kim SY, Seo JB, Do KH, et al. Coronary artery anomalies: classification and ECG-gated multi-detector row CT findings with angiographic correlation. RadioGraphics 2006; 26:317-334.

Manghat NE, Morgan-Hughes GJ, Marshall AJ, et al. Multidetector row computed tomography: imaging congenital coronary artery anomalies in adults. Heart 2005; 91:1515-1522.

McConnell MV, Stuber M, Manning WJ. Clinical role of coronary magnetic resonance angiography in the diagnosis of anomalous coronary arteries. J Cardiovasc Magn Reson 2000; 2:217-224.

Welker M, Salanitri J, Deshpande VS, et al. Coronary artery anomalies diagnosed by magnetic resonance angiography. Australas Radiol 2006; 50:114-121.

REFERENCES

1. Angelini P, Villason S, Chan A, et al. Normal and anomalous coronary arteries in humans. In Coronary Artery Anomalies, A Comprehensive Approach. Philadelphia, Lippincott Williams & Wilkins, 1999, pp 27-151.
2. Click RL, Holmes DR, Vlietstra RE, et al. Anomalous coronary arteries: location, degree of atherosclerosis and effect on survival—a report from the Coronary Artery Surgery Study. J Am Coll Cardiol 1989; 13:531-537.
3. Yamanaka O, Hobbs RE. Coronary artery anomalies in 126,595 patients undergoing coronary arteriography. Catheter Cardiovasc Diagn 1990; 21:28-40.
4. Levin DC, Fellows KE, Abrams HL. Hemodynamically significant primary anomalies of the coronary arteries: angiographic aspects. Circulation 1978; 58:25-34.
5. Liberthson RR, Dinsmore RE, Fallon JT. Aberrant coronary artery origin from the aorta: report of 18 patients, review of literature and delineation of natural history and management. Circulation 1979; 59:748-754.
6. Baltaxe HA, Wixson D. The incidence of congenital anomalies of the coronary arteries in the adult population. Radiology 1977; 122:47-52.
7. Chaitman BR, Lesperance J, Saltiel J, et al. Clinical, angiographic, and hemodynamic findings in patients with anomalous origin of the coronary arteries. Circulation 1976; 53:122-131.
8. Engel HJ, Torres C, Page HL. Major variations in anatomical origin of the coronary arteries: angiographic observations in 4,250 patients without associated congenital heart disease. Cathet Cardiovasc Diagn 1975; 1:157-169.
9. Garg N, Tewari S, Kapoor A, et al. Primary congenital anomalies of the coronary arteries: a coronary arteriographic study. Int J Cardiol 2000; 74:39-46.
10. Kimbiris D, Iskandrian AS, Segal BL, et al. Anomalous aortic origin of coronary arteries. Circulation 1978; 58:606-615.
11. Basso C, Maron BJ, Corrado D, et al. Clinical profile of congenital coronary artery anomalies with origin from the wrong aortic sinus leading to sudden death in young competitive athletes. J Am Coll Cardiol 2000; 35:1493-1501.
12. McConnell MV, Stuber M, Manning WJ. Clinical role of coronary magnetic resonance angiography in the diagnosis of anomalous coronary arteries. J Cardiovasc Magn Reson 2000; 2:217-224.
13. Virmani R, Burke AP, Farb A. Sudden cardiac death. Cardiovasc Pathol 2001; 10:275-282.
14. Cox ID, Bunce N, Fluck DS. Failed sudden cardiac death in a patient with an anomalous origin of the right coronary artery. Circulation 2000; 102:1461-1462.
15. Wesselhoeft H, Fawcett JS, Johnson AL. Anomalous origin of the left coronary artery from the pulmonary trunk: its clinical spectrum, pathology and pathophysiology, based on a review of 140 cases with seven further cases. Circulation 1968; 38:403-425.
16. Eckart RE, Scoville SL, Campbell CL, et al. Sudden death in young adults: a 25-year review of autopsies in military recruits. Ann intern Med 2004; 141:829-834.
17. Ropers D, Moshage W, Daniel WG, et al. Visualization of coronary artery anomalies and their anatomic course by contrast-enhanced electron beam tomography and three-dimensional reconstruction. Am J Cardiol 2001; 87:193-197.
18. Yoshimura N, Hamada S, Takamiya M, et al. Coronary artery anomalies with a shunt: evaluation with electron-beam CT. J Comput Assist Tomogr 1998; 22:682-686.
19. Post JC, van Rossum AC, Bronzwaer JG, et al. Magnetic resonance angiography of anomalous coronary arteries: a new gold standard for delineating the proximal course? Circulation 1995; 92:3163-3171.
20. Bunce NH, Lorenz CH, Keegan J, et al. Coronary artery anomalies: assessment with free-breathing three-dimensional coronary MR angiography. Radiology 2003; 227:201-208.
21. McConnell MV, Stuber M, Manning WJ. Clinical role of coronary magnetic resonance angiography in the diagnosis of anomalous coronary arteries. J Cardiovasc Magn Reson 2000; 2:217-224.
22. Taylor AM, Thorne SA, Rubens MP, et al. Coronary artery imaging in grown up congenital heart disease: complementary role of

magnetic resonance and x-ray coronary angiography. Circulation 2000; 101:1670-1678.
23. Shi H, Aschoff AJ, Brambs HJ, et al. Multislice CT imaging of anomalous coronary arteries. Eur Radiol 2004; 14:2172-2181.
24. van Ooijen PMA, Dorgelo J, Zijlstra F, et al. Detection, visualization and evaluation of anomalous coronary anatomy on 16-slice multidetector-row CT. Eur Radiol 2004; 14:2163-2171.
25. Schmid M, Achenbach S, Ludwig J, et al. Visualization of coronary artery anomalies by contrast-enhanced multi-detector row spiral computed tomography. Int J Cardiol 2006; 111:430-435.
26. Schmitt R, Froehner S, Brunn J, et al. Congenital anomalies of the coronary arteries: imaging with contrast-enhanced, multidetector computed tomography. Eur Radiol 2005; 15:1110-1121.
27. Deibler AR, Kuzo RS, Vohringer M, et al. Imaging of congenital coronary anomalies with multislice computed tomography. Mayo Clin Proc 2004; 79:1017-1023.
28. Datta J, White CS, Gilkeson RC, et al. Anomalous coronary arteries in adults: depiction at multi-detector row CT angiography. Radiology 2005; 235:812-818.
29. Roberts WC, Siegel RJ, Zipes DP. Origin of the right coronary artery from the left sinus of Valsalva and its functional consequences: analysis of 10 necropsy patients. Am J Cardiol 1982; 49:863-868.
30. Cheitlin MD, De Castro CM, McAllister HA. Sudden death as a complication of anomalous left coronary origin from the anterior sinus of Valsalva: a not-so-minor congenital anomaly. Circulation 1974; 50:780-787.
31. Chaitman BR, Lesperance J, Saltiel J, et al. Clinical, angiographic, and hemodynamic findings in patients with anomalous origin of the coronary arteries. Circulation 1976; 53:122-131.
32. Dodge-Khatami A, Mavroudis C, Backer CL. Anomalous origin of the left coronary artery from the pulmonary artery: collective review of surgical therapy. Ann Thorac Surg 2002; 74:946-955.
33. Wesselhoeft H, Fawcett JS, Johnson AL. Anomalous origin of the left coronary artery from the pulmonary trunk: its clinical spectrum, pathology and pathophysiology, based on review of 140 cases with seven further cases. Circulation 1968; 38:403-425.
34. Greenberg MA, Fish BG, Spindola-Franco H. Congenital anomalies of coronary artery: classification and significance. Radiol Clin North Am 1989; 27:1127-1146.
35. Vlodaver Z, Neufeld HN, Edwards JE. Pathology of coronary disease. Semin Roentgenol 1972; 7:376-394.
36. Danias PG, Stuber M, McConnell MV, et al. The diagnosis of congenital coronary anomalies with magnetic resonance imaging. Coron Artery Dis 2001; 12:621-626.
37. Sajja LR, Farooqi A, Shaik MS, et al. Dual left anterior descending coronary artery: surgical revascularization in 4 patients. Tex Heart Inst J 2000; 27:292-296.
38. Desmet W, Vanhaecke J, Vrolix M, et al. Isolated single coronary artery: a review of 50,000 consecutive coronary angiographies. Eur Heart J 1992; 13:1637-1640.
39. Smith JC. Review of single coronary artery with report of 2 cases. Circulation 1950; 1:1168-1175.
40. Ghahrani A, Iyengar R, Cunha D, et al. Myocardial infarction due to congenital coronary artery aneurysm (with successful saphenous vein bypass graft). Am J Cardiol 1972; 29:863.
41. Mohlenkamp S, Hort W, Ge J, et al. Update on myocardial bridging. Circulation 2002; 106:2616-2622.
42. Said SA, el Gamal MI, van der Werf T. Coronary arteriovenous fistulas: collective review and management of six new cases—changing etiology, presentation, and treatment strategy. Clin Cardiol 1997; 20:748-752.
43. McNamara JJ, Gross RE. Congenital coronary artery fistula. Surgery 1969; 65:59-69.

CHAPTER 34

Indications and Patient Selection in Obstructive Coronary Disease

Eva Maria Gassner and U. Joseph Schoepf

Since the advent of ECG-synchronized cardiac CT, this modality has become a rapidly evolving tool for noninvasive imaging of the coronary arteries.[1,2] Advances in technology with fast data acquisition, improvements in temporal resolution, and high spatial resolution have contributed to the widespread acceptance of this test in a number of clinical scenarios. On the other hand, because of the rapid succession of technologic innovations, several scanner generations are currently in simultaneous clinical use.[3] During the last decade, research has mainly been restricted to feasibility testing in tune with the rapid, roughly triennial, introduction of new multidetector-row CT (MDCT) scanner generations. Only recently do we see more emerging data of the greater impact of this potentially disruptive technology on the general field of health care. Albeit scarce, we see increasing evidence illustrating the cost-effectiveness of this test in the management of coronary heart disease.[4] After years during which technologic development was focused almost exclusively on improved image quality and increased spatial resolution, particular attention is now being paid to mechanisms of radiation protection.[5] Evidence-based guidelines have recently been implemented[2,4] to steer the appropriate use and to avoid overuse of this test. This contribution aims to summarize the current indications for the use of coronary CT angiography (CTA) for assessment of obstructive native coronary artery disease (CAD).

OVERVIEW OF EVIDENCE AND TRENDS

Significant obstructive CAD is defined as a diameter stenosis of 70% or more in at least one major epicardial artery and as a 50% reduction in the case of the left main coronary artery. At coronary CTA, the assessment for hemodynamically significant coronary artery stenosis is roughly analogous to that of conventional invasive coronary angiography, which in clinical reality is ordinarily based on visual assessment and subjective estimation of stenosis severity. More objective assessment with quantitative catheter angiography is typically not routinely performed and is reserved for equivocal cases or research applications. Similarly, routine clinical coronary CTA evaluation of stenosis severity is ordinarily performed visually and subjectively, although virtually every currently available image display and analysis software platform provides semiautomated measurement tools for stenosis grading. These allow quantification of stenosis severity based on the ratio of stenosed arterial lumen relative to adjacent prestenotic and poststenotic segments with normal luminal diameters, similar to the standards as established, for instance, for intravascular ultrasound.[6]

A number of meta-analyses present an overview of the diagnostic performance of ECG-gated coronary CTA,[7,8] and the number of studies is rapidly growing. One large analysis performed a systematic review of studies based on different scanner generations,[3] illustrating the continuously improving image quality but also the growing experience of observers, as demonstrated by the high percentage of segments considered assessable with more recent scanner generations. Most important, however, a consistent performance with regard to the well-established high negative predictive value of this test, and thus the reliable exclusion of significant stenosis, is observed across scanner generations.

At present, the use of 16-slice MDCT with a gantry rotation speed of less than 500 ms is considered to meet the minimal requirements for successful ECG-gated imaging of the coronary arteries.[2]

Data illustrating the performance of noninvasive coronary CTA frequently involve small groups of patients scheduled to undergo invasive coronary angiography. These study populations tend to show characteristics that are different from those of individuals referred in clinical routine, with high pretest probability and high prevalence of disease. Consequently, one point of criticism of many previous studies has been the potential of selection bias. By Bayes' theorem, the prevalence of disease in the study group has impact on the performance of a test because the finding is overrepresented in this group. On the other hand, the preselection implies that even in patients with high pretest likelihood, stenosis can reliably be ruled out, thus rendering this test sufficiently safe for exclusion of significant coronary artery stenosis in a symptomatic patient.

False-negative findings, however rare, do occur. With regard to the clinically relevant per-patient analyses, many studies report between one and three patients who are missed by coronary CTA who have stenosis of more than 50%, a number that is fairly consistent across scanner generations, including the recently introduced dual-source CT (DSCT) technology.[10] However the majority of missed stenoses were located in distal segments that are not amenable to revascularization.[2]

Noninvasive coronary CTA tends to overestimate disease. Main causes of false-positive findings are calcifications of the vessel wall and limited visualization of small-vessel lumens due to partial volume effects.[9] The average positive predictive value is therefore moderate. Although average positive predictive values are reported to be higher with 64-slice CT,[7] reports are ambiguous even with regard to the latest scanner types.[10] Thus, coronary CTA should still be mainly regarded as a reliable tool to rule out significant obstructive disease rather than a means to estimate the severity of detected lesions.

Early evidence with use of 16-slice MDCT was characterized by excluding small vessels (<1.5 mm or <2 mm) or vessel segments with heavy calcifications or motion artifact from analysis, an approach that is not clinically feasible. More recently, in the majority of studies using 64-slice scanners, the entire coronary tree is considered for assessment. The number of nonassessable segments in the available literature has dropped from a mean 12% with 16-slice CT to 4% with 64-slice CT.[7,8]

Some criticism also has been voiced about the study design of earlier studies based on consensus interpretation for identification of coronary obstruction. Studies increasingly account for observer variability, with consistently high agreement reported for studies with 64-slice MDCT, although obtained by highly experienced readers.

SEGMENT-BASED AND PATIENT-BASED ANALYSIS

For most practical purposes, the diagnostic performance for detection of stenosis is assessed on the basis of the modified 13- to 17-coronary segment model of the American Heart Association, providing a large sample size for statistics. In recent years, a patient-based analysis is additionally performed in the majority of investigations. Patient-based analyses are generally more suitable to determine the actual clinical value as a gatekeeper by differentiating individuals who need invasive work-up from those who do not. Results of per-patient analyses tend to be more accurate because patients found to have obstructive CAD are likely to have at least one stenosis in any location of the coronary tree (nesting effect).

Indications

Throughout the available literature and for all scanner generations, it has been consistently found that ECG-synchronized coronary CTA has the ability to reliably rule out significant stenosis on the basis of the exceedingly high negative predictive value of this test. Selection of patients who most likely would benefit from noninvasive imaging of the coronary arteries is based on existing evidence on coronary CTA, known performance of conventional diagnostic procedures, and potential impact on patient management and risk estimation.[4] Supported by broad consensus among experts, coronary CTA is recommended in symptomatic patients for the initial evaluation of chest pain in the setting of low to intermediate probability of CAD.[3,5] In this context, coronary CTA is considered to have incremental value in patient management to inform the indication for invasive coronary angiography (Fig. 34-1). Of note, this target group (i.e., symptomatic patients with low to intermediate probability of CAD) is still different from the study populations on which most of the currently accepted clinical evidence is based. Invasive coronary angiography is typically not performed in patients with low probability of CAD.[11] A few studies have closed this knowledge gap. Mejboom and colleagues[10] investigated symptomatic patients at different levels of pretest likelihood and demonstrated that the performance of coronary CTA is inversely related to the probability of CAD. Coronary CTA was more accurate in patients with low to intermediate likelihood (Figs. 34-2 and 34-3) than in groups with high probability. The limited value in the latter group was explained by the high prevalence of advanced disease with heavy calcifications.

Therefore, symptomatic patients with high pretest probability are not appropriate candidates for noninvasive coronary CTA because this test is unlikely to add incremental value in their diagnostic work-up. Rather, invasive coronary angiography with the option of direct intervention and revascularization is the more appropriate initial procedure in the management of such patients (Fig. 34-4).[9]

Asymptomatic Patients

Cardiac CT is insufficiently validated for the application in asymptomatic individuals and is not currently recommended for this group.[2,4] The characteristics of this test involving relatively high radiation doses and unclear cost/benefit currently do not support the use of coronary CTA as a screening modality.[2,9] Whether coronary CTA may in the future have a role for better risk stratification in asymptomatic individuals at high Framingham risk[12] or to detect silent CAD (e.g., in diabetic patients)[13] remains to be established.

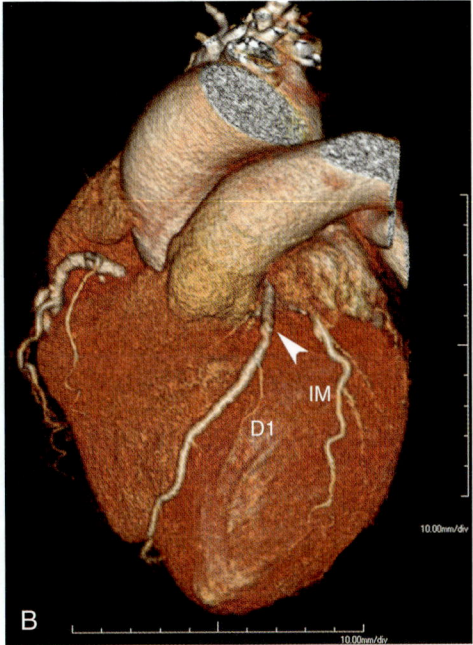

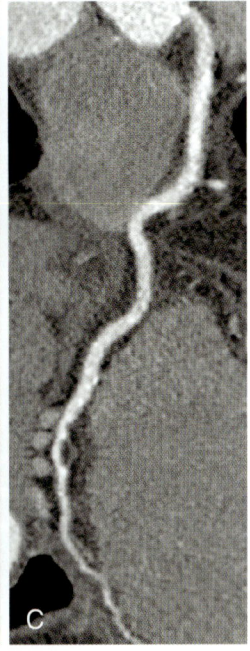

FIGURE 34-1 A 64-year-old woman presenting with atypical chest pain; intermediate pretest probability according to age, sex, and quality of the chest pain. Contrast-enhanced coronary CT angiogram, obtained at a heart rate of 70 beats/min, reveals minimal nonobstructive coronary atherosclerosis. **A,** Curved multiplanar reformation of the left anterior descending coronary artery shows a small mixed plaque deposit at the level of the mid vessel (*arrowhead*). **B,** Volume rendered display of the small plaque in segment 7 of the coronary artery tree (*arrowhead*). **C,** Curved multiplanar reformation of the right coronary artery displays minimal vessel wall irregularities. (IM, intermediate artery; D1, first diagonal branch).

Estimation of Cardiovascular Risk and Pretest Probability for Coronary Artery Disease

An asymptomatic individual's risk for future cardiovascular events is usually estimated on the basis of the traditional Framingham risk score, determining absolute and relative risk (compared with an age- and sex-adjusted low-risk group) of coronary heart disease.[14] Risk is stratified to determine the appropriate level of aggressiveness in risk modification for disease prevention.

Pretest probability, on the other hand, is estimated in symptomatic patients, based on the quality of the chest pain (typical, atypical, and noncardiac quality; Table 34-1). Beyond symptoms, probability depends on age and gender (Table 34-2) and, as in the Duke score, may also include risk factors.[12]

Role of Coronary CT Angiography in the Context of Other Noninvasive Tests

Exercise testing and stress echocardiography are firmly established in the diagnostic algorithm of CAD, supported by extensive population-based evidence. Noninvasive stress testing provides functional and clinical information about the significance of myocardial hypoperfusion. Treadmill testing is a readily available low-cost procedure and is the primary tool in the diagnostic work-up of patients with suspected CAD. Similar to noninvasive angiography, exercise testing performs most accurately in patients with intermediate likelihood for CAD.[13]

Stress echocardiography is indicated as a second-line tool for patients who are unable to exercise.[15] With recent developments in tissue Doppler imaging, improvements in the diagnostic performance of stress echocardiography have been reported. However, the modality is more sophisticated, and the diagnostic value depends on acoustic window and operator expertise. A considerable range of sensitivities and specificities is reported for both exercise testing and stress echocardiography to describe the accuracy of these tests for detection of significant CAD.[15] Of note, the diagnostic accuracy of stress testing is recognized to be decreased in women, resulting in a higher rate of post-test referrals to invasive coronary angiography for women.[16]

Given the variable performance of noninvasive stress testing, particularly in women, a group of symptomatic and asymptomatic individuals is left in whom the probability after stress testing remains indeterminate. According to the National Cardiovascular Data Registry, a considerable part of invasive angiography is indicated by false-positive results of stress tests.[17] Thus, most experts agree on the usefulness of coronary CTA in patients with inconclusive or uninterpretable stress test results.[2,4]

Patient-Related Considerations

Heavy Calcifications

Heavy calcifications tend to cause overestimation of the severity of lesions and are one of the most important sources of unassessable segments and false-positive findings at coronary CTA.[2] The presence of calcium causes

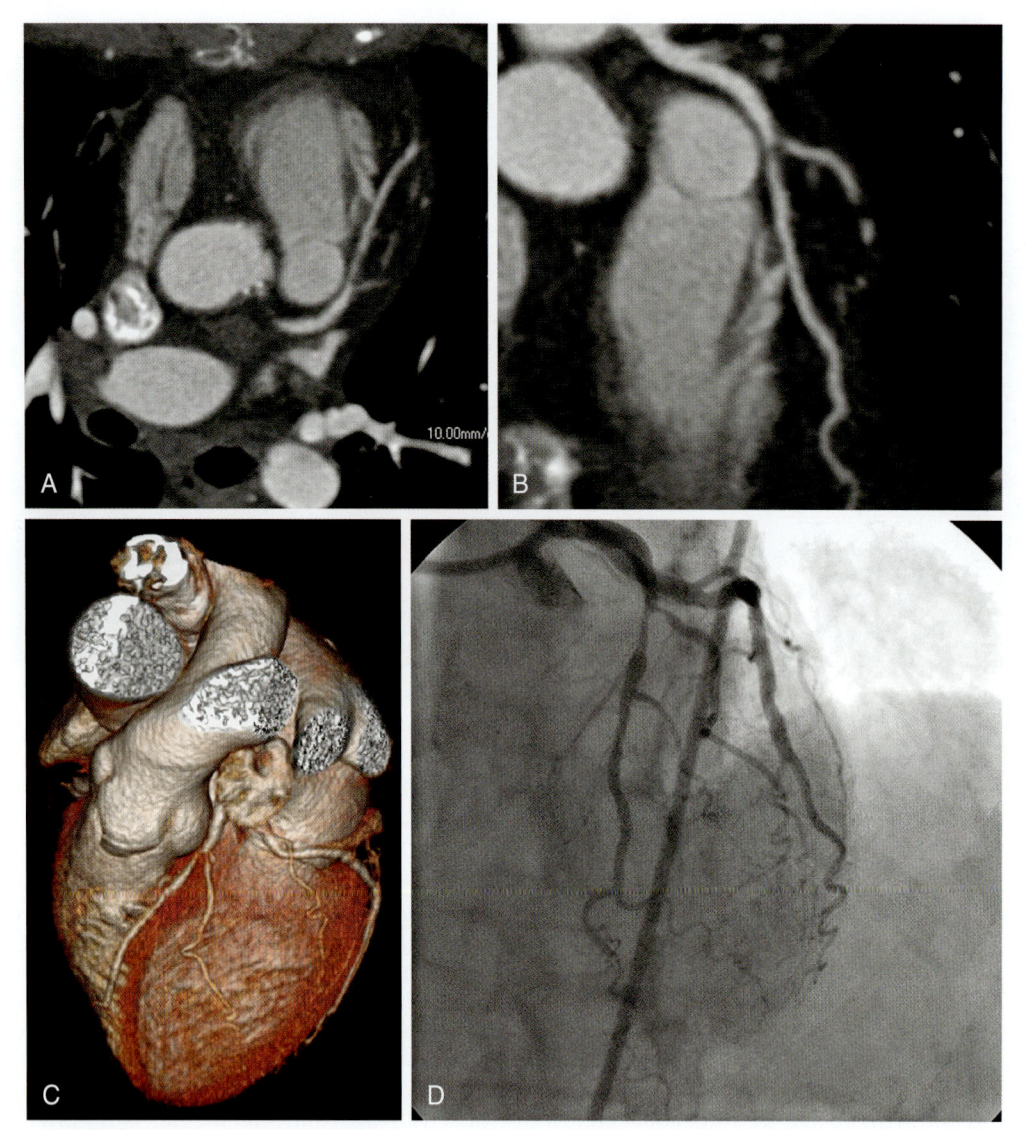

■ **FIGURE 34-2** A 56-year-old woman with typical chest pain, no risk factors; intermediate pretest probability; Agatston calcium score of 88 (75th age- and gender-corrected percentile); heart rate during scanning was 68 beats/min. **A,** Noninvasive coronary CTA with multiplanar reformation along the proximal left anterior descending coronary artery reveals high-grade stenosis, involving the D1 ostium. Also note the extensive, predominantly noncalcified aortic wall disease. **B,** Curved multiplanar reformation of the left anterior descending coronary artery. **C,** Volume rendered images show the stenosis at the orifice of D1. Note a small calcified plaque core at the ostium of D1. **D,** Invasive coronary angiogram confirming stenosis of the left anterior descending coronary artery at the D1 ostium.

"blooming" artifacts that consequently may obscure noncalcified plaque components and portions of the residual vessel lumen, which in extreme cases (Fig. 34-5) may interfere with coronary CTA interpretation. Although extensive calcifications are recognized as a major limiting factor, detailed data (e.g., with calcium score subclasses) illustrating the impact on diagnostic performance of coronary CTA remain rare.[18,19] Whereas calcifications are frequently reported to decrease the specificity of coronary CTA because of lesion overestimation, there appears to be no substantial negative effect on the overall clinically relevant high negative predictive value[20,21] because of the aforementioned nesting effect. Particularly with newer scanner generations with improved temporal and spatial resolution combined with advanced visualization tools, most experts agree that extensive calcifications should no longer be considered a contraindication to coronary CTA. Moreover, if it is used appropriately in the low- to intermediate-risk groups (see earlier), the prevalence of excessive calcifications in the target group should be within limits (Fig. 34-6).

The known relative limitations due to heavy calcifications are unlikely to be overcome soon because voxel size as a determinant factor of blooming artifacts is at the limits of the technically feasible spatial resolution at sustainable radiation dose. Improvements might be expected from

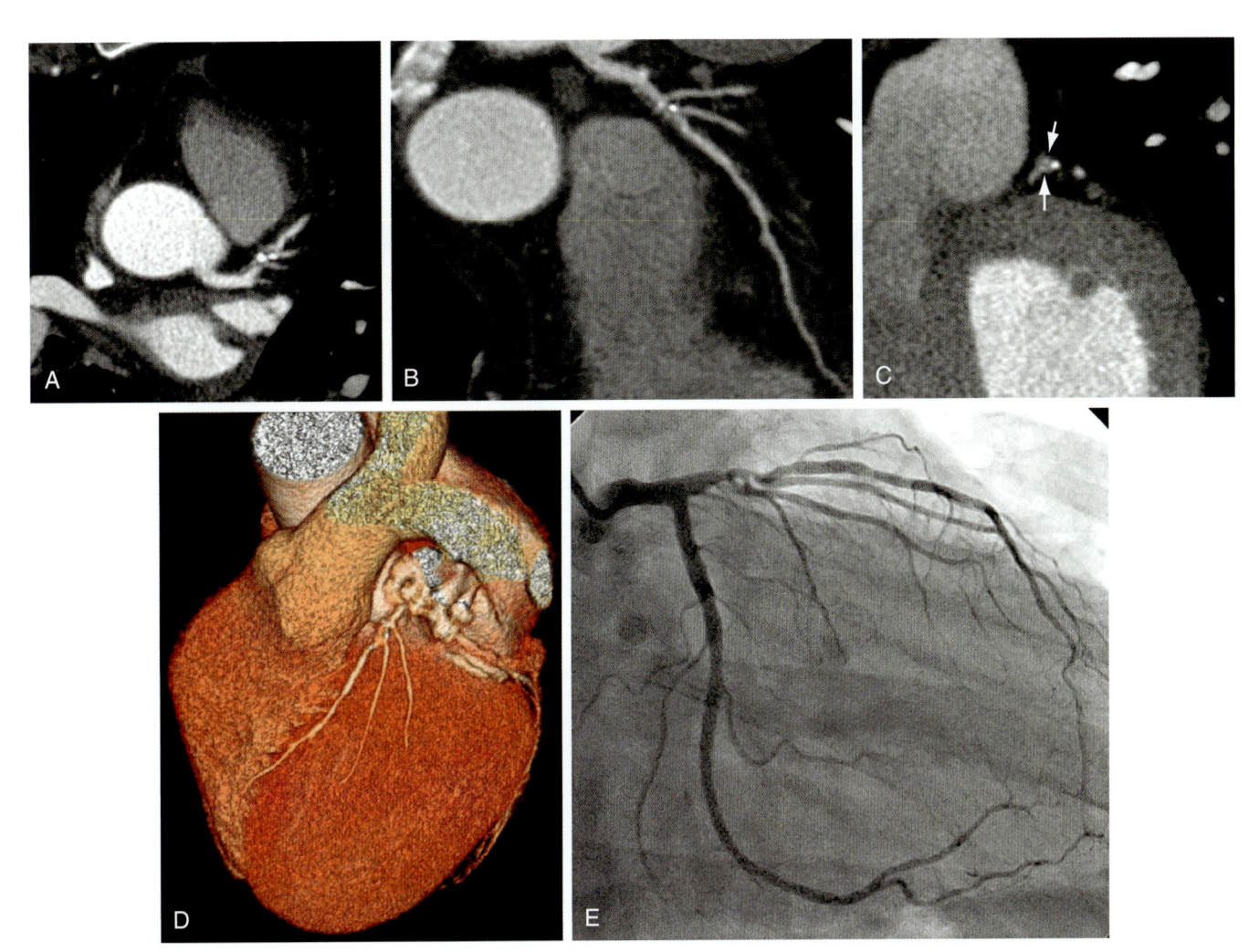

■ **FIGURE 34-3** A 60-year-old man presenting with atypical chest pain; intermediate pretest probability; calcium score of 38 (55th percentile). Coronary CTA shows complex stenosis of the proximal left anterior descending coronary artery with ostial involvement of the first and second diagonal branches. **A,** Multiplanar reformation along the proximal left anterior descending coronary artery. **B,** Curved multiplanar reformations display the mixed character of the underlying plaque. **C,** Cross section through the stenotic area. Large arrow points to the residual lumen; small arrow indicates a calcified nodule, subject to partial volume averaging. Note also a large high-attenuation deposit. **D,** Volume rendered image displaying involvement of the first and second diagonal branches. **E,** Invasive coronary catheter confirms the presence of left anterior descending coronary artery stenosis at the takeoff of D1 and D2.

limiting motion artifacts at the interface of calcium and surrounding structures by high temporal resolution. According to observations using DSCT technology, a high negative predictive value can be maintained in the presence of severe calcifications.[22]

Heart Rate and Heart Rate Variability

The need for a defined temporal window per heart cycle to acquire sufficient data for image reconstruction makes temporal resolution the most important factor to determine diagnostic accuracy. For imaging of the coronary arteries, the reconstruction interval is preferably placed in the relatively quiet mid-diastole. Because the duration of diastole shows a nonproportional shortening in relation to systole at higher heart rates, a stable sinus rhythm with heart rates below 65 beats/min is recommended by many authors for both 16-slice MDCT and single-source 64-slice CT scanners[23]; some guidelines propose a limit of 70 beats/min.[4] These relatively slow heart rates are ordinarily induced by pharmacologic rate control (e.g., β blockade), which may have the added benefit of reducing heart rate variability.[24] However, faster and more irregular heart rates are considered relative contraindications to coronary CTA, at least with 64-slice single-source CT, so that diagnostic image quality ordinarily can be obtained in cases in which pharmacologic rate control fails.[23]

Currently available DSCT scanners offer a temporal resolution of 83 ms, further widening the scope of patients who are eligible for this test. Most published studies agree

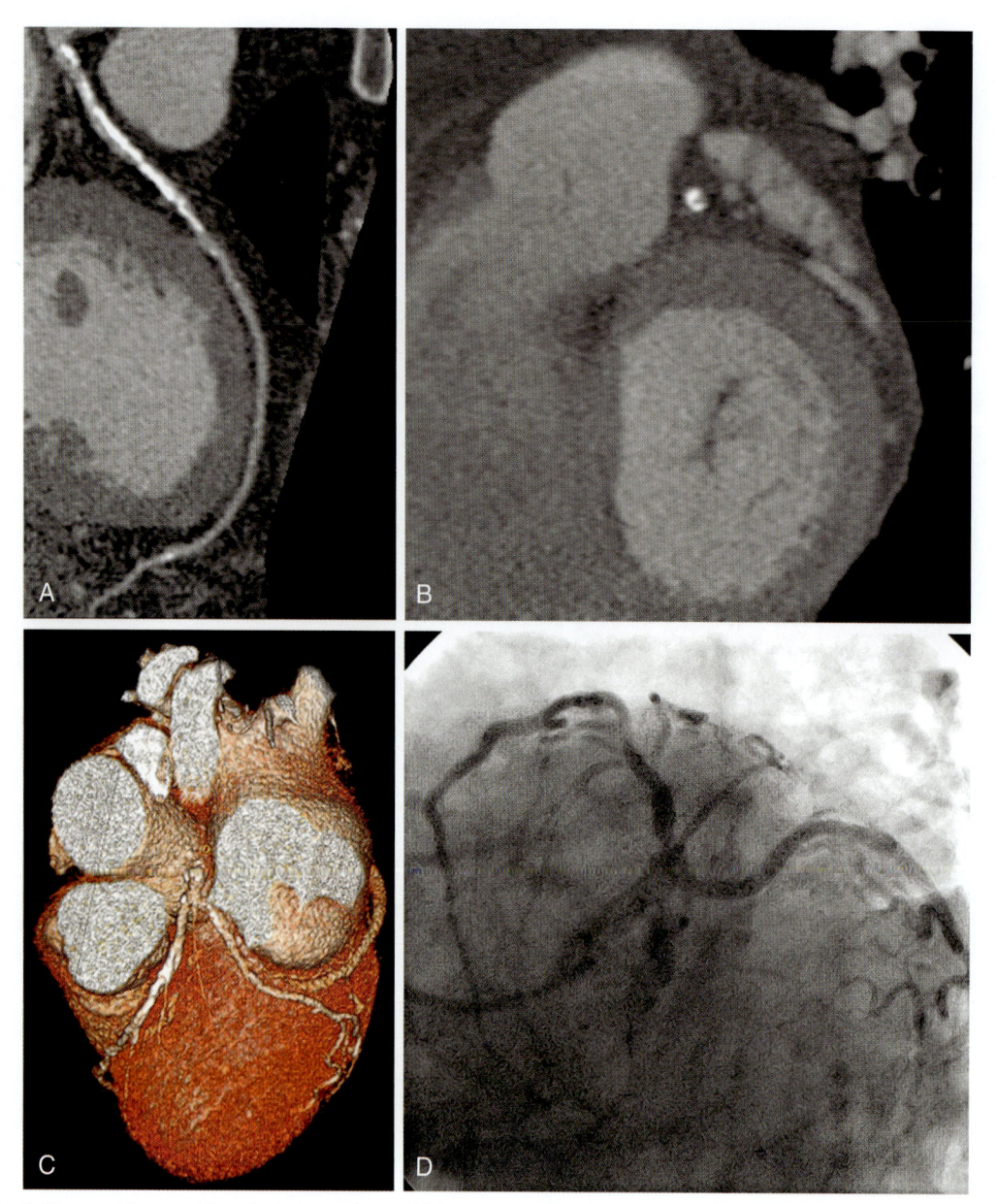

■ **FIGURE 34-4** A 73-year-old man with typical chest pain and high pretest probability. Calcium score of 1800 limits the diagnostic value of noninvasive coronary CTA. **A,** Curved multiplanar reformation of the left main artery and the left anterior descending coronary artery shows diffuse calcified disease partially obscuring the lumen, thereby precluding the accurate assessment of the degree of obstruction. **B,** Cross section through the left anterior descending coronary artery obtained perpendicular to the vessel course displays blooming artifacts due to circumferential calcification of the vessel wall. **C,** Volume rendering illustrates diffuse atherosclerotic disease changes. **D,** Conventional coronary angiography in left anterior oblique projection reveals a short-segment stenosis at the left anterior descending coronary artery ostium, not sufficiently characterized at coronary CTA.

TABLE 34-1 Clinical Classification of Chest Pain

Typical angina (definite)
 (1) Substernal chest discomfort with a characteristic quality and duration that is (2) provoked by exertion or emotional stress and (3) relieved by rest or nitroglycerin
Atypical angina (probable)
 Meets 2 of the above characteristics
Noncardiac chest pain
 Meets ≤1 of the typical angina characteristics

From Gibbons RJ, Chatterjee K, Daley J, et al. ACC/AHA/ACP-ASIM guidelines for the management of patients with chronic stable angina: executive summary and recommendations. A Report of the American College of Cardiology/American Heart Association Task Force on Practice Guidelines (Committee on Management of Patients with Chronic Stable Angina). Circulation 1999; 99:2829-2848.

that DSCT allows investigation of patients with high and irregular heart rates with diagnostic results so that pharmacologic heart rate control can be abandoned.[25] Recent investigations compared the performance of DSCT technology between groups with different heart rates and confirmed the robustness of this technology for exclusion of significant stenosis even at heart rates as high as 100 beats/min.[25] There is initial evidence that the high temporal resolution of recent-generation scanners along with the ability of ECG editing may expand the use of this technology to the population of patients with atrial fibrillation, which traditionally had been considered a contraindication to the successful use of coronary CTA (Fig. 34-7).[4]

TABLE 34-2 Pretest Probability of Coronary Artery Disease According to Age and Sex

Age (yr)	Gender	Typical/Definite Angina Pectoris	Atypical/Probable Angina Pectoris	Nonanginal Chest Pain	Asymptomatic
30-39	Men	Intermediate	Intermediate	Low	Very low
	Women	Intermediate	Very low	Very low	Very low
40-49	Men	High	Intermediate	Intermediate	Low
	Women	Intermediate	Low	Very low	Very low
50-59	Men	High	Intermediate	Intermediate	Low
	Women	Intermediate	Intermediate	Low	Very low
60-69	Men	High	Intermediate	Intermediate	Low
	Women	High	Intermediate	Intermediate	Low

High: greater than 90% pretest probability; intermediate: between 10% and 90% pretest probability; low: between 5% and 10% pretest probability; very low: less than 5% pretest probability.
From Gibbons RJ, Balady GJ, Beasley JW, et al. ACC/AHA guidelines for exercise testing: executive summary. A report of the American College of Cardiology/American Heart Association Task Force on Practice Guidelines (Committee on Exercise Testing). Circulation 1997; 96:345-354.

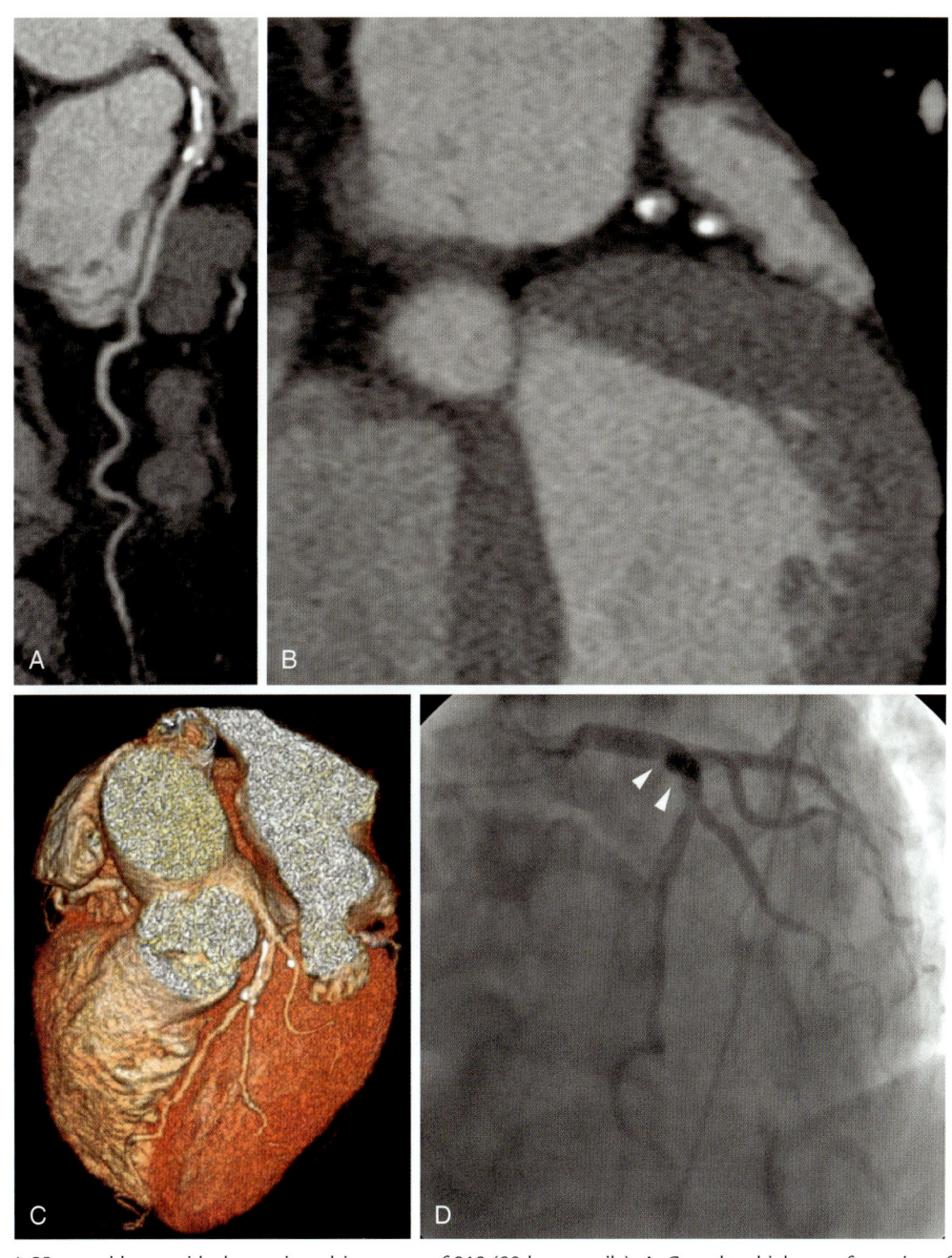

■ **FIGURE 34-5** A 55-year-old man with chest pain; calcium score of 919 (90th percentile). **A,** Curved multiplanar reformation of the left anterior descending coronary artery. Note contiguous calcified plaque of the proximal vessel. **B,** Cross section through the left anterior descending coronary artery and intermediate artery shows blooming at the interfaces of calcium and vessel lumen, resulting in overestimation of stenosis. **C,** Volume rendered image demonstrates the distribution of disease, extending from the origin of the left anterior descending coronary artery to the D1 ostium. Note the small plaque of the intermediate artery also seen in **B**. **D,** Invasive coronary angiography with intubation of the left system shows luminal irregularities of the left anterior descending coronary artery (*arrowheads*) without relevant stenosis.

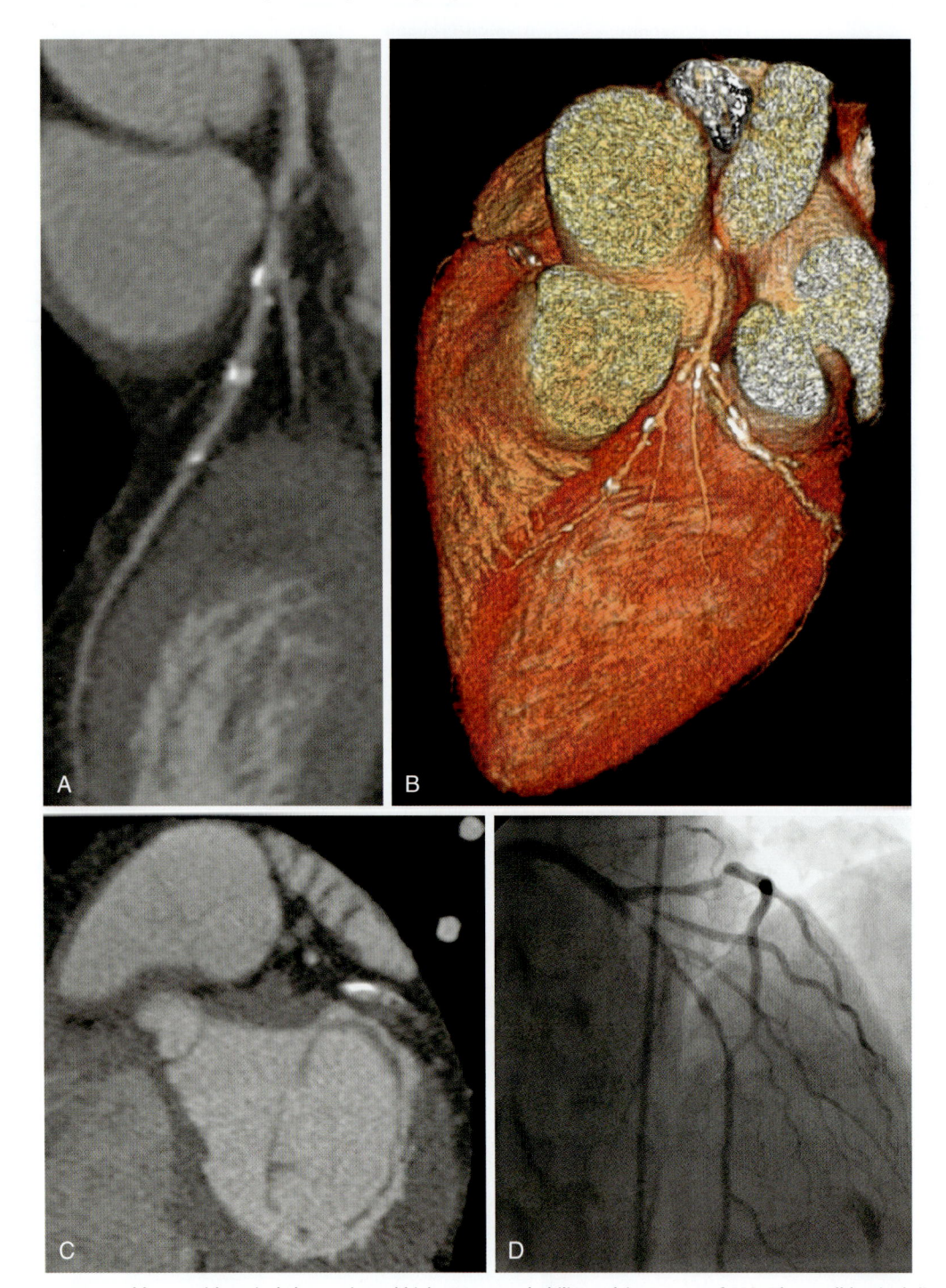

FIGURE 34-6 A 56-year-old man with typical chest pain and high pretest probability; calcium score of 528. The small luminal diameters are consistent with the patient's history of diabetes mellitus. **A,** Curved multiplanar reformation of the left anterior descending coronary artery. **B,** Volume rendering reveals high-grade stenosis caused by noncalcified plaque. **C,** Filiform luminal compromise demonstrated on multiplanar reformation in orthogonal orientation to the vessel course. **D,** Corresponding invasive coronary angiogram shows the short, severe stenosis of the proximal left anterior descending coronary artery.

Obesity

Obesity is defined as a body mass index (BMI) above 30, and extreme obesity by a BMI of 40 or more. In 2004, the prevalence of obesity among adults in the United States was 32%, with an upward trend.[26] Noninvasive visualization of the coronary arteries in obese patients represents a considerable challenge to ECG-gated coronary CTA. High image noise levels result in reduced spatial and contrast resolution (Fig. 34-8), with impaired evaluation of small vessels. Few studies evaluated the impact of obesity,

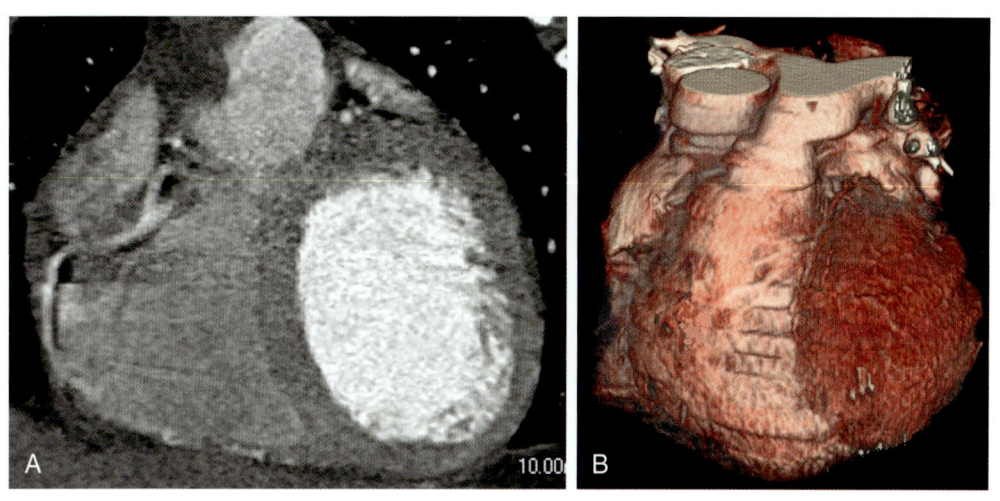

■ **FIGURE 34-7** High heart rate: 49-year-old woman with new-onset atrial fibrillation, referred for exclusion of coronary artery disease and contraindications to pharmacologic rate control. Images obtained on a 64-slice single-source CT system at a mean heart rate of 124 beats/min. **A,** Paracoronal multiplanar reformation shows misregistration artifacts in the course of the right coronary artery caused by premature beats. Note blurring of the right coronary artery and double contouring as a result of cardiac motion. **B,** Volume rendered image shows stair-step artifacts of the right myocardial contour.

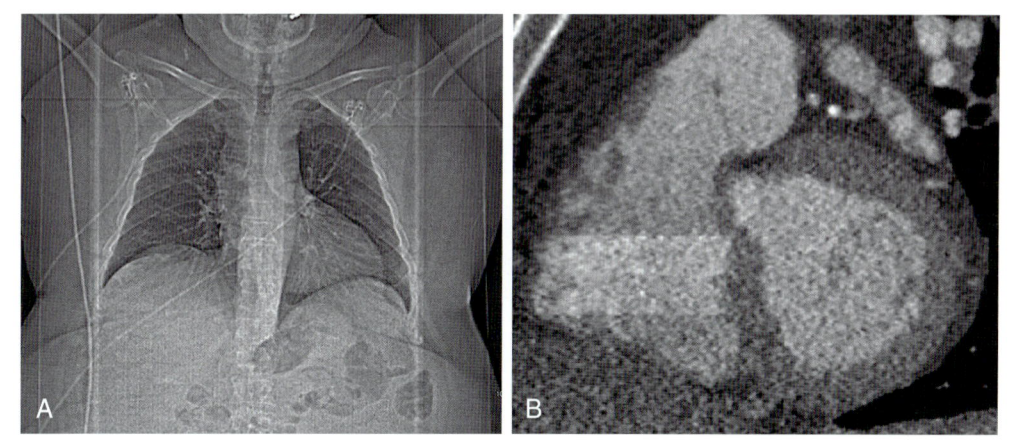

■ **FIGURE 34-8** Obese patient. **A,** Topogram (scout view) of a patient with a BMI of 38.3 (height, 1.98 m; weight, 150.3 kg). **B,** Paraxial multiplanar reformation through the left anterior descending coronary artery and intermediate artery. Image noise with reduced spatial and contrast resolution, combined with beam hardening artifacts from calcium deposits, results in considerable blooming and hazy delineation of the vessel lumen.

as defined by a BMI above 30, on the diagnostic accuracy of coronary CTA. Raff and coworkers[20] reported a reduced negative predictive value in a sample size of 35 patients. Strategies to reduce image noise comprise lowering of the pitch to accumulate data samples, increasing tube current, and modifying injection protocols with higher iodine concentration and high flow rates. Increasing kilovolt levels is not beneficial, given the loss of contrast resolution with high energy beams.[23] An expert paper proposes a BMI limit of 40 or lower for reasonable image quality of noninvasive coronary arteriography (Fig. 34-9).[4]

Renal Insufficiency

The amount of intravenous iodinated contrast medium required for noninvasive coronary CTA could be substantially reduced with the introduction of faster scanners with shorter scan duration in the range of 6 to 12 seconds, depending on scanner type and scan length. Because ECG-gated CT of the heart ordinarily represents an elective examination, an even more intense risk/benefit analysis is necessary before indicating coronary CTA in patients with elevated serum creatinine levels of above 1.8 mg/dL.[4]

EMERGING APPLICATIONS

Evaluation of Acute Chest Pain in the Emergency Department Setting

Acute chest pain is the second most common reason for emergency department visits. A particular diagnostic challenge is the subset of patients who present with

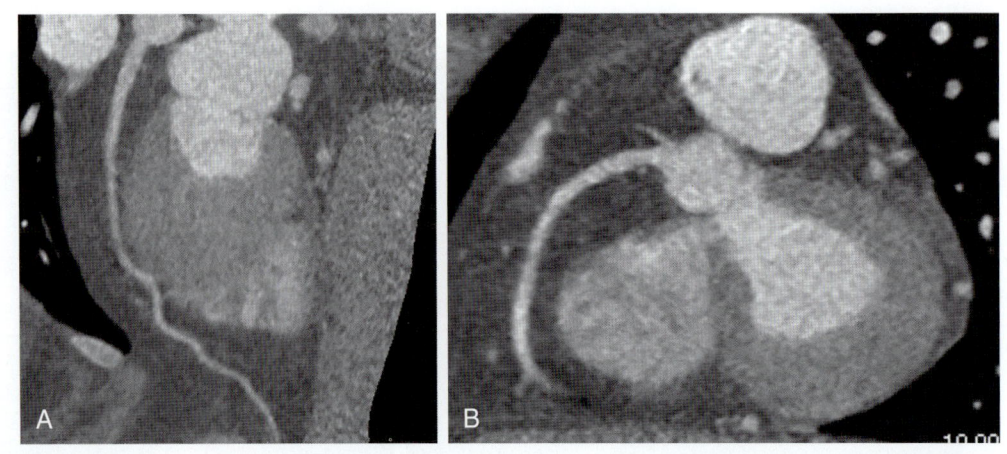

FIGURE 34-9 Obesity and high heart rate: 36-year-old woman with atypical chest pain and low pretest probability based on chest pain quality, age, and gender. Risk factors such as hyperlipidemia and history of smoking were present. BMI was 40. ECG-gated contrast-enhanced coronary CTA examination was performed with DSCT at a heart rate of 108 beats/min, without administration of β blockers. **A,** Curved multiplanar reformation of the left anterior descending coronary artery. **B,** Paracoronal multiplanar reformation shows the main course of the right coronary artery. Increased noise and mild blurring due to cardiac motion are present, but image quality is sufficient for noninvasive exclusion of CAD.

unspecific chest pain, with negative cardiac biomarkers, and without ECG changes. In this group of patients, there is a small but not negligible chance that the chest pain is of cardiac origin, constituting about 15% in this population according to current estimates.[27] To identify this minority, traditional clinical guidelines recommend observation for 12 hours[12] before resuming the diagnostic algorithm with a stress test. Fast scanners allow ECG-synchronized examination of the entire thorax with motion-free visualization of the cardiopulmonary vessels, enabling a "triple rule-out" protocol, that is, the exclusion of the major entities causing acute chest pain (obstructive CAD, acute aortic syndromes, pulmonary embolism).[28,29] Other noncardiac causes of acute chest pain that are amenable to diagnosis at coronary CTA include the full spectrum of thoracic CT findings in this setting, such as pneumothorax, pneumonia, pleuritis, hiatal hernia, other disorders of the upper gastrointestinal tract, and malignant neoplasms. For type A aortic dissection, ECG-synchronized examinations allow better identification of intimal tear sites and motion-free depiction of the flap, which may involve a coronary ostium or cause coronary dissection. Diagnostic pitfalls arising from the artifactual impression of aortic dissection secondary to cardiac motion artifacts along the aortic root can be successfully avoided. Overall, however, acute aortic syndromes appear to be the least commonly encountered pathologic process in the patients undergoing coronary CTA assessment for acute chest pain.

Cardiac causes of acute chest pain are exacerbated chronic obstructive CAD and acute coronary syndrome, with plaque rupture and thrombus formation (Fig. 34-10). Data illustrating the utility of ECG-synchronized thoracic CTA for acute chest pain are evolving and encouraging yet limited in number at this time.[30-32] Validation remains a problem related to the low prevalence of obstructive CAD in this population of patients. Even more than in the elective setting, the indication for noninvasive CTA in the emergency department must be stringent to avoid inappropriate application and overuse and must be restricted to patients with atypical chest pain with low to intermediate probability for CAD with negative biomarkers and ECG.[31] Also in this population, patient management should be primarily based on the high negative predictive value for ruling out significant stenosis, and patients with equivalent findings at CT should undergo the traditional work-up for acute chest pain.

Preoperative Evaluation

Noncardiac Surgery

Guidelines recommend stratification of perioperative risk based on patient-related predictors and surgical risk.[32] Preoperative invasive coronary angiography is routinely performed in patients with known cardiac conditions, such as heart failure, arrhythmia, or advanced valvular disease, to assess eligibility for and risk of surgery in such patients. Stress testing is recommended in the presence of less severe clinical risk factors before procedures that carry high (e.g., vascular surgery) or intermediate surgical risk. Noninvasive imaging with coronary CTA in the preoperative setting is not integrated in the current algorithm.[4] However, because the American College of Cardiology/American Heart Association Guidelines for Perioperative Evaluation recognize the limitations of exercise testing for detection of significant coronary stenosis,[32] preoperative spiral CTA might be considered to incrementally contribute for further work-up of patients with inconclusive stress test results before surgery.

Cardiac Surgery

A variety of studies investigated the performance of noninvasive coronary CTA in patients scheduled for heart valve surgery. In part, this relatively large evidence base

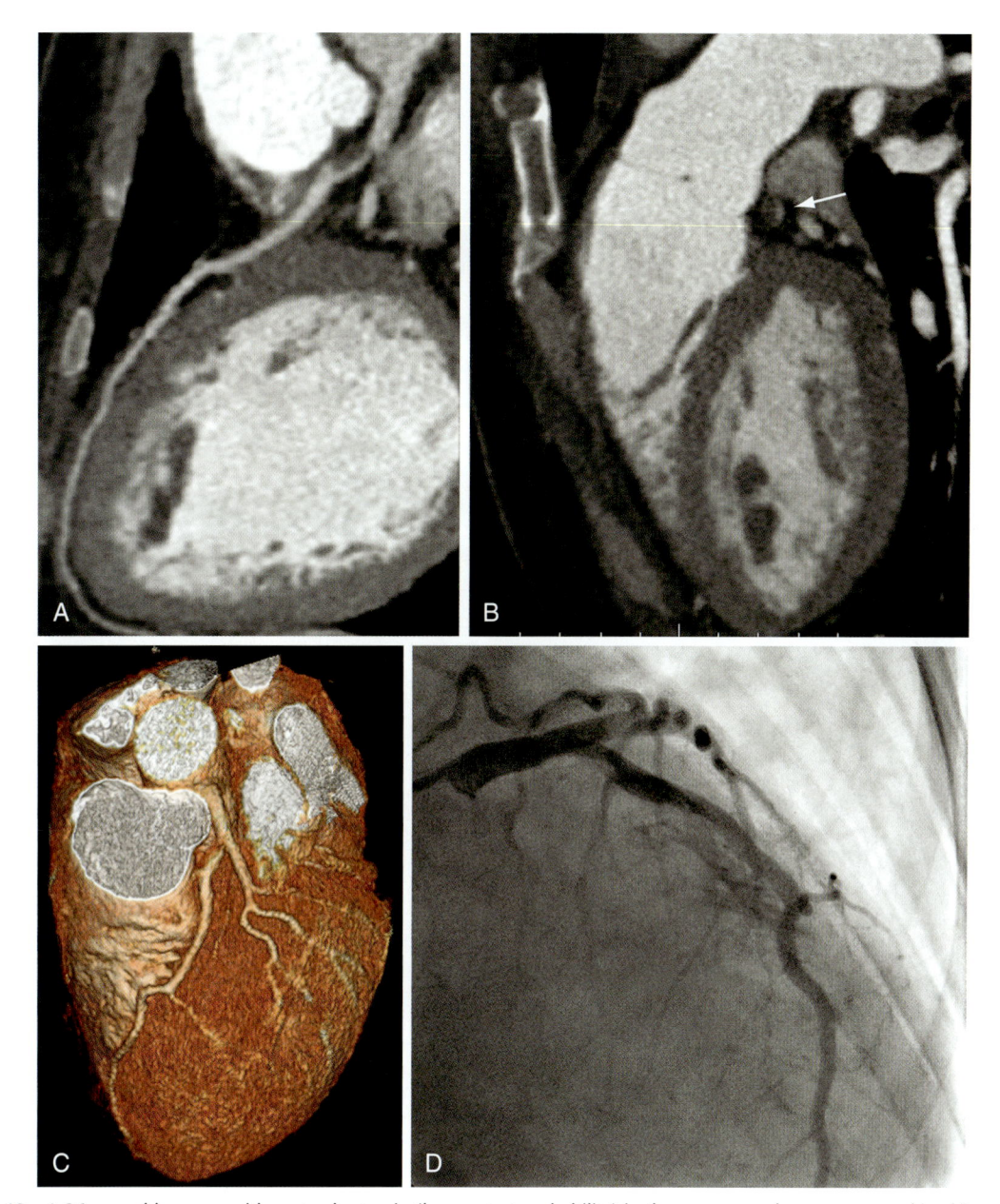

FIGURE 34-10 A 36-year-old woman with acute chest pain (low pretest probability) in the emergency department; smoking history. **A,** Curved multiplanar reformation of the left anterior descending coronary artery shows a partly vessel wall–adherent mass in the proximal left anterior descending coronary artery, suggestive of thrombus or embolus. Beyond the stenosis, no evidence of atherosclerotic disease is seen. **B,** Cross-sectional multiplanar reformation through the proximal left anterior descending coronary artery reveals the severity of luminal compromise. Note the structure in the apex of the left ventricle (*arrow*), which is hypoattenuating compared with the myocardium. The finding was reproducible on echocardiography and consistent with intraventricular thrombus with coronary embolization. **C,** Volume rendering demonstrates the left anterior descending coronary artery stenosis caused by a hypoattenuating mass compatible with thromboembolus. **D,** Conventional catheter angiography confirms high-grade proximal left anterior descending coronary artery obstruction.

might be due to the easily available reference standard because invasive coronary angiography is routinely performed before valve repair in the majority of patients.[33] The presence of concomitant CAD has considerable impact on perioperative risk. Among patients with degenerative aortic valve disease, the prevalence of CAD is as high as 50% (Fig. 34-11).[33] In patients with congenital valvular heart disease before surgery, current guidelines recommend preoperative invasive catheter angiography in a substantial portion of patients (men, ≥35 years; women, ≥35 years, with risk factors, and postmenopausal women).[33] Among the population of patients scheduled to undergo heart valve surgery, individuals with low to intermediate probability for CAD might also benefit from noninvasive assessment of the coronary arteries, although this has not yet been implemented in current guidelines.

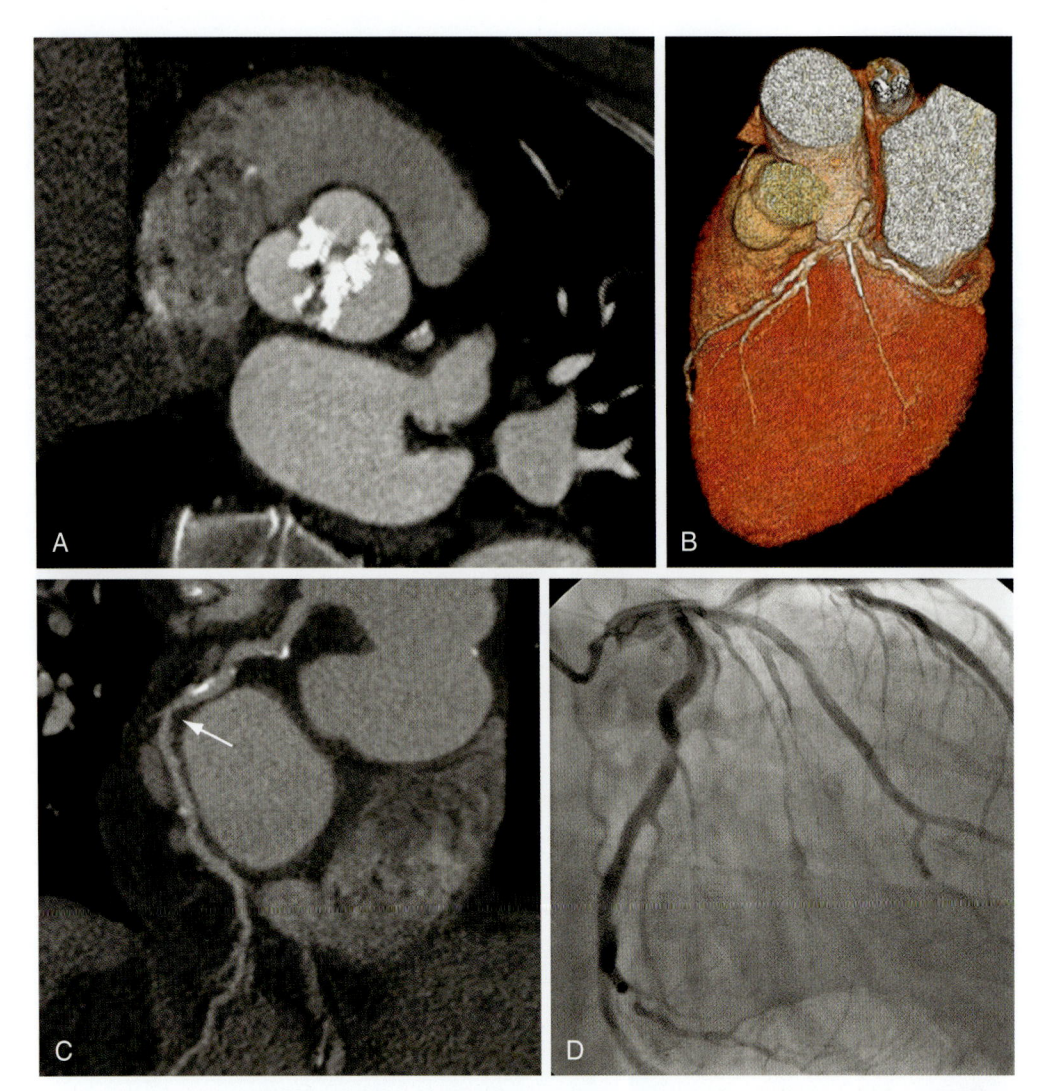

FIGURE 34-11 Aortic valve disease and CAD in a 59-year-old patient with risk factors (smoking, hyperlipidemia). **A,** Double oblique multiplanar reformation through the aortic valve shows heavily calcified leaflet margins. **B,** Volume rendering reveals extensive, predominantly calcified vessel wall changes of the left coronary system. **C,** Curved multiplanar reformation of the dominant circumflex artery shows significant stenosis at the takeoff of a marginal branch (*arrow*). **D,** On invasive catheter angiography, a relevant stenosis of the mid circumflex artery is seen. Up to 46% of patients scheduled for aortic valve repair undergo combined valve and bypass surgery. (*From Brown JW, Ruzmetov M, Parent JJ, et al. Does the degree of preoperative mitral regurgitation predict survival or the need for mitral valve repair or replacement in patients with anomalous origin of the left coronary artery from the pulmonary artery? J Thorac Cardiovasc Surg 2008; 136:743-748.*)

Vessel Wall Imaging

Coronary CTA allows unprecedented noninvasive imaging of the vessel wall comprising the entire coronary tree. During recent years, considerable efforts have been made to identify subjects at risk for future cardiovascular events. Calcium scoring has been established as a marker for atherosclerosis and has been advocated for cardiac risk stratification, but it shows only an approximate 20% of the total atherosclerotic plaque burden (Fig. 34-12).[2,34]

Invasive coronary angiography detects plaques that cause luminal compromise and cannot diagnose nonobstructive atherosclerotic disease. The high spatial and contrast resolution of intravascular ultrasound is unsurpassed, yet the modality, usually performed in combination with invasive coronary angiography, is expensive and invasive and requires considerable expertise.[6]

Several studies report on the feasibility of plaque characterization in comparison to intravascular ultrasound by defining CT attenuation criteria[35] for lipid-rich, collagen-rich, and calcified plaques. However, a considerable overlap in attenuation values was found in noncalcified (lipid-rich versus fibrous) lesions. The limited reproducibility of plaque characterization in subsequent publications is attributable to scanner-dependent spatial resolution, patient geometry, and luminal opacification.[36] Plaque characterization software has nonetheless become commercially available for routine applications, but its role in clinical routine is insufficiently established. The correlation between vessel wall disease and risk factors has attracted much scientific attention, but thus far the relationship between plaque characteristics and risk profiles remains inconclusive. Currently, noninvasive

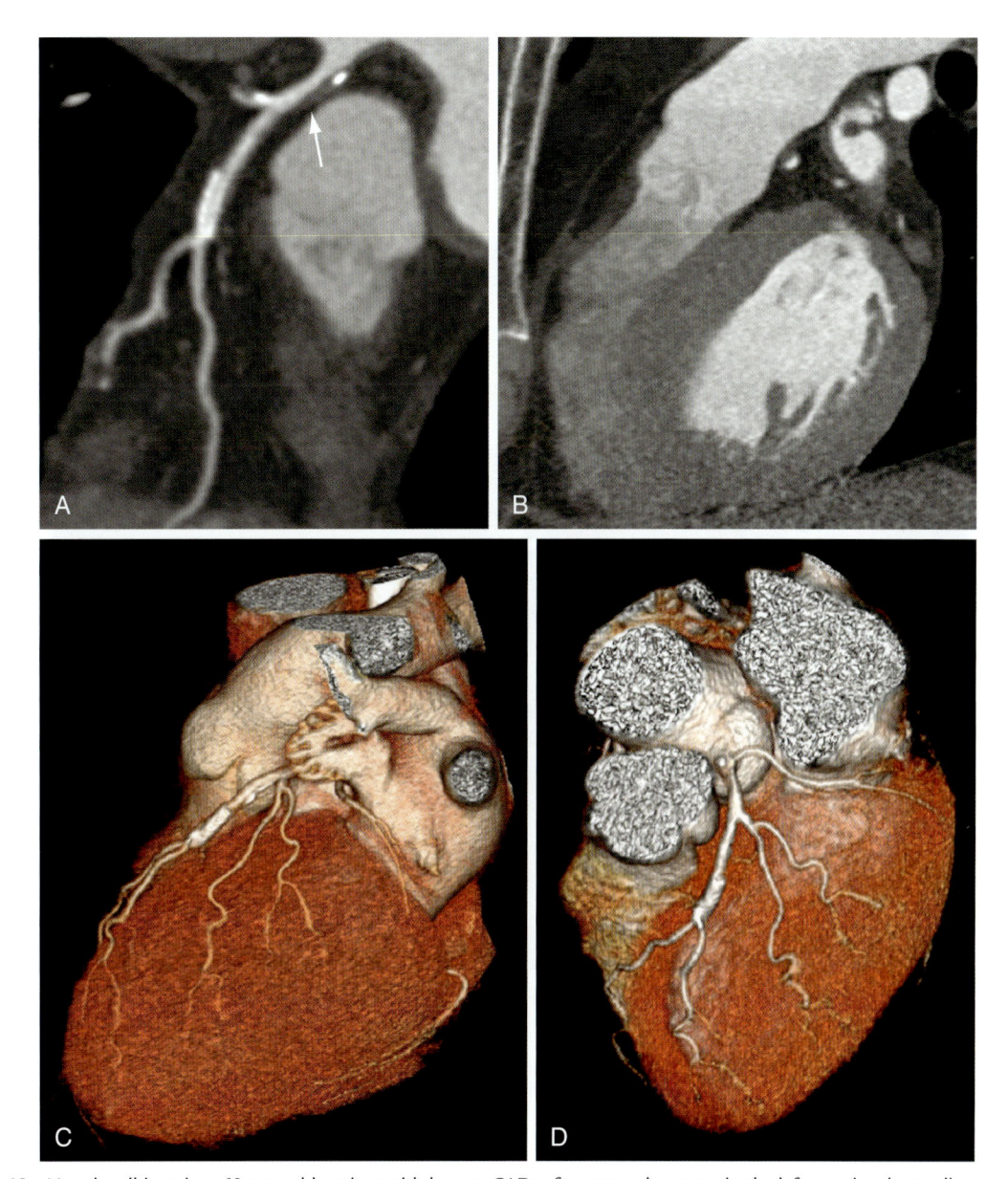

■ **FIGURE 34-12** Vessel wall imaging: 60-year-old patient with known CAD, after stent placement in the left anterior descending coronary artery and recurrent chest pain. **A,** Noninvasive coronary CTA displayed as curved multiplanar reformation of the left anterior descending coronary artery, showing the patent stent. Note diffuse, predominantly fibrolipomatous vessel wall thickening proximally to the stent (*arrow*), containing small calcified cores. **B,** Multiplanar reformation with cross section orthogonal to the vessel course reveals noncalcified eccentric wall thickening with positive vascular remodeling. **C,** Volume rendering shows a lateral view of the proximal left anterior descending coronary artery and reveals small calcified cores within the diffusely atherosclerotic vessel wall. **D,** Volume rendering displays the left main and proximal left anterior descending coronary artery with fibrolipomatous plaque.

coronary CTA has no established role for cardiac risk stratification, although initial data on the predictive value of this test are currently emerging. Considering the relatively high radiation exposure currently still associated with coronary CTA and the lack of evidence, coronary CTA for assessment of the vessel walls is currently considered useful only within established indications, for example, to inform the indication for aggressive risk modification in patients with atypical chest pain and nonobstructive atherosclerosis (Fig. 34-13). Cardiac CT is not considered appropriate as a screening test and is not established for monitoring of response to medical treatment,[4] although its use in such a manner for dedicated research applications has been described.

CONSIDERATIONS FOR PROCEDURE-RELATED RISKS

As with all medical testing, the specific risks of coronary CTA, such as adverse events related to contrast material and relatively high radiation dose, have to be weighed against the expected clinical benefit of performing coronary CTA. The lifetime risk for radiation-induced cancer is age and gender dependent.[5] In this context, one must

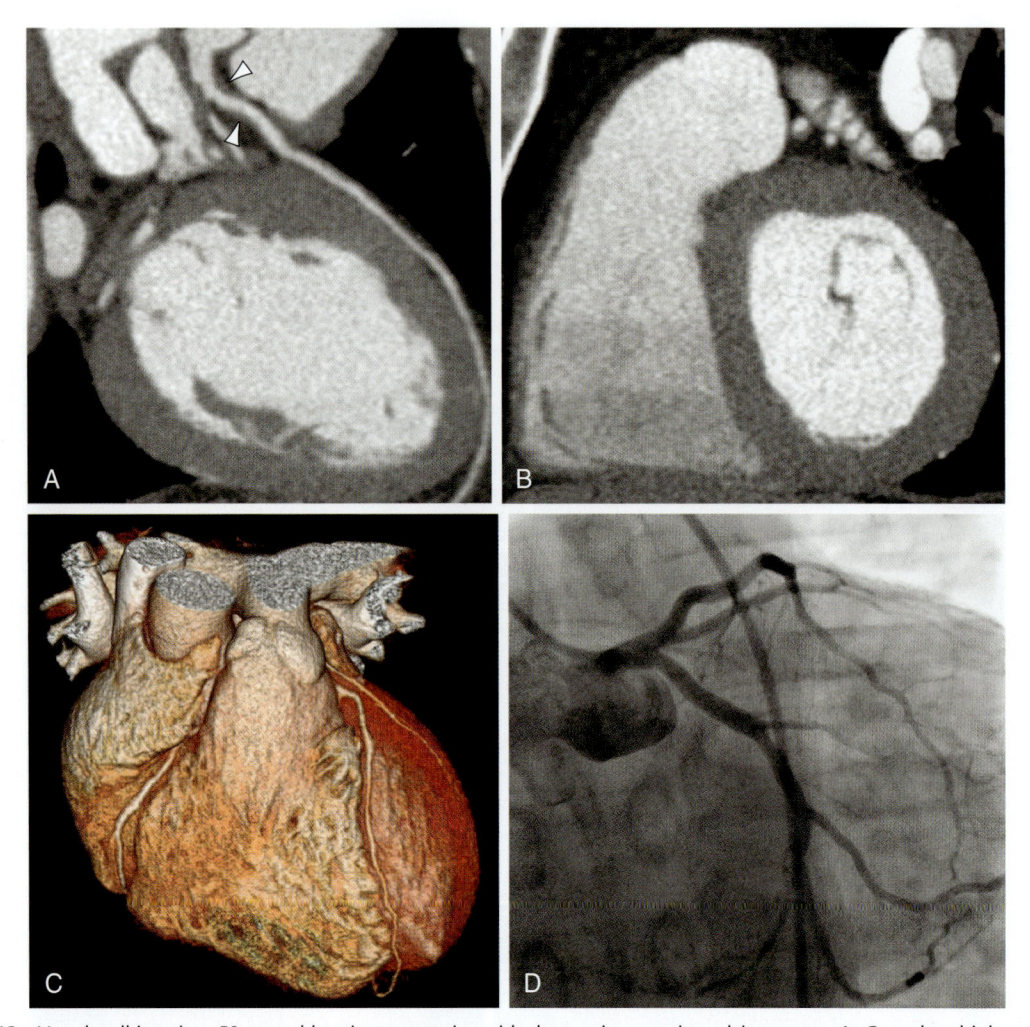

FIGURE 34-13 Vessel wall imaging: 50-year-old patient presenting with chest pain; negative calcium score. **A,** Curved multiplanar reformation of the left anterior descending coronary artery. Noncalcified wall thickening with smoothly bordered changes of the vessel caliber is seen (*arrowheads*). **B,** Cross section perpendicular to the course of the left anterior descending coronary artery reveals eccentric fibrolipomatous wall thickening associated with positive vascular remodeling. **C,** Volume rendering demonstrates nonobstructive luminal irregularities in the left and right coronary artery systems. **D,** Invasive catheter angiography underestimates the extent of noncalcified vessel wall involvement.

keep in mind that a population of patients with low to intermediate probability of CAD is more likely to be younger than the overall population of cardiovascular patients. Although female patients have lower age-related pretest likelihood for CAD compared with men, CAD is known to be under-diagnosed in the female population.[16] Women more frequently present with protean symptoms of atypical chest pain. This has the potential to lead to preferred use of coronary CTA in this group. Consequently, radiation exposure should be kept as low as reasonably achievable by use of all available tools for radiation protection.

KEY POINTS

- Coronary CTA is indicated in symptomatic patients with low to intermediate probability for obstructive CAD.
- Coronary CTA can reliably rule out significant coronary artery stenosis.
- Coronary CTA is not indicated in symptomatic patients with high pretest probability of CAD. This group of patients should primarily undergo invasive angiography.
- Coronary CTA is currently not considered to be indicated in asymptomatic individuals for risk stratification or for screening.
- Coronary CTA is recommended in patients with inconclusive or uninterpretable stress test results.
- The examination should provide incremental diagnostic benefit in management of the patient.
- Application in specific scenarios, such as exclusion of obstructive disease before general surgery and evaluation of acute chest pain in the emergency department, can be considered within the context of currently established indications (i.e., in individuals with low to intermediate pretest likelihood).
- Procedure-related risk, particularly age- and gender-dependent risk for radiation-induced cancer, must be weighed against the expected benefit.

SUGGESTED READINGS

Achenbach S. Computed tomography coronary angiography J Am Coll Cardiol 2006; 48:1919-1928.

Budoff MJ, Achenbach S, Blumenthal RS, et al. Assessment of coronary artery disease by cardiac computed tomography: a scientific statement from the American Heart Association Committee on Cardiovascular Imaging and Intervention, Council on Cardiovascular Radiology and Intervention, and Committee on Cardiac Imaging, Council on Clinical Cardiology. Circulation 2006; 114:1761-1791.

Flohr TG, Schoepf UJ, Ohnesorge BM. Chasing the heart. New developments for cardiac CT. J Thorac Imaging 2007; 22:4-16.

Gibbons RJ, Chatterjee K, Daley J, et al. ACC/AHA/ACP-ASIM guidelines for the management of patients with chronic stable angina: executive summary and recommendations. A Report of the American College of Cardiology/American Heart Association Task Force on Practice Guidelines (Committee on Management of Patients with Chronic Stable Angina). Circulation 1999; 99:2829-2848.

Hendel RC, Patel MR, Kramer CM, et al. ACCF/ACR/SCCT/SCMR/ASNC/NASCI/SCAI/SIR 2006 appropriateness criteria for cardiac computed tomography and cardiac magnetic resonance imaging: a report of the American College of Cardiology Foundation Quality Strategic Directions Committee Appropriateness Criteria Working Group, American College of Radiology, Society of Cardiovascular Computed Tomography, Society for Cardiovascular Magnetic Resonance, American Society of Nuclear Cardiology, North American Society for Cardiac Imaging, Society for Cardiovascular Angiography and Interventions, and Society of Interventional Radiology. J Am Coll Cardiol 2006; 48:1475-1497.

Hoffmann U, Ferencik M, Cury MC, Pena AJ. Coronary CT angiography. J Nucl Med 2006; 47:797-806.

Mahnken AH, Muhlenbruch G, Gunther RW, Wildberger JE. Cardiac CT: coronary arteries and beyond. Eur Radiol 2007; 17:994-1008.

Schoepf UJ, Zwerner PL, Savino G, et al. Coronary CT angiography. Radiology 2007; 244:48-63.

Schroeder S, Achenbach S, Bengel F, et al. Cardiac computed tomography: indications, applications, limitations, and training requirements: report of a Writing Group deployed by the Working Group Nuclear Cardiology and Cardiac CT of the European Society of Cardiology and the European Council of Nuclear Cardiology. Eur Heart J 2008; 29:531-556.

White CS, Kuo D. Chest pain in the emergency department: role of multidetector CT. Radiology 2007; 245:672-681.

REFERENCES

1. Becker CR, Knez A, Leber A, et al. Initial experiences with multi-slice detector spiral CT in diagnosis of arteriosclerosis of coronary vessels. Radiologe 2000; 40:118-122.
2. Budoff MJ, Achenbach S, Blumenthal RS, et al; American Heart Association Committee on Cardiovascular Imaging and Intervention; American Heart Association Council on Cardiovascular Radiology and Intervention; American Heart Association Committee on Cardiac Imaging, Council on Clinical Cardiology. Assessment of coronary artery disease by cardiac computed tomography: a scientific statement from the American Heart Association Committee on Cardiovascular Imaging and Intervention, Council on Cardiovascular Radiology and Intervention, and Committee on Cardiac Imaging, Council on Clinical Cardiology. Circulation 2006; 114:1761-1791.
3. Pugliese F, Mollet NR, Hunink MG, et al. Diagnostic performance of coronary CT angiography by using different generations of multisection scanners: single-center experience. Radiology 2008; 246:384-393.
4. Hendel RC, Patel MR, Kramer CM, et al. ACCF/ACR/SCCT/SCMR/ASNC/NASCI/SCAI/SIR 2006 appropriateness criteria for cardiac computed tomography and cardiac magnetic resonance imaging: a report of the American College of Cardiology Foundation Quality Strategic Directions Committee Appropriateness Criteria Working Group, American College of Radiology, Society of Cardiovascular Computed Tomography, Society for Cardiovascular Magnetic Resonance, American Society of Nuclear Cardiology, North American Society for Cardiac Imaging, Society for Cardiovascular Angiography and Interventions, and Society of Interventional Radiology. J Am Coll Cardiol 2006; 48:1475-1497.
5. Einstein AJ, Henzlova MJ, Rajagopalan S. Estimating risk of cancer associated with radiation exposure from 64-slice computed tomography coronary angiography. JAMA 2007; 298:317-323.
6. Mintz GS, Nissen SE, Anderson WD, et al. American College of Cardiology Clinical Expert Consensus Document on Standards for Acquisition, Measurement and Reporting of Intravascular Ultrasound Studies (IVUS). A report of the American College of Cardiology Task Force on Clinical Expert Consensus Documents. J Am Coll Cardiol 2001; 37:1478-1492.
7. Hamon M, Lepage O, Malagutti P, et al. Diagnostic performance of 16- and 64-section spiral CT for coronary artery bypass graft assessment: meta-analysis: Radiology 2008; 247:679-686.
8. Abdulla J, Abildstrom SZ, Gotzsche O, et al. 64-multislice detector computed tomography coronary angiography as potential alternative to conventional coronary angiography: a systematic review and meta-analysis. Eur Heart J 2007; 28:3042-3050.
9. Achenbach S. Computed tomography coronary angiography. J Am Coll Cardiol 2006; 48:1919-1928.
10. Weustink AC, Meijboom WB, Mollet NR, et al. Reliable high-speed coronary computed tomography in symptomatic patients. J Am Coll Cardiol 2007; 50:786-794.
11. Meijboom WB, van Mieghem CA, Mollet NR, et al. 64-slice computed tomography coronary angiography in patients with high, intermediate, or low pretest probability of significant coronary artery disease. J Am Coll Cardiol 2007; 50:1469-1475.
12. Ropers U, Ropers D, Pflederer T, et al. Influence of heart rate on the diagnostic accuracy of dual-source computed tomography coronary angiography. J Am Coll Cardiol 2007; 50:2393-2398.
13. Scanlon PJ, Faxon DP, Audet AM, et al. ACC/AHA guidelines for coronary angiography: executive summary and recommendations. A report of the American College of Cardiology/American Heart Association Task Force on Practice Guidelines (Committee on Coronary Angiography) developed in collaboration with the Society for Cardiac Angiography and Interventions. Circulation 1999; 99:2345-2357.
14. Gibbons RJ, Abrams J, Chatterjee K, et al; American College of Cardiology; American Heart Association Task Force on Practice Guidelines. Committee on the Management of Patients With Chronic Stable Angina. ACC/AHA 2002 guideline update for the management of patients with chronic stable angina—summary article: a report of the American College of Cardiology/American Heart Association Task Force on Practice Guidelines (Committee on the Management of Patients With Chronic Stable Angina). Circulation 2003; 107: 149-158.
15. Grundy SM, Pasternak R, Greenland P, et al. AHA/ACC scientific statement. Assessment of cardiovascular risk by use of multiple-risk-factor assessment equations: a statement for healthcare professionals from the American Heart Association and the American College of Cardiology. J Am Coll Cardiol 1999; 34:1348-1359.
16. Gibbons RJ, Balady GJ, Beasley JW, et al. ACC/AHA guidelines for exercise testing: executive summary. A report of the American College of Cardiology/American Heart Association Task Force on Practice Guidelines (Committee on Exercise Testing). Circulation 1997; 96:345-354.
17. Cheitlin MD, Armstrong WF, Aurigemma GP, et al; American College of Cardiology; American Heart Association; American Society of Echocardiography. ACC/AHA/ASE 2003 guideline update for the clinical application of echocardiography: summary article: a report of the American College of Cardiology/American Heart Association Task Force on Practice Guidelines. Circulation 2003; 108:1146-1162.
18. Mieres JH, Shaw LJ, Arai A, et al; Cardiac Imaging Committee, Council on Clinical Cardiology, and the Cardiovascular Imaging and Intervention Committee, Council on Cardiovascular Radiology and

Intervention, American Heart Association. Role of noninvasive testing in the clinical evaluation of women with suspected coronary artery disease: consensus statement from the Cardiac Imaging Committee, Council on Clinical Cardiology, and the Cardiovascular Imaging and Intervention Committee, Council on Cardiovascular Radiology and Intervention, American Heart Association. Circulation 2005; 111:682-696.
19. Brodoefel H, Burgstahler C, Tsiflikas I, et al. Dual-source CT: effect of heart rate, heart rate variability, and calcification on image quality and diagnostic accuracy. Radiology 2008; 247:346-355.
20. Raff GL, Gallagher MJ, O'Neill WW, Goldstein JA. Diagnostic accuracy of noninvasive coronary angiography using 64-slice spiral computed tomography. J Am Coll Cardiol 2005; 46:552-557.
21. Mahnken AH, Mühlenbruch G, Günther RW, et al. Coronary arteries and beyond. Eur Radiol 2007; 17:994-1008.
22. Pundziute G, Schuijf JD, Jukema JW, et al. Impact of coronary calcium score on diagnostic accuracy of multislice computed tomography coronary angiography for detection of coronary artery disease. J Nucl Cardiol 2007; 14:36-43.
23. Schoepf UJ, Zwerner PL, Savino G, et al. Coronary CT angiography. Radiology 2007; 244:48-63.
24. Leschka S, Wildermuth S, Boehm T, et al. Noninvasive coronary angiography with 64-section CT: effect of average heart rate and heart rate variability on image quality. Radiology 2006; 241:378-385.
25. Johnson TR, Nikolaou K, Wintersperger BJ, et al. Dual-source CT cardiac imaging: initial experience. Eur Radiol 2006; 16:1409-1415.
26. Ogden CL, Carroll MD, Curtin LR, et al. Prevalence of overweight and obesity in the United States, 1999-2004. JAMA 2006; 95:1549-1555.
27. Pope JH, Aufderheide TP, Ruthazer R, et al. Missed diagnoses of acute cardiac ischemia in the emergency department. N Engl J Med 2000; 342:1163-1170.
28. White CS, Kuo D. Chest pain in the emergency department: role of multidetector CT. Radiology 2007; 245:672-681.
29. Hoffmann U, Nagurney JT, Moselewski F, et al. Coronary multidetector computed tomography in the assessment of patients with acute chest pain. Circulation 2006; 114:2251-2260.
30. Rubinshtein R, Halon DA, Gaspar T, et al. Usefulness of 64-slice cardiac computed tomographic angiography for diagnosing acute coronary syndromes and predicting clinical outcome in emergency department patients with chest pain of uncertain origin. Circulation 2007; 115:1762-1768.
31. Goldstein JA, Gallagher MJ, O'Neill WW, et al. A randomized controlled trial of multi-slice coronary computed tomography for evaluation of acute chest pain. J Am Coll Cardiol 2007; 49:863-871.
32. Eagle KA, Berger PB, Calkins H, et al; American College of Cardiology/American Heart Association Task Force on Practice Guidelines (Committee to Update the 1996 Guidelines on Perioperative Cardiovascular Evaluation for Noncardiac Surgery). ACC/AHA guideline update for perioperative cardiovascular evaluation for noncardiac surgery—executive summary: a report of the American College of Cardiology/American Heart Association Task Force on Practice Guidelines (Committee to Update the 1996 Guidelines on Perioperative Cardiovascular Evaluation for Noncardiac Surgery). Circulation 2002; 105:1257-1267.
33. American College of Cardiology/American Heart Association Task Force on Practice Guidelines; Society of Cardiovascular Anesthesiologists; Society for Cardiovascular Angiography and Interventions; Society of Thoracic Surgeons, Bonow RO, Carabello BA, Kanu C, et al. ACC/AHA 2006 guidelines for the management of patients with valvular heart disease: a report of the American College of Cardiology/American Heart Association Task Force on Practice Guidelines (writing committee to revise the 1998 Guidelines for the Management of Patients With Valvular Heart Disease): developed in collaboration with the Society of Cardiovascular Anesthesiologists: endorsed by the Society for Cardiovascular Angiography and Interventions and the Society of Thoracic Surgeons. Circulation 2006; 114:e84-e231.
34. Rumberger JA, Simons DB, Fitzpatrick LA, et al. Coronary artery calcium area by electron-beam computed tomography and coronary atherosclerotic plaque area. A histopathologic correlative study. Circulation 1995; 92:2157-2162.
35. Leber AW, Knez A, Becker A, et al. Accuracy of multidetector spiral computed tomography in identifying and differentiating the composition of coronary atherosclerotic plaques: a comparative study with intracoronary ultrasound. J Am Coll Cardiol 2004; 43:1241-1247.
36. Cademartiri F, La Grutta L, Palumbo AA, et al. Coronary plaque imaging with multislice computed tomography: technique and clinical applications. Eur Radiol 2006; 16(Suppl 7):M44-M53.

CHAPTER 35

Interpretation and Reporting in Obstructive Coronary Disease

Tamar Gaspar

Since its introduction in the early 1970s, computed tomography (CT) has become a well-established imaging technology and the modality of choice for noninvasive evaluation of the aorta and pulmonary, carotid, renal, and peripheral arteries.

In CT angiography (CTA), the use of rapidly injected contrast agents raises the density in the blood pool, thereby allowing easy differentiation between the lumen, vessel walls, and surrounding tissues.

CT imaging of the coronary arteries became practical with the arrival of the 4-slice scanners. The ongoing advancement and innovation in CT technology over the years provided faster scans with improved temporal and spatial resolutions. As a result, the role of CT in the imaging of coronary arteries progressed from simple determination of the presence of arterial calcifications to demonstration of the atherosclerotic plaque itself and quantification of luminal stenoses.

DESCRIPTION OF TECHNICAL REQUIREMENTS

Challenges in noninvasive cardiac imaging by CT include small (typically 1 to 4 mm) and often tortuous vessels, complex and rapid cardiac motion, and variable, often unpredictable heart rates and respiratory motion. As a result, all cardiac scans are performed with ECG gating, either prospective or retrospective, to allow reconstruction of motion-free images.

CT scans of the heart should be fast and performed during a single, preferably short breath-hold to avoid breathing artifacts and to allow minimal contrast agent volume. Sub-second rotation time resulting in high temporal resolution is required to eliminate cardiac motion. High spatial resolution, preferably sub-millimeter, is necessary to adequately visualize small and complex anatomic structures such as the coronary arteries.

Adequate preparation of the patient is a must, and therefore a team made up of scheduling staff, technologist, physician, and nurse is required. Documentation of serum creatinine level and history of contrast allergy is essential at the time of scheduling. The risk of contrast nephropathy must be weighed against the benefits of the information gained by the procedure. Depending on the clinical indication, some degree of renal protection may be achieved with good hydration before and after injection of contrast material as well as the administration of N-acetylcysteine. In case of a known allergy to contrast material, and if the risk is acceptable to both patient and referring physician, pretreatment with corticosteroids may prevent reaction to the contrast agent.

The coronary arteries are best demonstrated when there is the least amount of motion. There are two relatively motionless phases during the cardiac cycle: diastasis in late diastole and isovolumic relaxation time in late systole. The diastasis period is longer; but at higher heart rates, it is almost eliminated. Isovolumic relaxation time, on the other hand, is shorter but unaffected by heart rate.

Lowering of the patient's heart rate is suggested on the basis of comparison of coronary artery visibility in patients with low versus high heart rates. Most studies so far have been performed on 4-, 16-, and 64-slice scanners and have shown a higher number of unassessable segments in patients with rapid heart rates compared with patients with lower heart rates. Furthermore, a low heart rate, with a longer cardiac cycle, enables the use of tube current modulation (with full x-ray output only during a fixed period in diastole), thus reducing radiation dose.

Preliminary experience with the latest generation of scanners (more than 64-slice and dual-source units) with improved temporal resolution shows promising results in patients with higher heart rates.

Heart rate can be controlled through the use of medication (e.g., oral or intravenous β blockers), by reassuring the patient (i.e., explaining the procedure, describing what to expect), and by rehearsing the breath-hold required during the scan. Practicing the breath-hold is also important to anticipate heart rate changes that may occur during the scan.

Sublingual nitroglycerin (if it is not contraindicated) should be administered immediately before the scan is started to improve vessel visualization. This is particularly important in women, smokers, diabetics, and patients who have had bypass graft surgery.

The radiation dose should be as low as possible with parameters adjusted to the patient's size and expected heart rate for optimal visualization. In very large patients, a lower pitch should be considered to allow increased radiation dose.

TECHNIQUES

Indications

In recent years, technologic advancements have improved the temporal and spatial resolution of scanners as well as reduced acquisition time, resulting in reliable assessments of the heart and coronary arteries.

Potential indications for coronary CTA are many and continue to evolve. Recently, the American College of Cardiology Foundation Quality Strategic Directions Committee Appropriateness Criteria Working Group, the American College of Radiology, and others have published a joint review on the appropriateness of cardiac CTA.[1] This report scored the appropriateness of cardiac CTA in several clinical applications on a scale from 1 to 9 based on the available literature. The information and experience available with cardiac CTA at this time are not robust enough to support categorical recommendations and guidelines. This is so because the technology continues to change rapidly, there are not enough prospective studies on different groups of patients, and there are no outcome studies on the prognostic value of cardiac CTA. Therefore, the appropriateness criteria are not guidelines but rather temporary recommendations until official guidelines are published.

Among the potential indications for cardiac CTA, there are four clinical groups. The first group includes patients with an indication for invasive catheterization when the procedure is anticipated to be technically demanding (e.g., ascending aortic aneurysm, atherosclerotic arch, anticoagulant therapy), patients with a prior incomplete catheterization, and patients with suspected coronary anomalies. For patients in this group, cardiac CTA may be the optimal imaging modality and in certain cases the only one.

The second group consists of patients with an intermediate pretest probability for obstructive coronary artery disease. This includes patients with atypical symptoms, acute chest pain of uncertain origin, and inconclusive stress test or thallium scan as well as candidates for valve or noncardiac surgery. The purpose of cardiac CTA in this group is to exclude significant coronary stenosis, and a normal scan may obviate the need for a catheter-based intervention.

The third group includes patients with known coronary artery disease (e.g., patients after stent placement or bypass grafting) who present with a specific question, such as stent or graft patency. This group of patients tends to have frequent complaints; traditional noninvasive tests have limited predictive accuracy, and invasive procedures are commonly employed. Here, exclusion of significant stenosis may prevent unnecessary catheter-based intervention.

The fourth group is controversial and consists of asymptomatic individuals at risk for coronary artery disease. On the one hand, CT is able to identify subclinical atherosclerosis, and the findings themselves may lead to improved compliance with preventive regimens. On the other hand, CTA involves administration of contrast material and radiation exposure, and we currently have not established an approach to dealing with such findings.

Contraindications

There are only a few contraindications to cardiac CTA, the main being a contraindication to administration of iodinated contrast agents. Injection of contrast material is mandatory for visualization of the coronary arteries.

Inability to follow breath-hold instructions (8 to 20 seconds, depending on the scanner used) may also be considered a contraindication. Breathing-induced motion artifacts may render a study unassessable.

Irregular heart rate is considered a relative contraindication, depending on scanner type and available algorithms for dealing with variable R–R intervals.

Excessive calcium within the wall of the coronary arteries is sometimes considered a contraindication to cardiac CTA. It may lead to overestimation of stenosis severity and prompt unnecessary intervention.

Technique Description

Cardiac CTA is a contrast-enhanced spiral study performed with ECG gating to eliminate cardiac motion. It is technically complex and requires high spatial resolution, high temporal resolution, good low-contrast resolution, intravascular contrast enhancement, and short scanning time. Advanced scanners have increased coverage, faster gantry rotation time, and sophisticated algorithms for reconstruction of partial scan data or combination of data from various phases (multicycle reconstruction) to further reduce temporal resolution.

Compared with invasive catheterization, cardiac CT evaluates the coronary arteries noninvasively, displays its wall as well as the lumen, and allows quantification and characterization of atherosclerotic plaques even before there is luminal narrowing.

Initially, scout images are acquired to determine anatomic span. For native coronary arteries, the CTA scan extends from the level of the carina to the base of the heart. In patients who have had bypass surgery, scans are

TABLE 35-1 Artifacts, Their Appearance and Causes, and Measures to Avoid Them

Artifact	Description	Cause	Solutions	Remarks
Blooming	High-contrast objects appear larger than they are as a result of partial volume effect May lead to false-positive interpretation (overestimation) of stenosis	Dense calcified plaques, stents, metallic clips	Use thin-slice acquisition Focus on axial slices and curved multiplanar reformation Measure calcium score before CTA Decrease pixel size (future)	Exacerbated by motion
Blurring (voluntary motion)	Smearing out of real attenuation values due to patient's motion	Movement or breathing of the patient during scan	Prescan instructions about the expected breath-hold and heat sensation Decreasing scan time Give oxygen (calm the patient)	May also lead to missing data
Blurring (involuntary motion)	Smearing out of real attenuation values due to cardiac motion	Heart rate variation during the scan	Look for different phases Use β blockers R-tag correction Decrease scan time (faster or shorter coverage) Warm contrast (iso-osmolar)	
Beam hardening	Dark bands or streaks due to absorption of the low-energy photons can appear adjacent to dense objects in the image	Dense calcified plaques, stents, metallic clips, dense contrast material	Filtration Focus on axial images and curved multiplanar reformation	
Streaks	Dense streaks projecting from object	Pacemakers, electrodes, stent, dense contrast material on right side	Use saline flash, multiple phase injection External metallic objects should be removed from field of view Sharp kernel reconstruction filter	
Stair-step	Data inconsistencies that are not recognized by the reconstruction algorithm Appear as steps in the edges of a multiplanar reformation or volume rendered reconstruction	Heart rate variation during the scan, breathing, motion of the patient	Look for different phases Use β blockers Pre-reconstruction alignment—R-tag correction (manual or automatic) Post-reconstruction alignment—choose different percentage of R-R interval for different segments of the vessel	Affects mainly the right coronary artery and circumflex artery
Poor contrast enhancement	Technical error in administration of the contrast agent (technical and patient-related factors)	Technical: timing, volume, speed, contrast extravasation Patient: heart failure, Valsalva maneuver, obesity	Instruct operator Update protocol Use high-density contrast agent Use automatic scan triggering Instruct patient	

started at the level of the clavicles. The scan is performed during a single breath-hold with timed injection of contrast material to achieve optimal enhancement of the coronary arteries.

Images are typically reconstructed from data acquired at 70% to 75% and 40% to 45% of the R-R interval. If needed, additional phases are reconstructed to find a "quiet" (motionless) phase.

Pitfalls and Solutions

In CT, the term *artifact* applies to any systematic discrepancy between the CT numbers in the reconstructed image and the true attenuation coefficients of the object. CT images are inherently prone to artifacts because the image is reconstructed from multiple independent detector measurements. The reconstruction algorithm assumes that all these measurements are consistent, so any error of measurement will usually be reflected as an error in the reconstructed image.[2,3]

Four types of artifact can occur: streaking, due to an inconsistency in a single measurement; shading, due to a group of channels or views deviating gradually from the true measurement; rings, which are due to errors in an individual detector calibration; and distortion, due to the helical reconstruction.

Artifacts can seriously degrade the quality of CT images, sometimes to the point of making them diagnostically unusable. Furthermore, accuracy of cardiac CTA for detection of stenoses depends highly on image artifacts,[3] which are a major cause of false-positive and false-negative interpretations.

To optimize image quality, it is necessary to understand why artifacts occur and how they can be prevented (Table 35-1). CT artifacts originate from a range of sources. Physics-based artifacts result from the physical processes involved in the acquisition of CT data. Patient-based artifacts are caused by such factors as movement of the patient or the presence of metallic materials inside or on the patient.

Careful preparation of the patient and optimum selection of scanning parameters are, therefore, important factors in avoiding CT artifacts.

Beam Hardening

An x-ray beam is composed of individual photons with a range of energies. As the beam passes through the patient,

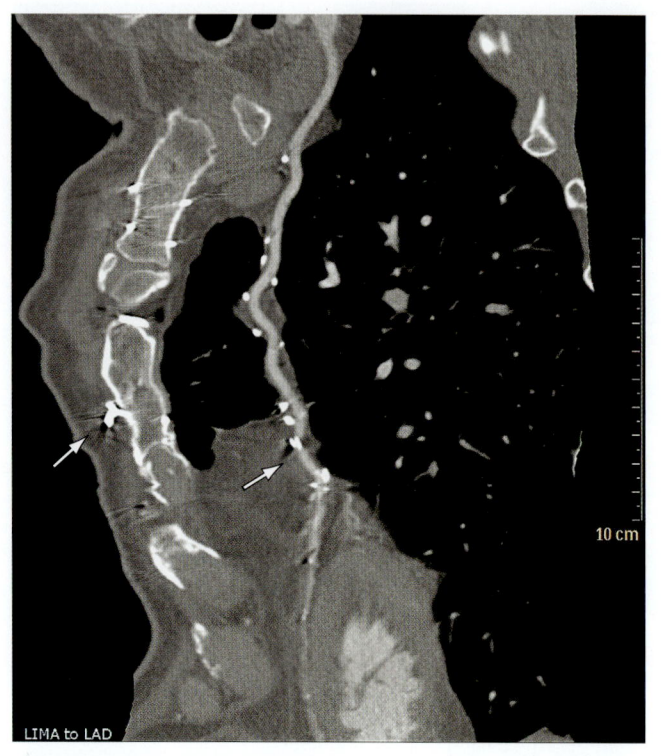

FIGURE 35-1 Beam hardening causes dark areas (*arrows*) adjacent to metallic sternal wires and surgical clips in this curved multiplanar reformation of a left internal mammary artery to left anterior descending coronary artery graft.

it becomes "harder"; its mean energy increases because the lower energy photons are absorbed. As a result of this effect, dark bands or streaks can appear on the image adjacent to dense objects such as calcifications, dense contrast material, or metallic clips (Fig. 35-1). Beam hardening can be minimized by filtration.

Partial Volume (Blooming)

CT numbers are based on attenuation coefficients for a voxel of tissue. If the voxel contains more than one tissue type, the CT number will be based on an average of the different tissues involved. For example, a dense calcified plaque or stent, lying off-center, may appear larger than it actually is in the reconstructed image because of partial volume effects and create an exaggerated luminal narrowing (Fig. 35-2). This problem is magnified if there are also motion artifacts (Fig. 35-3).

Partial volume artifacts can be best avoided by use of a thin-slice acquisition width and appropriate computer algorithms.

Metallic Materials (Streaks)

The presence of metal objects (such as pacemakers, electrodes, stents, and surgical clips) in the scan field can generate severe streak artifacts (Figs. 35-4 and 35-5). They occur because the metal object absorbs the radiation, resulting in incomplete projection profiles.

External metallic objects should be removed from the field of view when possible. Use of a sharp kernel reconstruction filter may help improve visualization of the vessel's lumen within metallic stents.

Patient Motion (Blurring)

Motion of the patient can cause misregistration artifacts, which usually appear as shading or streaking in the reconstructed image (Fig. 35-6). Steps can be taken to prevent voluntary motion (due to movement or breathing during the scan), but some involuntary motion may be unavoidable. Prescan instructions about the expected breath-hold are critical to minimize motion artifacts as well as to decrease scan time. Involuntary motion artifacts may be caused by heart rate irregularities during the scan and will appear as blurring or stair-step artifacts. Looking for a

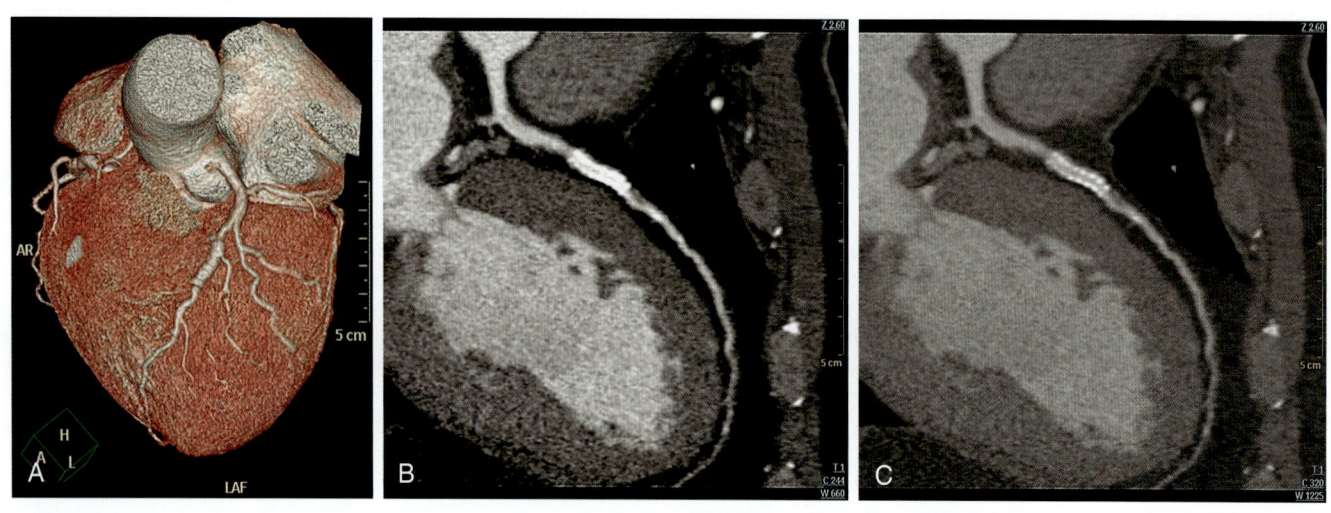

FIGURE 35-2 Partial volume effects cause this mid left anterior descending coronary artery stent to appear larger than it actually is in the volume rendered image (**A**) and curved multiplanar reformation (**B**), with overestimation of luminal narrowing. Use of a wider window with a higher center (**C**) may improve lumen visualization.

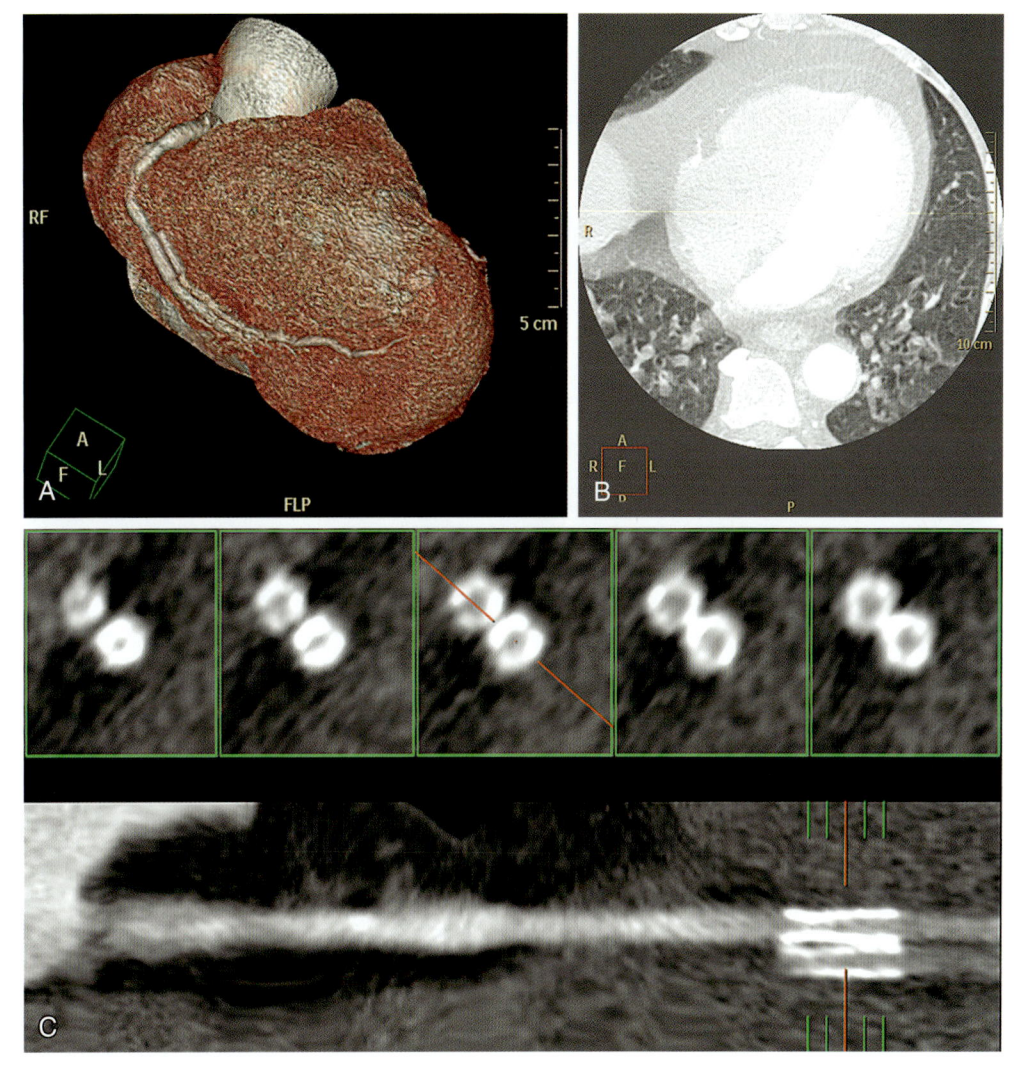

CHAPTER 35 • *Interpretation and Reporting in Obstructive Coronary Disease* 497

■ **FIGURE 35-3** Blooming artifacts are aggravated by motion, as seen in this patient with distal right coronary artery stent who was breathing during the scan. Volume rendered image (**A**), axial slice (**B**), and curved multiplanar reformation with cross-sectional images through the stent (**C**) show doubling of the stent as a result of motion (breathing).

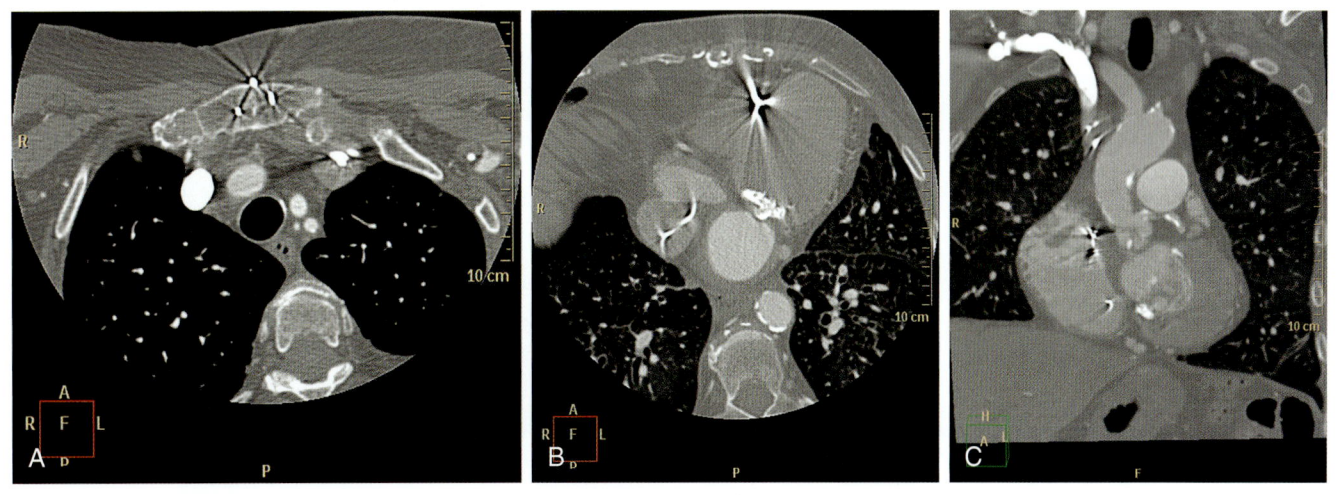

■ **FIGURE 35-4** Metal objects, such as surgical wires (**A**), pacemaker electrodes (**B**), and dense contrast material (**C**), can generate severe streak artifacts.

498   PART FOUR • *Coronary Artery Imaging*

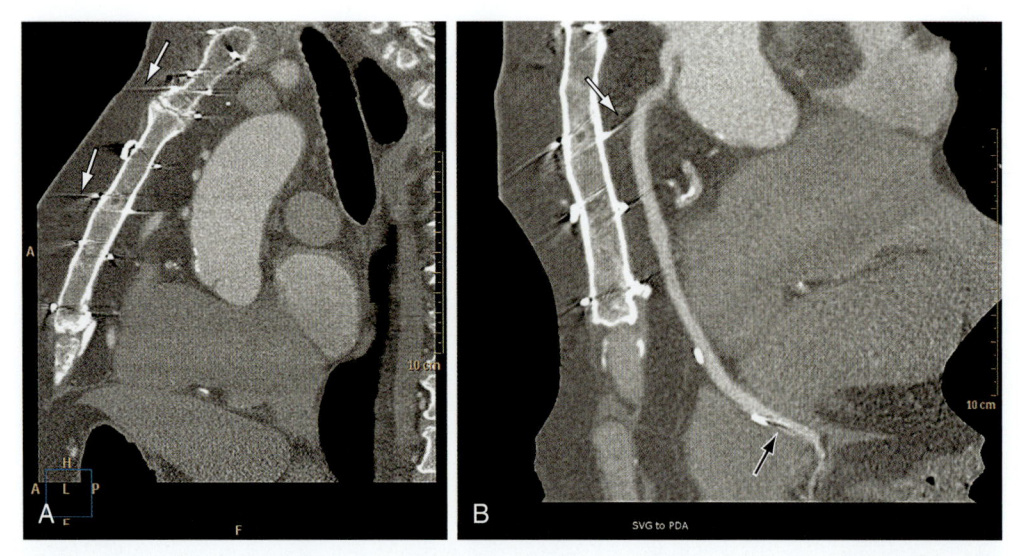

■ **FIGURE 35-5** Post-bypass metallic wires and clips can cause dense streak artifacts (*white arrows*) that may affect lumen visualization (**B**, *black arrow*) of adjacent vein graft.

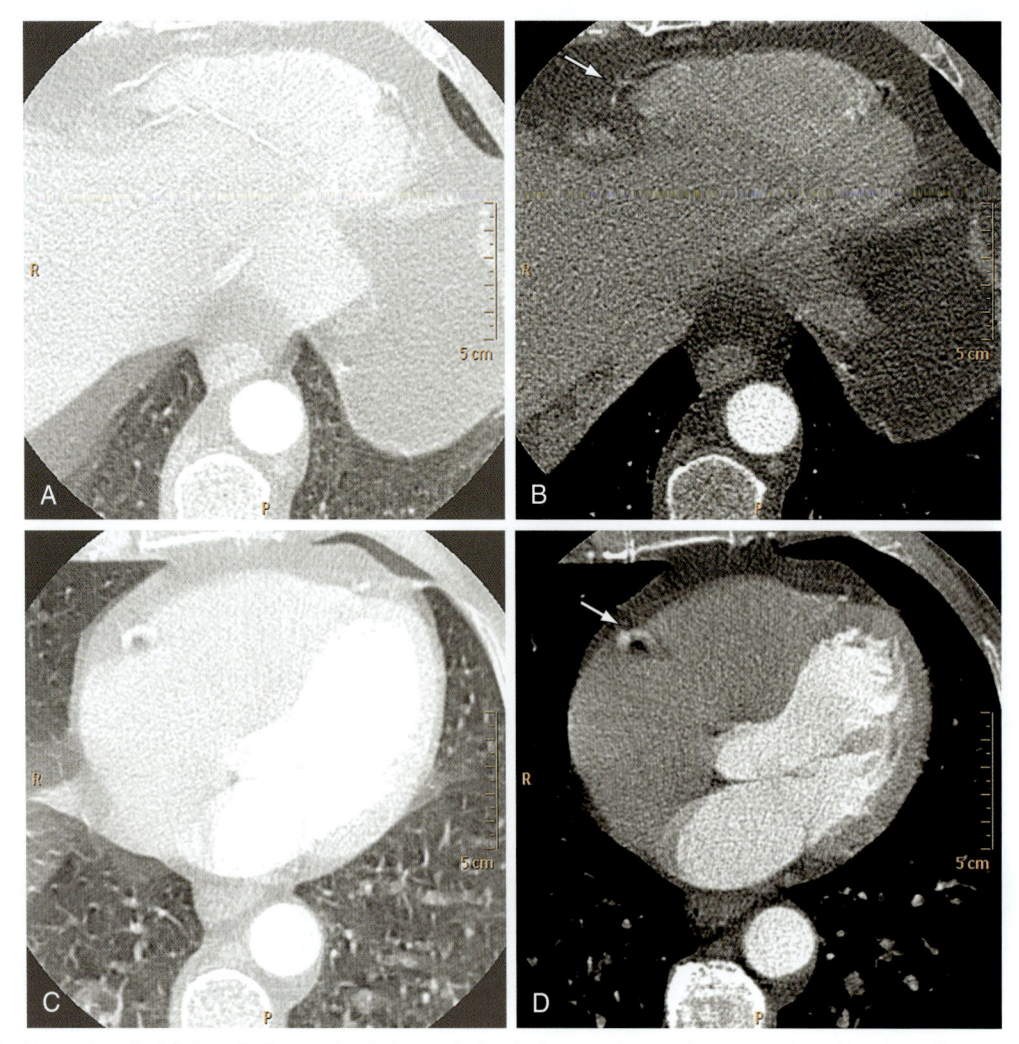

■ **FIGURE 35-6** Two pairs of axial slices (in lung and soft tissue windows) show motion artifacts due to breathing (**A** and **C**), causing blurring and streaking of the coronary arteries (**B** and **D**).

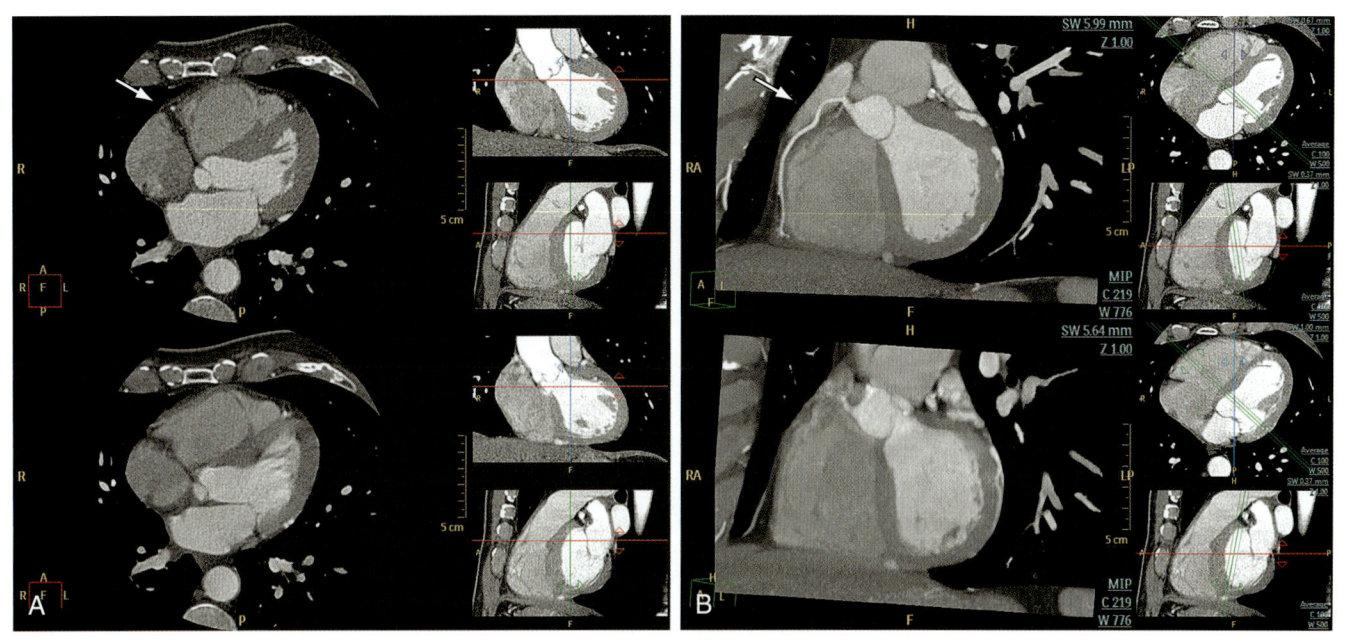

FIGURE 35-7 Involuntary motion artifacts may be caused by heart rate irregularities during the scan. The right coronary artery and, to a lesser extent, the circumflex artery are more susceptible to motion artifacts. Comparison of axial slices (**A**) and oblique coronal maximum intensity projection images (**B**) from phases 75% (*top*) and 0% (*bottom*) shows improved right coronary artery visualization with phase 75% (*arrows*).

motion-free phase can sometimes help improve visualization of the coronary arteries (Fig. 35-7).

Stair-Step Artifacts

Stair-step artifacts appear as horizontal lines through the image, visible especially around the edges of structures in multiplanar and three-dimensional reformatted images, when wide collimations and non-overlapping reconstruction intervals are used. They are less severe with helical scanning, which permits reconstruction of overlapping sections without the extra dose to the patient that would occur if overlapping axial scans were obtained. Stair-step artifacts are virtually eliminated in multiplanar and three-dimensional reformatted images from thin-section data obtained with today's multisection scanners.

In ECG-gated scans, an irregular R–R interval may cause data inconsistencies that are not recognized by the reconstruction algorithm, resulting in stair-step artifacts through the heart (Fig. 35-8).

Administration of β blockers to lower the heart rate and to try to stabilize it may prevent arrhythmia during the scan. Some manufacturers provide software for R-tag correction in case an arrhythmia has occurred (Fig. 35-9). Looking for a quiet phase of the cardiac cycle with minimal motion may help minimize cardiac motion–induced artifacts. If prospective gating with sequential (axial) acquisition mode is used, heart rate changes during the scan cause stair-step artifacts through the volume (Fig. 35-10).

Noise-Induced Artifacts

The number of photons striking the detector directly influences the noise. More photons means less noise and better image quality. Increased noise (as a result of inappropriate choice of radiation parameters, thin-slice reconstruction, and large patients) can cause streak artifacts and a grainy appearance to the image. Optimization of scan parameters may reduce image noise as well as add several thin sections together into a thicker slab.

Poor Vessel Enhancement

Poor contrast enhancement within the lumen of the coronary arteries impairs the ability to interpret the study because of poor contrast-to-noise ratio. Technical error in the administration of the contrast agent as well as patient-related factors may cause such poor enhancement. Technical errors are usually operator dependent and include extravasation of contrast material, inadequate volume or injection rate, and improper timing of the scan. A well-prepared operator can easily avoid such errors by updating scan protocols for different clinical settings and by using high-density contrast material with appropriate injection protocols. Use of automatic scan triggering, with accurate scan delay and scan parameters, may help avoid human errors. Patient-related factors include Valsalva maneuver, heart failure, and obesity. Instructing the patient before the scan as to the importance of cooperation always helps.

Incomplete Coverage

Incorrect planning of the scan range, due to either a technical error on the part of the operator or different breath-hold depth during the scan, causes incomplete coverage of the heart with missing data. This can be avoided by instructing the operator, using safety margins in plan-

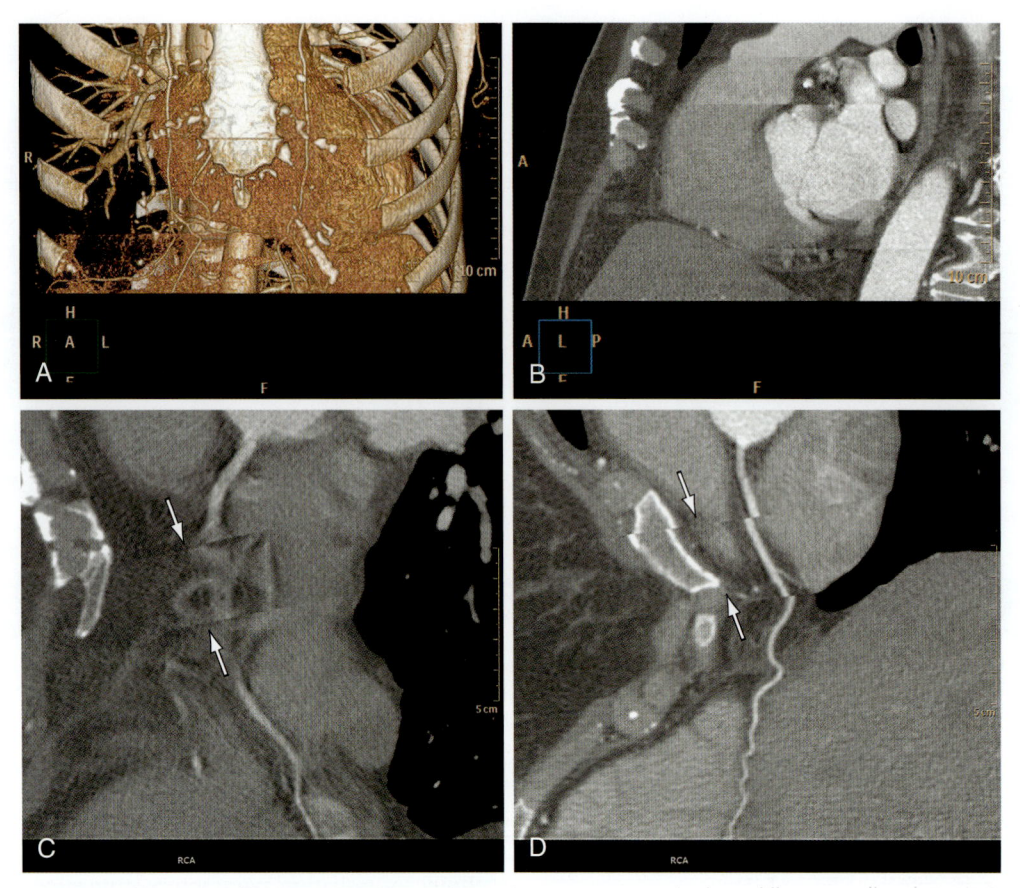

FIGURE 35-8 Stair-step artifacts caused by heart rate changes during the scan appear as horizontal lines extending through the heart in the three-dimensional (**A**) and multiplanar reformatted (**B**) images. On curved multiplanar reformation (**C**), there is a blurred segment (*between arrows*) representing a slab that was imaged during an arrhythmia. In another patient (**D**), with a milder change in heart rate during the scan, the segment (*between arrows*) is displaced but not blurred.

ning the scan, and rehearsing the breath-hold with the patient.

Image Interpretation

Postprocessing

Images can be reconstructed during different cardiac phases, allowing retrospective selection of the phase with the least motion artifacts.

For easier evaluation of the large amount of CT data and the complex anatomy of the coronary arteries, several postprocessing techniques are available. Image postprocessing requires modification of three-dimensional data to derive additional information or to hide unwanted information. The isotropic sub-millimeter voxel, available in all advanced scanners, improves the diagnostic quality of rendered images. Analysis of rendered images as well as of the axial slices has become a crucial component of cardiac CTA interpretation.

Axial Images

Axial images are the basic outcome images from a helical scan and include all the information acquired. In cardiac CTA, axial images should be reviewed in all cases and serve as a reference to confirm any pathologic change found or suspected on rendered images.

Multiplanar Reformation

In multiplanar reformation (MPR), a plane is defined within the three-dimensional volume of the scan, and only the data in this plane are displayed. MPR can be performed in either a straight plane or a curved plane (along a vessel's "centerline"). In performing MPR, the thickness of the selection is set to be as thin as the collimation allows. When a greater thickness is selected, a slab MPR is created, and it is usually rendered with maximum intensity projection (see later). MPR can be created in any plane; it is very fast and easy to use and provides images containing all available information (all Hounsfield unit values are retained). Curved MPR with cross-sectional images is the best method for stenosis assessment, particularly in patients with calcified lesions or stents (Fig. 35-11). It is possible to rotate the image around the centerline and to view any plaque from different rotational angles to differentiate between eccentric and concentric plaques. A major disadvantage of MPR is the dependence on manual orientation of the planes that may cause false-positive or false-negative interpretation of stenoses. Interactive viewing of these types of images from multiple viewing angles is therefore required. Furthermore, for each vessel branch, a separate MPR image is required, and only one branch can be displayed at a time. Advanced software is available to allow semiautomatic segmentation of the coronary arteries, to determine the vessel's centerline, and to reconstruct curved MPR as well as cross-sectional images.

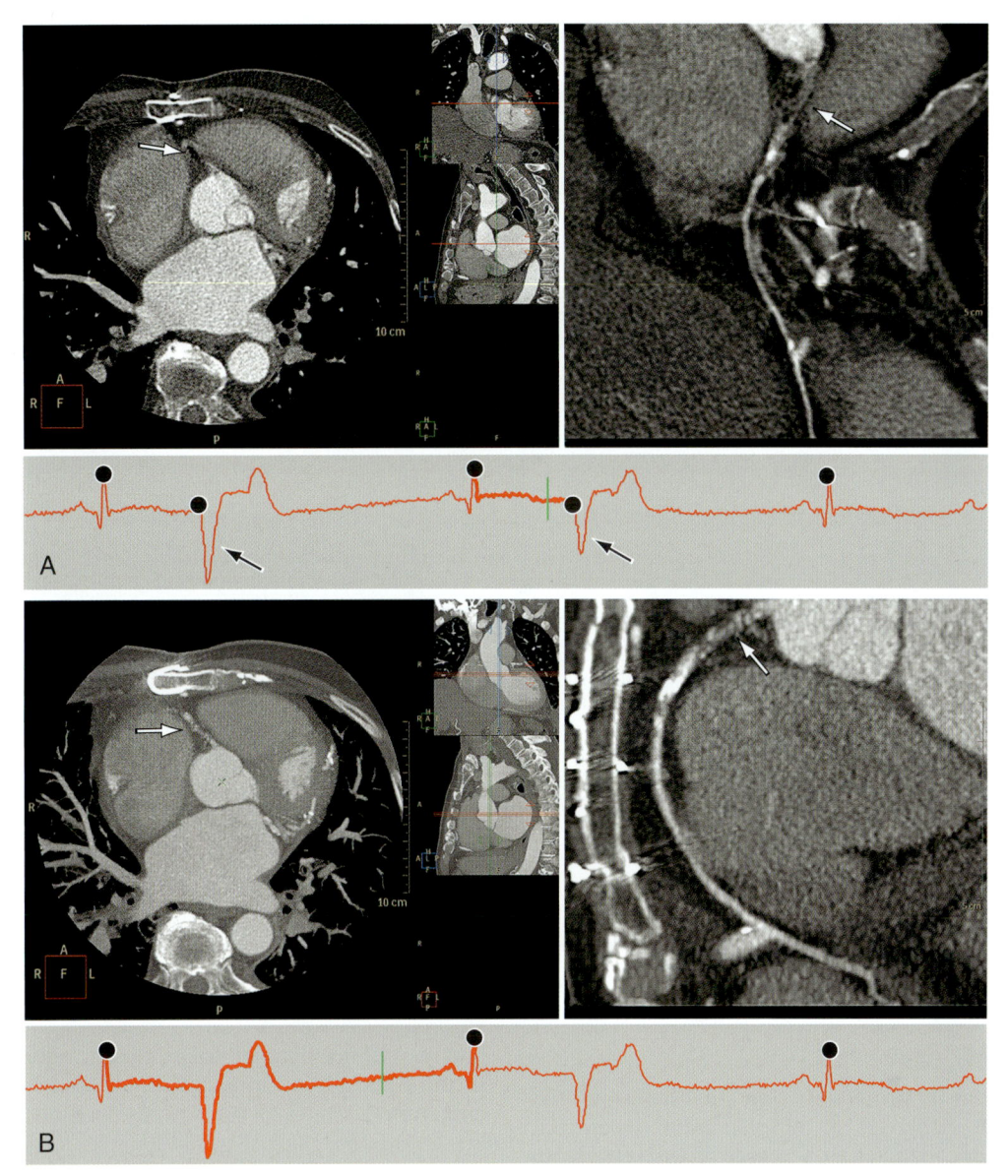

■ **FIGURE 35-9** **A,** On the right, there is blurring of the proximal right coronary artery (*white arrows*) due to premature beats (*black arrows*). **B,** After deletion of the tagging of the premature beats, the visualization of the proximal segment of the right coronary artery is improved, with obvious occlusion (*white arrows*).

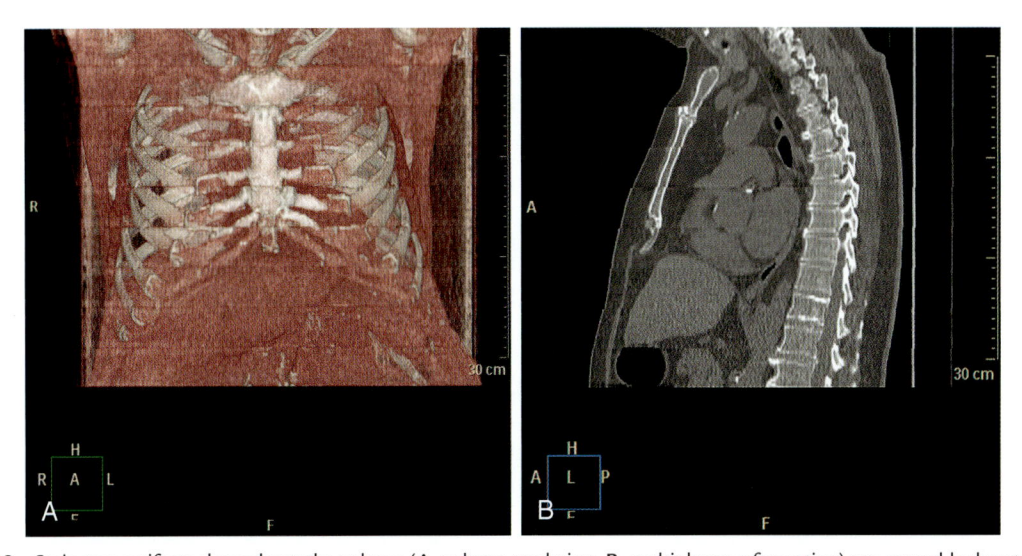

■ **FIGURE 35-10** Stair-step artifacts throughout the volume (**A,** volume rendering; **B,** multiplanar reformation) are caused by heart rate changes during a prospectively gated sequential (axial) acquisition for calcium scoring.

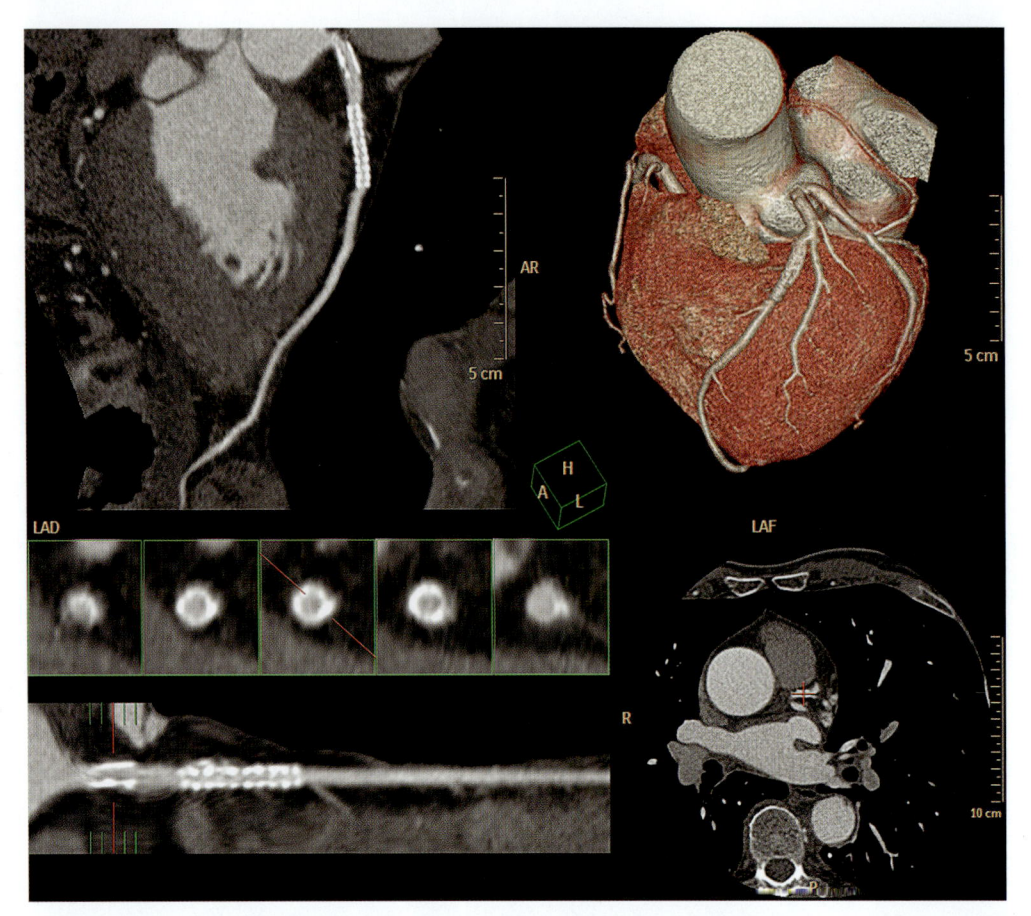

■ **FIGURE 35-11** Curved multiplanar reformation with cross-sectional images is the best method for stenosis assessment, particularly in patients with calcified lesions or stents.

Maximum Intensity Projection

In maximum intensity projection, only the highest attenuation voxels are displayed. A thin-slab MPR is selected (usually in a plane parallel to a vessel of interest) from which a maximum intensity projection image is rendered, and this slab can be moved through the volume. Maximum intensity projection images allow fast evaluation of vascular structures on CTA studies as initial screening of the luminal integrity of the vessel. It is easy to look for irregularities in the artery, with negative or positive remodeling. Because maximum intensity projection images demonstrate only part of the available data, small soft plaques may be obscured, especially with thicker slabs. We have found that a 4- to 6-mm slab is best for initial navigation and evaluation of the coronary tree. With dense material (such as calcifications and stents), this method is unsuitable because it may appear enlarged or thickened with overestimation of stenoses.

Volume Rendering

Volume rendering consists of all pixels above a certain threshold and therefore represents only part of the information. Instead of gray values, color can be attributed to the voxels according to their CT number. Volume rendering provides information about three-dimensional anatomy and orientation in relation to other structures. It allows comprehensive overview of lesion location and myocardial tissue at risk. Volume rendering is operator dependent and should not be used for stenosis evaluation, especially in the presence of dense materials (such as calcifications and stents).

Stenosis Assessment

The rapid evolution of multidetector CT (MDCT) technology has revolutionized cardiac CT, previously limited by cardiac motion, slow acquisition times, and insufficient resolution. Image quality and diagnostic performance have greatly improved with recent technical advances. Many studies have compared MDCT (4-, 16-, and 64-slice scanners) with invasive coronary angiography in the assessment of coronary artery narrowing.

The percentage of unassessable segments was more than 30% on a 4-slice scanner[4,5] and around 22% to 29% with 16-slice scanners.[6,7] One study stated that if these unassessable segments were excluded or considered negative, 25% of patients with a significant stenosis would have been missed.[7] With 64-MDCT, only 3% to 11% of coronary artery segments still cannot be evaluated.[8-11]

Sensitivities and specificities for detection of significant (>50%) coronary artery stenoses based on segmental analysis with 64-MDCT (with conventional x-ray coronary angiography as the standard of reference) have been found to be good to excellent, in the range of 76% to 99% and 95% to 97%, respectively.[11-15] However, these study outcomes are difficult to compare, mainly because of the different selection of patients and the prevalence of sig-

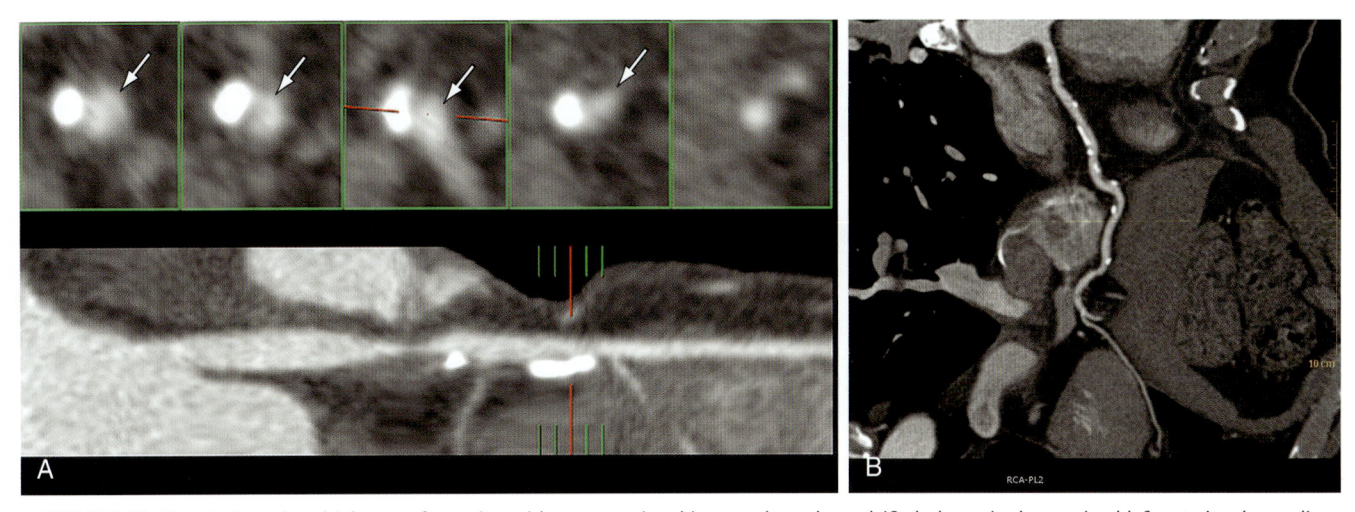

FIGURE 35-12 **A,** Curved multiplanar reformation with cross-sectional images through a calcified plaque in the proximal left anterior descending coronary artery. There is a visible lumen adjacent to the calcification (*arrows*); therefore, significant stenosis (>50%) can be excluded. **B,** In a different patient with multiple calcified plaques along the right coronary artery, it is possible to exclude significant stenosis on the basis of this curved multiplanar reformation.

nificant coronary artery disease. Moreover, these study results should be interpreted with care because of exclusion of unassessable segments from analysis as well as studies with reduced image quality. In an unselected population of patients referred for coronary catheterization with a high prevalence of risk factors, we found high specificity (95%) and negative predictive value (95%) and moderate sensitivity (72%) for significant coronary narrowing with use of a 40-slice scanner.[16] All studies found that cardiac CTA has a very high negative predictive value (95% or higher) for exclusion of significant coronary stenosis.

Accuracy for detection of stenoses depends highly on image quality and artifacts. False-positive and false-negative interpretations were attributed to image artifacts in 91% to 100% of cases,[10,12-14,17,18] mainly because of the presence of calcifications. Less frequent causes were motion artifacts and obesity, resulting in a poor contrast-to-noise ratio.

As mentioned, calcified plaques are a major cause of overestimation of stenosis, mainly with the older generation of scanners (4- and 16-slice scanners). It was recommended to perform a non–contrast-enhanced scan before the cardiac CTA and to avoid scanning patients with high calcium scores (usually above 400 to 600). In our experience, using the 64-slice scanner, with improved temporal and spatial resolution, it is possible to cope with most calcified plaques. Curved MPR with cross-sectional images through the plaque is the method of choice (Fig. 35-12). If a lumen is visible adjacent to a calcification (regardless of its size), significant stenosis (>50%) can be excluded.

Plaque Characterization

Acute coronary events are usually caused by rupture of atherosclerotic plaque (in most cases, nonobstructive plaque), platelet aggregation, and thrombosis with partial or complete occlusion of the arterial lumen. This is one of the reasons that many patients do not have symptoms before their first coronary event. When individuals at increased risk for acute coronary events are identified while still asymptomatic, initiation of preventive therapy, including antiplatelet, antihypertensive, and lipid-lowering medications as indicated, can substantially reduce the risk of coronary artery events. Traditionally, the classic risk factors have been used to identify individuals at risk (quantification of their risk by the Framingham score), but they have limited predictive accuracy. Cardiac CTA is a noninvasive imaging modality allowing identification, quantification, and to some extent characterization of the atherosclerotic process at a subclinical stage. Quantification of coronary calcium (calcium scoring) is an established method to estimate the coronary plaque burden, with a high predictive value for occurrence of future cardiac events in asymptomatic individuals, independently of the traditional risk factors.[19] However, the calcium score (calcified plaques) represents only about 20% of the total plaque burden,[20] and it is the noncalcified component of the plaque that is considered less stable and prone to rupture.

In its early stages, atherosclerotic plaque is usually accompanied by an outward growth of the vessel (termed positive remodeling), indicating a large plaque volume without lumen narrowing. Invasive coronary angiography, the clinical "gold standard" for coronary artery imaging, allows visualization of the lumen only and therefore is not suitable for plaque imaging. Intravascular ultrasound (IVUS) is considered the method of choice for plaque visualization. However, this is a highly invasive and expensive modality, therefore unsuitable for routine use and risk stratification. Cardiac CTA is a noninvasive modality, widely available, that enables visualization of both vessel wall and lumen.

The ability of CT to identify and to characterize nonobstructive plaque composition (calcified, noncalcified, and mixed) has been demonstrated before,[21,22] and Achenbach and coworkers[23] demonstrated vessel wall remodeling in high-quality 16-slice scans. Schroeder and associates[24] studied 12 patients and found that "hypoechoic" plaques on IVUS had a lower mean CT attenuation (14 ± 26 HU) compared with "fibrotic" plaques (91 ± 21 HU) or "calcified" plaques (419 ± 194 HU). Leber and colleagues[25] found a mean density of 49 ± 22 HU for soft plaque,

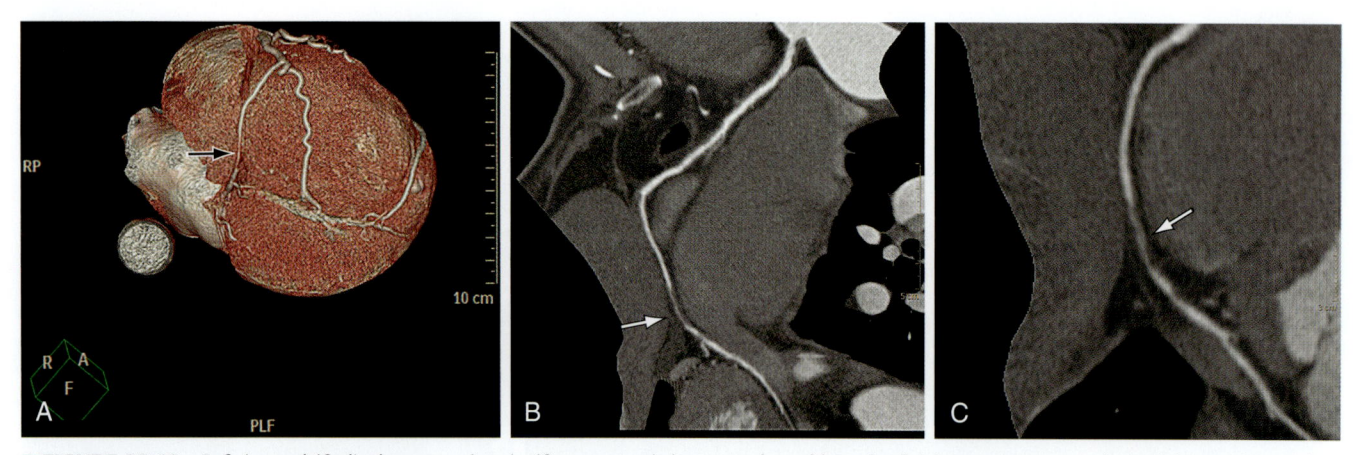

FIGURE 35-13 Soft (noncalcified) plaque causing significant stenosis in posterolateral branch of right coronary artery (*arrows*) in a patient with atypical chest pain and reversible perfusion defect in the lateral wall on thallium scan. **A**, Volume rendering. **B**, Curved multiplanar reformation. **C**, Enlarged section of the curve.

91 ± 226 HU for intermediate (fibrous) plaque, and 391 ± 156 HU for calcified plaque, as defined by IVUS. Even though CT is able to detect a variety of densities within the plaque, in our experience and that of others, there is substantial overlap between those groups. Furthermore, contrast enhancement within the vessel lumen may affect plaque enhancement, leading to variability in readings for any given plaque.

Comparing the performance of the 64-slice scanner with IVUS for noncalcified plaque detection, Leber and colleagues[26] found 84% sensitivity and 91% specificity, with good correlation between plaque and lumen area measured, especially in proximal segments of the coronary tree. Caussin and associates[27] found that 16-detector row CT can accurately assess certain vulnerable plaque characteristics, such as hypodense areas (representing lipid), eccentricity, arterial remodeling, and calcifications, in comparison to IVUS. However, detailed microanatomy and detection of inflammatory changes in unstable lesions are beyond the resolution of current CT scanners.

We compared the total coronary plaque burden (segmental analysis), visualized by cardiac CT, with the traditional risk factors in 97 patients who underwent invasive coronary angiography. We found that nonobstructive coronary plaques were better detected on cardiac CT (277 of 737) than on invasive coronary angiography (111 of 737). The overall plaque burden was significantly higher in patients with diabetes, hypertension, or longer history of coronary artery disease and correlated with the number of risk factors. Furthermore, we found that among symptomatic patients without evidence of calcifications in the coronary arteries, 20% had noncalcified plaques and 7% had significant stenosis on 64-slice cardiac CT.[28] Because the long-term prognostic significance of these findings is currently unknown, additional experience and especially follow-up are needed to determine whether the additional "effort" (radiation, contrast material, time) to detect noncalcified plaques is justified.

Reporting

A CTA report should be useful for the referring physician. It should begin with patient identification data and a brief clinical history as well as the indication for the current study. Next, a brief description of the procedural technique should be mentioned, including the type of scanner, type of contrast material and volume used, premedications (if given), and radiation dose.

Because the accuracy of cardiac CTA depends directly on image quality, it is very important to record the quality of the scan so that the referring physician will be able to assess its reliability. Address these questions: Is the scan assessable and reliable? What are the limitations of the scans? What are the reasons for artifacts? It is easy to answer these questions by a quick leaf through the axial slices or slab maximum intensity projection images of the best phase. If multiple phases are loaded, loop through all of them to choose the best phase and to assess integrity of the data. Changing into a "lung window" can help detect breathing artifacts. It is possible to look at the chest wall and cardiac margins in MPR or volume rendering techniques to assess for motion and stair-step artifacts. Assessment for cardiac motion is easier on an oblique MPR through the right coronary artery and circumflex artery, which are more susceptible to motion. If cardiac motion is detected, additional phases should be reconstructed, trying to find a motion-free phase (if the technologist is not trained to perform this assessment and to look for the best phase for the reader). Looking at the patient's ECG can help detect arrhythmia or heart rate changes during the scan and prompt an R-tag correction if necessary and if software is available. Comment about each unassessable segment (including location and reason). In a coronal MPR, it is easy to assess contrast density and uniformity throughout the aorta and coronary tree as well as noise level within the scan.

Report the calcium score level (if performed) and its clinical significance for the patient's gender and age. In the presence of a zero calcium score, even if the cardiac CTA quality is not optimal, the referring physician can be reassured of the very low likelihood of significant stenosis in a stable patient.

The next step is to report on each of the coronary artery segments visible (Fig. 35-13). Invasive angiography will usually visualize more distal segments than is possible with CTA, but vessels smaller than 1.5 mm are currently not suitable for an intervention (with stent placement or bypass grafting) anyway.

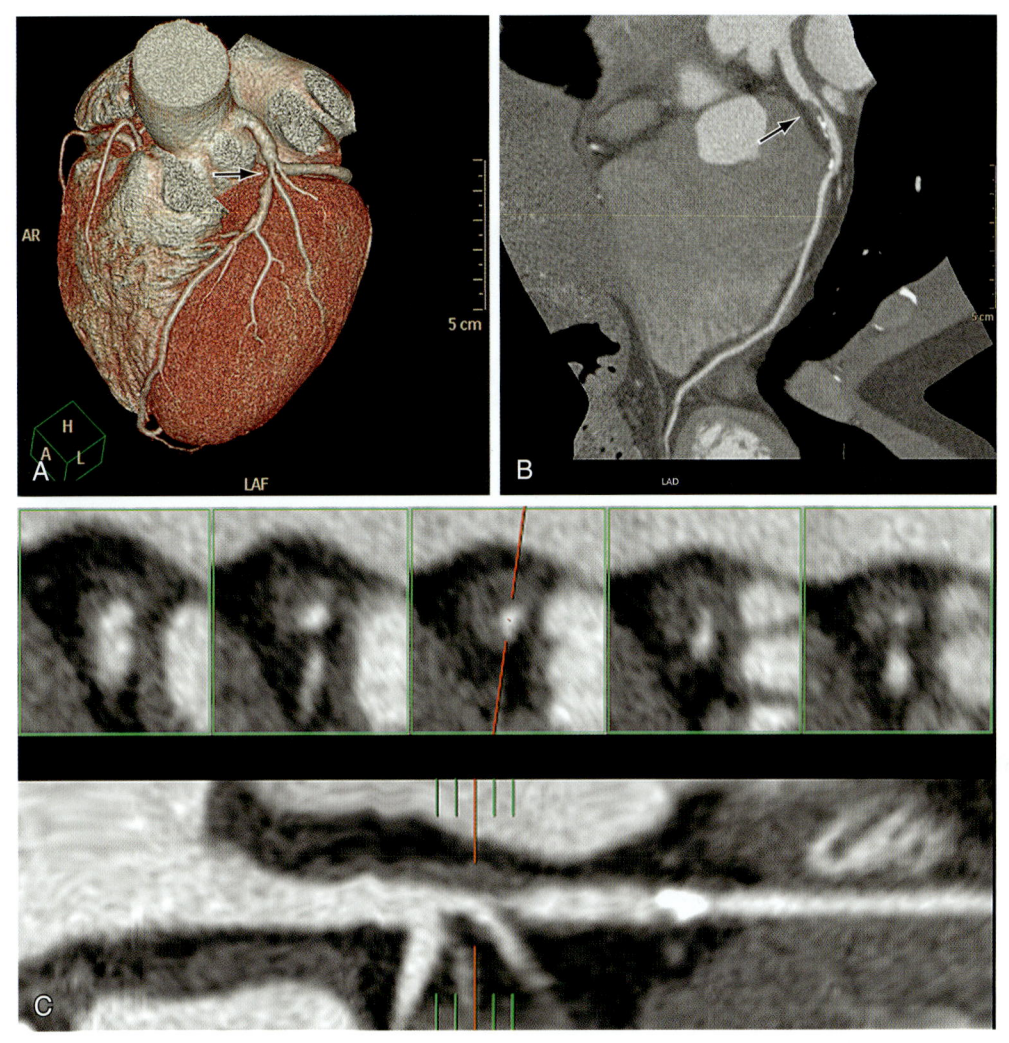

■ **FIGURE 35-14** Mixed plaque in the proximal left anterior descending coronary artery (*arrows*), shown by volume rendering (**A**), curved multiplanar reformation (**B**), and cross-sectional images (**C**), causing significant stenosis.

After the initial navigation with slab maximum intensity projection images to locate areas of suspected stenosis, we perform a curved MPR for each coronary artery and for each visible branch. Because CTA provides three-dimensional information, the view that shows the largest lumen is the correct one (Fig. 35-14). Invasive angiography, on the other hand, is a two-dimensional imaging modality that provides projections of the coronary tree, in which the tightest view is the correct answer. Therefore, it is important to look at every segment from different viewing angles (by rotating the MPR around the centerline) to appreciate correct lumen size. Plaques (especially calcified plaques) should be carefully evaluated in cross-sectional images to assess for a visible lumen adjacent to the calcification. Any abnormality should be confirmed in more than one phase to exclude artifacts.

Considering the spatial resolution of current scanners in relation to the size of the coronary arteries, in addition to the fact that cardiac motion may be reduced but not eliminated completely, cardiac CT cannot be expected to accurately quantify stenosis. Instead, cardiac CT should be used as a "filter" for patients with suspected coronary stenosis before invasive procedures.

For each lesion, it is important to indicate location (ostial, proximal, mid or distal, relation to branches), composition (noncalcified, mixed, or calcified plaque), eccentric or concentric, and evidence of remodeling.

Instead of giving precise stenosis percentage, we prefer to categorize each lesion into groups according to suspected severity of stenosis and clinical relevance (Table 35-2). Our categories include normal (when the vessel is smooth and there is no evidence of plaque), nonsignificant or mild stenosis (when there is some irregularity or plaques causing up to 40% stenosis), borderline lesions (when a lesion is suspected to cause 40% to 60% stenosis), and significant stenosis (when a lesion is suspected to cause more than 70% stenosis up to total occlusion). Alternatively, quartile gradations can be used, such as 0% to 25%, 26% to 50%, 51% to 75%, and 76% to 100%. Remember to underestimate stenosis caused by a calcified plaque (because of the blooming effect), and as long as a lumen is visible, significant stenosis can safely be excluded. The term *total occlusion* should be used only when no contrast material is visible distal to a stenosis because it is not possible to differentiate on CTA between antegrade and retrograde filling of a segment (Fig. 35-15). It is important

TABLE 35-2 Optional Categories for CTA Stenosis Assessment with Clinical Impression and Recommended Next Steps

Category	CTA Findings	Suspected Stenosis	Clinical Impression	Recommended Next Step
Normal	Vessel wall is smooth and there is no evidence of plaque	0%	There is no atherosclerosis	Nothing
Mild stenosis	Some vessel irregularity or nonobstructing plaques	1%-40%	Nonsignificant stenosis	Preventive medical treatment is required to control risk factors and to prevent future coronary events
Borderline lesion	Significant plaque causing borderline stenosis	40%-60%	Questionable significant stenosis; further investigation is needed	Noninvasive functional test (e.g., thallium scan or stress) echocardiography to assess myocardial perfusion
Significant stenosis	Lesion causing significant stenosis	>70%	Flow-limiting lesion causing reduced myocardial perfusion	Invasive angiography for treatment (in symptomatic patients)
Total occlusion	Lack of contrast enhancement within the segment distal to the lesion	100%	Calcifications indicate chronic or acute on chronic lesion	Consider invasive angiography to try to recanalize the segment

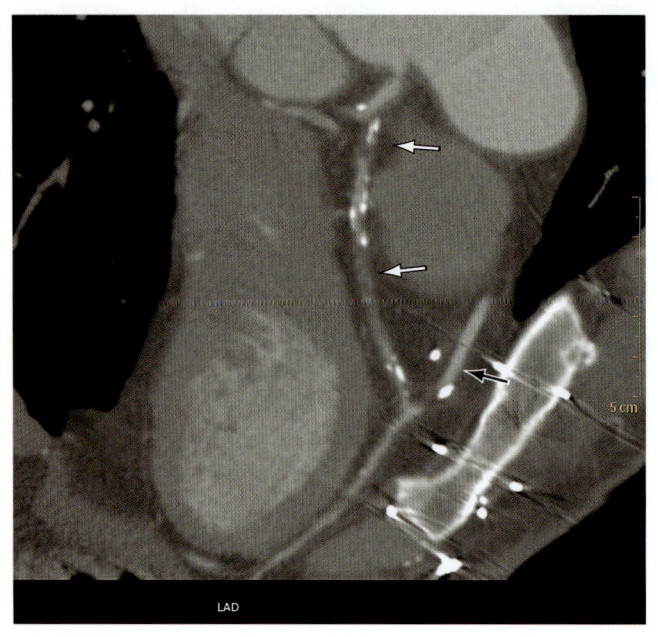

FIGURE 35-15 Total occlusion of the proximal and middle left anterior descending coronary artery (*white arrows*) with a left internal mammary artery to distal left anterior descending coronary artery graft (*black arrow*).

to comment on presence of calcifications within the occluded segment, indicating chronic or acute on chronic lesion, which may be more difficult to treat invasively. When a lesion is difficult to assess (because of artifacts or calcifications), use of a statement such as "stenosis cannot be excluded" may be reasonable.

After the findings and limitations based on scan quality are summarized, it is important to try to answer the questions that the referring physician is asking and to end with reasonable recommendations for the next step.

By dividing the lesions into the mentioned categories, it is easier for the referring physician to decide about the next step that needs to be taken. When the vessels are normal, this implies that no evidence of atherosclerosis is found. With mild stenosis, only preventive medical treatment is required to prevent future coronary events. In borderline lesions, it is clear that further investigation is needed, usually with a noninvasive functional test (myocardial perfusion scan or stress echocardiography). When a patient has obstructive coronary artery disease, an invasive procedure may be warranted for confirmation of stenosis severity and treatment (particularly if it is accompanied by symptoms and significant reversible perfusion defects on functional testing).

KEY POINTS

- With the ongoing advancement in CT technology, the role of CT in the imaging of coronary arteries progressed from simple determination of arterial calcifications to demonstration of the atherosclerotic plaque itself and quantification of luminal stenoses.
- Potential indications for coronary CTA are many and continue to evolve because the technology is constantly changing, there are not enough prospective studies on different groups of patients, and there are no outcome studies.
- Accuracy of cardiac CTA for detection of stenoses depends highly on image quality, and artifacts are a major cause of false-positive and false-negative interpretations.
- Sensitivity and specificity for detection of significant coronary artery stenosis with 64-MDCT compared with invasive angiography are good to excellent, with a very high negative predictive value for exclusion of significant disease. However, different selection of patients may affect these results.
- The percentage of unassessable segments dropped from more than 30% on a 4-slice scanner to only 3% to 11% with 64-slice scanners.
- Curved MPR with cross-sectional images is the best method for stenosis assessment, particularly in patients with calcified lesions or stents.

KEY POINTS—cont'd

- Cardiac CTA allows noninvasive identification, quantification, and to some extent characterization of the atherosclerotic plaque at a subclinical stage.
- Even though CT is able to detect a variety of densities within the plaque, there is substantial overlap between the groups, and contrast enhancement within the lumen may affect plaque density.
- A CTA report should include patient identification data, clinical history and indication for the study, procedural technique, scan quality, calcium score level, and lesions assessment.
- Cardiac CT cannot be expected to quantify stenosis accurately. Instead, cardiac CT should be used as a "filter" for patients with suspected coronary stenosis before invasive procedures, with categories based on suspected severity of stenosis and clinical relevance.

SUGGESTED READING

Kroft LJM, de Roos A, Geleijns J. Artifacts in ECG-synchronized MDCT coronary angiography. AJR Am J Roentgenol 2007; 189:581-591.

REFERENCES

1. Hendel RC, Patel MR, Kramer CM, Poon M. ACCF/ARC/SCCT/SCMR/ASNC/NASCI/SCAI/SIR 2006 appropriateness criteria for cardiac computed tomography and cardiac magnetic resonance imaging: a report of the American College of Cardiology Foundation Quality Strategic Directions Committee Appropriateness Criteria Working Group, American College of Radiology, Society of Cardiovascular Computed Tomography, Society for Cardiovascular Magnetic Resonance, American Society of Nuclear Cardiology, North American Society for Cardiac Imaging, Society for Cardiovascular Angiography and Interventions, and Society of Interventional Radiology. J Am Coll Cardiol 2006; 48:1475-1497.
2. Barrett JF, Keat N. Artifacts in CT: recognition and avoidance. Radiographics 2004; 24:1679-1691.
3. Kroft LJM, de Roos A, Geleijns J. Artifacts in ECG-synchronized MDCT coronary angiography. AJR Am J Roentgenol 2007; 189: 581-591.
4. Giesler T, Baum U, Ropers D, et al. Noninvasive visualization of coronary arteries using contrast-enhanced multidetector CT: influence of heart rate on image quality and stenosis detection. AJR Am J Roentgenol 2002; 179:911-916.
5. Nieman K, Rensing BJ, van Geuns RJ, et al. Usefulness of multislice computed tomography for detecting obstructive coronary artery disease. Am J Cardiol 2002; 89:913-918.
6. Heuschmid M, Kuettner A, Schroeder S, et al. ECG-gated 16-MDCT of the coronary arteries: assessment of image quality and accuracy in detecting stenosis. AJR Am J Roentgenol 2005; 184:1413-1419.
7. Garcia MJ, Lessick J, Hoffmann MHK. Accuracy of 16-row multidetector computed tomography for the assessment of coronary artery stenosis. JAMA 2006; 296:403-411.
8. Ferencik M, Nomura CH, Maurovich-Horvat P, et al. Quantitative parameters of image quality in 64-slice computed tomography angiography of the coronary arteries. Eur J Radiol 2006; 57:373-379.
9. Pannu HK, Jacobs JE, Lai S, Fishman EK. Coronary CT angiography with 64-MDCT: assessment of vessel visibility. AJR Am J Roentgenol 2006; 187:119-126.
10. Leshka S, Husmann L, Desbiolles LM, et al. Optimal image reconstruction intervals for non-invasive coronary angiography with 64-slice CT. Eur Radiol 2006; 16:1964-1972.
11. Nikolaou K, Knez A, Rist C, et al. Accuracy of 64-MDCT in the diagnosis of ischemic heart disease. AJR Am J Roentgenol 2006; 187: 111-117.
12. Mollet NR, Cademartiri F, van Mieghem CAG, et al. High-resolution spiral computed tomography coronary angiography in patients referred for diagnostic conventional coronary angiography. Circulation 2005; 112:2318-2323.
13. Leber AW, Knez A, von Ziegler F, et al. Quantification of obstructive and nonobstructive coronary lesions by 64-slice computed tomography: a comparative study with quantitative coronary angiography and intravascular ultrasound. J Am Coll Cardiol 2005; 46:147-154.
14. Raff GL, Gallagher MJ, O'Neill WW, Goldstein JA. Diagnostic accuracy of noninvasive coronary angiography using 64-slice spiral computed tomography. J Am Coll Cardiol 2005; 46:552-557.
15. Pugliese F, Mollet NRA, Runza G, et al. Diagnostic accuracy of non-invasive 64-slice CT coronary angiography in patients with stable angina pectoris. Eur Radiol 2006; 16:575-582.
16. Halon DA, Gaspar T, Adawi S, et al. Uses and limitations of 40 slice multi-detector row spiral computed tomography for diagnosing coronary lesions in unselected patients referred for routine invasive coronary angiography. Cardiology 2006; 108:200-209.
17. Leschka S, Alkadhi H, Plass A, et al. Accuracy of MSCT coronary angiography with 64-slice technology: first experience. Eur Heart J 2005; 26:1482-1487.
18. Ropers D, Rixe J, Anders K, et al. Usefulness of multidetector row spiral computed tomography with 64- × 0.6-mm collimation and 330-ms rotation for the non-invasive detection of significant coronary artery stenoses. Am J Cardiol 2006; 97:343-348.
19. Shaw LJ, Raggi P, Schisterman E, et al. Prognostic value of cardiac risk factors and coronary artery calcium screening for all-cause mortality. Radiology 2003; 228:826-833.
20. Rumberger JA, Simons DB, Fitzpatrick LA, et al. Coronary artery calcium area by electron beam computed tomography and coronary atherosclerotic plaque area: a histopathologic correlative study. Circulation 1995; 92:2157-2162.
21. Achenbach S, Moselewski F, Ropers D, et al. Detection of calcified and noncalcified coronary atherosclerotic plaque by contrast-enhanced, submillimeter multidetector spiral computed tomography. A segment-based comparison with intravascular ultrasound. Circulation 2004; 109:14-17.
22. Schoenhagen P, Tuzcu EM, Stillman AE, et al. Non-invasive assessment of plaque morphology and remodeling in mildly stenotic coronary segments: comparison of 16-slice computed tomography and intravascular ultrasound. Coron Artery Dis 2003; 14:459-462.
23. Achenbach S, Ropers D, Hoffmann U, et al. Assessment of coronary remodeling in stenotic and nonstenotic coronary atherosclerotic lesions by multidetector spiral computed tomography. J Am Coll Cardiol 2004; 43:842-847.
24. Schroeder S, Kopp AF, Baumbach A, et al. Noninvasive detection and evaluation of atherosclerotic coronary plaques with multislice computed tomography. J Am Coll Cardiol 2001; 37:1430-1435.

25. Leber AW, Knez A, Becker A, et al. Accuracy of multidetector spiral computed tomography in identifying and differentiating the composition of coronary atherosclerotic plaques. J Am Coll Cardiol 2004; 43:1241-1247.
26. Leber AW, Knez A, Ziegler F, et al. Quantification of obstructive and nonobstructive coronary lesions by 64-slice computed tomography—a comparative study with quantitative coronary angiography and intravascular ultrasound. J Am Coll Cardiol 2005; 46:147-154.
27. Caussin C, Ohanessian A, Ghostine S, et al. Characterization of vulnerable nonstenotic plaque with 16-slice computed tomography compared with intravascular ultrasound. Am J Cardiol 2004; 94:99-104.
28. Rubinshtein R, Gaspar T, Halon DA, et al. Prevalence and extent of obstructive coronary artery disease in patients with zero or low calcium score undergoing 64-slice cardiac multidetector computed tomography for evaluation of chest pain syndrome. Am J Cardiol 2007; 99:472-475.

CHAPTER 36

Coronary Artery Aneurysms

Jon C. George, Mariana Meyers, and Robert C. Gilkeson

DEFINITION

Coronary artery aneurysm (CAA) is defined as a dilation more than 1.5 times the diameter of adjacent normal segments.[1] It was first described by Morgagni in 1781[2,3]; the first case report was published by Bougon in 1812,[1,4] and the first documented case with angiography was published by Munker in 1958.[5,6] Before the advent of coronary angiography, CAAs were detected primarily at postmortem examination; however, most cases today are incidental findings on angiography.

PREVALENCE AND EPIDEMIOLOGY

The reported incidence of CAAs ranges from 0.2% to 4.9% among patients undergoing evaluation for coronary disease.[1,5] They occur predominantly in men at a ratio of almost 3:1.[4] CAAs are predominantly caused by atherosclerosis (52%). They may be single or multiple, may be focal or diffuse, and can involve various segments of the coronary circulation. They most commonly involve the right coronary artery (Fig. 36-1) followed by the left anterior descending (Fig. 36-2) and the left circumflex (Fig. 36-3) arteries.[4]

Atherosclerotic aneurysms of the left main coronary artery are rare, but have been reported.[7] Other important etiologies include congenital (17%), mycotic-embolic (11%), dissecting (11%), syphilitic (4%), and unclassified (5%).[4] Although most cases worldwide are secondary to atherosclerosis, systemic inflammatory diseases such as Takayasu arteritis (Fig. 36-4) and the mucocutaneous lymph node syndromes of Kawasaki disease (Fig. 36-5) account for many cases in East Asia.[8] Modern interventional techniques have also resulted in iatrogenic causes of CAAs. In the current era of percutaneous intervention, CAAs can be seen secondary to balloon angioplasty or stent deployment.[9] The increasing use of coronary artery bypass grafting techniques has resulted in numerous reports of saphenous vein graft aneurysms (Fig. 36-6), although they remain uncommon.

Although CAAs may be found at any age, atherosclerotic subtypes are predominant later in life, whereas congenital (Figs. 36-7 and 36-8), mycotic-embolic, and dissecting types are found in younger age groups. Multiple CAAs in childhood and adolescence are usually late complications of Kawasaki disease (Fig. 36-9).[10]

CAAs are associated with systemic syndromes of hyperlipidemia and hypertension, but a correlation between aneurysm size and cardiac risk factors has not been proven.[8,11] They have been shown to be more prevalent in patients with aortic aneurysms, which is corroborated by studies showing increased diameter indices of iliac arteries in patients with known CAA (Fig. 36-10).[12]

ETIOLOGY AND PATHOPHYSIOLOGY

CAA is likely a variant of obstructive coronary artery disease in most cases; however, its pathogenesis has not been fully elucidated. Systemic hypertension, inflammatory stimuli such as tobacco or increased inflammatory response in the vessel wall, hyperhomocysteinemia, and chronic Epstein-Barr virus infection are implicated as etiologic factors. Genetic predisposition or gene disruption, interference with normal cross-linking of collagen, and activation of matrix metalloproteinases are all possible factors implicated in the weakening of the vessel wall in aneurysmal disease.[8]

MANIFESTATIONS OF DISEASE

Clinical Presentation

Presentations of CAAs are almost always suggestive of coronary ischemia requiring further ischemic evaluations, which generally detect the anomaly.[3] Because CAAs are usually associated with obstructive atherosclerotic coronary disease, the clinical course depends on the severity of the associated stenosis,[3] and can culminate in myocardial infarction or sudden death complicated by

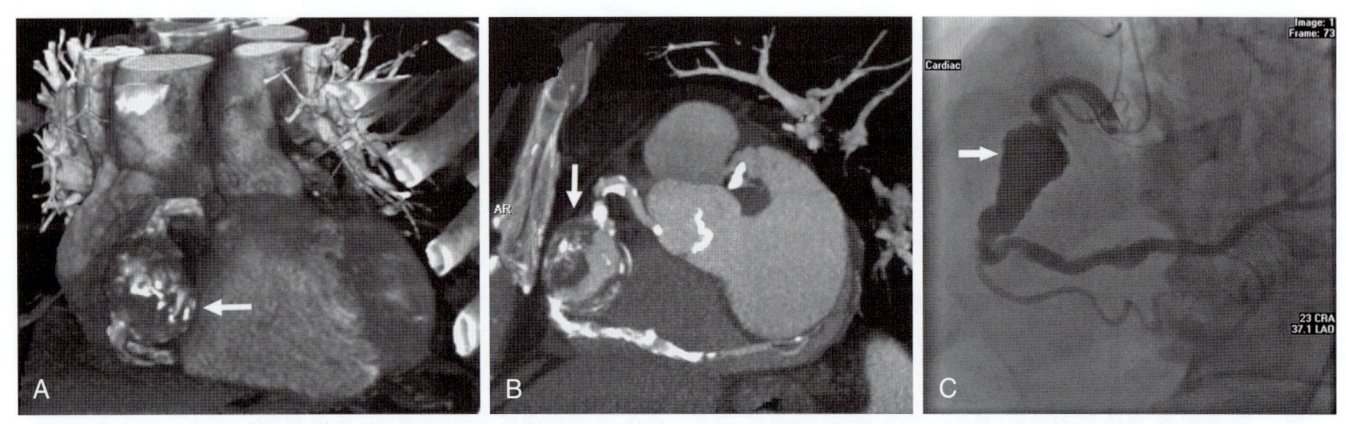

FIGURE 36-1 A 67-year-old patient with a right coronary artery (RCA) aneurysm presented for preoperative CT angiography evaluation. **A,** Coronal volume rendered image shows large calcified RCA aneurysm (*arrow*). **B,** Oblique sagittal maximum intensity projection better defines the full extent of the aneurysmal dilation (*arrow*) of the RCA. **C,** Conventional catheter angiography confirms aneurysmal dilation of the RCA (*arrow*).

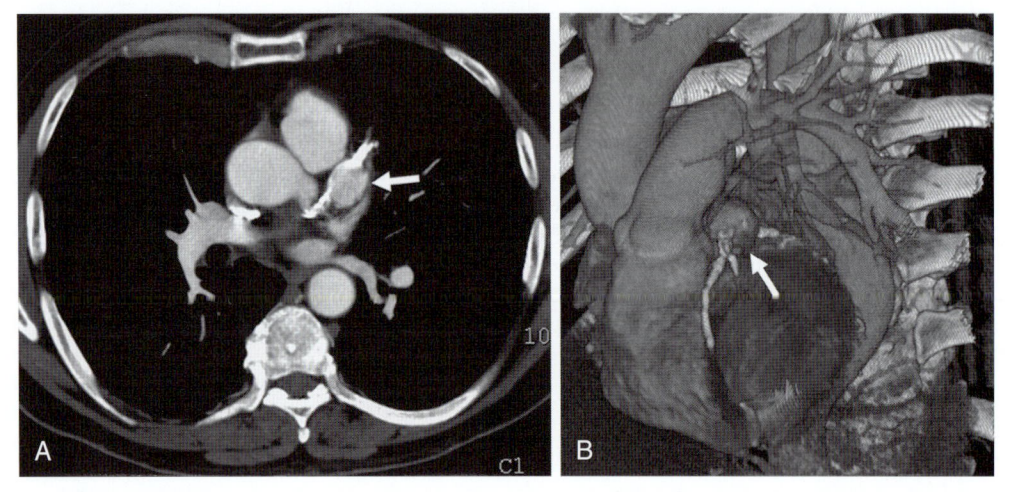

FIGURE 36-2 **A** and **B,** Coronary CT angiography shows focal aneurysm (*arrows*) of the left anterior descending coronary artery. **A,** Axial image. **B,** Coronal oblique volume rendered image.

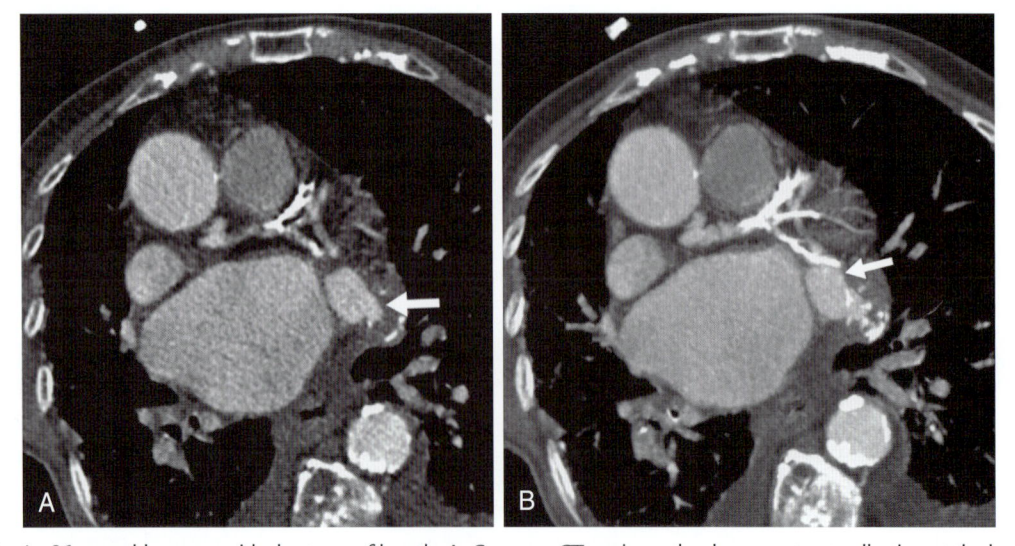

FIGURE 36-3 An 86-year-old woman with shortness of breath. **A,** Coronary CT angiography shows contrast collection at the level of the mitral annulus (*arrow*) consistent with aneurysm of the left circumflex coronary artery. **B,** Oblique maximum intensity projection CT angiography defines aneurysmal dilation of diffusely diseased circumflex artery (*arrow*).

CHAPTER 36 • *Coronary Artery Aneurysms* 511

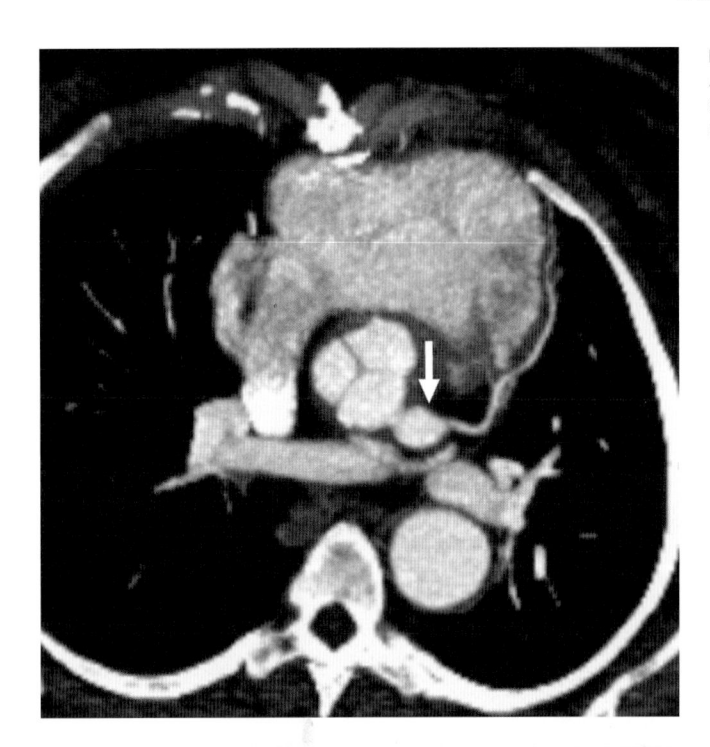

■ **FIGURE 36-4** A 21-year-old woman with history of Takayasu disease. Axial oblique maximum intensity projection from coronary CT angiography shows aneurysmal dilation of left main coronary artery (*arrow*).

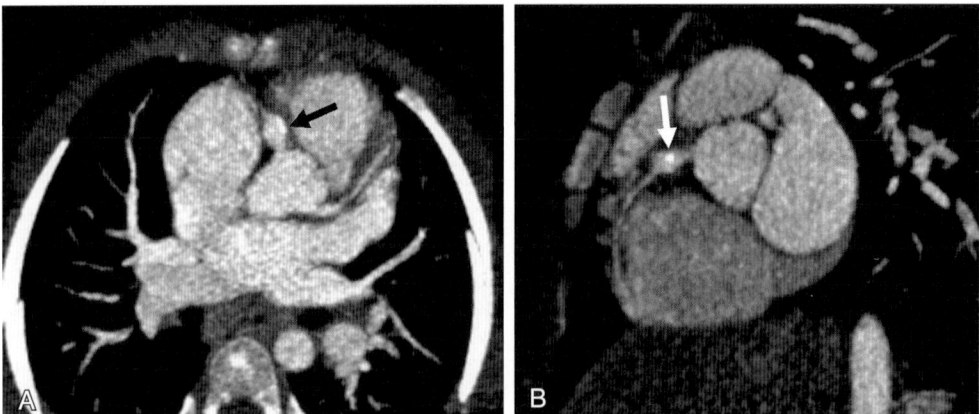

■ **FIGURE 36-5** An 8-month-old infant with Kawasaki disease. **A,** Axial maximum intensity projection CT angiography shows aneurysmal dilation of the right coronary artery (*arrow*). **B,** Sagittal oblique maximum intensity projection CT angiography confirms aneurysmal right coronary artery (*arrow*).

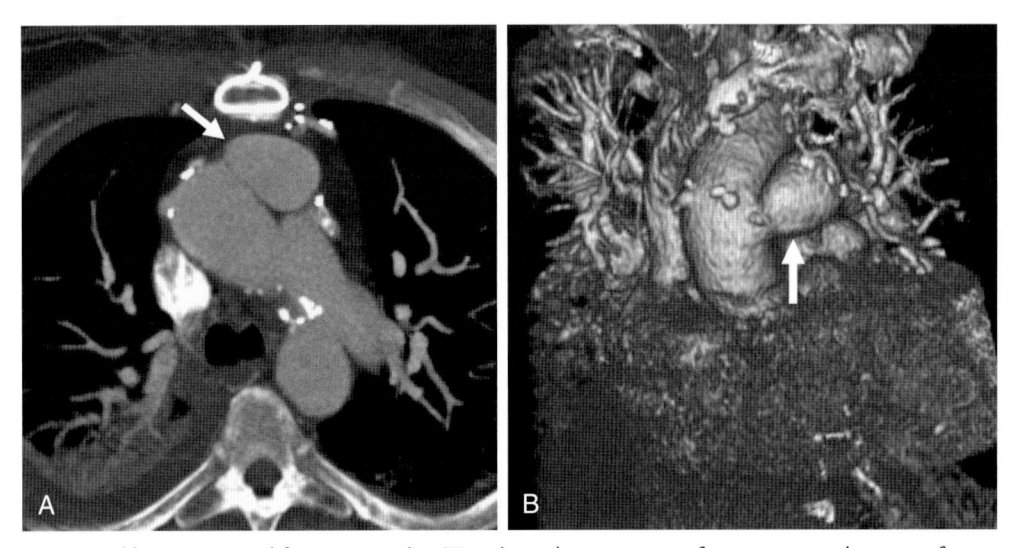

■ **FIGURE 36-6** A 76-year-old man presented for postoperative CT angiography assessment of coronary artery bypass graft patency. **A,** Axial oblique maximum intensity projection image shows a fusiform contrast collection (*arrow*) adjacent to the ascending aorta. **B,** Coronal volume rendered image confirms proximal pseudoaneurysm of a saphenous vein graft (*arrow*).

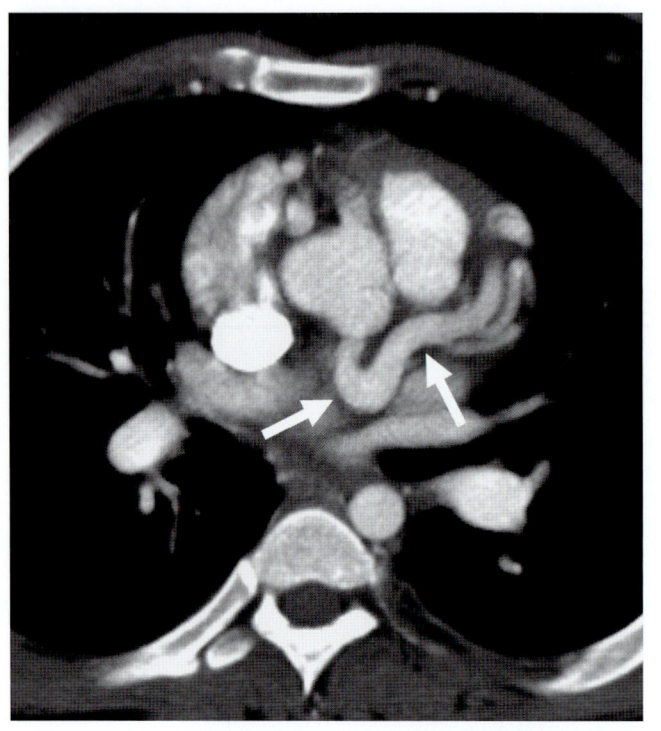

FIGURE 36-7 A 17-year-old patient with Down syndrome and uncorrected endocardial cushion defect. Axial maximum intensity projection CT shows diffuse coronary artery ectasia of the left coronary artery (*arrows*).

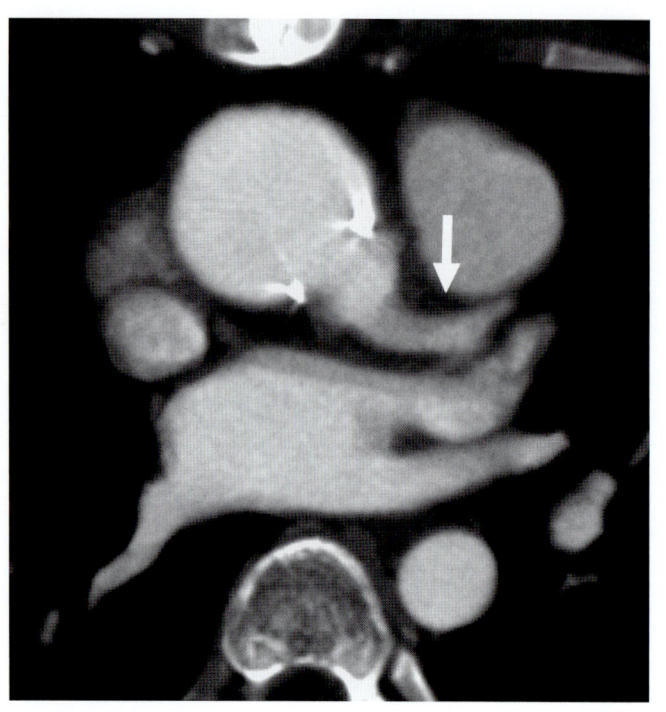

FIGURE 36-8 A 9-year-old child with congenital aortic stenosis. Axial maximum intensity projection CT shows fusiform dilation of the proximal left main coronary artery (*arrow*).

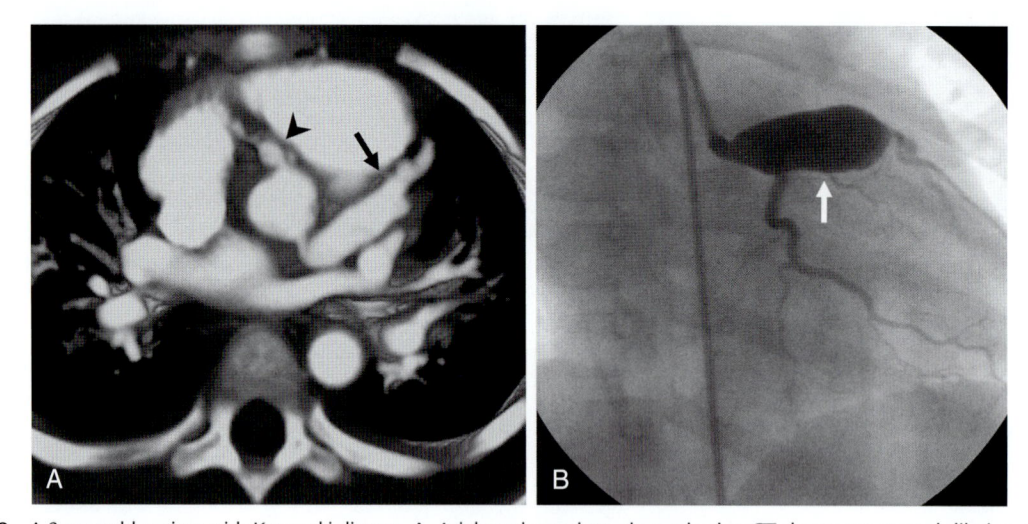

FIGURE 36-9 A 3-year-old patient with Kawasaki disease. **A,** Axial maximum intensity projection CT shows aneurysmal dilation of left anterior descending coronary artery (*arrow*). **B,** Catheter angiography confirms large LAD aneurysm (*arrow*).

thrombus formation, distal embolization, shunt formation, or rupture.[8] Exercise-induced angina pectoris or myocardial infarction may occur without significant coronary artery stenosis, however, and is usually attributed to distal microembolization of thrombus or microcirculatory dysfunction reflected by depressed coronary flow reserve in these patients.[8,13] The natural history and prognosis of this entity are unknown; however, observational studies have documented development of myocardial infarction with angiographically documented occlusion of the involved aneurysmal vessel.[3,5]

Imaging Techniques and Findings
Radiography

Although CAAs are commonly an incidental finding, rare cases of giant coronary aneurysms can cause a significant

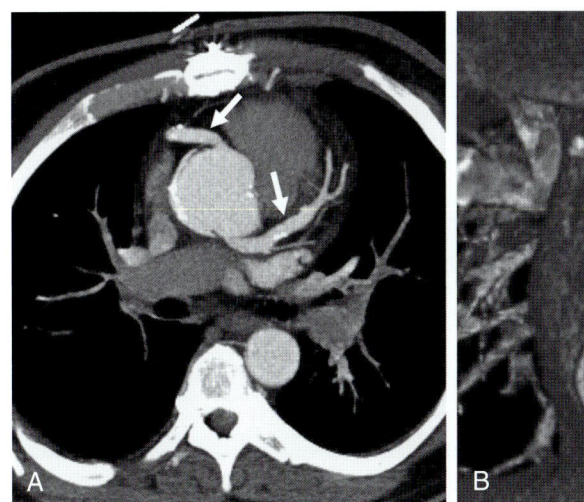

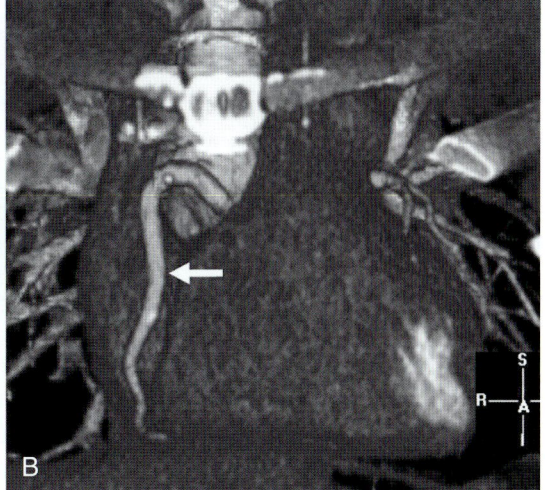

■ **FIGURE 36-10** A 50-year-old man with a history of dissecting aortic aneurysm and phenotypic features of Marfan syndrome. **A**, Axial oblique maximum intensity projection CT angiography shows diffuse aneurysmal dilation of the coronary arteries (*arrows*). **B**, Coronal volume rendered CT angiography image of the aneurysmal right coronary artery (*arrow*).

protrusion of the heart border on chest x-rays[14] or compression of cardiac chambers on echocardiography.[15]

Angiography

CAAs complicated by rupture or fistula formation (into a cardiac chamber) may create a continuous murmur on auscultation. The standard of reference for the diagnosis of CAAs is via a percutaneous approach with coronary angiography, which provides information about the size, shape, location, and number of aneurysms.[8] Evaluation and serial follow-up may require other diagnostic methods. Intravascular ultrasound further allows for distinguishing true and false aneurysms.[8]

Cardiac CT angiography enables a noninvasive alternative for initial diagnosis and follow-up. Its tomographic capabilities enable improved visualization of extraluminal pathology and important surrounding extravascular anatomy.[16] In suspected aneurysmal disease, standard cardiac CT angiography protocols are performed. Prospective ECG gating or retrospective ECG gating can be performed with dose modulation using 120 kV and 800 mAs (effective). An intravenous contrast agent is administered: 75 to 100 mL of 350 to 375 mg I/mL contrast agent, followed by 30 mL of saline. Studies are typically performed with an automated bolus tracking technique with the region of interest placed in the ascending aorta or with a timing bolus. Studies performed with retrospective gating are reconstructed at 10% intervals of the cardiac cycle. Although standard multiplanar reconstructions are performed for diagnosis, volume rendered reconstruction techniques can be helpful in preoperative planning.

DIFFERENTIAL DIAGNOSIS

Important differential diagnoses in the evaluation CAAs include benign and malignant mediastinal masses. CAAs may mimic cardiac/pericardial masses on standard CT acquisitions. CAAs need to be distinguished from focal aneurysms or pseudoaneurysms of the aorta and the sinuses of Valsalva. The imaging advances of retrospective ECG gating and three-dimensional reconstruction enable confident differentiation of CAAs from ventricular aneurysms.

TREATMENT OPTIONS

Medical

The management of CAAs can be medical, percutaneous, or surgical. If the patient is asymptomatic, and medical therapy is chosen, the regimen should include antiplatelet therapy with or without anticoagulation to prevent thromboembolic complications.[3,16] Risk factor modification with statins and antihypertensives may be beneficial in slowing the progression of atherosclerotic aneurysmal disease, but this has not been established.

Surgical/Interventional

Surgery is generally advised for large aneurysms associated with significant coronary stenosis, which includes ligation and bypass of the aneurysm.[17] Percutaneous approaches are increasingly being reported for moderate-sized aneurysms with associated coronary stenosis via polytetrafluoroethylene-covered balloon-expandable[18] or self-expandable stents.[19] Even complicated aneurysms with fistulization, when appropriate, can be addressed percutaneously with coil embolization (Fig. 36-11).[20]

KEY POINTS

- CAAs are uncommon but important complications of atherosclerotic heart disease.
- Kawasaki disease is the most common cause of CAAs in pediatric patients.
- Iatrogenic CAAs occur after catheter interventions and coronary artery bypass graft surgery.
- Retrospective ECG techniques are important in CAA evaluations.

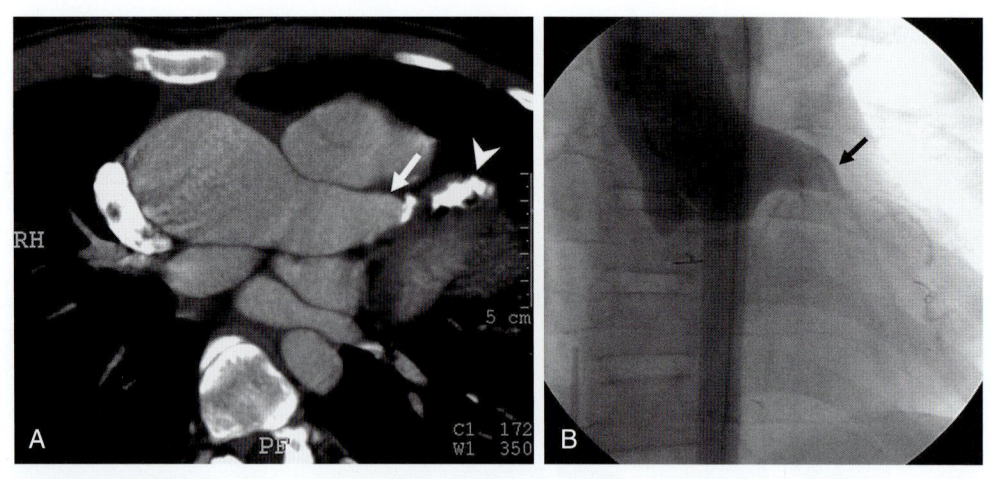

FIGURE 36-11 A 12-year-old child with a history of coronary artery–coronary sinus fistula after coil embolization. **A,** Axial maximum intensity projection CT image shows dilation of the left main and LAD arteries (*arrow*) with distal coil occlusion (*arrowhead*). **B,** Catheter angiography confirms occlusion of aneurysmal left main coronary artery (*arrow*).

SUGGESTED READINGS

Dell'Amore A, Sanna S, Botta L, et al. Giant atherosclerotic aneurysm of left internal mammary artery. Eur J Cardiothorac Surg 2006; 30: 557-558.

Kobulnik J, Hutchison SJ, Leong-Poi H. Saphenous vein graft aneurysm masquerading as a left atrial mass: diagnosis by contrast transesophageal echocardiography. J Am Soc Echocardiogr 2007; 20:1414.e1-1414.e 4.

REFERENCES

1. Swaye PS, Fisher LD, Litwin P, et al. Aneurysmal coronary artery disease. Circulation 1983; 67:134-138.
2. Morgagni JB. De sedibus et causis morborum per anatoment indagatis. Tomus Primus Liber II, Epist 27, Articlo 28. Venetiis, 1761.
3. Rath S, Har-Zahav Y, Battler A, et al. Fate of nonobstructive aneurysmatic coronary artery disease: angiographic and clinical follow-up report. Am Heart J 1985; 109:785-791.
4. Daoud AS, Pankin D, Tulgan H, et al. Aneurysms of the coronary artery: report of ten cases and review of literature. Am J Cardiol 1963; 11:228-237.
5. Dagalp Z, Pamir G, Alpman A, et al. Coronary artery aneurysms: report of two cases and review of the literature. Angiology 1996; 47:197-201.
6. Wilson CS, Weaver WF, Forker AD, et al. Bilateral arteriosclerotic coronary arterial aneurysms successfully treated with saphenous vein bypass grafting. Am J Cardiol 1975; 35:315-318.
7. Gowda RM, Dogan OM, Tejani FH, et al. Left main coronary artery aneurysm. Int J Cardiol 2005; 105:115-116.
8. Pahlavan PS, Niroomand F. Coronary artery aneurysm: a review. Clin Cardiol 2006; 29:439-443.
9. Bavry AA, Chiu JH, Jefferson BK, et al. Development of coronary aneurysm after drug-eluting stent implantation. Ann Intern Med 2007; 146:230-232.
10. Markis JE, Joffe DC, Cohn PF, et al. Clinical significance of coronary ectasia. Am J Cardiol 1976; 37:217-222.
11. Baman TS, Cole JH, Devireddy CM, et al. Risk factors and outcomes in patients with coronary artery aneurysms. Am J Cardiol 2004; 93:1549-1551.
12. Kahraman H, Ozaydin M, Varol E, et al. The diameters of the aorta and its major branches in patients with isolated coronary artery ectasia. Tex Heart Inst J 2006; 33:463-468.
13. Akyurek O, Berkalp B, Sayin T, et al. Altered coronary flow properties in diffuse coronary artery ectasia. Am Heart J 2003; 145:66-72.
14. Tanabe M, Onishi K, Hiraoka N, et al. Bilateral giant coronary aneurysms diagnosed non-invasively by dynamic magnetic resonance imaging. Int J Cardiol 2004; 94(2-3):341-342.
15. McGlinchey PG, Maynard SJ, Graham AN, et al. Giant aneurysm of the right coronary artery compressing the right heart. Circulation 2005; 112:e66-e67.
16. Plehn G, van Bracht M, Zuehlke C, et al. From atherosclerotic coronary ectasia to aneurysm: a case report and literature review. Int J Cardiovasc Imaging 2006; 22:311-316.
17. Harandi S, Johnston SB, Wood RE, et al. Operative therapy of coronary arterial aneurysm. Am J Cardiol 1999; 83:1290-1293.
18. Lee MS, Nero T, Makkar RR, et al. Treatment of coronary aneurysm in acute myocardial infarction with Angio-Jet thrombectomy and JoStent coronary stent graft. J Invasive Cardiol 2004; 16:294-296.
19. Burzotta F, Trani C, Romagnoli E, et al. Percutaneous treatment of a large coronary aneurysm using the self-expandable Symbiot PTFE-covered stent. Chest 2004; 126:644-645.
20. Jo SH, Choi YJ, Oh DJ, et al. Coronary artery fistula with a huge aneurysm treated by transcatheter coil embolization. Circulation 2006; 114:e631-e634.

CHAPTER 37

Imaging of Coronary Revascularization: Coronary Stents and Bypass Grafts

Jean Jeudy, Stephen Waite, and Joseph Jen-Sho Chen

NONINVASIVE EVALUATION OF CORONARY STENTS

Since Dr. Andreas Gruentzig performed the first successful percutaneous transluminal coronary angioplasty (PTCA) in 1977,[1] this procedure has become commonplace with more than 550,000 PTCA procedures performed in the United States in 2000. In the late 1980s Dr. Julio Palmaz invented the bare-metal stent (BMS). In 1993, randomized clinical trials demonstrated decreased angiographic restenosis rates (defined as >50% narrowing of a previously stented site) compared with PTCA alone—ushering in the era of elective stent implantation.[2] Currently, more than 80% of patients undergoing percutaneous coronary intervention also receive intracoronary stents (Fig. 37-1).[3] Intracoronary stent implantation is not, however, without risk with two major complications—occlusion secondary to thrombosis and restenosis.[4] Many patients undergo repeat angiography to ascertain the presence of these complications; however, given the invasive nature of coronary angiography and its potential complications, a noninvasive technique for detection of these complications would be clinically important.

In-Stent Restenosis and Thrombosis— Etiology, Prevalence, Pathophysiology

Restenosis after angioplasty can result from early vessel recoil, late constrictive remodeling (also called *negative remodeling*), and neointimal proliferation. Elastic recoil occurs nearly instantaneously, secondary to passive recoil of elastic media. Late constrictive remodeling occurs within 1 to 6 months and is secondary to increased collagen in the extracellular matrix and adventitial thickening.[1] Intracoronary stents prevent these mechanisms (acute recoil and constrictive remodeling) (Fig. 37-2).

Unfortunately, stent-induced vascular injury causes increased neointimal hyperplasia/proliferation. The pathophysiology includes proliferation and migration of smooth muscle cells and extracellular matrix formation.[1] In-stent restenosis, the principal problem after angioplasty, has a clinical incidence of 20% to 40% for bare-metal stents.[5,6] Although several characteristics of high-risk populations have been described as clinical predictors, the likelihood of restenosis in a particular patient remains largely unpredictable.[6,7]

Drug-eluting stents (DES) have revolutionized the treatment of coronary artery disease through marked reduction of in-stent restenosis.[8] The components of these stents can be divided into a platform (the stent), a carrier (usually a polymer), and an agent (a drug) to prevent restenosis (Fig. 37-3).[2] The advantage of using a stent as a delivery system is that it allows for local delivery of the drug and averts the need for higher systemic doses. The biology of vascular cells and the cell cycle is being used as a target to prevent restenosis and current agents used in drug-eluting stents all interfere with the cell cycle in some manner.[1] Numerous trials have established that sirolimus and paclitaxel drug-eluting stents markedly reduce the incidence of in-stent restenosis. DES have reduced restenosis rates to less than 10% at a 12-month follow-up.[6,9,10]

Although drug-eluting stents have significantly reduced restenosis events, its very effectiveness has led to increased rates of an uncommon but potentially very severe complication, in-stent thrombosis. To understand this phenomenon, it is important to be aware of risk factors for development of in-stent thrombosis. Persistent, slow coronary blood flow such as occurs with dissection or hypoperfusion, exposure of the blood to prothrombotic subendothelial constituents, such as tissue factor or to the stent itself, and failure to suppress platelet adhesion/aggregation at a time of prothrombotic risk predispose the patient to in-stent thrombosis.[11]

A probable explanation for an increased risk of thrombosis in DES compared to BMS after cessation of antiplatelet therapy is delayed arterial healing.[11] Normally after vascular injury, the vessel wall undergoes a number of changes including migration and hypertrophy of vascular smooth muscle cells. During this period, endothelial cells colonize the surface of the stent and regain their normal function.[12] DES cause incomplete neointimal coverage and delay endothelialization of the stent. Subsequently, there is eventual propagation of thrombi over the surface of the stent.

The reported incidence of thrombosis of bare-metal stents 1 month postprocedure has ranged from 0.5% to 2.5% in clinical trials. Bare-metal stent thrombosis usually occurs within the first 24 to 48 hours or much less commonly within the first month after stent placement. Eighty percent of stent thrombosis events have been found to occur within the first 2 days and events occurring more than 1 week after the procedure were rare.[13] Stent thrombosis within 1 year of implantation occurs with similar frequency between DES and BES; however beyond 1 year, there is a small but significant increased risk of very late stent thrombosis in DES.[14] Because of this increased risk, extension of antiplatelet therapy is recommended.

The decision to place a drug-eluting rather than a bare-metal stent therefore rests on clinical grounds and evaluation of the benefits and risks of these stents. The lower rate of repeat target revascularization with DES must be weighed against the cost of longer term antiplatelet therapy to prevent stent thrombosis, the risk of bleeding, and the complications of noncompliance with drug therapy (Fig. 37-4).

Clinical Presentation

Restenosis following angioplasty and stent implantation is classically considered a benign process in which the typical patient presents with exertional angina.[14] Importantly, however, an appreciable proportion of these patients present with an acute coronary syndrome. One study from the Cleveland Clinic demonstrated that 9.5% of patients with restenosis presented with acute myocardial infarction and 26.4% presented with unstable angina.[15]

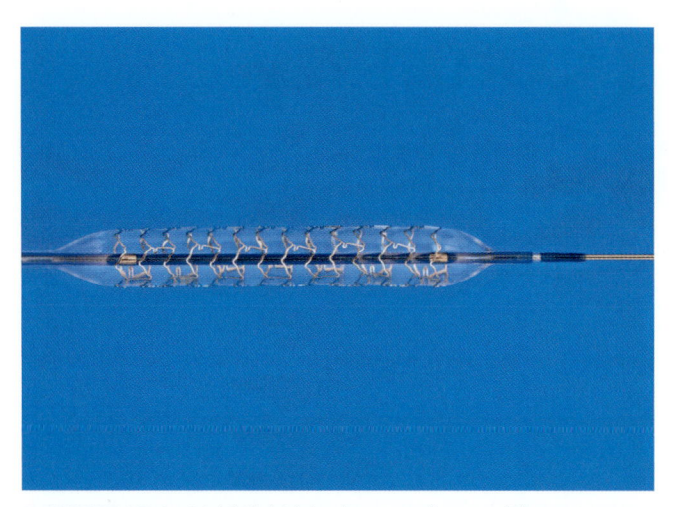

■ **FIGURE 37-1** Multi-Link Vision bare-metal stent. *(Photo courtesy Abbott Vascular, Abbott Park, Ill.)*

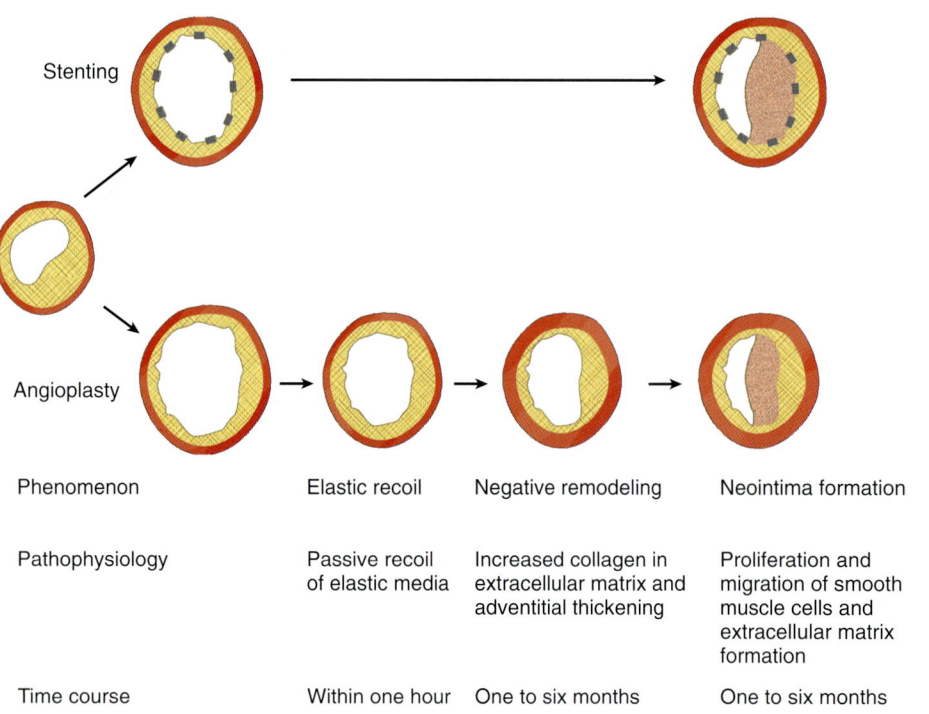

■ **FIGURE 37-2** Mechanisms contributing to coronary restenosis. Elastic recoil and negative remodeling contribute to stenosis but are controlled by coronary stenting. Stenting does, however, not reduce and indeed may promote neointimal proliferation. *(From Dobesh PP, Stacy ZA, Ansara AJ, et al. Drug-eluting stents: a mechanical and pharmacologic approach to coronary artery disease. Pharmacotherapy 2004; 24(11):1554-1577.)*

	Phenomenon	Elastic recoil	Negative remodeling	Neointima formation
	Pathophysiology	Passive recoil of elastic media	Increased collagen in extracellular matrix and adventitial thickening	Proliferation and migration of smooth muscle cells and extracellular matrix formation
	Time course	Within one hour	One to six months	One to six months

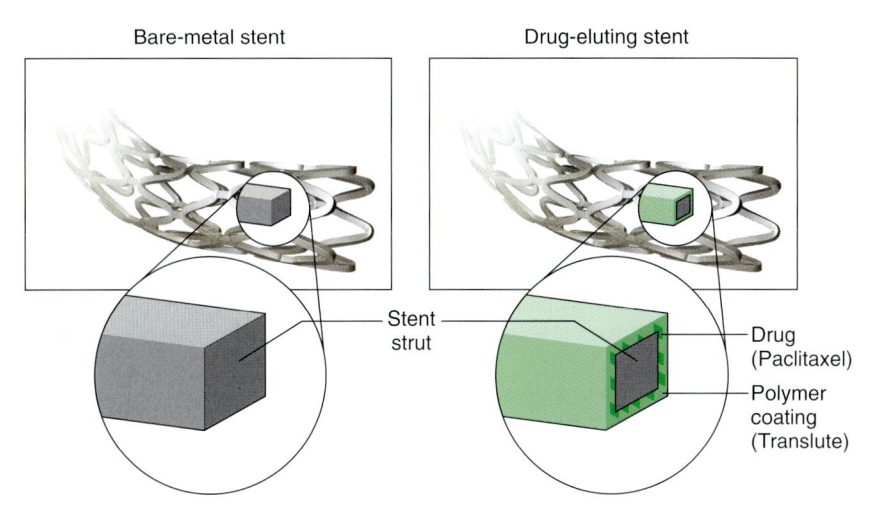

FIGURE 37-3 Schematic diagram of a bare-metal stent and a drug-eluting stent. A drug-eluting stent is coated with a polymer that allows consistent controlled release of a drug into the arterial wall.

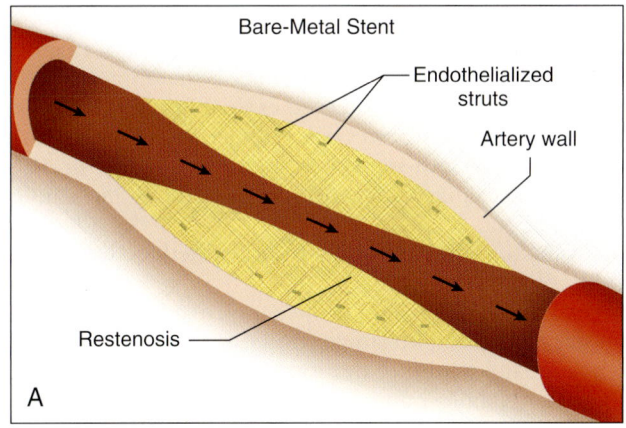

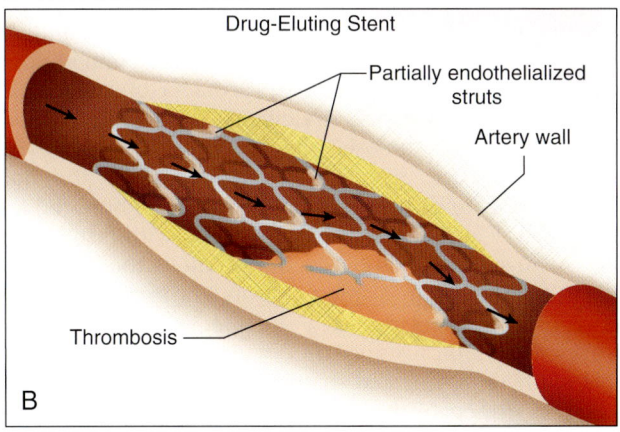

FIGURE 37-4 Illustration demonstrating potential complications of coronary stenting: Restenosis in a traditional bare-metal stent (**A**) and late thrombosis in a drug-eluting stent (**B**). *(Reprinted with permission from Curfman GD, Morrisey S, Jarcho JA, et al. Drug-eluting coronary stents—promise and uncertainty. N Engl J Med 2007, 8;356 (10):1059-1060. Copyright © 2007 Massachusetts Medical Society. All rights reserved.)*

Stent thrombosis is particularly concerning because of its potential catastrophic consequences. As stents are often placed in proximal segments of major coronary arteries, thrombotic occlusion usually manifests as severe ischemia or myocardial infarction. One study demonstrated that 70% of cases of stent thrombosis manifested as acute myocardial infarction.[8,16] Mortality rates are very high ranging from 11% to 15% for BMS thromboses and 25% to 45% with DES thrombosis. The higher mortality with DES thrombosis has been suggested to be secondary to a combination of abrupt thrombotic events and decreased collateral formation.[14] Again, the risk of coronary artery stent thrombosis and its frequent consequences of myocardial infarction or death are minimized by the use of dual antiplatelet therapy. Patient compliance is also an important issue when determining the type of stent to use.

Imaging Techniques and Findings

Radiography

To date, the majority of patients with chest pain after coronary artery stent placement undergo catheter angiography. This invasive method, however, has the disadvantage of moderate-to-high cost and the possibility of severe complications. Therefore, a noninvasive alternative for the assessment of stented segments in these patients would be highly desirable.[17] To that end, attempts have been made to noninvasively assess coronary artery stents with varying degrees of success.

Ultrasound

Transcatheter intravascular ultrasound (IVUS) imaging is another invasive technique in which a miniaturized ultrasound transducer, mounted on the tip of catheter, is inserted directly into a vessel to produce in-vivo real time assessment of the vascular lumen as well as plaque composition. IVUS has been used during stent placement with the promise that it will improve the clinical outcome of stent placement via reduction of incomplete expansion and incomplete apposition of the stent to the vessel wall. Also, IVUS allows for the measurement of minimal stent area which has been found to predict angiographic and clinical restenosis.[18]

MRI

The coronary arteries can be evaluated using cardiac MRI techniques; however, coronary magnetic resonance angiography (MRA) is currently not as easily performed or as fast as coronary computed tomographic angiography (CTA). A number of unsolved problems limit MRI reliability. Long acquisition times, the small size of the coronary arteries, and cardiac and respiratory artifacts causing nonevaluable segments hamper the clinical implementation of coronary MRA.[19]

Furthermore, although multiple studies have demonstrated that MRI performed less than 8 weeks after coronary stent placement is safe,[20-22] local susceptibility artifact leads to signal voids/artifacts at the site of the stent on MR images. These artifacts can be substantial and preclude direct MR evaluation of in-stent and persistent coronary patency.[23]

CT

Noninvasive assessment using computed tomography to assess in-stent stenosis has been attempted since the era of electron beam CT (EBCT). Early studies with EBCT could not directly visualize in-stent restenosis and quantification was not possible.[24,25]

Multidetector CT (MDCT) has several advantages over EBCT; of note, MBCT has increased spatial resolution and improved signal-to-noise ratio.[17] Early MDCT scanning with four-detector scanners were inadequate for stent interpretation with inability to visualize the majority of the stent lumen.[17,26] Subsequent studies using 16-, 40-, and 64-detector scanners have had mixed results. Most studies demonstrated high sensitivity and specificity but in general ignored nonevaluable segments from analysis. The number of stents found nonevaluable (up to 54% of 232 stents in a study by Gilard and colleagues), is a major limitation of this analysis. The negative predictive value was generally greater than 95%; however, the positive predictive value ranged from 29% to 78%.[6,27-34]

Hamon and colleagues performed a meta-analysis of 15 studies analyzing the diagnostic capabilities of 16-, 40-, and 64-detector CT scanners in comparison with invasive coronary angiography for detection of in-stent stenosis. 13% of 1175 stents in these studies were nonevaluable. After exclusion of these stents from analysis, they found a sensitivity of 84% and a specificity of 91%.[35] The positive-predictive value (PPV) was almost uniformly low secondary to nonevaluable stents being classified as in-stent restenosis (ISR) for statistical analysis. An additional meta-analysis of 16- to 64-detector row CT scanners performed by Sun and colleagues demonstrated similar results. Although there was the hope that 64-detector row CT scanners would be more accurate than slower 16-detector row CT scanners, both meta-analyses demonstrated equivalent sensitivity and specificity.[35,36] Kumbani and coworkers recently performed a meta-analysis of 14 studies solely using 64-detector row CT scanners for detection of ISR. Overall sensitivity was 91%, specificity was 91%, PPV was 68%, and the negative-predictive value (NPV) was 98%. Nine percent of 1447 stents were deemed nonevaluable with decreased performance with inclusion of these stents. Only five studies in the analysis included stents less than 3 mm.[37] Given that a large number of stents in the general population are less than 3 mm, this further decreases the utility of MDCT in nonselected stent patients.

A post-hoc analysis of 75 stents in 52 patients from the Core-64 trial, the first multicenter international, single-blinded study to determine the accuracy of 64-detector row CT MDCT, was performed to assess the accuracy of MDCT in detecting in-stent restenosis. This analysis demonstrated less favorable results than the previous meta-analyses. Only 48 of 75 stents (64%) were considered evaluable and there was an overall accuracy of 77.1% for detection of 50% in-stent restenosis of evaluable stents. The PPV and NPV was 57.1% and 80.5%, respectively. A quantitative approach using in-stent and peri-stent attenuation didn't improve accuracy. The researchers attribute the poor performance of MDCT to the fact that 80% of stents were <3 mm with secondary problems of calcifications, motion artifact, and blooming artifact.[38]

In general, there is increased evaluability and improved detection of in-stent restenosis with larger stents and unfavorable results with stents less than 3 mm diameter. High heart rates, calcification, and increased body mass index decreased the accuracy of MDCT.[32] When considered in the evaluation, thicker stent struts also reduced the evaluability of the stents.[36]

Dual-source CT scanners have improved temporal resolution compared with single source scanners and promise to potentially minimize motion artifacts that limit in-stent evaluation. Pugliese and associates evaluated a dual-source CT scanner for evaluation of instant restenosis in 100 patients with 178 stents. Nine of the stents were uninterpretable (all of which were smaller than 2.75 mm in diameter) secondary to high-density artifacts obscuring the stent lumen. Sensitivity, specificity, PPV, and NPV in detecting >50% restenosis was 94%, 92%, 77%, and 98%, respectively. The diagnostic performance of the dual source CT scanner at heart rates less than 70 bpm did not differ significantly from its performance with faster heart rates. The stent diameter was important as the sensitivity was 100% in >3 mm diameter stents but dropped to 84% in <2.75 mm stents. Similarly the specificity and the PPV dropped precipitously as the stent diameter decreased. This study demonstrated that the dual-source CT scanner was able to negate the effect of heart rate on evaluation of stent stenosis. The NPV was very good (97% to 98%), even in patients with fast heart rates. Stent diameter was the most important feature in this study.[39]

In the evaluation of the coronary arteries in a patient with history of percutaneous coronary intervention and stent placement, a clinical history with specific locations of stent placement is of utmost importance. Given that

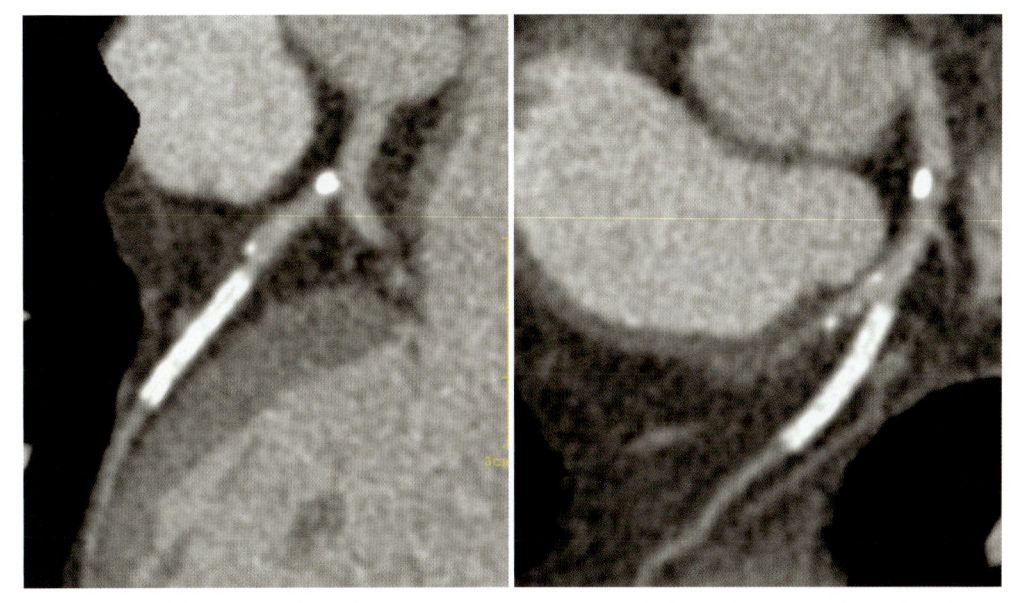

FIGURE 37-5 In-stent restenosis in the first diagonal coronary artery cannot be excluded secondary to significant blooming artifact. This artifact results from beam hardening and causes stent struts to appear thicker than they are with secondary underestimation of in-stent luminal diameter.

concentric calcification can mimic a stent and not all stents are uniformly recognized on MDCT;[40] a history of stent placement allows for a more accurate interpretation—understanding that even with the most current scanners, evaluation of in-stent restenosis remains challenging.

CT scanners with 64 or more detectors are, in general, currently considered the standard for coronary CTA because the reduced breath-holding time afforded by these scanners is better tolerated by patients owing to minimization of motion artifacts.[7,41] Metallic stents cause beam hardening on CT imaging resulting in stent struts appearing thicker (or "bloomed") than they really are with secondary overlap of the vessel lumen and underestimation of the in-stent luminal diameter. In addition, this artifact can cause streaky dark bands which can simulate stenosis (Fig. 37-5).[42] Calcification of the vessel wall near or at the outer surface of an implanted stent also contributes to beam hardening. Partial volume averaging is another artifact inherent in cross-sectional imaging and particularly problematic given the small caliber of the coronary arteries.[7,43]

Sharp filters and thin slices (0.5 to 0.6 mm) reduce blooming and partial volume averaging for improved assessment of stent patency.[44] Studies have demonstrated that dedicated edge-enhancing convolution kernels decrease severity of blooming artifacts, resulting in superior depiction of the stent lumen.[7] The disadvantages of these filters are an increase in image noise. The most appropriate filter must be chosen to account for this trade-off.

As with all cardiac CT examinations, reduction of cardiac motion, which exacerbates metal-related artifacts, as well as optimization of the contrast agent (fast speed of injection and high iodine concentration of contrast), improves in-stent evaluability. After the scan is performed, electrocardiographic (ECG) editing should be implemented in order to remove aberrant beats from the data set.

Analysis

When these technical factors are optimized and the data are obtained, the stent lumen should be evaluated using multiplanar reformation (MPR) and cross-sectional/short axis images. Appropriate display window settings must be considered to most accurately evaluate these images. Wide window settings (e.g., width 1500 HU) and center level of 300 HU have been recommended to further decrease image interpretation difficulties with blooming artifact.[7]

The first step in analyses is the determination of stent evaluability. If there is excessive blurring of the stent contour, motion artifact, or inadequate delineation between the stent and the surrounding fatty tissue or the in-stent lumen, the stents should be considered nonevaluable and should be reported to the clinician as such. As numerous papers have demonstrated, a significant number of stents are not evaluable and, therefore, cannot be commented on with any degree of accuracy.

When deemed evaluable, the in-stent lumen should be check for in-stent restenosis. The level and quality of enhancement should be ascertained and any in-stent filling defects should be noted. Homogeneous high attenuation in the stent similar to the attenuation in the proximal or distal reference vessel implies normal flow (Figs. 37-6 and 37-7). Different grades of restenosis similar to those used by Gasper and colleagues and Ehara and associates[27,34] can be used (Figs. 37-8 and 37-9), including mild neointimal proliferation (<50% stenosis), significant (>50% restenosis), severe (>75% stenosis)/possible occlusion, and definitive occlusion (100% occlusion).

The perigraft vasculature should also be analyzed as restenosis at stent borders and is reported to occur frequently.[45] No contrast distal to the stent indicates definitive occlusion.[46] The presence of contrast distal to the stent does not, however, exclude occlusion secondary to the possibility of collateral vasculature feeding the vessel segments distal to the occluded stent in a retrograde direction (Fig. 37-10). It has also been noted that with stent restenosis, the CT attenuation of vessels distal to the stent is decreased compared with the attenuation of the artery proximal to the stent; however, no specific cutoff point has been ascertained.[31]

The diagnosis of in-stent thrombosis is much rarer and requires a collaborative clinical history. This is a highly morbid event that results in Q-wave infarction and death in the majority of cases. It is likely to show complete occlusion on cardiac CTA and the angiographic definition is no flow or faint flow beyond the occlusion.[47]

Synopsis of Treatment Options

The treatment of in-stent restenosis is usually PTCA and adjunctive repeat stenting with DES. Prior to the availability of DES, one major focus of investigation was to treat restenosis with intracoronary radiation. DES, however, is the treatment of choice with greater efficacy. There is currently insufficient evidence to recommend any specific treatment for DES restenosis; however, repeat stenting with DES is currently performed in many institutions after IVUS evaluation and stent expansion by repeat balloon angioplasty.[11]

Emergency percutaneous coronary intervention to restore vessel patency is the treatment of choice for stent thrombosis, although intracoronary thrombolysis has also been used. Urgent coronary artery bypass graft (CABG) surgery should be considered as needed.

Reporting: Information to the Referring Physician

- Evaluability of stent for detection of in-stent thrombosis
- Presence of significant in-stent stenosis or occlusion

Conclusion

Coronary CTA can be considered to rule out in-stent restenosis in carefully selected patients such as in calm, thin patients with slow, stable heart rates who have large diameter stents.[48] Its routine use, however, is currently not recommended secondary to its low positive-predictive

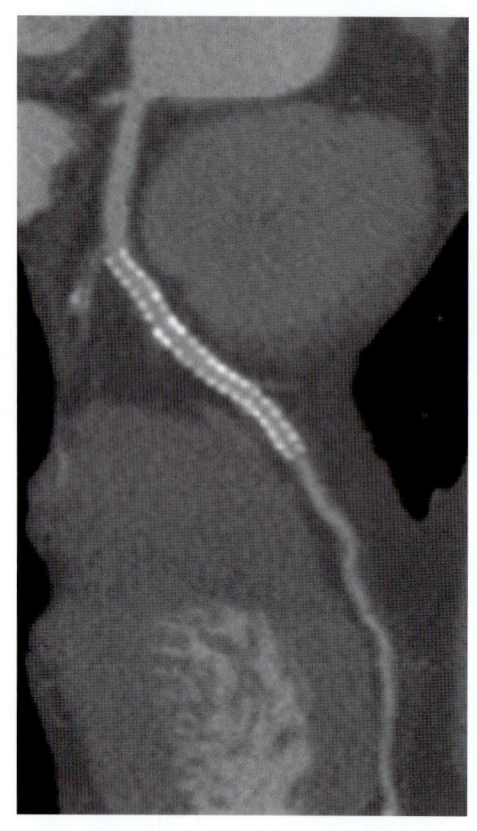

■ **FIGURE 37-6** Homogeneous contrast attenuation within LAD stent demonstrates lack of significant in-stent restenosis. *(Courtesy of Dr. Sablayrolles, Saint-Denis France.)*

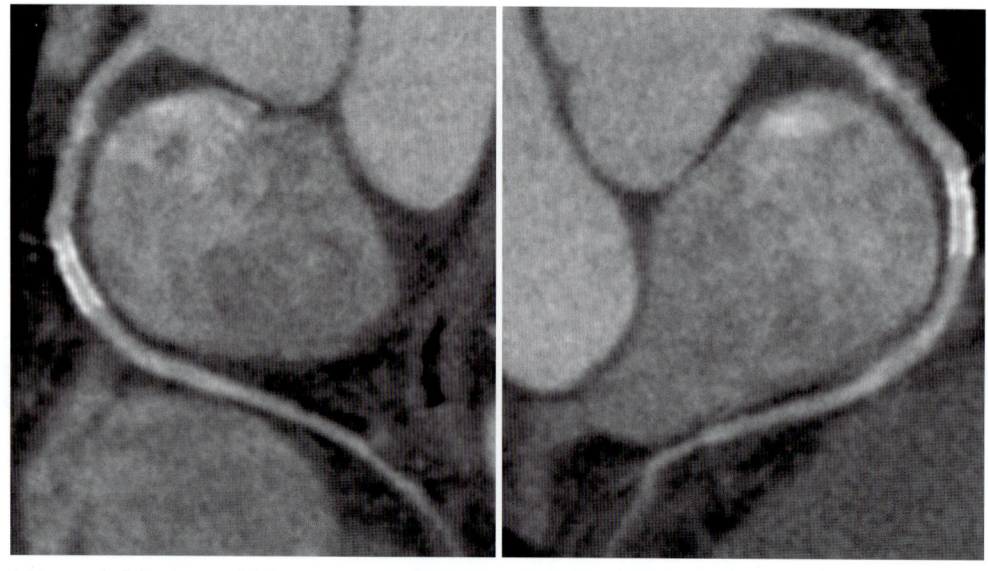

■ **FIGURE 37-7** RCA stent is fully patent with homogeneous enhancement throughout the stent and minimal blooming artifact. Furthermore, contrast enhancement in the RCA proximal and distal to the coronary stent is similar in attenuation, suggesting lack of significant in-stent restenosis.

CHAPTER 37 • *Imaging of Coronary Revascularization: Coronary Stents and Bypass Grafts*

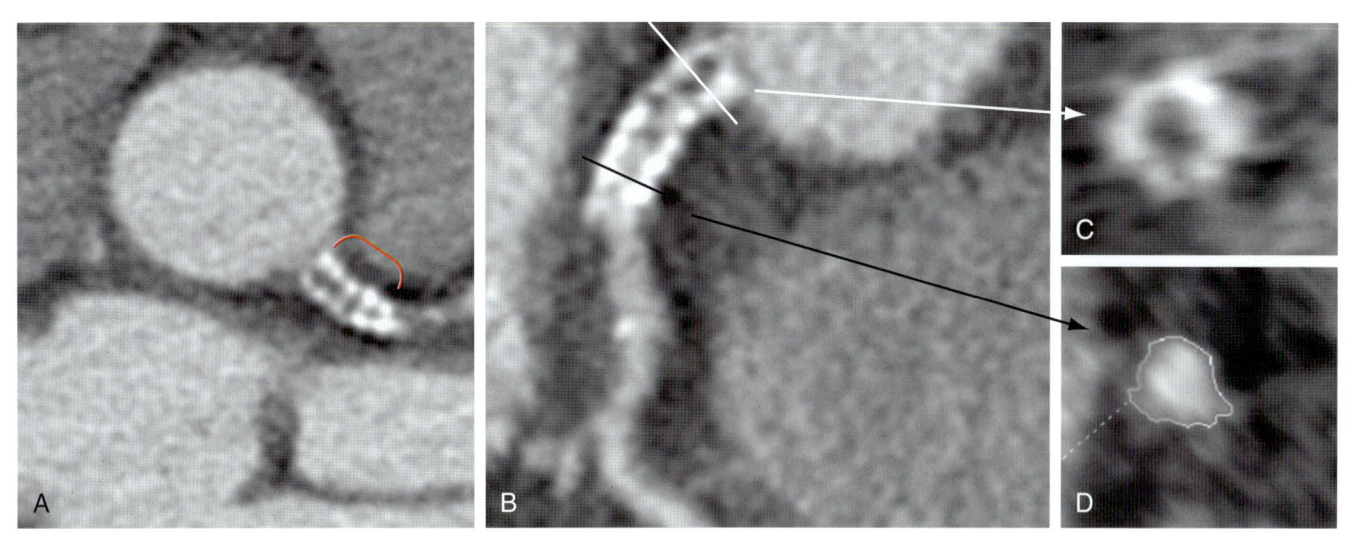

■ **FIGURE 37-8** A 56-year-old woman with chest pain after LIMA graft, s/p stent placement in the left main coronary artery. Axial CT (**A**) demonstrates a stent in the left main coronary artery (*brackets*). Long axis (**B**) and short axis images (**C**) demonstrate significant lack of contrast enhancement of the proximal portion measuring >75% of the vessel lumen (*white arrow*) consistent with severe in-stent restenosis or total occlusion. Distal flow does not exclude the possibility of total occlusion because collateral vasculature can supply distal segments. Compare this appearance to the normal distal in-stent appearance (**D**) with homogeneous enhancement. Finding was confirmed on conventional catheter angiography with 90% restenosis noted.

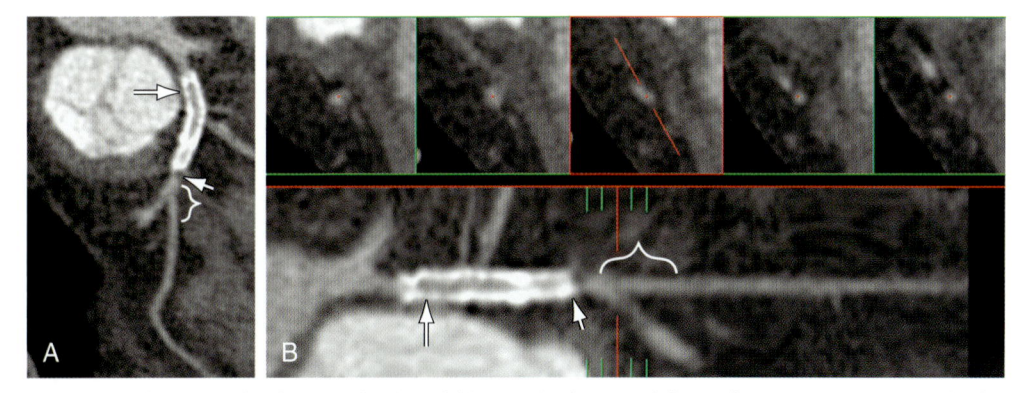

■ **FIGURE 37-9** Blooming artifact somewhat limits evaluation of this stent in the second diagonal coronary artery. Given this limitation, there is apparent decreased attenuation within the stent (*large arrow*) and in-stent restenosis (ISR) cannot be excluded. More concerning are foci of marked decreased attenuation seen on curved MPR (**A**) and computer-generated straightened MPR images (**B**) in the immediate persistent vasculature (*arrows*). There is also global decreased attenuation in the distal coronary vasculature (*bracket*). These findings are concerning for ISR and persistent occlusion with collateral vasculature reconstituting distal vasculature. Angiogram (*not shown*) demonstrated severe ISR and high-grade persistent stenosis but no occlusion.

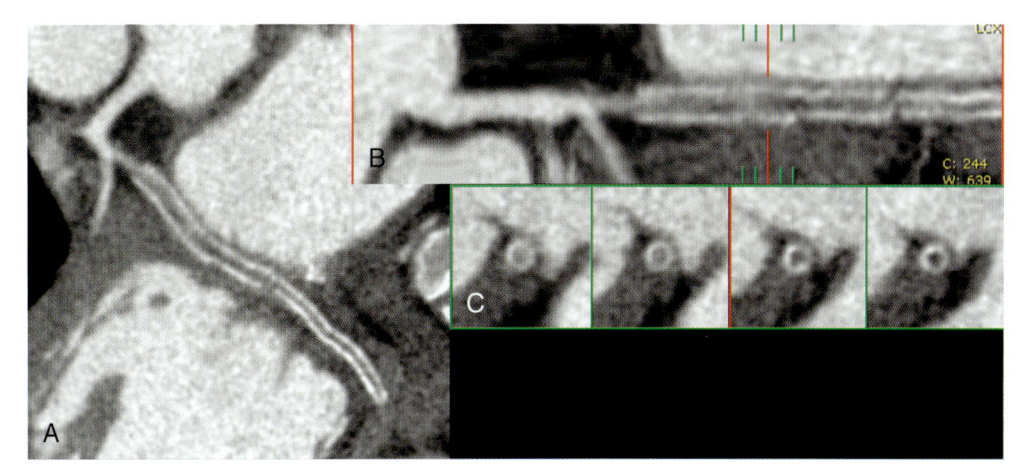

■ **FIGURE 37-10** Multiple stents in the left circumflex artery in this 70-year-old man with recurrent angina pectoralis. There is complete lack of contrast enhancement seen on curved MPR images (**A**) as well as computer generated "straightened" MPR images (**B**). Short axis views (**C**), perpendicular to the center long axis of the stent, confirms lack of contrast enhancement filling the entire lumen consistent with high-grade stenosis or total occlusion. Lack of contrast enhancement in the coronary artery distal to the stents confirms total occlusion.

value and frequent poor visualization of the lumen.[35,49,50] A multi-societal consensus statement that included the American College of Cardiology Foundation and American College of Radiology rates cardiac CT for the indication of evaluation of in-stent restenosis after percutaneous coronary intervention (PCI) as inappropriate, assigning it an appropriateness score of 2 on a 1 to 9 scale, with 9 being considered the highest reasonable and acceptable indication.[51] There is a consensus that only stents with diameter of over 3 mm are routinely interpretable. Unfortunately, in routine clinical settings many patients are treated with smaller stents. Even though the dual-source CT scanners can certainly reduce or possibly eliminate the limitation of motion artifacts, further increased spatial resolution appears necessary before reliable imaging of most stents for restenosis becomes suitably accurate for routine use.

CORONARY ARTERY BYPASS ASSESSMENT

Background

Surgical revascularization is well recognized as a modern achievement in therapy for advanced coronary artery disease. Although the concept of coronary bypass grafting for occlusive disease was originally proposed by Carrel in 1910,[52] Drs. Michael DeBakey and Edward Garrett are credited with the first successful saphenous vein graft (SVG) bypass in 1964. Performed as a salvage for a complicated left anterior descending coronary endarterectomy, the patient did well postoperatively and demonstrated continued patency of the SVG graft when restudied 8 years later.[53] That same year, Kolesov performed the first sutured mammary-artery-coronary bypass.[54] It wasn't until the end of the decade that broader acceptance and use of internal mammary grafting took place.

Within a decade from these initial advances, coronary bypass operations had a tremendous impact on therapy for atherosclerotic disease. The National Center for Health Statistics report 450,000 coronary revascularization procedures performed in 2006.[3] Continued improvements in operative techniques have allowed increasingly challenging patients to be operated on with success.

Selective conventional catheter coronary angiography is considered to be the reference standard for the assessment of CABG. However, recent advances in competing cross-sectional modalities—specifically, MDCT and MRI—represent minimally invasive alternatives with promising results for bypass patency evaluation.

Bypass Graft Conduits

The choice of conduits is highly dependent on the particular surgeon and institution. Primarily, the various conduits used for surgical revascularization can be divided into arterial and venous grafts.

Saphenous Vein Grafts

Saphenous venous grafts were first successfully used in a CABG operation in 1964.[55] Although resistant to spasm versus their arterial counterparts, the use of SVGs is limited by a higher occurrence of intimal hyperplasia and atherosclerotic changes after exposure to systemic blood pressure, resulting in lower graft patency rates.[56,57] Saphenous vein grafts are attached proximally from the ascending aorta to the coronary artery distal to the diseased coronary lesion(s). The SVG can be sutured directly to the anterior portion of the ascending aorta or can be attached with an anastomotic device.

Occlusive failures of saphenous vein grafts are well documented and have been extensively investigated.[58-63] A large angiographic study of bypass graft patency ($n = 5065$, 91% venous, 9% arterial) found 88% of grafts to be patent perioperatively, 81% to be patent at 1 year, and 75% of grafts to be patent at 5 years.[61] Further declines in patency to 50% were observed in 353 grafts examined more than 15 years after revascularization. Nevertheless, continued improvements in surgical techniques, combined with concomitant antiplatelet or anticoagulant agents, and lipid-lowering therapy have allowed SVGs to remain a main choice for surgical bypass.

Arterial Grafts

Despite early success with internal mammary grafts, widespread acceptance came nearly a decade later. Compared with the saphenous vein, the internal mammary artery (IMA) has unique biologic characteristics that enable it to resist atherosclerosis and maintain high patency rates. The IMA has a nonfenestrated internal elastic lamina and lacks vaso vasorum inside the vessel wall, which tends to protect against intimal hyperplasia and cellular migration.[63] In addition, the medial layer of IMA is thin and is limited in muscle cells, resulting in a decreased tendency for maladaptive vasoconstriction.[64]

Advantages of IMA conduits over SVGs include decreased postoperative mortality, improved cardiac event-free survival rates, and improved long-term patency rates well above 90% at 10 years.[62,63] Because of its proximity to the left anterior descending (LAD) artery and favorable patency rates, the left IMA (LIMA) is most commonly used as an in situ graft to revascularize the LAD or diagonal artery, supplying the anterior or anterolateral cardiac wall.

Other Arteries

The profound benefits afforded by IMA grafting have given foundation to utilization of arterial conduits as coronary bypass grafts including the right IMA, right gastroepiploic artery, radial artery, and inferior epigastric arteries. The use of right gastroepiploic and inferior epigastric arteries in CABG procedures has been limited because of the need to extend the median sternotomy to expose the abdominal cavity. Although the use of these arteries increases surgical time and technical difficulty of the surgery, these arteries can be used as a free graft to perform total arterial revascularization.[65,66] In rare instances, the right gastroepiploic artery may be used in situ for revascularization to the posterior descending artery.

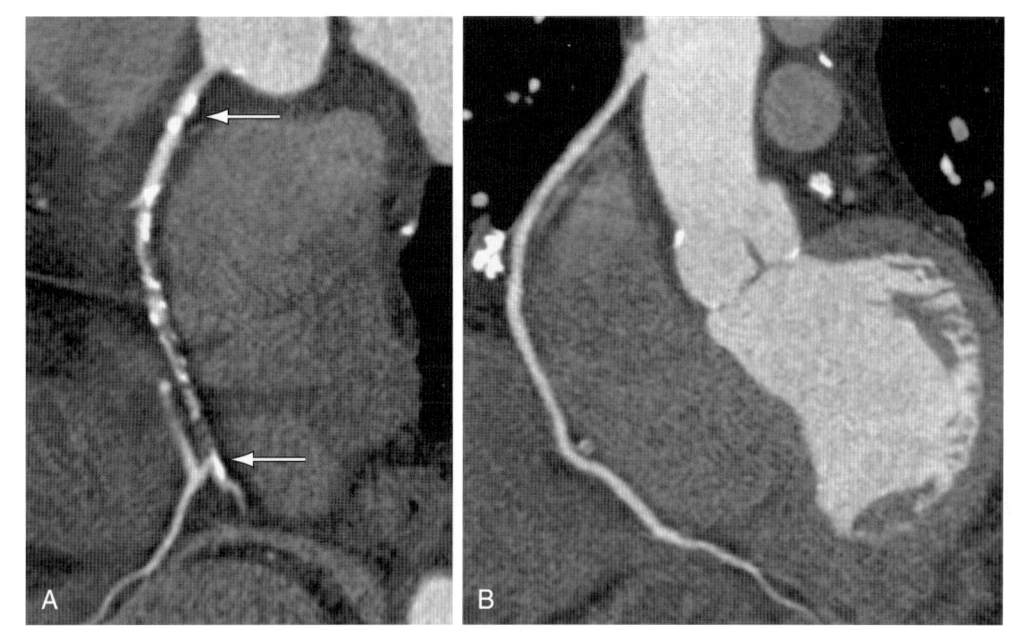

FIGURE 37-11 A 57-year-old male with diffuse disease of the right coronary artery. **A,** Multiplanar view of the native RCA demonstrated diffuse mixed calcified and soft coronary plaqu (*arrows*). **B,** Multiplanar image of a saphenous vein graft is observed arising from the ascending aorta with end-to-side anastomosis with the posterior descending artery.

Imaging Techniques and Findings

Catheter coronary angiography is still considered to be the gold standard for evaluation of severity of coronary artery disease. The procedure is not without risk of complications including pseudoaneurysm (1.2%), arrhythmia (1%), cerebrovascular accidents (0.3%), and myocardial infarction (0.2%). Noninvasive coronary imaging holds great potential utility in the pre-, peri-, and postoperative evaluation of bypass patients.

Computed Tomography

The ability of CT to characterize the patency of bypass grafts has been discussed since the 1990s[60,67-69] with first-generation (four- and eight-detector) MDCT scanners. A recent meta-analysis demonstrated that obstructive bypass graft disease can be detected by using at least a 16-detector row CT with a high diagnostic accuracy, with a sensitivity of 98%, a specificity of 97%, a positive-predictive value of 93%, and a negative-predictive value of 99%.[70]

The advent of ECG gating and improved subsecond data acquisition has given rise to near complete suppression of cardiac motion with superior subcentimeter spatial resolution. In particular, 64-detector row CT devices, available since 2005, have not only shown the ability to acquire high-quality images, but also have demonstrated impressive accuracy in evaluating coronary artery stenosis and bypass graft patency in a larger cohort of patients.[71]

The increased number of detectors lead to increased temporal resolution (e.g., 83 msec) and spatial resolution (e.g., $0.4 \times 0.4 \times 0.4$ mm^3) and reduction of both cardiac and respiratory motion artifacts, leading to improved ability to assess graft stenosis and occlusion.[13] Newer three-dimensional (3D) image processing algorithms and advanced volumetric visualization techniques can provide improved evaluation of grafts in multiple planes using various projections (Fig. 37-11).

Ropers and colleagues were among the first to compare bypass graft imaging with 64-detector MDCT compared to conventional catheter angiography and reported sensitivity of 97% and specificity of 98% of MDCT for detecting graft occlusion.[72] Other subsequent studies using 64-detector MDCT have reported sensitivity and specificity values of 93.3% and 100% and 91.4% and 100%, respectively, for graft occlusion and significant luminal stenosis (>50% luminal narrowing).[73-76]

The protocol for CT bypass imaging is similar to that for coronary CTA. One important difference is that the scan should be extended superiorly to include the origins of the internal mammary arteries. As is routine, heart rate control and proper breathing instructions are critical to performing a diagnostic study. Development of a new generation of scanner technology such as cardiac freeze-frame technique, dual-source CT, and flat-panel CT promise further improvements in temporal resolution and the ability to acquire slices with a gantry rotation time of about 100 ms, potentially reducing the problems of breath-holding, motion artifact, and artifacts related to variations of heart rate during the scan.[77] The role of bypass assessment with MDCT holds great potential to replace conventional catheter angiography in the near future as MDCT continues to evolve.

Magnetic Resonance Imaging

With the potential of multiplanar imaging, lack of radiation, and ability to evaluate physiologic parameters, MRI is an important adjunct to coronary imaging.

Coronary imaging with MRA can be performed using two-dimensional (2D) or 3D techniques. Cardiac synchronization with ECG gating is necessary to minimize degradation of images owing to cardiac motion. Motion of the diaphragm also presents a limitation. Different techniques, such as a breath-hold technique versus a free breathing with navigator echo-based technique, have been used to overcome these issues.[78] For a 2D coronary MRA using the breath-hold technique, the patient may be required to do many breath-holds for 16 to 20 seconds (and even longer for a 3D coronary MRA).[79,80]

Few studies have focused on the ability of MR to assess coronary bypass grafts. Brenner and coworkers evaluated 85 patients after an average of 7 days post CABG and were able to assess saphenous and arterial grafts with 94% specificity and 90% sensitivity.[81] Langerak and colleagues focused only on venous grafts and demonstrated a sensitivity and specificity of 65% to 82% and 82%, respectively, for the detection of a graft stenosis >50% and 73% and 80% to 87% for a graft stenosis >70%.[82]

Cardiac MRA is particularly limited in visualizing IMA bypass grafts. This is primarily due to the smaller diameters of arterial versus venous grafts (1 to 3 mm compared to the 3 to 6 mm), as well as the imaging artifacts arising from surgical metal clips. Several early studies failed to evaluate IMA grafts simply due to the suboptimal image quality.[83,84] Notwithstanding these results, Knoll and colleagues[85] and Wintersberger and associates[86] compared the assessment of IMA grafts with MRA versus conventional angiography. Both studies were able to determine IMA graft patency with MRI with a sensitivity of 94%

Despite these initial investigations, MR imaging of bypass grafts remains difficult in patients with atrial fibrillation and tachycardia. Furthermore, extremely agitated or claustrophobic patients cannot be examined. Whole heart SSFP coronary magnetic resonance angiography has emerged as another promising MR technique that has already shown promise in evaluating native coronary arteries.[87-90] However, its value in assessment of CABG is yet to be determined.

Analysis

Preoperative Planning

In many cases, preoperative MDCT evaluation may be helpful to identify the emergence, course, and size of native vessels and arterial conduits. An intramyocardial course of the LAD may alter or prevent some approaches of bypass grafting.

Postoperative Evaluation

Using either prospective or retrospective ECG gated techniques, CTA images are acquired in a limited field of view with axial images centered on the heart. Both 3D volume rendering and multiplanar reformatted images (MPR) are used to assess the bypass grafts, proximal and/or distal graft anastomoses, and the cardiac anatomy. In particular, curved planar images with center lines through the bypass grafts and native coronary arteries should be obtained.

It is important to follow the anatomic course of the bypass graft and note the patency of the graft at its expected target. The LIMA extends from its origin at the subclavian artery and courses through the anterior mediastinum along the right ventricular outflow tract after being separated surgically from its original position in the left parasternal region. Infrequently, sequential distal anastomoses, with side-to-side and end-to-side anastomoses to the diagonal and LAD arteries, respectively, or involving separate sections of the LAD artery, are performed (Figs. 37-12 and 37-13).

The right IMA (RIMA) is used less frequently than the LIMA. The RIMA can be placed as an in situ graft to revascularize the RCA or one of its branches. In cases in which both in situ IMAs are necessary to revascularize the left heart, either the LIMA is anastomosed to the left circumflex coronary artery (LCx) or side branches (i.e., obtuse marginal [OM] or diagonal branches) and the RIMA is attached to the LAD artery, or the LIMA is connected to the LAD artery and the RIMA is joined to the LCx artery or OM branches by extension through the transverse sinus of the pericardium. The RIMA can also be used as a composite or free graft. As a composite or "Y" graft, the RIMA is anastomosed proximally to LIMA, allowing total arterial revascularization instead of using a venous graft with LIMA.

On CTA, the LIMA is usually visualized as a small vessel in the left anterior mediastinum. As with other grafts, the distal anastomosis is typically difficult to visualize. Surgical clips are used routinely to occlude branch vessels of the IMA, and metallic artifact may limit assessment in some instances. The CTA appearance of the RIMA is similar to that of the LIMA.

Complications

Graft Thrombosis and Occlusion

Bypass graft failures are classified either as early or late following CABG surgery. During the early phase, usually within 1 month after CABG surgery, the most common cause of graft failure is thrombosis from platelet dysfunction at the site of focal endothelial damage during surgical harvesting and anastomosis.[91]

Additionally, other factors (such as the hypercoagulability state of the patient and the high-pressure distention or stretching of the venous graft, with its intrinsically weaker antithrombotic features) further initiate early venous graft failure, resulting in a 3% to 12% occlusion rate within 1 month postoperatively.[92]

Late-phase venous graft failure is due primarily to progressive changes related to systemic blood pressure exposure. One month after surgery, the venous graft starts to undergo neointimal hyperplasia.[92] Although this process does not produce significant stenosis, it is the foundation for later development of graft atheroma. Beyond 1 year, atherosclerosis is the dominant process, resulting in graft stenosis and occlusion (Fig. 37-14).

Arterial grafts, such as IMA grafts, are resistant to atheroma development. Late IMA graft failure is more commonly due to progression of atherosclerotic disease in the native coronary artery distal to the graft anastomosis (Fig. 37-15).[93]

CT angiography can delineate multiple findings associated with graft stenosis and occlusion. Calcified and noncalcified atherosclerotic plaque is readily identified, and the calculation of the extent of graft narrowing is

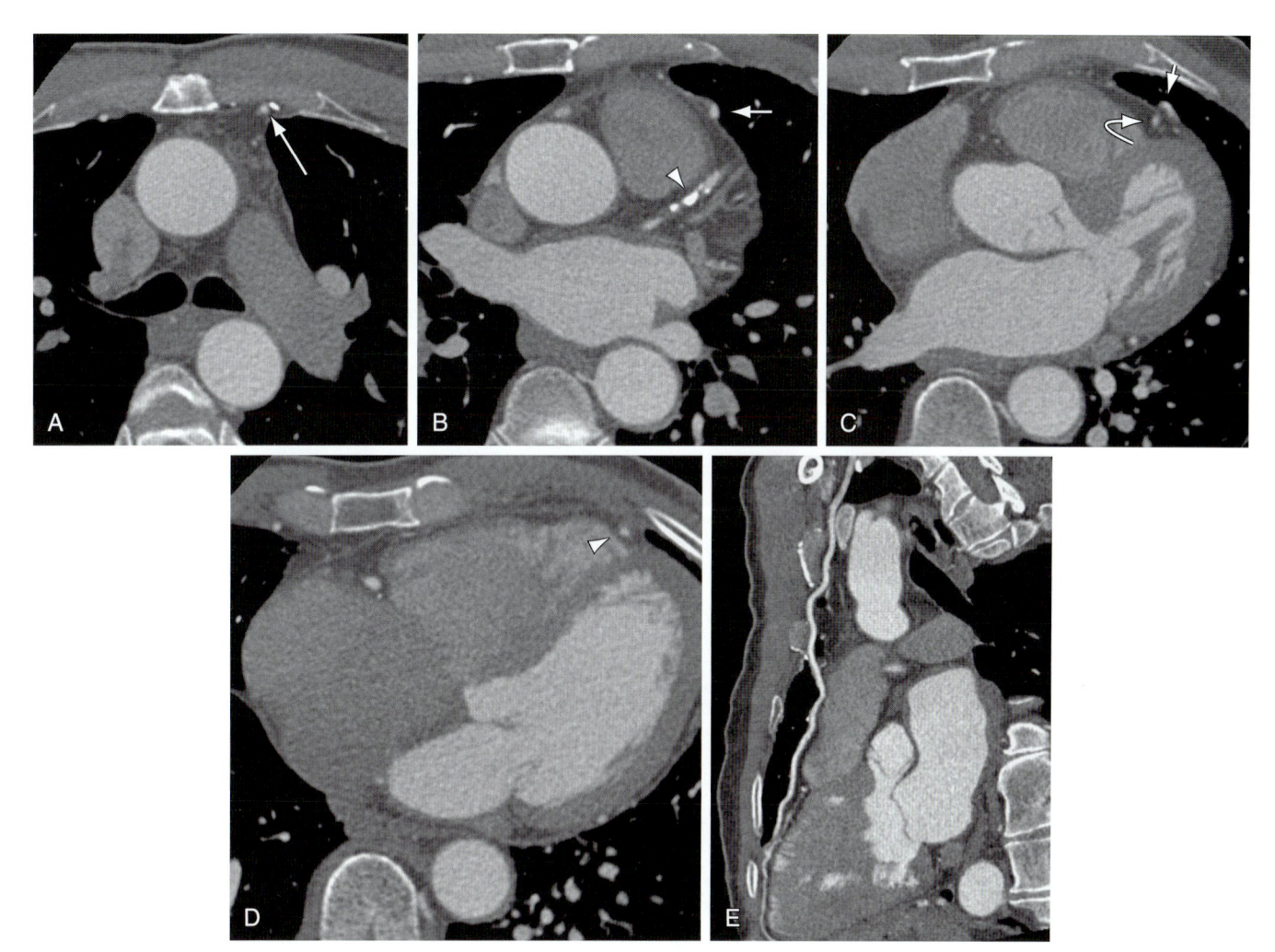

■ **FIGURE 37-12** A 64-year-old male with left internal mammary to left anterior descending coronary bypass. Sequential axial slices demonstrate the course of the LIMA graft running along its usual parasternal location (**A**, *arrow*) anterior to the heart (**B**, *arrow*). Note the mixed calcified and soft coronary plaque in the proximal LAD (*arrowhead*). The LIMA graft then courses along the apex of the heart to subsequently anastomose with the native LAD (**C**, *curved arrow*, and **D**, *arrowhead*). Additional multiplanar view provides full depiction of the course of the graft (**E**).

straightforward. Occlusion can be determined by nonvisualization of a vessel known to have been used for surgical grafting. In many instances, the most proximal part of an occluded aortocoronary graft fills with contrast, creating a small outpouching or "nubbin" from the ascending aorta, allowing a diagnosis (Fig. 37-16). A residual low attenuation structure, or "ghost", of part of the occluded graft may be visible. Acute or chronic graft occlusion can sometimes be differentiated by the diameter of the bypass graft (Fig. 37-17). In chronic occlusion, the diameter is usually reduced from scarring, as compared with acute occlusion in which the diameter is usually enlarged (Fig. 37-18).

Graft Aneurysm

There are two types of bypass graft aneurysms: true aneurysms and pseudoaneurysms. True aneurysms are usually found 5 to 7 years after CABG surgery and are related to atherosclerotic disease.[94] Alternatively, occurrences of pseudoaneurysms are more variable, although these lesions are usually found at the anastomotic site. Pseudoaneurysm cases that are found earlier may be related to infection or tension at the anastomotic site, resulting in suture rupture. In late-onset pseudoaneurysms, similar to true aneurysms, atherosclerotic changes likely played a role.[95]

Currently, there is no clear guideline for surgical repair. Measurement of an aneurysm >2 cm has been a cause for concern. Graft aneurysms can lead to various complications, including compression and mass effect on adjacent structures, thrombosis and embolization of the bypass graft leading to an acute coronary event, formation of fistula to the right atrium and ventricle, sudden rupture leading to hemothorax, hemopericardium, or death.[94]

Summary

Increasingly, the diagnosis of bypass graft patency and occlusion is feasible using noninvasive techniques. Although it is difficult to visualize smaller grafts, continued improvements in image quality promise greater spatial resolution and suppression of cardiac motion. With such improvements and continued research investigations, these noninvasive techniques may replace conventional angiography as a primary tool to visualize these conduits.

526   PART FOUR   ● Coronary Artery Imaging

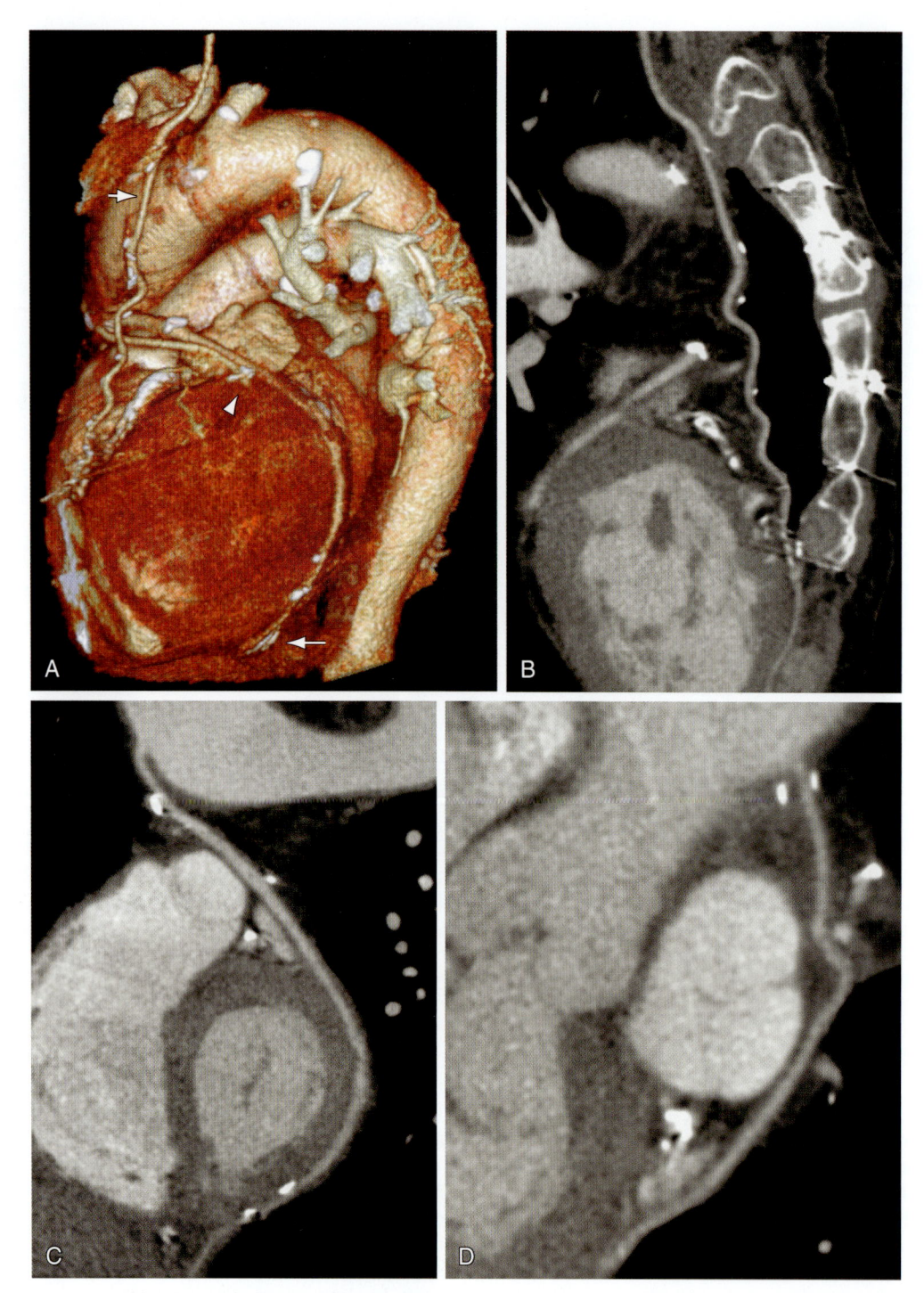

■ **FIGURE 37-13** A 63-year-old patient with three vessel bypass. Volume rendered (**A**) image of the heart demonstrates patent left internal mammary graft to LAD (*small arrow*), and saphenous venous graft (*large arrow*) arising from the ascending aorta to a posterolateral branch from the RCA. The radial artery graft is observed as a smaller caliber vessel arising from the ascending aorta and attached to a diagonal branch from the LAD (*arrowhead*). The entire course of the graft is best seen on the multiplanar reconstructions (**B, C, D**).

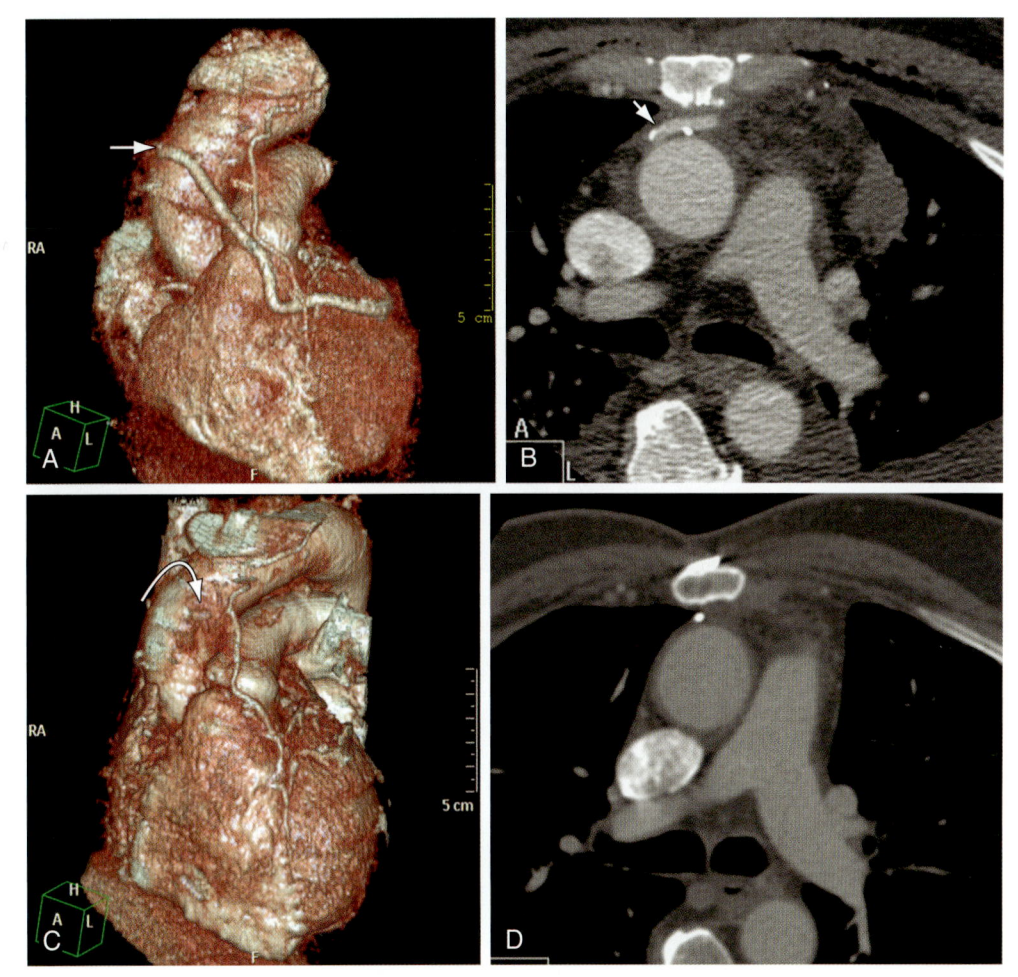

■ **FIGURE 37-14** A 63-year-old man with occlusion of a saphenous graft to diagonal-obtuse marginal graft (**A,B**). Perioperative study shows a patent aortocoronary graft: a saphenous vein to diagonal graft and sequential to the obtuse marginal artery (*arrow* on volume rendered image [**A**], and *arrow* on CT scan [**B**]) as well as a part of the left internal mammary graft. **C** and **D**, Study obtained 13 months later shows flow only to the left internal mammary graft (*curved arrow*); the saphenous graft has occluded.

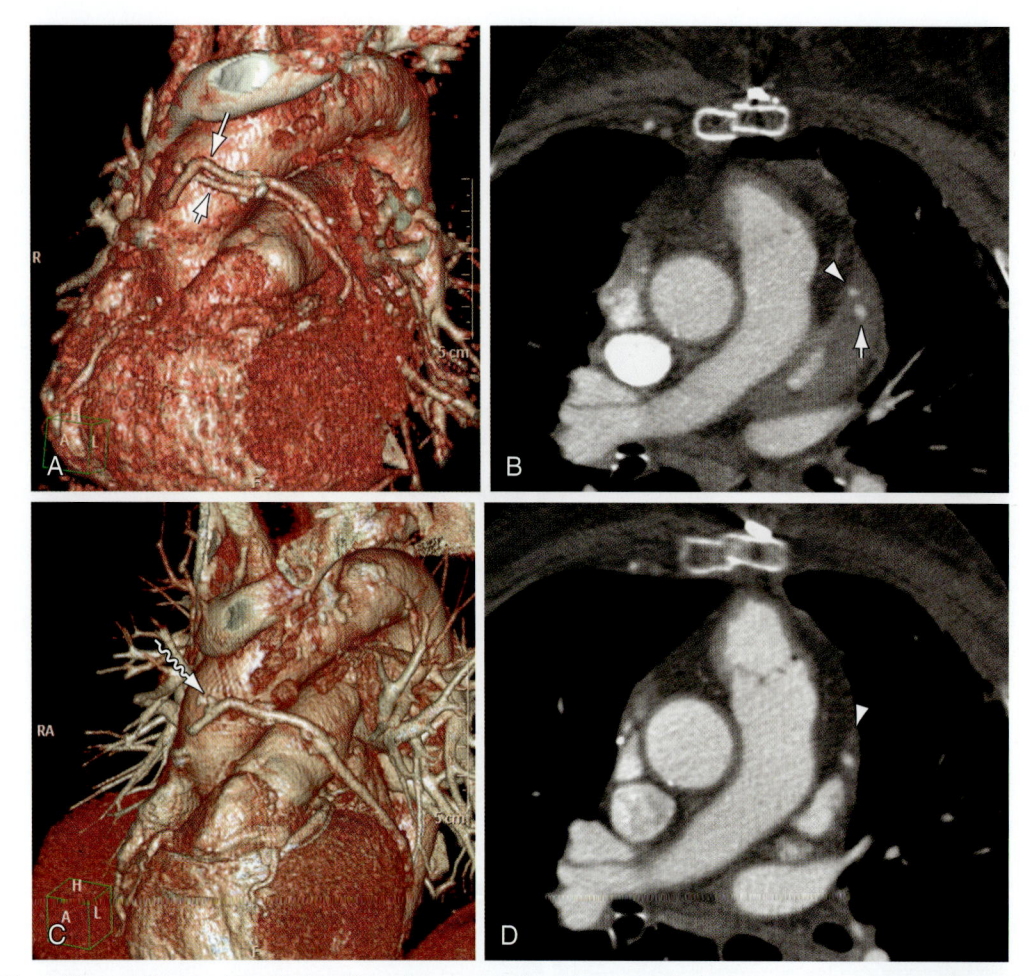

FIGURE 37-15 A 78-year-old man with occlusion of a radial artery graft to obtuse marginal artery. **A** and **B**, Perioperative study shows two patent aortocoronary grafts on volume rendered image: a saphenous vein to diagonal graft (*thin arrow* on volume rendering [VR] and *arrowhead* on CT scan) and a radial artery to obtuse marginal graft (*thick arrow* on VR and *thick arrow* on CT scan). **C** and **D**, Study obtained 11 months later shows flow only to the saphenous vein to diagonal graft (*squiggly arrow* on VR); the radial artery graft has occluded (*arrowhead* on CT scan).

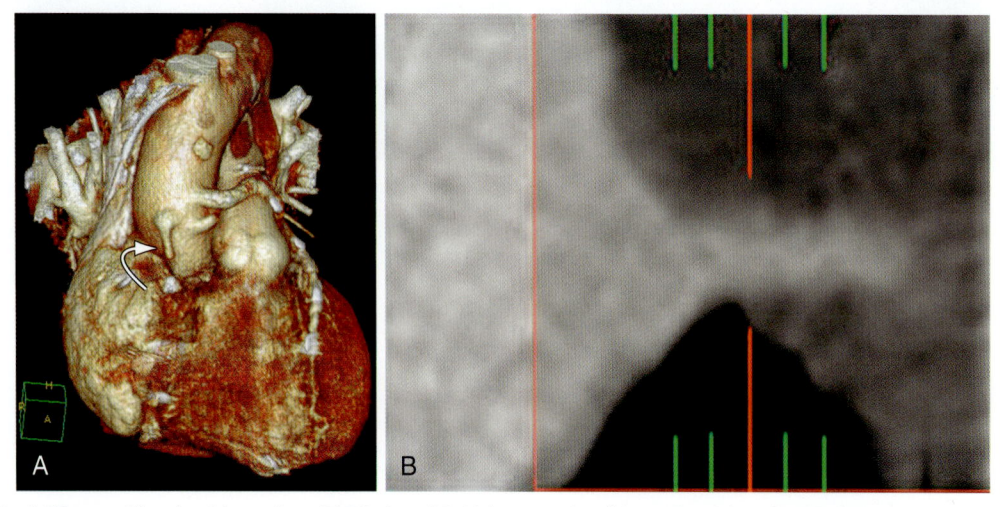

FIGURE 37-16 A 56-year-old male with previous CABG. **A** and **B**, Volume rendered (*curved arrow*) and MPR demonstrate a small focal outpouching of contrast, which is immediately truncated. We have noted this appearance as a "nubbin" sign related to graft occlusion.

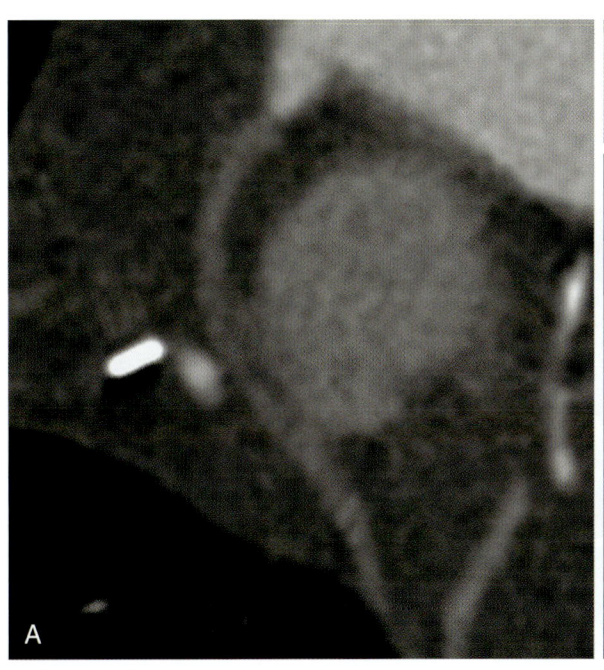

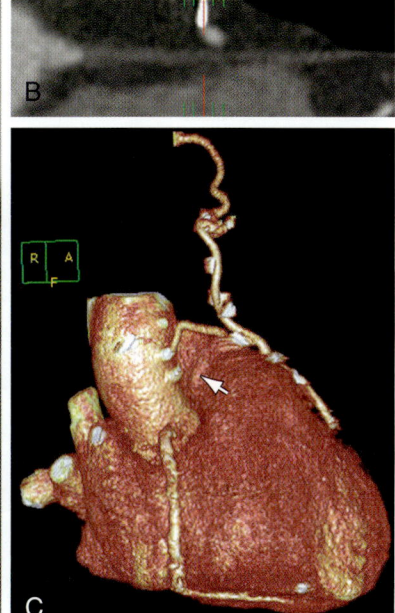

CHAPTER 37 • *Imaging of Coronary Revascularization: Coronary Stents and Bypass Grafts* 529

FIGURE 37-17 A 67-year-old patient with graft occlusion. **A** and **B**, Straight and curved MPRs of a saphenous vein graft demonstrating long segment decreased attenuation, later confirmed to be occlusion of the saphenous to diagonal branch conduit. We have noted this appearance as a "ghost" of the previous patent graft. **C**, Volume rendered image shows cutoff of the conduit (*arrow*).

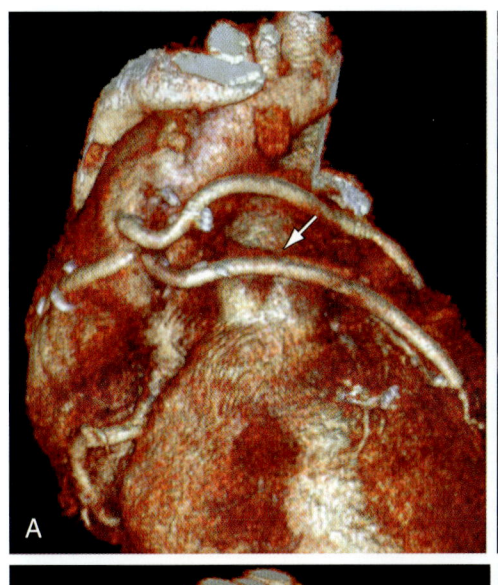

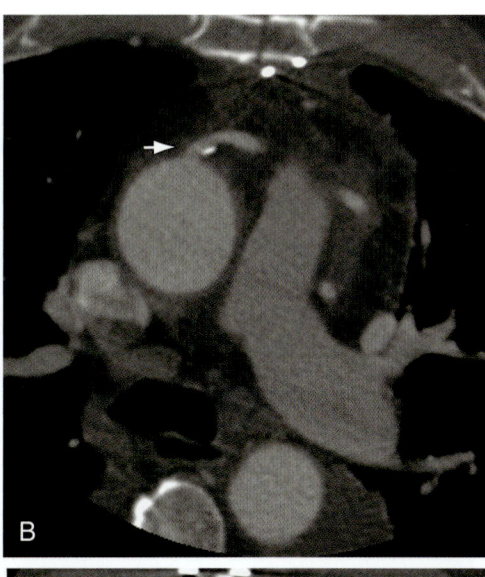

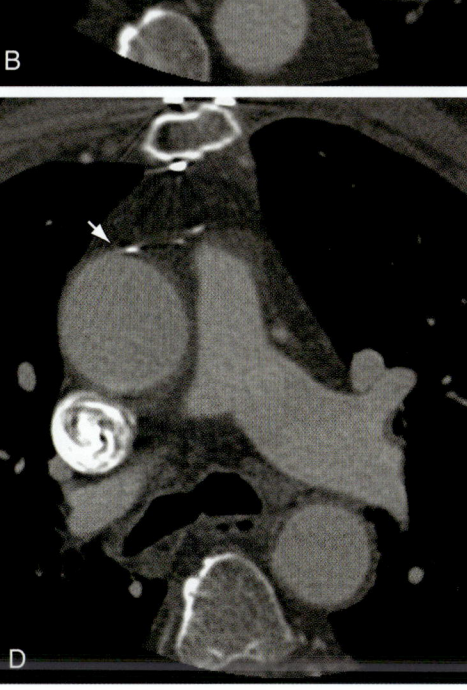

FIGURE 37-18 **A**, Volume rendered image demonstrating three-vessel bypass: saphenous graft to first diagonal branch, saphenous graft to first obtuse marginal branch, and saphenous graft to distal RCA. Axial CT scan (**B**) focuses on the origin of the saphenous to diagonal branch. The volume rendered image from a follow-up study performed 12 months later (**C**) demonstrates slightly decreased caliber of OM and RCA grafts with occlusion of SVG to diagonal branch (*arrow*). Note the decreased attenuation ("ghosting") observed on axial CT (**D**) in the region of the previous graft (*arrow*).

KEY POINTS

- Two major complications of coronary stent placements are in-stent thrombosis and restenosis.
- There is decreased rate of restenosis but potential for increased in-stent thrombosis with DES.
- The newer generations of CT scanners have demonstrated increased accuracy for detection of in-stent restenosis, however artifacts still prevent it from being routinely used except in select cases.
- Long-term patency of saphenous vein grafts is considerably less than with arterial grafts. The most common cause of early saphenous graft failure is thrombosis. Beyond 1 year, atherosclerosis is the dominant process, resulting in graft stenosis and occlusion.
- Arterial grafts such as IMA grafts, are resistant to atheroma development. Late IMA graft failure is more commonly due to progression of atherosclerotic disease in the native coronary artery distal to the graft anastomosis.
- Occlusion of bypass grafts may be visualized as diffuse low attenuation (ghosting), abrupt truncation of contrast in the proximal portion of the occluded graft (nubbin sign), or complete nonvisualization of the conduit.

SUGGESTED READING

Pugliese F, van Mieghem C, Meijboom WB, et al. Multidetector CT for visualization of coronary stents. Radiographics 2006; (3):887-904.

REFERENCES

1. Dobesh PP, Stacy ZA, Ansara AJ, Enders JM. Drug-eluting stents: a mechanical and pharmacologic approach to coronary artery disease. Pharmacotherapy 2004; (11):1554-1577.
2. Serruys PW, Kutryk MJB, Ong ATL. Coronary-artery stents. N Engl J Med 2006; 354(5):483-495.
3. Writing group members, Lloyd-Jones D, Adams R, Carnethon M, et al, for the American Heart Association Statistics Committee and Stroke Statistics Subcommittee. Heart Disease and Stroke Statistics—2009 Update: A Report from the American Heart Association Statistics Committee and Stroke Statistics Subcommittee. Circulation 2009; 119(3):e21-e181.
4. Schneider DB, Dichek DA. Intravascular stent endothelialization. A goal worth pursuing? Circulation 1997; 95(2):308-310.
5. Wolf F, Feuchtner GM, Homolka P, et al. In vitro imaging of coronary artery stents: are there differences between 16- and 64-slice CT scanners? Eur J Radiol 2008; 68(3):465-470.
6. Rixe J, Achenbach S, Ropers D, et al. Assessment of coronary artery stent restenosis by 64-slice multi-detector computed tomography. Eur. Heart J 2006; 27(21):2567-2572.
7. Pugliese F, Cademartiri F, van Mieghem C, et al. Multidetector CT for visualization of coronary stents. Radiographics 2006; 26(3):887-904.
8. Shimohama T, Honda Y, Fitzgerald PJ. The risks and benefits of drug-eluting stents. Am Heart Hosp J 2007; 5(3):146-150.
9. Morice M, Serruys PW, Sousa JE, et al. A randomized comparison of a sirolimus-eluting stent with a standard stent for coronary revascularization. N Engl J Med 2002; 346(23):1773-1780.
10. Raja SG, Dreyfus GD. Efficacy and safety of drug-eluting stents: current best available evidence. J Card Surg 2006; 21(6):605-612; discussion 613-614.
11. Cutlip D. Coronary artery stent thrombosis: general issues [Internet]. In Basow D, (ed). UpToDate. Up To Date. Waltham, Mass. 2009 [cited 2010 Jan 21] Available from: http://www.uptodateonline.com/online/content/topic.do?topicKey=correvas/7394&source=see_link
12. Stouffer G, Todd J. Percutaneous Transluminal Coronary Angioplasty: eMedicine Cardiology. Available from: http://emedicine.medscape.com/article/161446-overview
13. Cutlip D, Levin T. Intracoronary stent restenosis [Internet]. In Basow D, (ed). UpToDate. UpToDate, Waltham, Mass. 2009. Available from: http://www.uptodateonline.com/online/content/topic.do?topicKey=correvas/7394&source=see_link
14. Steinberg DH, Waksman R. Drug-eluting stent thrombosis vs. bare metal stent restenosis: finding the lesser of two evils. Am Heart Hosp J 2007; 5(3):151 154.
15. Chen MS, John JM, Chew DP, et al. Bare metal stent restenosis is not a benign clinical entity. Am. Heart J 2006; 151(6):1260-1264.
16. Harper RW. Drug-eluting coronary stents—a note of caution. Med J Aust 2007; 186(5):253-255.
17. Maintz D, Grude M, Fallenberg EM, et al. Assessment of coronary arterial stents by multislice-CT angiography. Acta Radiol 2003; 44(6):597-603.
18. Baim DS. Grossman's Cardiac Catheterization, Angiography, and Intervention. 7th ed. Philadelphia, Lippincott Williams & Wilkins, 2005.
19. Cademartiri F, Palumbo AA, Maffei E, et al. Noninvasive imaging of coronary arteries with 64-slice CT and 1.5T MRI: challenging invasive techniques. Acta Biomed 2007; 78(1):6-15.
20. Gerber TC, Fasseas P, Lennon RJ, et al. Clinical safety of magnetic resonance imaging early after coronary artery stent placement. J Am Coll Cardiol 2003; 42(7):1295-1298.
21. Schroeder AP, Houlind K, Pedersen EM, et al. Magnetic resonance imaging seems safe in patients with intracoronary stents. J Cardiovasc Magn Reson 2000; 2(1):43-49.
22. Syed MA, Carlson K, Murphy M, et al. Long-term safety of cardiac magnetic resonance imaging performed in the first few days after bare-metal stent implantation. J Magn Reson Imaging 2006; 24(5):1056-1061.
23. Manning WJ, Nezafat R, Appelbaum E, et al. Coronary magnetic resonance imaging. Magn Reson Imaging Clin N Am 2007; 15(4):609-637, vii.
24. Pump H, Möhlenkamp S, Sehnert CA, et al. Coronary arterial stent patency: assessment with electron-beam CT. Radiology 2000; 214(2):447-452.
25. Knollmann FD, Möller J, Gebert A, et al. Assessment of coronary artery stent patency by electron-beam CT. Eur Radiol 2004; 14(8):1341-1347.
26. Krüger S, Mahnken AH, Sinha AM, et al. Multislice spiral computed tomography for the detection of coronary stent restenosis and patency. Int J Cardiol 2003; 89(2-3):167-172.
27. Gaspar T, Halon DA, Lewis BS, et al. Diagnosis of coronary in-stent restenosis with multidetector row spiral computed tomography. J Am Coll Cardiol 2005; 46(8):1573-1579.

28. Schuijf JD, Bax JJ, Jukema JW, et al. Feasibility of assessment of coronary stent patency using 16-slice computed tomography. Am J Cardiol 2004; 94(4):427-430.
29. Carbone I, Francone M, Algeri E, et al. Non-invasive evaluation of coronary artery stent patency with retrospectively ECG-gated 64-slice CT angiography. Eur Radiol 2008; 18(2):234-243.
30. Sheth T, Dodd JD, Hoffmann U, et al. Coronary stent assessability by 64 slice multi-detector computed tomography. Catheter Cardiovasc Interv 2007; 69(7):933-938.
31. Das KM, El-Menyar AA, Salam AM, et al. Contrast-enhanced 64-section coronary multidetector CT angiography versus conventional coronary angiography for stent assessment. Radiology 2007; 245(2):424-432.
32. Nakamura K, Funabashi N, Uehara M, et al. Impairment factors for evaluating the patency of drug-eluting stents and bare metal stents in coronary arteries by 64-slice computed tomography versus conventional coronary angiography. Int J Cardiol 2008; 130(3):349-356.
33. Cademartiri F, Schuijf JD, Pugliese F, et al. Usefulness of 64-slice multislice computed tomography coronary angiography to assess in-stent restenosis. J Am Coll Cardiol 2007; 49(22):2204-2210.
34. Ehara M, Kawai M, Surmely J, et al. Diagnostic accuracy of coronary in-stent restenosis using 64-slice computed tomography: comparison with invasive coronary angiography. J Am Coll Cardiol 2007; 49(9):951-959.
35. Hamon M, Champ-Rigot L, Morello R, et al. Diagnostic accuracy of in-stent coronary restenosis detection with multislice spiral computed tomography: a meta-analysis. Eur Radiol 2008; 18(2):217-225.
36. Sun Z, Davidson R, Lin CH. Multi-detector row CT angiography in the assessment of coronary in-stent restenosis: a systematic review. Eur J Radiol 2009; 69(3):489-495.
37. Kumbhani DJ, Ingelmo CP, Schoenhagen P, et al. Meta-analysis of diagnostic efficacy of 64-slice computed tomography in the evaluation of coronary in-stent restenosis. Am J Cardiol 2009; 103(12):1675-1681.
38. Wykrzykowska JJ, Arbab-Zadeh A, Godoy G, et al. Assessment of in-stent restenosis using 64-MDCT: analysis of the CORE-64 Multicenter International Trial. AJR Am J Roentgenol 2010; 194(1):85-92.
39. Pugliese F, Weustink AC, Van Mieghem C, et al. Dual source coronary computed tomography angiography for detecting in-stent restenosis. Heart 2008; 94(7):848-854.
40. Gilard M, Cornily JC, Pennec PY, et al. Assessment of coronary artery stents by 16 slice computed tomography. Heart 2006; 92(1):58-61.
41. Raff GL, Gallagher MJ, O'Neill WW, Goldstein JA. Diagnostic accuracy of noninvasive coronary angiography using 64-slice spiral computed tomography. J Am Coll Cardiol 2005; 46(3):552-557.
42. Lewis BS, Halon DA. Integrating multidetector computed tomography into clinical practice: computed tomography scanning shows its metal. J Am Coll Cardiol 2007; 49(9):960-962.
43. Nakanishi T, Kayashima Y, Inoue R, et al. Pitfalls in 16-detector row CT of the coronary arteries. Radiographics 2005; 25(2):425-438; discussion 438-440.
44. Hoffmann U, Ferencik M, Cury RC, Pena AJ. Coronary CT angiography. J. Nucl. Med 2006; 47(5):797-806.
45. Schuijf JD, Pundziute G, Jukema JW, et al. Evaluation of patients with previous coronary stent implantation with 64-section CT. Radiology 2007; 245(2):416-423.
46. Oncel D, Oncel G, Karaca M. Coronary stent patency and in-stent restenosis: determination with 64-section multidetector CT coronary angiography—initial experience. Radiology 2007; 242(2):403-409.
47. Orford JL, Lennon R, Melby S, et al. Frequency and correlates of coronary stent thrombosis in the modern era: analysis of a single center registry. J Am Coll Cardiol 2002; 40(9):1567-1572.
48. Van Mieghem CAG, Cademartiri F, Mollet NR, et al. Multislice spiral computed tomography for the evaluation of stent patency after left main coronary artery stenting: a comparison with conventional coronary angiography and intravascular ultrasound. Circulation 2006; 114(7):645-653.
49. Herzog C, Zangos S, Zwerner P, et al. CT of coronary artery disease. J Thorac Imaging 2007; 22(1):40-48.
50. Schroeder S, Achenbach S, Bengel F, et al. Cardiac computed tomography: indications, applications, limitations, and training requirements: report of a Writing Group deployed by the Working Group Nuclear Cardiology and Cardiac CT of the European Society of Cardiology and the European Council of Nuclear Cardiology. Eur Heart J 2008; 29(4):531-556.
51. Hendel RC, Patel MR, Kramer CM, et al. ACCF/ACR/SCCT/SCMR/ASNC/NASCI/SCAI/SIR 2006 appropriateness criteria for cardiac computed tomography and cardiac magnetic resonance imaging: a report of the American College of Cardiology Foundation Quality Strategic Directions Committee Appropriateness Criteria Working Group, American College of Radiology, Society of Cardiovascular Computed Tomography, Society for Cardiovascular Magnetic Resonance, American Society of Nuclear Cardiology, North American Society for Cardiac Imaging, Society for Cardiovascular Angiography and Interventions, and Society of Interventional Radiology. J Am Coll Cardiol 2006; 48(7):1475-1497.
52. Carrel A. VIII. On the experimental surgery of the thoracic aorta and heart. Ann Surg 1910; 52(1):83-95.
53. Garrett HE, Dennis EW, DeBakey ME. Aortocoronary bypass with saphenous vein graft. Seven-year follow-up. JAMA 1973; 223(7):792-794.
54. Kolesov VI, Potashov LV. [Surgery of coronary arteries]. Eksp Khir Anesteziol 1965; 10(2):3-8.
55. Garrett HE, Dennis EW, DeBakey ME. Aortocoronary bypass with saphenous vein graft. Seven-year follow-up. JAMA 1973; 223(7):792-794.
56. Bourassa MG, Fisher LD, Campeau L, et al. Long-term fate of bypass grafts: the Coronary Artery Surgery Study (CASS) and Montreal Heart Institute experiences. Circulation 1985; 72(6 Pt 2):V71-78.
57. Campeau L, Lespérance J, Corbara F, et al. Aortocoronary saphenous vein bypass graft changes 5 to 7 years after surgery. Circulation 1978; 58(3 Pt 2):I170-175.
58. Bourassa MG. Fate of venous grafts: the past, the present and the future. J Am Coll Cardiol 1991; 17(5):1081-1083.
59. Campeau L, Enjalbert M, Lespérance J, et al. The relation of risk factors to the development of atherosclerosis in saphenous-vein bypass grafts and the progression of disease in the native circulation. A study 10 years after aortocoronary bypass surgery. N Engl J Med 1984; 311(21):1329-1332.
60. Engelmann MG, Knez A, von Smekal A, et al. Non-invasive coronary bypass graft imaging after multivessel revascularisation. Int J Cardiol 2000; 76(1):65-74.
61. FitzGibbon G, Kafka H, Leach A, et al. Coronary bypass graft fate and patient outcome: angiographic follow-up of 5,065 grafts related to survival and reoperation in 1,388 patients during 25 years. J Am Coll Cardiol 1996; 28(3):616-626.
62. Loop F, Lytle B, Cosgrove D, et al. Influence of the internal-mammary-artery graft on 10-year survival and other cardiac events. N Engl J Med 1986; 314(1):1-6.
63. Motwani JG, Topol EJ. Aortocoronary saphenous vein graft disease: pathogenesis, predisposition, and prevention. Circulation 1998; 97(9):916-931.
64. Cox JL, Chiasson DA, Gotlieb AI. Stranger in a strange land: the pathogenesis of saphenous vein graft stenosis with emphasis on structural and functional differences between veins and arteries. Prog Cardiovasc Dis 1991; 34(1):45-68.
65. Buche M, Schroeder E, Gurné O, et al. Coronary artery bypass grafting with the inferior epigastric artery. Midterm clinical and angiographic results. J Thorac Cardiovasc Surg 1995; 109(3):553-559; discussion 559-560.
66. Pym J, Brown PM, Charrette EJ, et al. Gastroepiploic-coronary anastomosis. A viable alternative bypass graft. J Thorac Cardiovasc Surg 1987; 94(2):256-259.
67. Nieman K, Oudkerk M, Rensing BJ, et al. Coronary angiography with multi-slice computed tomography. Lancet 2001; 357(9256):599-603.
68. Enzweiler CNH, Kivelitz DE, Wiese TH, et al. Coronary artery bypass grafts: improved electron-beam tomography by prolonging breath holds with preoxygenation. Radiology 2000; 217(1):278-283.
69. Ha J, Cho S, Shim W, et al. Noninvasive evaluation of coronary artery bypass graft patency using three-dimensional angiography obtained with contrast-enhanced electron beam CT. Am J Roentgenol 1999; 172(4):1055-1059.
70. Hamon M, Lepage O, Malagutti P, et al. Diagnostic performance of 16- and 64-section spiral CT for coronary artery bypass graft assessment: meta-analysis. Radiology 2008; 247(3):679-686.

71. Jones CM, Athanasiou T, Dunne N, et al. Multi-detector computed tomography in coronary artery bypass graft assessment: a meta-analysis. Ann Thorac Surg 2007; 83(1):341-348.
72. Ropers D, Ulzheimer S, Wenkel E, et al. Investigation of aortocoronary artery bypass grafts by multislice spiral computed tomography with electrocardiographic-gated image reconstruction. Am J Cardiol 2001; 88(7):792-795.
73. Ropers D, Pohle F, Kuettner A, et al. Diagnostic accuracy of noninvasive coronary angiography in patients after bypass surgery using 64-slice spiral computed tomography with 330-ms gantry rotation. Circulation 2006; 114(22):2334-2341; quiz 2334.
74. Onuma Y, Tanabe K, Chihara R, et al. Evaluation of coronary artery bypass grafts and native coronary arteries using 64-slice multidetector computed tomography. Am. Heart J 2007; 154(3): 519-526.
75. Meyer TS, Martinoff S, Hadamitzky M, et al. Improved noninvasive assessment of coronary artery bypass grafts with 64-slice computed tomographic angiography in an unselected patient population. J Am Coll Cardiol 2007; 49(9):946-950.
76. Malagutti P, Nieman K, Meijboom WB, et al. Use of 64-slice CT in symptomatic patients after coronary bypass surgery: evaluation of grafts and coronary arteries. Eur. Heart J 2007; 28(15):1879-1885.
77. Andreini D, Pontone G, Ballerini G, et al. Bypass graft and native postanastomotic coronary artery patency: assessment with computed tomography. Ann Thorac Surg 2007; 83(5):1672-1678.
78. Dhawan S, Dharmashankar KC, Tak T. Role of magnetic resonance imaging in visualizing coronary arteries. Clin Medicine Res 2004; 2(3):173-179.
79. Danias PG, Edelman RR, Manning WJ. Coronary MR angiography. Cardiol Clin 1998; 16(2):207-225.
80. Foo TK, Saranathan M, Hardy CJ, Ho VB. Coronary artery magnetic resonance imaging: a patient-tailored approach. Top Magn Reson Imaging 2000; 11(6):406-416.
81. Brenner P, Wintersperger B, von Smekal A, et al. Detection of coronary artery bypass graft patency by contrast enhanced magnetic resonance angiography. Eur J Cardiothorac Surg 1999; 15(4):389-393.
82. Langerak SE, Vliegen HW, de Roos A, et al. Detection of vein graft disease using high-resolution magnetic resonance angiography. Circulation 2002; 105(3):328-333.
83. Rubinstein RI, Askenase AD, Thickman D, et al. Magnetic resonance imaging to evaluate patency of aortocoronary bypass grafts. Circulation 1987; 76(4):786-791.
84. Theissen P, Sechtem U, Langkamp S, et al. [Noninvasive assessment of aortocoronary bypass using magnetic resonance tomography]. Nuklearmedizin 1989; 28(6):234-242.
85. Knoll P, Bonatti G, Pitscheider W, et al. [The value of nuclear magnetic resonance tomography in evaluating the patency of aortocoronary bypass grafts]. Z Kardiol 1994; 83(6):439-445.
86. Wintersperger BJ, Engelmann MG, von Smekal A, et al. Patency of coronary bypass grafts: assessment with breath-hold contrast-enhanced MR angiography—value of a non-electrocardiographically triggered technique. Radiology 1998; 208(2):345-351.
87. So NM, Lam WW, Li D, et al. Magnetic resonance angiography of coronary arteries with a 3-dimensional magnetization-prepared true fast imaging with steady-state precession sequence compared with conventional coronary angiography. Am Heart J 2005; 150(3): 530-535.
88. Maintz D, Ozgun M, Hoffmeier A, et al. Whole-heart coronary magnetic resonance angiography: value for the detection of coronary artery stenoses in comparison to multislice computed tomography angiography. Acta Radiol 2007; 48(9):967-973.
89. Katoh M, Spuentrup E, Stuber M, et al R. Flow targeted 3D steady-state free-precession coronary mr angiography: comparison of three different imaging approaches [Internet]. Invest Radiol 2009 Oct. Available from: http://www.ncbi.nlm.nih.gov/pubmed/19858729.
90. Sakuma H, Ichikawa Y, Chino S, et al. Detection of coronary artery stenosis with whole-heart coronary magnetic resonance angiography. J Am Coll Cardiol 2006; 48(10):1946-1950.
91. Fitzgibbon GM, Kafka HP, Leach AJ, et al. Coronary bypass graft fate and patient outcome: angiographic follow-up of 5,065 grafts related to survival and reoperation in 1,388 patients during 25 years. J Am Coll Cardiol 1996; 28(3):616-626.
92. Motwani JG, Topol EJ. Aortocoronary saphenous vein graft disease: pathogenesis, predisposition, and prevention. Circulation 1998; 97(9):916-931.
93. Douglas JS. Percutaneous approaches to recurrent myocardial ischemia in patients with prior surgical revascularization. Semin Thorac Cardiovasc Surg 1994; 6(2):98-108.
94. Memon A, Huang RI, Marcus F, et al. Saphenous vein graft aneurysm: case report and review. Cardiol Rev 2003; 11(1):26-34.
95. Dubois CL, Vandervoort PM. Aneurysms and pseudoaneurysms of coronary arteries and saphenous vein coronary artery bypass grafts: a case report and literature review. Acta Cardiol 2001; 56(4): 263-267.

PART FIVE

Congenital Heart Disease

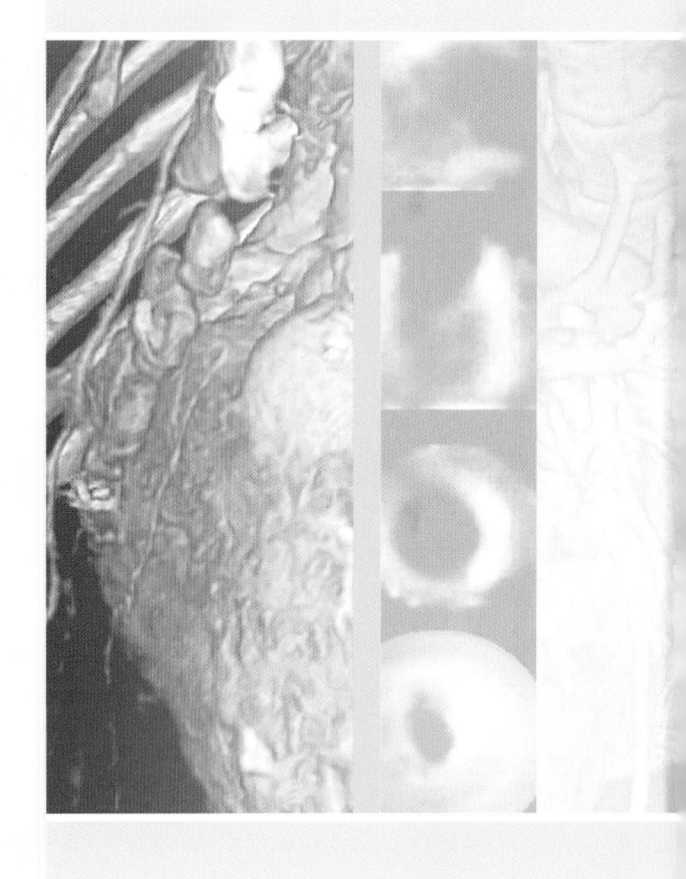

CHAPTER 38

Coarctation of the Aorta

Marilyn J. Siegel

Coarctation of the aorta is a narrowing of the proximal descending thoracic aorta. It can occur as an isolated lesion or in the presence of other congenital lesions, most commonly a bicuspid valve, patent ductus arteriosus, ventricular septal defects, or hypoplastic left heart. The severity of the coarctation and associated lesions determines the pathophysiology and clinical presentation. The clinical presentation varies from congestive heart failure in the newborn to asymptomatic hypertension or a murmur in older patients. Treatment options are surgical or interventional.

Definition

Coarctation refers to a stenosis of the proximal descending thoracic aorta that is almost always opposite the insertion of the ductus arteriosus—that is, at the junction of the distal aortic arch and the descending aorta just below the origin of the left subclavian artery (Fig. 38-1).[1-4]

Prevalence and Epidemiology

Coarctation of the aorta occurs in 3.2 of 10,000 births and accounts for 5% to 10% of all cases of congenital heart disease.[1-4] Coarctation is more common in white males than in white females, with a male-to-female ratio of 1.3 to 2.0:1.[3] Most cases are sporadic, but there may be a genetic inheritance.

Etiology and Pathophysiology

Coarctation is thought to be the result of a malformation of the aortic media, leading to a posterior infolding or shelf.[1,5,6] Most often, the shelf is discrete and opposite the ductus arteriosus. However, the malformation may be a long segment and circumferentially surround the aorta. In the latter form, there is typically diffuse tubular hypoplasia of the transverse arch and isthmus.[1,7,8]

Histologic examination shows thickened intima and media that protrude posteriorly and laterally into the aortic lumen. The ductus arteriosus or ligamentum arteriosus inserts anteromedially at the same level.[1]

The physiologic changes in cardiovascular function vary with the severity of the coarctation (severe or mild) and the presence of associated anomalies. In critical or severe coarctation, impedance to left ventricular outflow increases. The resultant hemodynamic changes include diminished stroke volume, increased left ventricular end-diastolic pressures, and elevated left atrial pressures. If there is associated aortic stenosis or a large ventricular septal defect, left ventricular systolic pressure and end-diastolic volume will further increase. The end result is heart failure and pulmonary edema. In addition to cardiac abnormalities, there are changes in vascular physiology. The diminished perfusion of the distal aorta and lower body leads to renal failure and bowel ischemia.

In milder forms of coarctation, the left ventricular myocardium hypertrophies to normalize myocardial wall stress and maintain normal systolic ventricular function. Left ventricular ejection fraction is often normal to increased. Collateral vessels also develop, which act as a source of lower body perfusion and help maintain normal flow to abdominal viscera.[1]

MANIFESTATIONS
Clinical Presentation

Critical or severe coarctation manifests in the first few days to first week of life. Symptoms include cyanosis (especially of the lower body), heart failure, shock, multi-organ failure and necrotizing enterocolitis.[1-5]

Milder forms of coarctation manifest later in life. Because left ventricular function is maintained and cardiac outflow is good, patients come to clinical attention because of hypertension or a heart murmur related to a bicuspid aortic valve.[1-4] Blood pressure in the upper extremities is typically higher than that in the lower extremities. However, if there is an aberrant right subclavian artery, the pressure in the right upper arm may be equal to or lower than that in the left upper arm.

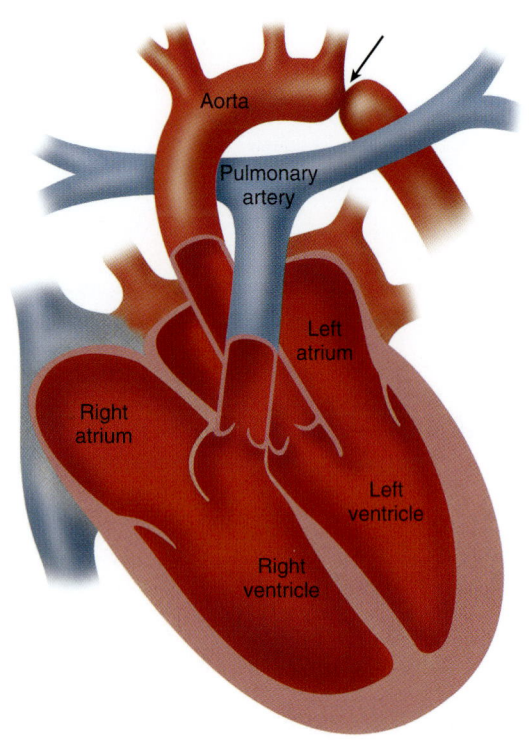

FIGURE 38-1 Diagram of aortic coarctation showing narrowing of the proximal descending aorta (*arrow*) just below the level of the left subclavian artery.

Imaging Studies

Indications and Algorithm

Imaging is performed to confirm the site, morphology and severity of the coarctation, extent of associated collateral circulation, any associated valvular lesions, and degree of left ventricular hypertrophy. The initial imaging examination is usually chest radiography and echocardiography. In uncomplicated cases, computed tomography (CT) or magnetic resonance imaging (MRI) is the study used to follow chest radiography to confirm the diagnosis of coarctation.

The identification of collateral flow is important in surgical planning. The aorta is cross-clamped during surgical repair if collateral flow is sufficient for lower body perfusion. If collateral formation is inadequate, the use of cardiopulmonary bypass for perfusion of the lower body may be indicated.

Techniques and Findings

Radiography

Plain radiographs are used to show cardiac size, pulmonary vascularity, size of the ascending and descending aorta, and rib notching.

Ultrasound

Two-dimensional echocardiography may show the site and extent of coarctation in young infants. Doppler imaging can help in determining the hemodynamic severity of the obstruction. In general, images in infants are of higher quality than those in older children and adults. In the latter populations, images of the distal arch may be suboptimal, requiring additional imaging with CT or MRI.[1,2,4]

Computed Tomography

CT can show anatomy of the coarctation, including the site, extent (i.e., size of the aortic arch) and severity, a bicuspid valve, collateral vessel formation, and left ventricular hypertrophy.

CT angiography is performed with a pulmonary embolism protocol using thin collimation (<1 mm), pitch lower than 1.5,[9,10] fast scan time, and a single breath-hold, when possible. In adolescents and adults, contrast medium is injected via a power injector at a high flow rate of 3 to 4 mL/sec using a contrast volume of 100 to 150 mL (280 to 320 mg I/mL). Scan delay time can be determined with an automatic bolus tracking system with the cursor over the aortic isthmus or empiric timing. Empiric timing, using a delay of 20 to 25 seconds after the start of the injection, is a default method if the bolus tracking fails to trigger. Electrocardiographic (ECG) gating is not needed for the evaluation of coarctation.

The volumetric data are reconstructed at 3- to 5-mm slice thickness for routine viewing and at 1- to 2-mm slice thickness for multiplanar reformatting and three-dimensional reconstructions. A standard reconstruction algorithm is used for reconstruction.

Special Considerations for Pediatric Patients

The contrast volume is 2 mL/kg (not to exceed 125 mL). Intravenous contrast medium can be administered with a power injector or manual (hand) injection. A power injector is used when a 22-gauge or larger cannula can be placed in an antecubital vein. For a 22-gauge catheter, flow rates are 1.5 to 2.5 mL/sec.[10,11] Flow rates for larger gauge catheters are similar to those described above. With a manual injection, the contrast is pushed as quickly as possible. Determination of the scan initiation time can be made by an empiric or bolus tracking method. In pediatric patients weighing less than 10 kg, an empiric scan delay of 12 to 15 seconds after the start of the intravenous contrast injection suffices.[10] In larger patients, the delay time is 15 to 25 seconds.

Magnetic Resonance Imaging

MRI, like CT, can accurately define the location, extent, and degree of aortic narrowing, collateral vessel formation, and valvular and ventricular morphology. In addition, MRI can provide an assessment of coarctation physiology, including information on blood flow and the pressure gradient across the stenosis.[1,3] Because MRI yields functional information and does not rely on ionizing radiation, many centers prefer this modality over CT, especially for children.

Noncontrast-enhanced methods, both black blood and bright blood techniques, and three-dimensional contrast-enhanced MR angiography (CEMRA) are routinely

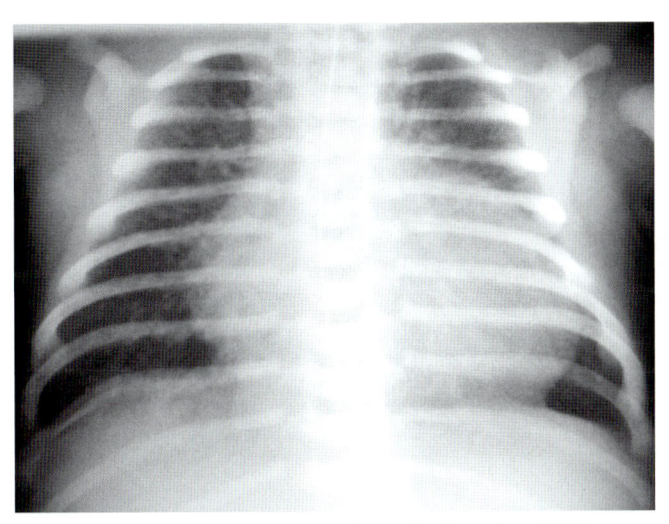

FIGURE 38-2 Anteroposterior radiograph of a 3-day-old infant shows moderate cardiomegaly and increased vascularity consistent with mild pulmonary edema.

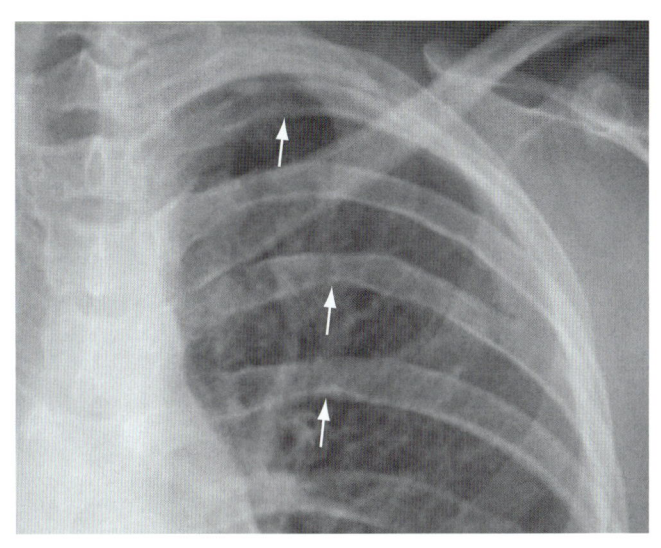

FIGURE 38-3 Chest radiograph shows rib notching (*arrows*) caused by erosion of the undersurface of the ribs by dilated intercostal vessels.

acquired. CEMRA is performed by acquiring a three-dimensional gradient-echo sequence following a rapid bolus of gadolinium. There are several ways to time contrast delivery. The best guess method is the simplest, the automated detection method is the most operator-independent,[12] and the timing run is the most reliable method.[13]

Velocity-encoded (VEC) phase contrast techniques are used to determine flow, peak flow rates, and the volume of flow per unit time (see Chapter 17, Fig. 17-8).[14,15] The pressure gradient across the obstruction is calculated with a modified Bernoulli equation (product of the cube of the peak velocity as measured in meters per second).

Angiography

Angiography is no longer needed for the diagnosis of uncomplicated coarctation if conventional noninvasive imaging can clearly delineate the anatomy and physiology.[1,4] If conventional studies are equivocal or indeterminate, or if there are possible associated intracardiac anomalies, angiography is performed.

Classic Signs

Chest Radiographs

In infants with critical coarctation, the chest radiograph demonstrates cardiomegaly and pulmonary edema (Fig. 38-2). In older children, the heart size is normal or slightly enlarged. There may be dilatation of the ascending aorta and a reverse 3 sign caused by aortic dilatation proximal and distal to the coarctation. Rib notching between the third and eighth ribs may be seen in older children, but rarely in children younger than 5 years (Fig. 38-3).[4]

Computed Tomography and Magnetic Resonance Imaging

The classic CT and MRI findings of coarctation are discrete short-segment aortic narrowing with an infolding or shelf-like appearance of the posterior wall (Fig. 38-4).[9,16-18] The isthmus and possibly the transverse arch will also be narrow in the diffuse form of coarctation (Fig. 38-5). In older individuals, other CT and MRI findings include dilatation of the aorta proximal to the coarcted segment, collateral vessel formation, and rib notching (Fig. 38-6). The common collateral pathways are the intercostal arteries (usually third through eighth) and internal thoracic arteries (Fig. 38-5; see Fig. 38-4B).[3] Other cardiac lesions, such as ventricular septal defect, bicuspid valve, and patent ductus arteriosus, may be seen.

Reconstructed images in the sagittal and parasagittal planes are best to show the location and extent of coarctation (see Fig. 38-4).[19] Coronal and sagittal reconstructions may help delineate rib notching and/or collateral vessel formation (see Fig. 38-6).

DIFFERENTIAL DIAGNOSIS

From Clinical Presentation

The differential diagnosis of coarctation in the neonate includes other lesions that cause critical obstruction of the left ventricle outflow tract, including the following: (1) interrupted aortic arch; (2) hypoplastic left heart; and (3) critical aortic stenosis.[5] Most neonates with critical left ventricular outflow obstruction present in the first few hours to first week of life with signs of shock and cardiac failure and radiographic findings of cardiomegaly and pulmonary edema.[5]

Interruption of the Aortic Arch

This is a rare anomaly, accounting for 1% to 1.5% of all critically ill infants with congenital heart disease.[4,20] This is a marked form of coarctation in which a segment of the aortic arch is completely absent. There are three types of interrupted arch based on the site of interruption:

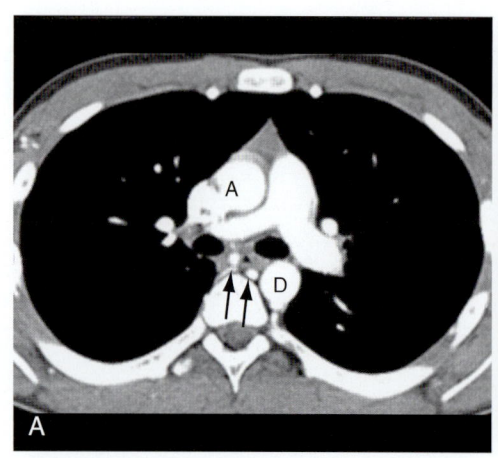

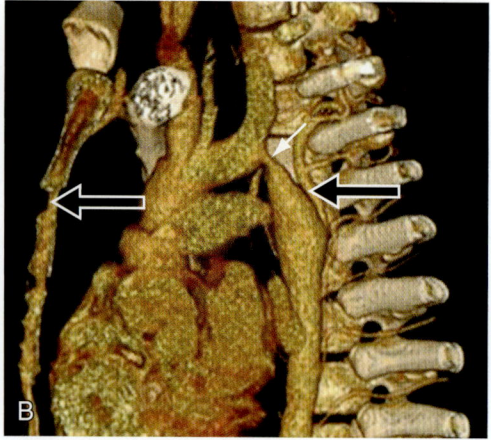

FIGURE 38-4 Focal coarctation. **A,** Axial CT image shows intercostal vertebral collateral vessels (*arrows*). The caliber of the ascending (A) and descending aorta (D) is equal. **B,** Sagittal volume rendered CT reconstruction demonstrates the characteristic narrowing (*small arrow*) of the aortic lumen just below the origin of the left subclavian artery (S) and aortic dilatation proximal and distal to the obstruction. Note also enlarged posterior intercostal (*black open arrow*) and internal mammary arteries (*white open arrow*). Of note, location and severity of the coarctation are best seen on reconstructed images.

Type A—distal to the left subclavian artery
Type B—between the left common carotid artery and the left subclavian artery
Type C—between the brachiocephalic trunk and the left carotid artery

A dilated patent ductus arteriosus usually supplies the descending aorta beyond the interruption (Fig. 38-7).[19,21] Associated cardiac defects include ventricular septal defect, bicuspid aortic valve, aortopulmonary window, truncus arteriosus, single ventricle subaortic stenosis.[3,4] CT and/or MRI can have a role in diagnosis.

Hypoplastic Left Heart Syndrome

This is a spectrum of left heart obstructive lesions characterized by underdevelopment of the mitral valve, left ventricle, aortic valve, and aorta. The right heart and main pulmonary artery are enlarged. Atrial and ventricular septal defects and patent ductus arteriosus are common associated defects.[22,23] Diagnosis is confirmed by echocardiography and cardiac angiography. CT and MRI usually have no role in preoperative assessment.

Critical Aortic Stenosis

This is a condition caused by fusion of the valve leaflets, resulting in a slit-like aortic orifice, severe outflow tract

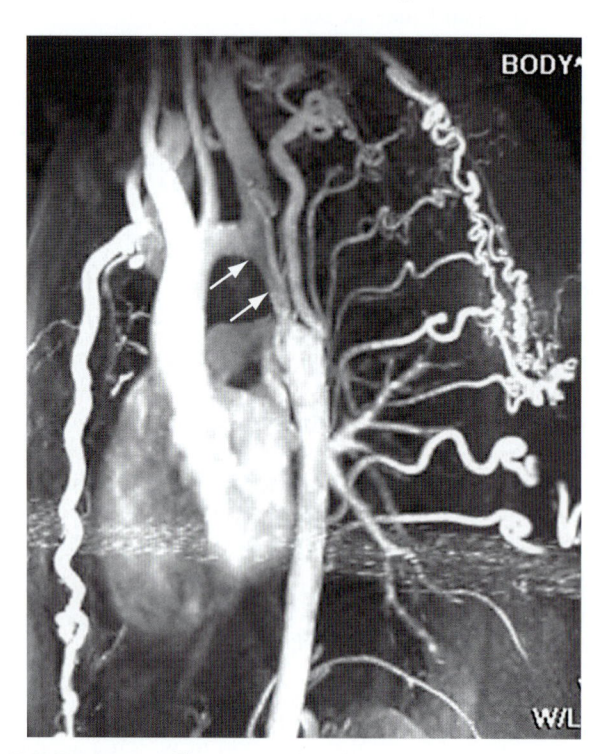

FIGURE 38-5 Diffuse coarctation. This sagittal view from a contrast-enhanced three-dimensional MR shows diffuse narrowing of the aortic isthmus (*arrows*) and enlarged internal thoracic artery and multiple enlarged intervertebral arteries.

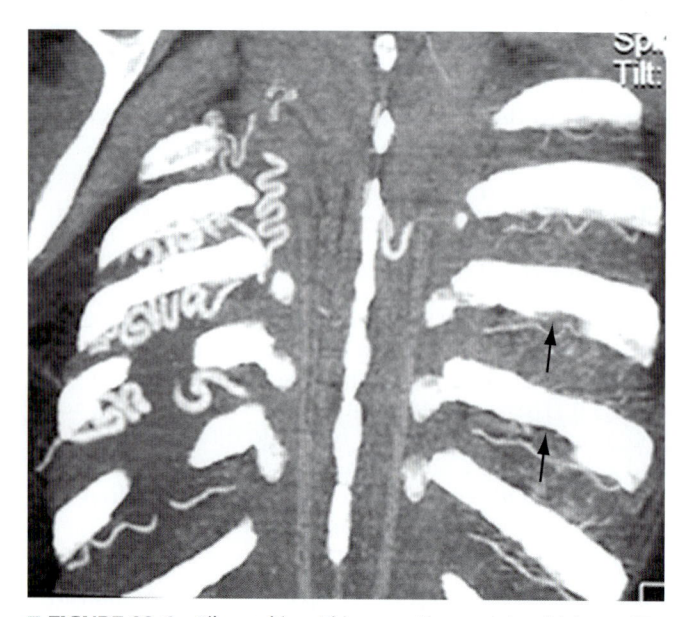

FIGURE 38-6 Rib notching. This posterior coronal multiplanar CT reformation shows erosions of the undersurfaces of several ribs (*arrows*) and collateral vessels.

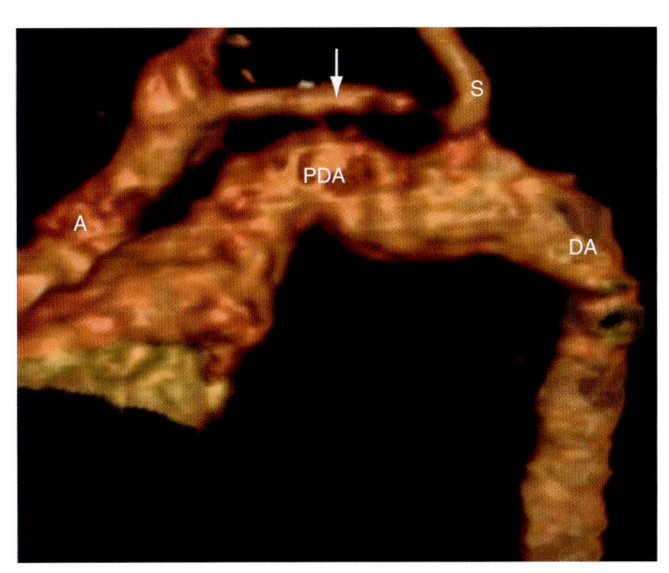

FIGURE 38-7 Interrupted aortic arch, type B. This three-dimensional volume rendered sagittal CT reconstruction shows a normal-caliber ascending aorta (A), hypoplastic transverse arch (*arrow*), and absence (i.e., interruption) of the aorta proximal to the left subclavian artery (S). A large patent ductus arteriosus (PDA) supplies the descending aorta (DA).

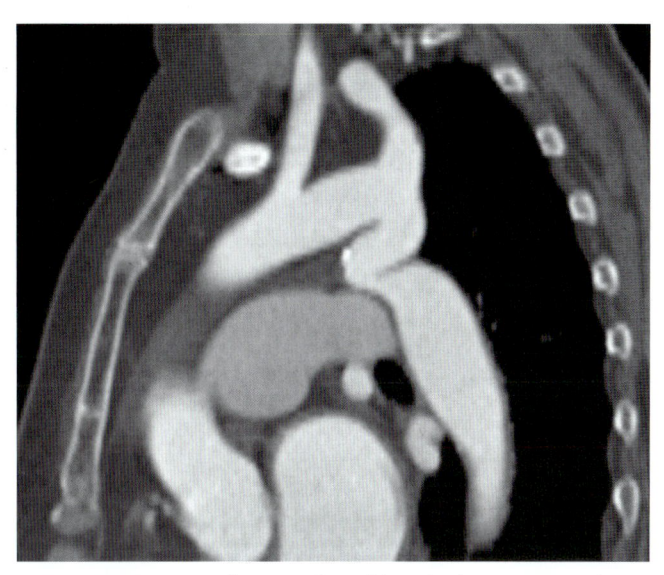

FIGURE 38-8 Pseudocoarctation. This sagittal CT reconstruction shows a tortuous proximal descending aorta with a focal kink below the origin of the left subclavian artery. Note the absence of collateral vessel formation.

obstruction, left ventricular hypertrophy, and ultimately cardiac failure and pulmonary edema.[5] Diagnosis is confirmed by echocardiography and cardiac catheterization. CT and MRI have no role in preoperative assessment.

There is almost no differential diagnosis of coarctation in older children and adults if there is a classic clinical history of upper extremity hypertension.

From Imaging Findings

The plain radiographic differential diagnosis of coarctation in the neonate includes any of the lesions discussed that are associated with cardiomegaly, heart failure, and pulmonary edema.

Pseudocoarctation is in the CT-MR differential diagnosis of coarctation in older patients. It is associated with an elongated, redundant aortic arch and appears as a buckle in the arch at the insertion of the site of the ligamentum arteriosum (Fig. 38-8). Luminal obstruction is absent. The blood pressures in the upper and lower extremities are almost always similar, although minor differences have been reported. There is no collateral circulation, which helps distinguish between pseudocoarctation and coarctation.

SYNOPSIS OF TREATMENT OPTIONS

Medical

In neonates with heart failure, prostaglandin E_1 is administered to reopen the ductus arteriosus and establish perfusion to the distal aorta and abdominal viscera. Treatment of congestive heart failure with digoxin and diuretics is also instituted. As soon as the patient condition improves, primary surgical repair is performed.[1,2,4]

Surgical and Interventional

Surgical management of the patient depends on the age of the patient, type of associated malformations, and morphology of the coarctation itself. Surgical procedures include the following:

1. Primary surgical repair, involving resection of the narrowed segment and an end-to-end anastomosis. This is the procedure of choice in neonates and young infants.
2. Subclavian flap aortoplasty, consisting of dividing the subclavian artery and inserting a flap of the vessel longitudinally into the aorta at the site of coarctation. It is no longer commonly performed because it requires sacrifice of the left subclavian artery, which may lead to claudication with exercise and diminished growth of the left arm.[24]
3. Patch aortoplasty in which the aorta is opened longitudinally, the fibrous shelf is excised, and a prosthetic patch is inserted to widen the aortic lumen. It is seldom used now because of the high incidence of late aneurysm formation.
4. Percutaneous balloon angioplasty with or without stent placement. It is used as treatment for residual stenosis or recoarctation after previous surgery[25,26] and for native coarctation in patients older than 12 months.[27,28] It has limited use in younger patients because restenosis is common.

The surgical mortality rate from a primary repair is less than 5% in neonates and less than 1% in older patients.[4] Late complications of surgical and interventional treatment include recoarctation or residual coarctation and aneurysm formation (Fig. 38-9).[29] The incidence of aneurysm formation is higher after angioplasty and patch graft repair than after primary surgical repair.[3]

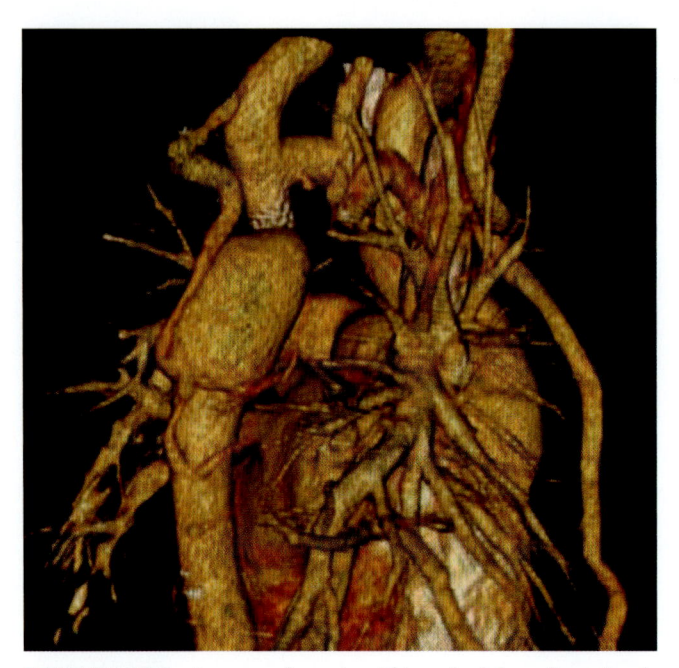

■ **FIGURE 38-9** Aneurysm formation. This sagittal three-dimensional volume rendered CT image shows dilation of the descending aorta at the site of balloon angioplasty.

What the Referring Physician Needs to Know

The site, extent (associated isthmus or arch hypoplasia) and severity of the coarctation, extent of collateral formation, number of aortic valve cusps, and left ventricular wall thickness should be reported. If MRI is performed, the gradient across the obstruction should be obtained

KEY POINTS

- Narrowing of proximal descending aorta with obstruction of blood flow
- Occurs as an isolated lesion or associated with other congenital lesions
- Clinical presentation varies from congestive heart failure in the newborn to asymptomatic hypertension or a murmur in older patients
- Classic plain radiographic findings—rib notching, reverse 3 sign
- CT and MRI findings—focal or diffuse narrowing, collateral vessel formation, rib notching, bicuspid valve, thick left ventricular wall
- Differential diagnosis—interrupted aortic arch, hypoplastic left heart, critical aortic stenosis, pseudocoarctation
- Surgical or interventional treatment

SUGGESTED READINGS

Gaca AM, Jaggers JJ, Dudley LT, Bisset GS. Repair of congenital heart disease: a primer—Part 2. Radiology 2008; 248:44-60.

Goo HW, Park I-S, Ko JK, et al. CT of congenital heart disease: normal anatomy and typical pathologic conditions. Radiographics 2003; 23:S147-S165.

Haramati LB, Glickstein FS, Issenberg HF, et al. MR imaging and CT of vascular anomalies and connections in patients with congenital heart disease. Radiographics 2002; 22:337-349.

Lee ED, Siegel MJ, Hildebolt CF, et al. Multidetector CT evaluation of pediatric thoracic aortic anomalies: comparison of axial, multiplanar, and three-dimensional images. AJR 2004; 182:777-784.

REFERENCES

1. Beekman RH. Coarctation of the aorta. In Alan HD, Gutgesell HP, Clark EB, Driscoll DJ (eds). Heart Disease in Infants, Children, and Adolescents, 6th ed. Philadelphia, Lippincott Williams & Wilkins, 2006, pp 988-1010.
2. Joshi VM, Sekhavat S. Acyanotic congenital heart defects. In Vetter VL (ed). Pediatric Cardiology: Requisites. St. Louis, Mosby, 2006, pp 79-96.
3. Kaemmerer H. Aortic coarctation and interrupted aortic arch. In Gatzoulis MA, Webb GD, Daubeney PEF (eds). Adult Congenital Heart Disease. Edinburgh, Churchill Livingstone, 2003, pp 253-264.
4. Park MK. Obstructive lesions. In Park MK (ed). Pediatric Cardiology for Practitioners, 5th ed. Philadelphia, Elsevier Mosby, 2008, pp 205-214.
5. Zeltser H, Tabbutt S. Critical heart disease in the newborn. In Vetter VL (ed). Pediatric Cardiology: Requisites. St. Louis, Mosby, 2006, pp 31-50.
6. Edwards JE, Christensen NA, Clagett OT, et al. Pathologic considerations in coarctation of the aorta. Mayo Clin Proc 1948; 23:324-332.
7. Ho SY, Anderson RH. Coarctation, tubular hypoplasia, and the ductus arteriosus: histologic study of 35 specimens. Br Heart J 1979; 41:268-274.
8. Bharati S, Lev M. The surgical anatomy of the heart in tubular hypoplasia of the transverse aorta (preductal coarctation). J Thorac Cardiovasc Surg 1986; 91:79-85.
9. Becker C, Soppa C, Fink U, et al. Spiral CT angiography and three-dimensional reconstruction in patients with aortic coarctation. Eur Radiol 1997; 7:1473-1477.
10. Siegel MJ. Heart. In: Siegel MJ (ed). Pediatric Body CT. Philadelphia, Lippincott Williams & Wilkins, 2007, pp 145-175.
11. Siegel MJ. CT angiography: optimizing contrast use in pediatric patients. Appl Radiol 2003; 32:S43-S49.
12. Foo TK, Saranathan M, Prince MR, Chenevert TL. Automated detection of bolus arrival and initiation of data acquisition in fast, three-dimensional, gadolinium-enhanced MR angiography. Radiology 1997; 203:275-280.
13. Earls JP, Rofsky NM, DeCorato DR, et al Breath-hold single-dose gadolinium-enhanced three-dimensional MR aortography: usefulness of a timing examination and MR power injector. Radiology 1996; 201:705-710.
14. Rebergen SA, van der Wall EE, Doornbos J, de Roos A. Magnetic resonance measurement of velocity and flow: technique, validation, and cardiovascular applications. Am Heart J 1993 126:1439-1456.
15. Varaprasathan GA, Araoz PA, Higgins CB, Reddy GP. Quantification of flow dynamics in congenital heart disease: applications of velocity-encoded cine MR imaging. Radiographics 2002 22:895-905.
16. Gilkeson RC, Ciancibello L, Zahka K. Multidetector CT evaluation of congenital heart disease in pediatric and adult patients. AJR 2003; 180:973-980.

17. Goo HW, Park I-S, Ko JK, et al. CT of congenital heart disease: normal anatomy and typical pathologic conditions. Radiographics 2003; 23: S147-S165.
18. Haramati LB, Glickstein FS, Issenberg HF, et al MR imaging and CT of vascular anomalies and connections in patients with congenital heart disease. Radiographics 2002; 22:337-349.
19. Lee Ed, Siegel MJ, Hildebolt CF, et al. Multidetector CT evaluation of pediatric thoracic aortic anomalies: comparison of axial, multiplanar, and three-dimensional Images. AJR 2004; 182:777-784.
20. Celoria CG, Patton RB. Congenital absence of the aortic arch. Am Heart J 1959; 58:407-413.
21. Cinar A, Haliloglu M, Karagoz T, et al. Interrupted aortic arch in a neonate: multidetector CT diagnosis. Pediatr Radiol 2004; 34:901-903.
22. Bardo DM, Frankel DG, Applegate KE, et al. Hypoplastic left heart syndrome. Radiographics 2001; 21:705-717.
23. Freedom RM, Black MD, Benson LN. Hypoplastic left heart syndrome. In Alan HD, Gutgesell HP, Clark EB, Driscoll DJ (eds). Heart Disease in Infants, Children, and Adolescents, 6th ed. Philadelphia, Lippincott Williams & Wilkins, 2006, pp 1011-1026.
24. Van Son JA, van Asten WN, van Lier HJ, et al. Detrimental sequelae on the hemodynamics of the upper limb after subclavian flap angioplasty in infancy. Circulation 1990; 81:996-1004.
25. Hijazi ZM, Fahey JT, Kleinman CS, Hellenbrand We. Balloon angioplasty for recurrent coarctation of the aorta. Intermediate and long-term results. Circulation 1991; 84:1150-1156.
26. Siblini G, Rao PS, Nouri S, et al. Long-term follow up results of balloon angioplasty of postoperative aortic recoarctation. Am J Cardiol 1998;81:61-67.
27. Fletcher SE, Nihill MR, Grifka RG, et al. Balloon angioplasty of native coarctation of the aorta: midterm follow-up and prognostic factors. J Am Coll Cardiol 1995; 25:73-734.
28. Mendelsohn AM, Lloyd TR, Crowley DC, et al. Late follow-up of balloon angioplasty in children with a native coarctation of the aorta. Am J Cardiol 1994; 25:696-700.
29. Shih M-CP, Tholpady A, Kramer CM, et al. Surgical and endovascular repair of aortic coarctation: normal findings and appearance of complications on CT angiography and MR angiography. AJR 2006; 187:W302-W312.

CHAPTER 39

Vascular Rings and Slings

Marilyn J. Siegel

Vascular rings and slings refer to a spectrum of arterial anomalies caused by abnormalities in development of the embryonic aortic arches.[1-4] Complications arise from compression of the trachea, esophagus, or both, leading to respiratory distress and dysphagia. The vast majority of rings and slings are found in infants and young children, but the anomalies can be seen in adults. Computed tomography (CT) and magnetic resonance imaging (MRI) provide accurate anatomic delineation of the vascular anomalies and compressed structures and are the imaging studies of choice to establish the diagnosis. Treatment is surgical intervention for symptomatic patients.

Definition

A vascular ring is a developmental abnormality of the primitive aortic arch in which the trachea and/or esophagus are surrounded by vascular and often ligamentous structures. Pulmonary sling, also known as anomalous left pulmonary artery, is a rare anomaly in which the lower trachea is partially surrounded by vascular structures.

The most common vascular rings are the double aortic arch, right aortic arch with aberrant left subclavian artery and left ligamentum arteriosus, left arch with aberrant right subclavian artery, and anomalous innominate artery.

Prevalence and Epidemiology

Vascular rings and slings represent approximately 1% of congenital cardiovascular anomalies,[3] although this incidence may be underestimated because some lesions are asymptomatic. Most cases are sporadic, but there may be a genetic inheritance in some arch anomalies. Microdeletions of chromosome 22q11, in particular, have been associated with various arch anomalies.[5]

Etiology and Pathophysiology

Persistence of a segment of arch that should have regressed or regression of a segment that should have normally persisted explains the development of most arch anomalies.

The theoretic embryonic double aortic arch model proposed by Edwards is most extensively used to demonstrate embryologic explanations for the variations in arch development.[6] This model classifies vascular rings by the side of the ductus arteriosus and the site of dissolution of the double arches (Fig. 39-1).

Vascular rings may be complete (true) or incomplete (Fig. 39-2).[3] In complete rings, the vascular structures entirely surround and compress the trachea and esophagus. These include the double aortic arch and right arch with aberrant retroesophageal left subclavian artery. In the double arch, an atretic segment of arch may complete the ring. With an aberrant left subclavian, a left ligamentum arteriosum connects the descending aorta and left pulmonary artery completing the ring.

In incomplete rings, the vascular anomalies do not entirely encircle the trachea and esophagus, but do cause mass effect on these structures. These include the left arch with aberrant right subclavian artery and anomalous innominate artery.[3] In the case of an aberrant right subclavian, the vessel itself or an aortic diverticulum (Kommerell diverticulum) at the takeoff of the artery compresses the posterior aspect of the esophagus. In anomalous innominate artery, the right innominate artery arises too far to the left from the arch and compresses the trachea anteriorly as it crosses the midline.

The mirror image right arch is a common vascular anomaly that comes to clinical attention because of associated cyanotic heart disease. It does not form a vascular ring and does not compress the trachea or esophagus.

MANIFESTATIONS

Clinical Presentation

Symptoms vary with the tightness of the ring around the trachea and/or esophagus, and hence the degree of tracheobronchial compression. Tight rings usually manifest in neonates or infants. Symptoms include stridor, cough, repeated pulmonary infections, cyanosis, and respiratory failure, and feeding difficulties.[1-4] Looser rings may be

CHAPTER 39 • Vascular Rings and Slings 543

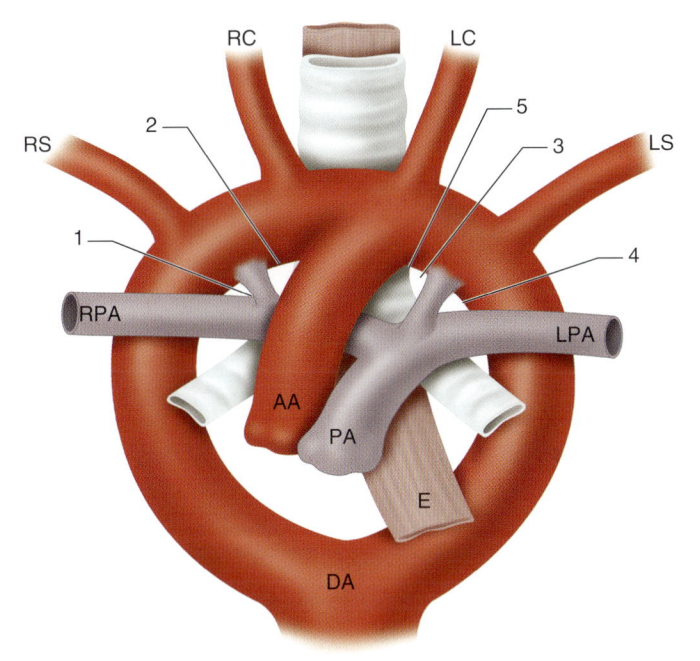

■ **FIGURE 39-1** Diagram of Edwards hypothetical double arch with bilateral ductus arteriosum. Breaks at 1 and 2 lead to left arch; breaks at 3 and 5 lead to right arch. A break at 1 with resorption of the right ductus results in normal anatomy. A break at 2 results in left arch with anomalous subclavian artery; typically, the right ductus resorbs (i.e., not a complete ring). A break at 4 results in right arch with mirror-image branching; the ductus courses from the innominate artery to the left pulmonary artery (not a complete ring). A break at 3 leads to right arch with aberrant subclavian artery; typically, the left ductus persists, coursing from the left subclavian to the left pulmonary artery and forming a vascular ring. A break at 5 differs in that the anomalous vessel is the innominate artery. AA, ascending aorta; DA, descending aorta; E, esophagus; LC, left carotid artery; LPA, left pulmonary artery; LS, left subclavian artery; PA, main pulmonary artery; RC, right carotid artery; RPA, right pulmonary artery; RS, right subclavian artery. *(Modified from Hernanz-Schulman M. Vascular rings: a practical approach to imaging diagnosis. Pediatr Radiol 2005; 35:961-979.)*

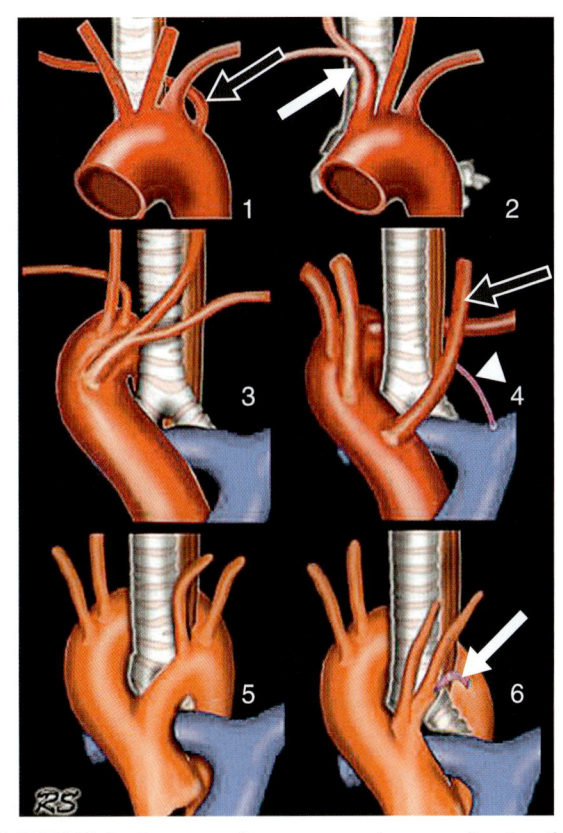

■ **FIGURE 39-2** Spectrum of common vascular anomalies. **1,** Left arch with aberrant right subclavian artery (*arrow*). Order of arterial branching is right carotid, left carotid, left subclavian, right subclavian. **2,** Anomalous right innominate artery (*arrow*). **3,** Right arch mirror image. Order of arterial branching is left innominate, right carotid, right subclavian. **4,** Right arch with aberrant left subclavian artery (*arrow*). Order of arterial branching is left carotid, right carotid, right subclavian, left subclavian. *Arrowhead* shows left ligamentum ductus arteriosum. **5,** Double aortic arch. **6,** Double arch with atretic segment (*arrow*). *(Courtesy of Dr. Robin Smithuis, Rijnland Hospital, Leiderdorp, the Netherlands.)*

discovered in older children or adults in whom mild dysphagia or choking on food prompts evaluation. Some asymptomatic rings will be discovered incidentally during an imaging study performed for other clinical indications. Rings that are asymptomatic early in life can become symptomatic later in life if the vascular structures become ectatic and compress the airway or esophagus.[2] Double aortic arches tend have more severe symptoms and present earlier than other rings.[7] Slings commonly manifest in neonates, producing respiratory compromise.

Imaging Studies

Indications and Algorithm

Imaging is performed to confirm the morphology of the ring or sling and the effect on adjacent structures. Chest radiography is usually the initial imaging examination. If the chest radiograph is abnormal or if there is high clinical concern of a vascular anomaly but a normal chest radiograph, CT or MRI is performed to confirm the diagnosis and provide detailed anatomy of the anomaly and its effect on adjacent structures.

Techniques and Findings

Radiography

Chest radiography is used to show the side of the aortic arch and compression of adjacent structures. If a right arch is identified, the likelihood of a vascular ring is high. If only a left arch is identified, a vascular ring is less likely, but not excluded.[2,8]

Ultrasound

Echocardiography or conventional sonography in infants, using a suprasternal or trans-sternal approach with the thymus as an acoustic window can identify the aortic arch and vascular branching pattern. Sonography, however, cannot provide detailed information about the arch anomaly and cannot delineate tracheal or esophageal compression. Its use also is limited in older patients because of a poor acoustic window. Thus, it is not routinely performed.

Computed Tomography

Computed tomography can provide accurate anatomic detail of the vascular anomalies and compressed trachea or esophagus. CT is especially useful for the evaluation of the tracheobronchial tree, simulating the surgical view.[1]

CT is performed using thin collimation (<1 mm), large pitch (<1.5), rapid scan time, and a single breath-hold, when possible. In adolescents and adults, contrast medium is injected via a power injector at a high flow rate of 3 to 4 mL/sec using a contrast volume of 100 to 150 mL (280 to 320 mg I/mL). Scan delay time is determined with an automatic bolus tracking system. The cursor is placed over the ascending aorta if aortic anomalies are suspected and over the main pulmonary artery if pulmonary sling is suspected. Electrocardiographic (ECG) gating is not needed. The volumetric data are reconstructed at a 3- to 5-mm slice thickness for routine viewing and at a 1- to 2-mm slice thickness for multiplanar reformatting and three-dimensional reconstructions. A standard reconstruction algorithm is used for reconstruction.[9-11] (See Chapter 38, Coarctation of the Aorta, for pediatric techniques.)

Magnetic Resonance Imaging

MRI, like CT, can accurately define the side of the arch and its relationship to adjacent structures. An advantage of MRI is that it does not use ionizing radiation.

MR studies are performed with head, knee, or phased-array coils according to body size. The imaging protocol includes at least a black blood sequence (T1-weighted spin-echo, fast-spin echo, and half-Fourier turbo spin-echo with double-inversion recovery pulse) or bright blood sequences (gradient-echo, segmented k-space fast gradient-echo, and steady-state free precession) and three-dimensional contrast-enhanced MR acquisition (CE-MRA). Black and bright blood sequences are obtained in at least the axial plane, but should also be obtained in a second imaging plane—either a sagittal or coronal orientation. CE-MRA is obtained in the coronal plane. A test dose of contrast is power-injected and the time of peak bolus is determined. The actual examination is performed with images acquired during peak bolus as determined by the test injection. Multiplanar reconstructions, maximum intensity projections, and three-dimensional volume rendered reconstructions are obtained to display the vessels optimally.

Angiography

Angiography is not required if CT or MRI is diagnostic.

Classic Signs

Double Aortic Arch

Chest radiographic findings include opacities lying on both sides of the tracheal air column, proximal tracheal indentation, and posterior esophageal indentation (Fig. 39-3). CT and MRI show the two arches arising from a single ascending aorta, with each arch giving rise to a subclavian and carotid artery before joining to form a single descending aorta, usually left-sided (Fig. 39-4).[1-4,12-16] The right arch is commonly larger and more cephalad than the left arch. In rare cases, one limb, often the left, is atretic, with a fibrous band completing the ring (Fig. 39-5).[17]

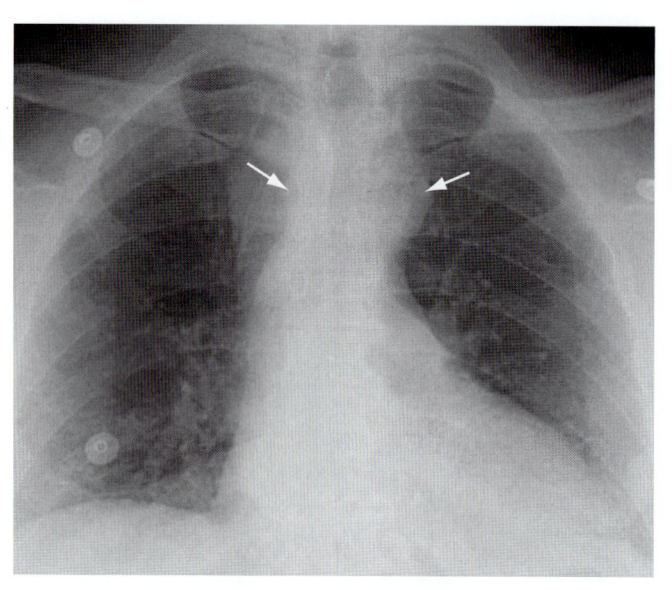

■ **FIGURE 39-3** Double aortic arch, 65-year-old woman. Chest radiograph shows bilateral paratracheal opacities (*arrows*), representing bilateral arches.

Right Aortic Arch with Aberrant Left Subclavian Artery

Chest radiographic findings include right-sided paratracheal opacity and tracheal indentation, posterior esophageal indentation, and absence of a normal left-sided aortic arch shadow (Fig. 39-6). CT and MRI findings are a right arch and left subclavian artery arising from the posterior aspect of the right arch (Fig. 39-7). A Kommerell diverticulum at the origin of the left subclavian artery from the aorta may be seen.[1-4,12-16]

Left Aortic Arch with Aberrant Right Subclavian Artery

This is an arch anomaly but not a vascular ring. A frontal chest radiograph may show an abnormal mediastinal contour at the level of the aortic arch, representing dilation of the origin of the aberrant artery (i.e., diverticulum of Kommerell; Fig. 39-8). A lateral chest radiograph can show posterior esophageal indentation. CT and MRI can confirm the diagnosis of anomalous origin of the right subclavian artery, which arises as the last branch off the aorta, rather than the first.[1-4,12-16] A Kommerell diverticulum and esophageal compression are other findings. Atherosclerotic changes and intramural thrombus formation can occur within this diverticulum (Fig. 39-9).

Innominate Artery Compression

Chest radiographic CT and MRI findings are anterior compression of the trachea.[1-4,12-16,18] The site of compression is usually at or just below the thoracic inlet (Fig. 39-10).

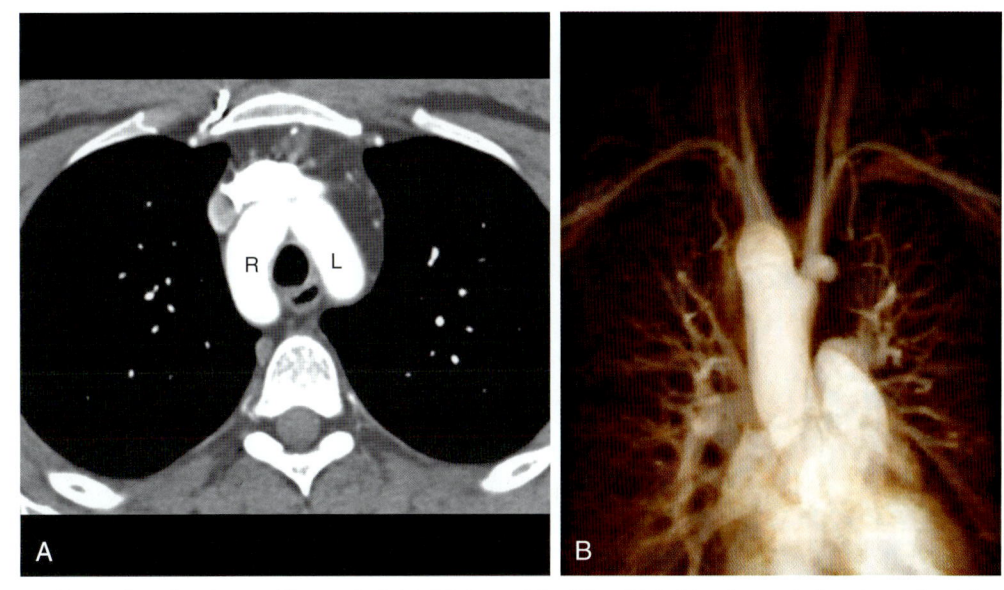

■ **FIGURE 39-4** Double aortic arch, 35-year-old man. **A,** Axial CT shows right (R) and left (L) arches encircling the trachea. The arches are of equal caliber. **B,** Coronal MRA shows two arches, each giving rise to a subclavian and carotid artery. The right arch is more cephalad than the left. (**B,** *Courtesy of Dr. Vamsi Narra, Mallinckrodt Institute of Radiology, St. Louis.*)

Anomalous Left Pulmonary Artery (Pulmonary Sling)

Chest radiographic findings include right-sided tracheal indentation and often hyperinflation of the right middle and lower lobes. CT and MRI show the left pulmonary artery arising from the right pulmonary artery, coursing over the right main bronchus, and crossing between the trachea and esophagus to reach the left hilum (Fig. 39-11).[1-4,12-16,19-21] When there are associated cartilaginous rings, long segment tracheal narrowing and a horizontal course of the main bronchi (i.e., T-shaped carina) will be noted.[22]

DIFFERENTIAL DIAGNOSIS

From Clinical Presentation

The clinical differential diagnosis of vascular ring includes other lesions that cause chronic stridor, wheezing, recurrent infections or dysphagia.

From Imaging Findings

These include a right arch with mirror-image branching. This anomaly is asymptomatic because there is no retro-

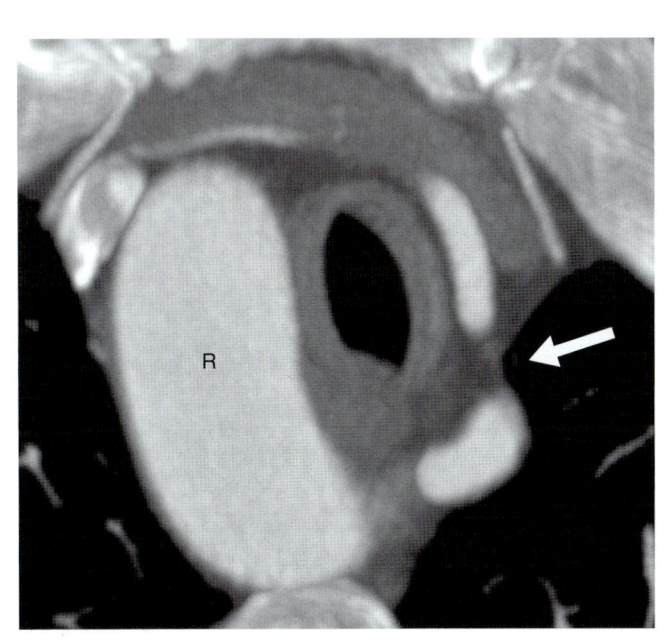

■ **FIGURE 39-5** Double aortic arch with hypoplastic component, 63-year-old man. This axial CT scan shows a dominant right arch (R) and area of atresia (*arrow*) in the smaller left arch.

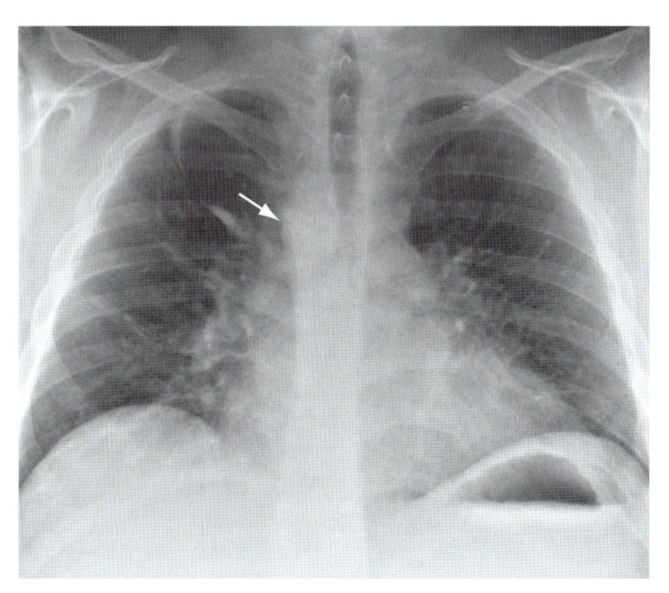

■ **FIGURE 39-6** Right aortic arch with aberrant left subclavian artery. This posterior anterior chest radiograph shows a right paratracheal opacity (*arrow*) indenting the tracheal air column. A left-sided arch shadow is absent.

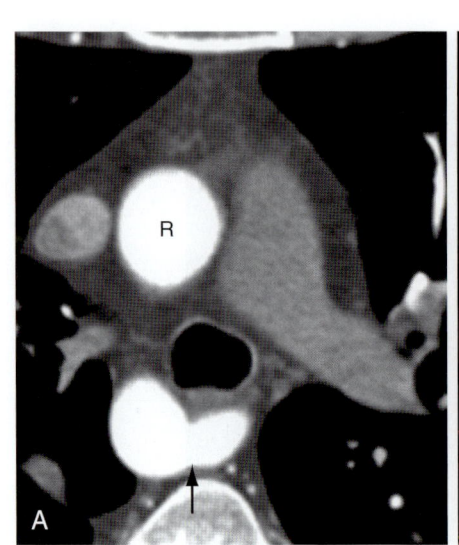

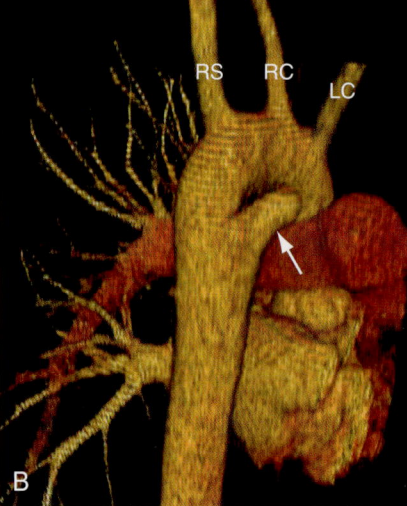

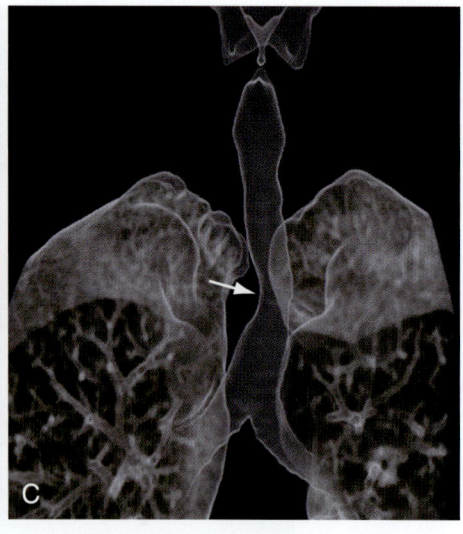

FIGURE 39-7 Right aortic arch with aberrant left subclavian artery, 55-year-old man. **A,** Axial CT scan demonstrates a right aortic arch (R) with aberrant left subclavian artery (*arrow*) crossing the mediastinum posteriorly. **B,** Coronal three-dimensional CT reconstruction. The left subclavian artery (*arrow*) is the last vessel arising from the aorta. Order of arterial branching is left carotid (LC), right carotid (RC), right subclavian (RS), and left subclavian. **C,** Coronal three-dimensional airway reconstruction shows focal compression of the trachea (*arrow*) by the anomalous subclavian artery.

esophageal vessel. Most patients come to clinical attention because of associated heart disease (98% of cases), particularly tetralogy of Fallot. The order of arterial branching is opposite that of normal (i.e., mirror image). The first branch is the left innominate artery, the second is the right carotid, and the last is the right subclavian.

SYNOPSIS OF TREATMENT OPTIONS

Medical

Vascular rings are usually not treated medically.

Surgical and Interventional

Surgical repair is performed for symptomatic patients. Others are treated conservatively.

1. Anomalous right subclavian artery—division of the ductus ligamentum arteriosum

FIGURE 39-8 Left aortic arch with aberrant right subclavian artery. This posterior anterior chest radiograph shows a left arch (*black arrow*) and mass-like right paratracheal opacity (*white arrow*) caused by the dilated aberrant artery.

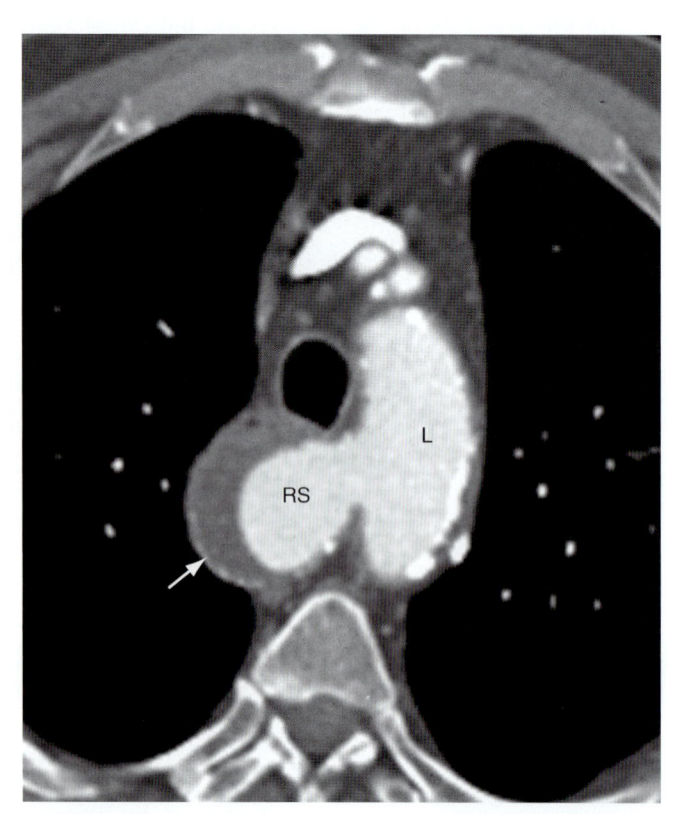

FIGURE 39-9 Left aortic arch with aberrant right subclavian artery (same patient as in Figure 39-8). This axial CT image shows a left aortic arch (L) and an aneurysm of the aberrant right subclavian artery (RS), which contains thrombus (*arrow*).

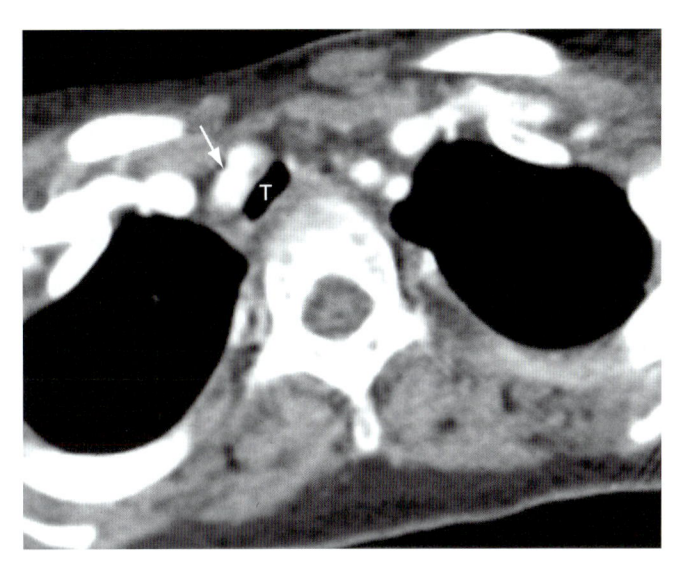

FIGURE 39-10 Innominate artery compression, 4-year-old boy. Anterior tracheal (T) compression by the right innominate artery (*arrow*) is seen just below the level of the thoracic inlet. (*From Siegel MJ. Great vessels. In Siegel MJ (ed). Pediatric Body CT. Philadelphia, Lippincott Williams & Wilkins, 2008, pp 121-144.*)

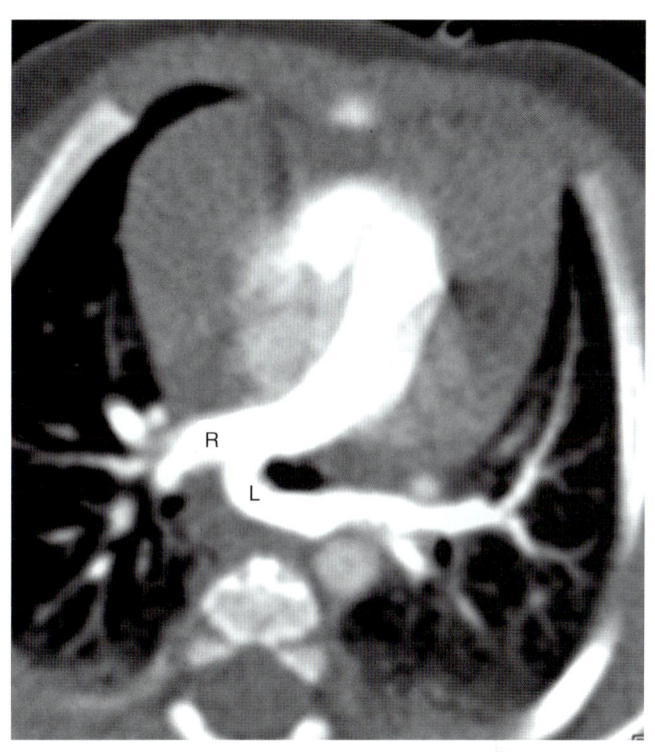

FIGURE 39-11 Pulmonary artery sling, 4-month-old girl. This axial CT scan demonstrates the left pulmonary artery (L) arising from the proximal right pulmonary artery (R) before crossing behind the trachea to reach the left lung. (*From Siegel MJ. Great vessels. In Siegel MJ (ed). Pediatric Body CT. Philadelphia, Lippincott Williams & Wilkins, 2008, pp 121-144.*)

2. Right arch with anomalous left subclavian artery—division of the ductus ligamentum arteriosum
3. Double arch—surgical division of the smaller arch
4. Innominate compression of the trachea—suspension of the innominate artery from the sternum
5. Pulmonary sling—division of the anomalous pulmonary artery and reanastomosis to the main pulmonary artery. Tracheoplasty in patients with complete cartilaginous rings

What the Referring Physician Needs to Know

- Position of the arch (right, left, bilateral); abnormalities of branching (anomalous subclavian artery, left pulmonary artery); tracheal or esophageal compression.

KEY POINTS

- Vascular ring—spectrum of arterial anomalies caused by errors in development of the embryonic aortic arches
- Most common vascular rings are double aortic arch, right aortic arch with aberrant left subclavian artery, left arch with aberrant right subclavian artery, and anomalous innominate artery
- Pulmonary sling—anomalous origin of left pulmonary artery from right pulmonary artery
- Complications of rings and slings relate to compression of esophagus and/or trachea
- Vast majority found in infants and young children
- Surgical intervention for symptomatic patients

SUGGESTED READINGS

Berdon WE. Rings, slings, and other things: vascular compression of the infant trachea updated from the mid-century to the millennium—the legacy of Robert E. Gross, MD, and Edward B.D. Neuhauser, MD. Radiology 2000; 216:624-632.

Goo HW, Park I-S, Ko JK, et al. CT of congenital heart disease: normal anatomy and typical pathologic conditions. Radiographics 2003; 23:S147-S165.

Hernanz-Schulman M. Vascular rings: a practical approach to imaging diagnosis. Pediatr Radiol 2005; 35:961-979.

Lee ED, Siegel MJ, Hildebolt CF, et al. Multidetector CT evaluation of pediatric thoracic aortic anomalies: comparison of axial, multiplanar, and three-dimensional images. AJR Am J Roentgenol 2004; 182:777-784.

Oddone M, Granata C, Vercellino N, et al. Multi-modality evaluation of the abnormalities of the aortic arches in children: techniques and imaging spectrum with emphasis on MRI. Pediatric Radiol 2005; 35:947-960.

Predey TS, McDonald V, Demos TC, Moncada R. CT of congenital anomalies of the aortic arch. Semin Roentgenol 1989; 14:96-111.

REFERENCES

1. Abrams D, Gerlis L, Daubeney P. Tracheoesophageal compression in congenital heart disease: vascular rings, pulmonary slings and other vascular abnormalities. In Gatzoulis MA, Webb GD, Daubeney PEF (eds). Adult Congenital Heart Disease. Edinburgh, Churchill Livingstone, 2003, pp 273-280.
2. Hernanz-Schulman, M. Vascular rings: a practical approach to imaging diagnosis. Pediatr Radiol. 2005; 35:961-979.
3. Park MK. Vascular ring. In Park MK (ed). Pediatric Cardiology for Practitioners, 5th ed. St. Louis, Mosby, 2008, pp 303-308.
4. Weinberg PM. Aortic arch anomalies. In Alan HD, Gutgesell HP, Clark EB, Driscoll DJ (eds). Heart Disease in Infants, Children, and Adolescents, 6th ed. Philadelphia, Lippincott Williams & Wilkins, 2006, pp 707-735.
5. Momma K, Matsuoka R, Takao A. Aortic arch anomalies associated with chromosome 22q11 deletion (CATCH 22). Pediatr Cardiol 1999; 20:97-102.
6. Edwards JE. Anomalies of the derivatives of the aortic arch system. Med Clin North Am 1948; 32:925-949.
7. Van Son JA, Julsrud PR, Hagler DJ, et al. Surgical treatment of vascular rings: the Mayo clinic experience. Mayo Clin Proc 1993; 68:1056-1063.
8. Pickhardt P, Siegel M, Gutierrez F. Vascular rings in symptomatic children: frequency of chest radiographic findings. Radiology 1997; 203:423-426.
9. Gilkeson RC, Ciancibello L, Zahka K. Multidetector CT evaluation of congenital heart disease in pediatric and adult patients. AJR 2003; 180:973-980.
10. Goo HW, Park I-S, Ko JK, et al. CT of congenital heart disease: normal anatomy and typical pathologic conditions. Radiographics 2003; 23: S147-S165.
11. Lee Ed, Siegel MJ, Hildebolt CF, et al. Multidetector CT evaluation of pediatric thoracic aortic anomalies: comparison of axial, multiplanar, and three-dimensional images. AJR 2004; 182:777-784.
12. Oddone M, Granata C, Vercellino N, et al. Multi-modality evaluation of the abnormalities of the aortic arches in children: techniques and imaging spectrum with emphasis on MRI. Pediatric Radiol 2005; 35:947-960.
13. Predey TS, McDonald V, Demos TC, Moncada R. CT of congenital anomalies of the aortic arch. Semin Roentgenol 1989; 14:96-111.
14. Remy-Jardin M, Remy J, Mayo JR, et al. Thoracic aorta. In Remy-Jardin M, Remy J, Mayo JR, et al. CT Angiography of the Chest. Philadelphia, Lippincott Williams & Wilkins, 2001, pp 29-50.
15. Siegel MJ. Great vessels. In Siegel MJ (ed). Pediatric Body CT. Philadelphia, Lippincott Williams & Wilkins, 2008, pp 121-144.
16. Van Dyke CW, White RD. Congenital abnormalities of the thoracic aorta presenting in the adult. J Thorac Imaging 1994; 9:230-245.
17. Schlessinger AE, Krishnamurthy R, Sena LM, et al. Incomplete double aortic arch with atresia of the distal left arch: distinctive imaging appearance. AJR 2005; 184:1634-1639.
18. Adler SC, Isaacson G, Balsara RK. Innominate artery compression of the trachea: diagnosis and treatment by anterior suspension. A 25-year experience. Ann Otol Rhinol Laryngol 1995; 104: 924-927.
19. Lee KH, Yoon CS, Choe KO, et al. Use of imaging for assessing anatomical relationships of tracheobronchial anomalies associated with left pulmonary artery sling. Pediatr Radiol 2001; 31:269-278.
20. Newman B, Meza MP, Towbin RB, Del Nido P. Left pulmonary artery sling: diagnosis and delineation of associated tracheobronchial anomalies with MR. Pediatr Radiol 1996; 26: 661-668.
21. Park HS, Im JG, Jung JW, et al. Anomalous left pulmonary artery with complete cartilaginous ring. J Comput Assist Tomogr 1997; 21:478-480.
22. Berdon WE: Rings, slings, and other things: vascular compression of the infant trachea updated from the mid-century to the millennium—the legacy of Robert E. Gross, MD, and Edward B.D. Neuhauser, MD. Radiology 2000; 216:624-632.

CHAPTER 40

Magnetic Resonance Imaging of the Aorta and Left Ventricular Function in Inherited and Congenital Aortic Disease

Heynric B. Grotenhuis, Jaap Ottenkamp, Lucia J.M. Kroft, and Albert de Roos

The aorta is not simply a tube or conduit but a highly complex part of the vascular tree originating from the left ventricular (LV) outflow tract and aortic valve and extending to its major thoracic and abdominal branches. Passing blood from the heart to the limbs and major organs is one functional aspect of the aorta; of equal importance is its capacity to distend and to recoil in response to pulsatile flow, thereby reducing afterload for the left ventricle and facilitating diastolic perfusion of the coronary arteries.

Intrinsic aortic wall abnormalities have been described in inherited connective tissue disorders such as Marfan syndrome and bicuspid aortic valve disease, but recent reports indicate similar aortic involvement in patients with classic congenital heart disease (CHD) entities, such as coarctation of the aorta, tetralogy of Fallot, and transposition of the great arteries, suggesting a degenerative process that results in structural weakness of the aortic wall.[1,2] The aortic media consists of smooth muscle and an extracellular matrix that is composed of ground substance, in which elastic fibers and collagen are embedded in a hydrated gel comprising glycosaminoglycans, proteoglycans, and adhesive glycoproteins.[1] Smooth muscle cells govern vasodilation and vasoconstriction, collagen provides inert aortic wall strength (stiffness), and elastin—with its low elastic modulus—is readily deformable, permitting phasic distention and recoil in response to pulsatile flow.[1] Current focus on the origin of aortic wall abnormalities has shifted toward these specific medial constituents and their crucial role in the structural and functional integrity of the aorta in affected groups of patients.[1]

In prototypical diseases such as Marfan syndrome and bicuspid aortic valve disease, loss of fibrillin 1 microfibrils has been reported to dissociate smooth muscle cells from the medial matrix components, resulting in accelerated cell death and matrix disruption (Fig. 40-1).[2] Matrix metalloproteinases, endogenous enzymes that degrade matrix components, become activated in fibrillin 1–deficient tissues, degrading the structural support of the aorta.[2] Similar focal abnormalities within the aortic media have recently been described in coarctation of the aorta, tetralogy of Fallot, and transposition of the great arteries.[1] Whether these aortic wall changes result from an intrinsic medial abnormality or are secondary to hemodynamic states before and after surgical repair (or both) is unknown.[1] Whatever the etiology of aortic wall disease given this heterogeneity, aortic dilation and reduced aortic elasticity will evolve when loss of structural support of the aortic wall progresses.[1,2]

With advancing age, ascending aortic elastic fibers will fragment, collagen and ground substance will increase, and the number of smooth muscle cells will decrease.[1,3]

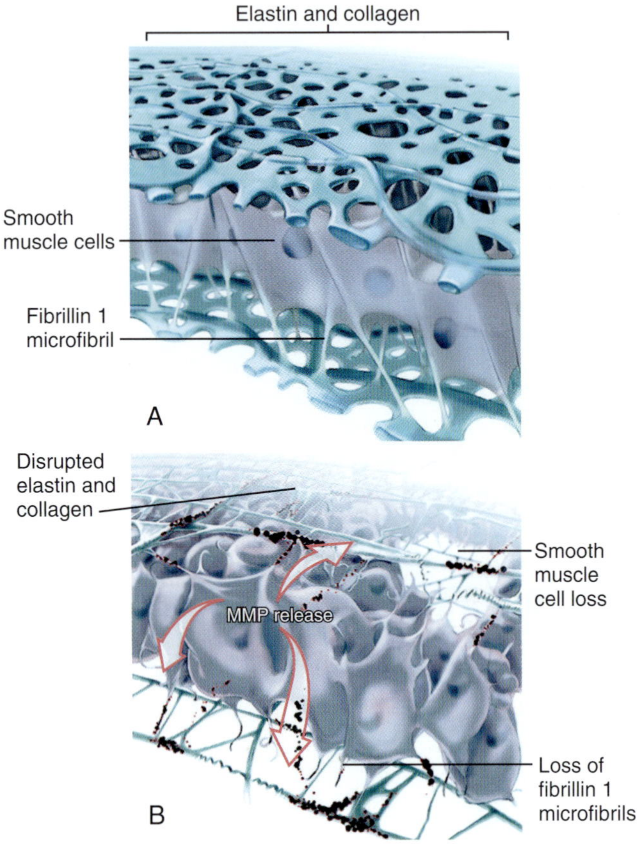

FIGURE 40-1 The elastic lamina of the aortic media provides structural support and elasticity to the aorta. In patients with a normal tricuspid valve (**A**), fibrillin 1 microfibrils tether smooth muscle cells to adjacent elastin and collagen matrix components. In patients with bicuspid aortic valve (**B**), deficient microfibrillar elements result in smooth muscle cell detachment, matrix metalloproteinase release, matrix disruption, cell death, and loss of structural support and elasticity. (From Fedak PW, Verma S, David TE, et al. Clinical and pathophysiological implications of a bicuspid aortic valve. Circulation 2002; 106:900-904.)

which in turn will increase myocardial oxygen demand by increasing LV afterload.[7] Arterial stiffening is also associated with impaired coronary perfusion, the presence of coronary artery disease, and LV dysfunction.[8]

As life expectancy of patients with CHD has much improved during the past decades, adult cardiologists will be increasingly confronted with the challenge of concomitant aortic sequelae. Therefore, noninvasive monitoring of aortic dimensions and elasticity, in conjunction with aortic valve competence and LV function, is clinically highly desirable in patients with potential aortic wall abnormalities. Echocardiography is widely used for routine assessment of the aortic root, aortic valve, and ventricular function, but it does not permit evaluation of the entire aorta.[4] Magnetic resonance imaging (MRI) provides advantages such as unlimited field of view within the entire thorax for accurate and reproducible assessment of aortic and cardiac anatomy and function.[5,9,10]

In this chapter, the five most common entities of inherited connective tissue disorders and classic CHD with intrinsic aortic wall abnormalities are discussed, including Marfan syndrome, bicuspid aortic valve disease, coarctation of the aorta, tetralogy of Fallot, and transposition of the great arteries, with description of the potential role of MRI in their evaluation and management of the aortic disease and associated LV disease.

MARFAN SYNDROME

Prevalence and Epidemiology

Marfan syndrome is a heritable connective tissue disorder resulting in a highly variable degree of premature aortic medial degeneration with a high risk of progressive aortic dilation and subsequent aortic dissection or rupture.[11,12] Marfan syndrome is caused by a mutation of the *FBN1* gene on chromosome 15 that codes for fibrillin 1, in the absence of which elastin is more readily degraded by matrix metalloproteinases and smooth muscle cells will dissociate from the medial matrix components.[1,4]

Pathophysiology and Follow-up

Aortic dilation is the most common cause of morbidity and mortality in patients with Marfan syndrome as dilation of the sinus of Valsalva is found in 60% to 80% of adult patients (Fig. 40-2).[13] The relative abundance of elastic fibers in the ascending aorta compared with other regions of the arterial tree, coupled with the repetitive stress of LV ejection, probably accounts for aortic dilation that usually occurs primarily in the aortic root.[13] Therefore, the majority of patients with Marfan syndrome present with enlargement of the ascending aorta or a type A dissection and only in very rare cases with a type B dissection involving the descending aorta.[11] Aortic dissection is associated with increasing aortic diameter but it may also occur in nondilated aortas.[11,12] Replacement of the aortic root with a composite graft conduit has been recommended before the diameter exceeds 5.0 to 5.5 cm.[11,12] Independent predictors of progressive aortic dilation that will prompt the recommendation for surgery when the aorta is smaller than 5.0 cm include rapid growth of the aortic diameter

In addition, arterial hypertension, atherosclerosis, and other cardiovascular risk factors such as smoking, hypercholesterolemia, and diabetes may lead to atheroma formation, which is associated with similar degenerative processes in the extracellular matrix and the vasa vasorum.[4] Therefore, the negative sequelae related to aging and numerous cardiovascular risk factors will have a superimposing impact on already existing aortic wall abnormalities.

Both reduced elasticity and dilation of the aorta have a detrimental effect on aortic valve function, especially if the aortic valve is already structurally malformed by being bicuspid or quadricuspid.[5,6] As aortic valve opening occurs in concert with root expansion during the beginning of systole, aortic elasticity is crucial for aortic valve dynamics.[5,6] Decreased aortic root elasticity increases leaflet stress and therefore predisposes to aortic valve dysfunction.[5,6] Aortic dilation contributes to aortic valve dysfunction by loss of coaptation of the aortic valve leaflets.[2,5] Moreover, with reduced aortic elasticity, the cushioning "windkessel" effect of the aorta is impaired. This leads to increased systolic blood pressure and pulse pressure,

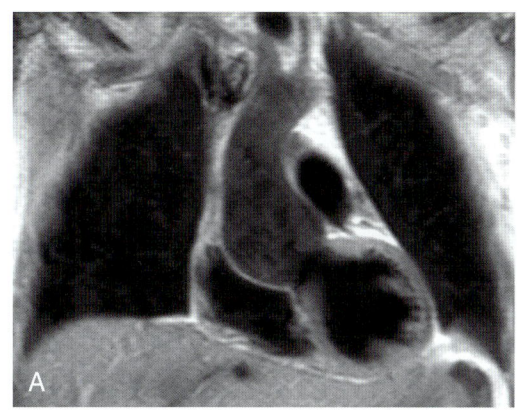

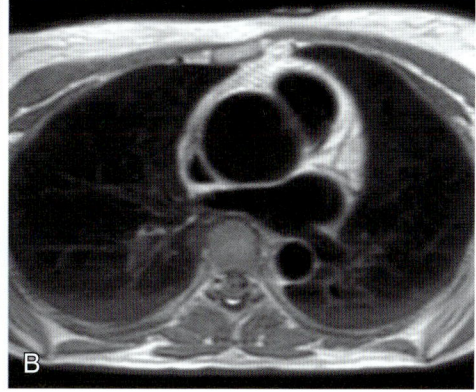

■ FIGURE 40-2 Coronal (A) and axial (B) black blood turbo spin-echo MR images in a 46-year-old woman with Marfan syndrome showing a pear-shaped aortic root (A) with dilation up to 5.1 cm.

(>1 cm/yr), family history of premature aortic dissection (<5 cm), greater than mild aortic regurgitation, and pregnancy or contemplated pregnancy.[11,12] Aortic regurgitation may result from distortion of the coaptation of the aortic valve cusps by the enlarged aortic root and occurs in 15% to 44% of patients.[11] Especially in young children, progression of findings is more important than absolute size of the aorta as a criterion for surgery.[11]

Recent MRI reports indicate that reduced aortic distensibility is an independent predictor of progressive aortic dilation in addition to aortic diameters.[12] Because elastin fragmentation in the aortic media is scattered in an irregular pattern along the aorta, regional distensibility may be sensitive in the detection of regional variations in aortic stiffness.[12] For optimal risk stratification, aortic stiffness may be taken into account in combination with aortic dimensions and the previously mentioned predictors of progressive aortic dilation.[4,12,13] MRI has been recommended for routine assessment of aortic diameters and stiffness in patients with Marfan syndrome as well as for the follow-up of aortic complications, such as intramural hematoma and aortic aneurysms.[4,11,12] Evaluation of aortic dilation should be performed every 6 months to determine the rate of progression, which can be extended to annual evaluation when the aortic size is stable over time.[11] MRI can also be used to adequately monitor the beneficial effect of administration of β blockers on the progression rate of aortic dilation and reduction of aortic complications.[11]

BICUSPID AORTIC VALVE DISEASE

Prevalence and Epidemiology

The bicuspid aortic valve (BAV) is the most common congenital cardiac malformation, occurring in 1% to 2% of the population.[14-16] BAV is the result of abnormal aortic cusp formation due to inadequate production of fibrillin 1 during valvulogenesis.[2,4] Adjacent cusps fuse to form a single aberrant cusp, larger than its counterpart yet smaller than two normal cusps combined.[2] BAV is probably the result of a complex developmental pathologic process rather than simply the fusion of two normal cusps.[2,14,16]

Pathophysiology and Follow-up

Aortic regurgitation is the most frequent (80%) complication in patients with BAV and usually occurs from cusp prolapse, fibrotic retraction, or dilation of the sinotubular junction, in many cases requiring aortic valve replacement.[2,4] BAV is also present in the majority of elderly patients with significant aortic stenosis, reflecting the propensity for premature fibrosis, stiffening, and calcium deposition in these abnormally functioning valves.[2,4] The vascular complications of BAV are less well understood and are associated with significant morbidity and mortality.[2,16] The histology of the ascending aortic wall in patients with BAV shows strong similarities with the fibrillin 1–deficient aortas of patients with Marfan syndrome, with accelerated degeneration of the aortic media due to loss of fibrillin 1 microfibrils as well as focal abnormalities within the aortic media, such as matrix disruption and smooth muscle cell loss (see Fig. 40-1).[1,14] Interestingly, BAV is present in more than 70% of patients with coarctation, and both conditions are by themselves and certainly in combination known to be associated with similar aortic wall abnormalities and concomitant aortic dilation.[1,14]

As a consequence of abnormal aortic wall composition in BAV, serious complications such as progressive aortic root dilation (50% to 60% of all patients with BAV; Fig. 40-3) and aneurysm formation may finally result in aortic dissection (5% of all patients with BAV).[16,17] Despite this lower incidence of aortic dissection than in Marfan syndrome (40%), BAV is the more common etiology in aortic dissection because Marfan syndrome is a much rarer entity (0.01% vs. 1% to 2% of patients with BAV).[2] Two different phenotypes of aortic dilation have been described. Dilation of the mid ascending aorta is most commonly present (70%) and is associated with aortic valve stenosis, suggesting a post-stenotic causative mechanism.[16] Aortic root dilation is much rarer (13%), being determined by male gender and degree of aortic regurgitation.[16] Aortic root replacement is generally more aggressively recommended for patients with BAV (i.e., 4 to 5 cm) than for those patients with a tricuspid aortic valve (i.e., 5 to 6 cm).[2] Subdivision into the two existing phenotypes may further refine the surgical approach by suggesting aortic root sparing when only dilation of the mid ascending aorta is present.[16]

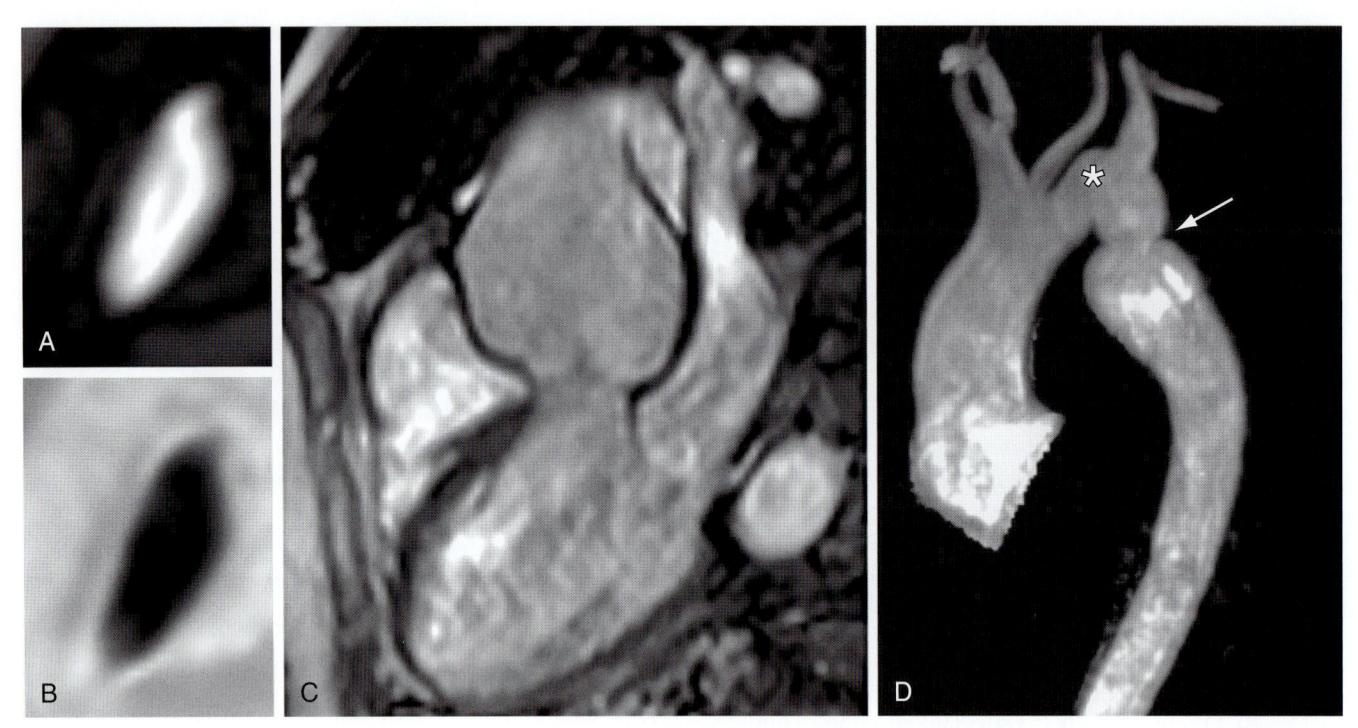

FIGURE 40-3 Phase contrast modulus (**A**) and phase (**B**) images of the bicuspid aortic valve, gradient-echo image of the aortic root (**C**), and gadolinium-chelate–enhanced MR angiography image of the thoracic aorta (**D**) in a 54-year-old woman with Turner syndrome. Note the combination of the slitlike bicuspid aortic valve with slit flow (**A, B**) and post-stenotic dilation that measured 4.6 cm (**C**) together with other aortic disease: aortic kinking (*asterisk*, **D**) and pseudocoarctation (*arrow*, **D**).

An MRI study reported frequent aortic root dilation and reduced elasticity in the entire aorta, suggesting not only that the proximal part of the aorta is affected in BAV but also that aortic wall lesions extend into the entire aorta.[18] Evaluation of the elastic properties of the ascending aorta might be useful to identify patients who are at risk of progressive aortic dilation, analogous to patients with Marfan syndrome.[12,18] Increased aortic stiffness was also associated with LV hypertrophy as a result of increased LV afterload.[18] Sustained LV hypertrophy is associated with reduced diastolic filling; therefore, as diastolic LV dysfunction is a major contributor to congestive heart failure, LV hypertrophy might pose a future risk for LV function in patients with BAV.[18] As many patients with BAV will require cardiac surgery during their lifetime, close monitoring of aortic dimensions, aortic elasticity, aortic valve competence, and LV function is mandatory during follow-up to allow timely intervention.[18]

COARCTATION OF THE AORTA

Prevalence and Epidemiology

Coarctation of the aorta accounts for 5% of all CHD and is defined as a congenital narrowing of the aorta, most commonly in a juxtaductal position just distal to the origin of the left subclavian artery.[19] A wide spectrum of narrowing of the aorta can be observed, from a discrete narrowing to a hypoplastic aortic arch, whether or not it is associated with an intracardiac defect such as a ventricular septal defect or aortic valve disease.[19] Classic symptoms are heart failure and an increased blood pressure proximal to the narrowing as well as a low perfusion status of the body distal to the coarctation.[19] Coarctation of the aorta is associated with a significantly increased cardiovascular morbidity and reduced life expectancy even after successful surgical correction at a young age.[7,12,20-22] Structural aortic wall abnormalities with reduced aortic elastic properties proximal and distal to the site of coarctation imply that coarctation of the aorta is a systemic vascular disease.[4,20] Neonates with coarctation were found to have reduced elastic properties of the aorta before and after successful operation, suggesting a primary defect.[22] Concomitant presence of BAV in 20% to 85% of patients with coarctation and the strong histologic similarity of aortic wall abnormalities between both entities are also suggestive of an inherited origin of aortic wall disease.[1,14,17]

Pathophysiology and Follow-up

After initially successful surgical repair, complications may occur, such as persistence of hypertension, recoarctation, aortic dilation, and aneurysm formation (Fig. 40-4).[20] Persistent resting hypertension and exercise-induced hypertension have been reported in 10% to 46% and 30% to 60%, respectively, being the most important postoperative cardiovascular events.[7,12] Hypertension in coarctation is accompanied by an increase in aortic medial collagen and a decrease in smooth muscle (increased stiffness) that may persist after successful repair and coincides with aortic abnormalities of a coexisting BAV.[1,4] In addition, late hypertension may be caused by functional recoarctation at the site of surgical repair due to decreased disten-

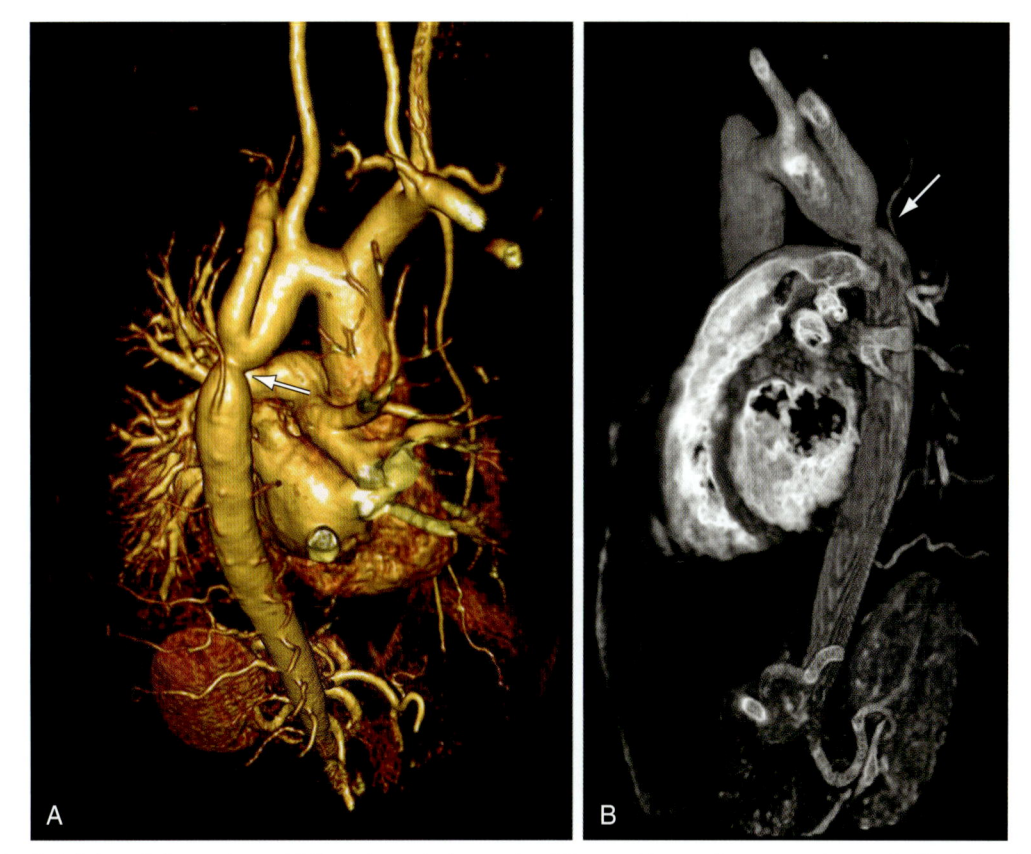

■ **FIGURE 40-4** Gadolinium-chelate–enhanced MR angiography images in a 34-year-old man after coarctation repair. Shaded surface full volume rendering display image (**A**) and selected volume rendering display image (**B**). Flow speed was significantly increased at the level of stenosis at residual coarctation or recoarctation (*arrow*, **A, B**). MRI phase contrast flow volume was 7.2 L/min as measured immediately distal from the level of the stenosis and 6.0 L/min measured at the level of the diaphragm. This indicates flow decrease from the proximal to the distal descending thoracic aorta that excludes hemodynamically significant collateral flow. Note the relative normal size of the intercostal arteries; no major collaterals were observed at MR angiography.

sibility.[23] Impaired LV function, increased LV mass, and concomitant adverse LV remodeling even in postoperative patients with normal blood pressure can be attributed to the reduced aortic elastic properties that result in increased LV afterload.[24] Furthermore, arterial hypertension and a resting pressure gradient are major contributing factors to early atherosclerotic development and should, therefore, be primary targets for therapy.[20]

Adults after surgical repair of coarctation, especially when it is associated with BAV, should be closely monitored for detection of recoarctation as well as for progressive aortic dilation.[20] Risk factors for these long-term aortic complications are the presence of BAV, advanced age, and hypertension.[4] Systematic MRI screening performed at 2- to 5-year intervals has been found to be the most "cost-effective" approach for the follow-up of patients after coarctation repair, with early detection of aortic complications such as recoarctation.[4,25] Spin-echo MRI is essential to detect abnormalities of the aortic wall and associated intracardiac abnormalities; contrast-enhanced three-dimensional MR angiography provides a highly accurate view of the entire reconstructed aorta, and this may obviate the need for invasive x-ray angiography by catheterization for planning of treatment (see Fig. 40-4).[21] A combination of anatomic and flow data obtained by MRI is able to predict a catheterization peak-to-peak gradient of 20 mm Hg or more, considered to be the reference standard for hemodynamic severity of recoarctation.[21] The combination of narrowest aortic cross-sectional area and heart rate–corrected mean flow deceleration in the descending aorta distinguishes between those who have transcatheter pressure gradients above and below 20 mm Hg, which can be used to determine the need for intervention.[21] Velocity-encoded MRI is also useful to determine presence and hemodynamics of collateral vessels, which maintain distal aortic perfusion, depending on the severity of the aortic obstruction.[26] Finally, promising utilities are MRI-guided balloon angioplasty and MRI-guided deployment of stents to repair aortic coarctation; studies have indicated that the combined use of MRI and x-ray imaging is effective for relief of stenosis with a significant reduction of radiation exposure.[27]

TETRALOGY OF FALLOT

Prevalence and Epidemiology

Tetralogy of Fallot (TOF) is the most commonly encountered cyanotic CHD entity with a frequency of nearly 10% of all CHD patients.[28] Anterior displacement of the outflow septum is the primary defect, resulting in a ventricular septal defect, overriding of the aorta, right ventricular outflow tract obstruction, and right ventricular hypertrophy.[28] Patients frequently encounter long-standing

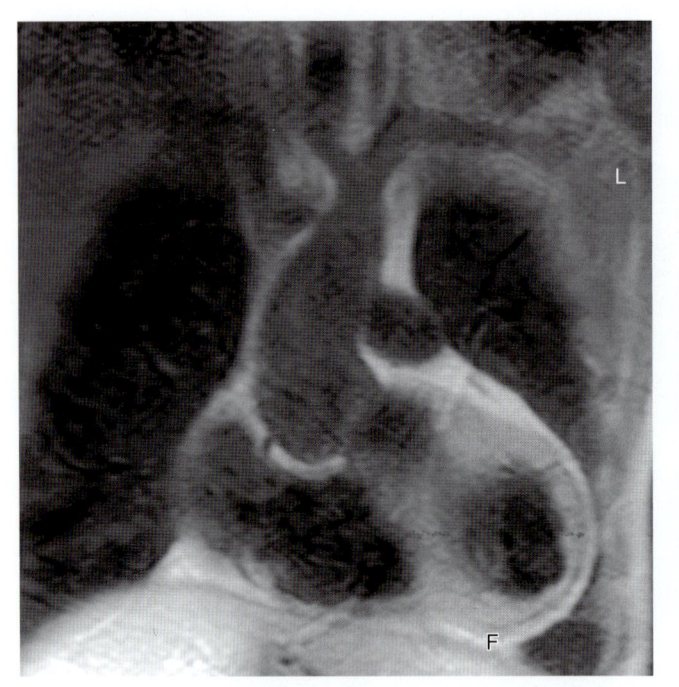

FIGURE 40-5 Coronal black blood turbo spin-echo MR image of the ascending aorta in a 16-year-old boy with tetralogy of Fallot showing a dilated ascending aorta with a maximum diameter of 4.0 cm. The patient had no aortic valve regurgitation.

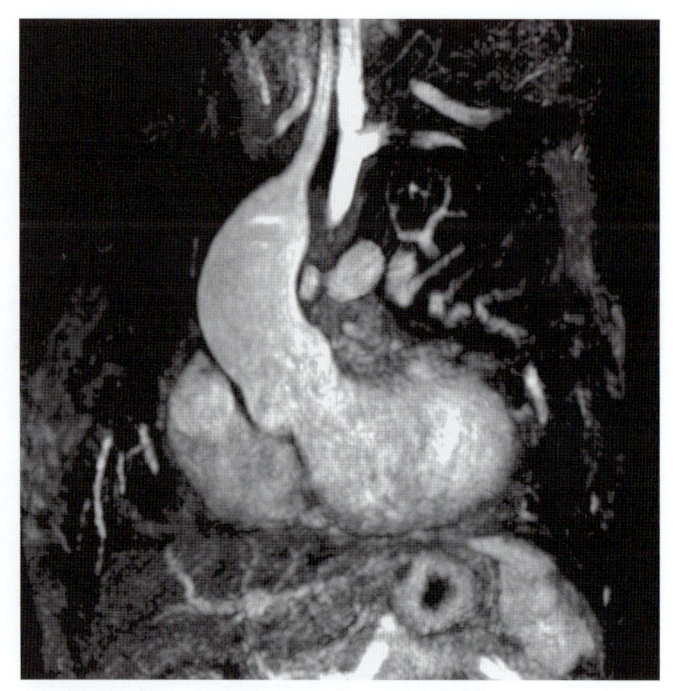

FIGURE 40-6 Coronal gadolinium-chelate–enhanced maximum intensity projection MR angiography image in a 36-year-old man with tetralogy of Fallot after previous repair. The aortic root and ascending aorta are dilated (aortic root, 4.8 cm; ascending aorta, 4.4 cm). The patient has slight aortic regurgitation (9%) and moderate biventricular function.

pulmonary regurgitation and associated impaired right ventricular function after primary TOF repair.[28]

Pathophysiology and Follow-up

Progressive dilation of the aortic root during long-term follow-up has also frequently been described after TOF repair, ranging in incidence between 15% and 88%, depending on definition of aortic root dilation (Figs. 40-5 and 40-6).[28-31] Two hypotheses have been postulated to explain this observation. First, increased blood flow from both ventricles to the overriding aorta before surgical repair is thought to be an underlying pathogenic mechanism, posing increased stress on the aortic wall.[1,28,30,31] This premise is supported by risk factors such as longer shunt-to-repair interval and a higher prevalence of pulmonary atresia among patients with TOF and aortic root dilation.[30,31] Second, histologic changes of the aortic media, such as noninflammatory loss of smooth muscle cells and fragmentation of the elastic fibers, resembling those observed in patients with Marfan syndrome and BAV, have been reported.[1,28]

The potential for complications of aortic root dilation that may necessitate surgical intervention is increasingly recognized in patients after TOF repair.[29] A study reported the progressive nature of aortic dilation in patients with TOF; aortic dilation increased at a rate of 1.7 mm/yr, in contrast to 0.03 mm/yr in healthy controls.[31] Also, more marked histologic changes were observed with increasing age, suggesting that aging coupled with volume overloading on top of intrinsic aortic wall abnormalities has an additional adverse effect on the aortic histology and thus on aortic dilation.[28] In addition, aortic regurgitation associated with progressive dilation of the aortic root is frequently present, and 15% to 18% of patients after TOF repair show mild degrees of aortic regurgitation (see Fig. 40-6).[31] Recent case reports of aortic dissection late after TOF repair in adults whose aortic roots exceeded 6 cm in diameter indicate that close monitoring of aortic dimensions is mandatory, especially when the ascending aorta is dilated.[32] Aortic root surgery may be considered for patients after TOF repair in case of progressive aortic regurgitation and aortic root dilation exceeding 5.5 cm, particularly when the primary indication for surgery is pulmonary valve replacement, and both procedures may be combined.[33] At present, there is no consensus on the administration of β blockers for prevention of progressive aortic root dilation or at what stage aortic root surgery should be considered in patients after TOF repair.[31]

TRANSPOSITION OF THE GREAT ARTERIES

Prevalence and Epidemiology

Transposition of the great arteries is defined as atrial situs solitus, normal (concordant) connection between atria and ventricles, and abnormal (discordant) ventriculoarterial connections.[34] The aorta arises from the right ventricle and the pulmonary artery arises from the left ventricle. It accounts for 4.5% of all congenital cardiac malformations.[34] The arterial switch operation (ASO) has become the preferred method of surgery for transposition of the great arteries.[35] Although this technique has significantly reduced the number of sequelae associated with surgical correction of transposition of the great arteries, comple-

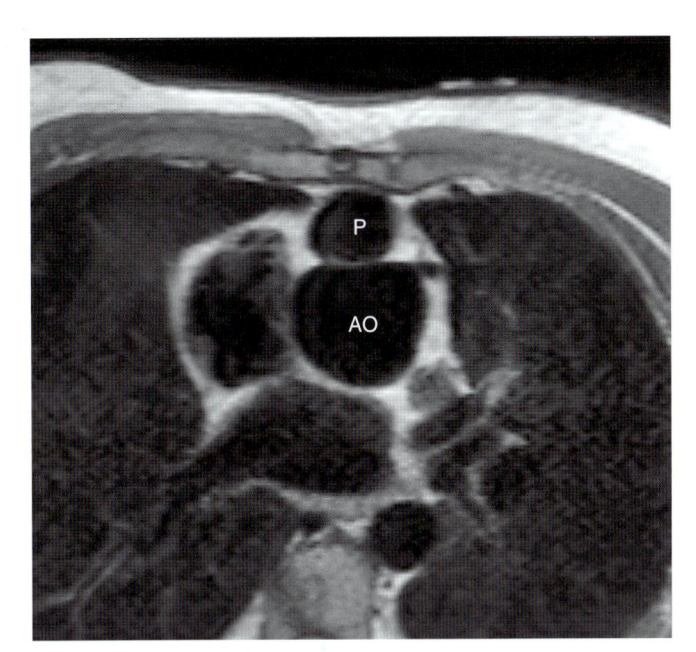

FIGURE 40-7 Oblique transverse black blood turbo spin-echo MR image of the ascending aorta in a 19-year-old man after the arterial switch operation with Lecompte maneuver. The dilated aortic root (AO) has a maximum diameter of 4.6 cm. Note the origin of the main coronary artery and the anterior position of the pulmonary artery (P) to the aorta.

TABLE 40-1 Cardiovascular Magnetic Resonance Scan Protocol

No.	Sequence Type	Scan Duration (minutes)
1	Scout images single-phase SSFP	1
2	Parallel imaging reference scan	1
3	Two-chamber LV multiphase SSFP (BH)	1
4	Four-chamber multiphase SSFP (BH)	1
5	Axial black blood TSE (BHs)	5-10
6	Oblique sagittal black blood along the aorta TSE (BHs)	5-10
7	Multislice, multiphase short-axis SSFP (BHs)	6
8	Oblique sagittal single-slice scout of the aorta for PWV (BH)	1
9	Flow mapping in ascending aorta and proximal descending aorta for PWV (FB)	4
10	Flow mapping in descending aorta for PWV (FB)	4
11	Flow mapping in descending aorta at level of diaphragm (FB), optional	4
12	Two sets of scout cine images of the aortic root (orthogonal) SSFP (BHs)	2
13	Minimal and maximal lumen area measurements at sinotubular junction SSFP (BHs)	4
14	Timing MRA aorta	4
15	MRA aorta (FB)	7
	Total scan duration time	50-60 minutes

BH, breath-hold; FB, free breathing; MRA, magnetic resonance angiography; PWV, pulse wave velocity; SSFP, steady-state free precession sequence; TSE, turbo spin-echo.

tion of the ASO may still predispose patients to aortic root dilation and aortic regurgitation.[35-37]

Pathophysiology and Follow-up

Intrinsic aortic wall disease has been reported in transposition of the great arteries due to abnormal aorticopulmonary septation, damage to the vasa vasorum, and surgical manipulations during the ASO, predisposing to aortic dilation, aneurysm formation, and even aortic dissection (Fig. 40-7).[35,38,39] In addition, aortic distensibility may be reduced by impaired aortic elastogenesis as well as by scar formation at the site of anastomosis.[35] High-grade medial abnormalities in the ascending aorta have already been observed during the neonatal period, suggesting that they are inherited analogous to prototypical extremes, such as in patients with Marfan syndrome or BAV.[1,35] Others concluded that aortic wall abnormalities develop because of structural differences in wall composition between the two great arteries; the former pulmonary arterial wall is exposed to higher systemic pressures after the ASO, posing increased stress on the neoaortic wall, which may ultimately lead to changes in structure and function of the neoaortic root.[39,40] Whether medial abnormalities are inherent or acquired remains therefore difficult to distinguish.[1]

A high incidence of aortic regurgitation has been reported after ASO (30% at 6 years after ASO) and is probably the result of a multifactorial process for which aortic root geometry, surgical techniques, and preoperative size discrepancy between the two great arteries are involved.[36,41] In addition, aortic regurgitation appears to be functionally correlated with aortic root dilation and reduced elasticity of the proximal aorta.[37] Whether the previous existence of a ventricular septal defect plays an additional role remains controversial, although its hemodynamic effect might contribute to a size discrepancy between the aorta and pulmonary artery.[35]

An MRI report described not only frequent aortic root dilation and aortic regurgitation but also a cascade of events ultimately leading to LV systolic dysfunction in patients after ASO.[37] Frequent aortic root dilation and reduced proximal aortic wall elasticity were associated with degree of aortic regurgitation. Aortic regurgitation subsequently led to increased LV dimensions, which consequently resulted in decreased LV ejection fraction. Therefore, LV systolic dysfunction as the endpoint in a sequence of events poses a prognostic risk for patients after ASO.[37] Further elucidation of the underlying pathogenic substrate of aortic wall abnormalities and its clinical repercussions for patients after ASO is required, however, because ASO is still a relatively new surgical procedure for patients with transposition of the great arteries.[37]

IMAGING TECHNIQUE AND FINDINGS

Magnetic Resonance Imaging of the Aorta: Techniques and Protocol

An overview of a typical imaging protocol is listed in Table 40-1. The focus of the protocol is on depiction of aortic dimensions and the vessel wall and assessment of aortic elasticity, aortic valve competence, and systolic LV function.

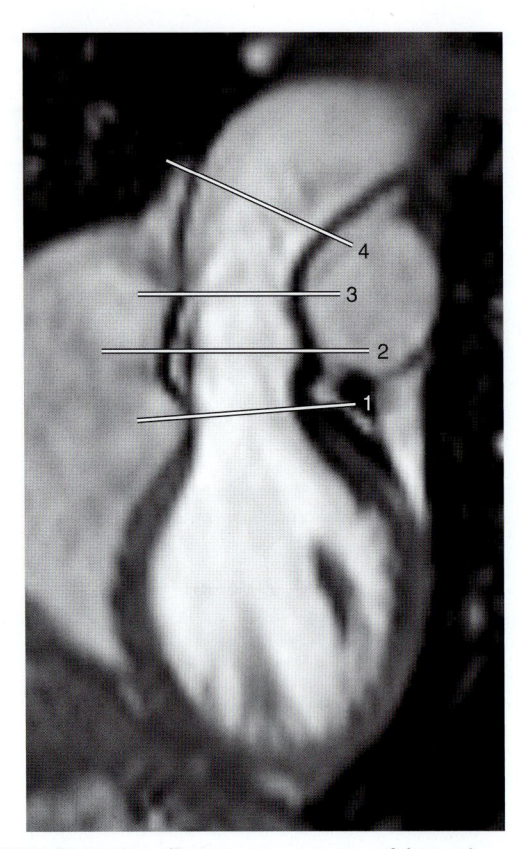

FIGURE 40-8 Four diameter measurements of the aortic root, by a steady-state free precession cine sequence, can be performed at the levels of the annulus of the aortic valve (1), the sinus of Valsalva (2), the sinotubular junction (3), and the ascending aorta at the crossing of the right pulmonary artery (4).

ness, which is represented by locally reduced aortic distensibility and increased regional pulse wave velocity.[45-48] Distensibility (mm Hg^{-1}) of the aortic root can be measured at the level of the sinotubular junction, for which two separate images are acquired for the maximal and minimal aortic lumen area, measured at the peak of aortic systolic flow and before the systolic flow curve (coinciding with the isovolumetric contraction phase), respectively (Fig. 40-9).[47] Pulse wave velocity can be measured for the aortic arch and the descending aorta,[45,46] for which velocity-encoded MRI is applied at the levels of the ascending aorta and proximal descending aorta and just above the bifurcation of the abdominal aorta (Fig. 40-10).[45,46] The addition of velocity-encoded MRI at the level of the diaphragm can be used to quantify collateral flow often present in patients with coarctation.[49]

Aortic Valve and Left Ventricular Function

Quantification of aortic flow with velocity-encoded MRI allows accurate calculation of aortic valve regurgitation fraction (as percentage from aortic forward flow).[47] Velocity-encoded MRI allows peak flow velocity assessment across stenotic lesions, such as aortic valve stenosis and coarctation, and thus an estimate of peak gradients by the simplified Bernoulli equation.[43] Systolic LV function can be assessed by a steady-state free precession cine sequence in the short-axis or axial orientation.[50] The end-diastolic volume (EDV) and end-systolic volume (ESV) are calculated after the endocardial contours are manually drawn at end-diastole and end-systole, respectively; epicardial borders may additionally be drawn for determination of LV mass.[50] Ejection fraction is calculated by dividing stroke volume (EDV − ESV) by EDV.

Aortic Anatomy and Dimensions

An axial stack of black blood turbo spin-echo images is acquired to generally outline cardiac and noncardiac anatomy. Aortic root dimensions can be assessed by double oblique transverse images perpendicular to the aorta, at the levels of the annulus of the aortic valve, the sinus of Valsalva, the sinotubular junction, and the ascending aorta at the crossing of the right pulmonary artery (Fig. 40-8). Oblique black blood turbo spin-echo images along the course of the aorta (see Figs. 40-2, 40-5, and 40-7) and contrast-enhanced three-dimensional MR angiography may be used to visualize aortic dimensions and the potentially complex nature of any coarctation lesion (see Figs. 40-3, 40-4, and 40-6) as well as for diagnosis and follow-up of aortic complications, such as aortic dissection, intramural hematoma, and aortic aneurysms.[42-45] Reference values of aortic dimensions are unfortunately scarce, especially for children, making individual follow-up even more valuable for depiction of aortic dilation and rate of progression.[43,46]

Aortic Elasticity

Intrinsic aortic wall abnormalities and progressive atherosclerotic disease are associated with increased aortic stiff-

---

KEY POINTS

- Intrinsic aortic wall abnormalities are present in inherited connective tissue disorders such as Marfan syndrome and bicuspid aortic valve disease, as well as in classic congenital lesions such as coarctation of the aorta, tetralogy of Fallot, and transposition of the great arteries.
- Determination of aortic pulse wave velocity and distensibility with MRI allows accurate assessment of regional and local aortic vessel wall condition, respectively.
- Both reduced elasticity and dilation of the aorta have a detrimental effect on aortic valve function.
- Reduced aortic elasticity gives rise to increased left ventricular afterload and is therefore associated with increased myocardial oxygen demand, impaired coronary perfusion, and the presence of coronary artery disease.

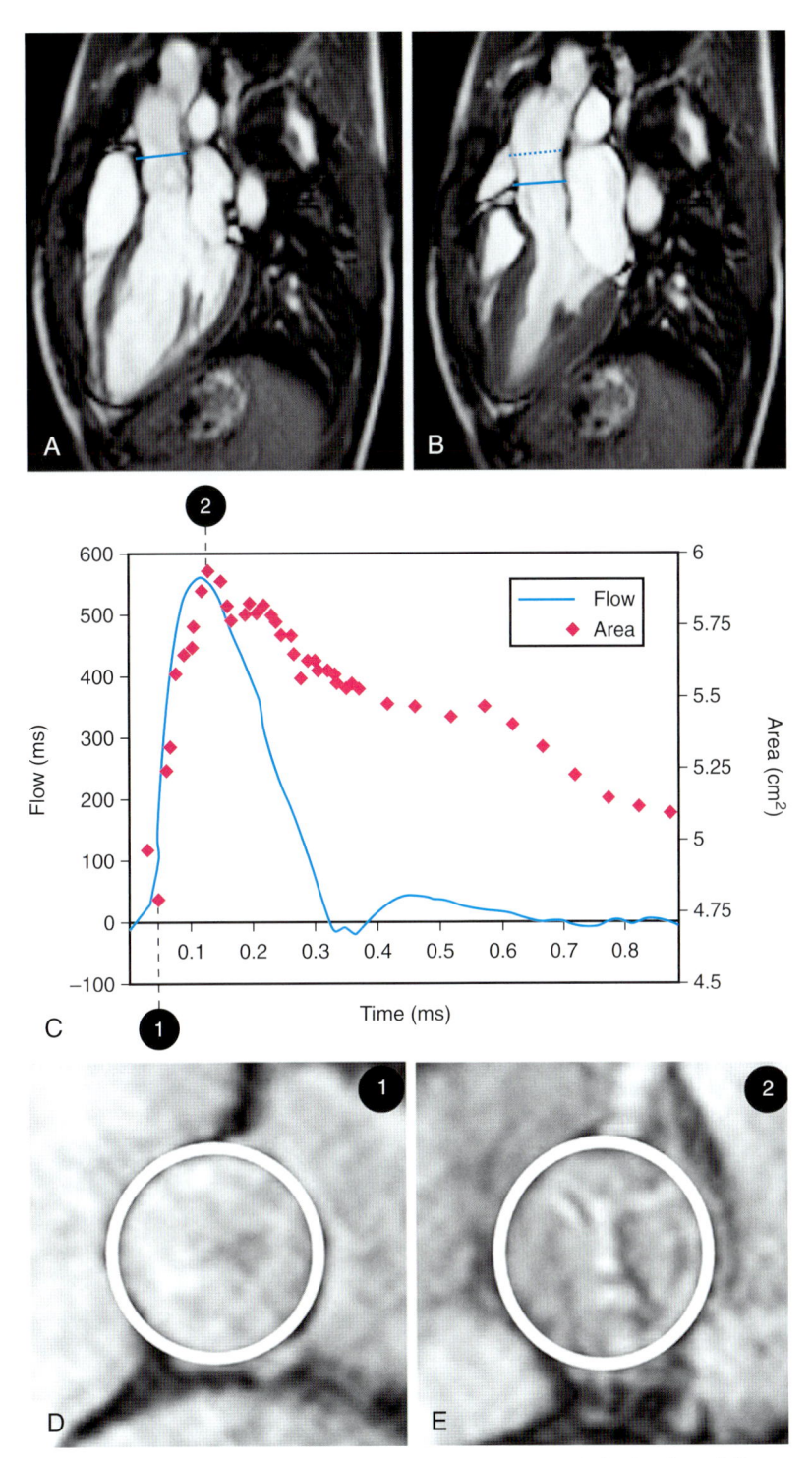

CHAPTER 40 ● *Magnetic Resonance Imaging of the Aorta and Left Ventricular Function*   557

FIGURE 40-9 **A** and **B** show slice positioning at minimal and maximal aortic flow, respectively, for distensibility measurements at the level of the sinotubular junction, thus correcting for through-plane motion of the aortic root during contraction. Note the difference in position of the aortic root in both images due to cardiac motion. Gate delay is 35 ms in **A** and 120 ms in **B**. An aortic flow curve—in a phase contrast study—and the corresponding lumen areas at the level of the sinotubular junction throughout the cardiac cycle of a healthy control are depicted in **C**. The minimal aortic lumen area (to be expected early in the cardiac cycle during the isovolumetric contraction phase) and the maximal aortic lumen area (to be expected when the peak of aortic flow passes through the ascending aorta) of the sinotubular junction are acquired to calculate distensibility (mm Hg^{-1}) by the following formula: $(A_{max} - A_{min})/A_{min} \times (P_{max} - P_{min})$, with A_{max} and A_{min} as maximal and minimal lumen area (mm^2) and P_{max} and P_{min} as systolic and diastolic blood pressure (mm Hg). The gated steady-state free precession images of **D** and **E** show the minimal and maximal aortic lumen areas, respectively.

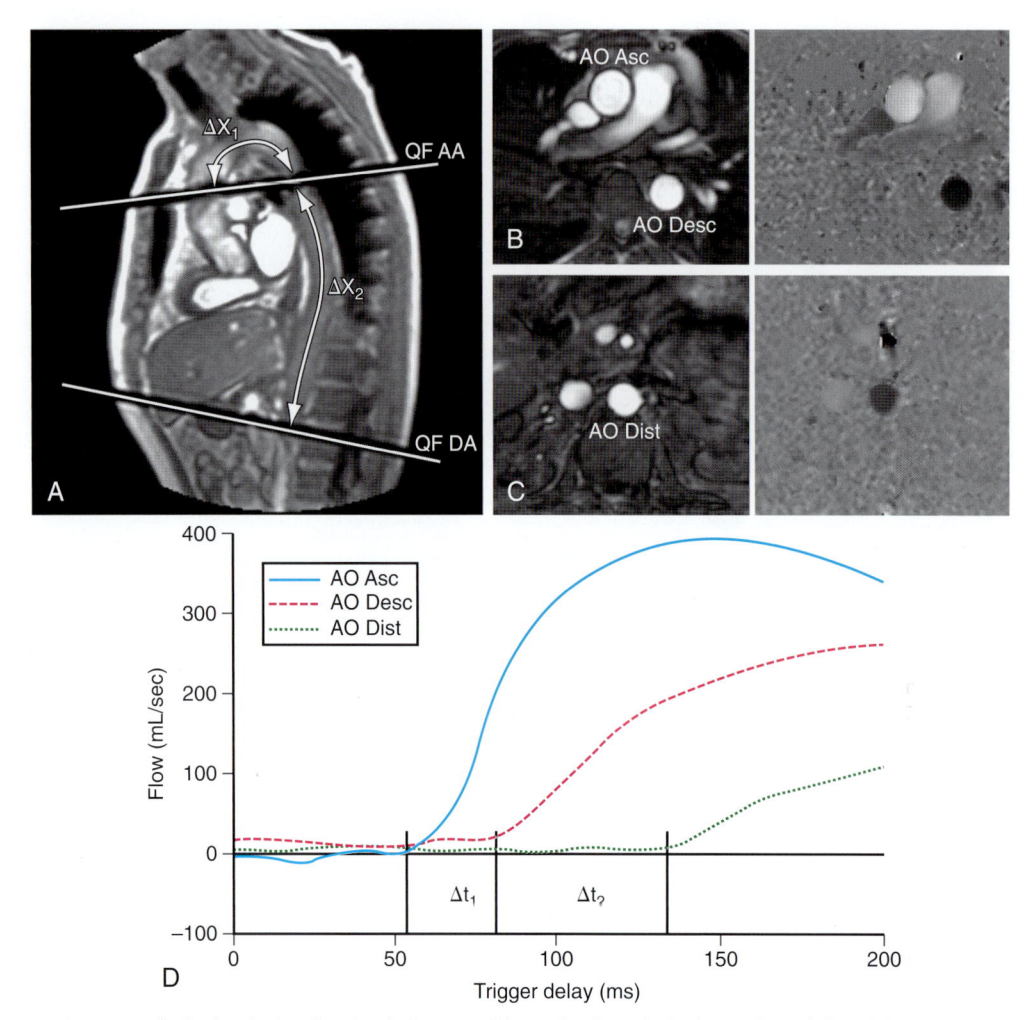

FIGURE 40-10 Pulse wave velocity is calculated as $\Delta X/\Delta t$ (expressed in m/s), where ΔX is the aortic path length between two imaging levels (ΔX_1 and ΔX_2) and Δt is the transit time between the arrival time of the aortic pulse wave (defined as the foot of the systolic upslope) in the flow graphs at these levels (Δt_1 and Δt_2). Sites for velocity-encoded MRI measurements are the ascending aorta and the proximal descending aorta in a single acquisition (**A, QF AA**) and the distal aorta above the aortic bifurcation (**A, QF DA**, distal aortic plane). On the corresponding velocity-encoded MR images, the arrival time of the aortic systolic pulse wave can be determined by measuring the through-plane flow (**B, C**). Arrival and transit times are determined in **D**.

SUGGESTED READINGS

Fedak PW, David TE, Borger M, et al. Bicuspid aortic valve disease: recent insights in pathophysiology and treatment. Expert Rev Cardiovasc Ther 2005; 3:295-308.

Milewicz DM, Dietz HC, Miller DC. Treatment of aortic disease in patients with Marfan syndrome. Circulation 2005; 111:e150-e157.

Niwa K, Perloff JK, Bhuta SM, et al. Structural abnormalities of great arterial walls in congenital heart disease: light and electron microscopic analyses. Circulation 2001; 103:393-400.

Nollen GJ, Mulder BJ. What is new in the Marfan syndrome? Int J Cardiol 2004; 97(Suppl 1):103-108.

Pemberton J, Sahn DJ. Imaging of the aorta. Int J Cardiol 2004; 97(Suppl 1):53-60.

Rosenthal E. Coarctation of the aorta from fetus to adult: curable condition or lifelong disease process? Heart 2005; 91:1495-1502.

Tan JL, Gatzoulis MA, Ho SY. Aortic root disease in tetralogy of Fallot. Curr Opin Cardiol 2006; 21:569-572.

Therrien J, Thorne SA, Wright A, et al. Repaired coarctation: a "cost-effective" approach to identify complications in adults. J Am Coll Cardiol 2000; 35:997-1002.

Ward C. Clinical significance of the bicuspid aortic valve. Heart 2000; 83:81-85.

Warnes CA. Transposition of the great arteries. Circulation 2006; 114:2699-2709.

REFERENCES

1. Niwa K, Perloff JK, Bhuta SM, et al. Structural abnormalities of great arterial walls in congenital heart disease: light and electron microscopic analyses. Circulation 2001; 103:393-400.
2. Fedak PW, Verma S, David TE, et al. Clinical and pathophysiological implications of a bicuspid aortic valve. Circulation 2002; 106:900-904.

3. Schlatmann TJ, Becker AE. Histologic changes in the normal aging aorta: implications for dissecting aortic aneurysm. Am J Cardiol 1977; 39:13-20.
4. Pemberton J, Sahn DJ. Imaging of the aorta. Int J Cardiol 2004; 97(Suppl 1):53-60.
5. Grotenhuis HB, Westenberg JJ, Doornbos J, et al. Aortic root dysfunctioning and its effect on left ventricular function in Ross procedure patients assessed with magnetic resonance imaging. Am Heart J 2006; 152:975-978.
6. Schmidtke C, Bechtel J, Hueppe M, et al. Size and distensibility of the aortic root and aortic valve function after different techniques of the Ross procedure. J Thorac Cardiovasc Surg 2000; 119:990-997.
7. Kim GB, Kang SJ, Bae EJ, et al. Elastic properties of the ascending aorta in young children after successful coarctoplasty in infancy. Int J Cardiol 2004; 97:471-477.
8. Arnett DK, Evans GW, Riley WA. Arterial stiffness: a new cardiovascular risk factor? Am J Epidemiol 1994; 140:669-682.
9. Mohrs OK, Petersen SE, Voigtlaender T, et al. Time-resolved contrast-enhanced MR angiography of the thorax in adults with congenital heart disease. AJR Am J Roentgenol 2006; 187:1107-1114.
10. van der Geest RJ, Reiber JH. Quantification in cardiac MRI. J Magn Reson Imaging 1999; 10:602-608.
11. Milewicz DM, Dietz HC, Miller DC. Treatment of aortic disease in patients with Marfan syndrome. Circulation 2005; 111:e150-e157.
12. Nollen GJ, Groenink M, Tijssen JG, et al. Aortic stiffness and diameter predict progressive aortic dilatation in patients with Marfan syndrome. Eur Heart J 2004; 25:1146-1152.
13. Nollen GJ, Mulder BJ. What is new in the Marfan syndrome? Int J Cardiol 2004; 97(Suppl 1):103-108.
14. Fedak PW, David TE, Borger M, et al. Bicuspid aortic valve disease: recent insights in pathophysiology and treatment. Expert Rev Cardiovasc Ther 2005; 3:295-308.
15. Warren AE, Boyd ML, O'Connell C, Dodds L. Dilation of the ascending aorta in pediatric patients with bicuspid aortic valve: frequency, rate of progression and risk factors. Heart 2006; 92:1496-1500.
16. Della CA, Bancone C, Quarto C, et al. Predictors of ascending aortic dilatation with bicuspid aortic valve: a wide spectrum of disease expression. Eur J Cardiothorac Surg 2007; 31:397-404.
17. Ward C. Clinical significance of the bicuspid aortic valve. Heart 2000; 83:81-85.
18. Grotenhuis HB, Ottenkamp J, Westenberg JJ, et al. Reduced aortic elasticity and dilatation are associated with aortic regurgitation and left ventricular hypertrophy in nonstenotic bicuspid aortic valve patients. J Am Coll Cardiol 2007; 49:1660-1665.
19. Rosenthal E. Coarctation of the aorta from fetus to adult: curable condition or lifelong disease process? Heart 2005; 91:1495-1502.
20. Meyer AA, Joharchi MS, Kundt G, et al. Predicting the risk of early atherosclerotic disease development in children after repair of aortic coarctation. Eur Heart J 2005; 26:617-622.
21. Nielsen JC, Powell AJ, Gauvreau K, et al. Magnetic resonance imaging predictors of coarctation severity. Circulation 2005; 111:622-628.
22. Vogt M, Kuhn A, Baumgartner D, et al. Impaired elastic properties of the ascending aorta in newborns before and early after successful coarctation repair: proof of a systemic vascular disease of the prestenotic arteries? Circulation 2005; 111:3269-3273.
23. Ong CM, Canter CE, Gutierrez FR, et al. Increased stiffness and persistent narrowing of the aorta after successful repair of coarctation of the aorta: relationship to left ventricular mass and blood pressure at rest and with exercise. Am Heart J 1992; 123:1594-1600.
24. Krogmann ON, Rammos S, Jakob M, et al. Left ventricular diastolic dysfunction late after coarctation repair in childhood: influence of left ventricular hypertrophy. J Am Coll Cardiol 1993; 21:1454-1460.
25. Therrien J, Thorne SA, Wright A, et al. Repaired coarctation: a "cost-effective" approach to identify complications in adults. J Am Coll Cardiol 2000; 35:997-1002.
26. Araoz PA, Reddy GP, Tarnoff H, et al. MR findings of collateral circulation are more accurate measures of hemodynamic significance than arm-leg blood pressure gradient after repair of coarctation of the aorta. J Magn Reson Imaging 2003; 17:177-183.
27. Krueger JJ, Ewert P, Yilmaz S, et al. Magnetic resonance imaging–guided balloon angioplasty of coarctation of the aorta: a pilot study. Circulation 2006; 113:1093-1100.
28. Tan JL, Davlouros PA, McCarthy KP, et al. Intrinsic histological abnormalities of aortic root and ascending aorta in tetralogy of Fallot: evidence of causative mechanism for aortic dilatation and aortopathy. Circulation 2005; 112:961-968.
29. Cheung YF, Ou X, Wong SJ. Central and peripheral arterial stiffness in patients after surgical repair of tetralogy of Fallot: implications for aortic root dilatation. Heart 2006; 92:1827-1830.
30. Niwa K. Aortic root dilatation in tetralogy of Fallot long-term after repair—histology of the aorta in tetralogy of Fallot: evidence of intrinsic aortopathy. Int J Cardiol 2005; 103:117-119.
31. Niwa K, Siu SC, Webb GD, Gatzoulis MA. Progressive aortic root dilatation in adults late after repair of tetralogy of Fallot. Circulation 2002; 106:1374-1378.
32. Rathi VK, Doyle M, Williams RB, et al. Massive aortic aneurysm and dissection in repaired tetralogy of Fallot; diagnosis by cardiovascular magnetic resonance imaging. Int J Cardiol 2005; 101:169-170.
33. Therrien J, Gatzoulis M, Graham T, et al. Canadian Cardiovascular Society Consensus Conference 2001 update: Recommendations for the Management of Adults with Congenital Heart Disease—Part II. Can J Cardiol 2001; 17:1029-1050.
34. Warnes CA. Transposition of the great arteries. Circulation 2006; 114:2699-2709.
35. Hwang HY, Kim WH, Kwak JG, et al. Mid-term follow-up of neoaortic regurgitation after the arterial switch operation for transposition of the great arteries. Eur J Cardiothorac Surg 2006; 29:162-167.
36. Formigari R, Toscano A, Giardini A, et al. Prevalence and predictors of neoaortic regurgitation after arterial switch operation for transposition of the great arteries. J Thorac Cardiovasc Surg 2003; 126:1753-1759.
37. Grotenhuis HB, Ottenkamp J, Fontein D, et al. Aortic elasticity and left ventricular function after arterial switch operation: MR imaging—initial experience. Radiology 2008; 249:801-809.
38. Murakami T, Nakazawa M, Momma K, Imai Y. Impaired distensibility of neoaorta after arterial switch procedure. Ann Thorac Surg 2000; 70:1907-1910.
39. Hourihan M, Colan SD, Wernovsky G, et al. Growth of the aortic anastomosis, annulus, and root after the arterial switch procedure performed in infancy. Circulation 1993; 88:615-620.
40. Schoof PH, Gittenberger-de Groot AC, de Heer E, et al. Remodeling of the porcine pulmonary autograft wall in the aortic position. J Thorac Cardiovasc Surg 2000; 120:55-65.
41. Haas F, Wottke M, Poppert H, Meisner H. Long-term survival and functional follow-up in patients after the arterial switch operation. Ann Thorac Surg 1999; 68:1692-1697.
42. Mohrs OK, Petersen SE, Voigtlaender T, et al. Time-resolved contrast-enhanced MR angiography of the thorax in adults with congenital heart disease. AJR Am J Roentgenol 2006; 187:1107-1114.
43. Pemberton J, Sahn DJ. Imaging of the aorta. Int J Cardiol 2004; 97(Suppl 1):53-60.
44. Milewicz DM, Dietz HC, Miller DC. Treatment of aortic disease in patients with Marfan syndrome. Circulation 2005; 111:e150-e157.
45. Nollen GJ, Groenink M, Tijssen JG, et al. Aortic stiffness and diameter predict progressive aortic dilatation in patients with Marfan syndrome. Eur Heart J 2004; 25:1146-1152.
46. Grotenhuis HB, Ottenkamp J, Westenberg JJ, et al. Reduced aortic elasticity and dilatation are associated with aortic regurgitation and left ventricular hypertrophy in nonstenotic bicuspid aortic valve patients. J Am Coll Cardiol 2007; 49:1660-1665.
47. Grotenhuis HB, Westenberg JJ, Doornbos J, et al. Aortic root dysfunctioning and its effect on left ventricular function in Ross procedure patients assessed with magnetic resonance imaging. Am Heart J 2006; 152:975-978.
48. Arnett DK, Evans GW, Riley WA. Arterial stiffness: a new cardiovascular risk factor? Am J Epidemiol 1994; 140:669-682.
49. Araoz PA, Reddy GP, Tarnoff H, et al. MR findings of collateral circulation are more accurate measures of hemodynamic significance than arm-leg blood pressure gradient after repair of coarctation of the aorta. J Magn Reson Imaging 2003; 17:177-183.
50. van der Geest RJ, Reiber JH. Quantification in cardiac MRI. J Magn Reson Imaging 1999; 10:602-608.

SECTION ONE

Acyanotic Heart Disease with Increased Vascularity

CHAPTER 41

Atrial Septal Defect

Amgad N. Makaryus and Lawrence M. Boxt

Atrial septal defect (ASD) is one of the most commonly recognized congenital cardiac anomalies in adults. Knowledge of the embryologic development of the atrial septum provides the basis for understanding the pathophysiology, anatomy, and clinical manifestations of ASD. ASD is rarely diagnosed in infancy, and it even less commonly results in significant symptoms in infants. Patients, especially patients with small or isolated defects, are usually asymptomatic through the first 3 decades of life, although more than 70% become impaired by the fifth decade. Early surgical closure of most types of ASD is recommended.[1]

DEFINITION

An ASD is characterized by a defect in the interatrial septum that allows pulmonary venous return to pass from the left to the right atrium (i.e., left-to-right shunt), resulting in right atrial and right ventricular chamber dilation. There are four types of ASD. The first type is an ostium secundum defect. This type of defect is located in the area of the fossa ovalis and is the most common type of ASD, accounting for 75% of all cases. Although it usually consists of a single defect, fenestrated defects have also been reported. Secundum ASD can be associated with partial anomalous pulmonary venous return (<10%) and mitral valve prolapse. A second type of ASD is an ostium primum defect, which accounts for 15% of ASDs; this defect is located in the lower part of the interatrial septum and commonly involves other "endocardial cushion" defects. It can be associated with a "cleft" anterior mitral valve leaflet, which results in mitral regurgitation, or defects in the atrioventricular or membranous interventricular septum. The third type of ASD is a sinus venosus defect, which accounts for 10% of ASDs and involves the junction of the superior vena cava with the left atrium. Anomalous right upper lobe pulmonary venous return is a common manifestation with this type of ASD. The last type of ASD is a coronary sinus ASD, which is the rarest type and results from direct communication of the coronary sinus and the left atrium. Persistent left superior vena cava is commonly associated with coronary sinus ASD.[1-4]

PREVALENCE AND EPIDEMIOLOGY

ASD accounts for 10% of all congenital heart disease, and for 22% to 40% of congenital heart disease in adults. ASD is twice as common in girls as in boys. Most ASDs occur sporadically as a result of spontaneous genetic mutations; however, hereditary forms have been reported. Associated extracardiac congenital defects are present in 25% of infants, and about 30% have an ASD in association with a hereditary syndrome, such as Down syndrome, Holt-Oram syndrome, and Noonan syndrome.[2]

ETIOLOGY AND PATHOPHYSIOLOGY

Ostium secundum ASD results from incomplete adhesion between the original ridge of tissue of the valve of the foramen ovale and the septum secundum. The patent foramen ovale usually results from abnormal resorption of the septum primum during the formation of the foramen secundum. Resorption in abnormal locations causes a fenestrated or netlike septum primum. An abnormally large foramen ovale can occur as a result of defective development of the septum secundum. The normal septum primum does not close this type of abnormal foramen ovale at birth. A combination of excessive resorption of the septum primum and a large foramen ovale produces a large ostium secundum ASD.[1,2]

Ostium primum ASD is caused by incomplete fusion of septum primum with the endocardial cushion. The defect lies immediately adjacent to the atrioventricular valves, either of which may be deformed and incompetent. In most cases, only the anterior leaflet of the mitral valve is displaced, and it is commonly cleft. The tricuspid valve is usually not involved. The defect is often large, and a "complete" atrioventricular canal defect may occur with an ASD associated with a ventricular septal defect.[1,2]

Sinus venosus ASD occurs when abnormal fusion between the embryologic sinus venosus and the atrium occurs. These defects generally lie high in the atrial septum near the entry of the superior vena cava, and are generally associated with anomalous right upper pulmonary venous return. An uncommon inferior type is associated with partial anomalous return of the right lower pulmonary vein. Anomalous drainage can be into the right atrium, the superior vena cava, or the inferior vena cava.[1,2]

Coronary sinus ASD is characterized by an unroofed coronary sinus and persistent left superior vena cava that drains into the left atrium. A dilated coronary sinus often suggests this defect. The diagnosis can be made explicitly by MRI, CT, echocardiography, or angiography by injecting contrast agent into the left upper extremity. Coronary sinus opacification, which precedes right atrial opacification, confirms the diagnosis.[1,2]

A small ASD results in trivial shunting and has no hemodynamic consequences. Larger defects are associated with substantial shunting, which may lead to volume overload of the right atrium, right ventricle, and pulmonary arteries. The magnitude of left-to-right shunting depends on the size of the ASD, the relative compliance of the two ventricles, and the pulmonary and systemic vascular resistance. If left untreated, the left-to-right shunting may result in pulmonary hypertension, right ventricular failure, decreased right ventricular compliance, and potentially right-to-left shunting (Eisenmenger syndrome). Eisenmenger syndrome secondary to ASD is rare in adults, however, occurring in about 5% of patients.[1,2]

MANIFESTATIONS OF DISEASE

Clinical Presentation

ASD generally goes unnoticed because patients are usually asymptomatic in the first and second decades of life. The most common manifestations of this condition are development of fatigue, dyspnea on exertion, and exercise intolerance generally during the third and fourth decades. The most common presenting symptom is dyspnea and easy fatigability. Other symptoms include palpitations, syncope, and heart failure. The development of palpitations related to supraventricular arrhythmia is the most common symptom in adults. Occasionally, patients may present with paradoxical embolization or recurrent respiratory infection. If left untreated, patients with hemodynamically significant ASD develop symptoms of right-sided heart failure, including jugular venous distention and lower extremity edema. Over time, pulmonary pressure increases because of increased pulmonary resistance, and the shunt may reverse with predominant right-to-left shunting (Eisenmenger syndrome).[3,4]

The cardiac examination is generally characterized by signs of right heart overload. Cardiac auscultation reveals a normal S_1, fixed splitting of S_2, and a systolic outflow murmur as a result of the increased flow into the main pulmonary artery. Shunting across the ASD does not produce a murmur. In patients with ostium primum ASD and a cleft anterior mitral valve leaflet, a mitral regurgitation murmur can be appreciated at the apex. The development of pulmonary hypertension results in narrowing of the splitting of S_2 and accentuation of the pulmonary closure component. The pulmonic systolic murmur decreases in intensity, and a diastolic pulmonic regurgitation murmur may appear. The development of Eisenmenger syndrome results in cyanosis and clubbing.[3,4]

Imaging Indications and Algorithm

Patients with clinical findings suggestive of right heart overload or failure should undergo imaging for the assessment of the presence of atrial level shunts secondary to an ASD. The initial imaging modality generally should be a chest radiograph. Radiography gives certain clues as noted subsequently for the presence or absence of an ASD. The next modality that gives the clinician a great deal of information is ultrasound imaging with transthoracic echocardiography (TTE). Ultrasonography gives anatomic and quantitative information about an ASD. If necessary, a patient may be sent for transesophageal echocardiography (TEE), which can give better anatomic visualization of the less common types of ASD, such as sinus venosus ASD and coronary sinus ASD.

If echocardiography does not provide adequate assessment of the ASD, CT may be performed; however, MRI is better at assessing ASD because it allows for quantitative assessment of shunts and determination of shunt fractions. Less commonly used modalities for the assessment of ASDs are nuclear medicine and angiography, which provide less anatomic information than the abovementioned modalities, but yield quantitative assessment of shunt fractions and hemodynamic pressure measurements in the case of invasive angiography. The algorithm for the work-up generally can be accomplished with echocardiography, but rarely, other imaging modalities, most commonly MRI or angiography, can be applied if discrepancies exist.[5]

Imaging Technique and Findings

Radiography

A plain chest radiograph (Fig. 41-1) is characterized by increased caliber of the main pulmonary artery segment and the hilar and parenchymal pulmonary arteries (i.e., shunt vascularity). Until pulmonary resistance increases, resulting in pulmonary hypertension, the parenchymal vessels extend farther toward the pleura than expected, and appear to taper normally. The pulmonary vessels are sharp. The left-to-right shunt volume loads the right heart, resulting in right atrial and ventricular dilation and clockwise (leftward) cardiac rotation. Increased pulmonary

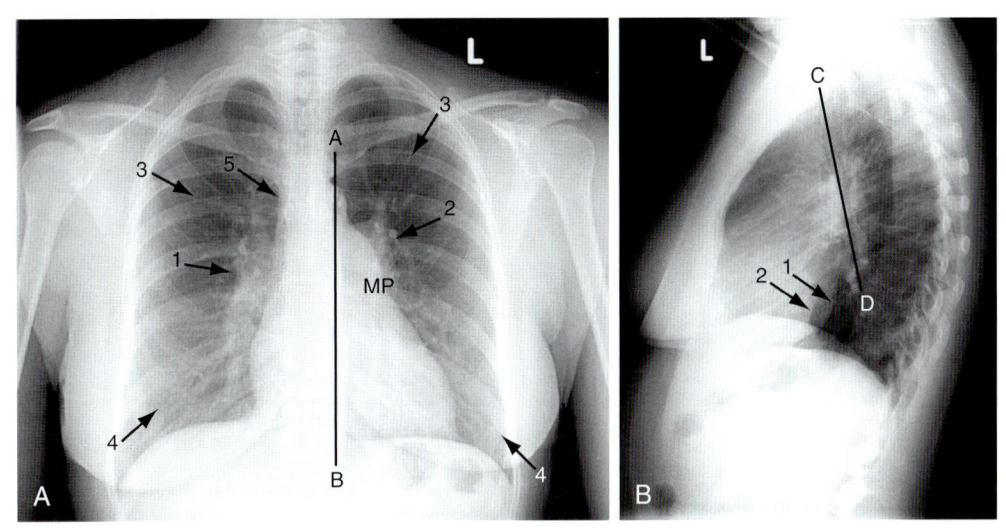

FIGURE 41-1 A 34-year-old woman with occasional shortness of breath. **A,** Posteroanterior radiograph shows shunt vascularity (i.e., enlargement of the main pulmonary artery segment [MP]), the hilar right (*1 arrow*) and left (*2 arrow*) pulmonary arteries, and the upper (*3 arrows*) and lower (*4 arrows*) pulmonary arteries. The vessels are sharp and extend farther toward the pleura than expected. Right heart enlargement causes clockwise (leftward) cardiac rotation, characterized by leftward displacement of the superior vena cava (*5 arrow*), causing narrowing of the superior mediastinum and displacement of the center of the heart (*AB line*) to the left of the midline. **B,** Lateral radiograph shows filling of the retrosternal space by the dilated main pulmonary artery and right heart, and no evidence of left heart enlargement. The left atrium is normal in volume; there is no mass in the superior retrocardiac space, and the tracheal air column (*CD line*) is not displaced. The left ventricle is normal; the posterior left ventricular border (*1 arrow*) does not extend significantly posterior to the inferior vena cava (*2 arrow*).

venous return is decompressed across the defect in the interatrial septum; the left atrium and ventricle are normal in size (Fig. 41-2). The typical chest film of a patient with ASD is shunt vascularity with right heart enlargement and a normal left heart.[4]

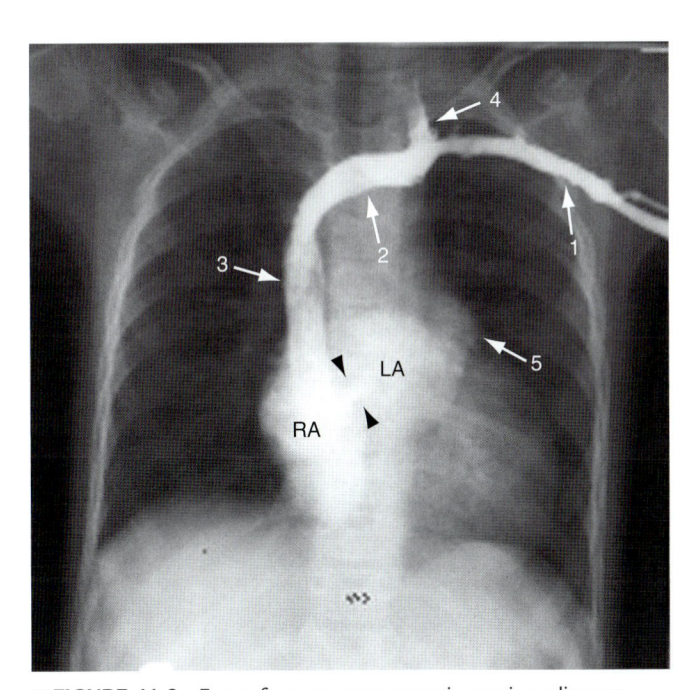

FIGURE 41-2 Frame from an anteroposterior angiocardiogram obtained after contrast injection from the left upper extremity. The left subclavian (*1 arrow*) and left brachiocephalic (*2 arrow*) veins and superior vena cava (*3 arrow*) have been opacified. There is reflux into the left internal jugular vein (*4 arrow*). Before complete opacification of the right heart border forming the right atrium (RA), there is reflux of contrast-enhanced blood across the atrial septum (*arrowheads*) into the left atrium (LA) and left atrial appendage (*5 arrow*).

When pulmonary resistance increases, causing pulmonary hypertension, the appearance of the chest film changes (Fig. 41-3). The central (extrahilar) pulmonary arteries remain enlarged, but the parenchymal pulmonary artery segments become vasoconstricted, producing the typical appearance of acute change of pulmonary artery caliber seen in pulmonary hypertension. Careful evaluation of the peripheral pulmonary artery segments reveals extension toward the pleura beyond that found in a normal examination, but in smaller caliber vessels. As long as the shunt is left-to-right, right heart enlargement and a normal left heart are seen. In the rare circumstance of shunt reversal, progressive right heart decompression and left heart enlargement may be seen.[4,5]

Ultrasonography

Echocardiography (Figs. 41-4 through 41-7) is generally the first-line assessment tool for the evaluation of ASD with TTE being the first method used. Echocardiography findings in the setting of ASD reveal evidence of right ventricular volume overload. TTE is the imaging study of choice for ostium primum or secundum ASD. Identification of a sinus venosus ASD usually requires TEE (see Fig. 41-6). Evaluation of the location, size, and direction of shunt can be performed by use of color flow Doppler and echocardiographic contrast agents. Important information such as estimated pulmonary artery pressure and the pressure of additional cardiac chambers can also be obtained. Accurate assessment of pulmonary-to-systemic flow (Qp/Qs) ratio can be obtained and corresponds to the shunt fraction. A Qp/Qs ratio of generally 1.5 to 2 indicates a significant left-to-right shunt. A patent foramen ovale generally does not cause a significant shunt, and Qp/Qs is generally around 1 to 1.05.[6]

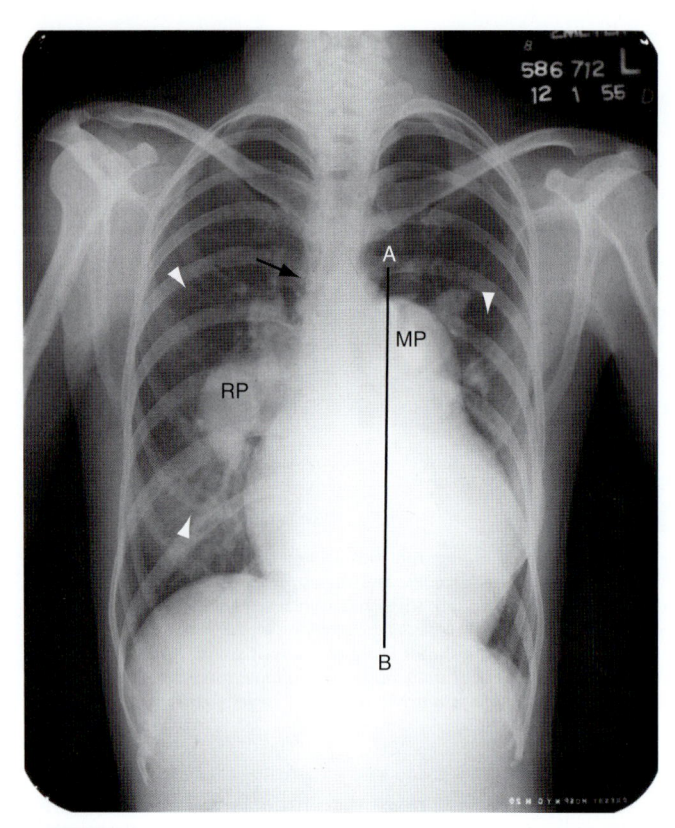

FIGURE 41-3 A 58-year-old woman with persistent shortness of breath. The main (MP) and hilar right (RP) pulmonary arteries are markedly dilated. Right heart enlargement is indicated by the narrow superior mediastinum (*arrow*) and the leftward rotation of the heart (*AB line*). The dilated left pulmonary artery is obscured by the rotated heart. The acute change in caliber of the pulmonary arteries from hilar to parenchymal branches (*arrowheads*) indicates pulmonary artery hypertension.

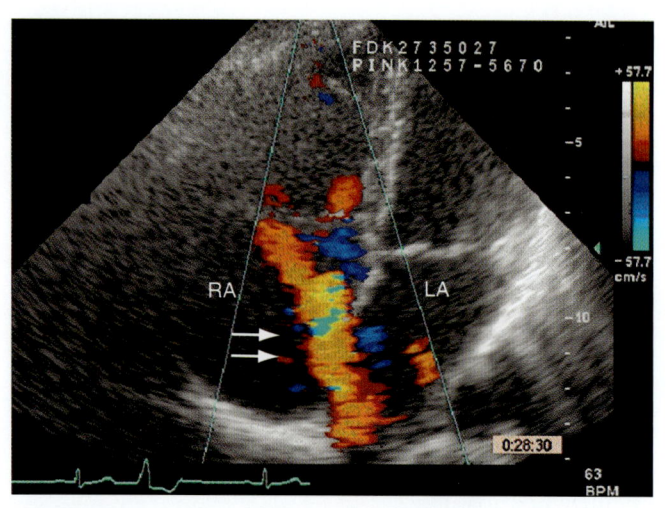

FIGURE 41-4 TTE in apical four-chamber view showing a left-to-right shunt across a secundum ASD (*arrows*) from the left atrium (LA) to the right atrium (RA).

TEE, although an invasive imaging modality, is an essential tool in the selection of patients who are candidates for percutaneous closure of secundum ASD. TEE allows for the sizing of the defect and the adequacy of the rim of tissue around the defect for proper attachment of the closure device. During the percutaneous closure, intracardiac echocardiography, which is now applied to many other percutaneous techniques, may be used for the guidance of the repair procedure.[6-8]

Computed Tomography

Findings on CT scans (Fig. 41-8), particularly multidetector CT scan, can be very specific; however, the CT scanner is less portable than the echocardiogram machine, and the radiation exposure related to the CT scan makes the assessment of ASD with CT less efficacious. Findings on CT include an incomplete interatrial septum, right heart enlargement, and pulmonary artery dilation. Size of the cardiac chambers can also be measured accurately. The three-dimensional capabilities of CT allow for the detection of anomalous pulmonary venous return associated with sinus venosus ASD.[9]

Magnetic Resonance Imaging

MRI (Figs. 41-9 through 41-12), especially cine MRI, has a sensitivity and specificity of greater than 90% in delineating septal defects. The high contrast that exists between the blood pool and cardiovascular structures because of the lack of signal from flowing blood using the spin-echo MRI technique or from the bright signal from blood using the gradient-echo (cine) MRI technique allows for excel-

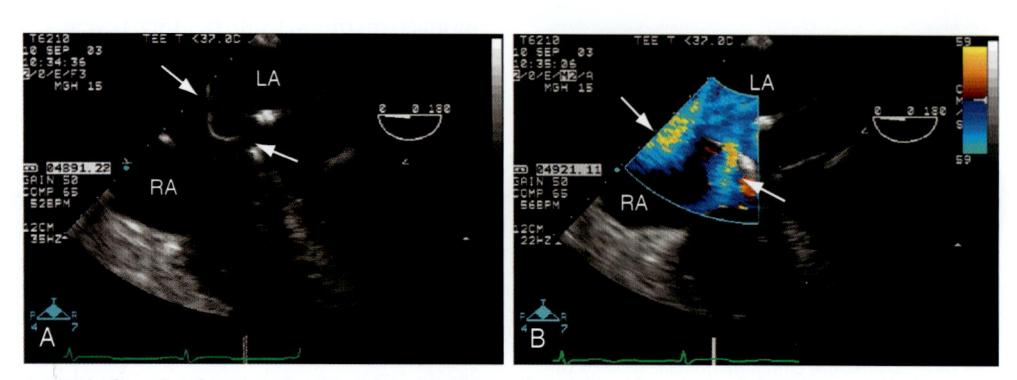

FIGURE 41-5 **A,** TEE in four-chamber view showing a fenestrated secundum ASD with two septal defects (*arrows*) between the left atrium (LA) and the right atrium (RA). **B,** TEE in the four-chamber view showing a left-to-right shunt across a fenestrated secundum ASD with two flow jets (*arrows*) from the LA to the RA.

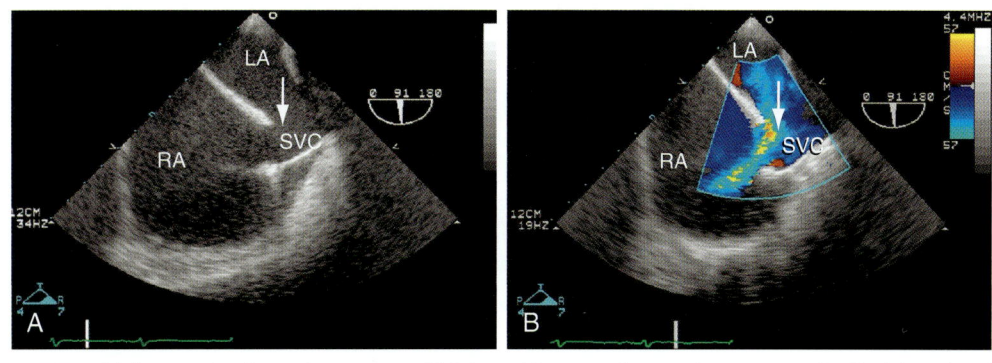

FIGURE 41-6 **A,** TEE at 91 degrees showing a sinus venosus ASD (*arrow*) between the superior vena cava (SVC), right atrium (RA), and left atrium (LA). **B,** TEE at 91 degrees showing color Doppler flow across a sinus venosus ASD (*arrow*) between the SVC, RA, and LA.

lent imaging capabilities. The three-dimensional capability of MRI allows for imaging to be performed in any plane, including planes parallel and perpendicular to the major axes of the ventricles.[10,11]

Ventricular volumes, mass, and function can be obtained by using cine MRI scans. Shunt volumes, valvular function, and pressure gradients, and blood flow and velocity across valves and conduits can be estimated using velocity-encoded phase contrast cine MRI. Gated cine MRI allows assessment of left and right ventricular function. MR angiography permits high-resolution three-dimensional evaluation of vessels and can noninvasively establish the presence of anomalous pulmonary veins.[12,13]

Nuclear Medicine and Positron Emission Tomography

Nuclear imaging is generally less useful in the assessment of ASD, but may be employed in some patients for assessing cardiac function. Equilibrium radionuclide angiography uses ECG gating to define the temporal relationship between the nuclear data and the components of the cardiac cycle. Several hundred heartbeats are sampled, quantified, and displayed in an endless-loop cine format for qualitative visual analysis and quantitative interpretation and analysis. The blood pool is labeled using a Tc 99m tracer. After a single labeling procedure, serial studies can be obtained for periods of 4 to 6 hours. Conventional scintillation cameras are used for these studies. The left anterior oblique view is used for qualitative analysis of global left ventricular ejection fractions and stroke volumes using a radioactivity count-based approach throughout the cardiac cycle.[14-16]

Right ventricular function is best evaluated using first-pass radionuclide angiography techniques. This technique involves sampling during the initial transit of the bolus through the central circulation. Analyzing right and left ventricular function independently during this brief transit is possible. Regional function also can be assessed from generated outlines of ventricular silhouettes. Tc 99m radiopharmaceuticals are also used for first-pass studies.

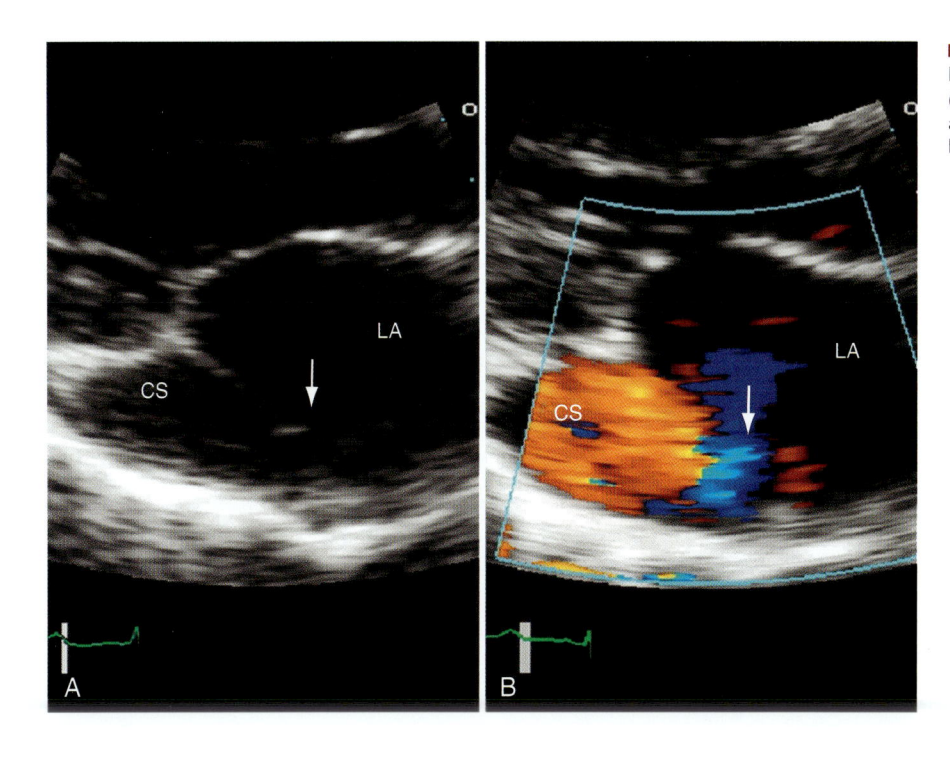

FIGURE 41-7 **A,** TTE in parasternal long-axis view showing a coronary sinus ASD (*left*) between the coronary sinus (CS) and left atrium (LA). **B,** Color Doppler flow is noted between the CS and LA (*arrow*).

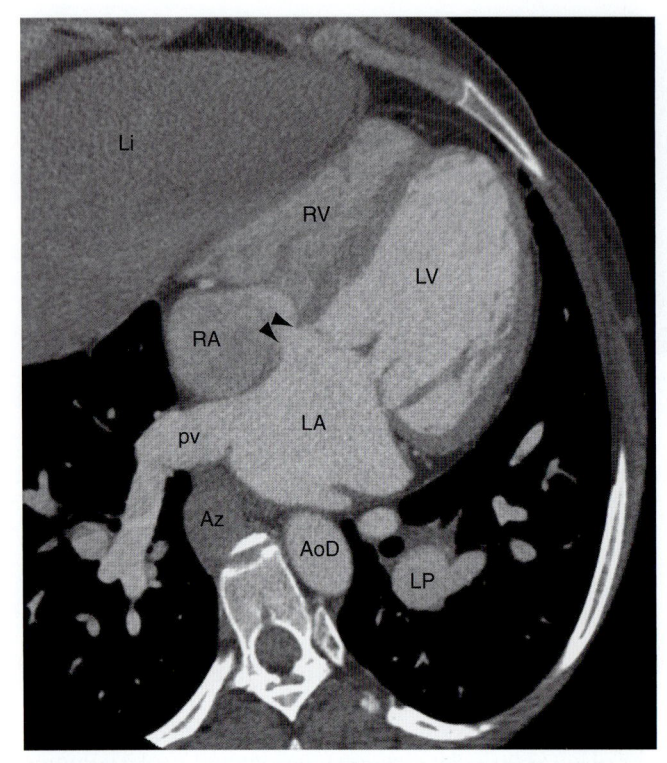

FIGURE 41-8 Contrast-enhanced CT scan from a 32-year-old woman with occasional shortness of breath, reconstructed in a four-chamber view. A break in the inferiormost and medialmost portion of the interatrial septum (*arrowheads*) allows communication between the left atria (LA) and right atria (RA). Notice the dilated left pulmonary artery (LP) and right lower lobe pulmonary vein (pv). The unopacified dilated azygos vein (Az) reflects the patient's heterotaxy syndrome (with interruption of the inferior vena cava and azygos continuation). The descending aorta (AoD), right (RV) and left (LV) ventricles, and liver (Li) are labeled.

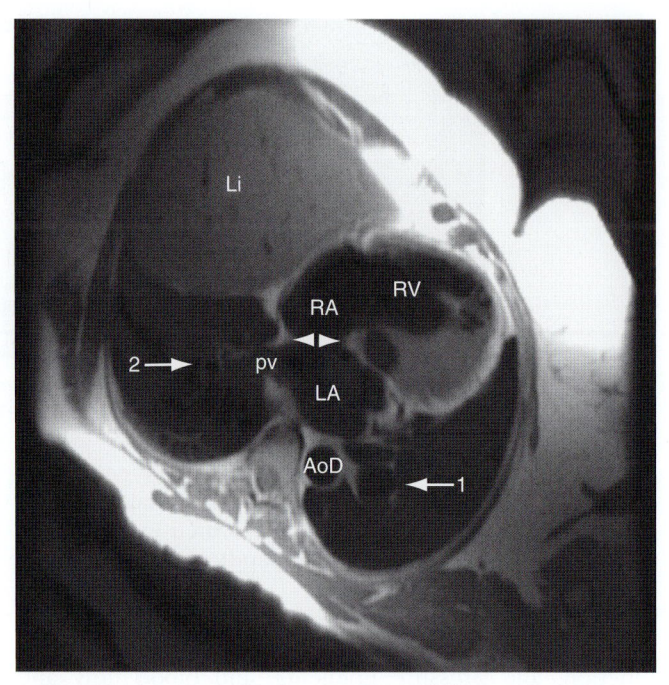

FIGURE 41-9 Four-chamber view using double inversion recovery fast spin-echo black blood MRI from an asymptomatic 36-year-old woman with a murmur. A large defect (*arrowheads*) in the interatrial septum allows communication between the right atria (RA) and left atria (LA). This represents a secundum ASD. The right ventricle (RV) is dilated. Note the dilated right lower lobe pulmonary vein (pv), and left (*1 arrow*) and right (*2 arrow*) pulmonary arteries. The descending aorta (AoD) and liver (Li) are labeled.

The finding of abnormal right ventricular ejection fraction in the absence of intrinsic right ventricular disease is excellent evidence of acquired pulmonary hypertension in the presence of an ASD.[14-16] Plain single photon emission computed tomography (SPECT) is not generally used in patients with ASD, but when it is performed, increased counts are seen in the right ventricle with dilation of the right ventricular cavity (Fig. 41-13).

Angiography

Invasive evaluation becomes necessary only when the results of noninvasive studies are inconclusive. When the aforementioned noninvasive techniques show the pres-

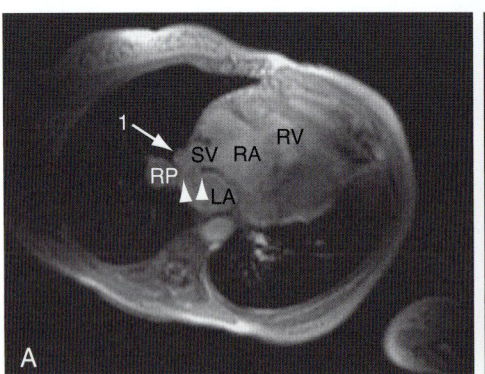

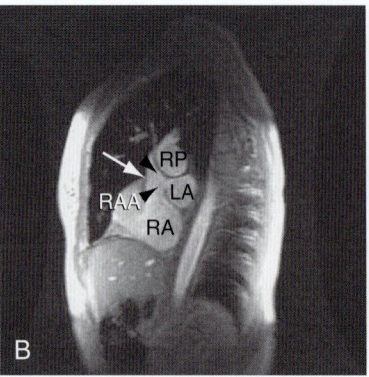

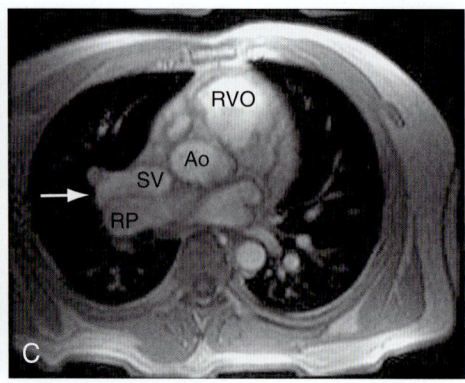

FIGURE 41-10 **A,** Oblique long-axis gradient-echo MR image at the base of the heart of a 23-year-old man with exercise intolerance. The left atrium (LA) communicates with the dilated right atrium (RA) across the defect (*arrowheads*) in the posterior wall of the superior vena cava (SV). Diagnosis of a sinus venosus ASD was made. The right ventricle (RV) lies anterior and inferior to the RA. The dilated right pulmonary artery (RP) and orifice of an anomalous right upper lobe pulmonary vein (*1 arrow*) draining into the superior vena cava are labeled. **B,** Left anterior oblique sagittal gradient-echo MR image shoes the defect (*arrowheads*) in the posterior wall of the superior vena cava (*arrow*) that allows communication among the superior vena cava, LA, and RA. The RA is dilated, resulting in convexity of the right atrial appendage (RAA). The RP is dilated as well. **C,** Axial gradient-echo MR image shows the right upper lobe pulmonary vein (*arrow*) to be anterior to the RP and to drain directly into the SV. The aortic root (Ao) and right ventricular outflow (RVO) are labeled.

CHAPTER 41 • Atrial Septal Defect 569

ence of an uncomplicated ASD in a child, routine cardiac catheterization is generally unnecessary. Invasive catheterization allows estimation of the magnitude of the shunt (Qp/Qs ratio) and measurement of the pulmonary artery pressure. Coronary angiography is recommended in patients with suspected coronary artery disease and in patients older than 40 years, especially if surgical repair of the ASD is planned. The diagnosis of ASD may also be confirmed by directly passing the catheter through the defect, and making serial oxygen saturation measurements to estimate the magnitude of the shunt. If high oxygen saturation is present in the superior vena cava, or if the catheter enters the pulmonary vein directly from the right atrium, an ASD of the sinus venosus type is likely present. In this case, partial anomalous pulmonary venous return is usually present and it affects the right upper pulmonary vein. Anomalous pulmonary venous return can also be seen with an ASD of the ostium secundum type.[17]

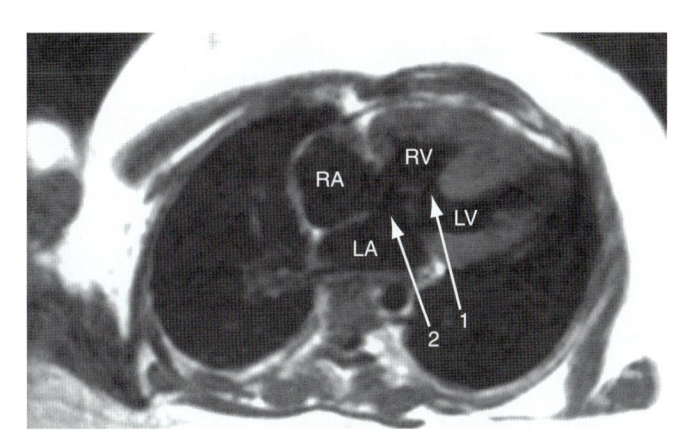

■ **FIGURE 41-11** Axial black blood MR image from a 23-year-old woman with complete atrioventricular canal and pulmonary hypertension. The medial (membranous) aspect of the interventricular septum (*1 arrow*) and the medial inferior (primum) aspect of the interatrial septum (*2 arrow*) are deficient. Notice the severe right ventricular (RV) hypertrophy and leftward cardiac rotation. The right atria (RA) and left atria (LA) and left ventricle (LV) are labeled.

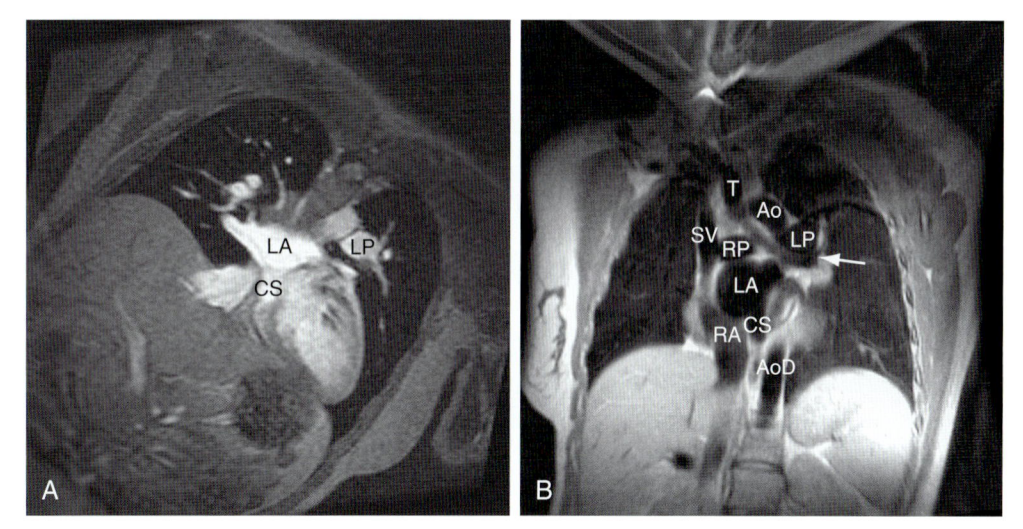

■ **FIGURE 41-12** **A,** MRI of a 23-year-old woman with palpitations. Steep four-chamber gradient-echo MR image shows communication between the inferior aspect of the left atrium (LA) and the superior aspect of the coronary sinus (CS). Note the dilated left pulmonary artery (LP). Diagnosis of a coronary sinus ASD was made. **B,** Left anterior oblique sagittal double inversion recovery fast spin-echo MRI acquisition through the defect. The floor of the LA communicates with the CS across the defect in the roof of the CS. The right atrium (RA), superior vena cava (SV), right pulmonary (RP) and left pulmonary (LP) arteries, trachea (T) and left bronchus (*arrow*), and aortic arch (Ao) and descending aorta (AoD) are labeled.

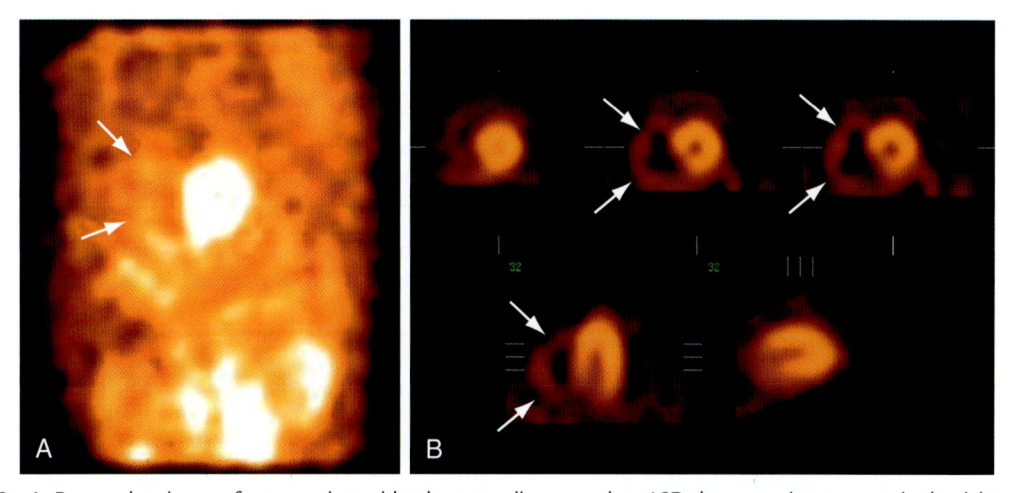

■ **FIGURE 41-13** **A,** Raw nuclear images from a patient with a long-standing secundum ASD show prominent counts in the right ventricle (*arrows*). **B,** Slice data nuclear images also show significant right ventricular dilation (*arrows*). *(Courtesy of Regina Druz, MD.)*

DIFFERENTIAL DIAGNOSIS
Clinical Presentation

The differential diagnosis for ASD may involve conditions such as pulmonary stenosis because of similarities in the physical examination. Partial anomalous pulmonary venous return without an associated ASD also results in a left-to-right shunt and may produce signs of right ventricular overload similar to ASD. Patients with pulmonary hypertension or shunts at other levels, such as a ventricular septal defect, may also produce murmurs and symptoms similar to those found in the presence of ASD.

Imaging Findings

From imaging findings, it is much easier to elucidate the differential diagnosis of ASD. Anatomic location of an ASD versus a ventricular septal defect can easily be differentiated. The degree of shunt can also be calculated and differentiated. Echocardiography is excellent at assessing degree of pulmonary hypertension through the assessment of pulmonary artery pressures.

SYNOPSIS OF TREATMENT OPTIONS
Medical

ASD is generally considered a surgical disorder, and no specific medical therapy is available. Patients with ASD-associated symptoms of heart failure may require heart failure therapy, however, including but not limited to diuretics, digitalis, and angiotensin-converting enzyme inhibitors. Patients with arrhythmias may require antiarrhythmic therapy.[18,19]

Surgical and Interventional

The decision to repair any kind of ASD is based on clinical and echocardiographic information, including the size and location of the ASD, the magnitude and hemodynamic impact of the left-to-right shunt, and the presence and degree of elevated pulmonary pressures. Closure is advised for an ASD with echocardiographic evidence of right ventricular overload or with a clinically significant shunt (Qp/Qs ratio >1.5). Lack of symptoms is not a contraindication for repair. In patients with interatrial septal aneurysm and secundum ASD, spontaneous closure may occur, and patients may be followed conservatively for a period before repair is advised.[20,21]

For children and adults, surgical mortality rates are approximately 1% for uncomplicated secundum ASD. Elective closure in patients with small defects is controversial because patients with small defects generally have a good prognosis, and the risk of cardiopulmonary bypass may not be warranted. The benefit of catheter closure of small secundum defects especially in these patients remains to be determined. Generally, long-term prevention of complications is best achieved when the ASD is closed before age 25 years, and when the systolic pressure in the main pulmonary artery is <40 mm Hg. Even in elderly patients with large shunts, surgical closure can be performed at low risk and with good results in reducing symptoms. Repair in patients older than 40 years does not eliminate the risk of atrial arrhythmias and cerebrovascular accidents.[18-21]

Closure of an ASD is not recommended in patients who have severe pulmonary hypertension or severe pulmonary vascular disease (Qp/Qs ratio ≥0.7) without a clinically significant shunt or in patients who have a reversed shunt with at-rest arterial oxygen saturations of less than 90% with little or no residual left-to-right shunt. In addition to the high surgical mortality and morbidity risk, closure of the defect in these patients worsens outcome.[18-21]

INFORMATION FOR THE REFERRING PHYSICIAN

Reports to referring physicians should document the type of ASD present—whether it is a primum, secundum, sinus venosus, or coronary sinus type of ASD. The size of the defect and the presence of tissue surrounding the defect and its size (this is important especially for the operator who plans to close an ASD percutaneously with a closure device) are generally useful for documentation. Another important component is an estimation of the degree of shunting by providing a Qp/Qs ratio. This ratio can easily be derived with echocardiography and cine phase contrast MRI. Finally, it is important to report associated cardiac malformations. An example is the association of primum ASD with a cleft mitral valve and the resulting mitral regurgitation, or the presence of anomalous pulmonary venous return associated with sinus venosus ASD.

> **KEY POINTS**
> - ASD is one of the most commonly recognized congenital cardiac anomalies in adults.
> - Knowledge of the embryologic development of the atrial septum provides the basis for understanding the pathophysiology, anatomy, and clinical manifestations of ASD.
> - Early surgical closure of most types of ASD is recommended.
> - Patients with clinical findings suggestive of right heart overload or failure should undergo imaging to assess the presence of atrial level shunts owing to an ASD.
> - The initial imaging modality generally should be a chest radiograph. Radiography gives certain clues for the presence or absence of an ASD.
> - The next and generally more definitive modality that gives the clinician a great deal of information is ultrasound imaging with TTE.
> - If necessary, a patient may be sent for TEE, which can give better anatomic visualization of the less common types of ASD and associated anomalies.
> - If ultrasound does not provide adequate assessment of the ASD, CT may be performed; however, MRI is better at assessing ASD because it allows for quantitative assessment of shunts and determination of shunt fractions.
> - Less commonly used modalities to assess ASD are nuclear medicine and angiography, which provide less anatomic information than the above-mentioned modalities, but do provide quantitative assessment of shunt fractions and hemodynamic pressure measurements in the case of invasive angiography.

SUGGESTED READINGS

Boxt LM. Magnetic resonance and computed tomographic evaluation of congenital heart disease. J Magn Reson Imaging 2004; 18:827-847.

Fayad LM, Boxt LM. Chest film diagnosis of congenital heart disease. Semin Roentgenol 1999; 34:228-248.

Lee T, Tsai IC, Fu YC, et al. MDCT evaluation after closure of atrial septal defect with an Amplatzer septal occluder. AJR Am J Roentgenol 2007; 188:W431-W439.

Sandhu SK. Transcatheter closure of the atrial septal defect in the elderly. J Invasive Cardiol 2007; 19:513-514.

Smallhorn JF. Cross-sectional echocardiographic assessment of atrioventricular septal defect: basic morphology and preoperative risk factors. Echocardiography 2001; 18:415-432.

Taylor AM, Stables RH, Poole-Wilson PA, et al. Definitive clinical assessment of atrial septal defect by magnetic resonance imaging. J Cardiovasc Magn Reson 1999; 1:43-47.

Wang ZJ, Reddy GP, Gotway MB, et al. Cardiovascular shunts: MR imaging evaluation. RadioGraphics 2003; 23(Spec No):S181-S194.

Webb G, Gatzoulis MA. Atrial septal defects in the adult: recent progress and overview. Circulation 2006; 114:1645-1653.

REFERENCES

1. Webb G, Gatzoulis MA. Atrial septal defects in the adult: recent progress and overview. Circulation 2006; 114:1645-1653.
2. Bedford D. The anatomical types of atrial septal defect: their incidence and clinical diagnosis. Am J Cardiol 1960; 6:568.
3. Hopkins WE. Atrial septal defect. Curr Treat Options Cardiovasc Med 1999; 1:301-310.
4. Krasuski RA. When and how to fix a "hole in the heart": approach to ASD and PFO. Cleve Clin J Med 2007; 74:137-147.
5. Espino-Vela J, Alvarado-Toro A. Natural history of atrial septal defect. Cardiovasc Clin 1971; 2:103-125.
6. Kowalski M, Hoffman P, Siudalska H, et al. Clinical and echocardiographic assessment of a right-to-left shunt across an atrial septal defect secondary to tricuspid regurgitation. Acta Cardiol 2001; 56:233-237.
7. Nanda NC, Ansingkar K, Espinal M, et al. Transesophageal three-dimensional echo assessment of sinus venosus atrial septal defect. Echocardiography 1999; 16:835-837.
8. Salem MI, Makaryus AN, Kort S, et al. Intracardiac echocardiography using the AcuNav ultrasound catheter during percutaneous balloon mitral valvuloplasty. J Am Soc Echocardiogr 2002; 15:1533-1537.
9. Berbarie RF, Anwar A, Dockery WD, et al. Measurement of right ventricular volumes before and after atrial septal defect closure using multislice computed tomography. Am J Cardiol 2007; 99:1458-1461.
10. Holmvang G, Palacios IF, Vlahakes GJ, et al. Imaging and sizing of atrial septal defects by magnetic resonance. Circulation 1995; 92:3473-3480.
11. Taylor AM, Stables RH, Poole-Wilson PA, et al. Definitive clinical assessment of atrial septal defect by magnetic resonance imaging. J Cardiovasc Magn Reson 1999; 1:43-47.
12. Wang ZJ, Reddy GP, Gotway MB, et al. Cardiovascular shunts: MR imaging evaluation. RadioGraphics 2003; 23(Spec No):S181-S194.
13. Piaw CS, Kiam OT, Rapaee A, et al. Use of non-invasive phase contrast magnetic resonance imaging for estimation of atrial septal defect size and morphology: a comparison with transesophageal echo. Cardiovasc Intervent Radiol 2006; 29:230-234.
14. Jimenez-Angeles L, Medina-Banuelos V, Valdes-Cristerna R, et al. Analysis of ventricular contraction by factorial phase imaging with equilibrium radionuclide angiography. Conf Proc IEEE Eng Med Biol Soc 2006; 1:1081-1084.
15. Chin BB, Metzler SD, Lemaire A, et al. Left ventricular functional assessment in mice: feasibility of high spatial and temporal resolution ECG-gated blood pool SPECT. Radiology 2007; 245:440-448.
16. Sharir T. Gated myocardial perfusion imaging for the assessment of left ventricular function and volume: from SPECT to PET. J Nucl Cardiol 2007; 14:631-633.
17. Yalonetsky S, Schwartz Y, Lorber A. Coronary angiography in patients undergoing transcatheter closure of interatrial shunt. J Invasive Cardiol 2007; 19:16-18.
18. Masura J, Gavora P, Podnar T. Long-term outcome of transcatheter secundum-type atrial septal defect closure using Amplatzer septal occluders. J Am Coll Cardiol 2005; 45:505-507.
19. Konstantinides S, Geibel A, Olschewski M, et al. A comparison of surgical and medical therapy for atrial septal defect in adults. N Engl J Med 1995; 333:469-473.
20. Formigari R, Di Donato RM, Mazzera E, et al. Minimally invasive or interventional repair of atrial septal defects in children: experience in 171 cases and comparison with conventional strategies. J Am Coll Cardiol 2001; 37:1707-1712.
21. Jones DA, Radford DJ, Pohlner PG. Outcome following surgical closure of secundum atrial septal defect. J Paediatr Child Health 2001; 37:274-277.

Ventricular Septal Defect

Amgad N. Makaryus and Lawrence M. Boxt

Ventricular septal defects (VSDs) are among the most common congenital cardiac disorders seen at birth, but are less frequently seen as isolated lesions in adulthood. The reason for this is that a VSD in an infant is usually either large and nonrestrictive, permitting equalization of pressures between the ventricles and leading to heart failure necessitating early surgical repair, or small and restrictive, closing spontaneously without intervention. A VSD can occur as an isolated lesion or in combination with other congenital cardiac anomalies. Blood flow across the defect is typically left to right, and depends on the size of the defect and the pulmonary vascular resistance.[1]

DEFINITION

A VSD is a defect in the interventricular septum. VSDs may occur anywhere, but are most commonly found at points of junction of the embryologic components of the septum (i.e., the main [or posterior] ventricular septum, the bulbar [or infundibular] septum, and the membranous septum). By dividing the septum into four components (membranous septum, inlet, trabecular septum, and outlet or infundibular septum), VSDs may be classified into four main categories according to their location and the appearance of the margins of defects.

Type I defects are also known as outlet defects. These defects comprise 5% of all VSDs and are located in the outlet portions of the left and right ventricles. The superior edge of the VSD is the joined annulus of the aortic and pulmonary valves. Because the aortic and pulmonary valves are in fibrous continuity, this type of defect may also be referred to as a supracristal, subpulmonary, infundibular, or conoseptal defect. This VSD is associated with prolapse of the unsupported aortic valve cusps and progressive aortic regurgitation.

Type II defects are also called infracristal, subaortic, perimembranous, or paramembranous defects. These defects are the most common type of VSD, constituting 75% of all cases. They occur around the membranous septum and are associated with a muscular defect. The defect is just inferior to the aortic valve, and the annulus of the tricuspid valve contributes to the rim of the defect.

Type III defects, also called atrioventricular (AV) canal, AV septal, or inlet septal defects, are located in the posterior region of the septum beneath the septal leaflet of the tricuspid valve. These defects account for 10% of all VSD types.

Type IV defects also account for 10% of all VSDs, and are called muscular defects. They may be single, but are commonly multiple. Most commonly, multiple defects occur in the apical trabecular septum.[1-5]

PREVALENCE AND EPIDEMIOLOGY

In the United States, VSD accounts for approximately 20% to 40% of all congenital cardiac malformations—approximately 1 to 2 cases per 1000 live births. Studies have shown that the prevalence of VSD has increased in the United States during the past 30 years. A twofold increase in the prevalence of VSD was reported by the U.S. Centers for Disease Control and Prevention from 1968 to 1980. This increase is primarily attributed to more sensitive detection through echocardiography.[6,7]

ETIOLOGY AND PATHOPHYSIOLOGY

Alcohol and illicit drug use have been identified as possible risk factors for VSD. There is a twofold increase in the risk of VSD associated with maternal cocaine use during pregnancy. Abnormal blood flow to the heart owing to the vasoconstricting effects of cocaine is a postulated reason for these increases.[5,6]

VSDs result from a lack of growth or a failure of alignment or fusion of the portions of the ventricular septum. Between weeks 4 and 8 of gestation, the single ventricular chamber is effectively divided into two. This division is accomplished with the fusion of the membranous portion of the ventricular septum, the endocardial cushions, and the bulbous cordis. The muscular portion of the ventricular septum grows cephalad as each ventricular chamber enlarges, eventually meeting with the right and left ridges of the bulbous cordis. The ridges fuse with the tricuspid and mitral valves and the endocardial cushions. The tricuspid valve is separated from the pulmonary valve by the infundibulum, but the mitral valve remains in fibrous continuity with the aortic valve. The endocardial cushions develop concomitantly and finally fuse with the bulbar ridges and the muscular portion of the septum. The fibrous tissue of the membranous portion of the interventricular septum makes the final closure and separates the two ventricles.[1-5]

The VSD permits a left-to-right shunt to occur at the ventricular level, causing increased pulmonary blood flow, right ventricular volume overload, and compromise of systemic cardiac output. These effects depend on the magnitude of the shunt, which is a function of the size of the VSD and the status of the pulmonary vascular bed. A small VSD with high resistance to flow permits only a small left-to-right shunt. A large interventricular communication allows a large left-to-right shunt. Measuring the ratio of pulmonary-to-systemic circulation (Qp/Qs ratio) is useful for determining the magnitude of the shunt. Over time, as pulmonary vascular resistance increases, right ventricular function is compromised. Eventually, irreversible damage may occur within the pulmonary vascular bed, leading to a reversal of the shunt and the development of increasing cyanosis (Eisenmenger syndrome).[1-5]

MANIFESTATIONS OF DISEASE

Clinical Presentation

The clinical significance of VSD depends on its size and location, and the level of pulmonary and left ventricular outflow resistance. A restrictive VSD produces a small shunt and does not cause significant hemodynamic derangement. In contrast, a large VSD may progressively lead to higher pulmonary resistance and, finally, to irreversible pulmonary vascular changes, producing Eisenmenger physiology with reversal of the shunt to a right-to-left shunt.[1,2]

A small VSD generally causes no symptoms, but respiratory distress and mild tachypnea may result from abnormal pulmonary compliance owing to left-to-right shunting. Because of compromised systemic output and vasoconstriction, infants with a moderately sized VSD may be pale and are often diaphoretic. Patients with a moderately sized VSD and decreased pulmonary compliance frequently have a history of upper respiratory tract infections.

Infants with a large left-to-right shunt often have heart failure and failure to thrive. Adults with a VSD complicated by pulmonary hypertension and shunt reversal (Eisenmenger syndrome) may present with exertional dyspnea, chest pain, syncope, hemoptysis, cyanosis, clubbing, and polycythemia. Patients may also develop bacterial endocarditis owing to turbulent blood flow through the VSD.

A VSD typically produces a harsh grade IV-VI holosystolic murmur. The murmur is best heard along the left sternal border, is usually louder at the third and fourth intercostal spaces, and is widely transmitted over the precordium with the production of a palpable thrill. The murmur of VSD does not radiate to the left axilla, as with mitral regurgitation, and does not increase in intensity with inspiration, as with tricuspid regurgitation. The smaller and more restrictive the VSD, the more turbulent the flow through the defect, and the louder the murmur. Large defects, with appreciable left-to-right shunts, have wide splitting of S_2, which varies with respiration. If pulmonary hypertension develops, the holosystolic murmur diminishes, and the thrill disappears. Cyanosis may become evident, and polycythemia follows. A pulmonary ejection sound may also be noted.[1-4]

Of patients with congenital VSD, 20% have additional cardiac abnormalities. Most abnormalities are detected at the initial assessment stage; however, aortic valve leaflet prolapse and pulmonary stenosis may also develop subsequently. Aortic regurgitation may result from the high-velocity flow beneath a poorly supported right aortic cusp near the VSD.[1]

Imaging Indications and Algorithm

Patients with clinical findings suggestive of right heart volume overload or failure should undergo imaging for the assessment of the presence of ventricular level shunt. The initial imaging modality should generally be a chest radiograph. Radiography gives certain clues as noted subsequently for the presence or absence of a VSD. The next modality that gives the clinician a great deal of information is ultrasound imaging with transthoracic echocardiography (TTE). Ultrasonography gives anatomic and quantitative information about a VSD. If necessary, a patient may be sent for transesophageal echocardiography (TEE), which can give better anatomic visualization of the less common types of VSD, and associated anatomic abnormalities.

If echocardiography does not provide adequate assessment, CT scanning may be performed, but MRI is currently presumed to be better for the assessment of VSD because it allows for quantitative assessment of shunts and determination of shunt fractions. Less commonly used modalities for the assessment of VSD are nuclear medicine and angiography, which provide less anatomic information than the previously mentioned modalities, but permit quantitative assessment of shunt fractions. Hemodynamic pressure measurements can be obtained by catheterization. The algorithm for the work-up generally can be accomplished with echocardiography, but rarely, other imaging modalities, most commonly MRI, but also angiography, can be performed if discrepancies exist.

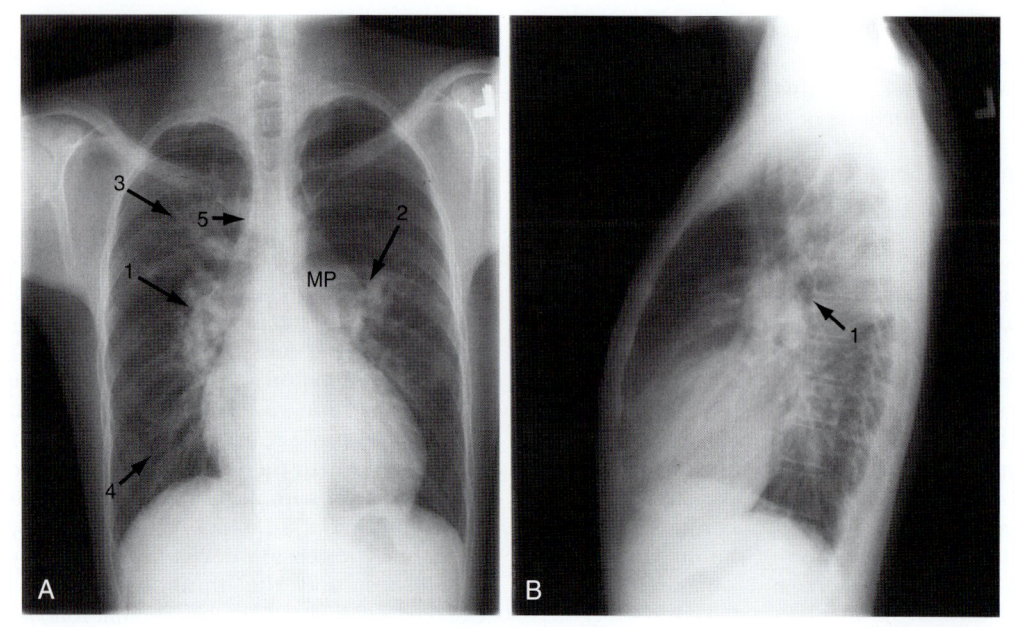

FIGURE 42-1 Chest examination in a 26-year-old man with a muscular VSD. **A,** Posteroanterior examination shows dilation of the main pulmonary artery (MP) and hilar right (*1 arrow*) and left (*2 arrow*) pulmonary arteries. The upper (*3 arrow*) and lower (*4 arrow*) lobe pulmonary arteries are sharp and dilated as well, indicating shunt vascularity. Narrowing of the superior mediastinum (*5 arrow*) and displacement of the heart toward the left indicate right heart volume loading. **B,** Lateral examination shows filling of the retrosternal space, indicating right heart and main pulmonary artery enlargement. The left bronchus (*1 arrow*) is displaced, and the inferior retrocardiac space is filled, indicating left atrial and ventricular enlargement.

Imaging Technique and Findings

Radiography

A small VSD usually manifests with no radiographic abnormality. With larger defects, chamber enlargement and pulmonary vascular changes are present, depending on the defect size and volume of the shunt. The typical plain film appearance of a patient with VSD is shunt vascularity associated with right and left ventricular and left atrial enlargement (Fig. 42-1). In young children, and especially in children with larger shunts, the plain film appearance is less specific. There is cardiac enlargement, but interstitial edema is superimposed on shunt vascularity, often giving the appearance of heart failure (Fig. 42-2). With increasing pulmonary resistance, right ventricular and pulmonary artery pressure increase, changing the appearance of the plain film to that of pulmonary hypertension (Fig. 42-3).[1]

Ultrasonography

Echocardiographic evaluation of VSD is a noninvasive modality that accurately delineates the morphology and associated defects (Figs. 42-4 through 42-6). Hemodynamic evaluation of the defect and the presence of elevated pulmonary artery pressure, insufficiency of the aortic valve, and distortion of the valve apparatus all are accurately evaluated by echocardiography. When limitations in image quality of TTE prevent adequate evaluation, TEE can be performed.[8-10]

Doppler echocardiography allows for the calculation of the Qp/Qs ratio, for estimation of gradients across the VSD, and for prediction of right-sided heart pressures. Combined color flow and pulsed Doppler assessments can provide substantial reliable information about the magnitude of left-to-right VSD flow and resistance, in most cases obviating an invasive catheter study. Echocardiography with color flow mapping is a more effective technique for detecting VSD than is cardiac catheterization. Contrast echocardiography also has been used to enhance the sensitivity and amplify the assessment of VSD by M-mode and two-dimensional techniques.[9]

A complete segmental echocardiographic study can provide accurate information about the size, location, and number of septal defects, and associated lesions. Perimembranous VSD is identified by septal dropout in the area adjacent to the septal leaflet of the tricuspid valve and below the right border of the aortic annulus. The subaortic VSD (type II) appears just below the posterior semilunar valve cusps, entirely superior to the tricuspid valve. The subpulmonary VSD (type I) appears as echo dropout within the outflow septum and extending to the pulmonary annulus. The inlet AV septal type of VSD (type III) extends from the fibrous annulus of the tricuspid valve into the muscular septum, and is often entirely beneath the septal tricuspid leaflet. Muscular VSD (type IV) is identified by echocardiography by echo-free septal areas located in the inlet, trabecular, or outlet portions.[8-11]

Computed Tomography

Dilated pulmonary arteries should alert the observer to the possibility of an intracardiac shunt (Fig. 42-7). When measured in the same axial section, the main pulmonary artery should be no greater in caliber than the ascending aorta. Dilated pulmonary arteries are a sign of increased

CHAPTER 42 • Ventricular Septal Defect 575

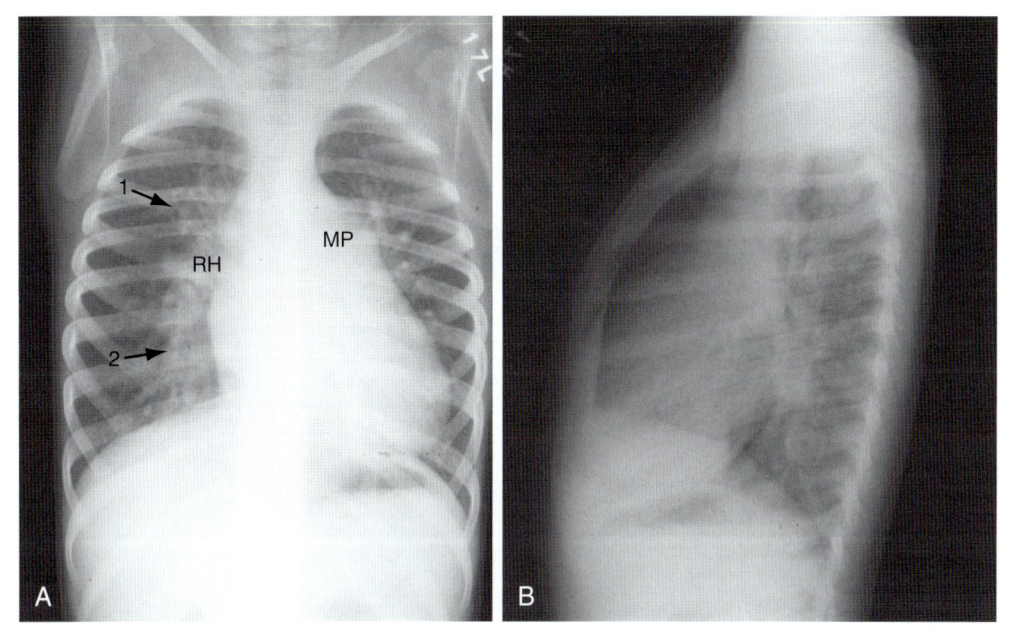

■ **FIGURE 42-2** Chest examination in a 6-year-old boy with a membranous VSD. **A,** Posteroanterior examination showing typical signs of shunt vascularity and cardiac enlargement. The main pulmonary artery (MP) and right hilar (RH) and upper lobe (*1 arrow*) and lower lobe (*2 arrow*) pulmonary arteries are enlarged. The left pulmonary artery lies posterior to the leftward rotated heart. The pulmonary arterial segments, although dilated, are unsharp (compare with the vessels in Fig. 42-1), typical of shunt vessels in young children. Right heart enlargement is indicated by the leftward displacement of the heart from the midline. **B,** Lateral examination shows filling of the retrosternal clear space (indicating right heart and pulmonary artery enlargement), and filling of the superior and inferior retrocardiac space, indicating left atrial and left ventricular enlargement.

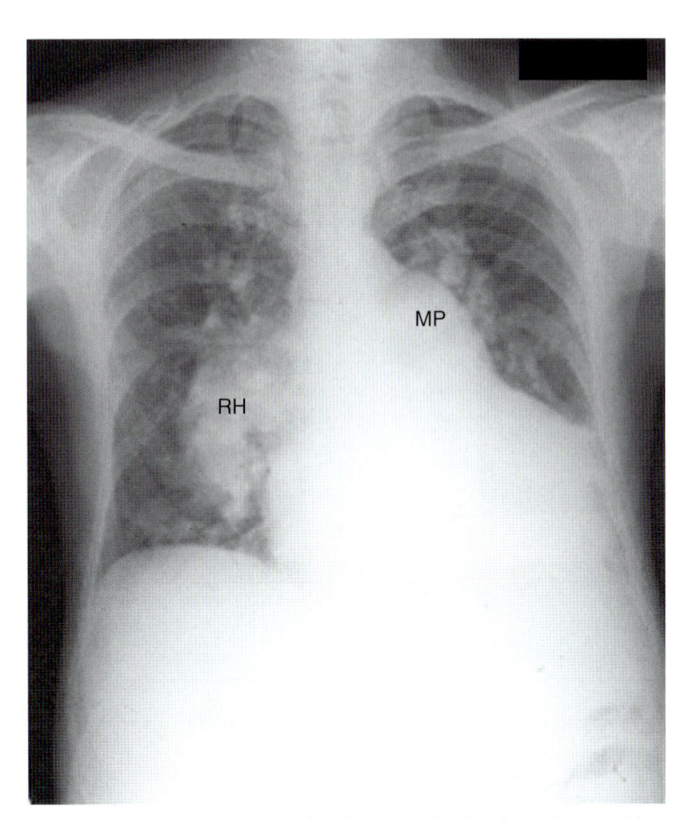

■ **FIGURE 42-3** Posteroanterior chest examination in a 38-year-old man with an unoperated membranous VSD. The main (MP) and right hilar (RH) pulmonary arteries are very dilated. The abrupt change in pulmonary arterial caliber from hilar to parenchymal vessel reflects vasoconstriction, associated with increased pulmonary artery resistance and pulmonary hypertension. The heart is enlarged and displaced toward the left, indicating right heart enlargement. The direction of the intracardiac shunting cannot be ascertained from the chest film.

pulmonary artery pressure and left-to-right shunting. Right-sided volume loading from the shunt is reflected in leftward cardiac rotation bringing the right ventricular free wall toward the left chest wall.[12] Right ventricular hypertension is reflected in varying degrees of free wall hypertrophy and septal flattening. In contrast to the left-to-right shunt in ASD, the right ventricle in VSD is volume and pressure loaded, resulting in flattening and reversal of normal septal curvature throughout the cardiac cycle (Fig. 42-8). The defect of a VSD is a gap in a portion of the interventricular septum. Type II defects are found in the posterior portion of the septum, just inferior to the aortic valve (Fig. 42-9). Partial closure and closure by formation of a membranous septal aneurysm are common. Muscular defects appear as a break in the continuity of the interventricular septum, allowing communication between left and right ventricles (Fig. 42-10).[13,14]

Magnetic Resonance Imaging

ECG gated MRI provides excellent anatomic delineation of the size and location of the VSD, and the presence and character of associated congenital malformations. Cine MRI acquisitions provide functional assessment of chamber function and shunt flow. MRI has a sensitivity and specificity of greater than 90% in delineating VSD. Black blood imaging (e.g., double inversion recovery fast spin-echo imaging) provides high-resolution visualization of defects (Figs. 42-11 through 42-13). Use of gradient-echo acquisition takes advantage of the high intrinsic contrast between the blood pool and shunt flow, and the three-dimensional capability of MRI for explicit demonstration of an intracardiac shunt in any anatomic plane (Figs. 42-14 and 42-15).[15] Myocardial mass and ventricular volumes and function can

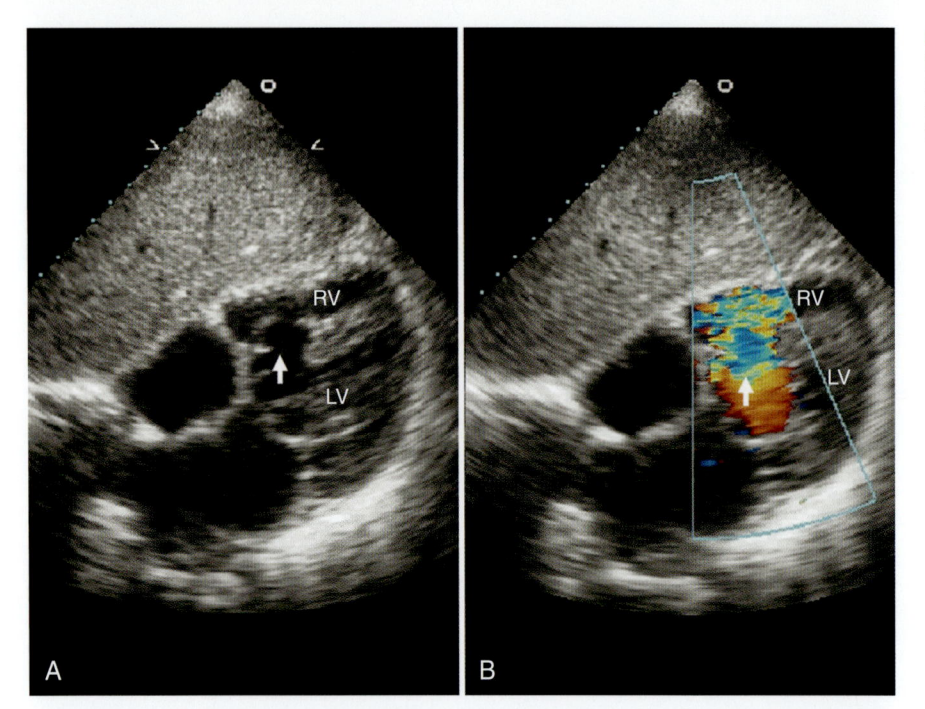

■ **FIGURE 42-4** **A,** TTE in subcostal four-chamber view shows a membranous VSD (*arrow*) between the left ventricle (LV) and right ventricle (RV). **B,** Color Doppler shows left-to-right shunt across the VSD (*arrow*).

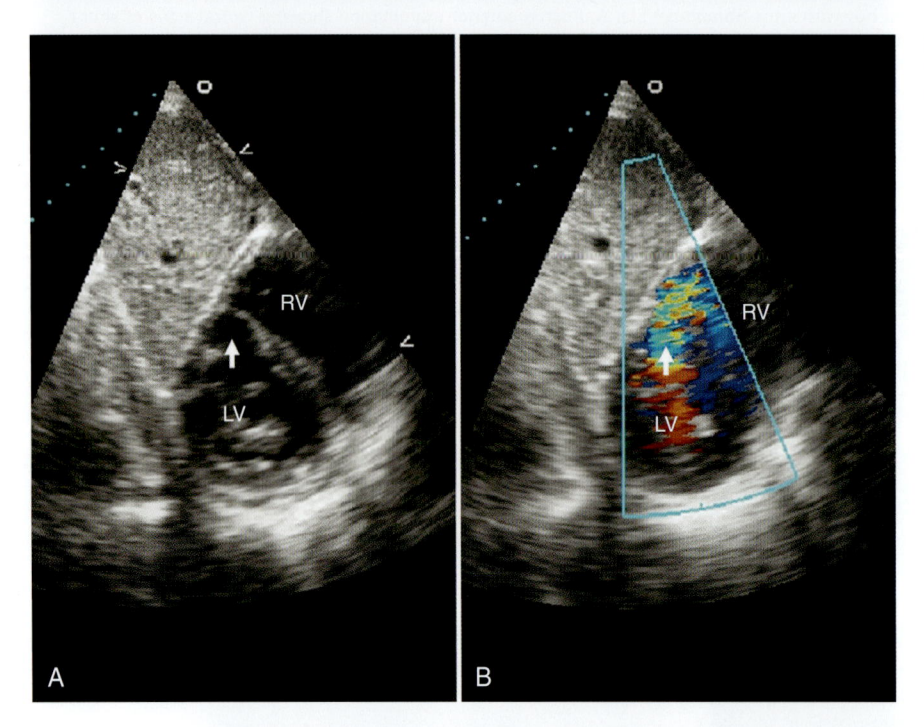

■ **FIGURE 42-5** **A,** TTE in subcostal short-axis view shows a VSD (*arrow*) between the left ventricle (LV) and right ventricle (RV). **B,** Color Doppler shows left-to-right shunt across the VSD (*arrow*).

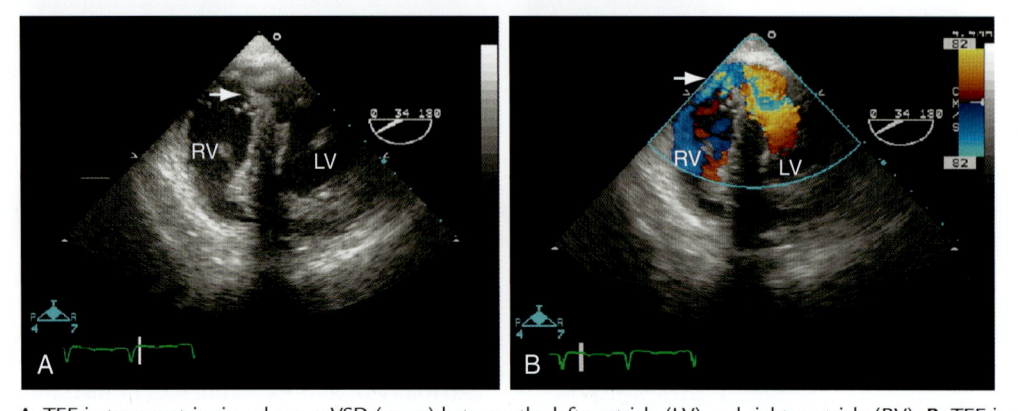

■ **FIGURE 42-6** **A,** TEE in transgastric view shows a VSD (*arrow*) between the left ventricle (LV) and right ventricle (RV). **B,** TEE in the transgastric view shows color Doppler flow across the VSD (*arrow*) between the left ventricle (LV) and right ventricle (RV).

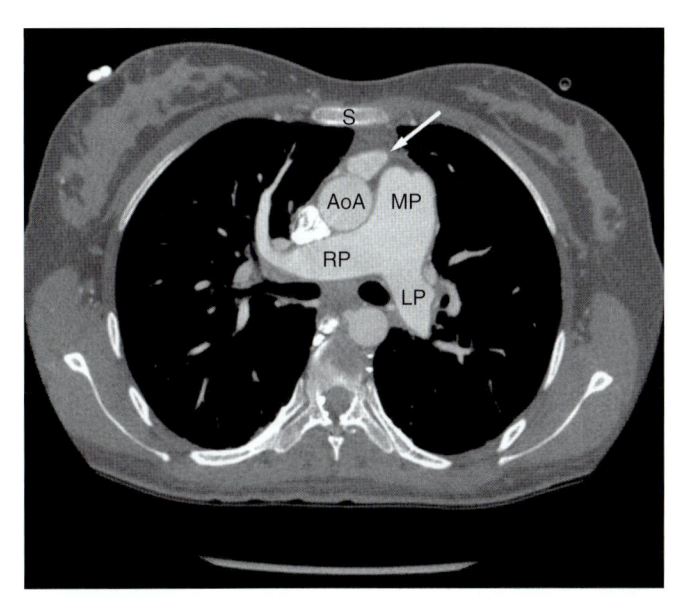

FIGURE 42-7 Axial acquisition image from contrast-enhanced CT scan in a 23-year-old woman with a membranous VSD. The main pulmonary artery (MP) is greater in caliber than the ascending aorta (AoA). The left (LP) and right (RP) pulmonary arteries are also enlarged. Right heart enlargement is indicated by the leftward rotation of the great arteries. The apex of the right atrial appendage (*arrow*) lies toward the left of the sternum (S).

angiography uses ECG gating to define the temporal relationship between the nuclear data and the components of the cardiac cycle. The left anterior oblique view is used for qualitative analysis of global left ventricular ejection fractions and stroke volumes using a radioactivity count-based approach throughout the cardiac cycle.[18-20]

Right ventricular function is best evaluated using first-pass radionuclide angiography techniques. Analyzing right and left ventricular function independently during this brief transit is possible. Regional function also can be assessed from generated outlines of ventricular silhouettes. Tc 99m radiopharmaceuticals are also used for first-pass studies. The finding of abnormal right ventricular ejection fraction in the absence of intrinsic right ventricular disease is evidence of acquired pulmonary hypertension in the presence of a VSD.[18-20]

Angiography

Although echocardiography and MRI generally obviate the need for invasive catheterization for the evaluation of VSD, catheterization can give accurate measurements of pulmonary vascular resistance, pulmonary reactivity, and volume of shunting. Response to pulmonary vasodilators can be determined and can guide therapy especially in patients in whom there is suspicion for the development of shunt reversal (Eisenmenger syndrome). Angiography can provide information on the location of a defect, number of defects, and degree of aortic insufficiency. The left ventriculogram (Fig. 42-17) in the long-axis view is the most useful projection for angiographic identification of a perimembranous VSD. The defect can be seen as a discontinuity of the chamber immediately beneath the anterior contour of the aortic valve. A muscular VSD (Fig. 42-18) is observed as a discontinuity in the septal wall away from the semilunar and AV valves.[1-4]

be obtained by planimetric analysis of gradient-echo acquisitions. Shunt volume, valvular function, pressure gradients, and blood velocity and flow across valves and conduits can be estimated using velocity encoded cine phase contrast imaging (Fig. 42-16).[16,17]

Nuclear Medicine and Positron Emission Tomography

Nuclear imaging is generally less frequently used in the assessment of VSDs, but may be employed in some patients for assessing cardiac function. Equilibrium radionuclide

In patients with left-to-right shunts, oxygen saturation is increased in the right ventricle compared with the right atrium because of shunting of highly oxygenated blood from the left ventricle into the right ventricle causing the

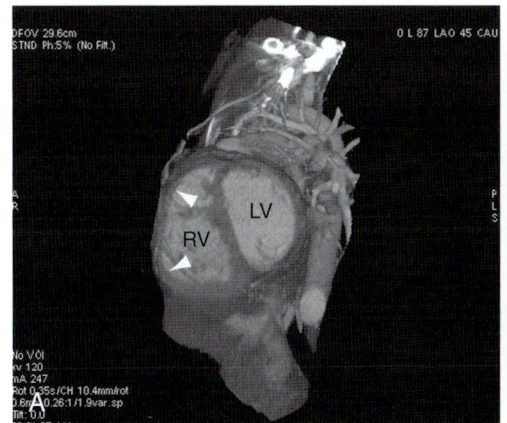

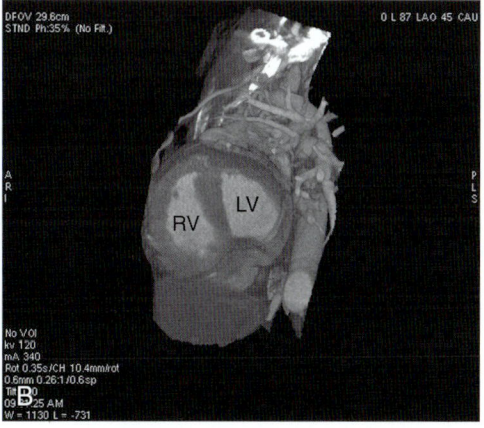

FIGURE 42-8 Short-axis reconstructions from contrast enhanced CT scan in a 23-year-old woman with a membranous VSD. **A,** End-diastolic image shows enlargement of the left (LV) and right (RV) ventricles. The RV free wall myocardium (*arrowheads*) is thickened, and the interventricular septum is flat. **B,** End-systolic image shows thickening of left (LV) and right (RV) ventricular myocardium. The interventricular septum remains flat.

578   PART FIVE   • *Congenital Heart Disease*

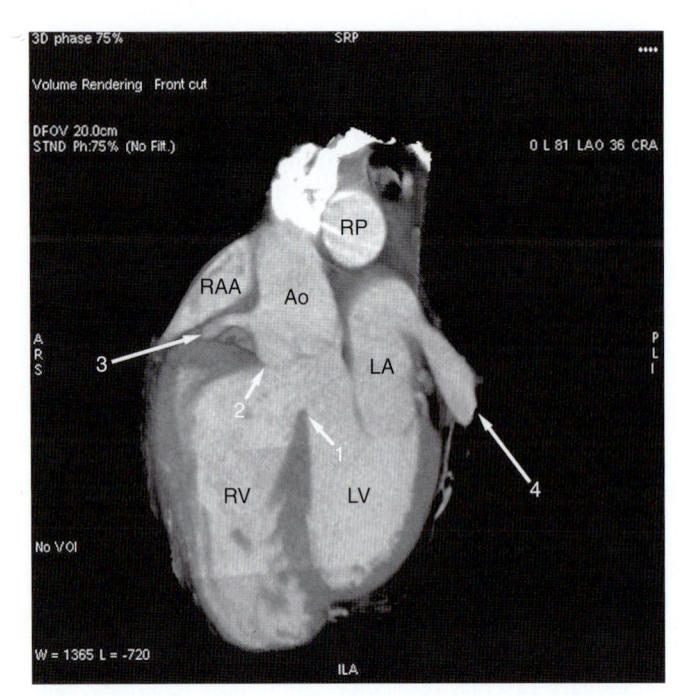

FIGURE 42-9 Horizontal long-axis reconstruction from contrast-enhanced CT scan of a 27-year-old man with a membranous VSD. The membranous septum should extend from the top of the muscular interventricular septum (*1 arrow*) to the aortic annulus (*2 arrow*). Because of the defect, there is free communication between the left ventricle (LV) and right ventricle (RV). Unsupported by the membranous septum, the aorta (Ao) is displaced anteriorly ("overriding aorta"), bearing a relationship with the left and right ventricles. The left atrium (LA), right atrial appendage (RAA), right pulmonary artery (RP), proximal right coronary artery (*3 arrow*), and left lower lobe pulmonary vein (*4 arrow*) are labeled.

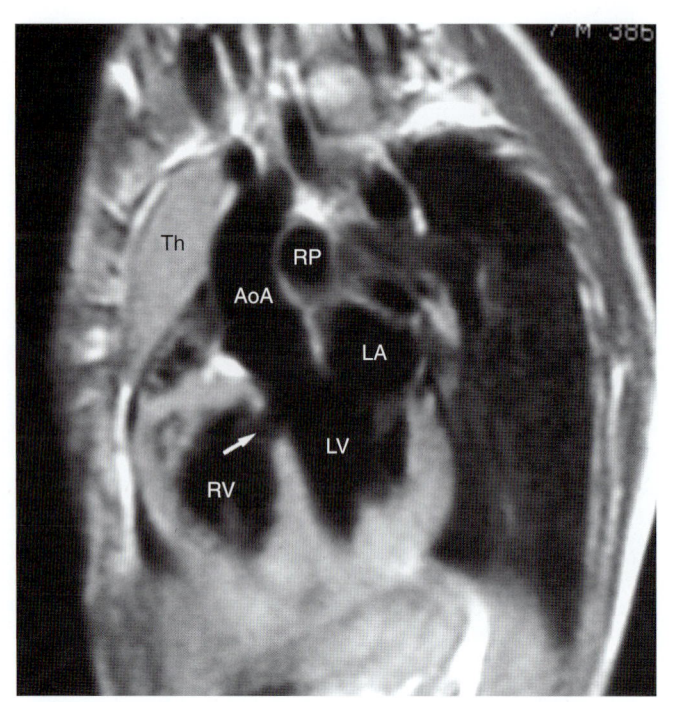

FIGURE 42-11 MRI of VSD. Left anterior oblique black blood image of a 7-year-old boy with posterior muscular VSD. The defect in the posterior muscular interventricular septum (*arrow*) allows communication between the left ventricle (LV) and right ventricle (RV). The thymus (Th), ascending aorta (AoA), transverse portion of the right pulmonary artery (RP), and left atrium (LA) are labeled.

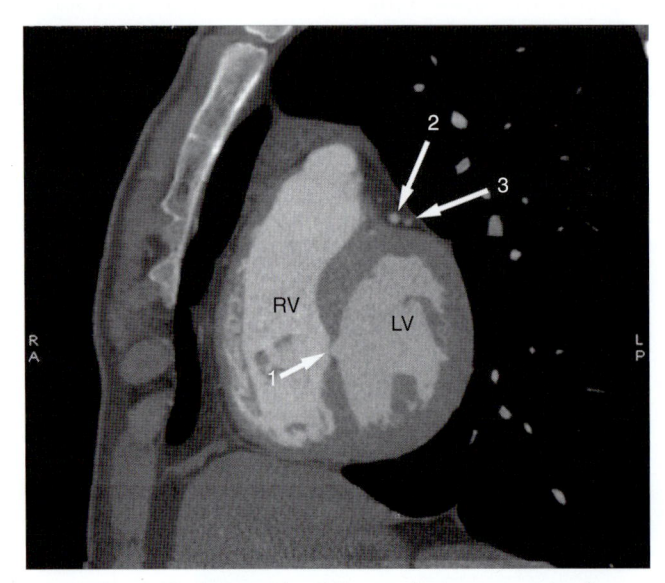

FIGURE 42-10 Left anterior oblique sagittal reconstruction from contrast-enhanced CT scan of a 20-year-old man with a previously stented coarctation of the aorta (not shown). A small, muscular VSD (*1 arrow*) appears as a discontinuity in the interventricular septum, allowing communication between the left ventricle (LV) and right ventricle (RV). The anterior descending coronary artery (*2 arrow*) and anterior interventricular vein (*3 arrow*) are viewed in cross-section.

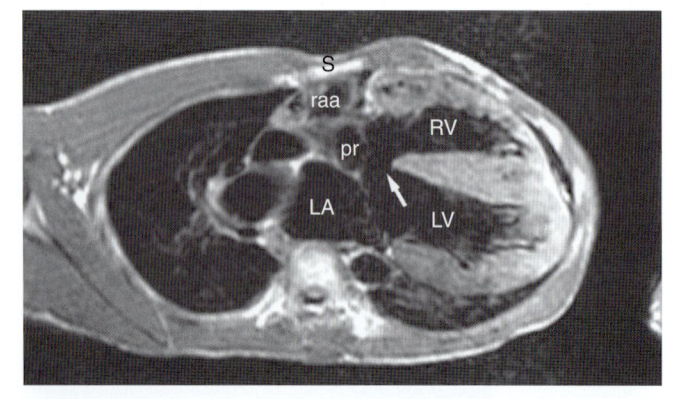

FIGURE 42-12 MRI of VSD. Horizontal long-axis double inversion recovery fast spin-echo image in a 23-year-old man with an unoperated membranous VSD. The heart is markedly enlarged. Anterior displacement of the posterior right (pr) aortic sinus of Valsalva reflects the overriding of the aorta over the VSD (*arrow*). Clockwise (leftward) cardiac rotation reflects right ventricular (RV) dilation. The dilated right atrial appendage (raa) lies posterior to the sternum (S). Notice the severe RV hypertrophy as well. The left ventricle (LV) and left atrium (LA) are also dilated.

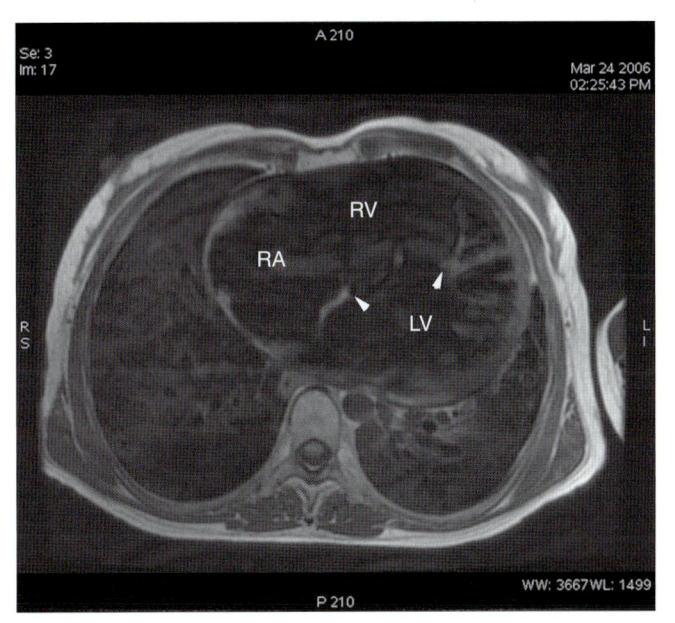

FIGURE 42-13 MRI of VSD. Axial double inversion recovery fast spin-echo image of a 22-year-old woman with heart failure. The heart is obviously enlarged. Clockwise cardiac rotation indicates right ventricular (RV) and right atrial (RA) dilation. The left ventricle (LV) is dilated as well. There is a large gap (*arrowheads*) in the interventricular septum, the site of a "Swiss cheese" (multiple) muscular VSD. Note the increased pulmonary parenchymal signal, indicating interstitial edema.

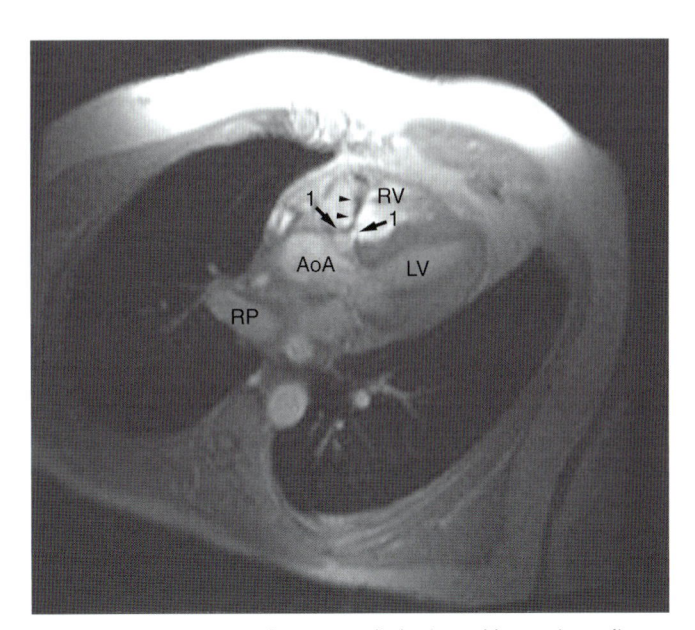

FIGURE 42-14 MRI of VSD. Systolic horizontal long-axis gradient-echo acquisition of a 24-year-old man with a partially occluded membranous VSD. The signal void jet of the shunt (*arrowheads*) extends from the membranous ventricular septal aneurysm (*1 arrows*) into the right ventricle (RV).

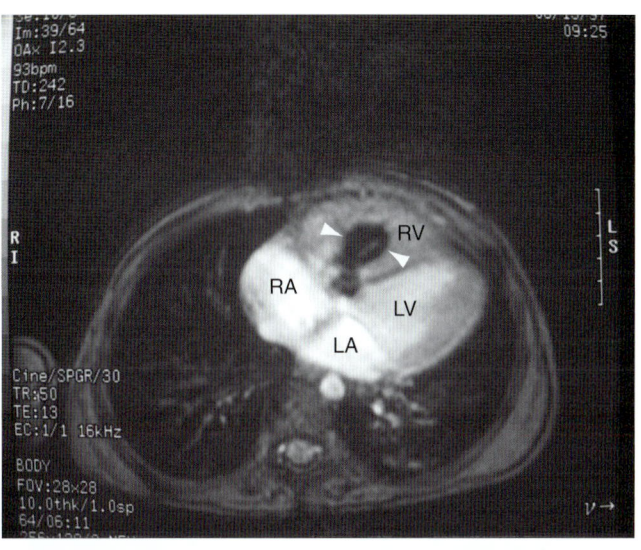

FIGURE 42-15 MRI of VSD. Systolic axial gradient-echo image in a 5-year-old girl with a membranous VSD. The broad signal void jet (*arrowheads*) extends from just beneath the aortic valve into the dilated right ventricle (RV). Note the clockwise cardiac rotation indicating RV dilation. The left ventricle (LV), left atria (LA) and right atria (RA), and dilated right pulmonary artery (RP) are labeled.

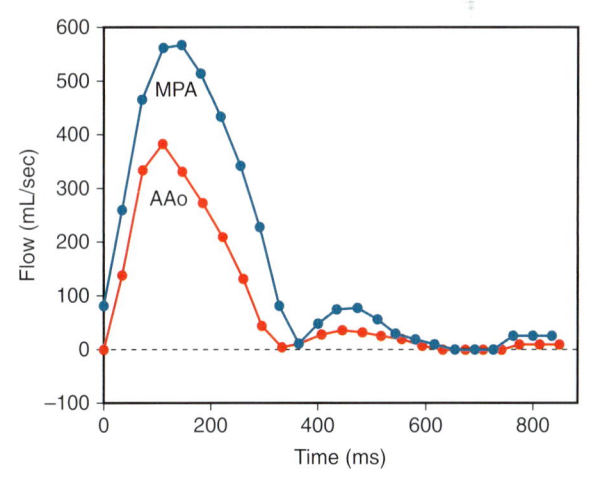

FIGURE 42-16 Graphic results from phase contrast analysis of flow in the main pulmonary artery (MPA) and ascending aorta (AAo) in a child with a VSD. The area beneath the MPA curve is 1.5 times the area beneath the AAo curve, indicating a Qp/Qs ratio of 1.5:1, reflecting the size of the left-to-right shunt. (*Courtesy of Laureen Sena, MD, Boston, MA.*)

so-called step-up. Cardiac catheterization also provides precise information about the magnitude of the left-to-right shunt, and estimates pulmonary artery pressures and resistance. A pulmonary vascular resistance of greater than 8 Wood units with pulmonary vasodilation testing during catheterization indicates inoperability.[1-4]

DIFFERENTIAL DIAGNOSIS

Clinical Presentation

The differential diagnosis for VSD may involve conditions such as pulmonary stenosis, patent ductus arteriosus, and subaortic stenosis because of similarities in the physical examination. Associated congenital defects, such as transposition of the great arteries, without an associated VSD may also produce signs of right-sided ventricular overload and increased pulmonary pressures similar to VSD. Patients with pulmonary hypertension or shunts at other levels, such as an atrial septal defect, may also produce murmurs and symptoms similar to those found in the presence of VSD.

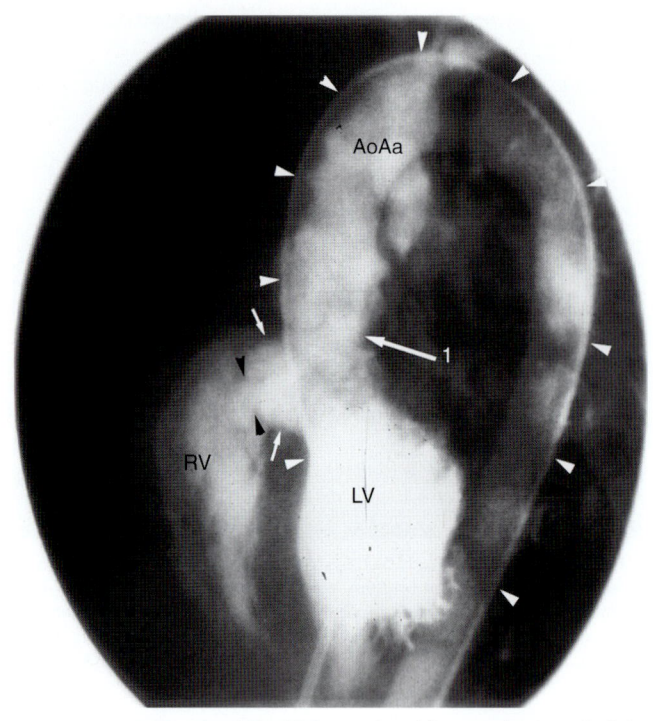

■ **FIGURE 42-17** Cranialized left anterior oblique projection of a left ventriculogram performed in a 3-year-old girl with a membranous VSD. The catheter (*white arrowheads*) has been threaded retrograde around the aortic arch (AoAa), across the aortic valve (*1 arrow*) and into the left ventricle (LV). Contrast medium passes through a residual defect (*black arrowheads*) in a membranous ventricular septal aneurysm (*short arrows*) into the right ventricle (RV). The intact muscular interventricular septum is the filling void between the two opacified ventricular cavities.

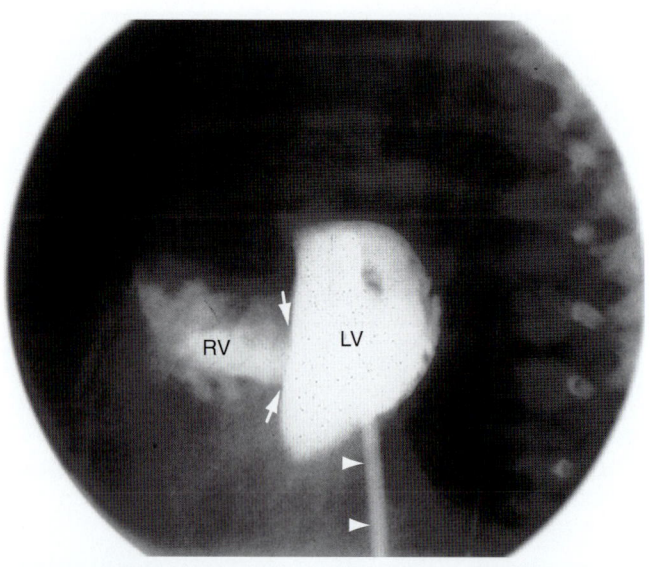

■ **FIGURE 42-18** Lateral left ventriculogram in a 7-month-old boy with D-transposition of the great arteries and a muscular VSD. The catheter (*white arrowheads*) has been threaded from the femoral vein to right atrium, across the interatrial septum, and into the left ventricle (LV). Contrast medium passes across the mid-septal muscular defect (*arrows*) into the right ventricle (RV). Note the flattened interventricular septum (the RV is hypertensive, pumping against systemic resistance).

Imaging Findings

From imaging findings, it is straightforward to formulate the differential diagnosis of VSD. Anatomic location of a VSD versus an atrial septal defect can easily be distinguished. The degree of shunt can also be calculated and differentiated. Echocardiography is excellent at assessing degree of pulmonary hypertension through the assessment of pulmonary artery pressures.

SYNOPSIS OF TREATMENT OPTIONS
Medical

The natural history of VSD encompasses a wide spectrum, ranging from spontaneous closure to congestive cardiac failure and death in early infancy. VSD is generally considered a surgical disorder, and no specific medical therapy is available. Patients with VSD-associated symptoms of heart failure may require heart failure therapy, however, including but not limited to diuretics, digitalis, and angiotensin-converting enzyme inhibitors. Patients with arrhythmias may require antiarrhythmic therapy. Medical management further includes endocarditis antibiotic prophylaxis for all patients.[1]

The medical treatment of infants with a VSD depends on the size of the VSD. A tiny defect (Roger disease) does not require any intervention. Medium and larger defects require various degrees of medical management and eventual surgical closure. The goals of therapy are to relieve symptoms, to minimize frequency and severity of respiratory infections, and to facilitate normal growth. Restricting the activities of a child with an isolated VSD is rarely necessary. Children with a VSD should be followed-up at least once or twice yearly to detect changes in the clinical picture that suggest the development of pulmonary vascular changes.[1,2]

Patients in whom the VSD is small do not require treatment because approximately 80% of such lesions get smaller or heal spontaneously. A VSD that either decreases in size or closes completely during the first year of life presents no future problems to the patient. Patients with VSD and pulmonary vascular disease who are deemed inoperable because of irreversibly elevated pulmonary vascular resistance require more intensive support and symptomatic therapy as cyanosis progresses and activity becomes more limited. Improvement in the symptoms associated with the polycythemia of Eisenmenger syndrome may be provided by partial exchange transfusion for red blood cell volume reduction.[1-3]

Surgical and Interventional

In patients with small and even some moderate VSDs with normal pulmonary artery pressure, there is a tendency for the VSD to become smaller and eventually close. Surgery is not indicated in these patients. For symptomatic patients, or patients with larger VSDs and elevated pulmonary resistance, surgical closure is indicated. The timing of surgery is very important, however. The ideal time to intervene is when the likelihood of spontaneous VSD closure is lowest, and the risk of irreversible pulmonary vascular disease and ventricular dysfunction is minimized. This is a narrow time frame, which is sometimes difficult to ascertain unless close follow-up is exercised.[1]

In type I VSD, the risk of irreversible aortic valve damage caused by cusp prolapse leads to earlier repair. With perimembranous and muscular defects, surgery may be delayed 1 year or more if the infant is thriving, and the pulmonary artery pressure is not elevated. Multiple VSDs present a different problem. If a large shunt is present and persists longer than 6 to 8 weeks, pulmonary artery banding and removal after age 2 years with an attempt at septation is reasonable. Banding is also a reasonable repair for a VSD complicated by straddling or overriding of the AV valves.[1]

Besides surgical repair, percutaneous transcatheter device occlusion of perimembranous and, in some instances, muscular VSD can be performed. This technique may be associated with further complications, including conduction anomalies and valve dysfunction. Treatment of patients with VSD and aortic regurgitation is controversial. In patients with a large, hemodynamically significant left-to-right shunt, repair of the VSD is indicated, but aortic regurgitation is repaired only if it is at least moderate in severity. If a type I VSD without aortic regurgitation is identified in early childhood, an argument for prophylactic closure of the VSD can be made to prevent the future potential complication of aortic valve incompetence. In the presence of moderate or severe aortic regurgitation, valve surgery would be required (valvuloplasty is preferred to valve replacement).[8]

INFORMATION FOR THE REFERRING PHYSICIAN

Reports to referring physicians should document the type of VSD present. The size of the defect and the presence of tissue surrounding the defect and its size (this is important especially for the operator who plans to close the defect percutaneously with a closure device) are generally useful for documentation. Another important component is an estimation of the degree of shunting by providing a Qp/Qs ratio. This ratio can easily be derived with echocardiography and cine phase contrast MRI. Finally, it is important to report on associated cardiac malformations.

KEY POINTS

- VSDs are among the most common congenital cardiac disorders seen at birth, but are less frequently seen as isolated lesions in adulthood.
- VSD can occur as an isolated lesion or in combination with other congenital cardiac anomalies.
- Blood flow across the defect is typically left to right, and depends on the size of the defect and the pulmonary vascular resistance.
- The clinical significance of the VSD depends on its size and location, the level of pulmonary pressure, and the left ventricular outflow resistance.
- The initial imaging modality should generally be a chest radiograph, which gives certain clues for the presence or absence of a VSD.
- The next modality that gives the clinician a great deal of information is TTE. Echocardiography gives anatomic and quantitative information about a VSD.
- The algorithm for the work-up generally can be accomplished with echocardiography, but occasionally, other imaging modalities, most commonly MRI, but also angiography, can be obtained if discrepancies exist.

SUGGESTED READINGS

Ammash NM, Warnes CA. Ventricular septal defects in adults. Ann Intern Med 2001; 135:812-824.
Boxt LM. MR imaging of congenital heart disease. Magn Reson Imaging Clin North Am 1996; 4:327-359.
Boxt LM. Magnetic resonance and computed tomographic evaluation of congenital heart disease. J Magn Reson Imaging 2004; 18:827-847.
Boxt LM, Rozenshtein AR. MR imaging of congenital heart disease. Magn Reson Imaging Clin North Am 2003; 11:27-48.
Fayad LM, Boxt LM. Chest film diagnosis of congenital heart disease. Semin Roentgenol 1999; 34:228-248.
Hagler DJ, Edwards WD, Seward JB, et al. Standardized nomenclature of the ventricular septum and ventricular septal defects, with applications for two-dimensional echocardiography. Mayo Clin Proc 1985; 60:741-752.
Minette MS, Sahn DJ. Ventricular septal defects. Circulation 2006; 114:2190-2197.
Moodie DS. Diagnosis and management of congenital heart disease in the adult. Cardiol Rev 2001; 9:276-281.
Soto B, Becker AE, Moulaert AJ, et al. Classification of ventricular septal defects. Br Heart J 1980; 43:332-343.
Wang ZJ, Reddy GP, Gotway MB, et al. Cardiovascular shunts: MR imaging evaluation. RadioGraphics 2003; 23(Spec No):S181-S194.

REFERENCES

1. Minette MS, Sahn DJ. Ventricular septal defects. Circulation 2006; 114:2190-2197.
2. Kanter KR. Management of infants with coarctation and ventricular septal defect. Semin Thorac Cardiovasc Surg 2007; 19:264-268.
3. Soto B, Bargeron LM Jr, Diethelm E. Ventricular septal defect. Semin Roentgenol 1985; 20:200-213.
4. Moodie DS. Diagnosis and management of congenital heart disease in the adult. Cardiol Rev 2001; 9:276-281.
5. Ammash NM, Warnes CA. Ventricular septal defects in adults. Ann Intern Med 2001; 135:812-824.
6. Ferencz C, Correa Villasenor A. Epidemiology of cardiovascular malformations: the state of the art. Cardiol Young 1991; 1:264-284.
7. Lewis DA, Loffredo CA, Correa-Villasenor A, et al. Descriptive epidemiology of membranous and muscular ventricular septal defects in the Baltimore-Washington Infant Study. Cardiol Young 1996; 6:281-290.
8. Tweddell JS, Pelech AN, Frommelt PC. Ventricular septal defect and aortic valve regurgitation: pathophysiology and indications for surgery. Semin Thorac Cardiovasc Surg Pediatr Card Surg Annu 2006; 147-152.

9. Helmcke F, de Souza A, Nanda NC, et al. Two-dimensional and color Doppler assessment of ventricular septal defect of congenital origin. Am J Cardiol 1989; 63:1112-1116.
10. Miller-Hance WC, Silverman NH. Transesophageal echocardiography (TEE) in congenital heart disease with focus on the adult. Cardiol Clin 2000; 18:861-892.
11. Sutherland GR, Godman MJ, Smallhorn JF, et al. Ventricular septal defects: two dimensional echocardiographic and morphological correlations. Br Heart J 1982; 47:316-328.
12. Schad N, Stark P. The radiologic features of cardiac rotation: a pictorial essay. J Thorac Imaging 1992; 3:81-87.
13. Berthaux XA, Brenot P, Angel C, et al. Multirow detector computed tomography assessment of intraseptal dissection and ventricular pseudoaneurysm in postinfarction ventricular septal defect. Circulation 2001; 104:497-498.
14. Romaguera R, Paya R, Ridocci F, et al. Ventricular septal defect as casual finding in non-invasive CT-angiography. Eur Heart J 2008; 29:1438.
15. Wang ZJ, Reddy GP, Gotway MB, et al. Cardiovascular shunts: MR imaging evaluation. RadioGraphics 2003; 23(Spec No):S181-S194.
16. Didier D, Higgins CB. Identification and localization of ventricular septal defect by gated magnetic resonance imaging. Am J Cardiol 1986; 57:1363-1368.
17. Brenner LD, Caputo GR, Mostbeck G, et al. Quantification of left to right atrial shunts with velocity-encoded cine nuclear magnetic resonance imaging. J Am Coll Cardiol 1992; 20:1246-1250.
18. Jimenez-Angeles L, Medina-Banuelos V, Valdes-Cristerna R, et al. Analysis of ventricular contraction by factorial phase imaging with equilibrium radionuclide angiography. Conf Proc IEEE Eng Med Biol Soc 2006; 1:1081-1084.
19. Chin BB, Metzler SD, Lemaire A, et al. Left ventricular functional assessment in mice: feasibility of high spatial and temporal resolution ECG-gated blood pool SPECT. Radiology 2007; 245:440-448.
20. Sharir T. Gated myocardial perfusion imaging for the assessment of left ventricular function and volume: from SPECT to PET. J Nucl Cardiol 2007; 14:631-633.

CHAPTER 43

Patent Ductus Arteriosus

Cylen Javidan-Nejad

Patent ductus arteriosus (PDA) is defined as incomplete closure and patency of the ductus arteriosus beyond functional closure after birth. The ductus arteriosus is a vessel that extends from the anterolateral aspect of the descending thoracic aorta to the superior aspect of the main pulmonary artery, close to the origin of the left pulmonary artery. Embryologically, it is a remnant of the distal left sixth aortic arch. A normal and vital structure in the fetus, it is necessary for diverting blood flow from the main pulmonary artery to the aorta, thereby bypassing the high-resistance pulmonary circulation.[1] This diversion is crucial to normal development of the right ventricle and results in passage of only 10% of the right ventricular cardiac output through the lungs. Premature closure of the ductus arteriosus in the fetus, as seen with maternal use of non-steroidal anti-inflammatory drugs (NSAIDs), leads to right ventricular failure and fetal hydrops (Fig. 43-1).[2]

The duct functionally closes in the first 18 hours of life in full-term healthy infants. However, it fully closes several weeks later, after which it is unable to regain its patency. In premature infants, patency can be seen up to 10 days after birth.[3,4] Some consider the patency abnormal only after 3 months of age. The patency causes a left to right shunt that increases pulmonary blood flow at the expense of systemic flow.[5] If untreated, based on the size of the PDA, pulmonary hypertension and Eisenmenger syndrome develop in children and adults (Fig. 43-2).[1]

MECHANISM OF PHYSIOLOGIC CLOSURE

Histologically, the wall of the ductus arteriosus is composed of the same three layers as those of the aorta or main pulmonary artery—the intima, media, and adventitia. The media of the ductus arteriosus is different in that the smooth muscle fibers have a spiral and longitudinal orientation, instead of a concentric one, as seen in the aorta and pulmonary artery.[1]

Relative low oxygen tension and high levels of prostaglandin E_2 (PGE_2) and prostacyclin (PGI_2), produced by the placenta, are responsible for the continued patency of the ductus arteriosus in the fetus. PGE_2 and PGI_2 interact with specific receptors in the smooth muscle layer of the media, leading to vasodilation.[6]

The process of closure begins at birth. The sudden increase of oxygen tension leads to influx of calcium and thereby muscle contraction in the smooth muscles of the media. Because of the metabolic breakdown of prostaglandins by the newly functioning lung and the absence of the placenta, the PGE_2 and PGI_2 levels fall, diminishing their vasodilation effect. Smooth muscle contraction in the ductus arteriosus wall shortens the ductus and causes luminal occlusion. In the following weeks, fibrosis ensues, leading to permanent sealing.[1,6] Perinatal hypoxia impedes the natural closure process. Pharmacologic treatment of PDA is based on muscular constriction in the middle of the ductus, leading to segmental ischemia and fibrosis.[3,6]

PREVALENCE AND EPIDEMIOLOGY

PDA can be isolate or part of a complex cardiac malformation.[7] The overall incidence in children born at term is 0.02% to 0.08%, which accounts for approximately 10% of all congenital heart disease. Most cases are sporadic. It is more common in premature and term infants with maternal rubella infection in the first trimester of pregnancy. Maternal use of amphetamine and phenytoin and fetal alcohol syndrome are also associated with PDA.[8] PDA is more frequent in certain genetic syndromes such as trisomy 21, trisomy 18, 4p– syndrome, Holt-Oram syndrome, Carpenter syndrome, and Char syndrome.[1,9]

The cause of isolated cases is unknown. The underlying cause of PDA in the setting of maternal rubella and genetic syndromes is structural abnormality of the ductus hindering normal closure after birth. The mechanism of PDA in infants born prematurely or infants who have experienced perinatal hypoxia is most likely physiologic factors impeding the normal constriction of the ductus arteriosus.

PDA is twice as common in females when it is isolated and sporadic; however, if associated with prematurity or prenatal infection, the frequency is equal between the genders.[9] A study by Mangones and colleagues,[10] which compared the prevalence of various congenital cardiovascular malformations by race and ethnicity, showed no racial preference for isolated PDA and an overall less frequency of congenital cardiac malformations in Hispanics. However, a previous study by Chavez and associates[11] described an increased prevalence of isolate PDA in African Americans.

ETIOLOGY AND PATHOPHYSIOLOGY

The magnitude of left to right shunting depends on the flow resistance of the ductus arteriosus and the pressure gradient between the aorta and pulmonary artery. The flow resistance depends mainly on the diameter and length of the narrowest portion of the ductus arteriosus. The pressure gradient between the two ends of the PDA depends on the pulmonary and systemic vascular resistance and the cardiac output. The larger the diameter of the narrowest portion of the ductus, the greater the impact of changes in the systemic and pulmonary resistance on the pressure gradient and, therefore, on the magnitude of shunting. If the narrow portion is small in caliber, thereby a restrictive shunt, then the length of the narrow portion is important. A longer length of the ductus is associated with a smaller magnitude of shunting.[1,6,8]

The left to right shunt causes overcirculation and fluid overload of the pulmonary bed, which lead to decreased lung compliance and increased work of breathing. The shunting also causes left heart volume overload and, if the ductus is moderate to large in size, the increased left atrial and left ventricular end-diastolic pressures can eventually lead to hypertrophy of the left ventricle. The wall tension of the hypertrophied left ventricle causes catecholamine release, which results in tachycardia and therefore a shorter diastolic time. On the other hand, the diastolic blood pressure of the aorta decreases because of blood passage through the ductus during diastole. This decreased diastolic pressure and shorter diastolic time causes decreased coronary perfusion and, when combined with increased myocardial tension and oxygen demand, may result in subendocardial ischemia, which can be detected by elevated troponin levels.[12]

When the pulmonary arteries are subjected to long-standing increased flow and high pressure, microvascular injury develops, which leads to intimal proliferation and arteriolar medial hypertrophy. This eventually causes fibrosis and obliteration of the pulmonary arterioles and capillaries, and pulmonary arterial hypertension ensues. As the pulmonary vascular resistance gradually increases and approaches or exceeds the systemic vascular resistance, ductal shunting reverses and becomes right to left. This is called Eisenmenger syndrome.[1,6,8]

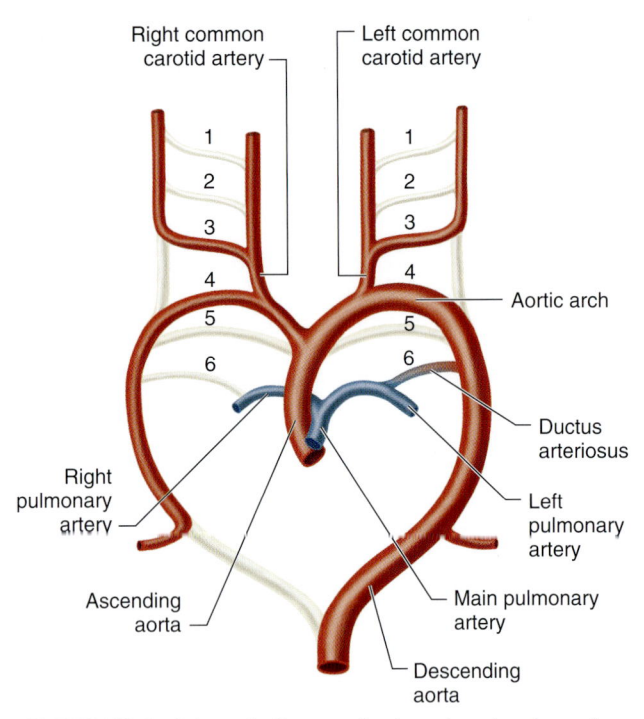

■ **FIGURE 43-1** Schematic diagram of embryonic arches shows that the ductus arteriosus arises from the distal aspect of the sixth embryonic arch. The *solid lines* display the embryonic arches from vasculature seen in normal newborns. The *thinner lines* refer to embryonic arches that eventually regress.

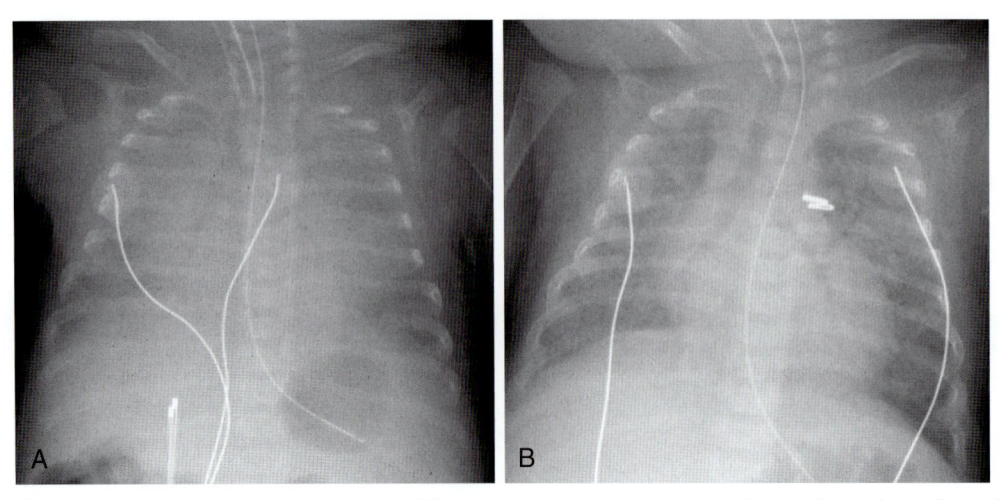

■ **FIGURE 43-2** Chest radiograph of newborn with respiratory failure and a large ductus arteriosus diagnosed on echocardiography. **A,** The child is intubated and on a respirator and there is diffuse pulmonary edema. **B,** Chest radiograph taken the same day after clipping the ductus arteriosus shows immediate improvement of the pulmonary edema. The child was extubated shortly afterward, with good spontaneous breathing.

Clinical Features

Age of clinical presentation and presence of and type of symptoms at the time of presentation depend on the size of the PDA and pulmonary vascular resistance. The clinical presentation can vary from no symptoms, where the shunt is diagnosed incidentally, to congestive heart failure and Eisenmenger syndrome. Many patients have exercise intolerance or the diagnosis of reactive airway disease.[1,8,13] Most patients compensate well, even with a moderate left to right shunt and remain asymptomatic during childhood. A well-tolerated PDA can become clinically significant when combined with effects of acquired conditions such as ischemic heart disease or calcific aortic stenosis. The hallmark physical finding is a machinery murmur, which is a continuous murmur detected at the left upper sternal border. If the shunt is moderate or large, the left ventricular impulse will be prominent and laterally displaced and the pulse pressure will be increased, resulting in a bounding peripheral pulse.

Eisenmenger syndrome presents with cyanosis and clubbing that may spare the fingers because the right to left shunting is distal to the subclavian arteries. This cyanosis may be more profound when systemic vascular resistance is decreased, such as after exercise or hot weather. On auscultation, there may be no murmur, a high-frequency diastolic decrescendo murmur of pulmonary regurgitation, and/or a holosystolic murmur from tricuspid valve regurgitation. Peripheral edema is a late manifestation caused by right ventricular dysfunction.[14,15]

MANIFESTATIONS OF DISEASE

Clinical Presentation

Grading

In adults, PDA is usually isolated and discovered incidentally on physical examination or during echocardiography screening. Grading of PDA is based on a combination of echocardiographic findings, physical findings on auscultation and examination, and presenting symptoms. In adults, PDA is categorized as four grades—silent, small, moderate, and large. A silent PDA is usually incidentally diagnosed on echocardiography. The patient is asymptomatic and has no audible heart murmur. A small PDA is associated with an audible continuous murmur in the left upper sternal border that radiates to the back. The patient has normal peripheral pulses and no pulmonary hypertension. In moderate PDA, there is an audible continuous murmur, wide, bouncy peripheral pulses caused by aortic regurgitation, and runoff of blood during diastole by the shunt. The left atrium and left ventricle are enlarged; the PDA is associated with pulmonary hypertension that is commonly reversible. A PDA is graded as large when signs of pulmonary hypertension have developed. The typical continuous murmur is absent. Differential cyanosis, in which the oxygen saturation of the feet is lower than that of the right arm, is typically seen. Grade 4 patients are mostly adults with Eisenmenger syndrome.[14,15]

Complications

The complications of PDA usually present in adulthood, when congestive heart failure presents in the third decade of life. This is caused by chronic left heart volume overload. Heart failure is associated with atrial flutter or fibrillation and is caused by left atrial dilation. This may be the first sign in these patients. Pulmonary hypertension or Eisenmenger syndrome is a manifestation of irreversible pulmonary vascular disease, seen with moderate and large PDA.[1,14,16]

Infective endarteritis is a significant health issue in countries where there are lower standards of health, inadequate oral hygiene, and less widespread antibiotic use. When endoarteritis develops, it occurs at the pulmonary end of the shunt, which can cause bland and septic emboli to the lungs. No systemic embolization occurs.[15,16]

The left recurrent laryngeal nerve passes in the triangular space created by the main pulmonary artery, aortic arch, and PDA. When pulmonary hypertension develops, the pulmonary artery becomes enlarged and this space narrows, which may cause impingement of the recurrent laryngeal nerve and development of unilateral vocal cord paralysis and hoarseness. This is a rare complication.[1]

Imaging Technique and Findings

Ultrasound

The diagnostic modality of choice for PDA is generally echocardiography, in which color Doppler is used to detect a PDA and used to estimate the degree of shunting. Gray-scale and M-mode echocardiography are useful for visualizing the geometry of the ductus, calculating left atrium and ventricle sizes, and quantifying the left ventricle systolic function. If Eisenmenger syndrome is present, there is a low-velocity right to left shunting, which is difficult to detect, even by color Doppler. In this case, secondary signs of septal flattening, right ventricular hypertrophy, and high-velocity pulmonary regurgitation are the findings that warrant a search for a PDA (Fig. 43-3).[1,15]

Radiography

On standard chest radiography, PDA only becomes evident when there is a moderate PDA. The left atrium and left ventricle are enlarged. In infants and children with a moderate or large PDA, shunt vascularity is seen. In patients who have Eisenmenger syndrome, the central pulmonary arteries are enlarged and there is peripheral pruning of the pulmonary arteries. In older patients, a calcification in the aortopulmonary window indicates a calcified ductus arteriosus or PDA. In such patients, the aorta may be enlarged because of the chronic right to left shunt (Fig. 43-4).[17]

Computed Tomography

Computed tomography angiography (CTA) is useful for demonstrating the PDA, especially when it is not detectable on echocardiography, but is suspected. CTA also helps in characterizing the morphology of PDA and determining whether it is calcified, both important factors in treatment planning. Other associated vascular anomalies, such as a vascular ring or the presence of other associated congenital heart disease, can be detected by CTA. Multidetector CT (MDCT) involves faster imaging with a smaller contrast bolus, allowing increased use of this modality in the assessment of mediastinal vascular anomalies and acquired disease. The quick scanning results in fewer motion artifacts and the ability to evaluate children and older patients. The higher spatial resolution and presence of multiple rows of detectors along the longitudinal axis of the patient allow better multiplanar-reformatted and surface-shaded three-dimensional images to be created. These are most useful for quickly displaying the anatomy of the vascular abnormality and its relationship with adjacent structures. The ease of use of MDCT and its excellent depiction of anatomy has rendered CTA a common first means of evaluating for vascular anomalies in the thorax. The disadvantage of CTA is the use of intravenous iodinated contrast, contraindicated for patients with renal failure and for those who are allergic to intravenous contrast (Fig. 43-5).[17-19]

Magnetic Resonance Imaging

Magnetic resonance imaging has the advantage of providing both anatomic and functional information without the use of ionizing radiation. Flow quantification across the PDA allows one to assess the direction of flow in addition to quantifying the velocity of flow across the ductus arteriosus. The shunt ratio can be quantified by comparing the flow across the pulmonary and aortic valves. MR angiography (MRA) also provides information about flow direction, presence of collateral vasculature, and the presence of a PDA and other vascular anomalies. The disadvantage of MRI and MRA is the inability to use them in patients with pacemakers, the need for sedation in infants and small children, the decreased sensitivity in depicting calcifications, and the long scanning time (Fig. 43-6).[17,20]

On both CT and MRI, PDA is seen as a tubular connection arising on the undersurface of the aortic arch, approximately 5 to 10 mm distal to the origin of the left subclavian artery.[19] It connects to the superior surface of the main pulmonary artery, close to the origin of the left pulmonary artery.[17] It is variable in length and shape; some are straight and some are tortuous (Fig. 43-7).[19] If the timing of imaging is optimized on CTA to opacify the pulmonary arteries, the left to right shunt can appear as negative contrast of nonopacified blood on the superior surface of the main pulmonary artery. On cine MRI, a signal void in the main pulmonary artery at the origin of the left pulmonary artery suggests the presence of a PDA. Three-dimensional MRA

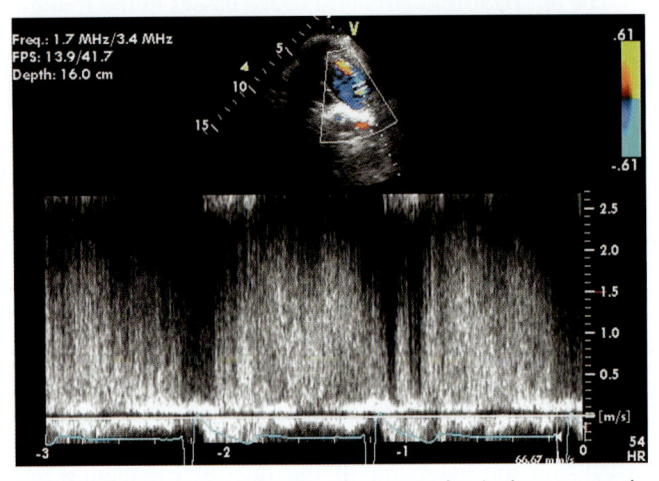

■ **FIGURE 43-3** Pulsed wave Doppler image taken in the parasternal short-axis view at the level of the main pulmonary artery. This demonstrates continuous flow during systole and diastole toward the pulmonic valve, consistent with a PDA.

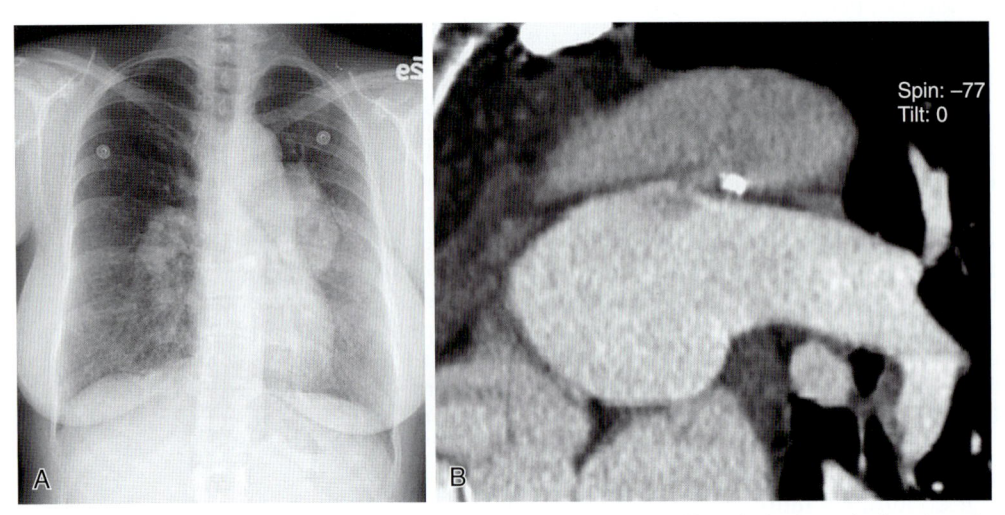

■ **FIGURE 43-4** Frontal chest radiograph of an adult who presented with chronic shortness of breath shows markedly enlarged pulmonary arteries and mild asymmetric pulmonary edema favoring the lower lungs. **A**, A linear calcification in the aortopulmonary window is a calcified PDA. This oblique CTA sagittal reformatted image of the chest shows calcification on the aortic side of the funnel-shaped PDA. **B**, Because scanning was performed during peak pulmonary arterial enhancement, the left to right shunting is depicted as a jet of contrast from the aorta. The pulmonary artery is seen as a blush of nonopacified blood (negative jet) in the opacified main pulmonary artery, close to the PDA.

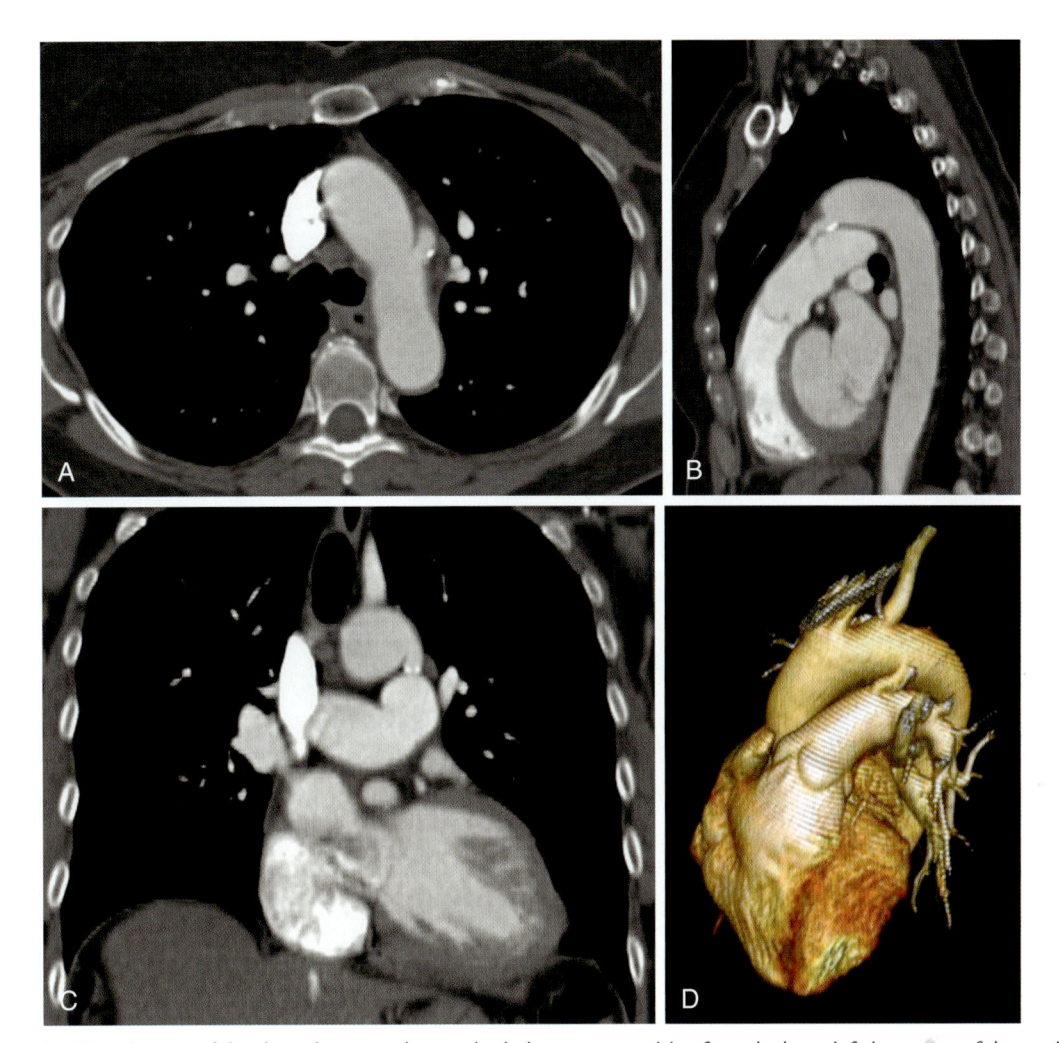

FIGURE 43-5 **A,** CT angiogram of the chest shows an abnormal tubular structure arising from the lateroinferior aspect of the aortic arch, representing a PDA. **B,** Oblique sagittal reformatted image well demonstrates the entire length of this partially calcified PDA. **C,** Coronal reformatted image can also display the course and caliber of the PDA. **D,** Volume rendered surface-shaded image of the heart and great vessels depicts the relationship of the PDA with the aorta and main pulmonary artery.

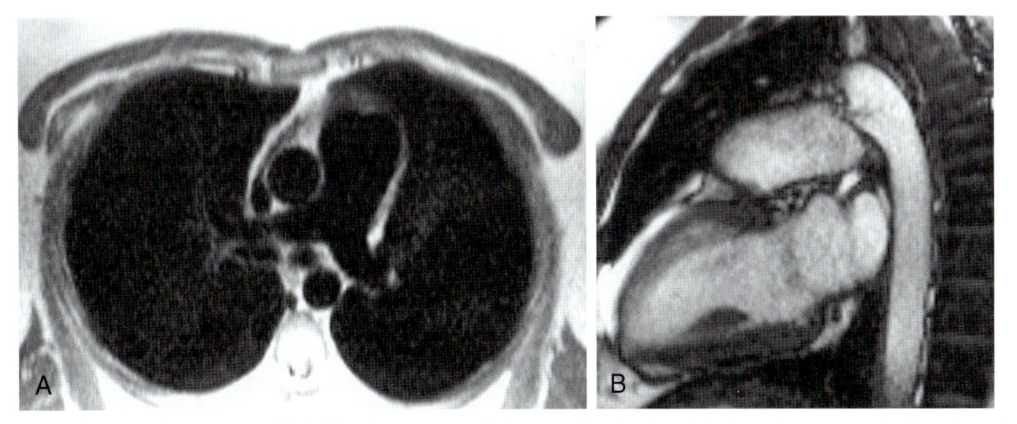

FIGURE 43-6 **A,** Double-inversion recovery black blood sequence MR image taken in the axial plane shows a markedly enlarged main pulmonary artery suggestive of pulmonary hypertension. **B,** This oblique sagittal cine balanced steady-state free precession (bSSFP) MR image of the aorta during systole shows a funnel-shaped PDA and a linear dephasing jet in the aorta, at the origin of the PDA. This is indicative of Eisenmenger physiology, in which supersystemic pulmonary arterial pressure causes right to left shunting.

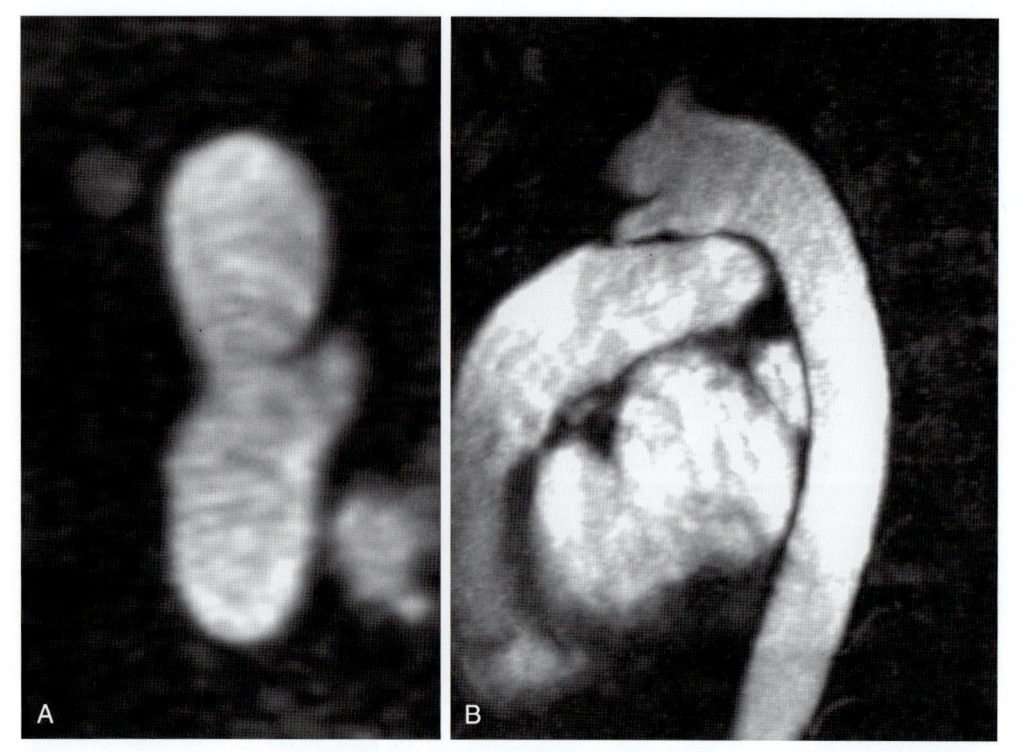

FIGURE 43-7 Maximum intensity projection (MIP) of MRA of the chest in axial **(A)** and oblique sagittal **(B)** projections display a large PDA in a 60-year-old woman who presented with atrial fibrillation.

in an oblique sagittal plane can reveal the ductus origin of the dephasing jet (Fig. 43-8).[17-19]

DIFFERENTIAL DIAGNOSIS
From Clinical Presentation
Aortopulmonary Window

Aortopulmonary window is a rare lesion in which there is a broad-based direct communication between the ascending aorta and pulmonary artery. It is caused by incomplete division of the embryonic common trunk. Clinically, it simulates the symptoms of PDA and radiographically it causes increased pulmonary vascularity on the chest radiographs of newborns who are acyanotic. With imaging, this entity can be distinguished from PDA by its location; the aortopulmonary window involves the ascending aorta and in PDA, it involves the proximal descending aorta at the isthmus.[15,21]

From Imaging Findings
Other Vascular Entities at the Aortic Isthmus

The differential diagnosis of PDA is composed of vascular lesions at the aortic isthmus, the point where the aortic arch joins the descending aorta (Fig. 43-9).[22] These include aortic spindle, ductus diverticulum, ductus aneurysm, diverticulum of Kommerell, traumatic pseudoaneurysm, atherosclerotic aneurysms and penetrating atherosclerotic ulcers, and mycotic or infectious pseudoaneurysms.

Aorta Spindle or Ductus Bump

Aortic spindle or ductus bump is a normal variant in which there is dilation of the descending thoracic aorta, just distal to the isthmus. It involves the aorta circumferentially and is smooth in outline. In newborns, such dilation is more prevalent when there is a normal decreased caliber of the aorta between the origins of the left subclavian artery and the ductus arteriosus, and dilation of the descending aorta distal to it. With closure of the ductus arteriosus and increased flow through the aortic arch, the narrowing of the isthmus resolves and this configuration usually disappears.[23] In adults, its frequency has been reported to be approximately 16% in adults and a ductus bump may be more prominent in older patients (Fig. 43-10).[24]

Ductus Diverticulum

Ductus diverticulum is defined as a focal convexity along the anterior undersurface of the isthmic region of the aortic arch, where the ligamentum arteriosum exists. Its frequency has been reported to be as high as 26%.[24] There are two theories about its origin. The first is that it is a remnant of the closed ductus arteriosus, where the unfused, nonatretic aortic end of the ductus creates the ductus diverticulum. The other theory is that it is a remnant of the right dorsal root.[25] The ductus diverticulum typically has gentle obtuse angles at its junction with the aortic wall and has smooth contours with symmetric shoulders as it gently slopes from the anteroinferior aorta. In a study of 200 normal aortograms, in which 51 ductus diverticula were found, Morse and coworkers[24] reported

CHAPTER 43 • *Patent Ductus Arteriosus* 589

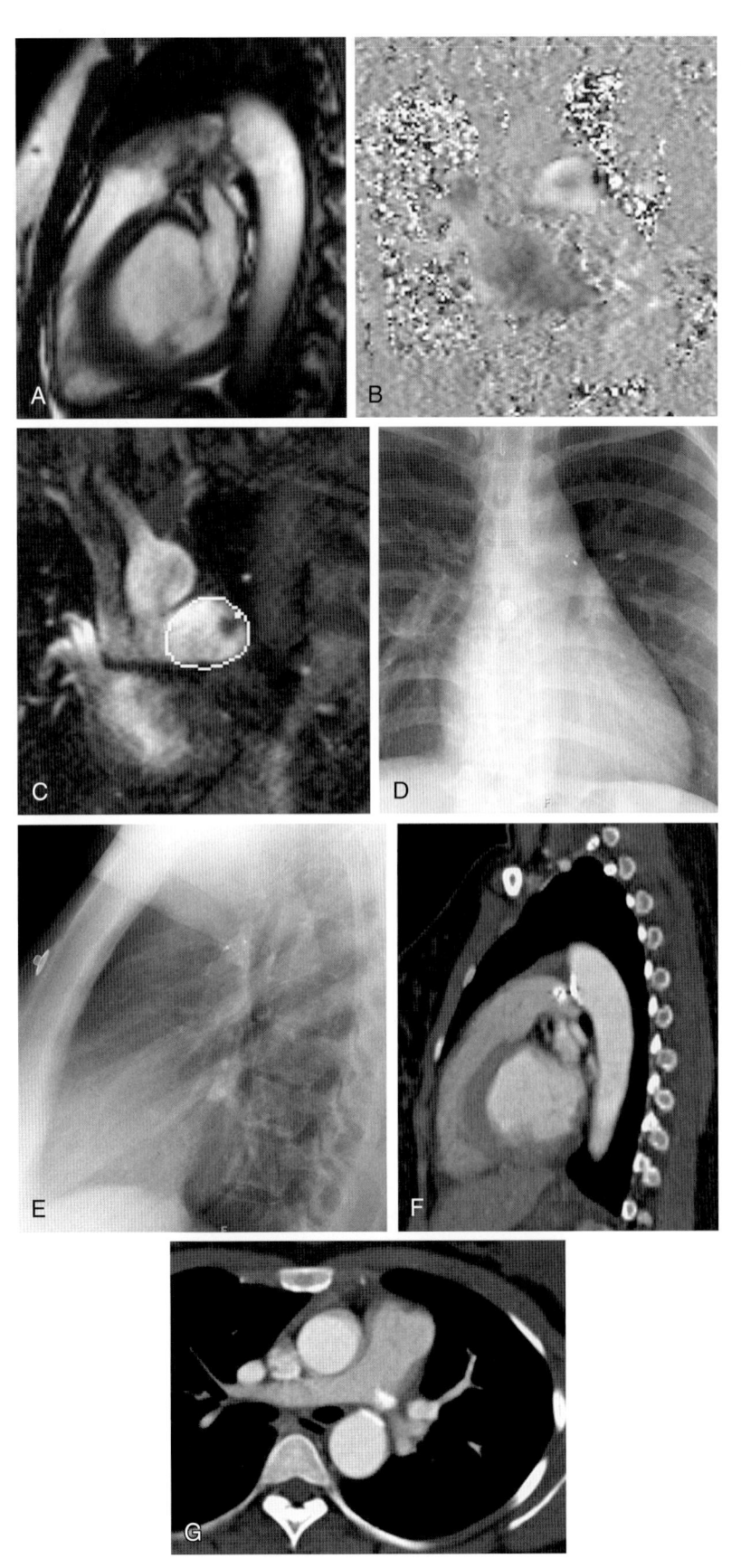

■ **FIGURE 43-8** A 29-year-old asymptomatic woman was found to have a cardiac murmur during a routine physical examination when she was pregnant. Echocardiography showed a PDA and mild left ventricular enlargement. MRI of the heart was performed to evaluate the anatomy further. **A,** Oblique sagittal balanced steady-state free precession (SSFP) images at the level of the main pulmonary artery show a dephasing jet directed from the aorta to the main pulmonary artery, consistent with a PDA with left to right shunting. There is a cloudlike area of low signal in the inferior aspect of the main pulmonary artery; there is an area of turbulence where the high-velocity jet is directed anteriorly and meets the normal flow of the main pulmonary artery, directed posteriorly. **B,** Phase-encoded MRI is used to assess the flow across the main pulmonary artery. **C,** Using this technique, while drawing a region of interest on magnitude images obtained simultaneously in the same plane, the peak velocity of the shunt and magnitude of flow across the main pulmonary artery can be assessed. The latter is compared with the flow across the proximal descending aorta to determine the degree of shunting. Several months after delivery, the patient underwent percutaneous closure of the PDA by an Amplatzer device. Frontal **(D)** and lateral **(E)** radiographs of the chest and oblique sagittal reformatted **(F)** and transaxial thick MIP **(G)** CTA images of the thorax demonstrate the Amplatzer device.

590 PART FIVE • *Congenital Heart Disease*

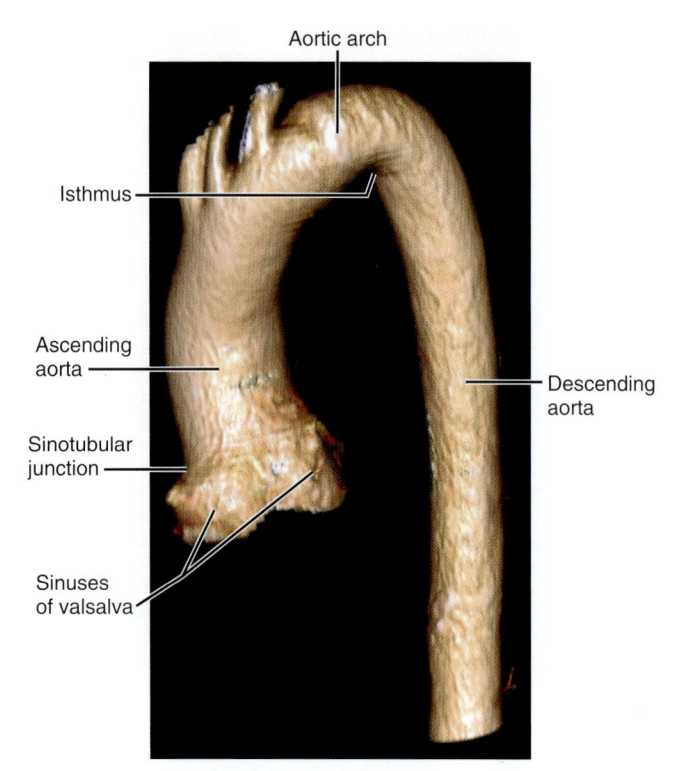

■ FIGURE 43-9 CTA volume rendered surface-shaded image of a normal aorta. The different segments of the aorta are delineated.

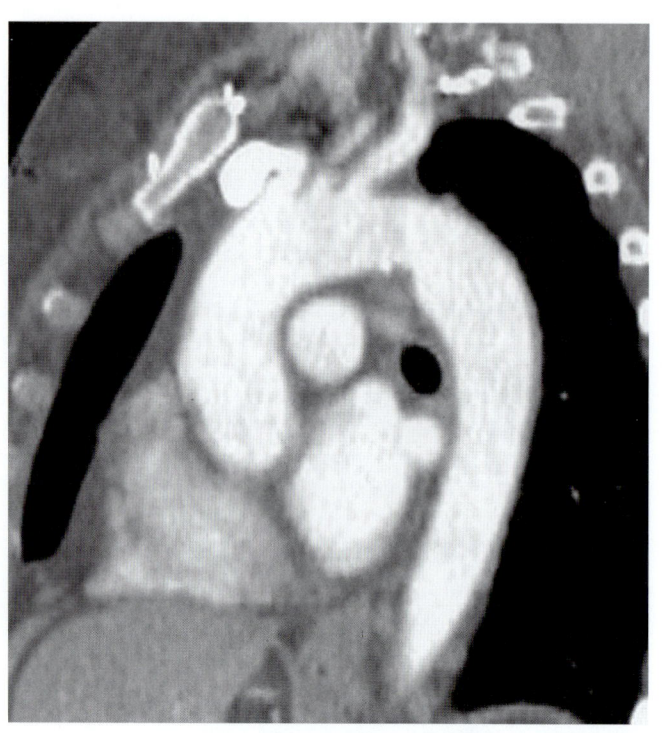

■ FIGURE 43-10 This oblique sagittal reformatted image of the aorta shows a fusiform mild dilation of the proximal descending aorta, immediately beyond the isthmus.

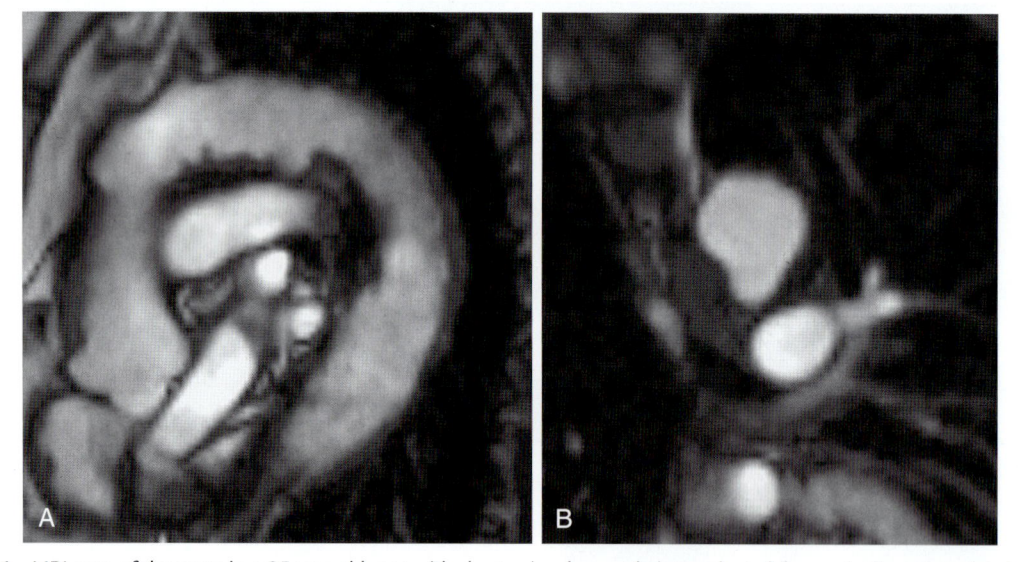

■ FIGURE 43-11 MRI scan of the aorta in a 35-year-old man with chest pain who was being evaluated for aortic dissection. A balanced steady-state free precession (bSSFP) MR sequence in the oblique sagittal **(A)** and coronal **(B)** planes shows a focal bulge along the inferior aspect of the distal aortic arch, in the region of the isthmus. This is a ductus diverticulum that was diagnosed incidentally.

that the inferior angle of the ductus diverticulum is always obtuse, but in 2% of cases the superior angle is acute. In that study, 75% of the diverticula had an anteromedial location and 25% had an anterolateral location. The main differential diagnosis of this entity is post-traumatic pseudoaneurysm, which is differentiated from a ductus diverticulum by its irregular contour and the acute angles it creates where it meets the anteroinferior aorta (Fig. 43-11).

Ductus Aneurysm

Ductal aneurysm is defined as saclike dilation of the ductus arteriosus in the absence of PDA. It is a rare lesion that

CHAPTER 43 • Patent Ductus Arteriosus   591

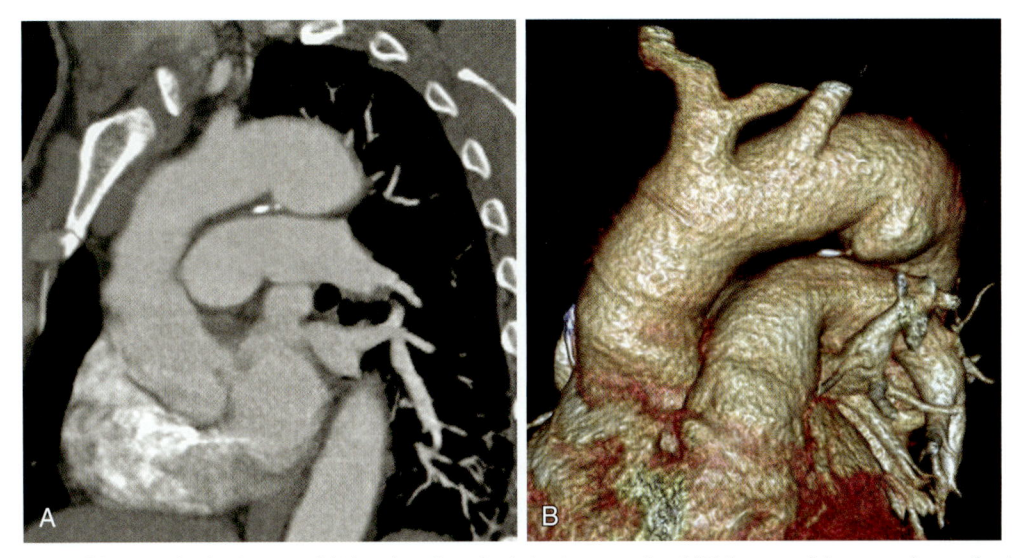

■ **FIGURE 43-12** CTA oblique sagittal reformatted **(A)** and surface-shaded volume rendered **(B)** images of the aorta show a focal aneurysm arising from the left inferolateral aspect of the distal aortic arch. This aneurysm connects to a calcified ductus arteriosus inferomedially.

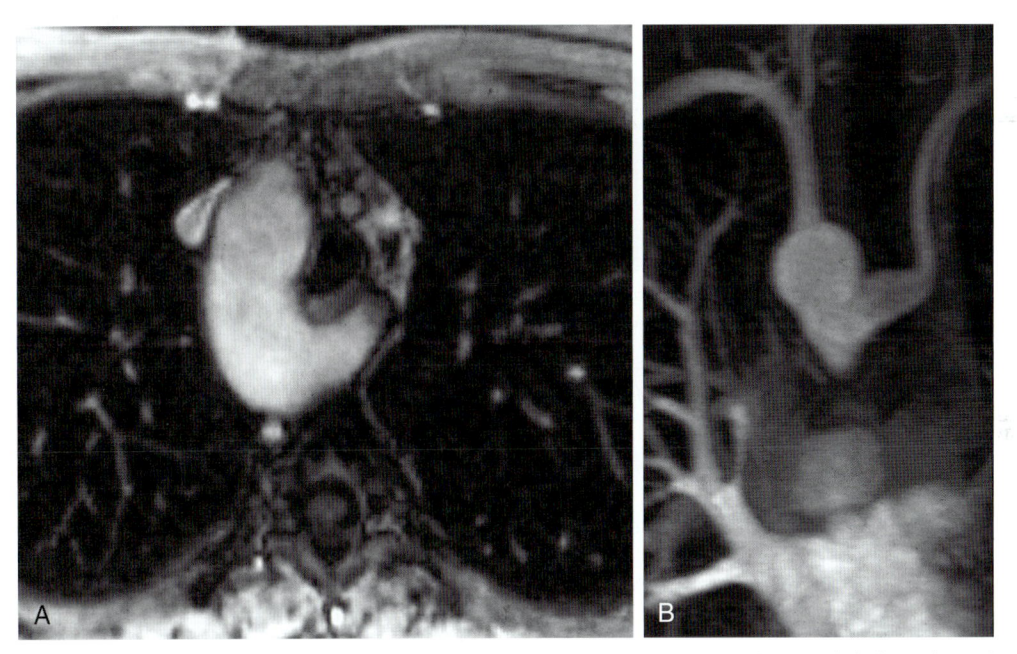

■ **FIGURE 43-13** Transaxial contrast-enhanced MRA images of the chest at the level of the aortic arch **(A)** and thick maximum intensity projection of the aorta in the coronal plane **(B)** show a right aortic arch and an aberrant left subclavian artery arising from the superolateral aspect of the proximal descending aorta and traveling posterior to the esophagus. There is an elongated focal dilation at the origin of the left subclavian artery, representing a diverticulum. This is the mirror image version of a diverticulum of Kommerell.

usually occurs spontaneously. It can sometimes occur after surgical repair of PDA. It is usually diagnosed in infancy because of its complications, when it could cause compression of the esophagus, bronchi, pulmonary arteries, or recurrent laryngeal nerve, thromboembolism, infection, and rupture.[26] In cases in which the aneurysm has developed spontaneously, the complication rate has been reported to be 31% in infants younger than 2 months old, 66% in infants and children between the ages of 2 months and 15 years, and 47% in adults. The complication rate is much greater when the aneurysm has developed after PDA repair, resulting in death in more than 90% of cases because of infection and rupture, when giant ductal aneurysms can be associated with aortic wall thinning. Prompt surgical resection of all ductal aneurysms should be considered to avoid potentially fatal complications (Fig. 43-12).[27]

Aneurysmal Original of Anomalous Right Subclavian Artery (Diverticulum of Kommerell)

Diverticulum of Kommerell is an ectatic infundibulum at the origin of an aberrant right subclavian artery. It is a remnant of the left dorsal aortic root. It arises along the lateral aspect of the distal aortic arch or proximal descending thoracic aorta and connects to the subclavian artery,

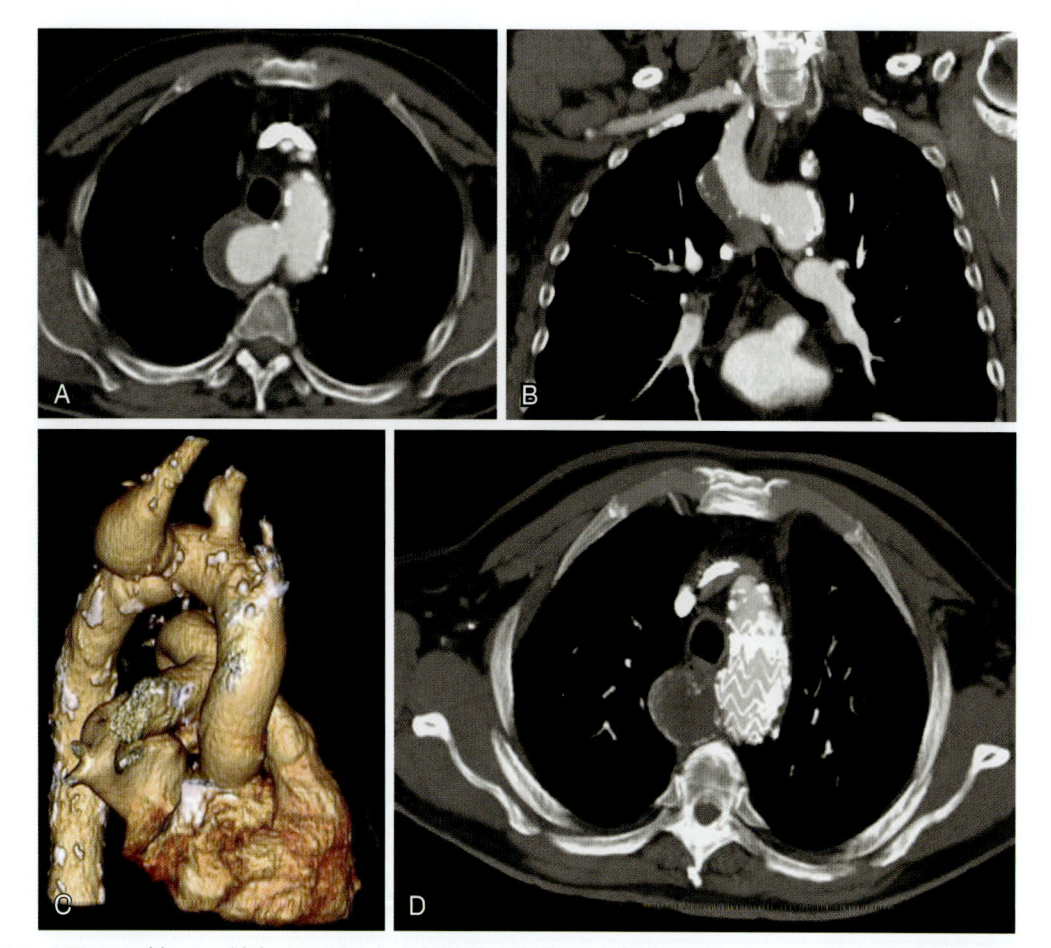

FIGURE 43-14 A 73-year-old man with known extensive atherosclerotic disease of the aorta underwent CTA to evaluate aneurysms of the descending thoracic and abdominal aorta. **A,** He was incidentally found to have a large, partially thrombosed aneurysm of the diverticulum of Kommerell. **B,** The right subclavian artery had connections to this aneurysm and has normal flow, best demonstrated on the coronal reformatted view. **C,** This surface-shaded volume rendered image also shows the large aneurysm arising from the right supralateral aspect of the distal aortic arch, close to the isthmus. The patient was treated by endovascular grafting. **D,** Subsequent CTA image of the aorta shows that the aneurysm has completely thrombosed.

differentiating it from a PDA, which arises from the anteroinferior aspect of the isthmus of the aorta (Fig. 43-13). This diverticulum can become aneurysmal and atherosclerotic, especially in older adults, causing mass effect on the posterior wall of the trachea and esophagus and causing difficulty swallowing, called dysphagia lusoria (Fig. 43-14).[18,22,28]

Traumatic Aortic Injury

Blunt chest trauma can cause acute aortic injury, which is commonly located at the aortic isthmus, because of the shearing injury to the aorta caused by its relative fixation by the ligamentum arteriosum. In most cases, traumatic aortic injury results in immediate mortality. Survival of those who have undergone imaging is mostly because of incomplete rupture of the layers of the aortic wall, where the aortic rupture is contained by the adventitia or periadventitial tissues. On cross-sectional imaging and aortography, a focal saccular aneurysm with a narrow neck is seen, usually located medially at the aortic isthmus. This pseudoaneurysm has an irregular shape and margin, creating acute angles with the wall of the aorta. Mediastinal hematoma and fat stranding, in addition to abnormal aortic contour and intimal flaps, are noted on CT and MRI. A pseudocoarctation in which there is abrupt tapering of the diameter of the descending aorta may occur (Fig. 43-15).[22,24]

Approximately 2.5% of patients who survive the initial trauma develop chronic pseudoaneurysms. These are usually detected incidentally, have rim calcifications and eccentric thrombus, and are located along the inferior aortic arch, at the isthmus. Because of risk of progressive enlargement and rupture, surgical treatment is a consideration (Fig. 43-16).[25]

Nontraumatic Aneurysm and Pseudoaneurysm

Other causes of aneurysm and pseudoaneurysms of the aorta at the isthmus and distal arch include penetrating atherosclerotic ulcers, mycotic aneurysm caused by invasion of the aorta by mediastinal neoplasm, and infectious aneurysms.

A penetrating atherosclerotic ulcer is caused by erosion of the aortic intima by an ulcerated atheromatous plaque, resulting in a hematoma in the media layer of the aortic

CHAPTER 43 • Patent Ductus Arteriosus 593

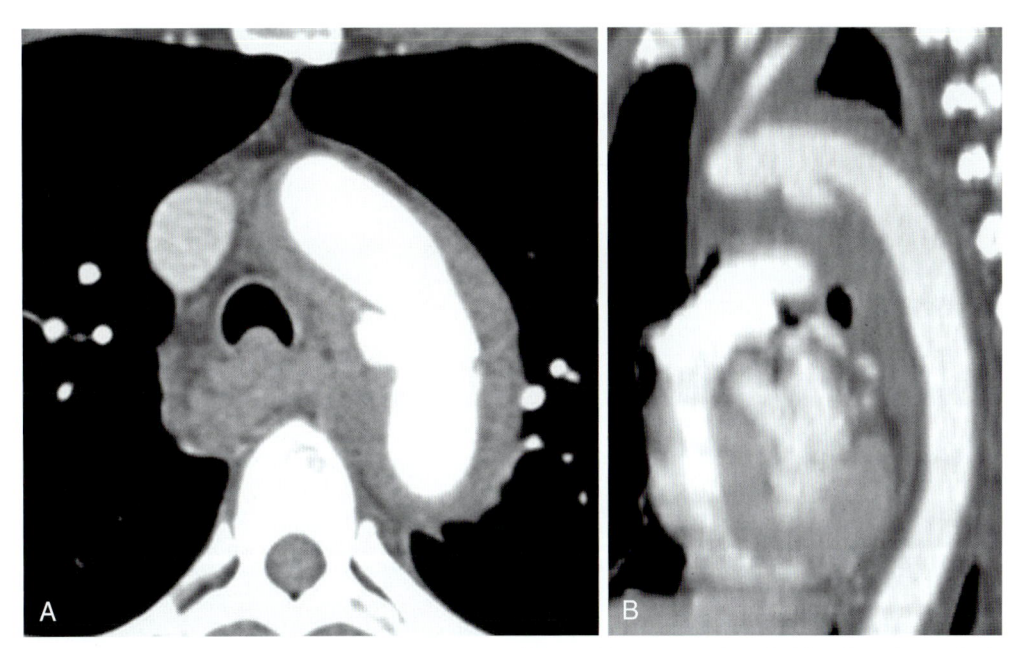

■ **FIGURE 43-15** This young man, who was involved in a severe motor vehicle accident, was evaluated with a thoracic CTA in the emergency department. The transaxial CT image of the chest at the level of the aortic arch (**A**) and sagittal reformatted CTA image (**B**) display a focal bulge located at the aortic isthmus, directed medially and inferiorly. Extensive hemorrhage surrounding the aorta confirms that this is acute aortic trauma, with a contained pseudoaneurysm.

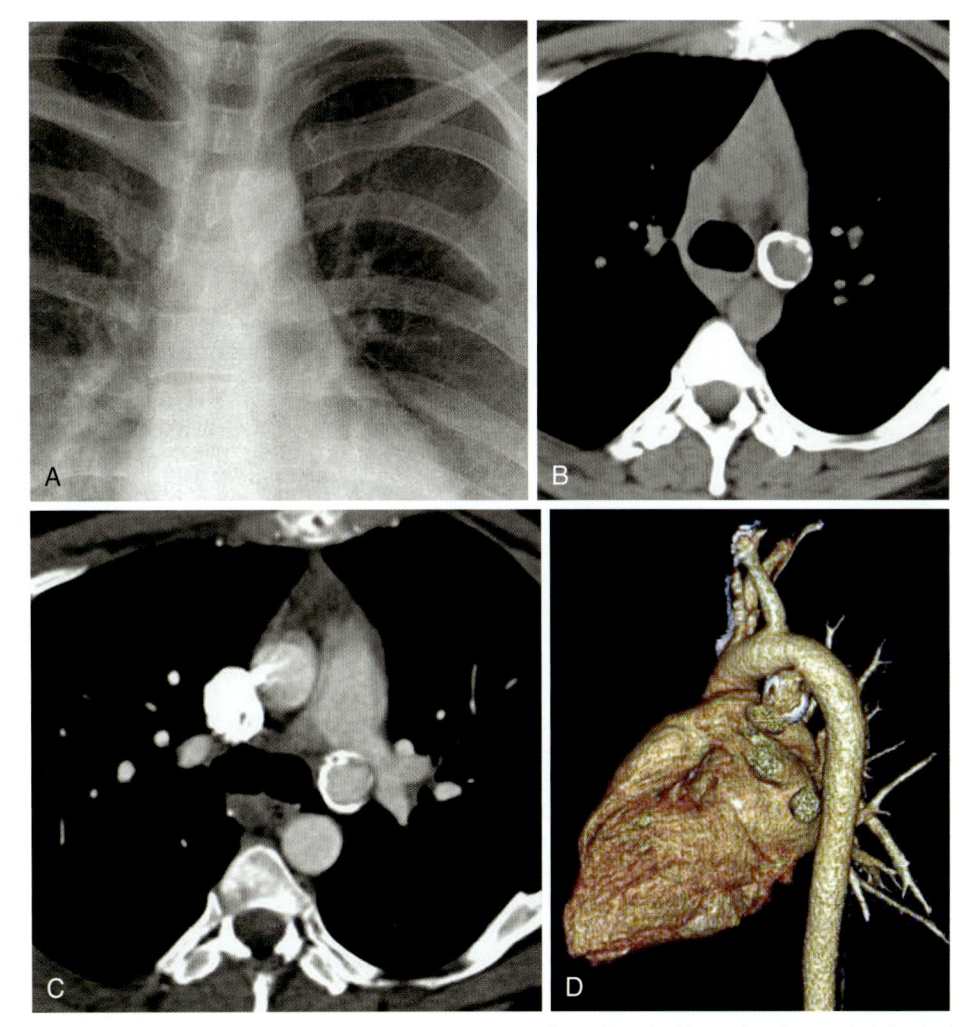

■ **FIGURE 43-16** A 27-year-old woman with chronic abdominal pain was initially evaluated with routine chest and abdominal radiography. **A,** An enlarged and coned-down image of the aortopulmonary window on a frontal chest radiograph shows an abnormal rounded contour, with faint peripheral calcification. **B,** A densely rim-calcified aneurysm at the aortic isthmus is seen in the same location on non-contrast enhanced CT of the chest. **C,** This transaxial image obtained after intravenous contrast administration displays complete opacification of this structure, indicating that this is an old post-traumatic pseudoaneurysm of the aorta, located at the insertion site of the ligamentum arteriosum. **D,** This volume-rendered surface-shaded image of the aorta shows the relationship of the aortic pseudoaneurysm with the aortic isthmus.

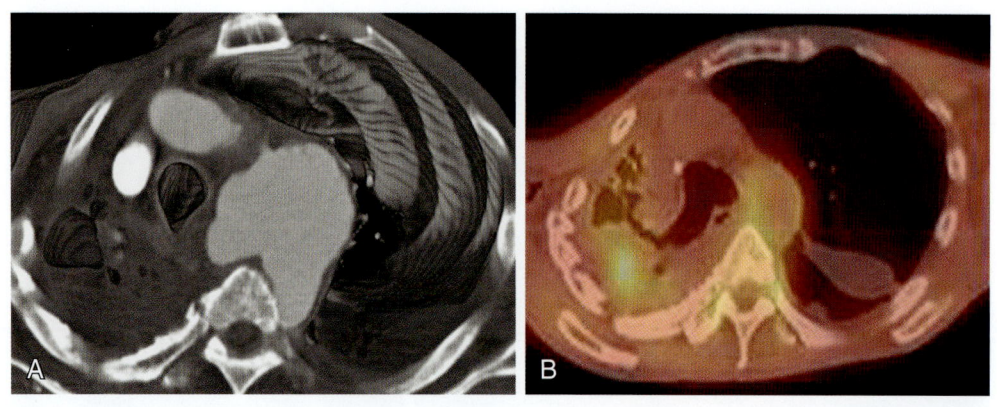

FIGURE 43-17 Mycotic aneurysm in patient with right upper lobe non–small cell lung cancer, invading the aorta. **A,** Thickened, volume rendered axial image displays the large aneurysm of the upper descending aorta. **B,** Transaxial positron emission tomography (PET)–CT image of the upper chest shows abnormal increased radiotracer uptake of the right upper lobe cancer, with associated volume loss.

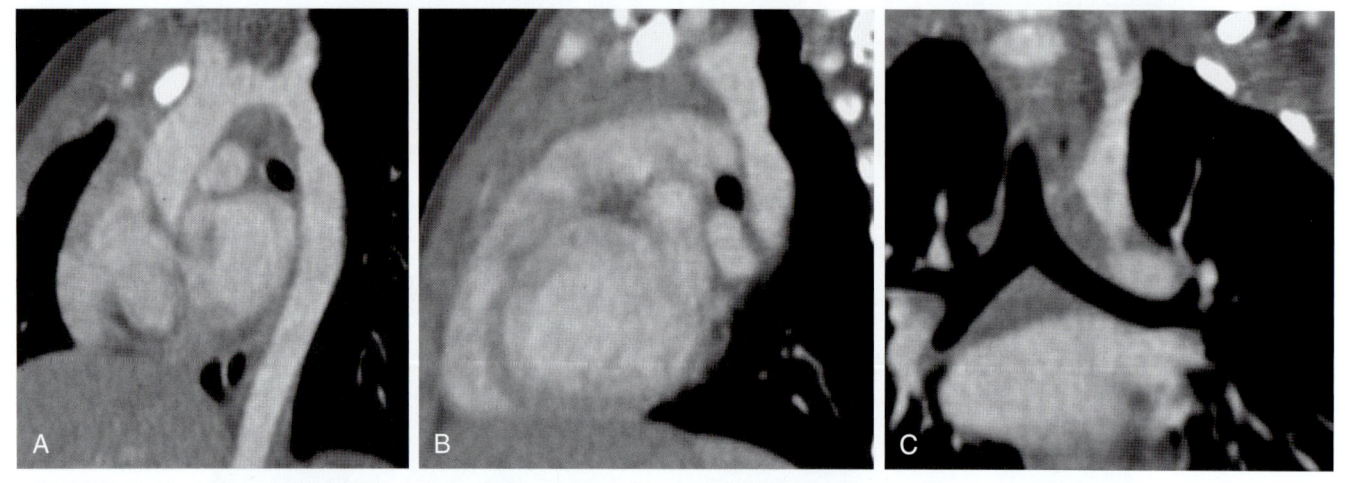

FIGURE 43-18 Oblique sagittal **(A)** and coronal **(B)** reconstructed images of CTA of the chest in a 4-year-old child show postductal coarctation of the aorta **(A)** with an associated small PDA **(B)**. **C,** Echocardiography calculated a peak gradient of 42 mm Hg across the coarctation and demonstrated left to right shunting of the PDA. The child was treated with coiling of the PDA and balloon dilation of the coarctation.

wall. It can be complicated by aneurysm, intramural hematoma or, less likely, rupture. It is more common in the older adults and, when present, there is evidence of atherosclerotic disease in the remainder of the arteries. It is more frequently seen in the descending thoracic aorta and abdominal aorta, where atherosclerosis is more prevalent.[22]

Infectious aneurysms of the aorta are rare and even more unusual in the thoracic aorta. In the chest, they are more common in the ascending aorta. The intima is very resistant to infection, so any condition that damages the aortic wall can predispose a person to infectious aneurysms. These conditions include contiguous bacterial endocarditis, an immunocompromised state, atherosclerosis, drug abuse, and aortic trauma. The infection may also be caused by local spread of an adjacent infection, such as infectious discitis. Because of the high mortality involved with this entity, early diagnosis is crucial. On CT and MRI, findings consist of a saccular aneurysm with eccentric thrombus and adjacent inflammation, fluid collection, abscess, or mediastinal soft tissue thickening or mass. The sudden development and rapid growth of mycotic aneurysms also help differentiate them from other causes of aneurysmal dilation of the aorta. Complications of leakage and periaortic hematoma are also well depicted by cross-sectional imaging. Because of the risk of rupture, mycotic aneurysms are treated by a combination of surgery, usually using endovascular grafts, and adjuvant antibiotic therapy (Fig. 43-17).[22,25,29]

Coarctation of Aorta

Coarctation and pseudocoarctation are also vascular entities that can occur at the isthmus. Coarctation of aorta can be associated with PDA in situations in which the stenosis is severe. The ductus arteriosus is a crucial pathway for flow in patients with severe postductal stenosis of the descending aorta, where the ductus arteriosus serves as a collateral pathway, resulting in a left to right shunt. Such children are acyanotic and have increased pulmonary vascularity on imaging studies. In newborns with preductal stenosis, the ductus arteriosus of the aorta provides flow to the descending aorta. CTA clearly depicts the vascular communications, aortic caliber, and collateral vasculature. MRI and MRA provide information on the degree of stenosis, for which a shunt gradient can be calculated, and the direction of blood flow through the collateral pathways (Fig. 43-18).[18,28]

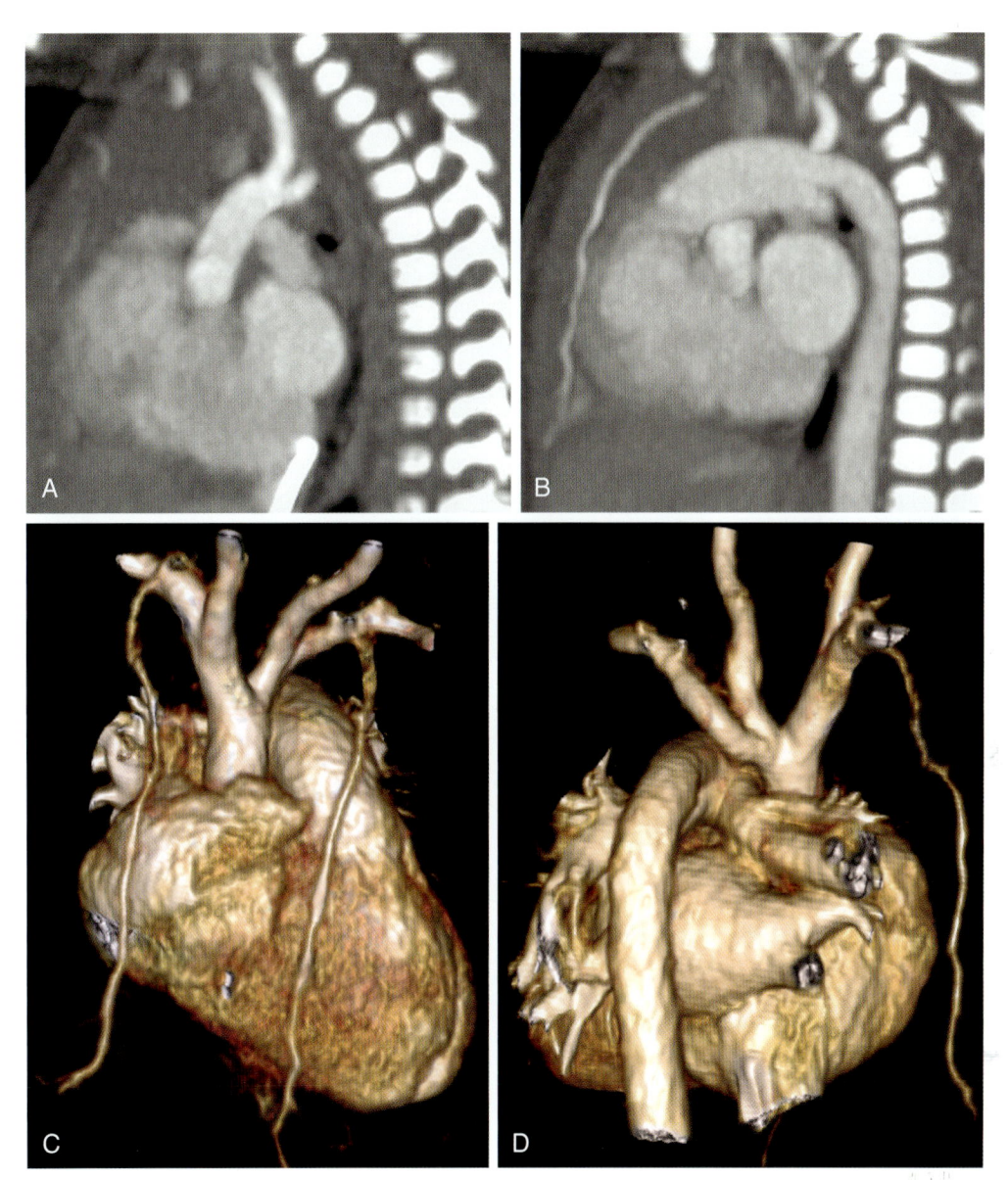

FIGURE 43-19 A 3-day-old newborn was found to have a PDA and an abnormal aorta on echocardiography. **A,** Oblique sagittal reformatted image of thoracic CTA, to evaluate the anatomy further, displays discontinuity of the aortic arch beyond the left subclavian artery. This represents a type A interrupted aorta. **B,** Similar reformatted image centered over the main pulmonary artery shows that the descending thoracic aorta receives blood flow from a markedly enlarged PDA. The enlarged internal mammary artery anteriorly provides collateral flow away from the ascending aorta. Surface-shaded volume rendered reconstructed images viewed anteriorly **(C)** and posteriorly **(D)** demonstrate the absence of the posterior aortic arch between the left subclavian artery and the aortic isthmus.

Interrupted Aortic Arch

Interrupted aortic arch is an advanced form of aortic coarctation in which there is absence or atresia of an aortic segment. A patent ductus arteriosus provides flow to the descending aorta. Enlarged systemic arterial collaterals help transfer blood from branches of the ascending aorta to the descending aorta. This anomaly is rare, comprising less than 1% of congenital heart defects. Based on the location of aortic atresia, this anomaly can be classified into three types: (1) type A is when the interruption occurs distal to the left subclavian artery (approximately 33% of cases); (2) in type B (65% of cases), the atresia is between the left carotid artery and left subclavian artery and approximately 50% of these patients have DiGeorge syndrome, especially if there is a right-sided aortic arch; and (3) in type C (<1% of cases), there is an interruption between the innominate artery and left common carotid artery. Based on where the right subclavian artery originates, this anomaly is further classified into subtypes. There is an increased incidence of interrupted aortic arch and ventricular septal defect. CTA and MRA of the chest clearly depict the PDA, the site of aortic interruption, distance between the proximal and distal segments, and narrowest diameter of the left ventricular outflow tract, all information that is needed to plan surgical repair (Fig. 43-19).[18,22,28]

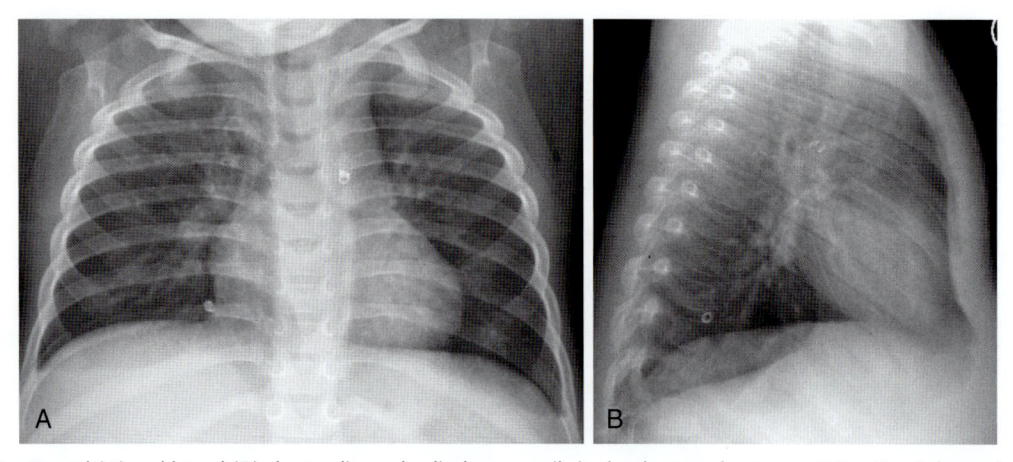

FIGURE 43-20 Frontal (**A**) and lateral (**B**) chest radiographs display two coils in the chest used to treat a PDA. One is located appropriately between the undersurface of the aortic arch and the superior aspect of the main pulmonary artery. The other has embolized into the segmental pulmonary arterial branch of the right lower lobe.

SYNOPSIS OF TREATMENT OPTIONS

Medical

All patients with PDA require lifelong prophylactic antibiotic treatment for infective endocarditis, even if the PDA is restrictive. Symptoms of congestive heart failure are treated with diuretics and digoxin, and atrial fibrillation and flutter are treated medically or by cardioversion. Adults with atrial fibrillation require lifelong anticoagulation. Before the development of permanent atrial dilation and ventricular failure, permanent closure of the PDA may reverse these symptoms. Patients who have developed pulmonary vascular disease are not candidates for procedures of definitive closure. These patients may benefit from vasodilating agents such as chronic oxygen, PGI_2, calcium channel blockers, endothelin antagonists, and phosphodiesterase type V inhibitors. An option for such patients is to close the duct partially by transcatheter techniques or surgery and medically treat with vasodilators. Permanent closure is considered after follow-up assessment reveals a decrease of pulmonary vascular resistance.[1,8,16]

Surgical and Interventional

Interruption of the left to right shunt is the goal of management. Closure is attempted in neonates by administration of indomethacin and similar NSAIDs. Definitive closure in children and adults is considered if they are symptomatic from the left to right shunting. Asymptomatic patients with moderate to large shunts should also be treated to prevent complications of heart failure and pulmonary hypertension. Because current methods of permanent closure are safe, effective, and associated with little morbidity, any child or young adult with PDA is routinely treated. The value of treatment of an incidentally discovered tiny PDA is not certain, especially for older adults.[16]

When Eisenmenger syndrome develops, permanent closure of the PDA may cause a hemodynamic strain, which could quickly spiral down to right ventricular failure. This is caused by the reliance on the left to right shunt to provide adequate flow to the pulmonary bed, despite high pulmonary vascular resistance and pulmonary artery pressure. Lung biopsy has been recommended in patients with a vascular resistance higher than 8 HRU/m^2 to determine whether such patients are candidates for permanent closure of PDA. Reactivity of pulmonary vessels to pulmonary vasodilating agents, and/or significant reduction of pulmonary artery pressure and resistance during test closure using a balloon catheter, suggest reversibility of the pulmonary vascular disease and positive outcome of PDA closure in patients with right to left shunting through the PDA.[15,16]

Permanent closure is achieved by transcatheter and surgical methods. Transcatheter occlusion is the treatment of choice for children and young adults. In patients who have increased pulmonary vascular resistance and the ductus arteriosus is calcified, transcatheter closure is preferred to surgical closure, which requires cardiopulmonary bypass and an anterior approach through a median sternotomy.[16]

Transcatheter closure involves advancing a catheter or delivery sheath across the ductus arteriosus, approaching it from the pulmonary artery or the aorta. A closure device is then positioned to occlude it. Various coils can be used, either those used for general vascular closure or those specific to PDA closure. If the PDA is moderate or large, an Amplatzer Duct Occluder device (AGA Medical, Plymouth, Minn) is preferred. Treatment is effective, so that assessment for complete closure at the time of follow-up has revealed a success rate exceeding 90% to 95%.[1,16] The most common complication, although uncommon, is device embolization, which is usually retrieved by an endovascular approach. Other complications are even more rare and constitute flow disturbance in the proximal left pulmonary artery or descending aorta from protrusion of the device, hemolysis from residual high-velocity shunting, and vein thrombosis caused by vascular access (Fig. 43-20).[16]

Surgical ligation or transection is reserved for patients who have a very large ductus, which may not be adequately occluded by occluder devices. If a large broad-based connection exists, patch closure under cardiopulmonary bypass is the surgical treatment of choice.[1,15]

SUMMARY

Patent ductus arteriosus accounts for 10% of congenital heart disease. In adults, it may go undiagnosed and be discovered incidentally, if small and restrictive, or after complications of congestive heart failure and pulmonary hypertension have developed if small or medium-sized and symptoms have been tolerated throughout the years. Because of the increased incidence of infectious endocarditis and ease of treatment by endovascular techniques, elective ligation is recommended if Eisenmenger phenomenon has not yet developed. Echocardiography is the modality of choice for diagnosis in infants and children. CT and MRI are good modalities to evaluate the presence of PDA in adults, assess the degree of shunting, and suggest the presence of expected complications. Various vascular entities at the aortic isthmus comprise the differential diagnosis of PDA. These can be well assessed by cross-sectional imaging, and the advent of MDCT has allowed creation of three-dimensional images that portray the vascular connections and their effects on adjacent mediastinal structures.

> **KEY POINTS**
>
> - Patent ductus arteriosus typically closes in the first few weeks after birth.
> - If the ductus remains patent after this initial period, the resulting left-to-right shunt can lead to pulmonary hypertension and Eisenmenger syndrome.
> - Echocardiography is the mainstay of imaging, but CT can better define anatomy and MRI can be used to assess function as well as structure.
> - Patent ductus arteriosus usually can be treated by transcatheter techniques, although surgery may be necessary in some patients.

REFERENCES

1. Schneider DJ, Moore JW. Patent ductus arteriosus. Circulation 2006; 114:1873-1882.
2. Goo HW, Park IS, Ko JK, et al. CT of congenital heart disease: normal anatomy and typical pathologic conditions. Radiographics 2003; 23: S147-S165.
3. Dattilo G, Tulino V, Tulino D et al. Letter to the editor: Interatrial defect and patent ductus arteriosus. Int J Cardiol 2009 Apr 28; Epub ahead of print.
4. Mandhan P, Brown S, Kukkady A, et al. Surgical closure of patent ductus arteriosus in preterm low birth weight infants. Congenit Heart Dis 2009; 4:34-37.
5. Tschuppert S, Doell C, Arlettaz-Mieth R, et al. The effect of ductal diameter on surgical and medical closure of patent ductus arteriosus in preterm neonates: size matters. J Thorac Cardiovasc Surg 2008; 135:78-82.
6. Chirvolu A, Jaleel MA. Pathophysiology of patent ductus arteriosus in premature neonates. Early Human Develop 2009; 85:143-146.
7. Tulino V, Dattilo G, Tulino D. et al. Letter to the editor: A recurrent patent ductus arteriosus. Int J Cardiol 2009 Mar 24; Epub ahead of print.
8. Neisch SR. Patent ductus arteriosus. eMedicine, July 23, 2009. Available at: http://emedicine.medscape.com/article/891096-overview. Accessed October 22, 2009.
9. Kaneko Y, Kobayashi J, Achiwa I, et al. Cardiac surgery in patients with trisomy 18. Pediatr Cardiol 2009; 30:729-734.
10. Mangones T, Manhas A, Vistainer P, et al. Prevalence of congenital cardiovascular malformations varies by race and ethnicity. Int J Cardiol 2009 Apr 2; Epub ahead of print.
11. Chávez GF, Cordero JF, Becerra JE. Leading major congenital malformations among minority groups in the United States, 1981-1986. MMWR Morb Mort Wkly Rep 1988; 37:17-24.
12. El-Khuffashaf, Molloy EJ. Influence of a patent ductus arteriosus on cardiac troponin T levels in preterm infants. J Pediatr 2008; 153:350-353.
13. Morgan JM, Gray HH, Miller GA, Oldershaw PJ. The clinical features, management and outcome of persistence of the arterial duct presenting in adult life. Int J Cardiol 1990; 27:193-199.
14. Wiyono SA, Witsenburg M, de Jaegere PPT, et al. Patent ductus arteriosus in adults—case report and review illustrating the spectrum of disease. Nether Heart J 2008; 16:255-259.
15. Brili SV, Toutouzas P. Patent arterial duct and aortopulmonary window. In Gatzoulis MA, Webb GD, Daubeney PE (eds). Diagnosis and Management of Adult Congenital Heart Disease. New York, Churchill Livingstone, 2003; pp 247-252.
16. Rapacciulo A, Losi MA, Borgia F, et al. Transcatheter closure of patent ductus arteriosus reverses left ventricular dysfunction in a septuagenarian. J Cardiovasc Med 2009; 10:344-348.
17. Goitein O, Fuhrman CR, Lacomis JM. Incidental finding on MDCT of patent ductus arteriosus: use of CT and MRI to assess clinical importance. AJR Am J Roentgenol 2005; 184:1924-1931.
18. Önbas O, Kantarci M, Koplay M, et al. Congenital anomalies of the aorta and vena cava: 16-detector-row CT imaging findings. Diagn Interv Radiol 2008; 13:163-171.
19. Haramati LB, Glickstein JS, Issenberg HJ, et al. MR imaging and CT of vascular anomalies and connections in patients with congenital heart disease: significance in surgical planning. Radiographics 2002; 22:337-349.
20. Debl K, Djavidani B, Buchner S, et al. Quantification of left to right shunting in adult congenital heart disease: phase-contrast cine MRI compared with invasive oximetry. Br J Radiol 2009; 82:386-391.
21. Chaudhari M, Hasan A. Distal aortopulmonary window: a morphological variation. Asian Cardiovasc Thorac Ann 2009; 17:413-414.
22. Yu T, Zhu X, Tang L, et al. Review of CT angiography of aorta. Radiol Clin North Am 2007; 45:461-483.
23. Fisher RG, Sanchez-Torres M, Whigham CJ, et al. "Lumps" and "bumps" that mimic acute aortic and brachiocephalic vessel injury. Radiographics 1997; 17:825-834.
24. Morse SS, Glickman MG, Greenwood LH, et al. Traumatic aortic rupture: false-positive aortographic diagnosis due to atypical ductus diverticulum. AJR Am J Roentgenol 1988; 150:793-796.
25. Agarwal PP, Chughtai A, Matzinger FRK, et al. Multidetector CT of thoracic aortic aneurysms. Radiographics 2009; 29:537-552.
26. Sachdeva R, Smith C, Greenberg BS, et al. Giant ductal aneurysm in an asymptomatic 4-year-old girl. Ann Thorac Surg 2009; 87:946-948.
27. Lund JT, Jensen MB, Hjelms E. Aneurysm of the ductus arteriosus. A review of the literature and the surgical implications. Eur J Cardiothorac Surg 1991; 5:566-570.
28. Fitoz S, Nuray Unsal N, Tekin M, et al. Contrast-enhanced MR angiography of thoracic vascular malformations in children. Int J Cardiol 2007; 123:3-11.
29. Van der Wal H, Van Geel PP, De Boer RA. Mycotic aneurysm of the aorta as an unusual complication of coronary angiography. Eur J Vasc Endovasc Surg 2008; 36:178-181.

SECTION TWO

Cyanotic Heart Disease with Increased Vascularity

CHAPTER 44

Transposition of the Great Arteries

Frandics P. Chan

Transposition of the great arteries (TGA) represents a spectrum of associated cardiac anomalies that share a common feature—ventriculoarterial discordance—meaning that the left ventricle (LV) is connected to the pulmonary trunk and the right ventricle (RV) is connected to the aorta. It is divided into two major types, complete transposition of the great arteries (CTGA) and congenitally corrected transposition of the great arteries (CCTGA). The primary lesion in CTGA is ventriculoarterial discordance alone, whereas CCTGA has both ventriculoarterial discordance and atrioventricular discordance, meaning that the connections between the two atria and two ventricles are also reversed. CTGA and CCTGA differ greatly in their clinical presentations, natural histories, management strategies, and imaging indications. They will be discussed separately in this chapter.

Historically, CTGA was first described by Matthew Baillie, a Scottish pathologist, in 1797. The first corrective surgery for CTGA was the atrial switch procedure developed by Senning[1] in 1959 and Mustard[2] in 1964. Atrial switching effectively converts a CTGA to a CCTGA, in which the RV pumps the systemic circulation. Although this circulation is compatible with life, the systemic RV is prone to early failure. To address the shortcomings of atrial switching, Jatene and colleagues[3] perfected the arterial switch procedure in 1975, in which the LV pumps the systemic circulation. It has become the preferred surgical treatment for CTGA. The Rastelli procedure[4] is used when the CTGA is associated with pulmonary stenosis. CCTGA was first described by the famous Bohemian pathologist Carl von Rokitansky in 1875. Early treatments focused on correcting secondary lesions, such as ventricular septal defect (VSD). In favor of an anatomically correct circulation, Ilbawi and associates[5] and others have advocated the double switch procedure, which combines the atrial switch and arterial switch procedures, or the atrial switch and Rastelli procedures. This procedure restores the LV as the systemic ventricle.

Definition and Classifications

CTGA is defined by ventriculoarterial discordance. It also can be described by the inlet-outlet features of the ventricles: the presence of subaortic infundibulum (Fig. 44-1), the absence of subpulmonary infundibulum, and mitral-pulmonary fibrous continuity (Fig. 44-2). Subaortic infundibulum implies a connection of the aorta to the infundibulum, which is a morphologic feature of the RV. The absence of subpulmonary infundibulum means that the pulmonary trunk is not connected to the RV. Because fibrous continuity of the inlet-outlet valves is a feature of the LV, a mitral-pulmonary fibrous continuity implies that the pulmonary trunk is connected to the LV.

CTGA is known by a number of other names. Because CTGA comprises 90% of all transposition cases, it is sometimes referred simply as transposition of the great arteries. Other designations are simple transposition and dextrotransposition of the great arteries (D-TGA). The letter D refers to D-loop of the ventricles and not the positional relationship of the great arteries. D-loop refers to the rightward folding of the heart tube during early embryologic development. This crucial event leads to the normal positions of the LV and RV at birth (Fig. 44-3). Usually, D-TGA corresponds with the physiology of CTGA, but this is not always the case. In situs inversus, the CTGA physiology corresponds to L-loop ventricles and CCTGA physiology corresponds to D-loop ventricles. To avoid confusion, it is best to use the terms *CTGA* and *CCTGA*, which correctly describe the underlying physiology.

There is no officially adopted classification for CTGA. Because the clinical presentation, prognosis, and treatment options are greatly influenced by the associated anomalies, it is useful to divide CTGA according to these anomalies into those with intact ventricular septum (CTGA-IVS), those with ventricular septal defect but without left ventricular outflow obstruction (CTGA-VSD),

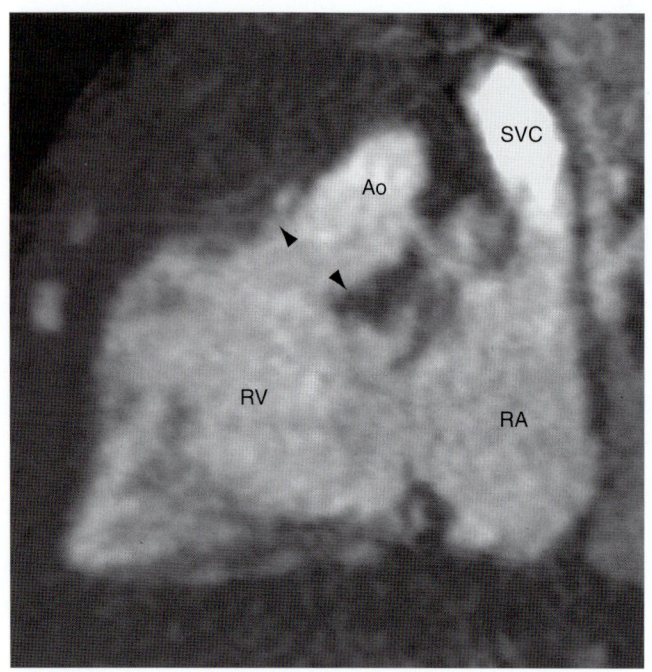

FIGURE 44-1 Cardiac-gated CTA of a newborn with CTGA. This RV inlet-outlet view shows a superior vena cava (SVC) draining into a right atrium (RA). The RA is connected to the right ventricle (RV), which in turn is connected to an anteriorly located aorta (Ao). The subaortic infundibulum and the surrounding conal muscle (*black arrowheads*) separate the aortic valve from the tricuspid valve.

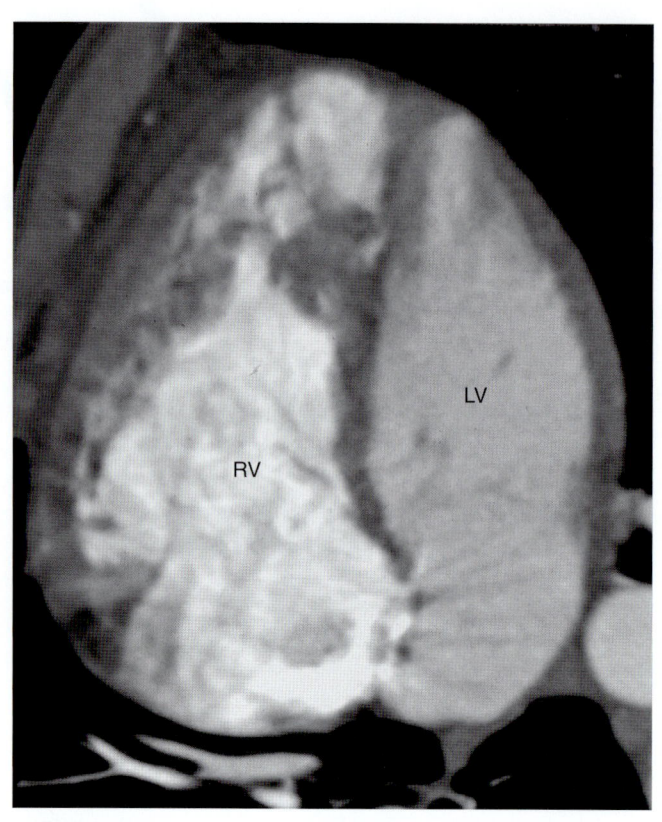

FIGURE 44-3 Cardiac-gated CTA of a patient with pulmonary hypertension. This four-chamber view shows coarse trabeculation in the RV, exaggerated by hypertrophy. The positions of the RV and LV are normal, consistent with D-loop.

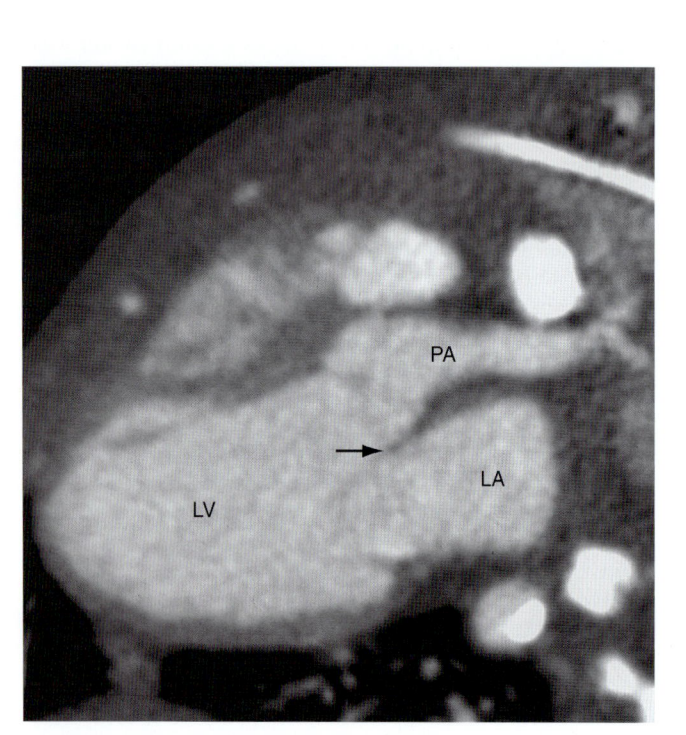

FIGURE 44-2 Cardiac-gated CTA of a newborn with CTGA. This LV inlet-outlet view shows the left atrium (LA) connected to the left ventricle (LV), which in turn is connected to the pulmonary trunk (PA). The absence of a subpulmonic infundibulum allows the pulmonary valve to be in contact with the mitral valve (*arrow*). They are said to be in fibrous continuity.

and those with ventricular septal defect and left ventricular outflow obstruction (CTGA-VSD-LVOTO).

CCTGA is defined by the presence of atrioventricular and ventriculoarterial discordance. Alternative names for CCTGA are corrected transposition, double discordance, and levotransposition of the great arteries (L-TGA). In a patient with normal situs, L-TGA implies L-loop ventricles (Fig. 44-4) and atrioventricular discordance, in addition to ventriculoarterial discordance. Like D-TGA, the term *L-TGA* is best avoided in favor of CCTGA.

Van Praagh proposed a three-letter scheme that labels the sidedness of the atrial, ventricular, and arterial segments,[6] and it has been used to categorize various anatomic manifestations of TGA. In this scheme, the first letter denotes the atrial situs, with S meaning solitus and I meaning inversus. The second letter denotes the ventricular loop, with D meaning D-loop, and L meaning L-loop. The third letter denotes the positions of the great arteries, with D meaning that the aortic root is on the right side of the pulmonary root (Fig. 44-5) and L meaning that the aortic root is on the left side of the pulmonary root (Fig. 44-6). In situs solitus and CTGA, the most common segmental anatomy is S, D, D, although S, D, L exists in a minority of cases. In situs inversus and CTGA, the most common pattern is I, L, L, which is the mirror image of S, D, D. In CCTGA, the segmental anatomy is usually S, L, L for situs solitus and I, D, D for situs inversus. Van Praagh and coworkers,[7] in a pathology series of CCTGA, reported one case of S, L, D.

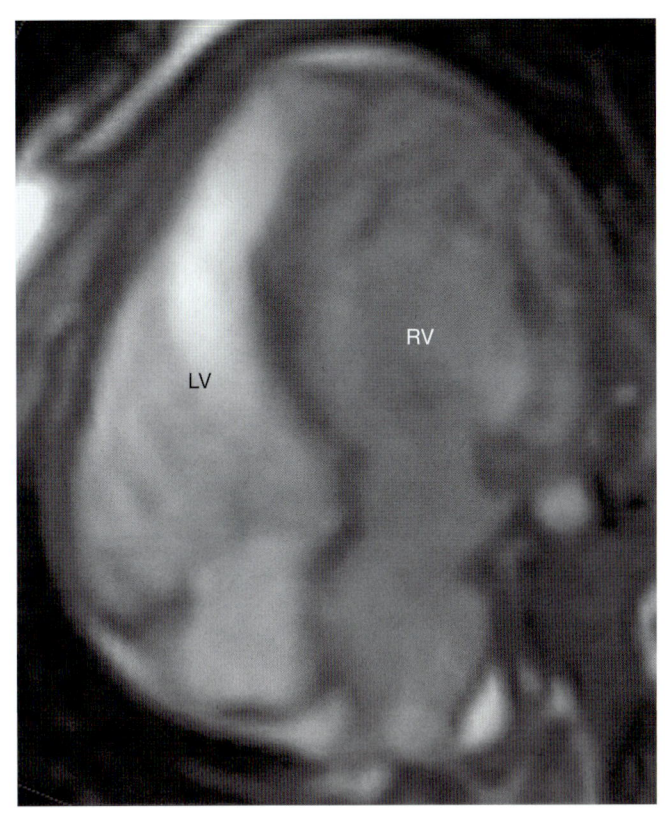

FIGURE 44-4 MRI steady-state free precession image of a patient with CCTGA. This four-chamber view shows that the positions of the right ventricle (RV) and the left ventricle (LV) are reversed, consistent with L-loop.

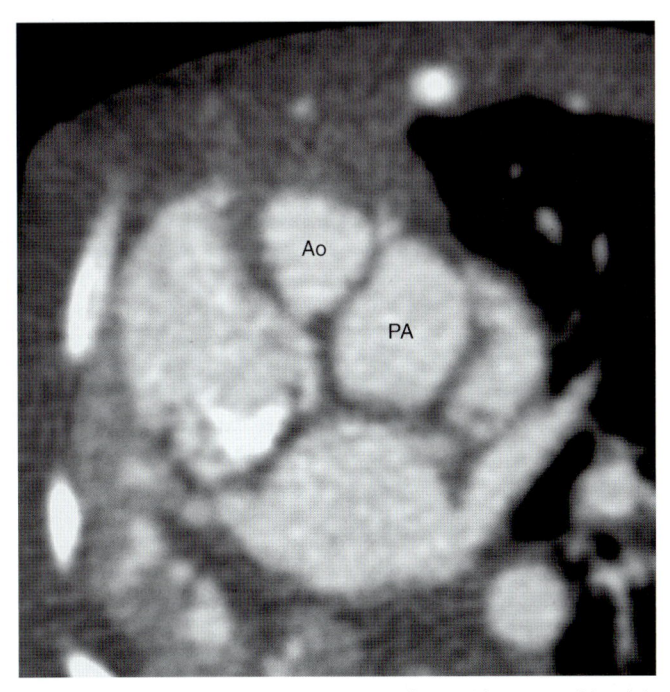

FIGURE 44-5 Cardiac-gated CTA a newborn with CTGA. This axial view shows that the aorta (Ao) is located anterior and to the right of the pulmonary artery (PA). The great arteries are in D-position.

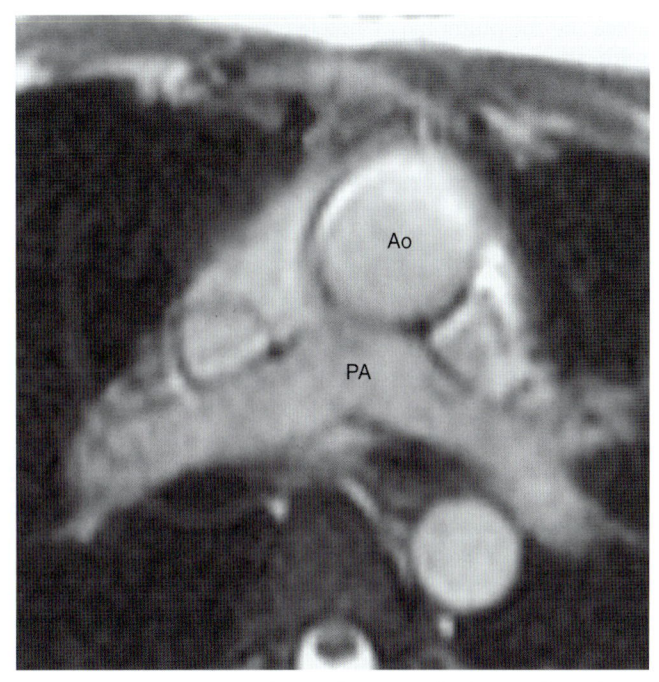

FIGURE 44-6 MRI steady-state free precession image of a patient with CCTGA. The position of the pulmonary trunk (PA) is implied at the junction between the left and right main pulmonary arteries. This axial view shows that the aorta (Ao) is anterior and to the left of the pulmonary trunk (PA). The great arteries are in L-position.

Epidemiology and Genetics

CTGA occurs in 5% to 7% of cases of congenital heart disease, with an incidence of 20 to 30/100,000 live births. It is the second most common cyanotic heart disease, behind tetralogy of Fallot, and it is the most common cyanotic heart disease that manifests in the neonatal period. There is no known racial predilection, but there is a 2:1 male predominance. CTGA has been reported in trisomies 18 and 21,[8] although the vast majority of cases have no identified genetic defect. Chromosomal 22q11 deletion, commonly found in conotruncal anomalies, is not associated with CTGA. Furthermore, the risk of recurrence in the offspring of individuals with CTGA is very low.[9] It has a greater incidence in mothers with diabetes. These observations suggest that genetics may play a less important role in the development of CTGA than environmental factors, possibly intrauterine hormonal disturbance or exposure to teratogens. CTGA is rarely associated with other extracardiac anomalies, with the possible exception of coarctation.

CCTGA occurs in 0.5% to 1.4% of cases of congenital heart disease. It is rare among congenital cardiac anomalies and is much less common than CTGA. Its incidence is on a par with Ebstein anomaly and interrupted aortic arch. Like CTGA, its inheritance pattern is multifactorial, without clear genetic association. There is a slight male predominance.

Etiology and Pathophysiology

Embryology

The embryology of CTGA is not well understood. The loss of the normal spiral relationship between the ascending aorta and the pulmonary trunk in CTGA suggests a problem with the process of conotruncal septation. In normal development during the fifth week of gestational age, two intertwined, spiraling flow streams in the conotruncus are thought to induce the proper spiraling septation that divides the conotruncus into the aorta and pulmonary trunk.[10] The spiraling flow streams may be disturbed, leading to abnormal conotruncal septation and CTGA. This may also explain why the infundibulum septum, formed during the same process, is often abnormal in CTGA.

The embryology of CCTGA, a rare condition, is also unknown. However, the origin of the reverse position of the ventricles can be traced to cardiac development during day 23 of gestational age. In normal development, the embryologic heart tube elongates and folds to the right side of midline. This leads to the normal positions of the ventricles at birth. If the heart tube folds to the left, the positions of the ventricles are reversed. In normal situs, where the atria are in their proper positions, a leftward folding of the heart tube leads to atrioventricular discordance, namely the left atrium (LA) connecting to the RV and the right atrium (RA) connecting to the LV.

Associated Cardiac Anomalies

In most cases of CTGA, the ventricular septum is intact. The most common associated anomaly is VSD, occurring in 40% to 45% of cases. Perimembranous VSD and muscular VSD are about equally common, followed by atrioventricular canal defect. The presence of a VSD is important for survival because it allows the mixing of oxygenated and deoxygenated blood in the otherwise disconnected pulmonary and systemic circulations. The second most common associated anomaly is left ventricular outflow tract (LVOT) obstruction, occurring in 25% of cases. The obstruction can be valvular at the pulmonary valve or subvalvular. In the latter, the cause of obstruction may be fibrous membrane, ring, shelf, septal muscular hypertrophy, septal aneurysm, or septal attachment of chordae tendineae of the mitral valve. In a mechanism similar to that of hypertrophic cardiomyopathy, LVOT obstruction may cause systolic anterior motion (SAM) of the mitral anterior leaflet, worsening the LVOT obstruction and causing mitral regurgitation. The physiologic effects of LVOT obstruction are decreased pulmonary flow and increased cyanosis. Uncommonly, coarctation coexists with CTGA in 5% of cases.

The relative positions of the great arteries in CTGA are variable. In normal anatomy, the aortic root is located posterior and to the right of the pulmonary root. In 90% of CTGA cases, the aortic root is located *anterior* and to the right of the pulmonary root. Uncommonly, in 10% of cases, the aortic root is located anterior and to the *left* of the pulmonary artery. This leads to the S, D, L designation in the Van Praagh segmental labeling scheme described earlier. Rarely, the aortic root can be posterior to the pulmonary root.

Knowledge of the coronary artery anatomy is crucial for the surgical management of CTGA. In CTGA, as in normal cardiac anatomy, the two main coronary arteries most often arise from the two aortic sinuses of Valsalva

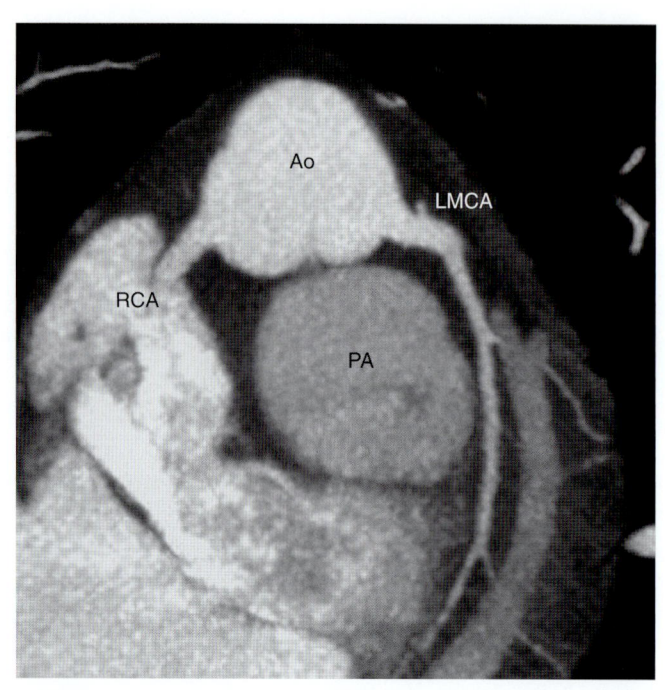

■ **FIGURE 44-7** Cardiac-gated CTA of a patient with CTGA. In this short-axis view, the aorta (Ao) and pulmonary trunk (PA) are in D-position. The left main coronary artery (LMCA) and the right coronary artery (RCA) arise from the aortic sinuses facing the pulmonary trunk. This is the most common coronary pattern for CTGA.

closest to, or facing, the pulmonary valve. In the most common coronary pattern for CTGA, which occurs in 67% of cases, the right coronary artery (RCA) originates from the right facing sinus and the left main coronary artery (LMCA) originates from the left facing sinus (Fig. 44-7). The LMCA then bifurcates into the left anterior descending (LAD) artery and left circumflex (LCx) artery, as expected. Less commonly, the LCx arises from the RCA in 22% of cases. Other variations include a single RCA (9.5%), a single LMCA (3%), reversed RCA and LMCA (3%), and others (Fig. 44-8).[11]

Only a small fraction (1% to 9%) of CCTGA cases are isolated without any associated anomalies.[12] The most common associations are VSD and pulmonary stenosis. VSD occurs in 60% to 80% of cases (Fig. 44-9). It can be of any type and the VSD can be multiple. Pulmonary stenosis occurs in 30% to 50% of cases, and it can be valvular or subvalvular. There is a frequent association with tricuspid abnormalities, which include dysplastic leaflets, Ebstein-like displacement of the leaflets, and a tricuspid valve straddling the ventricular septum. Other less common associated anomalies are atrial septal defect (ASD), patent ductus arteriosus (PDA), pulmonary atresia, mitral valve abnormalities, coarctation, and interrupted aortic arch. CCTGA manifests with dextrocardia in 25% of cases and situs inversus in 5% of cases.

An important feature of CCTGA is the abnormal development and position of the atrioventricular (AV) node. In normal anatomy, the AV node is located at a relatively posterior position near the tricuspid septal leaflet in an area known as the triangle of Koch. In CCTGA, this posterior AV node may be absent and replaced by an anterior AV node. This anterior node is fragile and can be damaged

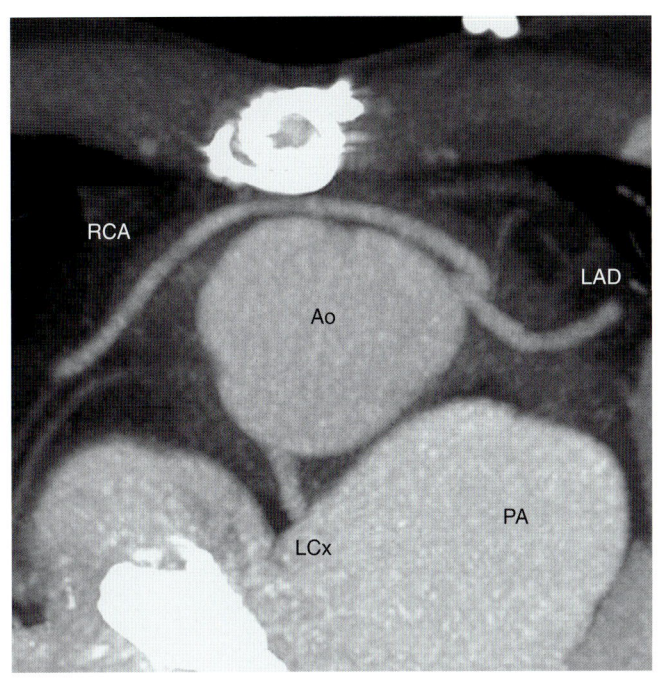

FIGURE 44-8 Cardiac-gated CTA of a patient with CTGA. This is an uncommon coronary pattern in which the right coronary artery (RCA) and left anterior descending artery (LAD) arise together from the left-facing sinus, whereas the left circumflex artery (LCx) arises alone from the posterior right-facing sinus. Transplantation of these coronary arteries in an arterial switch operation was thought to be impossible, and the patient underwent atrial switching.

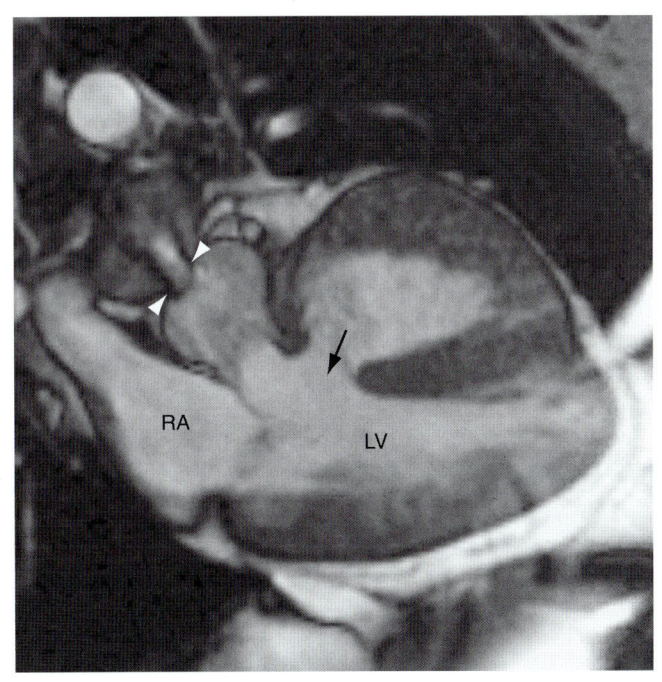

FIGURE 44-9 MRI steady-state free precession image of a patient with CCTGA. This LV inlet-outlet view shows a large ventricular septal defect (*arrow*) shunting flow into the left ventricle (LV) and then out the pulmonary artery. A pulmonary artery band is in place (*arrowheads*) to restrict this flow and prevent pulmonary vascular obstructive disease. Note that the right atrium (RA) is connected to the morphologic LV, consistent with atrioventricular discordance.

by fibrosis or surgical trauma, leading to heart block. In some cases, both the posterior and anterior AV nodes are present. Their expected locations must be recognized during surgery to avoid damage.

The aortic root position is typically anterior and to the left of the pulmonary root. Together with normal situs and L-loop ventricle, S, L, L is the most common segmental description for CCTGA. Variations in coronary anatomy are common, but the branching pattern of the coronary arteries generally follows the ventricles. Because the left ventricle is positioned on the right, the LMCA commonly arises from the right-facing sinus and travels to the right before branching into a LAD and a LCx. The latter lies in the right atrioventricular groove. Similarly, the RCA commonly arises from the left-facing sinus and lies in the left atrioventricular groove. Single coronary origin is also common.[13]

MANIFESTATIONS

Clinical Presentation

The early onset of cyanosis in CTGA can be understood from its unique physiology. In utero, the fetal circulation is composed of parallel pulmonary and systemic circulations. Two right-to-left shunts are established at the fossa ovalis of the atrial septum and at the PDA. Both shunts reduce pulmonary flow through the nonfunctioning lungs. The organ in which oxygen exchange occurs is the placenta, connected to the systemic circulation through the umbilical vein and arteries. Transposing the fetal great arteries produces no physiologic effect because they are connected by the PDA. This arrangement allows the fetus to grow normally.

At birth, the placenta no longer serves as the organ of oxygen exchange. During the transition from fetal to adult circulation, the fossa ovalis and PDA close, bringing the ventilated lungs into serial connection with the systemic circulation. CTGA, by conducting deoxygenated blood from the RV to the aorta and oxygenated blood from the LV to the pulmonary artery, disconnects the pulmonary circulation from the systemic circulation. This configuration is not viable.

In practice, some mixing of the oxygenated and deoxygenated blood occurs through shunts between the pulmonary and systemic circulations, providing some oxygen to the systemic organs. The degree of cyanosis depends on (1) the size and direction of these shunts and (2) the degree of obstruction to the pulmonary flow. In CTGA-IVS, the most common anatomic arrangement, shunting is limited and the neonate presents with cyanosis within hours of birth. Cyanosis worsens as the PDA closes in the first few days of life. Prognosis in this scenario is poor, with a 30% survival rate at 1 month. In CTGA-VSD, the VSD is usually large and mixing occurs freely at the ventricular level. Patients may present with mild cyanosis, even after the PDA closes. As the pulmonary resistance drops in the first week of life, a large shunting from the systemic RV to pulmonary LV may occur. This can lead to congestive heart failure and later pulmonary vascular obstructive disease. The latter is the cause of pulmonary hypertension and Eisenmenger syndrome. The survival rate at 1 year is 50%, which is better than that for CTGA-IVS. In CTGA-VSD-LVOTO, the LVOT obstruction limits flow to the pulmonary circulation. The physiology in this situation is similar to that of tetralogy of Fallot. Severe obstruction would lead to diminished pulmonary flow and worsening cyanosis. Little obstruction would lead to large shunting and the same outcome as CTGA-VSD. If the obstruction is balanced just right, the pulmonary circulation may be protected from harmful shunt flow at a level of tolerable cyanosis. The survival rate for CTGA-VSD-LVOTO is 50% at 3 years, with some surviving into adulthood. Left untreated, the overall survival rates for CTGA are 70% at 1 week, 50% at 1 month, and 10% at 1 year.[14]

The physiology and natural history for CCTGA are very different from those of CTGA. The addition of atrioventricular discordance reestablishes the physiologic circulations in which the oxygenated pulmonary venous blood flows into the aorta and the deoxygenated systemic venous blood flows to the pulmonary artery. Although the circulatory physiology is correct, the anatomy is abnormal because the RV is the systemic ventricle and the LV is the pulmonary ventricle; as a result, the pressure loads to the ventricles are reversed. Complications from CCTGA can be divided into those manifesting early and those manifesting late. Early complications are usually caused by the associated anomalies, such as VSD, pulmonary stenosis, and dysfunctional tricuspid valve. In patients with a large VSD, shunting from the systemic RV to the pulmonary LV can be large. The increased volume load can lead to congestive heart failure. Coexisting tricuspid valve abnormalities that cause significant tricuspid regurgitation will increase RV volume load and exacerbate the heart failure. Pulmonary stenosis can be beneficial by decreasing the pulmonary flow and reducing the RV to LV shunting. It also increases the left ventricular pressure and promotes a rightward shift of the ventricular septum. This configuration has the effect of reducing the tricuspid valve size and tricuspid regurgitation. Given these observations, pulmonary artery banding, a form of artificially induced pulmonary stenosis, is a valid palliative treatment for CCTGA. In the rare patients who do not have any associated anomaly, they may be asymptomatic throughout young adulthood.

Late complications of CCTGA are caused by RV failure and conduction abnormalities. The RV is not structurally homologous to the LV, and the RV has not been evolved to carry lifelong systemic pressure load. In men, RV failure commonly occurs during the fifth and sixth decades of life. In women, it may manifest during the first pregnancy. The pathophysiology of the RV failure is not well understood. Exercise studies have shown that the cardiac reserve of the system RV is less than the normal systemic LV. The right coronary system may not provide adequate perfusion to support the hypertrophic RV, leaving the systemic RV vulnerable to ischemia. RV with exuberant hypertrophy is particularly at risk because the perfusion per unit weight of tissue is decreased. The closed tricuspid valve, which normally operates against a 20 mm Hg systolic pulmonary pressure, must now hold against a 100 mm Hg systolic systemic pressure. This, together with the dysplastic and dysmorphic tricuspid leaflets that often accompany CCTGA, produces substantial regurgitation and volume load to the RV, causing further stress to the

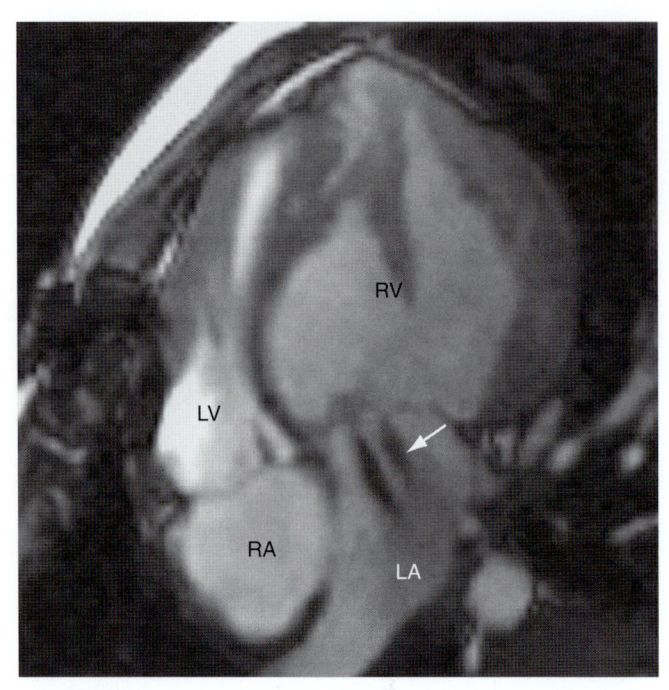

■ **FIGURE 44-10** MRI steady-state free precession image of a patient with CCTGA. This four-chamber view shows an enlarged systemic right ventricle (RV). The septum bulges into the left ventricle (LV), and there are multiple tricuspid regurgitant jets (*arrow*).

RV (Fig. 44-10). Patients without associated cardiac anomalies generally fare better, but both groups show substantial decline in RV function between ages 40 and 50 years. The probabilities of developing RV failure in patients with and without associated anomalies are 55% and 25%, respectively, at age 40, and 90% and 65% at age 50 years.[15]

The AV node is often abnormally developed in CCTGA. It is prone to fibrosis, even without surgical injury. There is a continuing risk of developing complete AV block at a rate of 2%/year. Overall, complete AV block is present in 12% to 33% of patients with CCTGA. Wolff-Parkinson-White syndrome from an accessory atrioventricular conduction pathway known as the bundle of Kent is present in 2% to 4% of patients. Other rhythm disorders include supraventricular tachycardia, atrial flutter, atrial fibrillation, and ventricular arrhythmia. Fortunately, sudden death from arrhythmia in CCTGA is rare.

DIFFERENTIAL DIAGNOSIS

From Clinical Presentation

Broadly speaking, CTGA may present with significant cyanosis, especially in CTGA-IVS, or congestive heart failure, as in CTGA-VSD. Chest radiography is helpful for separating those entities with diminished pulmonary vascularity, such as tetralogy of Fallot and Ebstein anomalies, from those with increased pulmonary vascularity, typically admixture lesions such as CTGA-VSD, truncus arteriosus, total anomalous pulmonary venous return without obstruction, tricuspid atresia, and single ventricle. Additional clinical features, physical findings, and hyperoxia and prostaglandin challenge testing can usually narrow down the diagnosis. An interesting sign of CTGA is the reverse differential cyanosis, manifested by higher oxygen saturation in the lower extremities than in the upper extremities. This is caused by oxygenated blood from the pulmonary artery shunting through the PDA to the descending artery and the lower extremities, while the deoxygenated blood from the aortic root supplies the cervical arteries. In patients with congestive heart failure, differential diagnoses include large left-to-right shunt such as truncus arteriosus, intrinsic systemic ventricular failure such as anomalous left coronary artery from the pulmonary artery (ALCAPA), and obstructive lesions such as critical aortic stenosis, interrupted aortic arch, and severe coarctation. Neonates born with profound cyanosis and metabolic acidosis at delivery may have CTGA-IVS with intact or restrictive atrial septum. The other consideration is hypoplastic left heart syndrome with intact atrial septum. Either case would require emergent balloon atrial septotomy to sustain life. Neonatal presentation of CCTGA is usually less dramatic. Ultimately, the precise diagnosis is established by imaging, usually with echocardiography.

From Imaging Findings

Both CTGA and CCTGA share the configuration of parallel ascending aorta and pulmonary trunk (Fig. 44-11). Distinguishing between the two types of transpositions requires additional imaging evidence. In CTGA, the ventricles are usually in their normal positions (see Fig. 44-3) and the aortic root tends to be on the right of the pulmonary root see (Fig. 44-5). In CCTGA, the ventricular positions are reversed (see Fig. 44-4) and the aortic root tends to be on the left of the pulmonary root (see Fig. 44-6). However, as discussed earlier, these signs are not completely reliable. It is better to trace the connections between the venous returns and great arteries. In CTGA, the pulmonary veins are ultimately connected to the pulmonary artery through the left ventricle and the venae cavae are connected to the aorta through the right ventricle. In CCTGA, blood flow from the pulmonary veins reaches the aorta through the right ventricle and blood flow from the venae cavae reaches the pulmonary trunk through the left ventricle.

Differentiation between CTGA and double-outlet right ventricle (DORV) can be challenging, especially when the DORV has a doubly committed large VSD. In DORV, more than 50% of both the aorta and pulmonary trunk should be aligned with the right ventricle. In contrast, CTGA has the aorta aligned mostly with the right ventricle and the pulmonary trunk aligned mostly with the left ventricle. When both outlet valves are separated from the inlet valves by intervening conal muscle, or bilateral conus, this is considered a sign of DORV (Fig. 44-12). In CTGA, the mitral valve remains in fibrous continuity with the pulmonary valve, without intervening conal muscle.

SYNOPSIS OF TREATMENT OPTIONS
Medical

Although palliative in nature, early medical therapy is crucial for stabilizing the cyanotic crisis in neonates with CTGA before definite surgery. The most important is the infusion of prostaglandin E_1 to keep the PDA from closing. The PDA allows oxygenated blood to enter the aorta from the pulmonary artery. Metabolic acidosis and oxygen desaturation may require intubation and mechanical ventilation. In patients with CCTGA, fixed lesions such as a large VSD, pulmonary stenosis, and tricuspid valve dysfunction will ultimately require surgical correction. Medical therapy is useful for the management of systemic RV failure. An angiotensin-converting enzyme (ACE) inhibitor may be given to reduce afterload, diuretics may be given to reduce preload, and digoxin may be given for its inotropic effect.

Surgical and Interventional

Surgery for Complete Transposition of the Great Arteries

In CTGA patients presenting with severe cyanosis, keeping the ductus arteriosus open may not be sufficient. Creating or enlarging the ASD to promote shunting at the atrial level is a valid palliative treatment. This is now performed at the bedside with an endovascular balloon atrial septostomy under echocardiography guidance. In this procedure, first described by Rashkind and Miller in 1966,[16] a balloon catheter with deflated balloon is passed from the right atrium, through the foramen ovale, to the left atrium. The balloon is inflated and forcibly retracted back to the right atrium, tearing the atrial septum to allow increased interatrial mixing. The goal is to increase systemic oxygen saturation to the 50% to 80% range. Although generally

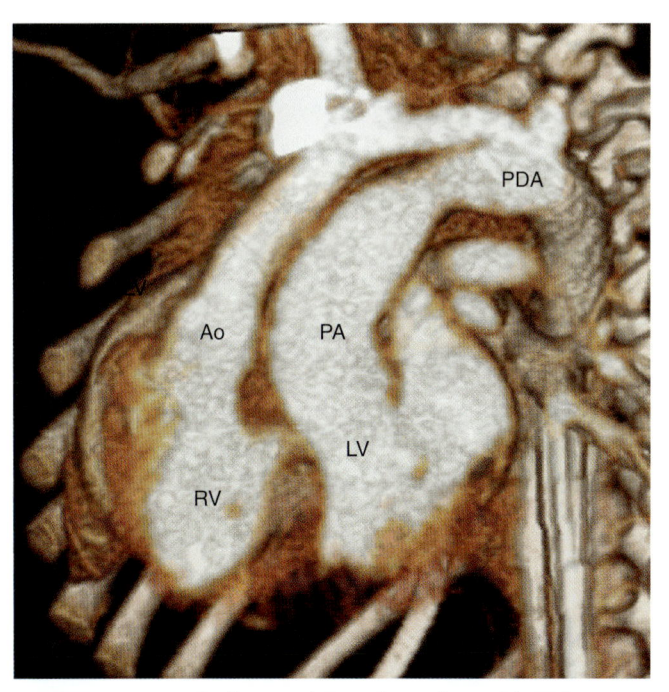

FIGURE 44-11 Cardiac-gated CTA of a newborn with CTGA. In both CTGA and CCTGA, the right ventricle (RV) is connected to the aorta (Ao) and the left ventricle (LV) is connected to the pulmonary artery (PA). The two great arteries lie in parallel. In this newborn patient, a patent ductus arteriosus (PDA) connects the two great arteries.

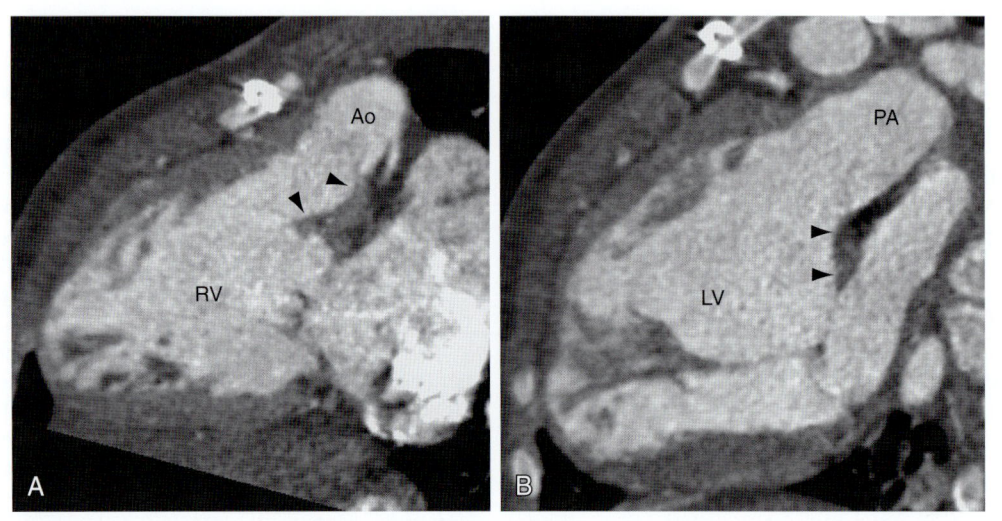

FIGURE 44-12 Cardiac-gated CTA of a patient diagnosed with double outlet right ventricle (DORV) with transposed great arteries. **A,** This RV inlet-outlet view shows discordant connection between the right ventricle (RV) and the aorta (Ao). Like CTGA, there is subaortic conal muscle (*arrowheads*). **B,** This LV inlet-outlet view shows discordant connection between the left ventricle (LV) and pulmonary artery (PA). Unlike CTGA, however, there is subpulmonic conal muscle (*arrowheads*). The presence of conal muscle under both great arteries classifies this as DORV.

safe and widely used, balloon septostomy has been associated with an increased risk of stroke.[17]

The preferred surgical correction of CTGA today is the arterial switch procedure, or the Jatene procedure, named after its creator, Adib Jatene.[3] Although conceptually straightforward, the arterial switch operation is technically difficult because of the need to transpose the tiny coronary arteries with the aorta. For this reason, the atrial switch procedure was developed first. Arterial switching became possible in the 1970s when a surgical technique was developed to reconnect the coronary arteries to the transposed aorta via coronary buttons. In this procedure, the ascending aorta and pulmonary trunk are transected. The coronary ostia, along with a large button of surrounding aortic wall, are excised from the aortic sinus of Valsalva. The proximal segments of the coronary arteries are freed from the surface of the heart to prevent tension or distortion after reimplantation. In a surgical manipulation called the Lecompte maneuver, the transected upper aorta is moved behind the pulmonary trunk so that the left and right main pulmonary arteries are now straddling the aorta (Fig. 44-13). The aorta is anastomosed to the proximal pulmonary trunk, creating a neoaorta. Openings are created at the appropriate positions on the neoaorta and the coronary buttons are sutured to these openings (Fig. 44-14). Finally, the transected pulmonary trunk, now located anteriorly to the aorta, is anastomosed to the proximal aorta. Any defects created by the coronary buttons are closed. If ASD and VSD are present, they are closed during the surgery.

The arterial switch procedure is usually performed during the first 2 to 4 weeks of life, during which the pulmonary LV remains hypertrophic enough to handle systemic pressure load after the switch. After the first month of life, pulmonary artery banding may be necessary to maintain the LV muscle mass. Contraindications for the arterial switch procedure include unfavorable coronary anatomy for reimplantation, aortic stenosis, pulmonary stenosis, and unfavorable VSD and ventricular sizes for two-ventricle repair. With increasing experience, contraindications to the arterial switch procedure have been relaxed. Some patients with coronary anatomy once thought not to be suitable for the arterial switch procedure who have undergone the atrial switch procedure are now referred for conversion to arterial switching.

The surgical outcome of the arterial switch procedure is favorable. Depending on the series, the surgical mortality is reported to be 2% to 5%.[18] Sudden death is uncommon. Late mortality related to coronary occlusion,

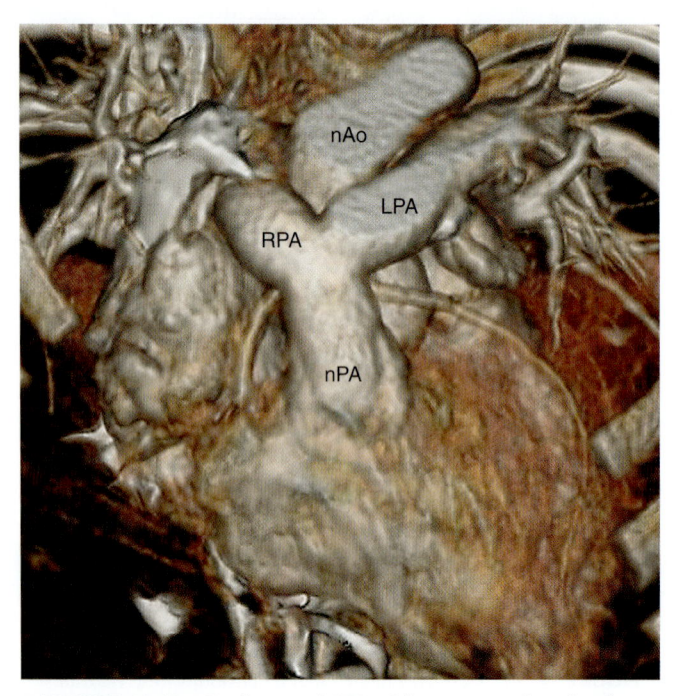

FIGURE 44-13 Cardiac-gated CTA of the great arteries after the Lecompte maneuver. In this volume rendered image, the neopulmonary trunk (nPA) is moved in front of the neoaorta (nAo). The left main pulmonary artery (LPA) and the right main pulmonary artery (RPA) straddle the neoaorta.

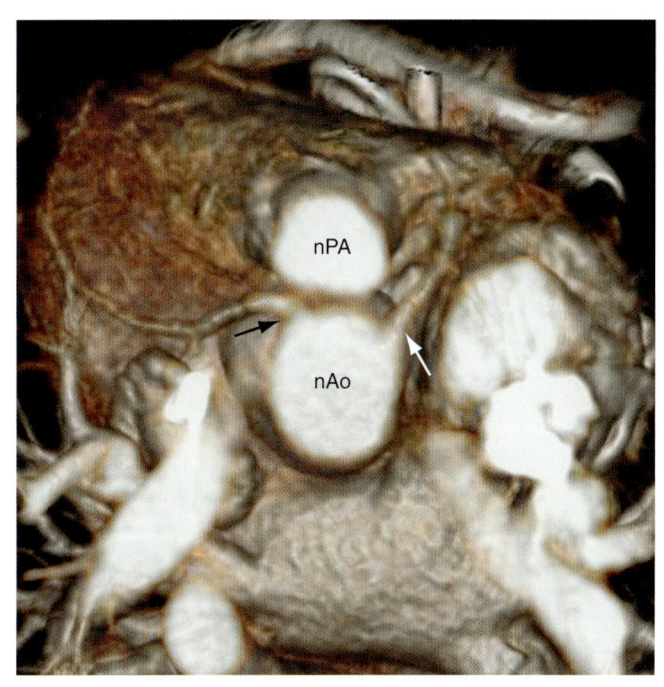

CHAPTER 44 • *Transposition of the Great Arteries* 609

■ **FIGURE 44-14** Cardiac-gated CTA of the transplanted coronary arteries. In this volume rendered image, the two main coronary arteries (*arrows*) have been transplanted from the neopulmonary artery (nPA) to the neoaorta (nAo).

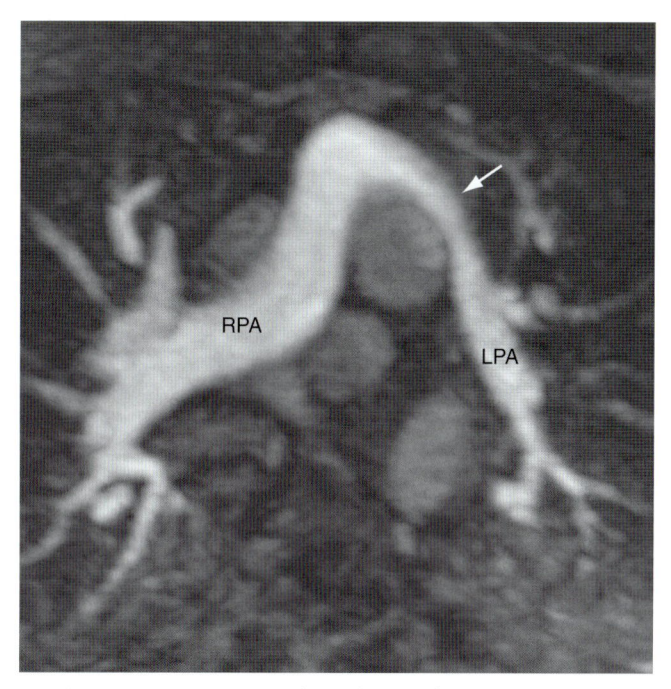

■ **FIGURE 44-15** Contrast-enhanced MRA of a patient who had an arterial switch procedure. The right pulmonary artery (RPA) is widely patent, whereas the left pulmonary artery (LPA) is stretched and compressed by the ascending neoaorta (*arrow*).

myocardial infarction, and left ventricular failure occurs in fewer than 1%. Survival rate is 88% at 10 years and unchanged at 15 years.[19] Because the coronary arteries are surgically manipulated, the long-term patency of the coronary arteries is of particular concern. In a series of 165 patients who underwent arterial switching, 7% had coronary occlusion, 5% developed more than 50% coronary stenosis, and 4% developed less than 50% coronary stenosis or coronary stretching.[20] The rate for surgical intervention for coronary obstruction was 2.4% in this series. Other complications include pulmonary stenosis in 5% to 25% of patients. The obstruction most often occurs at the left main pulmonary artery as it crosses the aorta (Fig. 44-15), followed by the right main pulmonary artery and the pulmonary valve compressed between the aorta and the sternum. Aortic regurgitation is detected in 16% of patients at 5-year follow-up, but only 4% had grade 2 or above, which is considered clinically significant.

The atrial switch procedure, having a less favorable outcome than the arterial switch procedure, is now reserved for special cases in whom the latter is contraindicated. It may also be seen in patients whose surgery predated the arterial switch procedure. The atrial switch operations developed by Senning and Mustard differ only on the methods of constructing the atrial baffle. Senning used native atrial septal tissue for the baffle construction[1] whereas Mustard used pericardium or Dacron material.[2] The postoperative anatomy and physiology of the two operations are the same. In this procedure, the normal atrial septum is resected. An atrial baffle is sutured to the atrial wall to create two compartments of very complex geometry. The posterior compartment collects flow from the pulmonary veins and channels it to the right ventricle (Fig. 44-16). The anterior compartment collects flow from the two cavae and channels it the left ventricle (Fig. 44-17). In effect, the atrial baffle creates an AV discordance, thereby converting the CTGA to a CCTGA.

Because the atrial baffle does not grow with the patient, the atrial switch procedure is performed later than the arterial switch procedure, typically at 1 month to 1 year

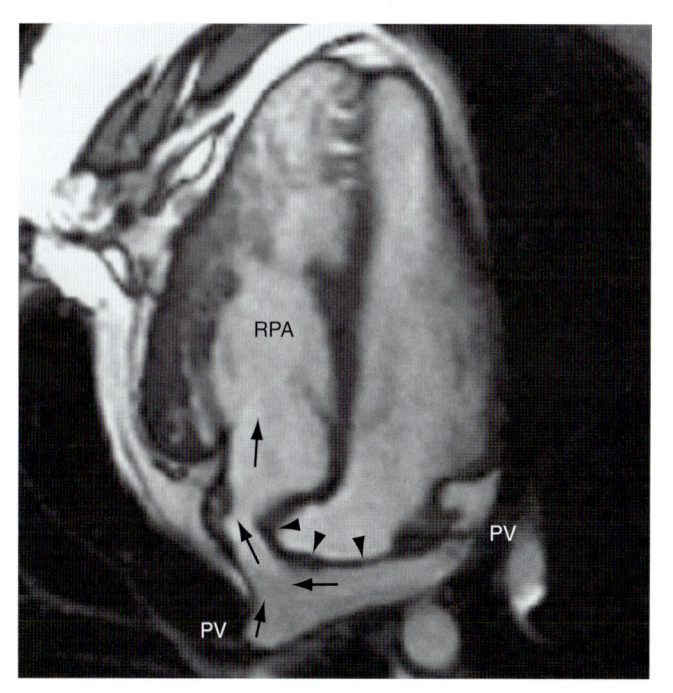

■ **FIGURE 44-16** MRI steady-state free precession image of a patient who had an atrial switch procedure. In this four-chamber view, a baffle (*arrowheads*) collects the pulmonary venous flow (*arrows*) in a posterior compartment and channels it into the right ventricle (RV). PV, pulmonary vein.

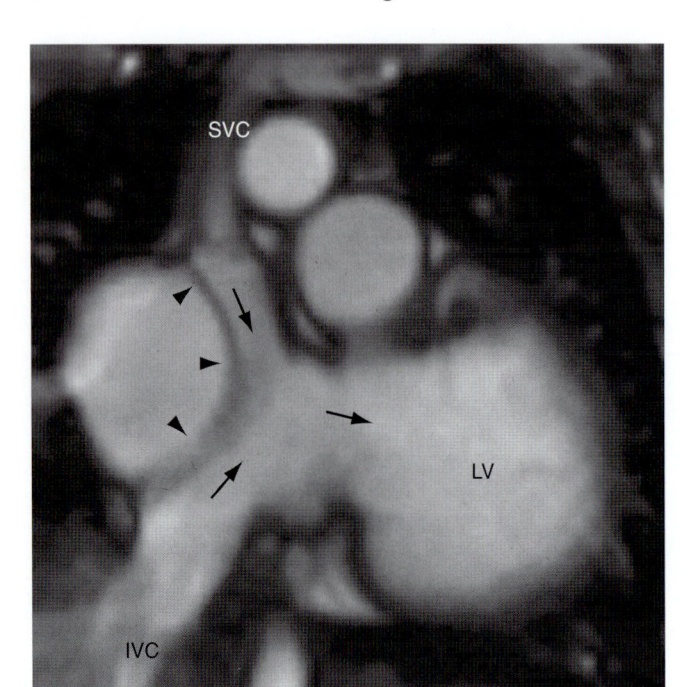

FIGURE 44-17 MRI steady-state free precession image of a patient who had an atrial switch procedure. In this oblique coronal view, the baffle (*arrowheads*) collects the caval flow (*arrows*) in an anterior compartment and channels it into the left ventricle (LV).

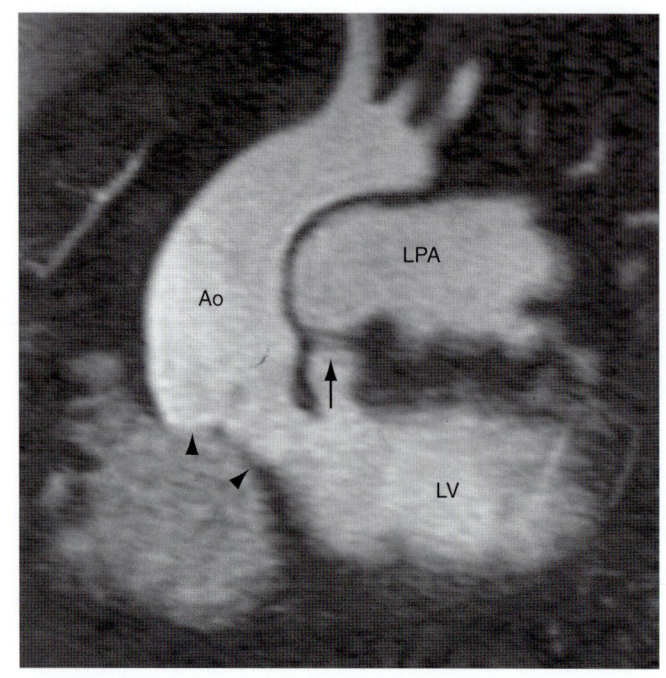

FIGURE 44-18 Contrast-enhanced MRA of a patient who had the Rastelli procedure. In this oblique coronal view, an intracardiac baffle (*arrowheads*) directs blood from the left ventricle (LV) to the aorta (Ao). The pulmonary trunk has been divided (*arrow*) from the branch pulmonary artery (LPA).

of age. The surgical mortality rate has been reported to be 1% to 10%, higher in patients with VSD.[21] Late mortality of 7% to 15% sudden death is significantly higher than that of the arterial switch procedure. Survival rate is 90% at 10 years and 76% to 80% at 20 years.[22] RV failure, as in CCTGA, is a late complication. Abnormal stretching of the atrial baffle may result in flow obstruction from channel narrowing or baffle leak from suture dehiscence. Although baffle leak is more common than flow obstruction, the former rarely requires reoperation. Flow obstruction typically occurs at the superior vena cava (SVC) channel (5% to 10%) and less commonly at the inferior vena cava (IVC) channel (1% to 2%). Pulmonary hypertension is associated with 7% of patients who had late repair of CTGA-VSD. Arrhythmia in postatrial switch patients is particularly troublesome. At 10 years, 50% of the patients develop bradyarrhythmia from sinus node dysfunction, requiring a pacemaker. Tachyarrhythmia may result from incisional atrial reentry tachycardia. Nearly 50% of patients experience one or more episodes of supraventricular tachycardia and 73% experience atrial flutter.

In CTGA patients with pulmonary stenosis, the Rastelli procedure is the indicated operation. In this procedure, the native pulmonary trunk is transected and the proximal trunk is surgically closed. An intracardiac baffle is placed in the RV to connect the VSD to the RVOT, effectively channeling the LV outflow to the transposed aorta (Fig. 44-18). An extracardiac valved pulmonary conduit is anastomosed to the RV after a ventriculostomy, and the conduit is connected to the distal pulmonary trunk, establishing the pulmonary flow (Fig. 44-19). After surgery, the LV becomes the systemic ventricle. A prerequisite for the Rastelli procedure is that the VSD must be large enough to conduct the left ventricular flow without obstruction.

Surgical enlargement of the VSD risks damaging the conduction system. Surgical mortality has been reported at less than 5%.[23] Survival rates are 82% at 5 years, 80% at 10 years, 68% at 15 years, and 52% at 20 years. Causes of late mortality include sudden death secondary to arrhythmia

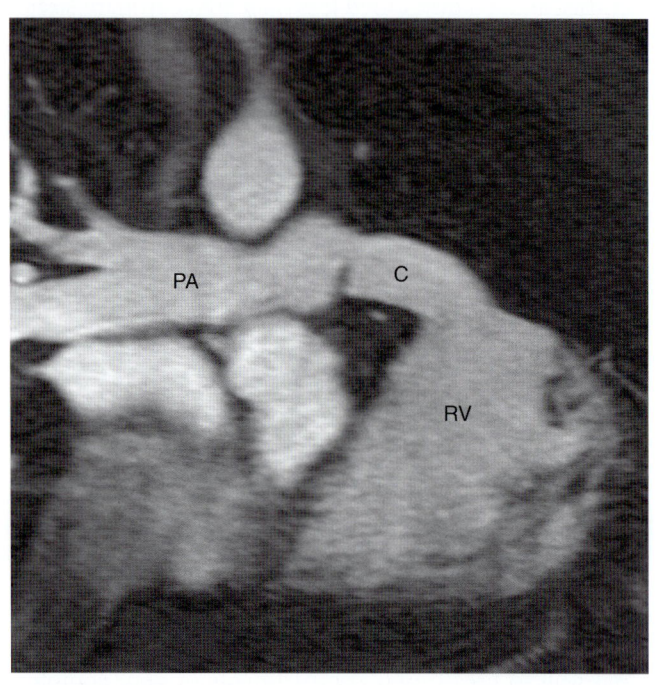

FIGURE 44-19 Contrast-enhanced MRA of a patient who had the Rastelli procedure. In this oblique sagittal view, an extracardiac pulmonary conduit (C) connects the right ventricle (RV) to the native pulmonary artery (PA).

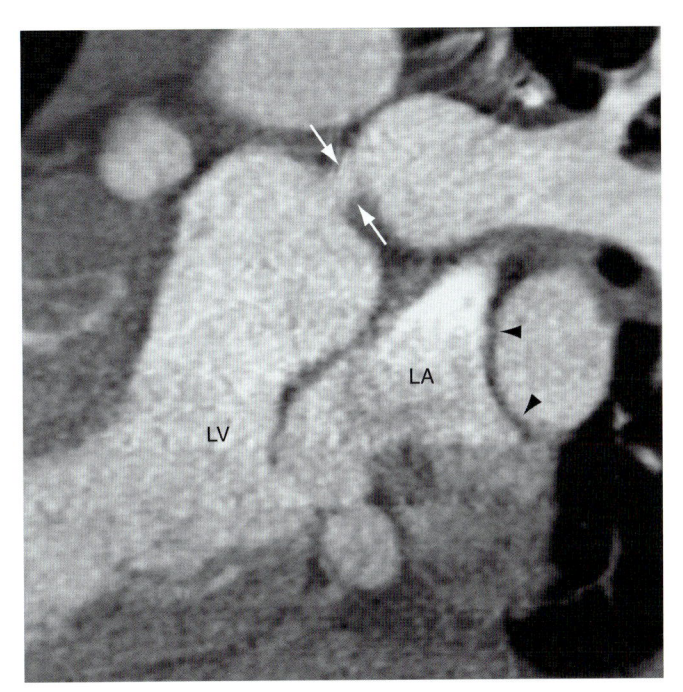

FIGURE 44-20 Cardiac-gated CTA of a patient who had pulmonary artery banding in preparation for a reverse switch procedure. In this oblique sagittal view, an atrial baffle (*arrowheads*) was placed previously in the atrium (LA) from an atrial switch procedure. A pulmonary artery band (*arrows*) creates a resistance to flow that the left ventricle (LV) must overcome with greater pressure.

and LV failure. Reoperation rate for the Rastelli procedure is high mainly because the pulmonary conduit develops pulmonary stenosis or regurgitation, requiring replacement every 10 to 20 years.

The Damus-Kaye-Stansel procedure is infrequently used in patients with TGA or Taussig-Bing anomalies. Indications are difficult coronary anatomy, subaortic stenosis, and absence of pulmonary stenosis.[24] In patients who had atrial switching, pulmonary artery banding may improve the systemic RV function by increasing LV pressure and shifting the ventricular septum to the right. In patients whose anatomy is amendable, a reverse switch procedure may be performed to convert the atrial switching to arterial switching. However, the pulmonary LV must first be conditioned, or trained, to handle the systemic pressure load. This is accomplished by raising the pulmonary resistance with a pulmonary artery band (Fig. 44-20) and forcing the LV to pump at a higher pressure. The band is gradually tightened until the LV pumps at near systemic pressure.

Surgery for Congenitally Corrected Transposition of the Great Arteries

In infants with CCTGA, palliative procedures are geared toward finding the right balance for the pulmonary flow. In patients with a large VSD, pulmonary artery banding is indicated to restrict the pulmonary flow and reduce the risk of developing pulmonary obstructive vascular disease. In patients with severe pulmonary stenosis and VSD, a Blalock-Taussig shunt is indicated to improve pulmonary flow and reduce cyanosis. Beyond palliation, operations are commonly performed to correct the anomalies other than CCTGA. These include VSD closure to remove shunting, resection to relieve pulmonary stenosis, and repair or annuloplasty of the tricuspid valve to reduce tricuspid regurgitation. The goals of these procedures are to reduce ventricular workloads and preserve ventricular functions. Compared with repairs of the same lesions in normal ventricles, the postoperative prognosis is worse for CCTGA. This may be related to conduction abnormality, worsening tricuspid regurgitation, and coronary anomalies inherent in CCTGA. Thirty-eight percent of postoperative patients develop complete AV block. Most patients undergo reoperation for atrioventricular valve regurgitations and pulmonary stenosis. The overall surgical mortality is 6%; the late survival rate is 55% to 85% at 10 years and 48% at 20 years.[25] Causes of death include reoperation, sudden death from arrhythmia, and progressive systemic RV failure.

In light of the long-term risk of RV failure, Ilbawi and colleagues[5] and others[26] have advocated the double switch procedure, which combines atrial and the arterial switching, as the definitive treatment for CCTGA. The purpose of this operation is to return the LV as the systemic ventricle. However, just as in the reverse switch procedure, the LV must be trained first to handle the systemic pressure load by pulmonary artery banding. The time required for LV training depends on the age of the patient, from a few weeks for infants to 1 year for older children. There is evidence that the LV responds poorly to training in patients older than 16 years.[27] The reported surgical mortality is 0% to 11%. Patients are also at risk for the complications associated with the atrial switch procedure. Although the immediate postoperative survival rate of the double switch procedure is good, it has yet to demonstrate long-term benefits over conventional operations that leave the RV as the systemic ventricle.[28]

IMAGING INDICATIONS AND REPORTING

Imaging for Complete Transposition of the Great Arteries

The manifestations of CTGA on chest radiographs are variable, from normal to shunt vascularity and increased heart size, depending on the size of the VSD. The classic cardiomediastinal silhouette of "egg on a string" is seen only in one third of cases (Fig. 44-21). Echocardiography is the definitive imaging modality. In the parasternal long-axis view, the LV is connected to the pulmonary trunk. In the short-axis view, the aorta is anterior and to the right of the pulmonary trunk. In the suprasternal view, the ascending aorta lies parallel to the pulmonary trunk. Echocardiography should assess for secondary lesions, such as ASD, VSD, and PDA, and the coronary anatomy, if possible. Doppler technique is used to detect any hemodynamically significant subvalvular and valvular stenoses of the outlet valves. Catheter angiography, CT, and MRI are generally not necessary for the initial diagnosis and management, except for the evaluation of the coronary anatomy when echocardiography is unclear. In rare cases, when the ventriculoarterial alignments and their relationship to

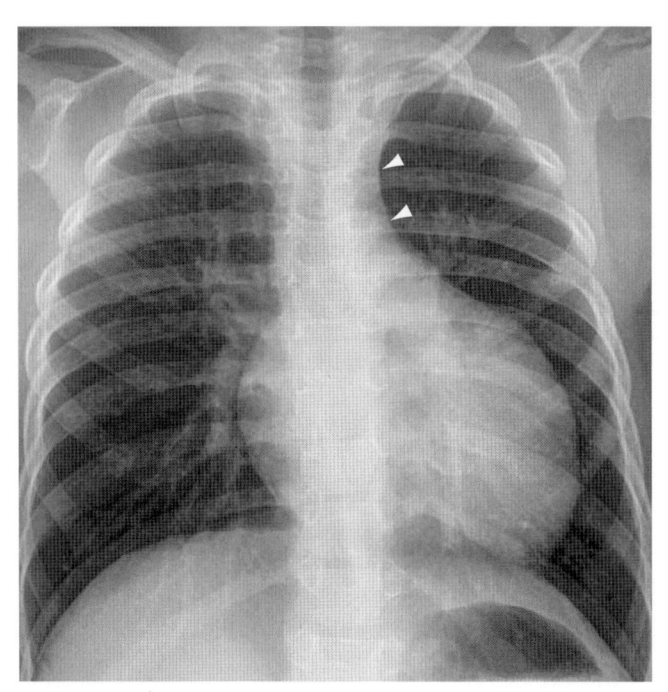

■ **FIGURE 44-21** Chest radiograph of a patient with CTGA corrected by atrial switching. The "egg on a string" appearance of CTGA refers to the enlarged cardiac silhouette, corresponding to the egg, and the narrowed mediastinal silhouette, corresponding to the string. The aortic arch and pulmonary trunk are absent from their normal positions (*arrowheads*), thereby leaving a thin mediastinum.

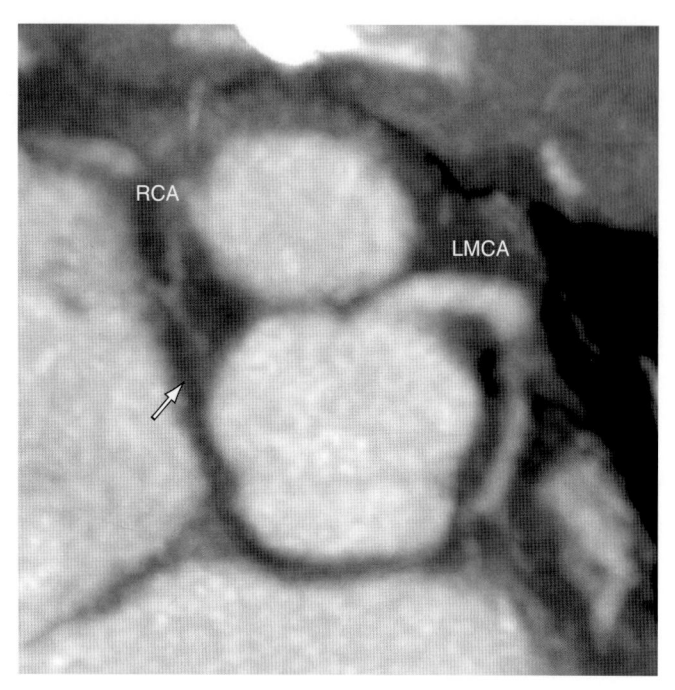

■ **FIGURE 44-22** Cardiac-gated CTA of the coronary arteries after an arterial switch procedure. The left main coronary artery (LMCA) is widely patent but the right coronary artery (RCA) is atretic and occluded at the origin (*arrow*).

the VSD are complex, three-dimensional imaging with cardiac-gated CT or MRI can be helpful for surgical planning.

In the early days, after the development of the arterial switch procedure, catheter coronary angiography was routinely performed in postoperative patients to assess coronary patency. With experience and improved surgical outcome, coronary angiography is now reserved for patients presenting with signs or symptoms of cardiac ischemia. Because the obstructions likely occur in the proximal coronary arteries where they have been surgically manipulated, the stenoses can be evaluated noninvasively with MRI or CT coronary angiography (Fig. 44-22). For patients with detected coronary stenoses, a stress test such as a stress myocardial perfusion study or stress echocardiography should be performed to determine the clinical significance of the lesions. On occasion, aortic regurgitation or pulmonary stenosis develops after the arterial switch operation. These complications, along with their ventricular responses, are monitored with echocardiography, supplemented by MRI quantifications of ventricular volumes and valvular regurgitant fractions if necessary.

After the atrial switch procedure, routine echocardiography is needed to assess the integrity of the atrial baffle and ventricular functions. Atrial baffle leak typically occurs at the suture site of the atrial baffle to the atrial wall and is readily detected by color Doppler duplex imaging. The baffle leak is usually small and does not require intervention. Of greater concern is any obstruction of the flow channels created by the atrial baffle. Doppler imaging may detect accelerated flow at the obstruction, which would require further evaluation by catheter measurement of pressure gradient. If hemodynamically significant, the obstruction can be relieved by stenting.

Assessment of ventricular functions is important because the systemic RV is prone to early failure. In echocardiography, special attention should be directed to the septal motion. Exaggerated leftward shift of the septum during systole reduces stroke volume of the RV and increases tricuspid annular size. The latter promotes tricuspid regurgitation and increases volume load to the RV. Furthermore, septal shift can narrow the LVOT, causing subpulmonic obstruction, SAM of the anterior leaflet of the mitral valve, and mitral regurgitation. These findings and their severity should be documented. In cases in which echocardiography is inadequate or precise quantifications of ventricular volumes and ejection fractions are desired, cardiac MRI is indicated.

After pulmonary artery banding for a planned reverse switch procedure, Doppler imaging is used to estimate the pressure gradient at the pulmonary band and the left ventricular systolic pressure from a mitral regurgitant jet. The latter helps monitor whether the trained left ventricle is ready to take on systemic pressure load. This pressure load should be confirmed by catheter measurement before surgery. In some centers, cardiac MRI is used to monitor the increase in the left ventricular mass during the LV training (Fig. 44-23). This is calculated as the epicardial volume of the LV minus the endocardial volume of the LV, multiplied by myocardial tissue density, 1.05 g/mL.[29] The goal of training is to attain an LV mass comparable to that of a normal systemic LV, estimated at 60 g/m^2 body surface area or higher.[30]

The imaging management of patients who have undergone the Rastelli procedure is similar to that of those who

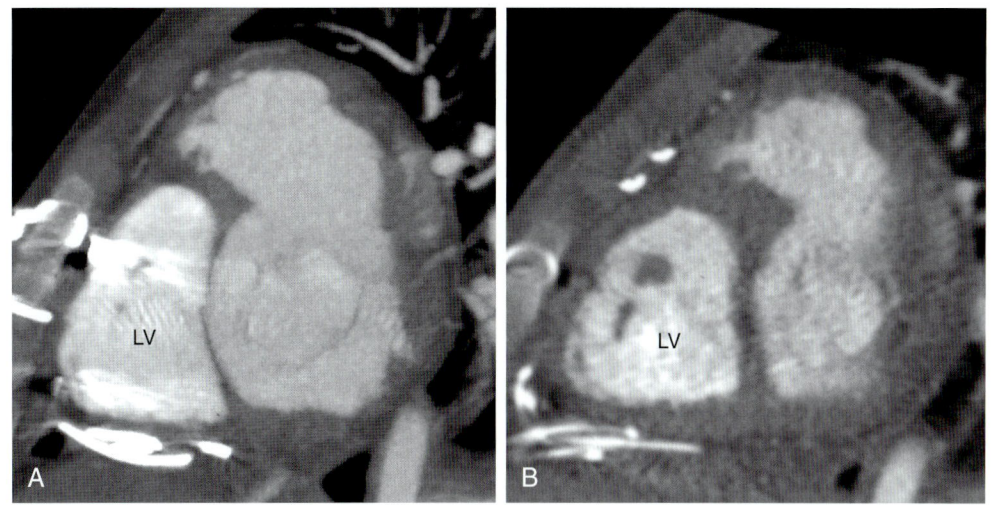

■ FIGURE 44-23 Cardiac-gated CTA of a patient who underwent pulmonary artery banding for left ventricle (LV) training. **A**, Before pulmonary artery banding, the wall of the pulmonary LV is thin in this short-axis view, especially at the septum. **B**, Two years after pulmonary artery banding, the wall of the pulmonary LV is significantly thickened.

had complete surgical repair for tetralogy of Fallot. Complications center on the pulmonary artery conduit, stenosis causing excessive pressure load to the RV (Fig. 44-24) and regurgitation causing excessive volume load to the RV. Echocardiography and MRI are indicated to monitor RV volume, RV ejection fraction, and pulmonary regurgitation severity. MRI has the advantage of providing accurate quantitative measurements of these parameters for serial comparison. As in the case of repaired tetralogy of Fallot, the goal is to postpone conduit replacement until these parameters suggest potentially irreversible deterioration of the RV function. The critical values of these parameters are under ongoing investigation. In addition, the intracardiac baffle created by the Rastelli procedure may leak or it may cause obstruction between the VSD and transposed aortic valve. Rarely, clots can form in the blind-ended pulmonary trunk. Dislodgment of these clots into the baffled channel causes systemic thromboembolism. These complications are typically evaluated with echocardiography.

Imaging for Congenitally Corrected Transposition of the Great Arteries

As in the case of CTGA, chest radiographic findings for CCTGA are variable and rarely diagnostic. Shunting through a VSD may produce shunt vascularity on the radiograph, and severe tricuspid regurgitation may cause significant RA enlargement. Dextrocardia is seen in 25% of cases. During early childhood, echocardiography is the definitive diagnostic test. Later in life, MRI may yield better visualization of the abnormal cardiac connections. Regardless of the imaging modality, the diagnosis of CCTGA depends on careful analysis of each cardiac segment and its connections.

First, the atrial situs is determined. The right atrium should have a broad-based, pyramidal atrial appendage and the left atrium should have a tubular, crenellated atrial appendage. The right main pulmonary artery should be anterior to the right mainstem bronchus and the left main pulmonary artery should course above the left mainstem bronchus. The right mainstem bronchus should be more vertically oriented than the left mainstem bronchus. The right lung should have three lobes and the left lung should have two lobes. If these features are left-right reversed, then the atrial situs is inversed and the positions of the morphologic left and right atria are reversed.

Second, the ventricular morphology is evaluated. A right ventricle typically has course trabeculations (see Fig. 44-3), a prominent moderator band, and separation of the

■ FIGURE 44-24 Gated CTA of a patient after the Rastelli operation. This volume rendering shows a pulmonary conduit (C) stenosis (*arrow*) at its anastomosis with the native pulmonary trunk (PA).

inlet-outlet valves (see Fig. 44-1). In contrast, a left ventricle has fine trabeculations except at the apex, absence of a moderator band, and fibrous continuity of the inlet-outlet valves without muscle in between (see Fig. 44-2). The diagnosis of CCTGA requires that the right atrium is aligned with the left ventricle and the left atrium aligned with the right ventricle, or atrioventricular discordance. In addition, it requires that the right ventricle be aligned with the aorta and the left ventricle is aligned with the pulmonary trunk, or ventriculoarterial discordance. Differentiation of the aorta and pulmonary trunk is usually straightforward by echocardiography and MRI.

Echocardiography should assess the presence and severity of lesions associated with CCTGA—VSD, pulmonary stenosis, and malformed tricuspid valve. Catheter measurements of the abnormal hemodynamics may be necessary. The hemodynamic significances of these lesions dictate the proper surgical interventions. If a double switch procedure is planned, imaging assessment of LV training is similar to the reverse switch procedure (see earlier). Later in life, when the LV is no longer responsive to training and double switch is not an option, echocardiography is used to monitor for signs and severity of RV failure. When medical management is maximized, cardiac transplantation is the final therapeutic option.

> **KEY POINTS**
>
> - Transposition of the great arteries (TGA) is broadly divided into complete transposition of the great arteries (CTGA) and congenitally corrected transposition of the great arteries (CCTGA).
> - CTGA is associated with VSD and pulmonary valvular and subvalvular stenoses.
> - The definitive surgical operations for CTGA are the arterial switch procedure (Jatene), atrial switch procedure (Mustard-Senning), and Rastelli procedure.
> - CCTGA is associated with VSD, pulmonary stenosis, and malformation of the tricuspid valve.
> - Current surgical procedures for CCTGA are geared toward correcting hemodynamic problems caused by the associated lesions.
> - The long-term benefit of the double switch procedure, a definitive surgery for CCTGA, is currently unknown.
> - Echocardiography is the primary diagnostic imaging modality for TGA. MRI is a useful supplemental imaging technique when echocardiography is inadequate or when accurate volume and flow quantifications are required for management decisions. Catheter angiography is reserved for coronary imaging and hemodynamic measurements.

SUGGESTED READINGS

Graham TP. Congenitally corrected transposition. In Gatzoulis MA, Webb GD, Daubeney PEF (eds). Diagnosis and management of adult congenital heart disease. Edinburgh. Churchill Livingstone, 2003, pp 379-387.

Hornung T. Transposition of the great arteries. In Gatzoulis MA, Webb GD, Daubeney PEF (eds). Diagnosis and management of adult congenital heart disease. Edinburgh, Churchill Livingstone, 2003, pp 349-362.

Warnes CA. Transposition of the great arteries. Circulation 2006; 114:2699-2709.

Yuh DD, Reitz BA. Cyanotic defects. In Reitz BA, Yuh DD (eds). Congenital Cardiac Surgery. New York, McGraw-Hill, 2002, pp 137-143.

REFERENCES

1. Senning A. Surgical correction of transposition of the great vessels. Surgery 1959; 45:966-980.
2. Mustard WT. Successful two-stage correction of transposition of the great vessels. Surgery 1964; 55:469-472.
3. Jatene AD, Fontes VF, Paulista PP, et al. Anatomic correction of transposition of the great vessels. J Thorac Cardiovasc Surg 1976; 72:364-370.
4. Rastelli GC, McGoon DC, Wallace RB. Anatomic correction of transposition of the great arteries with ventricular septal defect and subpulmonary stenosis. J Thorac Cardiovasc Surg 1969; 58:545-552.
5. Ilbawi MN, DeLeon SY, Backer CL, et al. An alternative approach to the surgical management of physiologically corrected transposition with ventricular septal defect and pulmonary stenosis or atresia. J Thorac Cardiovasc Surg 1990; 100:410-415.
6. Van Praagh R, Weinberg PM, Smith SD. Malpositions of the heart. In Adams FH, Emmanoulides GC, Riemenschneider TA (eds). Moss' Heart Disease in Infants, Children and Adolescents. Baltimore, Lippincott Williams & Wilkins, 1989, pp 530-580.
7. Van Praagh R, Papagiannis J, Grunenfelder J, et al. Pathologic anatomy of corrected transposition of the great arteries: medical and surgical implications. Am Heart J 1998; 135:772-785.
8. Pierpont ME, Basson CT, Benson DW Jr, et al. Genetic basis for congenital heart defects: current knowledge: a scientific statement from the American Heart Association Congenital Cardiac Defects Committee, Council on Cardiovascular Disease in the Young. Endorsed by the American Academy of Pediatrics. Circulation 2007; 115:3015-3038.
9. Burn J, Brennan P, Little J, et al. Recurrence risks in offspring of adults with major heart defects: results from first cohort of British collaborative study. Lancet 1998; 351:311-316.
10. Development of the cardiovascular and lymphatic systems. In Standring S (ed). Gray's anatomy: the anatomical basis of clinical practice, 39th ed. Edinburgh, Churchill Livingstone, 2005, pp 1029-1055
11. Wernovsky G, Sanders SP. Coronary artery anatomy and transposition of the great arteries. Coron Artery Dis 1993; 4:148-157.
12. Lundstrom U, Bull C, Wyse RK, Somerville J. The natural and "unnatural" history of congenitally corrected transposition. Am J Cardiol 1990; 65:1222-1229.
13. McKay R, Anderson RH, Smith A. The coronary arteries in hearts with discordant atrioventricular connections. J Thorac Cardiovasc Surg 1996; 111:988-997.
14. Liebman J, Cullum L, Belloc NB. Natural history of transpositon of the great arteries. Anatomy and birth and death characteristics. Circulation 1969; 40:237-262.
15. Graham TP Jr, Bernard YD, Mellen BG, et al. Long-term outcome in congenitally corrected transposition of the great arteries: a multi-institutional study. J Am Coll Cardiol 2000; 36:255-261.
16. Rashkind WJ, Miller WW. Creation of an atrial septal defect without thoracotomy. A palliative approach to complete transposition of the great arteries. JAMA 1966; 196:991-992.

17. McQuillen PS, Hamrick SE, Perez MJ, et al. Balloon atrial septostomy is associated with preoperative stroke in neonates with transposition of the great arteries. Circulation 2006; 113:280-285.
18. Castaneda AR, Trusler GA, Paul MH, et al. The early results of treatment of simple transposition in the current era. J Thorac Cardiovasc Surg 1988; 95:14-28.
19. Losay J, Touchot A, Serraf A, et al. Late outcome after arterial switch operation for transposition of the great arteries. Circulation 2001; 104:I121-I126.
20. Bonhoeffer P, Bonnet D, Piechaud JF, et al. Coronary artery obstruction after the arterial switch operation for transposition of the great arteries in newborns. J Am Coll Cardiol 1997; 29:202-206.
21. Trusler GA, Williams WG, Duncan KF, et al. Results with the Mustard operation in simple transposition of the great arteries 1963-1985. Ann Surg 1987; 206:251-260.
22. Wilson NJ, Clarkson PM, Barratt-Boyes BG, et al. Long-term outcome after the mustard repair for simple transposition of the great arteries: 28-year follow-up. J Am Coll Cardiol 1998; 32:758-765.
23. Kreutzer C, De VJ, Oppido G, et al. Twenty-five-year experience with rastelli repair for transposition of the great arteries. J Thorac Cardiovasc Surg 2000; 120:211-223.
24. DeLeon SY, Ilbawi MN, Tubeszewski K, et al. The Damus-Stansel-Kaye procedure: anatomical determinants and modifications. Ann Thorac Surg 1991; 52:680-687.
25. Yeh T Jr, Connelly MS, Coles JG, et al. Atrioventricular discordance: results of repair in 127 patients. J Thorac Cardiovasc Surg 1999; 117:1190-1203.
26. Devaney EJ, Charpie JR, Ohye RG, Bove EL. Combined arterial switch and Senning operation for congenitally corrected transposition of the great arteries: patient selection and intermediate results. J Thorac Cardiovasc Surg 2003; 125:500-507.
27. Winlaw DS, McGuirk SP, Balmer C, et al. Intention-to-treat analysis of pulmonary artery banding in conditions with a morphological right ventricle in the systemic circulation with a view to anatomic biventricular repair. Circulation 2005; 111:405-411.
28. Shin'oka T, Kurosawa H, Imai Y, et al. Outcomes of definitive surgical repair for congenitally corrected transposition of the great arteries or double outlet right ventricle with discordant atrioventricular connections: risk analyses in 189 patients. J Thorac Cardiovasc Surg 2007; 133:1318-1328.
29. Vinnakota KC, Bassingthwaighte JB. Myocardial density and composition: a basis for calculating intracellular metabolite concentrations. Am J Physiol Heart Circ Physiol 2004; 286:H1742-H1749.
30. Lorenz CH, Walker ES, Morgan VL, et al. Normal human right and left ventricular mass, systolic function, and gender differences by cine magnetic resonance imaging. J Cardiovasc Magn Reson 1999; 1:7-21.

CHAPTER 45

Truncus Arteriosus

Frandics P. Chan

Truncus arteriosus is an uncommon but potentially lethal congenital heart disease that manifests during the neonatal period or early infancy. It is defined by a common origin of the aorta and the pulmonary arteries, resulting from an incomplete embryologic septation and separation of the aorta and the pulmonary trunk. This congenital cardiac anomaly was first described in 1798 by Wilson.[1] In 1942, Lev and Saphir[2] proposed the anatomic criteria that defined truncus arteriosus. Since then, different classifications had been proposed by Collett and Edwards[3] in 1949, by Van Praagh and Van Praagh[4] in 1965, and by the Society of Thoracic Surgeons in 2000.[5]

DEFINITION

In common usage, the term *truncus arteriosus* implies persistent truncus arteriosus at birth. Synonyms are *common arterial trunk, truncus arteriosus communis,* and *common aorticopulmonary trunk.* Truncus arteriosus is defined by the anatomy: the aorta and the pulmonary arteries arise from a common trunk above a single truncal valve.

CLASSIFICATIONS

Historically, two major classification schemes for anatomic variations of the truncus arteriosus were proposed by Collett and Edwards[3] and by Van Praagh and Van Praagh.[4] The Collett and Edwards classification is strictly defined by the anatomic origins of the pulmonary arteries. It divides truncus arteriosus into four types, I to IV (Fig. 45-1). In Collett and Edwards type I, a common arterial trunk divides into an aorta and a short pulmonary trunk, which divides into the left and right branch pulmonary arteries. This is the most common configuration (48% to 68% of cases). In Collett and Edwards type II (29% to 48% of cases), the left and right branch pulmonary arteries arise close together from the common arterial trunk without a distinct pulmonary trunk. Collett and Edwards type III (6% to 10% of cases) is similar to type II except that the origins of the pulmonary arteries are far apart.

Collett and Edwards described a type IV configuration in which the pulmonary arteries arise from the descending aorta. These arteries are now known to be major aorticopulmonary collateral arteries associated with pulmonary atresia with ventricular septal defect (VSD) and not truncus arteriosus.

The Collett and Edwards classification developed in 1949 did not consider the roles of patent ductus arteriosus (PDA) and interrupted aortic arch, which are associated with truncus arteriosus and have prognostic and surgical implications. Subsequently, Van Praagh and Van Praagh[4] proposed a different classification with four types, 1 to 4 (Fig. 45-2). Each number may have a prefix letter *A* if a VSD is present (common) or *B* if a VSD is absent (rare). Van Praagh and Van Praagh type 1 is identical to Collett and Edwards type I, describing a short pulmonary trunk arising from the common arterial trunk. Van Praagh and Van Praagh type 2 describes separate origins of the left and right branch pulmonary arteries arising from the common arterial trunk, regardless of the distance separating their origins (Fig. 45-3). It corresponds to Collett and Edwards type II and type III. Van Praagh and Van Praagh type 3 describes one branch pulmonary artery arising from the common arterial trunk and the other connected to a ductus arteriosus or an aorticopulmonary collateral artery (Fig. 45-4). Van Praagh and Van Praagh type 4 describes the coexistence of a common arterial trunk and an interrupted or a severely hypoplastic aortic arch. The descending aorta is supplied by a PDA. Van Praagh and Van Praagh type 3 and type 4 have no correspondence in the Collett and Edwards classification.

Although the Van Praagh and Van Praagh classification provides a more refined description of truncus arteriosus, it does not completely serve the needs of surgeons. In 2000, the Society of Thoracic Surgeons proposed a uniform reporting system with modifiers that better describe anatomic features useful for surgical outcome studies.[5] In this system, cryptic numerical labels are replaced by descriptive phrases. Three major types are described: truncus arteriosus with confluent or near-confluent pulmonary arteries (corresponding to Van Praagh and Van Praagh

CHAPTER 45 • Truncus Arteriosus 617

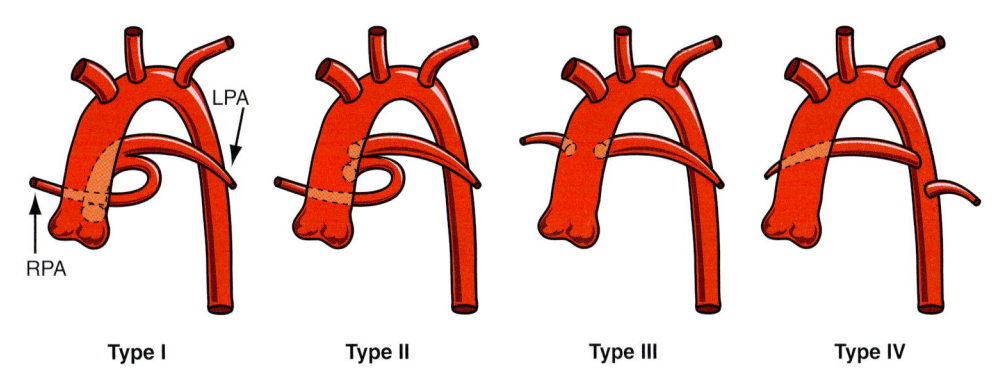

■ **FIGURE 45-1** Collett and Edwards classification: *type I*, a pulmonary trunk connects the common arterial trunk to the branch pulmonary arteries; *type II*, branch pulmonary arteries arise closely from the common arterial trunk; *type III*, branch pulmonary arteries arise far apart from the common arterial trunk; *type IV*, branch pulmonary arteries arise from the descending aorta. LPA, left pulmonary artery; RPA, right pulmonary artery.

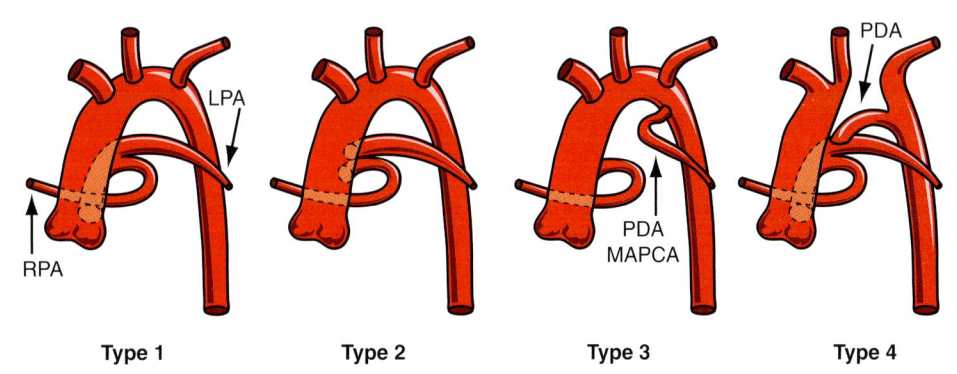

■ **FIGURE 45-2** Van Praagh and Van Praagh classification: *type 1*, a pulmonary trunk connects the common arterial trunk to the branch pulmonary arteries; *type 2*, branch pulmonary arteries arise anywhere from the common arterial trunk; *type 3*, one branch pulmonary artery connects to a PDA or major aorticopulmonary collateral artery (MAPCA); *type 4*, interrupted aortic arch. LPA, left pulmonary artery; RPA, right pulmonary artery.

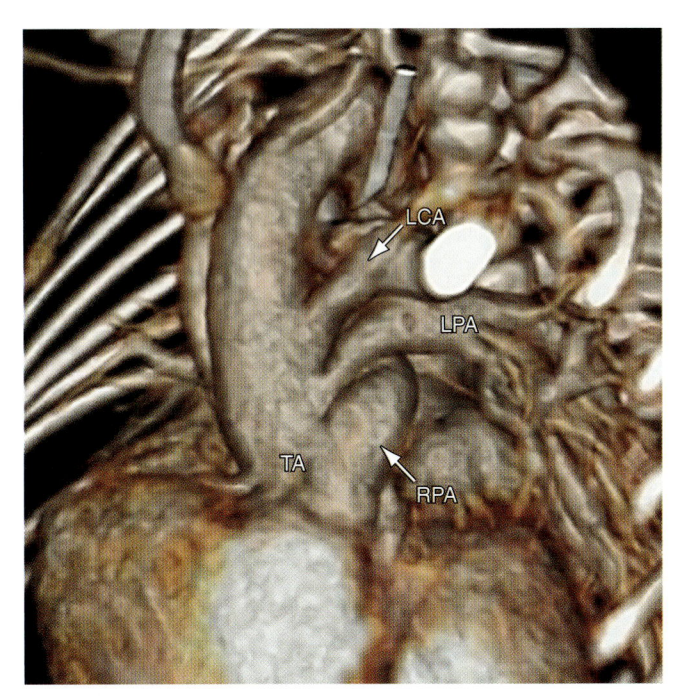

■ **FIGURE 45-3** ECG gated CT scan of a Van Praagh and Van Praagh type 2 truncus arteriosus. Volume rendered image shows the left pulmonary artery (LPA) and the right pulmonary artery (RPA) arising separately from the common arterial trunk (TA). The LPA is typically positioned above the RPA. The topmost branch is the left carotid artery (LCA).

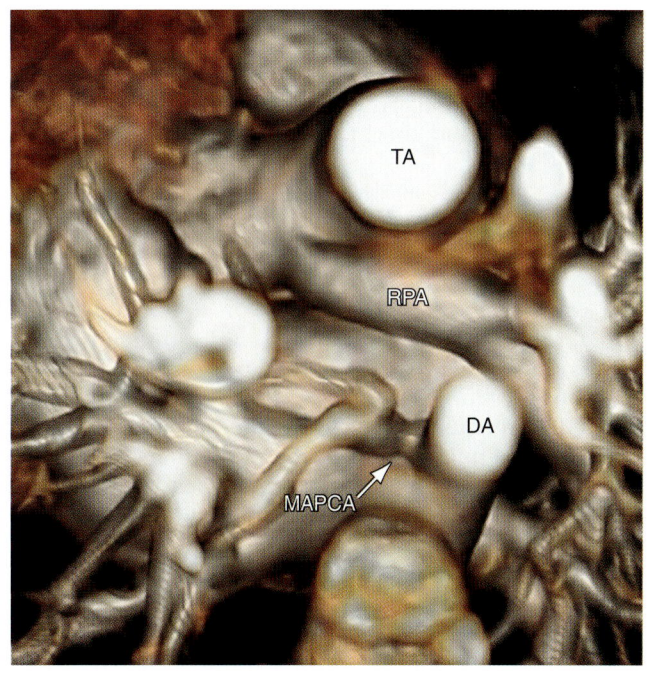

■ **FIGURE 45-4** ECG gated CT scan of a Van Praagh and Van Praagh type 3 truncus arteriosus. Volume rendered image shows the right pulmonary artery (RPA) arising from the common arterial trunk (TA). The left pulmonary artery is connected by a major aorticopulmonary collateral artery (MAPCA) to the descending aorta (DA).

type 1 and type 2), truncus arteriosus with absence of one pulmonary artery (corresponding to Van Praagh and Van Praagh type 3), and truncus arteriosus with interrupted aortic arch or coarctation (corresponding to Van Praagh and Van Praagh type 4). Additional modifiers describe the presence or absence of VSD, the number of truncal leaflets, the presence of truncal insufficiency or stenosis or both, coexisting coronary anomalies, any ventricular hypoplasia, the truncal valve position relative to the ventricles, and the presence or absence of thymus.

EPIDEMIOLOGY AND GENETICS

Truncus arteriosus occurs in 1% to 2% of infants born with congenital heart defects, or about 10 cases per 100,000 live births.[6] Among conotruncal anomalies, truncus arteriosus has a similar rate of occurrence as congenitally corrected transposition of the great arteries and double outlet right ventricle, but it is three times less common than complete transposition of the great arteries and four times less common than tetralogy of Fallot. There is no predilection by sex. Of patients with truncus arteriosus, 34% to 41% harbor a chromosome 22q11 deletion.[7] This deletion is also seen in a large proportion of patients with conotruncal developmental anomalies as found in DiGeorge syndrome, velocardiofacial syndrome, and interrupted aortic arch, suggesting the importance of this gene in the regulation of the embryologic development of the conotruncus. Today, this chromosomal deletion is readily detected with the fluorescence in situ hybridization technique.

Genetic screening is important because 22q11 deletion is inherited in an autosomal dominant fashion from one parent in 6% to 28% of cases.[8] This is important information for genetic family counseling. Knowledge of this deletion also heightens clinical suspicions for associated anomalies, including athymia, hypocalcemia, and nasopalatal malformation. Truncus arteriosus is also associated with trisomy 8 and chromosomal 10p deletion.[9]

ETIOLOGY AND PATHOPHYSIOLOGY

Embryology

The embryologic truncus arteriosus is a normal vascular structure that connects the conus cordis to the branchial arches from days 25 to 50 of gestational age. The conus cordis is destined to become the ventricular outflow tracts; the truncus arteriosus separates into the ascending aorta and the pulmonary trunk; and the branchial arches evolve into the branch pulmonary arteries and the aortic arch. For this reason, some authors prefer the term *persistent truncus arteriosus*.

In normal embryologic development, beginning in the fifth week of gestation, fusion of the endocardial cushions separates the atrioventricular canal into right and left openings, which are destined to become the tricuspid annulus and the mitral annulus. Through these two openings, blood flow develops into two intertwined, spiraling streams that flow out the conus cordis and the truncus arteriosus, or conotruncus for short. Between the two spiraling streams is a layer of stagnant blood. There is evidence that this layer of stagnant blood promotes the development of two ridges of tissue at opposing margins inside the conotruncus.[10] These two ridges grow toward each other until they meet and fuse. The fusion begins at the conotruncal junction. Similar to the closing of a zipper, the fusion proceeds upward through the truncus arteriosus, creating two spiraling lumens that become the ascending aorta and the pulmonary trunk. From this junction, the fusion also travels downward through the conus cordis until it meets the ventricular septum, separating the right and left ventricles. Separation of the systemic and the pulmonary circulations is completed by 9 weeks of gestation. Beginning in the seventh week, specialized tissue swellings from the conotruncal junction evolve into the aortic and the pulmonary semilunar valves; these are also completed by 9 weeks.

Persistent truncus arteriosus is the failure of development or fusion of the conotruncal ridges. This developmental anomaly has three major consequences. First, the incomplete septation of the conus cordis leaves a large VSD at the outflow region. Second, the failure to form separate aortic and pulmonary valves leave a single truncal valve. Third, the pulmonary and aortic blood flows are in free communication. All three defects lead to important hemodynamic derangements and their clinical manifestations.

Associated Cardiac Anomalies

Because the conus cordis is not partitioned properly below the truncal valve, a VSD usually exists at the infundibular septum beneath the truncal valve (Fig. 45-5). This

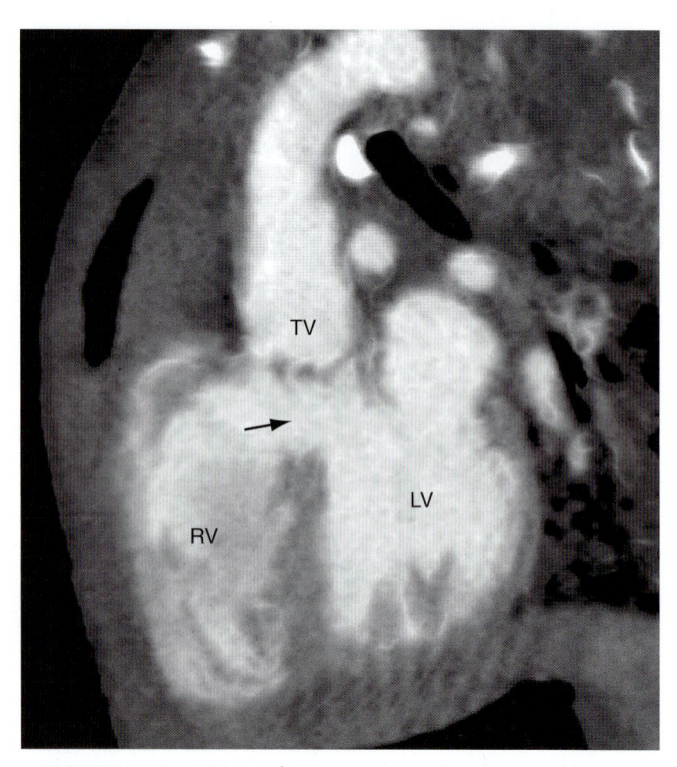

■ **FIGURE 45-5** ECG gated CT scan. Long-axis reformatted image shows a large subtruncal VSD (*arrow*). The truncal valve (TV) straddles the ventricular septum between the right ventricle (RV) and the left ventricle (LV).

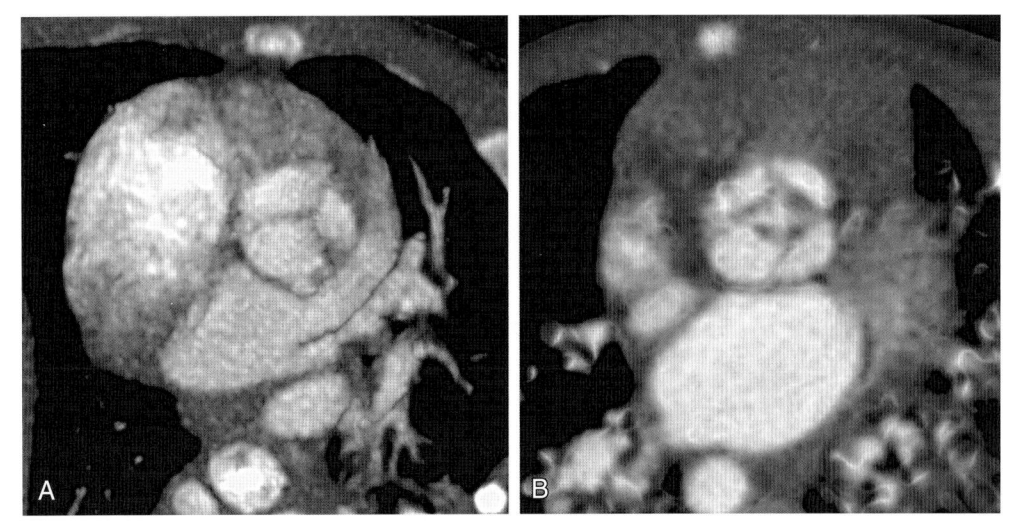

■ **FIGURE 45-6** ECG gated CT scan. **A** and **B,** Short-axis reformatted image shows a tricuspid truncal valve (**A**) and a quadricuspid truncal valve (**B**).

VSD is often large and nonrestrictive. The right ventricle, subjected to the systemic pressure generated by the left ventricle, becomes hypertrophic. In most instances (68% to 83%), the common arterial trunk and the truncal valve straddle the ventricular septum in a manner resembling the overriding aorta in tetralogy of Fallot or pulmonary atresia with VSD. Uncommonly (11% to 29%), the truncal valve aligns exclusively with the right ventricle. Rarely (4% to 6%), it aligns with the left ventricle. In the two latter situations, the VSD may be small or absent.

The truncal valve may have one to five leaflets. Tricuspid truncal valve (Fig. 45-6A) is the most common (69%), followed by quadricuspid valve (22%) (see Fig. 45-6B) and bicuspid valve (9%). The truncal valve has fibrous continuity with the mitral valve, similar to the normal relationship between the aortic valve and mitral valve. A muscle bridge usually separates the truncal valve from the tricuspid valve. Competency of the truncal valve has important implications to survival and surgical outcome. In most autopsy cases, the truncal valve leaflets are dysplastic and thickened with myxomatous degeneration. Truncal regurgitation is common, occurring in half of the cases. In 20% of cases, the truncal valve may be stenotic.[11] Severe regurgitation or stenosis heralds a poor prognosis.

In the most common situation, the truncal valve is tricuspid with a posterior cusp, a right anterior cusp, and a left anterior cusp. The right coronary artery usually arises from the right anterior cusp, and the left main coronary artery arises from the posterior cusp (Fig. 45-7A).[12] Variation from this pattern is extremely common, however, because the development of the proximal coronary arteries is closely coordinated with the development of the conotruncus. In a quadricuspid valve, the right and left coronary arteries most commonly originate from the opposing right and left cusps (see Fig. 45-7B). In pathology series, a single coronary artery was seen in 10% to 20% of cases,[13] and stenosis at the coronary ostium was found in 7% of cases.[14]

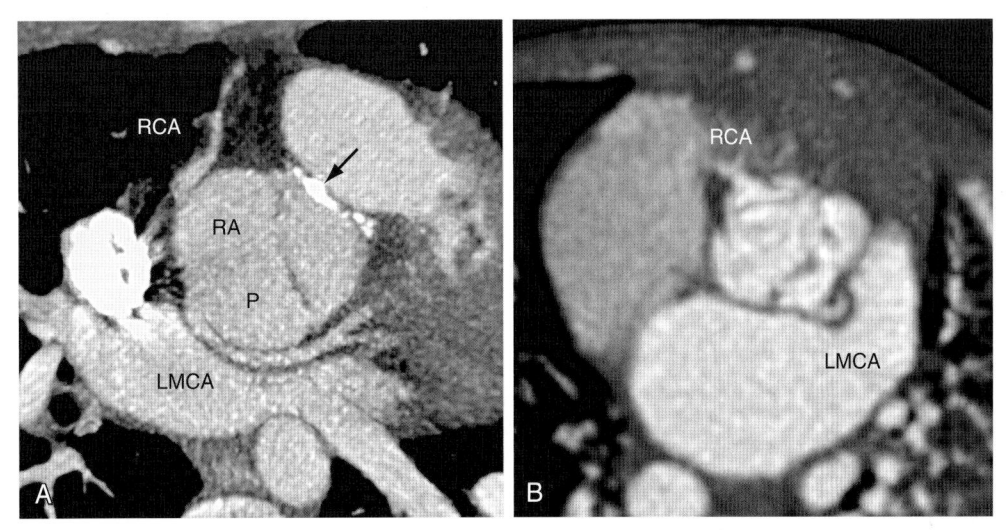

■ **FIGURE 45-7** ECG gated CT scan. **A,** Short-axis reformatted image shows the typical origins of the right coronary artery (RCA) from the right anterior cusp (RA) and the left main coronary artery (LMCA) from the posterior cusp (P). This patient had undergone surgical repair, and the VSD patch is calcified (*arrow*). **B,** The coronary arteries are shown originating from the opposite cusps of a quadricuspid valve.

Compared with a normal ascending aorta, the common arterial trunk usually appears large, but some can expand into an aneurysm. Histologic studies have shown tissue pathology similar to that of Marfan syndrome. The pathophysiology is unknown, but pulmonary hypertension may play a role. Truncus rupture and dissection have been reported.[15] The aortic arch is right-sided in one third of truncus arteriosus cases, usually with a mirror-image branching pattern of the cervical arteries. Aortic arch interruption is seen in 11% to 38% of cases. The most common interruption (84%) occurs between the left common carotid artery and the left subclavian artery (type B interrupted aortic arch).[16] In this configuration, the left and right carotid arteries are fed by the common arterial trunk, and the descending aorta and left subclavian artery are fed by the PDA. The right subclavian artery may be fed by either of these arteries depending on whether it has a normal or an aberrant origin. Less commonly (16%), the interruption occurs distal to the left subclavian artery (type A interrupted aortic arch). Interruption between the left and right carotid arteries (type C interrupted aortic arch) is rare.

The pulmonary arteries usually arise from the left posterior aspect of the common arterial trunk. When the branch pulmonary arteries arise from the common arterial trunk separately, the left branch pulmonary artery is often superiorly related to the right branch pulmonary artery (see Fig. 45-3). If a PDA is present, its size is inversely related to the aortic arch and the aortic isthmus. In the extreme case of aortic arch interruption, blood flow to the descending aorta is carried entirely by a large ductus arteriosus. Other cardiac anomalies associated with truncus arteriosus are secundum atrial septal defect, aberrant subclavian artery, persistent left superior vena cava, and tricuspid stenosis.

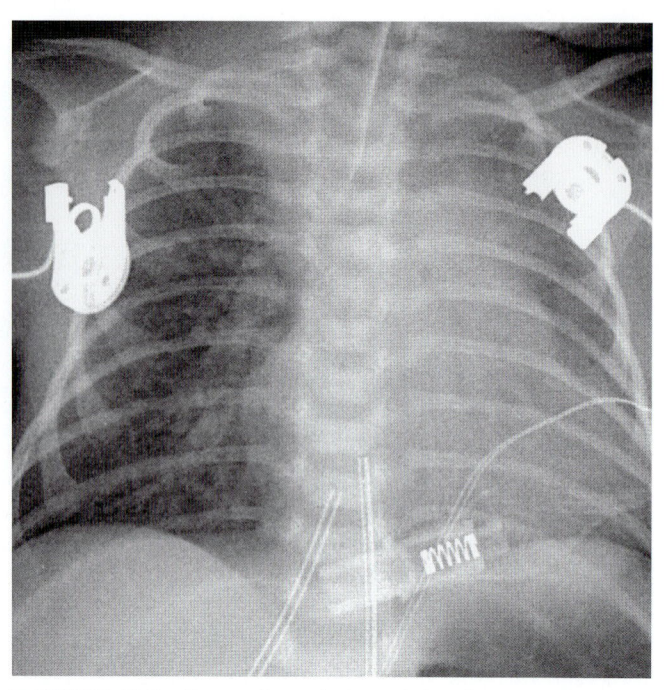

■ **FIGURE 45-8** Chest radiograph. Frontal view shows prominent peripheral pulmonary arteries from large pulmonary flow and diffuse ground-glass opacity from pulmonary edema.

MANIFESTATIONS OF DISEASE

Clinical Presentation

Although truncus arteriosus is classified as a cyanotic congenital heart disease with admixture of pulmonary and systemic venous blood, cyanosis is not a prominent feature, unless there is coexisting pulmonary artery stenosis. Instead, patients present with symptoms of heart failure a few days after birth and symptoms of pulmonary hypertension in the first year of life. These clinical presentations can be explained by the underlying hemodynamic derangements. In truncus arteriosus, because the pulmonary arteries and the aorta share a common origin, the pressures driving the pulmonary flow and the systemic flow are the same. Blood flow is equal to the arteriovenous pressure divided by vascular resistance. The shunt ratio, defined as pulmonary flow divided by systemic flow, is equal to systemic vascular resistance divided by pulmonary vascular resistance.

During the first week of life, the pulmonary vascular resistance decreases rapidly below the systemic vascular resistance. The shunt ratio can reach 5:1 or greater, which implies a pulmonary flow five times the systemic flow. This torrential pulmonary flow returns through the pulmonary veins into the left ventricle. Assuming that there is no shunting at the atrial level, the left ventricle must handle this amount of flow by stroking five times the volume of the right ventricle. The left ventricle is severely volume overloaded, leading to congestive heart failure. Chest radiography may show evidence for shunt vascularity and pulmonary edema (Fig. 45-8). If the truncal valve is incompetent, the regurgitant flow adds to the volume load, exacerbating the heart failure.

The lack of cyanosis after the first few days of life can be explained by the fact that the oxygenated pulmonary venous flow is much greater than the desaturated systemic venous flow. Despite admixture at the VSD and the common arterial trunk, the systemic oxygen saturation remains elevated. Left untreated, the large amount of pulmonary flow and the high pulmonary pressure induce remodeling in the pulmonary microvasculature, termed *pulmonary arteriopathy*. This condition irreversibly constricts flow, increasing pulmonary vascular resistance, leading to pulmonary hypertension and Eisenmenger syndrome in patients 6 to 8 months old.

The prognosis of truncus arteriosus without surgical repair is poor. The median age of survival ranges from 2 weeks to 3 months; mortality at 1 year of life is greater than 80%. Adult survivors have been reported, but are extremely rare.[17] As expected, early deaths are mostly due to heart failure and later mortality caused by pulmonary hypertension. Other factors that worsen prognosis are coexisting interrupted aortic arch, coarctation, truncal valve regurgitation, and truncal valve stenosis. Late survivors may have benefited from incidental pulmonary artery stenoses that protect the pulmonary vasculature from high flow and high pressure.

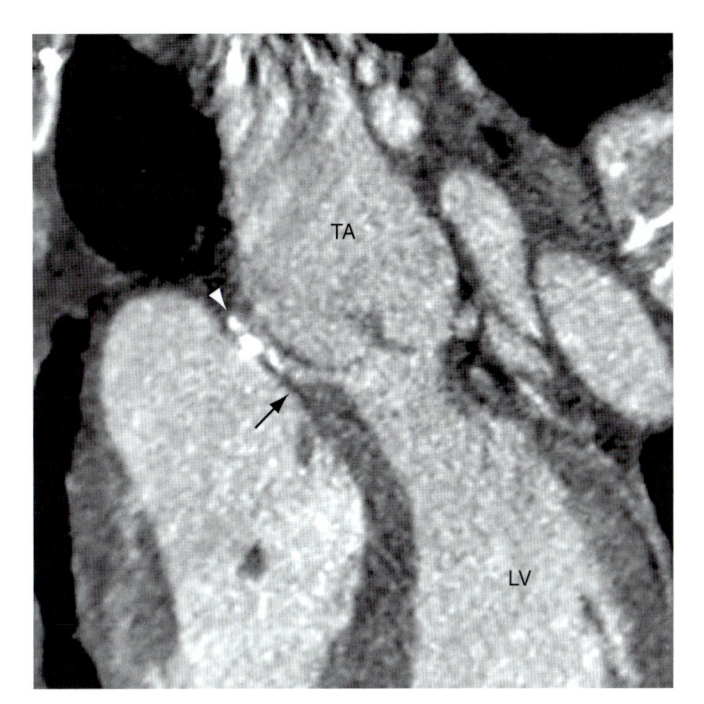

■ **FIGURE 45-9** ECG gated CT scan after surgical repair. Long-axis reformatted image shows a calcified VSD patch connecting the ventricular margin of the VSD (*arrow*) to the right ventricular margin of the truncal valve (*arrowhead*). The left ventricle (LV) is connected to the common arterial trunk (TA) exclusively.

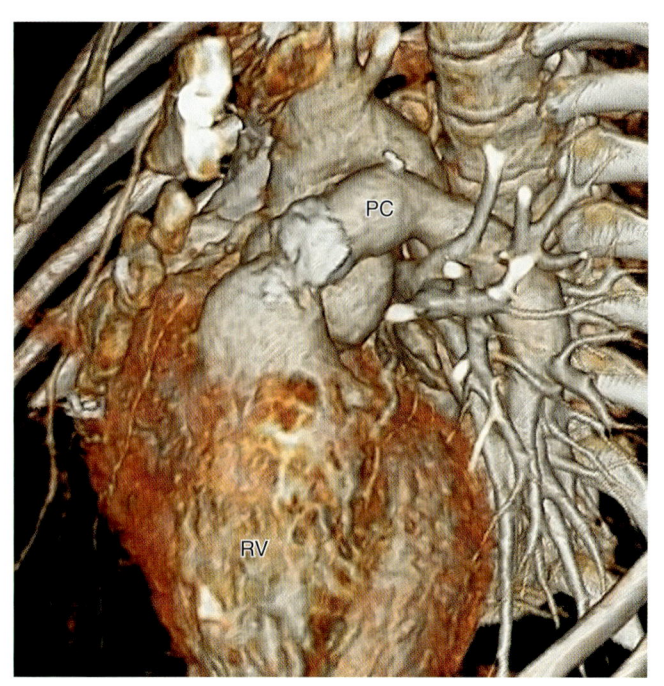

■ **FIGURE 45-10** ECG gated CT scan after surgical repair. Volume rendered image shows a valved pulmonary conduit (PC) connecting the right ventricle (RV) to the branch pulmonary arteries.

Imaging Indications and Algorithm

Imaging is discussed after surgical treatment because managing postoperative imaging is more common and important than diagnosing the original disease.

Differential Diagnosis

On imaging studies, truncus arteriosus and pulmonary atresia with VSD have very similar appearances. Both have a single outlet valve straddling the ventricular septum and the outlet valve connected to an ascending systemic great artery. In truncus arteriosus, there must be at least one pulmonary artery originating from this ascending great artery. In pulmonary atresia with VSD, the pulmonary circulation is supplied either by a PDA or by major aorticopulmonary collateral arteries from the coronary arteries, the cervical arteries, and the descending aorta. None of these should arise directly from the ascending great artery.

The term *hemitruncus* refers to an anatomy where one branch pulmonary artery arises from the aorta and the other branch pulmonary artery arises from the right ventricle. Separate aortic and pulmonary valves exist. The term *pseudotruncus* has been used to describe the large ascending aorta in pulmonary atresia with VSD. Embryologically, hemitruncus and pseudotruncus are not the results of abnormal conotruncal septation, and they are not considered a spectrum of truncus arteriosus. Congenital aorticopulmonary window is a rare anomaly in which a truncal septal defect allows communication between the ascending aorta and the pulmonary trunk. It differs from truncus arteriosus in that the aortic and pulmonary valves are formed and distinct.

TREATMENT OPTIONS

Because of the poor prognosis of truncus arteriosus and the early onset of pulmonary vascular disease, current treatment favors primary surgical repair within the first month of life.[18,19] Before the current era, pulmonary banding was performed to reduce pulmonary flow and the left ventricular volume load. Pulmonary banding was a palliative approach that did not require cardiopulmonary bypass, but its long-term outcome was generally unsatisfactory. The first complete repair was performed by McGoon and colleagues[20] in 1967 using an aortic homograft for the pulmonary connection.

The basic surgical approach for complete repair is the same today. After establishing cardiopulmonary bypass, the pulmonary arteries from the common arterial trunk or the aorta are identified and excised. Through a right ventriculotomy, the subtruncal VSD is visualized. A patch is sutured along the margin of the VSD and right ventricular side of the truncal annulus, connecting the common arterial trunk and the truncal valve to the left ventricle exclusively (Fig. 45-9). A valved pulmonary conduit is placed at the right ventriculotomy site and connected to the excised pulmonary arteries, establishing the pulmonary flow (Fig. 45-10). After surgery, the truncal valve effectively becomes the aortic valve, and the common arterial trunk becomes the ascending aorta. If the native truncal valve is dysfunctional and cannot be repaired, it is replaced with a prostatic valve. In cases with associated interrupted aortic arch or coarctation (Van Praagh and Van Praagh type 4), the arch is reconstructed to maintain continuity among the common arterial trunk, the cervical arteries, and the descending aorta.

Long-term prognosis after successful surgical repair is very good, with 80% survival rate at 20 years.[21] Major factors associated with postoperative complications and mortality are truncal valve abnormalities, interrupted aortic arch, nonconfluence or small pulmonary arteries, and coronary anomalies.[22] Of these, interrupted aortic arch seems to be of the greatest concern, with some series reporting early modality near 50%.[16,23] Reoperation, even after successful initial repair, is common. Most reoperations are done for the replacement of a malfunctioning pulmonary conduit. Other reasons for reoperation include the repair or replacement of an incompetent truncal valve, arterioplasty of branch pulmonary artery stenoses, and closure of residual VSD.[21]

IMAGING INDICATIONS AND REPORTING

The goals of imaging are to secure the early diagnosis of truncus arteriosus, to delineate vascular anatomy for surgical planning, to identify factors that adversely affect surgical outcome, and to evaluate complications that require reoperation. Fetal ultrasonography can diagnose truncus arteriosus, and this information may be useful for parental counseling during pregnancy.[24] In the neonatal period, echocardiography is the modality of choice for the diagnosis and characterization of truncus arteriosus.[25] In some centers, an echocardiographic diagnosis of uncomplicated truncus arteriosus is deemed sufficient for surgery without additional angiographic imaging. Color and gray-scale imaging at multiple imaging planes should be performed by an experienced operator, with special attention in differentiating truncus arteriosus, pulmonary atresia with VSD, and tetralogy of Fallot. Presurgical echocardiography should report (1) the alignment of the common arterial trunk with respect to the ventricles, (2) the size and location of the VSD, (3) the ventricular functions, (4) the morphology and function of the truncal valve, (5) the origins of the coronary arteries, (6) the origins of the pulmonary arteries, and (7) any anomaly of the aortic arch.

If echocardiography is unable to define the central pulmonary arteries, or if it detects aortic arch anomalies, these patients should undergo formal angiographic evaluation. This can be done with noninvasive MR angiography (which has the advantage of offering functional and anatomic information without the use of ionizing radiation) or CT angiography. The goals are to evaluate and report (1) any interrupted aortic arch or coarctation, (2) origins and patency of the cervical arteries, (3) existence and size of any PDA and aorticopulmonary collateral arteries, (4) location of the descending aorta, (5) origins and course of pulmonary arteries, and (6) any pulmonary artery stenosis.

For unoperated patients after 6 months of age, catheterization is necessary to measure pulmonary hemodynamics for signs of irreversible pulmonary vascular disease. In older children or adults, echocardiography may not adequately visualize all relevant cardiovascular structures. Echocardiography may be supplemented by MR angiography to evaluate the truncal anatomy, cine MRI to assess ventricular sizes and functions, and MRI phase contrast technique to quantify truncal regurgitation or stenosis.

Patients who have undergone complete surgical repair for truncus arteriosus are now surviving to adulthood in increasing numbers. Imaging goals for these patients are to detect postoperative complications and to help determine the optimal timing for reoperation. The two most important postoperative structures are the valved pulmonary conduit and the truncal valve. Regurgitation or stenosis of either or both valves has deleterious effects on the right and left ventricles. For these reasons, postoperative patients usually undergo routine surveillance with echocardiography. The problem with the valved pulmonary conduit after truncus arteriosus repair is analogous to the problem after tetralogy of Fallot repair. Surgical replacement of a failing pulmonary conduit is best timed just before the irreversible loss of right ventricular function because the new conduit would also deteriorate over time.[26] MRI, by quantifying right ventricular size and function, may be helpful in decision making.[27] These results may be applicable to truncus arteriosus. In addition, cardiac MRI can evaluate the truncal valve and the left ventricular function in the same study. The clinical role of MRI in the postoperative management of truncus arteriosus is of ongoing research interest.

Less commonly, new vascular lesions develop after surgery in the forms of pseudoaneurysm from a ruptured pulmonary conduit (Fig. 45-11); coarctation restenosis; branch pulmonary artery stenosis; and compression of the pulmonary arteries, veins, or airways by an aneurysmal common arterial trunk (Fig. 45-12).[28] These lesions are readily evaluated noninvasively by CT angiography or MR angiography.

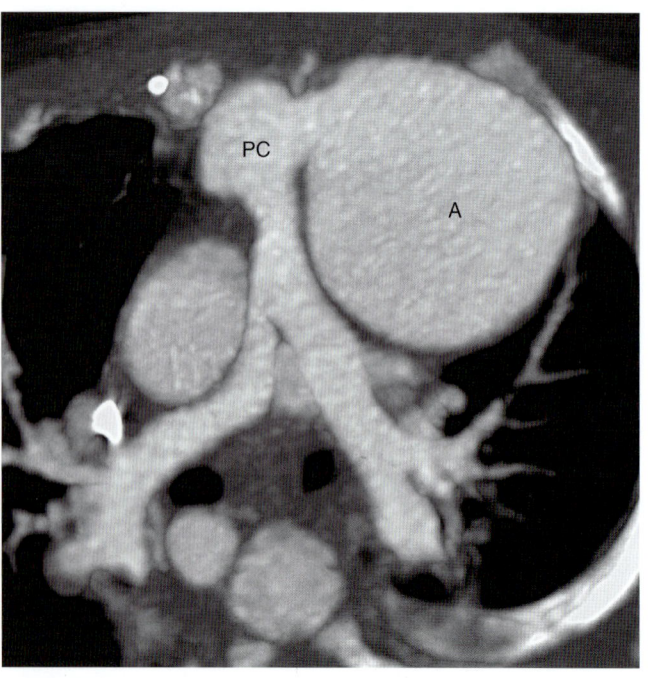

■ **FIGURE 45-11** ECG gated CT scan after surgical repair. Axial image shows a large, saccular pseudoaneurysm (A) arising from the proximal anastomosis of the pulmonary conduit (PC).

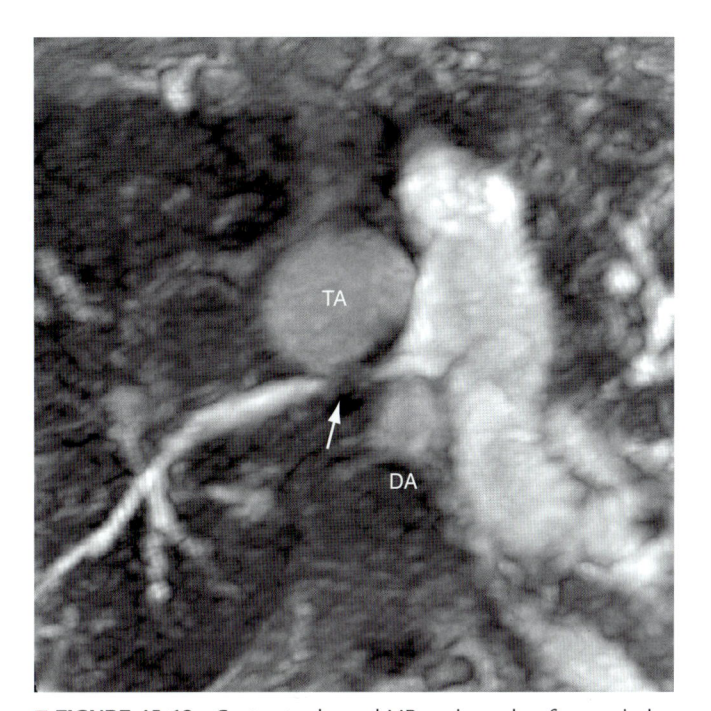

FIGURE 45-12 Contrast-enhanced MR angiography after surgical repair. Axial reformatted image shows that the common arterial trunk (TA) is more posteriorly located than usual, compressing the right branch pulmonary artery (*arrow*) against the descending aorta (DA).

KEY POINTS

- Truncus arteriosus is an uncommon congenital heart disease that is lethal within the first year of life.
- Neonatal patients with incomplete characterization of the pulmonary arteries or any aortic arch anomaly should undergo CT angiography or MR angiography.
- Childhood deaths are mainly caused by heart failure or early pulmonary hypertension.
- Adult survivors of truncus arteriosus have undergone surgical repair.
- Reoperation is commonly performed to replace the malfunctioning pulmonary conduit or truncal valve.
- MRI can be helpful in determining the optimal timing for pulmonary conduit replacement.

SUGGESTED READINGS

Connelly M. Common arterial trunk. In Gatzoulis MA, Webb GD, Daubeney PEF (eds). Diagnosis and Management of Adult Congenital Heart Disease. Edinburgh, Churchill Livingstone, 2003, pp 265-271.

Dorfman AL, Geva T. Magnetic resonance imaging evaluation of congenital heart disease: conotruncal anomalies. J Cardiovasc Magn Reson 2006; 8:645-659.

Larsen WJ. Development of the heart. In Human Embryology, 2nd ed. New York, Churchill Livingstone, 1997, pp 151-187.

McElhinney DB, Driscoll DA, Emanuel BS, et al. Chromosome 22q11 deletion in patients with truncus arteriosus. Pediatr Cardiol 2003; 24:569-573.

Tsai IC, Chen MC, Jan SL, et al. Neonatal cardiac multidetector row CT: why and how we do it. Pediatr Radiol 2008; 38:438-451.

REFERENCES

1. Wilson J. A description of a very unusual formation of the human heart. Phil Trans R Soc Lond (Biol) Part II 1798; 346-356.
2. Lev M, Saphir O. Truncus arteriosus communis persistens. J Pediatr 1943; 20:74.
3. Collett RW, Edwards JE. Persistent truncus arteriosus: a classification according to anatomic types. Surg Clin North Am 1949; 29: 1245-1270.
4. Van Praagh R, Van Praagh S. The anatomy of common aorticopulmonary trunk (truncus arteriosus communis) and its embryological implications: a study of 57 necropsy cases. Am J Cardiol 1965; 16:406-425.
5. Jacobs ML. Congenital heart surgery nomenclature and database project: truncus arteriosus. Ann Thorac Surg 2000; 69:S50-S55.
6. Hoffman JI, Kaplan S. The incidence of congenital heart disease. J Am Coll Cardiol 2002; 39:1890-1900.
7. Momma K, Matsuoka R, Takao A. Aortic arch anomalies associated with chromosome 22q11 deletion (CATCH 22). Pediatr Cardiol 1999; 20:97-102.
8. Digilio MC, Angioni A, De SM, et al. Spectrum of clinical variability in familial deletion 22q11.2: from full manifestation to extremely mild clinical anomalies. Clin Genet 2003; 63:308-313.
9. Pierpont ME, Basson CT, Benson DW Jr, et al. Genetic basis for congenital heart defects: current knowledge: a scientific statement from the American Heart Association Congenital Cardiac Defects Committee, Council on Cardiovascular Disease in the Young: endorsed by the American Academy of Pediatrics. Circulation 2007; 115:3015-3038.
10. Development of the cardiovascular and lymphatic systems. In Gray's Anatomy: The Anatomical Basis of Clinical Practice, 39th ed. Edinburgh, Churchill Livingstone, 2005, pp 1029-1055.
11. Elzein C, Ilbawi M, Kumar S, et al. Severe truncal valve stenosis: diagnosis and management. J Card Surg 2005; 20:589-593.
12. Chiu IS, Wu SJ, Chen MR, et al. Anatomic relationship of the coronary orifice and truncal valve in truncus arteriosus and their surgical implication. J Thorac Cardiovasc Surg 2002; 123:350-352.
13. de la Cruz MV, Cayre R, Angelini P, et al. Coronary arteries in truncus arteriosus. Am J Cardiol 1990; 66:1482-1486.
14. Butto F, Lucas RV Jr, Edwards JE. Persistent truncus arteriosus: pathologic anatomy in 54 cases. Pediatr Cardiol 1986; 7:95-101.
15. Gutierrez PS, Binotto MA, Aiello VD, et al. Chest pain in an adult with truncus arteriosus communis. Am J Cardiol 2004; 93:272-273.
16. Konstantinov IE, Karamlou T, Blackstone EH, et al. Truncus arteriosus associated with interrupted aortic arch in 50 neonates: a Congenital Heart Surgeons Society study. Ann Thorac Surg 2006; 81:214-222.
17. Silverman JJ, Scheinesson GP. Persistent truncus arteriosus in a 43 year old man. Am J Cardiol 1966; 17:94-96.

18. Rodefeld MD, Hanley FL. Neonatal truncus arteriosus repair: surgical techniques and clinical management. Semin Thorac Cardiovasc Surg Pediatr Card Surg Annu 2002; 5:212-217.
19. Thompson LD, McElhinney DB, Reddy M, et al. Neonatal repair of truncus arteriosus: continuing improvement in outcomes. Ann Thorac Surg 2001; 72:391-395.
20. McGoon DC, Rastelli GC, Ongley PA. An operation for the correction of truncus arteriosus. JAMA 1968; 205:69-73.
21. Henaine R, Azarnoush K, Belli E, et al. Fate of the truncal valve in truncus arteriosus. Ann Thorac Surg 2008; 85:172-178.
22. Brown JW, Ruzmetov M, Okada Y, et al. Truncus arteriosus repair: outcomes, risk factors, reoperation and management. Eur J Cardiothorac Surg 2001; 20:221-227.
23. Miyamoto T, Sinzobahamvya N, Kumpikaite D, et al. Repair of truncus arteriosus and aortic arch interruption: outcome analysis. Ann Thorac Surg 2005; 79:2077-2082.
24. Duke C, Sharland GK, Jones AM, et al. Echocardiographic features and outcome of truncus arteriosus diagnosed during fetal life. Am J Cardiol 2001; 88:1379-1384.
25. Sanders SP, Bierman FZ, Williams RG. Conotruncal malformations: diagnosis in infancy using subxiphoid 2-dimensional echocardiography. Am J Cardiol 1982; 50:1361-1367.
26. Ammash NM, Dearani JA, Burkhart HM, et al. Pulmonary regurgitation after tetralogy of Fallot repair: clinical features, sequelae, and timing of pulmonary valve replacement. Congenit Heart Dis 2007; 2:386-403.
27. Geva T. Indications and timing of pulmonary valve replacement after tetralogy of Fallot repair. Semin Thorac Cardiovasc Surg Pediatr Card Surg Annu 2006; 9:11-22.
28. Murashita T, Hatta E, Imamura M, et al. Giant pseudoaneurysm of the right ventricular outflow tract after repair of truncus arteriosus: evaluation by MR imaging and surgical approach. Eur J Cardiothorac Surg 2002; 22:849-851.

CHAPTER 46

Anomalous Pulmonary Venous Connections and Drainage

Laureen Sena and Neil Mardis

The development and drainage of the pulmonary veins is a complex and incompletely understood process. A variety of abnormalities form a spectrum of disease ranging from normal insertion of an abnormal number of veins to abnormal insertion of some or all of the pulmonary veins. In addition, one or more pulmonary veins may be obstructed, regardless of normal or abnormal insertion.

Controversy exists about the origin of the primordial pulmonary vein.[1] Regardless, it is generally accepted that a common pulmonary vein forms in the dorsal mesocardium and is progressively incorporated into the posterior wall of the left atrium. As the atrium expands and the common vein is absorbed, the four major branches (two left and two right) achieve their discrete insertions.

The primary diseases that fall within this spectrum include partial anomalous pulmonary venous connection, sinus venosus defect, total anomalous pulmonary venous connection, cor triatriatum, and pulmonary vein stenosis.

PARTIAL ANOMALOUS PULMONARY VENOUS CONNECTION

Definition

Partial anomalous pulmonary venous connection (PAPVC) represents failure of one or more of the pulmonary veins to be incorporated into the left atrium. The anomalous veins empty instead into the systemic circulation. By definition, at least one pulmonary vein must drain normally into the left atrium.

Prevalence and Epidemiology

The incidence of PAPVC at autopsy has been reported to range between 0.6% and 0.7%.[2,3] The clinical frequency is less, indicating that many cases remain asymptomatic. Ethnic and gender predilections are unknown, probably because of the relative infrequency of this process.

Etiology and Pathophysiology

The anatomic manifestations of PAPVC are varied. Anomalous connections can occur both above and below the diaphragm, generally to an ipsilateral systemic vein. The right-sided pulmonary veins most often drain into the embryologic derivatives of the right cardinal vein, usually the inferior vena cava (IVC) or superior vena cava (SVC). Anomalous left-sided veins typically empty into derivatives of the left cardinal vein, most often the left innominate vein or the coronary sinus. Anomalous veins may also connect through remnants of the primitive splanchnic plexus to contralateral systemic vessels, although this is less common. Connection of a pulmonary vein (usually the right upper lobe branch) to the posterior SVC at the junction of the right atrium due to a defect of the common wall between the SVC and the right upper lobe pulmonary vein represents a unique process known as a sinus venosus defect (see following section). Drainage of the right pulmonary veins to the IVC may be associated with systemic arterial supply and hypoplasia of the ipsilateral lung with secondary dextroposition of the heart. This condition, variably referred to as congenital venolobar syndrome or scimitar syndrome (Fig. 46-1), is often placed within the continuum of bronchopulmonary dysplasias.[4,5] A horseshoe lung refers to the fusion of the lower lobes across the midline without an intervening fissure. This anomaly is highly associated with scimitar syndrome, with up to 80% of patients with horseshoe lung also affected with PAPVC in some series.[5]

Manifestations of Disease

Clinical Presentation

Exertional dyspnea may occur; however, patients with PAPVC are most often asymptomatic. Chest radiographs performed for unrelated disease may suggest an anomalous vein (particularly with right-sided drainage to the

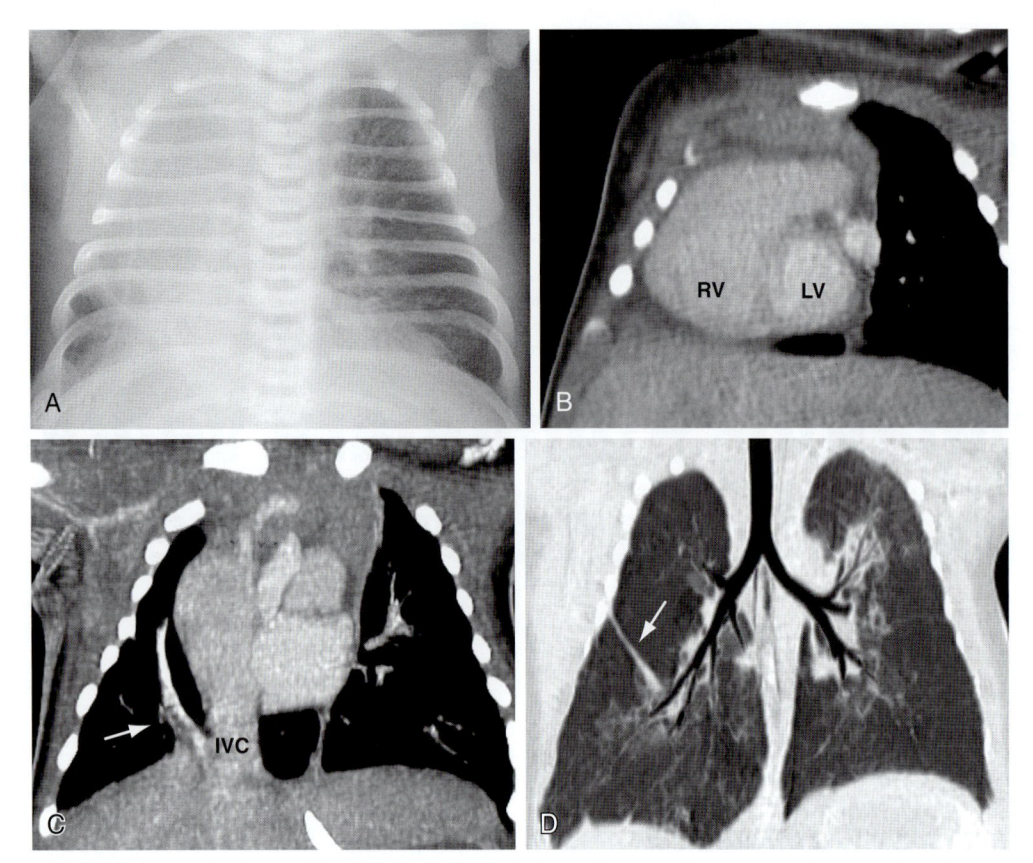

■ **FIGURE 46-1** Scimitar syndrome. Newborn with tachypnea. **A,** Frontal chest radiograph demonstrates dextrocardia with decreased aeration of the right lung. **B,** Subsequent coronal reformatted chest CT image shows shift of the heart into the right side of the chest with the left ventricle (LV) apex to the left and right ventricle (RV) to the right consistent with dextroposition or secondary dextrocardia. **C,** A posterior coronal reformatted image shows anomalous pulmonary venous drainage of the left lung to the IVC with a scimitar vein (*arrow*). **D,** Coronal minimum intensity projection image demonstrates that the right main stem bronchus bifurcates to support two lobes of the lung separated by a single fissure (*arrow*) consistent with absence of the right upper lobe.

IVC) and spur further evaluation. Likewise, an incidentally noted cardiac murmur may lead to imaging that reveals PAPVC. Because of variable association with other forms of congenital heart disease and situs anomalies, some cases of PAPVC may become apparent during the work-up of a separate entity.

Imaging Indications and Algorithm

The suggestion of anomalous venous return on chest radiography or echocardiography warrants further evaluation with cardiac CT angiography (CTA) or MRI. The choice of which cross-sectional modality to employ varies with institution. Patient factors (such as contraindications to MRI or contrast media) must also be considered. In addition, because of the increased frequency of PAPVC reported in patients with Turner syndrome, routine screening in this population may be warranted.[6]

Imaging Techniques and Findings

Radiography

Signs of right ventricular overload, including a lateralized or upturned cardiac apex on the frontal radiograph and filling in of the retrosternal clear space on the lateral view, may be evident. Increased pulmonary blood flow is often present; however, it is nonspecific. The abnormal vein itself may be visualized, as in anomalous pulmonary venous drainage of the right lung to the IVC, when the so-called scimitar vein (named for the crescent shape of the vessel likened to a Turko-Mongol saber; Fig. 46-2) can be visualized. As described previously, patients with scimitar syndrome display hypoplasia of the right lung and often some degree of cardiac dextroposition. Aberrant drainage into the SVC or azygos vein may result in dilation of these structures that is radiographically apparent. Anomalous left pulmonary veins emptying into the left innominate vein can create a bulbous appearance of the superior mediastinum (Fig. 46-3).

Ultrasonography

Echocardiography is often the first imaging modality employed to evaluate a child with suspected structural heart disease. Defining the pulmonary venous connections is an integral step in every echocardiographic examination. The pulmonary venous connections are often best demonstrated through a subxiphoid approach in infants. Suprasternal, parasternal, apical, and subcostal windows are often more revealing in older children. When not all of the pulmonary venous connections can be accounted for, a more detailed search for systemic connections is required. The presence of dilated systemic veins can be a clue to an unsuspected anomalous venous connection. Right ventricular volume overload resulting from PAPVC is well evaluated with echocardiography. Because of limitations in field of view of the pulmonary veins and left atrium from a transthoracic technique, transesophageal scanning may be needed for more detailed anatomic study of the pulmonary vein insertion.[7]

Computed Tomography

CTA timed to maximize left atrial and pulmonary venous opacification provides high spatial resolution images of the course and connections of anomalous pulmonary veins.[8] The isotropic acquisition of current multidetector CT scanners allows multiplanar reformation, maximum intensity projection, and volume rendered reconstruction. These techniques provide a degree of anatomic visualization previously available only with angiography. In addition, surrounding noncardiac structures, such as the lung parenchyma, are well demonstrated. This can aid in the characterization of an associated hypoplastic or horseshoe lung (see Fig. 46-1).

Magnetic Resonance

Cardiac MRI is another useful tool for the evaluation of PAPVC. MRI has been shown to be accurate in the evaluation of pulmonary vein anomalies and is often considered the method of choice for preoperative characterization of PAPVC (see Fig. 46-3).[9-11] Black blood images, like CTA, provide high spatial resolution for the evaluation of anatomic connections. Phase contrast cine images allow accurate quantification of pulmonary and systemic blood flow for shunt fraction calculation. Whereas the evaluation of lung parenchyma is less optimal than with CT, the lack of ionizing radiation and the functional information about the quantification of right ventricular volume overload and shunt fraction make MR superior for guiding clinical management.

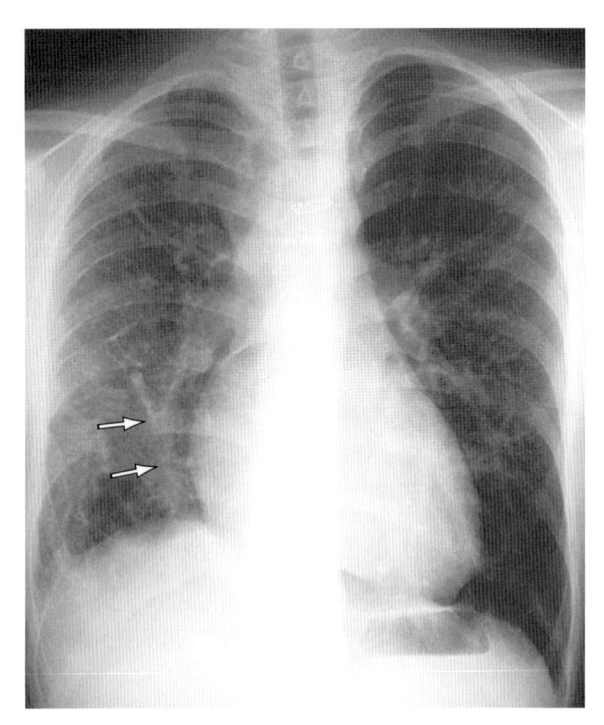

■ **FIGURE 46-2** Scimitar syndrome. Frontal chest radiograph of a 14-year-old boy demonstrates a scimitar vein (*arrows*) extending to the medial right hemidiaphragm with hypoplasia of the right lung.

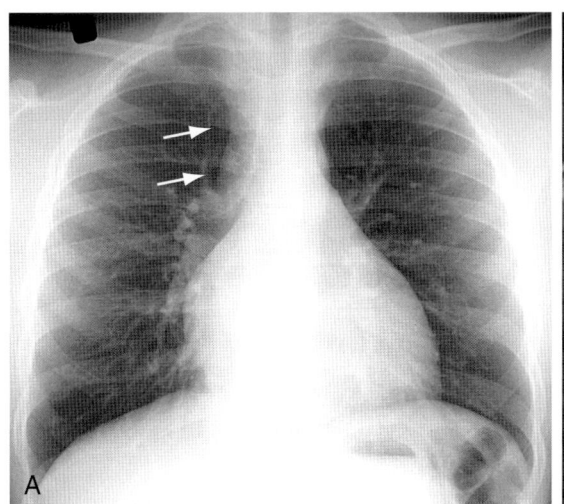

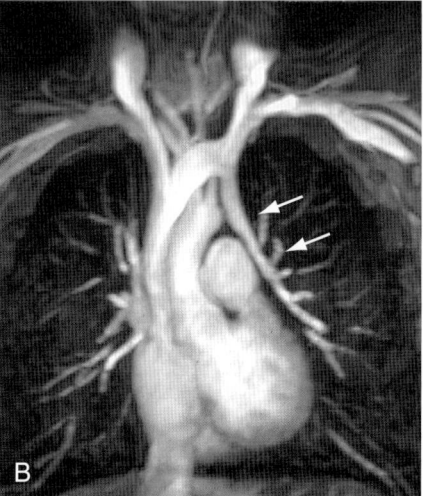

■ **FIGURE 46-3** PAPVC to the innominate vein. Frontal chest radiograph demonstrates thickening of the right paratracheal soft tissues (**A**, *arrows*) related to enlargement of the SVC due to shunting from anomalous venous connection of the left pulmonary veins (**B**, *arrows*) to the innominate vein as demonstrated on coronal maximum intensity projection image from MRA.

Nuclear Medicine/Positron Emission Tomography

Routine lung perfusion scintigraphy with technetium Tc 99m is not typically performed in patients suspected of having or known to have PAPVC. If there is pulmonary hypoplasia, as in scimitar syndrome or concurrent pulmonary venous stenosis, decreased perfusion may be noted secondary to ipsilateral pulmonary arterial hypoplasia.

Angiography

Angiography may be performed by either selective pulmonary artery injection with visualization of the anomalous vessel on the levophase or retrograde venous injection of the anomalous vessel itself. These techniques are employed less frequently with the advent of multidetector CTA and cardiac MRI.

Classic Signs

The "scimitar" sign, as described before, is a characteristic finding in right PAPVC. The "snowman" sign, although occasionally present in anomalous drainage of the left lung to the innominate vein, is less prominent and less often appreciated in partial than in supracardiac total anomalous pulmonary venous connection.

Differential Diagnosis

From Clinical Presentation

The major differential diagnosis from a clinical standpoint is that of an atrial septal defect (ASD). When they are symptomatic, patients with ASD or PAPVC can present with dyspnea on exertion. Murmurs in both conditions are related to increased blood flow across the pulmonary and tricuspid valves.

From Imaging Findings

Both CT and MR angiography are very helpful in patients who have echocardiographic findings suggesting right-sided heart volume overload but inconclusive evaluation of the pulmonary venous connection. Accurate delineation of the pulmonary venous connection can become limited in older and larger patients on transthoracic echocardiography and may require the transesophageal approach. CT and MR angiography provide noninvasive alternatives to transesophageal echocardiography and reliably depict the anomalous pulmonary veins connecting to the systemic venous system, thereby excluding other differential considerations.

Synopsis of Treatment Options

Medical

Patients who are not surgical candidates may require medical management for heart failure or arrhythmia. Definitive treatment, however, is achieved only through surgery.

Surgical/Interventional

Indications for surgical treatment are controversial. Generally speaking, all patients who are symptomatic and do not have a contraindication should be treated surgically. Specifically, the current consensus holds that if the Qp:Qs (shunt fraction) is greater than 1.5:1, surgical closure is performed. PAPVC with shunt ratios below 1.5:1 are usually well tolerated and can be clinically observed. The particular repair will vary according to the site of anomalous drainage and the coexistence of any other form of heart disease. Anomalous left pulmonary veins may be reanastomosed to the left atrial appendage. Right-sided anomalous veins are often anastomosed to the right atrium and connected to the left atrium with a patch or baffle through a preexisting or surgically created ASD. In general, surgical repair of PAPVC is associated with very good outcomes.[12] Patients with scimitar syndrome, however, often do poorly and suffer from high degrees of postoperative pulmonary venous stenosis related to baffle obstruction (Fig. 46-4).[12]

Reporting: Information for the Referring Physician

CTA and MRI reports should contain clear and detailed explanations of the drainage patterns of pulmonary veins. If MRI is performed, quantification of right ventricular end-diastolic volume, ejection fraction, and shunt fraction should be assessed. Additional information about associated cardiac and noncardiac (i.e., pulmonary parenchyma) anatomy is also important to the referring physician.

KEY POINTS

- PAPVC results from failure of at least one of the pulmonary veins to become incorporated into the left atrium.
- The anomalous pulmonary vein can connect to a variety of systemic veins, including the IVC, SVC, innominate and azygos veins, and coronary sinus.
- Patients with PAPVC can present with dyspnea on exertion or murmur related to right-sided heart enlargement and volume overload.
- CT or MR angiography is the noninvasive imaging method of choice for delineating anomalous pulmonary venous connections.
- MRI provides quantitative evaluation of right ventricular enlargement and shunt fraction, which are both needed to determine whether surgical repair is warranted.

SINUS VENOSUS DEFECT

Definition

A sinus venosus septal defect (SVD) most often represents an absence of the common wall between the right upper lobe pulmonary vein and the SVC or right atrium; it is also

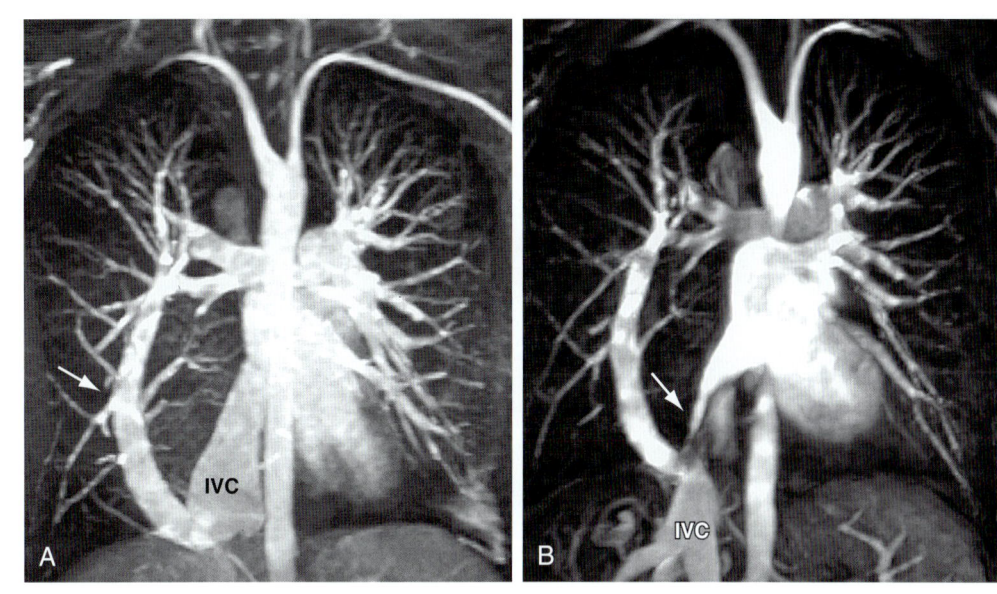

■ **FIGURE 46-4** Baffle obstruction after repair of scimitar syndrome; 24-year-old with exercise intolerance. Coronal maximum intensity projection (**A**) from MRA demonstrates anomalous pulmonary venous drainage (*arrow*) of the entire right lung to the IVC. After surgical construction of a baffle to connect the pulmonary venous drainage to the left atrium, coronal maximum intensity projection image from MRA (**B**) demonstrates complete baffle obstruction (*arrow*). The baffle also underwent dehiscence, allowing the scimitar vein to connect to the IVC, which is markedly dilated.

known as a superior type of SVD. Much less commonly, an inferior type of SVD can occur when the common wall between the right atrium and the right lower or middle pulmonary vein is absent, often associated with malposition of the septum primum.

Prevalence and Epidemiology

The SVD has been estimated to account for up to 10% of ASDs.[13] The exact prevalence is difficult to measure because of the often subclinical nature of the condition and the difficulty in detection with standard first-line cardiac imaging techniques (plain radiography and echocardiography). Most studies have found a female-to-male preponderance of roughly 2:1. No racial or ethnic predilection has been established.

Etiology and Pathophysiology

The lack of an intact intervening wall between a pulmonary vein and the SVC or right atrium results in "unroofing" of the pulmonary vein, thereby creating anomalous pulmonary venous drainage to the right atrium.[14] An interatrial connection posterior and superior to the fossa ovalis is commonly present. This does not represent an ASD, but rather it is a connection between the atria formed by the unroofed insertion of the pulmonary vein. Because of higher left-sided pressures, flow of blood can pass retrograde from the left atrium through the orifice of the pulmonary vein and then enter the SVC through the defect and continue to the right atrium, resulting in a left-to-right shunt. Additional anomalous connecting pulmonary veins to the SVC superior to the defect as well as other systemic veins may be present.

Manifestations of Disease

Clinical Presentation

The often large interatrial communication of an SVD results in a significant left-to-right shunt with increased pulmonary blood flow; some patients can be relatively asymptomatic while others may present with congestive heart failure.[13,14] Symptoms include dyspnea on exertion, palpitations, and angina.[13,15] As with conventional ASDs, SVD may be the cause of an otherwise unexplained stroke due to paradoxic embolization.[15]

Imaging Indications and Algorithm

As described with PAPVC, plain films and echocardiography are the initial and often the only necessary studies in the evaluation of SVD. If the diagnosis is still uncertain, cardiac MRI or CTA should be employed. Conventional angiography is rarely necessary in the preoperative work-up.

Imaging Techniques and Findings

Radiography

Plain film findings in SVD are nonspecific but include cardiomegaly with right-sided heart enlargement and increased pulmonary blood flow (Fig. 46-5).

Ultrasonography

Echocardiography demonstrates abnormal continuity between the right upper lobe pulmonary vein and the SVC in the superior type of SVD (Fig. 46-6). Right atrial and

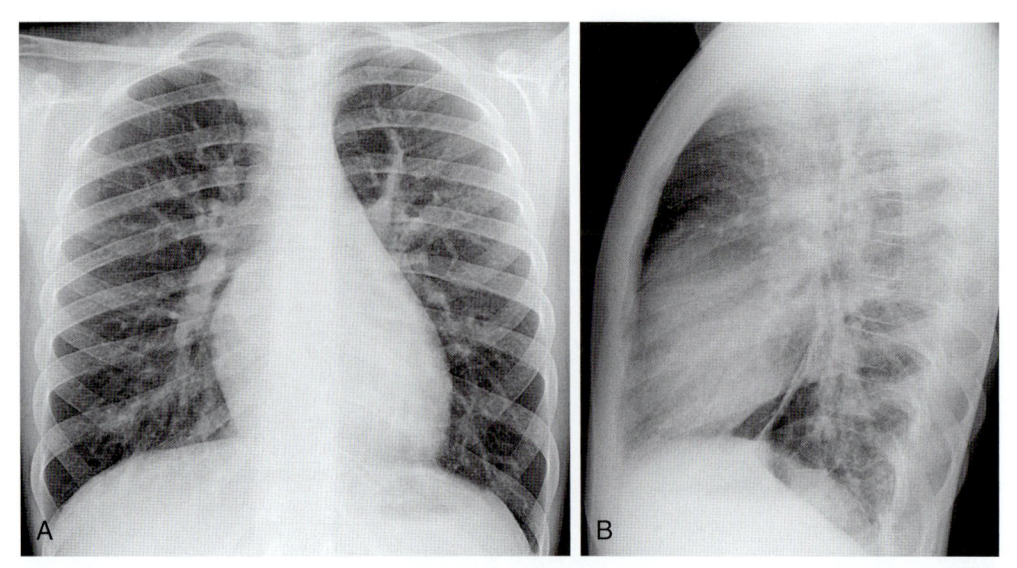

FIGURE 46-5 Sinus venosus septal defect. Frontal (**A**) and lateral (**B**) chest radiographs demonstrate cardiomegaly with increased pulmonary blood flow. Increased density filling the retrosternal clear space is present on the lateral view consistent with right ventricular dilation from the left-to-right shunt.

ventricular enlargement is present, and the atrial septum proper is intact.

Computed Tomography

Although there have been case reports,[16] no large case series has been published on the accuracy of CT in the evaluation of SVDs. That being said, the high spatial detail of CTA allows definition of the anomalous drainage.

Magnetic Resonance

Cardiac MR has been shown to be well suited for the evaluation of SVD.[17] In addition to defining the defect (Fig. 46-7), right ventricular volume and function and pulmonary-to-systemic blood flow ratio (shunt fraction) can be quantified. MR angiography (MRA) can also depict additional pulmonary veins that may be connecting anomalously to the SVC or other systemic veins.

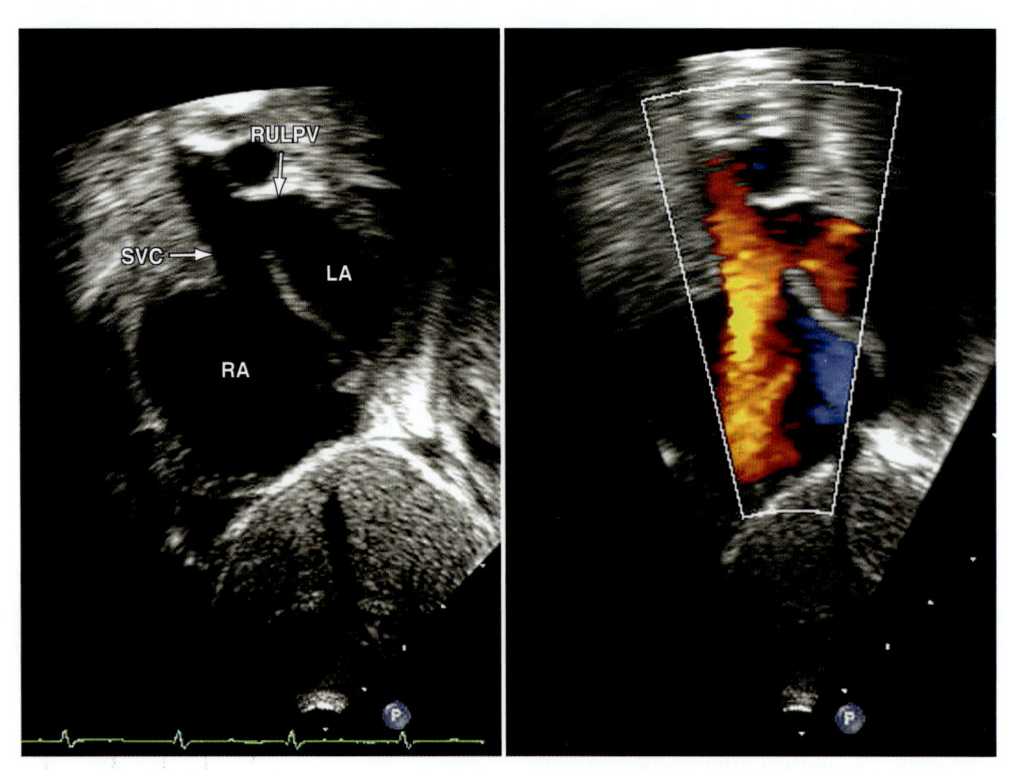

FIGURE 46-6 Sinus venosus defect. Long-axis spectral and color Doppler echocardiographic views of the SVC demonstrate absence of the posterior wall of the SVC so that the SVC communicates directly to the right upper lobe pulmonary vein (RULPV) that normally passes posteriorly. The right upper lobe pulmonary vein connects normally to the left atrium (LA), allowing blood to flow from the left to right atrium (RA) through the defect and the cardiac end of the SVC.

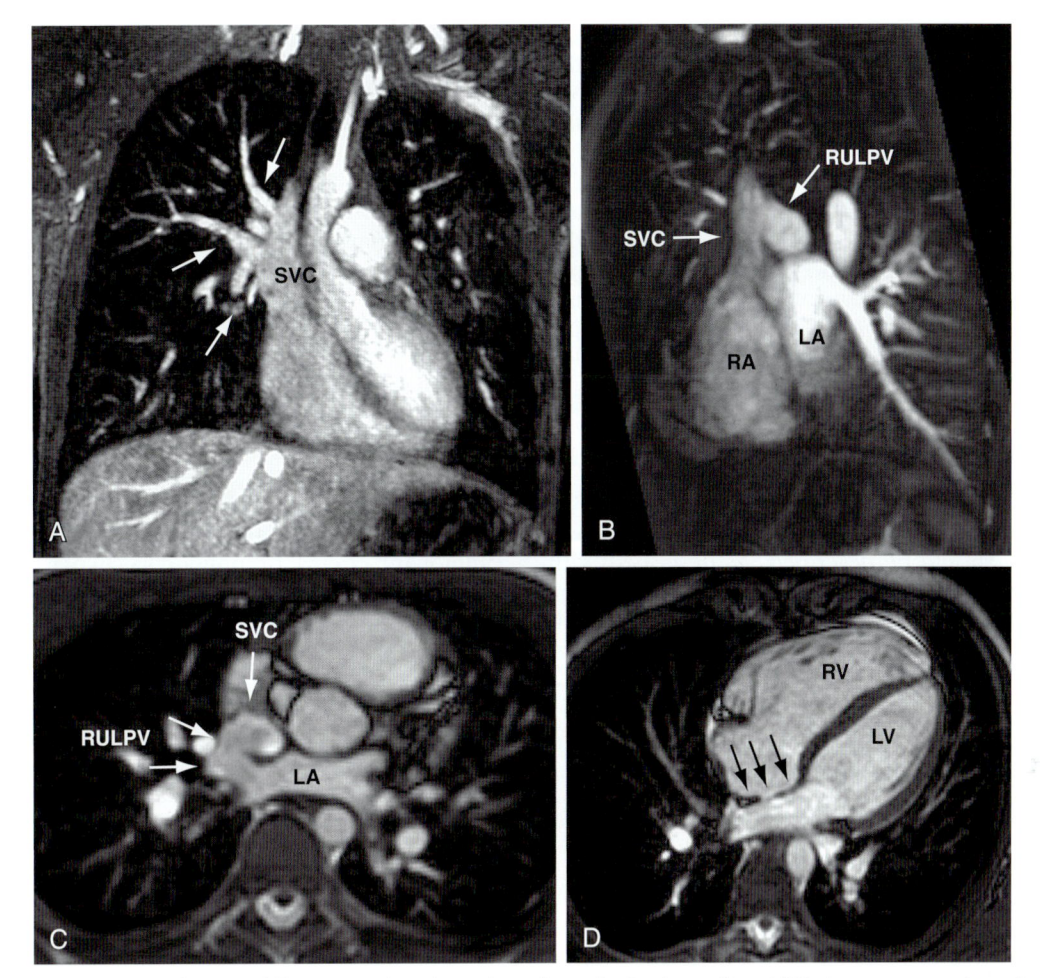

FIGURE 46-7 Sinus venosus defect. **A,** Oblique coronal maximum intensity projection image from MRA demonstrates at least three small pulmonary veins (*arrows*) draining from the right upper lobe from the right upper lobe to the SVC. **B,** Oblique sagittal maximum intensity projection image demonstrates the defect in the posterior wall of the SVC with the confluence of the right upper lobe pulmonary vein (RULPV). **C,** Axial steady-state free precession image through the left atrium demonstrates the defect in the wall between the SVC and right upper lobe pulmonary vein (RULPV) and normal connection of the right upper lobe pulmonary vein to the left atrium. **D,** Four-chamber steady-state free precession image shows dilation of the right ventricle due to the large left-to-right shunt between the atria through the SVD. The atrial septum proper (*arrows*) is intact.

Angiography

Angiographic findings of SVD are nonspecific, and this technique is not commonly employed in the preoperative evaluation.[18] The ability to pass a catheter into the anomalous vein through the right atrium implies PAPVC, although not necessarily an SVD.

Differential Diagnosis

From Clinical Presentation

ASDs and other forms of PAPVC are often difficult to distinguish clinically from SVDs.

From Imaging Findings

The main differential consideration is PAPVC. Whereas the distinction can often be difficult on transthoracic echocardiography, transesophageal echocardiography,[19] cardiac MR,[18] and CTA should allow exclusion of other entities.

Synopsis of Treatment Options

Medical

As with PAPVC, the definitive treatment of SVD is surgical. The SVD more often requires surgical repair because the shunt is usually larger with more severe right ventricular enlargement. Medical therapy aims to optimize cardiopulmonary status in anticipation of operative treatment.

Surgical/Interventional

The traditional means of SVD repair consists of a single patch closure of the defect that baffles the anomalous right upper lobe pulmonary vein back to the left atrium. This technique can be complicated by narrowing and obstruction of the SVC postoperatively. A second technique involves placement of a second patch to widen the SVC–right atrial junction to reduce the incidence of postoperative SVC narrowing,[20] but the sutures placed at the SVC–right atrial junction can lead to sinoatrial node dysfunction.[21] The Warden procedure involves transection of the cranial portion of the SVC above the anomalous venous connection and anastomosis of the SVC to the right atrial appendage. The connection of the right upper lobe pulmonary vein and the caudal end of the SVC is then patch closed. Because of the decrease in reported complications of obstruction and nodal dysfunction, the Warden technique has gained in popularity.[21,22]

Reporting: Information for the Referring Physician

In addition to pulmonary vein anatomy, the size and location of the SVD should be described. As described with PAPVC, right ventricular size and function should be assessed. The ratio of pulmonary-to-systemic flow (shunt fraction) should also be reported.

> **KEY POINTS**
>
> - The superior type of SVD is due to absence of the common wall between the right upper lobe pulmonary vein and the SVC.
> - The atrial septum proper is intact.
> - The SVD results in a left-to-right shunt between the atria and presents with symptoms related to right ventricular volume overload similar to ASD and PAPVC.
> - The shunt fraction associated with SVD tends to be very large, and surgical repair is usually clinically necessary.
> - MRI provides the most comprehensive imaging evaluation of SVD, including evaluation of additional anomalous draining veins.

COR TRIATRIATUM

Definition

When the pulmonary veins drain to an accessory chamber separated by a membrane from the remainder of the left atrium, the result is termed cor triatriatum.

Prevalence and Epidemiology

The reported incidence of cor triatriatum ranges between 0.1% and 0.4%.[23-25] No racial or gender predilections have been described.

Etiology and Pathophysiology

Like the previously described pulmonary vein anomalies, there is ample controversy surrounding the embryogenesis of cor triatriatum. The most commonly held theory is based on incomplete incorporation of the common primordial pulmonary vein into the left atrium. The common vein becomes a "third atrium" separated from the left atrium by a fibromuscular membrane. This accessory chamber typically receives all the pulmonary veins and connects to the left atrium through a stenotic orifice (classic cor triatriatum or cor triatriatum sinister). The common vein may also communicate with the right atrium (cor triatriatum dexter) or the systemic veins (cor triatriatum with PAPVC). Yet another variation is subtotal cor triatriatum, in which some of the pulmonary veins drain normally into the left atrium and others drain into an accessory chamber that then empties in any of the patterns previously described.[24]

Manifestations of Disease

Clinical Presentation

Clinical symptoms depend on the degree of stenosis affecting the orifice in the membrane dividing the accessory chamber and the true atrium and the presence or absence of a shunt (drainage into the right atrium or PAPVC). Symptoms are variable, ranging from none to pulmonary edema or pulmonary hypertension. Patients often have respiratory symptoms and recurrent pulmonary infections and are misinterpreted as having primary pulmonary disease.

Imaging Indications and Algorithm

Imaging indications are the same as those described in the previous sections.

Imaging Technique and Findings

Radiography

In addition to otherwise unexplained pulmonary edema, pulmonary artery enlargement may be seen secondary to pulmonary hypertension. The heart is often small; however, enlargement of the left atrium due to a dilated accessory chamber may be visualized (Fig. 46-8).

Ultrasonography

Echocardiography is often the only modality needed in the evaluation of cor triatriatum (Fig. 46-9). Visualization of the thin echogenic membrane is often best appreciated through a parasternal, apical, or subcostal approach. Supravalvular mitral stenosis due to a supramitral ring has an appearance similar to cor triatriatum and also results in venous obstruction. The two entities can be differentiated by the location and appearance of the membrane. The left atrial appendage and foramen ovale are located distal to the relatively thin curvilinear membrane of cor triatriatum, whereas the appendage and foramen are proximal to the stiff membrane of the supramitral ring. Right atrial dilation and ventricular dilation secondary to venous obstruction are nonspecific and are seen in both diseases.

Computed Tomography

CTA can demonstrate the accessory chamber[26] and, depending on the size of the membranous ostia, may allow differentiation of drainage to the left or right atrium. If the cor triatriatum is associated with partial anomalous venous connection, these aberrant pathways can be well

CHAPTER 46 • Anomalous Pulmonary Venous Connections and Drainage 633

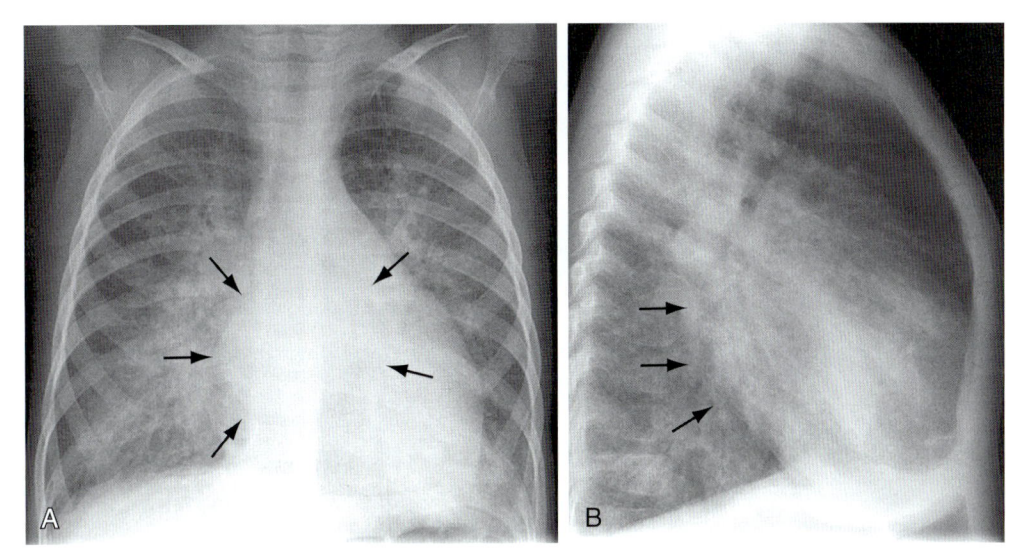

■ **FIGURE 46-8** Cor triatriatum. Frontal (A) and lateral (B) chest radiographs of a 6-year-old demonstrate cardiomegaly with pulmonary vascular congestion and edema. The left atrium appears enlarged on both views (*arrows*) but has an unusual round appearance on the frontal view.

demonstrated. As stated before, the requisite ionizing radiation and the relative lack of functional information pertaining to right-sided heart overload are drawbacks compared with MRI.

Magnetic Resonance

Like CTA, cardiac MRI allows excellent anatomic depiction of the accessory atrial chamber in cor triatriatum[27-30]

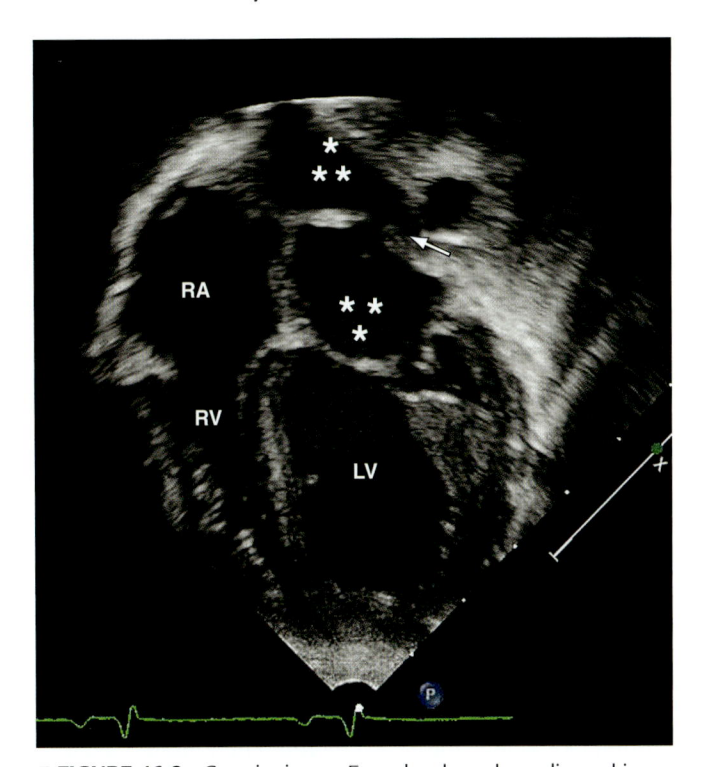

■ **FIGURE 46-9** Cor triatriatum. Four-chamber echocardiographic image demonstrates that the left atrium is divided into two chambers (*asterisks*) by an incomplete membrane. A restrictive opening (*arrow*) is present between the two chambers that obstructs the flow of blood between them.

(Fig. 46-10). Functional information about right-sided heart strain or overload may also be obtained. Flow from the high-pressure accessory chamber through the obstructed membrane into the low-pressure left atrium can produce visible turbulent jets or dephasing on cine images. Additional anomalies, such as PAPVC and the presence of an ASD, can be evaluated.

Angiography

Conventional angiography may demonstrate filling of the accessory chamber with a discrete membrane separating it from the true atrium. Contrast material may pool in this chamber for a prolonged period if the outflow obstruction is severe. Because the walls of the accessory chamber most likely form from the common pulmonary vein, they are noncontractile. Angiography, though, is often unsuccessful in discriminating between cor triatriatum, total anomalous pulmonary venous connection, and intrinsic pulmonary vein obstruction.[25,31,32]

Differential Diagnosis

From Clinical Presentation

The patient may present with respiratory symptoms, and primary pulmonary disease may be suspected. Other causes of pulmonary hypertension, either idiopathic or secondary to valvular or other congenital heart disease, should be considered.

From Imaging Findings

The main differential consideration in evaluating a chest radiograph in cor triatriatum is infracardiac total anomalous pulmonary venous connection with obstruction or other severe left-sided heart obstructive lesions, such as mitral stenosis.

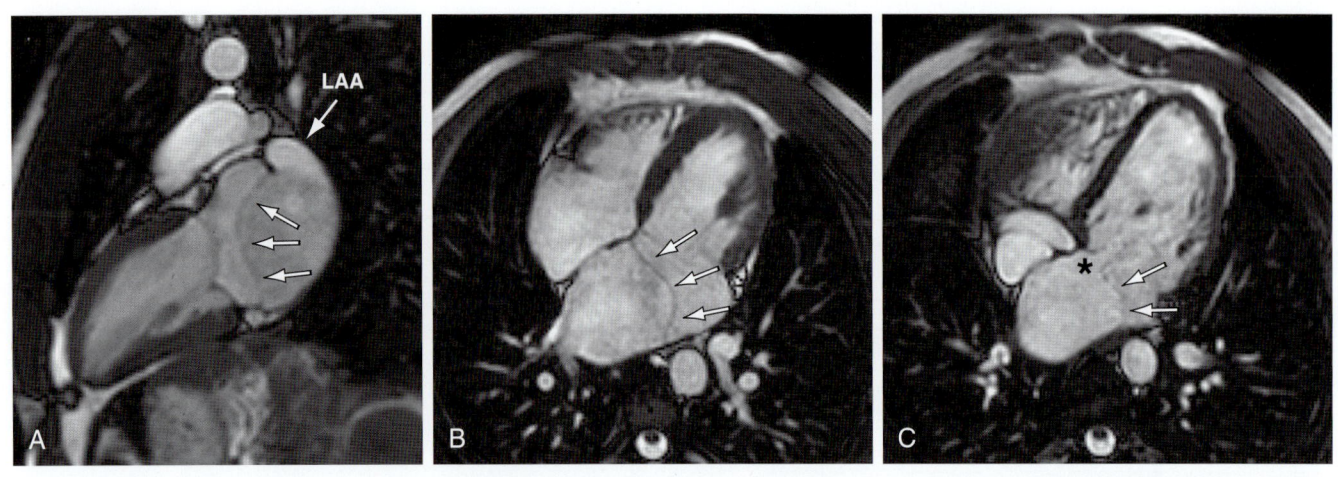

FIGURE 46-10 Cor triatriatum. Two-chamber (**A**) and four-chamber (**B** and **C**) steady-state free precession images demonstrate a thin membrane (*arrows*) dividing the left atrium into two chambers. Note that the membrane is located distal to the left atrial appendage (LAA). A restrictive defect in the membrane (*asterisk*) can be seen on a more inferior four-chamber image (**C**).

Synopsis of Treatment Options

Medical

Medical management of pulmonary venous congestion is necessary until the patient is stable for definitive surgical repair.

Surgical/Interventional

Resection of the cor triatriatum membrane with patch closure of any coexistent ASDs is the treatment of choice.[25,31,33-35] If the patient also has anomalous venous connections, these may be corrected.[34]

Reporting: Information for the Referring Physician

Accurate description of the size and drainage pattern of the accessory chamber in addition to clear descriptions of any associated anomalies is required. If functional information (as in cardiac MRI) has been obtained, it too should be included in the report.

KEY POINTS

- Cor triatriatum is present when the pulmonary veins drain to an accessory chamber separated by a membrane from the remainder of the left atrium.
- Cor triatriatum results in pulmonary venous obstruction leading to pulmonary edema and pulmonary hypertension.
- Cor triatriatum can be associated with an ASD and PAPVC.
- Echocardiography is often the only imaging modality needed for diagnosis before surgical repair.
- Both CT and MRI can depict the membrane separating the left atrium into two chambers and can also evaluate the pulmonary venous connections if prior echocardiography has been inconclusive.

TOTAL ANOMALOUS PULMONARY VENOUS CONNECTION

Definition

Drainage of all the pulmonary veins to any location other than the left atrium constitutes the entity known as total anomalous pulmonary venous connection (TAPVC). The pulmonary veins may drain to the right atrium, coronary sinus, or other systemic veins.

Prevalence and Epidemiology

TAPVC is generally estimated to represent not more than 2.0% of congenital heart disease.[36] For the most part, no strong gender prevalence has been noted.[37] The curious exception to this is total anomalous connection to the portal system, which affects males $3\frac{1}{2}$ times more often than females.[38] There is a common association of TAPVC with heterotaxy syndrome. More important, patients with heterotaxy and TAPVC (particularly those complicated by post-repair stenosis) are more likely to have poor outcomes.[39]

Etiology and Pathophysiology

As described before, failure of the normal incorporation of the common pulmonary vein into the dorsal wall of the left atrium with persistent connections of all pulmonary veins to systemic vessels, right atrium, or coronary sinus results in total anomalous venous connection. Various classification schemes for anomalous drainage patterns have been described. One commonly used classification put forth by Craig and Darling includes supracardiac drainage (type I), drainage at the cardiac level (type II), infracardiac drainage (type III), and mixed patterns (type IV).[40] The most frequently described connection is to the left innominate vein.[37] Other frequently encountered sites of drainage include the coronary sinus, the right atrium (secondary to malposition of the septum primum), the SVC, and the portal system. Patients with TAPVC often have a concurrent ASD, VSD, or patent ductus arteriosus (PDA).

Postnatal survival in patients with TAPVC is dependent on the presence of a shunt. In addition, many cases of TAPVC demonstrate some degree of pulmonary venous obstruction, especially the infradiaphragmatic type. Causes of venous obstruction include intrinsic abnormality of the vessel wall with medial hypertrophy, compression by adjacent structures, and narrowing at the level of the diaphragm or ductus venosus. The presence of venous obstruction portends a worse prognosis.[37]

Manifestations of Disease

Clinical Presentation

In the newborn with TAPVC, clinical symptoms and signs can be variable, depending on the presence and degree of obstruction to the pulmonary veins. When TAPVC is unobstructed, symptoms in the newborn infant are variable, depending on the size of the associated shunt and direction of flow. Symptoms and signs can range from mild cyanosis and murmur to severe pulmonary overcirculation with respiratory distress. On occasion, patients are so asymptomatic that the diagnosis is not made until they have reached adolescence or adulthood. Patients tend to present earlier with more severe symptoms when there is pulmonary venous obstruction. Tachypnea with gasping and intercostal retractions due to pulmonary edema develop within a few days of birth.

Imaging Indications and Algorithm

The nonspecific clinical findings of cyanosis or heart failure often lead to initial evaluation with chest radiography. Echocardiography is also commonly performed early in the setting of unexplained cardiopulmonary disease. Two-dimensional echocardiography with Doppler examination is often diagnostic; however, when not all of the pulmonary venous drainage can be accounted for because of limitations in echocardiographic windows, the next step should be cardiac MRI or CTA. The role of diagnostic angiography in the evaluation of TAPVC has greatly diminished with the increasing accuracy of two-dimensional and Doppler echocardiography and the widespread availability of MRI and CT.

Imaging Techniques and Findings

Radiography

When the pulmonary venous connection to the systemic circulation is unobstructed, cardiomegaly with right atrial and ventricular enlargement and increased pulmonary blood flow are present on the chest radiograph. Patients with total drainage to the left innominate vein may demonstrate the snowman sign, in which the upper portion of the snowman is derived from the vertical vein on the left, the enlarged innominate vein superiorly, and the enlarged SVC on the right. The cardiac silhouette constitutes the lower portion of the snowman (Fig. 46-11).

The chest radiograph appearance in patients with infradiaphragmatic obstructed TAPVC is very different. The heart size is normal or mildly enlarged, and there is normal

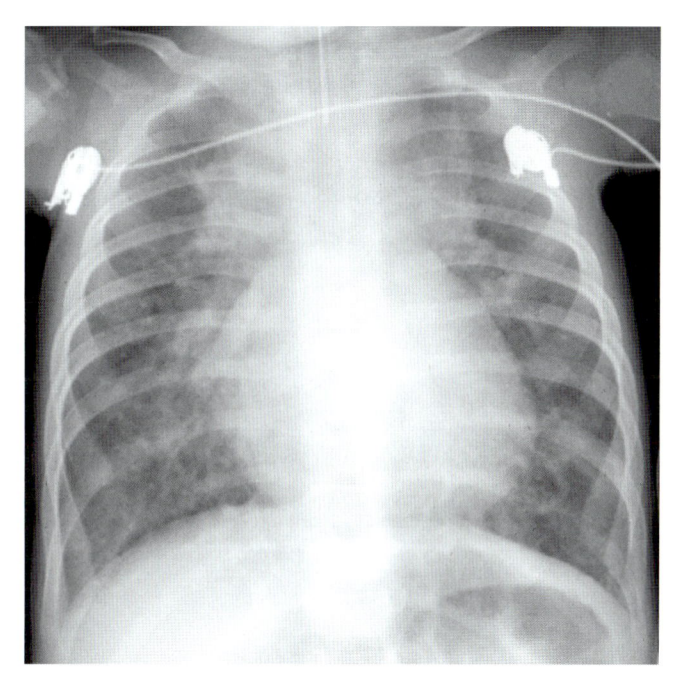

■ **FIGURE 46-11** Supracardiac TAPVC without obstruction. Frontal chest radiograph of an intubated patient demonstrates cardiomegaly and increased pulmonary blood flow. A classic snowman sign is seen with widening of the superior mediastinum.

pulmonary blood flow with a variable degree of pulmonary edema, depending on the degree of obstruction (Fig. 46-12).

Ultrasonography

The lack of pulmonary veins entering the left atrium together with signs of right ventricular volume overload establishes the diagnosis of TAPVC on echocardiography.

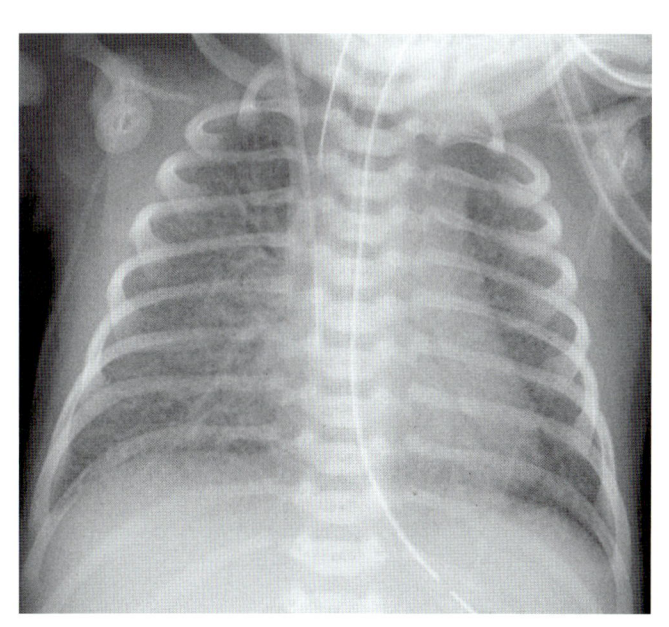

■ **FIGURE 46-12** Infracardiac TAPVC with obstruction. Frontal chest radiograph of an intubated patient demonstrates a mildly enlarged cardiac silhouette and pulmonary edema with a small right pleural effusion.

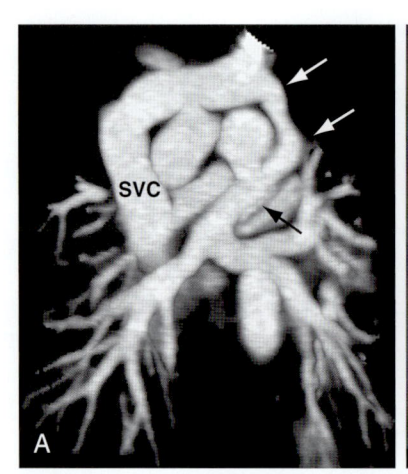

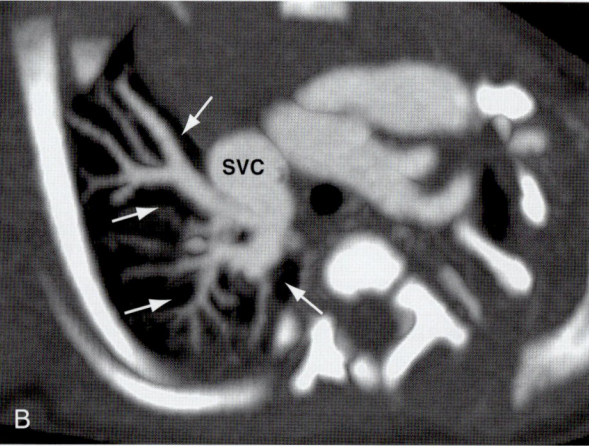

FIGURE 46-13 Mixed TAPVC. Coronal and axial oblique maximum intensity projection CTA images demonstrate anomalous venous drainage of the left lung and right lower lobe to a venous confluence to the innominate vein and SVC (**A**, *arrows*). The right upper lobe pulmonary venous drainage is directly to the SVC (**B**, *arrows*). *(Courtesy of Dr. Hyun Woo Goo).*

At this point, a detailed survey must be performed to account for all of the anomalous veins. The individual veins should be carefully examined with two-dimensional and color Doppler techniques. The size of the pulmonary veins at initial diagnosis has prognostic implications.[40] The orientation of aberrant vessels as well as presence or absence of obstruction should be clearly defined to aid surgical management. Because of the association with heterotaxy syndrome, the cardiac segmental anatomy and abdominal visceral morphology as well as intracardiac anomalies are also evaluated.

Computed Tomography

There are limited published data concerning the use of CTA for the evaluation of TAPVC. The small studies that have been performed indicate that the modality is capable of demonstrating the anatomy of the pulmonary veins in detail.[8,41-43] The course and size of the pulmonary veins can be determined with CTA, and the presence of venous obstruction is well demonstrated with isotropic multidetector-row CT acquisition with multiplanar reformats, maximum intensity projections, and volume rendered techniques (Fig. 46-13). Functional assessment (particularly in the neonatal period) is well evaluated by echocardiography. The pulmonary and abdominal visceral morphology is well demonstrated with CT, aiding in the evaluation of patients with concomitant heterotaxy.

Magnetic Resonance

In patients with TAPVC who have incomplete evaluation of all of the anomalous pulmonary venous connections by echocardiography, MRA can provide highly detailed comprehensive information.[9,44] The number of pulmonary veins and their sizes, courses, and drainage patterns are well depicted. As described before, the size of the pulmonary veins is clinically relevant in that those patients with smaller and obstructed anomalous veins tend to have a worse outcome[40] (Fig. 46-14). Improved MRA techniques now allow excellent spatial resolution to detect the presence or absence of venous obstruction. The anomalously draining veins should be carefully assessed for any intrinsic narrowing or extrinsic compression (i.e., from an adjacent pulmonary artery or bronchus). Functional evaluation by MRI is often unnecessary in the neonate and is usually performed by echocardiography. The cardiac segmental anatomy, intracardiac and great vessel connections, and abdominal visceral morphology in patients with heterotaxy can also be evaluated on MRI (Fig. 46-15).

Angiography

The increasing accuracy of two-dimensional echocardiography with Doppler examination, cardiac MRI, and CTA have eliminated the need for diagnostic angiography in the work-up of TAPVC. If it is performed, selective pulmonary angiography with attention to the levophase will demonstrate the anomalous venous channels (Fig. 46-16).

Classic Signs

The snowman sign or figure-eight appearance on chest radiography is the classic appearance of supracardiac TAPVC. This appearance may be difficult to appreciate on a radiograph of an infant, but it is more easily seen in older children with unrepaired TAPVC because of the progressive enlargement of the vessels carrying the anomalous pulmonary venous flow back to the right side of the heart.

Differential Diagnosis

From Clinical Presentation

An infant with TAPVC without venous obstruction may clinically appear similar to infants with any form of large shunt lesion (VSD, ASD, PDA, atrioventricular canal). Newborns or infants with TAPVC and venous obstruction are more likely to be cyanotic with severe tachypnea and retractions due to pulmonary edema.

CHAPTER 46 • Anomalous Pulmonary Venous Connections and Drainage

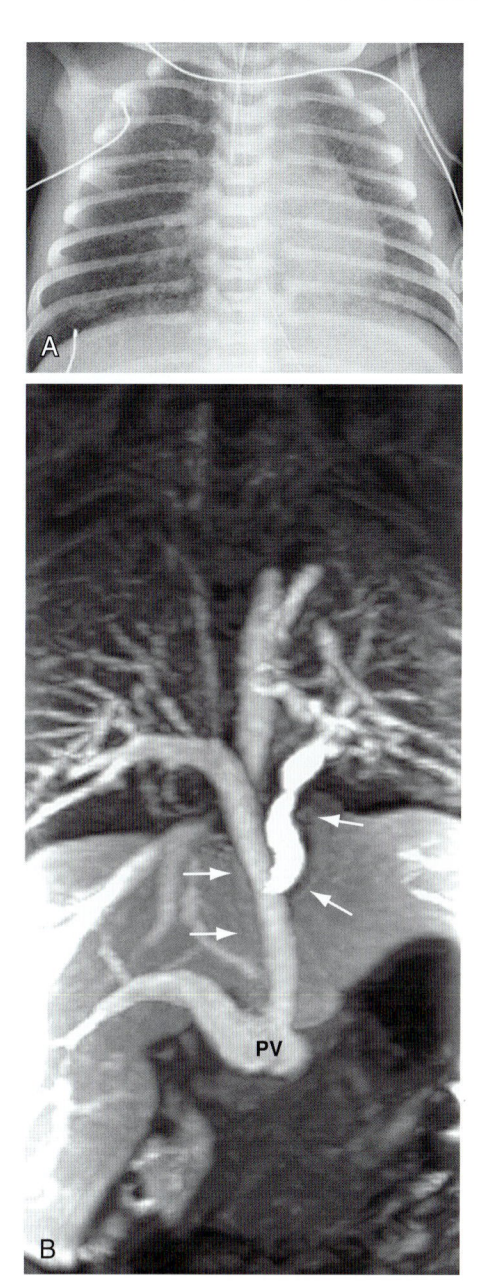

FIGURE 46-14 Infracardiac TAPVC with left-sided obstruction. **A,** Frontal chest radiograph of an intubated patient demonstrates a mildly enlarged cardiac silhouette with bilateral pulmonary edema, greater in the left lung than in the right lung. **B,** Coronal maximum intensity projection image from an MRA demonstrates infracardiac TAPVC to the portal vein. The left pulmonary veins connect to a densely enhancing venous confluence (*arrows*) that is severely obstructed. The right-sided pulmonary venous confluence is not obstructed to the portal vein (PV); however, there is obstruction to flow through the liver to the heart as the ductus venosus closes.

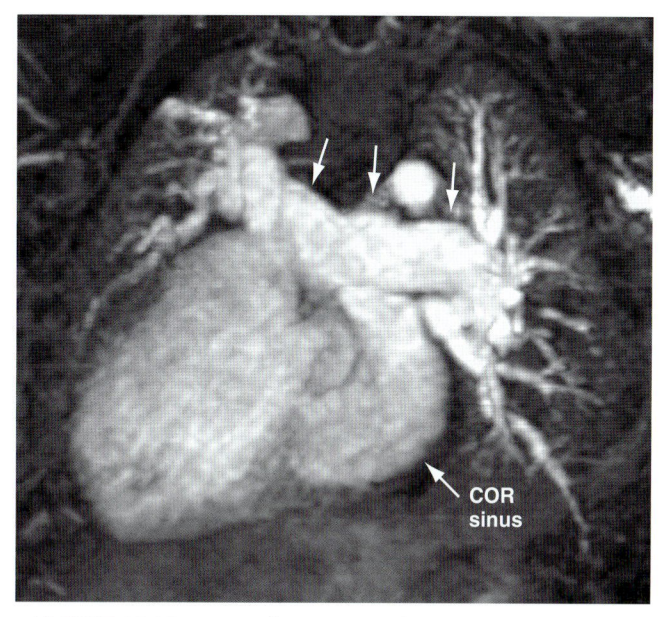

FIGURE 46-15 Intracardiac TAPVC to the coronary sinus. Oblique coronal maximum intensity projection image from MRA demonstrates an enlarged pulmonary venous confluence (*arrows*) from each lung joining to a dilated coronary sinus (*cor sinus*).

Synopsis of Treatment Options

Medical

Whereas medical therapy alone is insufficient for the treatment of TAPVC, therapy should be instituted before surgery to stabilize the patient in terms of metabolic acidosis and volume overload.

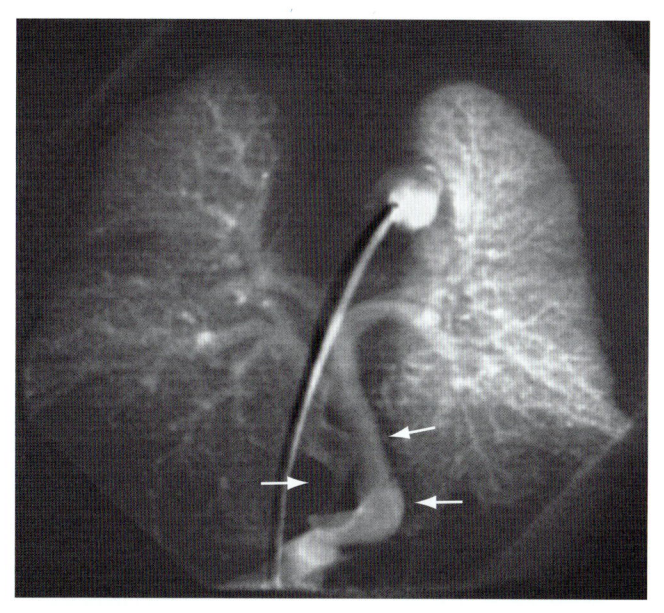

FIGURE 46-16 Infracardiac TAPVC to the portal vein. Levophase angiography image from a direct main pulmonary artery injection demonstrates two pulmonary vein confluences draining to the portal vein. The right-sided pulmonary vein confluence is smaller and more tortuous compared with the left (*arrows*).

From Imaging Findings

The lack of left-sided heart enlargement on the chest radiograph helps exclude shunt lesions such as VSD, PDA, and atrioventricular canal. Depiction of aberrant pulmonary venous drainage on more advanced imaging modalities essentially eliminates other differential considerations. The differential considerations are restricted to the type of TAPVC (i.e., supracardiac, cardiac, infracardiac, mixed).

Surgical/Interventional

The definitive treatment of TAPVC is surgical. In the case of supracardiac TAPVC draining to the left innominate vein, the common vein is anastomosed side-to-side with the left atrium, and the communication to the systemic veins as well as additional shunts, such as ASD or VSD, are closed. Other types of TAPVC are treated in a similar manner. Patients with preexisting venous obstruction and coexistent complex heart disease, especially single ventricle, have worse outcomes.[45,46] Other features that have been correlated with poor outcome include younger age and type II connection.[46] Pulmonary vein stenosis after repair is a common complication, particularly in patients with heterotaxy.

Reporting: Information for the Referring Physician

Detailed descriptions of the course and drainage sites of all pulmonary veins are crucial. Also, as stated before, the size of the individual pulmonary veins yields important prognostic information. Obstruction to venous drainage and signs of right ventricular volume overload or venous congestion on plain films implying infracardiac TAPVC should be clearly stated.

KEY POINTS

- TAPVC can be supracardiac, intracardiac, infracardiac, or mixed.
- The distinction between the obstructed and nonobstructed forms of TAPVC is important because the surgical repair of the obstructed veins is more difficult and patients tend to have a worse outcome with obstruction.
- Angiography with CT and MRI are important complementary imaging modalities when echocardiography is not able to completely delineate all of the anomalous pulmonary veins, especially with the mixed form of the disease.
- Associated obstruction to pulmonary venous drainage needs to be fully evaluated preoperatively.

SUGGESTED READINGS

Alphonso N, Norgaard MA, Newcomb A, et al. Cor triatriatum: presentation, diagnosis and long-term surgical results. Ann Thorac Surg 2005; 80:1666-1671

Darling RC, Rothney WB, Craig JM. Total pulmonary venous drainage into the right side of the heart: report of 17 autopsied cases not associated with other major cardiovascular anomalies. Lab Invest 1957; 6:44-64.

Kanter KR. Surgical repair of total anomalous pulmonary venous connection. Semin Thorac Cardiovasc Surg Pediatr Card Surg Annu 2006; 40-44.

Kim TH, Kim YM, Suh CH, et al. Helical CT angiography and three-dimensional reconstruction of total anomalous pulmonary venous connections in neonates and infants. AJR Am J Roentgenol 2000; 175:1381-1386.

Uçar T, Fitoz S, Tutar E, et al. Diagnostic tools in the preoperative evaluation of children with anomalous pulmonary venous connections. Int J Cardiovasc Imaging 2008; 24:229-235.

Valsangiacomo ER, Levasseur S, McCrindle BW, et al. Contrast-enhanced MR angiography of pulmonary venous abnormalities in children. Pediatr Radiol 2003; 33:92-98.

Wang ZJ, Reddy GP, Gotway MB, et al. Cardiovascular shunts: MR imaging evaluation. Radiographics 2003; 23:S181-S194.

Zylak CJ, Eyler WR, Spizarny DL, Stone CH. Developmental lung anomalies in the adult: radiologic-pathologic correlation. Radiographics 2002; 22:S25-S43.

REFERENCES

1. Webb S, Kanani M, Anderson RH, et al. Development of the human pulmonary vein and its incorporation in the morphologically left atrium. Cardiol Young 2001; 11:632-642.
2. Healy JE Jr. An anatomic survey of anomalous pulmonary veins: their significance. J Thorac Cardiovasc Surg 1952; 23:433-444.
3. Hughes C, Rumore P. Anomalous pulmonary veins. Arch Pathol 1944; 37:364-366.
4. Panicek DM, Heitzman ER, Randall PA, et al. The continuum of pulmonary developmental anomalies. Radiographics 1987; 7:747-772.
5. Freedom RM, Yoo SH, Goo HW, et al. The bronchopulmonary foregut malformation complex. Cardiol Young 2006; 16:229-251.
6. Moore JW, Kirby WC, Rogers WM, Poth MA. Partial anomalous pulmonary venous drainage associated with 45,X Turner's syndrome. Pediatrics 1990; 86:273-276.
7. Stümper O, Vargas-Barron J, Rijlaarsdam M, et al. Assessment of anomalous systemic and pulmonary venous connections by transoesophageal echocardiography in infants and children. Br Heart J 1991; 66:411-418.
8. Uçar T, Fitoz S, Tutar E, et al. Diagnostic tools in the preoperative evaluation of children with anomalous pulmonary venous connections. Int J Cardiovasc Imaging 2008; 24:229-235.
9. Masui T, Seelos KC, Kersting-Sommerhoff BA, Higgins CB. Abnormalities of the pulmonary veins: evaluation with MR imaging and comparison with cardiac angiography and echocardiography. Radiology 1991; 181:645-649.
10. Festa P, Ait-Ali L, Cerillo AG, et al. Magnetic resonance imaging is the diagnostic tool of choice in the preoperative evaluation of patients with partial anomalous pulmonary venous return. Int J Cardiovasc Imaging 2006; 22:685-693.
11. Greil GF, Powell AJ, Gildein HP, Geva T. Gadolinium-enhanced three-dimensional magnetic resonance angiography of pulmonary and systemic venous anomalies. J Am Coll Cardiol 2002; 39:335-341.
12. Alsoufi B, Cai S, Van Arsdell GS, et al. Outcomes after surgical treatment of children with partial anomalous pulmonary venous connection. Ann Thorac Surg 2007; 84:2020-2026.
13. Davia JE, Cheitlin MD, Bedynek JL. Sinus venosus atrial septal defect: analysis of fifty cases. Am Heart J 1973; 85:177-185.
14. Van Praagh S, Carrera ME, Sanders SP, et al. Sinus venosus defects—anatomic and echocardiographic findings and surgical treatment. Am Heart J 1994; 128:365-379.
15. Attenhofer Jost CH, Connolly HM, Danielson GK, et al. Sinus venosus atrial septal defect: long term postoperative outcome for 115 patients. Circulation 2005; 112:1953-1958.

16. Otsuka M, Itoh A, Haze K. Sinus venosus type of atrial septal defect with partial anomalous pulmonary venous return evaluated by multislice CT. Heart 2004; 90:901.
17. Valente AM, Sena L, Powell AJ, et al. Cardiac magnetic resonance imaging evaluation of sinus venosus defects: comparison to surgical findings. Pediatr Cardiol 2007; 28:51-56.
18. Kharouf R, Luxenberg DM, Khalid O, Abdulla R. Atrial septal defect: spectrum of care. Pediatr Cardiol 2008; 29:271-280.
19. Oliver JM, Gallego P, Gonzalez A, et al. Sinus venosus syndrome: atrial septal defect or anomalous venous connection? A multiplane transoesophageal approach. Heart 2002; 88:634-638.
20. Iyer AP, Somanrema K, Pathak S, et al. Comparative study of single- and double-patch techniques for sinus venosus atrial septal defect with partial anomalous pulmonary venous connection. J Thorac Cardiovasc Surg 2007; 133:656-659.
21. Stewart RD, Bailliard F, Kelle AM, et al. Evolving surgical strategy for sinus venosus atrial septal defect: effect on sinus node function and late venous obstruction. Ann Thorac Surg 2007; 84:1651-1655.
22. Warden HE, Gustafson RA, Tarnay TJ, Neal WA. An alternative method for repair of partial anomalous pulmonary venous connection to the superior vena cava. Ann Thorac Surg 1984; 38:601-605.
23. Van Praagh R, Corsini I. Cor triatriatum: pathologic anatomy and a consideration of morphogenesis based on 13 postmortem cases and a study of normal development of the pulmonary vein and atrial septum in 83 human embryos. Am Heart J 1969; 78:379-405.
24. Buchholz S, Jenni R. Doppler echocardiographic findings in 2 identical variants of a rare cardiac anomaly, "subtotal" cor triatriatum: a critical review of the literature. J Am Soc Echocardiogr 2001; 14:846-849.
25. Jegier W, Gibbons JE, Wiglesworth FW. Cor triatriatum: clinical, hemodynamic and pathological studies: surgical correction in early life. Pediatrics 1963; 31:255-267.
26. Chen K, Thng CH. Multislice computed tomography and two-dimensional echocardiographic images of cor triatriatum in a 46-year-old man. Circulation 2001; 104:2117.
27. Rumancik WM, Hernanz-Schulman M, Rutkowski MM, et al. Magnetic resonance imaging of cor triatriatum. Pediatr Cardiol 1988; 9:149-151.
28. Sakamoto I, Matsunaga N, Hayashi K, et al. Cine-magnetic resonance imaging of cor triatriatum. Chest 1994; 106:1586-1589.
29. Ibrahim T, Schreiber K, Dennig K, et al. Assessment of cor triatriatum sinistrum by magnetic resonance imaging. Circulation 2003; 108:e107.
30. Steen H, Merten C, Lehrke S, et al. Two rare cases of left and right atrial congenital heart disease: cor triatriatum dexter and sinister. Clin Res Cardiol 2007; 96:122-124.
31. Gheissari A, Malm JR, Bowman FO Jr, Bierman FZ. Cor triatriatum sinistrum: one institution's 28-year experience. Pediatr Cardiol 1992; 13:85-88.
32. Richardson JV, Doty DB, Siewers RD, Zuberbuhler JR. Cor triatriatum (subdivided left atrium). J Thorac Cardiovasc Surg 1981; 81:232-238.
33. Alphonso N, Norgaard MA, Newcomb A, et al. Cor triatriatum: presentation, diagnosis and long-term surgical results. Ann Thorac Surg 2005; 80:1666-1671.
34. Huang YK, Chu JJ, Chang JP, et al. Cor triatriatum sinistrum: surgical experience in Taiwan. Surg Today 2007; 37:449-454.
35. Oglietti J, Cooley DA, Izquierdo JP, et al. Cor triatriatum: operative results in 25 patients. Ann Thorac Surg 1983; 35:415-420.
36. Mehrizi A, Hirsch MS, Taussig HB. Congenital heart disease in the neonatal period: autopsy study of 170 cases. J Pediatr 1964; 65:721-726.
37. Delisle G, Ando M, Calder AL, et al. Total anomalous pulmonary venous connection: report of 93 autopsied cases with emphasis on diagnostic and surgical considerations. Am Heart J 1976; 91:99-122.
38. Lucas RV Jr, Adams P Jr, Anderson RC. Total anomalous pulmonary venous connection to the portal system: a cause of pulmonary venous obstruction. AJR Am J Roentgenol 1961; 86:561-575.
39. Foerster SR, Gauvreau K, McElhinney DB, Geva T. Importance of total anomalous pulmonary venous connection and postoperative pulmonary vein stenosis in outcomes of heterotaxy syndrome. Pediatr Cardiol 2008; 29:536-544.
40. Jenkins KJ, Sanders SP, Orav EJ, et al. Individual pulmonary vein size and survival in infants with totally anomalous pulmonary venous connection. J Am Coll Cardiol 1993; 22:201-206.
41. Kim TH, Kim YM, Suh CH, et al. Helical CT angiography and three-dimensional reconstruction of total anomalous pulmonary venous connections in neonates and infants. AJR Am J Roentgenol 2000; 175:1381-1386.
42. Shiraishi I, Yamagishi M, Iwasaki N, et al. Helical computed tomographic angiography in obstructed total anomalous pulmonary venous drainage. Ann Thorac Surg 2001; 71:1690-1692.
43. Sridhar PG, Kalyanpur A, Suresh PV, et al. Total anomalous pulmonary venous connection: helical computed tomography as an alternative to angiography. Indian Heart J 2003; 55:624-627.
44. Valsangiacomo ER, Levasseur S, McCrindle BW, et al. Contrast-enhanced MR angiography of pulmonary venous abnormalities in children. Pediatr Radiol 2003; 33:92-98.
45. Hancock Friesen CL, Zurakowski D, Thiagarajan RR, et al. Total anomalous pulmonary venous connection: an analysis of current management strategies in a single institution. Ann Thorac Surg 2005; 79:596-606.
46. Karamlou T, Gurofsky R, Sukhni EA, et al. Factors associated with mortality and reoperation in 377 children with total anomalous pulmonary venous connection. Circulation 2007; 115:1591-1598.

CHAPTER 47

Tetralogy of Fallot

S. Bruce Greenberg

Tetralogy of Fallot, the most common cyanotic congenital heart abnormality, is caused by a single anomaly—anterior conal septal malalignment. Despite the single defect causing the anomaly, a spectrum of clinical and imaging findings can occur depending on the extent of the conal septum deviation. A mild deviation results in minimal right ventricular outflow obstruction and severe deviation in outflow tract atresia. Patients range from "pink" to severely cyanotic. Imaging plays a major role in characterizing the extent of the abnormalities before palliative or corrective surgery. Improved surgical technique has led to improved survival with most patients surviving into adulthood. MRI and CT have an increasingly important role in the long-term follow-up of patients after initial repair.

DEFINITION

Anterior conal septum malalignment prevents fusion of the conal and ventricular septum resulting in the tetrad that characterizes tetralogy of Fallot: right ventricular tract obstruction, ventricular septal defect (VSD), overriding aorta, and right ventricular hypertrophy.

PREVALENCE AND EPIDEMIOLOGY

Tetralogy of Fallot is the most common congenital heart disease manifesting with cyanosis. The incidence is 0.06% of live births, and it constitutes 5% to 7% of all congenital heart disease.[1,2] Genetic syndromes are associated with tetralogy of Fallot in 20% of cases with 22q11 deletion and trisomy 21 being the most common.[3] Complete atrioventricular septal defects are present in 2% of patients with tetralogy of Fallot, especially patients with trisomy 21.[4] Alagille syndrome, VACTERL syndrome (*v*ertebral anomalies, *a*nal atresia, *c*ardiovascular anomalies, *t*racheoesophageal fistula, *e*sophageal atresia, *r*enal anomalies, *l*imb anomalies), and CHARGE syndrome (*c*oloboma of the eye, *h*eart defects, *a*tresia of the choanae, *r*etardation of growth and development, *g*enitourinary abnormalities; *e*ar abnormalities and deafness) are also associated with tetralogy of Fallot. Atrial septal defect is present in one third of patients with tetralogy of Fallot. Currently, 85% of children with tetralogy of Fallot survive to adulthood, increasing the prevalence of tetralogy of Fallot in adults.

In greater than 90% of children, right aortic arch and mirror-image branching are associated with congenital heart disease. Tetralogy of Fallot is the most common congenital heart disease associated with a right aortic arch. Approximately 90% of patients with a right aortic arch and mirror-image branching have tetralogy of Fallot. Of patients with tetralogy of Fallot, 25% have a right aortic arch, and most have a mirror-image branching pattern.

Aberrant subclavian arteries are associated in 5% to 8% of patients with tetralogy of Fallot. The prevalence of tetralogy of Fallot and anomalous subclavian artery is greater if associated with a right aortic arch or pulmonary atresia. Anomalous subclavian artery occurs in 24% of patients with tetralogy of Fallot, right aortic arch, and pulmonary atresia.[5]

Coronary artery anomalies are common, occurring in 5% to 12% of children with tetralogy of Fallot.[6,7] Coronary artery anomalies that result in major branches coursing anterior to the right ventricular outflow tract (RVOT) interfere with transannular patch angioplasty of the outflow tract.

ETIOLOGY AND PATHOPHYSIOLOGY

Tetralogy is the consequence of abnormal conotruncal development. Anterior conal septum deviation narrows the developing RVOT. The deviation may be minimal, causing little initial RVOT obstruction, or severe, resulting in pulmonary atresia. The abnormal position of the anterior conal septum prevents ventricular septal closure and results in a large VSD that does not spontaneously close. The aorta assumes a position overriding the VSD. The pressure within the ventricles equalizes, resulting in right ventricular hypertrophy. Right-sided obstruction classically involves the right ventricular infundibulum, but frequently also includes the pulmonary valve, pulmonary artery, and branch pulmonary arteries.

The pathophysiology varies with the degree of RVOT obstruction. A left-to-right shunt across the VSD might initially predominate if the RVOT obstruction is mild. Outflow tract obstruction is progressive leading to eventual right-to-left shunting and cyanosis. Pulmonary atresia or more severe RVOT obstruction occurs with immediate or early cyanosis.

MANIFESTATIONS OF DISEASE

Clinical Presentation

The initial presentation depends on the degree of right ventricular outflow obstruction. Infants may initially be acyanotic—so-called pink tetralogy. The VSD may act as a left-to-right shunt with pulmonary overcirculation. A murmur of VSD may be present. Cyanosis progresses during the first months of life owing to progressive RVOT obstruction. Infants typically present with cyanosis between 6 weeks and 6 months of age. Infants with severe RVOT obstruction can be ductal dependent and present earlier. Clubbing may be present. Outflow tract obstruction is associated with systolic murmurs.

The pulmonary infundibulum is prone to spasm, causing acute episodes of cyanosis referred to as "tet spells." Activity and acidosis stimulate these episodes, and squatting may relieve them. In children with right aortic arch, the large ascending aorta causes tracheal compression that can result in feeding or respiratory difficulty. Patients with tetralogy of Fallot and absent pulmonary valve present with severe dilation of the pulmonary artery and central pulmonary arteries that compress the trachea and bronchi. These patients can have severe respiratory distress. Polycythemia associated with cyanosis may lead to pulmonary or cerebral thrombosis.

A child with a palliative shunt has a continuous murmur similar to that heard in a child with a patent ductus arteriosus. After corrective surgery, symptoms may reflect continued right-sided obstruction or pulmonary regurgitation. Corrective surgery for tetralogy of Fallot requires enlargement of the RVOT and frequently a transannular patch, which results in pulmonary regurgitation.[8-10] Pulmonary regurgitation is initially well tolerated, but later is associated with fatigue. The right ventricle and its outflow tract progressively dilate. Right ventricular enlargement leads to distortion of the tricuspid valve annulus and tricuspid regurgitation, compromising right heart function further. ECG abnormalities with lengthening of the QRS complex can lead to arrhythmia that may result in sudden death. Diastolic dysfunction can progress to irreversible systolic dysfunction.[8] Revision of the RVOT with a valved conduit causes right ventricular remodeling and improved cardiac function. Pseudoaneurysms of the RVOT can follow corrective surgery with a transannular patch or pulmonary conduit.

Aortic root dilation and regurgitation are common in adults with tetralogy of Fallot and can lead to arterial medial abnormalities. Risk factors for aortopathy include patients with pulmonary atresia, right aortic arch, history of aorticopulmonary shunts, male sex, and chromosome 22q11 deletions.[11]

Imaging Indications and Algorithm

Echocardiography is the first and frequently the only imaging modality necessary before surgery for evaluation of tetralogy of Fallot. The intracardiac anomalies, potential critical coronary artery anomalies, and RVOT can be characterized by echocardiography. The branch pulmonary arteries and aortic arch anomalies are usually adequately evaluated on preoperative echocardiograms, but may require additional imaging—particularly if the branch pulmonary arteries are nonconfluent or severely hypoplastic, or major aorticopulmonary collateral arteries are present. The positions of the coronary arteries need to be established before surgery. MRI and CT are the second-line imaging modalities to complete preoperative evaluation if echocardiography is incomplete. Cardiac catheterization is no longer necessary before primary surgery.

After palliative or corrective surgery, echocardiography is more limited. The windows for echocardiography evaluation diminish with age. The importance of quantifying right ventricular size and function increases in importance. MRI has a more dominant role in the postoperative patient, particularly for the evaluation of pulmonary regurgitation. CT is useful when MRI is unavailable or contraindicated.

Imaging Technique and Findings

Radiography

Radiography plays a secondary role to echocardiography. The cardiac silhouette is frequently normal in size and configuration (Fig. 47-1). The classic radiographic appearance is a boot-shaped heart caused by elevation of the cardiac apex from right ventricular hypertrophy with a diminished or unapparent pulmonary artery segment (Fig. 47-2). The appearance of a boot-shaped heart can be mimicked if the central x-ray beam is caudal to the heart causing cephalic projection of the more anterior portion of the heart (Fig. 47-3). The pulmonary vascularity is

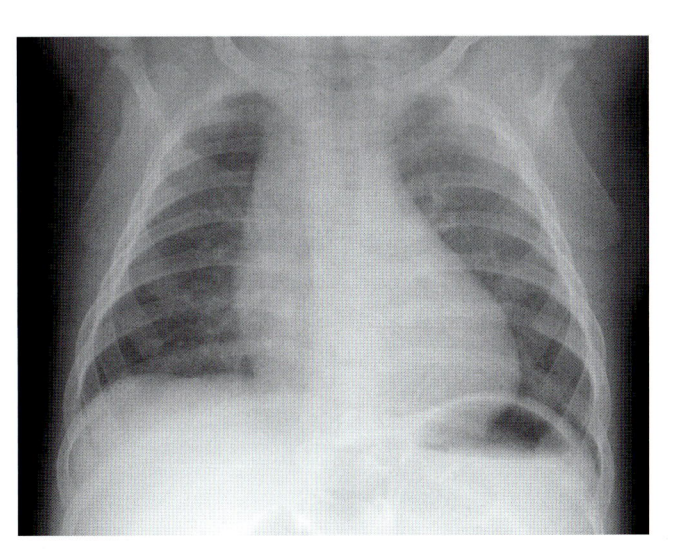

FIGURE 47-1 The heart is normal in appearance on this chest radiograph in a 5-month-old infant with tetralogy of Fallot. A right aortic arch is present.

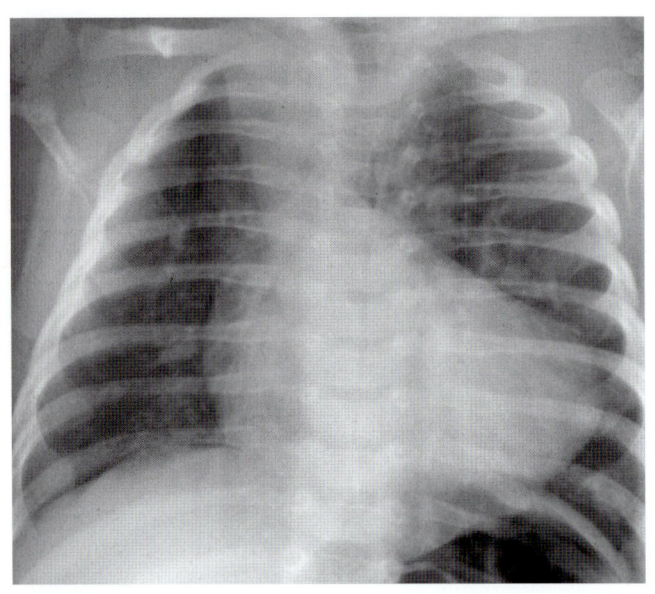

FIGURE 47-2 Tetralogy of Fallot in a 6-week-old infant shows elevation of the cardiac apex creating the classic boot-shaped heart. A right aortic arch is present.

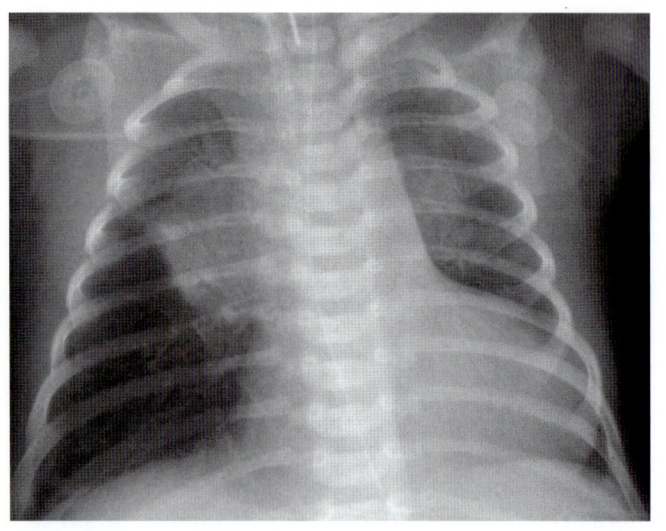

FIGURE 47-4 Chest radiograph in a 1-day-old infant with tetralogy of Fallot and absent pulmonary valve shows massive enlargement of the central pulmonary arteries.

diminished, but may be undetectable on a conventional radiograph if right ventricular obstruction is mild. A right aortic arch is visible in 25% of patients with tetralogy of Fallot. Direct visualization of the aortic arch and tracheal shift can be difficult to detect in infants and young children. The side of the aortic arch is reliably determined, however, by noting the increased density of the pedicles on the side of the aortic arch. Patients with tetralogy of Fallot and absent pulmonary artery have enlargement of the central pulmonary arteries (Fig. 47-4).

Ultrasonography

Echocardiography is definitive for the prenatal and postnatal diagnosis of tetralogy of Fallot.[12] A large VSD is identified in utero on the four-chamber view, but evaluation of the outflow tracts is necessary for the diagnosis because other conotruncal abnormalities can have a VSD and an overriding aorta. A large aorta overriding the VSD is present. The aorta is larger than the pulmonary artery. Doppler interrogation of the fetal RVOT shows elevated velocity. A left-to-right shunt through the ductus arteriosus suggests severe RVOT obstruction.[13]

Postnatal echocardiography characterizes all intracardiac features of tetralogy of Fallot. The VSD and aorta override are identified on the parasternal long-axis view (Fig. 47-5). The outflow tract must also be evaluated (Fig. 47-6) because truncus arteriosus and VSD with pulmonary atresia can have the same appearance. In contrast to double outlet right ventricle, the aortic override to the right ventricle is less than 50%, and aortic valve fibrous continuity with the mitral valve is preserved. The RVOT including the infundibulum, pulmonary valve, and pulmonary artery is measured for stenosis. The measured infundibular volume is small, and owing to reduced growth compared with somatic growth becomes progressively more stenotic.[14] Infants who require earlier surgical intervention have a greater reduction in infundibular volume. The pulmonary annulus can be hypoplastic and bicuspid. Hypoplasia with a z score less than 2 is an indication for a transannular patch. Branch pulmonary artery continuity and size is also determined. The position of the coronary arteries must be established. A coronary anomaly with a major coronary branch coursing anterior to the RVOT

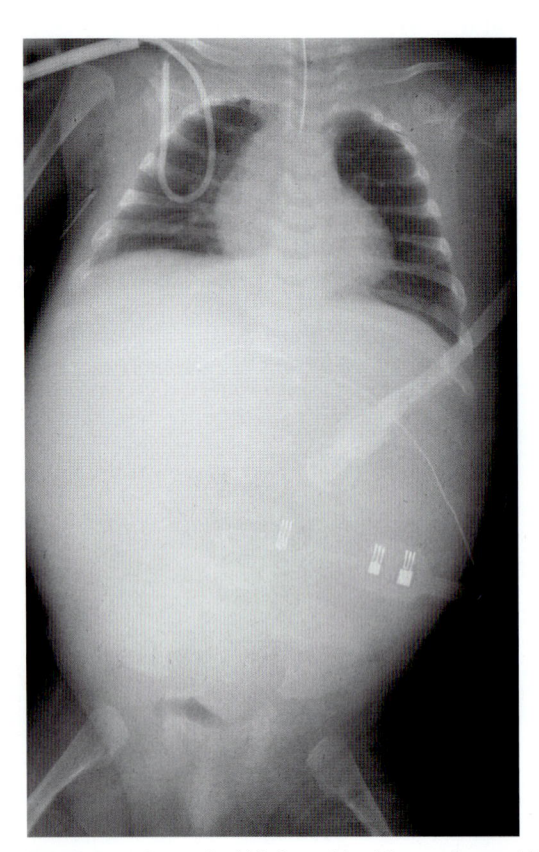

FIGURE 47-3 A 3-month-old infant with a history of necrotizing enterocolitis and no heart disease has a seemingly boot-shaped heart on the chest-abdomen examination owing to the x-ray beam being centered over the mid-abdomen.

■ **FIGURE 47-5** A, Parasternal long-axis echocardiogram shows the aorta overriding (*asterisk*) a large VSD. B, Parasternal short-axis echocardiogram shows anterior deviation of the anterior conal septum (*arrow*). *(Courtesy of Dr. Himesh Vyas, Arkansas Children's Hospital.)*

must be excluded before repair. CT or MRI may be necessary if the coronary arteries or pulmonary arteries are inadequately visualized.

Echocardiography is more limited after surgery because of mediastinal fibrosis. Palliative shunt stenosis or occlusion is difficult to image because of their positions. Branch pulmonary artery abnormalities are also more difficult to evaluate after surgery. Available windows diminish with patient age. Residual VSD, RVOT obstruction, and branch pulmonary artery stenosis can be detected. Pulmonary regurgitation is suggested by the presence of right ventricular enlargement. Color flow and spectral Doppler are helpful in detecting pulmonary regurgitation and residual VSD.

Computed Tomography

CT is a complementary imaging modality. Echocardiography is the primary imaging modality, and MRI is the preferred complementary imaging modality. The high diagnostic dose of ionizing radiation and the inability to detect flow patterns with CT make MRI the preferred complementary modality. Multidetector CT has an increasing role in the evaluation of tetralogy of Fallot in patients with contraindications to MRI, such as pacemakers or implantable cardioverter defibrillators. Multidetector CT is better than echocardiography and MRI for defining coronary artery abnormalities (Fig. 47-7) and can be used if echocardiography is inconclusive.[15,16] High spatial resolution allows for excellent demonstration of the RVOT and pulmonary arteries, allowing for noninvasive measurements of hypoplasia, focal stenosis,[17] or aneurysms (Fig. 47-8). CT is preferred to MRI to evaluate vascular stents (Figs. 47-9 and 47-10). Gated studies to measure cardiac function in patients with contraindications for MRI can be performed, but they require higher radiation dose gated techniques.[18]

Magnetic Resonance Imaging

MRI is the primary complementary imaging modality after echocardiography. The primary diagnostic findings of tetralogy of Fallot can be detected by MRI, but are adequately imaged by echocardiography. Although echocardiography is adequate for evaluation of intracardiac abnormalities, the branch pulmonary arteries and collateral arteries are better characterized by MRI (Fig. 47-11). MRI, notably using MR angiography, can characterize branch pulmonary confluence, absence, or stenosis, and the number and location of major aorticopulmonary collateral arteries. Palliative shunts are better visualized by MR angiography than echocardiography (Fig. 47-12).

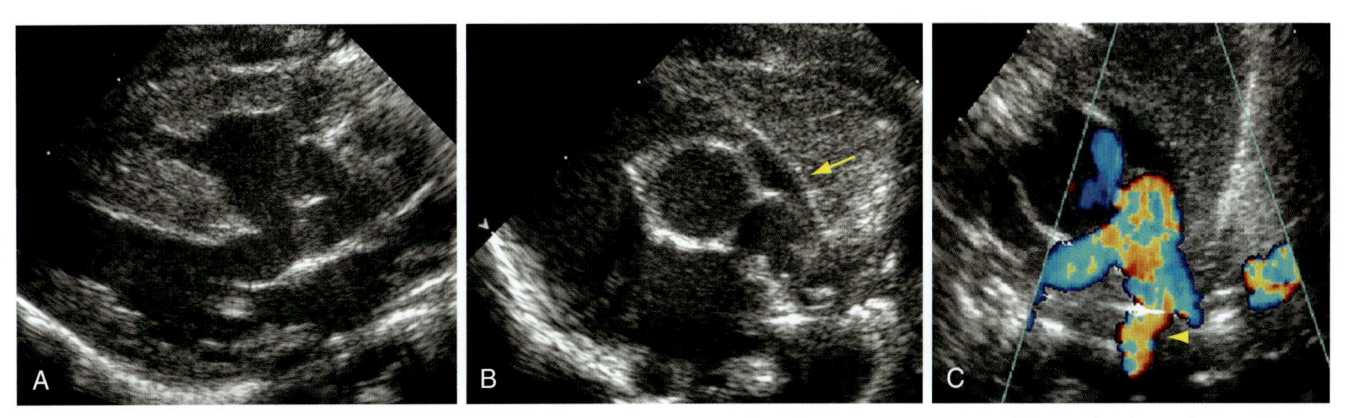

■ **FIGURE 47-6** A, Parasternal long-axis echocardiogram shows the aorta overriding a large VSD. B, Parasternal short-axis echocardiogram shows pulmonary atresia (*arrow*). C, Color flow Doppler image shows ductal dependent flow to the confluent branch pulmonary arteries. The ductus arteriosus is indicated by the *arrowhead*. *(Courtesy of Dr. Sadia Malik, Arkansas Children's Hospital.)*

644 PART FIVE • *Congenital Heart Disease*

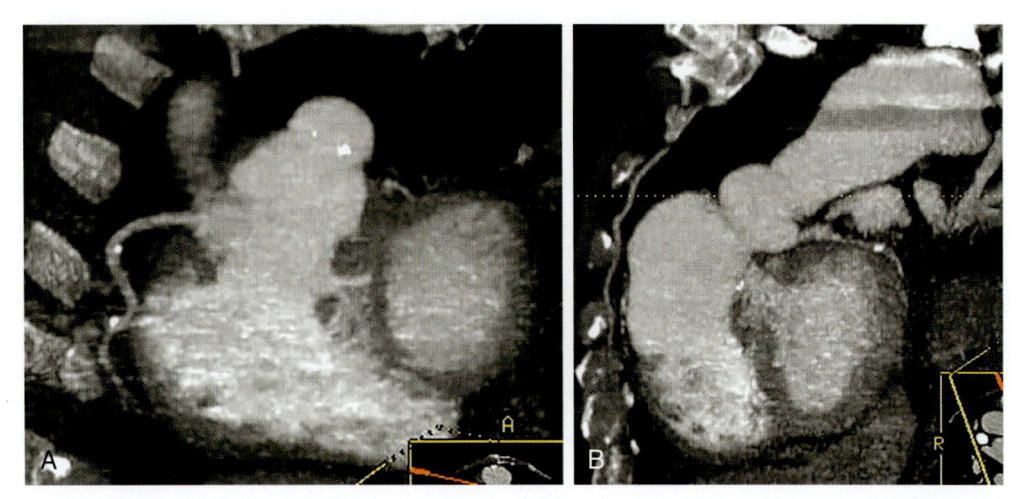

■ **FIGURE 47-7** A and B, CT shows right (**A**) and left (**B**) coronary artery calcifications in a 61-year-old patient with a history of tetralogy of Fallot. Pulmonary artery stenosis and poststenotic dilation are also present (**B**).

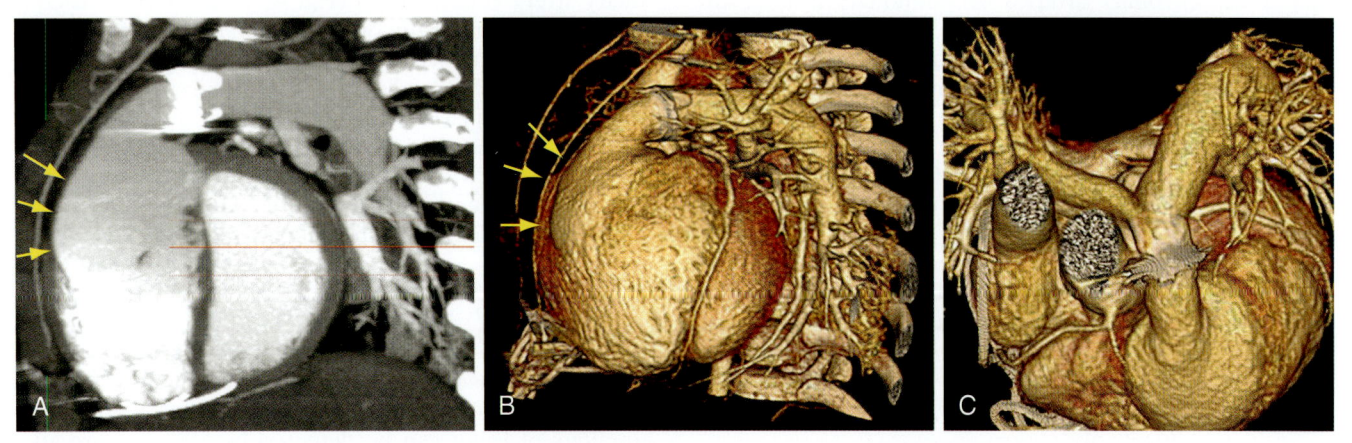

■ **FIGURE 47-8** A and B, CT in a 6-year-old patient after tetralogy of Fallot repair shows aneurysmal dilation of the RVOT caused by a large outflow tract patch (*arrows*) on multiplanar reformation (**A**) and three-dimensional volume rendering (**B**). C, A metal ring in the Hancock pulmonary conduit is present. Hypoplasia of the right pulmonary artery is present.

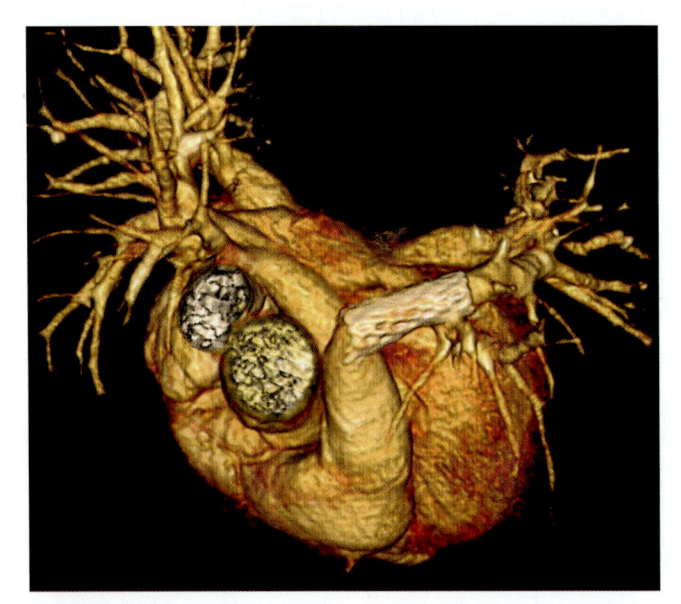

■ **FIGURE 47-9** Branch pulmonary artery stents are well visualized using multidetector CT in children after tetralogy of Fallot repair. Three-dimensional volume rendering shows left pulmonary artery stenosis distal to the stent in a 14-year-old patient.

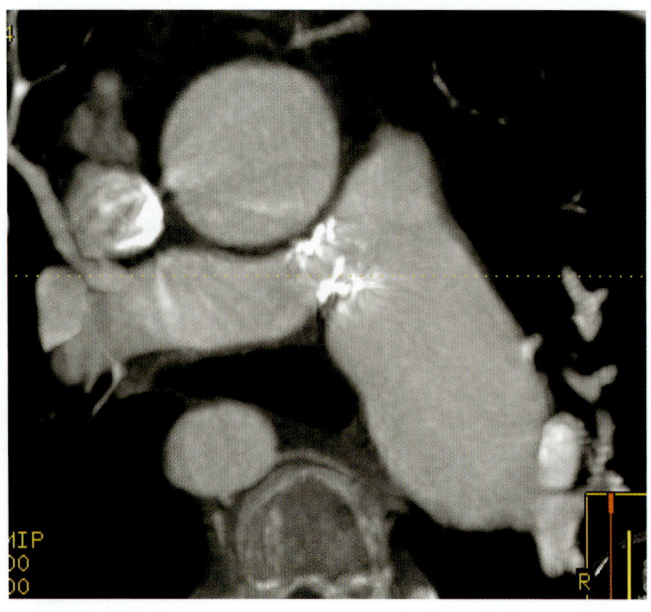

■ **FIGURE 47-10** Multiplanar reformation shows a widely patent right pulmonary artery stent in an 8-year-old child with stenosis of right pulmonary artery origin.

CHAPTER 47 • Tetralogy of Fallot 645

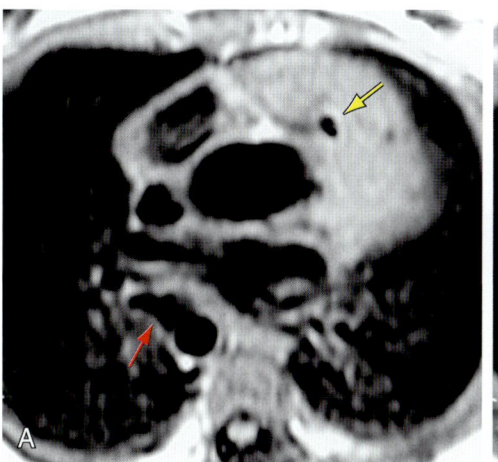

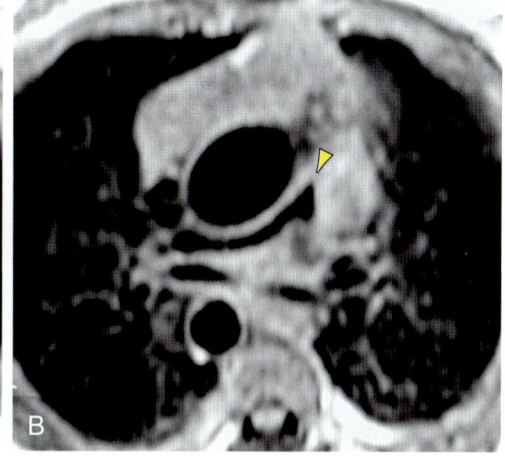

■ **FIGURE 47-11** A and B, Axial T1-weighted MRI (caudal [A] and cranial [B] images) in a 3-month-old infant with tetralogy of Fallot shows pulmonary atresia (*yellow arrow* in **A**). A large overriding aorta is present, and the aortic arch is on the right. The origin of a major aorticopulmonary collateral artery from the descending aorta (*red arrow* in **A**) is identified. Branch pulmonary artery confluence (*arrowhead* in **B**) is present.

Associated aortic arch anomalies that should be identified by echocardiography are more completely visualized by MR angiography (Fig. 47-13).[16]

MRI has a more dominant role in postoperative patients. Echocardiography windows become progressively more restricted and are particularly limited for evaluation of the right ventricle and branch pulmonary arteries. Complications of palliations, such as branch pulmonary artery stenosis (Fig. 47-14), distortion, or occlusion resulting from prior systemic pulmonary artery shunts, are well visualized by MR angiography. Complications of corrective surgery, including residual RVOT stenosis, pseudoaneurysm (Fig. 47-15), or dilation from pulmonary regurgitation, are well imaged by a combination of black and white blood imaging techniques or MR angiography.

Accurate right ventricular size quantification cannot be obtained by two-dimensional echocardiography because of the right ventricular shape and the poor available windows. MRI biventricular volume measurements using short-axis cine steady-state free precession white blood images to quantify right and left ventricular systolic function and the right ventricular regurgitant fraction are the gold standard (Fig. 47-16). Right ventricular enlargement and an elevated right ventricular regurgitant fraction are among the criteria used to determine the timing for further reoperation to place a valved pulmonary conduit. Criteria for determining the appropriate time for valved conduit surgery are evolving.[9]

Pulmonary regurgitation and late diastolic forward flow consistent with right ventricular diastolic dysfunction can be quantified using phase contrast MRI flow quantification (also known as velocity-encoded MRI) (Fig. 47-17).[19] A reduction in the normal E:A maximum flow amplitude ratio across the tricuspid valve detected by phase contrast MRI flow quantification across the tricuspid valve is also consistent with diastolic dysfunction and correlates with

■ **FIGURE 47-12** MR angiography volume rendering posterior view shows wide patency of a modified Blalock-Taussig shunt (*arrow*).

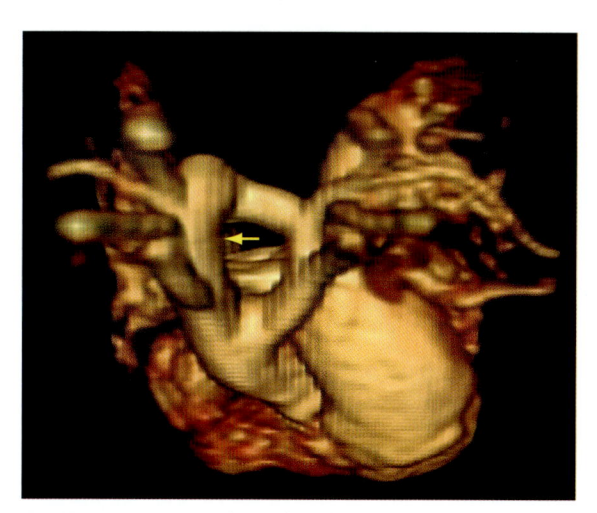

■ **FIGURE 47-13** MR angiography volume rendering cranial view shows a double aortic arch with a dominant right arch (*arrow*) in a 7-year-old patient with tetralogy of Fallot.

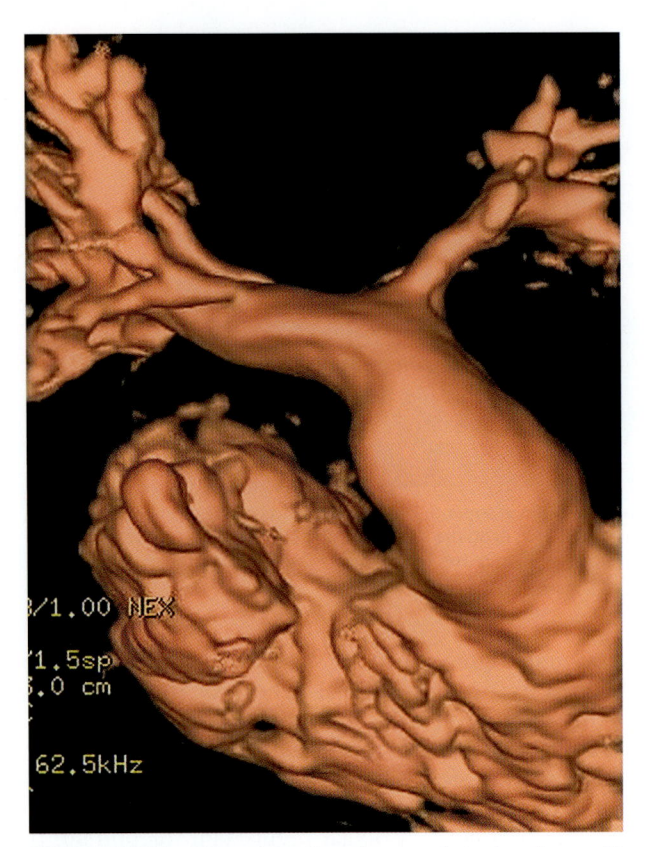

FIGURE 47-14 MR angiography volume rendering in a 5-year-old patient shows left pulmonary artery stenosis after tetralogy of Fallot repair.

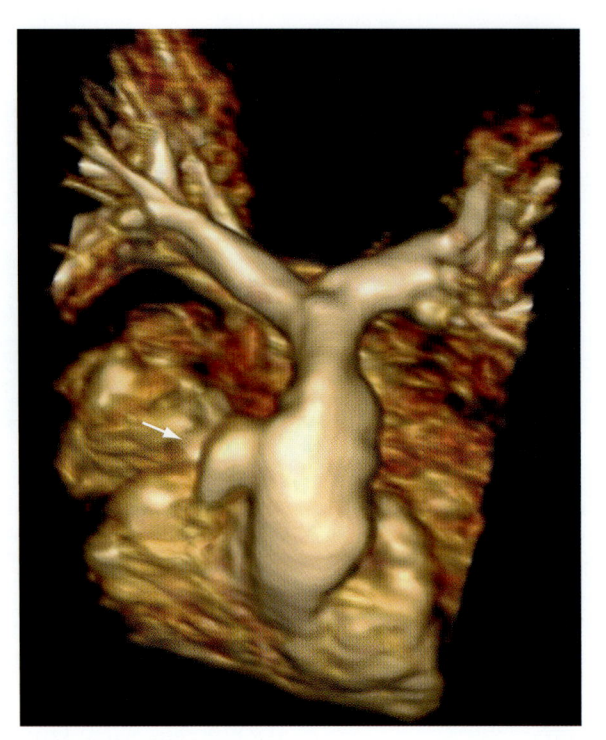

FIGURE 47-15 MR angiography volume rendering shows a right ventricular outflow pseudoaneurysm (*arrow*) projecting to the right of the RVOT in a 14-year-old patient.

right ventriculomegaly (Fig. 47-18).[20,21] Dobutamine stress MRI may unmask diastolic dysfunction not appreciated on rest imaging.[22] Delayed hyperenhancement imaging can show fibrosis in the RVOT and is associated with outflow tract dilation.[23]

Late aortopathy associated with tetralogy of Fallot can be evaluated by MR angiography (Fig. 47-19). Associated aortic valve regurgitation is quantified by phase contrast MRI flow quantification.

Angiography

Angiography was the historical gold standard for evaluation of pulmonary artery size and collateral pulmonary

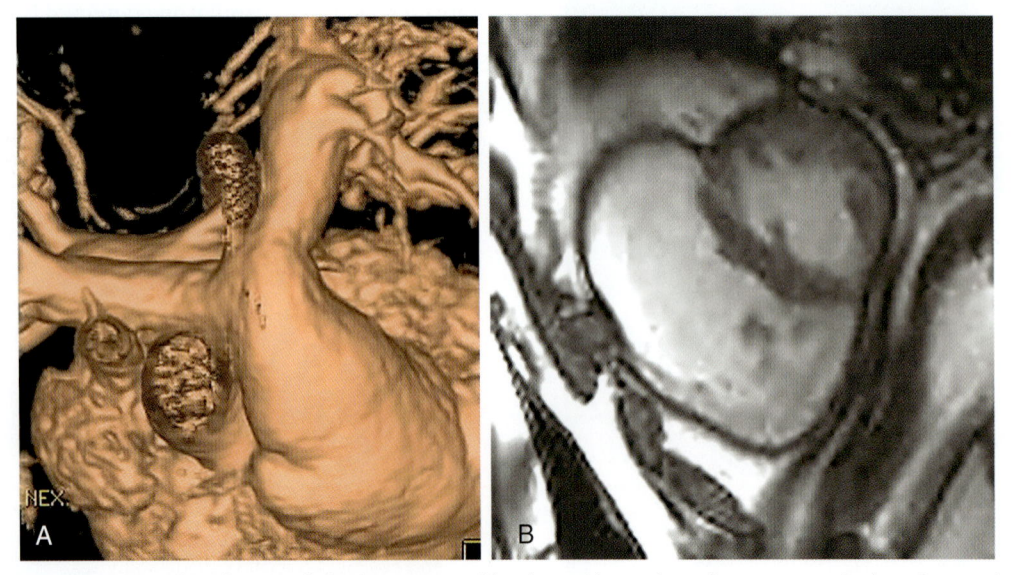

FIGURE 47-16 **A,** MR angiography volume rendering in a 40-year-old patient with massive pulmonary regurgitation after tetralogy of Fallot repair shows pulmonary artery and branch pulmonary aneurysmal enlargement. **B,** Short-axis cine imaging shows right ventricular enlargement and is used to quantify ventricular sizes. The right ventricular regurgitant fraction was 70%, and right ventricular end-diastolic volume index was 259 mL/m^2. Biventricular systolic dysfunction was also present.

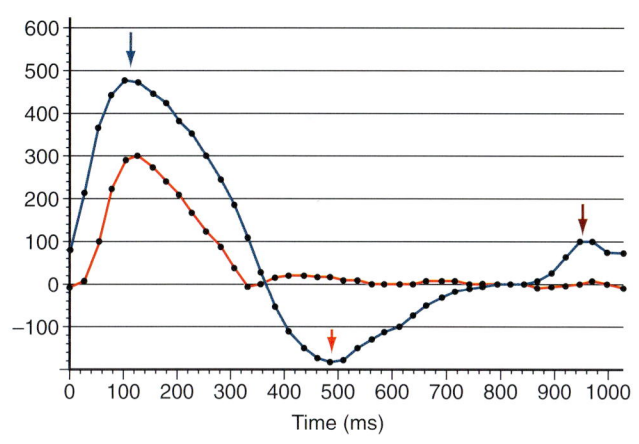

■ **FIGURE 47-17** Phase contrast MRI flow quantification of the aorta (*red*) and pulmonary artery (*blue*) in a 26-year-old patient showed initial increased systolic pulmonary artery flow (*blue arrow*) compared with the ascending aorta. Pulmonary regurgitation (*red arrow*) is severe (pulmonary regurgitant fraction = 30%). Late diastolic forward flow indicates right ventricular diastolic dysfunction (*dark red arrow*).

blood flow. These functions are now performed using noninvasive MR angiography or CT angiography. Catheterization still plays a role for interventions such as balloon angioplasty and stent placement within stenotic branch pulmonary arteries or coiling collateral arteries.

Classic Signs

The classic imaging sign of tetralogy of Fallot is the wooden shoe (*coeur en sabot*) or boot-shaped heart characterized on radiographs by elevation of the cardiac apex and pulmonary artery segment concavity. Right ventricular hypertrophy causes elevation of the cardiac apex. The greater the right ventricular hypertrophy, the more elevated the cardiac apex.[24]

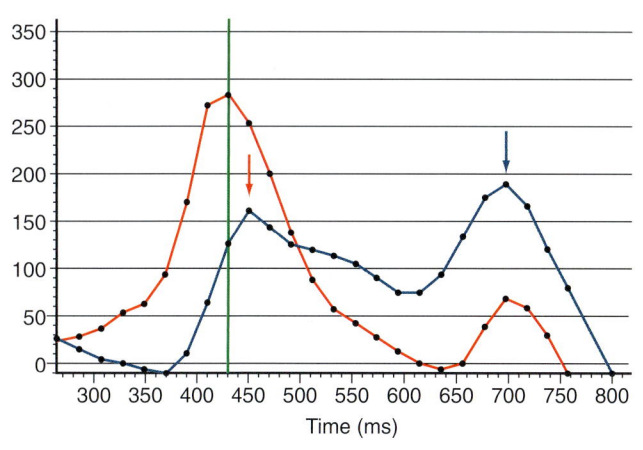

■ **FIGURE 47-18** A 10-year-old patient with a tetralogy of Fallot repair had a pulmonary regurgitant fraction of 42%. Right and left ventricular systolic function was normal. The right ventricular end-diastolic volume was twice that of the left ventricular end-diastolic volume. Phase contrast MRI flow quantification across the atrioventricular valves was performed. Mitral flow is shown in *red*, and tricuspid flow is shown in *blue*. The tricuspid E-wave amplitude (*red arrow*) is decreased compared with the A-wave (*blue arrow*) consistent with diastolic dysfunction.

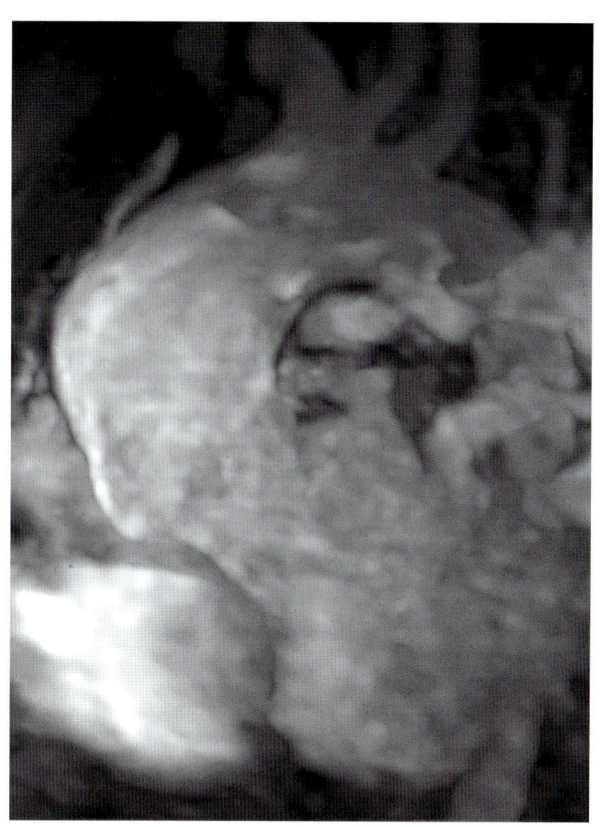

■ **FIGURE 47-19** A 37-year-old man with repaired tetralogy of Fallot had ascending aorta aneurysmal dilation that measured 5 cm. Aortic valve regurgitation was present (aortic valve regurgitant fraction = 18%).

DIFFERENTIAL DIAGNOSIS

Clinical Presentation

Tetralogy of Fallot is the most common cyanotic heart disease, but other anomalies manifest with cyanosis. D-transposition of the great arteries, truncus arteriosus, total anomalous venous return, and double outlet right ventricle all manifest with cyanosis, but are classified as admixture lesions that tend to manifest with large hearts and overcirculation. At birth, pulmonary overcirculation and cardiomegaly may be absent in patients with D-transposition because of elevated pulmonary pressures. Patients with tricuspid atresia also present with cyanosis, and similar to patients with tetralogy of Fallot are likely to have a normal-sized heart and decreased pulmonary circulation. Right ventricular hypertrophy is not present on an ECG because tricuspid atresia is characterized by absence of the right ventricle.

Imaging Findings

Echocardiography is diagnostic. The parasternal long-axis view shows the VSD and overriding aorta (see Fig. 47-5), which is common to other conotruncal anomalies such as truncus arteriosus. Imaging of the RVOT detects stenosis, determining the diagnosis. The chest radiograph may show a boot-shaped heart that is normal in size with decreased pulmonary vascularity. Admixture lesions typically have large hearts and overcirculation. Patients with

D-transposition of the great arteries clinically present early, and classic manifestations of cardiomegaly and increased pulmonary vascularity are absent. The chest radiograph in infants with D-transposition is initially normal with progressive enlargement and increased vascularity manifesting during the first week of life. Patients with truncus arteriosus frequently have a right aortic arch, but the cardiac silhouette is large and the pulmonary vascularity is increased compared with infants with tetralogy of Fallot. Patients with tricuspid atresia usually have normal-sized hearts and decreased pulmonary vascularity, but no elevation of the cardiac apex is present because the right ventricle is absent.

TREATMENT OPTIONS

Medical

Surgery is the primary treatment for tetralogy of Fallot. Ductal dependent infants require prostaglandin therapy to maintain ductal patency. Acute hypercyanotic spells ("tet spells") may be treated by calming the child and placing the child in a knee-chest or squatting position. This position increases peripheral resistance and increases pulmonary blood flow, which reduces cyanosis. Oxygen and sedatives may be necessary. β blockers help prevent tachyarrhythmias.

Surgical

Surgical palliation by systemic pulmonary shunts to increase pulmonary blood flow was initiated by Blalock in 1945. Blalock-Taussig, central, Potts, and Waterston shunts all have been used, but the most popular current palliative shunts are the modified Blalock-Taussig shunt and the central shunt. The modified Blalock-Taussig shunt uses a polytetrafluoroethylene tube graft to connect the brachiocephalic artery or subclavian artery to the ipsilateral branch pulmonary artery. A central shunt also uses a polytetrafluoroethylene tube graft, but connects the ascending aorta to the branch pulmonary artery confluence. Palliative shunts are outgrown as the child grows, but can be a bridge in time to allow sufficient growth before corrective surgery. Shunt complications include shunt occlusion, branch pulmonary artery stenosis, and branch pulmonary artery distortion.

Primary repair bypassing initial palliation is growing in popularity. Repair includes VSD closure and RVOT enlargement. RVOT reconstruction frequently requires a transannular pulmonary patch that creates pulmonary valve incompetence. Symptomatic infants with pulmonary hypoplasia can still be treated with initial palliation. Increased morbidity is associated with primary repair in the first 3 months of life, but survival is not adversely affected.[25] The ideal age for corrective surgery is 4 to 11 months in asymptomatic infants, but earlier repair is advocated in symptomatic infants.[2,26]

Long-term pulmonary regurgitation is associated with right ventricle, pulmonary artery, and branch pulmonary artery progressive dilation. Right heart dilation with associated complications can be prevented or reversed by placement of a valved conduit in the RVOT.[27] No criteria are universally accepted to determine the timing for valved conduit placement. A combination of clinical, ECG, and imaging criteria is used to determine the timing of valve replacement. Clinical criteria include exercise intolerance and signs of heart failure. ECG abnormalities include prolonged tachycardia. A QRS length greater than 180 ms is associated with sudden death.[28] MRI criteria noted by Geva[8] include pulmonary regurgitant fraction of 25% or greater combined with increased right ventricular size or decreased right ventricular systolic function.

Right ventricular remodeling occurs in children after placement of a valved conduit with a reduction in right ventricular size when the right ventricular end-diastolic volume index was ≥150 mL/m^2.[29] Right ventricular remodeling also occurs in adults, but Oosterhof and colleagues[30] found that right ventricular normalization did not occur if the right ventricular end-diastolic volume index was ≥160 mL/m^2 or the right ventricular end-systolic volume index was ≥82 mL/m^2. Studies in children and adults suggest that an optimal time exists for reoperation beyond which right ventricular remodeling is incomplete.

The aneurysmal size of the pulmonary artery and central branch pulmonary arteries in infants with tetralogy of Fallot and absent pulmonary valve requires additional surgical considerations. Surgical angioplasty to reduce the size of pulmonary arteries is essential to prevent airway compression.[31] A Lecompte maneuver can be helpful (Fig. 47-20).

INFORMATION FOR THE REFERRING PHYSICIAN

A segmental approach to reporting is essential to clarify all forms of congenital heart disease. Key preoperative findings for tetralogy of Fallot include the following:

1. VSD
2. Obstruction location and severity—RVOT, pulmonary valve, pulmonary artery, branch pulmonary arteries
3. Coronary artery position with special attention to RVOT
4. Aortic arch anomalies
5. Major aorticopulmonary collateral arteries—number and location

After palliative procedures, additional findings include the following:

1. Systemic pulmonary shunt—location, patency, stenosis
2. Branch pulmonary artery deformity
3. Pulmonary artery stents—integrity, patency, stenosis

After corrective surgery, additional findings include the following:

1. Residual or recurrent abnormalities—VSD or right ventricular outflow obstruction
2. Cardiac function to measure
   a. Pulmonary stenosis—echocardiography and phase contrast MRI flow analysis identify elevated RVOT velocity in RVOT and abnormal flow across tricuspid valve

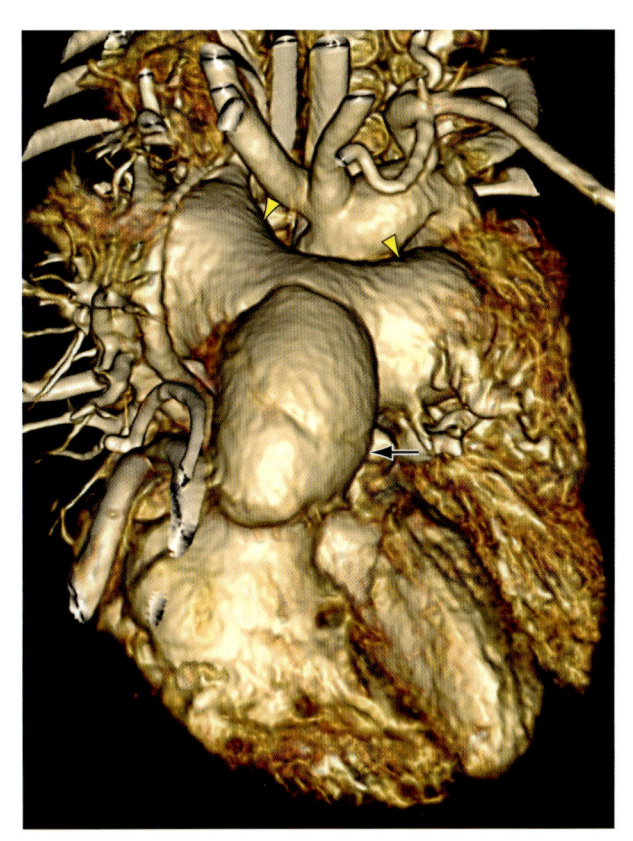

FIGURE 47-20 CT scan in a 2-month-old infant after repair of tetralogy of Fallot with absent pulmonary valve included a Lecompte maneuver and pulmonary angioplasty to reduce external compression of the airway by repositioning the central pulmonary arteries away from the airway and reducing their size. Despite the surgery, the pulmonary artery (*black arrow*) and branch pulmonary arteries (*yellow arrowheads*) remained aneurysmal and caused airway compression.

b. Pulmonary regurgitation—MRI or CT quantification of ventriculomegaly and right ventricular regurgitant fraction, and phase contrast MRI flow analysis of pulmonary regurgitation
c. Cardiac function
   i. Diastolic dysfunction—phase contrast MRI flow analysis of late diastolic forward flow in the pulmonary artery or a reduction in the E:A ratio across the tricuspid valve
   ii. Systolic dysfunction—MRI or CT quantification of right and left ventricular ejection fractions or cardiac indices

KEY POINTS

- Tetralogy of Fallot is the most common form of cyanotic congenital heart disease, but not monolithic in appearance, presentation, or treatment. It is the most common congenital heart lesion associated with a right aortic arch.
- MRI is crucial in follow-up because of limitations of echocardiography and the need to evaluate right heart size and function.
- CT is likely to play an increasingly important role in monitoring adults with tetralogy of Fallot. The indications are evolving, but include patients with contraindications to MRI, vascular stents, and concurrent acquired cardiopulmonary disease.

SUGGESTED READINGS

Anderson RH, Weinberg PM. The clinical anatomy of tetralogy of Fallot. Cardiol Young Suppl 2005; 1:38-47.
Bashore TM. Adult congenital heart disease: right ventricular outflow tract lesions. Circulation 2007; 115:1933-1947.
Boechat MI, Ratib O, Williams PL, et al. Cardiac MR angiography for assessment of complex tetralogy of Fallot and pulmonary atresia. RadioGraphics 2005; 25:1535-1546.
Boshoff D, Gewillig M. A review of the options for treatment of major aortopulmonary collateral arteries in the setting of tetralogy of Fallot with pulmonary atresia. Cardiol Young 2006; 16:212-220.
Dorfman AL, Geva T. Magnetic resonance imaging evaluation of congenital heart disease: conotruncal anomalies. J Cardiovasc Magn Reson 2006; 8:645-659.
Gaca AM, Jaggers JJ, Dudley LT, et al. Repair of congenital heart disease: a primer—part 2. Radiology 2008; 248:44-60.
Gregg D, Foster E. Pulmonary insufficiency is the nexus of late complications in tetralogy of Fallot. Curr Cardiol Rep 2007; 9:315-322.
Norton KI, Tong C, Glass RBJ, et al. Cardiac MR imaging assessment following tetralogy of Fallot repair. RadioGraphics 2006; 26:197-211.
Oosterhof T, Mulder BJM, Vliegen HW, et al. Cardiovascular magnetic resonance in the follow-up of patients with corrected tetralogy of Fallot: a review. Am Heart J 2006; 151:265-272.
Restivo A, Placidi GPS, Saffirio C, et al. Cardiac outflow tract: a review of some embryogenetic aspects of the conotruncal region of the heart. Anat Rec A Discov Mol Cell Evol Biol 2006; 288:936-943.

REFERENCES

1. Hoffman JIE, Kaplan S. The incidence of congenital heart disease. J Am Coll Cardiol 2008; 39:1890-1900.
2. Derby CD, Pizarro C. Routine primary repair of tetralogy of Fallot in the neonate. Expert Tev Cardiovasc Ther 2005; 3:857-863.
3. Michielon G, Marino B, Formigari R, et al. Genetic syndromes and outcome after surgical correction of tetralogy of Fallot. Ann Thorac Surg 2006; 81:968-975.
4. Uretzky G, Puga FJ, Danielson GK, et al. Complete atrioventricular canal associated with tetralogy of Fallot: morphologic and surgical considerations. J Thorac Cardiovasc Surg 1984; 87:756-766.
5. Ramaswamy P, Lytrivi ID, Thanjan MR, et al. Frequency of aberrant subclavian artery, arch laterality and associated intracardiac anomalies detected by echocardiography. Am J Cardiol 2008; 101:677-682.
6. Need LR, Powell AJ, del Nido P, et al. Coronary echocardiography in tetralogy of Fallot: diagnostic accuracy, resource utilization and surgical implications over 13 years. J Am Coll Cardiol 2000; 36:1371-1377.
7. Li J, Soukaias ND, Carvalho JS, et al. Coronary arterial anatomy in tetralogy of Fallot: morphological and clinical correlations. Heart 1998; 80:174-183.

8. Geva T. Indications and timing of pulmonary valve replacement after tetralogy of Fallot repair. Semin Thorac Cardiovasc Surg Pediatr Card Surg Annu 2006; 9:11-22.
9. Kadner A, Tulevski II, Bauerfeld U, et al. Chronic pulmonary valve insufficiency after repaired tetralogy of Fallot: diagnostics, reoperations and reconstruction possibilities. Expert Rev Cardiovasc Ther 2007; 5:221-230.
10. de Ruijter FTH, Weenink I, Hitchcock FJ, et al. Right ventricular dysfunction and pulmonary valve replacement after correction of tetralogy of Fallot. Ann Thorac Surg 2002; 73:1794-1800.
11. Niwa K. Aortic root dilatation in tetralogy of Fallot long-term after repair—histology of the aorta in tetralogy of Fallot: evidence of intrinsic aortopathy. Int J Cardiol 2005; 103:117-119.
12. Sivanandam S, Glickstein JS, Printz BF, et al. Prenatal diagnosis of conotruncal malformations: diagnostic accuracy, outcome, chromosomal abnormalities, and extracardiac anomalies. Am J Perinatol 2006; 23:241-245.
13. Shinebourne EA, Babu-Narayan SV, Carvalho JS. Tetralogy of Fallot: from fetus to adult. Heart 2006; 92:1353-1359.
14. Geva T, Ayres NA, Pac FA, et al. Quantitative morphometric analysis of progressive infundibular obstruction in tetralogy of Fallot. Circulation 1995; 92:886-892.
15. Wang XM, Wu LB, Sun C, et al. Clinical application of 64-slice spiral CT in the diagnosis of tetralogy of Fallot. Eur J Radiol 2007; 64:296-301.
16. Dogan OF, Karcaaltincaba M, Yorgancioglu C, et al. Demonstration of coronary arteries and major cardiac vascular structures in congenital heart disease by cardiac multidetector angiography. Heart Surg Forum 2007; 10:E90-E94.
17. Hayabuchi Y, Mori K, Kitagawa T, et al. Accurate quantification of pulmonary artery diameter in patients with cyanotic congenital heart disease using multidetector-row computed tomography. Am Heart J 2007; 154:783-788.
18. Leschka S, Oechslin E, Husmann L, et al. Pre- and postoperative evaluation of congenital heart disease in children and adults with 64-section CT. RadioGraphics 2007; 27:829-846.
19. Helbing WA, Niezen RA, Le Cessie S, et al. Right ventricular diastolic function in children with pulmonary regurgitation after repair of tetralogy of Fallot: volumetric evaluation by magnetic resonance velocity mapping. J Am Coll Cardiol 1996; 28:1827-1835.
20. Greenberg SB, Shah CC, Bhutta ST. Tricuspid valve magnetic resonance imaging phase contrast velocity-encoded flow quantification for follow up of tetralogy of Fallot. Int J Cardiovasc Imaging 2008; 24:861-865.
21. Paelinck BP, Lamb HJ, Bax JJ, et al. Assessment of diastolic function by cardiovascular magnetic resonance. Am Heart J 2002; 144: 198-2005.
22. van den Berg J, Wielopolski PA, Meijboom FJ, et al. Diastolic function in repaired tetralogy of Fallot at rest and during stress: assessment with MR imaging. Radiology 2007; 243:212-219.
23. Oosterhof T, Mulder BJ, Vliegen HW, et al. Corrected tetralogy of Fallot: delayed enhancement in right ventricular outflow tract. Radiology 2005; 237:868-871.
24. Ferguson EC, Krishnamurthy R, Oldham SAA. Classic imaging signs of congenital cardiovascular abnormalities. RadioGraphics 2007; 27:1323-1334.
25. Vohra HA, Adamson L, Haw MP. Is early primary repair for correction of tetralogy of Fallot comparable to surgery after 6 months of age? Interact Cardiovasc Thorac Surg 2008; 7:698-701.
26. Kantorova A, Zbieranek K, Sauer H, et al. Primary early correction of tetralogy of Fallot irrespective of age. Cardiol Young 2008; 18:153-157.
27. Gengaskul A, Harris L, Bradley TJ, et al. The impact of pulmonary valve replacement after tetralogy of Fallot repair: a matched comparison. Eur J Cardiothorac Surg 2007; 32:462-468.
28. Knauth AL, Gauvreau K, Powell AJ, et al. Ventricular size and function assessed by cardiac MRI predict major adverse clinical outcomes late after tetralogy of Fallot repair. Heart 2008; 94:211-216.
29. Buechel ER, Dave HH, Kellenberger CJ, et al. Remodeling of the right ventricle after early pulmonary valve replacement in children with repaired tetralogy of Fallot: assessment by cardiovascular magnetic resonance. Eur Heart J 2005; 26:2614-2615.
30. Oosterhof T, van Straten A, Vliegen HW, et al. Preoperative thresholds for pulmonary valve replacement in patients with corrected tetralogy of Fallot using cardiovascular magnetic resonance. Circulation 2007; 116:545-551.
31. Hraska V. Repair of tetralogy of Fallot with absent pulmonary valve using a new approach. Semin Thorac Cardiovasc Surg Pediatr Card Surg Annu 2005; 132-134.

CHAPTER 48

Ebstein Anomaly

Jeffrey C. Hellinger

The incidence of congenital heart disease ranges between 2.2 and 8.8/1000 live births.[1] Cyanotic lesions account for a low percentage of these defects, but result in a significant proportion of congenital heart morbidity and mortality, particularly if left untreated. Characterization of the pulmonary blood flow (PBF) and cardiac chamber morphology remains a fundamental step in evaluating suspected cyanotic congenital heart disease. This chapter will review cyanotic congenital heart disease with cardiomegaly and decreased PBF, specifically focusing on Ebstein anomaly.

EVALUATING THE CYANOTIC PATIENT

Clinical cyanosis is defined as tissue-threatening hypoxemia. If not promptly recognized and the cause is not correctly diagnosed and effectively treated, multisystem end-organ dysfunction will occur. Clinical workup and initial management will depend on prenatal diagnosis, obstetric course, comorbid symptoms, physical examination, and preliminary diagnostic imaging.

Initial diagnostic imaging in most algorithms begins with chest radiography. Single- and two-projection chest radiographs afford fundamental cyanotic cardiac disease evaluation, including heart size and contour, degree of pulmonary vascularity, and aortic arch sidedness. If the heart is enlarged, analysis should address which chambers may be dilated. In parallel, the airway, lung parenchyma, pleura, and thoracic skeleton are analyzed for alternative or comorbid noncardiovascular causes.

Recognition of cardiomegaly with decreased pulmonary vascularity on the chest radiograph signals that there is significant pulmonary inflow obstruction associated with intracardiac right-to-left shunting of venous deoxygenated blood away from the lungs and into the systemic circulation. Flow obstruction may occur at the tricuspid valve, infundibulum, pulmonary valve, or a combination thereof, whereas the shunting may occur at the atrial or ventricular septal levels. Specific anatomic pathologies include Ebstein anomaly, pulmonary atresia with ventricular septal defect, a severe variant of tetralogy of Fallot, isolated critical pulmonary stenosis, and pulmonary atresia with intact ventricular septum.

For anatomic obstructive lesions, the ductus arteriosus is often patent, providing retrograde flow into the pulmonary circulation. Bronchial arteries and other aortopulmonary collaterals (APCs) may also provide systemic perfusion into the pulmonary circulation. The degree of decreased PBF and size and involvement of the ventricular and atrial chambers will depend on the level of obstruction, level of shunting, collateral flow, right ventricular pressures, and tricuspid valve competence.

When further diagnostic imaging is required to evaluate cyanotic structural congenital heart lesions, decisions should reflect the cardiac imaging goals, presence of comorbid synchronous disorders in other body systems, and the patient's sedation, anesthesia risk, and radiosensitivity. Options include echocardiography, right and left heart catheterization with angiography, right heart catheterization with or without angiography, magnetic resonance imaging (MRI), and magnetic resonance angiography (MRA), and computed tomography angiography (CTA).

Echocardiography is ideal as the next step for most algorithms. It is portable, relatively inexpensive, and does not expose patients to ionizing radiation or iodinated contrast medium. Real-time two-dimensional, multiprojectional, transthoracic echocardiography with standard gray-scale and color Doppler techniques readily evaluates the cardiac chambers, interatrial and interventricular septa, valves, systemic and pulmonary venous connections, central pulmonary arteries, and thoracic aorta (including arch sidedness). In select applications, such as with valvular disease, three-dimensional echocardiography can offer greater structural detail. Concurrent with the structural analysis, flow, function, and hemodynamics are all assessed. Echocardiography, however, is operator-dependent, may have limited sonographic windows, and cannot evaluate peripheral thoracic vascular anatomy.

In the diagnostic algorithm at many centers, catheterization with angiography follows echocardiography. The objective is not primarily to confirm the anatomy, but rather to obtain flow and pressure dynamics directly.

However, this approach is invasive, exposes the patient to ionizing radiation, uses iodinated contrast medium and, in the current workflow, is not cost-effective. Radiation dose can be reduced and contrast medium obviated if the procedure is limited to a right heart catheterization without angiography.

MRI, MRA, and CTA are alternative noninvasive modalities to catheterization and may provide comprehensive evaluation of cardiac and pulmonary morphology and function, which is key to diagnosing the cyanotic patient with decreased pulmonary vascularity (Figs. 48-1 and 48-2). Both can generate cardiac chamber volume and qualitative and quantitative functional data. Image postprocessing can readily be facilitated for data sets from both modalities.

MRI and MRA are ideal because no ionizing radiation is required, there is no use of iodinated contrast medium, and only direct assessment of flow dynamics can be made. MRI and MRA examination times, however, may average 30 to 40 minutes, necessitating sedation or general anesthesia in the pediatric population. Furthermore, MRI does not afford comprehensive lung evaluation. Assessment of body systems outside of the thorax will add considerable examination time. During surveillance imaging, MRI and MRA may be contraindicated or nondiagnostic because of the presence of implanted devices and ferrous material.

A typical MRI protocol for evaluating cyanotic congenital heart lesions begins with standard bright and dark blood sequences. The goal is to survey and define the thoracic and upper abdominal cardiovascular and noncardiovascular morphology. Cine sequences should then be obtained for qualitative and quantitative cardiac chamber and valve functional analysis. Next, velocity maps are obtained for hemodynamic analysis, targeting at a minimum the ventriculoarterial valves and supravalvular segments. Regions of interest may also be placed on the branch pulmonary arteries, atrioventricular valves, central systemic veins, and pulmonary veins. Gadolinium-enhanced three-dimensional MRA is subsequently performed for further structural analysis. MRA is most useful for evaluating the pulmonary arteries, aorta, and systemic and pulmonary veins. Time-resolved MRA is advantageous in this instance because it provides real-time angiographic flow patterns.

Despite its dependence on ionizing radiation and iodinated contrast medium, CTA can be used for complete evaluation of the cyanotic cardiac disorders. Advantages include short examination times, maintenance of high diagnostic image quality in the presence of devices and metallic material, and nonthoracic cardiovascular and multisystem organ evaluation with the same bolus of contrast medium. With current CT scanner technology, sedation

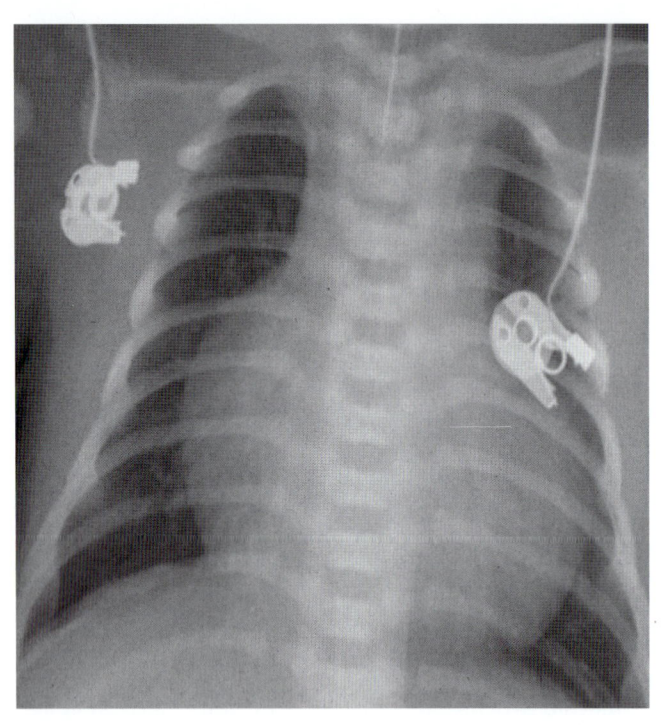

■ **FIGURE 48-1** A full-term neonate presented in respiratory distress on day 2 of life. An anteroposterior chest radiograph reveals an enlarged right atrium and ventricle associated with mild decreased pulmonary vascularity, consistent with a right-sided obstructive lesion. Echocardiography was subsequently performed, demonstrating critical pulmonary stenosis.

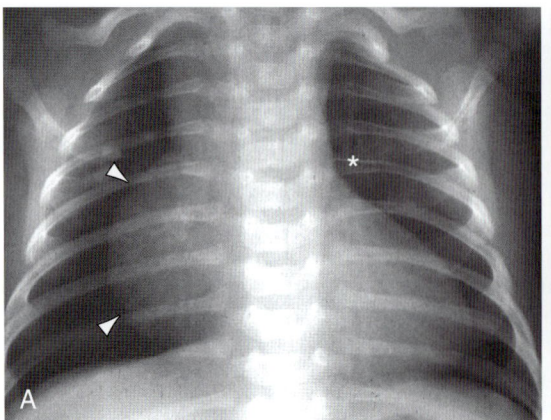

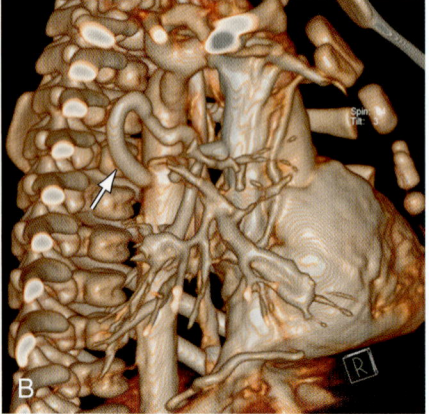

■ **FIGURE 48-2** The first few hours postdelivery of a term neonate was complicated by respiratory distress. **A,** An anteroposterior chest radiograph reveals moderate cardiomegaly with a dominantly enlarged right atrium (*arrowheads*), an absent main pulmonary artery segment (*asterisk*), and decreased peripheral pulmonary vascularity. Echocardiography confirmed pulmonary atresia with an intact ventricular septum. **B,** CTA (volume rendered image) was performed to map out the aortopulmonary collateral arteries (*arrow*).

and anesthesia often can be eliminated. As with all CTA applications, dose reduction strategies are the standard of care. Voltage and amperage should be reduced, balancing the expected diagnostic and image qualities. If possible, coverage should be targeted to the pertinent thoracic anatomy. For most pediatric applications, pertinent morphology can be evaluated in a single series without electrocardiographic gating. Noncontrast and delayed acquisitions are rarely required.

EBSTEIN ANOMALY

Ebstein anomaly is a rare cardiac disorder, accounting for 0.04% to 0.93% of congenital heart malformations.[1-4] The distinguishing pathology is dysplastic tricuspid valve leaflets, which extend into and attach to the right ventricle, rather than the annulus at the atrioventricular junction, leading to tricuspid valve incompetence. Usually, the septal and posterior leaflets are involved, with insertion at the margin of the inlet and trabecular right ventricular zones, either directly or by way of anomalous chordae tendinae and papillary muscles. The degree of septal and posterior leaflet displacement and abnormal morphology has wide variability.

In distinction to the septal and posterior leaflets, the anterior leaflet typically has dysplastic morphology, but maintains normal attachments. It is enlarged, with a sail appearance and fibrous strands, which may be muscularized. Rarely, the anterior leaflet may have abnormal displacement along the right ventricular anterior free wall, leading to tricuspid stenosis. In 10% of cases, the anterior leaflet may have downward displacement, obstructing the ventricular inlet, leading to an obstructing, imperforate tricuspid valve.[5,6]

Downward leaflet displacement divides the right ventricle into a basilar, atrialized inlet portion and a small functional true right ventricle. Both portions are typically dilated, with a loss of myocytes, leading to decreased contractility.[6] Less commonly, only the atrialized portion is dilated. The native functional right ventricle has reduced right ventricular (RV) filling capacity and cardiac output. RV preload volume is further reduced by virtue of the atrialized portion functioning as a false aneurysm such that as the native right atrium contracts, the abnormal segment above the functional right ventricle expands, collecting blood. In addition to these factors, tricuspid insufficiency and possible anterior leaflet stenosis or obstruction decrease forward flow, contributing to the diminished right ventricle filling volumes.

Hemodynamically, the decreased diastolic filling and myocardial contractility lead to diminished PBF, elevated right atrial and systemic venous pressures and, ultimately, right-sided failure. With elevated right atrial pressures, right-to-left shunting will occur across a patent foramen ovale (PFO) or secundum atrial septal defect (ASD), leading to cyanosis.[5,7] Increased pulmonary vascular resistance in the early neonatal period increases afterload, further exacerbating cyanosis in these patients.[8] As the intrapulmonary vascular resistance falls, cyanosis may improve.

Electrical conduction pathways may be abnormal with regard to the location and morphology of native pathways and the presence of accessory conduction pathways (Wolf-Parkinson-White; WPW). The conduction pathway abnormalities lead to dysrhythmias; the most common are atrial tachycardias and supraventricular and ventricular arrhythmias.[9,10]

In most cases of Ebstein anomaly, there is visceral situs solitus. The ASD or PFO has been confirmed by select angiography or autopsy to be present in at least 33% to 56% of patients.[9-11] Additional cardiac anomalies may be present in at least 22% of cases. Among these anomalies, common lesions include pulmonary stenosis (35%), ventricular septal defect (VSD; 21%), patent ductus arteriosus (PDA) (20%), and pulmonary stenosis with VSD (9%).

Clinical Manifestations

Ebstein anomaly shows almost equal distribution between males and females.[11] Depending on the degree of heart failure and shunting, and the occurrence of arrhythmias, patients may present as a neonate, infant, child, adolescent, or adult. Infants born with Ebstein anomaly are most commonly full term, with a weight between 2 and 4 kg.[12,13]

In addition to cyanosis, presenting symptoms may include dyspnea, palpitations, fatigue, epigastric or chest pain, and congestive heart failure. The neonate and infant may present with feeding intolerance, whereas children and older patients may use squatting to alleviate symptoms. Physical examination may be remarkable for a systolic and less commonly a diastolic murmur, systolic thrill, digital clubbing, and precordial deformity.[10]

Most patients with Ebstein anomaly have an abnormal electrocardiogram (ECG). Specific findings include an elevated P wave (indicative of right atrial enlargement), right bundle branch block, diminished right precordial lead voltage or dominant left ventricular voltage (indicative of a small right ventricle), notched QRS complex (secondary to delayed activation in the atrialized right ventricle), prolonged PR interval, and WPW (type B) pathway.[10]

Diagnostic Imaging

The degree of cardiomegaly on chest radiography is moderate to massive, with dominance of the right atrium (Fig. 48-3). This reflects the degree of elevated RV pressure and tricuspid insufficiency.[10] Cardiac size decreases with age, so that the mean cardiothoracic ratio is 0.73 as a neonate, 0.57 during infancy and childhood, and 0.55 during adolescence and adulthood.[11] Pulmonary vascularity may be normal to decreased, and directly correlates with the degree of valvular deformity, right-to-left shunting, and diminished right ventricular cardiac output.

Echocardiography, MRI, MRA, and CTA can all readily diagnose Ebstein anomaly. In a four-chamber projection, apical leaflet displacement into the right ventricle is identified by recognizing that it extends beyond the atrioventricular level of the mitral valve insertion (Fig. 48-4). Atrialized and native portions of the right ventricle are defined based on the insertion level. The size of the enlarged atrium, atrialized right ventricle, and small functional native right ventricle are characterized qualitatively

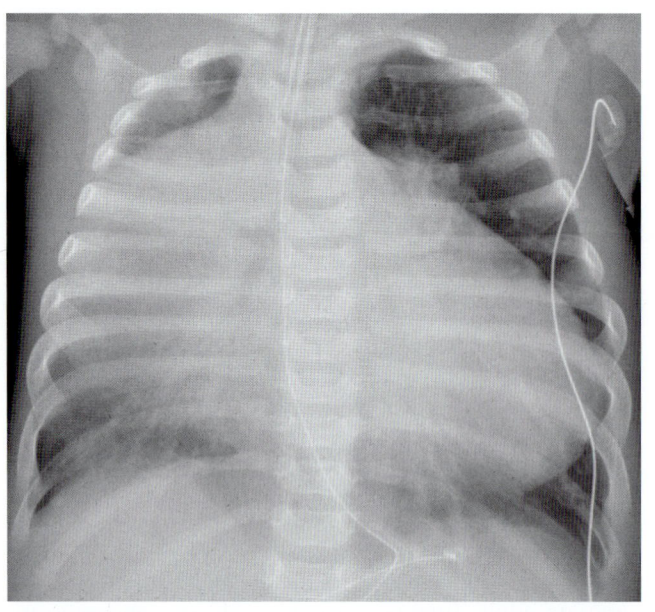

FIGURE 48-3 A 20-day-old neonate presented with respiratory difficulty and feeding intolerance. An anteroposterior chest radiograph demonstrates marked cardiomegaly, with a massively enlarged right atrium and ventricle. Echocardiography confirmed Ebstein anomaly.

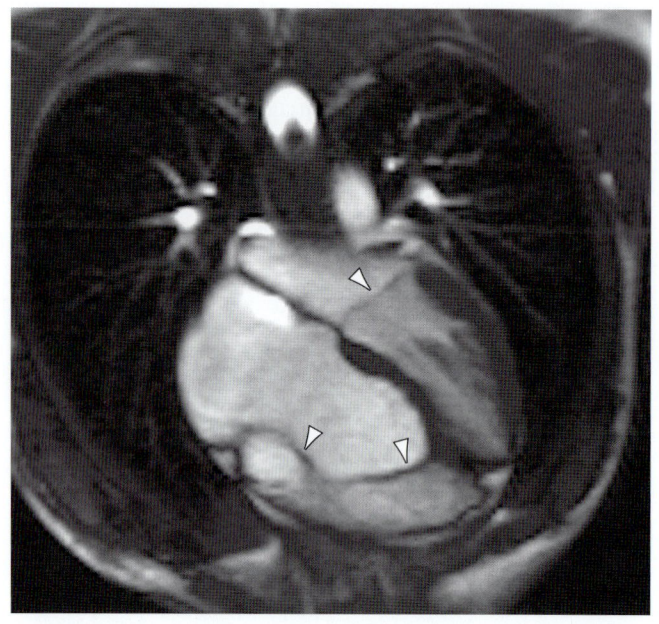

FIGURE 48-4 Cardiac MRI (four-chamber projection) in a patient with Ebstein anomaly demonstrates anterior displacement of the tricuspid apparatus (*black arrowheads*) relative to the normally positioned mitral valve (*white arrowhead*), resulting in atrialization of the right ventricle. Note the decreased size of the functional right ventricle.

and quantitatively. An atrial septal defect with right-to-left interatrial septal bowing is recognized with a short-axis or four-chamber projection.

Color Doppler echocardiography and cine or phase contrast MRI will confirm tricuspid insufficiency and right-to-left shunting. Retrospective or single-phase CTA can also define right-to-left shunting, but detection is dependent on the contrast medium bolus and acquisition timing.

Treatment

Conservative management is appropriate for patients who are asymptomatic, have no right-to-left shunting, and have only mild cardiomegaly.[14] Patients should be given prophylaxis for endocarditis, and patients who experience cardiac failure should be treated with diuretics and digoxin.

Arrhythmias can be treated with antiarrhythmic medications or with catheter ablation or surgery. Catheter ablation in patients with Ebstein anomaly has a lower rate of success than in patients with morphologically normal hearts.[15] Permanent pacemaker placement may be required in the setting of atrioventricular block or sinus node dysfunction.[16]

Surgery

Indications for surgery include symptoms such as paradoxic emboli, progressive increase in size of the right heart, compromise of systolic function, severe heart failure, or onset of tachyarrhythmias.[14] Biventricular reconstruction is appropriate for most patients. When a patient has severe biventricular dysfunction, heart transplantation should be considered.

REFERENCES

1. Samánek M, Vorísková M. Congenital heart disease among 815,569 children born between 1980 and 1990 and their 15-year survival: a prospective Bohemia survival study. Pediatr Cardiol 1999; 20: 411-417.
2. Campbell M. Incidence of cardiac malformations at birth and later, and neonatal mortality. Br Heart J 1973; 35:189-200.
3. Goetzová J, Benesová D. Congenital heart diseases at autopsy of still-born and deceased children in the Central Bohemian region. Cor Vasa 1981; 23:8-13.
4. Samánek M, Slavik Z, Zborilová B, et al. Prevalence, treatment, and outcome of heart disease in live-born children: a prospective analysis of 91,823 live-born children. Pediatr Cardiol 1989; 10:205-211.
5. Zuberbuhler JR, Allwork SP, Anderson RH. The spectrum of Ebstein's anomaly of the tricuspid valve. J Thorac Cardiovasc Surg 1979; 77:202-211.
6. Anderson KR, Zuberbuhler JR, Anderson RH, et al. Morphologic spectrum of Ebstein's anomaly of the heart: a review. Mayo Clin Proc 1979; 54:174-180.
7. Genton E, Blount SG Jr. The spectrum of Ebstein's anomaly. Am Heart J 1967; 73:395-425.
8. Jaquiss RD, Imamura M. Management of Ebstein's anomaly and pure tricuspid insufficiency in the neonate. Semin Thorac Cardiovasc Surg 2007; 19:258-263.
9. Watson H. Natural history of Ebstein's anomaly of tricuspid valve in childhood and adolescence: An international co-operative study of 505 cases. Br Heart J 1974; 36:417-427.
10. Bialostozky D, Horwitz S, Espino-Vela J. Ebstein's malformation of the tricuspid valve. A review of 65 cases. Am J Cardiol 1972; 29:826-836.
11. Radford DJ, Graff RF, Neilson GH. Diagnosis and natural history of Ebstein's anomaly. Br Heart J 1985; 54:517-522.

12. Shinkawa T, Polimenakos AC, Gomez-Fifer CA, et al. Management and long-term outcome of neonatal Ebstein anomaly. J Thorac Cardiovasc Surg 2010; 139:354-358.
13. Knott-Craig CJ, Overholt ED, Ward KE, et al. Neonatal repair of Ebstein's anomaly: indications, surgical technique, and medium-term follow-up. Ann Thorac Surg 2000; 69:1505-1510.
14. Attenhofer Jost CH, Connolly HM, Dearani JA, et al. Congenital heart disease for the adult cardiologist: Ebstein's anomaly. Circulation 2007; 115:277-285.
15. Hebe J. Ebstein's anomaly in adults: arrhythmias: diagnosis and therapeutic approach. Thorac Cardiovasc Surg 2000; 48: 214-219.
16. Allen MR, Hayes DL, Warnes CA, Danielson GK. Permanent pacing in Ebstein's anomaly. Pacing Clin Electrophysiol 1997; 20: 1243-1246.

CHAPTER 49

Complex Congenital Heart Disease

Kevin K. Whitehead, Stanford Ewing, and Mark A. Fogel

Complex congenital heart disease is obviously one of the most challenging issues faced by the health care provider who takes care of the pediatric patient with cardiac lesions. Taken as a group, this set of lesions represents only a small portion of congenital heart disease (CHD) and is rare in the population; nevertheless, these diseases take up a considerable amount of the physician's time. Hoffman and Kaplan[1] have reported the results of a meta-analysis of the literature and found the incidence of moderate to severe forms of congenital heart disease to be 6/1,000 live births, rising to 19/1,000 live births if potentially serious bicuspid aortic valves are included. Putting this in perspective, all forms of CHD represent 75/1,000 live births, including such lesions as tiny muscular ventricular septal defects. In addition, the New England Infant Cardiac Program[2] has reported that 3/1,000 live births need cardiac catheterization or surgery, or will die with CHD in early infancy (excluding premature infants with patent ductus arteriosus). This number rises to 5/1,000 live births who will need some type of specialized care during their lifetime. All these issues are a measure of the severity of the lesion. With improvements in diagnosis and treatment of CHD, along with a greater understanding of the anatomy and physiology, patients are living longer[3] and represent a growing patient base seen by adult cardiologists and internists. In 1980, there were an estimated 300,000 adults with CHD, whereas this rose to approximately 1 million in 2000. In 2020, the number is anticipated to be 1.4 million.

Complex CHD is an ill-defined entity because the word *complex* is ill defined. Is it complex in the anatomic relationships of the various portions of the cardiovascular system, physiologic or blood flow phenomenon, or care and management of these patients? For example, double-outlet right ventricle (DORV) with a subaortic ventricular septal defect and no outflow tract obstruction is clearly anatomically complex but, in the absence of associated lesions (e.g., mitral hypoplasia), the physiology is of a simple ventricular septal defect. There are obviously simple lesions such as atrial septal defects and complex ones such as truncus arteriosus and single ventricles; however, there is a grey zone in between. These lesions can be acyanotic, such as in DORV, or cyanotic, such as tetralogy of Fallot (TOF).

This chapter cannot be exhaustive in the treatment of complex CHD. Instead, it will focus in detail on imaging of four different lesions in this group—transposition of the great arteries, tetralogy of Fallot, single ventricle, and truncus arteriosus.

TRANSPOSITION OF THE GREAT ARTERIES

Definition

The classic transposition of the great arteries (TGA) consists of isolated ventriculoarterial discordance, with the aorta arising from the right ventricle and the main pulmonary artery arising from the left ventricle.[1,2,3] This results in separation of the systemic and pulmonary circulations, with limited mixing of oxygenated and deoxygenated blood. It usually refers to dextro-TGA (d-TGA; segmental anatomy {S,D,D}), in which the aortic valve is positioned anterior and to the right of the pulmonary valve. However, some refer to any segmental anatomy that results in this physiology as transposition. Occasionally, the conotruncus is further rotated so that the aorta is anterior and to the left of the pulmonary valve (segments {S,D,L}).

Prevalence and Epidemiology

The incidence of transposition of the great arteries is approximately 3 in 10,000 live births. It represents approximately 5% of all newborns with congenital heart disease.[1] It is rarely associated with syndromes or extracardiac malformations, but is more common in infants of diabetic mothers.

Etiology and Pathophysiology

D-TGA is in the spectrum of conotruncal alignment defects and is thought to result from abnormal positioning and rotation of the conotruncus during development. The exact cause or originating event during development is still unclear.

The basic defect is an abnormal rotation of the conotruncus so that the aorta sits over the right ventricle and the pulmonary artery sits over the left ventricle. Generally, the venous anatomy, atrial morphology, atrioventricular connections, and ventricular morphology are normal. The aorta is not in fibrous continuity with the mitral valve, but the pulmonary valve often is. The result is that oxygenated blood returning from the pulmonary veins to the left atrium and left ventricle is pumped back to the pulmonary arteries and lungs. The deoxygenated blood from the systemic veins returning to the right atrium and right ventricle is pumped to the aorta, resulting in profound cyanosis.

Systemic oxygen delivery is dependent on mixing between the two circulations. This can occur at three levels—atrial septal defect, ventricular septal defect (VSD), and patent ductus arteriosus.

In the absence of a VSD, the ductus generally shunts increasingly from the aorta to the pulmonary arteries as pulmonary vascular resistance decreases. In a steady state, the ductal shunt must be matched by a net left atrial to right atrial shunt, which provides for systemic oxygen delivery.

Aside from patent ductus arteriosus and atrial septal communication, the most common associations with d-TGA are VSDs. The VSD can be conoventricular, malalignment, or muscular. Malalignment ventricular septal defects are commonly posteriorly malaligned, and can result in significant left ventricular outflow tract (subpulmonary) obstruction. More rarely, there is anterior malalignment, which can, in turn, be associated with coarctation of the aorta, arch hypoplasia and, rarely, interruption of the aortic arch. Patients with an unrestrictive VSD generally have greater mixing and thus higher saturation.

Other less common associations with transposition of the great vessels include tricuspid atresia and straddling atrioventricular valves.

Manifestations of Disease

Clinical Presentation

The clinical presentation of transposition of the great vessels largely depends on the associated lesions. Patients with an intact ventricular septum will generally present with profound cyanosis in the first few hours to days of life as the ductus arteriosus closes and mixing is limited to the patent foramen, which is often restrictive. These patients require the immediate initiation of prostaglandins. If the foramen ovale is restrictive, these patients may require a balloon septostomy to improve left to right shunting.

Patients who have an unrestrictive VSD may not present with profound cyanosis, but with an arterial saturation from 70% to 90%. If undiagnosed, these patients may present later with overt heart failure caused by pulmonary overcirculation. Patients with significant subpulmonary obstruction may have physiology more similar to that of tetralogy of Fallot and present with varying degrees of cyanosis. Finally, patients with coarctation or arch obstruction may present with acidosis, shock, and reverse differential cyanosis.

Imaging Indications and Algorithm

The mainstay of imaging for unrepaired transposition of the great arteries is cardiac echocardiography; all infants suspected of transposition should undergo complete echocardiography when they are stabilized. This often includes the initiation of prostaglandins and a balloon atrial septostomy. For unstable patients, limited echocardiography should be carried out to confirm the diagnosis of transposition and evaluate the atrial septum to determine whether a restrictive atrial septum is present.

Beyond these initial requirements, a complete echocardiogram should focus on delineating the conotruncal anatomy, defining the coronary origins and proximal course, the patency, size and shunting of the ductus arteriosus, the presence and type of a ventricular septal defect, the presence of subarterial (usually subpulmonary) obstruction, and the aortic arch. In addition to defining the coronary anatomy, the exact relationship between the aorta and pulmonary artery should be delineated, as a more side by side relationship of the great vessels may make a Lecompte maneuver less desirable. Any questions left unanswered after complete echocardiography can be obtained by cardiac magnetic resonance imaging.

Imaging Techniques and Findings

Radiography

The classic radiographic findings of transposition of the great arteries include a narrow superior mediastinum (so-called egg on a string) caused by the anteroposterior orientation of the great vessels and inapparent thymus, increased pulmonary vascular markings, and cardiomegaly. However, these findings are rarely diagnostic and, in fact, were shown to be absent in the vast majority of newborns with d-TGA (Fig. 49-1).[4]

Ultrasound

Echocardiography can generally readily identify all the pertinent anatomic findings to manage patients with transposition of the great arteries. Subcostal imaging can readily identify the pulmonary artery arising from the left ventricle and the aorta arising from the right ventricle. The aorta can usually be identified by the coronaries and by its long length before branching (Fig. 49-2). The pulmonary artery branches early and the ductal arch should not be mistaken for the aorta (Fig. 49-3).

It is important to assess the atrial septum to determine whether it is restrictive (Fig. 49-4). In addition, the

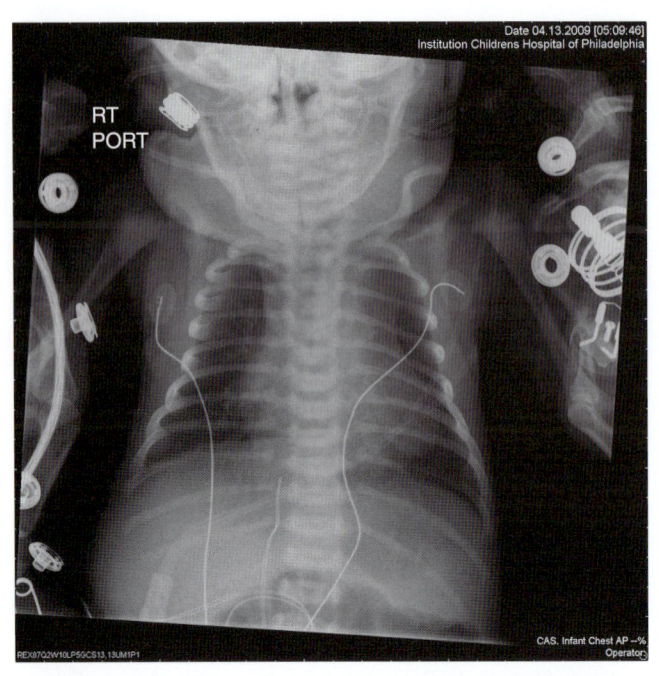

FIGURE 49-1 Chest radiograph from a patient with TGA shows mild cardiomegaly but lacks any of the classic findings, such as the narrow superior mediastinum or increased pulmonary vascular markings.

ventricular septum should be assessed to determine whether there are ventricular septal defects (Fig. 49-5). This is important for both preoperative management and surgical planning.

Computed Tomography

CT scanning does not play a routine role in transposition of the great arteries. There is generally no indication in unrepaired TGA. It may have some use in postoperative patients when an MRI cannot be performed (e.g., because of a stent or coil artifact, or pacemaker) to evaluate the coronary arteries or branch pulmonary arteries after an arterial switch operation.

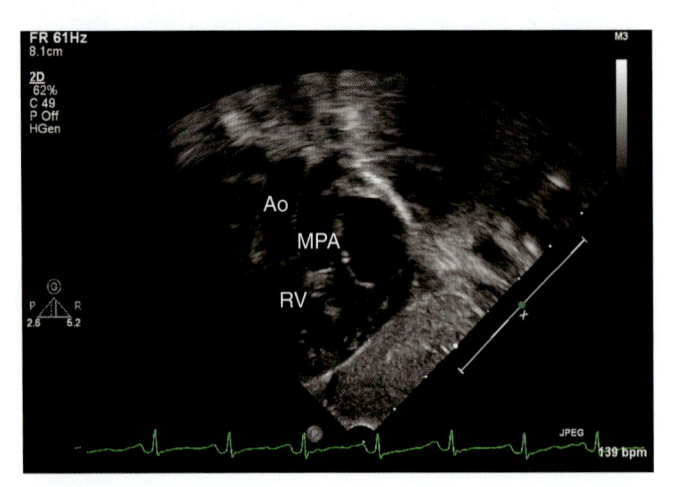

FIGURE 49-2 Subcostal imaging of unrepaired TGA demonstrating the parallel outflows, with the aorta arising from the right ventricle and the main pulmonary artery from the left ventricle.

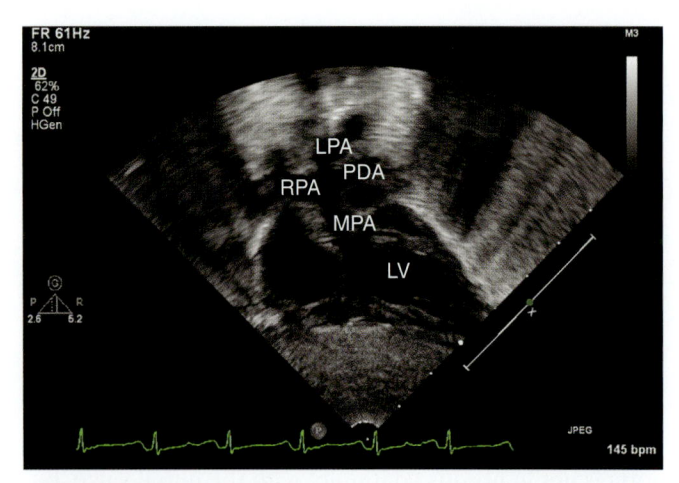

FIGURE 49-3 The pulmonary artery arises from the left ventricle in TGA and is readily identified by the early branching from subcostal. The duct is also readily identified.

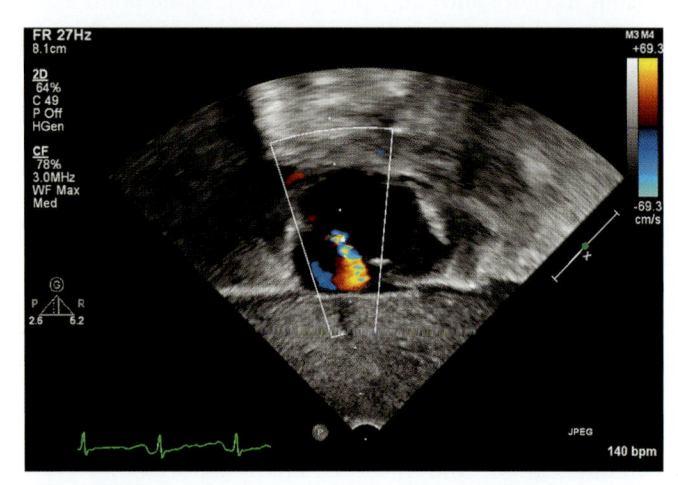

FIGURE 49-4 The patent foramen ovale in this TGA patient is small and mildly restrictive.

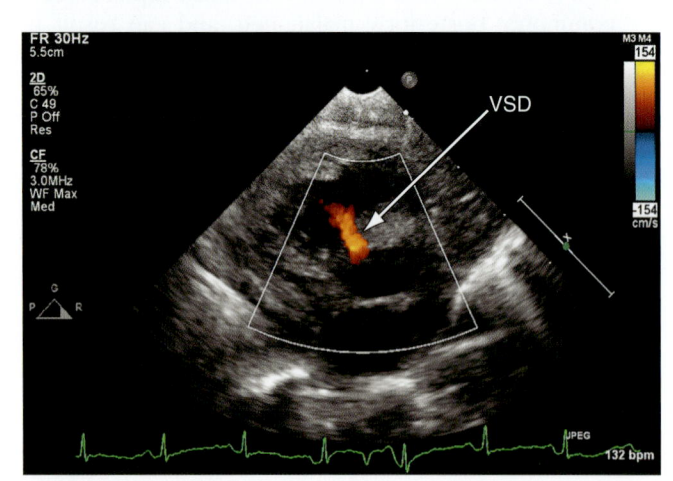

FIGURE 49-5 Small muscular VSD identified by color Doppler in a preoperative TGA patient.

Magnetic Resonance Imaging

Cardiac MRI plays a limited role in the initial management of d-TGA, generally when there are residual questions after complete echocardiography. Cardiac MRI may be useful in some situations in which the coronary anatomy

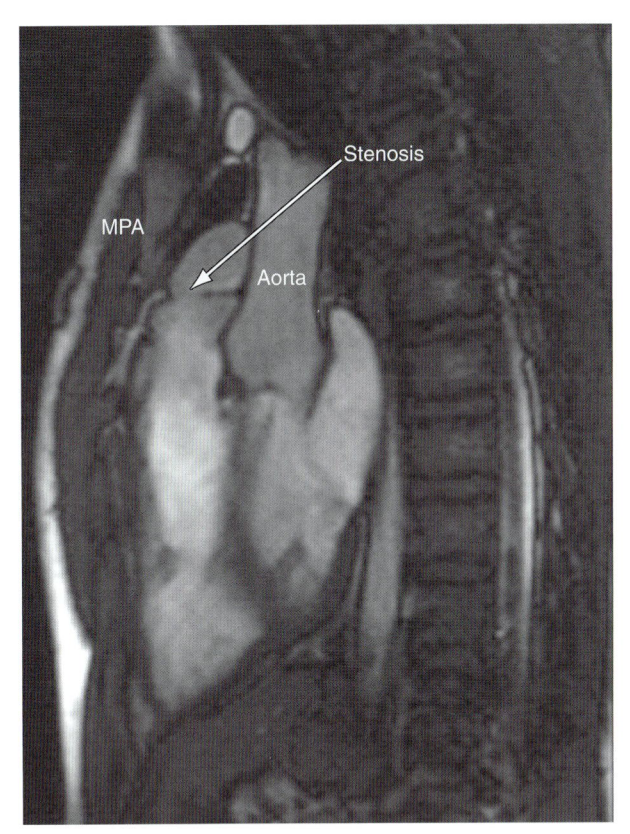

FIGURE 49-6 Moderate supravalvular narrowing is seen at the suture line in this TGA patient who has undergone an arterial switch procedure.

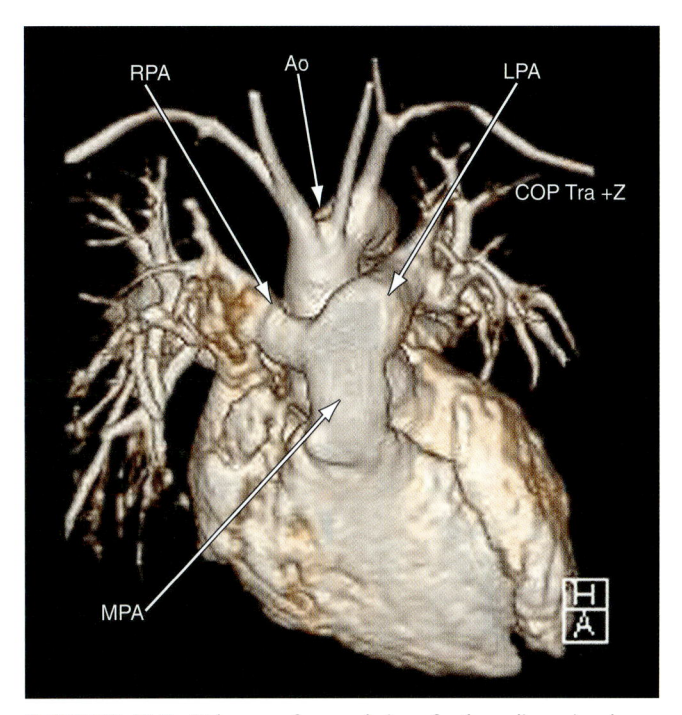

FIGURE 49-7 Volume surface rendering of a three-dimensional gadolinium acquisition from a TGA patient who has undergone an arterial switch. Note that the pulmonary arteries are draped over the aorta and, in this case, the right pulmonary artery is mildly stretched and narrowed.

is unusual and needs to be better evaluated prior to arterial switch.

MRI plays an important role in the postoperative management of TGA. The standard for the treatment of TGA is the arterial switch (Jatene procedure), in which the aorta and main pulmonary artery are transected and sewn to the pulmonary and aortic root, respectively. The pulmonary arteries are generally brought anteriorly and draped over the aorta. The coronary arteries are transferred separately with buttons of tissue from the aorta to avoid ostial stenosis. Several problems can result, for which cardiac MRI is well suited to investigate. Supravalvular stenosis can occur at either anastomosis site (Fig. 49-6). Cine and velocity mapping can be used effectively to define regions of stenosis and quantify the degree of acceleration. Three-dimensional gadolinium sequences can also be useful to define stenoses and their relationships to other structures (Fig. 49-7). Unilateral or occasionally bilateral branch pulmonary artery stenosis may occur from stretching the branch pulmonary arteries after the Lecompte maneuver. Insufficiency of either valve can result from distortion during surgery. Through-plane velocity mapping can be used to quantify the degree of insufficiency of the valves precisely. Furthermore, short-axis cine volume sets can quantify the ventricular size, ejection, and wall motion abnormalities to screen for the effects of valve regurgitation or coronary abnormalities. Whole heart sequences can be used to evaluate for ostial stenosis of the transferred coronaries (Fig. 49-8). Perhaps more importantly, MRI can be used to evaluate for perfusion defects secondary to coronary stenosis. Gadolinium perfusion imaging is generally performed at rest and during adenosine administration. Adenosine administration causes coronary vasodilation and accentuates perfusion abnormalities by "stealing" flow from regions of marginal coronary perfusion.

Older patients with transposition of the great vessels may have had an atrial switch (either a Mustard or Senning operation) in which the pulmonary venous return is

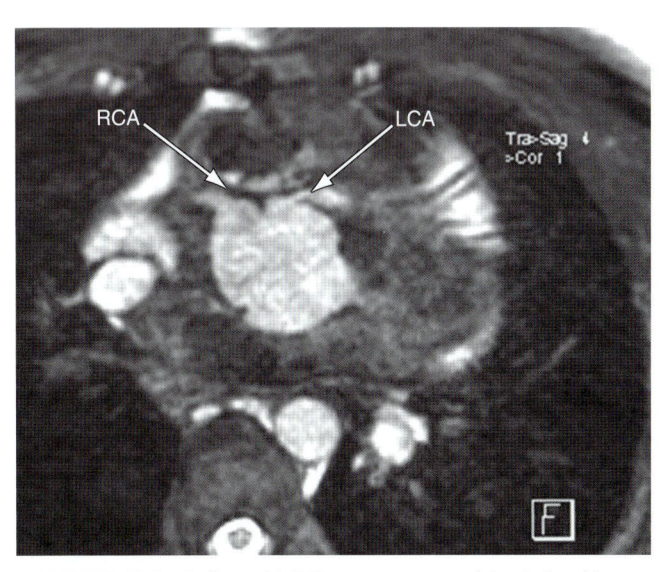

FIGURE 49-8 Patient with TGA status postarterial switch, with proximal narrowing of the left coronary artery as it runs underneath the RVOT conduit. Note that the coronary artery could be further compromised during stenting of the RVOT.

baffled to the right ventricle and the systemic veins baffled to the left ventricle. This makes the right ventricle the systemic ventricle and it is subject to dilation and failure, usually starting in the third or fourth decade of life. MRI plays a key role in evaluating ventricular function, perfusion, and viability of the systemic right ventricle, as well as assessing the baffle for stenosis or leaks.

See later, "Single Ventricle," for a more detailed description of the routine cardiac MRI examination.

Nuclear Medicine: Positron Emission Tomography

Perfusion imaging is useful in the postoperative management of patients undergoing an arterial switch procedure who have symptoms or clinical evidence of myocardial ischemia.

Angiography

Angiography is useful in evaluating for stenosis of the transplanted coronary arteries in patients who have undergone an arterial switch when there is suspicion clinically or from other imaging modalities. It also has a limited role preoperatively when the coronary anatomy is complex or cannot be delineated well noninvasively.

TETRALOGY OF FALLOT
Definition

Tetralogy of Fallot is defined as the constellation of a large anterior malalignment ventricular septal defect, an aorta that overrides the defect, subvalvular or valvular pulmonary stenosis, and right ventricular hypertrophy.

Prevalence and Epidemiology

The incidence of tetralogy of Fallot is approximately 4 in 10,000 live births, accounting for approximately 7% to 10% of cases of congenital heart disease.[5] It occurs equally in males and females, and represents one of the most common lesions requiring intervention in the first year of life. It occurs commonly in association with genetic defects, including Down syndrome, DiGeorge syndrome (22q11 microdeletion), and Alagille syndrome (Jag1 mutation).[6,7]

Etiology and Pathophysiology

While originally described by Fallot as a constellation of four findings,[8] it is now understood that the pathogenesis appears to be related to a single abnormality. The anterior malalignment VSD with normally related great vessels is responsible for the associated aortic override and right ventricular outflow tract obstruction, which classically results in right ventricular hypertrophy.

Certain associated conditions may be important to the management of tetralogy of Fallot. A right aortic arch occurs in approximately 25% of patients. Coronary anomalies are common (approximately 9%), including the left anterior descending (LAD) artery from the right coronary and single coronary.[9] Pulmonary atresia may occur, with or without the presence of major aortopulmonary collaterals. Patients may often have additional muscular VSDs, and it may occur in association with a complete common atrioventricular canal, especially in association with Down syndrome. Stenosis of the left pulmonary artery is common and, rarely, isolation of the pulmonary artery contralateral to the aortic arch may occur. A patent ductus arteriosus is common; when there is significant outflow tract obstruction, the duct may be tortuous.

Manifestations of Disease
Clinical Presentation

The presentation of these patients largely depends on the degree of outflow tract obstruction. Patients with severe obstruction present in the newborn period with profound cyanosis. Moderate obstruction may result in a relatively balanced circulation and, if not diagnosed prenatally, may be noticed during routine evaluation for a murmur. Patients with only mild outflow obstruction will present with a large left to right shunt, pulmonary overcirculation, and heart failure. Patients with moderate obstruction may be at risk for hypercyanotic spells ("tet spells"), which are caused by dynamic increases in the degree of right ventricular outflow tract obstruction, changes in the ratio of pulmonary to systemic vascular resistance, or a combination of the two.

Imaging Indications and Algorithm

Cyanotic newborns suspected of having tetralogy of Fallot should have prostaglandins initiated. A brief confirmatory echocardiogram may be obtained while this is being done, if available. As soon as the patient is stable, a complete echocardiogram should provide the information needed for initial management and surgical planning.

Imaging Techniques and Findings

Radiography

The classic radiographic finding is a boot-shaped heart, with an upturned apex (Fig. 49-9). Other findings may range from a normal heart size and decreased pulmonary blood flow to an increased heart size and increased pulmonary blood flow, depending on the degree of obstruction. A right aortic arch can be noted on the radiograph.

Ultrasound

The mainstay of the preoperative evaluation of tetralogy of Fallot is echocardiography. In addition to making the diagnosis (Fig. 49-10), the echocardiogram should focus on the degree and location (subpulmonary, valvular or supravalvular) of right ventricular outflow obstruction (Fig. 49-11), the presence of additional ventricular septal defects, the size and origin of the branch pulmonary arteries, the presence of aortopulmonary collaterals, the coronary origins and courses (with particular attention to whether the LAD or other major branch crosses the right ventricular outflow tract [RVOT]), the arch sidedness and

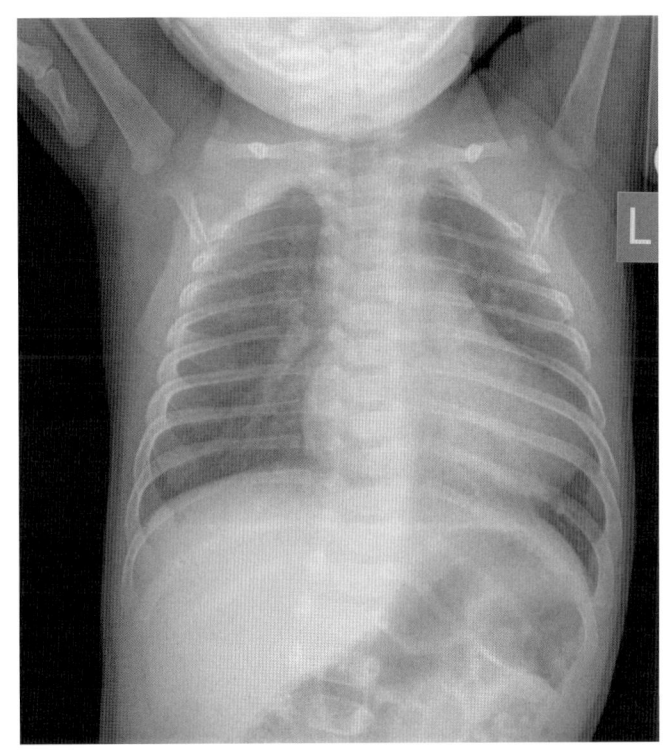

FIGURE 49-9 PA chest radiograph from an infant with tetralogy of Fallot demonstrating mild cardiomegaly with an upturned apex.

branching pattern, and the patency and course of the ductus arteriosus. With rare exception, these can be evaluated by routine transthoracic imaging.

Computed Tomography

The use of CT for the routine evaluation of tetralogy of Fallot should be limited. It is sometimes used in pulmonary atresia with major aortopulmonary collaterals to better define the collaterals in preparation for unifocalization, in which the collaterals are detached from the aorta and brought to a surgically created right ventricle (RV) to pulmonary artery (PA) conduit.

Magnetic Resonance Imaging

The preoperative use of cardiac MRI is limited to specific situations. In some cases, it may be useful to use respiratory and cardiac-gated, T2-prepared whole heart imaging to define the origins of the coronary arteries if they are not well seen by echocardiography. Gadolinium angiography is also useful to define aortopulmonary collaterals, and has been shown to be as effective as traditional angiography.[10]

MRI has become an important part of the postoperative management of tetralogy of Fallot. The repair for tetralogy of Fallot generally involves patch closure of the VSD and relief of the RVOT obstruction. Some patients may have an adequate pulmonary valve annulus and require only resection of an RV muscle bundle and/or pulmonary valvotomy. However, many will require a transannular patch. Patients in which a major coronary branch crosses the RVOT may require an RV to PA conduit, creating a double-barreled outflow. In patients who have had a transannular patch as part of the repair, pulmonary insufficiency may cause progressive RV dilation and decreased RV performance. In addition, left ventricular performance may decline, likely secondary to interactions with the left ventricle. Cardiac MRI can quantify the pulmonary regurgitation and right ventricular size, and is important in the monitoring of patients who have evidence of significant RV dilation by echocardiography or have poor echocardiographic windows (Figs. 49-12 and 49-13). MRI can also effectively evaluate residual RVOT obstruction or conduit stenosis, branch pulmonary artery stenosis, and pulmonary flow distribution to each lung (Fig. 49-14).

See later, "Single Ventricle," for a more detailed description of the routine cardiac MRI examination.

Nuclear Medicine: Positron Emission Tomography

Nuclear scintigraphy perfusion imaging has been used postoperatively in patients with TOF in the setting of branch pulmonary artery stenosis to quantify pulmonary blood flow distribution.[11] However, this has largely been supplanted by cardiac MRI velocity mapping.[12,13] It still may be useful for patients in whom a stent or coil artifact precludes assessment by MRI.

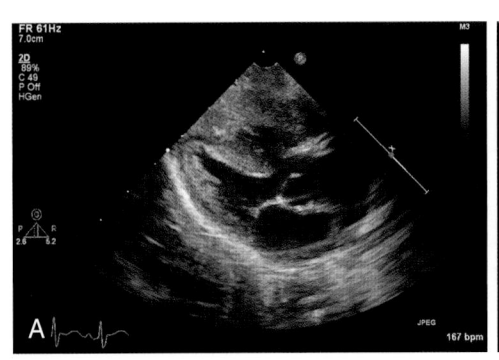

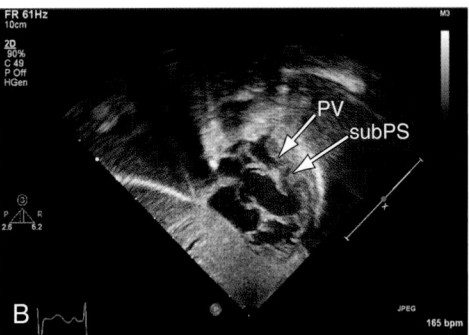

FIGURE 49-10 A, Parasternal long-axis view demonstrating a large anterior malalignment ventricular septal defect with the overriding aorta. B, Subcostal RAO view demonstrating anterior malalignment of the conal septum, causing moderate subpulmonary obstruction (subPS) as well as hypoplastic pulmonary valve (PV) annulus.

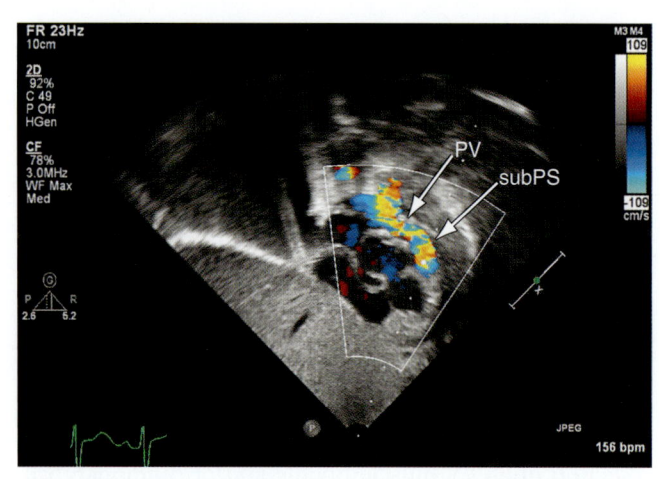

■ **FIGURE 49-11** Subcostal RAO with color Doppler showing acceleration of flow starting below the PV and demonstrating significant subpulmonary obstruction (subPS).

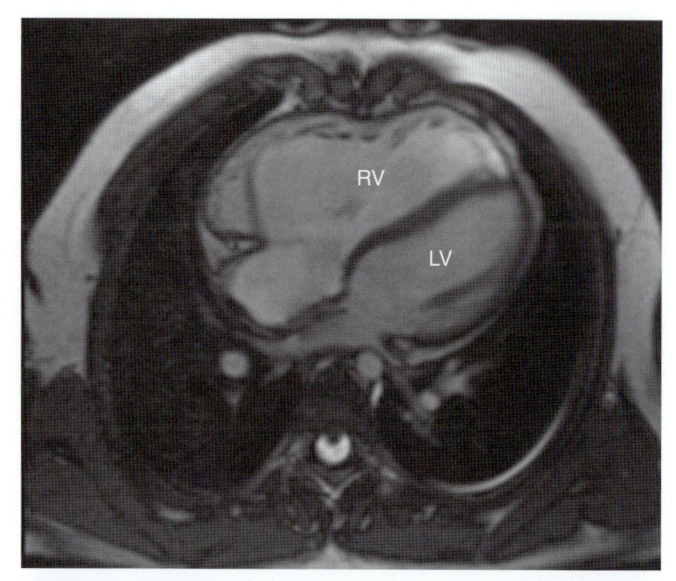

■ **FIGURE 49-12** Four-chamber view of a patient with tetralogy of Fallot with pulmonary insufficiency at end-diastole. This view is used to aid in setting up the short-axis stack to define the basal and apical slices.

Angiography

Angiography plays a limited role in the routine evaluation of tetralogy of Fallot. Selective aortic or coronary angiography may be useful for select patients with major aortopulmonary collaterals or unusual coronary patterns when the noninvasive images are inadequate.

TRUNCUS ARTERIOSUS

Definition

This definition, which has been in use since 1942, is a heart that has a single arterial trunk arising from it that supplies the systemic, pulmonary, and coronary circulations. The first known description, however, dates back to 1798.

There are two major classification schemes in use—those of Collett and Edwards[14] and Van Praagh.[15] These are invariably based on the position of the main pulmonary artery segment and branch pulmonary arteries, with the Van Praagh classification using types A and B to delineate whether a VSD is present (almost all have VSDs). Of the different forms, 92% of all patients fall into type 1A or 2A. The following are the definitions used in the Van Praagh classification with its differences and similarities with the Collett and Edwards classification noted; the Van Praagh classification takes into account aortic arch anomalies.

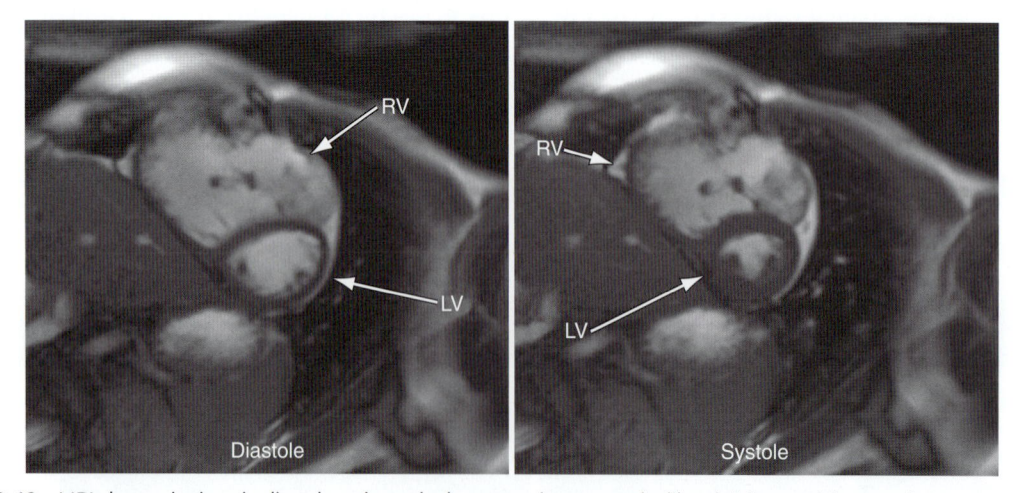

■ **FIGURE 49-13** MRI short-axis views in diastole and systole demonstrating a severely dilated right ventricle secondary to severe pulmonary insufficiency. Comparison of the systolic and diastolic frames shows a flattened interventricular septum during diastole, good LV ejection, and moderately decreased RV ejection. A complete axial stack can accurately quantify ventricular volumes, mass, and ejection to aid in the timing of valve replacement.

- Type 1A—proximal single arterial trunk with a distal main pulmonary artery segment, which is similar to Collett and Edwards type I.
- Type 2A—left and right branch pulmonary arteries originate from the trunk separately, with no main pulmonary segment present. This takes into account the Collett and Edwards type II (pulmonary arteries from the posterior part of the trunk) and type III (pulmonary arteries from the lateral walls of the trunk).
- Type 3A—the origin of one pulmonary branch artery is truncal and the contralateral artery is ductal or aortic in origin, or that lung is supplied entirely by collaterals.
- Type 4A—large ductus arteriosus supplying the descending aorta, with a coexisting hypoplastic or interrupted aortic arch (usually type B) supplying the innominate arteries.

The Collett and Edwards type IV is where the branch pulmonary arteries originate from the descending aorta.

Prevalence and Epidemiology

According to Hoffman and Kaplan,[1] the mean incidence of truncus arteriosus is 107 per million live births; it is thought to occur in 1% to 2% of patients with CHD at necropsy and represents approximately 0.7% of all congenital heart disease. The DiGeorge syndrome and patients with microdeletion of chromosome 22 have a high incidence of having truncus arteriosus. There is no race or gender predilection.

Etiology and Pathophysiology

Etiology

This rare lesion is caused by a failure in conotruncal septation of the embryonic truncus arteriosus and conus. The truncus is normally divided into the aorta and pulmonary artery by two ridges that appear in the 4- to 5-week-old embryo and that grow toward the midline. Cells from the neural crest directly contribute to this septation; one of the leading theories is that this malformation is a disruption in neural crest migration. Van Praagh and Van Praagh, however, believed this to be a form of tetralogy of Fallot.[15]

Pathophysiology

The pathophysiology is dominated by the consequences of the pulmonary circulation and systemic circulation in direct communication with each other. The pulmonary arteries are rarely obstructed, so the pulmonary vascular bed is directly exposed to systemic arterial level pressures similar to those of a large isolated ventricular septal defect with left to right shunting. However, unlike the ventricular septal defect, the pulmonary bed is exposed to systemic diastolic pressures as well, increasing the left to right shunt and acting as a runoff lesion similar to that of a patent ductus arteriosus. Relative flow to either circulation is determined by the relative resistances. Systemic oxygen saturations are only mildly decreased to approximately 90%.

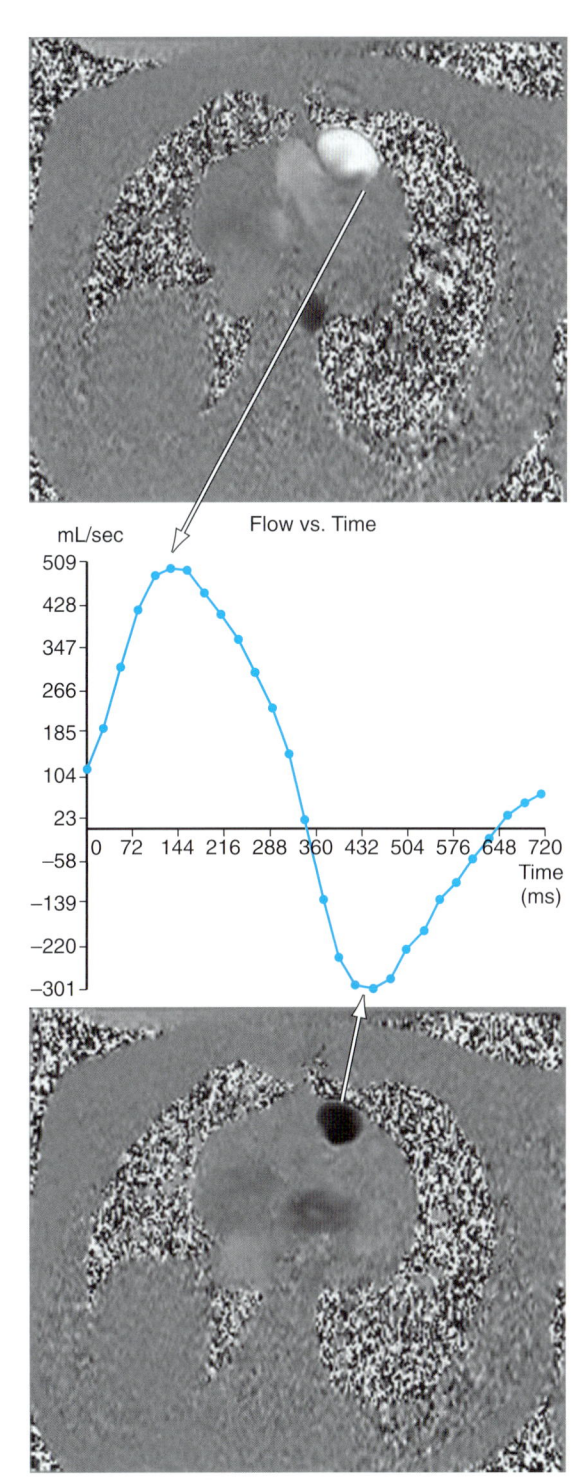

■ **FIGURE 49-14** Pulmonary insufficiency can be quantified by phase-encoded through-plane velocity mapping Forward flow is mapping in shades of white and reverse flow in shades of black. Manual or automated methods can be used to segment out only the pulmonary artery cross section. The flows in each pixel within the vessel are then summed to obtain the flow for that image. The total reverse and total forward flows can thereby be calculated, and the regurgitant fraction determined by dividing the reverse flow by the forward flow (35% in this example).

The truncal valve is commonly dysplastic and nodular, which may result in insufficiency (reported in approximately 50% of cases) or, less commonly, stenosis (reported in approximately one third of patients). The valve may have a variable number of leaflets, although the most common is trileaflet; quadricuspid valves have been reported in 9% to 24% and bicuspid valves have been reported in 6% to 23%. Because of the possibility of truncal valve insufficiency as well as the runoff physiology from the pulmonary arteries directly connected to the systemic circulation, coronary blood flow may be compromised. A widened pulse pressure may be seen.

As the patient ages and pulmonary vascular resistance drops, the patient may develop congestive heart failure from overcirculation of the pulmonary vascular bed.

There are associated cardiovascular malformations, such as abnormalities of the coronary arteries, a right aortic arch, persistent left superior vena cava, aberrant origin of the left subclavian, patent foramen ovale, partial and complete atrioventricular canal defects, mitral and tricuspid malformations, double-inlet or hypoplastic left ventricle, left pulmonary artery sling, and anomalous pulmonary venous connections.[16]

Manifestations of Disease

Clinical Presentation

Because pulmonary vascular resistance is high at birth, there may be no symptoms from the tiny left to right shunt; simply a murmur may be present. As noted, varying degrees of cyanosis may be present but the average systemic arterial saturation is 90%. As the pulmonary vascular resistance drops, signs of congestive heart failure will become evident, with symptoms of pallor, tachypnea, and poor feeding. There will be a widening of the pulse pressure as a direct result of increasing runoff into the pulmonary vascular bed. There is usually a loud systolic murmur and an ejection click from the abnormal truncal valve; a diastolic murmur may be present from truncal insufficiency.

Imaging Indications and Algorithm

Preoperatively, when the patient first presents for medical attention, one of the first examinations is chest radiography followed by echocardiography, with Doppler examination. This is generally, but not always, sufficient for the patient to undergo truncal repair. MRI is useful for certain situations preoperatively to evaluate the pulmonary arteries or the aortic arch. In the postoperative period and for subsequent follow-up, echocardiography and cardiac magnetic MRI are the mainstays of imaging. As the patient grows, echocardiography is less useful and cardiac MRI is relied on for imaging, although this varies among institutions. CT scanning is used when there is a contraindication to cardiac MRI. Some institutions use nuclear imaging to assess differential blood flow to the right and left lungs or if the myocardium is thought to be compromised. The following is a discussion of the indications for each imaging modality.

Imaging Techniques and Findings

Radiography

In the native state, the findings on chest radiography usually demonstrate cardiomegaly, with increased pulmonary blood flow after the first day or two of life. The heart continues to grow as pulmonary overcirculation increases, with enlargement of the left atrium. A right aortic arch may be seen.

Ultrasound

Echocardiography is the primary imaging modality used from in utero diagnosis through the middle of childhood. Generally, enough information may be obtained to go directly to surgery with only the echocardiographic information. The initial diagnosis is made by determining that one great vessel arises from the base of the heart and gives rise to the aorta, coronary arteries, and pulmonary arteries. The initial diagnosis is made from the subcostal and parasternal short-axis views be visualizing the anatomy. The VSD can readily be seen from the subcostal left anterior oblique and sagittal views, along with parasternal views; the apical four-chamber view can be used to identify additional ventricular septal defects (sweeps in short axis can also do this) in addition to atrioventricular valve morphology. Truncal valve regurgitation or stenosis can readily be seen in the subcostal left anterior oblique and sagittal views, along with parasternal views and the apical view angled superiorly. Truncal valve morphology is best seen in the parasternal short-axis view. The sidedness of the aortic arch, as well as the presence or absence of aortic arch interruption, can be determined from the suprasternal notch view. Additional lesions such as a left superior vena cava should also be sought. Ventricular function should be documented.

Color flow mapping is used to determine the physiology of truncal valve stenosis or insufficiency, along with Doppler examination, in regard to the exact systolic gradient and diastolic pressure half-time. Furthermore, color flow mapping sweeps in the short axis can determine the number of additional ventricular defects present. Atrioventricular valve insufficiency can also be determined using color flow techniques.

Postoperatively, narrowing of the reconstructed right ventricular outflow tract and pulmonary arteries needs to be assessed. Stenosis can be evaluated by color flow mapping and Doppler echocardiography can determine the gradient; this is best performed in the subcostal sagittal or parasternal short-axis views and, occasionally, in the apical view angled extremely anteriorly. Residual ventricular septal defects can be seen by short-axis sweeps. Assessment of the truncal valve, as in the preoperative assessment, must be made routinely (Figs 49-15 and 49-16).

Computed Tomography

Because of radiation considerations, CT scanning plays a limited role in the care of the patient with congenital heart disease, and truncus arteriosus is no different. It is done chiefly when there is a contraindication to MRI and, when

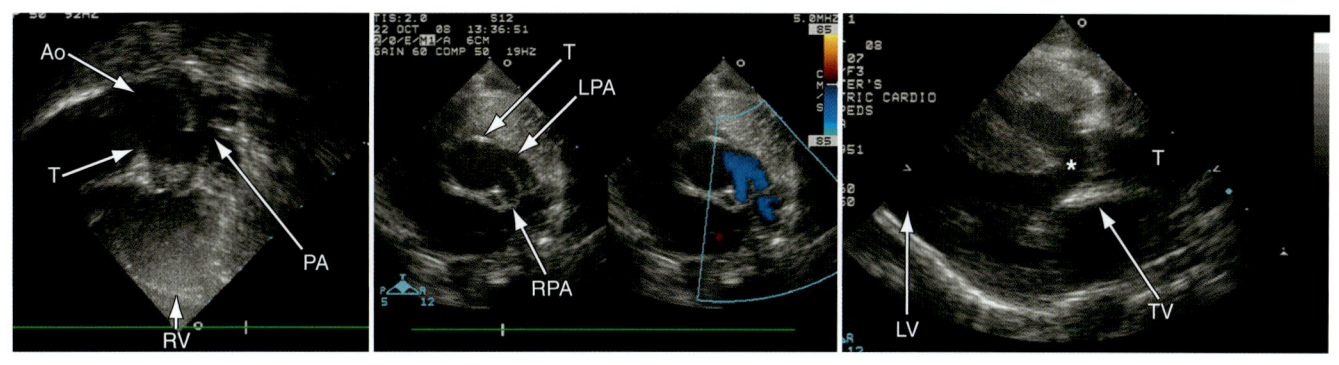

FIGURE 49-15 Echocardiographic images of a truncus arteriosus type II A from the apical (*left*), high parasternal short-axis (*middle*), and parasternal long-axis (*right*) views. The truncus arising from the base of the heart, with branching into the aorta (Ao) and pulmonary artery (PA), is seen. Note the thickened truncal valve (TV). The right pulmonary artery (RPA) and left pulmonary artery (LPA) takeoffs are easily seen from the truncus (T). The ventricular septal defect (*) and truncal valve (TV) are seen.

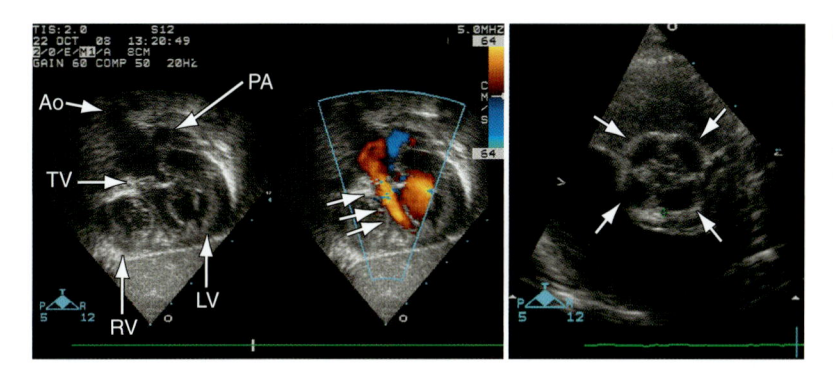

FIGURE 49-16 Echocardiographic images of a truncus arteriosus type II A from the subcostal (*left*) and parasternal short-axis (*right*) views. The truncus arising from the base of the heart, with branching into the aorta (Ao) and pulmonary artery (PA), is seen. By Doppler color flow, truncal insufficiency is seen (*arrows*). Quadricuspid truncal valve (*arrows*). TV, truncal valve.

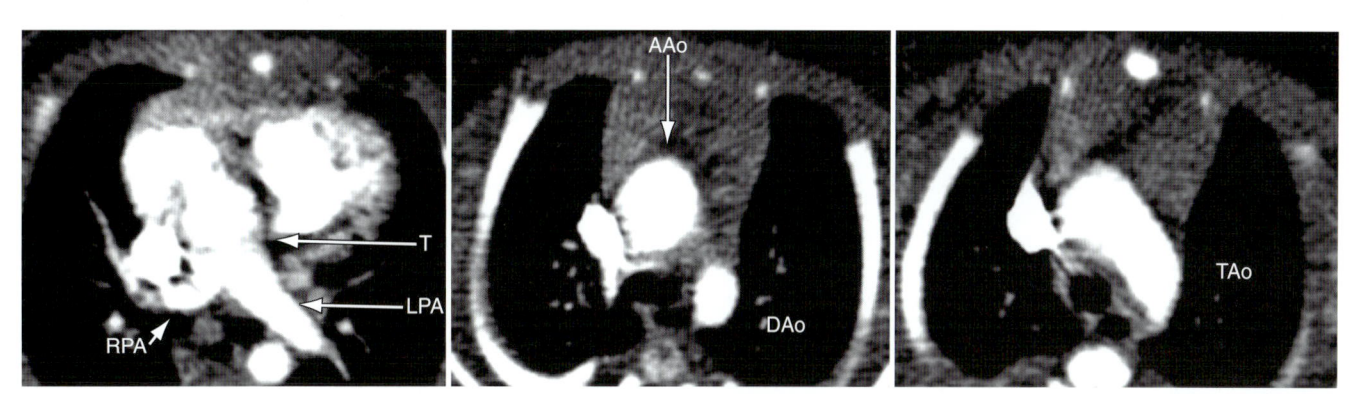

FIGURE 49-17 CT scans of a patient with truncus arteriosus, type IIA. *Left panel*, Axial images demonstrate the right pulmonary artery (RPA) and left pulmonary artery (LPA) originating from the truncus (T). *Middle panel*, Transverse aortic arch (TAo). *Right panel*, A superior cut, demonstrating the ascending (AAo) and descending (DAo) aorta.

used, it is generally carried out postoperatively to visualize the right ventricular outflow tract and branch pulmonary arteries along with the aortic reconstruction if the aortic arch was interrupted. Because of its very limited temporal resolution, except if absolutely needed, ventricular function is best determined by MRI or echocardiography (Figs. 49-17 to 49-19).

Magnetic Resonance Imaging

In the native state, the goal of MRI is to define the type of truncus arteriosus (including origin of pulmonary trunk, branches, and collaterals), functional abnormalities of the truncal valve (regurgitation, stenosis, morphology of the valve, number of cusps), alignment of the truncal valve with respect to the ventricular septum, brachiocephalic vessels, pulmonary veins, and aorta, associated cardiac anomalies, and mediastinal structures (hypoplasia or absence of thymus). This can be performed with the protocol outlined later (see later, "Single Ventricles"). Specifically, static steady-state free precession (SSFP), cine imaging, and gadolinium imaging can visualize the truncus arteriosus and branching pattern of the pulmonary arteries from this vessel. Determining aortic arch interruption or hypoplasia along with the presence of the ductus arteriosus can easily be done. Truncal valve insufficiency and

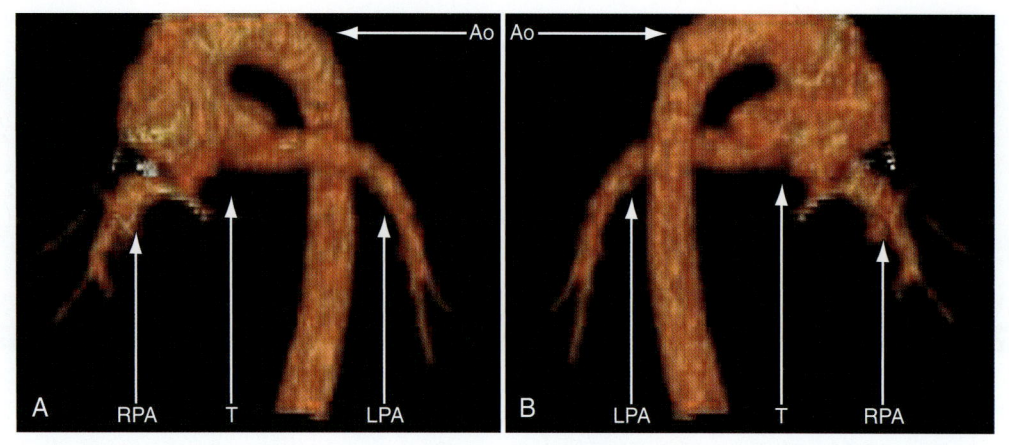

FIGURE 49-18 CT scan of a patient with truncus arteriosus, type IIA. Shown is a three-dimensional reconstruction of the truncus (T), right pulmonary artery (RPA), left pulmonary artery (LPA), and aorta (Ao) only from the off-axis anterior (**A**) and posterior (**B**) views.

stenosis should be assessed with cine and phase-encoded velocity mapping, which can quantify the regurgitant fraction. The Qp/Qs ratio may be assessed by placing velocity maps on each pulmonary artery and in the aortic arch distal to the takeoff of the main or branch pulmonary arteries. Velocity mapping at the level of the truncal valve not only quantifies truncal insufficiency, but is also used as an internal check on the data—sum of the net flows in the branch pulmonary arteries and aorta distal to the takeoff of the main and branch pulmonary arteries must equal the net flow across the truncal valve—as well as visualizing the number of leaflets. Cine is used to quantify ventricular performance and assess for any additional ventricular septal defects. T2-prepared coronary imaging can be used to identify any coronary artery abnormalities.

Postoperatively, MRI is used more often than in the preoperative state, especially as the patient gets older and the echocardiographic windows become poorer. Similar to echocardiography, imaging of the reconstructed right ventricular outflow tract and pulmonary arteries for stenosis is an important component of the examination and can be done with steady SSFP cine, three-dimensional gadolinium-enhanced MRI, and dark blood imaging. Residual VSDs can be seen by cine imaging. Assessment of the truncal valve, now the neoaorta, as in the preoperative assessment, must be made routinely with cine and velocity mapping in the right ventricular outflow tract, branch pulmonary arteries, and neoaorta. Delayed enhancement imaging is used to determine myocardial scar tissue. Follow-up of ventricular function by quantification by cine is routine (Figs. 49-20 to 49-24).

Nuclear Medicine: Positron Emission Tomography

This type of imaging is limited, as with CT, because of radiation concerns. It is generally used for relative flows to both lungs or for myocardial ischemia; however, this has been largely supplanted by cardiac MRI.

Angiography

During catheterization prior to surgery, angiography is used to delineate the coronary artery anatomy further, assess for additional ventricular septal defects, evaluate the distal pulmonary arteries, evaluate the aortic arch, or define associated abnormalities. Postoperatively, right ventricular outflow tract, pulmonary arteries, and residual VSDs may be visualized by angiography for assessment. Generally, this has been supplanted by echocardiography and cardiac MRI. The patient may be taken to the catheterization laboratory to assess the pulmonary vascular resistance if there is a question regarding the pulmonary vascular obstructive disease. Generally, angiography at this point is usually carried out during interventional procedures, such as angioplasty of the aorta or pulmonary arteries or device placement.

FIGURE 49-19 CT scan of a patient with truncus arteriosus, type IIA. Shown is a three-dimensional reconstruction of the truncus, right pulmonary artery (RPA), left pulmonary artery (LPA), and aorta (Ao) with the ventricles and atria as well as from the posterior view.

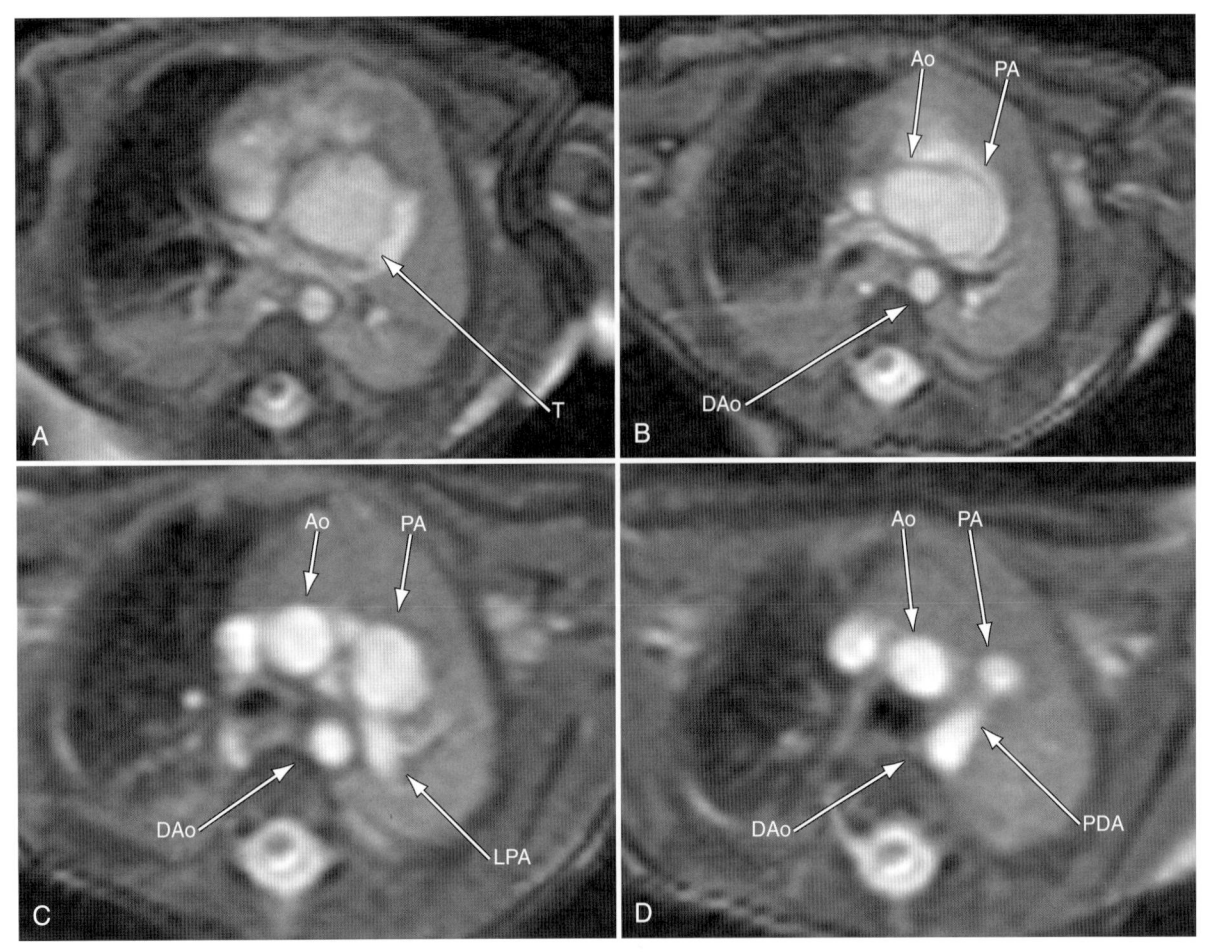

FIGURE 49-20 Cardiac MR images of a truncus arteriosus, type IVA, from selected static SSFP axial images. Images progress from inferior to superior, going from left to right and top to bottom. **A,** The truncus (T) is seen in cross section. **B,** Moving superiorly, the truncus begins to divide into the aorta (Ao) and pulmonary artery (PA). **C,** Further superiorly, the division is complete and the left pulmonary artery (LPA) is seen. **D,** Even more superiorly, a patent ductus arteriosus (PDA) is visualized. DAo, descending aorta.

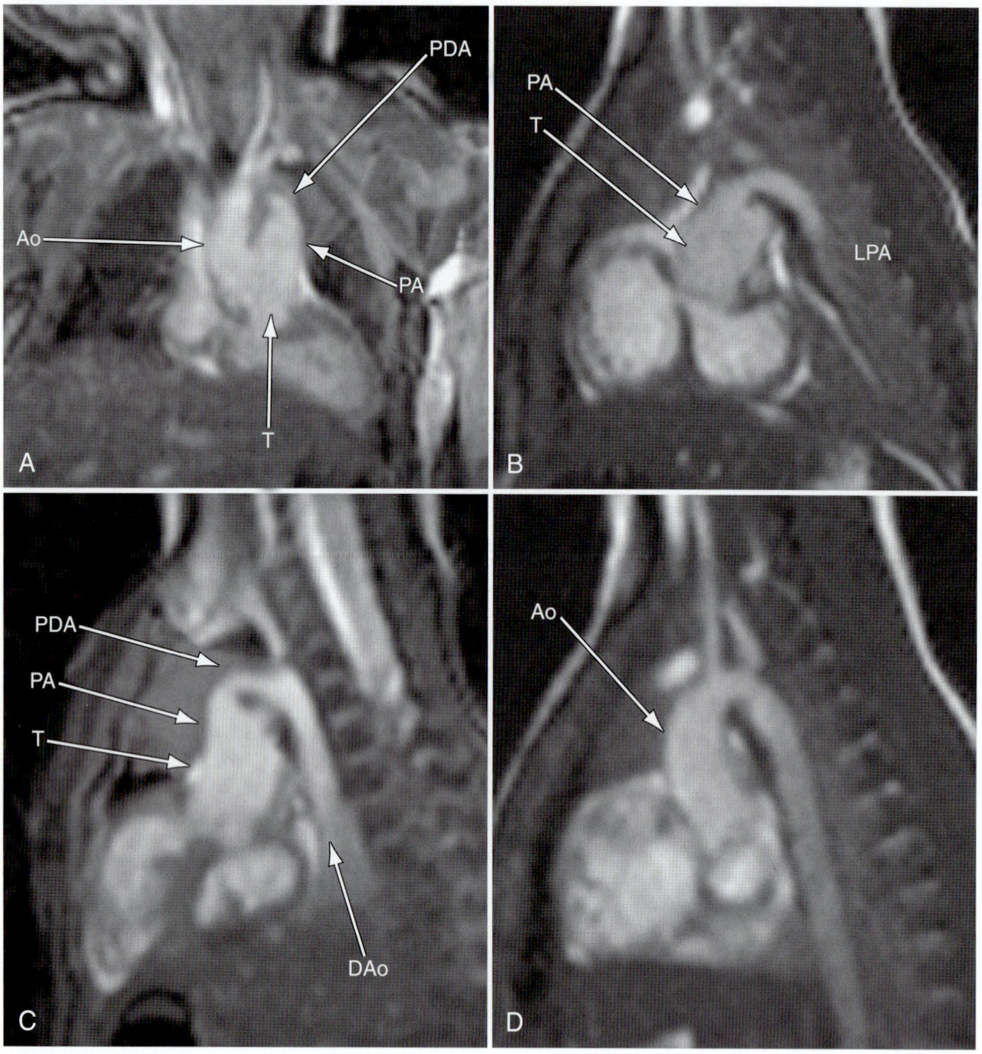

668 PART FIVE • *Congenital Heart Disease*

■ **FIGURE 49-21** Cardiac MR images of a truncus arteriosus, type IVA, from selected SSFP images in the off-axis coronal and off-axis sagittal views. **A,** This clearly demonstrates the division into aorta (Ao) and pulmonary artery (PA). **B-D,** These are sagittal images that progress from left to right as the panels progress from left to right. The lower left image demonstrates the PA takeoff from the truncus (T) and left pulmonary artery (LPA); the middle panel highlights the patent ductus arteriosus (PDA); the right panel clearly delineates the candy cane view of the aorta (Ao). DAo, descending aorta.

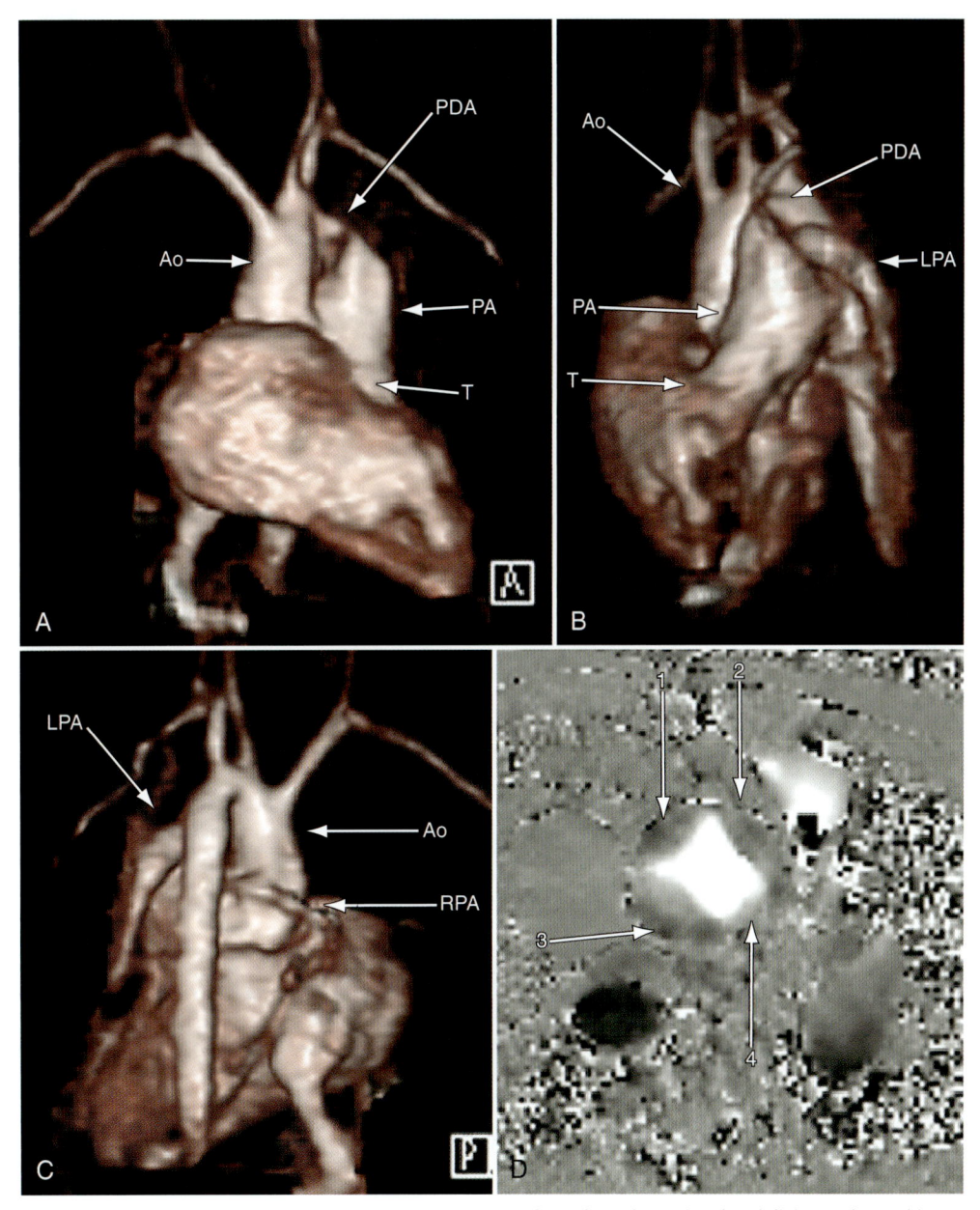

■ **FIGURE 49-22** **A-C,** Cardiac MR images of a truncus arteriosus, type IVA, from three-dimensional gadolinium-enhanced images and a phase contrast image of the truncal valve morphology (**D**) en face demonstrating a quadricuspid valve. The anterior (**A**) sagittal (**B**) view and the truncus viewed posteriorly (**C**). Note the small size of the right pulmonary artery (RPA). Ao, aorta; LPA, left pulmonary artery; PA, pulmonary artery; PDA, patent ductus arteriosus; RPA, right pulmonary artery; T, truncus.

670 PART FIVE • *Congenital Heart Disease*

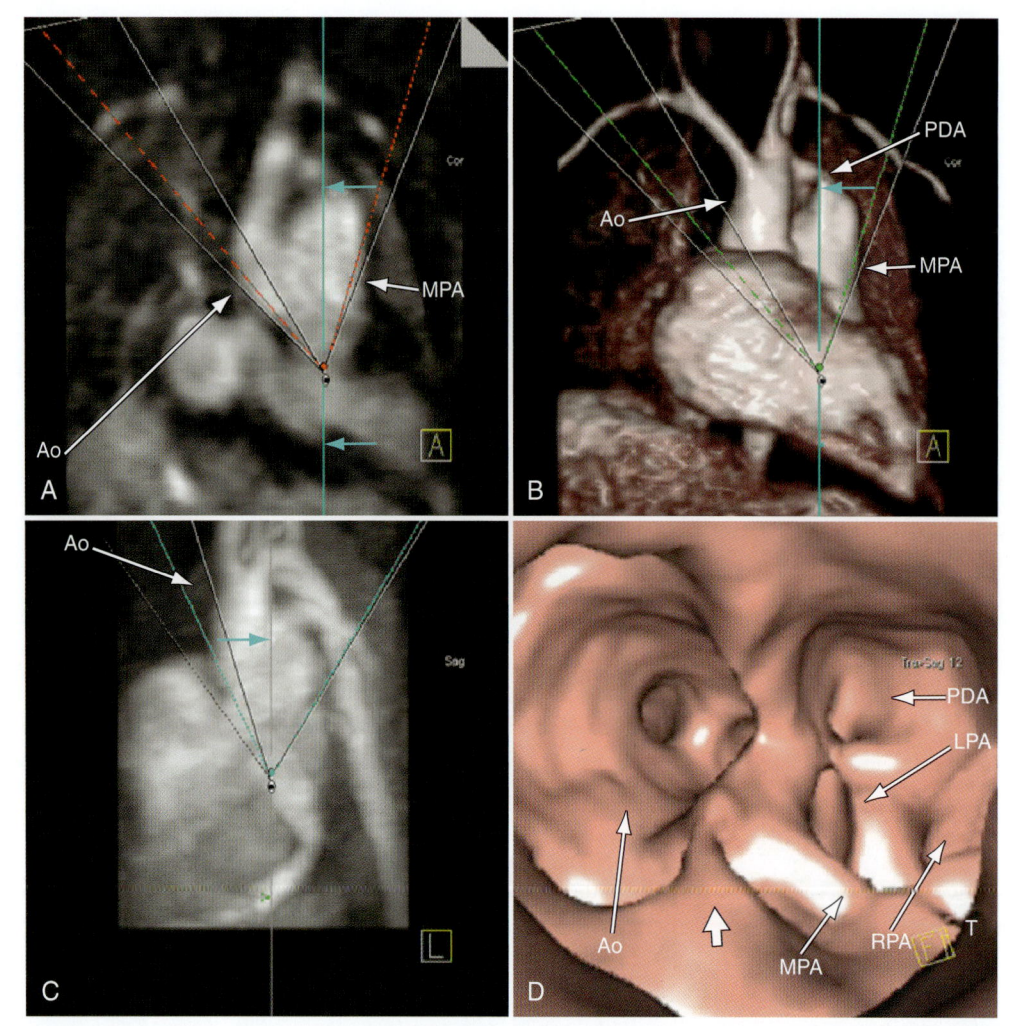

■ **FIGURE 49-23** Cardiac MR images of a truncus arteriosus, type IVA, from three-dimensional gadolinium-enhanced images highlighting an endoscopic fly-through (**D**). The multiplanar reconstruction image (**A**) in the coronal view visualizing the takeoff of the pulmonary artery from the truncus, the volume-rendered image (**B**) from the anterior view and the sagittal maximum intensity projection (**C**) all are used as orientation for the fly-through. Note how all the important structures such as the aorta (Ao), pulmonary artery (PA), right pulmonary artery (RPA), left pulmonary artery (LPA), and patent ductus arteriosus (PDA) can all be seen in one image—from inside the vessels.

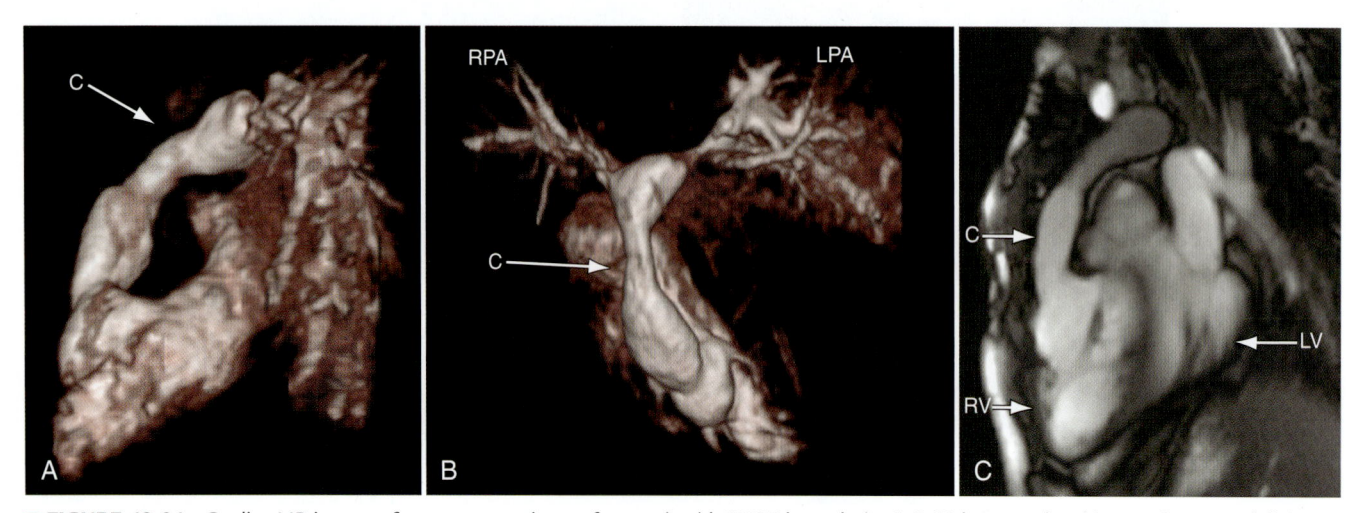

■ **FIGURE 49-24** Cardiac MR images of a truncus arteriosus after repair with RVOT hypoplasia. **A-B,** Volume-rendered images from a gadolinium injection highlighting the conduit (C); note the narrowing. **C,** SSFP cine of the conduit. LPA, left pulmonary artery; LV, left ventricle; RPA, right pulmonary artery; RV, right ventricle.

SINGLE VENTRICLE

Definition: Functional Single Ventricle

The simple definition of a functional single ventricle, sometimes called the univentricular heart, is a heart that has only one usable pumping chamber in the native state or with surgical correction. The detailed anatomy of functional single ventricles is highly variable; the ventricles can be of the RV or left ventricle (LV) morphologic type, can be D-looped or L-looped,[17] or can be a true single ventricle. A true single ventricle is defined as an atrioventricular (AV) valve to ventricle connection in which two AV valves or a common AV valve (excluding atresia) enters into one ventricle only in the presence of only one ventricular sinus. A functional single ventricle can be any type of ventricular arrangement, including a true single ventricle (e.g., two ventricles with multiple large ventricular septal defects, straddling AV valve with hypoplasia of one ventricle), in which the ventricle acts like a single pumping chamber and needs to be treated as such. Examples of single ventricles are hypoplastic left heart syndrome (HLHS; functional single RV), double-inlet left ventricle, and tricuspid atresia (functional single LV).

Prevalence and Epidemiology

Because this section deals with a series of lesions grouped under the rubric of single ventricle, it is difficult to be precise regarding the epidemiology. According to Hoffman and Kaplan,[1] the mean incidence of hypoplastic left heart complexes, hypoplastic right heart complexes, single ventricle, and tricuspid atresia is 266, 222, 106, and 79 per million live births, respectively.

Hypoplastic left heart syndrome, one of the most common cyanotic CHD lesions, has been reported to occur in 0.016% to 0.036% of all live births and in 1.4% to 3.8% of pathologic series,[18] with a male predominance (55% to 70%). Recurrence risk in siblings has been reported to be 0.5% and up to 13.5% for other forms of CHD. As a comparison, tricuspid atresia occurs in approximately 1 in 15,000 live births and has a prevalence in clinical series ranging from 0.3% to 3.7%, with no apparent gender predilection. In autopsy series, the rate is 2.9%.

Etiology and Pathophysiology

Etiology

As with prevalence, because functional single ventricle encompasses many disease states, there are a myriad of theories about the etiology of the lesions, which is beyond our scope here. Suffice it to say that from an embryologic standpoint, three theories have been presented, all with evidence to support their viewpoint. One is a flow-related phenomenon, in which blood is directed in an abnormal direction and results in the pathologic state. For example, in HLHS, if septum primum is deviated posteriorly, blood flow is directed away from the developing left-sided valves, LV, and aorta, causing these structures to be hypoplastic. A second theory is that the lesions are genetically determined based on the fact that some of these lesions are familial; as noted for HLHS, relatives of the affected patient have a higher incidence of cardiac disease than the general population. First-degree relatives of patients with HLHS have a 12% prevalence of cardiac abnormalities involving the left ventricular outflow tract. Multiple genetic syndromes have a high incidence of HLHS, such as Noonan, mosaic Turner, and Holt-Oram syndrome.[19] Finally, toxic or infectious causes are thought to result in these lesions.

Pathophysiology

In the native state, there is a unifying fundamental anatomic and physiologic concept that underlies all functional single ventricle—only one usable ventricle is present to pump blood effectively while the other is hypoplastic, or both ventricles are linked in such a way that separation of the circulations into two pumping chambers is impossible. Often associated with this is obstruction to the outflow or hypoplasia of one of the great vessels arising from the heart. Blood flow to the obstructed circulation is supplied in the neonatal period by flow in the patent ductus arteriosus, flow from the obstructed pulmonary valve that arises from the usable ventricle allowing just enough blood to enter the pulmonary circulation (e.g., double-outlet RV, pulmonary stenosis), or flow through a ventricular septal defect if one or both great vessels arises from the hypoplastic ventricle (e.g., tricuspid atresia with VSD and pulmonary stenosis). As an example of the blood flow in single ventricles in their native state, HLHS is instructive. In this lesion, systemic venous blood enters the right atrium, crossing the tricuspid valve to enter the RV, which pumps it to both lungs via the pulmonary arteries and to the systemic circulation via the patent ductus arteriosus. Blood from the lungs returns to the left atrium (usually) and crosses the atrial septum to mix with systemic venous blood; some blood crosses the hypoplastic mitral valve when patent and is pumped by the hypoplastic LV when present across the hypoplastic aortic valve when patent into the small ascending aorta, where it encounters flow from the ductus arteriosus.

Because staged reconstructive surgery for this lesion is so integral and is needed to understand the figures shown later in this section, it will be discussed under this heading of pathophysiology. The goal of this staged reconstruction is to separate the systemic and pulmonary circulations to allow for passive blood to flow into the pulmonary circulation while the functional single ventricle pumps blood to the systemic circulation.

Prior to bidirectional superior cavopulmonary connection (BSCC), no surgery may be needed, as in the case of tricuspid atresia with normally related great arteries and a restrictive ventricular septal defect or pulmonary stenosis. In this particular case, adequate but restricted pulmonary blood flow is maintained by the usable LV. The systemic venous return crosses an atrial septal defect, mixes with pulmonary venous return in the left atrium and LV, and is pumped to both circulations. Other patients, such as those with HLHS, need immediate surgery—the Norwood Stage I procedure[20]—which involves the following:

- Atrial septectomy
- Transection of the main pulmonary artery and anastomosis with the hypoplastic aorta with homograft augmentation of the arch, and
- Creation of a systemic to pulmonary artery shunt or Sano conduit.

In the case of HLHS, the LV and aorta are markedly hypoplastic and cannot support the systemic circulation. Prior to surgery, pulmonary venous flow crosses an atrial septal defect, mixes with systemic venous return in the right atrium and RV, and is pumped to the pulmonary and systemic circulation via antegrade flow in the patent ductus arteriosus. Some blood may cross the hypoplastic mitral valve and be pumped out the aorta. At this stage, whether or not surgical reconstruction is needed, the ventricle is volume overloaded because the single ventricle pumps blood to the systemic and pulmonary circulations in parallel.

At approximately 5 to 6 months of age, pulmonary vascular resistance has dropped enough so that the BSCC is performed, which can be done as a hemi-Fontan or bidirectional Glenn procedure. This creates a superior vena cava to pulmonary artery anastomosis and prevents blood from flowing into the atrium from the superior vena cava. Ligation of the systemic to pulmonary artery shunt is done at this time. The ventricle is thus volume-unloaded because it does not have direct access to the pulmonary circulation; instead, part of the systemic circulation's venous return (blood from the brain and upper body) is shunted into the lungs via the superior vena cava to pulmonary artery anastomosis. It is not clear from cardiac MRI data, however, that it remains volume-unloaded while the patient is in this physiologic state.[21,22] Because only part of the systemic venous return enters the lungs, cardiac output is maintained at the expense of cyanosis.

Finally, at about 2 years of age, the systemic and pulmonary circulations (with the possible exception of coronary venous flow) are finally separated by baffling inferior vena cava blood into the lungs via an intra-atrial baffle or extracardiac conduit, the Fontan completion.[23] This was formerly done as an atriopulmonary connection but it is now only of historical interest. The entire systemic venous return flows passively into the lungs and the ventricle is volume-unloaded again. To improve outcome, a communication is purposely created between the systemic and pulmonary venous pathways (a fenestration) to allow for right to left shunting when there is increased pulmonary vascular resistance. This allows for maintenance of the cardiac output at the expense of cyanosis, similar in concept to the bidirectional superior cavopulmonary connection. Usually the fenestrations close on their own.

Manifestations of Disease

Clinical Presentation

In general, almost all patients present early in life with cyanosis, but there are some who are congenitally optimally palliated and do not present until slightly later in infancy. There are a several ways that the single ventricle patient can present. Some demonstrate signs of congestive heart failure if pulmonary blood flow is unobstructed or pulmonary venous return is obstructed. Others can present in shock—for example, when the patent ductus arteriosus closes in HLHS, the diminutive LV and aorta alone cannot support the systemic circulation and decreased perfusion, pallor, diaphoresis, poor feeding, and tachypnea result. A murmur is typically heard on the physical examination. Electrocardiographic results are variable, depending on the lesion.

Imaging Indications and Algorithm

Imaging indications and algorithms depend on the stage of surgery. In general, when the patient first presents for medical attention, one of the first examinations is chest radiography, followed by echocardiography with Doppler examination. This is generally, but not always, sufficient for the patient to undergo the Norwood stage I operation, if needed. In the postoperative period and for subsequent follow-up with the other stages of surgery, echocardiography and cardiac MRI are the mainstays of imaging. Cardiac catheterization is useful for pressure measurements and for interventions such as angioplasty or stent placement; in general, a single-ventricle patient will undergo at least one, if not two, cardiac catheterizations in the pediatric age range. As the patient grows, echocardiography is less useful and cardiac MRI is relied on for imaging, although this varies among institutions. CT scanning is used when there is a contraindication to cardiac MRI. Some institutions use nuclear imaging to assess blood flow to both lungs or whether the myocardium is thought to be compromised. The following is a discussion of the indications for each imaging modality.

Imaging Techniques and Findings

Radiography

In the native state, the findings on chest radiography depend on the degree of pulmonary blood flow. With moderate restriction to blood flow, there may be near-normal pulmonary vascular markings and heart size. With severe pulmonary blood flow restriction, there is obvious decrease in pulmonary vascular markings with increased pulmonary blood flow, and the heart is enlarged with increased pulmonary vascular markings. In addition, for patients with heterotaxy syndromes, the tracheobronchial anatomy, stomach bubble, and sidedness of the liver may be assessed.

In the postoperative patient, the chest radiograph is used to assess heart size (e.g., pericardial effusion) and pulmonary vascular markings for assessment of pulmonary flow, pleural effusions, or ascites and to check for device placement (e.g. stent, coils) that may have been placed during cardiac catheterization (Fig. 49-25).

Ultrasound

Echocardiography is the primary imaging modality used from in utero diagnosis through the middle of childhood. The initial diagnosis is made by determining the relative sizes of the ventricles and the associated abnormalities of

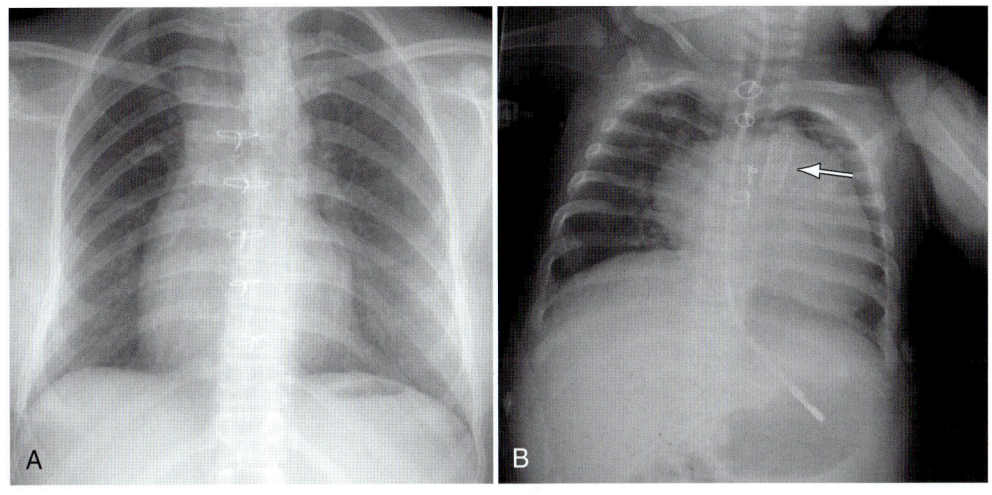

FIGURE 49-25 **A,** Chest radiograph from a patient with corrected transposition and tricuspid atresia with a right ventricular outlet chamber (after a Fontan procedure). The patient has dextrocardia. **B,** Neonate with hypoplastic left heart syndrome after stage I Norwood operation with obvious cardiomegaly. The patient had a small atrial septal defect and needed to have a stent placed in the atrial septal defect to remain open (*arrow*).

the atrioventricular and semilunar valves, along with the sizes of the great vessels.

Because functional single ventricles comprise a myriad of lesions, a systematic approach must be used. Systemic and pulmonary venous connections are defined; this is extremely important for this disease because the systemic venous connections will be manipulated during surgery. Is there an interrupted inferior vena cava with azygous continuation? Is there a left superior vena cava? Are there any anomalous veins noted? Atrial sidedness (for heterotaxy) and the status of the atrial septal defect (if present) are assessed; an intact atrial septum in the presence of HLHS is an emergency and requires an urgent procedure, surgery or catheterization. The atria to AV valve and AV valve to ventricle connections are visualized; the presence of an AV valve must be confirmed (e.g., tricuspid atresia) and how many (e.g., common AV valve). In conjunction with this is assessment of the sizes of the ventricles and determination of whether the child should undergo the single-ventricle procedure or a two-ventricle repair should be attempted. In addition, the echocardiographer must define whether the ventricles can be separated, even if both are of good size. Questions that must be answered include the following:

- How many ventricular septal defects are present and what are their sizes?
- Can all of them be closed?
- Are there overriding or straddling atrioventricular valves that will prevent a complete two-ventricle repair?

The ventricle to great artery connections must be assessed and the relative sizes of the great vessels must be determined. The size of the patent ductus arteriosus is also a question that the echocardiographer is often asked. Also, what is the sidedness of the aortic arch and the extent of aortic arch obstruction? Single-ventricle performance is an extremely important part of the examination and is assessed qualitatively.

Color flow mapping is used extensively to determine various parameters, such as detecting any anomalous veins and the direction and amount of flow across the atrial septal defect; it aids in determining systemic and pulmonary venous connections. In addition, color flow mapping is useful to assess semilunar and AV valve function (stenosis or insufficiency), as is determination of aortic arch obstruction. Flow patterns and direction across the patent ductus arteriosus are also important in determining the adequacy of systemic perfusion and can enter into the decision of whether to perform a one- or two-ventricle repair.

Postoperative assessment is also a key role of echocardiography in the patient's care; however, at different stages of reconstruction, it is important to focus on different structures. There are parameters such as ventricular function that are significant at all stages and one must endeavor to evaluate these as well. See later, "Magnetic Resonance Imaging," for important structures to image at each stage of surgical reconstruction (Figs. 49-26 to 49-28).

Computed Tomography

Because of radiation considerations, CT scanning plays a limited role in the care of the patient with CHD, and the single ventricle is no different. It is used chiefly when there is a contraindication to MRI. When used, it is usually done postoperatively to visualize the aortic reconstruction, pulmonary arteries, or systemic venous pathway. Because of the very limited temporal resolution, except if absolutely needed, ventricular function is best assessed by MRI or echocardiography.

Magnetic Resonance Imaging

At different stages of surgical reconstruction, certain structures and important points are different, but the overall goal remains the same—a complete assessment of anatomy, function, and physiology. At all stages, including

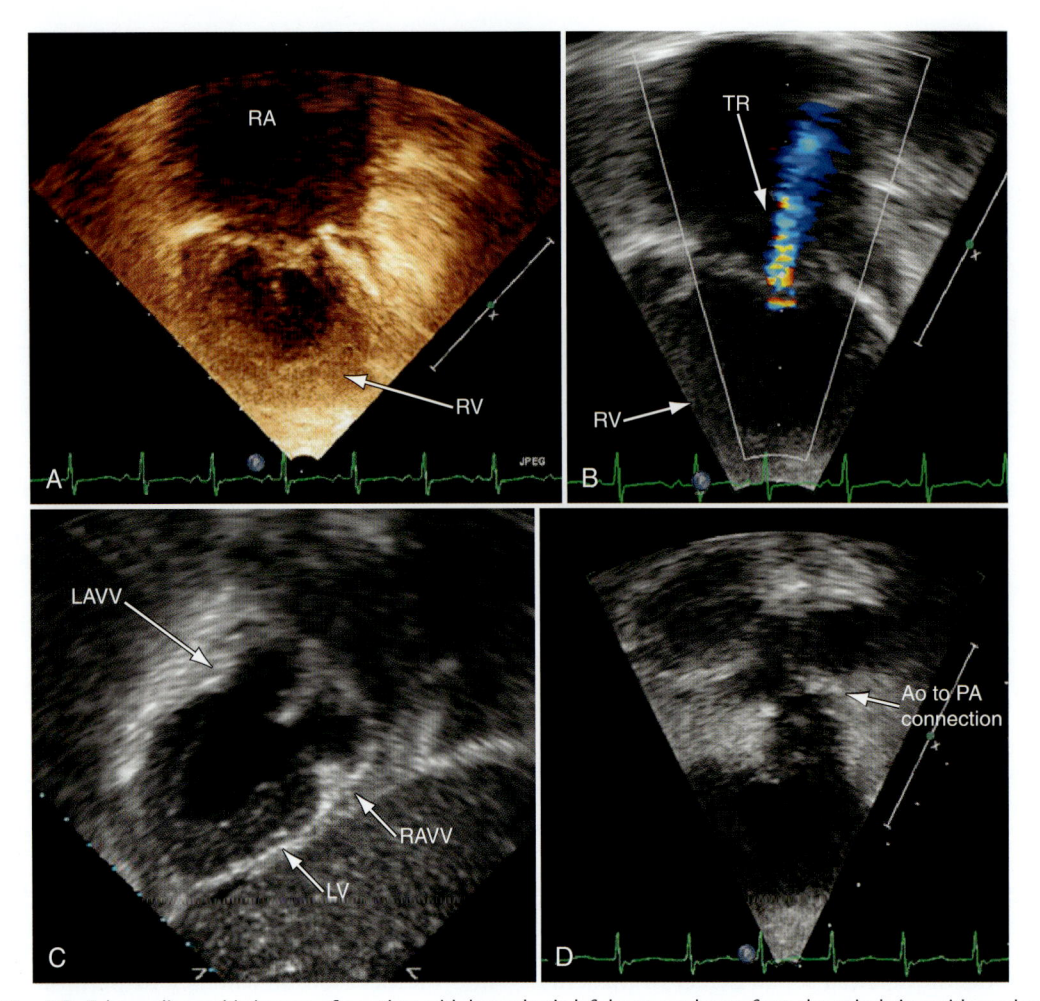

FIGURE 49-26 **A,B,** Echocardiographic images of a patient with hypoplastic left heart syndrome from the apical view with moderate tricuspid insufficiency (TR; **B**). Note how dilated is the right atrium (RA). **D,** Aortic to pulmonary (Ao to PA) anastomosis of the patient with hypoplastic left heart syndrome shown in the top panels. **C,** Patient with dextrocardia and double-inlet left ventricle from a subcostal view. LAVV, left atrioventricular valve; RAVV, right atrioventricular valve; RV, right ventricle.

the native state, the following is the minimum that should be included in an MRI examination:

- Aortic arch imaging
- Pulmonary artery imaging
- Pulmonary or systemic venous obstruction, including the status of the atrial septal defect
- Ventricular outflow tract obstruction
- Ventricular function
- Velocity mapping to assess for cardiac index, Qp/Qs ratio, relative flows to both lungs, and regurgitant fraction of the semilunar and, indirectly, AV valve.
- Anomalous venous structures

At each stage, the following are important to image.

Native State

A detailed assessment of the anatomy must be performed because much less is known about the patient's anatomy than at other stages. The presence of anomalous venous structures such as a left superior vena cava or visceral situs, and the presence or absence of an inferior vena cava, are all important. Assessment of ventricular function and valve insufficiency is also extremely important because some patients may have been compromised at birth.

After Stage I

Assessment of the aortic arch for obstruction as well as the aortic to pulmonary anastomosis and the aortic to pulmonary shunt (generally with dark blood imaging or possibly gadolinium) must be visualized. Turbulence in the shunt causing signal loss precludes cine imaging. An RV to pulmonary artery shunt should be evaluated in the same fashion. Qp/Qs is obtained by velocity mapping. The status of the atrial septal defect should be assessed and since this is a volume-loaded stage, ventricular function is also a key imaging goal.

After the Bidirectional Superior Cavopulmonary Connection

The major extra focus in this examination is the superior vena cava to pulmonary artery anastomosis—either the bidirectional Glenn or hemi-Fontan. This can be done

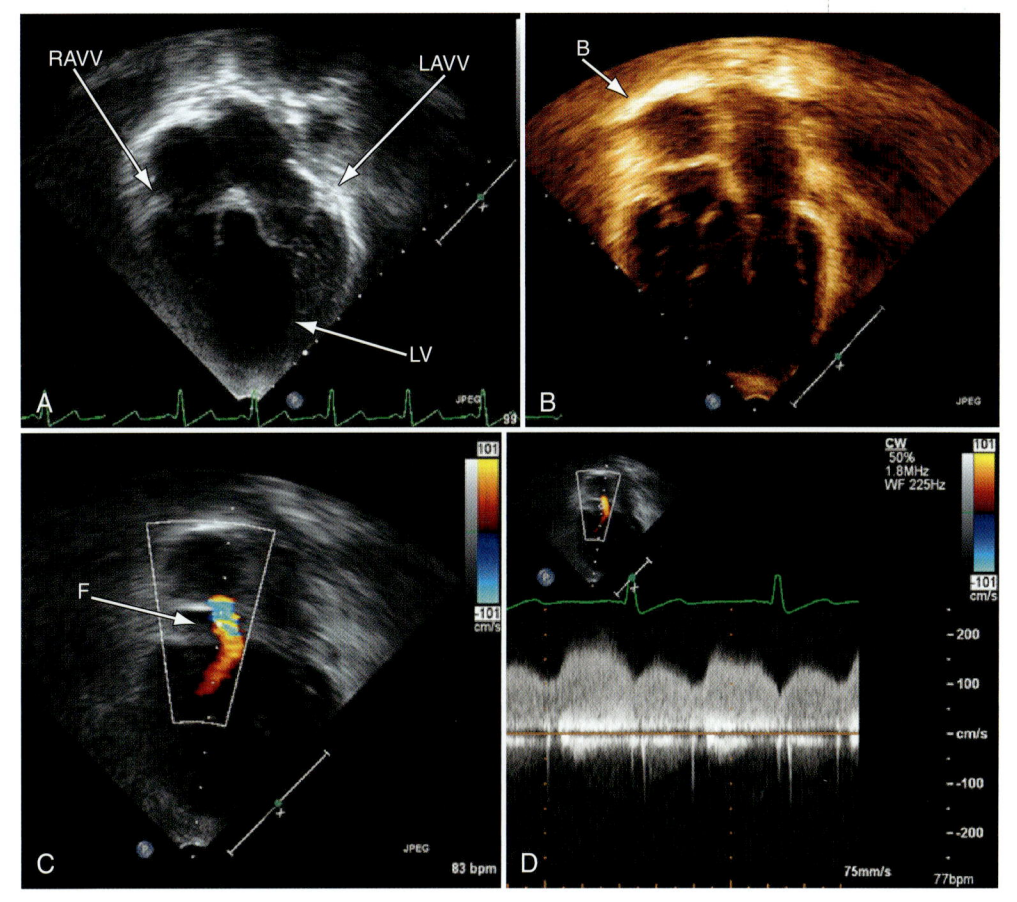

■ **FIGURE 49-27** Echocardiograph of a patient with a double-inlet left ventricle (apical view) after a bidirectional Glenn operation (**A**) and after Fontan operation (**B**). Note the Fontan baffle (**B**). **C,** Doppler color flow across a fenestration (F) in the baffle shunting from right to left. **D,** Doppler spectral recording of this flow. LAVV, left atrioventricular valve; LV, left ventricle; RAVV, right atrioventricular valve.

with cine or gadolinium (rarely dark blood) sequences. The Qp/Qs ratio can be calculated by flow in the superior vena cava or in both branch pulmonary arteries. However, recent data suggest that pulmonary vein mapping is much more appropriate because it also captures aortic collateral flow to the lungs,[22] much different from catheterization-derived data. If a hemi-Fontan procedure was performed, leaks into the atrium from the superior vena cava to pulmonary artery anastomosis should be assessed.

After the Fontan Procedure

The most important structure to image is the systemic venous pathway for thrombus, obstruction, and fenestration flow. Fontan patients generally have ventricular

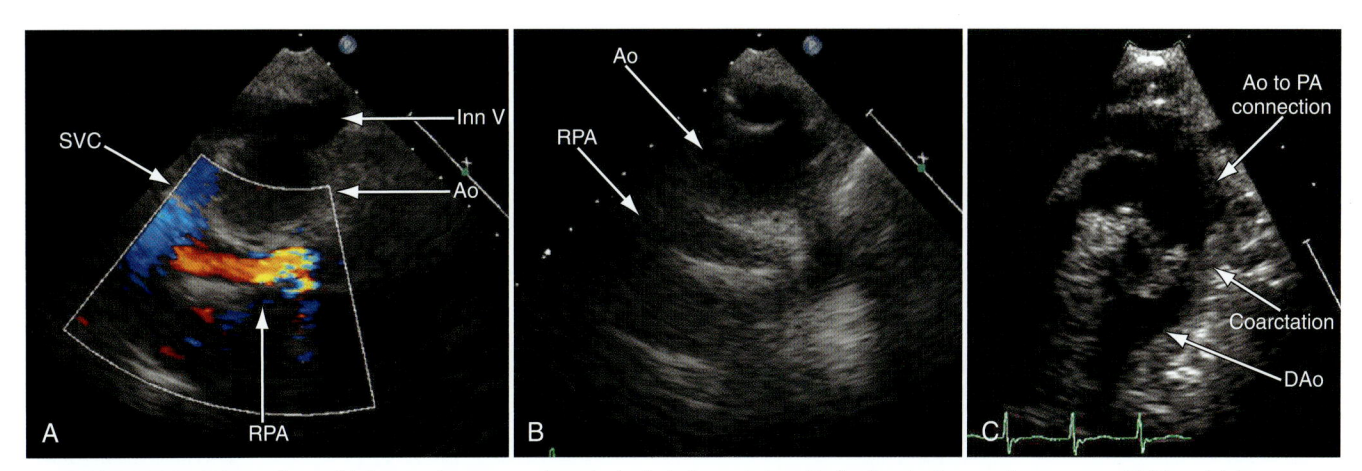

■ **FIGURE 49-28** Echocardiographic images (suprasternal notch view). **A,** Frontal view of color flow in the superior vena cava (SVC) and right pulmonary artery (RPA) of a single ventricle patient after bidirectional Glenn; the aorta (Ao) is seen in cross section. **B,** Off-axis sagittal view of the candy cane view of the Ao and the RPA; note how the large size of the ascending aorta. **C,** Also a candy cane view but demonstrates the hepatic to pulmonary (Ao to PA) anastomosis and a distal Ao arch obstruction. DAo, descending aorta; Inn V, innominate vein.

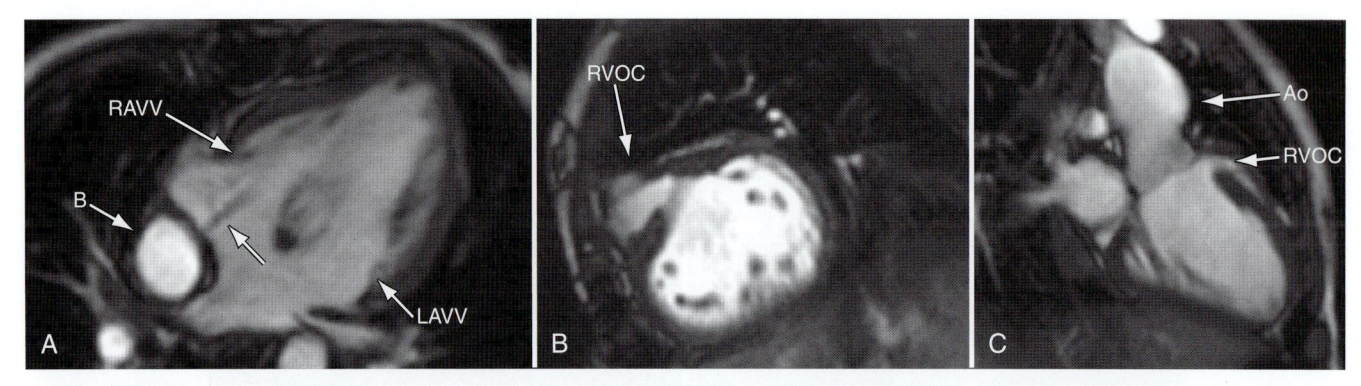

FIGURE 49-29 The cardiac MR image of a patient with double-inlet left ventricle from the apical view after Fontan operation (**A**). Note the Fontan baffle (B) and fenestration (*arrow*). **B,** Same patient as in short-axis view of the ventricle; note the right ventricular outflow chamber (RVOC). **C,** Left anterior oblique view of left ventricular tract through the ventricular septal defect of the RVOC to the aorta (Ao). B, baffle; LAVV, left atrioventricular valve; RAVV, right atrioventricular valve;

dysfunction, so evaluating ventricular performance such as end-diastolic volume, ejection fraction, and cardiac output is essential. Gadolinium-enhanced imaging can help determine the presence of collaterals and assess the aortic arch.

The MRI examination is typically performed in less than 1 hour, generally using the following step-wise procedure:

1. SSFP contiguous axial images. These survey the cardiovascular anatomy and are used as localizers for other imaging modalities in the study. An advantage to starting with this is that if the scan is terminated early because of technical problems or patient instability, a full anatomic volume data set has been obtained and can be reformatted to determine the important parts of the anatomy.
2. Reformatting of axial images. Multiplanar reconstruction of the axial images to localize subsequent imaging is carried out next.
3. Half-Fourier acquisition single-shot turbo spin-echo (HASTE) contiguous axial images. These are acquired while the imager performs reformatting of the images from step 1. They are also used to view structures that may contain diastolic turbulence.
4. Double-inversion dark blood imaging. This is used sparingly to image the systemic to pulmonary artery shunt, evaluate for clot or masses in the systemic venous pathway, or as an alternative to bright blood–cine CMR imaging of various important structures (e.g., pulmonary arteries and aortic arch).
5. Cine CMR. Generally, assessment of ventricular performance and answering other anatomic questions are evaluated by cine (e.g., the pulmonary arteries [long axis, cavopulmonary anastomosis], candy cane view of the aorta, systemic and pulmonary venous pathways).
6. Three-dimensional gadolinium imaging. This is used for three-dimensional viewing of the salient points of the anatomy. It provides the foundation for subsequent viability imaging 5 to 10 minutes later.
7. Velocity mapping. This is performed after gadolinium to add increased signal to the images. It is typically done across the branch pulmonary arteries, semilunar valves (if two are present), vena cavae, AV valves, and pulmonary veins. After stage I, flow in the systemic to pulmonary artery or RV to pulmonary artery shunt can be determined using high encoding velocity (VENC) MRI and echo time (TE).
8. Viability. This is determined in the ventricular short-axis and two-chamber long-axis views.
9. Special imaging. This is specific to the patient (e.g., selected coronary imaging if there is a question regarding the coronary arteries, assessment of regional wall motion abnormalities using myocardial tagging).

See Figures 49-29 to 49-32.

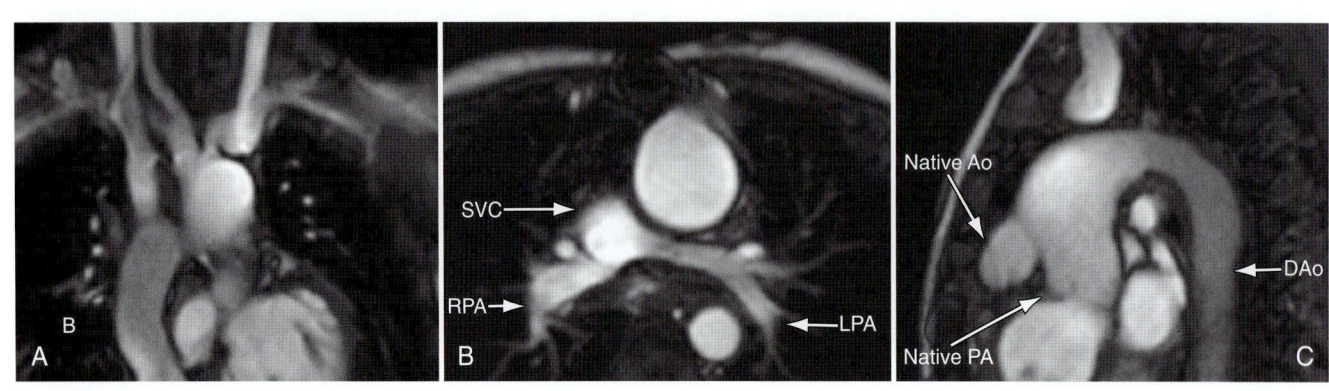

FIGURE 49-30 The cardiac MR image of a patient with hypoplastic left heart syndrome after a Fontan procedure. **A,** Off-axis coronal image of the Fontan baffle (B), the systemic venous pathway. **B,** Off-axis transverse image of the superior vena cava (SVC) to right pulmonary artery (RPA) anastomosis. **C,** "Candy cane" view of the aorta demonstrating the aortic to pulmonary anastomosis. Ao, aorta; DAo, descending aorta; LPA, left pulmonary artery; PA, pulmonary artery.

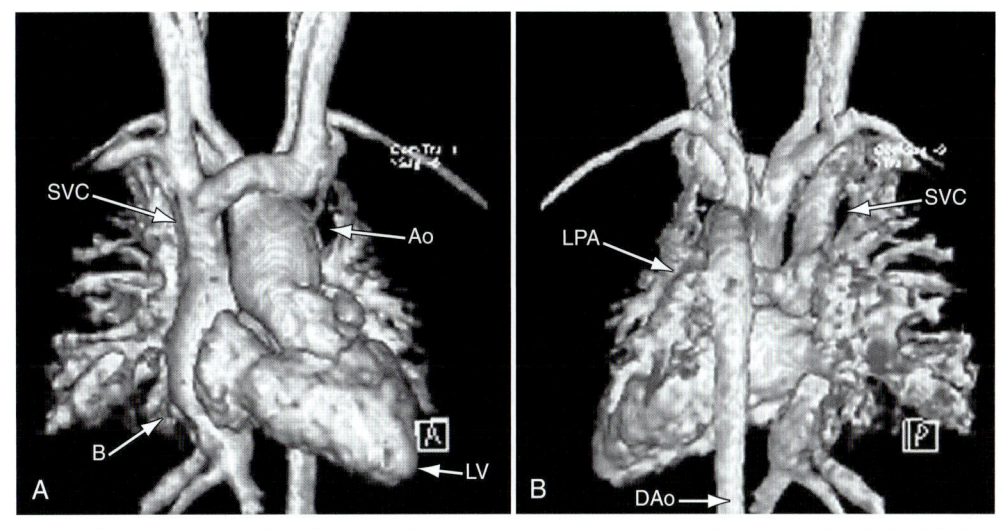

■ **FIGURE 49-31** This cardiac MR image is a three-dimensional volume rendered reconstruction of a patient with a double-inlet left ventricle after a Fontan operation. **A,** View of the heart from anterior. **B,** View of the heart from posterior. Note how well the Fontan baffle (B) can be visualized along with the superior vena cava (SVC) to pulmonary artery anastomosis. Ao, aorta; DAo, descending aorta; LPA, left pulmonary artery; LV, left ventricle.

Nuclear Medicine: Positron Emission Tomography

This type of imaging is limited, as with CT, because of radiation concerns. It is generally used for relative flows to both lungs or for myocardial ischemia, but this has been largely supplanted by cardiac MRI.

Angiography

During catheterization, angiography is used to assess all the structures listed earlier in the cardiac MRI subsection. Generally, in most cases, noninvasive means have been able to assess almost all important structures so angiography at this point is usually used during interventional procedures (e.g., angioplasty of the aorta or pulmonary arteries, device placement; Fig. 49-33).

LEVO-TRANSPOSITION OF THE GREAT ARTERIES

Definition

Levo-transposition of the great arteries (L-TGA) refers to a wide spectrum of structural heart disease, encompassing two-ventricle and single-ventricle hearts and dextro-, meso-, and levocardia. For the purposes of this section, L-TGA will consist of situs solitus and two good-sized ventricles in the setting of mesocardia or levocardia. The resultant setup gives rise to both AV and ventriculoarterial (VA) discordance (double discordance). The resultant anatomy results in physiologically corrected (atrioarterial concordance) flow so that systemic venous flow is directed to the lungs and pulmonary venous flow is directed to the body. Some have referred to this disorder as congenitally corrected TGA. Segmentation for this anatomy is classically {S,L,L} and includes situs solitus {S} to position the right atrium (RA) to the right, L-looping of the ventricles {L} to position the RV to the left, and L malposition of the great arteries to position the aorta (Ao) anterior and leftward to the PA. By definition, the PA arises from the LV and the Ao arises from the RV.[24]

Incidence and Epidemiology

The incidence of all forms of L-TGA is approximately 0.3 per 10,000 live births and represents approximately 0.5% to 1% of congenital heart disease. The vast majority of

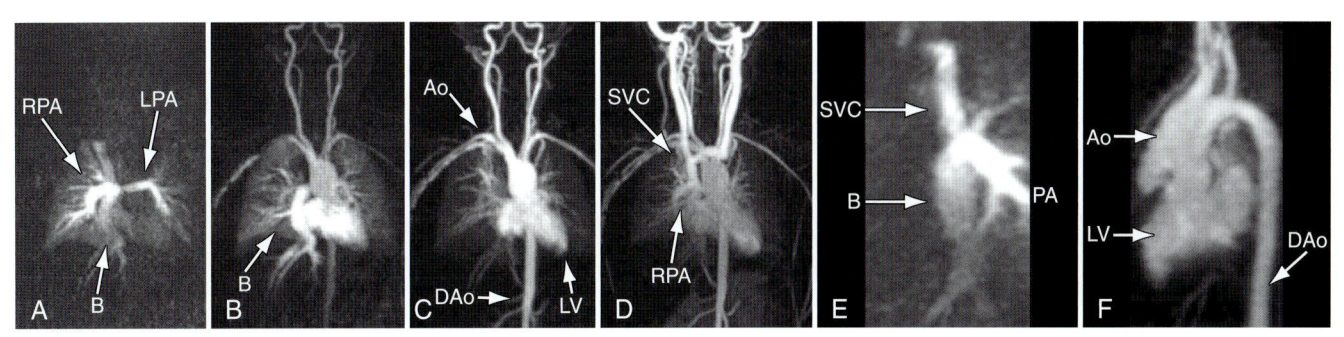

■ **FIGURE 49-32** This cardiac MR image is a three-dimensional time-resolved gadolinium injection peripherally reconstructed as a maximum intensity projection in the coronal and sagittal views. The patient has a double-inlet left ventricle (after a Fontan operation). Temporally, the injection proceeds from left to right. Note how the gadolinium can be tracked from the systemic venous phase (**A**) through the lungs (**B**) to the systemic arterial phase (**C**), and then back to the systemic venous phase (**D**). **E,** Systemic venous-pulmonary arterial phase. **F,** Systemic arterial phase. Ao, aorta; B, baffle; DAo, descending aorta; LPA, left pulmonary artery; LV, left ventricle; RPA, right pulmonary artery; SVC, superior vena cava.

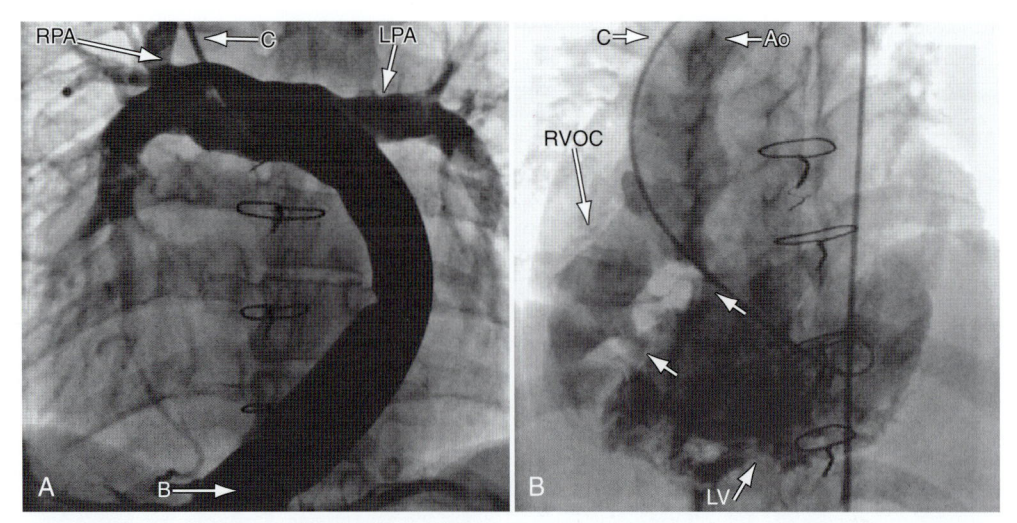

FIGURE 49-33 The patient has corrected transposition and tricuspid atresia with a right ventricular outlet chamber (RVOC) after a Fontan operation. **A,** The angiographic injection is into the Fontan baffle (B) in an anteroposterior view, revealing the right pulmonary artery (RPA) and left pulmonary artery (LPA). **B,** The catheter (C) is in the single left ventricle (LV) and is seen to course retrograde from the aorta (Ao) into the RVOC through one of two ventricular septal defects (*arrows*) into the LV.

patients with L-TGA have levocardia or mesocardia. In the setting of all ventricular inversions, 99% of patients will have L-TGA. In the setting of L-TGA, 99% of patients will have additional cardiac defects. There is a noted absence with right aortic arches and microdeletion of chromosome 22 in patients with this disorder.

Etiology and Pathophysiology

The cause of L-TGA is still under debate. There are ventricular inversion and conotruncal components. One theory has proposed L-looping of the ventricles along with inversion of the infundibulum (subaortic) and normal aortopulmonary septation (involving the cardiac neural crest), but absence of aortopulmonary rotation. Another theory has proposed that L-TGA involves not only L-looping with ventricular inversion but also suggests that the LV structures appear upside-down—there are posterolateral and anteromedial LV papillary muscles. This would help account for the inverted position of the dominant anterior AV node and the course of the AV bundle superior to a VSD. In contrast, normal looping of the ventricles gives rise to a posterior AV node and the course of the AV bundle is inferior to a VSD.[25]

As a result of physiologically corrected circulation, there is no cyanosis. The pathophysiology is related to the additional heart defects. These include tricuspid valve (TV) anomalies (e.g., dysplasia or Ebstein anomaly) in 90%, VSDs in 80%, and subpulmonary stenosis in 50% of patients. In general, significant TV dysplasia or Ebstein anomaly causes significant TV insufficiency, VSDs cause left-to-right shunt physiology, and subpulmonary stenosis causes RV hypertrophy.

Manifestations of Disease

Clinical Presentation

In the 1% of L-TGA patients in whom there are no other defects, the patient is often undiagnosed for years. They may then present with an abnormal chest radiograph or occasionally with supraventricular tachycardia (SVT) related to accessory pathways from Ebstein malformation. Otherwise, as noted, the dominant clinical feature will be related to the underlying associated heart defects. Common additional presenting abnormalities include abnormal RV shape and function and conduction abnormalities, with congenital complete AV block in 10% and progressive AV block in 20% of patients. All patients with third-degree AV block must be evaluated for L-TGA.

Rare associated defects that may also be significant in the presentation include AV valve straddle, a supravalvular TV ring, and a double aortic arch.

Imaging Indications and Algorithm

All patients with suspected L-TGA require a thorough imaging evaluation. Initial imaging should include a chest radiograph and transthoracic echocardiogram. Especially in the older child and in the adult, cardiac MRI is mandatory for anatomy and ventricular function. Especially if there are questions regarding the systemic or pulmonary veins or aortic arch anomalies, additional imaging is required. Further specialized imaging is based on individual patient requirements. Postoperative imaging is based on the specifics of each individual patient. If there are specific hemodynamic or pulmonary vascular resistance questions, the gold standard remains catheterization. MRI has emerged as an important adjunct for the estimation of hemodynamic data acquired noninvasively.

Imaging Techniques and Findings

Radiography

Typically, the AP chest radiograph shows situs solitus, levocardia or mesocardia with a prominent leftward and anterior aortic knob, a left aortic arch, a normal-sized cardiac silhouette and normal to increased pulmonary

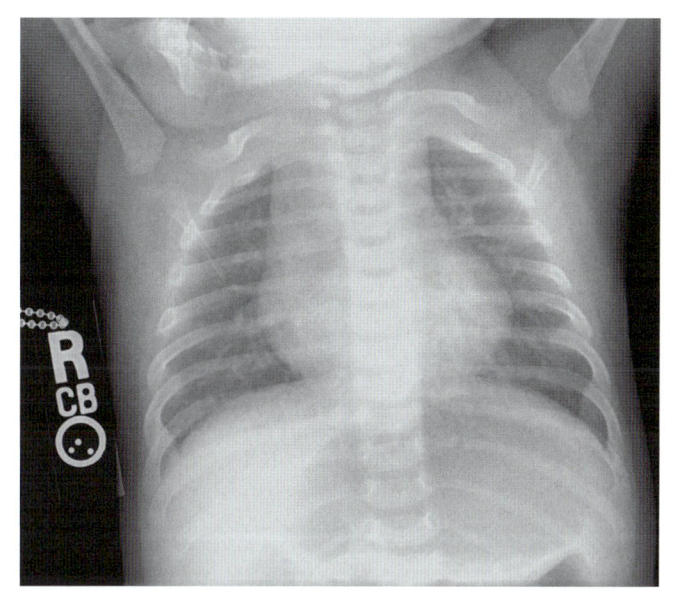

FIGURE 49-34 Newborn chest radiograph of a patient with L-TGA. Situs solitus is noted, with mesocardia. The left heart border has a distinctly RV shape, with mild upturning of the apex. The left hilum is full and represents the anterior and left aorta. Pulmonary vascular markings are mildly increased. A good-sized thymus appears to be present. As seen by echo, a double aortic arch was present, which was confirmed at cardiac catheterization.

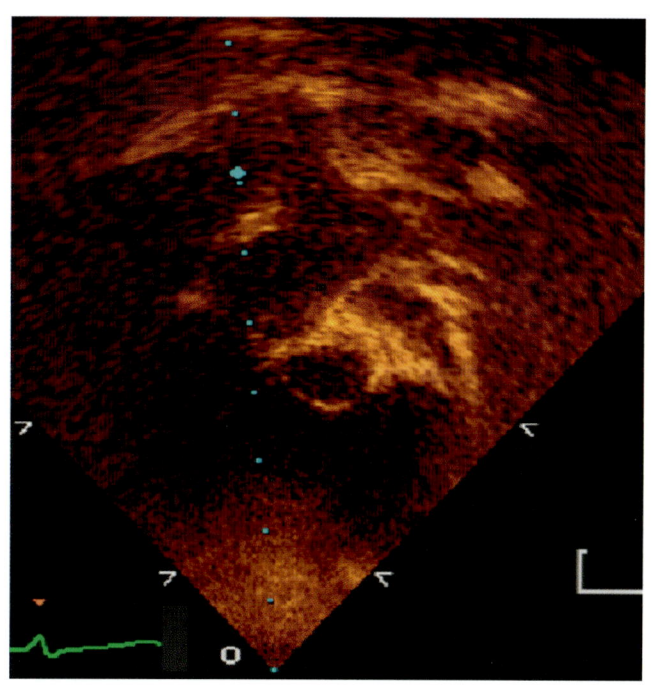

FIGURE 49-36 Modified apical four-chamber view showing the right-sided LV giving rise to the main pulmonary artery (MPA). The two branch PAs are seen coming off the MPA to form "pant legs." The outflow tract from the LV is unobstructed and the ventricular septum is intact.

vascular markings, depending on the size of the VSD (Fig. 49-34).

Ultrasound

Transthoracic echocardiography is a standard imaging procedure for L-TGA. All associated defects can be delineated with great accuracy, and echocardiography is superior for the evaluation of AV straddle. A careful search for common associated lesions should be undertaken, including delineation of TV anomalies, VSDs, and subpulmonary stenosis (Figs. 49-35 to 49-38).

Computed Tomography

CT has little place in congenital heart disease because of radiation exposure, even though it can demonstrate systemic and pulmonary venous connections, aortic arch and pulmonary artery anomalies, and aortopulmonary

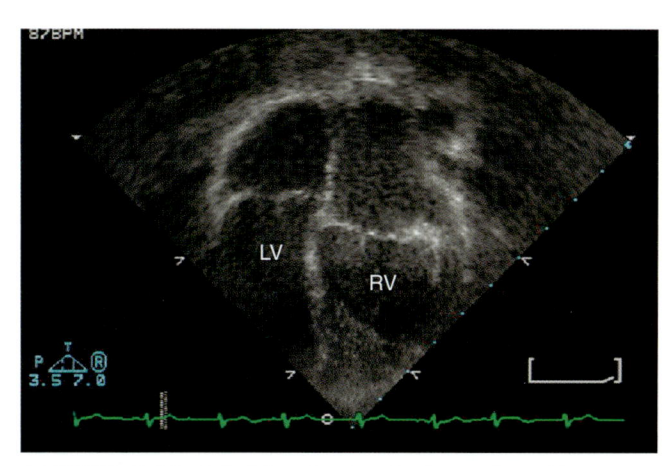

FIGURE 49-35 Apical four-chamber view in a patient with LTGA. **Right,** Finely trabeculated LV. **Left,** Coarsely trabeculated RV. The normal TV offset toward the RV is reversed with the L-looped RV. In addition, distance measurements of the septal TV leaflet downward displacement are consistent with mild Ebstein anomaly.

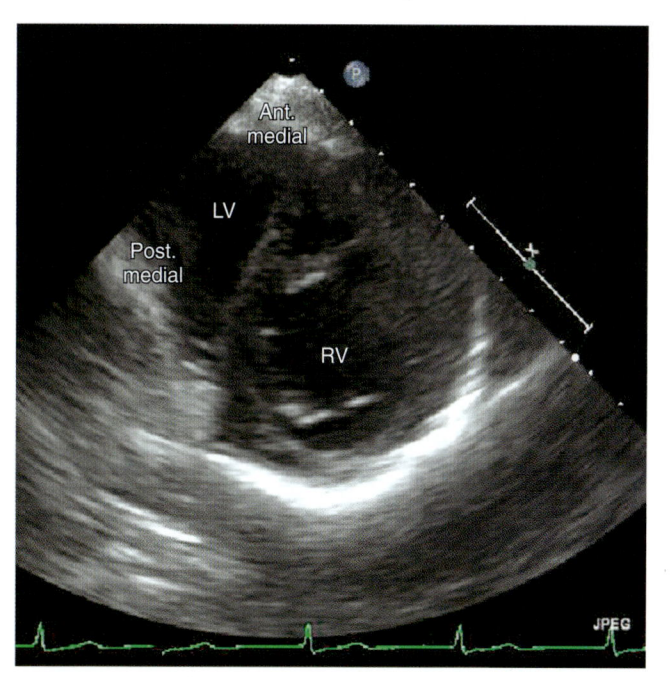

FIGURE 49-37 Parasternal short-axis view of a patient with L-TGA. The anterior papillary muscle (ant medial) is medial to the septum and the posterior papillary muscle (post lateral) is lateral to the septum. In this regard, the LV does appear to be upside down in its rightward placement.

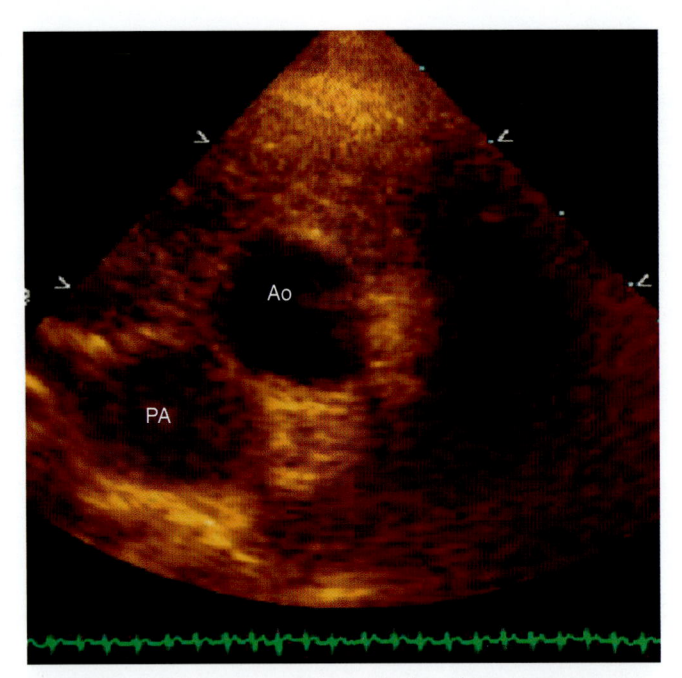

FIGURE 49-38 Parasternal short-axis view of the great artery relationship in LTGA. The aorta (Ao) is anterior and left with the pulmonary artery (PA) posterior and right. The left pulmonary artery courses posterior to the aortic arch in contrast to normally related great arteries and the right pulmonary artery courses posterior to the aortic arch.

collateral arteries. However, most of this can be determined by cardiac MRI without the significant radiation exposure, relegating the role of CT largely to situations in which MRI cannot be performed.

Magnetic Resonance Imaging

Cardiac MRI plays a particularly important role in the preoperative and postoperative management of patients with corrected TGA. In particular, for patients without repair or those who have had a repair in which the RV is still the systemic ventricle, cine MRI can help quantify ventricular size and performance. Deteriorating performance is often an indication to consider a double switch procedure (see later surgical section). Furthermore, by combining cine imaging with phase contrast velocity measurements of the RV outflow volume, the tricuspid regurgitant fraction can be accurately assessed. In addition, cardiac MRI plays a role in surgical planning for these patients with regard to anatomy and function.

It also plays an important role in the management of the late double switch, during which a pulmonary artery band is placed to retrain the left ventricle. Several centers have advocated monitoring the LV mass by serial cardiac MRI to ensure that the LV is properly trained before performing the double switch (Figs. 49-39 and 49-40).[26]

Additionally, respiratory-gated whole heart sequences are effective in defining the origins and proximal course of the coronary arteries preoperatively in preparation for a double switch when echocardiography cannot definitively delineate them. Viability can be used to assess for myocardial scarring.

Nuclear Medicine: Positron Emission Tomography

This imaging modality can be useful for evaluating cardiac perfusion defects in patients who have had an arterial switch procedure along with coronary button transfer. It is often combined with preexercise and postexercise imaging.

Cardiac Catheterization and Angiography

Angiography remains the gold standard for hemodynamic and pulmonary arterial and vascular resistance studies, but its role in the routine care of patients is limited. It often plays an important role in measuring LV pressures after a pulmonary artery band procedure to ensure, along with MRI LV mass measurements, that the LV has been properly retrained to withstand a double switch.

DOUBLE-OUTLET RIGHT VENTRICLE

Definition

DORV refers to a wide spectrum of structural heart disease, encompassing both two-ventricle and single-ventricle hearts and dextrocardia and levocardia. Included in this complex spectrum is heterotaxy, in which DORV is a predominant diagnosis. For the purposes of this section, DORV will consist of situs solitus and two good-sized ventricles in the setting of levocardia. The resultant setup gives rise to AV concordance, with both great arteries committed to the RV (bilateral subarterial conus). Essentially all DORVs have a VSD, 80% of which are malalignment in type. The remainder of VSDs are cono-ventricular but additional muscular VSDs are present in a small percentage of cases. The resultant anatomy gives rise to varying degrees of VSD physiology, with the VSD being the only outlet for the LV. VSDs have been classically divided into four categories according to their location to the great arteries: subaortic (nearly 50%), subpulmonary (8%), doubly committed, and noncommitted. The subpulmonary VSD in DORV is commonly referred to as the Taussig-Bing variant. A significant portion of DORVs will have subpulmonary stenosis (70%), with variable degrees of obstruction.

Typically, the spatial relation of the great arteries has also been important in the classification of DORV. This relation is usually divided into four types, according to the position of the aorta to the pulmonary artery: right and posterior, right and side by side, right and anterior, and left and anterior. Segmentation for DORV anatomy is classically {S,D,D} and includes situs solitus {S} to position the right atrium (RA) to the right, D-looping of the ventricles to position the right ventricle (RV) to the right, and D position of the great arteries to position the aorta (Ao) rightward to the pulmonary artery (PA). By definition, both great arteries arise from the RV and there is absence of aortic to mitral continuity.

Incidence and Epidemiology

The incidence of all forms of DORV is approximately 0.9 per 10,000 live births and represents approximately 1% to

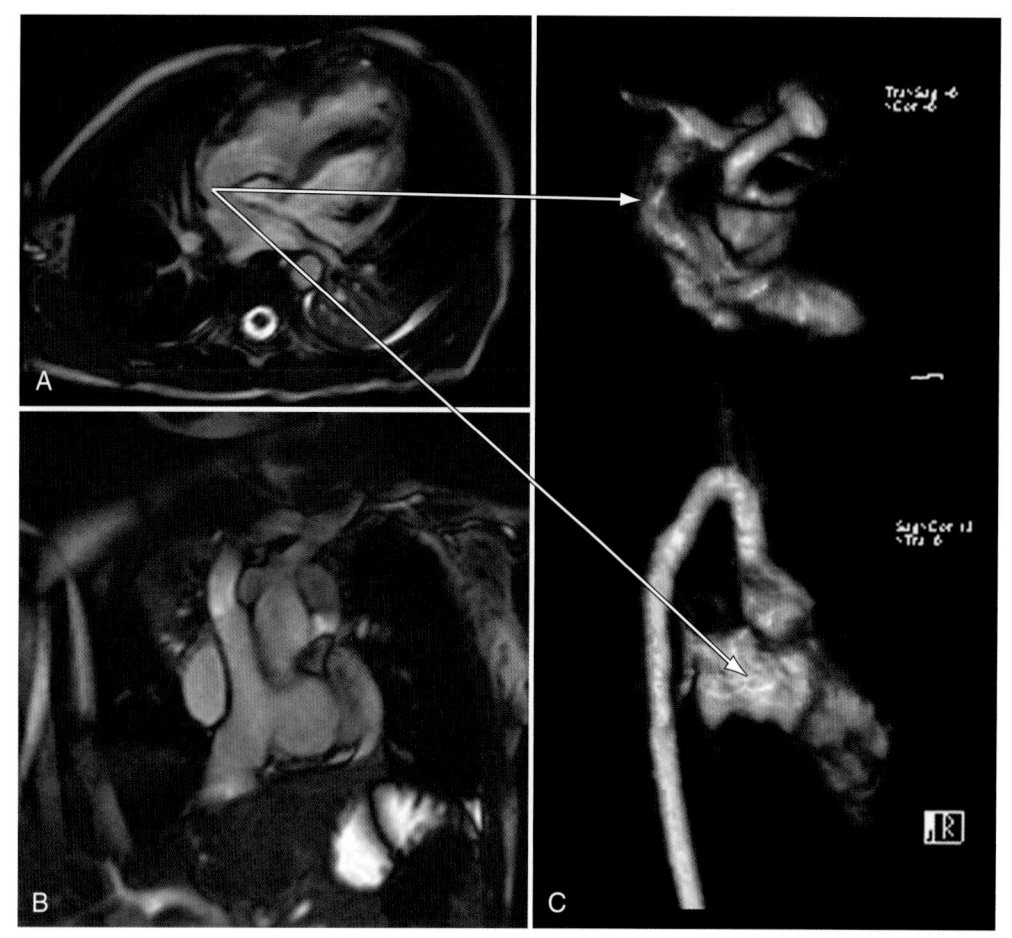

■ **FIGURE 49-39** MRI plays an important role in assessing the patient after a double switch. The complex pathways of the pulmonary venous pathway (**A**) and systemic venous pathway (**B**) can be assessed for obstruction or baffle leak by cine, although it can be challenging to image the entire pathway in a single cine. **C,** A time-resolved three-dimensional gadolinium sequence effectively isolates the pulmonary venous pathway, demonstrating that it is widely patent. This can be an important adjunct to cine imaging.

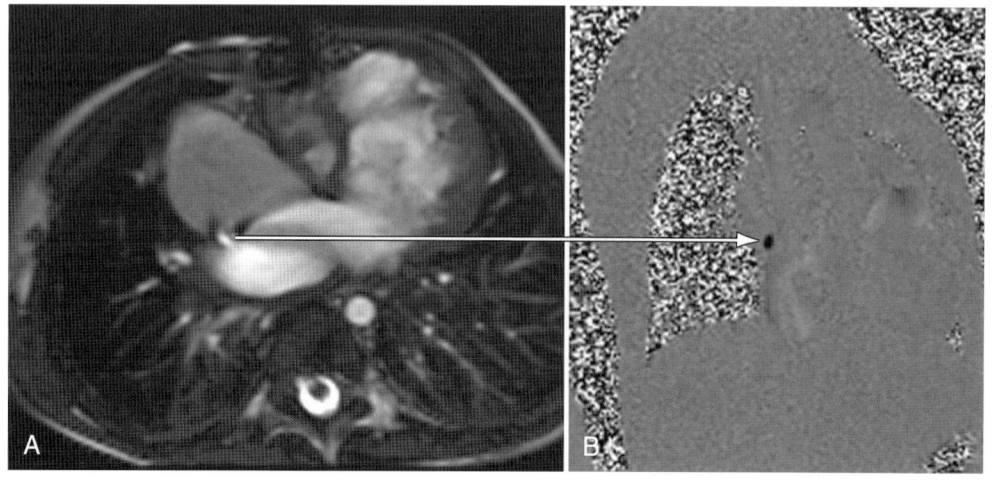

■ **FIGURE 49-40** Patient with LTGA who has undergone a double switch. **A,** The pulmonary venous pathway is markedly narrowed, causing turbulence artifact on this SSFP cine. **B,** Through-plane velocity mapping demonstrates significant acceleration. The peak measured velocity was 2 m/sec, confirming significant venous obstruction.

1.5% of congenital heart disease. The vast majority of patients with DORV have levocardia although DORV is seen frequently in patients with heterotaxy and dextrocardia. In the setting of all forms of DORV, more than 99% will have a VSD. There is a noted paucity of right aortic arches and microdeletion of chromosome 22 (<5%) in patients with DORV and levocardia.

Etiology and Pathophysiology

The cause of DORV is still under debate but overall is thought to be an abnormality of the conotruncus and mesenchymal tissue migration. In the developing embryo, the single arterial trunk sits over the bulbous cordis, which subsequently forms the RV. There is normal aortopulmonary septation (involving the cardiac neural crest) and the presence of aortopulmonary rotation; however, both great arteries remain over the RV. The amount of aortopulmonary rotation varies, resulting in varying positions of the aorta in relation to the pulmonary artery.

The pathophysiology of DORV is related primarily to the dominant cardiac defects and position of the VSD. A subaortic or noncommittal VSD manifests primarily left to right shunt physiology. In contrast, a subpulmonary VSD (Taussig-Bing DORV) results in pulmonary venous blood streaming across the VSD into the PA and manifests transposition physiology with cyanosis. A doubly committed VSD results in elements of shunt and transposition physiologies.

The conal septum plays an important role in DORV physiology. This septum is hypoplastic in doubly committed VSDs, resulting in unobstructed flow to either great artery. In contrast, malalignment VSDs often result in deviation of the conal septum toward a great artery. Deviation toward the PA results in tetralogy of Fallot physiology, whereas deviation toward the aorta results in coarctation physiology.

Manifestations of Disease

Clinical Presentation

Most DORVs present in the neonatal period with a hyperdynamic primordial impulse and murmurs. Otherwise, as noted, the dominant clinical feature will be related to the VSD position and deviation of the conal septum. As pulmonary vascular resistance falls over the first few days of life, one of three major patterns generally emerges. These include shunt physiology, transposition physiology, and coarctation physiology.

Imaging Indications and Algorithm

All patients with suspected DORV require a thorough imaging evaluation. Initial imaging should include chest radiography and transthoracic echocardiography. Especially in the older child and adult, cardiac MRI is mandatory for anatomy and ventricular function. If there are questions regarding the systemic or pulmonary veins or aortic arch anomalies, additional imaging is required. Further specialized imaging is based on individual patient requirements and may include transesophageal or three-dimensional real-time echocardiography to determine the feasibility of a two-ventricle repair. Postoperative imaging is individualized to each patient. If there is specific pulmonary vascular resistance or pressure-related questions, the gold standard remains catheterization. MRI has emerged as an important adjunct for the estimation of hemodynamic data acquired noninvasively.

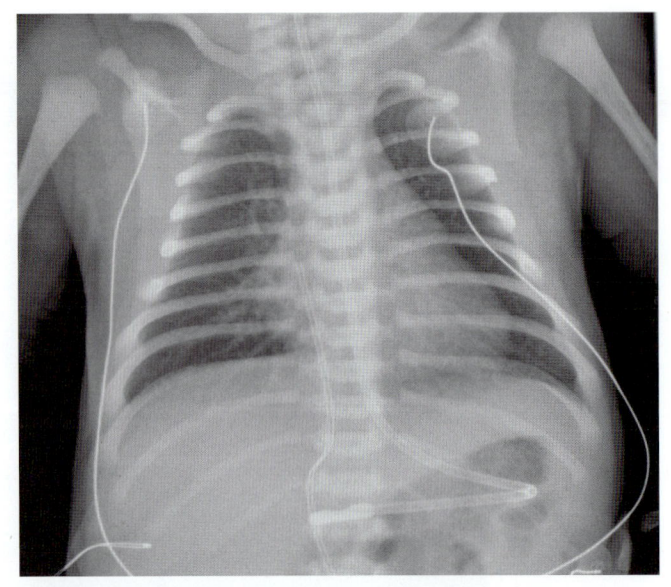

FIGURE 49-41 Chest radiograph in a patient with DORV. Situs solitus is noted, with levocardia and a normal heart size. The left heart border has a typical LV apex shape. The left upper heart border shows a prominent pulmonary artery segment. The trachea angles slightly to the right, consistent with a left aortic arch. There are high-normal pulmonary vascular markings. Minimal thymus tissue appears to be present.

Imaging Techniques and Findings

Radiography

Typically, the AP chest radiograph shows situs solitus, levocardia with a prominent heart size, a left aortic arch, and normal to increased pulmonary vascular markings, depending on the position of the VSD and conal septum deviation (Fig. 49-41).

Ultrasound

Transthoracic echocardiography remains one of the standard imaging techniques for DORV. Associated defects can be delineated and echocardiography is superior for the evaluation of AV straddle. A careful search for common associated lesions should be undertaken, including delineation of inlet and outlet anomalies, VSD location, subpulmonary or subaortic stenosis, and great artery caliber and narrowing. One important echo measurement for consideration of surgical management is the distance from the medial portion of the TV to the pulmonary valve annulus. Depending on the relation of the aorta to the PA, this distance can be accurately measured from subcostal views in varying planes. It represents the potential baffle pathway diameter to the aorta in a two-ventricle repair (Figs. 49-42 to 49-46).

CHAPTER 49 • *Complex Congenital Heart Disease* 683

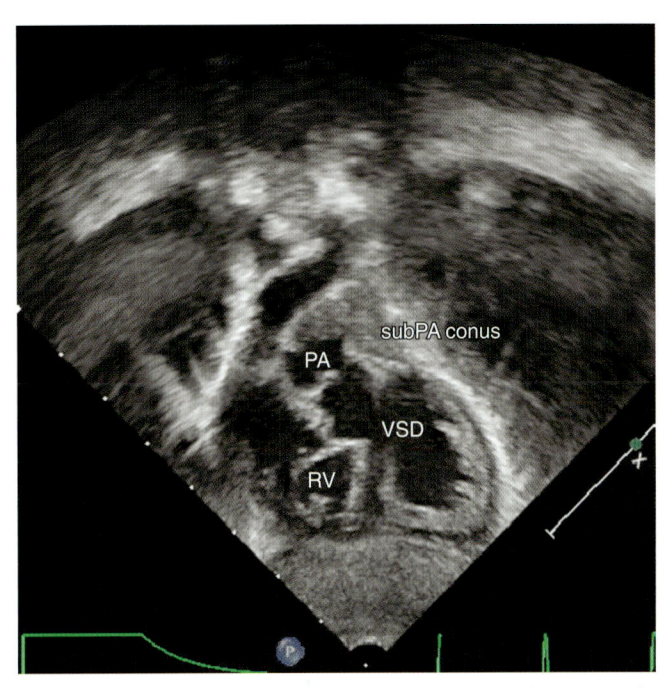

■ **FIGURE 49-42** Subcostal frontal view in a patient with DORV and a large malalignment VSD. The area of subpulmonary conus is identified. The VSD appears to be subpulmonary in this patient, consistent with the Taussig-Bing variant.

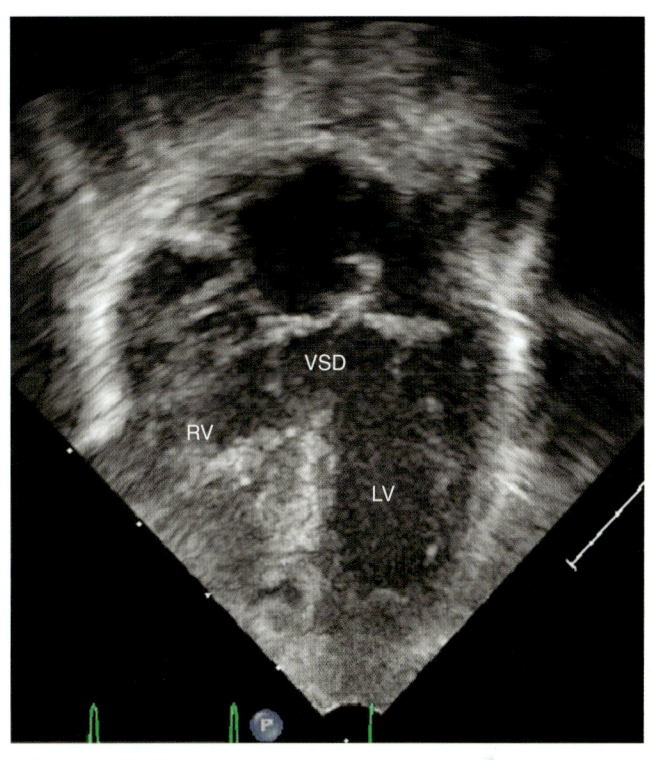

■ **FIGURE 49-44** Apical four-chamber in the same patient with DORV as shown in Figure 49-42. The VSD is large and nonrestrictive.

Computed Tomography

CT has little place in congenital heart disease because of radiation exposure, even though it can demonstrate systemic and pulmonary venous connections, aortic arch and pulmonary artery anomalies, and aortopulmonary collateral arteries. However, most of this can be obtained by cardiac MRI without the significant radiation exposure,

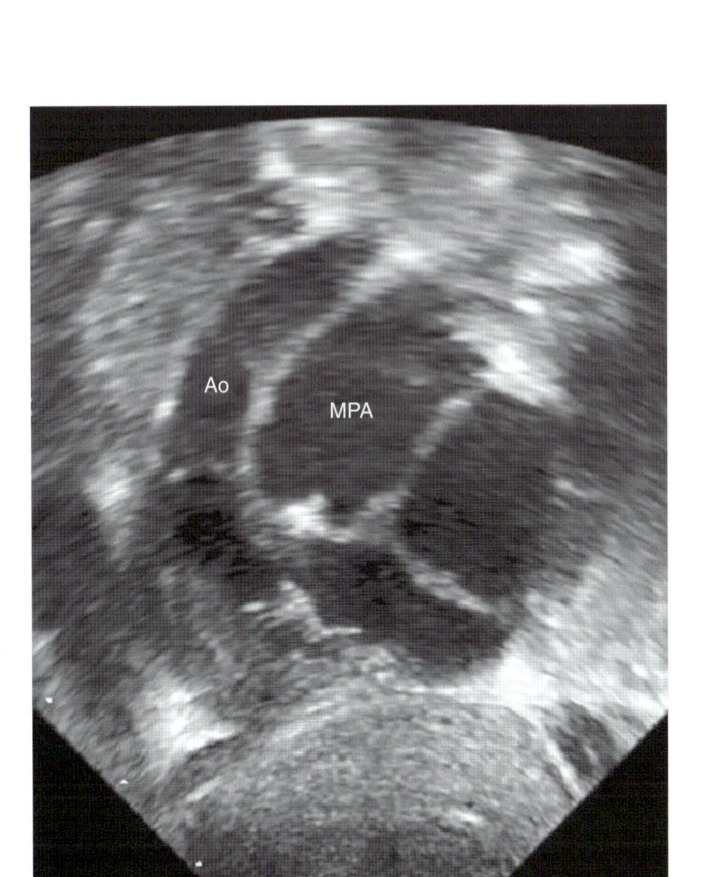

■ **FIGURE 49-43** Subcostal LAO view in the same patient with DORV as shown in Figure 49-42. The aorta is significantly smaller than the PA, despite the fact that the conal septum appears slightly deviated toward the PA.

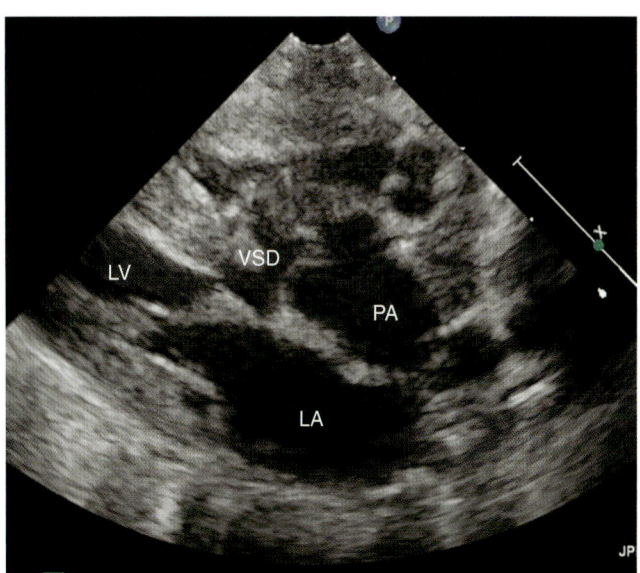

■ **FIGURE 49-45** Parasternal long-axis view in the same patient with DORV as shown in Figure 49-42. There is a modest subpulmonary conus present, forming mitral to pulmonary discontinuity. The VSD appears subpulmonary in this view also.

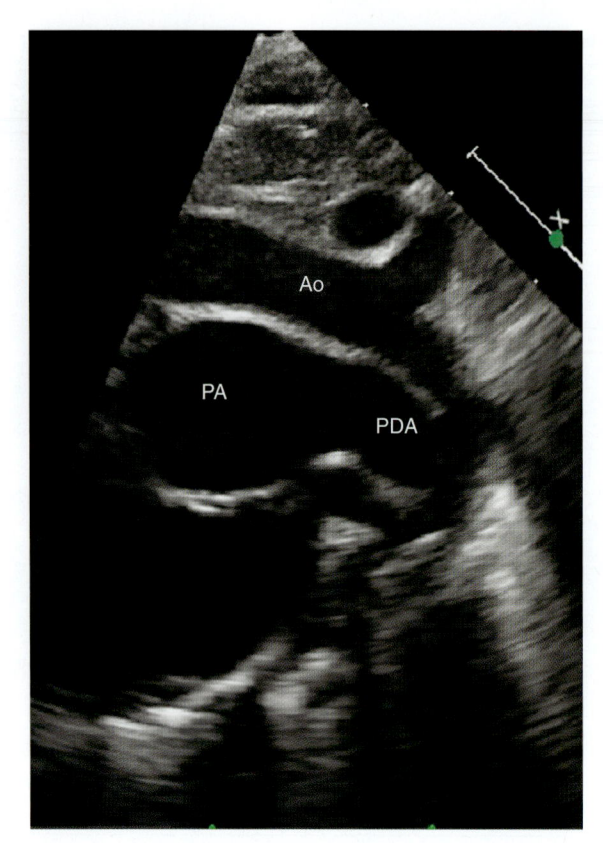

FIGURE 49-46 Suprasternal sagittal view in the same patient with DORV as shown in Figure 49-42. There is significant aortic arch hypoplasia, leading to a large patent ductus arteriosus (PDA). The arch will require augmentation at the time of surgery.

relegating the role of CT largely to situations in which MRI cannot be performed

Magnetic Resonance Imaging

MRI is complementary for imaging complex anomalies of the systemic and pulmonary venous connections, aortic arch and pulmonary artery anomalies, and calculation of cardiac output, regurgitant valve fractions, and systolic and diastolic volumes of the RV and LV (Fig. 49-47). Because DORV can take on many different types of physiology and anatomic variants, see the discussions of individual lesions for the use of MRI. It can also be useful for surgical planning.

Nuclear Medicine: Positron Emission Tomography

This imaging modality can be useful for evaluating cardiac perfusion defects in patients who have had an arterial switch procedure along with coronary button transfer. It is often combined with pre-exercise and postexercise imaging.

Angiography

Angiography remains the gold standard for pressure studies and pulmonary arterial and vascular resistance studies. It should be completed when definitive shunt or ventricular performance data, or full evaluation of the pulmonary artery tree, is required.

DIFFERENTIAL DIAGNOSIS

From Clinical Presentation

The clinical presentation and physical examination will allow differentiation among most forms of complex heart disease. The first differential is usually based on the presence or absence of cyanosis. Whereas cyanosis in the newborn can be seen with single-ventricle physiology and tetralogy of Fallot, profound cyanosis is highly suggestive of TGA or anomalous pulmonary venous connections with obstruction. Pulmonary stenosis with cyanosis can be differentiated by the presence of a loud outflow murmur, and often a thrill is palpated. Cyanosis in the absence of an outflow murmur is suggestive of transposition physiology or pulmonary atresia.

Another common presentation of complex congenital heart disease is pulmonary overcirculation. Patients with a large VSD and no significant outflow obstruction, such as in truncus arteriosus or tetralogy with only mild pulmonary obstruction, will present with increasing overcirculation over days to weeks as the pulmonary vascular resistance falls. This generally causes progressive tachypnea, tiring with feeding, and failure to thrive.

A third common presentation of complex heart disease is shock, manifested by poor peripheral pulses and perfusion, metabolic acidosis, and lethargy. It often manifests on the second or third day of life, and should be one of the first problems considered in an infant presenting with shock. It suggests a lesion with duct-dependent systemic circulation and can include hypoplastic left heart syndrome, critical aortic stenosis, coarctation of the aorta, interrupted aortic arch, and Taussig-Bing–type DORV. Suspicion of these conditions should elicit the immediate initiation of prostaglandins. Coarctation, interrupted arch (unless one or both subclavian arteries arise distal to the interruption), and HLHS with aortic stenosis will result in differential cyanosis, whereas HLHS with aortic atresia or critical aortic stenosis may not.

From Imaging Findings

TGA must be distinguished from other forms of cyanotic heart disease. In general, it can readily be identified by echocardiography or MRI by identifying the aorta arising from the right ventricle. The aorta is identified by its longer distance before branching and giving rise to the coronary arteries. It is also important to demonstrate that the pulmonary artery arises from the left ventricle to distinguish it from DORV and RV-aorta with pulmonary atresia.

Tetralogy of Fallot is identified by the features discussed—namely the normal segmental anatomy with an anterior malalignment VSD and some degree of RVOT obstruction. It should be distinguished from DORV by the absence of subaortic conus (i.e., muscle between the aortic valve and the mitral valve).

The major differential diagnosis of truncus arteriosus is with tetralogy of Fallot with pulmonary atresia. In general,

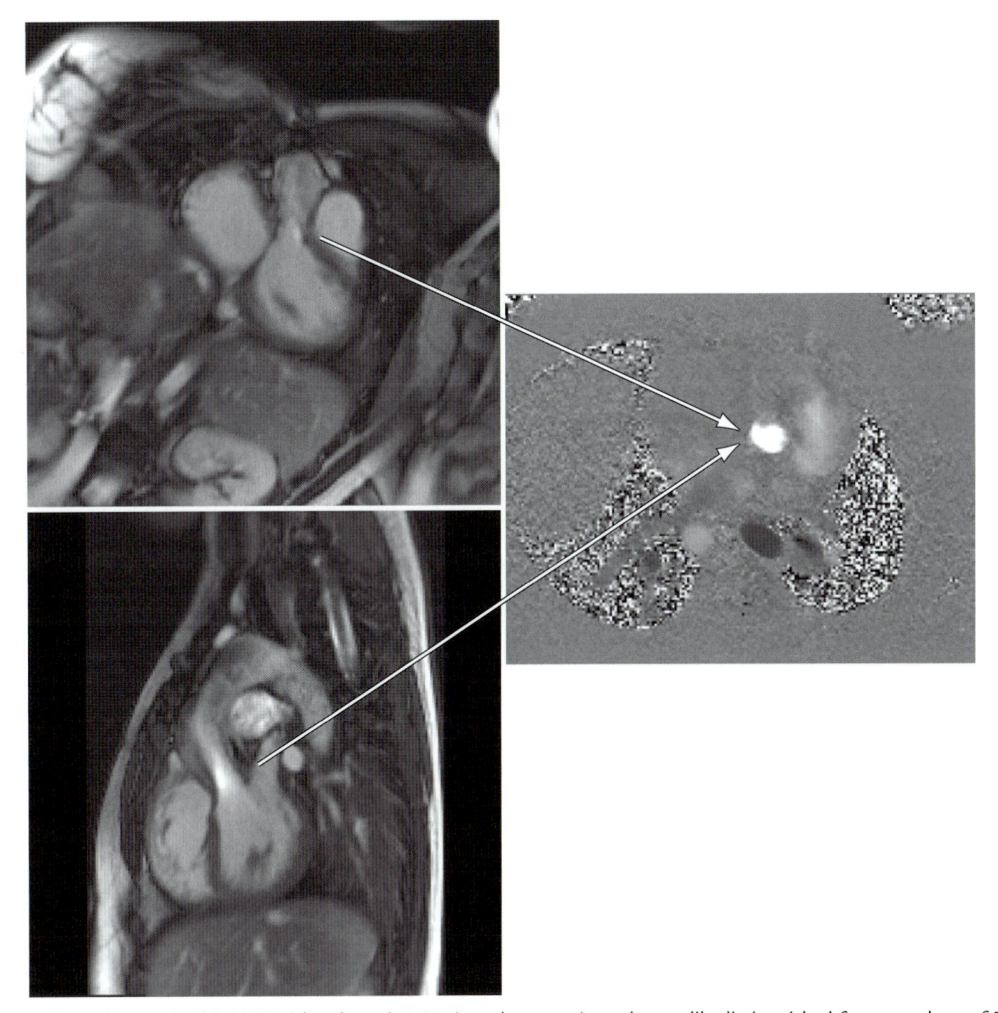

FIGURE 49-47 Patient with repaired DORV with subaortic VSD (tetralogy type) can be readily distinguished from tetralogy of Fallot by the elongated LVOT with a subaortic conus. In this patient, there is mild subaortic acceleration at the level of the conus, seen on the systolic images of orthogonal LVOT cines. This acceleration can be readily quantified by in-plane or through-plane (shown here) velocity mapping and the gradient can be estimated using the modified Bernoulli equation.

tetralogy of Fallot with pulmonary atresia does not have the pulmonary arteries originating from the ascending aorta, as in the Van Praagh classifications 1 to 3. In the case of the pulmonary arteries arising from the descending aorta (Edwards and Collett type 4), the Van Praagh classification would be considered tetralogy of Fallot with pulmonary atresia. Clues that may hint at the diagnosis of truncus arteriosus is the anatomy and morphology of the single semilunar valve (e.g., quadricuspid, dysmorphic) and the coronary artery anatomy, which is commonly abnormal. Hemitruncus is not a form of truncus arteriosus; it has two semilunar valves arising from the heart, with one branch pulmonary artery arising from the ascending aorta.

SYNOPSIS OF TREATMENT OPTIONS

Medical Treatment

In conditions in which there is a suspicion of duct-dependent pulmonary blood flow (e.g., severe pulmonary stenosis, pulmonary atresia without major aortopulmonary collaterals), prostaglandins should be initiated immediately. Suspicion of TGA with cyanosis should also prompt initiation of prostaglandins, although the patient must be watched carefully; this physiologic setup may increase pulmonary blood flow and close the flap valve of the foramen ovale, which actually decreases mixing. Other conditions with duct-dependent systemic circulation (e.g., HLHS, critical aortic stenosis, coarctation, interrupted aortic arch) should also prompt initiation of prostaglandins, ideally immediately after birth if a prenatal diagnosis is obtained. See individual sections.

Conversely, there are conditions with pulmonary overcirculation, which include tetralogy without significant RVOT obstruction (so-called "pink tet"), truncus arteriosus, and some forms of DORV without sufficient pulmonary stenosis. These can often be managed for several months with anticongestive medications such as furosemide and digoxin. Hypercaloric formulas and nasogastric supplements are sometimes required for adequate weight gain. It should be noted that truncus arteriosus and aortopulmonary window are very difficult to manage clinically and are at high risk for the development of early pulmonary vascular disease. Therefore, these conditions are generally repaired in the neonatal period at most centers.

Surgical and Interventional Treatment

The approach to surgical correction of truncus arteriosus type A1 and A2 is the separation of the right and left branch pulmonary arteries from the arterial trunk and association of those branch pulmonary arteries with the right ventricle by construction of an RVOT with a conduit. Reoperation because of conduit stenoses and regurgitation in the homograft is usually done as the child grows. The size of the conduit is, as would be expected, related to how quickly the conduit needs to be replaced, with earlier failure of smaller conduits. Aneurysms may develop at the location of surgical incisures. The openings created by the relocation of the branch pulmonary arteries are closed primarily or with a patch. The truncal valve regurgitation or stenosis is also addressed with valvuloplasty; however, future valve replacement may be needed. Patients should have their truncal valve monitored for progressive valve dysfunction. The VSD must also be closed, usually by a patch.

With aortic arch hypoplasia or interruption, as in type A4 truncus arteriosus, the aortic arch is reconstructed with direct anastomosis between the aortic arch and descending aorta or with conduit. A Lecompte maneuver may be performed as needed. There is, of course, a small risk of recurrent or residual obstruction or aneurysm formation.

The surgical options for single-ventricle, tetralogy of Fallot, and LTGA patients are discussed in their respective sections.

If the patient has L-TGA with an intact ventricular septum, no significant subpulmonary stenosis, and good TV and RV function, most centers advocate diligent observation. Surveillance intervals vary with age but generally would be twice yearly. Medium- and long-term RV function will determine eventual therapy. Natural history studies have shown that most patients begin to show symptoms of significant heart failure by the fourth or fifth decade of life, with worsening systemic right ventricular failure and tricuspid regurgitation.[27] This has prompted some centers to adopt a more aggressive approach, primarily performing a so-called double switch, consisting of an atrial switch and arterial switch operation with the goal of preventing right ventricular failure. Patients who are diagnosed at a later age, generally those without associated lesions, must first undergo pulmonary artery banding to retrain the left ventricle and prepare it for the increased workload of supporting the systemic circulation. This is often done in two stages, with a loose band first applied and then tightened at a later date once the left ventricle has acclimated. The pulmonary artery band itself can often improve symptoms by shifting the ventricular septum and reducing RV-LV interactions and tricuspid regurgitation, leading some to propose this as a palliative procedure. However, most advocate proceeding to a double switch as a long-term strategy, assuming the that LV tolerates the banding.[26]

For patients with L-TGA, large VSD, no evidence of subpulmonary stenosis, and good TV, surgery would be recommended, usually consisting of VSD patch closure along with an atrial switch and an arterial switch (a double switch). Postoperative surveillance intervals vary with age but generally would be twice yearly. For patients with L-TGA, large VSD, and significant subpulmonary stenosis, surgery would be recommended, usually consisting of a Rastelli operation (VSD baffle closure to the aorta) along with an atrial switch and an RV-PA valved homograft conduit.[28] Postoperative surveillance intervals vary with age but generally would be twice yearly. The RV-PA conduit will require future replacement. For patients with L-TGA and hemodynamically significant left-sided TV insufficiency, surgical intervention would be recommended. In general, direct surgical evaluation of the TV must be performed to determine if valvuloplasty or replacement benefits the patient the most. For some L-TGA patients, failed supraventricular tachycardia medical therapy will lead to an invasive electrophysiology study along with radiofrequency ablation of the accessory left-sided pathway. For L-TGA patients with symptomatic complete AV block, insertion of a dual-chamber pacemaker will be required.

Almost all patients with DORV require palliative or corrective surgery for optimal long-term survival. Exceptions to this would include concomitant lethal anomalies. For patients with DORV, subaortic VSD, and no significant pulmonary stenosis, surgery is usually performed in the neonatal period, usually consisting of VSD baffle closure to the aorta. Postoperative surveillance intervals vary with age but generally would be twice yearly. For patients with DORV, subaortic VSD, and significant pulmonary stenosis, surgery is usually performed in the infant period, usually consisting of VSD baffle closure to the aorta and relief of the subpulmonary stenosis. Postoperative surveillance intervals vary with age but generally would be twice yearly. For patients with DORV and subpulmonary VSD, surgery would be recommended early, usually consisting of VSD patch closure to align the PA with the LV, along with an arterial switch procedure. Aortic arch problems require attention at the same procedure. Postoperative surveillance intervals vary with age but generally would be twice yearly. For patients with DORV and a doubly committed VSD, surgery would be recommended early, usually consisting of VSD baffle closure to the aorta. Postoperative surveillance intervals vary with age but generally would be twice yearly. For patients with DORV and noncommitted VSD, the surgical pathway may involve complex palliation while waiting for possible corrective repair. For patients with complex DORV, including inlet abnormalities, AV valve straddle, unbalanced ventricles, and/or complex outlet anatomy, the surgical pathway often involves offering staged Fontan palliation or transplantion.[29]

KEY POINTS

- Dextrotransposition of the great arteries (DTGA) is defined as isolated ventriculoarterial discordance, with the aorta arising from the right ventricle and the main pulmonary artery arising from the left ventricle.
- The mainstay of preoperative imaging for DTGA is echocardiography. Care must be taken to evaluate the adequacy of the ASD and patent ductus arteriosus (PDA) for mixing, presence and type of VSD, coronary origins and proximal course in preparation for an arterial switch, precise relationship of the proximal great vessels and semilunar valves, presence of subarterial obstruction, and aortic arch.
- MRI plays an increasingly important role in postoperative imaging of complex congenital heart disease. In certain situations, preoperative imaging allows for precise quantification of ventricular volumes, mass and ejection, cardiac index, valvular regurgitation, valvular stenosis, main and branch pulmonary artery stenosis, residual arch obstruction, baffle leaks and residual septal defect (Qp/Qs ratio). It is also becoming the standard for identifying coronary perfusion defects (adenosine perfusion imaging) and screening for evidence of myocardial scar or fibrosis (delayed enhancement imaging).
- Preoperative imaging of tetralogy of Fallot is also routinely performed by echocardiography, defining the conotruncal anatomy, degree and location of RVOT obstruction, presence and location of additional VSDs, presence and location of any aortopulmonary collaterals, arch sidedness and branching pattern, and delineation of the proximal coronary arteries with particular attention to whether any major coronary branches cross the RVOT.
- Truncus arteriosus is defined as a heart with a single arterial trunk arising from it that supplies the systemic, pulmonary, and coronary circulations.
- The Edwards and Collett and Van Praagh classifications are the most widely used systems to classify truncus arteriosus.
- Almost all truncal lesions have associated ventricular septal defects. There is also truncal valve pathology, more commonly with regurgitation and less commonly with stenosis and abnormalities associated with the coronary arteries.
- The differential diagnosis of truncus arteriosus is with tetralogy of Fallot with pulmonary atresia. Hemitruncus is not a form of truncus arteriosus.
- Functional single ventricles are those hearts that have either one usable pumping chamber or two pumping chambers, which cannot be separated surgically.
- Two or three surgeries are needed to separate the systemic and pulmonary circulations. The first is a modified Blalock-Taussig shunt, Norwood stage I procedure, PA banding, or nothing (depending on the anatomy). The second is a bidirectional Glenn or hemi-Fontan procedure, and the final surgery is the Fontan operation.
- In the Fontan physiology, blood flows passively from the systemic veins into the lungs.
- Echocardiography and cardiac MRI are mainstays of imaging for these patients. Assessment of the various surgical manipulations at the different stages of surgery is key to successful repair.
- For L-TGA or corrected transposition, monitoring RV function is key. Some advocate a double switch, which consists of a Senning and arterial switch operation. A Rastelli-type operation may be needed for patients with pulmonic stenosis. Echocardiography and cardiac MRI are the mainstays of imaging.
- DORV is actually composed of many diseases. Patients may have ventricular septal defect, tetralogy of Fallot, TGA, or single-ventricle physiology. Different types of repairs are needed. Echocardiography and cardiac MRI are the mainstays of imaging.

REFERENCES

1. Hoffman JIE, Kaplan S. The incidence of congenital heart disease. J Am Coll Cardiol 2002; 39:1890-1900.
2. Fyler DC, Buckley LP, Hellenbrand WE. Report of the New England Regional Infant Cardiac Program. Pediatrics 1980; 65:377-461.
3. Perloff JK. Congenital heart disease in adults. A new cardiovascular subspecialty. Circulation 1991; 84:1881-1890.
4. Donnelly LF, Hurst DR, Strife JL, Shapiro R. Plain-film assessment of the neonate with D-transposition of the great vessels. Pediatric Radiology 1995; 25:195-197.
5. Centers for Disease Control and Prevention (CDC). Improved national prevalence estimates for 18 selected major birth defects—United States, 1999-2001. MMWR Morb Mortal Wkly Rep 2006; 54:1301-1305.
6. Goldmuntz E, Clark BJ, Mitchell LE, et al. Frequency of 22q11 deletions in patients with conotruncal defects. J Am Coll Cardiol 1998; 32:492-498.
7. Krantz ID, Smith R, Colliton RP, et al. Jagged1 mutations in patients ascertained with isolated congenital heart defects. Am J Med Genet 1999; 84:56-60.
8. Fallot E-LA. Contribution a l'anatomie pathologique de la maladie bleue (cyanose cardiaque). Marseille Médical 1888; 25:77-93; 138-158; 207-223; 341-354; 370-386; 403-420.
9. Dabizzi RP, Caprioli G, Aiazzi L, et al. Distribution and anomalies of coronary arteries in tetralogy of Fallot. Circulation 1980; 61:95-102.
10. Roche KJ, Rivera R, Argilla M, et al. Assessment of vasculature using combined MRI and MR angiography. Am J Roentgenol 2004; 182:861-866.
11. Ming-Ting W, Yi-Luan H, Kai-Sheng H, et al. Influence of pulmonary regurgitation inequality on differential perfusion of the lungs in tetralogy of Fallot after repair: a phase-contrast magnetic resonance imaging and perfusion scintigraphy study [abstract]. J Am Coll Cardiol 2007; 49:1880-1886.
12. Harris MA, Weinberg PM, Whitehead KK, Fogel MA. Usefulness of branch pulmonary artery regurgitant fraction to estimate the relative right and left pulmonary vascular resistances in congenital heart disease. Am J Cardiol 2005; 95:1514-1517.
13. Kang IS, Redington AN, Benson LN, et al. Differential regurgitation in branch pulmonary arteries after repair of tetralogy of Fallot: a phase-contrast cine magnetic resonance study. Circulation 2003; 107:2938-2943.
14. Collett RW, Edwards JE. Persistent truncus arteriosus: a classification according to anatomic types. Surg Clin North Am 1949; 29:1245-1270.
15. Van Praagh R, Van Praagh S. The anatomy of common aorticopulmonary trunk (truncus arteriosus communis) and its embryologic implications. A study of 57 necropsy cases. Am J Cardiol 1965; 16:406-425.
16. Jacobs ML. Congenital Heart Surgery Nomenclature and Database Project: truncus arteriosus. Ann Thorac Surg 2000; 69:S50-S55.

17. Van Praagh R. Terminology of congenital heart disease. Glossary and commentary. Circulation 1977; 56:139-143.
18. Edwards JE. Congenital malformations of the heart and great vessels. In Gould SE (ed). Pathology of the Heart. Springfield, Ill, Charles C Thomas, 1953, pp 406-407.
19. Natowicz M, Kelley RI. Association of Turner syndrome with hypoplastic left-heart syndrome. Am J Dis Child 1987; 141:218-220.
20. Norwood WI, Lang P, Hansen DD. Physiologic repair of aortic atresia–hypoplastic left heart syndrome. N Engl J Med 1983; 308:23-26.
21. Fogel MA, Weinberg PM, Chin AJ, et al. Late ventricular geometry and performance changes of functional single ventricle throughout staged fontan reconstruction assessed by magnetic resonance imaging. J Am Coll Cardiol 1996; 28:212-221.
22. Whitehead KK, Gillespie MJ, Harris MA, et al. Non-invasive quantification of systemic to pulmonary collateral flow: a major source of inefficiency in patients with superior cavopulmonary connections. Circ Cardiovasc Imaging 2009; 2:405-411.
23. Fontan F, Baudet E. Surgical repair of tricuspid atresia. Thorax 1971; 26:240-248.
24. Allen HD, Gutgesell HP, Clark EB, Driscoll DJ. Moss and Adams' Heart Disease in Infants, Children, and Adolescents, 7th ed. Lippincott Williams & Wilkins, 2008, pp 1087-1227.
25. Kuehl KS, Loffredo CA. Genetic and environmental influences on malformations of the cardiac outflow tract. Expert Rev Cardiovasc Ther 2005; 3:1125-1130.
26. Duncan BW, Mee RB, Mesia CI, et al. Results of the double switch operation for congenitally corrected transposition of the great arteries. Eur J Cardiothorac Surg 2003; 24:11-19.
27. Graham TP, Jr., Bernard YD, Mellen BG et al. Long-term outcome in congenitally corrected transposition of the great arteries: a multi-institutional study. J Am Coll Cardiol 2000; 36:255-261.
28. Konstantinov IE, Williams WG. Atrial switch and Rastelli operation for congenitally corrected transposition with ventricular septal defect and pulmonary stenosis. Oper Tech Thorac Cardiovasc Surg 2003; 8:160-166.
29. Lecompte Y, Batisse A, DiCarlo D. Double-outlet right ventricle: a surgical synthesis. Adv Card Surg 1993; 4:109-136.

CHAPTER 50

Magnetic Resonance Imaging in the Postoperative Evaluation of the Patient with Congenital Heart Disease

Alison Knauth Meadows, Karen G. Ordovas, Charles B. Higgins, and Gautham P. Reddy

In recent years, advances in pediatric cardiovascular surgery, catheter-based interventional therapies, intensive care, and medical management have dramatically changed the landscape of the field of congenital heart disease (CHD). The complexity of the anatomy and physiology of patients surviving with CHD is increasing exponentially; the majority will survive to adulthood, and the need for reintervention is common. This changing field is placing new demands on imaging to plan medical management as well as to identify the need for and timing of reintervention. A number of imaging modalities are available to the clinician and imaging specialist when it comes to these evaluations. Given its ability to assess both anatomy and function, magnetic resonance imaging (MRI) holds a unique and growing position among these.

Echocardiography has been and remains a mainstay of imaging in CHD. Despite its importance in rapid diagnosis and follow-up, it has limitations in the evaluation of the postoperative patient with CHD. Postoperative scar, chest wall deformities, overlying lung tissue, and large body size as the patient ages often result in suboptimal transthoracic echocardiographic windows. Transesophageal echocardiography, although providing improved acoustic windows, is limited by its small field of view and more invasive nature, often requiring deep sedation or general anesthesia.

Cardiac catheterization, employing x-ray fluoroscopy and contrast angiography, has an expanding role in minimally invasive interventions, but its role as a diagnostic procedure is rapidly diminishing. This is in part due to its limitation as a two-dimensional projection imaging technique with poor soft tissue contrast and the substantial ionizing radiation exposure involved; also, both diagnostic analysis and functional analysis are often better performed with noninvasive imaging techniques.

Computed tomography (CT) has been useful in evaluating vascular anatomy, and with the advent of high-resolution CT and cardiac gating, it has emerged as a useful tool for assessment of intracardiac anatomy, coronary artery anatomy, and myocardial function. Nevertheless, the temporal resolution of cardiac CT remains limited, and advances in CT imaging technology have often come with increases in exposure to ionizing radiation.

MRI has emerged during the past few decades as an alternative, complementary, and frequently superior imaging modality for the investigation of anatomy and function in the postoperative CHD patient. It has many advantages over other imaging modalities. It does not require the use of iodinated contrast agents and does not involve exposure to ionizing radiation. This is particularly important in a population of patients who have been and continue to be exposed to large doses of contrast agent and radiation during hemodynamic and interventional catheterization. In addition, many of these patients are children, who are more susceptible to the adverse effects of radiation. Major advances in MRI hardware and software, including advanced coil design, faster gradients, new pulse sequences, and faster image reconstruction techniques, allow rapid, high-resolution imaging of complex anatomy and accurate, quantitative assessment of function.

This chapter highlights the MRI techniques frequently employed to evaluate the anatomy and physiology of the postoperative CHD patient. It provides information about the general application of MRI in this population of patients as well as sample protocols and guidelines for its use in the more commonly encountered lesions referred for MRI.

POSTOPERATIVE ASSESSMENT

A number of MRI techniques are useful to the examination of the anatomy and physiology of the postoperative CHD patient. These techniques are detailed in Chapters 13 to 17. Here, their importance to this population is highlighted.

Cine Magnetic Resonance Imaging

ECG-gated gradient-echo sequences can be employed to provide multiple images throughout the cardiac cycle in prescribed anatomic locations. Display of these images in a cine mode permits visualization of the dynamic motion of the heart and vessels.[1-3] Cine MRI techniques, at a minimum, allow assessment of anatomy. More important, such techniques allow qualitative and quantitative assessment of function. Specifically, cine MRI permits quantification of chamber volumes, myocardial mass, and ventricular function. Further, cine MRI allows qualitative assessment of focal and global wall motion abnormalities, qualitative and quantitative assessment of valve disease (including the mechanism and severity of valve regurgitation and the location and severity of valve stenoses), identification and quantification of intracardiac and extracardiac shunts, and visualization of other areas of flow turbulence.

Cine MRI is the principal tool used to quantitatively assess ventricular function. Such techniques, both fast gradient-echo[4-7] and balanced steady-state free precession,[1,2] have been extensively evaluated and validated.[8,9] Briefly, evaluation of function begins with obtaining a series of contiguous cine slices along the short axis of the ventricles, extending from base to apex. The prescription of such slices should be performed from a true four-chamber view at end-diastole to ensure coverage of the entire ventricular mass (Fig. 50-1). These images are played back in a cine loop, and the end-systolic and end-diastolic phases are chosen. The endocardial borders are traced at both time points, and the epicardial borders are traced at one of the two time points (Fig. 50-2). Ventricular volumes are then calculated as the sum of the traced volumes (area × slice thickness). Myocardial mass is calculated as the myocardial muscle volume × 1.05 g/mm³ (density of myocardium). From these data, ventricular

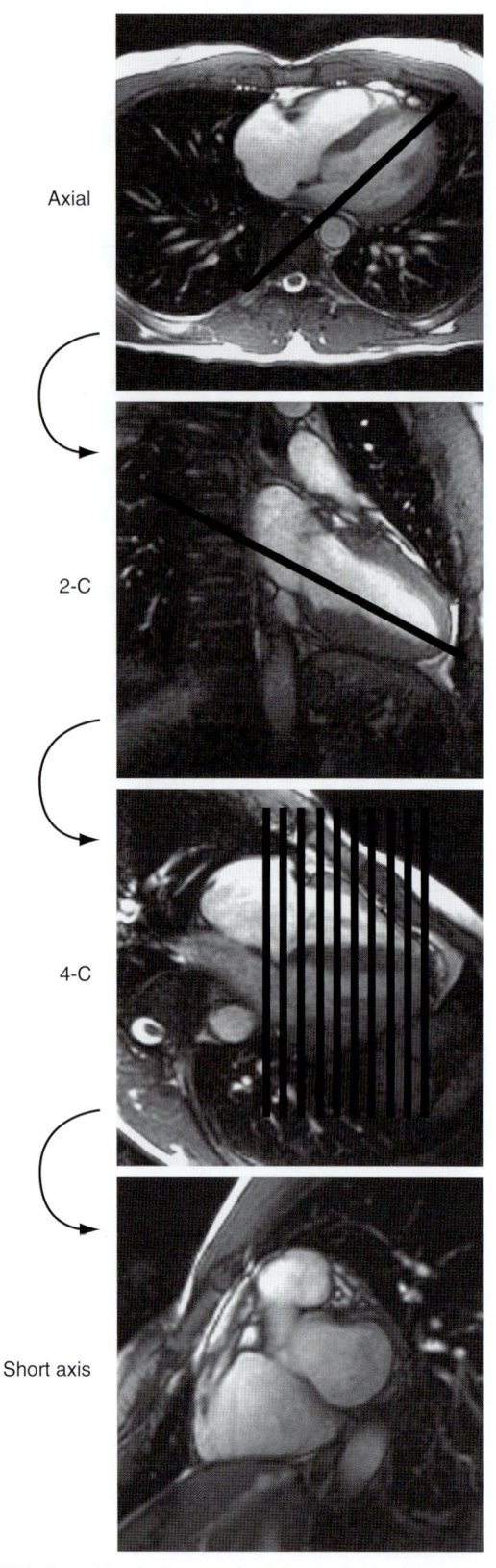

■ **FIGURE 50-1** To obtain a stack of short-axis cine images, a two-chamber (2-C) view is prescribed from an axial cine, then a four-chamber (4-C) view is prescribed from the two-chamber cine, then a short-axis stack is prescribed from the four-chamber cine at end-diastole.

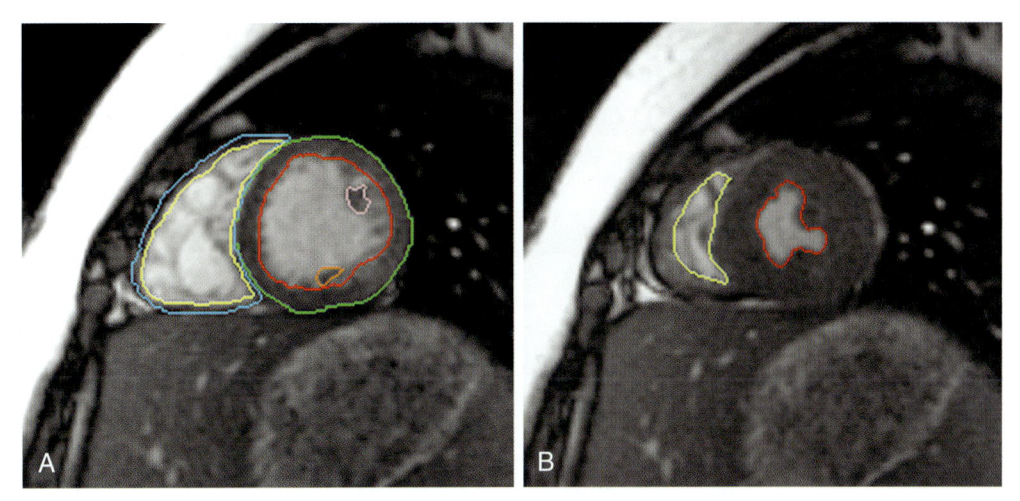

FIGURE 50-2 Single image from a stack of short-axis cine images at end-diastole (**A**) and end-systole (**B**). Right and left ventricular endocardial contours are drawn at end-systole, and endocardial and epicardial contours are drawn at end-diastole. It is from these data that chamber volumes, myocardial mass, and ventricular function are derived.

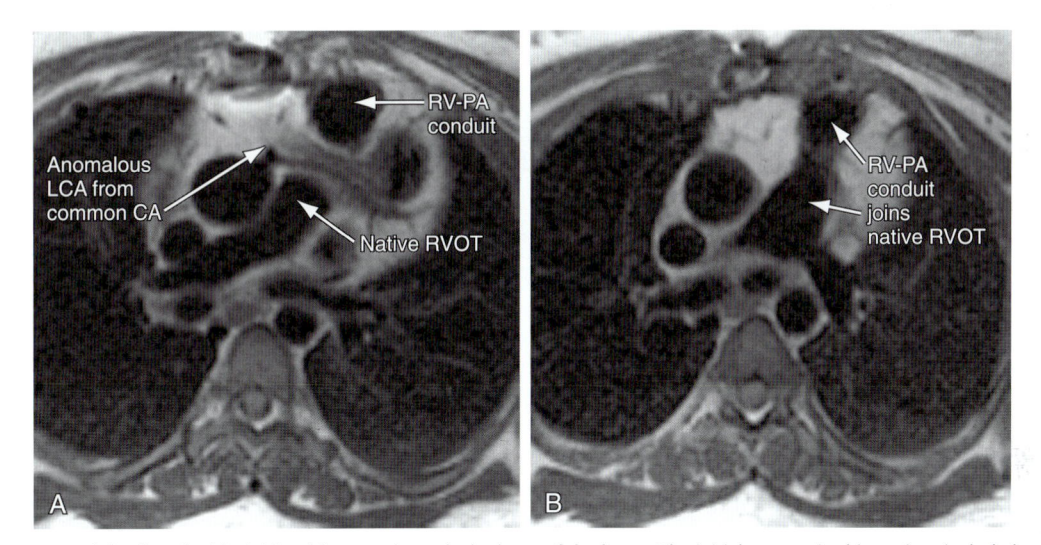

FIGURE 50-3 Two axial spin-echo black blood images through the base of the heart. The initial surgery in this patient included a right ventricle-to-pulmonary artery conduit, which subsequently became stenotic. Unknown to this patient's caregivers was the fact that the indication for a conduit rather than a transannular patch was an anomalous left coronary artery (LCA) from the right that traversed the right ventricular outflow tract (RVOT). This was important for the management of her conduit stenosis as a percutaneous stent placement may have caused coronary compression. The aorta (Ao), native pulmonary artery (native RVOT), right ventricle-to-pulmonary artery conduit (RV-PA conduit), and anomalous coronary artery are identified (**A**). CA, coronary artery. The connection of the conduit and native pulmonary artery is demonstrated (**B**).

end-diastolic volume, end-systolic volume, stroke volume, ejection fraction, myocardial mass, and mass-to-volume ratio can be calculated for both the right and left ventricles. Most computer workstation software packages for cardiac MRI analysis provide semiautomated postprocessing tools to maximize efficiency.

Spin-Echo (Black Blood) Imaging

ECG-gated spin-echo sequences (black blood imaging) represent another important tool for imaging in the postoperative CHD patient. Despite providing only static information, black blood imaging has many benefits in this population. It allows assessment of anatomy with thin slices, high spatial resolution, and excellent blood-myocardium and blood-vessel wall contrast (Fig. 50-3).

Black blood techniques are superb for evaluation of the spatial relationship between cardiovascular and other intrathoracic structures, such as the chest wall and the tracheobronchial tree. These features hold particular relevance in delineation of complicated postsurgical cardiac anatomy. Such techniques are also less susceptible to artifact from metallic implanted devices, such as stents, coils, occluder devices, clips, and sternal wires, which are commonly seen in the postoperative CHD patient.

Flow Quantification

Electrocardiography-gated gradient-echo sequences with flow-encoding gradients are used to quantify the velocity and flow of blood (Fig. 50-4).[10] These sequences are referred to as velocity-encoded cine MRI or phase contrast

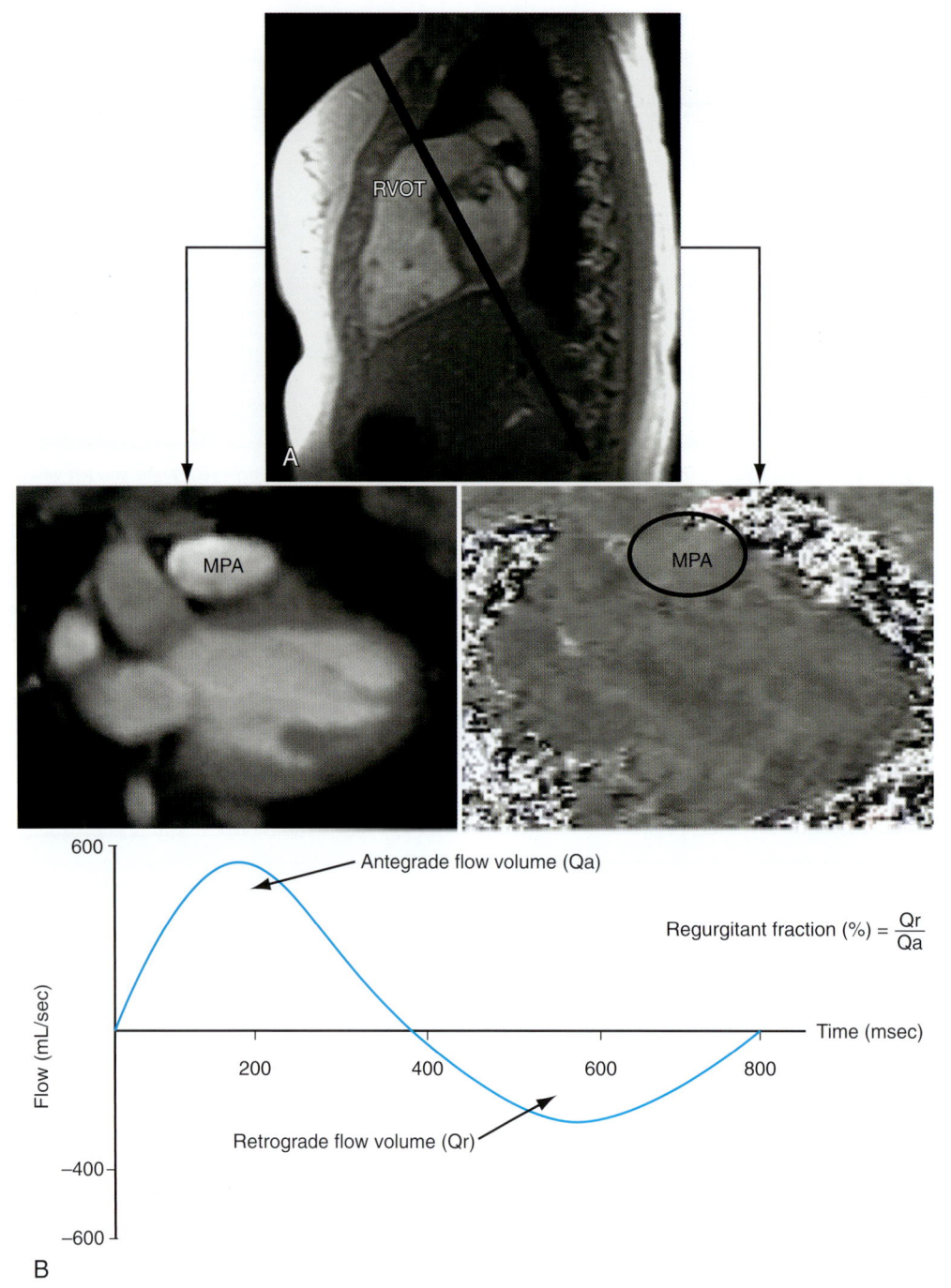

FIGURE 50-4 From an image in the plane of the right ventricular outflow tract (RVOT), an imaging plane is chosen to capture the cross section of the main pulmonary artery (**A**). Velocity-encoded cine MRI is then performed in this plane to produce a magnitude (*bottom left*) and phase (*bottom right*) image (**A**). A region of interest encompassing the main pulmonary artery (MPA) is chosen for each image in the cardiac cycle. From these data, net flow is obtained. Flow is then displayed, allowing the calculation of peak velocity, net forward flow, and regurgitant fraction (**B**).

MRI. Two-dimensional velocity-encoded cine MRI sequences are commonly used in clinical practice. They can be used to quantify cardiac output, pulmonary-to-systemic flow ratio (shunt), valvular regurgitation, differential lung perfusion, and coronary flow reserve. They can be used to observe the location and severity of flow obstruction. In addition, velocity-encoded cine MRI assessment of flow is useful for corroboration of volumetric data obtained with cine imaging to ensure the interpreting physician that the data obtained are accurate.

Newer velocity-encoded cine MRI sequences allow resolution of velocity vectors in three directions, with spatial coverage of a three-dimensional volume, temporally resolved throughout the cardiac cycle. Such techniques have been coined seven-dimensional flow encoding.[11,12] These techniques have the advantage of providing complete spatial and temporal resolution of velocity with a higher signal-to-noise ratio than in two-dimensional methods. Postprocessing tools permit the construction of vector field plots that highlight the intracardiac and intravascular nature of flow. Although they are currently limited by long scan durations, faster imaging techniques will likely allow such methods to reach clinical practice in the near future.

Gadolinium-Enhanced Three-Dimensional Angiography

Three-dimensional magnetic resonance angiography (MRA) sequences are typically not ECG-gated and thus do not allow optimal assessment of intracardiac structures. Regardless, such techniques provide excellent depiction of arterial and venous vascular structures (Fig. 50-5). In the population of postoperative CHD patients, three-dimensional MRA fills a significant diagnostic role. It can be used to diagnose systemic arterial anomalies, such as aortopulmonary collaterals, shunts, vascular rings, and coarctation. It is useful in the diagnosis of pulmonary arterial abnormalities, such as focal and diffuse stenoses and abnormal distal arborization patterns. Three-dimensional MRA methods are also useful for investigation of systemic and pulmonary venous abnormalities, both congenital anomalies and postoperative abnormalities. Finally, three-dimensional MRA is useful for evaluation of the relation between vascular and other thoracic structures. With the development of faster imaging techniques, ECG-gated three-dimensional MRA sequences are becoming more practical, allowing evaluation of intracardiac anatomy and acquisition of time-resolved three-dimensional MRA data sets.[13]

Coronary Artery Imaging, Perfusion Imaging, and Myocardial Viability

Coronary artery abnormalities and ischemia are important issues to be investigated in postoperative CHD patients. Not only is this population of patients aging sufficiently to develop atherosclerotic coronary artery disease, they also commonly have congenitally abnormal or postoperatively acquired coronary artery lesions. It is not uncommon to find an anomalous origin or course of the left or right coronary artery, postsurgical coronary obstruction (i.e., after arterial switch for transposition of the great arteries), coronary artery thrombus (Fig. 50-6), or abnormal fistulous connections (i.e., pulmonary atresia with intact ventricular septum and right ventricle–dependent coronary circulation). Identification of such abnormalities is often critical to planning of reintervention or medical management. There is growing evidence to support that myocardial delayed hyperenhancement in a number of subsets of postoperative CHD patients is predictive of poor outcome, including patients with tetralogy of Fallot (Fig. 50-7).[14,15] Delayed hyperenhancement has been observed in other postoperative patients with CHD as well, the significance of which is being explored and elucidated.[16,17] In summary, although it is still not as robust as routine coronary artery angiography with x-ray fluoroscopy or ECG-gated CT

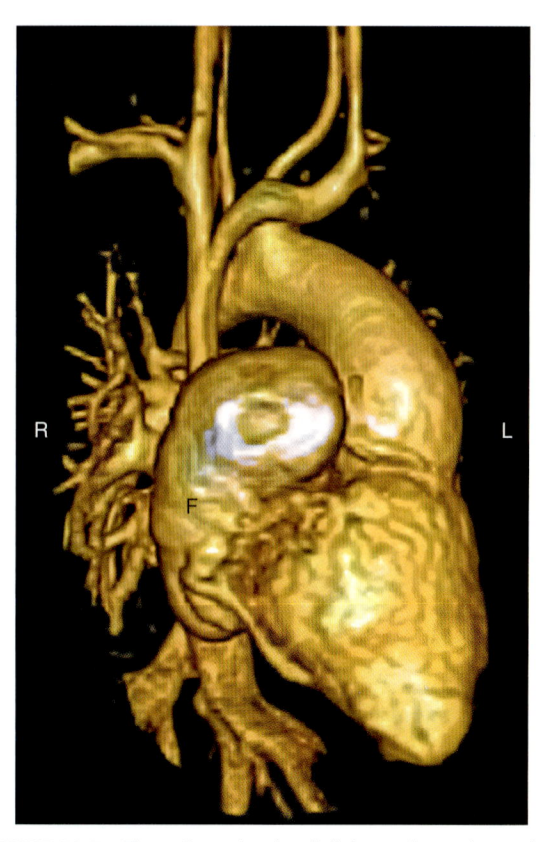

■ **FIGURE 50-5** Three-dimensional gadolinium-enhanced MRA in a patient with single ventricle after the Fontan procedure. The image is displayed as a three-dimensional volume rendered reconstruction. A dilated Fontan pathway (F) is visualized.

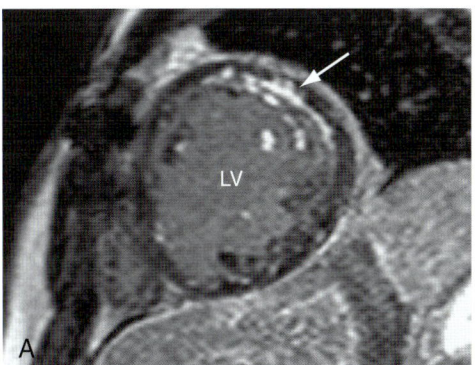

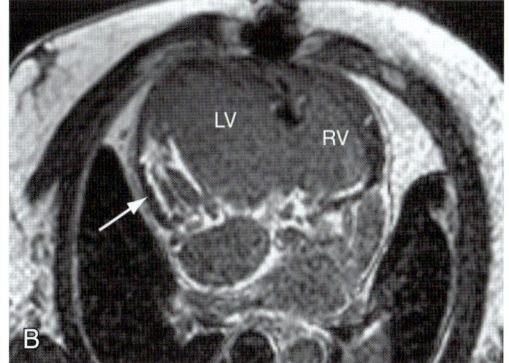

■ **FIGURE 50-6** Short-axis (**A**) and four-chamber (**B**) cine images revealing delayed hyperenhancement (*arrow*) in the left circumflex distribution in this patient with {S,L,L} double-inlet left ventricle (LV).

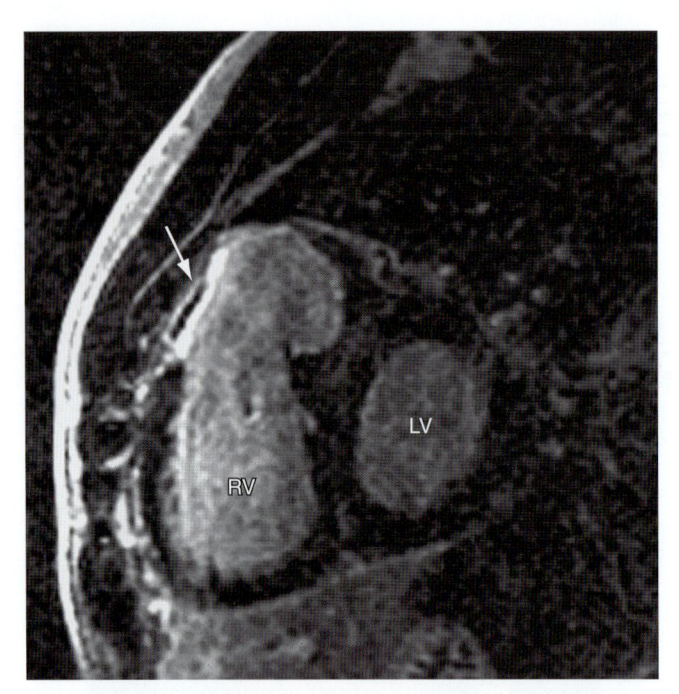

FIGURE 50-7 In this short-axis view of the right ventricular outflow tract, delayed hyperenhancement is present at the location of the ventriculotomy and transannular patch (*arrow*). The right ventricle (RV) and left ventricle (LV) are labeled for orientation.

angiography at investigating distal coronary artery lesions, MRI can image proximal coronary arteries well,[18-21] evaluate myocardial perfusion and viability,[22-26] and allow stress testing,[27-30] all noninvasively without exposure to contrast agents and ionizing radiation.

CLINICAL PRESENTATION

The clinical presentation indicating need for MRI varies across this broad population of patients. MRI is often requested strictly for monitoring of the effects of residual hemodynamic burdens to guide recommendations for additional interventions. Other times, a postoperative CHD patient has an urgent issue related to vascular obstruction, valve obstruction or insufficiency, abnormalities in ventricular function, or coronary ischemia. This is detailed in the following algorithms.

IMAGING INDICATIONS AND ALGORITHMS

The indications for MRI in the postoperative CHD patient are evolving and expanding as MRI technology advances and this population becomes more complex. In general, MRI is indicated in this population when transthoracic echocardiography is insufficient to provide adequate diagnostic information, as an alternative to invasive and costly diagnostic catheterization, and when the unique capabilities of MRI can be exploited.

MRI is commonly applied to the evaluation of patients who have undergone either palliation or repair with the following CHD: tetralogy of Fallot, transposition of the great arteries, coarctation of the aorta, and single-ventricle lesions. For each of these anomalies, the congenital heart lesion is described, the types of repair are detailed, the common residual hemodynamic burdens are summarized, sample MRI protocols are outlined, and recommendations for baseline and follow-up MRI evaluation are suggested.

IMAGING TECHNIQUE AND FINDINGS
Tetralogy of Fallot

Tetralogy of Fallot (TOF), the most common form of cyanotic CHD, accounts for approximately 10% of all CHD and represents a large portion of postoperative CHD patients. This malformation consists of one embryologic abnormality, namely, anterior malalignment of the infundibular septum, leading to four constant features: malalignment ventricular septal defect, subvalvular (infundibular) and valvular pulmonary stenosis, overriding aorta, and right ventricular hypertrophy. Patients with TOF compose a varied group ranging from TOF with pulmonary atresia and multiple aortopulmonary collateral vessels to TOF with mild pulmonary stenosis.

Repair is also varied and has evolved during the past few decades. Early repair in the first few months of life is now possible and recommended as standard of care. Older patients referred for MRI will likely have undergone initial palliation to augment pulmonary blood flow (e.g., Blalock-Taussig, Waterston, or Potts shunt) with later definitive repair. The goals of definitive repair are to close the ventricular septal defect and to relieve right ventricular outflow tract obstruction (placement of a right ventricle–to–pulmonary artery conduit in patients with pulmonary atresia, placement of a transannular patch in those with severe pulmonary stenosis, or infundibular muscle resection in those with mild pulmonary stenosis).

Increasingly rare, imaging specialists will continue to see patients with only palliated TOF, pulmonary atresia, and multiple aortopulmonary collaterals. The goal of MRI in these patients is to delineate the anatomy of the pulmonary vascular bed and aortopulmonary collaterals. In this way, MRI can aid in determination of a patient's candidacy for definitive repair.

Postoperative Management

Most patients with repaired TOF will have a certain degree of pulmonary regurgitation or stenosis, which has been shown to result in right ventricular dilation and dysfunction. In addition, progressive right ventricular dilation often leads to tricuspid valve annular stretch and ultimately regurgitation, which perpetuates continued right ventricular dilation. In addition, many patients with repaired TOF will have abnormal peripheral pulmonary vasculature and residual aortopulmonary collaterals, all of which contribute to their hemodynamic burden. Multiple studies in the recent literature have demonstrated that right ventricular dilation and dysfunction, as determined by MRI, predict adverse outcomes such as symptoms of right-sided heart failure, major arrhythmic events, and even death.[31] Right ventricular dilation and dysfunction will often be detected by MRI before the onset of obvious clinical symptoms. In addition, delayed hyperenhance-

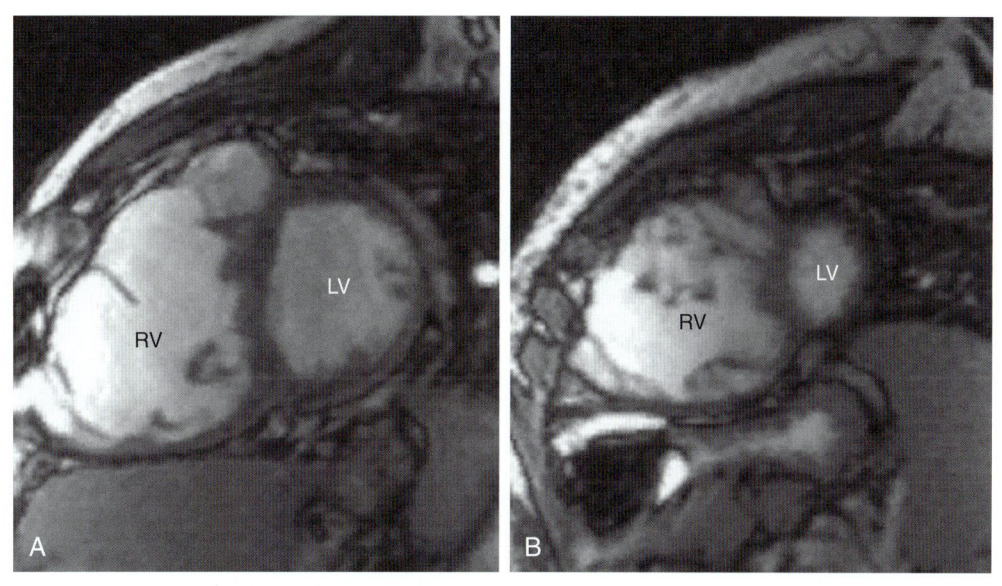

FIGURE 50-8 Cine images at one location in the short-axis plane of the ventricles in a patient with repaired tetralogy of Fallot at end-diastole (**A**) and end-systole (**B**). The right ventricle (RV) is severely enlarged. Analysis demonstrated severely depressed function. LV, left ventricle.

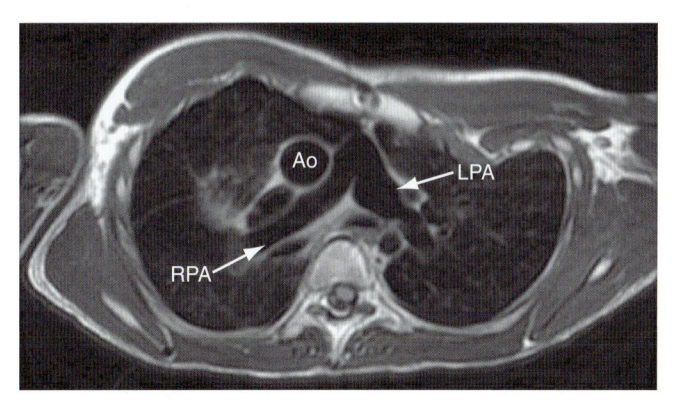

FIGURE 50-9 Black blood imaging at the level of the branch pulmonary arteries in a patient with tetralogy of Fallot. The right pulmonary artery (RPA) is mildly hypoplastic and the left pulmonary artery (LPA) is dilated. Ao, aorta.

ment has been shown to correlate with adverse outcomes in patients with repaired TOF.[32]

For these reasons, MRI is useful in this population to delineate anatomy; to identify distal pulmonary vascular lesions; to identify the location and severity of pulmonary stenosis; to quantify pulmonary regurgitation; to quantify right and left ventricular mass, volumes, and function; and to identify regions of myocardial scar.

MRI for a patient with TOF may include the following:

- Four-chamber cine MRI for qualitative assessment of atrial and ventricular chamber size and identification of tricuspid valve regurgitation.
- Short-axis cine MRI to quantify biventricular mass, volume, and function (Fig. 50-8).
- Axial black blood MRI for assessment of chambers as well as branch pulmonary arteries and an overall look at coronary artery anatomy (Fig. 50-9; see also Fig. 50-3A).
- Three-dimensional MRA can be useful for identification of arch abnormalities, including right aortic arch and branch vessel abnormalities; for delineation of aortopulmonary collaterals; and for identification of postsurgical abnormalities, such as stenotic or absent subclavian arteries in the setting of previous palliative shunts.
- Flow quantification. Velocity-encoded cine MRI is performed to quantify flow and degree of obstruction, if present. A two-dimensional plane is chosen across the main pulmonary artery for quantification of right ventricular stroke volume and pulmonary regurgitation (as a net volume as well as a percentage of the stroke volume; see Fig. 50-4). In addition, a two-dimensional plane can be prescribed in the plane of the right ventricular outflow tract to obtain a peak velocity and to quantify a peak pressure gradient if echocardiographic assessment proved insufficient.
- Delayed hyperenhancement to look for myocardial scar (see Fig. 50-7).

At many institutions, MRI has become the standard of care for initial delineation of anatomy, monitoring for residual hemodynamic lesions, and surgical planning in patients with unrepaired and repaired TOF. A baseline study should be obtained in late childhood when sedation no longer is necessary (i.e., 6 to 8 years of age). Serial MRI evaluation should be performed every 1 to 4 years on the basis of initial findings and clinical symptoms (i.e., more frequently if there is pulmonary stenosis, moderate to severe pulmonary regurgitation, significant right ventricular dilation or dysfunction, left ventricular dysfunction, or clinical symptoms). If there is pulmonary stenosis, MRI should be paired with echocardiography.

Transposition of the Great Arteries

D-Transposition of the great arteries (D-TGA), in which the aorta arises anteriorly and rightward from the right

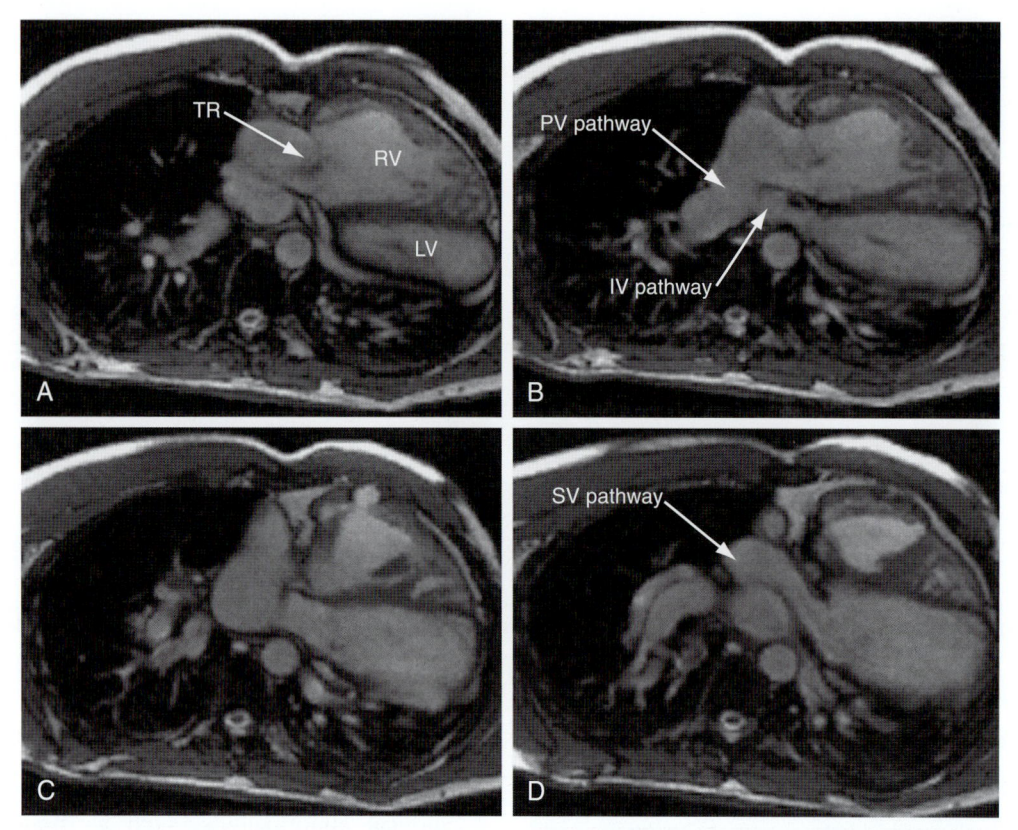

FIGURE 50-10 Four steady-state free precession images in a four-chamber plane demonstrating the pulmonary venous and systemic venous pathways (PV pathway, SV pathway, and IV pathway) in a patient with D-transposition of the great arteries after a Mustard (atrial switch) procedure. Note the right ventricular dilation and hypertrophy typical of the systemic right ventricle (RV). Also note the jet indicating tricuspid regurgitation (TR).

ventricle and the pulmonary artery arises posterior and leftward from the left ventricle, is the most common form of TGA (accounting for 5% to 7% of all children born with CHD) and is a common form of cyanotic CHD (second only to TOF). This circulation is typically not compatible with life unless surgery is performed to redirect deoxygenated flow to the lungs and oxygenated flow to the body. Until the mid-1980s, this defect was surgically corrected with an atrial-level switch (Senning or Mustard procedure). The arterial switch (Jatene procedure) became popular in the mid-1980s and remains the standard of care in this population of patients.

Postoperative Management

After an atrial-level switch, patients suffer a number of residual hemodynamic burdens. The most important of these is systemic right ventricular failure as the right ventricle is not morphologically designed to handle a systemic afterload. Right ventricular dilation and failure are often accompanied by tricuspid (systemic atrioventricular valve) regurgitation, which leads to worsening right ventricular dilation and dysfunction. Patients who have undergone an atrial-level switch also suffer systemic or pulmonary venous baffle obstruction and baffle leaks with either right-to-left or left-to-right shunting, depending on the anatomy.

Patients who have undergone an arterial switch have the benefit of having a left ventricle as the systemic pumping chamber but still retain a number of potential hemodynamic burdens, such as supra-aortic and suprapulmonary stenoses at the suture lines, branch pulmonary artery stenoses secondary to stretch of the pulmonary arteries across the ascending aorta, and coronary ostial occlusions at the site of coronary artery reimplantation.

MRI for a patient with D-TGA who has undergone an atrial-level switch procedure may include the following:

- Four-chamber cine MRI to evaluate ventricular function, atrial pathways, and atrioventricular valve regurgitation (Fig. 50-10).
- Short-axis cine MRI to quantify biventricular mass, volume, and function. Images should extend coverage from the ventricles through the atrial pathways.
- Baffle cine MRI. Axial plane and coronal oblique planes through the superior vena cava and inferior vena cava pathways are useful for diagnosis of obstruction to flow. These images will often display baffle leaks (although the absence of a baffle leak on MRI does not rule out a baffle leak) (Fig. 50-11).
- Flow quantification. Velocity-encoded cine MRI sequence is performed to assess flow. First, two-dimensional planes across the cross-sectional area of the ascending aorta and main pulmonary artery are obtained to quantify pulmonary-to-systemic flow ratio (if there is any concern for baffle leak). Velocity-encoded cine MRI sequences can be planned in the plane of the atrioventricular valves to assess the degree of tricuspid regurgitation.

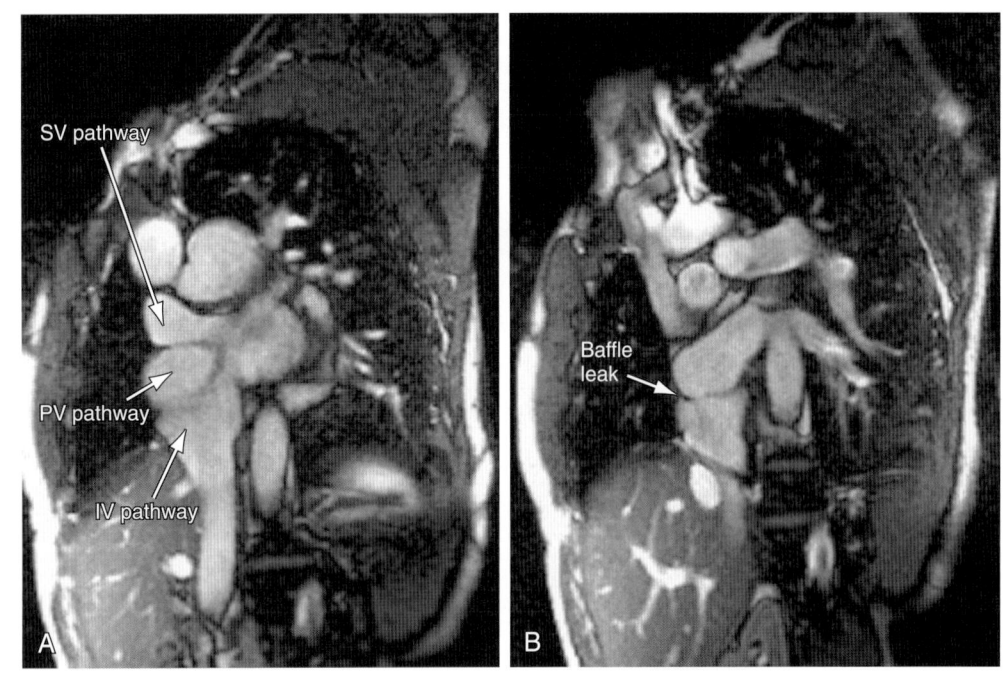

■ **FIGURE 50-11** **A,** Coronal oblique steady-state free precession stack demonstrating the superior (SV pathway) and inferior (IV pathway) limbs of the systemic venous baffle draped like a "pair of pants" over the pulmonary venous pathway (PV pathway). **B,** Of note, there is evidence of a baffle leak in the inferior limb of the baffle with left-to-right flow.

- Delayed hyperenhancement to look for myocardial scar.

Guidelines for MRI in patients with D-TGA who have undergone an atrial-level switch procedure include a baseline investigation and serial follow-up evaluation. The information uniquely provided by MRI includes quantitative systemic right ventricular function, visualization of the synchrony (or asynchrony) of ventricular contraction, atrioventricular valve regurgitation, systemic venous or pulmonary venous pathway obstruction, and baffle leaks (with cine imaging and quantification of systemic-to-pulmonary flow ratio). Depending on systemic right ventricular function, other anatomic and physiologic abnormalities, and clinical symptoms, MRI should be repeated every 2 to 4 years to monitor these.

MRI for a patient with D-TGA who has undergone an arterial switch procedure may include the following:

- Short-axis cine MRI to quantify biventricular mass, volume, and function.
- Axial cine MRI to assess for supra-aortic and suprapulmonary valve stenoses.
- Axial black blood imaging to provide better spatial resolution and more anatomic detail, complementing the axial cine MRI.
- Three-dimensional MRA if there is any concern about vascular abnormalities.
- Coronary artery, stress perfusion, and delayed hyperenhancement imaging can be used if there is any concern about coronary ostial obstruction.

MRI is useful for baseline and serial evaluation of patients with D-TGA who have undergone arterial switch. The information uniquely provided by MRI includes evaluation of the great vessels (supra-aortic and suprapulmonary stenosis and branch pulmonary artery obstruction). In addition, the coronary artery ostia and proximal coronary arteries can be evaluated. Stress MRI (dipyridamole, adenosine, or dobutamine) can additionally allow evaluation of perfusion defects and coronary flow reserve. Finally, MRI offers an assessment of ventricular function. Depending on baseline findings and clinical symptoms, MRI can be repeated serially.

Coarctation of the Aorta

MRI is useful for delineation of anatomy and physiology in patients after repair of coarctation of the aorta.[33,34] This can be monitored with serial MRI to identify the need for and to ensure appropriate timing of reintervention.

Coarctation of the aorta is a common form of CHD. Simple coarctation of the aorta accounts for 5% to 8% of all patients born with CHD and is a component of many more complex lesions. In coarctation of the aorta, ductal tissue surrounds the aortic isthmus, and with ductal closure, there is constriction leading to arch obstruction. If it is diagnosed in the newborn period, surgical repair with resection of the obstruction and end-to-end anastomosis is the preferred therapy. If it is diagnosed later in life, catheter-based intervention with balloon dilation or stenting of the obstruction can be performed as an alternative to surgery. Patients with native or repaired coarctation of the aorta often suffer aortic complications, such as restenosis, aneurysm formation of the ascending aorta or repair site, dissection, systemic hypertension with left ventricular hypertrophy, and early coronary artery disease. These complications are often asymptomatic and go unrecognized until it is too late.

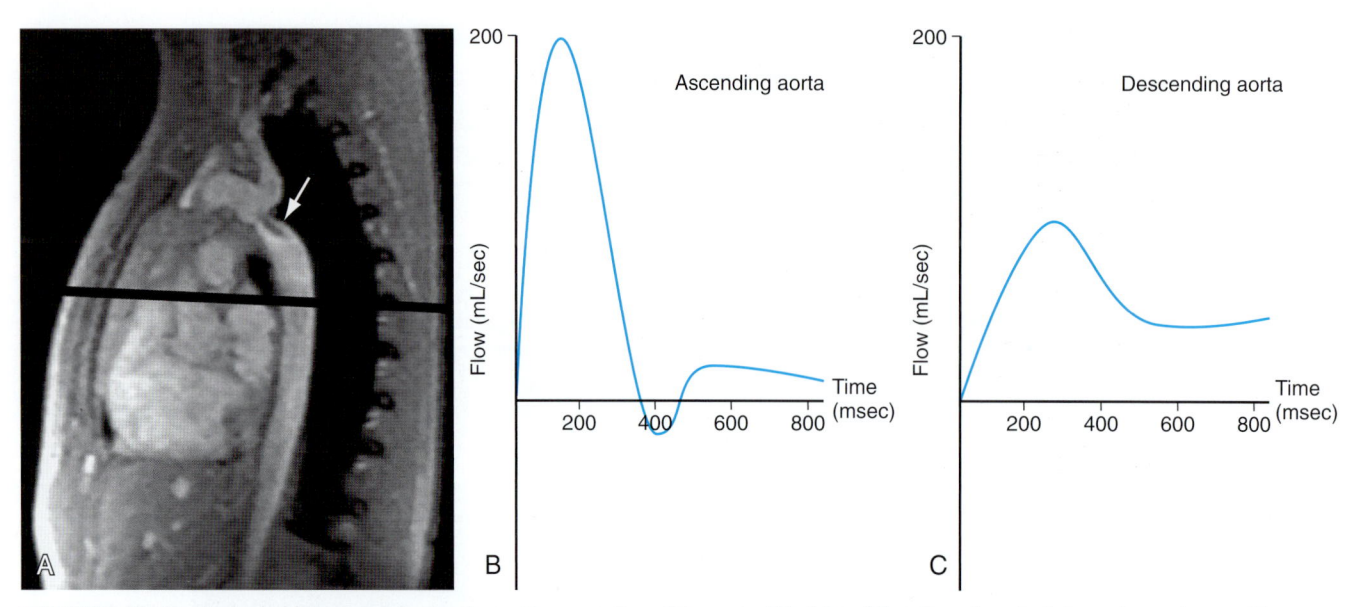

FIGURE 50-12 Sagittal oblique image in a patient with coarctation of the aorta (**A**). A jet of flow (*arrow*) at the isthmus is consistent with obstruction. The flow curves demonstrate the flow in the ascending aorta (**B**) and descending aorta (**C**). The delayed onset of systolic flow, damped rate of return to baseline, and persistent flow during diastole seen in the descending aorta are suggestive of significant obstruction.

Echocardiographic assessment is often limited by poor acoustic windows. Although CT angiography provides anatomic detail, it is unable to characterize flow and the effect of the obstruction on the myocardium. MRI can noninvasively enhance our understanding of coarctation severity, and clinical assessment combined with MRI as a primary imaging modality can be more cost-effective than an approach using echocardiography as a primary imaging modality.[35,36]

Postoperative Management

The initial goal of a cardiac MRI examination in a patient after repair of coarctation of the aorta is delineation of the anatomy. This includes anatomic characterization of recurrent or residual obstruction, relationship of the obstruction to other arch vessels (which is necessary for planning of surgical or catheter-based interventions), arch anatomy (e.g., aortic root or ascending aorta dilation, hypoplasia of the arch, post-stenotic dilation of the descending aorta, aneurysm at site of repair), and number of collateral vessels. The second goal is to evaluate the effect of the obstruction or resultant systemic hypertension on the myocardium, including left ventricular myocardial mass and left ventricular function. The final goal is to ascertain the physiologic severity of the obstruction by evaluating the nature of flow at the obstruction and in the descending aorta.

MRI for a patient with repaired coarctation of the aorta may include the following:

- Short-axis cine MRI for quantification of biventricular mass, volume, and function.
- Arch cine MRI. Sagittal oblique plane in the long axis of the aorta should be obtained, the so-called candy cane view. This allows visualization of the jet of turbulent flow at the coarctation of the aorta, thus providing a qualitative assessment of the severity of the obstruction (Fig. 50-12A).
- Black blood imaging in the sagittal oblique plane can be of additional value. This is particularly useful when there is a previously placed stent or if finer spatial resolution is required.
- Three-dimensional MRA to assess arch anatomy. It is from these images that cross-sectional areas can be measured, arch anatomy can be delineated, and collaterals can be defined. These findings are critical to planning of medical, catheter-based, or surgical interventions (Fig. 50-13).
- Flow quantification. Velocity-encoded cine MRI sequences are performed to assess flow. First, a two-dimensional plane across the cross-sectional area of the ascending aorta is obtained. If prescribed well, this often yields not only flow in the ascending aorta but also flow in the descending aorta just distal to the obstruction. It is also useful to obtain flow in the descending aorta at the level of the diaphragm. Delayed onset of systolic flow, damped rate of return to baseline, persistent flow during diastole, and augmentation of flow secondary to collaterals are suggestive of significant obstruction (Fig. 50-12B).

In general, MRI should be used to evaluate anyone older than 6 years after repair of coarctation of the aorta with concern for recurrent or residual obstruction, aneurysm formation, or systemic hypertension. MRI should be used in younger children if questions remain after echocardiography. In patients who have undergone apparently successful repair, MRI should be obtained at baseline in late childhood when sedation is no longer necessary (i.e., 6 to 8 years of age). It should be repeated every 6 months to 5 years, depending on initial findings.

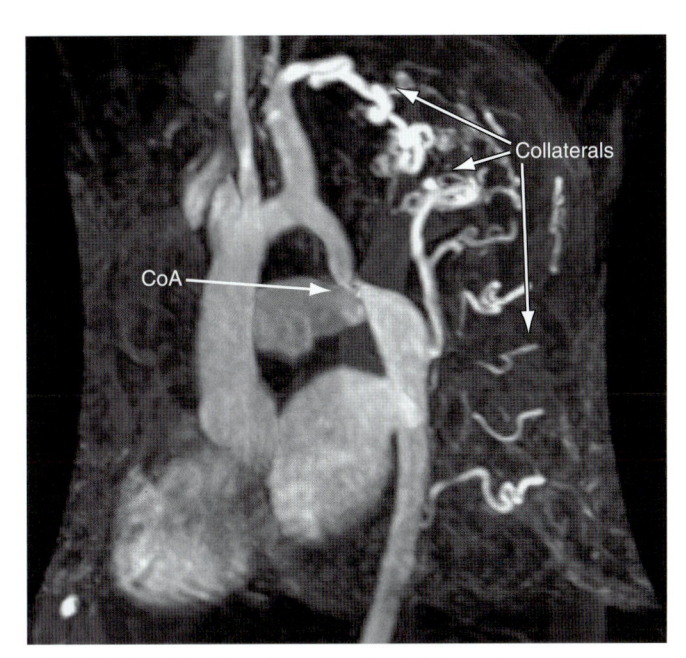

FIGURE 50-13 Three-dimensional gadolinium-enhanced MRA in a patient with coarctation of the aorta (CoA). Images are displayed as a maximum intensity projection image. Both the region of coarctation of the aorta and the collaterals are identified (*arrows*).

Single Ventricle After Fontan Palliation

Patients born with complex CHD and single-ventricle physiology (i.e., tricuspid atresia, hypoplastic left heart syndrome, pulmonary atresia with intact ventricular septum) represent a spectrum of disease severity, depending on their initial anatomy. In the current era, they typically undergo several surgical procedures during the first several years of life to provide a stable cardiopulmonary physiology. The first of these procedures is usually performed in the neonatal period and is directed at recruiting the single ventricle as the systemic pumping chamber and providing controlled pulmonary blood flow. The subsequent procedures involve sequential conversion to a physiology of separated systemic and pulmonary circulations with passive pulmonary blood flow (elimination of intracardiac "mixing"). The final circulation is named the Fontan circulation after the French surgeon who developed and first performed it in humans.[37] This palliation improves the patient's cardiovascular efficiency and provides nearly normal systemic arterial oxygen saturations, but the physiology remains abnormal.

Postoperative Management

These patients suffer many complications. First, as a result of the passive nature of pulmonary blood flow, they develop high right-sided filling pressures, dilated Fontan pathways, and atrial arrhythmias. As a result of high filling pressures, they often form systemic-to-pulmonary venous collaterals, which lead to cyanosis. As a result of sluggish pulmonary blood flow, they have poor left-sided preload and diminished output despite normal contractility. They often have single right ventricles that ultimately fail in the face of systemic afterload. They may have valvular disease that increases the pressure or volume load of the single ventricle. All of this inevitable pathophysiology must be monitored to ensure timely medical, catheter-based, and surgical interventions that may improve the patient's clinical status.

The goal of a cardiac MRI evaluation of patients with single-ventricle physiology is first the delineation of anatomy. This postsurgical anatomy is often complex and often unexpected. The second goal is the characterization of physiology, including valvular disease, myocardial function, and flow assessment. A cardiac MRI protocol for such a patient may include the following:

- Axial cine MRI. Images should extend from the diaphragm to the arch vessels to begin to assess cardiac and vascular anatomy. These images help guide the remainder of the cardiac MRI examination.
- Short-axis cine MRI to quantify ventricular mass, volume, and function.
- Black blood imaging may be helpful if anatomy is in question or if there are metallic devices in place causing artifact on cine imaging.
- Flow quantification. Velocity-encoded cine MRI imaging is performed to assess flow. First, two-dimensional planes are prescribed across the aorta as well as the vessels supplying blood flow to the pulmonary vascular bed (i.e., right and left branch pulmonary arteries, main pulmonary artery in the setting of an old-style Fontan circulation in which the main pulmonary artery is connected to the right atrium). Two-dimensional flow assessment across the atrioventricular valves as well as the superior and inferior venae cavae is often helpful for assessment of atrioventricular valve regurgitation and for corroboration of other flow and volumetric data. A seven-dimensional flow technique may prove useful in this anatomy and physiology as it can obtain flow in all vessels in a single acquisition.
- Three-dimensional MRA is often useful for assessment of arterial and venous vascular anatomy, including identification of collateral vessels.
- Delayed hyperenhancement to look for myocardial scar.

Guidelines for the use of cardiac MRI in the setting of palliated single-ventricle physiology need to be tailored to the individual patient. If there are no concerns early, baseline cardiac MRI should be obtained in late childhood when sedation is no longer necessary (i.e., 6 to 8 years of age). Serial examinations should be performed, the frequency of which should be dictated by clinical status. Obviously, if there are concerns earlier (i.e., valvular disease, myocardial dysfunction, arterial or venous abnormalities, baffle leaks), MRI can be performed under sedation or general anesthesia.

KEY POINTS

- The field of CHD is advancing rapidly, and as a result, patients with complex disease are surviving and patients in general are living longer.
- Despite repair, postoperative CHD patients uniformly have residual hemodynamic burdens that need to be monitored carefully. Reintervention is often necessary. Choice of appropriate timing for reintervention is often challenging.
- MRI is ideally suited as a primary noninvasive imaging modality, given its ability to provide accurate and reproducible anatomic and functional information. Multiple MRI techniques can be combined to provide a complete evaluation of anatomy and function, including cine (steady-state free precession) imaging, black blood (spin-echo) imaging, flow quantification (velocity-encoded cine) MRI, gadolinium-enhanced three-dimensional MRA, coronary artery imaging, perfusion imaging, and viability (delayed hyperenhancement) MRI.
- The postoperative CHD patients presenting for MRI most commonly include those with tetralogy of Fallot, transposition of the great arteries, coarctation of the aorta, or single ventricles after Fontan repair.
- MRI has advanced significantly during the past 3 decades and continues to advance at a rapid rate. Real-time imaging, MRI-guided interventions, myocardial tagging assessment of wall strain, and seven-dimensional flow techniques will reach the clinical armamentarium in the near future, making MRI an even more useful tool in evaluation and management of this population of patients.

SUGGESTED READINGS

Gutierrez FR, Ho ML, Siegel MJ. Practical applications of magnetic resonance in congenital heart disease. Magn Reson Imaging Clin N Am 2008; 16:403-435.

Kellenberger CJ, Yoo SJ, Buchel ER. Cardiovascular MR imaging in neonates and infants with congenital heart disease. Radiographics 2007; 27:5-18.

Knauth Meadows A, Ordovas K, Higgins CB, Reddy GP. Magnetic resonance imaging in the adult with congenital heart disease. Semin Roentgenol 2008; 43:246-258.

Valente AM, Powell AJ. Clinical applications of cardiovascular magnetic resonance in congenital heart disease. Cardiol Clin 2007; 25:97-110.

REFERENCES

1. Plein S, Bloomer TN, Ridgway JP, et al. Steady-state free precession magnetic resonance imaging of the heart: comparison with segmented k-space gradient-echo imaging. J Magn Reson Imaging 2001; 14:230-236.
2. Carr JC, Simonetti O, Bundy J, et al. Cine MR angiography of the heart with segmented true fast imaging with steady-state precession. Radiology 2001; 219:828-834.
3. Weiger M, Pruessmann KP, Boesiger P. Cardiac real-time imaging using SENSE. SENSitivity Encoding scheme. Magn Reson Med 2000; 43:177-184.
4. Hernandez RJ, Aisen AM, Foo TK, Beekman RH. Thoracic cardiovascular anomalies in children: evaluation with a fast gradient-recalled-echo sequence with cardiac-triggered segmented acquisition. Radiology 1993; 188:775-780.
5. Furber A, Balzer P, Cavaro-Menard C, et al. Experimental validation of an automated edge-detection method for a simultaneous determination of the endocardial and epicardial borders in short-axis cardiac MR images: application in normal volunteers. J Magn Reson Imaging 1998; 8:1006-1014.
6. Bax JJ, Lamb H, Dibbets P, et al. Comparison of gated single-photon emission computed tomography with magnetic resonance imaging for evaluation of left ventricular function in ischemic cardiomyopathy. Am J Cardiol 2000; 86:1299-1305.
7. Bellenger NG, Marcus NJ, Davies C, et al. Left ventricular function and mass after orthotopic heart transplantation: a comparison of cardiovascular magnetic resonance with echocardiography. J Heart Lung Transplant 2000; 19:444-452.
8. Pennell DJ. Ventricular volume and mass by CMR. J Cardiovasc Magn Reson 2002; 4:507-513.
9. Lorenz CH. The range of normal values of cardiovascular structures in infants, children, and adolescents measured by magnetic resonance imaging. Pediatr Cardiol 2000; 21:37-46.
10. Varaprasathan GA, Araoz PA, Higgins CB, Reddy GP. Quantification of flow dynamics in congenital heart disease: applications of velocity-encoded cine MR imaging. Radiographics 2002; 22:895-905; discussion 905-896.
11. Markl M, Alley MT, Pelc NJ. Balanced phase-contrast steady-state free precession (PC-SSFP): a novel technique for velocity encoding by gradient inversion. Magn Reson Med 2003; 49:945-952.
12. Markl M, Chan FP, Alley MT, et al. Time-resolved three-dimensional phase-contrast MRI. J Magn Reson Imaging 2003; 17:499-506.
13. Zhang H, Maki JH, Prince MR. 3D contrast-enhanced MR angiography. J Magn Reson Imaging 2007; 25:13-25.
14. Babu-Narayan SV, Kilner PJ, et al. Ventricular fibrosis suggested by cardiovascular magnetic resonance in adults with repaired tetralogy of Fallot and its relationship to adverse markers of clinical outcome. Circulation 2006; 113:405-413.
15. Oosterhof T, Mulder BJ, Vliegen HW, de Roos A. Corrected tetralogy of Fallot: delayed enhancement in right ventricular outflow tract. Radiology 2005; 237:868-871.
16. Harris MA, Johnson TR, Weinberg PM, Fogel MA. Delayed-enhancement cardiovascular magnetic resonance identifies fibrous tissue in children after surgery for congenital heart disease. J Thorac Cardiovasc Surg 2007; 133:676-681.
17. Prakash A, Powell AJ, Krishnamurthy R, Geva T. Magnetic resonance imaging evaluation of myocardial perfusion and viability in congenital and acquired pediatric heart disease. Am J Cardiol 2004; 93:657-661.
18. Weber OM, Martin AJ, Higgins CB. Whole-heart steady-state free precession coronary artery magnetic resonance angiography. Magn Reson Med 2003; 50:1223-1228.
19. Weber OM, Pujadas S, Martin AJ, Higgins CB. Free-breathing, three-dimensional coronary artery magnetic resonance angiography: comparison of sequences. J Magn Reson Imaging 2004; 20:395-402.
20. Spuentrup E, Katoh M, Buecker A, et al. Free-breathing 3D steady-state free precession coronary MR angiography with radial k-space sampling: comparison with cartesian k-space sampling and cartesian

21. Danias PG, Roussakis A, Ioannidis JP. Diagnostic performance of coronary magnetic resonance angiography as compared against conventional x-ray angiography: a meta-analysis. J Am Coll Cardiol 2004; 44:1867-1876.
22. Plein S, Radjenovic A, Ridgway JP, et al. Coronary artery disease: myocardial perfusion MR imaging with sensitivity encoding versus conventional angiography. Radiology 2005; 235:423-430.
23. Nagel E, Klein C, Paetsch I, et al. Magnetic resonance perfusion measurements for the noninvasive detection of coronary artery disease. Circulation 2003; 108:432-437.
24. Kim RJ, Fieno DS, Parrish TB, et al. Relationship of MRI delayed contrast enhancement to irreversible injury, infarct age, and contractile function. Circulation 1999; 100:1992-2002.
25. Weinsaft JW, Klem I, Judd RM. MRI for the assessment of myocardial viability. Cardiol Clin 2007; 25:35-56, v.
26. Simonetti OP, Kim RJ, Fieno DS, et al. An improved MR imaging technique for the visualization of myocardial infarction. Radiology 2001; 218:215-223.
27. Akhtar M, Ordovas K, Martin A, et al. Effect of chronic sustained-release dipyridamole on myocardial blood flow and left ventricular function in patients with ischemic cardiomyopathy. Congest Heart Fail 2007; 13:130-135.
28. Jahnke C, Nagel E, Gebker R, et al. Prognostic value of cardiac magnetic resonance stress tests: adenosine stress perfusion and dobutamine stress wall motion imaging. Circulation 2007; 115:1769-1776.
29. Ingkanisorn WP, Kwong RY, Bohme NS, et al. Prognosis of negative adenosine stress magnetic resonance in patients presenting to an emergency department with chest pain. J Am Coll Cardiol 2006; 47:1427-1432.
30. Kim RJ, Chen EL, Lima JA, Judd RM. Myocardial Gd-DTPA kinetics determine MRI contrast enhancement and reflect the extent and severity of myocardial injury after acute reperfused infarction. Circulation 1996; 94:3318-3326.
31. Knauth AL, Gauvreau K, Powell AJ, et al. Ventricular size and function assessed by cardiac MRI predict major adverse clinical outcomes late after tetralogy of Fallot repair. Heart 2008; 94:211-216.
32. Geva T, Sandweiss BM, Gauvreau K, et al. Factors associated with impaired clinical status in long-term survivors of tetralogy of Fallot repair evaluated by magnetic resonance imaging. J Am Coll Cardiol 2004; 43:1068-1074.
33. Bogaert J, Kuzo R, Dymarkowski S, et al. Follow-up of patients with previous treatment for coarctation of the thoracic aorta: comparison between contrast-enhanced MR angiography and fast spin-echo MR imaging. Eur Radiol 2000; 10:1847-1854.
34. Pujadas S, Reddy GP, Weber O, et al. Phase contrast MR imaging to measure changes in collateral blood flow after stenting of recurrent aortic coarctation: initial experience. J Magn Resonance Imaging 2006; 24:72-76.
35. Nielsen JC, Powell AJ, Gauvreau K, et al. Magnetic resonance imaging predictors of coarctation severity. Circulation 2005; 111:622-628.
36. Therrien J, Thorne SA, Wright A, et al. Repaired coarctation: a "cost-effective" approach to identify complications in adults. J Am Coll Cardiol 2000; 35:997-1002.
37. Fontan F, Baudet E. Surgical repair of tricuspid atresia. Thorax 1971; 26:240-248.

PART SIX

Ischemic Heart Disease

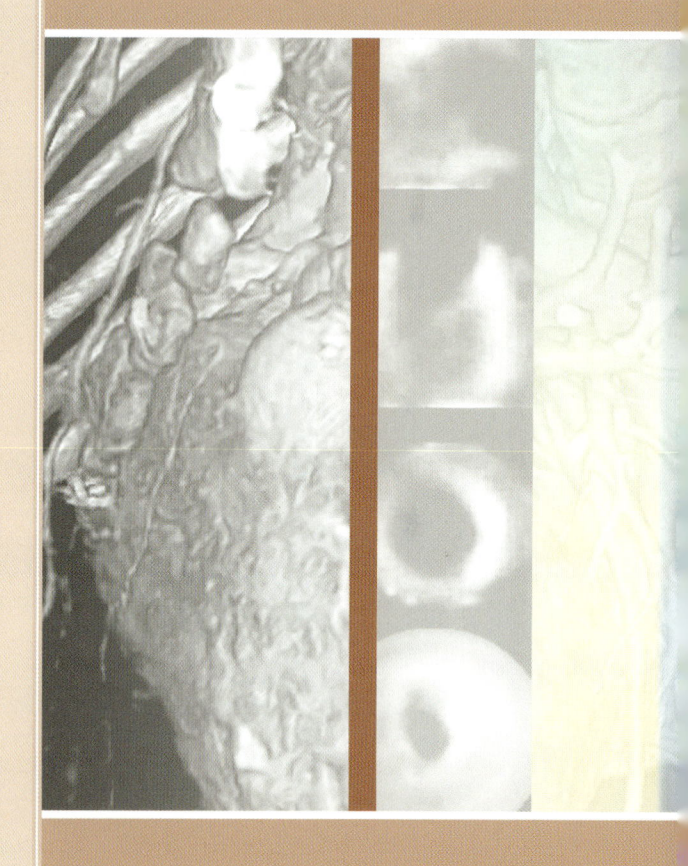

CHAPTER 51

Atherosclerotic Coronary Artery Disease

Allen Burke, Gaku Nakazawa, and Charles S. White

Imaging of coronary atherosclerosis has depended on coronary angiography as the gold standard since Sones and Shirey developed the technique at the Cleveland Clinic in the 1960s.[1] As pathologic studies have described the stages of atherosclerosis and identified underlying plaque components in areas of thrombosis, the limitations of angiography, which outlines the vessel lumen, have emerged. Currently, we are on the brink of new methods of coronary imaging. Noninvasive transthoracic imaging now rivals angiography for the detection of luminal stenosis, and new catheter-based techniques such as intravascular ultrasound (IVUS) promise to identify the lipid component of plaques. Although the in vivo demonstration of vulnerable plaques, allowing for prevention of plaque progression, is yet elusive, it may be only a matter of time before coronary angiography is replaced by noninvasive techniques as the primary tool for coronary atherosclerotic imaging.

DEFINITION

Atherosclerosis is an intimal arterial reaction to injury that results in the accumulation of smooth muscle cells and extracellular matrix with the potential obstruction of the lumen. Typically, the interaction between endothelial injury, inflammation, lipid influx, angiogenesis, thrombosis, and cell death results in the pathologic hallmark of atherosclerosis—the *atheroma,* or core of cellular debris left by remnants of smooth muscle cells, macrophages, and red blood cells. The nature of the atheroma and the components of the fibrous tissue overlying the necrotic core influence the likelihood of plaque rupture, which is the underlying cause for a large proportion of acute myocardial infarctions (MIs). A small subset of patients with obstructive coronary lesions lack atheroma formation, however, and their coronary lesions may be related to thrombosis secondary to plaque erosion (see later).

PREVALENCE AND EPIDEMIOLOGY

Coronary atherosclerosis is prevalent in developed countries, with obstructive lesions occurring frequently in individuals older than 50 years. The prevalence is affected by age, gender, genetic predisposition, and acquired risk factors. Although there is a downward trend in the prevalence of heart disease (largely caused by coronary atherosclerosis), it remains the leading cause of death in the United States. The prevalence of coronary heart disease from 1999 to 2004 in the U.S. population, as estimated by the National Center for Health Statistics and National Heart, Lung and Blood Institute, was 22.8% for men and 15.4% for women 60 to 79 years old. Approximately 10% of men 50 to 70 years old who die of noncardiac causes have obstructive coronary lesions at autopsy.[2]

ETIOLOGY AND PATHOPHYSIOLOGY

Atherosclerosis is the result of reaction to arterial injury that begins at the endothelial lining. As imaging of the vessels becomes more sophisticated, the identification of atherosclerotic plaque composition will become as important as degree of stenosis, which is at the limit of the capability of current modalities such as angiography. There is a great morphologic heterogeneity of atherosclerotic plaque, which reflects the stage of progression and the variety of pathways involved after intimal injury. Inflammatory, thrombotic, proliferative, and apoptotic pathways typically result in lipid accumulation, which is currently the major target of newer imaging strategies.

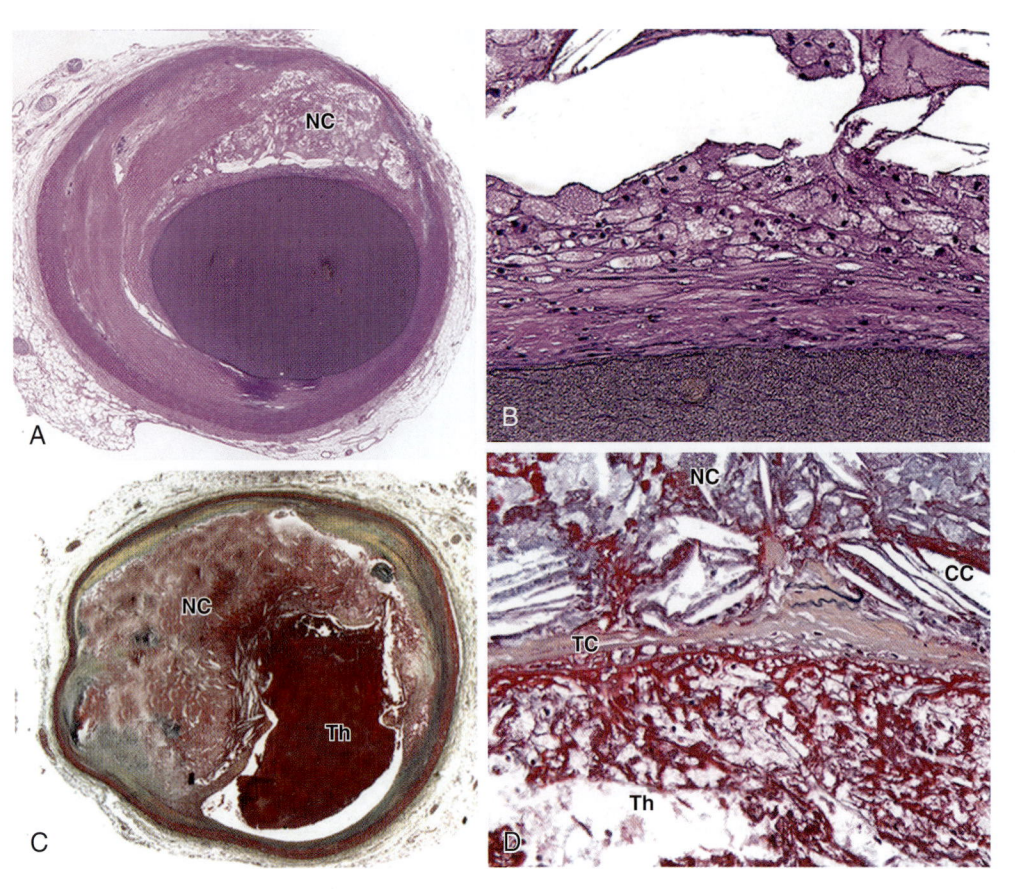

FIGURE 51-1 Atheromatous plaque progression. **A,** Thin cap atheroma, with a necrotic core (NC) characterized by cholesterol clefts (free cholesterol). **B,** Higher magnification of the thin cap, with numerous foam cells and portions of cholesterol crystals at the top of the image. **C,** Large necrotic core (NC) with abundant intraplaque hemorrhage and luminal thrombus (Th). **D,** Higher magnification of the rupture site. CC, cholesterol crystal (cleft); NC, necrotic core; TC, thin cap; Th, thrombus.

Stages of Atherosclerotic Plaque Progression: Atheromatous versus Nonatheromatous

The heterogeneity of coronary atherosclerotic plaques is characterized by two major mechanisms of plaque progression: atheromatous, which is the most common, and relatively non–lipid-rich, or nonatheromatous. In most men, and men and women older than 50 years, atheromatous plaques dominate in most coronary lesions. In younger patients, especially women, obstructive coronary disease may occur in the absence of significant cell death and necrotic core formation. The identification of the two types of plaque is crucial if imaging techniques evolve that specifically target the identification of lipid-rich necrotic core.

Atheromatous Plaque Progression

The classic stages of plaque progression, as defined by the American Heart Association (AHA), involve the formation of the necrotic core. A more recent modification of this staging schema[3] outlines development of atheroma. The normal human intima contains a small cushion of smooth muscle cells and matrix, which is present from birth and accentuated at branch points; this lesion has been termed *adaptive* or *diffuse intimal thickening*. Later in life, with intimal injury, there is influx of lipids, much of which is oxidized; at this stage (*pathologic intimal thickening*), there is typically influx of small numbers of foamy macrophages, generally luminal in location to the lipid pools. The progression of the pathologic intimal thickening to fibroatheroma (AHA class II-III) is key in the development of lipid-rich plaques that result in symptoms owing to tendency to rupture and thrombose. The features of fibroatheroma include a core of necrotic material (Fig. 51-1), which is composed of apoptotic cell debris–derived smooth muscle cell membranes, macrophages, and red blood cells. Much current imaging technology is focused on the identification of necrotic material because this is the precursor lesion of the most common substrate for coronary atherothrombosis.

Thin Cap Atheroma and the Vulnerable Plaque

The expansion of the atheroma, or necrotic core of the lipid-rich atherosclerotic plaque, results in thinning of the overlying fibrous cap (see Fig. 51-1). An arbitrary fibrous cap thickness of 65 µm has been designated as the criterion for the "vulnerable" plaque or thin cap fibroatheroma.[4] The characteristics of thin cap atheroma that render it prone to rupture are unknown, but likely involve physical factors, such as size of the necrotic core, and biologic factors, such as proteolytic enzyme activity within the thinned cap. The goal of imaging to detect thin cap fibroatheroma and distinguish it from fibroatheroma with thicker caps remains elusive, but may eventually enable the prophylactic treatment of lesions prone to rupture with the aim of preventing atherothrombosis.

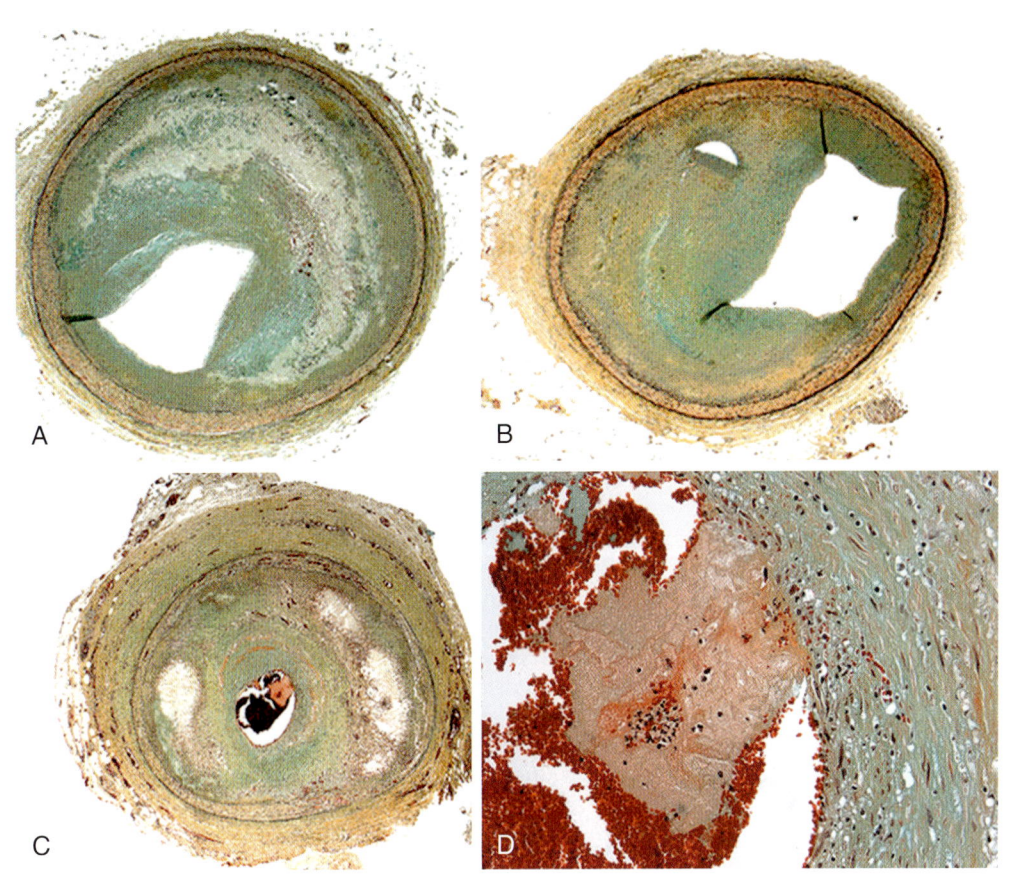

FIGURE 51-2
Nonatheromatous plaque progression. **A,** Significant stenosis with areas rich in extracellular lipid (clear areas), which is composed largely of esterified cholesterol and phospholipid, but no necrotic core formation. **B,** Significant stenosis without abundant lipid (from the same patient). **C,** Thrombus overlying a smooth muscle cell–rich plaque, with cleared areas indicative of lipid pools (pathologic intimal thickening), but little or no necrotic core formation. **D,** Higher magnification of the plaque erosion, showing the platelet-rich thrombus in the lumen.

Nonatheromatous Plaque Progression

In autopsy studies, approximately 15% of patients who die of coronary artery disease (CAD) lack lipid-rich atheromatous lesions. Nevertheless, these patients develop significant luminal narrowing, and luminal thrombus may occur by mechanisms other than rupture of the thin fibrous cap. The major alternative mechanism of atherothrombosis (Fig. 51-2), termed *plaque erosion,* is of unclear etiology.[5] Erosion may result from endothelial injury that results directly in thrombosis, either via coronary spasm or via interaction with matrix receptors. Because plaque erosion thrombi may be small and nonocclusive, they result in layering of smooth muscle cell–rich plaque that expands without a requisite necrotic core, often with little outward expansion (positive remodeling). Although the goal of imaging remains the detection of lipid-rich plaques, a subset of potentially lethal lesions are not detected by modalities that target lipid.

Life Cycling of the Atherosclerotic Plaque

Because coronary imaging seeks to identify lipid-rich plaques, especially plaques with large necrotic cores, mention of the life cycle of lipid-rich lesions and the effect of successive ruptures on plaque composition is relevant. One outcome of plaque rupture, after slowly enlarging core and thinning of the fibrous cap, is occlusive thrombus that organizes as a total occlusion and results in acute coronary syndrome. Much more common after acute rupture is a subocclusive thrombus with healing. The outcome of subocclusive plaque rupture is often plaque enlargement and outward expansion (remodeling) of the arterial wall. The thickening of the fibrous cap that occurs after healed rupture is roughly represented by the AHA class V plaque. Autopsy studies have shown multiple old rupture sites at sites of acute rupture, resulting in compartmentalization of the plaque into areas of lipid core and fibrous healing.[6] The site of future rupture may not have a single large lipid compartment, but a heterogeneous makeup that includes fibrous tissue. The consequences for imaging are unclear at this time.

Calcification and Coronary Atherosclerosis: Implications for Imaging

Calcification is a reliable marker for the presence of atherosclerotic plaque because there are no other processes in the coronary arteries that result in calcium deposition. Calcium scoring is a reliable marker for atherosclerotic plaque burden, although in younger patients severe obstructive lesions can occur in the absence of any calcification (see Chapter 32). Calcification is not a marker of plaque instability, however. Solid calcification can be the result of diffuse deposition in fibrous tissue in stable plaques, whereas more stippled calcification, reflective of necrotic core calcification in more heterogeneous plaques, may be more suggestive of an unstable plaque.[7]

MANIFESTATIONS OF DISEASE

Clinical Presentation

The major clinical presentations of coronary atherosclerosis are stable angina, acute coronary syndromes (ST segment elevation MI and non–ST segment elevation MI), congestive heart failure, and sudden death. Acute coronary syndromes are discussed Chapter 52. Coronary lesions in sudden death are quite heterogeneous because the mechanisms of ventricular arrhythmias vary. In stable angina, there is generally stable plaque with significant obstruction, whereas unstable syndromes are characterized by intraluminal thrombus. In unstable angina or non–ST segment elevation MI, typically nonocclusive thrombi are present, whereas ST segment elevation MI is associated with larger, often occlusive thrombi. Coronary artery lesions in ischemic cardiomyopathy are typically diffuse and multiple, and there is significant myocardial damage generally with transmural healed MI.

Imaging Indications and Algorithm

Currently, angiography is the gold standard for imaging atherosclerotic coronary disease, and other imaging techniques are investigational. CT scanning for coronary calcium is used as identification for coronary risk (see Chapter 32), and IVUS is indicated for the evaluation of graft vascular disease in heart transplant recipients.

The indication for coronary angiography varies by clinical setting. The AHA has set forth algorithms for coronary angiography that are stratified by specific patient groups.[8] Patients in whom coronary arteries should be evaluated by angiography include patients with symptoms of stable angina, nonspecific chest pain, unstable angina, recurrence of ischemia after revascularization, and acute MI, and patients undergoing perioperative risk assessment for noncardiac surgery. Patients with valvular heart disease in whom surgery is contemplated, patients undergoing cardiac surgery for other indications including congenital heart disease, and patients with unexplained congestive heart failure may also be candidates for coronary angiography. There are no currently accepted indications for coronary artery imaging other than angiography, although noninvasive modalities, especially multislice CT, are on the brink of being established as a viable option for the identification of coronary artery stenoses (see later).

Imaging Technique and Findings

Radiography

Radiography is of no diagnostic use in imaging of coronary arteries, although coronary calcification in large quantities may be visible.

Angiography

Catheter-based invasive coronary angiography is the gold standard for diagnosing significant (≥50% diameter stenosis) CAD. Despite various, less invasive tests to detect CAD, including stress imaging studies, 35% of patients referred for catheter-based angiography have no significant stenoses, stressing the need for better noninvasive tests. The rate of false-negative results of coronary angiography is not well appreciated, however; one of the few anatomic correlations showed that angiography significantly underestimates lesions in 44% of cases.[9] Degree of stenosis as measured by coronary CT angiography shows little correlation between functional severity as measured by fractional flow reserve.[10] These findings suggest that angiography is not ideal for identifying coronary stenosis, and that the mere detection of luminal narrowing by even more sophisticated methods may not be as important as functional studies or imaging techniques that show lesion characteristics.

The need to identify functional characteristics of coronary lesions is borne out by follow-up studies. Although the incidence of progression of thin cap atheroma is unknown, at least 6% of patients undergoing percutaneous coronary intervention develop progression of disease requiring intervention for a different target lesion within 1 year.[11] The major predictors of plaque progression are multivessel disease, prior percutaneous coronary intervention, and age younger than 65 years. It has also been shown that 17% of acute MI patients with multiple complex angiographic lesions undergo percutaneous coronary intervention of nonculprit lesions within 1 year.[12] These data underscore the need for identifying plaques in high-risk patients who would benefit from prophylactic intervention.

Ultrasonography

Transthoracic or transesophageal ultrasonography has little utility for the detection of intracoronary stenoses. Catheter-based techniques are beginning to establish themselves, however, as valuable imaging modalities for coronary lesions. Despite the invasive nature of IVUS, the technique may be coupled with angiography and percutaneous coronary intervention, other invasive measures, in the evaluation of patients with stable angina and acute coronary syndromes.

IVUS is the preferred imaging method for the detection of graft vascular disease. Allograft arteriosclerosis differs from native atherosclerosis in that lesions are typically concentric, which limits the usefulness of angiography for determining the extent of intimal disease.

Conventional IVUS has limited use in de novo coronary atherosclerosis because its resolution of 150 to 300 μm is inadequate for the visualization of plaque components, although the current consensus document on IVUS describes the classification of atherosclerotic plaque based on the echogenicity.[13] "Soft plaques" have a low echogenicity and represent high lipid content with or without a necrotic core, whereas "fibrous plaques" have an intermediate echogenicity between soft (echolucent) and high echogenic calcific plaques, which is attributable to a fibrous tissue. Vessel calcification appears as high echogenicity, which causes distal shadowing and obscures visualization of the intima, especially if the calcification is superficial. IVUS is considered more accurate than angiography in the detection of overall coronary plaque burden,

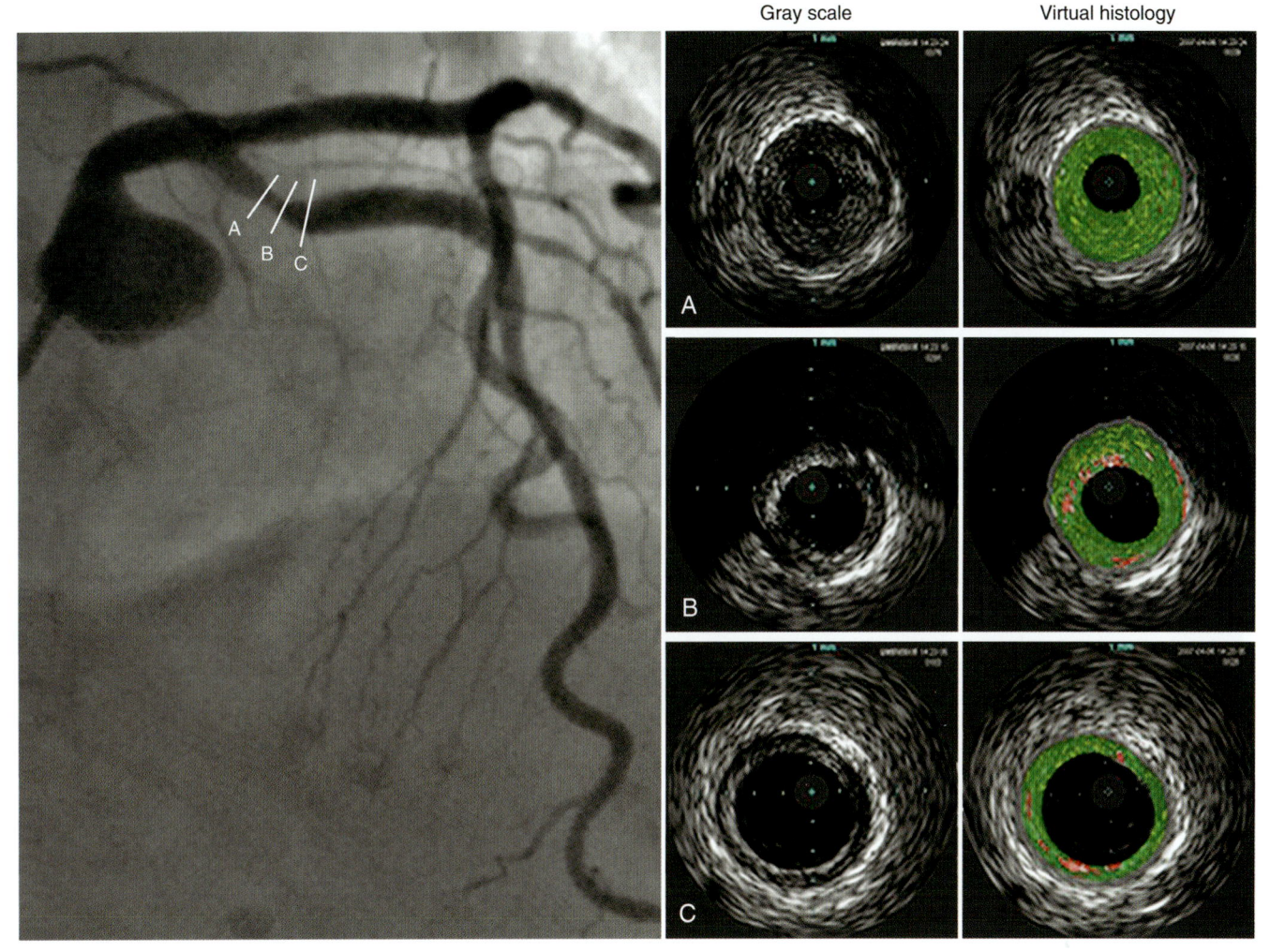

FIGURE 51-3 IVUS-VH correlating angiogram (*left*) with gray-scale IVUS images (**A-C,** *center*) with corresponding reconstruction using back-scatter data. Colors are coded for different plaque components (*green,* fibrous; *greenish yellow,* fibrofatty; *red,* necrotic core; *white,* calcification). A-C correspond to areas of stenosis in the angiogram at left.

a capability that renders it useful to assess progression of disease, an end point used in clinical trials.[14]

There are several methods of potentially improving the imaging resolution of IVUS to detect lipid-rich plaques and possibly even thin cap fibroatheroma. The use of radiofrequency back-scattered ultrasound signals (IVUS-IB) allows for the detection of lipid-rich plaque, which has been shown to decrease after short-term aggressive statin therapy.[15] Similarly, virtual histology IVUS (IVUS-VH) refers to spectral analysis of ultrasound back-scatter radiofrequency signals.[16] After the spectral signature of four tissue types (fibrous, fibrofatty, necrotic core, and calcium) is determined (Fig. 51-3), the data are programmed into software. The technique has been validated ex vivo and in vivo, using directional coronary atherectomy specimens. IVUS-VH image acquisition requires ECG gating and motorized catheter pullback, ideally at 0.5 mm/s.

Currently, IVUS-VH cannot distinguish thin cap fibroatheromas based on measurements of cap thickness, although IVUS-derived thin cap fibroatheromas have been described as focal, necrotic core–rich plaques in contact with the lumen and a percent atheroma volume of 40% or greater.[16] IVUS-VH defines plaque rupture as "a ruptured capsule with an underlying cavity or plaque excavation by atheromatous extrusion with no visible capsule."[17] Based on these criteria, the numbers and distribution of thin cap fibroatheromas and acute plaque ruptures have been estimated in patients with acute coronary syndromes and stable angina pectoris.[17]

Limitations of IVUS-VH include distinguishing necrotic core from calcification and calcium-induced back-scatter artifacts. The degree of calcification in large cores is quite variable, ranging from microscopic calcification of macrophages to irregular blocks of calcium, often involving adjacent fibrous structures. This feature of necrotic core—variability in the degree and type of calcium deposition, often within a single lesion—renders interpretation of radiofrequency data difficult. The accuracy of IVUS-VH in identifying types of vulnerable plaques, including thin cap atheromas, small fissures within nonocclusive thrombi, and overt ruptures with occlusive thrombi, is still undetermined.

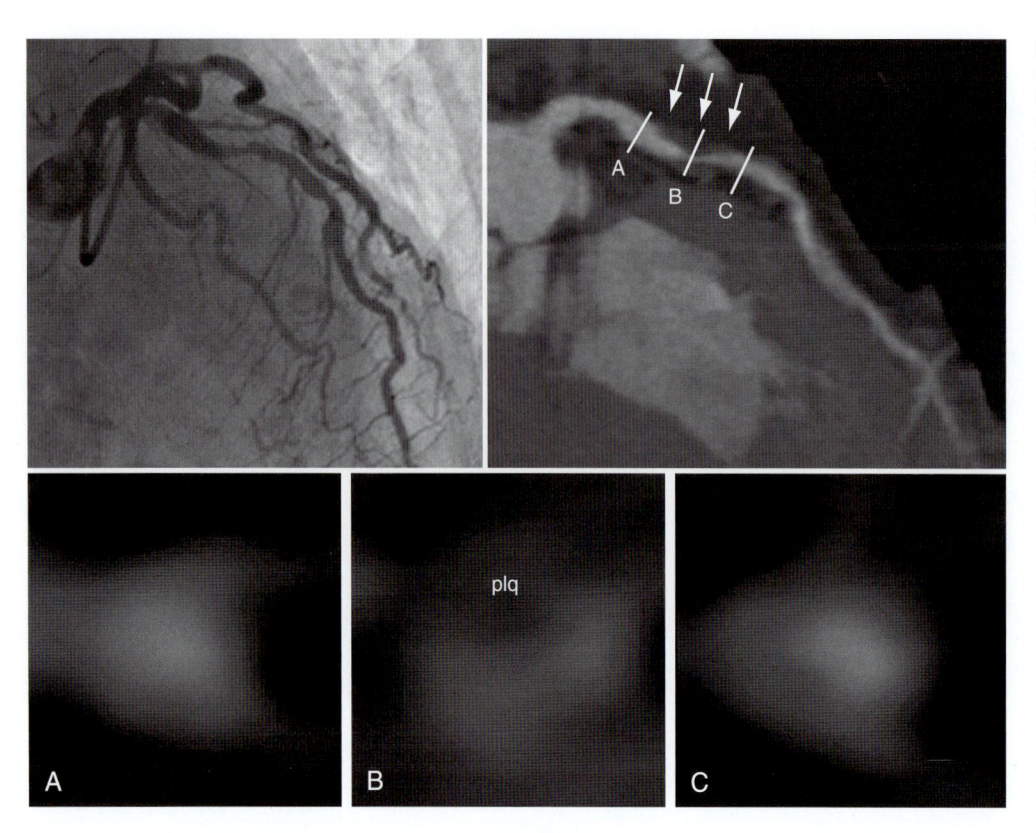

FIGURE 51-4 Angiogram and corresponding CT angiogram show luminal stenosis (*arrows*) of the left anterior descending artery, with cross-sectional reconstructions of the proximal (**A**), stenosis with plaque (plq) (**B**), and distal (**C**) segments.

Computed Tomography

Electron-beam CT was established in the 1980s as a method to detect coronary calcium (see Chapter 32). Current techniques of multidetector CT coupled with angiography (coronary CT angiography) allow the imaging of arteries to detect luminal plaque (Fig. 51-4).

The difficulties inherent in CT imaging of coronary arteries include the small caliber of the coronary arteries combined with cardiac and respiratory motion. Using currently available 64-detector CT scanners, spatial resolution is 0.4 mm^3, and temporal resolution duration of the reconstruction window during end-diastolic phase is 165 to 200 ms. In the sequential mode, the table moves, slice by slice; in the spiral mode, there is continuous acquisition while patient moves at a constant speed.

The signal is gated to capture images during middiastole to end-diastole using prospective triggering for sequential acquisition; retrospective gating is used for spiral acquisition with data collected throughout the cardiac cycle. For a normal size heart (10- to 12-cm window), acquisition time is 10 seconds, given 400-ms rotation time and 64 rows or slices. An intravenous bolus of high-concentration iodinated contrast agent allows differentiation of lumen from wall and plaques; a β blocker is administered for heart rate greater than 70 beats/min, and nitroglycerin is given to promote coronary vasodilation.

In studies of high-risk patients, multidetector CT has been compared with angiography in the detection of significant coronary stenoses (Fig. 51-5). Using the 17-coronary segment model of the AHA, the number of evaluable segments was greater than 95%, with a sensitivity of 90%, specificity of 95%, positive predictive value of 80%, and negative predictive value of almost 99%.[18] Plaque quality, quantity, and morphology such as remodeling have also been assessed by multidetector CT compared with IVUS data.[19,20] Because of the improvement in multidetector CT technology, plaque characterization is becoming possible. At this point, multidetector CT to assess plaque composition, specifically thin cap atheroma, is still experimental, however.

Limitations of multidetector CT for the detection of coronary stenoses include "blooming" artifact overestimating stenoses in areas of calcification, with a marked blooming artifact in areas of intracoronary stents. Another drawback of multidetector CT is radiation exposure of 20 mSv and reduced efficacy in patients who are in atrial fibrillation. For the detection of coronary artery bypass graft patency, multidetector CT is considered to have high sensitivity and specificity. Newer CT scanners have become available more recently and include a 320-slice scanner, which permits acquisition of the heart in a single rotation, and dual-source 64-slice CT scanner, which allows for increased temporal resolution to 83 ms. The capability of these scanners to improve on noninvasive visualization of coronary plaque is as yet unknown.

Magnetic Resonance Imaging

Challenges to MRI of coronary arteries are similar to the challenges of multidetector CT, and include small caliber of the vessels, cardiac and respiratory motion artifact, vessel tortuosity, and signal differential from fat and myo-

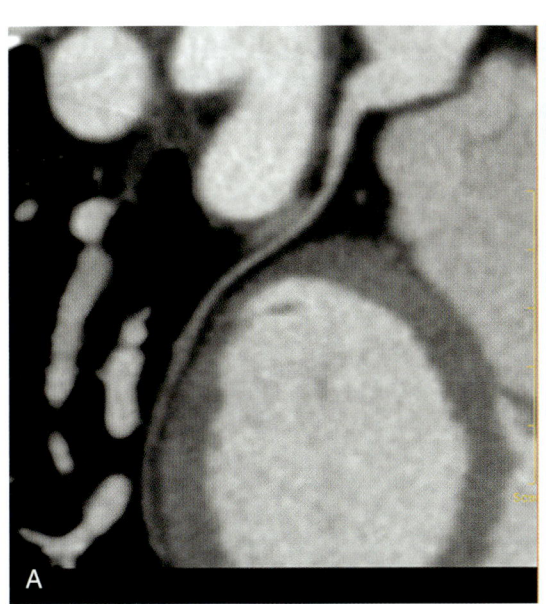

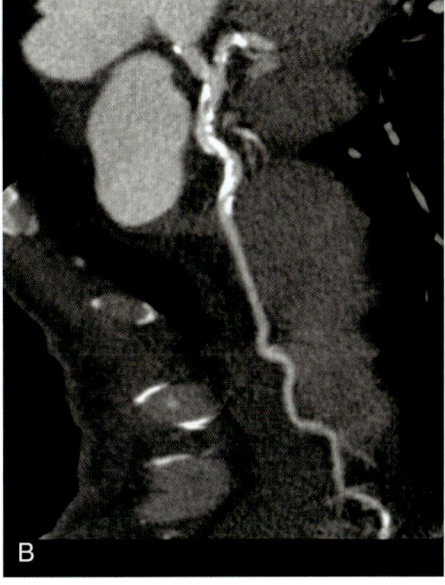

FIGURE 51-5 A and B, CT angiogram showing lack of stenosis in the circumflex and obtuse marginal branch (**A**), and significant stenosis with calcification of the left anterior descending artery (**B**).

cardium. Coronary MRI is currently limited to evaluation of proximal and mid vessel segments, which are the sites of more than 95% of unstable coronary plaques, as found in autopsy studies.[3] Motion artifact affecting signal resolution is almost twice as great for the right compared with the left coronary artery and is minimal immediately before atrial contraction. In contrast to multidetector CT, there is no limitation because of gantry rotation, and gating can be tailored to the individual patient; signal duration is 80 ms for 60 to 70 beats/min. Respiratory motion can be limited by breath-holding, averaging for free breathing and navigator gating. The spatial resolution is theoretically similar to angiography at approximately 200 to 500 μm, but is limited by signal-to-noise ratio and duration of signal acquisition.

Imaging sequences in coronary MRI may involve black blood (fast spin-echo and double-inversion recovery fast spin-echo) or bright blood (segmented k-space gradient-echo and steady-state free precession), with either two-dimensional (breath-hold) or three-dimensional (prolonged breath-hold or free-breathing navigator) imaging. Signal-to-noise ratio is improved by frequency-selected prepulses for fat in T1 and T2 preparation prepulses, or magnetization transfer contrast to increase contrast with myocardium. Contrast-enhanced MRI is widely used for carotid, aortic, renal, and peripheral arteries; timing constraints for coronary imaging have limited the applications of clinically available extracellular agents such as gadolinium, which requires single-breath imaging.

For segmented k-space gradient-echo MRI, rapidly moving laminar blood flow is bright, whereas stagnant flow or turbulence is dark. Stenoses show varying severity of signal voids, which correlate with the degree of luminal compromise.

There is wide variation in reports of coronary MRI compared with angiography. In a multicenter trial using navigator-gated three-dimensional MR angiography, Kim and colleagues[21] reported an overall accuracy of 72% for diagnosing CAD. They reported 100% sensitivity for detection of left main or three-vessel coronary disease, and 100% negative predictive value for diagnosing left main and three-vessel coronary disease. Most segmental data suggest, however, that the predictive values for coronary MR angiography are not as high as with multidetector CT, and there are insufficient data to support clinical coronary MR angiography for the routine identification of coronary disease for chest pain or screening high-risk patients. One exception may be in patients with presumed nonischemic cardiomyopathy, in whom obstructive coronary lesions are excluded using cardiac MR angiography in conjunction with absence of segmental abnormalities on perfusion and viability studies.

Cardiac MR angiography shows promise in the detection of coronary artery bypass graft obstruction, which is excluded by two contiguous transverse images that are patent along the expected course (signal void for spin-echo and bright signal for gradient-echo). There is some evidence that there is less calcification-induced artifact in the detection of significant stenoses compared with multidetector CT.[22] Intracoronary stents result in image-degrading signal voids, which depend on the stent material and MRI sequence; stainless steel stents have prominent artifacts, in contrast to tantalum stents, which are not yet approved for coronary use. Assessment of blood flow and direction proximal and distal to the stent provides indirect evidence of stent patency.

Nuclear Medicine

Nuclear imaging approaches use molecular tags that have the potential for functional assessment of vulnerable plaques. Although highly sensitive and specific for their specific targets, these techniques lack spatial resolution; they are currently being studied in the carotid and aortic circulation. Spatial limitations can be significantly improved by coregistration of positron emission tomography (PET) images with CT in the newer combined PET/CT scanners. The major targets for nuclear imaging approaches have been related to inflammation, apoptosis, and oxidative stress.

Single photon emission computed tomography (SPECT) is performed using a gamma camera rotated around the patient, using single, dual, or triple headed instruments to obtain three-dimensional images. Cardiac SPECT uses ECG gating to minimize motion artifact. Current applications for cardiac SPECT are limited to myocardial perfusion imaging, generally using Tc 99m attached to a compound such as sestamibi, a lipophilic cation that distributes in the myocardium proportionally to myocardial blood flow (see Chapters 20 to 22). Gated cardiac SPECT can be used to assess regional and global wall motion and the ejection fraction.

On an investigational level, SPECT may be used for functional imaging of coronary arteries. Tc 99m-HYNIC-annexin V has been shown in animal studies to bind apoptotic cells, and shows a correlation with macrophage content in advanced atherosclerotic lesions. In humans, annexin V imaging has been limited to larger vessels, such as the carotid arteries, to identify macrophage-rich lesions. Similarly, oxidized phospholipids are concentrated in unstable plaques and can be radiolabeled with oxidation-specific epitopes. Imaging of unstable carotid plaques with the use of SPECT is under investigation. Other functional imaging targets for atherosclerosis include radiolabeled apo-B analogues, endothelin, and aminomalonic acid.

PET has some advantages over gamma camera technology, including increased resolution and the range of radionuclides that emit positrons, such as ^{11}C, ^{18}F, and ^{3}H, which can label biochemical and metabolic substrates. Currently, PET/CT scanners are used in the evaluation of obstructive coronary disease with pharmacologic stress (typically adenosine infusion). Cardiac PET/CT using rubidium 82 or ammonia N 13 is emerging as an alternative to SPECT in selected patients because it has higher spatial resolution, accurate attenuation correction, and quantitative capabilities. The images show perfusion defects reflecting coronary stenoses, and as such PET/CT does not specifically image the coronary arteries. Additionally, PET/CT using the most common clinical radioisotope, ^{18}FDG (half-life 110 minutes) (^{18}FDG-PET), can assess myocardial viability. An ^{18}FDG defect may be due to scar or hibernating myocardium, but segmental or global myocardial uptake indicates viability.

PET/CT is typically used for tumor imaging by tagged metabolites such as ^{18}FDG (^{18}FDG-PET). ^{11}C radiopharmaceuticals can also be used, but because of the short half life of ^{11}C (20 minutes), it is mostly restricted to research settings. The standard applications are oncologic, in the imaging detection of metabolically active tumors and metastases, and neurologic, in the diagnosis of dementias and seizure foci. ^{18}FDG-PET for oncologic use has shown uptake in the aorta and carotid plaques in areas of atherosclerotic inflammation and in vascular grafts.[23] There are limitations for the use of ^{18}FDG-PET or hybrid ^{18}FDG-PET/CT in coronary imaging, however, because of a lack of resolution for smaller vessels and the high myocardial uptake of ^{18}FDG. Other positron-emitting tracers, such as radiolabeled ligands that recognize macrophage receptors, including the benzodiazepine receptor ligand [^{3}H]PK 11195, also show promise in imaging atherosclerotic plaques.

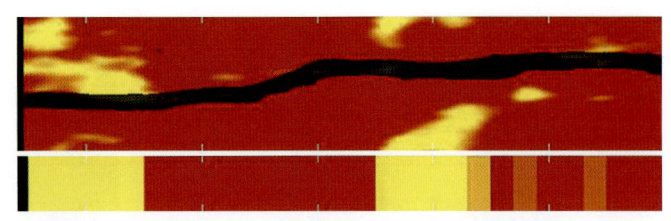

■ **FIGURE 51-6** NIRS of coronary artery. False color map of the artery wall. The color indicates probability that a lipid-rich plaque of interest is present at each location along the length (x-axis, in mm) and circumference (y-axis, in degrees) of the scanned artery (red = low probability; yellow = high probability). This display is termed a *chemogram*. (Courtesy of Simon Dixon, MD, William Beaumont Hospital, Troy, MI.)

Investigational Catheter-Based Imaging Techniques

Emerging technologies with the greatest resolution for coronary imaging are catheter-based. In addition to IVUS-VH, optical coherence tomography (OCT) offers resolution of 10 μm. OCT measures back-reflection of infrared light, analogous to IVUS, which measures reflected sound. OCT provides an image with high resolution, and is highly sensitive to the presence of lipid, including lipid within foam cell macrophages. Because of the high resolution, thin cap fibroatheroma would be expected to be detected by this modality. Acquisition rates are high, and there are no transducers within the catheters. Attenuation by blood and surface foam cells and lack of penetration of deeper regions of plaque remain obstacles to the current use of OCT as a diagnostic tool. Scattering of the signal because of blood necessitates displacing blood during imaging.[24]

Near-infrared spectroscopy (NIRS) (Fig. 51-6) is a technique that can be adapted to a catheter-based system. In contrast to OCT, these wavelengths are able to penetrate blood, can scan the circumference of the artery, and are performed at a sufficient speed to overcome interference owing to cardiac motion. The resulting spectra can be processed by an algorithm to map out lipid-rich segments of the plaque. NIRS catheter-based systems for the detection of lipid-rich plaque are currently investigational.

DIFFERENTIAL DIAGNOSIS
Clinical Presentation

The differential diagnosis of chest pain related to coronary occlusion includes musculoskeletal and gastrointestinal disease. Patients with typical cardiac pain, with ST segment abnormalities, who have normal coronary arteries by angiography are diagnosed with syndrome X, or atypical angina. Patients with syndrome X may have coronary spasm or microvascular disease, and are often women with comorbid conditions such as hypertension and diabetes.

Imaging Findings

Obstructive lesions in the coronary arteries are assumed to represent atherosclerotic plaque because few other pathologic processes result in coronary blockages in adults. In children, the most common cause of coronary lesions is Kawasaki disease, an idiopathic form of vasculitis that is likely an autoimmune disease. Rarely, coronary vasculitis may occur in adults, often as an extension of aortitis, such as Takayasu disease, in which the narrowing is generally limited to the ostium. Diffuse coronary vasculitis in adults is rare, and may be a reflection of autoimmune disease, such as lupus erythematosus, or idiopathic coronary vasculitis. In such patients, imaging findings would differ from atherosclerosis, in that lesions are typically concentric, similar to the lesions seen in allograft immune disease (transplant graft vasculopathy).

TREATMENT OPTIONS

Medical

Medical therapy for CAD includes risk factor modification, lipid lowering with statin drugs, and treatment for comorbid conditions such as hypertension and diabetes. Patients with ischemic cardiomyopathy are treated for congestive heart failure. Acute MI is treated with thrombolytic therapy (see Chapter 52).

Surgical/Interventional

Invasive treatment for coronary atherosclerosis includes thrombolytic therapy with stenting for acute MI and bypass surgery (see Chapter 52). For patients with stable disease, percutaneous intervention with stenting is typically the first-line treatment, especially in patients with focal stenosis and absence of left main disease. There is a current debate between use of bare metal stents and drug-eluting stents; the latter are approved for limited indications, and used on an off-label basis for acute coronary syndromes, distal vessel stenoses, and left main disease. There is no question that drug-eluting stents result in decreased rates of restenosis; however, there may be a slight increase in late stent thrombosis after 1 year compared with bare metal stents.

It remains to be seen if novel plaque imaging technologies allow for stratification of patients who would benefit best from one type of stent versus another—drug-eluting stent versus bare metal stent. Pathologic studies have shown that restenosis and late stent thrombosis rates may be affected by underlying plaque morphology, especially the degree of inflammation and necrotic core within the intima.[25,26]

Coronary artery bypass graft surgery has been a standard surgical treatment for CAD, especially with multivessel and left main disease. Newer technologies that minimize morbidity include off-pump methods and minimally invasive surgery. There are similar survival rates between percutaneous intervention and bypass surgery in patients with three-vessel disease.[27,28]

KEY POINTS

- Although angiography remains the gold standard for identifying stenosis in coronary arteries, CT angiography provides an alternative noninvasive approach in selected patients with similar sensitivity and specificity.
- Identification of stenoses in itself does not predict future unstable events (i.e., thrombosis). The goal of coronary artery imaging is to identify the "vulnerable plaque."
- Nuclear medicine technologies including PET and SPECT detect functional deficit caused by CAD, but they do not provide anatomic details of coronary stenoses.
- ^{18}FDG-PET and SPECT labeled with functional targets are currently investigational in functional plaque imaging, primarily of carotid and aorta, but may be applicable in the future to coronary circulation.
- Catheter-based imaging techniques, such as IVUS-VH and NIRS, are promising as complements to angiography because they provide data on composition of plaques including thin cap atheroma, a type of vulnerable plaque.

SUGGESTED READINGS

Ben-Haim S, Israel O. PET/CT for atherosclerotic plaque imaging. Q J Nucl Med Mol Imaging 2006; 50:53-60.

Burke AP, Joner M, Virmani R. IVUS-VH: a predictor of plaque morphology? Eur Heart J 2006; 27:1889-1890.

Burke AP, Virmani R, Galis Z, et al. 34th Bethesda Conference: Task force #2—what is the pathologic basis for new atherosclerosis imaging techniques? J Am Coll Cardiol 2003; 41:1874-1886.

Chien C, Feng YF, Arora RR. Advances in computed tomography-based evaluation of coronary arteries: a review of coronary artery imaging with multidetector spiral computed tomography. Rev Cardiovasc Med 2007; 8:53-60.

Choi SH, Chae A, Chen CH, et al. Emerging approaches for imaging vulnerable plaques in patients. Curr Opin Biotechnol 2007; 18:73-82.

Davies JR, Rudd JH, Weissberg PL. Molecular and metabolic imaging of atherosclerosis. J Nucl Med 2004; 45:1898-1907.

De Feyter PJ, Meijboom WB, Weustink A, et al. Spiral multislice computed tomography coronary angiography: a current status report. Clin Cardiol 2007; 30:437-442.

de Roos A, Kroft LJ, Bax JJ, et al. Applications of multislice computed tomography in coronary artery disease. J Magn Reson Imaging 2007; 26:14-22.

Kolodgie FD, Burke AP, Farb A, et al. The thin-cap fibroatheroma: a type of vulnerable plaque: the major precursor lesion to acute coronary syndromes. Curr Opin Cardiol 2001; 16:285-292.

Manning WJ, Nezafat R, Appelbaum E, et al. Coronary magnetic resonance imaging. Magn Reson Imaging Clin N Am 2007; 15:609-637.

Meijs MF, Meijboom WB, Cramer MJ, et al. Computed tomography of the coronary arteries: an alternative? Scand Cardiovasc J 2007; 41:277-286.

Schuijf JD, Jukema JW, van der Wall EE, et al. The current status of multislice computed tomography in the diagnosis and prognosis of coronary artery disease. J Nucl Cardiol 2007; 14:604-612.

REFERENCES

1. Proudfit WL, Shirey EK, Sones FM Jr. Selective cine coronary arteriography: correlation with clinical findings in 1,000 patients. Circulation 1966; 33:901-910.
2. Rosamond W, Flegal K, Furie K, et al. Heart disease and stroke statistics—2008 update: a report from the American Heart Association Statistics Committee and Stroke Statistics Subcommittee. Circulation 2008; 117:e25-e146.
3. Virmani R, Kolodgie FD, Burke AP, et al. Lessons from sudden coronary death: a comprehensive morphological classification scheme for atherosclerotic lesions. Arterioscler Thromb Vasc Biol 2000; 20:1262-1275.
4. Burke AP, Farb A, Malcom GT, et al. Coronary risk factors and plaque morphology in men with coronary disease who died suddenly. N Engl J Med 1997; 336:1276-1282.
5. Farb A, Burke AP, Tang AL, et al. Coronary plaque erosion without rupture into a lipid core: a frequent cause of coronary thrombosis in sudden coronary death. Circulation 1996; 93:1354-1363.
6. Burke AP, Kolodgie FD, Farb A, et al. Healed plaque ruptures and sudden coronary death: evidence that subclinical rupture has a role in plaque progression. Circulation 2001; 103:934-940.
7. Burke AP, Taylor A, Farb A, et al. Coronary calcification: insights from sudden coronary death victims. Z Kardiol 2000; 89(Suppl 2):49-53.
8. Scanlon PJ, Faxon DP, Audet AM, et al. ACC/AHA guidelines for coronary angiography: executive summary and recommendations: a report of the American College of Cardiology/American Heart Association Task Force on Practice Guidelines (Committee on Coronary Angiography) developed in collaboration with the Society for Cardiac Angiography and Interventions. Circulation 1999; 99: 2345-2357.
9. Staiger J, Adler CP, Dieckmann H, et al. Postmortem angiographic and pathologic-anatomic findings in coronary heart disease: a comparative study using planimetry. Cardiovasc Intervent Radiol 1980; 3:139-143.
10. Wijpkema JS, Dorgelo J, Willems TP, et al. Discordance between anatomical and functional coronary stenosis severity. Neth Heart J 2007; 15:5-11.
11. Glaser R, Selzer F, Faxon DP, et al. Clinical progression of incidental, asymptomatic lesions discovered during culprit vessel coronary intervention. Circulation 2005; 111:143-149.
12. Goldstein JA, Demetriou D, Grines CL, et al. Multiple complex coronary plaques in patients with acute myocardial infarction. N Engl J Med 2000; 343:915-922.
13. Mintz GS, Nissen SE, Anderson WD, et al. American College of Cardiology Clinical Expert Consensus Document on Standards for Acquisition, Measurement and Reporting of Intravascular Ultrasound Studies (IVUS). A report of the American College of Cardiology Task Force on Clinical Expert Consensus Documents. J Am Coll Cardiol 2001; 37:1478-1492.
14. Bose D, von Birgelen C, Erbel R. Intravascular ultrasound for the evaluation of therapies targeting coronary atherosclerosis. J Am Coll Cardiol 2007; 49:925-932.
15. Kawsasaki M, Sano K, Okubo M, et al. Volumetric quantitative analysis of tissue characteristics of coronary plaques after statin therapy using three-dimensional integrated backscatter intravascular ultrasound. J Am Coll Cardiol 2005; 45:1846-1953.
16. Rodriguez-Granillo GA, Garcia-Garcia HM, McFadden EP, et al. In vivo intravascular ultrasound-derived thin-cap fibroatheroma detection using ultrasound radiofrequency data analysis. J Am Coll Cardiol 2005; 46:2038-2042.
17. Hong MK, Mintz GS, Lee CW, et al. A three-vessel virtual histology intravascular ultrasound analysis of frequency and distribution of thin-cap fibroatheromas in patients with acute coronary syndrome or stable angina pectoris. Am J Cardiol 2008; 101:568-572.
18. Rubinshtein R, Halon DA, Gaspar T, et al. Usefulness of 64-slice multidetector computed tomography in diagnostic triage of patients with chest pain and negative or nondiagnostic exercise treadmill test result. Am J Cardiol 2007; 99:925-929.
19. Leber AW, Becker A, Knez A, et al. Accuracy of 64-slice computed tomography to classify and quantify plaque volumes in the proximal coronary system: a comparative study using intravascular ultrasound. J Am Coll Cardiol 2006; 47:672-677.
20. Achenbach S, Moselewski F, Ropers D, et al. Detection of calcified and non-calcified coronary atherosclerotic plaque by contrast-enhanced, submillimeter multidetector spiral computed tomography: a segment-based comparison with intravascular ultrasound. Circulation 2004; 109:14-17.
21. Kim WY, Danias PG, Stuber M, et al. Coronary magnetic resonance angiography for the detection of coronary stenoses. N Engl J Med 2001; 345:1863-1869.
22. Liu X, Zhao X, Huang J, et al. Comparison of 3D free-breathing coronary MR angiography and 64-MDCT angiography for detection of coronary stenosis in patients with high calcium scores. AJR Am J Roentgenol 2007; 189:1326-1332.
23. Tawakol A, Migrino RQ, Bashian GG, et al. In vivo 18F-fluorodeoxyglucose positron emission tomography imaging provides a noninvasive measure of carotid plaque inflammation in patients. J Am Coll Cardiol 2006; 48:1818-1824.
24. Manfrini O, Mont E, Leone O, et al. Sources of error and interpretation of plaque morphology by optical coherence tomography. Am J Cardiol 2006; 98:156-159.
25. Farb A, Weber DK, Kolodgie FD, et al. Morphological predictors of restenosis after coronary stenting in humans. Circulation 2002; 105:2974-2980.
26. Finn AV, Joner M, Nakazawa G, et al. Pathological correlates of late drug-eluting stent thrombosis: strut coverage as a marker of endothelialization. Circulation 2007; 115:2435-2441.
27. Hannan EL, Wu C, Walford G, et al. Drug-eluting stents vs. coronary-artery bypass grafting in multivessel coronary disease. N Engl J Med 2008; 358:331-341.
28. Yang JH, Gwon HC, Cho SJ, et al. Comparison of coronary artery bypass grafting with drug-eluting stent implantation for the treatment of multivessel coronary artery disease. Ann Thorac Surg 2008; 85:65-70.

CHAPTER 52

Acute Coronary Syndrome

Joseph Jen-Sho Chen and Charles S. White

Acute coronary syndrome (ACS) is usually diagnosed in the emergency department based on history, physical examination, abnormalities on ECG, and elevations of cardiac serum biomarkers. According to the American Heart Association (AHA) and American College of Cardiology (ACC), high-risk patients recognized as having ACS should undergo early invasive coronary angiography and angiographically directed revascularization.[1] The ultimate goal is to reperfuse and salvage any viable myocardium immediately. Other imaging modalities play minimal role in the evaluation of these patients. ACS is just one of many possible diagnoses when patients present to the emergency department with acute chest pain, however. Other considerations range from acute life-threatening conditions, such as pulmonary embolism, tension pneumothorax, or aortic dissection, to conditions with less morbidity and mortality, such as gastroesophageal reflux or costochondritis.

Acute chest pain accounts for approximately 6 million emergency department visits annually, and is the second most common reason for patients to present to the emergency department in the United States.[2] Although most emergency department physicians and cardiologists have a low threshold for diagnosing ACS, 2% to 5% of patients are misdiagnosed and discharged inappropriately.[3] In these patients, the mortality rate is 1.7 to 1.9 times greater than in patients who are hospitalized. Most patients who are inappropriately discharged with ACS have a nondiagnostic initial assessment. Various noninvasive imaging modalities are available to evaluate patients with acute, but indeterminate, chest pain in the emergency department.

DEFINITION

ACS refers to any group of clinical symptoms compatible with acute myocardial ischemia. Acute myocardial ischemia is precipitated by coronary artery disease (CAD), resulting in chest pain owing to the lack of blood supply to the myocardium. When patients present with chest pain, an ECG is usually performed. The ECG may show myocardial infarction (MI) with or without ST segment elevation. Patients with ischemia-related discomfort but without ST segment elevation are classified as having either unstable angina or non–ST segment elevation myocardial infarction (NSTEMI). Unstable angina is unexpected chest pain or discomfort that usually occurs while at rest. The discomfort may be more severe and prolonged than typical angina, or may be an initial episode of angina. NSTEMI usually progresses to subendocardial acute MI. Patients who have ST segment elevation myocardial infarction (STEMI) are likely to go on to develop a transmural acute MI. ACS is a spectrum of clinical diagnoses, ranging from unstable angina to NSTEMI to STEMI. Other conditions may mimic ACS, and these need to be excluded.

PREVALENCE AND EPIDEMIOLOGY

In the most recent National Hospital Discharge Survey by the National Center for Health Statistics, there were approximately 1.4 million unique hospitalizations because of ACS in the United States in 2005.[4] ACS is a major cause of morbidity and mortality in Western countries. The prevalence of ACS increases with age and predominates in men among patients younger than 70 years. In patients older than 70 years, the incidence occurs with equal frequency in men and women. Other risk factors that predispose patients to ACS include diabetes mellitus, smoking, hypertension, hypercholesterolemia, hyperlipidemia, a prior cerebrovascular event, inherited metabolic or connective tissue disorder, cocaine or amphetamine use, and occupational stress.

ETIOLOGY AND PATHOPHYSIOLOGY

Atherosclerosis is the most common culprit leading to acute myocardial ischemia because it decreases the blood supply to a portion of myocardium. At first, even in the setting of atherosclerotic coronary plaques, the coronary arteries permit adequate blood flow to counterbalance myocardial demand. As myocardial demand increases, such as during exercise or stress, the decrease in blood supply may become clinically significant, resulting in angina. Initially, the angina may develop during exertion and resolve at rest, and this is termed *stable angina*.

Many atherosclerotic plaques are composed of rich foam cells (lipid-laden macrophages), inflammatory cells, and a thin fibrous cap. Such plaques are susceptible to sudden rupture or erosion, exposing the thrombogenic surfaces of the plaques, and allowing platelet aggregation and thrombus formation to occur. Distal microembolization of thrombi may also result. These events usually are not limited to one particular coronary artery, but affect other coronary arteries as well.

Less common causes of acute myocardial ischemia include intense focal epicardial coronary spasm (Prinzmetal angina), cardiac emboli, and arterial inflammation caused by or related to infection. Rarely, myocardial ischemia may occur secondary to increased myocardial demand, particularly sepsis, fever, tachycardia, thyrotoxicosis, or anemia. These precipitating conditions usually occur in patients who have underlying stable CAD.

MANIFESTATIONS OF DISEASE
Clinical Presentation

The typical presentation is characterized by substernal tightness, pressure, squeezing, or heaviness with or without pain radiating to the neck or arm. The chest pain, or angina, can be new in onset and can cause marked limitation of physical activity. The pain may be initiated either at rest or during exertion. Unstable angina may last more than 20 minutes during rest or be signified by a change compared with previous angina, with increasing length, frequency, or onset with less exertion. Atypical chest pain, such as epigastric pain or stabbing or pleuritic chest pain, is a common manifestation of myocardial ischemia. Symptoms other than chest pain, such as dyspnea, nausea or vomiting or both, palpitations, syncope, or cardiac arrest, also can be observed. Atypical presentations are more common in patients who are older, diabetic, and female.

Physical examination findings are frequently unremarkable. Signs of hypotension or congestive heart failure, such as new murmurs, gallops, or rales, may be present.

ECG findings of ST segment or T wave changes and elevated serum cardiac biomarkers, especially cardiac troponins, indicate ACS. The results of ECG are often nonspecific, however, and serum cardiac biomarkers, such as creatine kinase MB (CK-MB) isoenzyme and cardiac troponins, may not be useful in patients who present to the emergency department less than 4 to 5 hours after the onset of their symptoms.

Imaging Indications and Algorithm

Although complicated algorithms exist for classifying risk with regard to indications for noninvasive imaging, chest pain can be categorized into three general groups. The first group comprises patients with life-threatening conditions, in particular high-risk patients diagnosed with ACS based on the history and physical examination, ECG findings, and elevated troponins. These patients immediately undergo coronary angiography and angiographically directed revascularization. Emergent medical and surgical intervention is also required for other life-threatening conditions, such as pulmonary embolism, aortic dissection, and tension pneumothorax.

The second group comprises patients who present with acute chest pain that does not require immediate invasive intervention or imaging, such as gastroesophageal reflux disease or costochondritis. These patients are usually triaged and discharged quickly with a recommendation for outpatient follow-up.

The third group comprises patients who usually present to the emergency department with acute chest pain that is indeterminate for ACS because of a nondiagnostic history, physical examination, or ECG. These patients are considered a diagnostic challenge and often require further noninvasive imaging, including chest radiography, echocardiography, multidetector CT, MRI, and radionuclide perfusion imaging as part of further work-up.

Imaging Technique and Findings
Radiography

Conventional chest radiography is the imaging modality used initially for screening noncardiac etiologies of acute chest pain, including pneumonia, pneumothorax, or rib fractures. Chest pain of cardiac origin also can be indirectly evaluated using chest radiography. Coronary arterial stenosis may be hinted by coronary artery calcification, which is seen in the "coronary triangle"—the mid-upper portion of the left cardiac silhouette on the frontal chest radiograph. In addition, circumferential calcifications may be seen within the expected location of myocardial wall, suggesting prior MI (Fig. 52-1). On the lateral chest radiograph, "tram-track" hyperdensities along the aortic arch correspond to atherosclerotic calcifications in the aorta, which can be independently correlated with coronary heart disease.[5]

Atherosclerotic calcifications overlying the borders of the heart may also indicate previous episodes of MI.[6,7] Specifically, hyperdensity or calcifications of the left heart border, often curvilinear, may signify prior infarction of the left ventricular anterolateral wall. Focal outpouching of the left heart border may also represent postinfarct myocardial pseudoaneurysm or aneurysm.[8]

Chest radiography may not only indicate coronary heart disease and prior MI, but it may also be indicative of acute myocardial ischemia. Acute myocardial ischemia may manifest as mild to severe congestive heart failure, ranging from cephalization of blood flow to the upper lobes on erect chest radiography to diffuse interstitial or alveolar pulmonary edema.

Ultrasonography

In risk stratifying and evaluating patients who present to the emergency department with acute chest pain, stress echocardiography is a versatile imaging modality. The prognostic information obtained is equivalent to radionuclide perfusion imaging and may be used to exclude ACS.[9,10] Stress echocardiography provides functional and

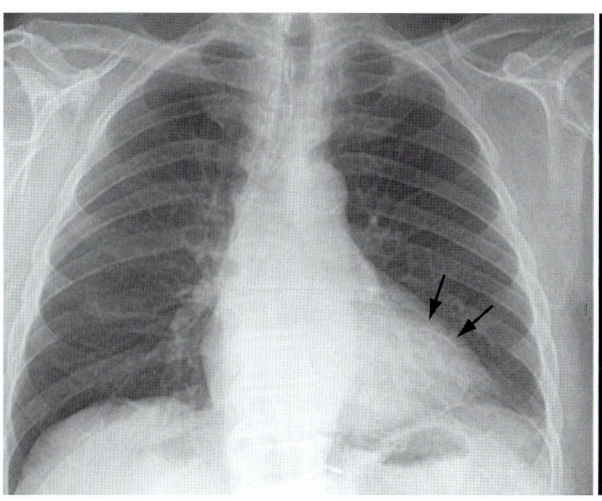

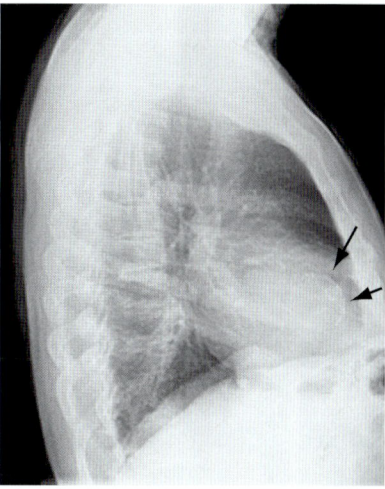

FIGURE 52-1 A 58-year-old man presented to the emergency department with chest pain. Posteroanterior and lateral chest radiographs show a circumferential thin band of calcification (*arrows*) in the left mid-anterior myocardium, likely representing prior MI.

anatomic information by evaluating baseline ventricular function (e.g., ejection fraction, wall motion), valvular function, aortic root morphology, and pericardial anatomy. If a study shows reduction in ejection fraction or wall motion abnormality, especially as an interval change from previous assessment, the findings suggest myocardial ischemia.

Stress echocardiography has limitations in the acute emergency department setting. Patients who have had interval resolution of their acute chest pain symptoms, nontransmural or small MI, or other structural abnormality of the heart may not have wall motion abnormalities or reduced ejection fraction, and may have false-negative results. In addition, causes of chest pain outside the heart are often not well evaluated by echocardiography. Conversely, the portability of stress echocardiography is beneficial, although its use may be limited by dependence on operator experience and restricted availability during off-hours.

Computed Tomography

In recent years, CT has become a noninvasive alternative to invasive coronary angiography in addition to its long-standing role in more general evaluation of the thorax. As the number of detectors has increased from 4 to 320, and gantry rotation speeds have increased, the spatial and temporal resolution for cardiac imaging acquisition has dramatically improved. The current generation of multidetector CT scanners provides accurate anatomic assessment of the coronary vasculature, allowing visualization to at least the third generation of coronary vessels. Compared with invasive coronary angiography, multiple studies have found multidetector CT to have sensitivity of 83% to 99%, specificity of 86% to 98%, positive predictive value of 66% to 93%, and negative predictive value of 97% to 99% in the evaluation of significant coronary arterial stenosis.[11]

Cardiac multidetector CT approaches the capability of invasive coronary angiography, the gold standard, in its ability to evaluate coronary arterial stenosis. Multidetector CT has several additional capabilities that can be valuable to emergency department physicians and cardiologists (Figs. 52-2 to 52-5). Cardiac multidetector CT can be used to assess the quantity and composition of atherosclerotic plaques and, potentially, to differentiate stable from unstable plaques.[12,13] Cardiac multidetector CT also can evaluate myocardial function by assessing left ventricular wall motion and ejection fraction on the basis of images obtained throughout the different phases of the cardiac cycle.[14] Dynamic imaging can be performed to assess perfusion of the myocardium.

Before actual multidetector CT imaging, oral or intravenous β blockers, particularly metoprolol, are administered to reduce heart rate and prevent beat-to-beat variability, with the purpose of reducing motion artifacts and improving image quality. Cardiac images are typically acquired when the patient is breath-holding during mid-inspiration to allow smooth flow of nonionic intravenous contrast agent into the right atrium, resulting in homogeneous enhancement of the heart. With breath-holding, an anatomic triggering mechanism is used to allow rapid injection of intravenous contrast agent. ECG gating is crucial for optimal image acquisition and reconstruction of evenly spaced phases of the cardiac cycle. The reconstructed images are performed in a limited field of view, with the axial images centered on the heart. In the "triple rule-out" chest pain protocol, which is directed at excluding pulmonary embolism and aortic dissection in addition to CAD, an additional large field of view reconstruction, usually at 70% or 80% of the R–R interval, is obtained.

Currently, two protocols—comprehensive or triple rule-out multidetector CT of the chest and dedicated coronary CT angiography—are available when a patient presents to the emergency department with acute chest pain, depending on the specific clinical suspicion related to the chest pain. The comprehensive or triple rule-out protocol images the entire chest. In a patient who has acute, but nonspecific chest pain, a triple rule-out protocol may be used to evaluate life-threatening diagnoses other than ACS, particularly pulmonary embolism and aortic dissection, in addition to the coronary arteries. The dedicated coronary CT angiography protocol is more appropriate when the patient's presentation strongly suggests a coronary etiology for the chest pain. By using a limited field of view and excluding structures superior to the aortic arch and

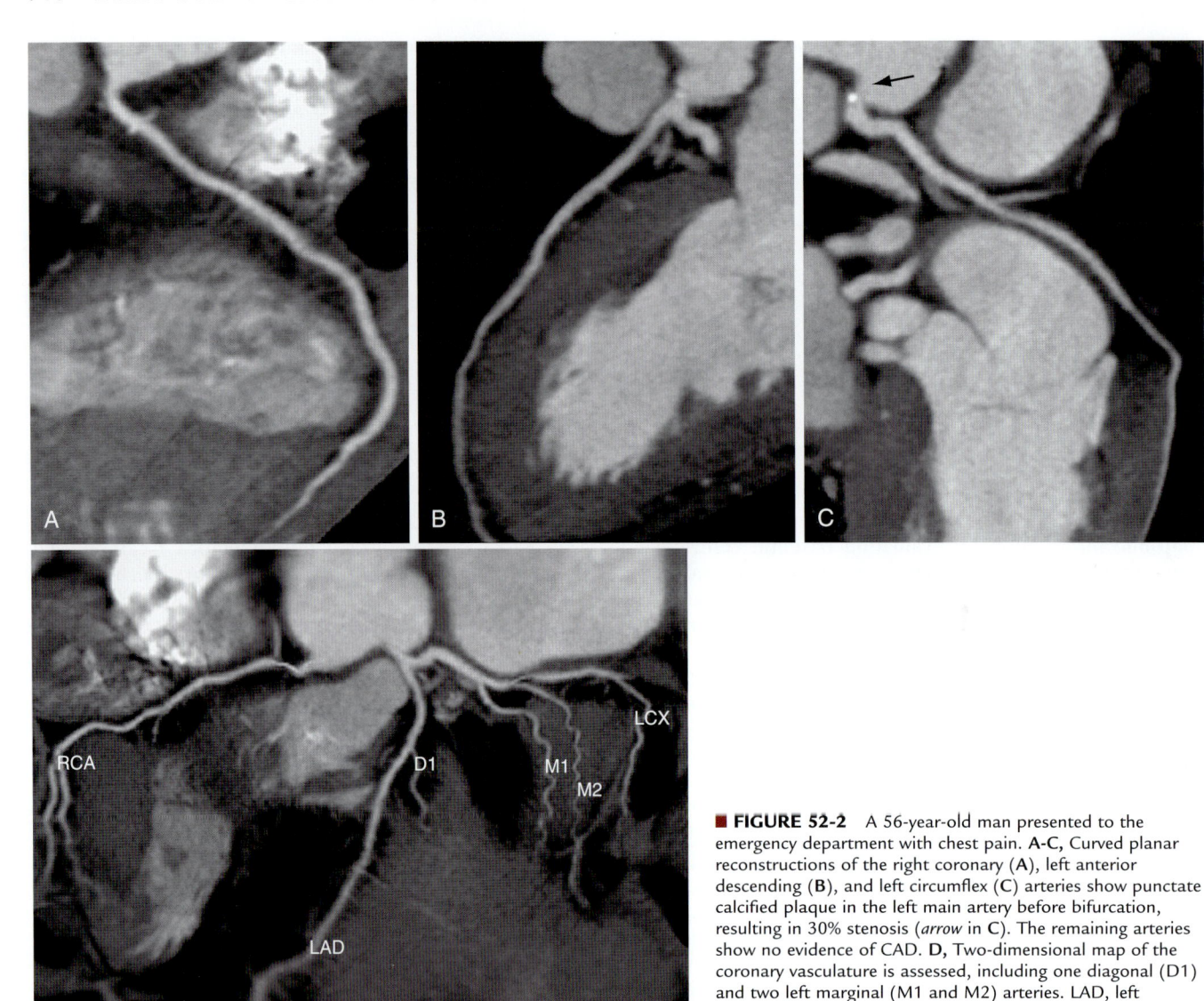

FIGURE 52-2 A 56-year-old man presented to the emergency department with chest pain. **A-C,** Curved planar reconstructions of the right coronary (**A**), left anterior descending (**B**), and left circumflex (**C**) arteries show punctate calcified plaque in the left main artery before bifurcation, resulting in 30% stenosis (*arrow* in **C**). The remaining arteries show no evidence of CAD. **D,** Two-dimensional map of the coronary vasculature is assessed, including one diagonal (D1) and two left marginal (M1 and M2) arteries. LAD, left anterior descending; LCX, left circumflex; RCA, right coronary artery.

FIGURE 52-3 A 43-year-old man presented to the emergency department with chest pain. **A-C,** Curved planar reconstructions of the left anterior descending (**A**), left circumflex (**B**), and right coronary (**C**) arteries show no evidence of CAD.

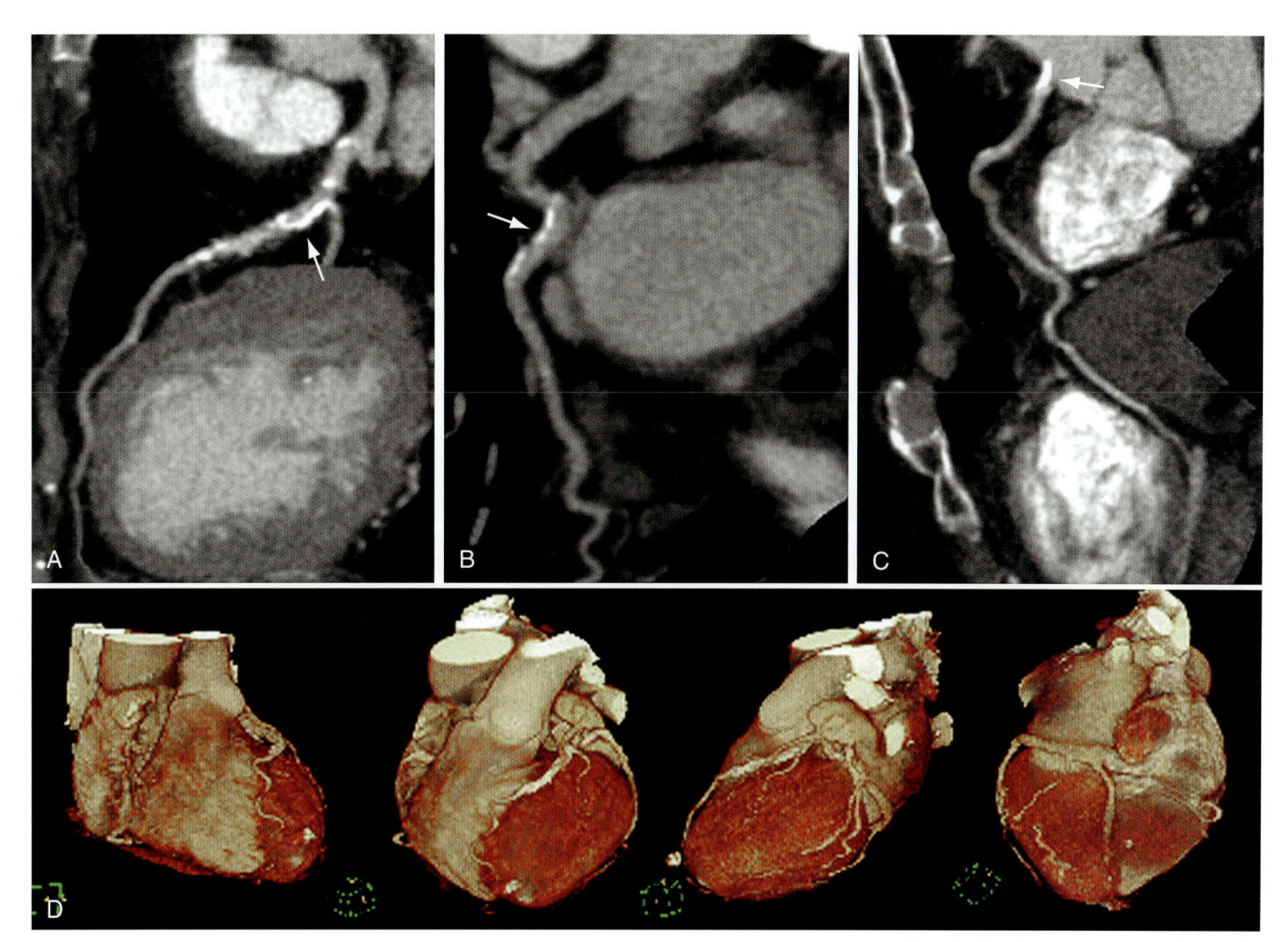

FIGURE 52-4 A 78-year-old man presented to the emergency department with atypical chest pain and was diagnosed with three-vessel CAD with predominantly calcified plaques. **A-C,** Using curved planar reconstructions, a 50% to 70% stenosis involving the proximal and mid left anterior descending artery (*arrow* in **A**), and a 30% to 50% stenosis in the proximal left circumflex artery (*arrow* in **B**) are seen. The right coronary artery also shows a proximal lesion with a 30% to 50% stenosis (*arrow* in **C**). **D,** Volumetric reconstructions show scattered atherosclerotic changes of the vessels. A right dominant posterior descending artery is also seen.

inferior to the cardiac apex, the dedicated protocol reduces image acquisition time and radiation dose, and provides the best possible resolution of the coronary arteries.

Images of a standard multidetector CT scan of the chest are acquired from the thoracic inlet to the upper portion of the abdomen without the use of ECG gating and with a wide field of view. The dedicated coronary CT angiography protocol requires the use of ECG gating and a limited field of view. A major challenge of the triple rule-out protocol is the fusion of these two methods. Currently in our institution, the triple rule-out protocol is obtained using ECG gating and an unrestricted field of view. Images are acquired in a caudocephalic direction, the reverse of dedicated coronary CT angiography, with the goal of minimizing artifacts caused by respiration. For optimal image quality, a slightly larger volume of intravenous contrast agent is administered to maintain simultaneous peak contrast levels in the coronary and pulmonary arteries (Table 52-1).

Several preliminary studies have shown dedicated coronary CT angiography to be a useful noninvasive imaging modality in the evaluation of patients with acute chest pain in the emergency department. In one study, all patients received standard of care assessment to rule out ACS, including invasive coronary angiography.[15] Patients also underwent CT angiography to assess the presence of coronary atherosclerotic plaque and significant coronary artery stenosis (≥50%). Compared with standard of care, coronary CT angiography had 100% sensitivity and 82% specificity. The absence of coronary plaque and significant arterial stenosis excluded ACS in 100% of patients.

The use of the comprehensive or triple rule-out multidetector CT protocol has also been studied in patients with acute chest pain in the emergency department. In a separate study of this algorithm, all patients underwent a triple rule-out multidetector CT scan immediately after a serum creatinine value and an initial history, physical examination, and ECG were obtained.[16] After CT, patients proceeded to receive the standard of care evaluation and treatment. One month after discharge, medical records were reviewed by consensus. Overall, the sensitivity, specificity, positive predictive value, and negative predictive value for CAD were 83%, 96%, 83%, and 96%,

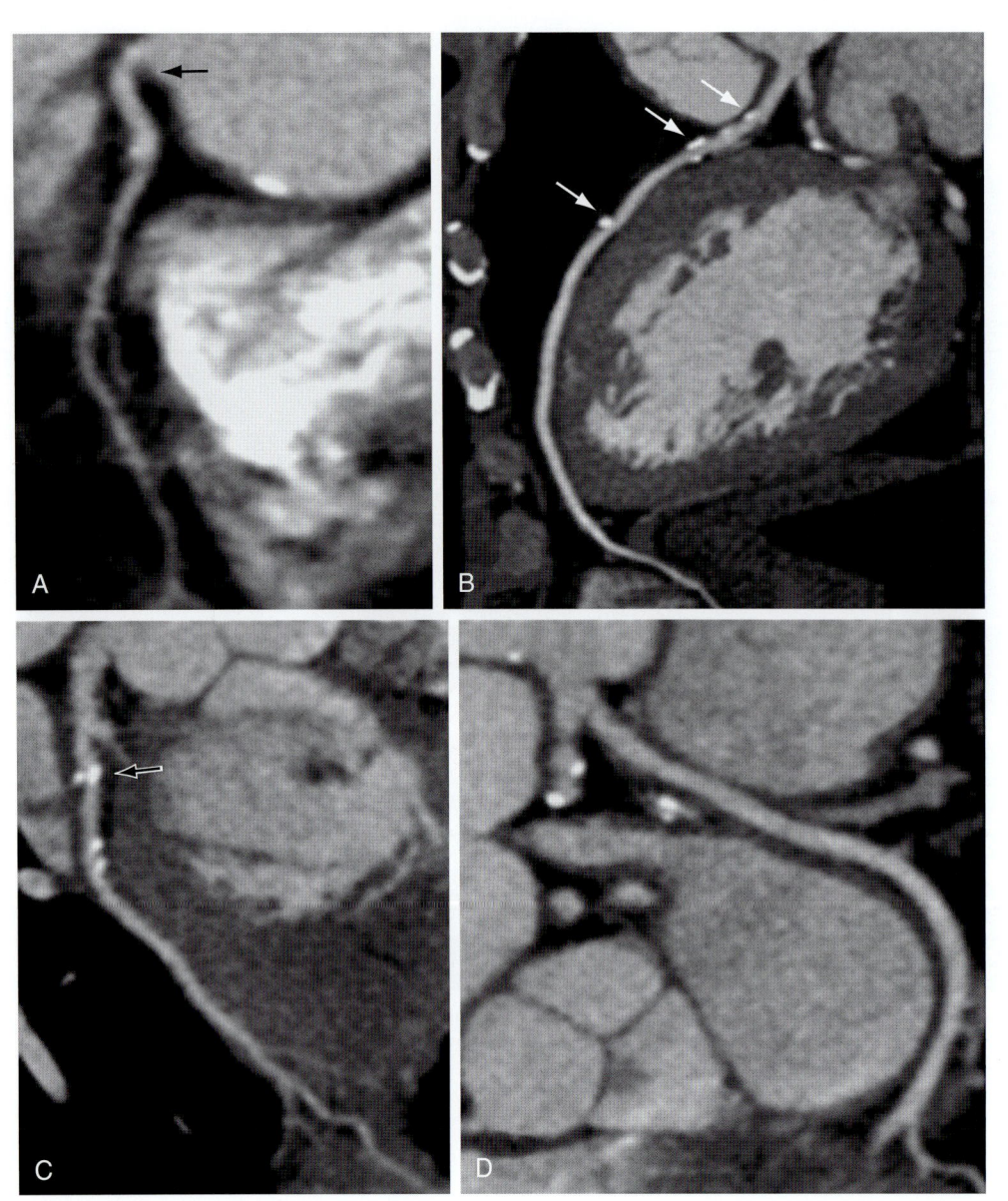

FIGURE 52-5 A 56-year-old man presented to the emergency department with chest pain and shortness of breath. **A,** Curved planar reconstruction of the right coronary artery shows small and nondominant mild calcified plaque at the ostium (*arrow*). **B,** Scattered foci of calcified plaque formation involve the proximal, mid, and distal left anterior descending artery, resulting in 30% stenoses (*arrows*). **C,** A calcified plaque (*arrow*) in the proximal first obtuse marginal branch results in significant narrowing with several smaller calcified plaques distally. **D,** The left circumflex artery shows no evidence of disease.

TABLE 52-1	Sample Protocol Parameters for 64-Detector Multidetector CT for Acute Chest Pain Evaluation	
Protocol	Dedicated CT Angiography	Triple Rule-Out
kVp	120	120
mAs/slice	800	600
Field of view	220	400
Thickness (mm)	0.67	0.9
Increment (mm)	0.33	0.45
Rotation time (sec)	0.4	0.4
Direction	Cephalocaudal	Caudocephalad
Time (sec)	9-10	15-18
Injection protocol	6 mL/sec (80 mL contrast), then 5 mL/sec (50 mL contrast/saline), then 5 mL/sec (50 mL saline)	5 mL/sec (80 mL contrast), then 2 mL/sec (50 mL contrast), then 2 mL/sec (50 mL saline)
Bolus tracker	Ascending aorta	Descending aorta

respectively. If noncardiac etiologies were also assessed, the sensitivity and positive predictive value increased to 87%. Comprehensive multidetector CT has the potential to evaluate cardiac and noncardiac causes of acute chest pain.

Another study has shown cardiac multidetector CT to be just as accurate in detecting and excluding ACS as the current standard of care using radionuclide perfusion imaging.[17] In addition, the median diagnostic time and cost of care were significantly reduced. Cardiac multidetector CT can be as safe and efficacious as the standard of care, and the efficiency (diagnostic time and cost of care) is improved in evaluating emergency department patients with acute chest pain.

To date, there are several limitations to the widespread adoption of cardiac multidetector CT in the emergency department. First, the postprocessing of data after image acquisition is time-consuming and labor-intensive, restricting its use during off hours. Second, the radiation burden is still high (often >10 mSv), even with the use of current

CHAPTER 52 • Acute Coronary Syndrome

TABLE 52-2 University of Maryland Triage for Cardiac Multidetector CT Studies

Risk Category for ACS	CT Interpretation	Clinical Guideline
High	Coronary calcification (Agatston score) >400 Hard or soft plaque Stenosis >70% in any vessel Stenosis >50% in left main artery	Admission
Medium	Coronary calcification 100-400 Stenosis 30%-70% in any vessel	Cardiology consultation
Low	Coronary calcification <100	Follow-up with preventive cardiology
Negative	Normal study	Follow-up with primary care provider

technologies, such as ECG-controlled tube current modulation, which can potentially reduce the exposure. Radionuclide perfusion imaging (8 to 10 mSv) and invasive coronary angiography also have substantial radiation doses, however. Third, although the triage of a negative result in cardiac multidetector CT is straightforward, the course of a positive result is less certain and remains to be defined (Table 52-2). Finally, a larger, multi-institutional clinical study using cardiac multidetector CT to evaluate ACS is still required to establish the role of multidetector CT in acute chest pain assessment.

Magnetic Resonance Imaging

MRI can be used to assess myocardial function, perfusion, and viability.[18] Myocardial function assessment is based on the evaluation of myocardial wall motion. Assessments of myocardial perfusion and viability require intravenous administration of gadolinium contrast material and acquisition of dynamic images during the immediate and delayed (10 to 15 minutes) phases. These findings can facilitate the detection of myocardial ischemia, postischemic stunning or hibernation, and MI. In one study, cardiac MRI detected and diagnosed ACS with a sensitivity of 84% and specificity of 85%.[19]

Cardiac assessment using MRI is primarily based on myocardial wall motion and perfusion and viability images obtained after contrast administration. If wall motion abnormality is observed, but the perfusion and viability (delayed) images are normal, the myocardium may have endured an ischemic insult, a situation termed *myocardial stunning*. If wall motion and the perfusion (immediate postgadolinium) images are abnormal, but no abnormal uptake of the contrast material is seen in the viability (delayed) images, postischemic hibernation is diagnosed. If viability images show uptake of gadolinium within the myocardium, as shown by high signal intensity, the finding is consistent with MI (Fig. 52-6).

Compared with radionuclide myocardial imaging and stress echocardiography, MRI is able to overcome some disadvantages. The anatomic and functional assessments of the myocardium are better because of improved spatial and temporal resolution. In addition, cardiac MRI may be available 24 hours a day, particularly in larger centers. In addition, there is no radiation dose exposure because no ionizing radiation is used in MRI, in contrast to radionuclide myocardial perfusion. The disadvantages of MRI include the greater length of time for image acquisition, distance of the scanner from the emergency department in most departments, and lack of expertise at many facilities. From a practical standpoint, cardiac MRI is more often used to assess chronic myocardial ischemia or infarction than acute chest pain.

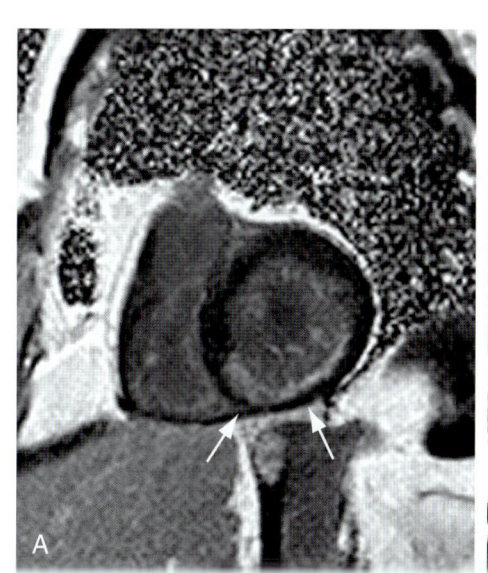

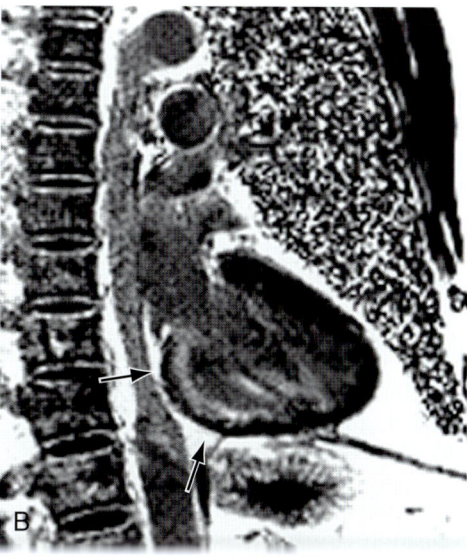

■ **FIGURE 52-6** A 60-year-old man presented to the emergency department with chest pain. **A** and **B**, MRI viability images in short-axis (**A**) and vertical long-axis (**B**) views of the left ventricle show delayed contrast enhancement involving the mid to basal portion of the inferior, subendocardial wall of the left ventricle (*arrows*), consistent with subendocardial infarct of the myocardium.

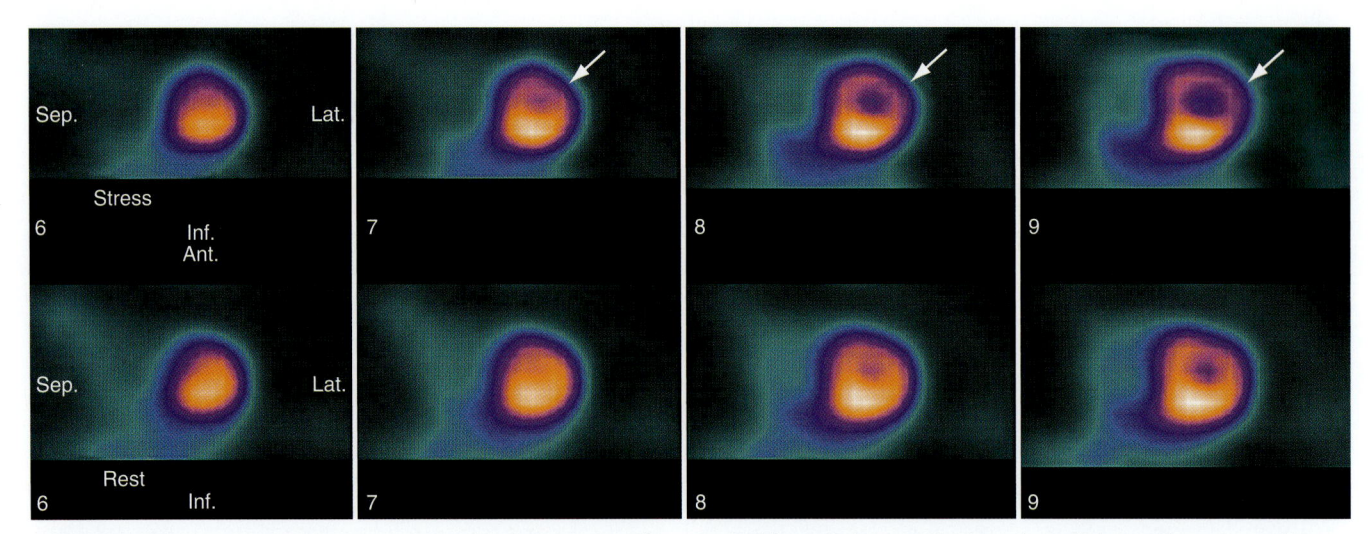

FIGURE 52-7 A 55-year-old woman presented to the emergency department with atypical chest pain. Stress images show radiotracer uptake defect in the apical anterior/anterolateral myocardium (*arrows*). On rest images, the uptake defect is reversed, and the myocardial uptake of the radiotracer is normal, suggesting reversible myocardial ischemia.

Nuclear Medicine

In patients with low to intermediate risk of ACS, radionuclide or myocardial perfusion imaging is typically a part of a cardiac evaluation protocol for risk stratification.[20] Either during or immediately after an acute episode of chest pain, Tc 99m tetrofosmin or sestamibi is injected. Image acquisition is obtained using single photon emission computed tomography (SPECT) 45 to 60 minutes after injection of the radionuclide. Two sets of images are acquired to reflect myocardial blood flow at the time of the injection: one set of images with adenosine infusion or exercise stress and a second set of images at rest.

Radionuclide perfusion imaging is a powerful imaging modality in the diagnosis of ACS. The sensitivity, specificity, and negative predictive value are 92%, 71%, and 99%, respectively.[21] As a result, a negative radionuclide perfusion study in a patient with acute chest pain in the emergency department suggests minimal or no risk of an adverse cardiac event.[22] Myocardial perfusion imaging can also be used for prognosis and risk stratification for future cardiac events.[23] If a perfusion defect is shown, the patient is at higher risk of having a cardiac event during hospitalization or at follow-up.

The main purpose of myocardial perfusion study is to assess the myocardial function by evaluating inducible perfusion abnormality, myocardial viability, and regional and global myocardial wall motion. Inducible perfusion abnormality is diagnosed if the uptake of radiotracer in a certain region of the myocardium is reduced during stress imaging. During the rest images, the myocardium takes up the radiotracer normally, suggesting the ischemic territory is reversible, and the perfusion abnormality is inducible by stress (Fig. 52-7). Conversely, if the radiotracer is not taken up by the myocardium during the rest images, the myocardium is considered nonviable. Abnormality in wall motion can also be evaluated by visualizing the decrease or lack of contractility in the region of myocardial ischemia and infarct.

Although radionuclide perfusion is a powerful component of the acute chest pain evaluation armamentarium, there are several drawbacks that hinder its widespread use. Radionuclide perfusion imaging is restricted in its ability to assess the myocardial structure and anatomy because of technical limitations in spatial resolution and photon attenuation. In addition, isotope preparation, decay, and licensing, and restrictive availability during off-hours limit its use. In most hospitals, any radionuclide perfusion study requires transporting a potentially unstable patient because nuclear medicine departments are rarely located adjacent to the emergency department.

Angiography

Cardiac catheterization and coronary angiography are currently the standard in the evaluation of high-risk patients with ACS. Cardiac catheterization provides a measure of intracardiac pressure, oxygen saturation, and cardiac output. Left ventricular function can also be evaluated. Coronary angiography remains the gold standard for delineating coronary anatomy and diagnosing CAD. Coronary angiography is used to assess the site, severity, and morphology of lesions and provides a qualitative measurement of coronary blood flow. Collateral vessels can also be identified.

Percutaneous coronary intervention (PCI) using angioplasty and stent placement to revascularize the myocardium may be performed in the same setting. Compared with thrombolytic therapy, PCI is associated with a lower mortality, lower reinfarction rate, and lower frequency of stroke.[24,25] PCI also restores flow to the occluded coronary artery with greater speed and frequency and with a high success rate.[26]

Classic Signs

Obstruction to coronary flow and myocardial wall motion and perfusion abnormalities may be evident using one or more of the previously described techniques.

DIFFERENTIAL DIAGNOSIS

The differential diagnoses that should be considered other than ACS, especially if the patient presents to the emergency department with atypical chest pain, can be categorized as either life-threatening conditions or conditions with less morbidity and mortality. Life-threatening diagnoses include aortic dissection or leaking aneurysm, cardiac tamponade, cardiomyopathies, esophageal rupture, hypertensive emergencies, perforated gastric ulcer, pneumothorax, and pulmonary embolism. Less emergent conditions include anxiety, asthma, costochondritis, esophagitis, gastroenteritis, myocarditis, and pericarditis. Many life-threatening conditions cannot be diagnosed solely based on clinical presentation. Various imaging modalities are essential to differentiate and treat these conditions emergently.

TREATMENT OPTIONS

Medical

ACC/AHA guidelines recommend all initial therapy be implemented in the emergency department based on an institution-specific, written protocol.[27] Patients presenting to the emergency department with symptoms suggestive of an acute myocardial event should be evaluated within 10 minutes after arrival. Early assessment includes confirmation of hemodynamic stability and securing the airway, breathing, and circulation; obtaining a 12-lead ECG; and administering oxygen to maintain saturation greater than 90%, intravenous analgesia (most commonly morphine sulfate), oral aspirin (162 to 325 mg), and sublingual nitroglycerin (0.4 mg per 5 minutes for a total of three doses) if not contraindicated. Initial history, physical examination, and laboratory work are also necessary.

All patients with suspected or definite ACS should be admitted to the hospital. High-risk patients should be admitted to a coronary care unit. Patients with a low risk for major complications can be admitted to a telemetry unit. Resuscitative medical therapy and equipment should be readily available, including lidocaine, atropine, an external or internal pacemaker, and a defibrillator.

In patients with acute STEMI whose onset of symptoms is of less than 12 hours' duration, reperfusion therapy with primary PCI or thrombolysis is essential. If PCI is unavailable, thrombolytic therapy (combination of heparin plus tissue plasminogen activator or streptokinase or both) must be administered promptly (in <30 minutes) in patients without contraindications for thrombolysis. If there is a relative delay in performing primary PCI (>60 minutes), thrombolytic therapy is also recommended. In patients with unstable angina or NSTEMI, thrombolytic therapy should not be administered.

Several medications should also be given to all patients with ACS and without contraindications, regardless of reperfusion therapy, including clopidogrel, glycoprotein IIb/IIIa inhibitors, β blockers, and calcium channel blockers. Angiotensin-converting enzyme inhibitors and angiotensin receptor blockers may also be given. If a patient is to undergo reperfusion therapy, data have shown that clopidogrel (300 or 600 mg) and glycoprotein IIb/IIIa inhibitors reduce thrombotic complications.

Surgical/Interventional

The ACC/AHA Task Force recommends the use of PCI with possible stent placement for any patient with acute STEMI who presents within 12 hours of onset of symptoms, and who can undergo the procedure within 90 minutes of presentation.[27] For unstable angina and NSTEMI, only high-risk patients should undergo early PCI management. High-risk indicators include (1) recurrent angina at rest or with low-level activity despite intensive medical therapy; (2) elevated cardiac troponin levels; (3) new, or presumably new, ST segment depression; (4) recurrent angina or ischemia with heart failure; (5) high-risk findings on noninvasive stress testing; (6) depressed left ventricular function (ejection fraction <40%) on noninvasive study; (7) hemodynamic instability; (8) sustained ventricular tachycardia; (9) PCI within the previous 6 months; and (10) previous coronary artery bypass graft (CABG) surgery.[28] Otherwise, medical management is recommended.

As described in the most recent ACC/AHA practice guideline, CABG surgery may offer a survival advantage compared with medical management in patients with unstable angina and left ventricular dysfunction, especially in patients with three-vessel CAD.[29] There is as yet no medical evidence, however, to suggest CABG surgery is better than PCI in patients with unstable angina. No study has shown that CABG surgery should be performed in patients with NSTEMI or STEMI in the acute setting.

INFORMATION FOR THE REFERRING PHYSICIAN

Standard methods of reporting the various imaging modalities exist with templates having been developed for each technique. Images can also be placed in the report. Notwithstanding the necessity of a complete written report, it is often essential for direct communication to occur between the imaging physician and the referring physician because of the acuteness of the situation.

KEY POINTS

- ACS is a life-threatening illness that must be distinguished from other causes of chest pain in the emergency department.
- Multiple imaging techniques are used to make the distinction, including chest radiography, echocardiography, radionuclide studies, multidetector CT, and MRI.
- Invasive angiography with intervention may be necessary in patients with definite ACS and in patients in whom the diagnosis is uncertain.

SUGGESTED READINGS

Anderson JL, Adams CD, Antman EM, et al: ACC/AHA 2007 guidelines for the management of patients with unstable angina/non-ST-elevation myocardial infarction: a report of the American College of Cardiology/American Heart Association Task Force on Practice Guidelines (Writing Committee to Revise the 2002 Guidelines for the Management of Patients with Unstable Angina/Non-ST-Elevation Myocardial Infarction) developed in collaboration with the American College of Emergency Physicians, the Society for Cardiovascular Angiography and Interventions, and the Society of Thoracic Surgeons endorsed by the American Association of Cardiovascular and Pulmonary Rehabilitation and the Society for Academic Emergency Medicine. J Am Coll Cardiol 2007; 50:e1.

Antman EM, Anbe DT, Armstrong PW, et al: ACC/AHA guidelines for the management of patients with ST-elevation myocardial infarction—executive summary: a report of the American College of Cardiology/American Heart Association Task Force on Practice Guidelines (Writing Committee to Revise the 1999 Guidelines for the Management of Patients with Acute Myocardial Infarction). Circulation 2004; 110:588.

Hoffmann U, Pena AJ, Cury RC, et al: Cardiac CT in emergency department patients with acute chest pain. RadioGraphics 2006; 26:963.

Jeudy J, White CS: Evaluation of acute chest pain in the emergency department: utility of multidetector computed tomography. Semin Ultrasound CT MR 2007; 28:109.

Kuo D, Dilsizian V, Prasad R, et al: Emergency cardiac imaging: state of the art. Cardiol Clin 2006; 24:53.

Thilo C, Auler M, Zwerner P, et al: Coronary CTA: indications, patient selection, and clinical implications. J Thorac Imaging 2007; 22:35.

White CS, Kuo D: Chest pain in the emergency department: role of multidetector CT. Radiology 2007; 245:672.

REFERENCES

1. Braunwald E, Antman EM, Beasley JW, et al: ACC/AHA 2002 guideline update for the management of patients with unstable angina and non-ST-segment elevation myocardial infarction—summary article: a report of the American College of Cardiology/American Heart Association task force on practice guidelines (Committee on the Management of Patients With Unstable Angina). J Am Coll Cardiol 2002; 40:1366.
2. McCaig LF, Nawar EW: National Hospital Ambulatory Medical Care Survey: 2004 emergency department summary. Adv Data 2006; 372:1.
3. Pope JH, Aufderheide TP, Ruthazer R, et al: Missed diagnoses of acute cardiac ischemia in the emergency department. N Engl J Med 2000; 342:1163.
4. Rosamond W, Flegal K, Furie K, et al: Heart disease and stroke statistics—2008 update: a report from the American Heart Association Statistics Committee and Stroke Statistics Subcommittee. Circulation 2008; 117:e25.
5. Iribarren C, Sidney S, Sternfeld B, et al: Calcification of the aortic arch: risk factors and association with coronary heart disease, stroke, and peripheral vascular disease. JAMA 2000; 283:2810.
6. MacGregor JH, Chen JT, Chiles C, et al: The radiographic distinction between pericardial and myocardial calcifications. AJR Am J Roentgenol 1987; 148:675.
7. Margolis JR, Chen JT, Kong Y, et al: The diagnostic and prognostic significance of coronary artery calcification: a report of 800 cases. Radiology 1980; 137:609.
8. Higgins CB, Lipton MJ, Johnson AD, et al: False aneurysms of the left ventricle: identification of distinctive clinical, radiographic, and angiographic features. Radiology 1978; 127:21.
9. Sicari R, Pasanisi E, Venneri L, et al: Stress echo results predict mortality: a large-scale multicenter prospective international study. J Am Coll Cardiol 2003; 41:589.
10. Kontos MC, Arrowood JA, Jesse RL, et al: Comparison between 2-dimensional echocardiography and myocardial perfusion imaging in the emergency department in patients with possible myocardial ischemia. Am Heart J 1998; 136:724.
11. Raff GL, Gallagher MJ, O'Neill WW, et al: Diagnostic accuracy of noninvasive coronary angiography using 64-slice spiral computed tomography. J Am Coll Cardiol 2005; 46:552.
12. Kunimasa T, Sato Y, Sugi K, et al: Evaluation by multislice computed tomography of atherosclerotic coronary artery plaques in non-culprit, remote coronary arteries of patients with acute coronary syndrome. Circ J 2005; 69:1346.
13. Leber AW, Knez A, von Ziegler F, et al: Quantification of obstructive and nonobstructive coronary lesions by 64-slice computed tomography: a comparative study with quantitative coronary angiography and intravascular ultrasound. J Am Coll Cardiol 2005; 46:147.
14. Yamamuro M, Tadamura E, Kubo S, et al: Cardiac functional analysis with multi-detector row CT and segmental reconstruction algorithm: comparison with echocardiography, SPECT, and MR imaging. Radiology 2005; 234:381.
15. Hoffmann U, Nagurney JT, Moselewski F, et al: Coronary multidetector computed tomography in the assessment of patients with acute chest pain. Circulation 2006; 114:2251.
16. White CS, Kuo D, Kelemen M, et al: Chest pain evaluation in the emergency department: can MDCT provide a comprehensive evaluation? AJR Am J Roentgenol 2005; 185:533.
17. Goldstein JA, Gallagher MJ, O'Neill WW, et al: A randomized controlled trial of multi-slice coronary computed tomography for evaluation of acute chest pain. J Am Coll Cardiol 2007; 49:863.
18. Al-Saadi N, Nagel E, Gross M, et al: Noninvasive detection of myocardial ischemia from perfusion reserve based on cardiovascular magnetic resonance. Circulation 2000; 101:1379.
19. Kwong RY, Schussheim AE, Rekhraj S, et al: Detecting acute coronary syndrome in the emergency department with cardiac magnetic resonance imaging. Circulation 2003; 107:531.
20. Heller GV, Stowers SA, Hendel RC, et al: Clinical value of acute rest technetium-99m tetrofosmin tomographic myocardial perfusion imaging in patients with acute chest pain and nondiagnostic electrocardiograms. J Am Coll Cardiol 1998; 31:1011.
21. Kontos MC, Jesse RL, Schmidt KL, et al: Value of acute rest sestamibi perfusion imaging for evaluation of patients admitted to the emergency department with chest pain. J Am Coll Cardiol 1997; 30:976.
22. Wackers FJ, Brown KA, Heller GV, et al: American Society of Nuclear Cardiology position statement on radionuclide imaging in patients with suspected acute ischemic syndromes in the emergency department or chest pain center. J Nucl Cardiol 2002; 9:246.
23. Bulow H, Schwaiger M: Nuclear cardiology in acute coronary syndromes. Q J Nucl Med Mol Imaging 2005; 49:59.
24. A clinical trial comparing primary coronary angioplasty with tissue plasminogen activator for acute myocardial infarction. The Global Use of Strategies to Open Occluded Coronary Arteries in Acute Coronary Syndromes (GUSTO IIb) Angioplasty Substudy Investigators. N Engl J Med 1997; 336:1621.
25. Keeley EC, Boura JA, Grines CL: Primary angioplasty versus intravenous thrombolytic therapy for acute myocardial infarction: a quantitative review of 23 randomised trials. Lancet 2003; 361:13.
26. Berger PB, Bell MR, Holmes DR Jr, et al: Time to reperfusion with direct coronary angioplasty and thrombolytic therapy in acute myocardial infarction. Am J Cardiol 1994; 73:231.
27. Antman EM, Anbe DT, Armstrong PW, et al: ACC/AHA guidelines for the management of patients with ST-elevation myocardial infarction—executive summary: a report of the American College of Cardiology/American Heart Association Task Force on Practice Guidelines (Writing Committee to Revise the 1999 Guidelines for the Management of Patients with Acute Myocardial Infarction). Circulation 2004; 110:588.
28. Anderson JL, Adams CD, Antman EM, et al: ACC/AHA 2007 guidelines for the management of patients with unstable angina/non-ST-elevation myocardial infarction: a report of the American College of Cardiology/American Heart Association Task Force on Practice

Guidelines (Writing Committee to Revise the 2002 Guidelines for the Management of Patients with Unstable Angina/Non-ST-Elevation Myocardial Infarction) developed in collaboration with the American College of Emergency Physicians, the Society for Cardiovascular Angiography and Interventions, and the Society of Thoracic Surgeons endorsed by the American Association of Cardiovascular and Pulmonary Rehabilitation and the Society for Academic Emergency Medicine. J Am Coll Cardiol 2007; 50:e1.

29. Eagle KA, Guyton RA, Davidoff R, et al: ACC/AHA 2004 guideline update for coronary artery bypass graft surgery: a report of the American College of Cardiology/American Heart Association Task Force on Practice Guidelines (Committee to Update the 1999 Guidelines for Coronary Artery Bypass Graft Surgery). Circulation 2004; 110:e340.

CHAPTER 53

Magnetic Resonance and Computed Tomographic Imaging of Myocardial Perfusion

Ricardo C. Cury, Anand Soni, and Ron Blankstein

Ischemic heart disease is a broad term that includes many different disease processes related to coronary atherosclerosis and its downstream consequences. On a continuum, it encompasses silent myocardial ischemia, chronic stable angina, acute coronary syndromes (ACS), and ischemic cardiomyopathy. All of these disease processes typically share the same underlying mechanism of reduced myocardial perfusion from obstructive coronary plaque, which results in myocardial ischemia or myocardial infarction (MI) from oxygen deprivation.

Data from the National Health and Nutrition Examination Survey (1999-2004, National Heart, Lung and Blood Institute) estimate the prevalence of coronary heart disease to be 16 million individuals in the United States, and incidence of new and recurrent coronary events to be 1.2 million per year.[1] Data from 44 years of follow-up in the original Framingham Heart Study cohort and 20 years of their offspring surveillance show the lifetime risk of developing coronary heart disease for individuals 40 years old to be 49% in men and 32% in women.[2] With mortality statistics claiming that one out of every five deaths is the result of coronary artery disease (CAD),[1] there is a clear need for improved diagnostic imaging strategies for detecting coronary heart disease and myocardium vulnerable to scenarios of reduced perfusion.

Myocardial ischemia is caused by inadequate coronary perfusion as a result of either an increase in myocardial oxygen requirements or a reduced supply of oxygen-carrying blood. Typically, myocardial ischemia is the result of atherosclerotic CAD. Initially, atherosclerotic vascular disease starts as atheromatous fatty streak buildup within the arterial wall, but in which there is no reduction in coronary blood flow (also known as "positive" remodeling) and patients remain asymptomatic. With further disease progression, there is mild to moderate buildup in plaque, which poses no limits to coronary perfusion at rest or stress, but poses the risk of being "unstable" and abruptly rupturing. If these plaques rupture, the thrombotic consequences can result in near-complete or complete coronary occlusion with severe acute reduction of myocardial perfusion; this is the framework for ACS. Lastly, atherosclerotic plaque may be large enough nearly to obstruct the coronary lumen (also known as "negative" remodeling). This lesion tends to cause reduced myocardial perfusion at times of stress and provides the basis for stable angina.

The clinical presentation of ischemic heart disease is incredibly diverse and includes asymptomatic or silent ischemia, chronic angina, unstable angina or infarction (i.e., ACS), new-onset or chronic heart failure, or sudden cardiac death. Although symptomatic patients are often identified by symptoms related to angina or heart failure, patients who have silent ischemia represent a diagnostic dilemma because they are less likely to be referred for testing. Patients who are particularly susceptible to silent ischemia include diabetics, elderly patients, and patients with prior MI or surgical revascularization.[3]

Noninvasive imaging is a crucial component in the evaluation of patients with suspected ischemic heart disease. Figure 53-1 illustrates an algorithm for the management of patients with potential ischemic heart disease. For patients presenting with a possible ACS who have a

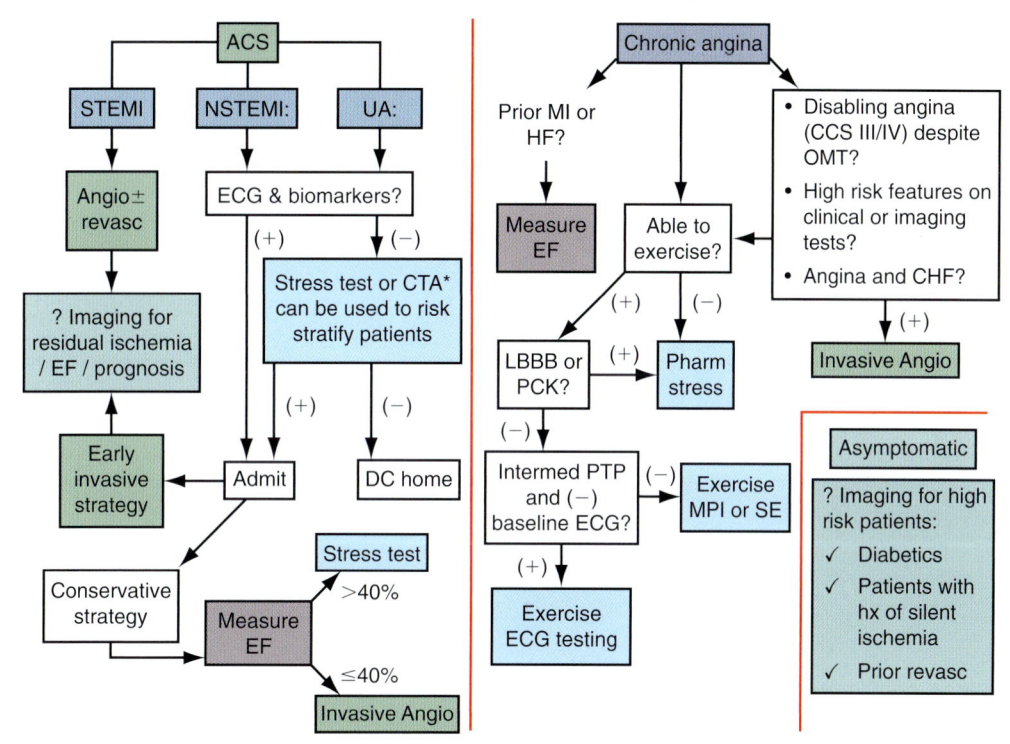

FIGURE 53-1 Algorithm for management of patients with suspected ischemic heart disease. CCS, Canadian Classification System; CHF, congestive heart failure; CTA, CT angiography; DC, discharge; EF, ejection fraction; HF, heart failure; LBBB, left bundle branch block; OMT, optimal medical therapy; Pharm stress, pharmacologic stress testing; PTP, pretest probability; SE, stress echocardiogram; UA, unstable angina. (Data from Anderson JL, Adams CD, Antman EM, et al. ACC/AHA 2007 guidelines for the management of patients with unstable angina/non ST-elevation myocardial infarction: a report of the American College of Cardiology/American Heart Association Task Force on Practice Guidelines [Writing Committee to Revise the 2002 Guidelines for the Management of Patients with Unstable Angina/Non ST-Elevation Myocardial Infarction]: developed in collaboration with the American College of Emergency Physicians, the Society for Cardiovascular Angiography and Interventions, and the Society of Thoracic Surgeons: endorsed by the American Association of Cardiovascular and Pulmonary Rehabilitation and the Society for Academic Emergency Medicine. Circulation 2007; 116:e148-e304; and Gibbons RJ, Abrams J, Chatterjee K, et al. ACC/AHA 2002 guideline update for the management of patients with chronic stable angina—summary article: a report of the American College of Cardiology/American Heart Association Task Force on Practice Guidelines [Committee on the Management of Patients with Chronic Stable Angina]. Circulation 2003; 107:149-158.)

negative ECG and biomarkers (e.g., troponin), a stress test can be used to identify high-risk patients who would benefit from being admitted to the hospital for further evaluation and testing. The American College of Cardiology/American Heart Association guidelines for the management of unstable angina/non–ST segment elevation MI suggest that coronary CT angiography is a reasonable alternative to stress testing in patients with low to intermediate probability of CAD in whom initial ECG and initial biomarkers are unremarkable.[4]

Patients who are admitted with an ACS can be treated with an early invasive or early conservative strategy. High-risk patients have been shown to benefit from early interventions, and warrant early referral for invasive angiography. For low-risk patients, and in particular women, a conservative strategy that uses noninvasive testing is recommended.[4]

For patients with chronic stable angina, the American College of Cardiology/American Heart Association guidelines[5] suggest that ejection fraction should be measured for all patients with a history of MI or signs suggesting heart failure. In the presence of a systolic murmur suggestive of aortic stenosis, mitral regurgitation, or hypertrophic cardiomyopathy, an echocardiogram should be obtained.

As is shown in Figure 53-1, all patients with chronic angina (i.e., stable angina) should have an evaluation for the presence of ischemic heart disease. This evaluation can be accomplished by ECG exercise testing, noninvasive stress imaging, or invasive angiography. Higher risk patients or patients with abnormal baseline ECG should be referred for an imaging-based test. The goal of such a test is to identify the extent, severity, and location of ischemia and when possible provide information about prognosis.

The role of cardiac imaging for the detection of silent ischemia is controversial. Patients with diabetes may benefit from such a strategy because they have a high risk of cardiovascular-related mortality, are more likely to have silent ischemia, and are less likely to survive an MI than nondiabetic patients.[6] Nevertheless, the cost-effectiveness of screening all such at-risk patients with nuclear perfusion imaging is controversial.[7]

The detection of myocardial perfusion abnormalities is mainly used to identify patients with CAD, to evaluate the hemodynamic significance of epicardial coronary stenosis, and to enhance clinical decisions regarding treatment options. Myocardial perfusion imaging (MPI) assessment is frequently performed using rest and stress studies to detect myocardial ischemia (reversible defects) and myocardial infarct (fixed defects).

At present, multiple noninvasive imaging modalities are used in evaluating myocardial perfusion, including single photon emission computed tomography (SPECT), posi-

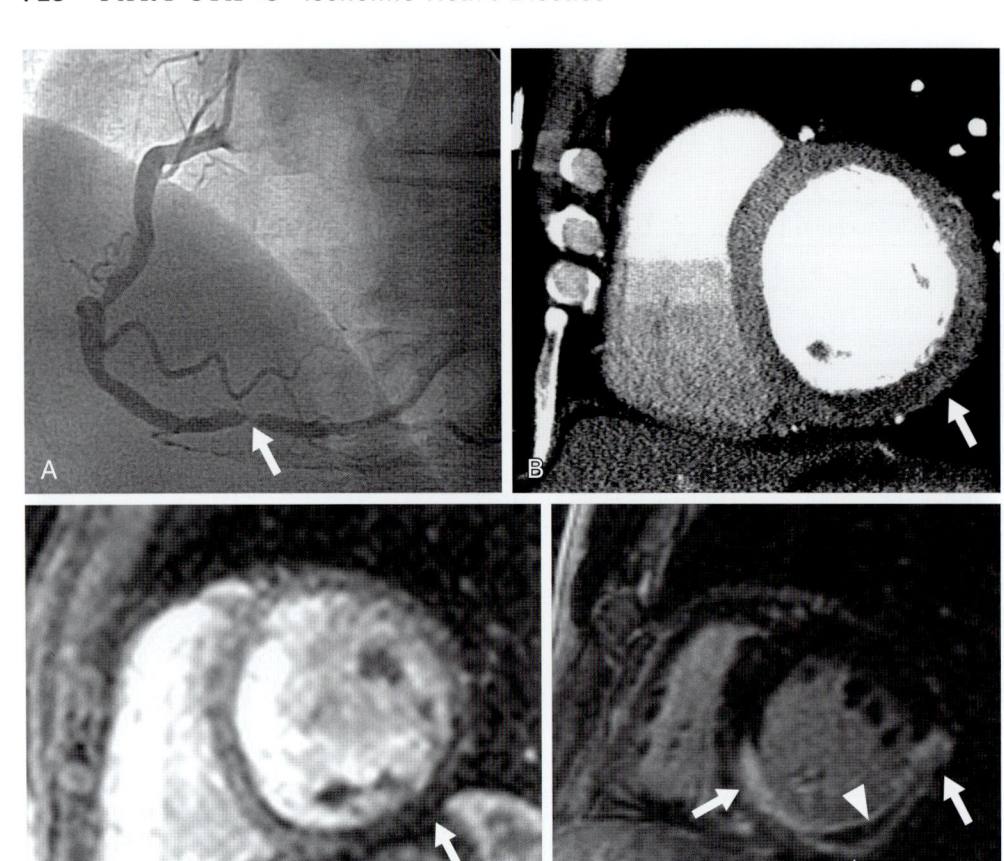

FIGURE 53-2 A 55-year-old man presented with ST segment elevation MI. **A,** Invasive coronary angiography revealed a significant high-grade stenosis of the distal right coronary artery (*arrow*). The patient underwent cardiac CT and MRI 3 days later. **B,** Short-axis CT image showed a perfusion defect (*arrow*) in mid-inferior and inferolateral wall of the left ventricle. **C,** MRI first-pass perfusion showed a resting perfusion defect in the same corresponding territory (*arrow*). **D,** MDE MRI showed a large area of hyperenhancement (*arrows*) in the mid-inferior, inferolateral, and inferoseptal walls of the left ventricle with a greater than 50% transmurality. The hyperenhancement pattern was based in the subendocardium and was consistent with a large MI. Within the infarct, a smaller region of no hyperenhancement (*arrowhead*) was noted that corresponds to a region of no reflow (also known as microvascular obstruction).

tron emission tomography (PET), echocardiography, and MRI. Although SPECT has been well shown to assess rest and stress perfusion accurately, and provides useful prognostic data based on a patient's burden of ischemia and infarct, it is limited by its low spatial resolution and attenuation artifacts, which can lead to equivocal studies. [18]FDG-PET has the ability to evaluate myocardial ischemia using radiotracers such as ammonia N 13 or rubidium 82, but has limitations regarding availability. MRI shows promise in the evaluation of myocardial ischemia with first-pass perfusion imaging, and large-scale multicenter trials are just beginning to be released. CT has the best spatial resolution of any imaging modality, and many emerging studies are suggesting it may have an important role for the future evaluation of myocardial perfusion and infarct detection.

This chapter focuses on the evaluation of MRI and CT for the assessment of myocardial perfusion (Figs. 53-2 and 53-3). The advantages and disadvantages of other imaging modalities are discussed and compared with MRI and CT, and these imaging modalities are put in clinical perspective with descriptions of how and when they can facilitate the diagnosis and management of patients suspected to have CAD or with known CAD.

MAGNETIC RESONANCE IMAGING

The goal of stress myocardial perfusion MRI is to visualize the first pass of gadolinium contrast agent within the left ventricle blood pool into the myocardium during rest and stress. Stress is achieved with pharmacologic vasodilation with either adenosine or dipyridamole. Under vasodilatory stress, myocardial blood flow should increase four to five times except in areas of obstructive epicardial CAD, where downstream vascular beds are already maximally vasodilated. These coronary territories obtain lower peak myocardial signal intensity on contrast administration compared with resting conditions, and a myocardial perfusion defect is visualized.

Preclinical and Clinical Evaluation

Numerous animal studies have shown good correlation of MRI perfusion with tissue perfusion as measured by radioactive microspheres.[8,9] Notable studies included work by Wilke and colleagues and Klocke and associates,[8] in which porcine and canine models of left circumflex coronary artery stenosis were created that showed that MRI can detect different degrees of myocardial perfusion under adenosine stress.

Subsequently, Lee and colleagues[9] used a canine model of left circumflex coronary artery stenosis and compared perfusion MRI with Tc 99m sestamibi and thallium 201. They showed that MRI could detect perfusion defects with a left circumflex coronary artery stenosis of 50% or greater, whereas SPECT perfusion defects were detected only with left circumflex coronary artery stenosis of 85% or greater.

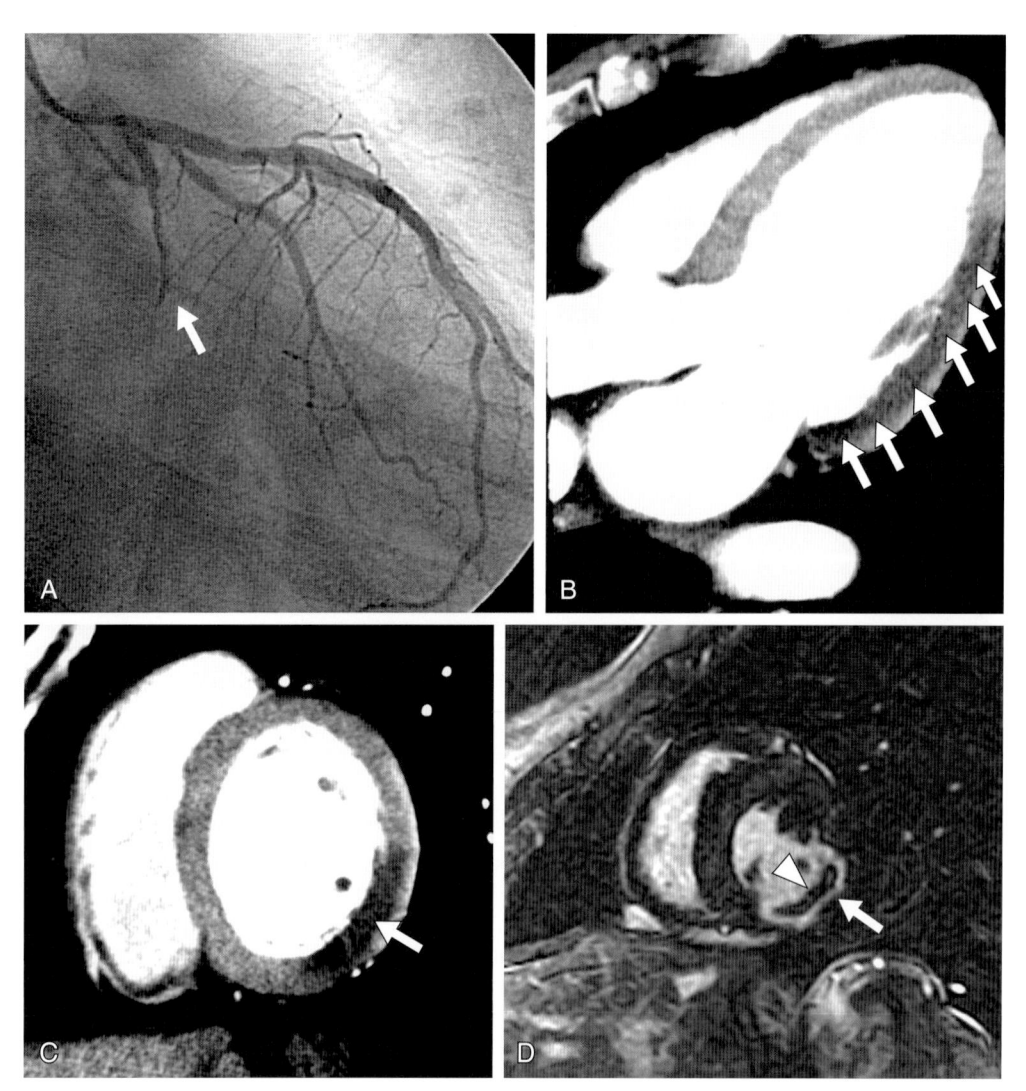

■ FIGURE 53-3 A 40-year-old man was transferred from an outside hospital with MI. **A,** During invasive coronary catheter angiography, he was found to have a complete occlusion of the left circumflex coronary artery (*arrow*). **B** and **C,** Short-axis (**B**) and long-axis (**C**) CT images showed a large perfusion defect of the entire lateral wall (*arrows*). **D,** First-pass perfusion MRI confirms this and shows a large perfusion defect of the inferolateral wall (*arrow*). MDE MRI shows the extent of the MI. Within the area of hyperenhancement, there is a substantial central area that lacks hyperenhancement, representing microvascular obstruction (*arrowhead*).

Multiple clinical human studies testing the diagnostic accuracy and performance of stress perfusion MRI were performed comparing MRI with nuclear imaging and conventional coronary angiography. Table 53-1 summarizes published data with x-ray angiography as the reference standard. Nandalur and associates[10] performed a meta-analysis of all stress MRI studies with two main techniques in use, perfusion imaging and imaging of stress-induced wall motion abnormalities, from January 1990 to January 2007 with a total of 37 studies involving 2191 patients. All studies used catheter x-ray angiography as the reference standard. Fourteen studies ($N = 754$ patients) using stress-induced wall motion abnormalities imaging showed 83% sensitivity and 86% specificity on a patient level. Perfusion imaging showed a sensitivity of 91% and specificity of 81% on a patient level (disease prevalence 57.4%).

Two more recent studies by Cury and associates[11] and Klem and coworkers[12] (see Table 53-1) sought to improve the diagnostic accuracy of stress perfusion MRI by using a comprehensive imaging approach of first-pass contrast administration for myocardial perfusion at rest and stress with the addition of myocardial delayed enhancement (MDE) imaging for infarct detection and characterization. Our group showed that this combined approach has 87% sensitivity, 89% specificity, and 88% accuracy, and was superior to rest/stress perfusion MRI alone, which has 81% sensitivity, 87% specificity, and 85% accuracy, having invasive coronary angiography as the reference standard. Klem and coworkers[12] showed similar results—that stress perfusion and MDE MRI can better detect inducible ischemia and fixed defects compared with stress/rest perfusion MRI. MDE MRI also provides the benefit of improved identification of regions of no reflow or microvascular obstruction, which is readily identified on MDE as regions of no hyperenhancement within the hyperenhancing infarction (see Figs. 53-2 and 53-3).

In another study evaluating patients presenting to the emergency department with acute chest pain, Ingkanisorn and colleagues[13] evaluated the diagnostic value of adenosine stress myocardial perfusion MRI in 135 patients who presented to the emergency department with chest pain and a negative initial troponin value. The main study outcome was the detection of any evidence of significant CAD. Patients were contacted at 1 year to determine the

TABLE 53-1 Diagnostic Accuracy of Stress Perfusion Magnetic Resonance Imaging Studies, Having Invasive Coronary Angiography as the Reference Standard

Author	Year	Journal	Patients (N)	Stenosis (%)	Sensitivity (%)	Specificity (%)
Al-Saadi	2000	Circulation	34	≥75	90	83
Bertschinger	2001	J Magn Reson Imaging	14	≥50	85	81
Schwitter	2001	Circulation	48	≥50	87	85
Panting	2001	J Magn Reson Imaging	22	>50	79	83
Ibrahim	2002	J Am Coll Cardiol	25	>75	69	89
Chiu	2003	Radiology	13	>50	92	92
Ishida	2003	Radiology	104	≥70	90	85
Nagel	2003	Circulation	84	≥75	88	90
Wolff	2004	Circulation	75	≥70	93	75
Giang	2004	Eur Heart J	80	≥50	93	75
Paetsch	2004	Circulation	79	>50	91	62
Plein	2004	J Am Coll Cardiol	68	≥70	88	83
Plein	2005	Radiology	92	≥70	88	82
Klem	2006	J Am Coll Cardiol	100	≥70	89	87
Cury	2006	Radiology	47	≥70	87	89
Rieber	2006	Eur Heart J	43	≥50	88	90
Cheng	2007	J Am Coll Cardiol	61	≥50	3.0 T = 98; 1.5 T = 90	3.0 T = 76; 1.5 T = 67
Schwitter	2008	Eur Heart J	234	≥50	85	67

incidence of significant CAD, defined as significant coronary artery stenosis (>50%) on invasive coronary angiography, abnormal correlative stress test, new MI, or death. Adenosine myocardial perfusion MRI abnormalities had 100% sensitivity and 93% specificity for detection of significant CAD, and an abnormal MRI added significant prognostic value in predicting a future diagnosis of CAD, MI, or death over clinical risk factors. No patients with a normal adenosine myocardial perfusion MRI had a subsequent diagnosis of CAD or an adverse outcome.

The first multicenter trial involving 18 centers in Europe and the United States (MR-IMPACT trial) comparing stress myocardial perfusion MRI with SPECT imaging and invasive coronary angiography was published more recently.[14] When comparing perfusion MRI at 0.1 mmol/kg versus the entire SPECT population, the receiver operating curve analysis showed a better performance for perfusion MRI (n = 42, area under the curve [AUC] 0.86 ± 0.06) versus SPECT (n = 212, AUC 0.67 ± 0.05; P = .013 vs. MRI). The MRI performance at 0.1 mmol/kg was also superior in patients with multivessel disease (n = 32 and n = 161 for MRI and SPECT, AUC 0.89 ± 0.06 vs. 0.70 ± 0.05; P =.006). Overall, the authors concluded that the comparison of stress perfusion MRI with the entire SPECT population suggests superiority of MRI over SPECT, which warrants further evaluation in larger trials. These results are in concordance with a prior study from Ishida and associates[14a] that also showed superiority of MRI over SPECT in a single-center trial.

MRI offers an impressive range of information (i.e., function, anatomy, viability, perfusion, and advanced research applications) that is pertinent to the clinical evaluation and subsequent management of patients presenting with acute chest pain. The technique has inherent benefits in terms of its lack of exposure to ionizing radiation and use of nephrotoxic iodinated contrast agents. Initial studies have shown its utility in the setting of acute chest pain. In addition, it has become the gold standard for imaging in the setting of myocardial injury and MI. In the future, MRI may be the imaging study of choice in the evaluation of patients with acute chest pain or MI.

COMPUTED TOMOGRAPHY

Although multiple, more recent single-center and multi-center studies[15] have established the diagnostic accuracy of cardiac CT for the detection of coronary artery stenosis, the functional significance of many coronary artery lesions identified by such techniques (or by invasive coronary angiography) is often unknown.[16] MPI and angiography have the potential to provide complementary information by imaging ischemia and atherosclerosis. The potential of obtaining this information from a single imaging modality is very attractive.

This section presents a brief overview of the animal and human studies showing the use of CT perfusion during rest and stress. Because most of the initial animal studies employed an infarct model to assess perfusion defects, they showed the use of CT in accurately characterizing rest perfusion defects that are found in infarcted myocardium. In the process of characterizing such resting perfusion defects further, the use of MDE imaging was found to be useful in distinguishing nonviable (i.e., typically infarcted) from viable myocardium. As a natural extension of the ability to assess perfusion, more recent human and animal studies have used adenosine stress perfusion to identify ischemia. Current animal studies in this field use a "stenosis model" to identify lesions that are non-flow-limiting at rest, but are significant during stress. Only more recently have small human studies been conducted showing the feasibility of using multidetector CT to characterize perfusion during adenosine stress.

Animal Studies: Rest Perfusion

The ability of CT to detect acute MI in explanted hearts and experimental animal models dates back to the late 1970s.[17] More recently, multidetector CT has been used

TABLE 53-2 Multidetector Computed Tomography Rest and Stress Perfusion: Animal Studies

Study	Model	Imaging	Results	Conclusions
Hoffmann, 2004[18]	7 pigs; acute MI via LAD balloon occlusion	Multidetector CT vs. TTC and microsphere blood flow	Area: CT (ED): 16.1 ± 4.8%; CT (ES): 17 ± 6.4%; TTC: 13.6 ± 6% (*One animal had nonevaluable images owing to high heart rate)	Multidetector CT permits detection and further characterization of acute MI
Mahnken, 2006[19]	5 pigs; acute MI via LAD balloon occlusion	Multidetector CT vs. first-pass MRI vs. TTC	Area: multidetector CT: 19.3 ± 4.5%; MRI: 17.2 ± 4%; TTC: 18.7 ± 5.7%	Showed potential for semiquantitative evaluation of myocardial perfusion using multidetector CT
George, 2006[22]	8 dogs; LAD stenosis (non-flow-limiting at rest, but flow-limiting during stress)	64 × 0.5 mm multidetector CT rest and stress perfusion vs. ex vivo staining	Myocardial SD was 92.3 ± 39.5 HU in stenosed vs. 180.4 ± 41.9 HU in remote territories ($P < .001$); there was a significant linear association of the SD ratio with MBF in the stenosed territory ($R = 0.98$, $P = .001$)	Adenosine-augmented multidetector CT MPI provides semiquantitative measurements of myocardial perfusion during first-pass multidetector CT imaging in a canine model of LAD stenosis
George, 2007[24]	6 dogs with moderate to severe LAD stenosis	64 × 0.5 mm dynamic multidetector CT stress perfusion (adenosine 140 μg/kg/min) vs. microsphere-derived MBF	Myocardial upslope-to-left ventricular upslope and myocardial upslope-to-left ventricular maximum ratio strongly correlated with MBF ($R^2 = 0.92$, $P < .0001$ and $R^2 = 0.87$, $P < .0001$); absolute MBF derived by model-based deconvolution analysis modestly overestimated MBF; overall, multidetector CT-derived MBF strongly correlated with microspheres ($R = 0.91$, $P < .0001$)	Multidetector CT MBF measurements using upslope and model-based deconvolution methods correlate well with microsphere MBF

ED, end diastole; ES, end systole; LAD, left anterior descending artery; MBF, myocardial blood flow; SD, signal density.

to assess myocardial perfusion in animal models of total coronary occlusion.[18,19] Table 53-2 lists some of the main studies that characterized myocardial perfusion in animal models under rest and stress conditions.

Hoffmann and coworkers[18] used four-slice multidetector CT and performed a quantitative analysis of CT attenuation and compared that with microsphere-determined blood flow and triphenyltetrazolium chloride (TTC)–stained tissue samples. The quantitative analysis by multidetector CT showed significant differences in the mean CT attenuation of infarct and reference areas (32.1 ± 8.5 Hounsfield units [HU] vs. 75.6 ± 16.7 HU; $P < .001$), and this correlated with changes in microsphere-determined blood flow. The volume of perfusion defect was similar to volume of tissue that lacked TTC staining (17 ± 6.4% vs. 13.6 ± 6%), with slight overestimation of infarct size by multidetector CT.

Mahnken and colleagues[19] used a similar porcine model to assess the ability of multidetector CT to evaluate rest myocardial perfusion versus first-pass perfusion MRI with TTC staining serving as the gold standard. In their protocol, they used dynamic multidetector CT imaging by acquiring 64 scans at the apical level with a prospectively acquired ECG triggered examination protocol. Hypoenhanced regions on multidetector CT corresponded directly to perfusion defects visualized on MRI and areas of MI seen on TTC staining. The hypoenhanced regions detected by multidetector CT were again slightly larger than areas of acute MI as detected by MRI and TTC staining.

These studies exploited the ability of multidetector CT to visualize areas of myocardial hypoattenuation, indicative of decreased myocardial perfusion. Areas of decreased myocardial perfusion in the setting of MI can represent either myocardial necrosis with microvascular obstruction or areas of infarction with preserved microvascular obstruction. Direct comparisons of multidetector CT delayed enhancement with TTC showed excellent correlation with infarct morphology, transmurality, and infarct volume ratios. Additionally, analogous to MRI, multidetector CT hypoenhanced identified regions of microvascular obstruction at 5 minutes after contrast agent injection in the delayed enhancement images that compared well with thioflavin S–derived measurements.

Human Studies of Rest Perfusion

Table 53-3 summarizes several key human studies of stress and rest myocardial perfusion using multidetector CT. Nikolaou and colleagues[20] attempted to correlate rest multidetector CT to stress perfusion MRI and MDE MRI in 30 patients with chronic infarcts or suspected CAD or both. In this retrospective study, all patients previously underwent multidetector CT (16 detectors) and MRI within 10 ± 16 days. Multidetector CT was able to detect 13 of 17 perfusion defects correctly (sensitivity 76%, specificity 92%, accuracy 83%); however, when considering only the 6 perfusion defects not associated with chronic MI, the sensitivity decreased to 50%—not surprising given that multidetector CT was performed under resting conditions, whereas stress perfusion MRI used vasodilator-induced hyperemic blood flow. Comparing multidetector CT versus MDE MRI for detection of infarct resulted in a

TABLE 53-3 Multidetector Computed Tomography Rest and Stress Perfusion: Human Studies

Study	Population	Imaging	Results	Conclusion
Nikolaou, 2005[20]	30 patients	CE multidetector CT (rest)	CT vs. MDE MRI: 10/11 infarcts identified (SN 91%, SP 79%)	Rest CT can detect chronic infarctions, but has a poor sensitivity for detecting perfusion defects in noninfarcted regions
	11 chronic MI, 19 known or suspected CAD Retrospective	Stress perfusion MRI MDE MRI	CT vs. stress perfusion MRI: 13/17 perfusion defects identified (SN 76%, SP 92%)	
Nieman, 2006[21]	CE multidetector CT retrospectively evaluated for patients with recent MI (<7 days, $n = 16$), long-standing MI (>12 mo, $n = 13$), or no MI ($n = 13$)	Multidetector CT measurement of attenuation (HU) at consecutive transmural locations of injured and normal remote myocardium	Significantly lower CT attenuation with long-standing MI (-13 ± 37 HU) vs. acute MI (26 ± 26 HU) vs. normal controls (73 ± 14 HU; $P < .001$); attenuation difference between infarcted and remote myocardium was larger in patients with long-standing MI than in patients with recent MI (89 ± 41 HU and 55 ± 33 HU; $P < .001$)	Recent and long-standing MIs may be differentiated by CT based on myocardial CT attenuation values and ventricular dimensions
Mahnken, 2005[25]	28 patients with reperfused STEMI	16-multidetector CT early and delayed enhancement (15 min); MDE MRI	Infarct size on MRI $31.2 \pm 22.5\%$ compared with $33.3 \pm 23.8\%$ for delayed enhancement multidetector CT and $24.5 \pm 18.3\%$ for early perfusion deficit multidetector CT	Late enhancement multidetector CT seems to be as reliable as delayed contrast-enhanced MRI in assessing infarct size and myocardial viability in acute MI
Gerber, 2006[26]	16 patients with acute MI	CE multidetector CT (rest)	Concordance of early hypoenhanced regions (92%, $\kappa = 0.54$, $P < .001$) and late hyperenhanced regions (82%, $\kappa = 0.61$, $P < .001$)	CE multidetector CT can characterize acute and chronic MI with contrast patterns similar to CE MRI, providing important information on infarct size and viability
	21 patients with chronic left ventricular dysfunction	Delayed multidetector CT (10 min post contrast) First-pass MRI MDE MRI		
George, 2006[22]	17 patients with positive MPI and chest pain referred for invasive angiography	64×0.5 mm multidetector CT Rest perfusion Stress perfusion using adenosine (140 μg/kg/min) infusion	For identifying ≥50% stenosis by CT angiography and ICA, multidetector CT SN 83%, SP 100% (vs. SN 67% and SP 80% for MPI)	Adenosine stress CT can accurately assess coronary atherosclerosis and its physiologic significance in patients with chest pain
George, 2007[23]	19 patients with positive SPECT	256×0.5 mm multidetector CT Rest perfusion Stress perfusion using adenosine (140 μg/kg/min) infusion	Compared with ≥50% stenosis by CT angiography, multidetector CT SN 85%, SP 77% (vs. SN 69% and SP 74% for SPECT) Compared with a gold standard combining ≥50% stenosis by CT angiography and SPECT perfusion defect SN 78%, SP 90%	256 multidetector CT enables combination of noninvasive CT angiography and perfusion with high accuracy and at radiation levels similar to currently used dual isotope nuclear techniques

CE, contrast enhanced; ICA, invasive coronary angiography; SN, sensitivity; SP, specificity; STEMI, ST segment elevation myocardial infarction.

sensitivity of 91%, specificity of 79%, and accuracy of 83%. The attenuation values in the 10 infarcted areas correctly detected by multidetector CT were significantly lower than in noninfarcted areas of myocardium (53.7 ± 33.5 HU vs. 122.3 ± 25.5 HU; $P < .01$). In the volumetric assessment of infarct size, a strong correlation between the volumes of 16-multidetector CT and MDE MRI was found ($r = 0.98$), but 16-multidetector CT tended to underestimate the infarct volume as assessed by cardiac MRI by 19% ($P < .01$).

More recently, Nieman and coworkers[21] retrospectively tested the hypothesis that 64-multidetector CT can differentiate recent (<7 days) versus old (>12 months) MI. They found significantly lower CT attenuation values in patients with long-standing MI (−13 ± 37 HU) than patients with acute MI (26 ± 26 HU) and normal controls (73 ± 14 HU; $P < .001$). The attenuation difference between infarcted and remote myocardium was larger in patients with long-standing MI than in patients with recent MI (89 ± 41 HU and 55 ± 33 HU; $P < .001$), probably owing to fatty replacement. As anticipated, long-standing MI was associated with wall thinning and ventricular dilation, whereas recent MI was not ($P > .05$).

Stress Multidetector Computed Tomography to Identify Ischemia

George and colleagues[22] performed rest and adenosine-mediated stress multidetector CT on a canine model of left anterior descending artery stenosis and were able to achieve lesions that were non–flow-limiting at rest but flow-limiting during pharmacologic stress. They were able to identify perfusion defects in noninfarcted myocardium. By using microspheres to measure myocardial blood flow, they were able to show that the myocardial signal density ratio (myocardial signal density/left ventricular blood pool signal density) corresponded well with microsphere-derived myocardial blood flow.

Preliminary human studies investigating the feasibility and accuracy of multidetector CT stress myocardial perfusion have been presented only more recently. In 19 patients with an abnormal SPECT study, George and colleagues[23] used 256-detector multidetector CT to assess for subendocardial perfusion defects during rest and intravenous adenosine infusion. When compared with 50% or greater stenosis by CT angiography, the sensitivity and specificity of multidetector CT stress MPI were 85% and 77% compared with 69% and 74% sensitivity and specificity of SPECT. When compared with a gold standard combining 50% or greater stenosis by CT angiography with a SPECT perfusion defect, the 256-row multidetector CT was 78% sensitive and 90% specific. Although these findings represent preliminary work, they suggest that ischemia can be detected with a modest sensitivity and reasonably high specificity.

Most of the multidetector CT studies reviewed in this section are small, and many of the imaging approaches are continuously being improved. Currently, there are no widely accepted multidetector CT protocols for properly imaging the myocardium in patients with suspected myocardial ischemia.

INDICATIONS

Magnetic Resonance Imaging

The indication for stress perfusion MRI is the evaluation of myocardial ischemia in the assessment of chest pain syndrome in patients with low to moderate pretest probability of having CAD. Patients with a high pretest likelihood of significant disease should proceed directly to invasive coronary angiography. These indications are similar to nuclear MPI with SPECT or PET and stress echocardiography. The improved spatial and temporal resolution of MRI compared with SPECT makes MRI a superior imaging modality with fewer false-positive results.

Computed Tomography

Although clinical data are currently too limited to advocate use of CT as a primary modality to assess MI or to evaluate for perfusion defects, in patients already undergoing CT for evaluation of coronary anatomy, rest perfusion defects—when present—can be very helpful in identifying areas of infarcted myocardium.

CONTRAINDICATIONS

Magnetic Resonance Imaging

The contraindications for myocardial perfusion MRI are similar to contraindications for other MRI examinations. The most common contraindications include periorbital metallic fragments or intracranial aneurysm clips, magnetically activated implanted devices, insulin pumps, neurostimulators, and cochlear implants. Because stress MRI involves gadolinium administration, decreased renal function is also a contraindication because of the rare occurrence of nephrogenic systemic fibrosis. Other contraindications include the inability to cooperate with breath-holding exercises and claustrophobia.

Computed Tomography

Contraindications for CT include renal insufficiency and known allergy to iodinated contrast agents. Because CT is associated with a low level of exposure to ionizing radiation, individuals who may potentially be more susceptible to adverse effects of radiation (e.g., young women) may be viewed as having a relative contraindication.

TECHNIQUE DESCRIPTION

Magnetic Resonance Imaging

Patients are monitored during the entire MRI scan with continuous ECG recording, vital signs, and pulse oximetry. A standard stress perfusion MRI protocol consists of the following steps; the entire examination takes approximately 40 minutes.

1. *Localization.* Localization of the heart position in the axial, sagittal, and coronal planes of the chest are obtained using a nongated breath-hold steady-state free precession (SSFP) pulse sequence. After localization of

the left ventricle, paraseptal long-axis, short-axis, and four-chamber cine views are obtained.
2. *Adenosine stress scan.* Adenosine infusion is started at 0.14 mg/kg/min over 6 minutes. Five minutes into the adenosine infusion, 0.1 mmol/kg of gadolinium-chelate contrast agent is injected at 5 mL/s followed by 15 mL of saline. Five seconds after initiation of contrast agent injection, the stress perfusion MRI sequence is acquired during one breath-hold in the short-axis view in 8 to 10 locations in the left ventricle to monitor the wash-in of the gadolinium through the myocardium.
3. *Left ventricular functional images.* Left ventricular function is assessed over 8 to 10 short-axis slices using ECG-gated breath-holding SSFP pulse sequences.
4. *Resting perfusion scan.* Another 0.1 mmol/kg of gadolinium-chelate contrast agent is injected at 5 mL/s followed by 15 mL of saline. Five seconds after initiation of contrast injection, a rest perfusion MRI sequence is acquired during one breath-hold in the short-axis view in 8 to 10 locations in the left ventricle to monitor the wash-in of the gadolinium through the myocardium.
5. *Myocardial delayed enhancement.* MDE imaging is obtained 7 to 10 minutes after the aforementioned scans in the left ventricular short-axis and long-axis views to determine the presence and extent of MI.

Computed Tomography

There are no standard techniques for the assessment of myocardial perfusion using CT. In our center, an 18-gauge intravenous catheter is placed for contrast injection for all CT examinations. If stress perfusion is planned, a second intravenous catheter (20-gauge) is placed for adenosine administration. The patient is brought to the CT suite, and standard ECG monitoring leads are connected. For studies involving rest or stress perfusion assessment, we do not administer any intravenous nitroglycerin or β blockers.

Rest Perfusion

When information on early perfusion is desired, the timing of image acquisition should be obtained by adding at least 2 to 4 seconds to the measured time of peak aortic root contrast enhancement. Images acquired during this phase can be used to visualize early phase myocardial hypoenhancement indicative of a myocardial perfusion defect.

Stress Perfusion

Stress perfusion images are acquired during intravenous adenosine administration (0.14 mg/kg/min) with a contrast agent administration rate of 4 to 5 mL/s. Images are typically obtained after 3 minutes of adenosine infusion (0.14 mg/kg/min), and the drug is administered until the end of the acquisition. The administration of adenosine requires careful monitoring of the patient's heart rhythm because transient heart block and hypotension may occur.

Myocardial Delayed Enhancement

To perform a delayed enhancement scan, scanning is performed 5 to 10 minutes after contrast agent injection. To minimize radiation exposure, we suggest that prospective triggering be used, and that the prior available imaging series be used to reduce the scan length as much as possible to decrease scan time. Use of lower kilovolt peak (100 kVp) and wider detector collimation is also helpful in this regard. Lower kilovolt peak is also advantageous because it increases contrast resolution.

PITFALLS AND SOLUTIONS
Magnetic Resonance Imaging

Dark rings that occur mainly in the septum (Gibbs artifacts) are the main artifact in stress perfusion MRI, and are due to high susceptibility of gadolinium contrast agent in the right and left ventricles. Otherwise, myocardial perfusion MRI is a reliable examination. The major issue with execution of the protocol is patient participation and cooperation with breath-holding. There are pulse sequence–specific imaging artifacts that an experienced operator needs to recognize and correct, but generally this modality is faster, more reliable, and less subject to imaging artifact and false-positive results compared with nuclear perfusion imaging.

Computed Tomography

CT-based evaluation of myocardial perfusion offers the advantage of superb spatial resolution, but it has lower image contrast resolution, especially compared with MRI. In addition, artifacts may appear as areas of hypoenhancement and be falsely interpreted as perfusion defects. CT artifacts may occur because of cardiac motion or image noise. A particular artifact that can lead to an area of decreased attenuation is beam hardening—decreased mean energy of x-ray beams when they pass through a dense object. Although beam hardening is usually caused by metallic objects such as clips, it may be caused by areas of dense contrast enhancement in natural structures such as the ventricles.

When a multiphase series is available, a true perfusion defect persists throughout multiple different phases of the cardiac cycle and is visualized in systole and diastole. Correlation of perfusion data with functional images is also helpful in improving the specificity of the CT examination.

IMAGE INTERPRETATION
Postprocessing
Magnetic Resonance Imaging

Comprehensive MR image analysis first needs to assess perfusion defects on stress imaging. Comparison with resting perfusion is mandatory to assess reversibility, similar to nuclear imaging. A perfusion defect under vasodilator stress in a coronary territory that appears normal at rest indicates a significant epicardial coronary artery stenosis. A stress perfusion defect that remains "fixed" at rest may indicate a chronic infarction or artifact. MDE images then become vital because a fixed perfusion defect

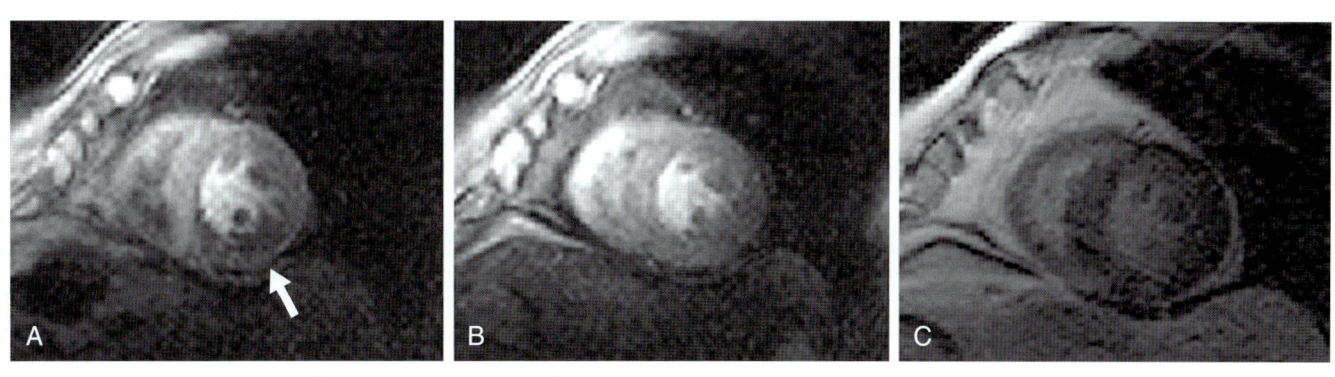

■ **FIGURE 53-4** A 48-year-old obese woman presented with chest pain. **A** and **B**, First-pass perfusion MRI reveals a perfusion defect (*arrow*) in the inferior wall during adenosine stress (**A**), which is not present during the rest images (**B**) confirming inducible ischemia in the right coronary artery distribution. **C**, MDE MRI reveals that there is no evidence of hyperenhancement and no infarct in the inferior wall. The lack of hyperenhancement in the affected region is consistent with viable myocardium, and suggests that the patient is very likely to benefit from a myocardial revascularization procedure.

owing to infarction would have a matched area of hyperenhancement on delayed images.

The absence of significant hyperenhancement on MDE (Fig. 53-4) is consistent with viable myocardium, and suggests that the patient would likely benefit from myocardial revascularization (i.e., percutaneous coronary intervention or coronary artery bypass graft surgery). Lastly, left ventricular systolic function and wall motion under stress are assessed. A wall motion abnormality in a coronary territory that matches perfusion defects is further evidence of ischemic myocardium. The diagnosis of CAD is made in the presence of a stress-induced perfusion defect or if an MI is detected on MDE images.

Computed Tomography

Postprocessing of cardiac CT images is quick and simple. The operator must choose the area of interest for reconstruction and the desired phase in the cardiac cycle (for retrospectively gated studies). Although perfusion images can be viewed in any phase, typically they are interpreted in mid-diastole (i.e., 65% to 75%). Although each vender has different reconstruction kernels, we suggest the use of a smoother reconstruction algorithm (i.e., B20 kernel) to reduce image noise. Occasionally, ectopic beats (either premature atrial contractions or premature ventricular contractions) may result in step artifacts owing to misregistration of data during reconstruction. Review of the ECG rhythm strip can identify such abnormal beats, and "ECG editing" (i.e., manipulation of tracings) can sometimes be very useful in reducing such artifacts.

The initial evaluation of perfusion is performed by reconstruction of short-axis images viewed in thick (i.e., 8 mm) multiplanar reformation. Increasing reconstruction slice thickness increases the voxel size, and decreases image noise and improves low contrast resolution. Optimal visualization of perfusion defects can be achieved by setting a narrow window width and narrow window level (e.g., window, 200; level, 100)

As discussed earlier, stress images should be compared with the corresponding rest images to determine whether defects are reversible or fixed. This comparison requires the reader to ensure the appropriate alignment (i.e., coregistration) of rest and stress images. In other words, it is essential to compare an image acquired in rest with the exact image acquired during stress.

REPORTING

Current data favor MRI for the assessment of myocardial perfusion under stress for detection of myocardial ischemia and delayed enhancement for detection of MI. MRI has the capability of detecting inducible ischemia under stress imaging with high diagnostic accuracy compared with invasive coronary angiography and may be superior to SPECT.

Although clinical data are currently too limited to advocate use of CT as a primary modality to assess myocardial perfusion, in patients already undergoing coronary CT angiography for evaluation of coronary anatomy, rest perfusion defects—when present—can be helpful in identifying areas of infarcted myocardium. Within such areas, levels of attenuation values, in combination with other morphologic features such as wall thinning, dilation, or wall motion abnormalities, can be helpful in distinguishing between acute and chronic infarcts, and suggest whether viable myocardium is present. Current CT research involving stress perfusion and delayed enhancement is expected to define further the future role of these developing techniques.

The conclusion from these various studies is that a comprehensive stress perfusion MRI protocol should include (1) stress perfusion MRI for myocardial ischemia under coronary vasodilation; (2) rest perfusion MRI to assess for "reversibility" of perfusion defects; (3) cine MRI for left ventricular morphology, function, and wall motion; and (4) MDE MRI for infarct detection and characterization. Given the high volume of stress MPI studies performed in the United States each year, comprehensive myocardial imaging using MRI has a very promising future in clinical practice.

KEY POINTS

- Myocardial perfusion CT can assess areas of perfusion defects at rest that represent myocardial infarct.
- CT evaluation of coronary arteries, myocardial perfusion, and myocardial function is possible with 64-detector multidetector CT.
- Stress myocardial perfusion MRI has shown superiority over SPECT in assessing inducible ischemia and myocardial infarct.
- MRI provides comprehensive functional assessment of patients with suspected or known CAD through stress/rest MPI, cine left ventricular function assessment, and MDE imaging.

SUGGESTED READINGS

Berman DS, Hachamovitch R, Shaw LJ, et al. Roles of nuclear cardiology, cardiac computed tomography, and cardiac magnetic resonance: assessment of patients with suspected coronary artery disease. J Nucl Med 2006; 47:74-82.

Cury RC, Nieman K, Shapiro MD, et al. Comprehensive cardiac CT study: evaluation of coronary arteries, left ventricular function, and myocardial perfusion—is it possible? J Nucl Cardiol 2007; 14:229-243.

Gershlick AH, de Belder M, Chambers J, et al. Role of non-invasive imaging in the management of coronary artery disease: an assessment of likely change over the next 10 years. A report from the British Cardiovascular Society Working Group. Heart 2007; 93:423-431.

Jerosch-Herold M, Muehling O, Wilke N. MRI of myocardial perfusion. Semin Ultrasound CT MR 2006; 27:2-10.

Kellman P, Arai AE. Imaging sequences for first pass perfusion—a review. J Cardiovasc Magn Reson 2007; 9:525-537.

Mahnken AH, Mühlenbruch G, Günther RW, et al. Cardiac CT: coronary arteries and beyond. Eur Radiol 2007; 17:994-1008.

Nieman K, Shapiro MD, Ferencik M, et al. Reperfused myocardial infarction: contrast-enhanced 64-section CT in comparison to MR imaging. Radiology 2008; 247:49-56.

Pennell DJ. Cardiovascular magnetic resonance and the role of adenosine pharmacologic stress. Am J Cardiol 2004; 94:26D-31D.

REFERENCES

1. Rosamond W, Flegal K, Friday G, et al. Heart disease and stroke statistics—2007 update: a report from the American Heart Association Statistics Committee and Stroke Statistics Subcommittee. Circulation 2007; 115:e69-e171.
2. Lerner DJ, Kannel WB. Patterns of coronary heart disease morbidity and mortality in the sexes: a 26-year follow-up of the Framingham population. Am Heart J 1986; 111:383-390.
3. Deedwania PC, Carbajal EV. Silent myocardial ischemia: a clinical perspective. Arch Intern Med 1991; 151:2373-2382.
4. Anderson JL, Adams CD, Antman EM, et al. ACC/AHA 2007 guidelines for the management of patients with unstable angina/non ST-elevation myocardial infarction: a report of the American College of Cardiology/American Heart Association Task Force on Practice Guidelines (Writing Committee to Revise the 2002 Guidelines for the Management of Patients with Unstable Angina/Non ST-Elevation Myocardial Infarction): developed in collaboration with the American College of Emergency Physicians, the Society for Cardiovascular Angiography and Interventions, and the Society of Thoracic Surgeons: endorsed by the American Association of Cardiovascular and Pulmonary Rehabilitation and the Society for Academic Emergency Medicine. Circulation 2007; 116:e148-e304.
5. Gibbons RJ, Abrams J, Chatterjee K, et al. ACC/AHA 2002 guideline update for the management of patients with chronic stable angina—summary article: a report of the American College of Cardiology/American Heart Association Task Force on Practice Guidelines (Committee on the Management of Patients with Chronic Stable Angina). Circulation 2003; 107:149-158.
6. Bax JJ, Bonow RO, Tschope D, et al. The potential of myocardial perfusion scintigraphy for risk stratification of asymptomatic patients with type 2 diabetes. J Am Coll Cardiol 2006; 48:754-760.
7. Beller GA. Noninvasive screening for coronary atherosclerosis and silent ischemia in asymptomatic type 2 diabetic patients: is it appropriate and cost-effective? J Am Coll Cardiol 2007; 49:1918-1923.
8. Klocke FJ, Simonetti OP, Judd RM, et al. Limits of detection of regional differences in vasodilated flow in viable myocardium by first-pass magnetic resonance perfusion imaging. Circulation 2001; 104:2412-2416.
9. Lee DC, Simonetti OP, Harris KR, et al. Magnetic resonance versus radionuclide pharmacological stress perfusion imaging for flow-limiting stenoses of varying severity. Circulation 2004; 110:58-65.
10. Nandalur KR, Dwamena BA, Choudhri AF, et al. Diagnostic performance of stress cardiac magnetic resonance imaging in the detection of coronary artery disease: a meta-analysis. J Am Coll Cardiol 2007; 50:1343-1353.
11. Cury RC, Cattani CA, Gabure LA, et al. Diagnostic performance of stress perfusion and delayed-enhancement MR imaging in patients with coronary artery disease. Radiology 2006; 240:39-45.
12. Klem I, Heitner JF, Shah DJ, et al. Improved detection of coronary artery disease by stress perfusion cardiovascular magnetic resonance with the use of delayed enhancement infarction imaging. J Am Coll Cardiol 2006; 47:1630-1638.
13. Ingkanisorn WP, Kwong RY, Bohme NS, et al. Prognosis of negative adenosine stress magnetic resonance in patients presenting to an emergency department with chest pain. J Am Coll Cardiol 2006; 47:1427-1432.
14. Schwitter J, Wacker CM, van Rossum AC, et al. MR-IMPACT: comparison of perfusion-cardiac magnetic resonance with single-photon emission computed tomography for the detection of coronary artery disease in a multicentre, multivendor, randomized trial. Eur Heart J 2008; 29:480-489.
14a. Ishida N, Sakuma H, Motoyasu M, et al. Non-infarcted myocardium: correlation between dynamic first-pass contrast-enhanced myocardial MR imaging and quantitative coronary angiography. Radiology 2003; 229:209-216.
15. Miller Jr RC, Dewey M, et al. Coronary artery evaluation using 64-row multidetector computed tomography angiography (CORE-64): results of a multicenter, international trial to assess diagnostic accuracy compared with conventional coronary angiography. Presented at American Heart Association 30th Annual Scientific Sessions, Orlando, November 3-7, 2007.
16. Hacker M, Jakobs T, Matthiesen F, et al. Comparison of spiral multidetector CT angiography and myocardial perfusion imaging in the noninvasive detection of functionally relevant coronary artery

lesions: first clinical experiences. J Nucl Med 2005; 46:1294-1300.
17. Higgins CB, Sovak M, Schmidt W, et al. Uptake of contrast materials by experimental acute myocardial infarctions: a preliminary report. Invest Radiol 1978; 13:337-339.
18. Hoffmann U, Millea R, Enzweiler C, et al. Acute myocardial infarction: contrast-enhanced multi-detector row CT in a porcine model. Radiology 2004; 231:697-701.
19. Mahnken AH, Bruners P, Katoh M, et al. Dynamic multi-section CT imaging in acute myocardial infarction: preliminary animal experience. Eur Radiol 2006; 16:746-752.
20. Nikolaou K, Sanz J, Poon M, et al. Assessment of myocardial perfusion and viability from routine contrast-enhanced 16-detector-row computed tomography of the heart: preliminary results. Eur Radiol 2005; 15:864-871.
21. Nieman K, Cury RC, Ferencik M, et al. Differentiation of recent and chronic myocardial infarction by cardiac computed tomography. Am J Cardiol 2006; 98:303-308.
22. George RT, Silva C, Cordeiro MA, et al. Multidetector computed tomography myocardial perfusion imaging during adenosine stress. J Am Coll Cardiol 2006; 48:153-160.
23. George RT, Arbad-Zadeh A, Miller JM, et al. Adenosine stress 64- and 256-row detector computed tomography angiography and perfusion imaging: a pilot study evaluating the transmural extent of perfusion abnormalities to predict atherosclerosis causing myocardial ischemia. Circ Cardiovasc Imaging 2009; 2:174-182.
24. George RT, Jerosch-Herold M, Silva C, et al. Quantification of myocardial perfusion using dynamic 64-detector computed tomography. Invest Radiol 2007; 42:815-822.
25. Mahnken AH, Koos R, Katoh M, et al. Assessment of myocardial viability in reperfused acute myocardial infarction using 16-slice computed tomography in comparison to MRI. J Am Coll Cardiol 2005; 45:2042-2047.
26. Gerber BL, Belge B, Legros GJ, et al. Characterization of acute and chronic myocardial infarcts by multidetector computed tomography: comparison with contrast enhanced magnetic resonance. Circulation 2006; 113:823-833.

CHAPTER 54

Nuclear Medicine Imaging of Myocardial Perfusion

Olga James, Kenneth J. Nichols, and Bennett Chin

Radionuclide myocardial perfusion imaging (MPI) is a well-established, highly accurate, and reproducible noninvasive method to diagnose and assess functionally significant coronary artery disease (CAD). Extensive development and validation have brought this modality to the forefront of quantitative, noninvasive assessment of CAD. High accuracy and reproducibility have also contributed to its widespread adoption as a gold standard to quantify myocardial ischemia. MPI also provides important information regarding myocardial viability and prognosis.

The basic principles of MPI have been validated in animal models and clinical trials over the past several decades.[1-4] Accepted clinical guidelines for use, technical aspects of quality control, and protocols for MPI stress testing and imaging for positron emission tomography (PET) and single photon emission computed tomography (SPECT) have been summarized in joint statements from the American Heart Association, American Society of Nuclear Cardiology, and American College of Cardiology,[5] and the European Association of Nuclear Medicine and the European Society of Cardiology.[6] This chapter highlights and summarizes the current clinical aspects of MPI. Emphasis is placed on describing the rationale and principles of MPI. The authors acknowledge variations in clinical practice based on local expertise and preference; however, space limitations do not permit a detailed discussion of all issues.

The first section reviews current clinical MPI using SPECT. Topics include radiotracers, instrumentation, procedures, and data analysis, including quantification and interpretation. Test performance and prognosis are reviewed under the general topic of interpretation. Assessment of myocardial viability with MPI also is briefly summarized (this is discussed more extensively in Chapter 55). Gated MPI to assess ventricular function is discussed in Chapter 56. Planar imaging produces lower image contrast and is reserved for special circumstances such as claustrophobic patients or patients unable to undergo SPECT imaging. An extensive review has been published.[7] The second section reviews MPI with PET. The same general outline is followed in an abbreviated format with salient differences discussed between PET and SPECT.

MYOCARDIAL PERFUSION IMAGING WITH SPECT

Technical Aspects

Radiotracers

SPECT radionuclides in widespread clinical use include thallium 201 and Tc 99m radiotracers. Thallium 201 is a cyclotron-generated, monovalent cation with biologic properties analogous to those of potassium (K^+). After intravenous administration, thallium 201 rapidly diffuses from the blood pool into the extravascular space where it is highly extracted by myocytes via the Na^+,K^+-ATPase pump. The initial myocardial uptake of thallium 201 is proportional to myocardial blood flow (MBF) and extraction fraction. Thallium 201 has the advantage of a high extraction fraction (approximately 85% to 88%), which is maintained up to MBF of approximately 2.5 mL/min/g. Myocardial territories distal to physiologically significant stenoses (i.e., ischemic myocardial regions) are unable to compensate sufficiently at stress with increased blood flow, and a perfusion defect can be detected as a relative reduction in radiotracer activity in this territory.

After administration, thallium 201 begins to redistribute significantly as it equilibrates with the extracellular concentration. In ischemic territories of lower MBF at rest, lower washout of radiotracer also contributes to equilibration. This more uniform myocardial radiotracer distribution at delayed (typically 4 hours) time points ("redistribution") is deemed "reversible" compared with stress perfusion, and a functionally significant coronary stenosis can be noninvasively diagnosed. Previous studies have verified that administration of a small reinjection of thallium 201 of 37 MBq (1 mCi) at rest improves the detection of viable myocardium.[8] This is a widely accepted clinical procedure to enhance the detection of viable myocardium.

The major disadvantages of thallium 201 are related to its physical properties compared with the properties of Tc 99m radiotracers. The long physical radiotracer half-life (73 hours) limits the administered activity to 148 to 167 MBq (4 to 4.5 mCi) per day because of radiation dose considerations (148 MBq [4 mCi] of activity delivers 24 mSv [2.4 rem] of whole body radiation dose equivalent). Because of radiation dose limitations, low photon flux contributes to lower true count images compared with Tc 99m radiotracer studies. The photopeak of thallium 201 (69 to 83 keV; 95% abundance) is also relatively low; this increases the amount of radiation absorbed and the scatter fraction. Also, spatial resolution and energy resolution of gamma camera imaging is better for the higher 140 keV gamma ray energy of Tc 99m than for the lower energies of thallium 201. The combination of these effects, especially in large patients, adversely affects thallium 201 image quality and can make interpretation difficult.

Tc 99m-sestamibi and Tc 99m-tetrofosmin are the most commonly used clinical MPI radiotracers. Common properties include high lipophilicity, relatively high first-pass extraction, and insignificant radiotracer redistribution. Conceptually, they can be viewed as radiotracer "microspheres" that define MBF at the time of administration with no significant washout or redistribution at delayed imaging. Their first-pass extraction fractions are lower than that of thallium 201. Their linear relationships with blood flow are maintained up to MBF rates of approximately 2 mL/min/g. Theoretically, this can result in reduced sensitivity for detection of CAD; however, large clinical studies have shown similar overall accuracies compared with examinations performed with thallium 201. These radiotracers enter myocytes by passive diffusion, the diffusion rate of which is proportional to the regional myocardial flow. They are then sequestered in the mitochondria because of the electrochemical gradient, which is maintained in viable myocytes.

An advantage of Tc 99m radiotracers is the short half-life (6.02 hours). This short half-life permits a higher administered activity (approximately 8 to 10 times higher; 14 mSv [1.4 rem] for 1.11 GBq [30 mCi] activity), higher photon flux, and, consequently, higher count images compared with thallium 201. In addition, the higher photopeak of 140 keV results in less soft tissue attenuation, less scatter, and improved spatial resolution. These factors contribute to improved image quality compared with thallium 201, and reduce the time required for image acquisition. This is particularly important because ECG gating with Tc 99m radiotracers is commonly performed. Reduced imaging time also reduces patient discomfort and the likelihood of motion artifacts, which may compromise image quality. Tc 99m is also commercially available from generators, which are widely available at a low cost.

Tc 99m-sestamibi is a lipophilic cationic compound. Tc 99m-tetrofosmin is a diphosphine lipophilic cationic complex of Tc 99m. Tetrofosmin is reported to have faster clearance from the liver and lungs; however, the clinical significance with respect to improved diagnostic accuracy has yet to be established. A large retrospective study has shown that Tc 99m-tetrofosmin scans are essentially equivalent to Tc 99m-sestamibi in determining prognosis in high-risk patients.[9] Examples of normal Tc 99m-sestamibi studies are shown in Figures 54-1 and 54-2. A gated study showing the utility of aiding in identifying a breast attenuation artifact is shown in Figure 54-3.

Instrumentation

Clinical gamma cameras used in SPECT have until more recently been similar in design and performance. The overall system resolution is limited by the lowest resolution component of the entire system. The limiting factor in clinical SPECT spatial resolution is collimator design. Typical Tc 99m full-width half-maximum SPECT spatial resolution is approximately 8 to 9 mm. This resolution can be improved by using "ultra-high" resolution collimation, but at the expense of reduced photon collection efficiency (i.e., lower camera sensitivity). For the same imaging time, higher resolution parallel hole collimation results in lower acquired counts. This can be compensated for by increasing imaging time.

A modest improvement in image resolution may not be deemed necessary if the diagnostic accuracy is not significantly improved, particularly if increasing imaging time results in a higher frequency of patient motion artifacts. Advanced instrumentation and software are currently being tested, with the goal of reducing imaging time while preserving image quality. The specific details of typical clinical instrumentation, including gamma cameras, collimators, and quality assurance (QA), have been well described in a detailed review article.[10]

Techniques in SPECT

Indications

The American College of Cardiology Foundation and the American Society of Nuclear Cardiology jointly published guidelines for appropriateness criteria.[11] The indications deemed most appropriate were those in which patients presented with intermediate or high pretest probabilities in the categories described subsequently. MPI as a screening tool in very low pretest probability patients is generally considered inappropriate.

Appropriate patient populations include the following categories: (1) detection of CAD in symptomatic or asymptomatic patients (chest pain, newly diagnosed heart failure or diastolic dysfunction, newly diagnosed arrhythmias including atrial fibrillation and ventricular fibrillation); (2) risk assessment in patients with intermediate or high pretest probability of CAD; (3) risk assessment in patients with known coronary disease; and (4) evaluation of myocardial viability. Although other indications may be warranted, the above-listed indications were judged to be most appropriate in most referred cases. Typical MPI patterns are shown in Figures 54-4 through 54-6.

Stress | **Delayed**

HLA

VLA

SA

Bull's-eye

History
71-year-old man with atypical chest pain

Exercised Bruce protocol 7 minutes
Peak heart rate 154 (103% MPHR)
Appropriate BP response
No chest pain

Negative ECG

Findings
Intermediate size, mild inferior - fixed

Impression
Inferior tissue attenuation

■ **FIGURE 54-1** Normal Tc 99m-sestamibi exercise MPI shows inferior diaphragm attenuation in a male patient. Decreased activity inferiorly is typically mild, gradually increasing in severity from apex to base (*arrows*). BP, blood pressure; HLA, horizontal long axis; MPHR, maximum predicted heart rate; SA, short axis; VLA, vertical long axis.

Stress | **Delayed**

HLA

VLA

SA

Bull's-eye

History
58-year-old woman with atypical chest pain

Exercised Bruce protocol 6 minutes
Peak heart rate 148 (91% MPHR)
Appropriate BP response
No chest pain

Negative ECG

Findings
Small, mild severity anterior - fixed

Impression
Anterior tissue attenuation

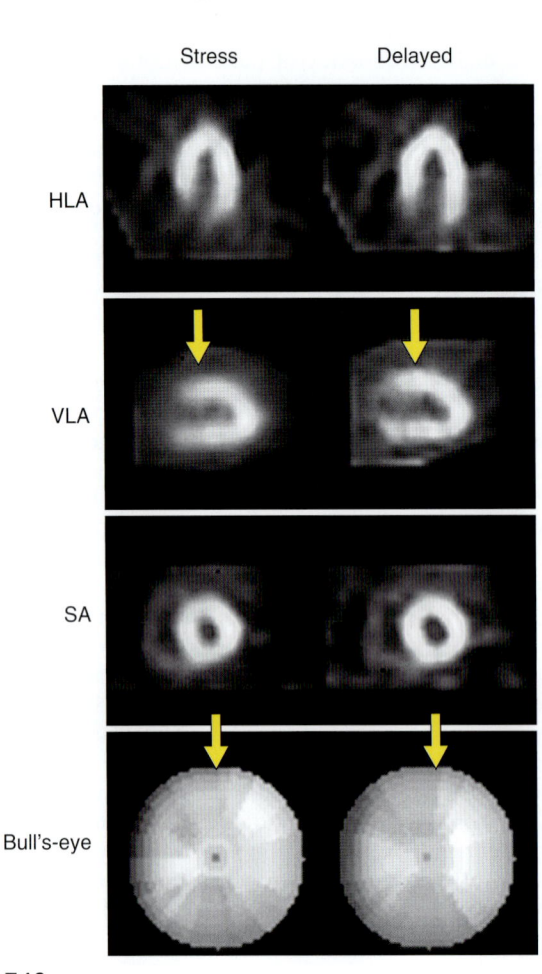

■ **FIGURE 54-2** Normal Tc 99m-sestamibi exercise MPI shows anterior breast attenuation in a female patient. Decreased activity anteriorly is typically mild, may gradually increase in severity from apex to base (*arrows*), and may not follow the typical coronary distribution of a perfusion defect in the left anterior descending artery territory. BP, blood pressure; HLA, horizontal long axis; MPHR, maximum predicted heart rate; SA, short axis; VLA, vertical long axis.

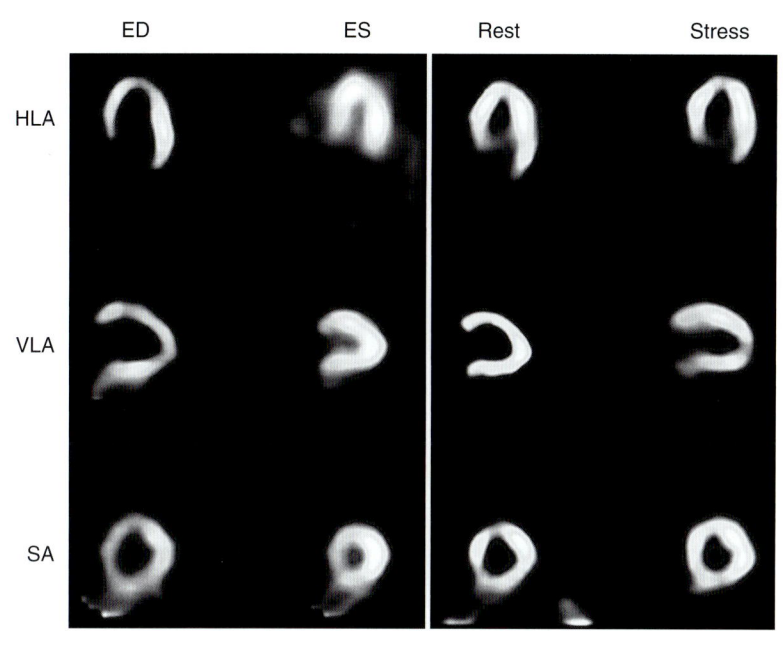

FIGURE 54-3 Normal Tc 99m-sestamibi exercise MPI shows anterior breast attenuation in a female patient. The rest gated study shows normal wall motion and normal wall thickening anteriorly. The rest perfusion study (ungated, *second panel, left column*) shows mild decreased activity anteriorly that does not involve the apex (noncoronary distribution for a left anterior descending artery stenosis). The stress perfusion study (ungated, *second panel, right column*) shows no perfusion defect on stress imaging. ED, end-diastole; ES, end-systole; HLA, horizontal long axis; SA, short axis; VLA, vertical long axis.

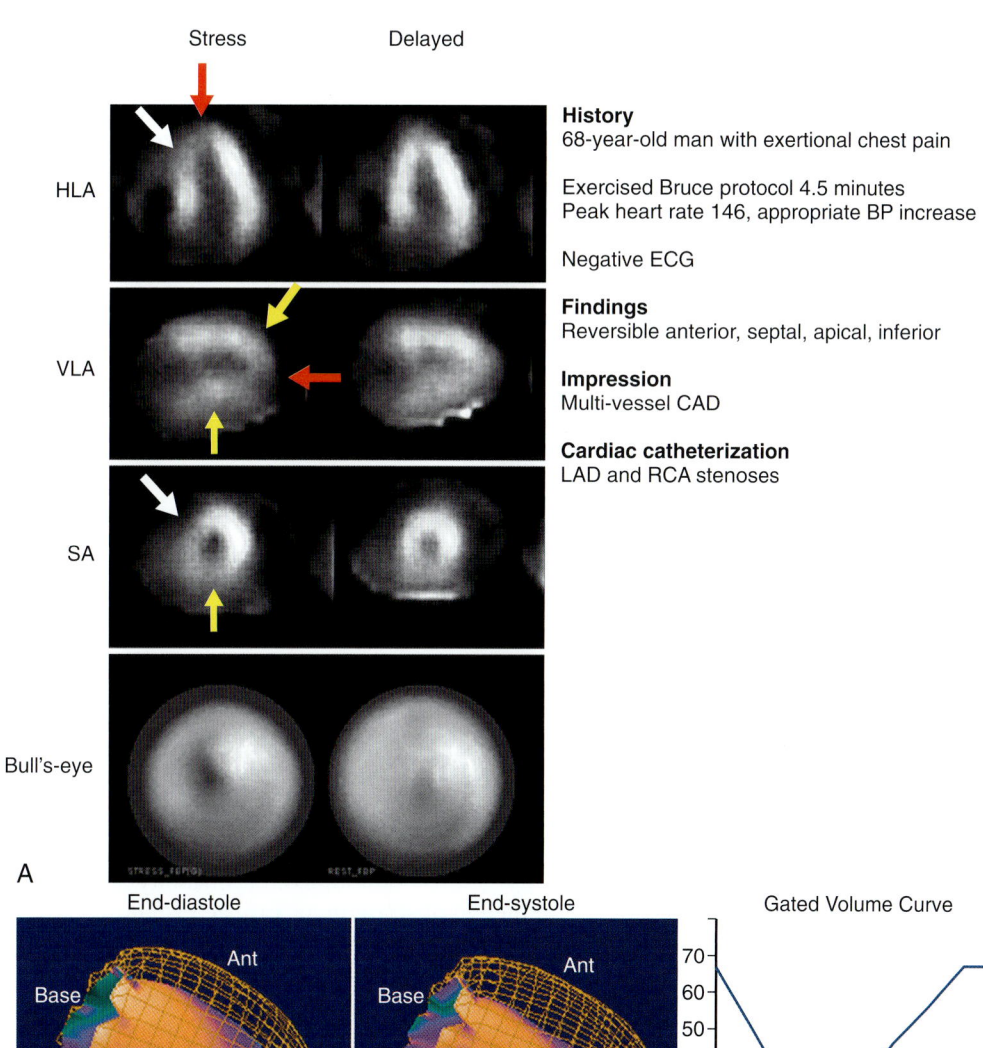

History
68-year-old man with exertional chest pain

Exercised Bruce protocol 4.5 minutes
Peak heart rate 146, appropriate BP increase

Negative ECG

Findings
Reversible anterior, septal, apical, inferior

Impression
Multi-vessel CAD

Cardiac catheterization
LAD and RCA stenoses

FIGURE 54-4 Myocardial ischemia. **A,** Tc 99m-sestamibi exercise-induced myocardial ischemia in the left anterior descending coronary artery (LAD) distribution confirmed at cardiac catheterization. Moderate and severe distal anterior (*large yellow arrow*), anteroseptal (*white arrows*), apical (*red arrows*), inferoseptal, and inferior (*small yellow arrows*) defects are not present on resting delayed images (mild inferior diaphragm attenuation also present). Bull's-eye confirms reversibility of defects. LAD and right coronary artery (RCA) stenoses were confirmed at cardiac catheterization. BP, blood pressure; HLA, horizontal long axis; SA, short axis; VLA, vertical long axis. **B,** Gated Tc 99m-sestamibi MPI shows normal wall motion despite multivessel CAD. End-diastolic (*left*) and end-systolic (*middle*) volumes show concentric left ventricular contraction in all regions. Volume curves (*right*) show normal left ventricular end-diastolic and end-systolic volumes, and normal left ventricular ejection fraction of 58%.

FIGURE 54-5 MI. **A,** Tc 99m-sestamibi adenosine pharmacologic stress study shows MI without ischemia. The left ventricular cavity is markedly dilated. Severe distal anterior (*small white arrows*), anteroseptal (*small yellow arrow*), apical (*red arrows*), septal (*large yellow arrow*), and inferoseptal and inferior (*large white arrow*) defects are present on stress and rest images (i.e., fixed defects). Bull's-eye confirms irreversibility of defects. HLA, horizontal long axis; ICD, implantable cardioverter-defibrillator; LV, left ventricle; SA, short axis; VLA, vertical long axis. **B,** Gated Tc 99m-sestamibi MPI shows markedly abnormal wall motion with severe global hypokinesis. End-diastolic (*left*) and end-systolic (*middle*) volumes show severe global hypokinesis in all regions. Volume curves (*right*) show abnormal left ventricular end-diastolic and end-systolic volumes, and abnormal left ventricular ejection fraction of 16%.

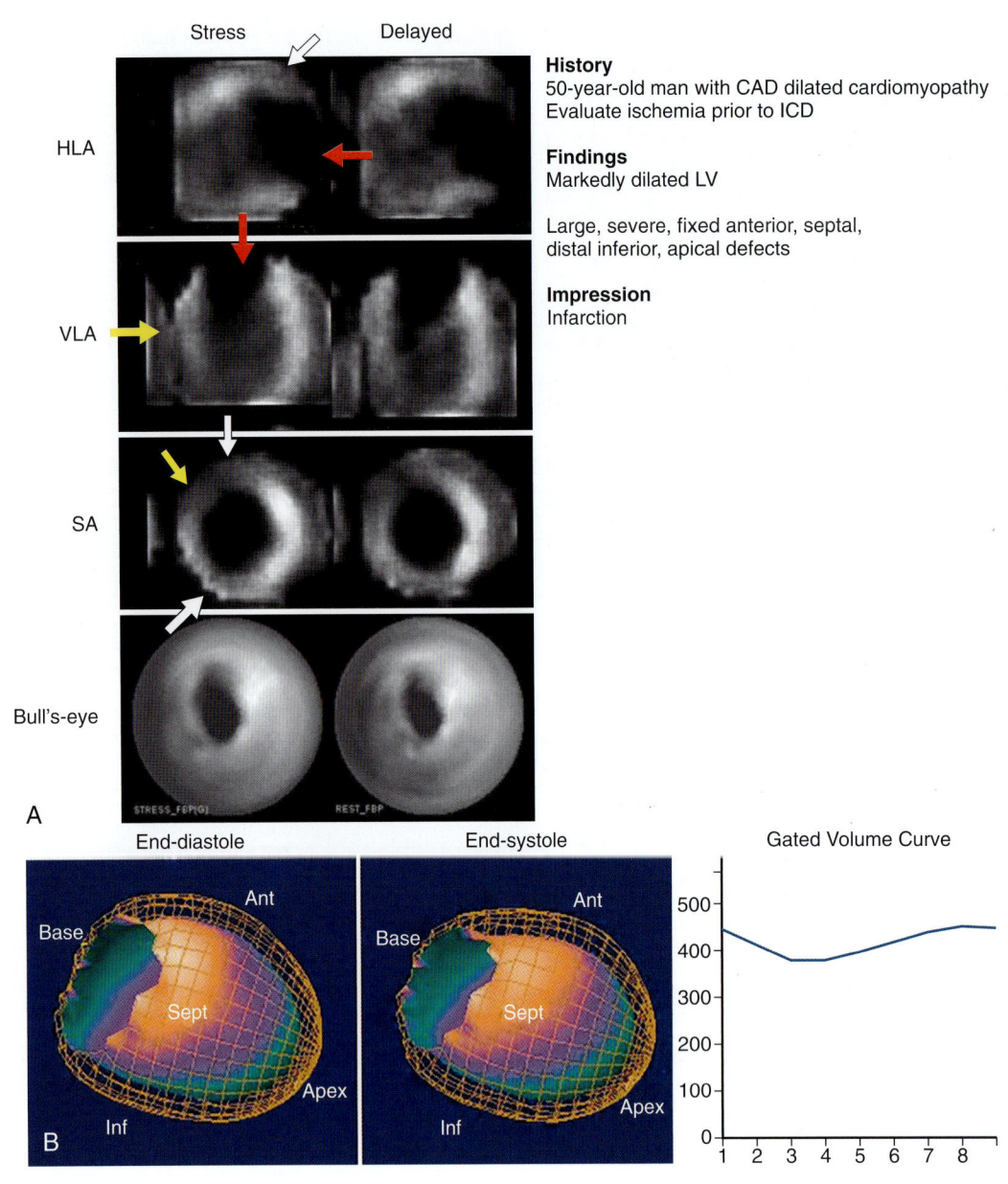

History
50-year-old man with CAD dilated cardiomyopathy
Evaluate ischemia prior to ICD

Findings
Markedly dilated LV

Large, severe, fixed anterior, septal, distal inferior, apical defects

Impression
Infarction

A unique clinical scenario for MPI is in the evaluation of acute coronary syndromes in patients presenting to the emergency department.[12] In patients without a history of prior myocardial infarction (MI) and an intermediate probability of CAD, the sensitivity for detection is very high. In this population actively having chest pain at the time of radiotracer administration, the negative predictive value of normal MPI is 99% to 100%. If the chest pain has resolved at the time of radiotracer administration, test sensitivity is modestly reduced, and current guidelines recommend repeating radiotracer administration within 2 hours of symptom abatement.[12] Because Tc 99m perfusion agents do not have significant redistribution for 6 hours, imaging can be performed after resolution of chest pain and still reflects the myocardial perfusion at the time administration. In patients presenting to the emergency department with chest pain that has resolved, and in whom recent myocardial injury has been excluded by a chest pain protocol including ECG and cardiac enzymes, a subsequent stress MPI study can be safely performed to exclude functional CAD.

Another unique use of MPI is for risk assessment. A large body of knowledge has shown that the defect size and severity, and the amount of reversibility by MPI are highly predictive of subsequent cardiac events. The negative predictive value of a normal or mildly abnormal study is also very high; these patients have a cardiac mortality of less than 1% per year, which is approximately the same as that of the general population. A highly abnormal study with severe and extensive perfusion abnormalities can have a cardiac event rate of 6% to 8% per year. This significantly higher incidence of adverse cardiac events, including subsequent MI, can have an impact on subsequent clinical management decisions.

As previously mentioned, an important specific indication is for the evaluation of myocardial viability. In most

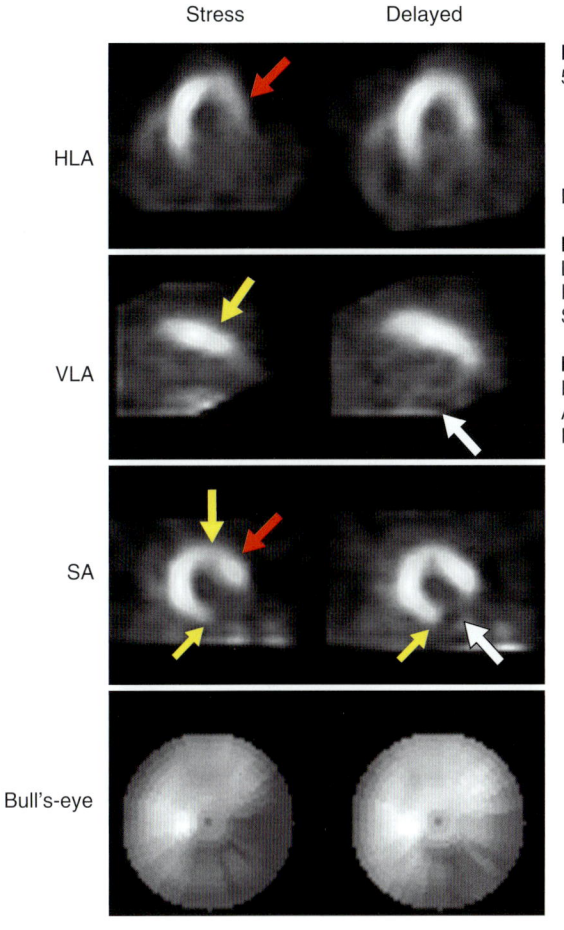

FIGURE 54-6 MI and myocardial ischemia. Tc 99m-sestamibi stress study shows MI and myocardial ischemia. Severe distal inferolateral (IL) and inferior defect is fixed (*white arrows*). Anterior (*large yellow arrows*) and anterolateral (AL) (*red arrows*) mild defects are reversible. Inferoseptal region (*small yellow arrows*), at the periphery of the infarct, shows partial improvement (compare stress with rest images). Bull's-eye confirms reversibility and irreversibility of defects. HLA, horizontal long axis; LAD, left anterior descending coronary artery; LADD, left anterior descending diagonal coronary artery; LCx, left circumflex coronary artery; RCA, right coronary artery; SA, short axis; VLA, vertical long axis.

cases, SPECT MPI can accurately assess myocardial viability with a resting thallium 201 study followed by redistribution imaging, or with a stress-redistribution-reinjection thallium 201 protocol.

Contraindications

The contraindications for stress MPI are the same as those for exercise and pharmacologic stress testing without the radionuclide component with the additional concerns related to radiation exposure and radionuclide administration (e.g. pregnant or nursing woman). The radionuclides are administered in tracer quantities, and thus, they have no known pharmacologic side effects. Contraindications for exercise stress testing are well established and include ongoing MI or myocardial ischemia, unstable angina, hypotension, and unstable cardiovascular conditions which could result in exercise induced cardiac fatality. Additional relative contraindications may include those which limit the patient's ability to exercise such as stroke, severe debilitation, severe peripheral vascular disease or underlying respiratory disease limiting exercise capacity, and altered mental status. Contraindications for pharmacologic stress testing are related to the specific pharmacologic stress agents administered, and are described in the next section under pharmacologic stress testing.

Pitfalls and Solutions

Quality Assurance

A QA program for gamma camera SPECT operation is essential to avoid artifacts, which could result in misinterpretation of test results. Proof of the establishment and diligent adherence to an equipment QA program is an integral part of laboratory accreditation by the American College of Radiology and the Intersocietal Commission for the Accreditation of Nuclear Medicine Laboratories. Conventional planar and specific SPECT and PET imaging QA procedures should be performed and recorded periodically. Daily QA includes ensuring correct isotope energy peak, and "daily floods" to assess gamma camera imaging field uniformity. Weekly QA includes resolution and linearity checks with "bar phantoms." Many manufacturers include software that can automatically compute planar measurements including differential and integral flood field uniformity and intrinsic linear resolution from bar phantoms.[10]

SPECT requires additional calibrations and gamma camera measurement to avoid artifacts specifically related to tomographic imaging. Calibrations to correct for the center of rotation and high count extrinsic (with a collimator) flood field uniformity are typically acquired on a weekly or quarterly basis. SPECT imaging of multipurpose thermoplastic (Plexiglas) phantoms is also highly recommended on a quarterly basis, and is mandated by laboratory accrediting agencies. These phantoms have solid "cold" spheres of differing sizes, and are filled with background radioactivity. The phantom assesses three-dimensional spatial resolution, uniformity, and tomographic image contrast. Full QA testing is also typically performed with initial equipment acceptance testing, and after each major servicing or software upgrade to ensure proper functioning. Errors in center of rotation or nonuniformities in the flood field may result in loss of spatial resolution (blurring), or SPECT artifacts ("ring"), or both, which could affect clinical interpretation of images and can be particularly troublesome in MPI.

Many SPECT systems include attenuation correction components, using radioactive scanning line sources, low-end CT devices, or diagnostic-quality CT. These attenuation-correcting devices require their own set of daily, weekly, and annual QA procedures. Likewise, PET and PET/CT scanners have specific QA requirements, as specified by the equipment manufacturers and as mandated by laboratory accreditation agencies. Typical PET and PET/CT QA procedures have been reviewed in a more recent publication.[10]

Description of Techniques and Protocols

Radionuclide Imaging Protocols

Stress Protocols—Pharmacologic versus Exercise Protocols

The most common types of stress protocols in the United States are exercise treadmill and pharmacologic stress test. Exercise stress testing is preferred over pharmacologic testing because it allows a more physiologic assessment of the patient's functional capacity and symptoms and the hemodynamic response to stress. Additionally, exercise generally results in lower radiotracer uptake in the gastrointestinal tract, improving image quality. The pharmacologic agents routinely used in clinical practice are adenosine, dipyridamole, and dobutamine. Pharmacologic stress tests can be performed on patients who cannot tolerate physical exercise. Patients with left bundle branch block, a known cause of false-positive septal perfusion defects with exercise, may undergo stress testing performed with dipyridamole to decrease the potential for this artifact. Other limiting factors in exercise stress testing are physical deconditioning, peripheral vascular disease, history of stroke, lower extremity amputation, and severe chronic obstructive pulmonary disease.

Exercise Protocols

In normal individuals, peak exercise increases heart rate and myocardial oxygen demand. At peak exercise, MBF typically increases approximately three to four times over that of rest. In patients with significant CAD, this mechanism fails to increase blood flow adequately distal to an obstructive lesion, resulting in an imbalance between oxygen supply and demand.

Before exercise, patients should have nothing per mouth after midnight, and be instructed to wear loose, comfortable clothing. We recommend abstinence from caffeinated substances because of the possibility that a pharmacologic stress test may be needed if an inadequate maximal heart rate is reached during maximal exercise stress testing. Intravenous access is obtained typically in the antecubital vein, ECG leads are securely placed, and the patient's hemodynamic status is closely monitored and recorded throughout the procedure. The radiotracer is administered at peak or target heart rate while exercising. Hemodynamic and ECG monitoring are continued for at least 5 minutes into the recovery period, or until symptoms or ECG changes resolve. Patients with good functional capacity can typically exercise on the Bruce protocol, which rapidly increases in speed and incline. Patients who are older or debilitated may use a modified Bruce exercise protocol, which more gradually increases in speed and incline to achieve target heart rate. In individuals with significant limitations of physical tolerance or in patients 3 to 5 days post-MI, a Naughton protocol or other low-level exercise protocol may be used at the physician's discretion.

Pharmacologic Protocols—Adenosine

Adenosine is a coronary vasodilator commonly used in combination with MPI.[13] This is a purine base, endogenously produced by myocardial smooth muscle and vascular endothelium. It is derived through extracellular dephosphorylation of adenosine triphosphate (ATP) and adenosine diphosphate (ADP). There are four known receptor subtypes specific for adenosine. A2A is considered a cardiac specific receptor, through which coronary vasodilation is initiated after intravenous adenosine administration.

Adenosine causes a vasodilation without direct chronotropic or inotropic responses in myocardium. Secondary hemodynamic changes in response to vasodilation include a modest decrease in systolic and diastolic blood pressure, and a compensatory increase in heart rate with modest increase in cardiac output. The coronary vasodilation increases MBF three to five times above that of baseline resting MBF in normal coronary vessels; this is comparable to the increase in MBF with maximal exercise. Coronary arterial segments distal to a significant coronary artery lesion (i.e., stenoses ≥70%) typically are vasodilated as a basal condition to maintain normal blood flow at rest. Adenosine causes vasodilation and an increase in blood flow to territories with normal coronary arteries, but cannot comparably increase flow to regions distal to stenoses that are already dilated in a resting condition. A relative perfusion abnormality can be seen in regions distal to a stenosis.

Adenosine has a very short half life of 10 to 15 seconds and is administered at the rate of 140 μg/kg/min over 4 minutes. Protocols using either 6 minutes or 3 to 4 minutes are equally effective. The stress radiotracer is administered after 4 minutes of infusion to define coronary blood flow at maximal vasodilation. Side effects are similar to dipyridamole, but also include atrioventricular block. The most common side effects are intermittent atrioventricular block, flushing, chest pain, and dyspnea. Because of the very short physiologic half-life, these side effects are very short-lived and resolve within 1 to 2 minutes of discontinuation.

Pharmacologic Protocols—Dipyridamole

Dipyridamole is also a commonly used vasodilator for MPI stress testing.[14] It is an indirect vasodilator that acts by blocking the cellular metabolism of adenosine. This results in a high local interstitial concentration, which subsequently results in coronary vasodilation. Dipyridamole is infused at a rate of 142 µg/kg/min over 4 minutes. The most common side effects include headache, flushing, hypotension, nausea, and chest discomfort. Because of a relatively longer biologic half-life of dipyridamole, the radiotracer is administered at 6 minutes after the start of the dipyridamole infusion. In addition, side effects may last for several minutes, but can be rapidly reversed by intravenous infusion of aminophylline, which acts by competitively inhibiting adenosine binding to its receptors.

Compared with adenosine, dipyridamole is equally effective in producing coronary vasodilation, and has a lower overall incidence of side effects, including induction of atrioventricular block. Dipyridamole can be used in patients with prolonged P-R interval and in elderly patients with poor tolerance to side effects.

Contraindications to Vasodilator Stress Testing

Vasodilators are contraindicated in patients with severe chronic obstructive pulmonary disease and asthma, particularly patients currently receiving treatment with β-agonists. Because high levels of adenosine block the β-agonist activity of bronchodilators, patients with chronic or reactive airways disease may experience bronchoconstriction and respiratory compromise. Unstable angina, persistent hypotension with systolic blood pressure less than 90 mm Hg, high-grade atrioventricular block without a pacemaker, uncontrolled arrhythmias, and severe aortic stenosis are also contraindications. Patients who have consumed caffeine or taken xanthine derivatives (e.g., theophylline, aminophylline) before testing have a potential for a false-negative result from inadequate vasodilation. Because xanthines block adenosine receptors, these should be discontinued at least 24 hours before vasodilator stress testing.

Pharmacologic Protocols—Dobutamine

Dobutamine is a β-adrenergic agent with a biologic half-life of 2 minutes. It acts by increasing myocardial contraction and heart rate, which subsequently increases myocardial oxygen demand and blood flow.[15] It is considered an alternative stress agent when an exercise or pharmacologic vasodilator study cannot be performed. Intravenous administration starts at an initial dose of 5 to 10 µg/kg/min for 3 minutes, with subsequent increases to doses of 20 µg/kg/min, 30 µg/kg/min, and 40 µg/kg/min in 3-minute stages, or until the goal of reaching 85% of maximal heart rate target is achieved. At approximately 1 to 2 minutes after target heart rate is achieved, the radiopharmaceutical is administered intravenously.

Severe hypotension, ventricular tachycardia and hemodynamically unstable sustained supraventricular tachycardia, and atrial fibrillation with rapid ventricular response are indications for termination of dobutamine. Other side effects of dobutamine include chest pain, dyspnea, palpitations, hypertension, anxiety, nausea, and vomiting. Contraindications to dobutamine include ventricular tachycardia, atrial fibrillation with rapid ventricular response, uncontrolled hypertension, hypotension, hypertrophic obstructive cardiomyopathy or aortic stenosis with severe left ventricular outflow obstruction, recent aortic dissection, and coronary artery dissection.

SPECT Imaging Protocols

Several protocols using thallium 201, Tc 99m, or both radiotracers have been well studied and characterized with respect to accuracy. Although modest differences exist, overall accuracy of the most common protocols is comparable. When using same-day protocols with Tc 99m radiotracers, however, the resting study should be performed first to avoid "false-positive" fixed defects.[16] If stress imaging is performed first, the higher MBF at stress combined with a relatively high stress radiotracer injection activity may lead to overestimation of MI because the subsequent resting images also reflect stress tracer distribution. If the resting study is performed first, the subsequent stress activity is much higher (approximately three times higher), and the increased blood flow at stress (approximately 2.5 to 3 times higher) produces a higher "weighting" on the stress images; this effectively reduces the contribution of the previous resting activity on the stress images. The number of potential false-negative results for ischemia is small because the resting activity has a relatively small contribution to the stress imaging.

Acquisition Protocols

The following protocols are suggested guidelines for an average-sized 70-kg man. For larger patients, increasing administered activity, imaging time, or both may partially compensate for the loss in detected true counts and subsequent decrease in image quality. Generally, the multi-headed gamma camera parameters for acquisition are similar for thallium 201 and Tc 99m radiotracers. Similar parameters include acceptance energy window (15% to 20% symmetric); low-energy, high-resolution collimation; 180 degrees orbit (45 degrees right anterior oblique to 45 degrees left posterior oblique); number of projections (60 to 64); matrix size (64 × 64); time per projection (20 to 30 seconds); and ECG frames per cardiac cycle (8 to 16). Stress and rest imaging time is currently approximately 20 to 30 minutes.

ECG gating permits the acquisition of separate time bin data sets with respect to the phase of the ECG cycle. By acquiring and reconstructing separate data sets within the ECG cycle, a dynamic set of images can be reconstructed to reflect the various phases of contraction and permit evaluation of ventricular function. This can be performed routinely without adversely increasing imaging time or compromising patient comfort. The gated images are reconstructed and displayed in cine format for evaluation as described subsequently. A limitation of this technique is the requirement of a relatively regular rhythm over the imaging period. In patients with atrial fibrillation or other markedly irregular rhythms, the ventricular function from gating cannot be reliably assessed. Routine patient-specific QA procedures include verification of the successful transmission of the correct heart rate information to the data acquisition computer system. Common imaging protocols include the following.

Same-Day Rest-Stress Tc 99m Radiotracer Protocol

Rest imaging typically begins 15 minutes to 1 hour after a resting injection of 370 MBq (10 mCi). Stress imaging begins approximately 15 minutes to 1 hour after the stress injection of 1.11 GBq (30 mCi). The time interval between radiotracer administration and the beginning of imaging varies. Delayed imaging may favor improved liver clearance; however, earlier imaging may reduce bowel activity.

Two-Day Protocol Rest-Stress Tc 99m Radiotracer Protocol

This protocol is very similar to the above-described 1-day protocol. This protocol may be used in patients with a higher body mass index who may require a higher resting activity for adequate image quality. The 24-hour delay allows the relatively higher resting Tc 99m activity to decay and avoid interference with the stress perfusion.

Stress-Redistribution Thallium 201 Protocol

An initial stress activity of 93 to 130 MBq (2.5 to 3.5 mCi) is administered intravenously at peak exercise. Stress imaging begins immediately after the recovery phase before significant redistribution. Indirect signs of stress-induced ventricular dysfunction (abnormal lung uptake and left ventricular dilation) can also be seen early after stress. Resting-redistribution images are acquired at approximately 4 hours after the initial stress. As discussed previously, a 37-MBq (1-mCi) resting reinjection activity is commonly administered just before imaging to enhance the detection of viable myocardium.

To improve total count statistics, thallium 201 imaging may be slightly longer than Tc 99m imaging. Typical imaging protocols include imaging on multidetector gamma cameras for approximately 30 minutes. Another option to increase counting statistics is to use a high-sensitivity, low-resolution collimator. Finally, increasing the width of the photopeak acceptance window to 30%, and including the higher energy window at 167 keV, can also increase counts, although at the expense of diminished spatial resolution and a larger fraction of scattered radiation.

Dual Isotope Acquisition with Thallium 201 and Tc 99m Protocol

The rest study for this protocol is first performed with 93 to 130 MBq (2.5 to 3.5 mCi) of thallium 201 followed immediately by imaging. The stress study is performed with 1.11 GBq (30 mCi) of Tc 99m radiotracer administered at peak stress. An advantage of this protocol is the short time interval between the initial resting injection and the stress study. Photopeak overlap is avoided because thallium 201 has a lower photopeak.

The major disadvantage of this protocol relates to differences in final image quality. Thallium 201 has a lower photopeak energy, for which gamma cameras have inferior energy resolution and spatial resolution compared with higher gamma ray energies. The lower thallium 201 images also contain a larger percentage of Compton-scattered gamma rays than do images acquired at higher energies. These factors, combined with lower administered activity at lower resting blood flow, all contribute to overall lower true counts and the need for greater degree of filtering. Care is taken specifically to process these different radiotracer studies with specific protocols. These differences also need to be taken into account during interpretation of these studies.

Image Interpretation

Postprocessing

Tomographic images typically are reconstructed from the raw projection data with filtered back-projection and low-pass filtering. The degree of low-pass filtering depends on the counting statistics and noise. New algorithms have become commercially available that replace filtered back-projection by iterative reconstruction techniques, some versions of which incorporate depth-dependent collimator imaging characteristics and attenuation correcting data, both of which may improve overall image quality, particularly for low count perfusion images.

After tomographic reconstruction, the stress and rest images are normalized to the peak activity within the myocardium. This normalization permits a consistent comparison of regions within the myocardium, and it allows for a relative comparison between the stress and rest studies despite differences in absolute counts between studies.

An important aspect of MPI is quantification of defect size and severity. After normalization, this quantification can be performed automatically by computer analysis. Because the normal radiotracer distribution may vary depending on the patient population (e.g., breast attenuation in women and diaphragm attenuation in men), tomographic images are matched to the appropriate normal database cohort. Myocardial perfusion tomograms are processed automatically to generate a two-dimensional parametric display (bull's-eye plot) from the three-dimensional count distribution. This display provides a rapid overview of three-dimensional myocardial perfusion for comparison between stress and rest count distributions.

Automated boundary detection programs define endocardial and epicardial borders of the myocardium. Applied to all cycles of gated studies, the left ventricular volumes provide measurements of global and regional left ventricular function and ejection fraction. Several groups and manufacturers have implemented their algorithms into commercially available software. Because of differences in physical modeling assumptions, algorithm implementation, and boundary detection methods, different software packages have different normal values and may produce significantly different results.[17] Direct comparisons between values produced from different software packages should be performed carefully and should take into account algorithm differences, including the use of algorithm-specific databases of normal limits.

Interpretation

Interpretation of projection images ("raw data") is essential for proper interpretation of the tomographic images. Projection data typically are first viewed in cine format to identify potential causes of decreased activity or artifacts. Identifying patient motion during image acquisition is an important step in identifying artifacts that could potentially be misinterpreted as perfusion defects. The effect of patient motion is often very difficult to predict with respect to location or appearance on reconstructed images. An artifactual perfusion defect may appear with misalignment of the ventricular walls, association with extracardiac activity adjacent to the defect, or a defect in a noncoronary distribution.

If there is a concern that an apparent perfusion defect may represent an artifact owing to patient motion, repeat imaging (Tc 99m radiotracers or resting thallium 201) should be considered to clarify the issue. Although motion correction software may reduce the effect of patient motion, software may be unable to eliminate completely the effect of patient motion on the final reconstructed tomographic images. Any application of motion-correcting software must be reviewed carefully to verify that the algorithm performed the intended correction appropriately, as part of routine patient-specific QA. Generally, vertical motion errors are detected and corrected more reliably than horizontal and bulk body motion errors. An example of a motion artifact is shown in Figure 54-7.

Another common artifact is due to soft tissue attenuation. In women, breast attenuation can result in either a uniform or a nonuniform decrease in detected counts, most commonly in the anterior or anterolateral left ventricular wall region. Similarly, inferior decreased activity from diaphragm attenuation may be seen with a relatively high frequency in men. "Diaphragmatic creep" is an artifact caused by the changing position of the heart immediately after strenuous exercise stress and during the recovery phase. Because deep respiratory excursion gradually subsides after exercise, the location and orientation of the heart may change while imaging after exercise stress. The resulting tomographic images, which are a composite of various positions, may show a lower activity in the inferior wall because of this cardiac motion artifact. Assessment of the projection images for changes in heart position through imaging can determine if the potential for this artifact is present in an individual study.

Three physiologic parameters can be assessed from the projection data. The first is left ventricular cavity size. It is possible to appreciate markedly decreased counts within the left ventricular cavity, and a relatively large cavity compared with the myocardial thickness indicates left ventricular dilation. Measurements of ventricular size from the computer-generated boundaries may also confirm left ventricular enlargement. In patients with prior apical infarction and left ventricular dysfunction, ungated images may show a markedly decreased left ventricular cavity activity because of abnormally and severely decreased wall motion adjacent to infarction. In patients with an area of severely decreased activity at the apex because of prior infarction, severely decreased wall motion or dyskinesis may contribute to an almost entirely absent apical defect of attenuating blood pool ("black hole sign"; Fig. 54-8) that is associated with a higher incidence of apical aneurysm.

The second physiologic sign is increased lung uptake. This increased lung uptake has been well described in thallium 201 myocardial perfusion studies as a poor prognostic indicator, which reflects left ventricular dysfunction. The increase in lung uptake, defined as greater than 50% of the peak myocardial activity, is an indicator of abnormally prolonged pulmonary transit time. Patients with either exercise-induced or resting left ventricular dysfunction have increased pulmonary transit time, and prolonged exposure of the radiotracer to the lungs results

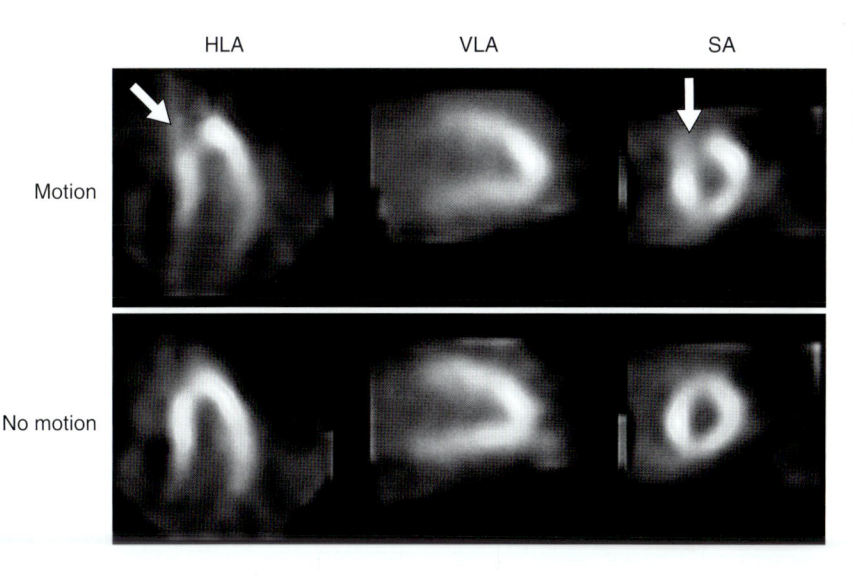

FIGURE 54-7 Motion artifact causing a defect owing to patient motion during image acquisition. *Top row,* Initial images acquired with significant patient motion suggest an anteroseptal defect (*arrow*) with misalignment of the ventricular walls and extracardiac activity outside of the normal myocardial boundaries (HLA view). *Bottom row,* Repeat imaging without patient motion shows normal perfusion. HLA, horizontal long axis; SA, short axis; VLA, vertical long axis.

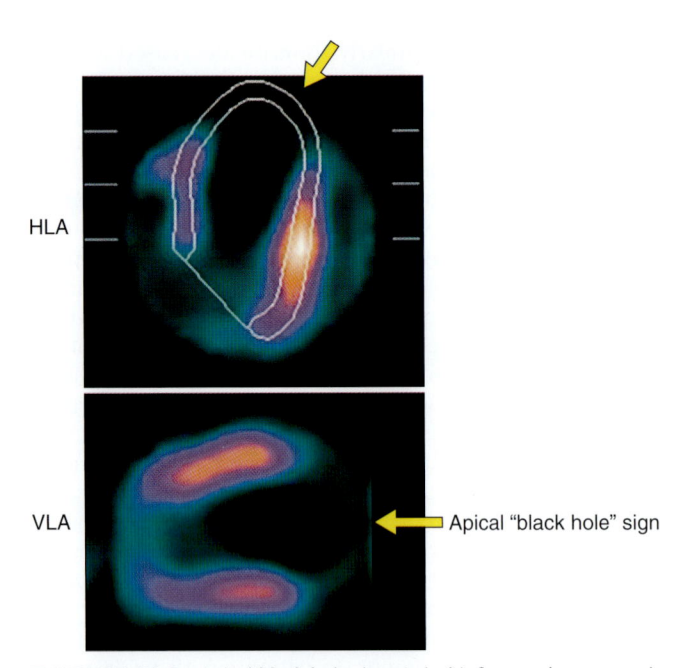

FIGURE 54-8 Apical black hole sign. Apical infarct and aneurysm in a patient with a history of CAD, ischemic cardiomyopathy, large anterior apical MI, and left ventricular aneurysm resection. Tc 99m-sestamibi stress study shows severe fixed apical defect (*arrow*; black hole sign). The severe left ventricular apical cavity dilation is compatible with residual left ventricular aneurysm. HLA, horizontal long axis; VLA, vertical long axis.

in increased lung uptake, which can be assessed visually. This may be seen in patients with prior MI and elevated left ventricular end-diastolic pressure, or exercise-induced left ventricular dysfunction when the pulmonary transit time is increased. These findings may also be seen with Tc 99m radiotracers; however, because Tc 99m imaging may be performed at a time considerably later than the stress testing, some degree of lung clearance may occur, and increased lung uptake may not be apparent on subsequent imaging.

The third physiologic sign relates to right ventricular uptake. In normal patients, right ventricular myocardium is thin and may not be seen reliably because of partial volume effects. In patients with elevated right ventricular pressures or unusually thickened myocardium, abnormal right ventricular size or uptake may also be detected, in at least the thickest parts of the right ventricle, if not the entire right ventricle. These may be indirect signs of right ventricular hypertrophy, volume overload, or pressure overload.

When interpreting and reporting MPI, important aspects include perfusion defect size, severity, and reversibility. Although a visual interpretation may be accurate with respect to the presence or absence of coronary disease, quantitative information has prognostic significance. The size and severity of the perfusion defect are predictive of cardiac events, including MI and cardiac death.[18] These are important for risk stratification and patient management. Small, mild defects are associated with low cardiac mortality of less than 1% per year.[19] Severe defects and extensive ischemia are associated with significantly higher cardiac events and worse short-term prognosis. In addition, the short-term outcome for cardiac events in patients with mild ischemia is worse for patients undergoing revascularization.[20] In contrast, the short-term cardiac event rate for patients with severe defects is lower for patients undergoing revascularization compared with medical management. Quantitative measures of myocardial perfusion scintigraphy may determine the most appropriate subsequent therapy in patients with known CAD.[20]

As discussed in Chapter 55, global and regional left ventricular function are very important parameters for clinical management. Left ventricular functional assessment by left ventricular ejection fraction is highly predictive of mortality. Regional functional assessment may also influence clinical management. A segment of dysfunctional myocardium with preserved viability may be important from the perspective of potential revascularization.

Other Artifacts and Normal Variants

Apical Thinning

The thickness of the myocardium in the apex varies from patient to patient. Physiologic thinning of the myocardium at the apex may show an apparent relative decrease in radiotracer uptake, however, because of partial volume effects.

Left Bundle Branch Block

Reversible septal perfusion defects can be seen in patients with left bundle branch block who undergo exercise stress MPI. This phenomenon has been attributed to asynchronous septal relaxation, which is out of phase with diastolic filling of the remainder of the ventricle. Perfusion defects related to left bundle branch block usually do not involve the apex. Septal asynchrony is more profound with higher heart rates, and it may appear as a reversible perfusion defect. Use of vasodilator stress has been reported to reduce the frequency of this artifact. More recently, the evaluation of patients with left bundle branch block by MPI has been enhanced considerably by the additional computations of ventricular asynchrony made possible by three-dimensional phase distributions measured from gated MPI count distributions.

Long Membranous/Short Muscular Septum

The length of the muscular septum varies among individuals. Absence of uptake in the basal membranous portion of the septum results in the appearance of a short basal septum.

Misregistration of SPECT and Computed Tomography

With the introduction of fast multislice CT, it is possible that a similar "artifactual" defect could be seen on SPECT if corrected with high temporal resolution CT. Cardiac PET studies have shown clearly potential artifactual "perfusion" defects owing to misalignment of the PET emission and the transformed CT transmission image used for attenuation correction. This is due to differences in the respiratory cycle during CT and the average PET emission diaphragm position. Data for a single high-resolution CT transaxial slice can be acquired in a fraction of a second, whereas PET emission data typically are acquired over several minutes to 15 to 30 minutes. Cardiac PET data may be ECG gated, but data are not currently gated with respiratory cycle information. The frequency of misalignment is high (42% in a retrospective study[21]); however, impact on the emission corrected images is still under investigation.

Test Accuracy

Detection of Coronary Artery Disease

Stress perfusion scintigraphy with SPECT has the highest accuracy among all imaging modalities in the noninvasive detection of functionally significant CAD. Overall, the diagnostic accuracy is approximately 85% to 90%, with sensitivity and specificity varying depending on the patient population and methodology of the study. In women with functionally significant CAD (>70% stenosis), gated Tc 99m-sestamibi reported diagnostic sensitivity is 80%, and specificity is 92%.[22] Other studies have reported higher sensitivities and specificities of 90% and 93%.[3,23]

Myocardial Viability

Using the stress-redistribution-reinjection thallium 201 protocol, areas of reversible ischemia can be identified as viable. A resting-redistribution thallium 201 study can assess regions of low resting blood flow and residual viable myocardium ("hibernating myocardium"). Resting images obtained immediately after injection represent MBF. Any perfusion defects seen on initial imaging caused by low resting blood flow show slower washout and "redistribution" compared with defects with normal resting blood flow. This normalization ("reversibility") of resting perfusion defects on delayed imaging indicates viable myocardium. If a severe perfusion defect on initial rest imaging does not improve on the redistribution study ("fixed"), this correlates well with infarction.

A more recent study comparing rest-redistribution thallium 201 with myocardial delayed hyperenhancement by MRI confirmed high quantitative correlation of infarct size ($r = 0.90$).[24] Thallium 201 rest-redistribution also correlates well with viability by ^{18}FDG-PET.[8] Despite being "fixed" perfusion defects, mild and moderate (<50% decreased counts compared with normal areas) defects are considered viable. Viable regions by thallium 201 showed a 98% concordance with viability by ^{18}FDG-PET. Only a relatively small proportion (approximately 30%) of severe fixed defects by thallium 201 showed discordant viability by ^{18}FDG-PET.[8] This detection of myocardial viability can determine the suitability of a candidate for revascularization.

Rest-redistribution and stress-redistribution-reinjection thallium 201 with SPECT are considered highly accurate in evaluating myocardial viability; however, PET has better spatial resolution and attenuation correction, and is generally considered superior for this indication. MRI has shown comparable results for viability determination, and is able to determine the extent of subendocardial infarction with better spatial resolution.[25]

MYOCARDIAL PERFUSION IMAGING WITH PET

Clinical Indications

The currently approved indications for PET in nuclear medicine include MPI and myocardial viability assessment. The major advantages of PET over SPECT include the routine use of attenuation correction, higher detection sensitivity, and superior spatial resolution. PET perfusion radiotracers are currently relatively expensive, however, and have shorter physical half-lives compared with SPECT radiotracers. Although absolute quantification of MBF is possible, dynamic imaging and modeling are technically demanding, and have not been considered essential for clinical diagnostic imaging.

Patients with a high body mass index are especially well suited for PET because of (1) routine use of high-quality attenuation correction, and (2) higher photon detection sensitivity, owing to a lower proportion of photon scatter and tissue attenuation compared with SPECT. In addition, PET scans generally contain more than 100 times as many counts as do SPECT scans, particularly for three-dimensional data acquisitions, as opposed to two-dimensional PET data acquisitions. An example of an ammonia N 13 dipyridamole PET study is shown in Figure 54-9.

The major clinical disadvantages of PET currently relate to the available myocardial perfusion radiotracers (expense, availability, cost, and physical properties). These physical factors result in numerous technical differences compared with SPECT, which are discussed briefly here.

Technical Aspects

PET Myocardial Perfusion Imaging Radiotracers

Numerous radiotracers have been validated to evaluate myocardial perfusion. The two most commonly used are ammonia N 13 and rubidium 82. Other validated PET myocardial perfusion radiotracers, such as ^{15}O water and ^{11}C compounds with high first-pass extraction fraction, are currently investigational and not approved for clinical use. Although data indicate superiority of these as perfusion tracers, they have physical half-lives of only 122 seconds (^{15}O water) and 20 minutes (^{11}C), requiring an on-site cyclotron for synthesis, and these tracers currently are impractical for widespread clinical use.

PET has been well established as an accurate means for the evaluation of myocardial viability. The presence of preserved myocardial metabolism by ^{18}FDG is highly accurate in the detection of myocardial viability, and its use is briefly discussed here. Aspects of PET imaging involving highly sophisticated radiotracer compartmental modeling quantification are not discussed. Although well validated in many prior studies, these are not routinely used in clinical practice.

Ammonia N 13

The very short physical half-life of ammonia N 13 (10 minutes) requires an on-site cyclotron and radiochemical

FIGURE 54-9 Normal ammonia N 13 PET myocardial perfusion pharmacologic stress imaging with dipyridamole. Note excellent spatial resolution and more uniform radiotracer distribution compared with traditional SPECT Tc 99m-sestamibi imaging (see Figs. 54-1 and 54-2), despite the patient's high body mass index (BMI) of 50. BP, blood pressure; HLA, horizontal long axis; LAD/D1, first diagonal branch of the left anterior descending artery; PTCA, percutaneous transluminal coronary angioplasty; SA, short axis; VLA, vertical long axis.

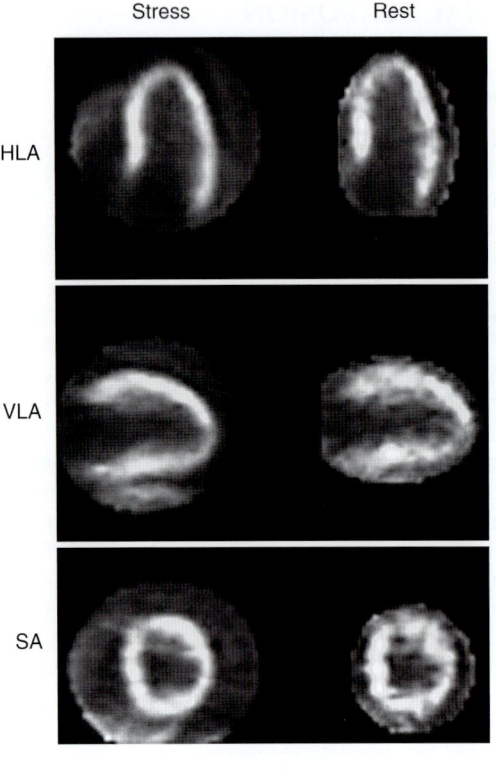

History
49-year-old woman with CAD s/p PTCA, s/p stent LAD/D1, recurrent chest pain
BMI = 50

Dipyridamole pharmacologic stress
Appropriate BP response
No chest pain

Negative ECG

Findings
Normal perfusion

Impression
Normal study. No dipyridamole-induced ischemia or decreased coronary flow reserve

synthesis. The first pass extraction fraction of ammonia N 13 is very high at approximately 95%. This compound rapidly crosses the intravascular capillary membrane into the interstitial space and into myocytes by passive diffusion. It is rapidly metabolized by ATP-dependent processes and trapped intracellularly. The uptake and retention can be altered by metabolic changes within the myocardium. Although ammonia N 13 is widely considered an excellent indicator of MBF, the dependence on the metabolic state of the myocyte may theoretically limit its ability to indicate absolute blood flow. The radiation dose from ammonia N 13 is 1.7 mSv (0.17 rem) for an injected activity of 740 MBq (20 mCi).

Rubidium 82

Rubidium 82 is a monovalent cationic analogue of potassium. It is commercially produced and available from a strontium (strontium 82) generator. Strontium 82 has a relatively long physical half-life (25.5 days); however, rubidium 82 has a very short physical half life (75 seconds). The strontium 82 generator requires replacement approximately every 4 weeks. Rubidium 82 is extracted from plasma with a very high efficiency through the Na^+,K^+-ATPase pump. The myocardial extraction fraction of rubidium 82 is similar to that of thallium 201, but is less than that of ammonia N 13. The extraction can be reduced by severe acidosis, hypoxia, and ischemia. The initial radiotracer uptake is a function of blood flow, metabolism, and myocardial cell integrity. The radiation dose is 2.2 mSv (0.22 rem) for an injection of 1.85 GBq (50 mCi) of activity.

Description of Technique and Protocols

The general procedures for PET MPI are outlined next. Differences in physical properties of the PET radiotracers necessitate differences in protocols to optimize imaging.

Stress Protocols

For ammonia N 13, an exercise protocol can be performed. The very short half-life of ammonia N 13 requires close coordination of isotope production, exercise testing, and imaging, however, if treadmill exercise is performed, the cyclotron, exercise facility, and PET imaging facility must be in close proximity. For rubidium 82, pharmacologic stress is typically performed in place of exercise stress because of the very short physical half-life of the isotope.

Resting perfusion is performed first. Because the physical half-lives of PET radiotracers are short, background resting perfusion does not significantly contribute to the subsequent stress radiotracer distribution. For ammonia N 13, a 740-MBq (20-mCi) activity typically is injected followed by approximately 10 minutes of imaging. For rubidium 82, a typical activity of 1.48 to 2.22 GBq (40 to 60 mCi) is administered followed by approximately 5 minutes of imaging. ECG gating can be performed with both radiotracers to assess left ventricular wall motion and left ventricular function.

PET Image Acquisition

The typical imaging time for acquiring PET myocardial perfusion emission data is approximately 10 minutes for ammonia N 13 and 5 minutes for rubidium 82. The attenuation correction scan, either the PET transmission scan or the CT transmission scan, should be acquired in close temporal proximity to the emission study. A single transmission scan can be performed to correct the rest and stress emission scans if the emission scans are done in close temporal proximity, and there is little chance of patient motion. If there is a question of patient motion between the two scans, separate transmission scans can be acquired to correct each emission scan separately. For attenuation correction, older PET scanners used a transmission scan with a positron-emitting source (e.g., ^{68}Ga or ^{137}Cs). More recent PET scanners, optimized primarily for whole body ^{18}FDG-PET oncology applications, have incorporated sophisticated multidetector CT devices, which are used for attenuation correction and colocalization. Cardiac PET emission data from these PET scanners use attenuation correction data acquired using the CT scanners, transformed to attenuation maps for 511-keV gamma ray emission.

Image misregistration between the PET emission and the CT transmission scans is a potential cause of artifacts, the clinical impact of which is currently under investigation. Because of the high temporal resolution of CT and the short imaging time during which the CT scan is acquired, the depth of respiration during CT scanning may significantly differ compared with the average diaphragm position during the PET emission scan. This mismatch could potentially result in inaccurate attenuation correction, and a mismatch could potentially be misinterpreted as a perfusion defect. Several methods to correct for this mismatch are currently under investigation; inspection of the degree of mismatch is recommended as part of QA before interpretation of these studies.

For most clinical studies, relative quantification of perfusion and function with PET is performed in a manner that is very similar to that performed with SPECT. The attenuation-corrected PET scans result in a more uniform normal perfusion pattern with PET. Overall, the diagnostic accuracy of PET is higher than that of SPECT. Because of attenuation correction, higher sensitivity, and better spatial resolution, PET may be particularly useful in large patients, and in patients with severe attenuation artifacts.

Myocardial Viability

The diagnostic accuracy of ^{18}FDG-PET in the evaluation of myocardial viability is well established.[26,27] Revascularization improved left ventricular function in 85% of segments with preservation of ^{18}FDG uptake; no functional improvement was seen in 92% of segments with matched absence of blood flow and ^{18}FDG uptake.[26] More recently, ^{18}FDG-PET myocardial viability used to select revascularization candidates was associated with significantly lower in-hospital death rate, improved 12-month survival, and reduced complicated perioperative recovery.[28] Fluorine 18 is a positron imaging isotope with a physical half-life of 110 minutes. ^{18}FDG is a glucose analogue, which is transported intracellularly via glucose transporters. It is subsequently phosphorylated to FDG-6-phosphate, and trapped intracellularly without further metabolism because of its stereochemistry. The radiation dose of typical injected activity of 370 MBq (10 mCi) of ^{18}FDG is approximately 11 mSv (1.1 rem).

When myocardial tissue is subjected to oxygen demands that exceed limited blood flow, myocardial ischemia results in a shift of metabolism from free fatty acids to glycolysis. To maintain myocardial viability, energy consumption is reduced, and myocardial contraction is decreased. Because of this, ^{18}FDG uptake is high in residual viable myocardium.

Myocardial viability with regional dysfunction may be present in a spectrum of overlapping physiologic scenarios ranging from decreased to normal resting MBF. This complex issue is currently evolving as further studies report new data. Classically, hibernating myocardium by PET is defined by reduced resting MBF with preserved myocardial metabolism evidenced by ^{18}FDG uptake. If resting perfusion is normal, intermittent episodes of myocardial ischemia produced by episodes of increased oxygen demand may produce a condition termed *stunning*. This repetitive, intermittent stress-induced ischemia may be sufficient to produce chronic myocardial dysfunction. In this clinical scenario, resting perfusion by PET may be normal, and there may be preservation of ^{18}FDG uptake in regions of myocardial dysfunction. A matched reduction in blood flow and metabolism is considered nonviable myocardium or infarction. An example of a myocardial viability study is shown in Figure 54-10.

PITFALLS AND SOLUTIONS

A potential limitation of imaging with ^{18}FDG is difficulty in diabetic patients with elevated serum glucose levels. In preparation for the ^{18}FDG study, oral glucose loading is typically performed to increase endogenous insulin levels and increase ^{18}FDG uptake in the myocardium. In diabetics, elevated serum glucose levels may interfere with adequate uptake in the myocardium. To overcome this issue, a sliding scale of intravenous insulin administration may be used. Alternatively, some European protocols use pharmacologic interventions, such as Acipimox, which reduces peripheral free fatty acid levels by inhibiting lipolysis; this indirectly stimulates glucose use. Another limitation is spatial resolution. MRI with inherently better spatial resolution is currently superior to PET in detecting subendocardial MI.

FUTURE DIRECTIONS

The more recent availability of rapid acquisition CT and combined PET/CT and SPECT/CT instrumentation provides the possibility of assessing coronary artery calcifications and coronary anatomy. The technical factors potentially limiting coronary angiography with CT include (1) coronary artery calcification interfering with intraluminal assessment; (2) cardiac motion degrading image quality in patients with high heart rates; (3) radiation dosimetry considerations; and (4) reconstruction streak artifacts caused by high-attenuation structures, such as metallic surgical clips or defibrillators. In contrast to radionuclide techniques that provide information regarding functional significance of stenosis, coronary CT reveals information

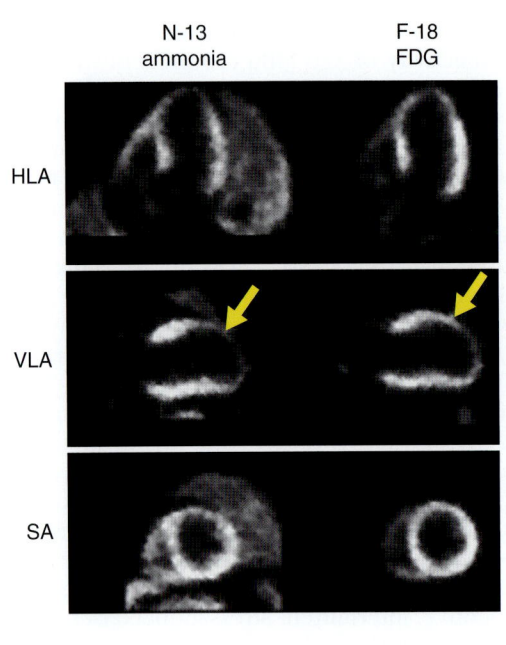

FIGURE 54-10 ^{18}FDG and ammonia N 13 PET myocardial viability study. Small region of decreased perfusion on ammonia N 13 and preserved metabolism on ^{18}FDG in distal anterior wall indicate hibernating myocardium (*arrows*). Large, severe, matched apical lesion is from an MI. Other regions show preserved resting perfusion and metabolism indicating viable myocardium, despite global hypokinesis. *Left column,* ammonia N 13 resting perfusion. *Right column,* ^{18}FDG metabolism. HLA, horizontal long axis; LV, left ventricular; LVEF, left ventricular ejection fraction; SA, short axis; VLA, vertical long axis.

History
51-year-old man with 3 vessel CAD, Global LV hypokinesis, reduced LVEF = 25%

Findings
Small mismatched distal anterior region with decreased flow and preserved metabolism

Large severe apical matched defect

Resting perfusion and metabolism in all other areas are normal

Impression
Small hibernating distal anterior region – viable
Large apical infarction – nonviable
All other regions – viable

---

regarding subclinical CAD. Combined PET/CT to assess CAD and the correction techniques for its limitations are currently active areas of investigation.[29,30]

CONCLUSION

SPECT and PET radionuclide techniques are the most accurate, widely available, quantitative methods to assess CAD and myocardial viability noninvasively. Quantitative data, including left ventricular function, and defect size and severity, are also prognostic. MPI with SPECT is excellent in identifying and defining viable myocardium in most cases; however, PET and MRI are generally considered more sensitive and accurate.

KEY POINTS

- Myocardial perfusion scintigraphy is well established as the most accurate noninvasive method to diagnose, assess, and quantify extent of functionally significant coronary artery disease.
- Myocardial perfusion scintigraphy, in conjunction with ECG gating, provides a quantitative assessment of ventricular function.
- Myocardial perfusion scintigraphy can determine myocardial viability with high accuracy.
- Quantitative myocardial perfusion scintigraphy provides prognostic information with respect to future cardiac events and mortality.

SUGGESTED READINGS

Baggish AL, Boucher CA. Radiopharmaceutical agents for myocardial perfusion imaging. Circulation 2008; 118:1668-1674.

Di Carli MF, Dorbala S, Meserve J, et al. Clinical myocardial perfusion PET/CT. J Nucl Med 2007; 48:783-793.

Hendel RC, Berman DS, Di Carli MF, et al. Appropriate use criteria for cardiac radionuclide imaging. A Report of the American College of Cardiology Foundation Appropriate Use Criteria Task Force, the American Society of Nuclear Cardiology, the American College of Radiology, the American Heart Association, the American Society of Echocardiography, the Society of Cardiovascular Computed Tomography, the Society for Cardiovascular Magnetic Resonance, and the Society of Nuclear Medicine. Circulation 2009; 119:e561-e587.

Russell RR 3rd, Zaret BL. Nuclear cardiology: Present and future. Curr Probl Cardiol 2006; 31:557-629.

Shaw LJ, Narula J. Risk assessment and predictive value of coronary artery disease testing. J Nucl Med 2009; 50:1296-1306.

Zoghbi GJ, Dorfman TA, Iskandrian AE. The effects of medications on myocardial perfusion. J Am Coll Cardiol 2008; 52:401-416.

REFERENCES

1. Gerson MC. Cardiac Nuclear Medicine, 3rd ed. New York, McGraw-Hill, 1997.
2. Iskandrian AE, Garcia EV. Nuclear Cardiac Imaging: Principles and Applications, 3rd ed. New York, Oxford University Press, 2003.
3. Zaret BL, Beller G. Clinical Nuclear Cardiology: State of the Art. St Louis, Mosby, 1993.
4. Heller GV, Hendel R. Nuclear Cardiology: Practical Applications. New York, McGraw Hill, 2004.
5. Klocke FJ, Baird MG, Lorell BH, et al. ACC/AHA/ASNC guidelines for the clinical use of cardiac radionuclide imaging—executive summary: a report of the American College of Cardiology/American Heart Association Task Force on Practice Guidelines (ACC/AHA/ASNC Committee to Revise the 1995 Guidelines for the Clinical Use of Cardiac Radionuclide Imaging). Circulation 2003; 108:1404-1418.
6. Hesse B, Tagil K, Cuocolo A, et al. EANM/ESC procedural guidelines for myocardial perfusion imaging in nuclear cardiology. Eur J Nucl Med Mol Imaging 2005; 32:855-897.

7. Peter LT, Frans JT. Myocardial perfusion planar imaging (abstract). J Nucl Cardiol 2006; 13:c91-c96.
8. Dilsizian V, Perronefilardi P, Arrighi JA, et al. Concordance and discordance between stress-redistribution-reinjection and rest-redistribution thallium imaging for assessing viable myocardium—comparison with metabolic-activity by positron emission tomography. Circulation 1993; 88:941-952.
9. Borges-Neto S, Tuttle RH, Shaw LK, et al. Outcome prediction in patients at high risk for coronary artery disease: comparison between Tc-99m tetrofosmin and Tc-99m sestamibi. Radiology 2004; 232: 58-65.
10. Nichols KJ, Bacharach SL, Bergmann SR, et al. Instrumentation quality assurance and performance. J Nucl Cardiol 2006; 13: e25-e41.
11. Brindis R. ACCF/ASNC appropriateness criteria for single-photon emission computed tomography myocardial perfusion imaging (SPECT MPI)—a report of the American College of Cardiology Foundation Quality Strategic Directions Committee Appropriateness Criteria Working Group and the American Society of Nuclear Cardiology. J Am Coll Cardiol 2005; 46:1587-1605.
12. Wackers FJT, Brown KA, Heller GV, et al. American Society of Nuclear Cardiology position statement on radionuclide imaging in patients with suspected acute ischemic syndromes in the emergency department or chest pain center. J Nucl Cardiol 2002; 9:246-250.
13. Verani MS. Pharmacological stress with adenosine for myocardial perfusion imaging. Semin Nucl Med 1991; 21:266-272.
14. Botvinick EH, Dae MW. Dipyridamole perfusion scintigraphy. Semin Nucl Med 1991; 21:242-265.
15. Geleijnse ML, Elhendy A, Fioretti PM, et al. Dobutamine stress myocardial perfusion imaging. J Am Coll Cardiol 2000; 36:2017-2027.
16. Taillefer RF, Gagnon AF, Laflamme LF, et al. Same day injections of Tc-99m methoxy isobutyl isonitrile (hexamibi) for myocardial tomographic imaging: comparison between rest-stress and stress-rest injection sequences. Eur J Nucl Med 1989; 15:113-117.
17. Arik W, Piotr JS, Mathews BF, et al. Quantitative myocardial-perfusion SPECT: comparison of three state-of-the-art software packages (abstract). J Nucl Cardiol 2008; 15:27-34.
18. Hachamovitch R, Hayes SW, Friedman JD, et al. Stress myocardial perfusion single-photon emission computed tomography is clinically effective and cost effective in risk stratification of patients with a high likelihood of coronary artery disease (CAD) but no known CAD. J Am Coll Cardiol 2004; 43:200-208.
19. Metz LD, Beattie MF, Hom RF, et al. The prognostic value of normal exercise myocardial perfusion imaging and exercise echocardiography: a meta-analysis. J Am Coll Cardiol 2007; 49:227-237.
20. Hachamovitch RF, Hayes SW, Friedman JD, et al. Comparison of the short-term survival benefit associated with revascularization compared with medical therapy in patients with no prior coronary artery disease undergoing stress myocardial perfusion single photon emission computed tomography. Circulation 2003; 107:2900-2907.
21. Goetze S, Wahl RL. Prevalence of misregistration between SPECT and CT for attenuation-corrected myocardial perfusion SPECT. J Nucl Cardiol 2007; 14:200-206.
22. Taillefer R, DePuey EG, Udelson JE, et al. Comparative diagnostic accuracy of Tl-201 and Tc-99m sestamibi SPECT imaging (perfusion and ECG-gated SPECT) in detecting coronary artery disease in women. J Am Coll Cardiol 1997; 29:69-77.
23. Beller GA, Zaret BL. Contributions of nuclear cardiology to diagnosis and prognosis of patients with coronary artery disease. Circulation 2000; 101:1465-1478.
24. Fieno DS, Louise EJT, Piotr S, et al. Quantitation of infarct size in patients with chronic coronary artery disease using rest-redistribution Tl-201 myocardial perfusion SPECT: correlation with contrast-enhanced cardiac magnetic resonance (abstract). J Nucl Cardiol 2007; 14:59-67.
25. Schinkel AF, Poldermans DF, Elhendy AF, et al. Assessment of myocardial viability in patients with heart failure. J Nucl Med 2007; 48:1135-1146.
26. Tillisch J, Brunken R, Marshall R, et al. Reversibility of cardiac wall-motion abnormalities predicted by positron tomography. N Engl J Med 1986; 314:884-888.
27. Saha GB, MacIntyre WJ, Brunken RC, et al. Present assessment of myocardial viability by nuclear imaging. Semin Nucl Med 1996; 26:315-335.
28. Haas F, Haehnel CJ, Picker W, et al. Preoperative positron emission tomographic viability assessment and perioperative and postoperative risk in patients with advanced ischemic heart disease. J Am Coll Cardiol 1997; 30:1693-1700.
29. Di Carli MF, Hachamovitch R. Hybrid PET/CT is greater than the sum of its parts: relationship between CT coronary angiography and stress perfusion imaging in patients with suspected ischemic heart disease assessed by integrated PET-CT imaging. J Nucl Cardiol 2008; 15:118-122.
30. Di Carli MF, Dorbala S, Curillova Z, et al. Relationship between CT coronary angiography and stress perfusion imaging in patients with suspected ischemic heart disease assessed by integrated PET-CT imaging. J Nucl Cardiol 2007; 14:799-809.

ual
CHAPTER 55

Magnetic Resonance and Computed Tomographic Imaging of Myocardial Function

Kristin Mercado and Raymond Kwong

The work-up of ischemic heart disease necessitates an accurate and reproducible method of assessing cardiac function. The importance of cardiac function analysis in the evaluation of coronary artery disease (CAD) lies in the diagnostic and prognostic implications and, consequently, its usefulness in guiding medical therapy. Being the reference standard technique, MRI can quantify global systolic function and detect regional abnormalities in wall motion and help establish the diagnosis of CAD. In addition, pharmacologic stress imaging protocols using function or perfusion MRI have been shown to provide a sensitive detection of CAD.[1] CT seems promising in at least some of these applications,[2] although it is currently limited by the temporal resolution and scarce clinical validation data. Exercise stress imaging using MRI has been performed, although its feasibility in assessing patients with or suspected to have ischemic heart disease has been shown only in select, highly experienced sites.[3]

Prognosis after myocardial infarction (MI) has been correlated with the extent of myocardial necrosis and the degree of contractile dysfunction of the left ventricle.[4] In patients with MI and chronic left ventricular (LV) dysfunction, LV ejection fraction and LV volumes are important prognostic parameters.[5] The extent of late myocardial hyperenhancement on MRI and regional contractile improvement in response to low-dose dobutamine stress MRI can accurately predict recovery of function after MI, identify myocardial viability, and effectively guide coronary revascularization therapy.[6-9]

Although still experimental, growing evidence suggests that assessment of diastolic functional parameters is possible using current CT and MRI techniques. A time/volume curve per heart cycle is calculated on multidetector CT, from which determination of the peak filling rate (PFR) and the ratio of time to peak filling rate to R–R interval (tPFR/RR) have been evaluated as parameters of LV diastolic function. The early-to-late diastolic filling ratio (E/A) on Doppler echocardiography has been found to correlate positively with PFR ($r = 0.54$) and negatively with tPFR/RR ($r = -0.57$) on multidetector CT.[10] Using MRI, a time/volume curve can likewise be derived, and diastolic function is expressed as PFR, early and active PFR (PFR_E and PFR_A), and their ratios. Diastolic parameters using echocardiography and MRI have been shown to vary by gender and age. Aging results in a decrease in LV distensibility that increases the early diastolic filling time, allowing the ventricle more time to fill, and increases the contribution of the atrial kick to LV filling. Although Doppler echocardiography provides peak velocities, MRI provides absolute peak filling rates from the time/volume curves. These data are also obtainable from radionuclide ventriculography; however, MRI has the advantage of significantly higher spatial resolution.[11]

Another more advanced MRI technique that has been studied in the evaluation of diastolic function involves the use of a high temporal resolution velocity-mapping technique that is able to identify previously undetectable myocardial motion patterns. This method has been shown to be comparable to tissue Doppler imaging—a well-established method that allows noninvasive assessment of diastolic function. Tissue Doppler imaging is limited, however, by limitations in acoustic window, low velocity resolution, lack of spatial information, and effect of the angle of insonation on myocardial velocities. Other established MRI methods for quantifying wall motion, such as tagging, phase contrast velocity mapping (tissue phase mapping), and displacement encoding with stimulated echoes (DENSE), can also be used to extract parameters such as strain or radial and circumferential velocity components, which are measures of diastolic function.[12]

Various imaging modalities are available to assess ventricular systolic function. Direct left ventriculography may be used, but it is rarely employed for the sole purpose of determining LV function because of its invasive nature. Among noninvasive imaging modalities, echocardiography is the most widely used because of its ease, relatively low cost, and widespread availability. Nuclear scintigraphy including gated single photon emission computed tomography (SPECT) and positron emission tomography can assess global and regional LV function, although their accuracies in this regard have been challenged by low spatial and temporal resolution. Radionuclide ventriculography provides accurate and reproducible assessment of global LV function. More recently, multidetector CT has been used in the evaluation of global and regional systolic LV function.[13,14] Among all noninvasive imaging modalities, MRI has been shown to be the most accurate and reproducible modality for the evaluation of global and regional systolic LV function.[15]

TABLE 55-1 Indications for Magnetic Resonance Imaging in Coronary Artery Disease

Indication	Class*
Assessment of Global Ventricular (Left and Right) Function and Mass	I
Detection of CAD	
Regional LV function at rest and during dobutamine stress	II
Assessment of myocardial perfusion	II
Coronary MR angiography (CAD)	III
Coronary MR angiography (anomalies)	I
Coronary MR angiography of bypass graft patency	II
MRI flow measurements in coronary arteries	Inv
Arterial wall imaging	Inv
Acute and Chronic MI	
Detection and assessment	I
Myocardial viability	I
Ventricular septal defect	III
Mitral regurgitation (acute MI)	III
Ventricular thrombus	II
Acute coronary syndromes	Inv

*Indication class: I, provides clinically relevant information and is usually appropriate; may be used as first-line imaging technique; usually supported by substantial literature; II, provides clinically relevant information and is frequently useful; other techniques may provide similar information; supported by limited literature; III, provides clinically relevant information, but is infrequently used because information from other imaging techniques is usually adequate; Inv, potentially useful, but still investigational.
From Pennell DJ, et al. Clinical indications for cardiovascular magnetic resonance (CMR): consensus panel report. Eur Heart J 2004; 25:1940-1965.

INDICATIONS AND APPLICATIONS OF MAGNETIC RESONANCE IMAGING AND COMPUTED TOMOGRAPHY IN THE EVALUATION OF ISCHEMIC HEART DISEASE

Magnetic Resonance Imaging

Improvements in MRI have introduced new methods for evaluating CAD and its consequences. MRI often provides additional data that may be unavailable from other noninvasive imaging modalities, such as echocardiography, nuclear scintigraphy, and CT. Table 55-1 lists indications for MRI in CAD based on the European Consensus Panel report. Not included in this list are less common techniques, such as T2* measurements and T2-weighted edema imaging, which are being increasingly used in more experienced centers for assessment of cardiomyopathy of unknown etiology.

Computed Tomography

CT is increasingly being used in diagnosis of CAD. Because of its prognostic implications, the quantification of coronary artery calcification is a growing clinical application. Arad and colleagues[17] were the first to report attempts to predict cardiac events with coronary calcium as detected by electron-beam CT, showing increased risk of cardiovascular events with higher Agatston scores. Coronary calcium scoring is discussed in Chapter 32.

Contrast-enhanced CT angiography of the coronary arteries is another application of multidetector CT used in the delineation of coronary anatomy and the detection of vascular stenosis. This technique has been used in the detection of CAD in patients at risk, and has been found to correlate with findings on invasive angiography.[18]

Multidetector CT was initially primarily used for detection of coronary artery stenosis and assessment of cardiac morphology, but more recently has been shown to be useful for cardiac function.[10,13,14] Considering the need for administration of contrast material, radiation exposure, and limited temporal resolution (80 to 250 ms), use of multidetector CT exclusively for analysis of cardiac function parameters does not seem clinically prudent at present. If the data are already obtained across all phases of the cardiac cycle during a standard coronary CT angiography evaluation, however, the combination of noninvasive coronary artery imaging and assessment of cardiac function with multidetector CT is a suitable approach because it enables a more comprehensive cardiac work-up in patients with suspected CAD.

Quantification of cardiac function using multidetector CT has been shown to be in good agreement with echocardiography, invasive cine ventriculography, SPECT, and MRI as the reference standard.[19] In addition, CT provides a useful alternative to MRI in the evaluation of ischemic heart disease in patients in whom MRI is contraindicated (e.g., patient has a periorbital metallic foreign body or metallic device; see Chapter 19 on MR safety for more information). Table 55-2 compares the advantages and disadvantages of the use of CT versus MRI in the evaluation of CAD.

TABLE 55-2 Advantages and Disadvantages of Magnetic Resonance Imaging and Computed Tomography

	MRI	Multidetector CT

Advantages	No ionizing radiation
	No exposure to iodinated contrast media
	Better temporal and spatial resolution
	Better validation in clinical assessment of the following:
	    Myocardial perfusion-ischemia
	    Ventricular mass, volumes, and global systolic function
	    Regional myocardial function
	    MI
	    Valvular function and flow quantification
	    Diastolic function
	Stress testing clinically available
		Widely available
		Ease and rapidity of performance
		Not contraindicated in patients with cardiac devices
		Single breath-hold acquisition eliminates motion artifact
		Better quality of images in the assessment of coronary artery anatomy
		Can be used clinically to assess the following (although with less validation studies compared with MRI):
		    Ventricular mass, volumes and global systolic function
		    Regional myocardial function
		    MI

Disadvantages	Less availability Relatively more complex and lengthy examination Contraindicated in patients with noncompatible biometallic implants, pacemakers or implantable cardioverter defibrillators Claustrophobic patients Risk of nephrogenic systemic fibrosis in patients with renal dysfunction exposed to gadolinium contrast medium	Valvular function Diastolic function Stress testing and assessment of myocardial perfusion-ischemia possible, but clinical experience is scant Radiation exposure Risk of contrast medium allergy Risk of worsening renal function from iodinated contrast dye exposure

ASSESSMENT OF CARDIAC FUNCTION

Global Systolic Function

Magnetic Resonance Imaging

Anatomic Planning and Standard Views

To produce high accuracy and reproducibility, standard imaging planes need to be used in quantifying ventricular function. The axes of the heart are defined using transverse, coronal, and sagittal views obtained as three-plane or individual scout images or through the use of real-time imaging techniques. We present one of many approaches to localize quickly and obtain the standard imaging planes for this purpose using cine MRI. Coronal images are used to define the transverse mid-ventricular slices (i.e., oblique axial images or "quasi" four-chamber view*). The short-axis views of the left ventricle can be defined by prescribing views perpendicular to the line between the center of the mitral valve and apex on the "quasi" four-chamber view. Slices are obtained from the base of the left ventricle at the level of the mitral annulus to the apex, allowing for full LV coverage for proper calculation of LV volumes, ejection fraction, and mass.

The four-chamber view (also known as horizontal long-axis view) is planned from a mid-ventricular short-axis view of the left ventricle in which a line is drawn across the center of the left ventricle to the acute margin of the right ventricle (defined by the junction between the right ventricular (RV) free wall and the diaphragmatic surface of the right ventricle). The two-chamber view (also known as vertical long-axis view) can also be planned on the mid-ventricular short-axis view, and is defined by a line through the center of the left ventricle that is perpendicular to the anterior and inferior wall. This view should include the apex, so it is recommended that the four-chamber view be used as a second localizer. The three-chamber view is planned on the basal short-axis view at the level where the mitral valve opening and LV outflow tract is visualized. The slice is defined by a line drawn through the center of the left ventricle and the LV outflow tract (and aortic root), preferably cutting through the LV apex. These views (short-axis, two-chamber, three-chamber, and four-chamber) are similar to the views achieved in transthoracic echocardiography.

RV function is typically evaluated using the previously described LV views to limit total imaging time. A more detailed evaluation of RV structure and function, of particular importance in the evaluation of arrhythmogenic RV dysplasia, requires the acquisition of additional views. Standard transverse views from cranial to caudal slices are roughly perpendicular to the RV outflow tract, RV free wall, and RV inflow. To visualize the diaphragmatic segment of the right ventricle, a slice planned on a coronal scout, generating an oblique sagittal view through the long axis of the RV outflow tract, should be acquired.[20]

Sequences

Evaluation of cardiac function involves the use of multiphase, or cine, MRI that employs fast gradient-echo imaging with k-space segmentation to acquire images during end-inspiration breath-holding, which minimizes respiratory motion artifact.[21] It is generally accepted that a temporal resolution of 50 ms is required to "freeze" end-systolic motion accurately to quantify ventricular volumes and calculate ejection fraction accurately. Segmented k-space breath-hold cine imaging has an in-plane spatial resolution that typically ranges from 1.5 to 2 mm^2, slice thickness of 5 to 10 mm, temporal resolution of 30 to 50 ms, and scan times of 8 to 16 s/slice. The k-space

---

*Because this view is derived from a coronal image, it represents a single oblique view. A "true" four-chamber view requires a double-oblique prescription.

segmentation allows for shorter acquisition times and enables the acquisition of a complete set of multiphase images per slice within a breath-hold. Generally, blood appears bright and myocardium appears gray in these cine gradient-echo images; however, the specific appearance of blood, myocardium, and blood flow depends on whether spoiled gradient-recalled-echo or steady-state free precession (SSFP) is used for signal generation within the segmented k-space structure.[15]

The current standard for quantification of ventricular volumes and function involves the use of SSFP gradient-echo sequences. The SSFP technique has assumed different names from different MRI scanner vendors: true fast imaging with steady-state precession (TrueFISP), fast imaging employing steady-state acquisition (FIESTA), and balanced fast field echo (FFE). Before the development of high-performance gradient systems, earlier methods involved the use of gradient-echo (e.g., fast low-angle shot [FLASH], fast gradient-echo, FFE). Using these methods, longitudinal magnetization is converted to transverse magnetization by means of radiofrequency (RF) excitation and is sampled. This is followed by spoiling of the residual transverse magnetization using any of the following methods: long repetition time (TR), RF spoiling, or application of spoiler gradients.

The use of spoiler gradients is the most commonly employed method, and involves extending the duration of the readout gradient beyond the sampling of the echo and before the next RF pulse. The prolonged application of the gradient results in accelerated dephasing of the residual transverse magnetization.[22] Because residual magnetization is spoiled, signal intensity is not maximized. To improve image quality, SSFP imaging of the heart was later developed, which offers specific advantages to cardiac imaging. This method results in improved signal-to-noise and contrast-to-noise ratios.[23] With SSFP, residual transverse magnetization is refocused, not spoiled, before the next RF pulse, and signal intensity is maximized. With this method, magnetization is in a steady state, so the RF pulses are applied throughout the acquisition.

SSFP was not practical before the development of high-performance gradient systems because it is prone to dark-band artifacts caused by off-resonance effects when the repetition time is longer than 4 to 5 ms. With the introduction of high-performance gradient systems, 1.5 T MRI systems can now routinely achieve repetition times at less than 2 ms, however, and acquire artifact-free SSFP motion imaging of the heart. Although SSFP sequences have shorter acquisition times, improved contrast, and improved signal-to-noise properties, it has some limitations. Because SSFP generally uses shorter echo times (i.e., TE) and is to some degree inherently motion compensated, this technique is less sensitive to show the signal loss (also known as intravoxel dephasing) from turbulent blood flow abnormalities owing to valvular dysfunction compared with older cine techniques such as fast gradient-echo pulse sequences.

SSFP is extremely sensitive to field inhomogeneities, of particular importance at 3.0 T, where repeated local shimming or frequency manipulation may be necessary to improve image quality. Traditional fast gradient-echo pulse sequences should be used for the detection of subtle flow abnormalities in valvular heart disease, or when field inhomogeneities result in significant artifacts with SSFP.[22] The energy deposition associated with continuous application of RF pulses to maintain steady-state magnetization is higher, and specific absorption rate limits may be reached during SSFP, particularly with higher performance gradient scanners.

Myocardial contractility and regional function can be evaluated further through the use of cine MRI with tagging in conjunction with segmented k-space cine gradient-echo imaging, also known as spatial modulation of magnetization. To evaluate diastolic function, the tagging pulse may be applied in late systole, with images acquired throughout diastole. Quantification of wall motion and myocardial strain can be determined based on displacement of the tagged regions.[22] To overcome the time-consuming aspect of tag analysis, harmonic phase analysis and DENSE techniques have been developed to improve the postprocessing duration.[24-26]

Image Analysis

Quantification of myocardial mass, ventricular volumes and dimensions, stroke volume, and ejection fraction is currently done using volumetric data computed from tracings of contiguous short-axis images obtained using cine SSFP pulse sequences. It is important to identify correctly the most basal extent of the ventricle because this determines the LV volumes and the LV ejection fraction.[27] Manual planimetry of LV endocardial and epicardial borders is performed during end-systole and end-diastole on each of the short-axis slices (Fig. 55-1). Because of the time required to do manual planimetry, automatic and semiautomatic methods have been developed. In studies comparing manual, automatic, and semiautomatic techniques in animals that were sacrificed for ex vivo measurements, it was determined that manual contours were closer to ex vivo measurements than automatic contours, however, which overestimates true volume.[28,29] After border detection, cardiac volumes are calculated by multiplying the blood pool area (defined by the endocardial border) by the slice thickness and summing all the slices. Myocardial mass is computed from the difference between the volumes determined from the endocardial and epicardial borders multiplied by the specific gravity of the myocardium (1.05 g/cm^3).[15]

Cine MRI enables the accurate description of segmental wall motion and quantitation of contractile function. The excellent contrast between the endocardium and blood pool improves measurement of wall thickness, end-diastolic and end-systolic volumes, and LV ejection fraction. The assumption of a uniform LV shape in the calculation of global functional parameters, as is practiced in other noninvasive imaging modalities such as echocardiography, carries potential errors. Errors resulting from these assumptions are magnified when the LV shape is deformed, such as in dilated cardiomyopathy or after MI. Because cine MR images are acquired in a tomographic set of planes, and no specific assumptions regarding LV geometry are necessary, volumetric measurements made from MRI generally provide more precise quantification of myocardial function.[15]

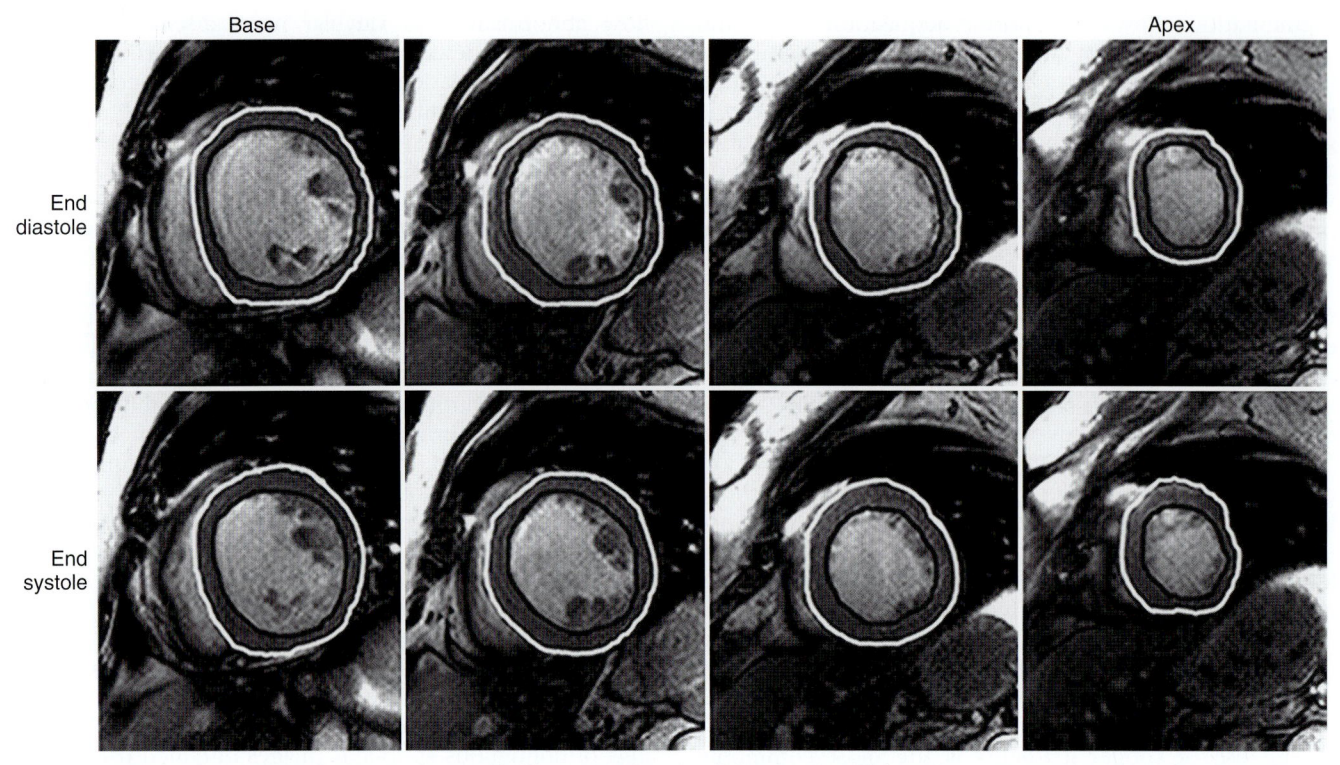

FIGURE 55-1 LV global systolic function is quantified by tracing the epicardial and endocardial borders on short-axis images. *(From Kwong R. Cardiovascular Magnetic Resonance Imaging. Totowa, NJ, Humana Press, 2007.)*

Computed Tomography

Techniques

Ventricular volume and function is quantified using multiplanar reformations of the retrospectively ECG gated data set obtained for coronary artery imaging. Multiphase reconstructions are performed throughout the entire cardiac cycle in increments of 5% or 10%, with 20 heart phases or 10 heart phases that are obtained and can be displayed as a cine loop. Temporal resolution varies from 80 to 250 ms, depending on the patient's heart rate, hardware, and algorithm used for reconstruction.[13,30] The selection of planes aligned with the axes of the heart is essential in the accurate analysis of global and regional LV function. These orientations are initially obtained from the axial plane, where a line transecting the apex and the midline of the base of the left ventricle yields a standard two-chamber view. Using this second image reference, the line transecting the apex and base of the left ventricle generates a longitudinal horizontal plane four-chamber view. From these longitudinal views of the heart, a series of short-axis planes can be obtained (Fig. 55-2).

End-diastolic and end-systolic frames are selected, and endocardial borders can be automatically detected, although these usually require some manual adjustment (Fig. 55-3). Quantification of LV volumes and LV ejection fraction is obtained from the entire three-dimensional data set with software analysis using the same summation principles applied in the evaluation of cardiac function in MRI as described in the previous section. As with MRI, a tomographic set of planes is acquired, and no assumptions are made concerning LV geometry, resulting in an accurate assessment of functional parameters.

In a study of 50 patients, Yamamuro and colleagues[13] compared LV ejection fraction values estimated with multidetector CT, echocardiography, and SPECT using MRI as a standard, and found that functional analysis with multidetector CT had good correlation with MRI and was more accurate than analysis with two-dimensional echocardiography or ECG gated SPECT.[13] Other investigators have confirmed the accuracy of assessment of LV ejection fraction and excellent correlation of functional parameters obtained by multidetector CT compared with cine MRI.[31] Because of the limitations with insufficient temporal resolution in functional analysis using multidetector CT, Brodoefel and coworkers[32] assessed the performance of a dual-source CT system compared with cine MRI. With the improvement of temporal resolution to 42 to 83 ms, dual-source CT enables improved accuracy in the assessment of global functional parameters.

Left Ventricular Function

Magnetic Resonance Imaging

Normal Values

Several reports of MRI-based normal values for LV function have been published. Normal values using earlier fast gradient-echo techniques differ from SSFP-derived values.[11,33,34] SSFP imaging sequences have higher temporal resolution and improved myocardial–blood pool differentiation compared with the earlier gradient-echo techniques, leading

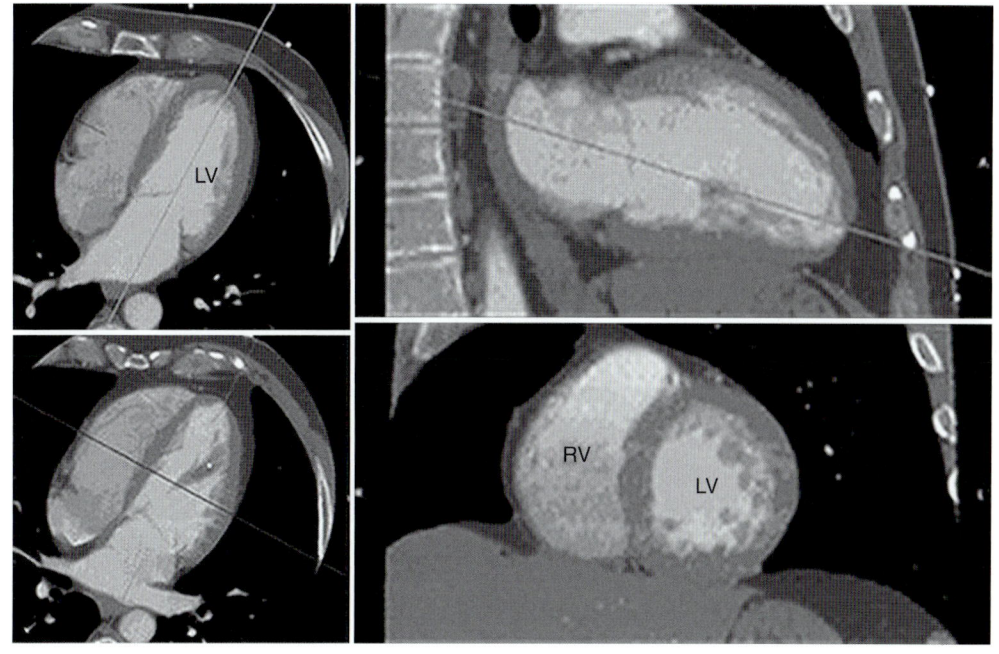

FIGURE 55-2 Method of obtaining short-axis and long-axis views of the ventricle through multiplanar reconstruction of axial CT images. LV, left ventricle; RV, right ventricle.

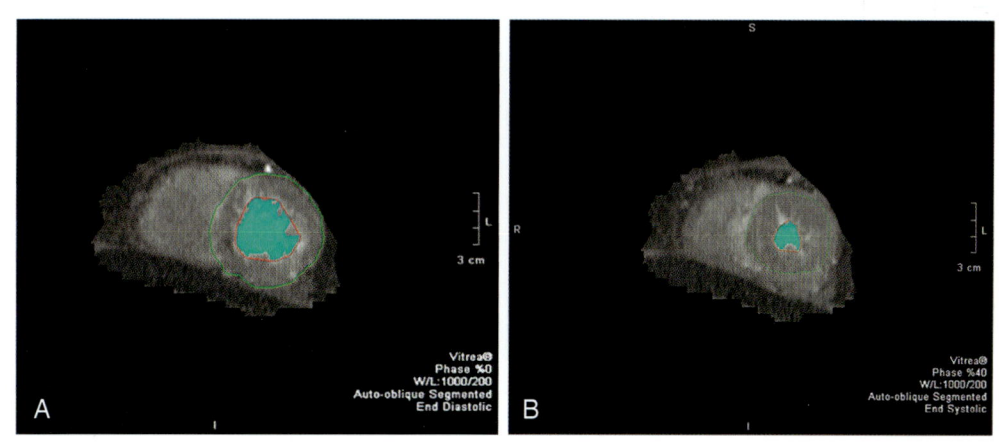

FIGURE 55-3 A and B, LV volumes and LV ejection fraction are calculated from end-diastolic (A) and end-systolic (B) tracings in short-axis planes.

to less blurring and thinner appearance of myocardial walls. As a result, calculated LV mass is smaller and measured LV volumes are larger using SSFP.[34]

Although there is general agreement that normal values should be indexed to body size, some debate exists whether to normalize for height or body surface area (BSA). Some authors recommend normalization for height because this is genetically determined, whereas adjustment for BSA benefits obese patients.[33]

Gender-specific MRI reference values for normal LV anatomy and function in a healthy adult population were derived from a representative sample of 318 Framingham Heart Study Offspring participants free of clinically overt cardiovascular disease. These patients underwent MRI examination using fast gradient-echo sequences. The following parameters were measured: LV end-diastolic volume (EDV) and end-systolic volume (ESV), mass, LV ejection fraction, and linear dimensions (wall thickness, cavity length). All volumetric (EDV, ESV, LV mass) and unidimensional measures were significantly greater in men than in women, and remained greater after adjustment for subject height. Volumetric measures were greater in men than in women after adjustment for BSA, but there were increased linear dimensions in women after adjustment for BSA. In particular, end-diastolic dimension indexed to BSA was greater in women than in men. There were no gender differences in global LV ejection fraction. The range of values derived from this study is provided in Table 55-3.

More recently, cine SSFP MRI has been used to define ranges for normal LV volumes and systolic and diastolic function. These were normalized to gender, BSA, and age. The determination of normality or the severity of abnormality depends on the use of appropriate reference ranges normalized to all three variables. Values derived from this study are presented in Tables 55-4, 55-5, and 55-6.[11]

TABLE 55-3 Means and 95% Upper Limits for Raw, Height-Adjusted, and Body Surface Area–Adjusted Left Ventricular Variables

	Raw				
	Men		Women		
Variables	Mean	95% Upper Limit	Mean	95% Upper Limit	P Value*
LV mass (g)	155.1	201.4	103	134	.0001
LV EDV (mL)	114.9	169	84.4	116.5	.0001
LV ESV (mL)	36.3	65	25.1	40.9	.0001
PWT (mm)	9.9	11.2	8.7	9.8	.0001
IVS (mm)	10.1	11.7	8.9	10.1	.0001
EDD (mm)	50.2	58.5	45.6	51.1	.0001
Two-chamber length (mm)	82.3	93.8	73.2	83.7	.0001
Four-chamber length (mm)	81.9	93	71.7	81.5	.0001
LV EF	0.69	0.77	0.70	0.79	.1019

	Raw/Height				
	Men		Women		
Variables	Mean	95% Upper Limit	Mean	95% Upper Limit	P Value*
LV mass (g/m)	88.6	114	63.6	81.9	.0001
LV EDV (mL/m)	65.6	93.6	52.1	70.3	.0001
LV ESV (mL/m)	20.7	35.5	15.5	24.5	.0001
PWT (mm/m)	5.6	6.5	5.4	6.1	.0013
IVS (mm/m)	5.8	6.9	5.5	6.4	.0134
EDD (mm/m)	28.7	33.1	28.2	31.8	.1616
Two-chamber length (mm/m)	47.1	52.1	45.1	49.8	.0009
Four-chamber length (mm/m)	46.9	53	44.3	49.3	.0001

	Raw/BSA				
	Men		Women		
Variables	Mean	95% Upper Limit	Mean	95% Upper Limit	P Value*
LV mass (g/m^2)	77.9	95	60.8	74.7	.0001
LV EDV (mL/m^2)	57.6	79.5	49.8	65.5	.0001
LV ESV (mL/m^2)	18.1	30.8	14.8	24	.0001
PWT (mm/m^2)	5	6	5.2	6.3	.0523
IVS (mm/m^2)	5.1	6.2	5.3	6.4	.0564
EDD (mm/m^2)	25.3	29.7	27.1	31.8	.0004
Two-chamber length (mm/m^2)	41.3	46.8	43.5	48.4	.0005
Four-chamber length (mm/m^2)	41.5	47.7	42.7	47.8	.0867

*P values are from the test of difference in means between genders for each of the LV variables.
EDD, end-diastolic dimension; EF, ejection fraction; IVS, interventricular septum thickness; PWT, posterior wall thickness.
From Salton CJ, et al. Gender differences and normal left ventricular anatomy in an adult population free of hypertension: a cardiovascular magnetic resonance study of the Framingham Heart Study Offspring cohort. J Am Coll Cardiol 2002; 39:1055-1060.

TABLE 55-4 Left Ventricular Volumes, Systolic Function, and Mass (Absolute and Indexed to Body Surface Area) by Age Decile (Mean, 95% Confidence Interval) in Men

	20-29 yr	30-39 yr	40-49 yr	50-59 yr	60-69 yr	70-79 yr
Absolute Values						
EDV (mL), SD 21	167 (126, 208)	163 (121, 204)	159 (117, 200)	154 (113, 196)	150 (109, 191)	146 (105, 187)
ESV (mL), SD 11	58 (35, 80)	56 (33, 78)	54 (31, 76)	51 (29, 74)	49 (27, 72)	47 (25, 70)
SV (mL), SD 14	109 (81, 137)	107 (79, 135)	105 (77, 133)	103 (75, 131)	101 (73, 129)	99 (71, 127)
EF (%), SD 4.5	65 (57, 74)	66 (57, 75)	66 (58, 75)	67 (58, 76)	67 (58, 76)	68 (59, 77)
Mass (g), SD 20	148 (109, 186)	147 (109, 185)	146 (108, 185)	146 (107, 184)	145 (107, 183)	144 (106, 183)
Indexed to BSA						
EDV/BSA (mL/m^2), SD 9	86 (68, 103)	83 (66, 101)	81 (64, 99)	79 (62, 97)	77 (60, 95)	75 (58, 93)
ESV/BSA (mL/m^2), SD 5.5	30 (19, 41)	29 (18, 39)	27 (17, 38)	26 (15, 37)	25 (14, 36)	24 (13, 35)
SV/BSA (mL/m^2), SD 6.1	56 (44, 68)	55 (43, 67)	54 (42, 66)	53 (41, 65)	52 (40, 64)	51 (39, 63)
Mass/BSA (g/m^2), SD 8.5	76 (59, 93)	75 (59, 92)	75 (58, 91)	74 (57, 91)	73 (57, 90)	73 (56, 89)

EF, ejection fraction; SD, standard deviation; SV, stroke volume.

TABLE 55-5 Left Ventricular Volumes, Systolic Function, and Mass (Absolute and Indexed to Body Surface Area) by Age Decile (Mean, 95% Confidence Interval) in Women

	20-29 yr	30-39 yr	40-49 yr	50-59 yr	60-69 yr	70-79 yr
Absolute Values						
EDV (mL), SD 21	139 (99, 179)	135 (94, 175)	130 (90, 171)	126 (86, 166)	122 (82, 162)	118 (77, 158)
ESV (mL), SD 9.5	48 (29, 66)	45 (27, 64)	43 (25, 62)	41 (22, 59)	39 (20, 57)	36 (18, 55)
SV (mL), SD 14	91 (63, 119)	89 (61, 117)	87 (59, 115)	85 (57, 113)	83 (56, 111)	81 (54, 109)
EF (%), SD 4.6	66 (56, 75)	66 (57, 75)	66 (58, 76)	67 (58, 76)	69 (60, 78)	69 (60, 78)
Mass (g), SD 18	105 (69, 141)	106 (70, 142)	107 (71, 143)	108 (72, 144)	109 (73, 145)	110 (74, 146)
Indexed to BSA						
EDV/BSA (mL/m^2), SD 8.7	82 (65, 99)	79 (62, 96)	76 (59, 93)	73 (56, 90)	70 (53, 87)	67 (50, 84)
ESV/BSA (mL/m^2), SD 4.7	28 (19, 37)	27 (17, 36)	25 (16, 34)	24 (14, 33)	22 (13, 31)	21 (12, 30)
SV/BSA (mL/m^2), SD 6.2	54 (42, 66)	53 (40, 65)	51 (39, 63)	50 (37, 62)	48 (36, 60)	47 (34, 59)
Mass/BSA (g/m^2), SD 7.5	62 (47, 77)	62 (47, 77)	63 (48, 77)	63 (48, 78)	63 (48, 78)	63 (49, 78)

EF, ejection fraction; SD, standard deviation; SV, stroke volume.

TABLE 55-6 Left Ventricular Volumes, Systolic Function, and Mass (Absolute and Indexed to Body Surface Area) by Age Decile (Mean, 95% Confidence Interval) in All Subjects

	20-29 yr	30-39 yr	40-49 yr	50-59 yr	60-69 yr	70-79 yr
Absolute Values						
EDV (mL), SD 21	153 (112, 193)	149 (108, 189)	144 (104, 185)	140 (100, 181)	136 (96, 177)	132 (91, 172)
ESV (mL), SD 10	53 (32, 73)	50 (30, 71)	48 (28, 69)	46 (26, 67)	44 (24, 65)	42 (21, 62)
SV (mL), SD 14	100 (72, 128)	98 (70, 126)	96 (68, 124)	94 (66, 122)	92 (64, 120)	90 (62, 118)
EF (%), SD 4.6	66 (57, 74)	66 (57, 75)	67 (58, 76)	67 (58, 76)	68 (59, 77)	69 (60, 77)
Mass (g), SD 19	127 (90, 164)	127 (90, 164)	127 (90, 164)	127 (90, 164)	127 (90, 164)	127 (90, 164)
Indexed to BSA						
EDV/BSA (mL/m^2), SD 8.8	84 (67, 101)	81 (64, 98)	79 (62, 96)	76 (59, 93)	74 (57, 91)	71 (54, 88)
ESV/BSA (mL/m^2), SD 5.1	29 (19, 39)	28 (18, 38)	26 (16, 36)	25 (15, 35)	24 (14, 34)	22 (12, 32)
SV/BSA (mL/m^2), SD 6.2	55 (43, 67)	54 (42, 66)	52 (40, 65)	51 (39, 63)	50 (38, 62)	49 (37, 61)
Mass/BSA (g/m^2) SD 8.1	69 (53, 85)	69 (53, 85)	69 (53, 84)	68 (53, 84)	68 (52, 84)	68 (52, 84)

EF, ejection fraction; SD, standard deviation; SV, stroke volume.

Computed Tomography

Normal Values

Normal adult values had been established by electron-beam CT in the mid-1980s for LV myocardial mass (98 ± 18 g/m^2), EDV (73 ± 19 mL/m^2), ESV (24 ± 8 mL/m^2), and stroke volume (48 ± 11 mL/m^2).[35] Although most of the earlier validation studies were performed using electron-beam CT, many have been adapted and validated using multidetector CT.

Right Ventricular Function

Magnetic Resonance Imaging

Normal Values

Tandri and associates[36] examined 500 subjects free of cardiovascular disease who were participants in the Multi-Ethnic Study of Atherosclerosis. The endocardial borders of the right ventricle were manually traced on short-axis images, and RV volumes were calculated using summation-of-disks method. RV dimensions were measured on four-chamber gradient-echo images and in the short-axis plane. Except for the ejection fraction, all unadjusted RV parameters were significantly greater in men than in women. RV volumes and linear dimensions each correlated significantly with height and BSA. Gender differences remained after adjustment for subject height. After adjustment for BSA, volumetric variables remained significantly greater in men than in women. Table 55-7 presents gender-specific normal values for the adult right ventricle by MRI. Cardiovascular MRI measures of RV volumes and linear dimensions differ significantly according to gender and body size. These values are useful in distinguishing RV health from diseases that result in abnormal RV structure and function.

More recent advances in MRI include improved image quality with SSFP sequences and advanced postprocessing of high temporal resolution ventricular function. SSFP cine imaging with three-dimensional modeling was performed on 120 healthy subjects, yielding a set of normal RV reference values normalized to age, sex, and BSA. These RV functional parameters are listed in Tables 55-8, 55-9, and 55-10.[11]

Identification of RV dysfunction is of particular importance in the assessment of ischemic heart disease. It has

TABLE 55-7 Gender-Specific Raw, Height-Adjusted, and Body Surface Area–Adjusted Right Ventricular Variables

Variable	Men Mean ± SD	Men Upper Limits 5%	Men Upper Limits 95%	Women Mean ± SD	Women Upper Limits 5%	Women Upper Limits 95%	P Value
Raw							
EDV (mL)	142.4 ± 31.1	96	201	110.2 ± 24	77	155	.0001
ESV (mL)	54.3 ± 16.9	28	85	35.1 ± 2.5	18	57	.0001
Stroke volume (mL)	88.3 ± 21.6	57	125	75 ± 17.9	51	106	.0001
Short-axis end-diastolic diameter (mm)	35.3 ± 6.8	25	46.2	31.6 ± 1.7	21	39.1	.0001
Four-chamber end-diastolic diameter (mm)	39.1 ± 5.2	31	48.5	36.5 ± 1.2	27	45.1	.0001
Four-chamber length (mm)	72.9 ± 8.8	59	88.1	67 ± 2.9	51	80	.0001
Ejection fraction	0.62 ± 0.1	0.5	0.75	0.69 ± 0.1	0.58	0.81	.0001
Right atrial diameter (mm)	43 ± 5.6	33	52	39.7 ± 1.6	31	49.1	.0001
Raw/Height							
EDV (mL/m)	73.3 ± 13.7	51.9	98.1	64.9 ± 11.3	46.4	83.3	.0001
ESV (mL/m)	28 ± 8.1	15.8	43.4	20.6 ± 6.7	10.8	32.6	.0001
Stroke volume (mL/m)	45 ± 10	28.3	63.2	44.3 ± 8.1	32	57.9	.1021
Short-axis end-diastolic diameter (mm/m)	18.2 ± 3.3	13.5	23.2	18.1 ± 3.2	12.5	23.4	.5539
Four-chamber end-diastolic diameter (mm/m)	22.6 ± 2.9	16.2	24.8	21.8 ± 3.1	16	27.9	.8292
Four-chamber length (mm/m)	49 ± 2.4	30	46.6	39 ± 5.4	29.2	47.7	.2927
Right atrial diameter (mm/m)	22.4 ± 1.5	18	29	23.4 ± 3.3	18.2	9	.0759
Raw/BSA							
EDV (mL/m^2)	82 ± 16.2	56.7	100.9	68.6 ± 14	48.7	94.5	.0001
ESV (mL/m^2)	31.2 ± 9.2	16.5	48.3	21.7 ± 7.5	10.4	34	.0001
Stroke volume (mL/m^2)	50.7 ± 11	34.1	70.3	46.8 ± 9.9	32.3	63	.0981
Short-axis end-diastolic diameter (mm/m^2)	18 ± 3.2	15	25	19 ± 3.3	13.5	24.8	.4161
Four-chamber end-diastolic diameter (mm/m^2)	20.2 ± 2.6	17	28	22.3 ± 3.3	17	27.7	.6790
Four-chamber length (mm/m^2)	37.8 ± 4.6	34	51	40.9 ± 5	32	49	.0135
Right atrial diameter (mm/m^2)	24.9 ± 3	19	30	24.2 ± 3.6	18	30	.0378

From Tandri H, et al. Normal reference values for the adult right ventricle by magnetic resonance imaging. Am J Cardiol 2006; 98:1660-1664.

TABLE 55-8 Right Ventricular Volumes, Systolic Function, and Mass (Absolute and Normalized to Body Surface Area) by Age Decile (Mean, 95% Confidence Interval) in Men

	20-29 yr	30-39 yr	40-49 yr	50-59 yr	60-69 yr	70-79 yr
Absolute Values						
EDV (mL), SD 25.4	177 (127, 227)	171 (121, 221)	166 (116, 216)	160 (111, 210)	155 (105, 205)	150 (100, 200)
ESV (mL), SD 15.2	68 (38, 98)	64 (34, 94)	59 (29, 89)	55 (25, 85)	50 (20, 80)	46 (16, 76)
SV (mL), SD 17.4	108 (74, 143)	108 (74, 142)	107 (73, 141)	106 (72, 140)	105 (71, 139)	104 (70, 138)
EF (%), SD 6.5	61 (48, 74)	63 (50, 76)	65 (52, 77)	66 (53, 79)	68 (55, 81)	70 (57, 83)
Mass (g), SD 14.4	70 (42, 99)	69 (40, 97)	67 (39, 95)	65 (37, 94)	63 (35, 92)	62 (33, 90)
Normalized to BSA						
EDV/BSA (mL/m^2), SD 11.7	91 (68, 114)	88 (65, 111)	85 (62, 108)	82 (59, 105)	79 (56, 101)	75 (52, 98)
ESV/BSA (mL/m^2), SD 7.4	35 (21, 50)	33 (18, 47)	30 (16, 45)	28 (13, 42)	25 (11, 40)	23 (8, 37)
SV/BSA (mL/m^2), SD 8.2	56 (40, 72)	55 (39, 71)	55 (39, 71)	54 (38, 70)	53 (37, 69)	52 (36, 69)
EF/BSA (%/m^2), SD 4	32 (24, 40)	32 (25, 40)	33 (25, 41)	34 (26, 42)	35 (27, 42)	35 (27, 43)
Mass/BSA (g/m^2), SD 6.8	36 (23, 50)	35 (22, 49)	34 (21, 48)	33 (20, 46)	32 (19, 45)	31 (18, 44)

EF, ejection fraction; SD, standard deviation; SV, stroke volume.

been reported that in post-MI patients, reduction in RV function to less than 40% was strongly associated with mortality.[37]

Computed Tomography

Currently, there are no widely established normal values for RV volumes and function using multidetector CT in normal volunteers because evaluation of cardiac function using this modality is performed using data obtained from coronary CT angiography in patients originally referred for suspected CAD. It has been shown that enlarged RV dimensions detected on multidetector CT carry a worse prognosis in other diseases, such as pulmonary embolism.[38]

Kim and colleagues[39] assessed RV EDV, ESV, ejection fraction, and mass using multidetector CT compared with first-pass radionuclide angiography (FPRA). The mean RV ejection fraction (47 ± 7%) measured by multidetector CT showed good correlation with RV ejection fraction

TABLE 55-9 Right Ventricular Volumes, Systolic Function, and Mass (Absolute and Normalized to Body Surface Area) by Age Decile (Mean, 95% Confidence Interval) in Women

	20-29 yr	30-39 yr	40-49 yr	50-59 yr	60-69 yr	70-79 yr
Absolute Values						
EDV (mL), SD 21.6	142 (100, 184)	136 (94, 178)	130 (87, 172)	124 (81, 166)	117 (75, 160)	111 (69, 153)
ESV (mL), SD 13.3	55 (29, 82)	51 (25, 77)	46 (20, 72)	42 (15, 68)	37 (11, 63)	32 (6, 58)
SV (mL), SD 13.1	87 (61, 112)	85 (59, 111)	84 (58, 109)	82 (56, 108)	80 (55, 106)	79 (53, 105)
EF (%), SD 6	61 (49, 73)	63 (51, 75)	65 (53, 77)	67 (55, 79)	69 (57, 81)	71 (59, 83)
Mass (g), SD 10.6	54 (33, 74)	51 (31, 72)	49 (28, 70)	47 (26, 68)	45 (24, 66)	43 (22, 63)
Normalized to BSA						
EDV/BSA (mL/m^2), SD 9.4	84 (65, 102)	80 (61, 98)	76 (57, 94)	72 (53, 90)	68 (49, 86)	64 (45, 82)
ESV/BSA (mL/m^2), SD 6.6	32 (20, 45)	30 (17, 43)	27 (14, 40)	24 (11, 37)	21 (8, 34)	19 (6, 32)
SV/BSA (mL/m^2), SD 6.1	51 (39, 63)	50 (38, 62)	49 (37, 61)	48 (36, 60)	46 (34, 58)	45 (33, 57)
EF/BSA (%/m^2), SD 5.2	37 (27, 47)	38 (27, 48)	38 (28, 49)	39 (29, 49)	40 (30, 50)	41 (31, 51)
Mass/BSA (g/m^2), SD 5.2	32 (22, 42)	30 (20, 40)	29 (19, 39)	27 (17, 37)	26 (16, 36)	24 (14, 35)

EF, ejection fraction; SD, standard deviation; SV, stroke volume.

TABLE 55-10 Right Ventricular Volumes, Systolic Function, and Mass (Absolute and Normalized to Body Surface Area) by Age Decile (Mean, 95% Confidence Interval) in All Subjects

	20-29 yr	30-39 yr	40-49 yr	50-59 yr	60-69 yr	70-79 yr
Absolute Values						
EDV (mL), SD 23.5	159 (113, 206)	154 (107, 200)	148 (102, 194)	142 (96, 188)	136 (90, 182)	130 (84, 177)
ESV (mL), SD 14.3	62 (34, 90)	57 (29, 85)	53 (25, 81)	48 (20, 76)	44 (16, 72)	39 (11, 67)
SV (mL), SD 15.3	98 (68, 128)	96 (66, 126)	95 (65, 125)	94 (64, 124)	93 (63, 123)	92 (61, 122)
EF (%), SD 6.2	61 (49, 73)	63 (51, 75)	65 (53, 77)	67 (54, 79)	68 (56, 81)	70 (58, 83)
Mass (g), SD 12.6	62 (37, 87)	51 (27, 76)	49 (24, 74)	47 (22, 72)	45 (20, 70)	43 (18, 67)
Normalized to BSA						
EDV/BSA (mL/m^2), SD 10.6	88 (67, 108)	84 (63, 105)	80 (60, 101)	77 (56, 98)	73 (52, 94)	70 (49, 90)
ESV/BSA (mL/m^2), SD 7	34 (20, 48)	31 (17, 45)	29 (15, 42)	26 (12, 40)	23 (10, 37)	21 (7, 35)
SV/BSA (mL/m^2), SD 7.2	54 (39, 68)	53 (38, 67)	52 (38, 66)	51 (37, 65)	50 (36, 64)	49 (35, 63)
EF/BSA (%/m^2), SD 4.6	34 (25, 43)	35 (26, 44)	36 (27, 45)	37 (27, 46)	37 (28, 46)	38 (29, 47)
Mass/BSA (g/m^2), SD 6	34 (22, 46)	33 (21, 45)	31 (20, 43)	30 (18, 42)	29 (17, 41)	28 (16, 39)

EF, ejection fraction; SD, standard deviation; SV, stroke volume.

($44 \pm 6\%$) measured by FPRA. A significant difference in the mean RV ejection fraction was found between cardiac multidetector CT and FPRA, with an overestimation of $2.9 \pm 5.3\%$ by multidetector CT versus FPRA. Multidetector CT is relatively simple and allows the RV volume and mass to be assessed, and the RV ejection fraction obtained by multidetector CT correlates well with that measured by FPRA.

Using semiautomated contour detection software, Koch and associates[40] determined RV EDV and ESV from short-axis CT multiplanar reconstruction (MPR) created at every 10% of the R-R interval. End-systolic and end-diastolic axial images were transformed to three-dimensional images to determine the volumes by using a threshold-supported reconstruction algorithm. CT-derived RV parameters were compared with parameters obtained using SSFP cine MRI in the short-axis orientation. Mean RV EDV (155.4 ± 54.6 mL) and ESV (79.1 ± 37 mL) determined with MPR correlated well with MRI values (151.9 ± 53.7 mL and 75 ± 36 mL). RV stroke volume (76.2 ± 20.2 mL for MPR CT, 76.9 ± 20.7 mL for MRI) showed a good correlation, and RV ejection fraction ($50.8 \pm 8.4\%$ for MPR CT, $51.9 \pm 7.4\%$ for MRI) showed a moderate correlation. Threshold-supported three-dimensional reconstructions revealed insufficient correlations with MRI. MPR-based semiautomated analysis of cardiac 16-detector row CT allows for RV functional analysis and correlates well with MRI findings. Threshold value–supported three-dimensional reconstructions did not show adequate MRI correlation because of inhomogeneities of RV contrast enhancement.

Regional Myocardial Function

Nomenclature

In the evaluation of myocardial segments, the American Heart Association recommends a 17-segment model of the left ventricle for standardized description that is applicable to all cardiac imaging modalities, including CT and MRI (Figs. 55-4 and 55-5). Identification of abnormalities in particular myocardial segments enables the approximate localization of coronary disease to the corresponding artery supplying the affected territory (Fig. 55-6).

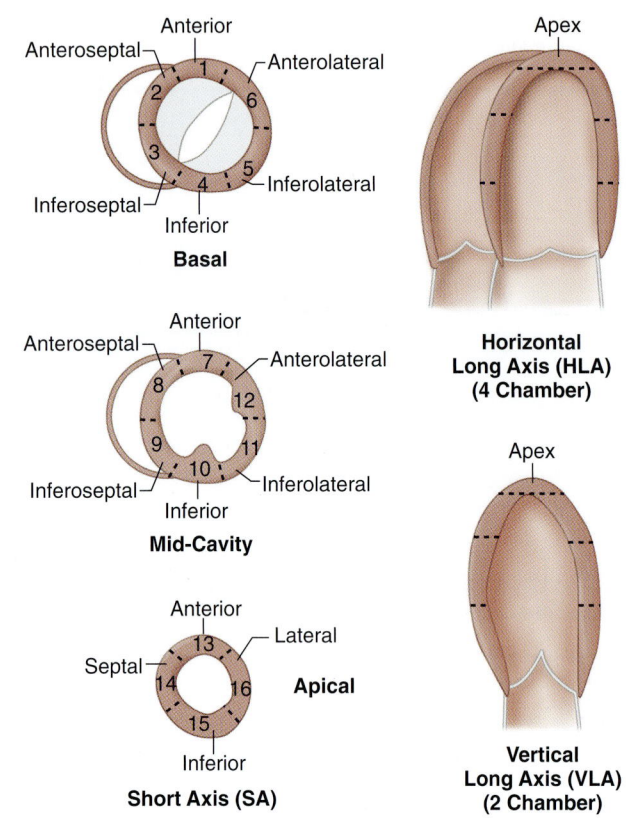

FIGURE 55-4 Diagram of vertical long-axis (VLA, approximating the two-chamber view), horizontal long-axis (HLA, approximating the four-chamber view), and short-axis (SA) planes showing the name, location, and anatomic landmarks for selection of the basal (tips of the mitral valve leaflets), mid-cavity (papillary muscles), and apical (beyond papillary muscles, but before cavity ends) short-axis slices for the recommended 17-segment system. All imaging modalities should use these same landmarks, when available, for slice selection. *(From Cerqueira MD, et al. Standardized myocardial segmentation and nomenclature for tomographic imaging of the heart. A statement for healthcare professionals from the Cardiac Imaging Committee of the Council on Clinical Cardiology of the American Heart Association. Circulation 2002; 105:539-542.)*

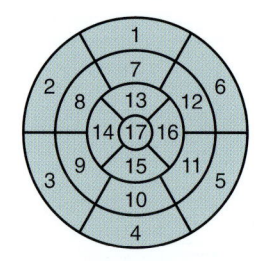

1. Basal anterior
2. Basal anteroseptal
3. Basal inferoseptal
4. Basal inferior
5. Basal inferolateral
6. Basal anterolateral
7. Mid anterior
8. Mid anteroseptal
9. Mid inferoseptal
10. Mid inferior
11. Mid inferolateral
12. Mid anterolateral
13. Apical anterior
14. Apical septal
15. Apical inferior
16. Apical lateral
17. Apex

FIGURE 55-5 Circumferential polar plot of the 17 myocardial segments and the recommended nomenclature for tomographic imaging of the heart. *(From Cerqueira MD, et al. Standardized myocardial segmentation and nomenclature for tomographic imaging of the heart. A statement for healthcare professionals from the Cardiac Imaging Committee of the Council on Clinical Cardiology of the American Heart Association. Circulation 2002; 105:539-542.)*

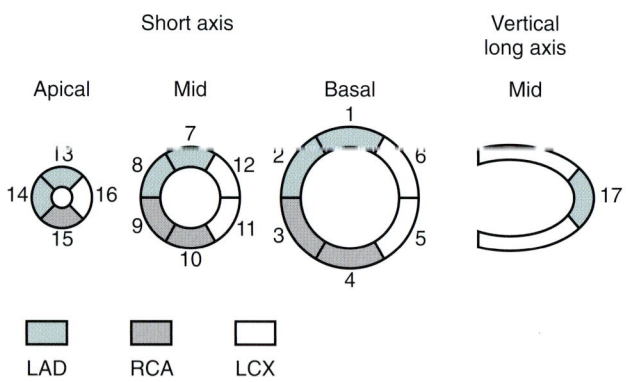

FIGURE 55-6 Assignment of the 17 myocardial segments to the territories of the left anterior descending coronary artery (LAD), right coronary artery (RCA), and left circumflex coronary artery (LCX). *(From Cerqueira MD, et al. Standardized myocardial segmentation and nomenclature for tomographic imaging of the heart. A statement for healthcare professionals from the Cardiac Imaging Committee of the Council on Clinical Cardiology of the American Heart Association. Circulation 2002; 105:539-542.)*

Magnetic Resonance Imaging

Techniques

Although various MRI techniques can be used to evaluate regional myocardial function, cine SSFP pulse sequences are the most commonly used with visual assessment of regional wall motion as normal, hypokinetic, akinetic, or dyskinetic. Other, more quantitative methods of assessing regional function are currently available, however. MRI is used not only in imaging anatomic details, but also can be used to evaluate the movement and deformation of soft tissues such as ventricular myocardium, and can provide measurements of tissue motion at high resolution. Displacement imaging is particularly useful in assessing the contractile function of myocardial segments. The technique involves measuring the change of position of tissue elements over time starting from a reference time point, similar to tracking the three-dimensional movement of implanted radiopaque markers in cine fluoroscopy. Instead of using extraneous markers, controlled modulations of various aspects of tissue proton magnetization produce grids that are used as noninvasive markers. Advanced phase modulation techniques allow all pixels of an image to be tracked simultaneously and give high-density measurements of tissue motion.

Displacement fields are the basis for computing functional maps of myocardial strain, strain rates, and torsion. *Strain* represents local deformation and is often calculated from the differences in displacement vectors of adjacent pixels. *Torsion* and *twist* of the ventricle refer to the rotation of the ventricular wall around its longitudinal axis, and torsion maps are obtained by calculating the rotation of individual pixels.[15]

Early displacement-imaging methods used modulation of image intensity. Zerhouni and coworkers[42] proposed the concept of myocardial *tagging* for quantifying regional myocardial function. Radial and linear grids of low signal

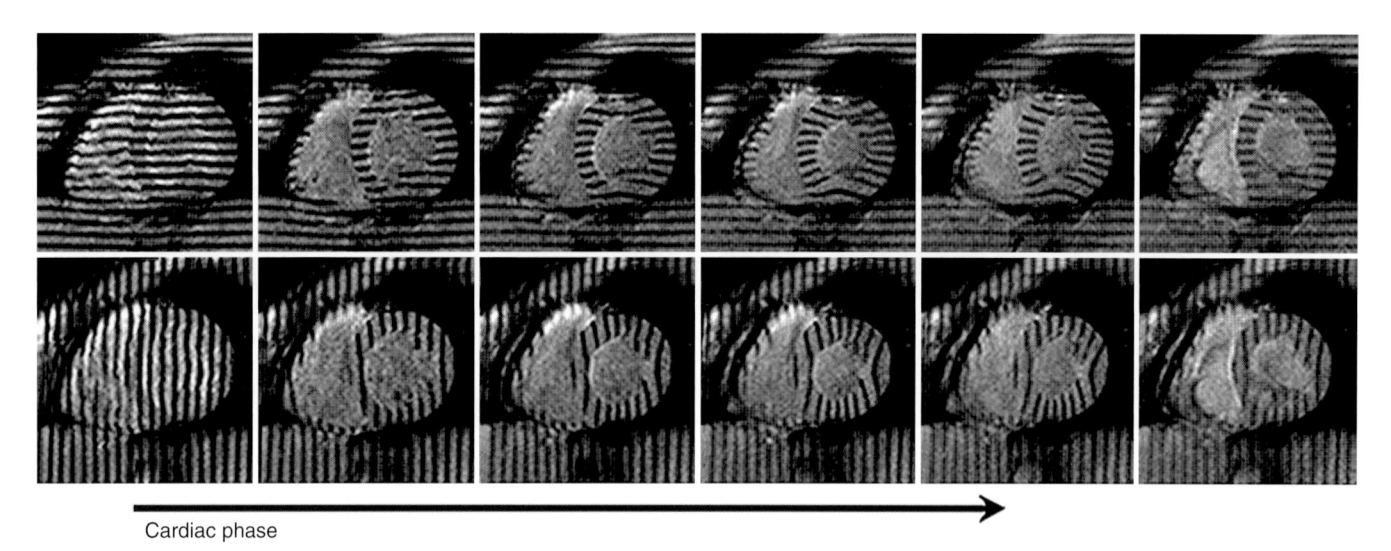

FIGURE 55-7 Multiphase myocardial tagging of a mid-ventricular slice using two sets of orthogonal line tags. The tag lines bend as the heart contracts, revealing intramyocardial motion. Tag fading over time because of T1 relaxation is evident near the end of the cardiac cycle. *(From Kwong R. Cardiovascular Magnetic Resonance Imaging. Totowa, NJ, Humana Press, 2007.)*

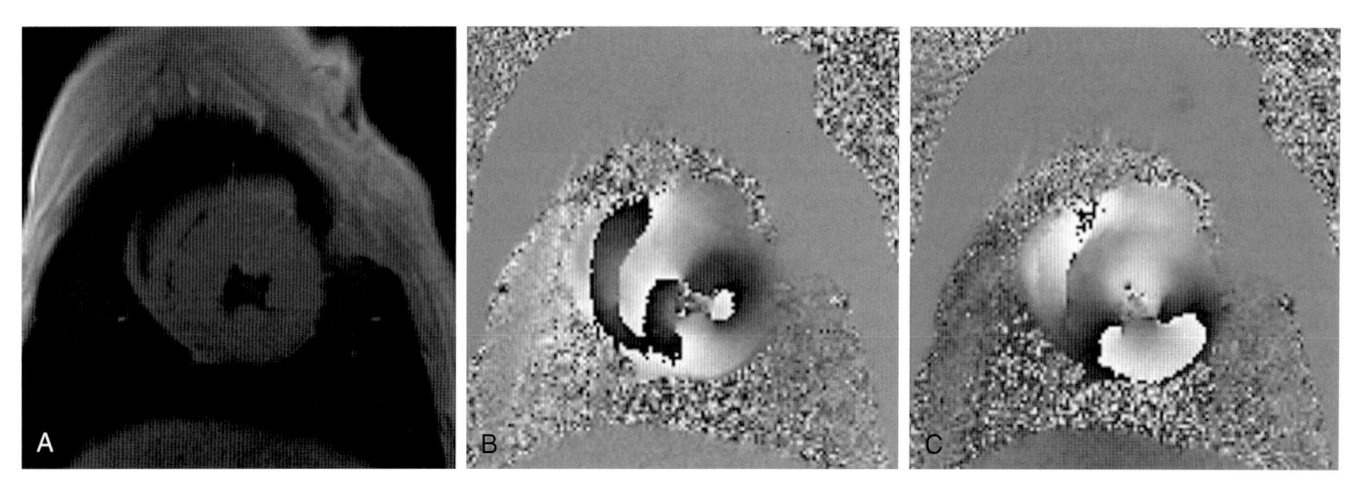

FIGURE 55-8 **A,** Magnitude DENSE image contains only anatomic information. **B,** This phase image contained data with respect to motion along the *x*-axis. **C,** This phase image contains data with respect to motion along the *y*-axis. *(From Kwong R. Cardiovascular Magnetic Resonance Imaging. Totowa, NJ, Humana Press, 2007.)*

intensity were created by nulling the magnetization in those locations, which are called *tags*. Tags persist for a period comparable to the T1 relaxation time and move with the underlying tissue. The displacement vectors of tag intersect points can be quantified by directly identifying their positions in the magnitude images (Fig. 55-7).

Aside from image intensity, the phase of the MRI signal can be modulated to allow tracking of individual pixels.[43,44] The benefit of using phase-based methods is the ability to measure the displacement vector of each pixel. Aletras and associates[25] developed a technique to improve the spatial and temporal resolution of a conventional phase contrast velocity encoding myocardial motion method for use with more rapid pulse sequences. This technique has the advantages of tagging and phase velocity mapping sequences because it can measure larger displacements over longer periods with greater spatial resolution. This method, known as DENSE, has gained increasing clinical utility as a versatile imaging tool. A typical DENSE magnitude image is shown in Figure 55-8A, which provides no motion information. A DENSE phase image is shown in Figure 55-8B; this phase image shows motion along the *x*-axis. Because of regional contraction, the myocardium shows values other than gray, which reflects zero motion. For two-dimensional in-plane motion measurements, another DENSE phase map with encoding along the *y*-axis is acquired (Fig. 55-8C).

The combination of the two phase maps generates a displacement plot (Fig. 55-9) in which each arrowtail corresponds to the position of a pixel at the beginning of systole, and each arrowhead corresponds to the final position at end-systole. Because each pixel carries its own displacement information, there are numerous measurements made within the myocardium.

Myocardial strain can be computed from DENSE displacement images and is provided along the circumferential and radial directions. These strain maps show the degree of myocardial shortening in the circumferential

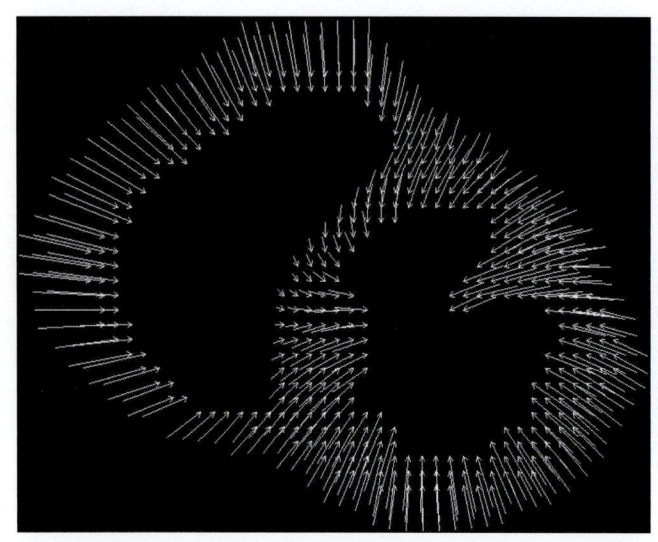

FIGURE 55-9 Two-dimensional displacement arrow plots derived from the phase maps shown in Figure 55-8. (From Kwong R. Cardiovascular Magnetic Resonance Imaging. Totowa, NJ, Humana Press, 2007.)

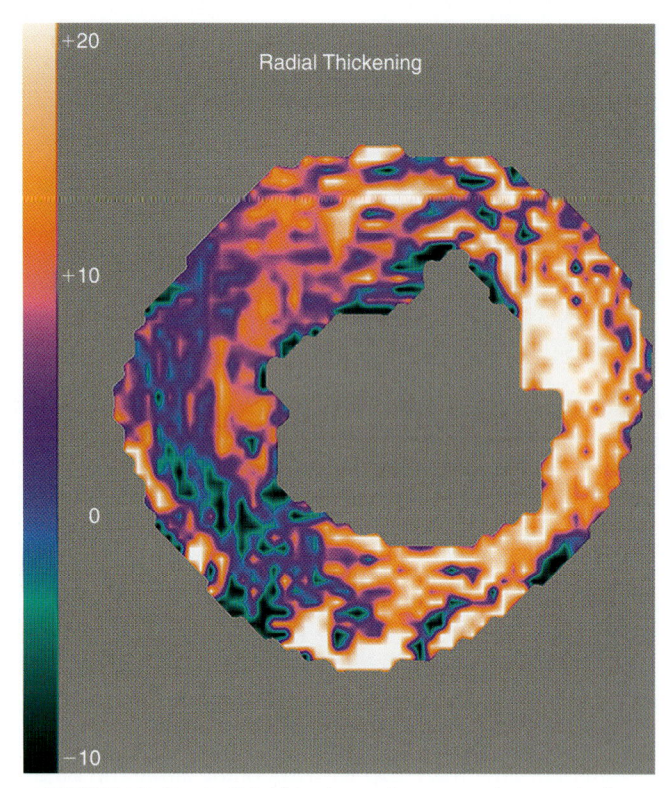

FIGURE 55-10 Radial thickening strain computed automatically from the displacement plot of Figure 55-9. White zones correspond to normally contracting myocardium, and black zones show contractile abnormalities.

Displacement imaging with DENSE is a relatively new concept in MRI that enables quantitative assessment of regional function in the heart. In concept, it is the same as cine fluoroscopy using radiopaque markers. It is a major improvement over the invasive techniques, however, and with the development of pixel-by-pixel measurements provides high-density in-plane data and can cover the whole heart.

In combination with T2-weighted imaging to assess for myocardial edema after ischemia-reperfusion injury, DENSE allows a full assessment of not only the area at risk, but also the degree and extent of myocardial salvage (Fig. 55-11).[45] Application in human studies is now possible to assess infarct size and area of myocardial salvage, determine quantitatively whether novel medical or intervention treatments can be beneficial, and evaluate the success of reperfusion strategies with a noninvasive technique.

Compared with other noninvasive imaging modalities, MRI is a true three-dimensional modality with unmatched soft tissue contrast and image resolution. Translation of the superior image quality into a more accurate assessment of cardiac function requires that analysis goes beyond visual inspection of the images to more detailed and quantitative results using techniques such as MRI displacement imaging and phase tagging.[15]

Computed Tomography

Multidetector CT has been studied in the assessment of regional wall motion. A study by Haraikawa and colleagues[46] included 20 patients with various kinds of heart disease. All patients underwent contrast-enhanced multidetector CT and biplane left ventriculography (LVG). Using a retrospective ECG gating technique, 10 phases over one cardiac cycle were extracted. Wall motion was scored. The scores obtained by multidetector CT were compared with scores obtained by LVG. Wall motion could be assessed in all segments of the 20 patients using interactive multiplanar animation. Of 140 segments in 20 patients, scores in 118 were concordant between multidetector CT and LVG.

Yamaguchi and coworkers[10] evaluated regional cardiac function using multidetector CT and quantitative gated SPECT (QGS) compared with LVG, and evaluated parameters of LV diastolic function using multidetector CT. Regional cardiac function was evaluated using shortening fraction. The PFR and tPFR/RR on multidetector CT were measured as parameters of LV diastolic function. The shortening fractions by multidetector CT and LVG were evaluated using a seven-segment model (*1*, anterobasal; *2*, anterolateral; *3*, apical; *4*, diaphragmatic; *5*, posterobasal; *6*, septal; *7*, posterolateral), and were found to be correlated in almost each segment ($r = 0.64$ to 0.88) except the anterobasal segment ($r = 0.34$), whereas the shortening fractions by QGS and LVG were not correlated in more segments. The shortening fractions by QGS and LVG were not correlated in the myocardial infarcted segments. Multidetector CT is more useful in detecting regional cardiac function compared with QGS, and parameters of diastolic function could also be measured by multidetector CT.

direction and its degree of thickening along the radial direction as a result of local contractile action. Normally contracting myocardium would exhibit strain of about 20% along both directions (white part of the scale), and abnormal myocardium would exhibit reduced strain (black part of the scale) (Fig. 55-10).

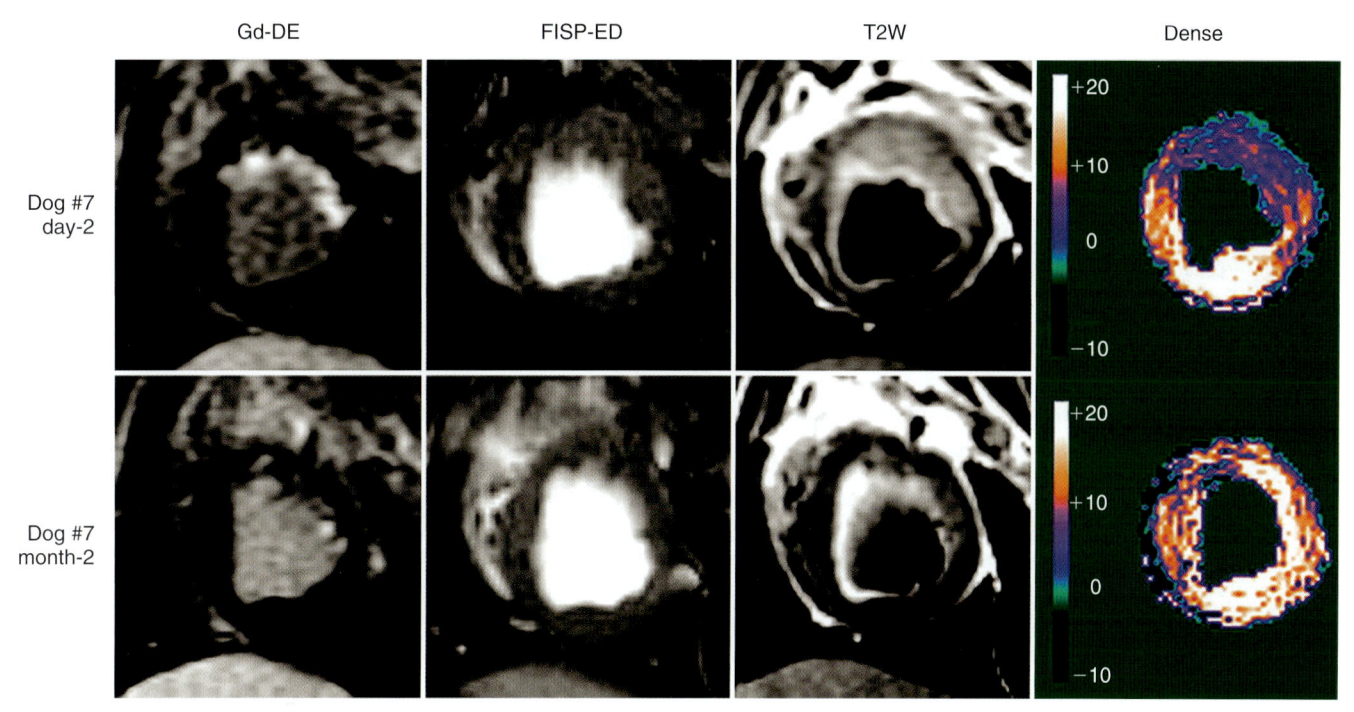

FIGURE 55-11 T2-weighted (T2W) image in the top row (day 2 post-MI) shows a hyperintense area (representing edema/area at risk) that is nearly transmural, whereas the infarcted area was only subendocardial, as seen using a gadolinium-enhanced MDE technique. T2W hyperintense zone corresponded well to the hypokinetic zone on the DENSE systolic strain maps in the right column (radial thickening). Two months after MI (*bottom row*), the T2W abnormality was nearly completely resolved, and systolic strain had normalized (color scale = −10% to +20% strain). Normal strain is in the orange-white zone; blue-green represents severely hypokinetic-to-dyskinetic segments. (*From Aletras AH, et al. Retrospective determination of the area at risk for reperfused acute myocardial infarction with T2-weighted cardiac magnetic resonance imaging: histopathological and displacement encoding with stimulated echoes (DENSE) functional validations. Circulation 2006; 113:1865-1870.*)

Belge and colleagues[31] showed that regional end-diastolic and end-systolic wall thicknesses by multidetector CT were highly correlated, but significantly lower than by MRI (8.3 ± 1.8 mm vs. 8.8 ± 1.9 mm and 12.7 ± 3.4 mm vs. 13.3 ± 3.5 mm). Values of regional wall thickening by multidetector CT and MRI were similar (54 ± 30% vs. 51 ± 31%) and correlated well. Retrospectively gated multidetector CT can accurately estimate regional LV wall thickening compared with cine MRI. In a pilot study by Fischbach and coworkers,[14] segmental LV wall motion obtained by multidetector CT was assessed using a 17-segment model, and compared with SSFP cine MRI. Multidetector CT correctly identified 252 out of 266 (94.7%) normal segments and 189 out of 214 (88.3%) segments with decreased wall motion, yielding a sensitivity of 88% and specificity of 95% for identification of wall motion abnormalities. LV wall motion scores were identical in 86.7% of 480 segments. Multidetector CT had a tendency to underestimate the degree of wall motion impairment. Interobserver agreement was lower in multidetector CT (66.5%) than in MRI (89.1%).

Normokinetic segments are reliably identified with multidetector CT. Sensitivity for the accurate detection of regional wall motion abnormalities may be enhanced only by upgrading temporal resolution.[14] With the improvement of temporal resolution between 42 ms and 83 ms, some investigators showed the utility of dual-source CT not only in the accurate assessment of global functional parameters, but also in the quantification of time-dependent variables, providing a more reliable evaluation of regional wall motion.[32]

EVALUATION OF CARDIAC FUNCTION DURING STRESS

Magnetic Resonance Imaging

The use of MRI in the detection of CAD and the assessment of its hemodynamic significance is a growing clinical application. The availability of rapid gradient systems and resultant short imaging times allows for high-resolution cine imaging of the heart at rest and with faster heart rates during stress conditions. Endocardial border definition using standard cine SSFP MRI pulse sequences is superior to even state-of-the-art echocardiographic image quality.[15]

Stress Agents

Exercise stress MRI has been performed on healthy subjects in highly experienced centers or in an experimental setting; however, its application and feasibility in detection of ischemic heart disease needs to be exhibited further.[3] Physical exercise within the magnet leads to degradation of image quality from motion artifacts, and currently pharmacologic stress is preferred.[16] Various pharmacologic stress agents are available, which include the vasodilators adenosine and dipyridamole and the inotropic agent dobutamine. Although vasodilator stress has been reported to induce ischemic wall motion abnormalities, a low diagnostic sensitivity for the detection of epicardial CAD has been reported using any cine imaging technique during vasodilator stress.[47]

Dobutamine stress MRI is well established as a technique for identifying ischemia-induced wall motion abnormalities in CAD, with developed guidelines for clinical practice.[1] In a head-to-head comparison of dobutamine stress echocardiography and high-dose dobutamine/atropine stress MRI (DSMRI), with x-ray coronary angiography as the standard of reference in a large patient cohort, Nagel and associates[48] showed a high accuracy of DSMRI for the detection of inducible wall motion abnormalities related to epicardial coronary stenosis in patients with suspected CAD. Diagnostic accuracy was 86% (sensitivity 86%, specificity 86%), which was superior to dobutamine stress echocardiography (76% accuracy). In patients with limited echocardiographic image quality, Hundley and colleagues[49] reported a similar diagnostic performance of DSMRI (accuracy 83%, sensitivity 83%, specificity 83%). The gain in diagnostic accuracy is high in patients with inadequate acoustic windows or limited echocardiographic image quality despite the use of second-harmonic imaging.

Results obtained from dobutamine stress testing have important prognostic implications. Normal dobutamine stress function carries a good prognosis, whereas the presence of inducible ischemia signifies an increased risk for cardiovascular events.[50]

Dobutamine Stress Magnetic Resonance Imaging Protocol

We present in this section the current DSMRI imaging protocol used in our center. We use a standard high-dose dobutamine/atropine regimen similar to stress echocardiography. Cine MRI scans are acquired in the diagnostic standard views (apical, mid, and basal short-axis view; four-chamber, two-chamber, and three-chamber view) at rest and during each stage of progressive dobutamine infusion at 3- to 5-minute intervals at doses of 10 μg/kg/min, 20 μg/kg/min, 30 μg/kg/min, and 40 μg/kg/min. If the age-predicted target heart rate ($[220 - age] \times 0.85$) is not achieved at the maximal dobutamine dose, a maximal dose of 2 mg of atropine is administered in 0.25-mg increments every 1 to 2 minutes. We prefer to administer atropine at the early part of the 30 μg/kg/min infusion stage, when the inotropic effect of dobutamine has been reached so that atropine aliquots can help achieve the desired target heart rate sooner than depending on progressive dobutamine alone. Termination criteria are identical to those of dobutamine stress echocardiography: achievement of target heart rate, systolic blood pressure decrease more than 40 mm Hg, blood pressure increase greater than 240/120 mm Hg, intractable symptoms, new or worsening wall motion abnormalities in at least two adjacent left ventricular segments, or complex cardiac arrhythmias.[1]

In addition to the assessment of ischemia, DSMRI can be used in identifying viable myocardium after MI. This evaluation is based on the contractile response to low-dose dobutamine stimulation. Dobutamine stimulates recruitment of hibernating myocardium at a dose of 10 to 20 μg/kg/min, which can be seen as an improvement of the contractile response of a given myocardial region that is dysfunctional at rest. In addition, in myocardial regions subtended by a stenotic coronary artery, a "biphasic response" can be observed with a wall motion abnormality at rest, improvement at low-dose dobutamine, and deterioration at high-dose dobutamine when myocardial ischemia develops.

Although debate remains, there have been reports of specific clinical settings when DSMRI was compared with gadolinium-enhanced scar imaging (i.e., myocardial delayed enhancement [MDE] imaging), and it was found that low-dose dobutamine is superior in predicting recovery of function after revascularization.[1] This observation was most pronounced in segments with nontransmural scar. It has been suggested that the reason for this phenomenon is that even though scar imaging depicts the area of myocardial necrosis, it does not assess the functional state of the surrounding (potentially viable) epicardial myocardium, and its capability for the prediction of functional recovery of nontransmurally scarred myocardium is limited.[15] The use of MRI in the detection of myocardial viability is discussed further in Chapter 57.

Diagnostic Criteria

The standard 17-segment model as described in the previous section is used in the evaluation of stress-induced perfusion and wall motion abnormalities. Perfusion imaging may be performed with any of the pharmacologic stress agents mentioned. The principle behind first-pass myocardial perfusion imaging is that differences in myocardial blood flow can be assessed by direct visualization of enhancement from a first-pass transit of a gadolinium contrast agent.[22] The use of MRI in the evaluation of myocardial perfusion is discussed further in Chapter 54.

Regional wall motion is graded by visual assessment because quantification has not been shown to be superior to visual assessment. Each of the 17 myocardial segments needs to be assessed at all times. For image interpretation, multiple synchronized cine loop display is used to view one or more imaging planes at each dose level simultaneously. Segmental wall motion is classified as normokinetic, hypokinetic, akinetic, or dyskinetic and assigned a grade of 1 to 4. The sum of points divided by the number of analyzed segments generates a wall motion score. A wall motion score of 1 indicates normal contraction, whereas a higher score indicates wall motion abnormalities. With increasing doses during dobutamine stress, a lack of augmentation in the wall motion or systolic wall thickening and a reduction of the wall motion or thickening are regarded as pathologic findings.[15]

Other MRI techniques have been used to assess CAD during DSMRI. Tagging methods have shown increased sensitivity for diagnosis of CAD.[51,52] Objective analysis of myocardial wall motion using tagging would be expected to reduce observer interpretation variability, which remains an issue in dobutamine stress echocardiography. The application of this MRI technique in a large clinical trial is anticipated.[16] An example of the application of tagging in the analysis of myocardial function during dobutamine stress is shown in Figure 55-12.

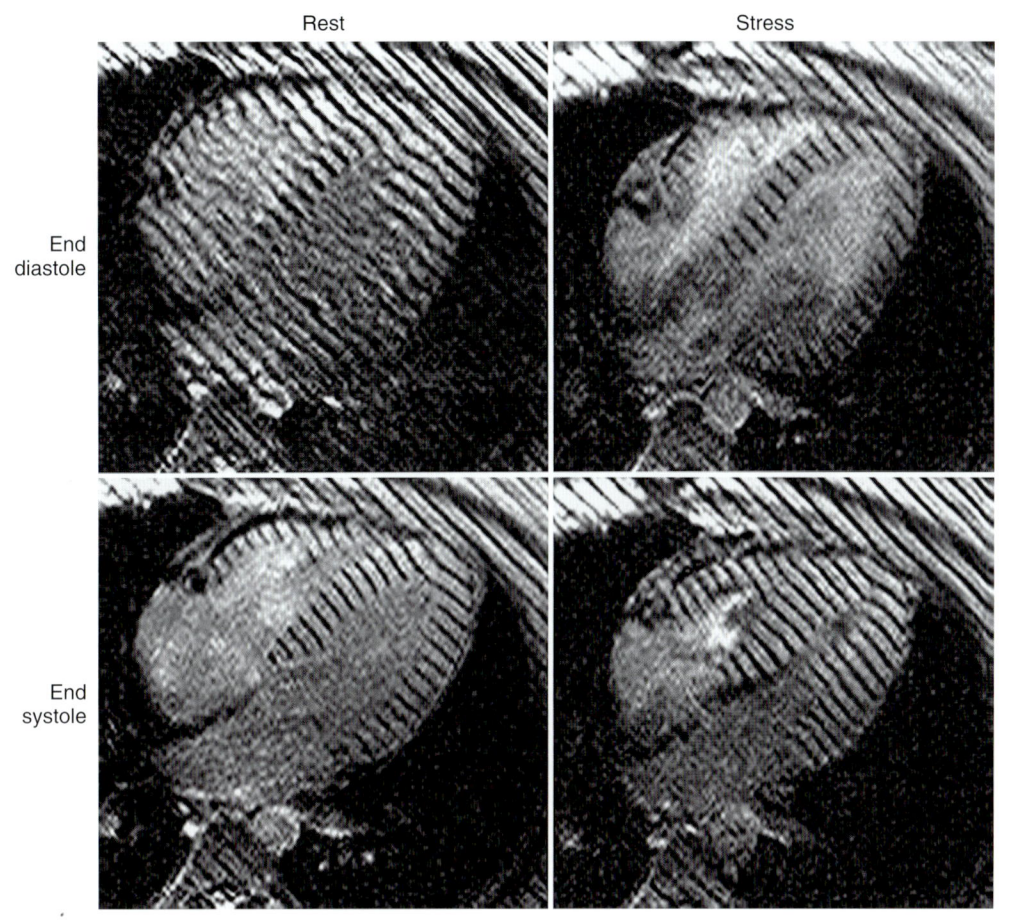

FIGURE 55-12 Long-axis myocardial tagging at rest (*left*) and during high-dose dobutamine stress (*right*). Improved myocardial motion is detected at end-systole with dobutamine (*bottom right*) compared with rest (*bottom left*). (From Kwong R. Cardiovascular Magnetic Resonance Imaging. Totowa, NJ, Humana Press, 2007.)

Computed Tomography

The clinical application of stress imaging techniques using multidetector CT is still in development. George and colleagues[2] showed the use of adenosine-augmented multidetector CT myocardial perfusion imaging in providing semiquantitative measurements of myocardial perfusion during first-pass multidetector CT in a canine model of left anterior descending coronary artery stenosis.[2] This technique of identifying the presence of CAD using adenosine stress multidetector CT is yet to be validated in humans. The detection of stress-induced regional wall motion abnormalities with either exercise or dobutamine is not currently possible using multidetector CT because of limited temporal resolution.

Late enhancement imaging using multidetector CT has been used in the evaluation of myocardial viability, providing useful information in the prediction of LV remodeling and prognosis after MI.[6] In a small pilot study of patients with acute MI, late enhancement multidetector CT has been shown to correlate well with late enhancement MRI in assessing infarct size and myocardial viability.[7] Further clinical validation and investigation of the prognostic implication of multidetector CT in various clinical settings need to be prospectively studied. CT applications in the assessment of myocardial perfusion and viability are discussed further in Chapters 54 and 57.

REFERENCES

1. Nagel E, et al. Stress cardiovascular magnetic resonance: consensus panel report. J Cardiovasc Magn Reson 2001; 3:267-281.
2. George RT, et al. Multidetector computed tomography myocardial perfusion imaging during adenosine stress. J Am Coll Cardiol 2006; 48:153-160.
3. Jekic M, et al. Cardiac function and myocardial perfusion immediately following maximal treadmill exercise inside the MRI room. J Cardiovasc Magn Reson 2008; 10:3.
4. Sanz G, et al. Determinants of prognosis in survivors of myocardial infarction: a prospective clinical angiographic study. N Engl J Med 1982; 306:1065-1070.
5. White HD, et al. Left ventricular end-systolic volume as the major determinant of survival after recovery from myocardial infarction. Circulation 1987; 76:44-51.
6. Sato A, et al. Early validation study of 64-slice multidetector computed tomography for the assessment of myocardial viability and the

prediction of left ventricular remodelling after acute myocardial infarction. Eur Heart J 2008; 29:490-498.
7. Mahnken AH, et al. Assessment of myocardial viability in reperfused acute myocardial infarction using 16-slice computed tomography in comparison to magnetic resonance imaging. J Am Coll Cardiol 2005; 45:2042-2047.
8. Kim RJ, et al. The use of contrast-enhanced magnetic resonance imaging to identify reversible myocardial dysfunction. N Engl J Med 2000; 343:1445-1453.
9. Baer FM, et al. Dobutamine magnetic resonance imaging predicts contractile recovery of chronically dysfunctional myocardium after successful revascularization. J Am Coll Cardiol 1998; 31:1040-1048.
10. Yamaguchi K, et al. Accurate estimation of regional and global cardiac function in old myocardial infarction patients by multidetector-row computed tomography. J Med Invest 2007; 54(1-2):72-82.
11. Maceira AM, et al. Normalized left ventricular systolic and diastolic function by steady state free precession cardiovascular magnetic resonance. J Cardiovasc Magn Reson 2006; 8:417-426.
12. Jung B, et al. Detailed analysis of myocardial motion in volunteers and patients using high-temporal-resolution MR tissue phase mapping. J Magn Reson Imaging 2006; 24:1033-1039.
13. Yamamuro M, et al. Cardiac functional analysis with multi-detector row CT and segmental reconstruction algorithm: comparison with echocardiography, SPECT, and MR imaging. Radiology 2005; 234:381-390.
14. Fischbach R, et al. Assessment of regional left ventricular function with multidetector-row computed tomography versus magnetic resonance imaging. Eur Radiol 2007; 17:1009-1017.
15. Kwong R. Cardiovascular Magnetic Resonance Imaging. Totowa, NJ, Humana Press, 2007.
16. Pennell DJ, et al. Clinical indications for cardiovascular magnetic resonance (CMR): consensus panel report. Eur Heart J 2004; 25:1940-1965.
17. Arad Y, et al. Predictive value of electron beam computed tomography of the coronary arteries: 19-month follow-up of 1173 asymptomatic subjects. Circulation 1996; 93:1951-1953.
18. Miller J, Rochitte C, Dewey M. Coronary artery evaluation using 64-row multidetector computed tomography angiography (CORE-64): results of a multicenter, international trial to assess diagnostic accuracy compared with conventional coronary angiography. American Heart Association 30th Annual Scientific Sessions, Orlando, 2007.
19. Orakzai SH, et al. Assessment of cardiac function using multidetector row computed tomography. J Comput Assist Tomogr 2006; 30:555-563.
20. Nagel E. Cardiovascular Magnetic Resonance. Berlin, Steinkopff Verlag Darmstadt, 2004.
21. Atkinson DJ, Edelman RR. Cineangiography of the heart in a single breath hold with a segmented turboFLASH sequence. Radiology 1991; 178:357-360.
22. Lee V. Cardiovascular Magnetic Resonance: Physical Principles to Practical Applications. Philadelphia, Lippincott Williams & Wilkins, 2006.
23. Carr JC, et al. Cine MR angiography of the heart with segmented true fast imaging with steady-state precession. Radiology 2001; 219:828-834.
24. Osman NF, et al. Cardiac motion tracking using CINE harmonic phase (HARP) magnetic resonance imaging. Magn Reson Med 1999; 42:1048-1060.
25. Aletras AH, et al. DENSE: displacement encoding with stimulated echoes in cardiac functional MRI. J Magn Reson 1999; 137:247-252.
26. Kim D, et al. Myocardial tissue tracking with two-dimensional cine displacement-encoded MR imaging: development and initial evaluation. Radiology 2004; 230:862-871.
27. Marcus JT, et al. The influence of through-plane motion on left ventricular volumes measured by magnetic resonance imaging: implications for image acquisition and analysis. J Cardiovasc Magn Reson 1999; 1:1-6.
28. Francois CJ, et al. Left ventricular mass: manual and automatic segmentation of true FISP and FLASH cine MR images in dogs and pigs. Radiology 2004; 230:389-395.
29. Shors SM, et al. Accurate quantification of right ventricular mass at MR imaging by using cine true fast imaging with steady-state precession: study in dogs. Radiology 2004; 230:383-388.
30. Pons-Llad G. Atlas of Non-invasive Coronary Angiography by Multidetector Computed Tomography. New York, Springer Publishing, 2006.
31. Belge B, et al. Accurate estimation of global and regional cardiac function by retrospectively gated multidetector row computed tomography: comparison with cine magnetic resonance imaging. Eur Radiol 2006; 16:1424-1433.
32. Brodoefel H, et al. Dual-source CT with improved temporal resolution in assessment of left ventricular function: a pilot study. AJR Am J Roentgenol 2007; 189:1064-1070.
33. Salton CJ, et al. Gender differences and normal left ventricular anatomy in an adult population free of hypertension: a cardiovascular magnetic resonance study of the Framingham Heart Study Offspring cohort. J Am Coll Cardiol 2002; 39:1055-1060.
34. Alfakih K, et al. Normal human left and right ventricular dimensions for MRI as assessed by turbo gradient echo and steady-state free precession imaging sequences. J Magn Reson Imaging 2003; 17:323-329.
35. Guiliani ER. Mayo Clinic Practice of Cardiology, 3rd ed. St Louis, Mosby, 1996.
36. Tandri H, et al. Normal reference values for the adult right ventricle by magnetic resonance imaging. Am J Cardiol 2006; 98:1660-1664.
37. Larose E, et al. Right ventricular dysfunction assessed by cardiovascular magnetic resonance imaging predicts poor prognosis late after myocardial infarction. J Am Coll Cardiol 2007; 49:855-862.
38. Quiroz R, et al. Right ventricular enlargement on chest computed tomography: prognostic role in acute pulmonary embolism. Circulation 2004; 109:2401-2404.
39. Kim TH, et al. Evaluation of right ventricular volume and mass using retrospective ECG-gated cardiac multidetector computed tomography: comparison with first-pass radionuclide angiography. Eur Radiol 2005; 15:1987-1993.
40. Koch K, et al. Assessment of right ventricular function by 16-detector-row CT: comparison with magnetic resonance imaging. Eur Radiol 2005; 15:312-318.
41. Reference deleted in proofs.
42. Zerhouni EA, et al. Human heart: tagging with MR imaging—a method for noninvasive assessment of myocardial motion. Radiology 1988; 169:59-63.
43. Reese TG, Wedeen VJ, Weisskoff RM. Measuring diffusion in the presence of material strain. J Magn Reson B 1996; 112:253-258.
44. Chenevert TL, et al. Elasticity reconstructive imaging by means of stimulated echo MRI. Magn Reson Med 1998; 39:482-490.
45. Aletras AH, et al. Retrospective determination of the area at risk for reperfused acute myocardial infarction with T2-weighted cardiac magnetic resonance imaging: histopathological and displacement encoding with stimulated echoes (DENSE) functional validations. Circulation 2006; 113:1865-1870.
46. Haraikawa T, et al. Assessment of left ventricular wall motion using 16-channel multislice computed tomography: comparison with left ventriculography. Radiat Med 2006; 24:159-164.
47. Paetsch I, et al. Comparison of dobutamine stress magnetic resonance, adenosine stress magnetic resonance, and adenosine stress magnetic resonance perfusion. Circulation 2004; 110:835-842.
48. Nagel E, et al. Noninvasive diagnosis of ischemia-induced wall motion abnormalities with the use of high-dose dobutamine stress MRI: comparison with dobutamine stress echocardiography. Circulation 1999; 99:763-770.
49. Hundley WG, et al. Utility of fast cine magnetic resonance imaging and display for the detection of myocardial ischemia in patients not well suited for second harmonic stress echocardiography. Circulation 1999; 100:1697-1702.
50. Hundley WG, et al. Magnetic resonance imaging determination of cardiac prognosis. Circulation 2002; 106:2328-2333.
51. Kuijpers D, et al. Dobutamine cardiovascular magnetic resonance for the detection of myocardial ischemia with the use of myocardial tagging. Circulation 2003; 107:1592-1597.
52. Power TP, et al. Breath-hold dobutamine magnetic resonance myocardial tagging: normal left ventricular response. Am J Cardiol 1997; 80:1203-1207.

CHAPTER 56

Nuclear Medicine Imaging of Ventricular Function

Bennett Chin and Kenneth J. Nichols

Left ventricular (LV) function is an important, well-established indicator of patient prognosis. Radionuclide imaging techniques are established as the most highly reproducible methods to assess LV ejection fraction non-invasively. Comprehensive textbooks have summarized the results of studies over several decades showing the high reproducibility and accuracy of gated equilibrium blood pool scintigraphy and radionuclide angiography in determining LV and right ventricular (RV) ejection fraction measurements.[1-4] Cardiac mortality is strongly associated with impaired ventricular function as assessed by decreased LV ejection fraction. Additionally, identifying dysfunctional segments in viable myocardium is crucial in clinical management. Numerous studies have shown an almost threefold higher incidence of cardiac mortality in medically treated patients with viable compared with nonviable myocardium.[5] The identification of focal dysfunctional segments is highly relevant to clinical management.

The introduction of Tc-99m radiotracers has made gated myocardial perfusion imaging (MPI) readily available, easily feasible, and now a standard technique requiring little additional effort or cost.[6] Because MPI is the most commonly performed procedure in nuclear cardiology, evaluation of LV function in nuclear cardiology is most often performed in conjunction with MPI. Similarly, assessment of ventricular function by gated MPI can be performed with positron emission tomography (PET).[7]

Gated equilibrium blood pool imaging is a well-established technique commonly used to assess ventricular function quantitatively in oncology patients receiving cardiotoxic chemotherapy. High reproducibility, technical simplicity, and availability, make this study the procedure of choice in evaluating LV function sequentially. Although first-pass radionuclide angiocardiography is a well-established and elegant technique to determine ejection fraction, equilibrium blood pool imaging provides the ability to view ventricular function from multiple planar projections, or in a fully three-dimensional manner using single photon emission computed tomography (SPECT).

For quantitative, functional analysis of the right ventricle by RV ejection fraction, first-pass angiocardiography currently remains the method of choice because planar equilibrium blood pool imaging cannot separate underlying or adjacent blood pool structures sufficiently for an accurate determination of RV ejection fraction. Newer techniques, such as tomographic ECG gated blood pool (GBP) imaging, are becoming more widespread as quantitative software programs are being developed and validated. These newer techniques have the potential to evaluate simultaneously and quantitatively RV and LV size and function, with high spatial and temporal resolution. Elegant first-pass techniques have been developed to evaluate intraventricular shunts quantitatively; the need for these is relatively uncommon, and they are described elsewhere.[1]

This chapter describes the most commonly performed radionuclide techniques to assess ventricular function. First, gated SPECT MPI is discussed. These principles are generally applicable to gated PET assessment of ventricular function. As PET MPI becomes more prevalent in the future, this technique is expected to become increasingly important. Next, equilibrium GBP imaging is reviewed briefly. Finally, RV functional evaluation with first-pass radionuclide angiocardiography is discussed.

LEFT VENTRICULAR FUNCTIONAL ASSESSMENT FROM GATED MYOCARDIAL PERFUSION IMAGING

ECG gating to assess ventricular function is now a standard, integral part of MPI. The quantitative evaluation of LV ejection fraction has exhibited high reproducibility and accuracy. Compared with CT, LV ejection fraction assessed by SPECT is not significantly different, although absolute values for end-diastolic volume and end-systolic volume

771

are different with SPECT.[8] As expected, LV functional impairment quantified by SPECT is associated with a poor prognosis, including cardiac death. LV ejection fraction less than 45% and LV end-systolic volume greater than 70 mL were associated with approximately 8% to 9%/yr cardiac death rate compared with approximately 1%/yr for LV ejection fraction 45% or greater and end-systolic volume 70 mL or less.[9] Although perfusion defect reversibility is most predictive of future myocardial infarction, LV ejection fraction is the strongest predictor of mortality.[10]

Several studies have shown the clinical utility with improved specificity by identifying normal wall motion and wall thickening in areas of decreased activity because of tissue attenuation. This improvement in specificity may be particularly important in women because of breast attenuation artifacts. The gating information also assists in improving the degree of certainty when interpreting studies as definitely normal or definitely abnormal.[6,11] In a prospective study of 115 women, gated Tc 99m sestamibi significantly improved specificity (92%) compared with the same study without gating (84%; $P = .0004$) or with thallium 201 without gating (59%).[12]

In addition, gating improves sensitivity for detection of coronary artery disease (CAD) in the subset of patients with multivessel disease ("balanced disease") who have transient, stress-induced wall motion abnormalities that are not detected by MPI alone.[13] Additional wall motion information significantly increased the sensitivity for detection of multivessel CAD without adversely affecting specificity.[14] In this study, the sensitivity for multivessel disease was significantly increased from 46% to 60%, and sensitivity for three-vessel disease significantly increased from 10% to 25%.[14] Principles of gated MPI with SPECT are similar to gating with PET radiotracers such as ammonia N 13 or rubidium 82, providing regional and global wall motion information.[15,16] The more recent development of combined PET/CT and SPECT/CT instrumentation may also permit additional, independent, high spatial resolution CT assessment of regional myocardial function.[17]

Electrocardiogram Gated Acquisition

Analogous to traditional methods of acquiring planar gated studies, the ECG is used to bin counts from the various phases of the cardiac cycle temporally during data acquisition. Because of count limitations, most studies currently use eight time frames per cardiac cycle. In patients with irregular rhythms, such as atrial fibrillation, ventricular function may be better assessed with methods that do not rely on data from multiple, averaged heartbeats (e.g., echocardiography). If gated MPI is used, the averaged data may be subject to inaccuracies because of misplacement of counts within the cardiac cycle, and careful inspection of the ECG and gating data is necessary to ensure that appropriate beats with similar RR intervals are included for analysis.[18,19]

Data Processing, Reconstruction, and Analysis

In most cases, appropriate binning of the data into the various phases of the cardiac cycle results in accurate representation of LV function. Tomographic images are typically reconstructed with filtered back-projection, and sophisticated edge detection programs are used to define ventricular boundaries. From these volumes, time-activity curves are generated, indices of ventricular function are derived, and a cine display is generated for visual assessment of regional and global LV function.

Well-developed programs to evaluate LV wall motion have been commercially available for several years.[20-22] Generally, these use boundary detection algorithms, count densities, or a combination of variables to define the endocardial and epicardial borders for LV volume calculations. Another important parameter is LV wall thickening. Detected activity within the myocardium depends on radioactive concentration and volume (or thickness) of the myocardium. When small objects (LV myocardial wall thickness) are below twice the full-width half-maximum of the system resolution, detected activity within the ventricular wall appears lower than the true activity because of partial volume effects.[23] Because myocardial wall thickness is susceptible to the partial volume effect, a higher wall thickness at end-systole corresponds to higher detected activity by SPECT. The degree of regional wall thickening is related to the change in detected regional myocardial wall activity. Detected activity at end-diastole typically is lower than that at end-systole because of differences in ventricular wall thickness. Some algorithms assume there is an exact linear relationship between myocardial wall thickening and percent systolic count increases.

Cardiac volume and myocardial thickening can be appreciated visually for cine display formats of individual tomographic slices and computer-generated derived surface renderings. In addition, quantitative, physiologic indices are derived from tomographic volumes and from counts within the myocardium. Fourier analysis is applied to the time-activity curve of each data element in the volume (voxel) to generate parametric images of contraction. Fourier analysis forms the basis of phase and amplitude analysis by which the pattern of myocardial contraction and regional wall motion is assessed quantitatively. More recently, high correlation of LV ejection fraction measurements was reported between techniques in hybrid instrumentation combining high-resolution 64-slice CT with SPECT; mean values were not significantly different.[8]

As described earlier, the primary potential benefits of concurrent wall motion assessment include (1) improved specificity in cases of fixed regions of decreased activity (improving detection of attenuation artifacts), and (2) improved sensitivity in detection of multivessel CAD or three-vessel disease (i.e., detection of abnormal wall motion in patients with "balanced disease"). With respect to increased specificity, this may be particularly beneficial in women with severe anterior breast attenuation, and in men with severe inferior diaphragmatic attenuation. The presence of completely normal wall motion and wall thickening is strong evidence that large transmural infarction has not occurred. Although small subendocardial infarction may not be detected with gated perfusion imaging, normal wall motion and normal LV function are good prognostic indicators, which can greatly aid in the assessment of prognosis.

With respect to sensitivity, exercise-induced LV dysfunction has shown improvement in sensitivity for detection of multivessel CAD over perfusion information alone; it also provides further information regarding the clinical significance of known disease. This information may be clinically important in patients with multivessel CAD, who are among the patients most likely to benefit from further therapy.

PITFALLS AND SOLUTIONS

Potential limitations of this technique should also be mentioned. In patients with prior infarction, boundaries in regions of low or absent tracer uptake may be difficult to define accurately. Although edge detection algorithms are in most cases beneficial, in some cases the extremely low activity renders myocardial boundary definition very difficult and susceptible to computer boundary definition errors. In a canine experimental model, boundary detection and reproducibility were adversely affected by prior infarction, low tracer dose administration, and high background activity.[24] Additionally, in patients with small LV cavities (e.g., small women), the endocardial borders may be difficult to identify, and an underestimation of LV cavity size at end systole may lead to artifactually high LV ejection fraction values.[6]

As with all ECG gated techniques, arrhythmias may also interfere with appropriate data collection, and ECG data should be inspected carefully. Differences in boundary detection algorithms exist in different software packages, and volumes and LV ejection fraction values may differ from one algorithm to the next because of variability in data analysis methods. Comparing ejection fraction or volume calculations produced by more than one nuclear cardiology software package, or comparing against values obtained from another imaging modality such as MRI, should be performed carefully and should take into account methodologic differences, including the normal limits specific to each algorithm.[25]

LV function assessed with MPI is a well-established method that has high prognostic significance. Gated MPI provides functional information highly predictive of cardiac mortality; this is independent of MPI data, which is also predictive of future cardiac events, including myocardial infarction. Gating improves the sensitivity in the detection of multivessel CAD and increases specificity or normalcy rate in patients with attenuation artifacts, such as anterior breast attenuation in women and LV inferior wall attenuation in men.

TECHNIQUES

Equilibrium Gated Blood Pool Imaging

Planar GBP imaging with Tc 99m–labeled red blood cells (RBCs) is a well-established and validated technique with the highest reproducibility for LV ejection fraction among all noninvasive imaging procedures. Several factors contribute to this high reproducibility: (1) Tc-99m RBC labeling efficiency is high, (2) LV ejection fraction is calculated by counts within boundaries that are defined by automated detection algorithms, and (3) high count images can be obtained within a short imaging time.

Indications

This technique has been well established as the clinical method of choice to assess objectively oncology patients at risk of developing cardiotoxicity from chemotherapy.[26] Although echocardiography is rapid and results in little patient discomfort, its low quantitative reproducibility obviates its use in standard chemotherapeutic monitoring. Radionuclide gated equilibrium blood pool imaging similarly provides rapid assessment with little discomfort, but the high quantitative reproducibility, technical simplicity, and widespread availability, combined with relatively low cost, make this the method of choice for quantitative assessment of LV function in this population.

Technique Description

All three methods of radiolabeling RBCs with Tc-99m pertechnetate (in vivo, modified in vivo, and in vitro) result in high radiolabeling efficiency that is typically approximately 85% to 90% or greater. Although the in vivo method typically produces the lowest (>85%) radiolabeling efficiency, it is the simplest and provides excellent contrast sufficient for reproducible LV ejection fraction measurements in most cases. For the in vivo method, stannous pyrophosphate is first administered intravenously to reduce the hemoglobin within the RBCs. Approximately 10 to 20 minutes afterward, Tc-99m pertechnetate is administered intravenously, effectively binding to the reduced hemoglobin.

If a quantitative measurement of RV ejection fraction is desired, the radiotracer can be administered with the gamma camera in the right anterior oblique projection using a "gated list mode" acquisition. This acquisition acquires and stores the precise location of all detected photons and when they occurred with respect to the ECG trigger throughout the acquisition. After acquisition, these data are retrospectively processed by rebinning the data into the appropriate phases of the ECG cycle. Typically, the data obtained during radiotracer bolus transit through the right ventricle occurs in approximately three to five heartbeats (or ECG cycles). The rebinned data from these heartbeats are combined to obtain sufficient counts for quantitative analysis. Approximately 20 to 30 minutes afterward, planar equilibrium blood pool images are obtained in the anterior, best septal separation (left anterior oblique 45 degrees [LAO 45]), and left lateral positions to evaluate ventricular wall motion and LV ejection fraction.

The anterior view evaluates anterior and apical segments. The best septal separation view (typically LAO 45) displays septal, inferoapical, and lateral walls. The left lateral view shows anterior, inferior, and apical regions. The best septal separation (LAO 45) has the least amount of overlapping blood pool from adjacent structures. This view is used to calculate LV ejection fraction according to the following formula:

$$\text{LV ejection fraction} = 100\% \times (\text{LVED} - \text{LVES})/\text{LVED}$$

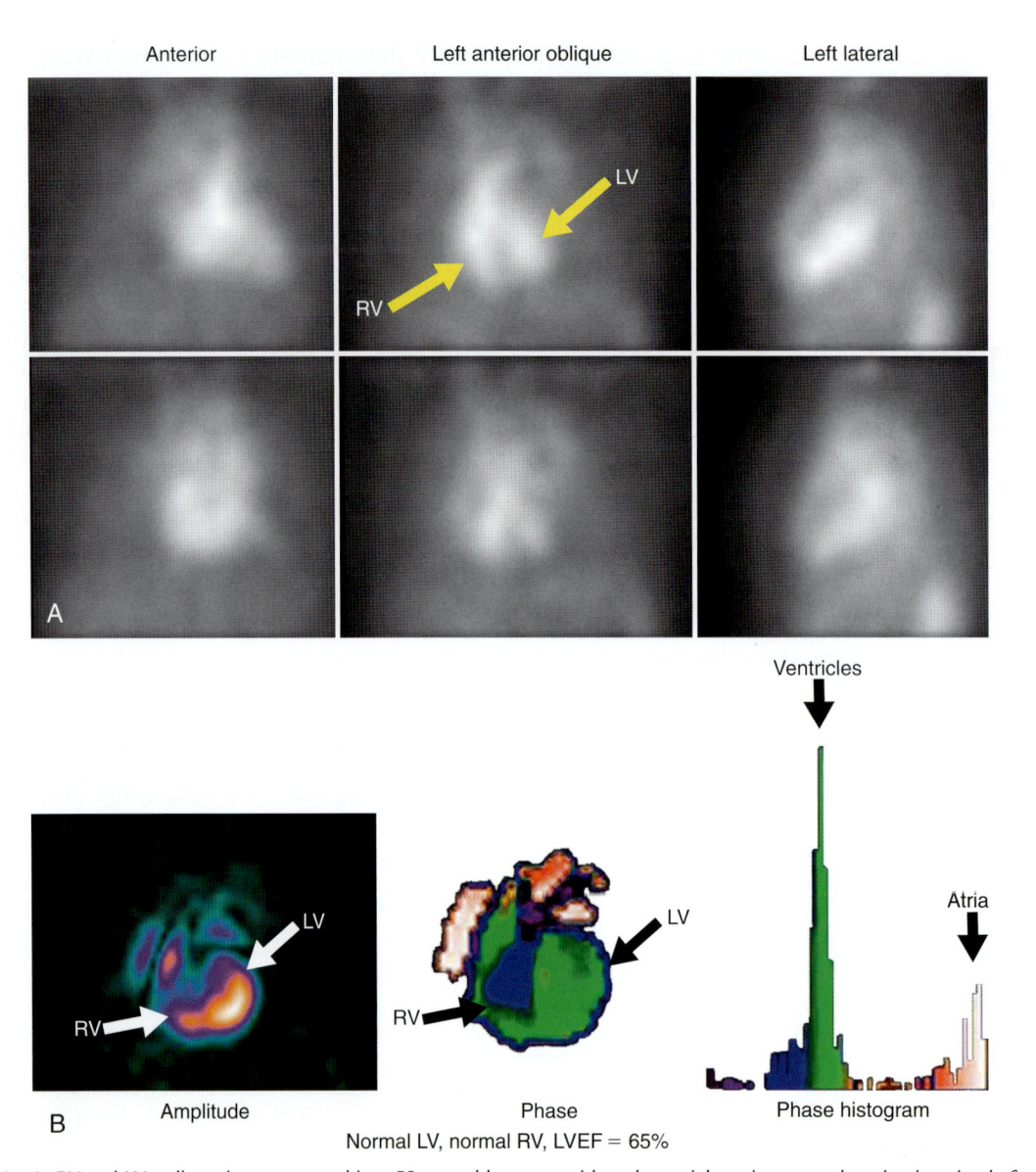

FIGURE 56-1 **A,** RV and LV wall motion are normal in a 58-year-old woman with endometrial carcinoma undergoing imaging before chemotherapy. LV ejection fraction (LVEF) = 65%. End-diastolic (*top row*) and end-systolic (*bottom row*) images show normal ventricular sizes and normal end-systolic volumes. **B,** Parametric amplitude image (*left image*) of the planar LAO 45 acquisition shows high and relatively uniform change in counts in RV and LV regions. The parametric phase image (*middle image*) shows relatively uniform peak activity in the ventricles, indicating a uniform contraction pattern. The histogram of phase shows a narrow and uniform ventricular phase; this is out of phase compared with the atrial voxels.

for background-corrected end-diastolic and end-systolic counts, where LVED is LV end-diastolic volume counts and LVES is LV end-systolic volume counts after background correction.

Background counts typically are determined using an extraventricular region defined from the lateral to inferolateral LV wall. The normal LV ejection fraction is defined as 50% or greater. Reproducibility data show that greater than 5% difference in LV ejection fraction constitutes a statistically significant difference. Curve fitting with Fourier analysis is performed for each voxel in the best septal separation view (typically LAO 45); this provides parametric phase and amplitude images representing the onset and magnitude of contraction. These aid in image processing by defining ventricular boundaries and valve planes; they also aid in image interpretation by providing an objective method to assess the pattern of contraction and regional asynchrony (Figs. 56-1 and 56-2).

RV wall motion can be assessed visually (Fig. 56-3); however, planar images do not permit accurate or reproducible RV ejection fraction calculations because of the adjacent structures that overlap the right ventricle. This issue can be addressed by calculating RV ejection fraction from a gated first-pass list mode radionuclide angiogram or by tomographic methods, as described later. Specific pathologic entities (e.g., atrial septal defect, ventricular septal defect) can also affect ventricular size and function as seen on GBP imaging and have been described elsewhere in detail.[1]

Tomographic blood pool imaging has shown high correlation of RV ejection fraction with planar first-pass techniques.[27] More recently, automated analysis software for

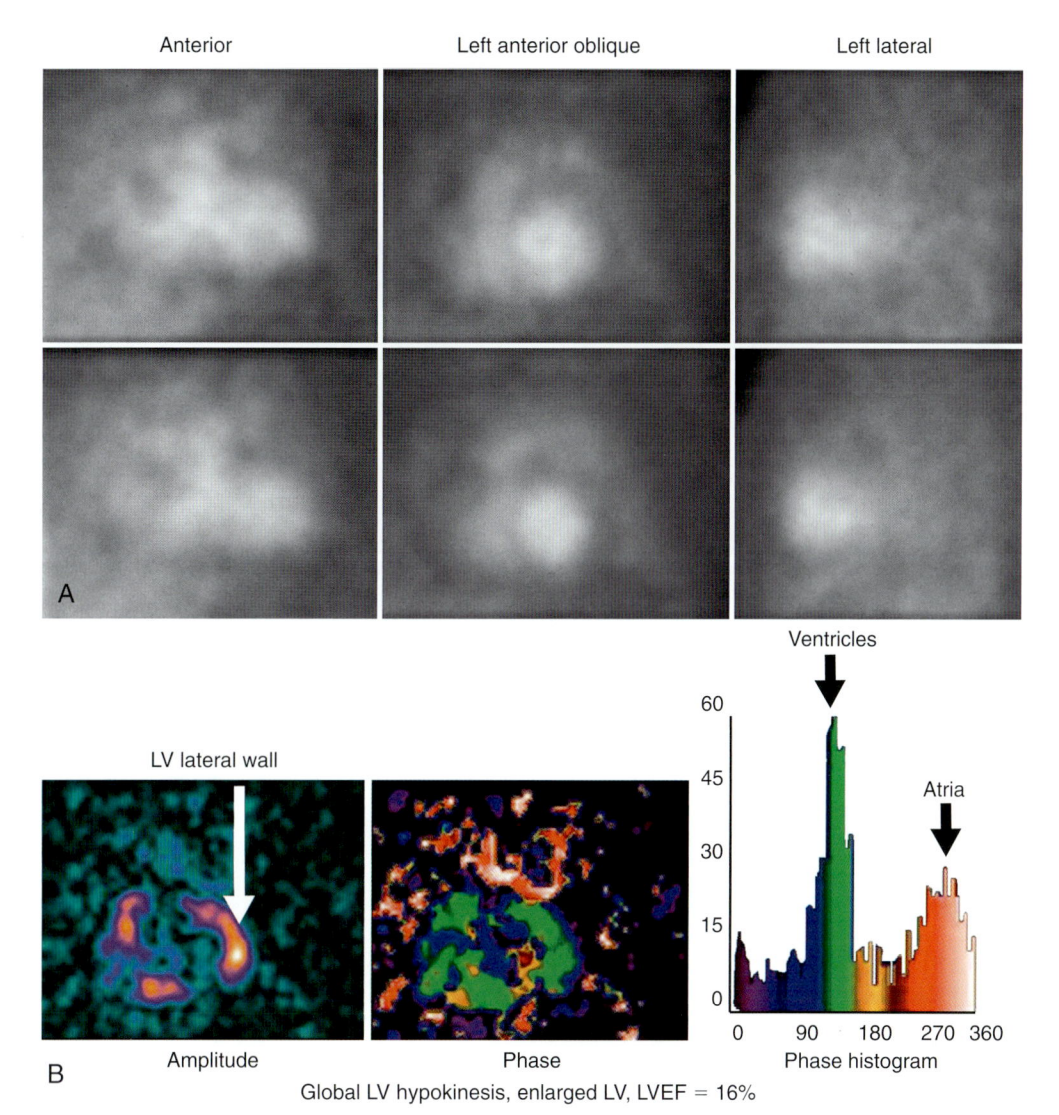

■ **FIGURE 56-2** **A,** Severe RV and LV global hypokinesis in 55-year-old man with obesity and severe CAD who is also status post myocardial infarctions, coronary artery bypass graft surgeries, and multiple stents. The left ventricle and right ventricle are dilated, and their respective end-systolic volumes are abnormally increased. Images appear "noisy" because of scatter from soft tissue attenuation. LV ejection fraction (LVEF) = 16%. End-diastolic (*top row*) and end-systolic (*bottom row*) images show markedly enlarged ventricular cavities and abnormally high end-systolic volumes. **B,** Parametric amplitude image (*left image*) of the planar LAO 45 acquisition shows low ventricular change in counts for RV and LV regions. Best region of LV contraction is the lateral wall (*arrow*); most of the LV cavity shows near-absent change in counts. The parametric phase image (*middle image*) shows relatively nonuniform peak activity in the ventricles, indicating a nonuniform contraction pattern. The histogram of phase shows a wide and nonuniform ventricular phase; this is out of phase compared with the atrial voxels.

tomographic GBP imaging has confirmed high accuracy and reproducibility in the assessment of RV function as confirmed by MRI and echocardiography.[21,28] Because of the increasing incidence of heart failure, accurate biventricular functional assessment may become increasingly important in clinical practice and investigations.

Advantages of tomography include higher contrast, three-dimensional localization, potential for higher accuracy with respect to ventricular volume and wall motion measurements, and simultaneous assessment of the right and left ventricles. These advantages are particularly useful in assessing the right ventricle because of its irregular shape, which is difficult to model using simple assumptions (Fig. 56-4). It has been shown more recently that LV and RV measurements of function are highly reproducible by tomographic blood pool techniques.[29] Consequently, interest has re-emerged in the use of GBP SPECT to identify candidates with ventricular asynchrony who may benefit from cardiac resynchronization therapy. GBP SPECT incorporates analysis of RV and LV contraction phase information, in contrast to gated MPI phase analysis, which currently measures only contraction phases for the left ventricle, but not for the right ventricle.[30]

First-Pass Radionuclide Angiography

Clinical Indications

The current primary clinical application for first-pass angiography is to evaluate quantitatively RV function. As briefly mentioned earlier, RV ejection fraction calculations cannot be accurately performed using planar gated

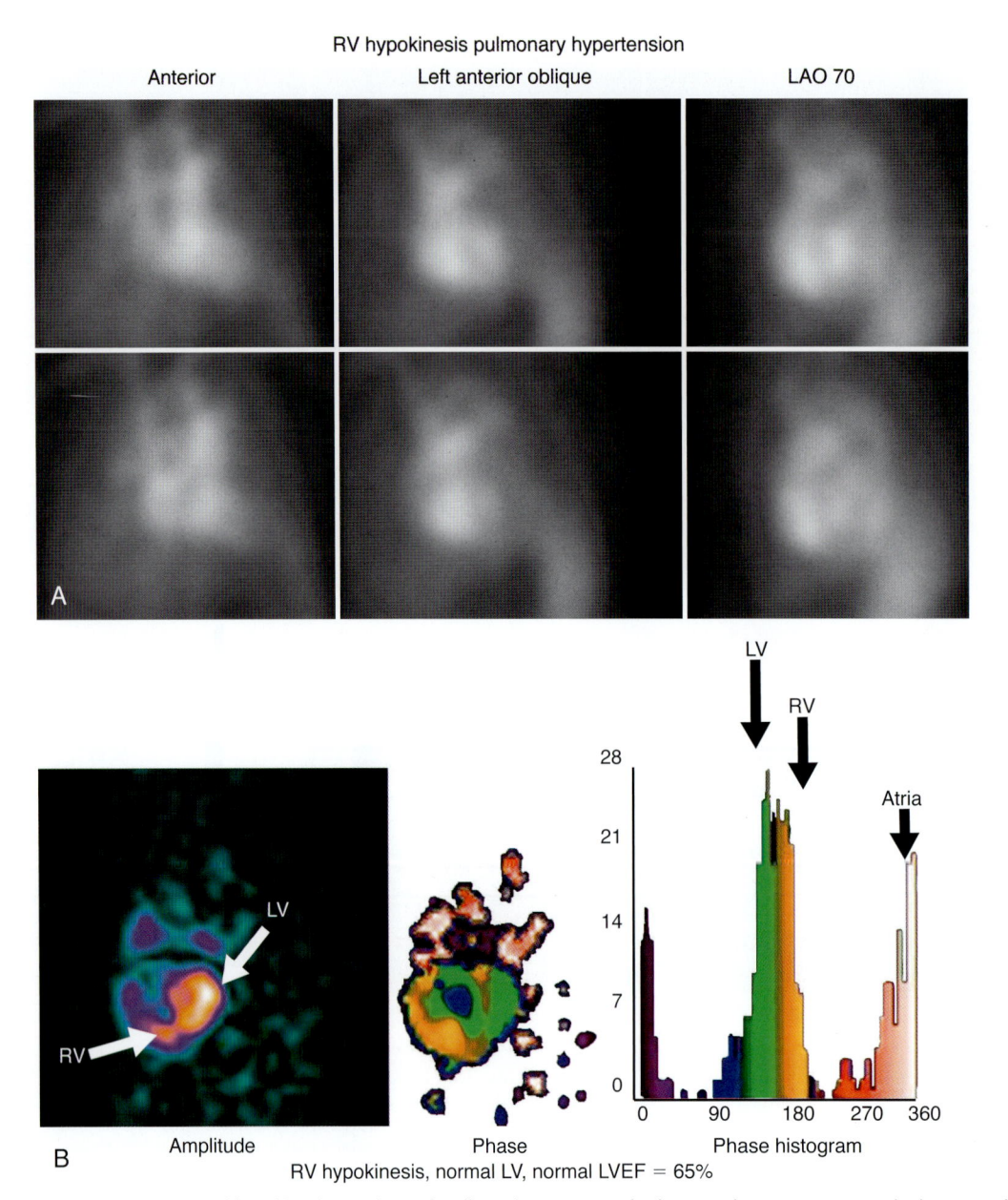

FIGURE 56-3 **A,** RV enlargement and hypokinesis; LV size and wall motion are normal. The RV enlargement rotates the best septal separation view to left anterior oblique 70 degrees (LAO 70). LV ejection fraction (LVEF) = 74%. End-diastolic (*top row*) and end-systolic (*bottom row*) images show markedly enlarged RV cavity at end-diastole and end-systole. LV cavity is normal in size at end-diastole and end-systole. **B,** The parametric amplitude image (*left image*) of the planar LAO 70 acquisition shows relatively lower ventricular change in counts for the right ventricle. The LV change in counts is high, relatively uniform, and normal. The parametric phase image (*middle image*) shows relatively uniform peak activity in the left ventricle, indicating a uniform contraction pattern. The right ventricle is also uniform, but is slightly delayed compared with the left ventricle. The histogram of phase shows a wide ventricular phase with the right ventricle slightly delayed compared with the left ventricle; these are both out of phase compared with the atrial voxels.

equilibrium blood pool techniques. First-pass techniques are elegant, quantitative methods to assess intraventricular shunts. In the past, first-pass techniques used in conjunction with exercise protocols were used to diagnose CAD noninvasively by detection of stress-induced wall motion abnormalities. Generally, first-pass techniques provide relatively lower counts, however, and are more technically challenging to perform compared with tomographic GBP techniques. They are much less commonly used in clinical practice because of the relatively uncommon prevalence specifically requiring their use, and the emergence of alternative techniques, such as contrast echocardiography, which may provide sufficient information for clinical management.

Technical Aspects

Data Acquisition

The technical details of acquisition are extensive and have been reviewed more recently.[5] To perform planar gated first-pass imaging, an ECG gated list mode acquisition is used in conjunction with Tc-99m pertechnetate injection of 740 to 1110 MBq (20 to 30 mCi). Because this is the

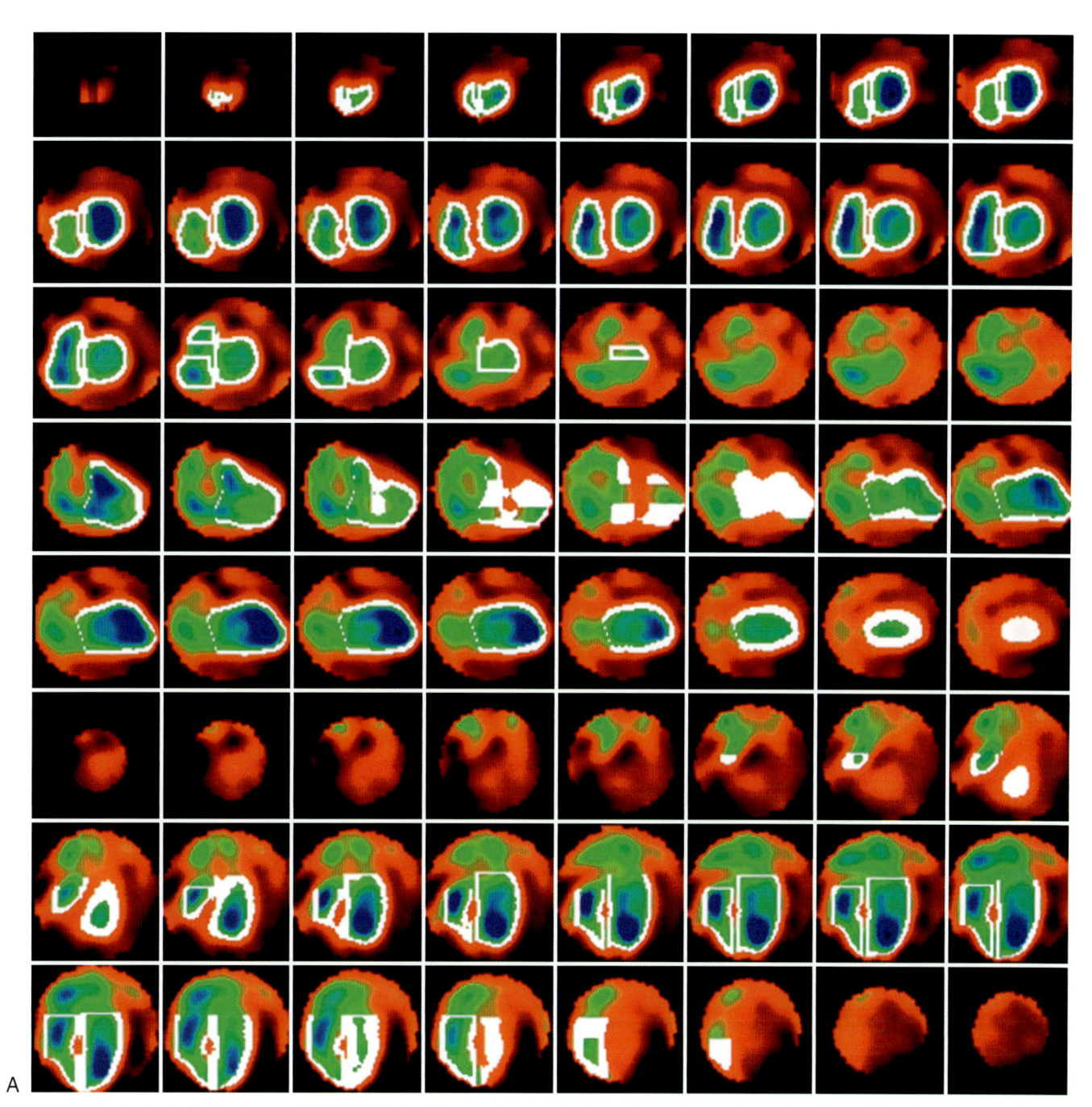

■ **FIGURE 56-4** **A,** Markedly abnormal GBP SPECT of a 75-year-old man with heart failure. Boundaries outline RV and LV regions for analysis. The left ventricle and right ventricle are prominent in size. Short-axis from apex to base (*rows 1 to 3*); vertical long-axis from right ventricle to left ventricle (*rows 4 and 5*); and horizontal long-axis from inferior to anterior (*rows 6 to 8*).

Continued

same radionuclide activity used for GBP imaging, this study can be combined with the aforementioned GBP study to obtain RV ejection fraction and LV ejection fraction measurements. For the first-pass acquisition, the gamma camera is placed in the shallow right anterior oblique (20 to 30 degrees) position to maximize the likely separation of the right atrium and RV outflow tract. The radiotracer is injected over several seconds to allow more heartbeats for RV analysis. A large peripheral vein (antecubital or external jugular) is used, and radiotracer administration is followed by a saline flush.

First-pass images for RV evaluation typically are acquired as high temporal resolution list mode data. The bolus is viewed in cine mode to select the appropriate frames for analysis. RV analysis requires isolation of the specific heartbeats (typically three to six beats) during which the bolus first traveled through the right ventricle. For this imaging application, the very low background activity produces high image contrast and reduces the effect of boundary variability on the RV ejection fraction calculation. The selected heartbeat data are binned with respect to the phase of the ECG cycle, and background-corrected

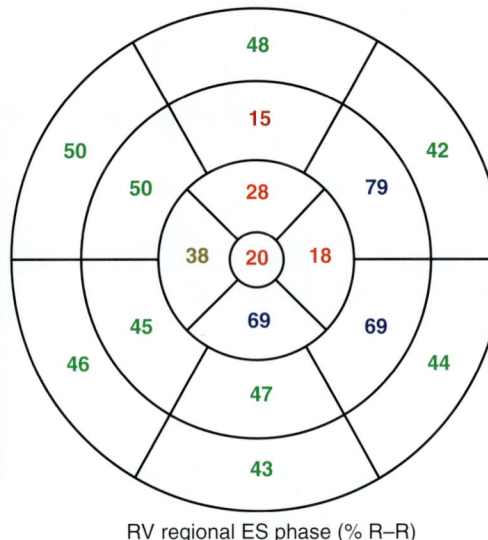

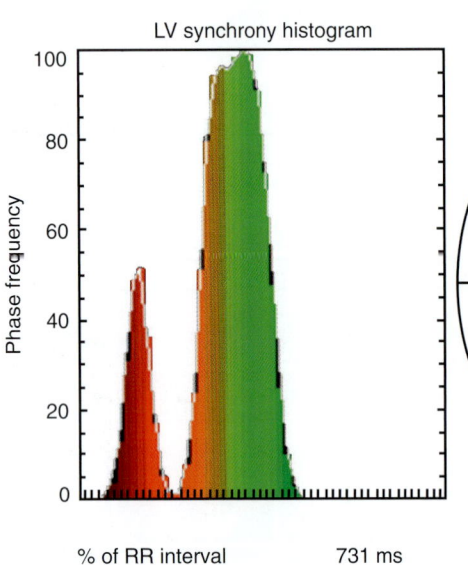

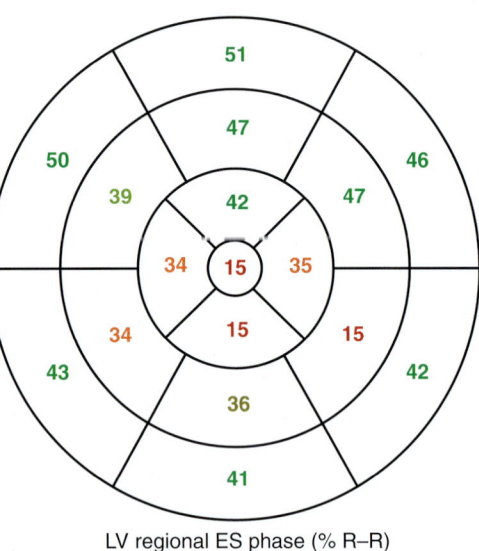

FIGURE 56-4, cont'd B, Quantitative analysis of GBP SPECT. Analysis shows LV apical dyskinesis, which was confirmed by MRI (not shown). LV ejection fraction by GBP SPECT is 21%, and LV ejection fraction by MRI was 23%. Right ventricle (*top row*) and left ventricle (*bottom row*) regional analyses. Phase histogram (*left column*) and polar plots (*right column*) of regional segmental analysis. Phase histogram (*left column*) shows multiple, wide peaks for right ventricle and left ventricle indicating abnormal contraction. A single narrow peak would indicate normal contraction. Polar plots (*right column*) show regional measurements of phase with a wide variation indicating asynchronous contraction. ES, end-systolic. (*Courtesy of K. Nichols, PhD.*)

RV end-diastolic and end-systolic counts are used to determine the RV ejection fraction. Spatially smoothed data are displayed in cine format for visual and quantitative analysis (Fig. 56-5).

Analogous to equilibrium GBP processing, the data from each voxel are fit by Fourier analysis to determine regional phase and amplitude. These data are displayed with the selected first-pass data in cine format to aid in boundary definition and for visual analysis. A disadvantage of the first-pass technique is the low number of counts acquired; this can lead to less visually appealing images and potentially to higher variability in boundary definition. In addition, this method is subject to technical variability if a good bolus through the right ventricle cannot be attained. This situation may be due to poor peripheral intravenous access, right heart failure, or other physiologic issues that may not be amenable to improvement with technique. Administering a higher activity to compensate for this variability is generally not recommended because of radiation dose considerations and gamma camera crystal count rate limitations.

Image Interpretation

The technical aspects of the study, including data acquisition, image processing, and variability in patient physiology, can have a significant impact on final accuracy and interpretation. The first step in interpretation is review of

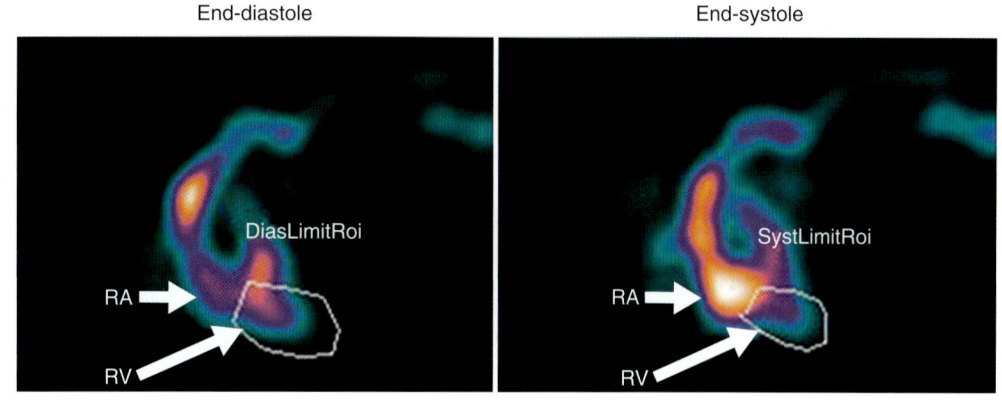

FIGURE 56-5 RV assessment. End-diastole (*left*) and end-systole (*right*). Normal planar first-pass images are obtained in the right anterior oblique 20 degrees orientation in list-mode, proper RV frames are selected and rebinned according to phase of the ECG cycle, and spatial smoothing is applied for cine analysis. Further processing is similar to gated equilibrium blood pool studies. RV ejection fraction (RVEF) is normal at 45%. Semiautomated boundary definitions are aided by amplitude and phase analysis. RA, right atrial.

raw data. Assessment is performed for adequacy of the bolus, tracer transit, counting statistics, ECG rhythm, and number and quality of beats selected for processing. For data analysis, the regions of interest, background region, and parametric phase and amplitude images are inspected. Images displayed in cine format are assessed for chamber size, wall motion, and ejection fraction. RV ejection fraction of 45% or greater is considered normal.[1]

CONCLUSION

Gated MPI SPECT routinely provides quantitative assessment of regional and global LV function. This assessment improves accuracy of image interpretation by increasing specificity in cases of attenuation and increasing sensitivity for multivessel CAD. In addition, functional information is highly prognostic for mortality. Equilibrium GBP scintigraphy provides the most reproducible, accurate, technically feasible, and low-cost method to assess LV function sequentially; this is currently the method of choice to assess potential cardiotoxicity from chemotherapy in oncology patients. Tomographic GBP SPECT is an emerging technique to provide quantitatively accurate regional and global function for the right ventricle and the left ventricle.

The radionuclide first-pass technique is a well-validated method to assess RV ejection fraction accurately and quantitatively; however, it requires technical attention to detail to maintain high accuracy and reproducibility. In addition, unavoidable physiologic factors, such as right heart failure, may adversely affect the technical quality of this study. These technical factors do not adversely affect tomographic gated equilibrium SPECT, and this modality is promising as a method of choice to evaluate RV and LV function simultaneously and quantitatively.

KEY POINTS

- ECG gating, in conjunction with MPI SPECT, provides accurate and reproducible assessment of LV function; these benefits are without additional cost in acquisition time and without additional radiation exposure.
- Planar ECG gated equilibrium blood pool imaging is established as the most accurate and reproducible method to evaluate LV function.
- Planar radionuclide first-pass techniques provide accurate and reproducible measurements of RV function; however, this technique may be subject to factors that adversely affect technical quality.
- ECG gated equilibrium blood pool imaging with SPECT is an emerging technique to quantify RV and LV function with the potential for high accuracy and reproducibility, and without the technical limitations of the first-pass technique.

SUGGESTED READINGS

Gerson MC. Cardiac Nuclear Medicine, 3rd ed. New York, McGraw-Hill, 1997.

Iskandrian AE, Garcia EV. Nuclear Cardiac Imaging: Principles and Applications, 3rd ed. New York, Oxford University Press, 2003.

Lima RSL, Watson DD, Goode AR, et al. Incremental value of combined perfusion and function over perfusion alone by gated SPECT myocardial perfusion imaging for detection of severe three-vessel coronary artery disease. J Am Coll Cardiol 2003; 42:64-70.

Nakajima K, Higuchi T, Taki J, et al. Accuracy of ventricular volume and ejection fraction measured by gated myocardial SPECT: comparison of 4 software programs. J Nucl Med 2001; 42:1571-1578.

Nichols KJ, Van Tosh A, Wang Y, et al. Validation of gated blood-pool SPECT regional left ventricular function measurements. J Nucl Med 2009; 50:53-60.

Phelps ME. PET: Molecular Imaging and Its Biological Applications. New York, Springer, 2004.

Sharir T, Germano G, Kavanagh PB, et al. Incremental prognostic value of post-stress left ventricular ejection fraction and volume by gated myocardial perfusion single photon emission computed tomography. Circulation 1999; 100:1035-1042.

REFERENCES

1. Gerson MC. Cardiac Nuclear Medicine, 3rd ed. New York, McGraw-Hill, 1997.
2. Iskandrian AE, Garcia EV. Nuclear Cardiac Imaging: Principles and Applications, 3rd ed. New York, Oxford University Press, 2003.
3. Zaret BL, Beller G. Clinical Nuclear Cardiology: State of the Art and Future Directions. St Louis, Mosby, 1993.
4. Heller GV, Hendel R. Nuclear Cardiology: Practical Applications. New York, McGraw Hill, 2004.
5. Friedman JD, Berman DS, Borges-Neto S, et al. First-pass radionuclide angiography (abstract). J Nucl Cardiol 2006; 13:e42-e55.
6. Go V, Bhatt MR, Hendel RC. The diagnostic and prognostic value of ECG-gated SPECT myocardial perfusion imaging. J Nucl Med 2004; 45:912-921.
7. Phelps ME. PET: Molecular Imaging and Its Biological Applications. New York, Springer, 2004.
8. Schepis T, Gaemperli O, Koepfli P, et al. Comparison of 64-slice CT with gated SPECT for evaluation of left ventricular function. J Nucl Med 2006; 47:1288-1294.
9. Sharir T, Germano G, Kavanagh PB, et al. Incremental prognostic value of post-stress left ventricular ejection fraction and volume by gated myocardial perfusion single photon emission computed tomography. Circulation 1999; 100:1035-1042.
10. Sharir T, Germano G, Kang XP, et al. Prediction of myocardial infarction versus cardiac death by gated myocardial perfusion SPECT: risk stratification by the amount of stress-induced ischemia and the post-stress ejection fraction. J Nucl Med 2001; 42:831-837.
11. DePuey EG, Rozanski A. Using gated technetium-99m-sestamibi SPECT to characterize fixed myocardial defects as infarct or artifact. J Nucl Med 1995; 36:952-955.
12. Taillefer R, DePuey EG, Udelson JE, et al. Comparative diagnostic accuracy of Tl-201 and Tc-99m sestamibi SPECT imaging (perfusion and ECG-gated SPECT) in detecting coronary artery disease in women. J Am Coll Cardiol 1997; 29:69-77.
13. Shirai N, Yamagishi H, Yoshiyama M, et al. Incremental value of assessment of regional wall motion for detection of multivessel coronary artery disease in exercise Tl-201 gated myocardial perfusion imaging. J Nucl Med 2002; 43:443-450.
14. Lima RSL, Watson DD, Goode AR, et al. Incremental value of combined perfusion and function over perfusion alone by gated SPECT myocardial perfusion imaging for detection of severe three-vessel coronary artery disease. J Am Coll Cardiol 2003; 42:64-70.
15. Kanayama S, Matsunari I, Kajinami K. Comparison of gated N-13 ammonia PET and gated Tc-99m sestamibi SPECT for quantitative analysis of global and regional left ventricular function. J Nucl Cardiol 2007; 14:680-687.
16. Khorsand A, Graf S, Eidherr H, et al. Gated cardiac N-13-NH3 PET for assessment of left ventricular volumes, mass, and ejection fraction: Comparison with electrocardiography-gated F-18-FDG PET. J Nucl Med 2005; 46:2009-2013.
17. Di Carli MF, Dorbala S, Meserve J, et al. Clinical myocardial perfusion PET/CT. J Nucl Med 2007; 48:783-793.
18. Nichols K, Dorbala S, DePuey EG, et al. Influence of arrhythmias on gated SPECT myocardial perfusion and function quantification. J Nucl Med 1999; 40:924-934.
19. Nichols K, Yao SS, Kamran M, et al. Clinical impact of arrhythmias on gated SPECT cardiac myocardial perfusion and function assessment. J Nucl Cardiol 2001; 8:19-30.
20. Faber TL, Cooke CD, Folks RD, et al. Left ventricular function and perfusion from gated SPECT perfusion images: an integrated method. J Nucl Med 1999; 40:650-659.
21. Nichols K, Lefkowitz D, Faber T, et al. Echocardiographic validation of gated SPECT ventricular function measurements. J Nucl Med 2000; 41:1308-1314.
22. Germano G, Kiat H, Kavanagh PB, et al. Automatic quantification of ejection fraction from gated myocardial perfusion SPECT. J Nucl Med 1995; 36:2138-2147.
23. Galt JR, Garcia EV, Robbins WL. Effects of myocardial wall thickness on SPECT quantification. IEEE Trans Med Imaging 1990; 9:144-150.
24. Vallejo E, Dione DP, Bruni WL, et al. Reproducibility and accuracy of gated SPECT for determination of left ventricular volumes and ejection fraction: experimental validation using MRI. J Nucl Med 2000; 41:874-882.
25. Nakajima K, Higuchi T, Taki J, et al. Accuracy of ventricular volume and ejection fraction measured by gated myocardial SPECT: comparison of 4 software programs. J Nucl Med 2001; 42:1571-1578.
26. Gurusher SP, Diwakar J. Monitoring chemotherapy-induced cardiotoxicity: role of cardiac nuclear imaging (abstract). J Nucl Cardiol 2006; 13:415-426.
27. Chin BB, Bloomgarden DC, Xia WS, et al. Right and left ventricular volume and ejection fraction by tomographic gated blood-pool scintigraphy. J Nucl Med 1997; 38:942-948.
28. Nichols KJ, Saouaf R, Ababneh A, et al. Validation of SPECT equilibrium radionuclide angiographic right ventricular parameters by cardiac magnetic resonance imaging (abstract). J Nucl Cardiol 2002; 9:153-160.
29. Nichols K, Van Tosh A, De Bondt P, et al. Normal limits of gated blood pool SPECT count-based regional cardiac function parameters. Int J Cardiovasc Imaging 2008; 24:717-725.
30. Chen J, Henneman MM, Trimble MA, et al. Assessment of left ventricular mechanical dyssynchrony by phase analysis of ECG-gated SPECT myocardial perfusion imaging. J Nucl Cardiol 2008;15:127-136.

CHAPTER 57

Magnetic Resonance Imaging of Myocardial Viability

Zelmira Curillova and Raymond Kwong

Heart failure is a complex clinical syndrome with high hospitalization and mortality rates. The incidence of heart failure approaches 10 per 1000 in the population older than 65 years.[1] The most common etiology of heart failure in developed countries is coronary artery disease. In patients with left ventricular (LV) dysfunction, it is of great therapeutic and prognostic importance to differentiate irreversibly damaged scarred myocardium, dysfunctional but viable myocardium (hibernating or stunned), and LV dysfunction from causes not related to coronary artery disease. The assessment of myocardial viability is important to guide the management of patients with ischemic LV dysfunction when clinicians must weigh the risks and benefits of coronary revascularization in regard to the increased perioperative morbidity and mortality in this patient population.[2,3]

The meta-analysis by Allman and colleagues[4] assessed the prognostic value of viability assessment across various nuclear and echocardiographic techniques. Determining the presence and extent of myocardial viability is crucial in guiding clinical decision making and influencing patient outcomes. Patients with significant viability assigned to be treated medically had higher rates of cardiac mortality (16% vs. 3.2% per year) and nonfatal myocardial infarction (MI) (12.2% vs. 6% per year) than patients who were assigned to undergo coronary revascularization. In patients without significant myocardial viability, there was no difference in annual mortality or nonfatal MI rates between coronary revascularization and medical therapy (7.7% vs. 6.2% and 10.2% vs. 8%).[4] These findings underscore the importance of noninvasive assessment of viability in guiding appropriate treatment decision making.

VIABILITY DEFINITIONS

Dysfunctional but viable myocardium in patients with ischemic cardiomyopathy can be divided into two general categories: myocardial stunning and hibernation. These two processes likely coexist and lead to varying degrees of LV dysfunction depending on the severity of coronary stenosis, coronary vasomotor tone, hemodynamic states, and duration of ischemic episodes. *Myocardial stunning* is defined by nonpermanent contractile dysfunction resulting from transient ischemia without injury. *Hibernation* is a state of chronically impaired resting myocardial function resulting from reduced coronary blood flow.

Stunned and hibernating myocardium can benefit from restoration of blood supply. Rahimtoola[5] first reported the process of myocardial hibernation, and it was then observed that LV dysfunction resulting from myocardial hibernation is not an irreversible process. The process of myocardial hibernation is a dynamic process that involves a continuum of downregulation of myocyte metabolism, reduction in contractile elements, and dedifferentiation of myocardial cells with preserved cell membrane integrity. The following processes have been observed in hibernating myocardium: loss of sarcomeres, sarcoplasmic reticulum, and T tubules; intracellular buildup of glycogen; atrophic mitochondria; accumulation of extracellular matrix and fibrosis; and expression of fetal proteins.[6]

There are various noninvasive techniques to image myocardial viability. The traditional nuclear techniques include single photon emission computed tomography (SPECT) perfusion using thallium 201 or Tc 99m sestamibi or tetrofosmin radiotracers. The detection of viable myocardium with these radiotracers is based on the presence of intact cell membrane or intact mitochondria. [18]FDG is used as a radiotracer in positron emission tomography (PET) or SPECT to detect preserved glucose metabolism in the myocytes. Echocardiography assesses myocardial contractile reserve with low-dose (5 to 15 µg/kg/min) dobutamine infusion. This chapter explores the role of MRI and CT in assessment of myocardial viability.

MAGNETIC RESONANCE IMAGING ASSESSMENT OF MYOCARDIAL VIABILITY

Several MRI techniques exist to assess myocardial viability. Common clinical techniques include assessment of LV end-diastolic wall thickness on resting cine MRI, myocardial contractile reserve and ischemia by dobutamine stress MRI (dobutamine MRI), and transmural extent of MI by contrast-enhanced myocardial delayed enhancement (MDE) imaging. Other MRI techniques, such as quantification of myocardial contractile reserve with MRI tagging[7,8] and MR spectroscopy for assessment of high-energy phosphates metabolism (e.g., quantification of concentration and ratio of adenosine triphosphate and phosphocreatine using ^{31}P spectroscopy within a small volume of myocardium), are currently not in wide clinical use and are beyond the scope of this chapter.[9,10]

Wall Thickness

In the presence of extensive chronic MI, wall thinning develops in the infarct zone because of infarct resorption and fibrotic contracture. Although autopsy studies have shown that wall thinning is frequently associated with transmural scar,[11,12] end-diastolic wall thickness (EDWT) measured in millimeters has limited prediction for functional recovery after revascularization, which serves as the most common surrogate reference method for myocardial viability. Baer and coworkers[13] compared resting MRI with [18]FDG-PET in 35 patients. Regions with EDWT less than 5.5 mm had significantly reduced [18]FDG uptake compared with regions with thickness 5.5 mm or greater that had preserved [18]FDG uptake. The same investigators also tested the predictive value of EDWT for functional recovery after revascularization. A EDWT cutoff of 5.5 mm had 94% sensitivity, but only 52% specificity for predicting segmental functional recovery after revascularization.[14]

The low specificity of LV wall thinning can be attributed to the fact that myocardial segments even with preserved wall thickness can have substantial transmural scar. In addition, EDWT is a structural variable that does not assess physiologic response of the myocardium, and there is a wide variation of EDWT among individuals and among different myocardial segments in the same individual.[15] Kim and Shah[15] showed that regional wall thinning may occur early after MI even in the absence of transmural necrosis, and that the thinned myocardium can still improve its contractile function.

Dobutamine Magnetic Resonance Imaging Contractile Reserve

Improvement in wall thickening or contractile reserve in response to inotropic challenge such as a low-dose dobutamine infusion (5 to 15 µg/kg/min) has been well validated for assessment of myocardial viability in echocardiography and MRI literature.[14,16-20] There are several advantages of MRI over the conventional echocardiography for detecting contractile reserve. Widely used cine steady-state free precession provides excellent spatial resolution and tissue contrast between the blood pool and LV myocardium. In contrast to echocardiography, which is limited by acoustic windows, MRI is able to provide multiplanar image acquisition for improved volumetric coverage of the heart. The quantification of LV volumes, mass, and ejection fraction with MRI does not require any geometric assumptions and is highly reproducible.[21]

Schmidt and colleagues[22] assessed resting EDWT (5.5 mm cutoff), dobutamine-induced wall thickening of greater than 2 mm, and presence of normalized [18]FDG uptake greater than 50% on PET in 40 patients with chronic MI to predict segmental functional recovery. The sensitivity and specificity for segmental functional recovery were 100% and 53% for resting EDWT 5.5 mm or greater alone, 96% and 87% for dobutamine-induced contractile reserve, and 100% and 73% for preserved [18]FDG (>50%) uptake. These findings indicate that dichotomizing a threshold value of resting EDWT or [18]FDG uptake is less accurate than the physiologic assessment of low-dose dobutamine challenge. This point is supported further by a study reported by Wellnhofer and associates,[20] which showed higher specificity of dobutamine MRI compared with transmural extent of late hyperenhancement on MDE imaging to predict functional recovery, especially with 1% to 74% transmural extent of late hyperenhancement.

Contractile response during low-dose dobutamine challenge is specific, yet is only moderately sensitive in detecting segmental viability. Kaandorp and coworkers[23] reported a weighted mean sensitivity and specificity for predicting functional recovery of 73% and 83% after pooling nine previously published dobutamine MRI studies. The relatively low sensitivity of dobutamine MRI can be attributed to the fact that in the presence of severe coronary stenosis, viable myocardial segments fail to show augmentation of segmental thickening because of rapid development of ischemia even with low dobutamine doses. We choose to infuse low-dose dobutamine using 5-minute per stage protocol. This prolonged infusion allows building up of the inotropic effects of the dobutamine, and the resultant display of augmentation of segmental thickening may enhance the sensitivity in detection of segmental viability.

Hyperenhancement on Myocardial Delayed Enhancement Imaging

The basis for development of MDE imaging was an observation that the differential between normal and infarcted myocardium can be accentuated by the use of gadolinium-chelate contrast agents on T1-weighted images.[24] Gadolinium shortens the T1 relaxation time of tissues with increased gadolinium content. Nevertheless, the limitation in image quality had restricted the clinical application of contrast-enhanced MRI until recent years. The proposed mechanism of hyperenhancement on MDE (also known as *late gadolinium enhancement*) is related to a relatively large molecular size of conventional extracellular gadolinium-chelate contrast agents that is made metabolically inert by the chelation and unable to cross the cell membrane of a normal myocyte. When the cell membrane is damaged (e.g., acute MI), or if there is an increase in the extracellular space between myocytes (e.g., acute interstitial edema or chronic fibrosis), there is accumulation of gadolinium-chelate contrast agent in the extracellular space, and its washout is delayed after the injection (Fig. 57-1).

Areas of abnormal myocardium (e.g., infarcted, fibrotic, inflamed, or infiltrated myocardium) have elevated per-voxel gadolinium concentration and have a brighter signal (i.e., hyperenhancement) relative to normally enhancing myocardium, which appears nulled (i.e., dark) on the T1-weighted inversion recovery imaging sequence used for MDE imaging.[25] Using this technique in a clinical setting of coronary artery disease, dysfunctional myocardium with normal nulled signal intensity suggests myocardial stunning or hibernation. In acute or chronic MI, myocardial hyperenhancement characteristically involves the subendocardium or progresses to involve the entire transmural extent in myocardial segments subtended by a coronary arterial territory (Fig. 57-2). Apart from illustration of myocardial hyperenhancement consistent with MI, other specific patterns of hyperenhancement (mid-wall, epicardial, focal, or diffuse) can also provide potential differentiation of other etiologies of cardiomyopathy, such as myocarditis, nonischemic idiopathic dilated cardiomyopathy, cardiac sarcoidosis, cardiac amyloidosis, or endomyocardial fibrosis (Fig. 57-3).[26]

Many animal and human studies have validated the use of this technique to detect the presence of or the extent of MI. Kim and colleagues[27] used the inversion recovery MDE technique in 18 dogs with experimental MI and showed that MDE imaging accurately depicts the extent of histologically defined necrosis. The signal intensity of the infarcted myocardium was on average three to six times higher than the signal intensity of the normal myocardium during the acute and convalescence phases of infarction, allowing sensitive delineation of the transmural extent of myonecrosis. These authors also showed high agreement between the extent of scar tissue on MDE and histologic extent of necrosis across all time points during infarct healing (Fig. 57-4).[27]

Kim and colleagues[28] went on to study the use of gadolinium-enhanced MDE MRI in 50 patients with LV dysfunction before undergoing surgical or percutaneous revascularization. They showed that the likelihood of improvement in segmental myocardial contractility after revascularization decreased progressively with the increased transmural extent of the myocardial hyperenhancement on MDE (Fig. 57-5). The major advantage contrast-enhanced MDE MRI had over other imaging

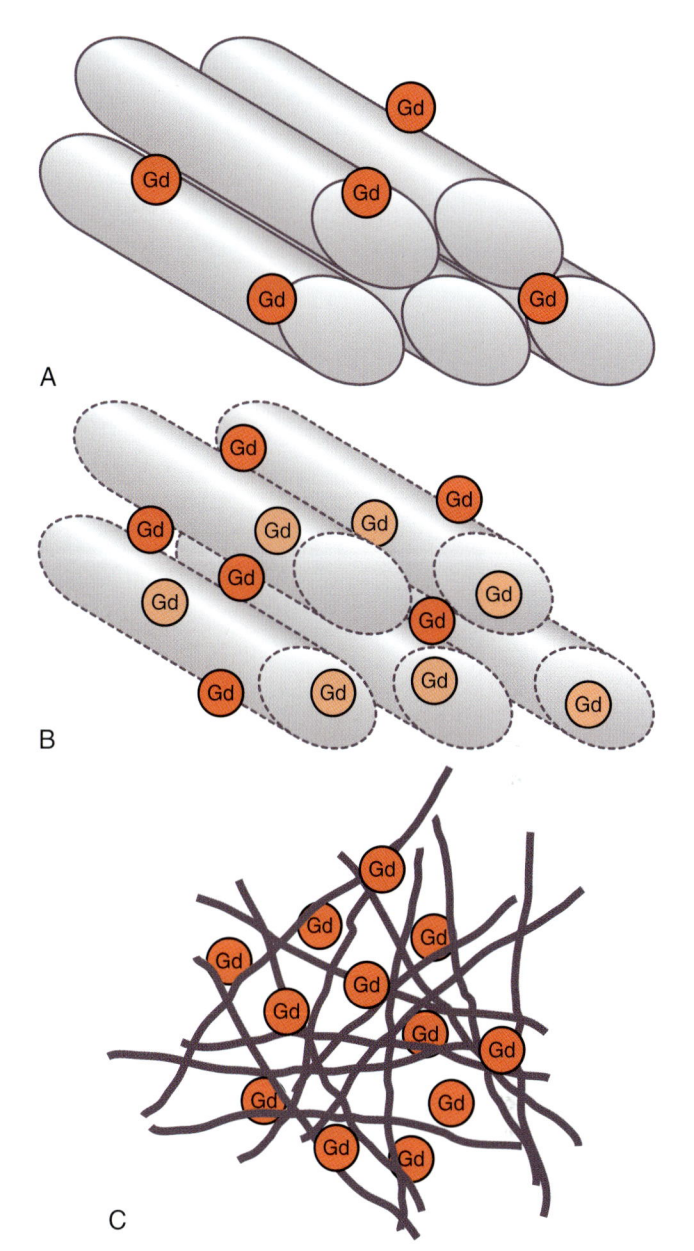

FIGURE 57-1 Diagram of potential mechanisms for hyperenhancement on MDE MRI. The actual mechanisms for hyperenhancement on MDE imaging have yet to be determined. Differing theories have been proposed, however, for hyperenhancement that is noted clinically in acute versus chronic MI. **A**, In healthy myocardium, intact cell membranes preclude gadolinium-chelate contrast medium (Gd) from entering the otherwise tightly arranged myocytes, and Gd remains primarily extracellular in the interstitial space. Normally, there is no significant Gd retention on delayed imaging, and myocardial signal is typically homogeneously nulled on MDE imaging. **B**, With acute MI, myocyte cell membranes rupture, enabling the intracellular entry of Gd into the swollen myocytes, resulting in an increased concentration of Gd and hyperenhancement on MDE imaging. The concomitant edema and increase in interstitial space associated with acute MI may also contribute to the retention of interstitial Gd and hyperenhancement. **C**, With chronic MI, myocardial scarring occurs. Myocytes are replaced with collagen matrix and an increased interstitial space, which has been proposed as the underlying cause for an increased concentration of Gd and hyperenhancement on delayed imaging.

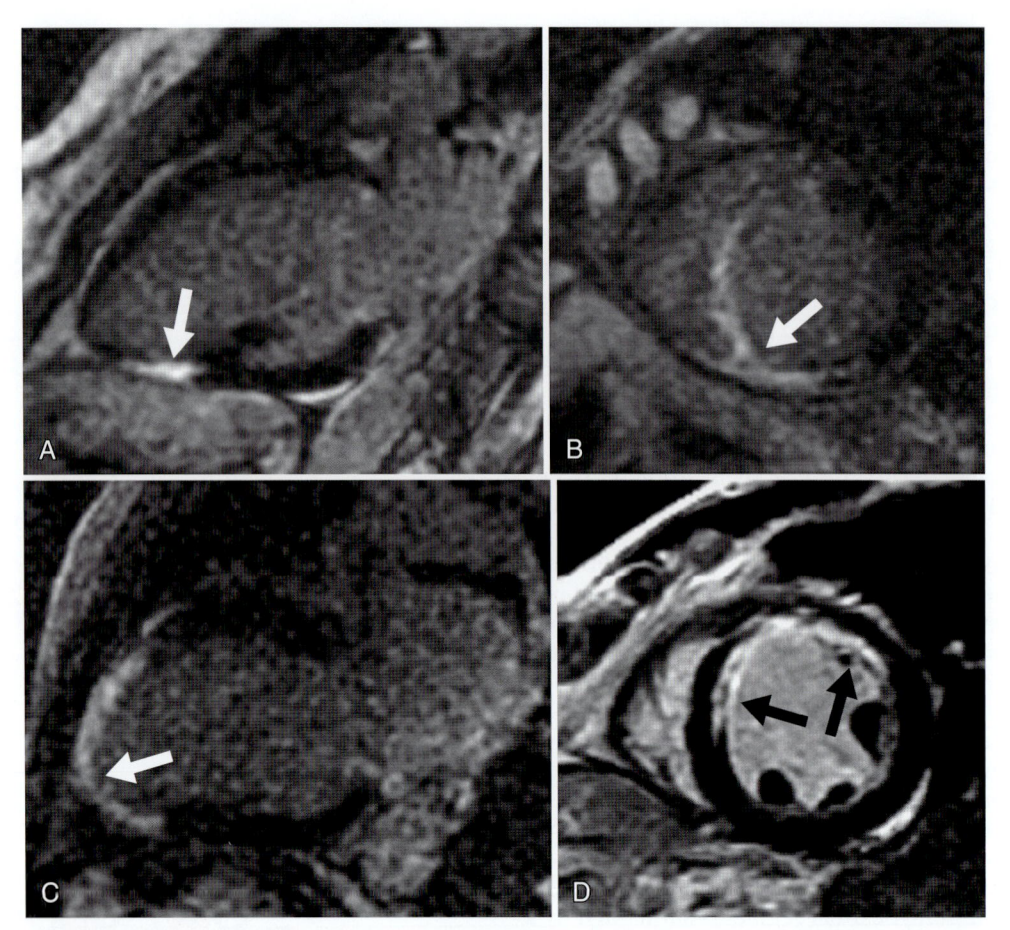

FIGURE 57-2 Hyperenhancement on MDE using MRI in four different patients. **A-C,** Transmural hyperenhancement (*arrows*) represents significant MI with little viable myocardium (**A,** inferior wall MI; **B,** inferior and inferoseptal wall MI; **C,** apical MI). **D,** Less severe hyperenhancement (*arrows*) limited to the subendocardium (anteroseptal, anterior, and anterolateral MI)—that is, less than full thickness or transmural hyperenhancement—corresponds with residual viable myocardium in the affected regions that is represented by the proportion of normal (nonhyperenhancing) nulled or dark myocardium. Generally, the less transmurality of hyperenhancement (e.g. <25%) corresponds with higher likelihood for functional improvement after a myocardial revascularization procedure.

modalities is the ability to assess the presence of subendocardial micromyonecrosis and the transmural extent of MI because of the excellent spatial resolution of this technique (1 to 3 mm in-plane).

Ricciardi and associates[29] studied a small group of patients without history of infarction who had elevated creatine kinase-MB enzyme after percutaneous coronary intervention. They found that MDE MRI detected discrete areas of myonecrosis that were not detected by cine wall motion imaging. Wagner and colleagues[30] compared the detection of MI by gadolinium-enhanced MDE MRI and SPECT in 12 dogs. Both imaging modalities detected all segments with greater than 75% transmural extent of MI. Gadolinium-enhanced MRI detected 92% of segments with less than 50% transmural infarction, whereas SPECT detected only 28% of those segments (Fig. 57-6).[30]

Klein and coworkers[31] directly compared MDE MRI with ^{18}FDG-PET in 31 patients with severe LV dysfunction. They found that myocardial hyperenhancement on MDE imaging correlated well with areas of PET scar defined as matched decrease in perfusion and metabolism. Of segments defined as viable by PET, 11% showed some degree of subendocardial hyperenhancement, reflecting the stronger capability of MRI in detecting small subendocardial infarction than PET because of its higher spatial resolution.

COMPUTED TOMOGRAPHY FOR ASSESSMENT OF MYOCARDIAL VIABILITY

Multidetector CT is a noninvasive imaging technique primarily used for evaluation of coronary artery anatomy and coronary stenoses. Coronary multidetector CT provides a three-dimensional volumetric data set of the entire heart after injection of iodinated contrast medium, and the data can be reconstructed at multiple phases of the cardiac cycle, able to provide additional functional information, such as LV volumes, mass, and ejection fraction. In small pilot clinical studies, comparison with MRI showed a good correlation in measuring LV volumes and global LV ejection fraction.[32,33]

Another emerging application of multidetector CT is evaluation of myocardial perfusion and viability. Similar to MRI, multidetector CT images are acquired during administration of an intravenous bolus of contrast agent. Similar to MRI first-pass perfusion technique, the hypoperfused

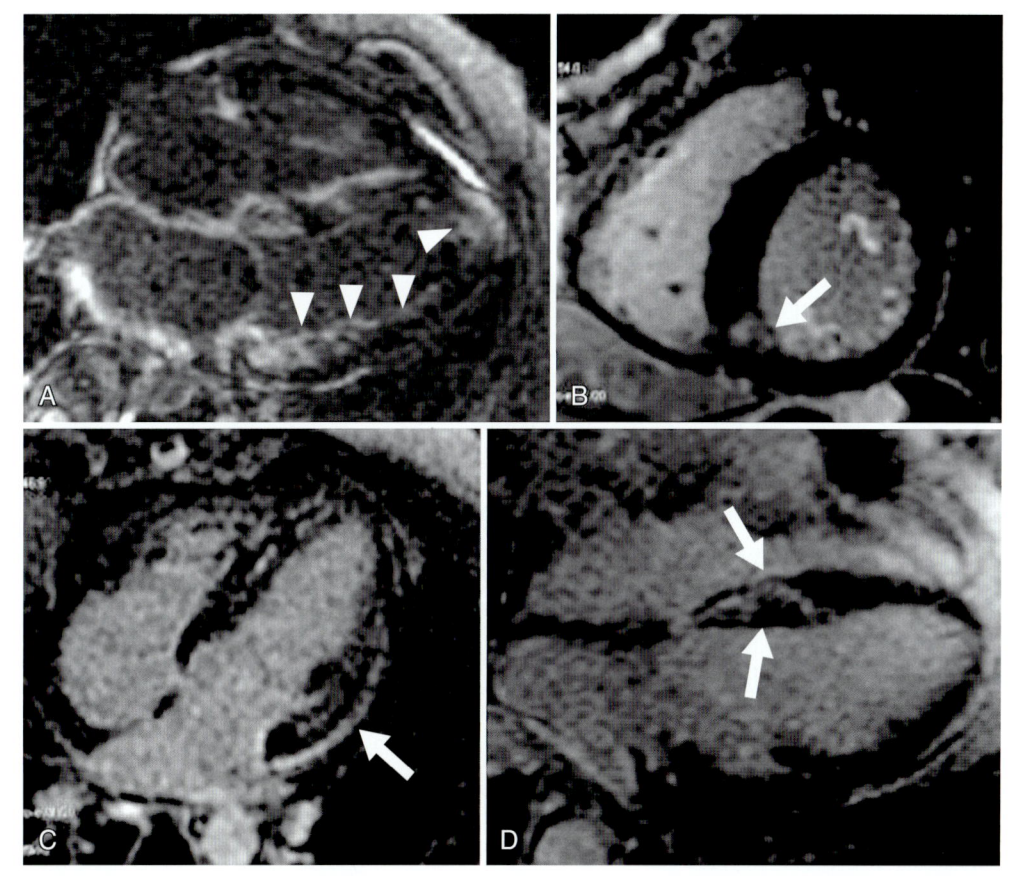

■ **FIGURE 57-3** Patterns of hyperenhancement on MDE using MRI in four patients with nonischemic cardiomyopathy. **A-D,** Cardiac amyloidosis (**A,** diffuse subendocardial hyperenhancement [*arrowheads*]), hypertropic cardiomyopathy (**B,** mid-myocardial hyperenhancement [*arrow*]), myocarditis (**C,** subepicardial hyperenhancement [*arrow*]), and cardiac sarcoidosis (**D,** mid-myocardial hyperenhancement [*arrows*]). These patterns are distinct from the hyperenhancement of MI that is based primarily in the subendocardial region or subendocardium outward, a distribution consistent with the end-vessel territory of the coronary circulation.

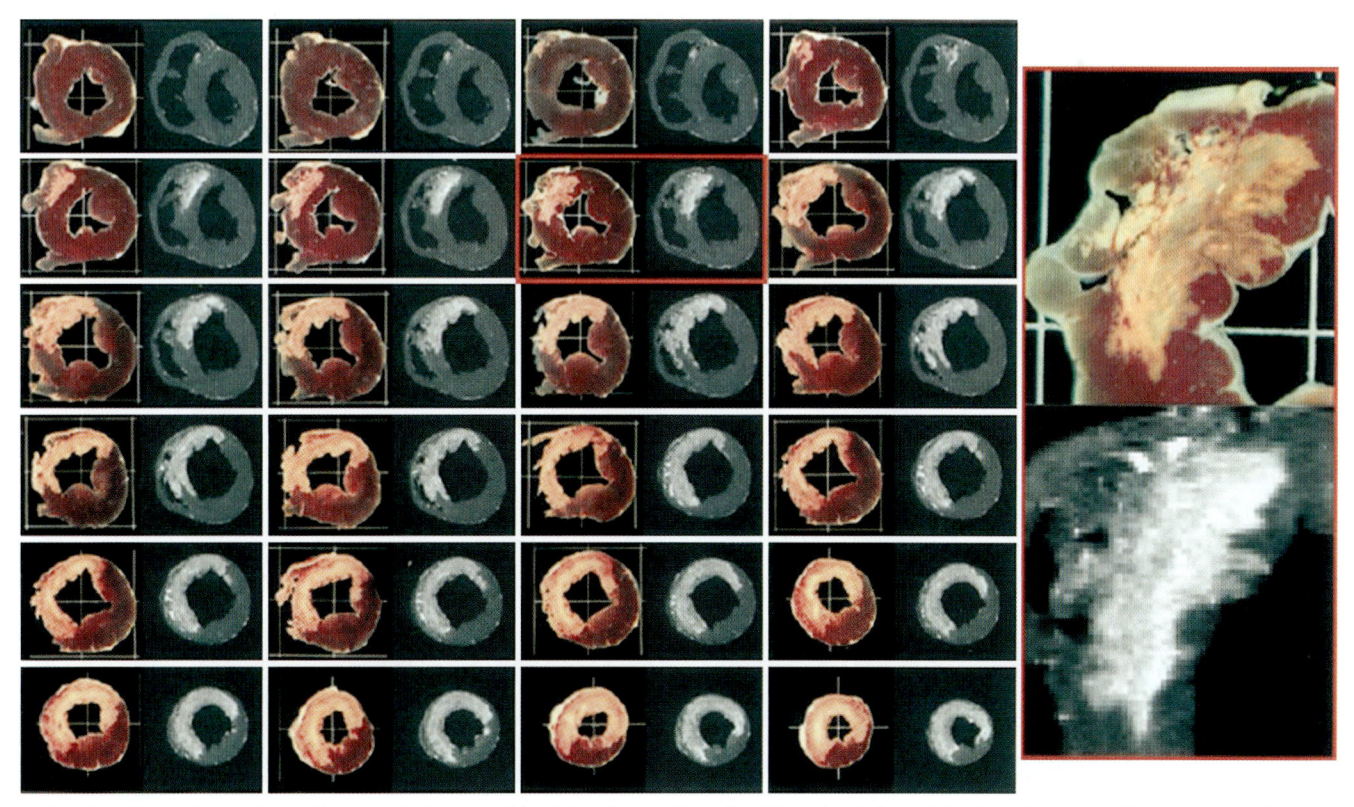

■ **FIGURE 57-4** Comparison of ex vivo MR images with triphenyltetrazolium chloride–stained slices of the heart in an animal 3 days after infarct. Slices are arranged from base to apex starting at the top. On the right is a magnified view. *(From Kim RJ, Fieno DS, Parrish TB, et al. Relationship of MRI delayed contrast enhancement to irreversible injury, infarct age, and contractile function. Circulation 1999; 100:1992-2002.)*

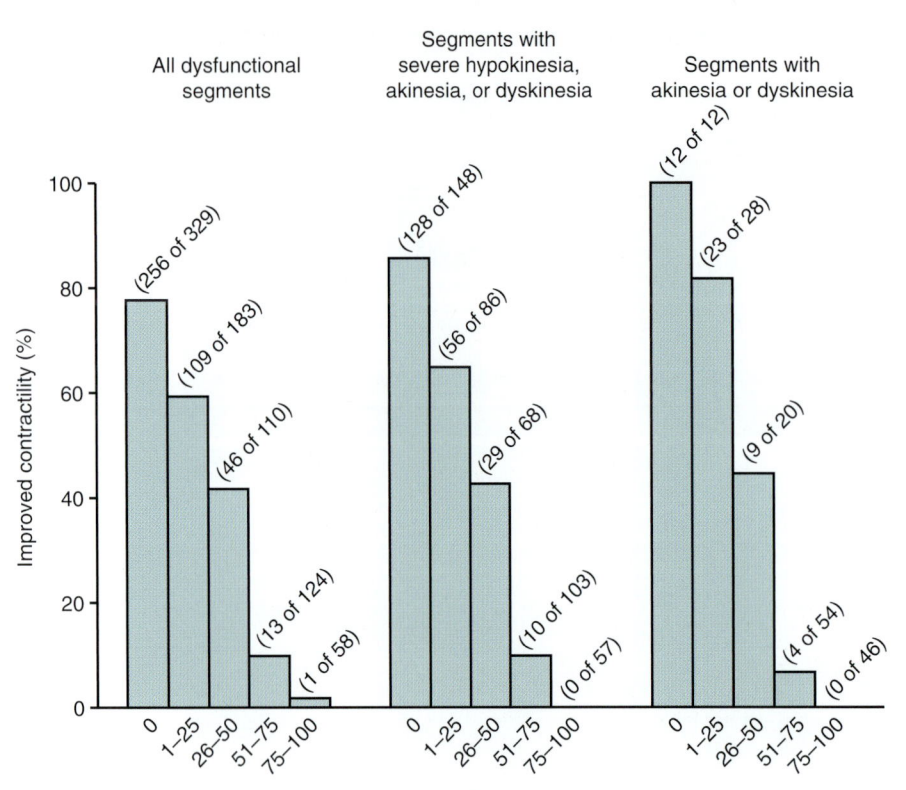

FIGURE 57-5 Relationship between the transmural extent of hyperenhancement on MDE imaging before revascularization and the likelihood of increased contractility after revascularization. *(From Kim RJ, Wu E, Rafael A, et al. The use of contrast-enhanced magnetic resonance imaging to identify reversible myocardial dysfunction. N Engl J Med 2000; 343:1445-1453.)*

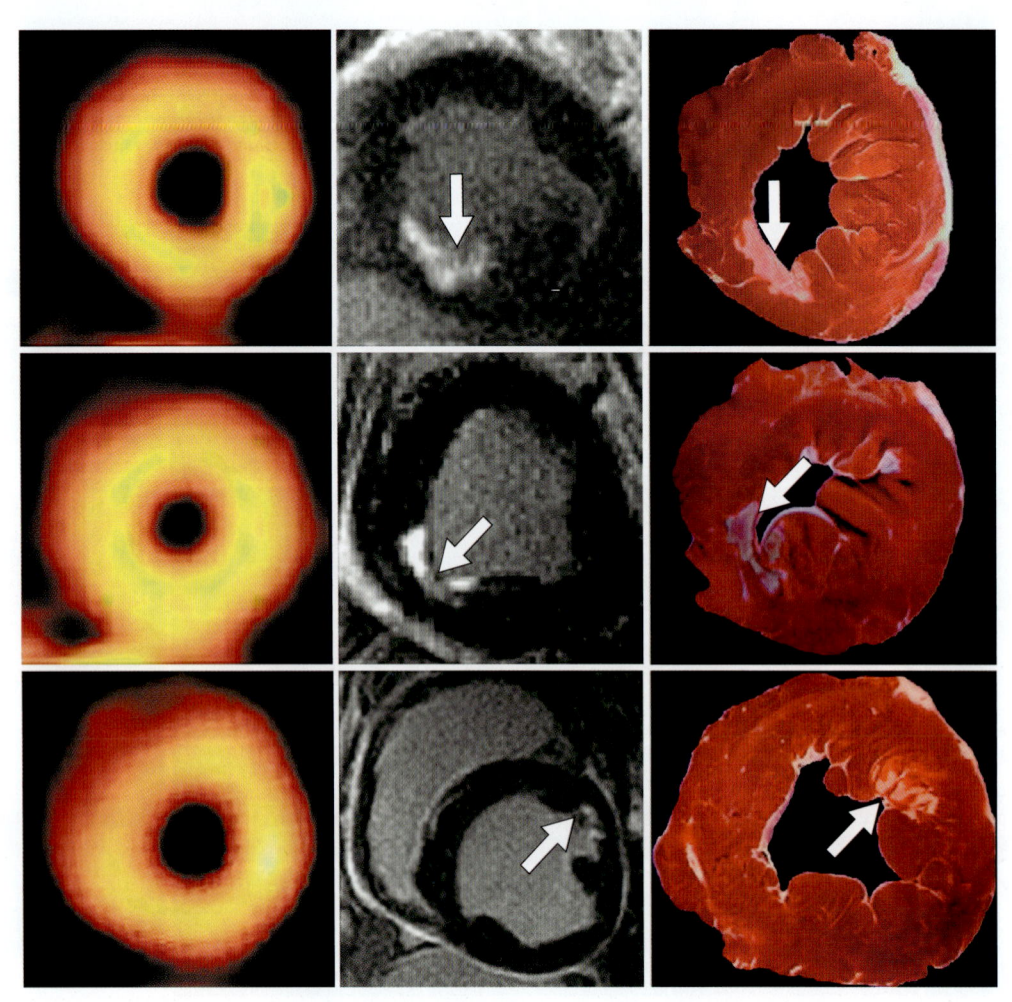

FIGURE 57-6 Short-axis views from three dogs with subendocardial infarcts. From *left to right*, SPECT, MDE MRI, and histology with triphenyltetrazolium chloride staining. *(From Wagner A, Mahrholdt H, Holly TA, et al. Contrast-enhanced MRI and routine single photon emission computed tomography [SPECT] perfusion imaging for detection of subendocardial myocardial infarcts: an imaging study. Lancet 2003; 361:374-379.)*

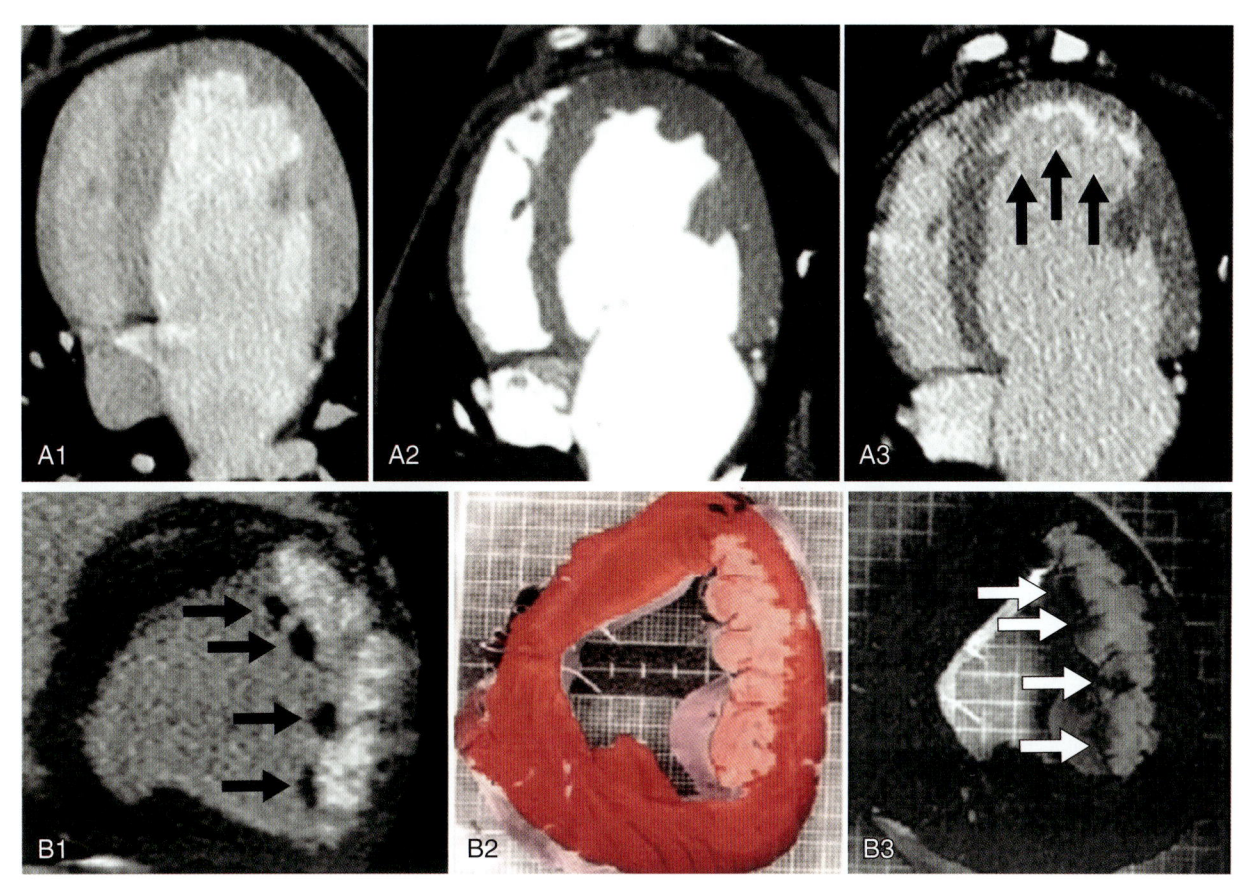

■ **FIGURE 57-7** **A,** Typical contrast-enhanced multidetector CT myocardial images: *A1,* at baseline (preinfarct) obtained 5 minutes after contrast agent administration; *A2,* postinfarct during first-pass contrast agent injection; and *A3,* postinfarct 5 minutes after contrast agent injection. The infarcted region is represented by subendocardial anterior hyperenhancing region (*arrows*). **B,** Multidetector CT and histopathologic staining comparison of infarct morphology: *B1,* reconstructed short-axis multidetector CT slice 5 minutes after contrast agent injection showing a large anterolateral infarct (hyperenhancing region) with discrete endocardial regions of microvascular obstruction (*arrows*); *B2,* triphenyltetrazolium chloride–stained slice; and *B3,* triphenyltetrazolium chloride and thioflavine S staining of the same slice confirming the size and location of the microvascular obstruction. *(From Lardo AC, Cordeiro MA, Silva C, et al. Contrast-enhanced multidetector computed tomography viability imaging after myocardial infarction: characterization of myocyte death, microvascular obstruction, and chronic scar. Circulation 2006; 113:394-404.)*

areas on dynamic contrast-enhanced multidetector CT have lower attenuation compared with normally perfused myocardial segments.[34] Nieman and associates[35] investigated the ability of multidetector CT to differentiate recent and chronic MI based on CT attenuation measured in Hounsfield units (HU). Significantly lower CT attenuation values on the CT perfusion images were found in patients with long-standing MI (−13 ± 37 HU) than in patients with acute MI (26 ± 26 HU) or normal controls (73 ± 14 HU).

Using MDE multidetector CT in animal models of acute and chronic MI, Lardo and coworkers[36] could identify the infarct size and its transmural extent when compared with histology (Fig. 57-7). The peak hyperenhancement of infarcted regions occurred approximately 5 minutes after contrast injection (see Fig. 57-7A1-A3). Acute and chronic infarcts by multidetector CT were characterized by hyperenhancement on MDE imaging, whereas regions of microvascular obstruction were characterized by hypoenhancement. Lessick and colleagues[37] evaluated sensitivity of myocardial early perfusion defects and late enhancement with multidetector CT in 26 patients with acute MI to predict myocardial functional recovery. They concluded that in segments abnormal at baseline, the lack of functional recovery was related to the presence and size of the defect on early perfusion and late enhancement.

LIMITATIONS

There are contraindications for MRI in patients with hazardous metallic implants, such as cardiac defibrillators or pacemakers. Patients with claustrophobia can be premedicated with a low-dose sedative, or in more severe cases, intravenous conscious sedation can be used. The image quality of MRI is limited in patients unable to lie still, patients unable to maintain breath-holding, or patients with irregular heart rate (e.g., atrial fibrillation or frequent ectopy). Alternative MRI techniques can be used in patients with breath-holding difficulties, such as navigator respiratory gating or single-shot MDE imaging provided by some MRI vendors. Administration of gadolinium-chelates has been associated with rare cases of nephrogenic systemic fibrosis, especially in patients with renal dysfunction.

Cardiac CT is a fast imaging technique, but has the associated concerns of ionizing radiation exposure and iodinated contrast agent use. The radiation dose for 64-slice coronary multidetector CT was reported to range from 15 to 21 mSv without the ECG gated dose modulation and 9 to 14 mSv with dose modulation. Organ-specific radiation doses are reported to range from 42 to 91 mSv for the lungs and 50 to 80 mSv for female breast, findings associated with non-negligible lifetime attributable risk of cancer.[38] Other limitations of multidetector CT relate to use of iodinated contrast medium with increased risk of contrast-induced nephropathy or allergic reaction. Similar to MRI, the CT image quality is limited in patients unable to maintain breath-holding or in patients with fast or irregular heart rate. There is currently a paucity of data on validation and prognostic implications of CT-based perfusion and MDE imaging.

> **KEY POINTS**
>
> - Cardiac MRI is the current standard in detection of infarction and quantification of infarct size.
> - Cardiac MRI provides accurate prediction of segmental and global recovery of ventricular function as benefits from coronary revascularization.
> - Myocardial enhancement patterns provide unique information in tissue characteristics and diagnostic value in patients with cardiomyopathy.

SUGGESTED READINGS

Kim RJ, Pennell DJ. Cardiovascular magnetic resonance imaging. Heart Failure Clinics 2009; 5:3.

Kwong RY (ed). Cardiovascular Magnetic Resonance Imaging. Totowa, NJ, Humana Press, 2008.

REFERENCES

1. Rosamond W, Flegal K, Furie K, et al. Heart disease and stroke statistics—2008 update: a report from the American Heart Association Statistics Committee and Stroke Statistics Subcommittee. Circulation 2008; 117:e25-e146.
2. Alderman EL, Fisher LD, Litwin P, et al. Results of coronary artery surgery in patients with poor left ventricular function (CASS). Circulation 1983; 68:785-795.
3. Pepper J. Surgery for hibernation. Heart (British Cardiac Society) 2004; 90:144-145.
4. Allman KC, Shaw LJ, Hachamovitch R, et al. Myocardial viability testing and impact of revascularization on prognosis in patients with coronary artery disease and left ventricular dysfunction: a meta-analysis. J Am Coll Cardiol 2002; 39:1151-1158.
5. Rahimtoola SH. The hibernating myocardium. Am Heart J 1989; 117:211-221.
6. Maes A, Flameng W, Nuyts J, et al. Histological alterations in chronically hypoperfused myocardium: correlation with PET findings. Circulation 1994; 90:735-745.
7. Geskin G, Kramer CM, Rogers WJ, et al. Quantitative assessment of myocardial viability after infarction by dobutamine magnetic resonance tagging. Circulation 1998; 98:217-223.
8. Sayad DE, Willett DL, Hundley WG, et al. Dobutamine magnetic resonance imaging with myocardial tagging quantitatively predicts improvement in regional function after revascularization. Am J Cardiol 1998; 82:1149-1151, A1110.
9. Yabe T, Mitsunami K, Inubushi T, et al. Quantitative measurements of cardiac phosphorus metabolites in coronary artery disease by 31P magnetic resonance spectroscopy. Circulation 1995; 92:15-23.
10. Bottomley PA, Weiss RG. Non-invasive magnetic-resonance detection of creatine depletion in non-viable infarcted myocardium. Lancet 1998; 351:714-718.
11. Dubnow MH, Burchell HB, Titus JL. Postinfarction ventricular aneurysm: a clinicomorphologic and electrocardiographic study of 80 cases. Am Heart J 1965; 70:753-760.
12. Fishbein MC, Maclean D, Maroko PR. The histopathologic evolution of myocardial infarction. Chest 1978; 73:843-849.
13. Baer FM, Voth E, Schneider CA, et al. Comparison of low-dose dobutamine-gradient-echo magnetic resonance imaging and positron emission tomography with [18F]fluorodeoxyglucose in patients with chronic coronary artery disease: a functional and morphological approach to the detection of residual myocardial viability. Circulation 1995; 91:1006-1015.
14. Baer FM, Theissen P, Schneider CA, et al. Dobutamine magnetic resonance imaging predicts contractile recovery of chronically dysfunctional myocardium after successful revascularization. J Am Coll Cardiol 1998; 31:1040-1048.
15. Kim RJ, Shah DJ. Fundamental concepts in myocardial viability assessment revisited: when knowing how much is "alive" is not enough. Heart (British Cardiac Society) 2004; 90:137-140.
16. Anselmi M, Golia G, Cicoira M, et al. Prognostic value of detection of myocardial viability using low-dose dobutamine echocardiography in infarcted patients. Am J Cardiol 1998; 81(12A):21G-28G.
17. Sandstede JJ, Bertsch G, Beer M, et al. Detection of myocardial viability by low-dose dobutamine cine MR imaging. Magn Reson Imaging 1999; 17:1437-1443.
18. Dendale PA, Franken PR, Waldman GJ, et al. Low-dosage dobutamine magnetic resonance imaging as an alternative to echocardiography in the detection of viable myocardium after acute infarction. Am Heart J 1995; 130:134-140.
19. Baer FM, Theissen P, Crnac J, et al. Head to head comparison of dobutamine-transesophageal echocardiography and dobutamine-magnetic resonance imaging for the prediction of left ventricular functional recovery in patients with chronic coronary artery disease. Eur Heart J 2000; 21:981-991.
20. Wellnhofer E, Olariu A, Klein C, et al. Magnetic resonance low-dose dobutamine test is superior to SCAR quantification for the prediction of functional recovery. Circulation 2004; 109:2172-2174.
21. Grothues F, Smith GC, Moon JC, et al. Comparison of interstudy reproducibility of cardiovascular magnetic resonance with two-dimensional echocardiography in normal subjects and in patients with heart failure or left ventricular hypertrophy. Am J Cardiol 2002; 90:29-34.
22. Schmidt M, Voth E, Schneider CA, et al. F-18-FDG uptake is a reliable predictor of functional recovery of akinetic but viable infarct regions as defined by magnetic resonance imaging before and after revascularization. Magn Reson Imaging 2004; 22:229-236.
23. Kaandorp TA, Lamb HJ, van der Wall EE, et al. Cardiovascular MR to access myocardial viability in chronic ischaemic LV dysfunction. Heart (British Cardiac Society) 2005; 91:1359-1365.
24. McNamara MT, Tscholakoff D, Revel D, et al. Differentiation of reversible and irreversible myocardial injury by MR imaging with and without gadolinium-DTPA. Radiology 1986; 158:765-769.
25. Simonetti OP, Kim RJ, Fieno DS, et al. An improved MR imaging technique for the visualization of myocardial infarction. Radiology 2001; 218:215-223.
26. McCrohon JA, Moon JC, Prasad SK, et al. Differentiation of heart failure related to dilated cardiomyopathy and coronary artery disease using gadolinium-enhanced cardiovascular magnetic resonance. Circulation 2003; 108:54-59.
27. Kim RJ, Fieno DS, Parrish TB, et al. Relationship of MRI delayed contrast enhancement to irreversible injury, infarct age, and contractile function. Circulation 1999; 100:1992-2002.

28. Kim RJ, Wu E, Rafael A, et al. The use of contrast-enhanced magnetic resonance imaging to identify reversible myocardial dysfunction. N Engl J Med 2000; 343:1445-1453.
29. Ricciardi MJ, Wu E, Davidson CJ, et al. Visualization of discrete microinfarction after percutaneous coronary intervention associated with mild creatine kinase-MB elevation. Circulation 2001; 103:2780-2783.
30. Wagner A, Mahrholdt H, Holly TA, et al. Contrast-enhanced MRI and routine single photon emission computed tomography (SPECT) perfusion imaging for detection of subendocardial myocardial infarcts: an imaging study. Lancet 2003; 361:374-379.
31. Klein C, Nekolla SG, Bengel FM, et al. Assessment of myocardial viability with contrast-enhanced magnetic resonance imaging: comparison with positron emission tomography. Circulation 2002; 105:162-167.
32. Grude M, Juergens KU, Wichter T, et al. Evaluation of global left ventricular myocardial function with electrocardiogram-gated multidetector computed tomography: comparison with magnetic resonance imaging. Invest Radiol 2003; 38:653-661.
33. Belge B, Coche E, Pasquet A, et al. Accurate estimation of global and regional cardiac function by retrospectively gated multidetector row computed tomography: comparison with cine magnetic resonance imaging. Eur Radiol 2006; 16:1424-1433.
34. Hoffmann U, Millea R, Enzweiler C, et al. Acute myocardial infarction: contrast-enhanced multi-detector row CT in a porcine model. Radiology 2004; 231:697-701.
35. Nieman K, Cury RC, Ferencik M, et al. Differentiation of recent and chronic myocardial infarction by cardiac computed tomography. Am J Cardiol 2006; 98:303-308.
36. Lardo AC, Cordeiro MA, Silva C, et al. Contrast-enhanced multidetector computed tomography viability imaging after myocardial infarction: characterization of myocyte death, microvascular obstruction, and chronic scar. Circulation 2006; 113:394-404.
37. Lessick J, Dragu R, Mutlak D, et al. Is functional improvement after myocardial infarction predicted with myocardial enhancement patterns at multidetector CT? Radiology 2007; 244:736-744.
38. Einstein AJ, Henzlova MJ, Rajagopalan S. Estimating risk of cancer associated with radiation exposure from 64-slice computed tomography coronary angiography. JAMA 2007; 298:317-323.

CHAPTER 58

Nuclear Medicine Imaging of Myocardial Viability

Steven A. Messina and Vasken Dilsizian

Coronary artery disease (CAD) remains the number one cause of mortality in the United States, responsible for nearly half of daily deaths.[1] The lifetime risk of developing CAD after 40 years of age is 49% for men and 32% for women.[2] In developed nations, the leading cause of left ventricular (LV) dysfunction (i.e., heart failure) is CAD.[3] Retrospective analysis of 13 randomized multicenter heart failure trials showed that CAD was present in approximately 70% of the greater than 20,000 enrolled patients.[4] Over the past decade, the number of patients presenting with heart failure has increased exponentially. It has been estimated that 4.7 million patients in the United States have chronic heart failure, with 550,000 new cases per year, resulting in 1 million hospitalizations.

Heart failure is the leading cause of morbidity, mortality, and hospitalization in patients older than 60 years and is the most common Medicare diagnosis-related group.[5] The diagnostic and therapeutic costs associated with heart failure are estimated to be more than $29 billion per year.[1] The long-term prognosis for patients with heart failure remains poor, despite advances in different therapies. More recent data from the Framingham Heart Study showed 5-year mortality rates of 59% for men and 45% for women with heart failure in the period from 1990-1999.[6] Mortality rates increase in older patients with heart failure.

Etiologies for LV systolic dysfunction in patients with ischemic cardiomyopathy include (1) transmural scar, (2) nontransmural scar, (3) repeatedly stunned myocardium, (4) hibernating myocardium, and (5) remodeled myocardium. Established treatment options for ischemic cardiomyopathy include medical therapy, revascularization, and cardiac transplantation. Revascularization procedures include percutaneous coronary interventions (e.g., endovascular stent placement) and coronary artery bypass graft (CABG) surgery. Although patients with heart failure resulting from noncoronary etiologies may best benefit from medical therapy or heart transplantation, coronary revascularization has the potential to improve ventricular function, symptoms, and long-term survival in patients with heart failure symptoms secondary to CAD and ischemic cardiomyopathy.

DEFINITION OF MYOCARDIAL VIABILITY

Before the 1980s, the conventional wisdom was that impaired LV function at rest in patients with CAD was an irreversible process. This clinical dogma was shown to be not always true when observational studies in patients with LV dysfunction undergoing coronary artery revascularization exhibited improvement in regional and global LV function.[7] To explain the subsequent improvement in function, the concept of viability was introduced. Dysfunctional but viable myocardium has the potential to recover function after revascularization, whereas the revascularization of dysfunctional scar tissue does not result in improvement of function. There are several mechanisms of adaptation that the myocardium follows to maintain viability during temporary or sustained reductions in coronary blood flow.

Dysfunctional but viable myocardium has been broadly categorized as either stunned or hibernating myocardium. *Stunned myocardium* refers to the state of delayed recovery of regional ventricular contractile dysfunction after a transient period of ischemia that has been followed by restoration of perfusion (Fig. 58-1).[8,9] Resulting dysfunction may persist for hours to days, but generally improves with time. *Hibernating myocardium* refers to an adaptive rather than an injurious response of the myocardium to impaired coronary flow reserve (repetitive ischemia and stunning) and reduced resting coronary blood flow (Fig. 58-2).[7,9] Hibernation and stunning are categorized as different pathophysiologic states; however, these states most often exist concomitantly as a continuum in patients with dysfunctional but viable myocardium.

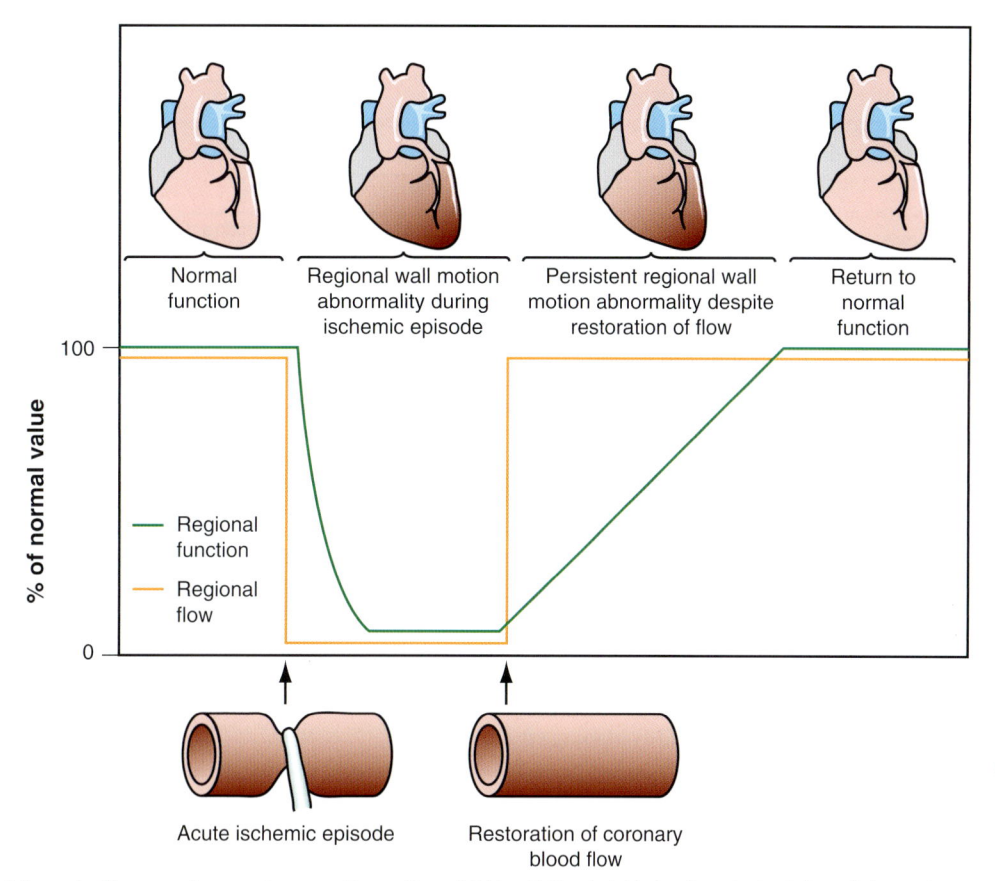

■ **FIGURE 58-1** Schematic diagram of stunned myocardium. *(From Dilsizian V, Narula J. Nuclear investigation in heart failure and myocardial viability. In Dilsizian V, Narula J [eds]. Atlas of Nuclear Cardiology, 3rd ed. Philadelphia, Current Medicine, 2009, pp 201-224.)*

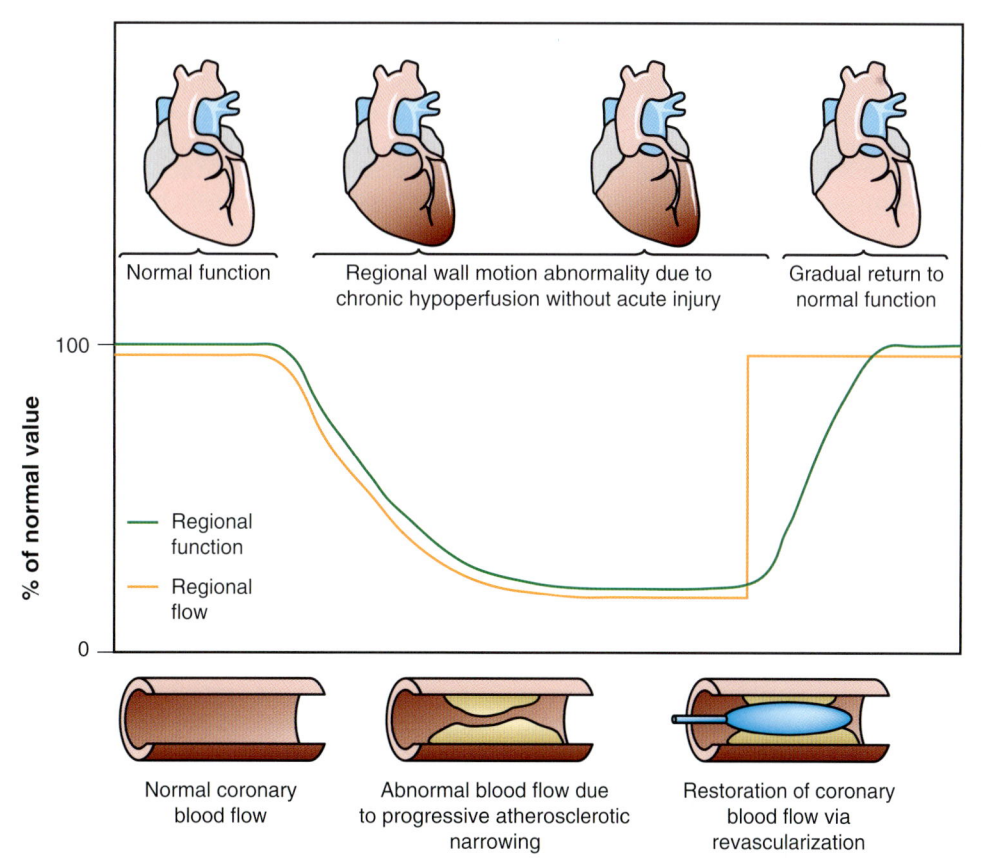

■ **FIGURE 58-2** Schematic diagram of hibernating myocardium. *(From Dilsizian V, Narula J. Nuclear investigation in heart failure and myocardial viability. In Dilsizian V, Narula J [eds]. Atlas of Nuclear Cardiology, 3rd ed. Philadelphia, Current Medicine, 2009, pp 201-224.)*

There is extensive evidence delineating the adaptations of the myocardium to reduced blood flow. Signs of energy depletion and downregulation of energy turnover have been described in hibernating myocardium.[10] These alterations of energy metabolism likely cause and perpetuate contractile dysfunction, continued tissue degeneration, and subsequent cardiomyocyte loss. These responses to regional hypoperfusion are thought to preserve the minimal amount of energy needed to protect the structural and functional integrity of the cardiac myocyte. Myocardial biopsy specimens have shown disorganization of the cytoskeletal proteins, dedifferentiation (expression of more fetal proteins), and changes in the extracellular matrix with evidence of reparative fibrosis with basement membrane thickening and increased collagen fibrils and fibroblasts. Hibernating myocardium showed a loss of contractile filaments (sarcomeres), an accumulation of glycogen in the spaces previously occupied by the myofilaments, nuclei with uniformly distributed chromatin, small mitochondria, and a nearly absent sarcoplasmic reticulum.[11] Additional histologic studies analyzed myocardial biopsy specimens obtained during revascularization procedures, confirming that segments with recovery after revascularization contained viable myocytes compared with the large extent of fibrosis detected in irreversibly damaged myocardium.[12]

Myocardial Ischemia

Imbalance between oxygen supply and oxygen demand, which is determined by regional myocardial perfusion and the rate and force of myocardial contraction, is termed *ischemic myocardium*. Myocardial ischemia alters myocardial substrate metabolism. As blood flow and oxygen supply decline, oxidative metabolism decreases, and glycolysis increases. As ischemia continues, glycolytic metabolism becomes overwhelmed with excess production of lactate. During states of mild ischemia, lactate continues to be removed from the myocardium by the residual blood flow, but rapidly accumulates in tissue, with a further reduction in blood flow, during more severe states of ischemia. Subsequently, increased tissue concentrations of lactate and hydrogen ions impair glycolysis, leading to loss of transmembrane ion concentration gradients, disruption of cell membranes, and cell death.[13]

Cell death after myocardial ischemia and reperfusion can be the consequence of apoptosis and necrosis. The induction of either apoptosis or necrosis is regulated by similar biochemical intermediates, including alterations in high-energy phosphates, intracellular calcium accumulation, and reactive oxygen species. The reduction of contractile function associated with hibernation is thought to be a protective response of the myocardium to meet minimal metabolic requirements with the reduced supply of oxygen and substrates, leading to the situation of perfusion contraction matching, preventing apoptosis and cell death.[14] Histologic analysis of hibernating myocardium shows myocytes in a stable noncontractile state with intact cell membranes and cellular metabolism with little or no evidence of apoptosis.[15] In contrast to programmed cell death, or apoptosis, the term *programmed cell survival* has been used to describe the commonality between myocardial stunning, hibernation, and ischemic preconditioning, despite their distinct pathophysiology (Fig. 58-3).[16]

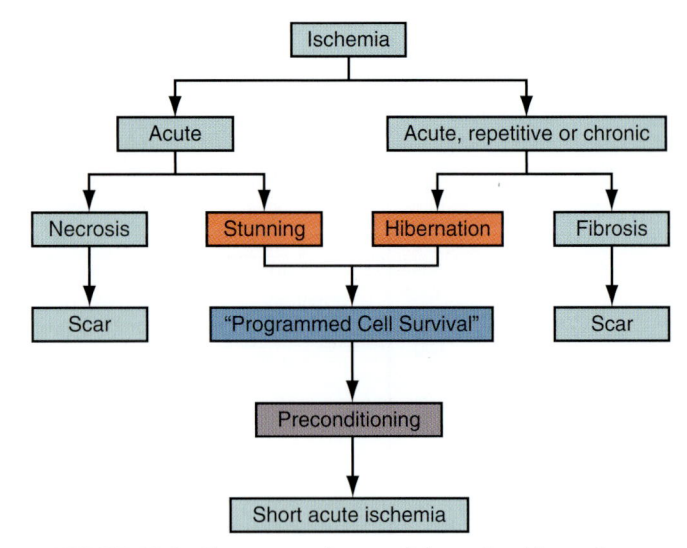

■ **FIGURE 58-3** Phenomena of myocardial stunning, hibernation, and ischemia preconditioning are part of the spectrum of myocardial ischemia and reperfusion resulting in programmed cell survival. These natural pathophysiologic responses, which compensate for ischemia, can be used to differentiate ischemic tissue from healthy tissue. (*From Taegtmeyer H. Modulation of responses to myocardial ischemia: metabolic features of myocardial stunning, hibernation, and ischemic preconditioning. In Dilsizian V [ed]. Myocardial Viability: A Clinical and Scientific Treatise. Armonk, NY, Futura, 2000, pp 25-36.*)

Injury as a result of myocardial ischemia can be categorized as a continuum from fully viable, through partially viable (admixture of scarred and viable tissue), to nonviable or scarred. Not all myocardium involved in an infarction is dead or irreversibly damaged. The process of infarction starts at the endocardium and spreads toward the epicardium. The extent of myocardial infarction (MI) can be reduced when the affected vascular territory is reperfused (spontaneously, pharmacologically, or mechanically), or when the area of MI is sufficiently collateralized. Even completed infarcts vary in their transmural extent, and the epicardium is usually the most likely site of viable myocardium. The likelihood of recovery of function after revascularization is related to the extent of myocyte injury and the amount of fibrosis (Fig. 58-4).[17,18]

Potential End Points Used in Myocardial Viability Studies

Viable myocardium has several characteristics, including cell membrane integrity, intact mitochondria, preserved glucose metabolism, preserved fatty acid metabolism, intact resting perfusion, and inotropic reserve. The objective of myocardial viability assessment is to identify patients prospectively with potentially reversible LV dysfunction. Reversible LV dysfunction may be due to transient myocardial ischemia (stunning) or chronic hypoperfusion (hibernation). The end points used in viability studies after revascularization include improvement in regional LV function (segments), improvement in global LV function as assessed by LV ejection fraction, improvement in symptoms (New York Heart Association

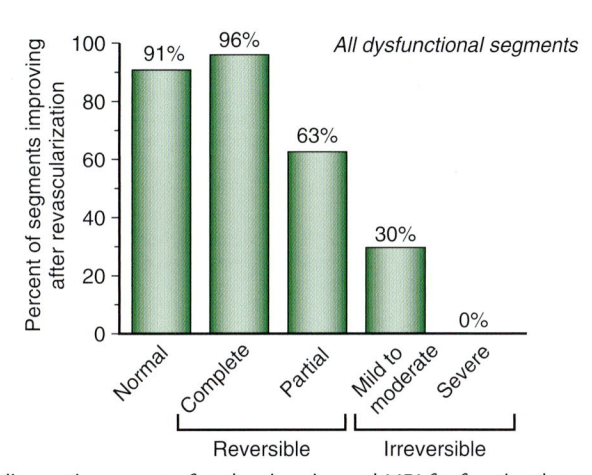

FIGURE 58-4 Comparison of diagnostic accuracy of nuclear imaging and MRI for functional recovery after revascularization. Relationships between recovery of function after revascularization with contrast-enhanced MRI and two thallium protocols optimized for viability detection: rest-redistribution and stress-redistribution-reinjection imaging. Regardless of the imaging modality applied, the data suggest that recovery of function after revascularization is a continuum, and is coupled to the ratio of viable to scarred myocardium within dysfunctional myocardial segments. The extent of infarct size on MRI or percent thallium defect on SPECT correlated with decreasing likelihood of functional recovery after revascularization. (From Dilsizian V. Cardiac magnetic resonance versus SPECT: are all non-infarct myocardial regions created equal? J Nucl Cardiol 2007; 14:9-14.)

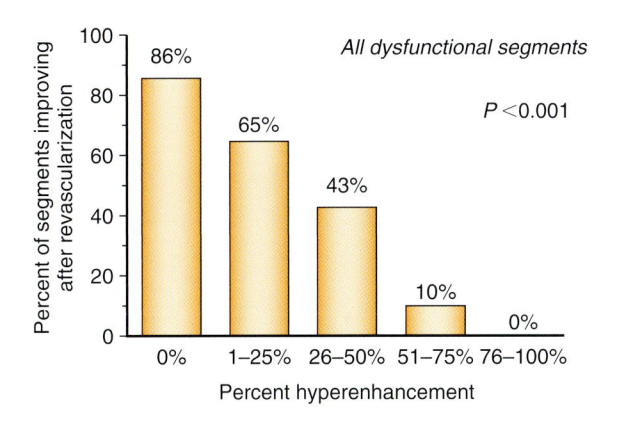

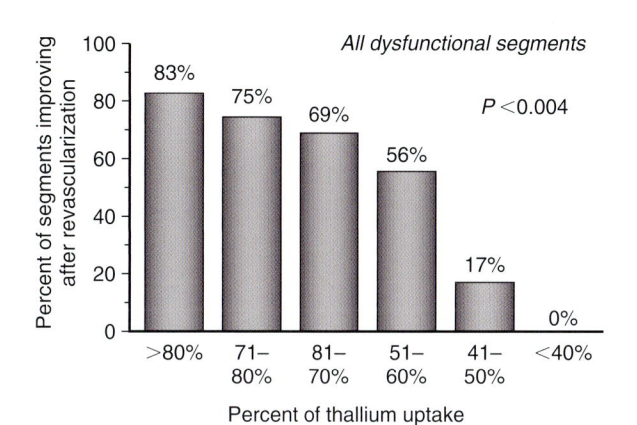

functional class), improvement in exercise capacity (metabolic equivalents), reverse LV remodeling (LV volumes), prevention of sudden death (ventricular arrhythmias), and long-term prognosis (survival).

Patients with severe LV dysfunction who undergo CABG surgery or percutaneous coronary interventions can have a considerable risk of procedure-related morbidity and mortality.[18,19] Identification of patients with the potential for improvement in LV ejection fraction and survival is needed to justify the higher risk of therapeutic intervention in these patients. Revascularization of viable myocardium has been shown to improve significantly regional and global contractile function.[20-22] Improvement in regional contractile function is seen in approximately one third of dysfunctional segments, and an improvement in LV ejection fraction is seen in approximately 40% of patients.[21,23] Revascularization of viable myocardium has also been shown to improve significantly symptoms and New York Heart Association functional class.[24] The magnitude of improvement in heart failure symptoms after CABG surgery is linearly related to the preoperative extent of myocardial viability (Fig. 58-5).[24]

Revascularization may also be associated with many favorable clinical effects even in the absence of ventricular functional improvement. Benefits can include relief of chest pain or heart failure symptoms, improved exercise tolerance related to diminished inducible ischemia or improved diastolic function, stabilization (or reversal) of LV remodeling, stabilization of the electrophysiologic milieu, and prevention of MI.[25-27] Besides improvement in LV ejection fraction, revascularization of viable myocardium may have a beneficial effect on the prevention of arrhythmias and sudden cardiac death, which may also improve longevity. One study showed that the long-term survival rates of patients who underwent CABG surgery were similar regardless of whether LV ejection fraction increased after revascularization.[28] Chronic LV dysfunction can result from nontransmural necrosis in combina-

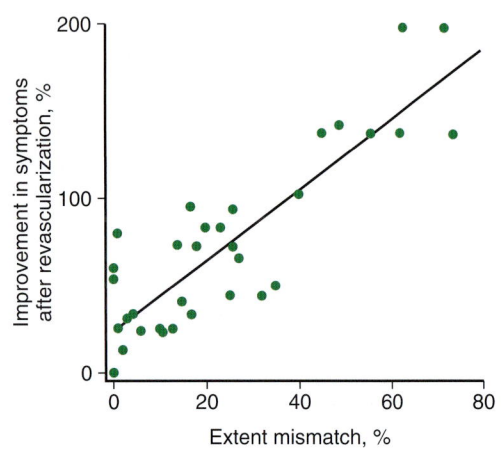

FIGURE 58-5 Relationship between the anatomic extent of perfusion:metabolism PET mismatch pattern (expressed as percent of the left ventricle) and the change in functional status after revascularization (expressed as percent improvement from baseline). Patients with myocardial viability (mismatch pattern) who underwent revascularization manifested a significant improvement in heart failure symptoms and exercise tolerance. The scatterplot shows that the greatest improvement in heart failure symptoms occurs in patients with the largest mismatch defects on quantitative analysis of PET images. (From Di Carli MF, Asgarzadie F, Schelbert HR, et al. Quantitative relation between myocardial viability and improvement in heart failure symptoms after revascularization in patients with ischemic cardiomyopathy. Circulation 1995; 92:3436-3444.)

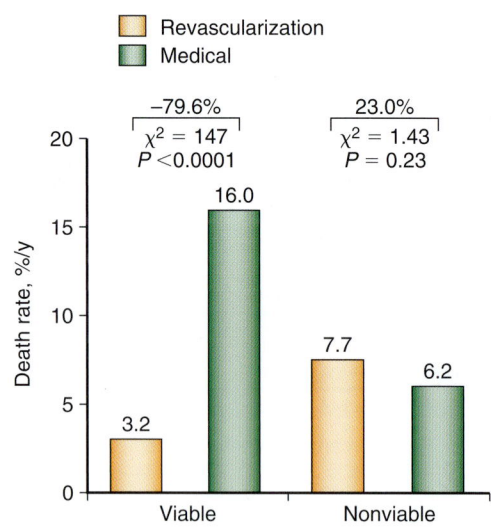

FIGURE 58-6 Prognostic implications of myocardial viability testing derived from meta-analysis of 3088 patients with CAD and LV dysfunction who underwent viability testing. Death rates for patients with and without myocardial viability treated by revascularization or medical therapy are shown. In patients with viable myocardium, there is a 79.6% reduction in mortality among patients who were treated with revascularization ($P < .0001$). In contrast, in patients without evidence of viable myocardium, there was no significant difference in mortality with revascularization versus medical therapy. (Adapted from Allman KC, Shaw LJ, Hachamovitch R, et al. Myocardial viability testing and impact of revascularization on prognosis in patients with coronary artery disease and left ventricular dysfunction: a meta-analysis. J Am Coll Cardiol 2002; 39:1151-1158.)

tion with viable (normal) myocardium. The subendocardial layer contributes significantly to contraction, and subendocardial necrosis of greater than 20% of the myocardial wall results frequently in akinesia.

Revascularization of these regions may not significantly improve contractile function. The prevention of remodeling and arrhythmias may be of critical clinical relevance, however. In such patients, preserved viability in the outer layers of the myocardium could prevent progressive LV dilation, despite the lack of any improvement in resting function after revascularization. The prevention or reversal of adverse LV remodeling seems to be an important determinant of long-term natural history outcomes, and strategies that prevent or reverse remodeling generally have very favorable effects on that natural history.[29]

A meta-analysis of the prognostic value of viability testing and the impact of therapeutic choice on survival showed a significant association between revascularization and improved survival rate in patients with LV dysfunction and evidence of myocardial viability independent of the imaging technique used.[30,31] Additionally, these studies identified a 3.2% annual death rate in patients who had viable myocardium and underwent revascularization compared with a 16% annual death rate in patients who had viable myocardium and were treated medically (Fig. 58-6). Medical treatment of heart failure has improved substantially with the introduction of angiotensin-converting enzyme (ACE) inhibitors, angiotensin II receptor blockers, and spironolactone. Patients with chronic ischemic LV dysfunction with viable myocardium have a poor prognosis when treated with medical therapy alone, however.[32]

NUCLEAR IMAGING TECHNIQUES FOR IDENTIFYING MYOCARDIAL VIABILITY

Prospective assessment of myocardial viability in dysfunctional myocardium involves assessment of perfusion, sarcolemmal membrane integrity, intact mitochondria, preserved metabolism (glucose and fatty acid), and contractile reserve. These characteristics can be evaluated with scintigraphic techniques using single photon emission computed tomography (SPECT) or positron emission tomography (PET). A principal advantage of nuclear techniques is in the synergy that exists between the modality—radionuclide tracers that, by their nature, reflect physiologic processes at the cellular level—and the underlying pathophysiologic states being investigated. Perfusion can be evaluated by Tc 99m–labeled radiotracers or by thallium 201. Cell membrane integrity can be evaluated by thallium 201, and intact mitochondria can be verified with Tc 99m–labeled tracers. Preserved glucose metabolism can be evaluated with ^{18}FDG, and free fatty acid metabolism can be assessed by iodine 123–labeled fatty acids, for which beta-methyliodophenylpentadecanoic acid (BMIPP) has gained the most widespread clinical use in Japan.

Single Photon Emission Computed Tomography

Tc 99m Labeled Radiotracers

Tc 99m labeled flow tracers, such as Tc 99m sestamibi and Tc 99m tetrofosmin, are lipophilic cationic complexes, which are taken up by myocytes across mitochondrial membranes and at equilibrium are retained within the mitochondria because of a large negative transmembrane potential. The initial uptake and retention of sestamibi and tetrofosmin (whether injected at rest or during stress) are flow-dependent and reflect cell membrane integrity and mitochondrial function. Myocardial ischemia interferes with mitochondrial K⁺-ATP channel activation, changing its mitochondrial membrane potential, and finally reducing cellular radiotracer uptake.[33]

Tc 99m labeled perfusion tracers emit higher energy photons (yielding better image quality), and the shorter half-life time allows the administration of higher dosage, with less radiation exposure to the patient. Accumulation and retention of these tracers are related to energy-dependent processes that maintain mitochondrial membrane polarization; myocardial uptake and retention of sestamibi and tetrofosmin may also be a marker of cellular viability. In contrast to thallium, however, these tracers do not exhibit significant redistribution with time.

Experimental studies have shown that myocardial retention of Tc 99m sestamibi and Tc 99m tetrofosmin requires cellular viability.[34] Histopathologic studies have shown that tissue viability is a continuum, and that there is a nearly linear relationship with sestamibi uptake and the percentage of normal (viable) myocardium in dysfunctional regions.[35] The most commonly used clinical viability criterion is the percentage of tracer uptake (frequently 50% to 60%) in dysfunctional segments. Most frequently, Tc 99m labeled tracers are injected under resting conditions, and the dysfunctional segments with tracer uptake of 50% to 60% are considered viable.[36] Regional Tc 99m sestamibi or Tc 99m tetrofosmin activity has been shown to be closely correlated with the redistribution phase of rest-redistribution thallium 201 study, indicating myocardial viability (Fig. 58-7).[37,38]

Using Tc 99m perfusion tracers for the assessment of viability is not without limitations. In particular, photon attenuation may result in lower regional activities, particularly in the inferior and septal walls, which could result in false-negative results. In the case of a nontransmural infarction, false-positive results may also become a concern because these dysfunctional segments could show 50% or greater uptake of radiotracer, yet not recover function after revascularization. The addition of ECG gated SPECT is valuable in its ability to enhance artifact identification by differentiating scarred tissue from attenuation artifacts because these artifacts reveal normal wall motion and thickening, decreasing false-positive perfusion studies by incorporating regional wall motion data in the interpretation of perfusion imaging.

Studies have suggested that sestamibi may underestimate myocardial viability, particularly in patients with severe LV dysfunction.[39-41] Despite using quantitative techniques, studies have reported that rest sestamibi imaging underestimates myocardial viability compared with ¹⁸FDG-PET. Potential factors affecting the accuracy of sestamibi in assessing viability were determined by comparing the results of sestamibi SPECT and ¹⁸FDG-PET in patients with varying degrees of LV dysfunction. The concordance between sestamibi and ¹⁸FDG was 64% in patients with severe LV dysfunction and 78% in patients with mild to moderate LV dysfunction.[42] In particular, only 42% of regions with blood flow–metabolism mismatch patterns by PET (the pattern most predictive of functional recovery after revascularization) were identified as viable by quantitative sestamibi SPECT.

Tc 99m Labeled Radiotracers with Nitrate Administration

Nitrates (intravenous, oral, or sublingual) enhance collateral blood flow and radiotracer uptake in hypoperfused myocardial regions that are subtended by severely stenosed coronary arteries. In most nitrate-enhanced studies, two sets of images are obtained: a resting image and a nitrate-enhanced image. Defect reversibility after nitrate administration (i.e., a defect filling in) is considered to be indicative of viability. Nitrate-enhanced Tc 99m perfusion tracer uptake compared with baseline is thought to be a better estimate of coronary flow reserve. Several investigators have used improvement in the regional concentration of a flow tracer injected after nitrate administration as a marker of viability.[43,44]

A retrospective analysis of studies using Tc 99m labeled flow tracers to assess improvement in regional function after revascularization showed a mean overall sensitivity and specificity of 81% and 66%.[45] Most of these studies used a resting image, and segments were classified as viable when activity exceeded a certain threshold. Nitrate-enhanced studies, when analyzed separately, showed a higher accuracy, with a sensitivity of 86% and a specificity of 83% (Fig. 58-8).[46] Studies that investigated functional outcomes showed an improvement of LV ejection fraction from 47% to 53% in patients with viable myocardium, whereas the LV ejection fraction did not change in patients without viable myocardium (40% vs. 39%). When gated SPECT regional function was added to nitrate enhancement, the accuracy of the technique for predicting recovery of function after revascularization was even higher.[47,48]

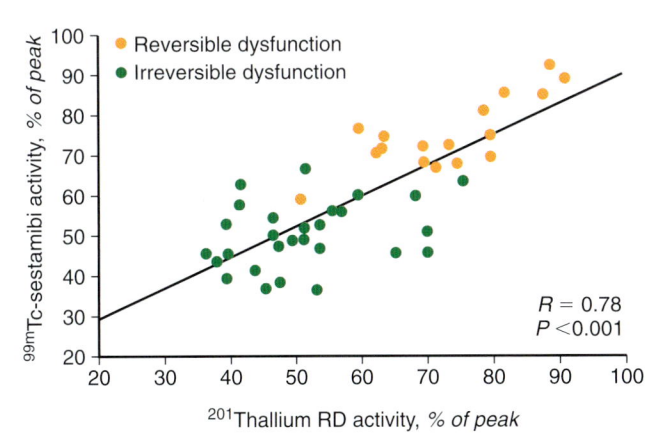

FIGURE 58-7 Scatterplot showing correlation of quantitative regional activities of thallium (at redistribution [RD] imaging after rest injection) on the *abscissa* and regional activities of sestamibi (at rest) on the *ordinate* among segments with significant regional dysfunction in patients undergoing revascularization. (Modified from Udelson JE, Coleman PS, Metherall J, et al. Predicting recovery of severe regional ventricular dysfunction: comparison of resting scintigraphy with 201Tl and 99mTc-sestamibi. Circulation 1994; 89:2552-2561.)

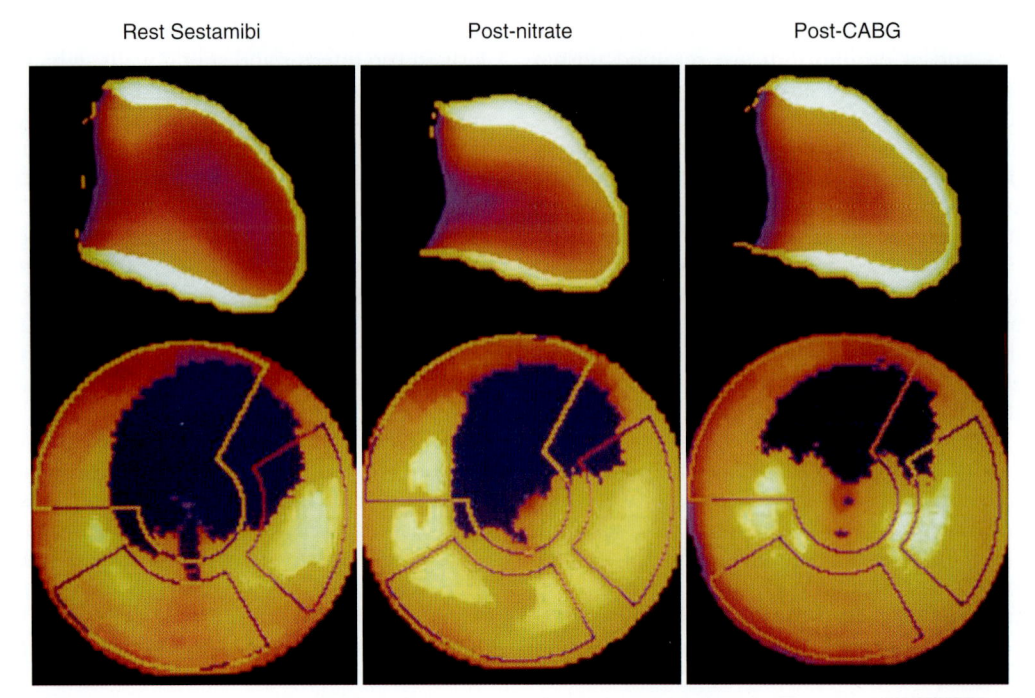

■ **FIGURE 58-8** In this patient example with anterior MI and single-vessel left anterior descending coronary artery (LAD) disease, baseline images before revascularization (*left panel*) show anteroapical akinesis and global LV ejection fraction of 38% on first-pass radionuclide angiography associated with a large anterior and apical sestamibi perfusion defect (63% of the LAD vascular territory) on the bull's-eye image at rest. Sestamibi images acquired after nitrate infusion (*middle panel*) show improvement in the anteroapical wall motion associated with an increase in global LV ejection fraction to 42% and a decrease in the extent of sestamibi perfusion defect size to 42% of the LAD vascular territory. After revascularization of the LAD with coronary artery bypass graft (CABG) surgery (*right panel*), there is improvement in the anteroapical wall motion at rest, increase in global LV ejection fraction to 45%, and decrease in the extent of sestamibi perfusion defect to 38% of the LAD vascular territory. (*Adapted from Dilsizian V. SPECT and PET myocardial perfusion imaging: tracers and techniques. In Dilsizian V, Narula J [eds]. Atlas of Nuclear Cardiology, 3rd ed. Philadelphia, Current Medicine, 2006, pp 37-60.*)

In patients with chronic CAD and nitrate-enhanced Tc 99m perfusion studies, superior survival was shown in patients with complete revascularization compared with patients treated with medical therapy and patients who underwent incomplete revascularization. The most important prognostic predictor of future cardiac events was the number of nonrevascularized dysfunctional regions with viable tissue on sestamibi imaging. That is, patients who had viable myocardium but who did not receive adequate revascularization had poorer prognosis.[49]

Thallium 201

Cardiac imaging with thallium 201 is predicated on the principle that myocardial perfusion and cell membrane integrity need to be preserved for radiotracer uptake and accumulation in the myocyte. Thallium 201 is a monovalent potassium analogue that is actively transported by the energy-dependent Na^+,K^+-ATPase pump through the intact sarcolemmal membrane. The initial uptake of thallium 201 is mainly determined by perfusion, whereas delayed retention is dependent on cell membrane integrity. Myocardial thallium 201 uptake represents myocardial perfusion and cellular viability.

Thallium 201 enters myocytes primarily by active transport, and regional myocardial concentration of thallium 201 depends on regional blood flow, extraction, and clearance. First-pass extraction of thallium 201 from blood is almost 85% even in hypoperfused regions of myocardium, and subsequent retention is unaltered, unless there is irreversible sarcolemmal membrane injury. In viable myocardium, thallium 201 is continuously exchanged between the myocardium and the bloodstream, with the rate of exchange in proportion to the difference in thallium 201 concentration between the myocardium and the blood. As expected, after the administration of thallium 201, the myocardial concentration is greatest in the areas of myocardium with the highest blood flow. Thallium 201 concentration trends toward an equilibrium within viable myocardium on delayed imaging. This phenomenon is termed *redistribution*. A thallium 201 perfusion defect that is reversible is considered indicative of ischemic but viable myocardium.

Experimental studies have shown that extraction of thallium 201 across the cell membrane is unaffected by hypoxia, chronic hypoperfusion (hibernation), or post-ischemic dysfunction (stunning), unless irreversible injury (scarred myocardium) is present. Necrotic myocardium cannot retain thallium 201, and, despite its initial uptake, thallium 201 washout is accelerated in necrotic tissue.[50,51] Because thallium 201 is not actively taken up in regions of fibrotic or scarred myocardium, a defect on rest images that persists on redistribution images (termed *irreversible* or *fixed defect*) represents a pattern of scarred myocardium.

Thallium 201 has been used and investigated extensively for identifying myocardial viability and hibernation, and was the first radiotracer to be used for this purpose.[52]

Rest 30 min

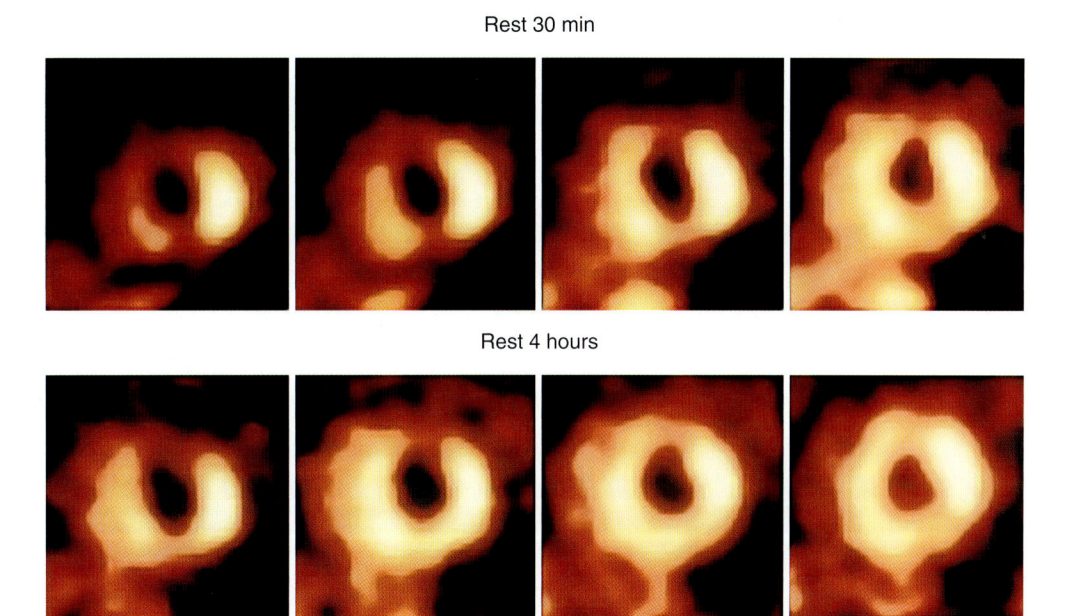

Apex ──────────────────────────────▶ Base

■ **FIGURE 58-9** Rest-redistribution short-axis thallium 201 tomograms are displayed from a patient with CAD. There are extensive thallium 201 abnormalities in the anteroapical, anteroseptal, and inferior regions on the initial rest images. On 3- to 4-hour redistribution images, the anteroapical region remains fixed (scarred myocardium), whereas the inferior and anteroseptal regions show significant reversibility, suggestive of viable myocardium. *(Adapted from Dilsizian V. SPECT and PET myocardial perfusion imaging: tracers and techniques. In Dilsizian V, Narula J [eds]. Atlas of Nuclear Cardiology, 3rd ed. Philadelphia, Current Medicine, 2009, pp 37-60.)*

Despite the excellent flow kinetics and biologic properties, however, the low-energy gamma ray emission and long half-life of thallium 201 are potential limitations, leading to attenuation of photons, particularly in patients with a large body habitus, and higher radiation exposure compared with Tc 99m labeled perfusion tracers.

Myocardial perfusion scan clinical protocols can be used with thallium 201 with an injection of a tracer either during stress (exercise or pharmacologic) or at rest with subsequent late imaging after the redistribution of the radiotracer. The initial acquisition soon after thallium 201 injection primarily reflects delivery of the tracer through blood flow. The delayed redistribution images acquired 4 to 24 hours after radiotracer injection are a marker of sarcolemmal integrity and myocardial K^+ space and Na^+,K^+-ATPase function, which reflects tissue viability.[50,53] Delayed thallium 201 imaging for assessment of myocardial viability relies on properties of thallium 201 that allow for redistribution. Thallium 201 redistribution images represent a balance between thallium 201 washout and continued thallium 201 uptake via the active Na^+,K^+-ATPase transport system over time, and redistribution images reflect the distribution volume of thallium 201 as representative of the myocardial K^+ space. In normal myocardium, the rate of thallium 201 washout is greater than the rate of uptake, resulting in a net thallium washout, which is potentiated further in infarcted myocardium. Redistribution imaging allows time for thallium 201 washout from necrotic myocardium, and for thallium 201 wash-in or redistribution into viable tissue.

Redistribution of thallium 201 after stress depends partly on the blood levels of thallium 201. Some ischemic but viable myocardial regions may show no redistribution on either early (3- to 4-hour) or late (24-hour) redistribution imaging, unless blood levels of thallium 201 are increased. Reinjection of 1 mCi of thallium 201 at rest immediately after either stress early (3- to 4-hour) redistribution or stress late (24-hour) redistribution studies boosts the blood level of thallium 201, potentiating the differentiation of hypoperfused and scarred myocardium from hypoperfused but viable myocardium.[54]

Thallium 201 Protocols for Viability Assessment

Numerous thallium 201 protocols are used clinically for the detection of myocardial viability. The following two protocols are optimized for viability detection: (1) rest-redistribution (Fig. 58-9)[46,55] and (2) stress–4-hour redistribution–reinjection imaging (Fig. 58-10).[54] The former assesses myocardial viability alone,[56] whereas the latter assesses myocardial ischemia and viability.[54] A pooled analysis of rest-redistribution and stress-redistribution-reinjection thallium studies reported high sensitivity (80% to 90%) and modest specificity (54% to 80%) for the prediction of recovery of regional function after revascularization.[45] These conclusions must be viewed, however, in the context of the limitations of pooled data analysis. When taking into consideration regions with reversible defects (ischemia) and success of revascularization (re-examining regional perfusion or vessel patency after revascularization), stress-redistribution-reinjection thallium 201 imaging yields excellent positive and negative predictive accuracy (both 80% to 90%) for recovery of function after revascularization (Fig. 58-11).[56]

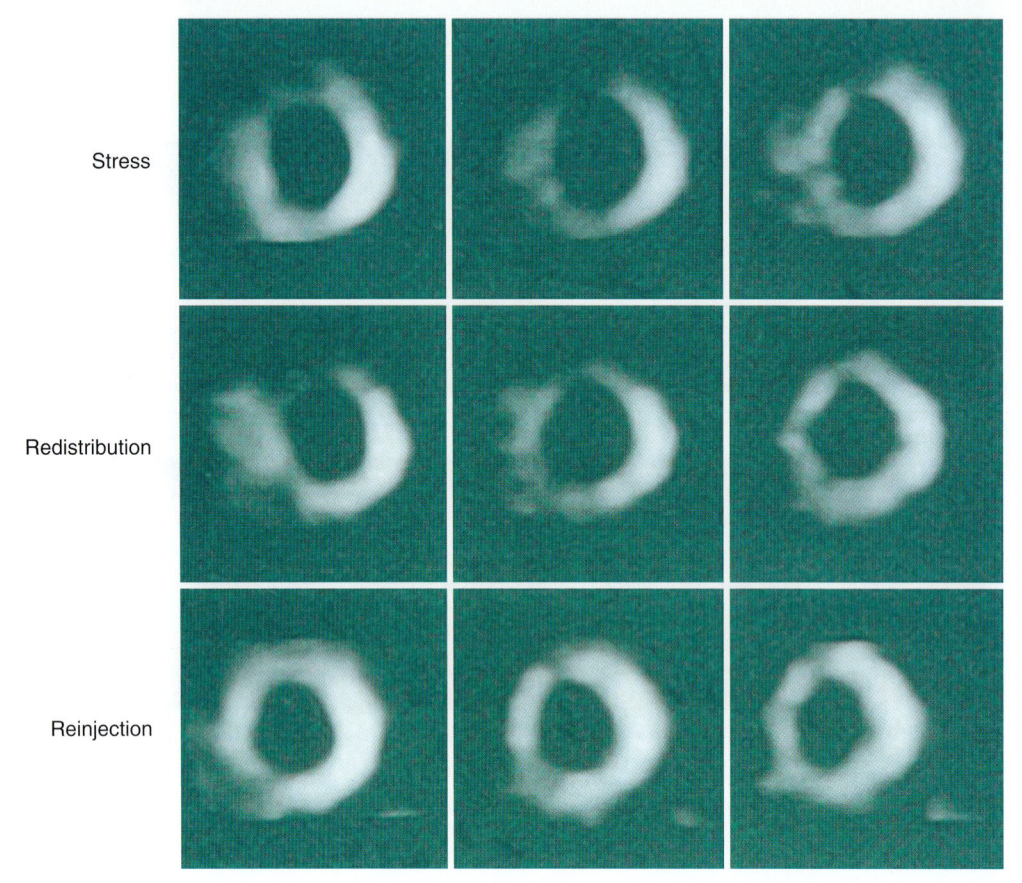

■ **FIGURE 58-10** Short-axis thallium 201 tomograms during stress, redistribution, and reinjection imaging in a patient with CAD. There are extensive thallium 201 abnormalities in the anterior and septal regions during stress that persist on redistribution images, but improve markedly on reinjection images. *(From Dilsizian V, Rocco TP, Freedman NM, et al. Enhanced detection of ischemic but viable myocardium by the reinjection of thallium after stress-redistribution imaging. N Engl J Med 1990; 323:141-146. Copyright 1990 Massachusetts Medical Society. All rights reserved.)*

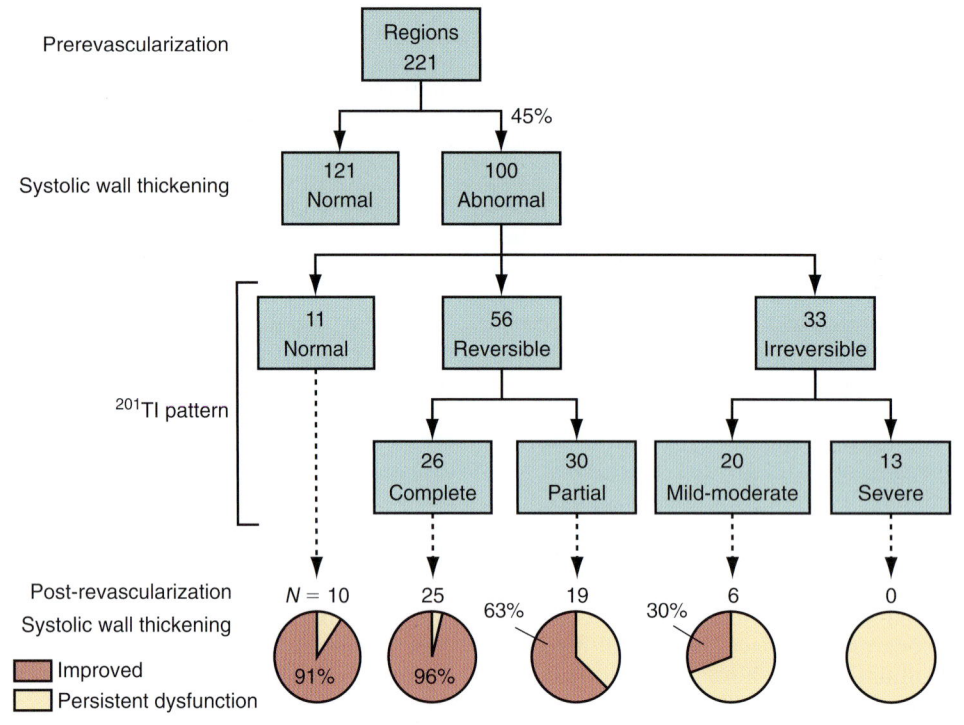

■ **FIGURE 58-11** Flow diagram showing postrevascularization functional outcome of asynergic regions in relation to prerevascularization thallium 201 patterns of stress-induced reversible and mild to moderate irreversible thallium 201 defects using stress-redistribution-reinjection thallium 201 protocol. The probabilities of functional recovery after revascularization were greater than 90% in normal or completely reversible defects, 63% in partially reversible defects, 30% in mild to moderate irreversible defects, and 0% in severe irreversible defects. Asynergic regions with reversible defects (complete or partial) on the prerevascularization thallium study were shown to be more likely to improve function after revascularization compared with asynergic regions with mild to moderate irreversible defects (79% vs. 30%; $P < .001$). Even at a similar mass of viable myocardial tissue (as reflected by the final thallium content), the presence of inducible ischemia (reversible defect) was associated with an increased likelihood of functional recovery. *(Adapted from Kitsiou AN, Srinivasan G, Quyyumi AA, et al. Stress-induced reversible and mild-to-moderate irreversible thallium defects: are they equally accurate for predicting recovery of regional left ventricular function after revascularization? Circulation 1998; 98:501-508.)*

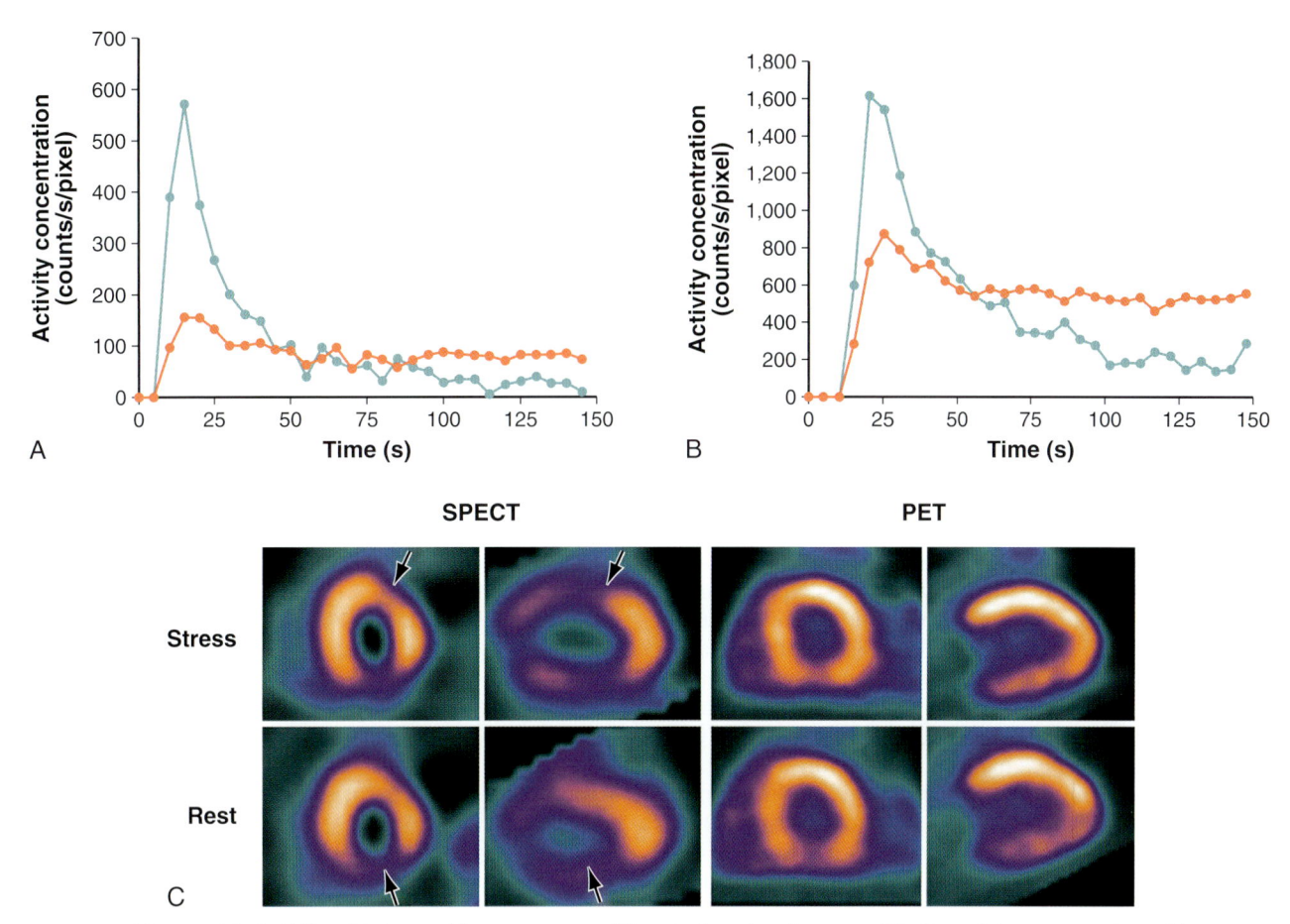

■ **FIGURE 58-12** **A** and **B**, Rubidium 82 time-activity curves at rest (**A**) and after adenosine stress (**B**). *Green circles* represent the activity concentration in the left atrium, and *orange circles* represent the activity concentration in myocardial tissue. Although the first few minutes after infusion of rubidium 82 are not usually included in clinical acquisition protocols, it is precisely this period that is of interest if myocardial perfusion is to be quantified. Dynamic imaging of the heart during this time allows analysis of the rubidium 82 concentration in arterial blood and myocardial tissue as a function of time. **C**, Disparity between myocardial perfusion SPECT and rubidium 82 PET studies is shown. Clinically indicated adenosine dual-isotope gated SPECT images (*left panel*) without attenuation correction show regional Tc 99m sestamibi perfusion defect in anterior and inferior regions (*arrows*). On the rest thallium 201 images, the anterior defect became reversible, whereas the inferior defect persisted. Corresponding rubidium 82 PET myocardial perfusion tomograms were performed in the same patient (*right panel*). PET images were acquired after an infusion of adenosine and 30 mCi of rubidium 82 (*top*) and at rest after another infusion of 30 mCi of rubidium 82 (*bottom*). Rubidium 82 PET images show normal distribution of the radiotracer in all myocardial regions, without evidence for reversible or fixed defects to suggest myocardial ischemia or infarction. Although the high-energy positrons of rubidium 82 degrade spatial resolution, and the short half-life increases statistical noise, high-quality images free from attenuation artifacts can be produced with rubidium 82 PET with only 30 mCi injected dose. *(Adapted from Lodge MA, Braess H, Mahmood F, et al. Developments in nuclear cardiology: transition from single photon emission computed tomography to positron emission tomography-computed tomography. J Invasive Cardiol 2005; 17:491-496.)*

Positron Emission Tomography

PET has several technical advantages over gamma-technique SPECT, such as higher counting sensitivity, higher spatial resolution, routine use of more accurate attenuation correction, and absolute quantification of myocardial perfusion flow and metabolism. The principal PET radiopharmaceuticals used in cardiac applications include rubidium 82, N-13 ammonia, and oxygen 15–water for myocardial perfusion imaging and ^{18}FDG to evaluate glucose metabolism to elucidate myocardial viability. PET myocardial perfusion tracers N-13 ammonia, oxygen 15–water, and rubidium 82 each have their own unique properties that may make one preferable over another in certain applications. Clinical assessment of relative perfusion most commonly is performed with N-13 ammonia or rubidium 82 (both have received U.S. Food and Drug Administration [FDA] approval).

Rubidium 82 is a PET perfusion radiotracer and is a cation and an analog of K^+ (similar to thallium 201). The extraction of rubidium 82 from the plasma into myocardial cells is flow-dependent, whereas the washout of rubidium 82 depends on sarcolemmal membrane integrity and the Na^+,K^+-ATPase pump. Uptake and retention of rubidium 82 are a function of blood flow and of myocardial cell integrity (Fig. 58-12).[57] The half-life of rubidium 82 is only 75 seconds, with peak energy of 3.3 MeV. It is eluted from a commercially available strontium 82 generator.

N-13 ammonia consists of neutral ammonia (NH_3) in equilibrium with its charged ammonium ($^+NH_4$) ion. The neutral NH_3 molecule readily diffuses across plasma and cell membranes. Inside the cell, it re-equilibrates with its ammonium form, which is trapped in glutamine via the enzyme glutamine synthase.[58] The first-pass trapping of

N-13 ammonia at rest is high; however, it decreases with higher flow rates. N-13 ammonia localizes in the myocardium and does not persist in the cardiac blood pool. These preferable characteristics allow better quantification of regional myocardial tracer distribution.

In contrast to N-13 ammonia, oxygen 15–water diffuses freely across plasma membranes, and with a high first-pass extraction and metabolically inert characteristics, it is theoretically better suited for blood flow measurement. The relatively short half-lives of N-13 ammonia (10 minutes) and oxygen 15–water (2 minutes) necessitate an on-site cyclotron. Oxygen 15–water does not exhibit a plateau effect at high flow rates. Additionally, the tracer persists in the cardiac blood pool and is present in the cardiac chambers and the myocardium, resulting in poor contrast, requiring subtraction of cardiac blood pool for the accurate semiquantitative and quantitative assessment. Because of these limitations, some investigators have reported heterogeneity of flow measurements.[59]

Estimates of myocardial blood flow by oxygen 15–water may differ from estimates by N-13 ammonia in dysfunctional myocardium. The properties of N-13 ammonia are such that a quantified average of transmural myocardial blood flow is obtained, whereas the oxygen 15–water technique measures flow only in the fraction of the myocardium that is able to exchange water rapidly and not in scar tissue.[59,60] Some investigators have explored the ability of oxygen 15–water to assess myocardial viability through the modification of the blood flow information (Fig. 58-13).[61] Rather than reliance on the net transmural blood flow, the volume of perfusable and nonperfusable tissue within a myocardial region was measured.[60,61] When this perfusable tissue index method of oxygen 15–water was tested in patients with acute and chronic ischemic heart disease, the determination of myocardial viability was comparable to that obtained using N-13 ammonia and ^{18}FDG metabolism.[61,62]

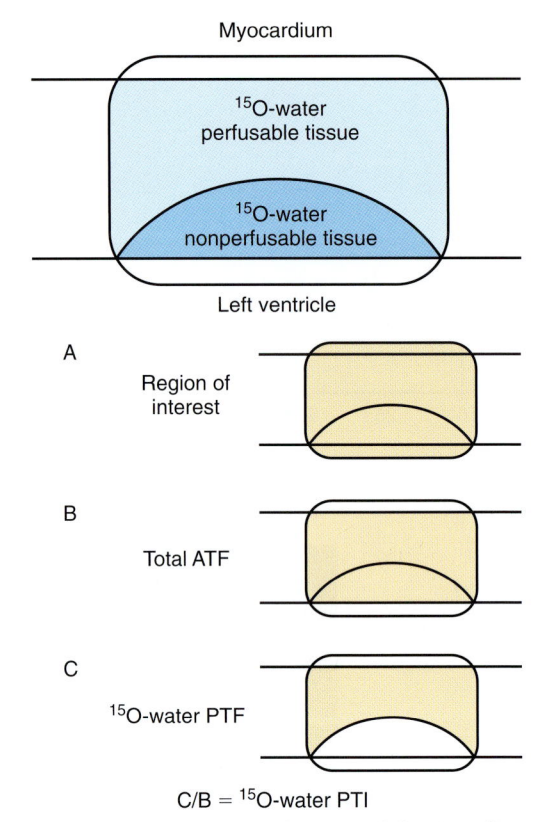

■ **FIGURE 58-13** **A,** Schematic of a myocardial region of interest containing a mixture of oxygen 15–water perfusable and nonperfusable tissue. **B,** Total anatomic tissue fraction (ATF) represents the total extravascular tissue and contains perfusable and nonperfusable tissue components. **C,** Oxygen 15–water perfusable tissue fraction (PTF) for the region of interest that is calculated from the oxygen 15–water data set and identifies the mass of tissue within the region of interest that is capable of rapid trans-sarcolemmal exchange of water. The nonperfusable or necrotic region is excluded from this parameter. Oxygen 15–water perfusable tissue index is calculated by dividing oxygen 15–water PTF (**C**) by the total ATF (**B**), and represents the fraction of the total anatomic tissue that is perfusable by water. (From Yamamoto Y, de Silva R, Rhodes CG, et al. A new strategy for the assessment of viable myocardium and regional myocardial blood flow using 15O-water and dynamic positron emission tomography. Circulation 1992; 86:167-178; with permission from the American Heart Association.)

TECHNIQUE DESCRIPTIONS

Myocardial Metabolism

Fatty Acid Radiotracer Imaging

Under aerobic conditions, the heart uses predominantly fatty acids for energy production. Fatty acids are actively taken up by myocardial cells, where they are activated by binding to coenzyme A. The fatty acids may be used for the synthesis of lipids, or they may undergo β-oxidation in the mitochondria. The myocyte in the failing heart exhibits altered metabolic activity characterized by downregulation of fatty acid oxidation, increased glycolysis and glucose oxidation, reduced respiratory chain activity, and an impaired reserve for mitochondrial oxidative flux. Fatty acid metabolism would be an invaluable tool.

PET and SPECT fatty acid radiotracers have been developed, but none has received approval from the FDA. The clearance of tracers that are metabolically active is complex; these tracers comprise one component that reflects turnover of myocardial lipids and β-oxidation, and a second component that reflects turnover of the lipid and triglyceride pool. From an imaging standpoint, tracers that are trapped but *not* metabolized are preferable, and methylated iodinated long-chain fatty acids have been developed.

Radioiodine-labeled branched-chain fatty acid BMIPP allows the assessment of fatty acid metabolism using SPECT technology and has been extensively investigated. BMIPP is taken up by the myocyte and undergoes ATP-dependent thioesterification, but does not undergo significant mitochondrial β-oxidation (Fig. 58-14).[63] As a result, BMIPP is trapped in the intracellular lipid pool. BMIPP tracks myocardial fatty acid uptake and is retained within the myocardium for longer periods, facilitating imaging. BMIPP has been studied in conjunction with perfusion radiotracers, including thallium 201, Tc 99m sestamibi, and Tc 99m tetrofosmin. Clinically, BMIPP uptake can be concordantly reduced with regional perfusion (BMIPP-perfusion match) or relatively decreased (BMIPP-perfusion mismatch). Areas with a BMIPP-perfusion mismatch have been shown to correlate with ischemia (reversible defects) on stress-redistribution thallium 201 imaging.[64]

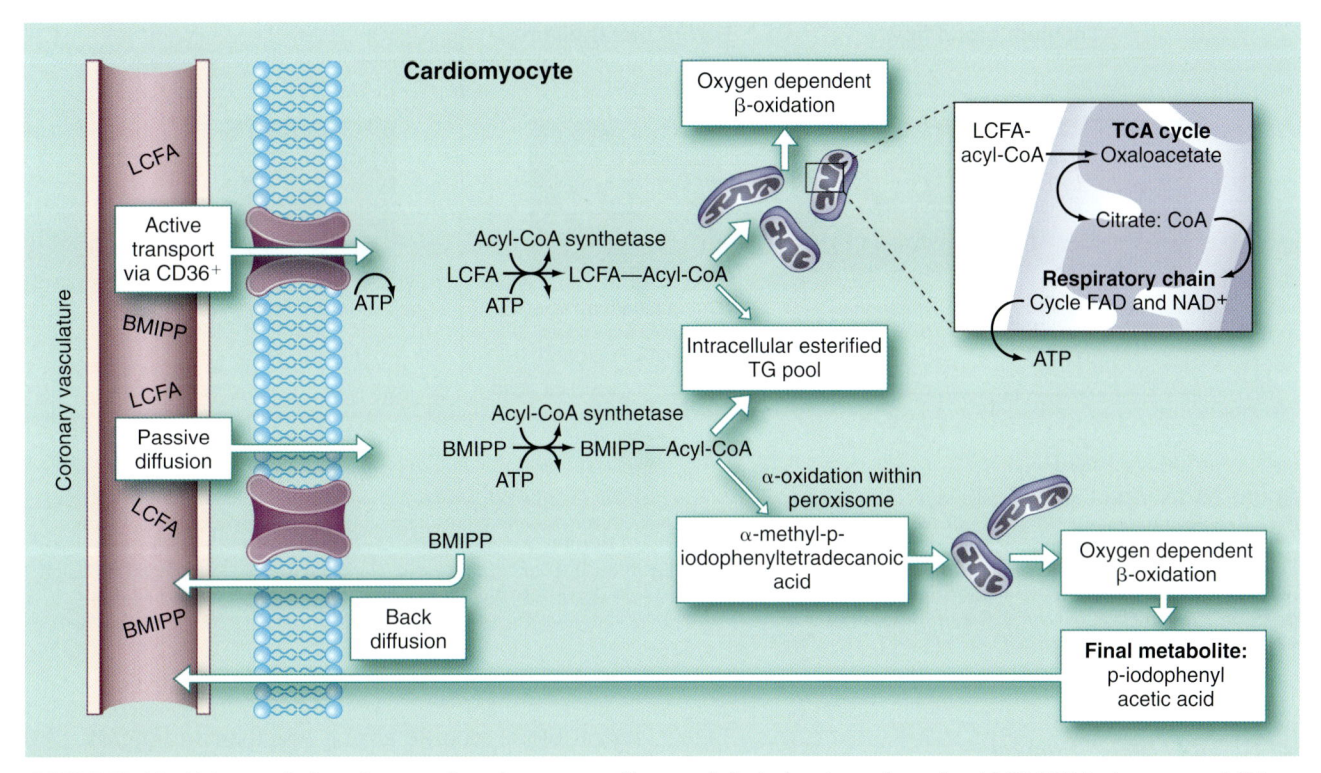

■ **FIGURE 58-14** Major metabolic pathways and regulatory steps of beta-methyliodophenylpentadecanoic acid (BMIPP) in the myocyte. LCFA, long-chain fatty acid; TCA, tricarboxylic acid; TG, triglyceride. *(From Messina SA, Aras O, Dilsizian V. Delayed recovery of fatty acid metabolism after transient myocardial ischemia: a potential imaging target for "ischemic memory." Curr Cardiol Rep 2007; 9:159-165.)*

Similarly, regions with BMIPP-perfusion mismatch (cold metabolic signal relative to perfusion) have been shown to correlate with ^{18}FDG metabolic activity (hot metabolic signal relative to perfusion)—hence viability—on PET. Comparative studies support the concept that regions with BMIPP-perfusion mismatch represent areas of jeopardized, but viable myocardium. After a transient ischemic event, prolonged and persistent metabolic disturbances in fatty acid metabolism can occur for 30 hours—termed *ischemic memory* (Fig. 58-15).[64] Corollary findings have been shown with glucose metabolism (Fig. 58-16).[65-67] Such metabolic stunning, as assessed by BMIPP, has been observed in patients undergoing clinically indicated myocardial perfusion SPECT studies and in patients presenting with acute coronary syndrome.[64,68]

^{18}FDG

PET imaging of myocardial metabolism is most often performed with ^{18}FDG. ^{18}FDG is a glucose analogue with an ^{18}F substituted for hydroxyl (–OH) group that is taken up by the myocyte and accumulates intracellularly after initial phosphorylation by 6-hexokinase. The clinical utility of ^{18}FDG for differentiating viable from scarred myocardium with PET was first described in the 1980s.[20,69] Under aerobic conditions, the heart uses predominantly fatty acids for energy production. During conditions of myocardial ischemia, fatty acid metabolism is diminished, and glucose uptake is enhanced as the myocardium energy requirements are primarily met by glucose metabolism. As ischemia persists, increased tissue concentrations of lactate and hydrogen ions impair glycolysis, eliminating the only source of energy for the myocyte. This elimination leads to loss of transmembrane ion concentration gradients, disruption of cell membranes, and cell death. Residual glucose metabolism in dysfunctional myocardium indicates the presence of viable but functionally compromised myocardium.

^{18}FDG-PET Clinical Protocols

Uptake and distribution of ^{18}FDG in the myocardium are influenced by the dietary state of the patient. In the fasting state, fatty acids are the primary source of myocardial energy production, with glucose accounting for only 30% of the energy derived from oxidative metabolism. In the fed state, plasma insulin levels increase, glucose metabolism is stimulated, and tissue lipolysis is inhibited. Fatty acid delivery to the myocardium is reduced, and glucose use by the myocardium becomes prevalent. Most clinical protocols involve fasting the patient for 6 to 12 hours, and administering a standardized glucose load orally or intravenously, making glucose the preferred fuel substrate for myocardial metabolism.

In patients with diabetes mellitus (in whom supplemental intravenous insulin was not administered), only 58% of ^{18}FDG images were of adequate quality for interpretation.[70] Four common standardization schemes have been proposed to overcome this limitation: (1) oral glucose loading, (2) intravenous glucose loading, (3) hyperinsulinemic-euglycemic clamping, and (4) use of nicotinic acid derivative.

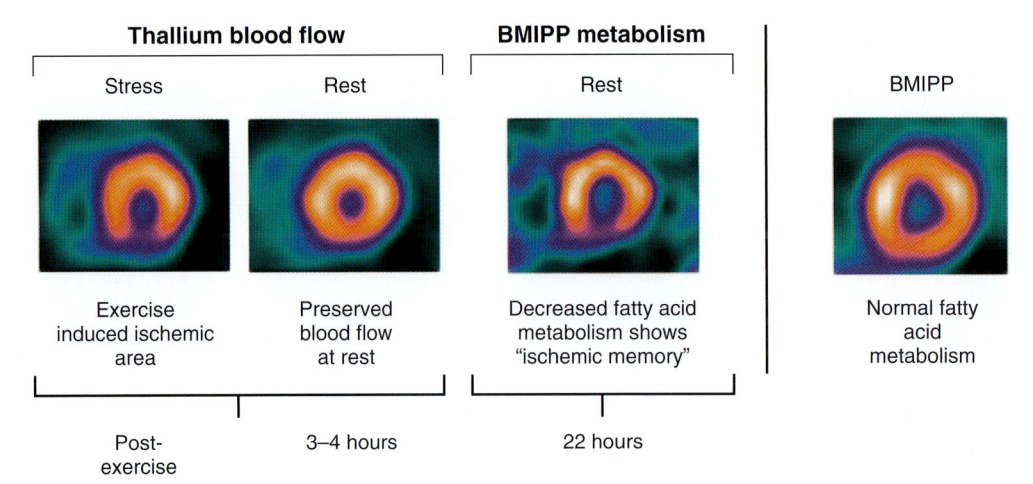

FIGURE 58-15 SPECT showing delayed recovery of regional fatty acid metabolism after transient exercise-induced ischemia, termed *ischemic memory*. Representative stress (*left*) and rest reinjection (*middle*) short-axis thallium tomograms show a reversible inferior defect consistent with exercise-induced myocardial ischemia. Beta-methyliodophenylpentadecanoic acid (BMIPP)–labeled SPECT (*center*) injected and acquired at rest 22 hours after exercise-induced ischemia shows persistent metabolic abnormality in the inferior region despite complete recovery of regional perfusion at rest, as evidenced by thallium reinjection image. The tomogram on the *far right* shows retention of BMIPP in the heart of a normal adult for comparison. *(Adapted from Dilsizian V, Bateman TM, Bergmann SR, et al. Metabolic imaging with beta-methyl-p-[(123)I]-iodophenyl-pentadecanoic acid identifies ischemic memory after demand ischemia. Circulation 2005; 112:2169-2174.)*

Oral Glucose Loading Protocol

First, the fasting blood glucose of the patient is checked. If the fasting blood glucose level is less than 100 mg/dL, 50 g of glucose is administered orally followed by a repeat blood glucose measurement 30 to 45 minutes later. If the repeat blood glucose level is less than 140 mg/dL, ^{18}FDG dose is injected, and images of the heart are subsequently obtained. If the blood glucose level after glucose administration is greater than 140 mg/dL, and if it remains greater than 140 mg/dL on repeat testing, or continues to increase over time, intravenous boluses of regular insulin are

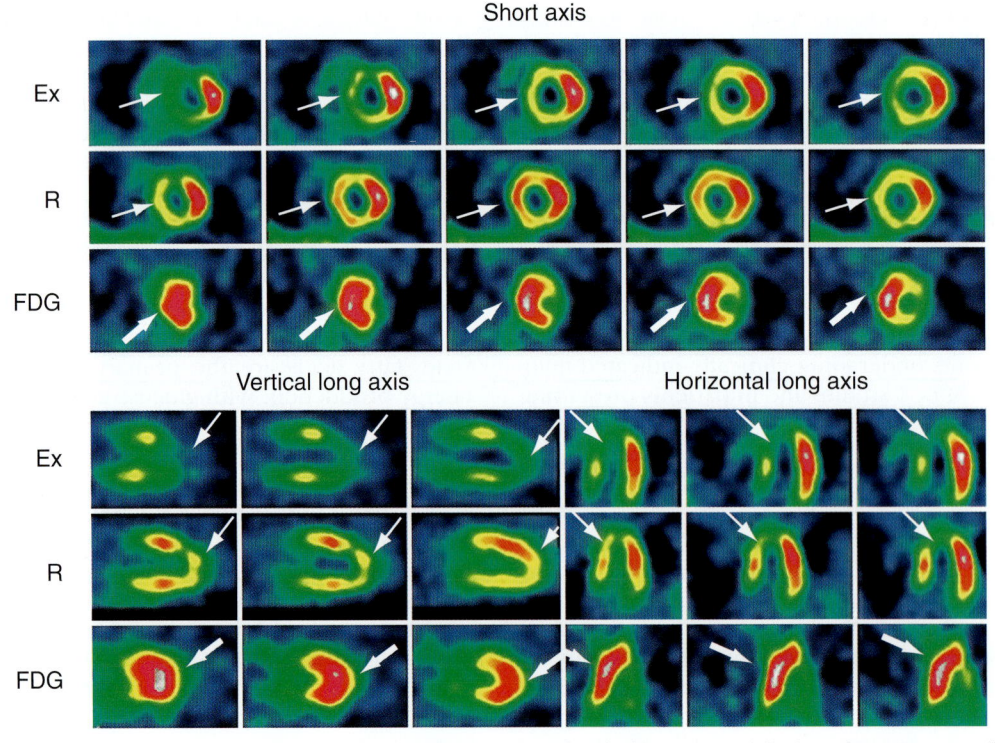

FIGURE 58-16 Simultaneous myocardial perfusion and metabolism imaging after dual intravenous injection of Tc 99m sestamibi and ^{18}FDG at peak exercise. Dual isotope simultaneous acquisition was carried out 40 to 60 minutes after the exercise study was completed. Rest Tc 99m sestamibi imaging was carried out separately. In this patient with angina and no prior MI, there is evidence for extensive reversible perfusion defect (*arrows*) in the anterior, septal, and apical regions. Coronary angiography showed 90% stenosis of the left anterior descending and 60% of the left circumflex coronary arteries. The corresponding ^{18}FDG images show intense uptake in the regions with reversible sestamibi defects reflecting the metabolic correlate of exercise-induced myocardial ischemia. Ex, exercise study; R, rest study. *(Adapted from He ZX, Shi RF, Wu YJ, et al. Direct imaging of exercise-induced myocardial ischemia with fluorine-18-labeled deoxyglucose and Tc-99m-sestamibi in coronary artery disease. Circulation 2003; 108:1208-1213.)*

administered to reduce blood glucose to less than 140 mg/dL or observe a significant decrease in blood glucose level (even if the glucose level is still >140 mg/dL), and ^{18}FDG is injected at that time. The most common approach is to administer an intravenous bolus of regular insulin (according to a predetermined sliding scale) and recheck the plasma glucose level every 15 minutes (administering additional boluses of insulin if necessary) until it is less than 140 mg/dL, at which point ^{18}FDG is injected, and image acquisition is resumed.

Patients with clinical or subclinical diabetes mellitus can pose a problem because, owing to some degree of insulin resistance, the subsequent endogenous insulin release after glucose administration is often blunted. Decisions regarding the morning insulin dose (whether it is withheld or only half of the dose is administered), the amount of oral glucose administered, and consequent doses of intravenous insulin required to reduce the blood glucose level should be tailored for the individual diabetic patient. It has been reported that with the use of supplemental insulin, 88% of patients with diabetes could undergo successful imaging with ^{18}FDG.[70]

Intravenous Glucose Loading Protocol

An intravenous glucose loading protocol involves administration of regular insulin (8 U) and a 10-g dextrose intravenous bolus, followed by an infusion of insulin (1.7 U/kg/min) and dextrose (10 mg/kg/min) for 60 minutes. Blood glucose is checked every 10 minutes. If blood glucose is 100 to 200 mg/dL at 20 minutes, ^{18}FDG is administered. If the blood glucose level is greater than 200 mg/dL, small intravenous boluses of regular insulin are given until the value is less than 200 mg/dL. ^{18}FDG is administered at that time. To prevent hypoglycemia, 20% dextrose infusion is started (2 to 3 mg/kg/hr) at 60 minutes and continued during image acquisition.

This protocol becomes problematic in patients with clinical or subclinical diabetes mellitus because the increase in plasma insulin levels after glucose loading may be attenuated. Consequently, tissue lipolysis is not inhibited, and free fatty acid levels in the plasma remain high. High plasma free fatty acid levels inhibit myocardial glucose uptake, and ^{18}FDG images may be of poor quality and may not accurately reflect myocardial viability.

Hyperinsulinemic-Euglycemic Clamping

To better standardize metabolic conditions during the ^{18}FDG study, other investigators have proposed the use of hyperinsulinemic-euglycemic clamping.[71] In this procedure, insulin and glucose are infused simultaneously to achieve a stable plasma insulin level of 100 to 120 IU/L and a normal plasma glucose level. The rate of glucose infusion (20% dextrose solution with potassium chloride) is adjusted intermittently on the basis of frequently measured plasma glucose levels. Although the hyperinsulinemic-euglycemic clamp technique provides excellent image quality compared with oral glucose loading, it is tedious and impractical for routine clinical studies. It has been reported that the clamp technique does not reduce the interindividual variability of ^{18}FDG measurements compared with the oral glucose loading technique.[71]

Nicotinic Acid Derivative

More recently, the use of nicotinic acid derivative (e.g., acipimox) has been proposed as an alternative to the hyperinsulinemic-euglycemic clamp technique.[72] Approximately 2 hours before ^{18}FDG injection, a single dose of 250 mg of acipimox is given orally followed by glucose loading. With this technique, ^{18}FDG image quality was shown to be comparable to that obtained after the clamp technique in the same patient population.[73] Acipimox has not received FDA approval, however.

^{18}FDG-PET Mismatch and Match Patterns

Functional Recovery

^{18}FDG-PET provides a biologic marker of cellular viability, which is considered to be one of the most accurate noninvasive techniques for identifying viable myocardium before revascularization. In clinical practice, ^{18}FDG is often combined with a flow tracer to assess the presence or absence of myocardial metabolism in hypoperfused myocardial regions. Preserved or enhanced glucose use in dysfunctional myocardial regions with concomitant reduction of blood flow (termed *mismatch defect*) is indicative of hibernating but viable myocardium (Fig. 58-17).[74] Decreased (or absent) glucose use in dysfunctional myocardial regions with concomitant reduction of blood flow (termed *match defect*) is indicative of scarred myocardium.

In combination with myocardial perfusion, gated ^{18}FDG-PET permits evaluation of regional myocardial metabolism and regional and global LV function. When perfusion and metabolism examinations are done in conjunction for the assessment of myocardial viability, the positive and negative predictive accuracies for a mismatch and match defect are 80% to 90% for reversibility or lack of improvement of contractile dysfunction after revascularization.[17,20] Meta-analysis of studies with ^{18}FDG used to predict improvement in regional function after revascularization showed improvement of mean LV ejection fraction from 37% to 47% in patients with viable myocardium (mismatch defect), whereas in patients without viable myocardium (matched defect), the mean LV ejection fraction remained unchanged (39% vs. 40%).[75] Some myocardial regions with flow-metabolism mismatch may have prior subendocardial infarction, however, with an admixture of scarred and viable myocardium. Depending on the extent of the subendocardial damage, some of these mismatch regions may not recover contractile function after revascularization.

Prognosis

Numerous studies have evaluated the prognostic value of ^{18}FDG-PET with regard to future cardiac events. In patients with prior MI but stable CAD, ^{18}FDG uptake was shown to be the most important independent predictor of future cardiac events.[76] In combined data analysis, the incidence

■ **FIGURE 58-17** PET showing perfusion-metabolism mismatch in hibernating heart tissue as an example of preserved cardiometabolic reserve. **A,** Rubidium 82–labeled PET in short-axis view shows markedly decreased perfusion defects in the apical, inferior, inferolateral, and septal regions of the left ventricle at rest, which extends from distal to basal slices. **B,** Images acquired under glucose-loaded conditions, labeled with ^{18}FDG, show perfusion-metabolism mismatch pattern (the scintigraphic hallmark of hibernation) in all abnormally perfused myocardial regions at rest. An exception is the anteroseptal region, which shows matched perfusion-metabolism pattern (compatible with scarred myocardium). *(Adapted from Taegtmeyer H, Dilsizian V. Imaging myocardial metabolism and ischemic memory. Nat Clin Pract Cardiol 2008; 5:S42-S48.)*

of cardiac death over 1 to 2 years was 24% in patients with mismatch pattern treated with medical therapy alone compared with 10% in patients without mismatch pattern.[77] The long-term survival was shown to be significantly decreased to 10% in patients with mismatch pattern (viable myocardium) who underwent revascularization compared with 42% in patients with viable myocardium who were treated with medical therapy alone.[30]

These long-term studies have shown a strong relationship between blood flow–metabolism mismatch pattern and subsequent development of MI or cardiac death. Critical clinical management decisions must be made in patients with high perioperative mortality imposed by the severity of LV dysfunction on one hand, and having the potential for significant improvement in symptoms, functional status, and survival after a successful revascularization on the other hand. In patients selected for revascularization on the basis of PET perfusion-metabolism mismatch classified predominantly as having viable myocardium, 1-year and 5-year survival is reported to be 70% to 80%. In contrast, when patients were managed conservatively despite the mismatch, survival was only 40% to 50%. In patients with predominantly nonviable myocardium by PET, there was no survival benefit of revascularization compared with medical therapy.[78,79]

Many studies have established the necessity for a critical or threshold mass of viable myocardium necessary for improvement in global LV function after revascularization. Using ^{18}FDG-PET, in patients with two or more viable segments in a 15-segment LV model, LV ejection fraction improved from 30 ± 11% to 45 ±14%.[20] In patients with ischemic cardiomyopathy (mean LV ejection fraction 28 ± 6%), the magnitude of improvement in heart failure symptoms after CABG surgery was correlated with the preoperative extent of viable myocardium as determined by PET perfusion-metabolism mismatch (see Fig. 58-5).[24] Patients with evidence of viability involving 18% or more of the LV myocardium had the greatest improvement in functional status (Fig. 58-18).[24] A direct correlation between the magnitude of preserved myocardial viability and the magnitude of improvement in functional status suggests that the extent of dysfunctional ischemic viable myocardium in heart failure patients can be used as a potential marker of the symptomatic benefit that would accrue as a result of revascularization. Because revascularization in patients with significant LV dysfunction is high risk, the data suggest a role for viability imaging results in prognostication and providing a signal of the potential benefit to inform the risk-benefit equation, guiding patient selection.

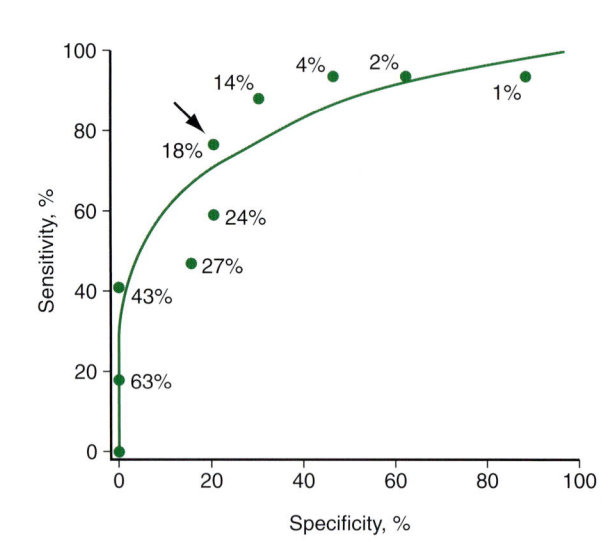

■ **FIGURE 58-18** Receiver operating characteristic curve for different anatomic extent of perfusion-metabolism mismatch to predict a change (at least one grade) in functional status after revascularization. When the extent of PET mismatch involves >18% or greater of the LV mass, the sensitivity for predicting a change in functional status after revascularization is 76%, and the specificity is 78% (area under the fitted curve = 0.82). The prognostic significance of mismatch in randomized, prospective study is the subject of ongoing investigation. *(From Di Carli MF, Asgarzadie F, Schelbert HR, et al. Quantitative relation between myocardial viability and improvement in heart failure symptoms after revascularization in patients with ischemic cardiomyopathy. Circulation 1995; 92:3436-3444.)*

^{18}FDG-SPECT

Despite the inherent resolution differences between PET and SPECT, ^{18}FDG-SPECT shows a good agreement (94%) with ^{18}FDG-PET.[80] As with PET studies, metabolic activity measured by ^{18}FDG-SPECT is generally interpreted in conjunction with a perfusion tracer. Dual-isotope simultaneous acquisition SPECT protocols have been developed, with ^{18}FDG and Tc 99m perfusion tracer injected and acquired simultaneously, capitalizing on the capabilities of gamma cameras to monitor two energy peaks, assessing myocardial perfusion and glucose use and perfusion in a single acquisition.[65,66]

Future Opportunities for Molecular Imaging

The composition and volume of the extracellular matrix is altered in heart failure, as manifested by interstitial, perivascular, and replacement fibrosis. These changes contribute to further impairment of LV diastolic relaxation and compliance, LV contractile dysfunction, and reduction in coronary flow reserve. Myocardial fibrosis in chronic heart failure is a dynamic process that is determined by a balance between collagen synthesis, its degradation by matrix metalloproteinases (MMPs), and the regulation of the latter by another group of glycoproteins, tissue inhibitors of metalloproteinases that bind to and inactivate MMPs. The dynamic nature of the structural changes in LV remodeling is emphasized by their potential for reversibility in response to appropriate interventions, such as coronary revascularization, biventricular pacing, or administration of pharmacologic agents that inhibit the renin-angiotensin-aldosterone or the β-adrenergic systems.

The myocardial extracellular matrix represents a dynamic balance between the synthesis and degradation of collagen with a stable yet dynamic turnover in the normal heart. In the setting of LV remodeling, increased myocardial collagen turnover not only allows repair of damaged tissue, but also permits the muscle fiber slippage and rearrangement that precede chamber enlargement and disfiguration. Myocardial collagen degradation is regulated through the action of MMPs. Indium 111 radiolabeled and Tc 99m radiolabeled ligands have been synthesized and used to show increased MMP activity in infarcted myocardium by planar and SPECT imaging in a murine model.[81]

Targeting Apoptosis

Continuing cell loss, through apoptotic and necrotic pathways, contributes to adverse LV remodeling in heart failure.[82] The various components of the apoptotic pathway have been well characterized, and potential molecular targets for noninvasive imaging of apoptosis have been identified. Activation of the apoptotic pathway leads to translocation of phosphatidylserine, a phospholipid normally confined to the inner aspect of the cell membrane, to the cell surface. After externalization, phosphatidylserine is bound to the phosphatidyl-binding protein annexin-V. The latter has a high affinity for binding to phosphatidylserine, and fluorescein-labeled annexin V has been used routinely for histologic assessment of apoptosis. Tc 99m labeled annexin-V has identified cell loss after acute MI.[83] In vivo imaging of apoptosis is a technique that may prove to be a valuable prognostic tool to follow patients with heart failure after revascularization or those on conservative therapy.

Targeting the Renin-Angiotensin System

The renin-angiotensin system (RAS), an adept regulator of human physiology, is frequently activated early in heart failure, and linked to LV remodeling and myocardial fibrosis through its primary effector peptide angiotensin II. Increased ACE has been seen in association with myocardial fibrosis, and inhibition of RAS modulates LV remodeling in heart failure. It is now known that the various components of RAS are locally produced in the heart, and that knowledge of the tissue expression of these enzymes and peptides could have important implications for the proper management of patients with heart failure.[84,85] The discovery of the tissue RAS and its ability for local production of effector hormones (autocrine effects) has encouraged the development of PET tracers targeting ACE.[86]

To date, five radiolabeled ACE inhibitors have been developed, all exhibiting specific binding to the active ACE site, although certain tracers bind with higher affinity to tissue ACE than others.[86-91] In explanted hearts of patients with ischemic cardiomyopathy, ^{18}F-fluorobenzoyl-lisinopril was shown to bind specifically to myocardial tissue ACE, with the highest activity in regions adjacent to infarcted myocardium (Fig. 58-19).[86] Specific ACE binding was approximately 2-fold higher than the nonspecific binding, and ACE binding in peri-infarct segments was about 1.3-fold greater than binding in remote, noninfarcted segments. A similar pattern of nonuniform distribution was observed with type 1 angiotensin II receptor (AT_1R) immunoreactivity. In addition, increased ACE activity and AT_1R immunoreactivity were seen in the juxtaposed areas of replacement fibrosis, consistent with their observed roles in the development of scars and remodeling of the collagen matrix in ischemic cardiomyopathy.

Lisinopril also has been successfully labeled with Tc 99m, with near-quantitative active site binding and inhibition in rats.[89] If reproduced in humans, the in vivo application of these imaging techniques with either PET (for ^{18}F-fluorobenzoyl-lisinopril) or SPECT (for Tc 99m lisinopril) would allow serial monitoring of tissue ACE activity in patients with heart failure and LV remodeling.

Targeting Autonomic Innervation

Heart failure is a hyperadrenergic state characterized by elevated plasma norepinephrine levels that result in downregulation and uncoupling of cardiac β-adrenergic receptors. The latter contributes to progressive impairment of LV systolic function by altering postsynaptic signal transduction. Altered sympathetic tone in heart failure is also directly linked to disease progression, prognosis, and risk of sudden death. Noninvasive strategies to determine the state of cardiac autonomic regulation are of significant clinical interest.

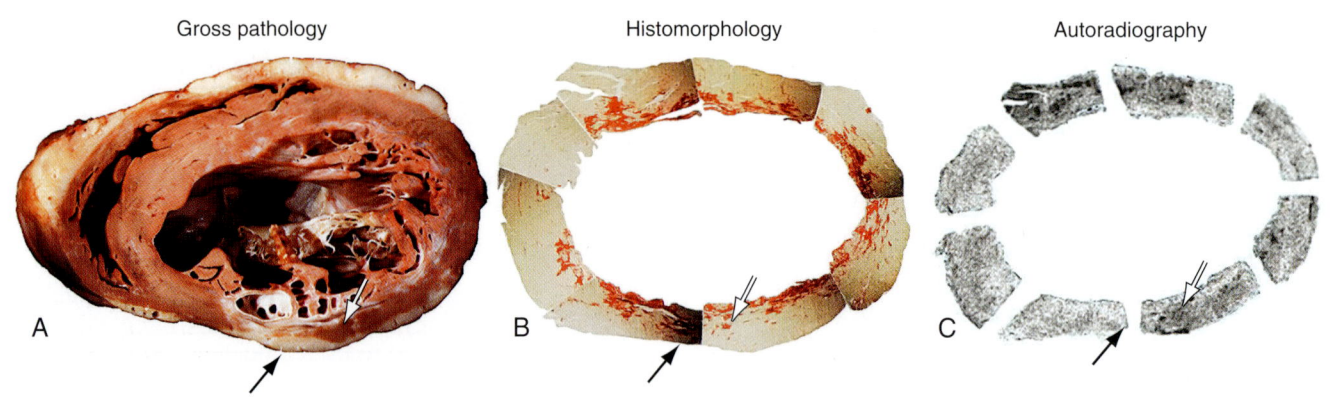

■ **FIGURE 58-19** Presence and distribution of ACE activity in relation to collagen replacement as assessed by Picrosirius red stain in human heart tissue removed from a cardiac transplant recipient with ischemic cardiomyopathy. **A-C,** Gross pathology of a mid-ventricular slice (**A**) with corresponding contiguous mid-ventricular slices stained with Picrosirius red stain (**B**) and [^{18}F]fluorobenzyl-linsinopril (FBL) autoradiographic images (**C**) are shown. FBL binding to ACE is nonuniform in infarct, peri-infarct, and remote noninfarct segments. Increased FBL binding (*white arrows*) can be seen in the segments adjacent to the collagen replacement (*black arrow*). *(Adapted from Dilsizian V, Eckelman WC, Loredo ML, et al. Evidence for tissue angiotensin-converting enzyme in explanted hearts of ischemic cardiomyopathy using targeted radiotracer technique. J Nucl Med 2007; 48:182-187.)*

Several radiolabeled catecholamines or catecholamine analogues have been successfully used in conjunction with SPECT and PET for the evaluation of myocardial autonomic innervation. The most commonly used SPECT tracer is the radiolabeled norepinephrine analogue iodine 123–metaiodobenzylguanidine (MIBG), which competes with norepinephrine for reuptake in presynaptic vesicles, and has been successfully used to assess cardiac presynaptic sympathetic innervation. After an ischemic myocardial injury, dissociation between recovery of myocardial perfusion and myocardial innervation, as determined with MIBG, has been shown (Fig. 58-20).[92] Despite considerable myocardial salvage after coronary artery reperfusion, MIBG images obtained 2 weeks after MI and reperfusion show a persistent area of myocardial denervation within the left ventricle. This area is comparable to the area of ischemic myocardium at risk, as determined by myocardial perfusion SPECT during the acute ischemic event.[92]

Such modifications of cardiac neuronal function have an important role in the pathophysiology of heart failure and arrhythmias. Mortality is significantly higher in heart failure patients with presynaptic sympathetic denervation, as assessed by MIBG, compared with patients with preserved MIBG uptake.[93] More recent studies suggest that such characterization of the sympathetic denervation of the heart could be useful for selecting heart failure patients for β-adrenergic receptor blocker therapy.[94] Another synthetic norepinephrine analogue, ^{11}C-meta-hydroxyephedrine, has also been used as a PET tracer and has the

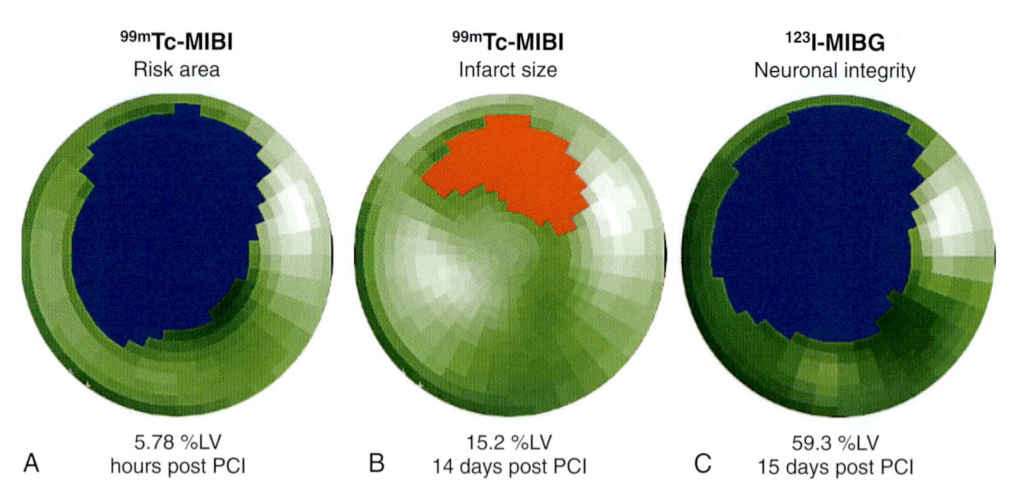

■ **FIGURE 58-20** Neuronal damage in ischemic myocardium detected by MIBG. SPECT polar maps from a patient with acute anterior MI and reperfusion show the presence and extent of Tc 99m sestamibi myocardial perfusion and MIBG myocardial innervation. **A,** The first polar map shows the area of myocardial hypoperfusion (area of risk) in the emergency department, which was calculated to be 58% of the left ventricle. **B,** Myocardial perfusion image repeated 14 days after the acute event shows significant interim salvage of myocardium with only 15% of residual defect in the left ventricle. **C,** Despite the considerable amount of myocardial salvage after coronary artery reperfusion, MIBG images obtained 1 day after the repeat perfusion study (day 15 after the acute myocardial injury) show persistent area of myocardial denervation within the left ventricle that is comparable to the area of ischemic myocardium at risk determined by myocardial perfusion SPECT during the acute ischemic event. These findings suggest that there is a dissociation between recovery of myocardial perfusion after an ischemic myocardial injury and myocardial innervation. Recovery of myocardial innervation after an acute myocardial injury lags significantly behind myocardial perfusion. *(From Matsunari I, Schricke U, Bengel FM, et al. Extent of cardiac sympathetic neuronal damage is determined by the area of ischemia in patients with acute coronary syndromes. Circulation 2000; 101:2579-2585.)*

advantage over MIBG of higher sensitivity and spatial resolution.[95] In addition, PET allows for quantification and measurement of the tracer kinetics. Combined imaging with other presynaptic PET tracers, such as ^{11}C-epinephrine and ^{11}C-phenylephrine, could allow comprehensive evaluation of the norepinephrine uptake, storage, and metabolism in presynaptic nerve terminals.

CONCLUSION

The concept of myocardial viability was first validated with nuclear medicine imaging modalities in the late 1970s. Numerous PET and SPECT techniques continue to be crucial for clinical evaluation and stratification of patients for subsequent treatment decision making for intervention. The prevalence of CAD and resultant mortality and morbidity continues to burden the health care system. Regardless of the technique employed, extensive evidence shows the importance of identifying myocardial viability in patients with ischemic LV dysfunction before treatments and intervention to offer the patient the best chance for prolonged survival and improved quality of life.

As the details of heart failure on a cellular level are delineated, more focus will be placed on the development of molecular imaging targets, which will prove to be more powerful tools for diagnosis, treatment, and prognosis of patients with CAD. Nuclear imaging techniques will continue to play a crucial role in the identification of myocardial viability and diagnosis of CAD, and prove invaluable in the basic research on development and validation of new modalities in the future.

KEY POINTS

- The concept of myocardial viability first arose after observational studies in patients with LV dysfunction who subsequently exhibited improvement in regional and global LV function after coronary artery revascularization.
- There is a significant association between revascularization and improved survival rate in patients with LV dysfunction and evidence of myocardial viability independent of the imaging technique used.
- Dysfunctional but viable myocardium has been broadly categorized as stunned or hibernating myocardium. Stunned myocardium refers to the state of delayed recovery of regional ventricular contractile dysfunction after a transient period of ischemia that has been followed by restoration of perfusion. Hibernating myocardium refers to an adaptive rather than an injurious response to impaired coronary flow reserve (repetitive ischemia and stunning) and reduced resting coronary blood flow.
- Prospective assessment of myocardial viability in dysfunctional myocardium involves assessment of perfusion, sarcolemmal membrane integrity, intact mitochondria, preserved metabolism (glucose and fatty acid), and contractile reserve, which can be assessed with scintigraphic techniques using SPECT or PET.
- [18]FDG-PET provides a biologic marker of cellular viability, which is considered to be one of the most accurate noninvasive techniques for identifying viable myocardium before revascularization.
- Continuing apoptotic and necrotic myocyte loss can lead to adverse LV remodeling in heart failure, and associated contributory pathways offer numerous targets for the continued development of molecular imaging techniques.

SUGGESTED READINGS

Allman KC, Shaw LJ, Hachamovitch R, et al. Myocardial viability testing and impact of revascularization on prognosis in patients with coronary artery disease and left ventricular dysfunction: a meta-analysis. J Am Coll Cardiol 2002; 39:1151-1158.

Di Carli MF, Asgarzadie F, Schelbert HR, et al. Quantitative relation between myocardial viability and improvement in heart failure symptoms after revascularization in patients with ischemic cardiomyopathy. Circulation 1995; 92:3436-3444.

Dilsizian V, Narula J. Nuclear investigation in heart failure and myocardial viability. In Dilsizian V, Narula J (eds). Atlas of Nuclear Cardiology, 3rd ed. Philadelphia, Current Medicine, 2009, pp 201-224.

Lodge MA, Braess H, Mahmood F, et al. Developments in nuclear cardiology: transition from single photon emission computed tomography to positron emission tomography-computed tomography. J Invasive Cardiol 2005; 17:491-496.

REFERENCES

1. Rosamond W, Flegal K, Friday G, et al. Heart disease and stroke statistics—2007 update: a report from the American Heart Association Statistics Committee and Stroke Statistics Subcommittee. Circulation 2007; 115:e69-e171.
2. Lloyd-Jones DM, Larson MG, Beiser A, et al. Lifetime risk of developing coronary heart disease. Lancet 1999; 353:89-92.
3. Bax JJ, van der Wall EE, Harbinson M. Radionuclide techniques for the assessment of myocardial viability and hibernation. Heart 2004; 90(Suppl 5):v26-v33.
4. Gheorghiade M, Bonow RO. Chronic heart failure in the United States: a manifestation of coronary artery disease. Circulation 1998; 97:282-289.
5. Massie BM, Shah NB. Evolving trends in the epidemiologic factors of heart failure: rationale for preventive strategies and comprehensive disease management. Am Heart J 1997; 133:703-712.
6. Levy D, Kenchaiah S, Larson MG, et al. Long-term trends in the incidence of and survival with heart failure. N Engl J Med 2002; 347:1397-1402.
7. Rahimtoola SH. The hibernating myocardium. Am Heart J 1989; 117:211-221.
8. Braunwald E, Kloner RA. The stunned myocardium: prolonged, postischemic ventricular dysfunction. Circulation 1982; 66:1146-1149.
9. Dilsizian V, Narula J. Nuclear investigation in heart failure and myocardial viability. In Dilsizian V, Narula J (eds). Atlas of Nuclear Cardiology, 3rd ed. Philadelphia, Current Medicine, 2009, pp 201-224.
10. Elsasser A, Muller KD, Skwara W, et al. Severe energy deprivation of human hibernating myocardium as possible common pathomechanism of contractile dysfunction, structural degeneration and cell death. J Am Coll Cardiol 2002; 39:1189-1198.

11. Depre C, Vanoverschelde JL, Gerber B, et al. Correlation of functional recovery with myocardial blood flow, glucose uptake, and morphologic features in patients with chronic left ventricular ischemic dysfunction undergoing coronary artery bypass grafting. J Thorac Cardiovasc Surg 1997; 113:371-378.
12. Maes A, Flameng W, Nuyts J, et al. Histological alterations in chronically hypoperfused myocardium: correlation with PET findings. Circulation 1994; 90:735-745.
13. Camici P, Ferrannini E, Opie LH. Myocardial metabolism in ischemic heart disease: basic principles and application to imaging by positron emission tomography. Prog Cardiovasc Dis 1989; 32:217-238.
14. Braunwald E, Rutherford JD. Reversible ischemic left ventricular dysfunction: evidence for the "hibernating myocardium." J Am Coll Cardiol 1986; 8:1467-1470.
15. Dispersyn GD, Ausma J, Thone F, et al. Cardiomyocyte remodelling during myocardial hibernation and atrial fibrillation: prelude to apoptosis. Cardiovasc Res 1999; 43:947-957.
16. Taegtmeyer H. Modulation of responses to myocardial ischemia: metabolic features of myocardial stunning, hibernation, and ischemic preconditioning. In Dilsizian V (ed). Myocardial Viability: A Clinical and Scientific Treatise. Armonk, NY, Futura, 2000, pp 25-36.
17. Schinkel AF, Poldermans D, Vanoverschelde JL, et al. Incidence of recovery of contractile function following revascularization in patients with ischemic left ventricular dysfunction. Am J Cardiol 2004; 93:14-17.
18. Dilsizian V. Cardiac magnetic resonance versus SPECT: are all non-infarct myocardial regions created equal? J Nucl Cardiol 2007; 14:9-14.
19. Passamani E, Davis KB, Gillespie MJ, et al. A randomized trial of coronary artery bypass surgery: survival of patients with a low ejection fraction. N Engl J Med 1985; 312:1665-1671.
20. Tillisch J, Brunken R, Marshall R, et al. Reversibility of cardiac wall-motion abnormalities predicted by positron tomography. N Engl J Med 1986; 314:884-888.
21. Bonow RO, Dilsizian V. Thallium-201 for assessment of myocardial viability. Semin Nucl Med 1991; 21:230-241.
22. Meluzin J, Cerny J, Frelich M, et al. Prognostic value of the amount of dysfunctional but viable myocardium in revascularized patients with coronary artery disease and left ventricular dysfunction. Investigators of this Multicenter Study. J Am Coll Cardiol 1998; 32:912-920.
23. Bax JJ, Visser FC, Poldermans D, et al. Relationship between preoperative viability and postoperative improvement in LVEF and heart failure symptoms. J Nucl Med 2001; 42:79-86.
24. Di Carli MF, Asgarzadie F, Schelbert HR, et al. Quantitative relation between myocardial viability and improvement in heart failure symptoms after revascularization in patients with ischemic cardiomyopathy. Circulation 1995; 92:3436-3444.
25. Bonow RO. Identification of viable myocardium. Circulation 1996; 94:2674-2680.
26. Udelson JE. Steps forward in the assessment of myocardial viability in left ventricular dysfunction. Circulation 1998; 97:833-838.
27. Dilsizian V. Myocardial viability: contractile reserve or cell membrane integrity? J Am Coll Cardiol 1996; 28:443-446.
28. Samady H, Elefteriades JA, Abbott BG, et al. Failure to improve left ventricular function after coronary revascularization for ischemic cardiomyopathy is not associated with worse outcome. Circulation 1999; 100:1298-1304.
29. Udelson JE, Konstam MA. Relation between left ventricular remodeling and clinical outcomes in heart failure patients with left ventricular systolic dysfunction. J Card Fail 2002; 8:S465-S471.
30. Allman KC, Shaw LJ, Hachamovitch R, et al. Myocardial viability testing and impact of revascularization on prognosis in patients with coronary artery disease and left ventricular dysfunction: a meta-analysis. J Am Coll Cardiol 2002; 39:1151-1158.
31. Bourque JM, Hasselblad V, Velazquez EJ, et al. Revascularization in patients with coronary artery disease, left ventricular dysfunction, and viability: a meta-analysis. Am Heart J 2003; 146:621-627.
32. Emond M, Mock MB, Davis KB, et al. Long-term survival of medically treated patients in the Coronary Artery Surgery Study (CASS) Registry. Circulation 1994; 90:2645-2657.
33. Holmuhamedov EL, Jovanovic S, Dzeja PP, et al. Mitochondrial ATP-sensitive K+ channels modulate cardiac mitochondrial function. Am J Physiol 1998; 275:H1567-H1576.
34. Takahashi N, Reinhardt CP, Marcel R, et al. Myocardial uptake of ^{99m}Tc-tetrofosmin, sestamibi, and ^{201}Tl in a model of acute coronary reperfusion. Circulation 1996; 94:2605-2613.
35. Dakik HA, Howell JF, Lawrie GM, et al. Assessment of myocardial viability with 99mTc-sestamibi tomography before coronary bypass graft surgery: correlation with histopathology and postoperative improvement in cardiac function. Circulation 1997; 96:2892-2898.
36. Bonow RO, Dilsizian V. Thallium-201 and technetium-99m-sestamibi for assessing viable myocardium. J Nucl Med 1992; 33:815-818.
37. Udelson JE, Coleman PS, Metherall J, et al. Predicting recovery of severe regional ventricular dysfunction: comparison of resting scintigraphy with ^{201}Tl and ^{99m}Tc-sestamibi. Circulation 1994; 89:2552-2561.
38. Matsunari I, Fujino S, Taki J, et al. Quantitative rest technetium-99m tetrofosmin imaging in predicting functional recovery after revascularization: comparison with rest-redistribution thallium-201. J Am Coll Cardiol 1997; 29:1226-1233.
39. Dilsizian V, Arrighi JA, Diodati JG, et al. Myocardial viability in patients with chronic coronary artery disease: comparison of ^{99m}Tc-sestamibi with thallium reinjection and ^{18}F-fluorodeoxyglucose. Circulation 1994; 89:578-587.
40. Soufer R, Dey HM, Ng CK, et al. Comparison of sestamibi single-photon emission computed tomography with positron emission tomography for estimating left ventricular myocardial viability. Am J Cardiol 1995; 75:1214-1219.
41. Arrighi JA, Ng CK, Dey HM, et al. Effect of left ventricular function on the assessment of myocardial viability by technetium-99m sestamibi and correlation with positron emission tomography in patients with healed myocardial infarcts or stable angina pectoris, or both. Am J Cardiol 1997; 80:1007-1013.
42. Dilsizian V. Technetium-99m labeled myocardial perfusion tracers: blood flow or viability agents? In Dilsizian V (ed). Myocardial Viability: A Clinical and Scientific Treatise. Armonk, NY, Futura, 2000, pp 315-348.
43. Bisi G, Sciagra R, Santoro GM, et al. Rest technetium-99m sestamibi tomography in combination with short-term administration of nitrates: feasibility and reliability for prediction of postrevascularization outcome of asynergic territories. J Am Coll Cardiol 1994; 24:1282-1289.
44. Leoncini M, Marcucci G, Sciagra R, et al. Nitrate-enhanced gated technetium 99m sestamibi SPECT for evaluating regional wall motion at baseline and during low-dose dobutamine infusion in patients with chronic coronary artery disease and left ventricular dysfunction: comparison with two-dimensional echocardiography. J Nucl Cardiol 2000; 7:426-431.
45. Bax JJ, Poldermans D, Elhendy A, et al. Sensitivity, specificity, and predictive accuracies of various noninvasive techniques for detecting hibernating myocardium. Curr Probl Cardiol 2001; 26:147-186.
46. Dilsizian V. SPECT and PET myocardial perfusion imaging: tracers and techniques. In Dilsizian V, Narula J (eds). Atlas of Nuclear Cardiology, 3rd ed. Philadelphia, Current Medicine, 2009, pp 37-60.
47. Bisi G, Sciagra R, Santoro GM, et al. Technetium-99m-sestamibi imaging with nitrate infusion to detect viable hibernating myocardium and predict postrevascularization recovery. J Nucl Med 1995; 36:1994-2000.
48. Sciagra R, Bisi G, Santoro GM, et al. Comparison of baseline-nitrate technetium-99m sestamibi with rest-redistribution thallium-201 tomography in detecting viable hibernating myocardium and predicting postrevascularization recovery. J Am Coll Cardiol 1997; 30:384-391.
49. Sciagra R, Pellegri M, Pupi A, et al. Prognostic implications of Tc-99m sestamibi viability imaging and subsequent therapeutic strategy in patients with chronic coronary artery disease and left ventricular dysfunction. J Am Coll Cardiol 2000; 36:739-745.
50. Pohost GM, Zir LM, Moore RH, et al. Differentiation of transiently ischemic from infarcted myocardium by serial imaging after a single dose of thallium-201. Circulation 1977; 55:294-302.
51. Granato JE, Watson DD, Flanagan TL, et al. Myocardial thallium-201 kinetics during coronary occlusion and reperfusion: influence of method of reflow and timing of thallium-201 administration. Circulation 1986; 73:150-160.
52. Akins CW, Pohost GM, Desanctis RW, et al. Selection of angina-free patients with severe left ventricular dysfunction for myocardial revascularization. Am J Cardiol 1980; 46:695-700.

53. Kiat H, Berman DS, Maddahi J, et al. Late reversibility of tomographic myocardial thallium-201 defects: an accurate marker of myocardial viability. J Am Coll Cardiol 1988; 12:1456-1463.
54. Dilsizian V, Rocco TP, Freedman NM, et al. Enhanced detection of ischemic but viable myocardium by the reinjection of thallium after stress-redistribution imaging. N Engl J Med 1990; 323:141-146.
55. Ragosta M, Beller GA, Watson DD, et al. Quantitative planar rest-redistribution ^{201}Tl imaging in detection of myocardial viability and prediction of improvement in left ventricular function after coronary artery bypass surgery in patients with severely depressed left ventricular function. Circulation 1993; 87:1630-1641.
56. Kitsiou AN, Srinivasan G, Quyyumi AA, et al. Stress-induced reversible and mild-to-moderate irreversible thallium defects: are they equally accurate for predicting recovery of regional left ventricular function after revascularization? Circulation 1998; 98:501-508.
57. Lodge MA, Braess H, Mahmood F, et al. Developments in nuclear cardiology: transition from single photon emission computed tomography to positron emission tomography-computed tomography. J Invasive Cardiol 2005; 17:491-496.
58. Schelbert HR, Phelps ME, Huang SC, et al. N-13 ammonia as an indicator of myocardial blood flow. Circulation 1981; 63:1259-1272.
59. Nitzsche EU, Choi Y, Czernin J, et al. Noninvasive quantification of myocardial blood flow in humans: a direct comparison of the [13N]ammonia and the [15O]water techniques. Circulation 1996; 93:2000-2006.
60. Iida H, Rhodes CG, de Silva R, et al. Myocardial tissue fraction: correction of partial volume effects and measure of tissue viability. J Nucl Med 1991; 32:2169-2175.
61. Yamamoto Y, de Silva R, Rhodes CG, et al. A new strategy for the assessment of viable myocardium and regional myocardial blood flow using ^{15}O-water and dynamic positron emission tomography. Circulation 1992; 86:167-178.
62. Gerber BL, Melin JA, Bol A, et al. Nitrogen-13-ammonia and oxygen-15-water estimates of absolute myocardial perfusion in left ventricular ischemic dysfunction. J Nucl Med 1998; 39:1655-1662.
63. Messina SA, Aras O, Dilsizian V. Delayed recovery of fatty acid metabolism after transient myocardial ischemia: a potential imaging target for "ischemic memory." Curr Cardiol Rep 2007; 9:159-165.
64. Dilsizian V, Bateman TM, Bergmann SR, et al. Metabolic imaging with beta-methyl-p-[(123)I]-iodophenyl-pentadecanoic acid identifies ischemic memory after demand ischemia. Circulation 2005; 112:2169-2174.
65. He ZX, Shi RF, Wu YJ, et al. Direct imaging of exercise-induced myocardial ischemia with fluorine-18-labeled deoxyglucose and Tc-99m-sestamibi in coronary artery disease. Circulation 2003; 108:1208-1213.
66. Dou KF, Yang MF, Yang YJ, et al. Myocardial 18F-FDG uptake after exercise-induced myocardial ischemia in patients with coronary artery disease. J Nucl Med 2008; 49:1986-1991.
67. Dilsizian V. FDG Uptake as a surrogate marker for antecedent ischemia. J Nucl Med 2008; 49:1909-1911.
68. Kawai Y, Tsukamoto E, Nozaki Y, et al. Significance of reduced uptake of iodinated fatty acid analogue for the evaluation of patients with acute chest pain. J Am Coll Cardiol 2001; 38:1888-1894.
69. Marshall RC, Tillisch JH, Phelps ME, et al. Identification and differentiation of resting myocardial ischemia and infarction in man with positron computed tomography, 18F-labeled fluorodeoxyglucose and N-13 ammonia. Circulation 1983; 67:766-778.
70. Gropler RJ. Methodology governing the assessment of myocardial glucose metabolism by positron emission tomography and fluorine 18-labeled fluorodeoxyglucose. J Nucl Cardiol 1994; 1:S4-S14.
71. Knuuti MJ, Nuutila P, Ruotsalainen U, et al. Euglycemic hyperinsulinemic clamp and oral glucose load in stimulating myocardial glucose utilization during positron emission tomography. J Nucl Med 1992; 33:1255-1262.
72. Knuuti MJ, Yki-Jarvinen H, Voipio-Pulkki LM, et al. Enhancement of myocardial [fluorine-18]fluorodeoxyglucose uptake by a nicotinic acid derivative. J Nucl Med 1994; 35:989-998.
73. Bax JJ, Veening MA, Visser FC, et al. Optimal metabolic conditions during fluorine-18 fluorodeoxyglucose imaging: a comparative study using different protocols. Eur J Nucl Med 1997; 24:35-41.
74. Taegtmeyer H, Dilsizian V. Imaging myocardial metabolism and ischemic memory. Nat Clin Pract Cardiol 2008; 5:S42-S48.
75. Maddahi J, Schelbert H, Brunken R, et al. Role of thallium-201 and PET imaging in evaluation of myocardial viability and management of patients with coronary artery disease and left ventricular dysfunction. J Nucl Med 1994; 35:707-715.
76. Tamaki N, Kawamoto M, Takahashi N, et al. Prognostic value of an increase in fluorine-18 deoxyglucose uptake in patients with myocardial infarction: comparison with stress thallium imaging. J Am Coll Cardiol 1993; 22:1621-1627.
77. Schelbert HR. ^{18}F-deoxyglucose and the assessment of myocardial viability. Semin Nucl Med 2002; 32:60-69.
78. Eitzman D, al Aouar Z, Kanter HL, et al. Clinical outcome of patients with advanced coronary artery disease after viability studies with positron emission tomography. J Am Coll Cardiol 1992; 20:559-565.
79. Di Carli MF, Davidson M, Little R, et al. Value of metabolic imaging with positron emission tomography for evaluating prognosis in patients with coronary artery disease and left ventricular dysfunction. Am J Cardiol 1994; 73:527-533.
80. Srinivasan G, Kitsiou AN, Bacharach SL, et al. [18F]fluorodeoxyglucose single photon emission computed tomography: can it replace PET and thallium SPECT for the assessment of myocardial viability? Circulation 1998; 97:843-850.
81. Su H, Spinale FG, Dobrucki LW, et al. Noninvasive targeted imaging of matrix metalloproteinase activation in a murine model of postinfarction remodeling. Circulation 2005; 112:3157-3167.
82. Grazette LP, Rosenzweig A. Role of apoptosis in heart failure. Heart Fail Clin 2005; 1:251-261.
83. Hofstra L, Liem IH, Dumont EA, et al. Visualisation of cell death in vivo in patients with acute myocardial infarction. Lancet 2000; 356:209-212.
84. Paul M, Poyan MA, Kreutz R. Physiology of local renin-angiotensin systems. Physiol Rev 2006; 86:747-803.
85. Shirani J, Narula J, Eckelman WC, et al. Novel imaging strategies for predicting remodeling and evolution of heart failure: targeting the renin-angiotensin system. Heart Fail. Clin 2006; 2:231-247.
86. Dilsizian V, Eckelman WC, Loredo ML, et al. Evidence for tissue angiotensin-converting enzyme in explanted hearts of ischemic cardiomyopathy using targeted radiotracer technique. J Nucl Med 2007; 48:182-187.
87. Hwang DR, Eckelman WC, Mathias CJ, et al. Positron-labeled angiotensin-converting enzyme (ACE) inhibitor: fluorine-18-fluorocaptopril: probing the ACE activity in vivo by positron emission tomography. J Nucl Med 1991; 32:1730-1737.
88. Lee YHC, Kiesewetter DO, Lang L, et al. Synthesis of 4-[18F]fluorobenzoyllisinopril: a radioligand for angiotensin converting enzyme (ACE) imaging with positron emission tomography. J Labelled Cpd Radiopharm 2001; 44:S268-S270.
89. Femia FJ, Maresca KP, Hillier SM, et al. Synthesis and evaluation of a series of 99mTc(CO)3+ lisinopril complexes for in vivo imaging of angiotensin-converting enzyme expression. J Nucl Med 2008; 49:1-8.
90. Fyhrquist F, Tikkanen I, Grönhagen-Riska C, et al. Inhibitor binding assay for angiotensin-converting enzyme. Clin Chem 1984; 30:696-700.
91. Matarrese M, Salimbeni A, Turolla EA, et al. ^{11}C-Radiosynthesis and preliminary human evaluation of the disposition of the ACE inhibitor [11C]zofenoprilat. Bioorg Med Chem 2004; 12:603-611.
92. Matsunari I, Schricke U, Bengel FM, et al. Extent of cardiac sympathetic neuronal damage is determined by the area of ischemia in patients with acute coronary syndromes. Circulation 2000; 101:2579-2585.
93. Merlet P, Valette H, Dubois-Rande JL, et al. Prognostic value of cardiac metaiodobenzylguanidine imaging in patients with heart failure. J Nucl Med 1992; 33:471-477.
94. Fukuoka S, Hayashida K, Hirose Y, et al. Use of iodine-123 metaiodobenzylguanidine myocardial imaging to predict the effectiveness of beta-blocker therapy in patients with dilated cardiomyopathy. Eur J Nucl Med 1997; 24:523-529.
95. Raffel DM, Jung YW, Gildersleeve, DL, et al. Radiolabeled phenethylguanidines: novel imaging agents for cardiac sympathetic neurons and adrenergic tumors. J Med Chem 2007; 50:2078-2088.

CHAPTER 59

Postoperative Imaging of Ischemic Cardiac Disease

Praveen Jonnala, Swati Deshmane, and Mayil S. Krishnam

Congestive heart failure, the most common admitting diagnosis for patients older than 65 years in the United States,[1] continues to increase in incidence and prevalence, with more than 500,000 new cases of chronic heart failure diagnosed yearly. The most common cause of heart failure is ischemic cardiomyopathy; the second most common cause is dilated cardiomyopathy. The diagnosis, management, treatment, and rehabilitation of patients suffering from ischemic heart disease represent a large percentage of health care costs. Current interventions for management and treatment of end-stage ischemic heart disease include aggressive medical management, extracorporeal circulatory support, percutaneous left ventricular assist device placement, implantable ventricular assist device placement, coronary artery revascularization, mitral valve repair or replacement, scar ablation, passive epicardial restraint, surgical ventricular restoration, and heart transplantation. Combinations of these surgical interventions are sometimes used, depending on the patient's needs.

In this chapter, we cover common surgical options (other than coronary artery bypass graft surgery) for ischemic heart disease and its complications. These surgeries include the ventricular restoration procedure (Dor procedure), cardiac assist device, and heart transplantation. Although mitral valve repair involving mitral annuloplasty is considered an option in the treatment of patients with ischemic or nonischemic dilated cardiomyopathy, it is not widely practiced. This surgery is considered for patients with secondary mitral regurgitation (normal mitral valve anatomy) due to a dilated ventricle from ischemic or other causes that results in displacement of papillary muscles and dilation of the mitral annulus.

PREVALENCE, EPIDEMIOLOGY, AND BACKGROUND

Of 5.3 million Americans suffering from heart failure, about 2.8 million will die within a year. Between 2000 and 4000 Americans are on waiting lists for heart transplants at any given time, and according to the United Network for Organ Sharing, approximately 2000 heart transplants are performed every year. About 10% to 20% of patients on the heart transplant waiting list die while awaiting the opportunity for receipt of a transplant. According to the United Network for Organ Sharing, 5-year post–heart transplantation survival rates for heart status 1A, 1B, and 2 are 68.7%, 72.7%, and 74%; 1-year survival rates for heart status 1A, 1B, and 2 are 85.7%, 87.3%, and 90.6%.

For patients obtaining ventricular assist devices as a bridge to transplantation or destination therapy, 1-year survival rates have been reported to be 52% compared with 25% for a medically treated cohort of patients; the 2-year survival rate is 23% compared with 8% for a medically treated cohort of patients.[2]

In one study including 1198 patients, 5-year survival rates of patients undergoing surgical ventricular restoration with concomitant coronary artery bypass graft or mitral valve surgery were 69.9% ± 4.7% for New York Heart Association (NYHA) class III patients.[3] Results of the STICH (Surgical Treatment for Ischemic Heart Failure) trial, a recently completed randomized surgical versus medical trial, will help clarify indications for coronary revascularization, surgical ventricular restoration, and medical therapy. Alternative therapies to heart transplantation will continue to be important because of the yearly increasing gap between demand and supply of hearts.

Ventricular Assist Device

The ventricular assist device (VAD) is an implantable electromechanical cardiovascular support device for patients with heart failure to improve cardiac output and thereby to achieve adequate circulatory status and to maintain effective end-organ perfusion. Common indications are cardiogenic shock due to myocardial infarction, postcardiotomy cardiogenic shock, and bridge to heart transplantation for patients with ischemic heart failure. It may be used permanently as a destination therapy for patients who are not eligible for heart transplantation. A temporary percutaneous left VAD (LVAD) can provide support during complex percutaneous coronary interventions. Contraindications to VAD placement include very short stature and emaciated, thin patients.

Examples of short-term temporary percutaneous LVADs are the CardiacAssist, Inc., TandemHeart; Abiomed Impella, Abiomed BVS 5000; Medtronic Bio-Medicus Bio-Pump; Terumo Sarns Centrifugal System; St. Jude Medical Lifestream centrifugal pump; Levitronix CentriMag LVAS; and intra-aortic balloon pump counterpulsation.

Long-term VADs include pulsatile (first-generation) and nonpulsatile (second-generation) devices and can provide support for 6 to 12 months, with much longer reported durations (even up to 2 to 3 years). In general, nonpulsatile devices, such as the MicroMed DeBakey VAD pump unit, MicroMed DeBakey HeartAssist 5 pump (for pediatric and adult implantation), Thoratec HeartMate II VAD, and Jarvik 2000, are continuous flow pumps that require some baseline native cardiac reserve in case of device mechanical failure. These are simpler to implant and also smaller and quieter than pulsatile devices.

The first-generation pulsatile devices, such as WorldHeart Levacor VAD, Thoratec HeartMate XVE, WorldHeart Novacor LVAS, Thoratec IVAD (implantable ventricular assist device), and Thoratec PVAD (paracorporeal ventricular assist device), are not continuous flow pumps and simulate the cardiac cycle.

Three total artificial hearts are the SynCardia Systems, Inc., CardioWest Total Artificial Heart; the Abiomed AbioCor system; and the Arrow LionHeart LVAS. Newer generation nonpulsatile VADs include the Berlin Heart INCOR LVAD; Ventracor VentrAssist system; Thoratec HeartMate III, HeartWare HVAD, and MVAD; Terumo DuraHeart LVAS; and Cleveland Clinic Foundation CorAide blood pump.

Surgical Ventricular Restoration: Dor Procedure

The ventricular restoration procedure (Dor procedure or endoventricular circular patch plasty) is an established surgical option for patients with ischemic dilated cardiomyopathy with left ventricle aneurysms and akinetic or dyskinetic myocardial segments. It can be used as an alternative treatment because of limitations of cardiac transplantation and VADs, such as donor organ shortage and financial restraints.

The Dor procedure involves excision of akinetic or dyskinetic and nonviable myocardium of the left ventricle and patch repair of the distal left ventricular cavity, thus restoring the normal elliptical shape of the left ventricle from a spherical dilated heart. The opening of the ventricle is closed by Dacron patch or stitches.[4] The restoration of ventricular volume reduces the stress on the ventricular wall, reduces myocardial oxygen consumption, and increases wall contractility and compliance.[5] Associated mitral valve regurgitation or intraventricular thrombi are corrected simultaneously. Before surgery, appropriate coronary revascularization procedures, including grafting of the left anterior descending coronary artery, which supplies a high portion of the septum, should be performed.[5] Perioperatively, appropriate ventricular volume is restored in the septal and anterior wall without deforming the chamber that will result in neither restrictive nor dilated cardiomyopathy. Care is also taken to achieve an optimal postoperative ventricular short-axis/long-axis ratio; otherwise, mitral regurgitation can result.

The first reported surgery to treat left ventricle aneurysms by Cooley and colleagues involved excision of the thinned segment with linear closure of the free edges.[6] Alternative approaches were developed by Dor and Jatene; an intraventricular patch was placed to exclude akinetic and nonresectable areas. The Dor procedure, or endoventricular circular patch plasty, was first performed in 1985.[4] Some of the criteria for the Dor procedure are ischemic dilated cardiomyopathy involving one third or more of the ventricular perimeter that causes a spherical dilated left ventricle with akinetic or dyskinetic portions of the septum and anterior wall with end-diastolic volume above 100 mL/m^2, reduced ejection fraction (<20%), left ventricular regional asynergy (>35%), and symptomatic patient (angina, heart failure, arrhythmias, and inducible ischemia). Contraindications to the procedure are systolic pulmonary artery pressure above 60 mm Hg without associated mitral regurgitation, severe right ventricular dysfunction, and regional asynergy without ventricular dilation.

Cardiac Transplantation

Cardiac transplantation has been established as the most reliable permanent treatment option for patients with deteriorating heart failure due to ischemic dilated cardiomyopathy despite maximum medical therapy and other revascularization techniques. The most commonly performed type is orthotopic cardiac transplantation, in which the recipient heart is removed except for the posterior aspect of the atrial cuffs. The donor heart is then attached to the recipient's atria, and the donor's ascending aorta and main pulmonary artery are anastomosed end to end to the severed ends of the recipient's ascending aorta and main pulmonary artery, respectively.[7]

Indications include severe ventricular dysfunction with a life expectancy between 12 and 18 months and lack of improvement in ejection fraction from medical therapy or resynchronization therapies. The criteria include NYHA classification III or IV status, age younger than 65 to 70 years, and reproducible $\dot{V}O_2$ max of less than 14 mL/kg per minute.

Patients with nonischemic causes of heart failure, such as hypertensive heart disease, myocarditis, idiopathic cardiomyopathy, valvular heart disease, congenital heart disease, and peripartum cardiomyopathy, can also benefit from cardiac transplantation.[8] Contraindications to heart transplantation may include AIDS, active systemic infection, malignant disease, irreversible pulmonary hypertension, irreversible secondary organ failure, comorbid life-threatening conditions, active substance abuse, psychiatric history likely to result in noncompliance, cachexia or obesity, chronic obstructive pulmonary disease, renal insufficiency, continued smoking, and severe osteoporosis.

Heterotopic cardiac transplantation is performed in patients with potentially reversible cardiac dysfunction, high pulmonary vascular resistance, or small donor hearts.[9] The donor heart is placed anterior to the right lung along the right side of the native heart, and the two left atria are anastomosed, resulting in a common left atrium. The orifices of the donor inferior vena cava and right pulmonary veins are closed. The donor ascending aorta is anastomosed to the recipient aorta in end-to-side fashion, and the donor main pulmonary artery is combined with a Dacron graft, resulting in an end-to-side anastomosis with the recipient main pulmonary artery. The donor superior vena cava and right atrium are connected to the native right atrium, allowing systemic venous return to pass into either the native or the donor right ventricle. Chambers involved in functioning include the right ventricle of the recipient and the left ventricle of the donor.

POSTOPERATIVE ASSESSMENT

Imaging is paramount in assessment of postoperative patients for complications of these surgical procedures. Immediate complications include hematoma, effusions, pneumothorax, and pulmonary embolism. Delayed and late complications include mediastinitis, conduit thrombosis in the VAD, intracardiac thrombus, mitral regurgitation, restricted left ventricular cavity, and patch dehiscence in the Dor procedure; and pulmonary infections, anastomotic dehiscence, aortic pseudoaneurysms, allograft rejection, coronary arteriopathy, and post-transplantation lymphoproliferative disorder in cardiac transplantation.

Radiography, echocardiography, and computed tomography (CT) are used for immediate postoperative imaging of the VAD, surgical ventricular restoration, and cardiac transplantation, depending on the indication and postoperative complications. Cardiac magnetic resonance imaging (MRI) with delayed enhancement technique is the best imaging modality to assess transplanted patients for rejection; however, cardiac CT and catheter angiography are particularly useful for evaluation of coronary arteriopathy.

General Surgery-Related Complications

Mediastinal hematoma, pericardial hematoma, pleural effusions, pneumothorax, hemothorax, pneumoperitoneum and hemoperitoneum, basal lung atelectasis, aspiration, and infectious pneumonia are common complications related to these procedures in the immediate postoperative period. It is not uncommon to identify malpositioning of support tubes and catheters or a foreign body such as a surgical sponge on the portable radiographs. Median sternotomy complications, such as mediastinitis and sternal wound infections, may occur. These patients are prone to pulmonary embolism during the perioperative and immediate postoperative period. Perioperative bleeding is a result of prolonged surgical time under extracorporeal circulation and hypothermia, use of anticoagulants and antiplatelets drugs, vascular injury to the surgical bed, associated malnourishment, and hepatic dysfunction due to low-flow state and congestive hepatopathy.[1]

Specific Complications

Ventricular Assist Device

Right-sided heart failure may be due to adverse effects of the LVAD on the interventricular septum, increased pulmonary pressure due cardiopulmonary bypass or massive blood transfusions, and right coronary artery disease.[1] After the perioperative period, infection related to the VAD, thromboembolism with infarction, and limited reliability of the VAD remain the most important concerns. Patients with a VAD are more susceptible to infection because of tracking along subcutaneous drivelines for connecting batteries and controllers, leading to entry and exit site infection, driveline infection, or pump infection. Pump infection may require removal of the device and hence is of the greatest concern.[1] Thrombus can sometimes be seen in the cardiac chambers or inflow and outflow cannulas. Thromboembolism and resultant infarction of lung, brain, or systemic organs may occur after VAD placement, although the HeartMate device is believed to have less chance for this development because of the textured surface of the blood-containing chamber by a polyurethane diaphragm, which leads to pseudointima formation.[10] Aortic dissection at the level of the ascending aorta can result from high-velocity blood injected against the aortic wall. Device reliability depends on the type of device; it is 1 to 3 years for pulsatile pumps and about 5 years for miniaturized axial flow pumps. However, because the VAD does not fail catastrophically, further treatment by device exchange or transplantation can be warranted.[1]

Dor Procedure

Specific complications associated with surgical ventricular restoration are suture line or patch dehiscence, excessive reduction in left ventricular volume resulting in mitral regurgitation, and restrictive or constrictive physiology.[11] Intracardiac thrombus that is adherent to the patch at the left ventricle apex is a noted complication of this procedure.

Cardiac Transplantation

Early postoperative complications (between 0 and 30 days) are related to surgical complications, including cardiac ischemia, pulmonary edema, and anoxic brain injury and thromboembolic events. Intermediate postoperative complications (between 1 month and 12 months) mainly include acute allograft rejection and infection. Allograft rejection is manifested usually between 2 and 12 weeks after transplantation.[9] The time of greatest immunosuppression is during the first 3 months after transplantation. Bacterial (predominantly aerobic gram-negative rods), viral, and fungal infections occur within the first month and often affect the lungs.

Mediastinal infection can lead to weakening of suture lines and cause aortic dissection and pseudoaneurysm formation. Late complications (after 12 months) resulting in death include transplant-associated coronary artery accelerated graft atherosclerosis, malignant disease, infection, transplant rejection, aortic allograft rejection, and cerebral infarctions.[12]

Coronary allograft vasculopathy or atherosclerosis is caused by immune-mediated and nonimmunologic injury,[7] which affects half of patients within 5 years of transplantation and is characterized by diffuse concentric intimal thickening of both proximal and distal coronary arteries. The major risk factors for late mortality from coronary allograft vasculopathy include ischemic heart disease, younger recipient age (but older than 20 years), black race, cigarette use within 6 months of listing for transplantation, older donor age, and development of coronary artery disease during the first post-transplant year.[13] Malignant neoplasms are likely to be secondary to long-term immunosuppression and include lymphomas, acute leukemia, visceral tumors, Kaposi sarcoma, gynecologic cancers, primary lung carcinoma, skin cancer (predominantly squamous cell cancer), and post-transplant lymphoproliferative disorder.[9]

Other complications are related to long-term corticosteroid use and immunosuppression. These include osteoporosis, vertebral insufficiency fractures, and lipomatosis.[8]

CLINICAL PRESENTATION

Perioperative bleeding and air accumulation can draw early attention on serial radiographs or by symptoms such as acute-onset breathlessness and dyspnea in the immediate postoperative period.

Patients with mediastinitis are often unwell and may have fever, tachycardia, chest discomfort, sternal tenderness, and leukocytosis. Discharge from the sternotomy wound with delayed healing may be indirect evidence of ongoing sternal osteomyelitis or a mediastinal infection or collection.[9]

Fever or lethargy may be the first indicator of internal systemic infection. If it is associated with breathlessness, productive cough, and pleuritic chest pain, it can be a warning symptom of community-acquired or opportunistic pulmonary infections, which are quite common in the postoperative period because of immunosuppression. Patients with infective (mycotic) pseudoaneurysms may be asymptomatic or may present with fever, lethargy, and chest pain.[9] Pulmonary embolism is typically manifested with sudden-onset breathlessness, chest pain, tachycardia, and hypoxia.

Focal neurologic deficits or sudden-onset peripheral vascular ischemia may indicate a thromboembolic phenomenon; imaging is recommended to assess for intracardiac thrombus, especially in patients with the Dor procedure. In patients with a VAD, contrast-enhanced CT is preferred to assess for intraconduit thrombus formation.

Sudden-onset chest pain may be a common manifestation of a variety of causes, such as aortic dissection, intramural hematoma, aortic pseudoaneurysm formation, coronary atherosclerosis, pulmonary embolism, new-onset myocardial infarction, ventricular wall perforation, and cardiac arrhythmias. Cross-sectional imaging, such as CT and echocardiography, is essential for early diagnosis and treatment of these conditions.

In heart transplantation, a common complication in the postoperative period is impending rejection, which may be asymptomatic or can be manifested by dyspnea, palpitation, fatigability, weakness, syncope and signs suggestive of hypotension, worsening of cardiac function, and increasing heart failure.[9]

Clinical manifestations of coronary vasculopathy include myocardial infarction, graft failure, arrhythmias, and sudden death. It starts distally in small coronaries and progresses proximally to epicardial vessels without formation of collaterals.[7] Because of the difficulty in preventing this complication and the clinically silent presentation, routine surveillance has been advocated for detection and early intervention by revascularization procedures.[7]

New-onset back pain in patients receiving corticosteroids should suggest osteoporosis, vertebral fractures, intervertebral diskitis, or internal malignant disease with bone metastases. Gastrointestinal complications, such as peptic ulcer, diverticulitis, and organ perforation, may go unnoticed because of the effect of corticosteroids, which may mask signs and symptoms.[8] A high index of clinical suspicion and appropriate timely imaging would help in identifying these serious pathologic processes.

IMAGING INDICATIONS AND ALGORITHM

Radiography

Portable anteroposterior radiography is used for assessment of postoperative normal appearances of cardiac transplantation, cardiac assist devices, and surgical ventricular restoration and of immediate surgery-related complications (intrathoracic air collections, hematoma, pulmonary edema, and pneumonia). Chest radiographs also play an important role in follow-up of these patients for late complications, such as pneumonia, cardiac failure, and opportunistic infections (e.g., *Aspergillus* infection). A posteroanterior view taken at maximum inspiration is recommended in stable patients, in whom lateral radiographs may or may not add additional information.

Echocardiography

Echocardiography is a simple and useful modality in the evaluation of pericardial effusion, hematoma, cardiac tamponade, and intracardiac thrombus. Serial echocardiography (once or twice a year) is used to monitor allograft and valvular function as well as for diagnosis of moderate rejection. Intravascular ultrasound competes with ECG-gated coronary CT angiography (CTA) and routine angiography for surveillance of cardiac allograft vasculopathy. Intravascular ultrasound allows visualization of the lumen and arterial wall thickness; however, unlike CTA, it is an invasive examination.

Perioperative echocardiography is an important aspect of VAD placement planning and assessment. Transesophageal echocardiography and transthoracic echocardiography are done by use of gray-scale, color flow, pulsed wave Doppler, and continuous wave Doppler imaging. Right and left ventricle functional analysis is also readily performed. Intracardiac thrombus, functional parameters of the left ventricle (including end-diastolic volume, shape, and size), and excursion and coaptation of the mitral valve apparatus after surgical ventricular restoration are also readily assessed by echocardiography.

Computed Tomography

Multidetector CT (MDCT) is the ideal and most rapid modality, with high spatial resolution for imaging of complications (such as pulmonary embolism, infected mediastinal collection, vascular injury) and for differentiation of atelectasis from infectious consolidation, opportunistic infections such as those due to *Aspergillus,* and conduit patency in cardiac assist devices. Contrast-enhanced CT pulmonary angiography is the technique of choice to evaluate for pulmonary embolism.

Axial images should be reconstructed at 1.5-mm slice thickness to increase the sensitivity and specificity for identification of segmental and subsegmental pulmonary embolism. Non–contrast-enhanced 3-mm images through the chest and upper abdomen are recommended for all indicated patients in the immediate postoperative period to assess for hematoma. Contrast-enhanced CT aortic angiography might be useful for vascular injury, such as iatrogenic dissection. For good contrast opacification of the aorta to be achieved, the region of interest is placed at the aortic arch for bolus tracking. For angiography, 80 to 100 mL of nonionic water-soluble contrast material at 3 mL/sec is sufficient. ECG-gated CTA is preferred for evaluation of aortic root disease, such as dissection or intramural hematoma. ECG-gated coronary CTA can be performed for annual surveillance to evaluate transplant coronary arteries for vasculopathy. An oral or intravenous β blocker is essential to keep the patient's heart rate below 70 beats/min at 16- and 64-slice MDCT scanners, but this may be alleviated in dual-source CT. For coronary CTA, acquisition is performed from carina to diaphragm at 0.6-mm collimation with 80 to 100 mL of contrast material given at 5 mL/sec. For better contrast opacification of coronary arteries, the region of interest is placed in the ascending aorta at the level of the main pulmonary artery for bolus tracking. Images can be reconstructed at 0.75-mm slice thickness at 50% overlap between images.

Although prospective triggering can be used, retrospective gating currently is widely used; prospective triggering is associated with less radiation but does not provide multiphase reconstruction as the retrospective gating method does, which is essential for interrogation of a doubtful coronary artery segment for the presence or absence of concentric narrowing. ECG-gated CT competes with MRI and echocardiography in assessing ventricular volumes and function, which is important in determining success of surgical ventricular restoration procedures. Post-transplantation ECG-gated CT is also useful to delineate complex anatomy and anastomoses as well as for imaging of complications. Coronary calcium scoring may be helpful for screening, and the retrospective ECG-gated technique is useful for assessment of cardiac function.

Magnetic Resonance Imaging

Although MRI plays very little role in postoperative assessment of ischemic cardiac disease, it has an important role in preoperative assessment and in a few other conditions when the issue of MRI incompatibility is ruled out.

Cardiac function and morphology are adequately assessed by cine steady-state free precession (SSFP) MRI, and validation studies have shown strong agreement between MRI and echocardiography for determination of myocardial mass, end-systolic volumes, end-diastolic volumes, and ejection fractions. MR spectroscopy, first-pass perfusion techniques, and postcontrast inversion recovery techniques add important information to the commonly performed multiplanar cine sequences. Ideally, SSFP cine images through the left ventricle for function, HASTE and SSFP axial images through the chest for morphology of mediastinal vessels, and postcontrast delayed T1 gradient-recalled-echo images for myocardial enhancement are important to assess the transplanted heart for rejection or coronary arteriopathy. Thoracic MR angiography supplemented with postcontrast two-dimensional or three-dimensional gradient-echo images may be employed as indicated to assess the patency of the vascular anastomosis at the aorta, pulmonary artery, superior vena cava, and inferior vena cava.

Post-transplantation changes in the myocardium from rejection and coronary artery vasculopathy can be best identified with cardiac MRI with delayed enhancement technique. In addition to this sequence, a T2 edema sequence, such as triple-inversion recovery turbo spin-echo, is useful to evaluate for myocardial edema or inflammation in rejection. Cardiac perfusion MRI is a noninvasive method that can correlate tissue blood flow changes with graft vasculopathy. First-pass perfusion is performed in short-axis planes with T1-weighted gradient-echo imaging and a small bolus of gadolinium contrast. With two or three slices, signal intensity curves can be generated throughout the left ventricle. Cardiac MRI, especially the first-pass perfusion technique, is a better modality than other imaging techniques to identify wall-adherent intracardiac thrombus.

The left ventricular end-systolic volume index measurement before and after treatment and the relationship of the post-treatment end-systolic volume index to subsequent outcomes, left ventricle shape, contractile function, and wall tension indices are also assessed by MR after ventricular restoration.

The high spatial and temporal resolution of MRI allows better morphologic assessment than with two-dimensional echocardiography. Postoperative complications of suture dehiscence and myocardial infarction are better diagnosed on MRI. VADs present challenges to MRI systems because of their ferromagnetic properties. A prototype cannula that replaces the stainless steel wire-reinforced cannula has been tested in vitro on the 3T MRI system.[14]

Nuclear Medicine/Positron Emission Tomography

Nuclear medicine imaging studies are used in assessing cardiac function after transplantation and related complications such as rejection. Chronic rejection, or cardiac graft vasculopathy, can be diagnosed with serial myocardial perfusion scans. The added advantage of a stress-rest perfusion study includes determination of reversible ischemia. Identification of regional perfusion defects is often difficult because of the balanced ischemia patterns related to the diffuse nature of the distal arterial narrowings. Gated studies can reveal abnormal diastolic function. Dobutamine single photon emission computed tomography (SPECT) thallium 201 study has sensitivity, specificity, and negative predictive value of 89%, 71%, and 96%, respectively.[15] The positron emission tomography (PET) scan, like the gated SPECT study, can show perfusion defects indicative of vasculopathy, and PET also quantifies myocardial blood flow.

Other tracers are also used. Indium In 111 pentetreotide uptake may predict impending rejection 1 week before endomyocardial biopsy. Technetium Tc 99m annexin V uptake correlates with areas of myocyte apoptosis, or programmed cell death.[16] Gallium Ga 67, ^{18}FDG-PET, and ^{111}In-labeled white blood cell examinations are used to assess complications such as fevers of unknown origin, post-transplantation lymphoproliferative disorder, and infections.

Blood pool radionuclide angiography with ^{99m}Tc-labeled red blood cells is an alternative to echocardiography or functional cardiac CTA in patients with VADs, who may be prohibited from MRI scanners. Left ventricular ejection fractions, volumes, and cardiac outputs are calculated. ^{111}In-labeled white blood cells can noninvasively confirm suspected postoperative infections.

Gated myocardial perfusion studies and PET provide similar value to patients having undergone surgical ventricular restoration and coronary artery bypass graft operations.

Angiography

Before LVAD implantation, angiography is used to assess right ventricular blood supply as well as right atrial pressures and pulmonary vascular resistance. Right atrial pressures greater than 20 mm Hg and a transpulmonary gradient greater than 16 mm Hg should cause consideration for biventricular VAD support. Routine right-sided heart catheterizations of the post-VAD patient are done to assess pulmonary vascular resistance at 1, 3, and 6 months after surgery. Left- and right-sided heart studies are done on the basis of the echocardiographic diagnosis of inflow valve regurgitation or outflow graft obstruction.

Preoperative ventriculography is sensitive for the diagnosis of dyskinesia related to left ventricle aneurysms. Angiographic assessment of target vessels for revascularization is necessary before coronary artery bypass and surgical ventricular restoration operations. Postoperative angiographic findings should parallel the morphologic and functional changes that have been documented on MRI studies after surgical ventricular restoration.

Because cardiac allograft vasculopathy is the major cause of long-term mortality after cardiac transplantation, and because of the lack of symptoms such as chest pain secondary to denervation of the transplanted heart, yearly coronary angiography has been the diagnostic study of choice to evaluate for this serious complication. This is often combined with intravascular ultrasound as well.[7]

IMAGING TECHNIQUE AND FINDINGS

Ventricular Assist Device

Preoperative and Perioperative Assessment of VAD

Perioperative transesophageal and transthoracic echocardiography is used to diagnose patent foramen ovale, which becomes clinically symptomatic after LVAD placement because of decreased left atrial pressures. Valvular assessment is also done as aortic valve leaflets stay closed with some types of LVADs, but other types, such as the Jarvik 2000 and HeartMate II, are associated with intermittent opening. If preoperative aortic stenosis is diagnosed, the axial types of LVADs could be less efficient because of decreased forward output, whereas aortic regurgitation can worsen after LVAD placement because of increased flow in the ascending aorta. Aortic valvular disease as well as mitral stenosis can be addressed at the time of LVAD placement, which can decrease outflow into the LVAD pump. The diagnosis of preoperative tricuspid regurgitation is important because of the relatively high chance of right-sided heart failure after LVAD placement.

Postoperative Appearance of VAD

Plain radiography and CT can be used for proper visualization of the VADs (Figs. 59-1 and 59-2). Normal appearance of VADs depends on the type of device and the components of the device. The HeartMate LVAD pump is placed preperitoneally or in an intra-abdominal location and is seen on plain abdominal radiographs in the left upper quadrant.[10] The inflow cannula contains a porcine bioprosthetic valve and is seen in the left ventricle apex aligned with the mitral valve. The outflow cannula also contains a porcine bioprosthetic valve and is attached to a Dacron patch of approximately 12 to 15 cm, which in turn inserts into the ascending aorta. The device is connected to an external portable console that provides pneumatic or electric power through a driveline in the fascial tunnel in the left lower quadrant. The Pierce-Donachy Thoratec VAD is placed external to the patient.[10] In a right VAD, the inflow cannula is inserted in the right atrium or ventricle, and the outflow cannula along with a Dacron graft is placed into the pulmonary artery.

A commonly used short-term circulatory assist device, the intra-aortic counterpulsation balloon device, is optimally positioned just distal to the left subclavian artery to prevent occlusion of extracerebral cranial arteries.

Inflow and outflow cannulas are assessed for proper alignment, thrombus, kinks, and obstructions by transesophageal and transthoracic echocardiography. In axial flow pumps, peak velocities in outflow cannulas are between 1 and 2 m/sec. Inflow valve regurgitation is a common cause of LVAD dysfunction in long-term LVAD support and, along with outflow valve regurgitation, can be diagnosed by echocardiography.

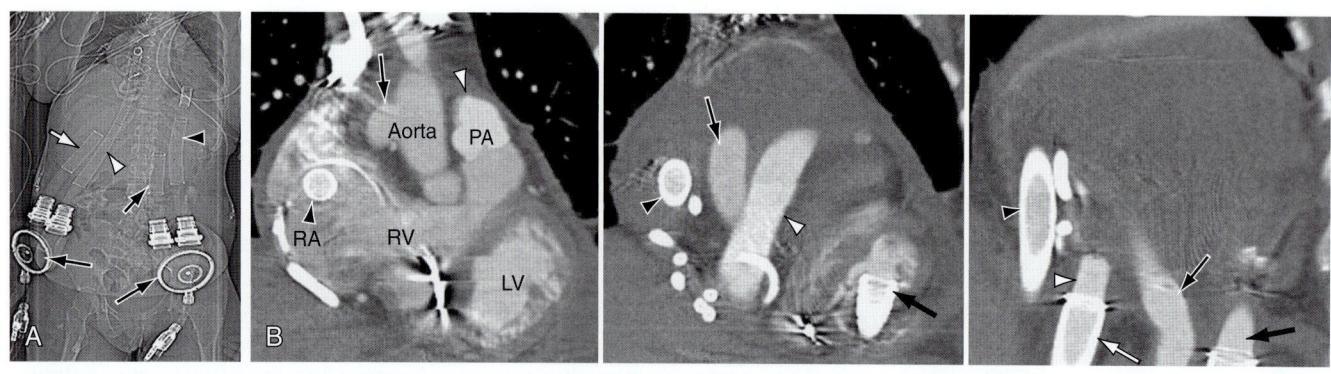

FIGURE 59-1 A 65-year-old patient with history of ischemic cardiomyopathy after biventricular cardiac assist device placement. **A,** Scout tomogram shows the outflow tract cannula (*small black arrow*) and left ventricle inflow cannula (*black arrowhead*) of the left VAD. The outflow cannula is connected to the ascending aorta through a long nonopaque Dacron graft. The right VAD is seen as the right inflow cannula connecting with the right atrium (*white arrowhead*) and right outflow cannula (*white arrow*), which is connected to the pulmonary artery through a nonopaque Dacron graft. Electronic pumps of both assist devices are noted outside the patient's body (*long black arrows*). **B,** Coronal reformatted images of contrast-enhanced chest CT show the normal course of a patent right inflow cannula (*all panels, black arrowheads*), right outflow cannula (*right panel, white arrow*) to main pulmonary artery through the Dacron graft portion (*all panels, white arrowheads*), left ventricular inflow cannula (*right and middle panels, thick black arrows*), and left outflow cannula (Dacron portion, *all panels, short black arrows*) to ascending aorta.

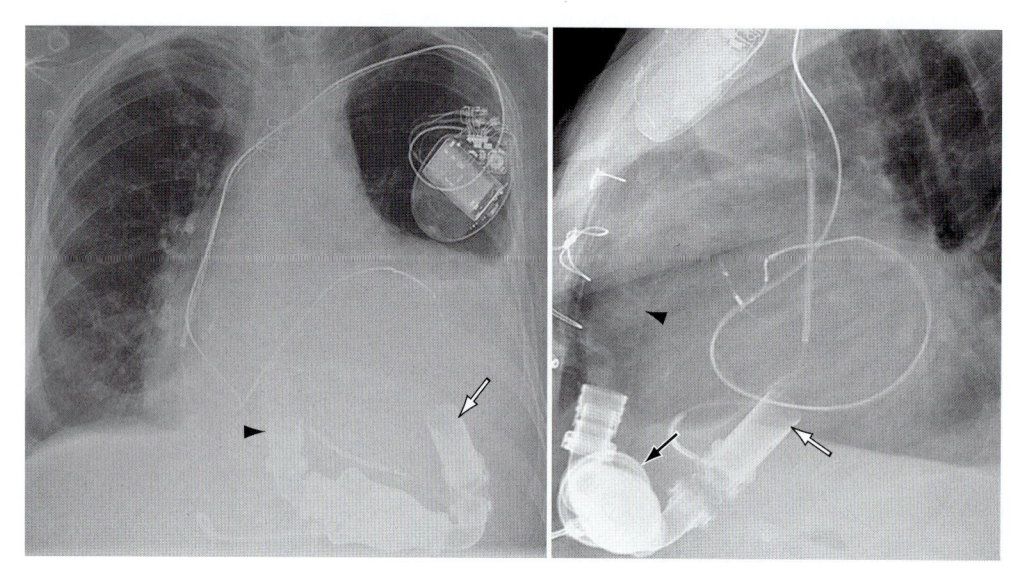

FIGURE 59-2 A 58-year-old patient with left VAD for ischemic dilated cardiomyopathy. Frontal and lateral chest radiographs show inflow cannula (*white arrow*) aligned with mitral valve and outflow cannula (*arrowhead*). Dacron graft bridging outflow cannula and ascending aorta is seen as faint shadow (*arrowhead, lateral radiograph*). Cardiomegaly, automatic implantable cardioverter-defibrillator, left pleural effusion, and assist device pump (*black arrow*) are noted.

Imaging of Postoperative Complications of VAD

Perioperative bleeding in the operative field as well as in potential spaces such as pleura, pericardium, and peritoneum is best seen on CT as a hypodense collection with the attenuation value of blood (30 to 50 HU) (Fig. 59-3). Right-sided heart failure[1] is manifested as cardiomegaly and enlarged azygos vein on chest radiography. Echocardiography and CT are more diagnostic and show dilated right atrium, right ventricle, and systemic veins with decreased right ventricular function. Arterial phase contrast-enhanced CT may show reflux of contrast material into enlarged hepatic veins and dilated suprahepatic and hepatic inferior vena cava. On plain radiographs, pneumothorax and pneumomediastinum appear as radiolucencies in the pleural space or around the cardiac shadow in the mediastinum, respectively, and there may be associated surgical emphysema. CT can demarcate air better as very low density of air attenuation. Infection related to the VAD can be seen on contrast-enhanced CT as mixed-density collections with peripheral wall enhancement tracking along subcutaneous drivelines leading to entry and exit sites. Thrombus can be seen as a nonenhancing low-density mass on contrast-enhanced CT in the cardiac chambers and inflow and outflow cannulas (Fig. 59-4B). Thromboemboli can result in segmental infarcts, which are seen as peripheral wedge-shaped low densities without enhancement on CT in lung, brain, or systemic organs. Pulmonary emboli are seen as hypovascular intraluminal filling defects within the branch pulmonary arteries.

CT has high sensitivity and specificity for identification of intramural hematoma and aortic dissection (Fig. 59-4A).

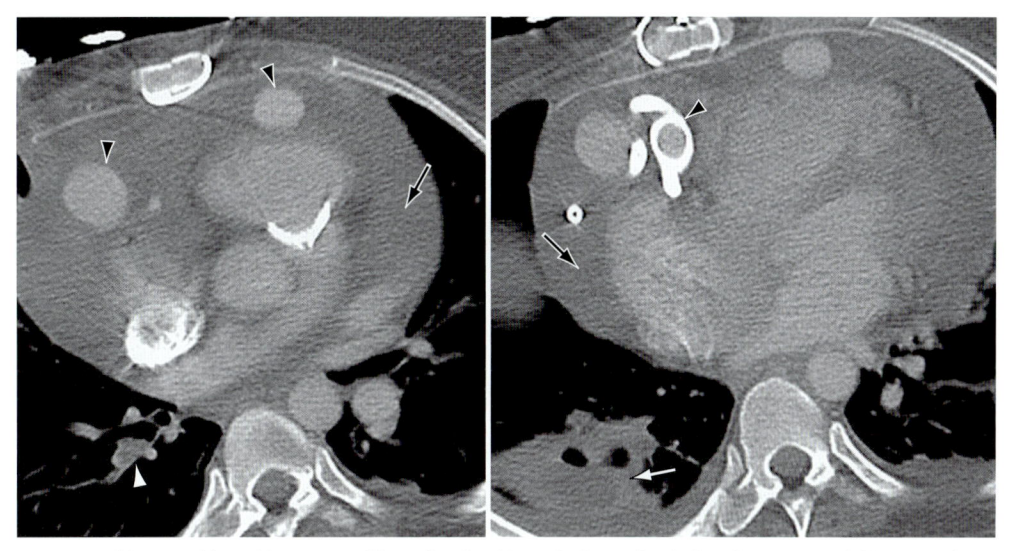

CHAPTER 59 • *Postoperative Imaging of Ischemic Cardiac Disease* 817

■ **FIGURE 59-3** A 60-year-old man with sudden onset of hypoxia after biventricular assist device placement. Axial images of CTA of chest show hypodense embolus in the segmental right lower lobe pulmonary arteries (*white arrowhead* [*left panel*]) with resultant peripheral cavitating infarction (*white arrow* [*right panel*]). Moderate pericardial (*black arrows*) and bilateral pleural collections are noted. Three of the four cannulas are seen on these images (*black arrowheads*). The left ventricle inflow cannula is not shown here.

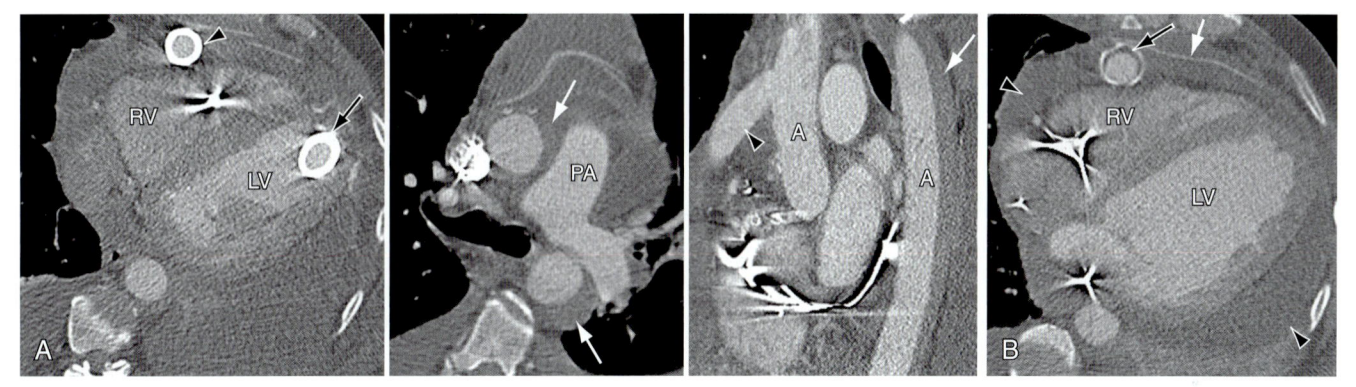

■ **FIGURE 59-4** A 60-year-old patient with left VAD for ischemic dilated cardiomyopathy undergoing chest CTA for severe chest pain. **A,** Axial (*left and middle panels*) and sagittal (*right panel*) images show crescentic mural density in both the ascending and the descending aorta (*white arrows*); these findings are consistent with iatrogenic type A intramural hematoma. The left ventricle inflow cannula (*black arrow*) and outflow cannula (*black arrowhead*) to the aorta from the assist device pump are patent. **B,** Axial postcontrast CTA image in the same patient shows a nonocclusive low-density peripheral thrombus within the aortic outflow cannula (*black arrow*). Note the hyperdense Silastic membrane in the anterior mediastinum (*white arrow*). Note moderate pericardial effusion or resolving hematoma.

On contrast-enhanced CT and contrast-enhanced MRI, aortic dissection appears as two contrast-filled channels separated by a hypodense or hypointense intimal flap in the aorta. Intramural hematoma is seen as mural high density on non–contrast-enhanced CT and low density on contrast-enhanced CTA, but the perfused lumen has a smooth margin with no intimal flap.

Focal accumulation of blood around the left VAD outflow or right VAD inflow can be seen as a focal bulge on the postoperative chest radiograph or CT scan.[10] Active bleeding can be seen as an extravascular collection of contrast material.

Ventricular Restoration Procedure (Dor Procedure)

Postoperative Appearance

Functional assessment of the left ventricle after surgical ventricular restoration is readily done by echocardiography. Baseline evaluation consists of left ventricular systolic and diastolic dysfunction assessment, cardiac hemodynamics, and valvular regurgitation. It is compared with the 4- and 24-month follow-up studies to judge success of surgical ventricular restoration.

Radiography may show decreased cardiac size after the surgery due to resection of the left ventricle aneurysm and resection of akinetic and dyskinetic myocardium. Cardiac CT or chest CT with contrast may show surgical material at the newly created left ventricle apex, normal elliptical shape of the left ventricle, interval decrease in size of the cardiac silhouette, and patch repair of aneurysm at the left ventricle apex (Fig. 59-5).

Imaging of Postoperative Complications

The postoperative appearance of blood and air accumulation (hemothorax, hemopericardium, pneumothorax, pneumomediastinum) is the same as described for the VAD. Abnormally reduced ventricular size may be seen on

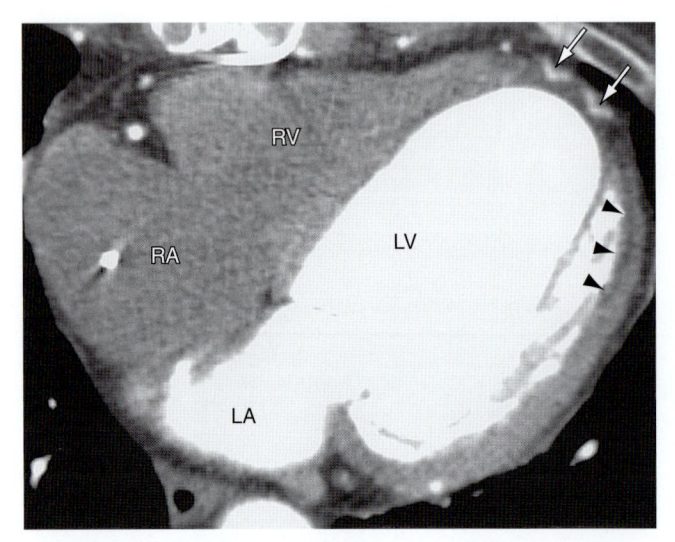

FIGURE 59-5 A 67-year-old patient after a surgical ventricular restoration procedure for ischemic dilated cardiomyopathy. Axial image from coronary CTA shows reconstructed left ventricle and postsurgical material (*arrows*) in the neo–left ventricle apex. The left ventricular cavity maintains its shape and is not severely compromised in size. No thrombus is noted in the left ventricle apex. Incidental note is made of a segmental subendocardial perfusion defect within the lateral wall of the distal left ventricular myocardium (*arrowheads*), denoting remote infarction. (*Courtesy of Carol Wu, MD.*)

echocardiography and contrast-enhanced CT. Echocardiography and cardiac CT and MR may readily show abnormal left ventricular volumes due to small size of the left ventricle from inadvertent removal of the affected myocardium. Wall motion abnormalities due to prior infarction are seen on echocardiography, MR, and cardiac CT. Mitral regurgitation is seen as a flow void jet directed toward the left atrium during systole on cine SSFP MRI. Perfusion defects and delayed enhancement may be seen on ECG-gated cardiac CT and MR as a result of prior infarction.

Late constrictive pericarditis can be seen as pericardial thickening of more than 4 mm with or without associated pericardial effusion on CT or MRI. Intracardiac thrombus is seen as low density on CT and low signal on MR. Calcification within the thrombus indicates chronicity of the clot, which is better observed on contrast-enhanced CT.

Suture line or patch dehiscence may lead to pseudoaneurysm formation, which is better seen on CT and MR as a dyskinetic contrast-filled outpouching from the left ventricle apex. Color Doppler echocardiography may show turbulent flow at the origin of the pseudoaneurysm.

Cardiac Transplantation

Postoperative Appearance

Radiographic findings after orthotopic cardiac transplantation include enlarged cardiac silhouette (Figs. 59-6 to 59-8); double right atrial contour; and resolving findings of pneumomediastinum, pneumothorax, pneumopericardium, subcutaneous emphysema, and mediastinal widening up to the first 20 days after surgery.[9] Mediastinal lipomatosis due to steroid therapy can lead to delayed mediastinal widening of relatively low density.[9] Pericardial effusions are rarely seen because of the disproportionately larger pericardial sac or cyclosporine immunotherapy.

CT findings include high and redundant main pulmonary artery[17] due to size discrepancy of the recipient and donor pulmonary arteries, size discrepancy between the recipient and donor ascending aorta anastomoses, large space between recipient superior vena cava and donor ascending aorta, space between donor ascending aorta and main pulmonary artery, and prominent left atrium with waist or indentation at atrial anastomoses. The remnant donor superior vena cava is usually placed medial to the recipient's superior vena cava and posterior to the donor ascending aorta.[9] If the size discrepancies between donor and recipient aorta and pulmonary arteries are significant, a radiosynthetic patch is used to bridge the difference; this can be imaged as radiodense material encircling the aorta or pulmonary artery on CT.

Radiographic findings of heterotopic transplants include markedly enlarged cardiac silhouette due to the position of the donor heart along with the recipient heart. Normal post-transplantation echocardiographic findings can include mitral regurgitation, tricuspid regurgitation, and dumbbell-shaped atria.

Not infrequently, stenoses and waists at anastomoses are seen and indicate either size mismatches or stenoses.

Imaging of Postoperative Complications

The most definitive diagnosis of acute allograft rejection is made with endomyocardial biopsy, with its associated risks of bleeding, pneumothorax, hemothorax, vascular access complications, right ventricular wall perforation, coronary artery fistula, cardiac arrhythmias, and pseudoaneurysm formation. Noninvasive diagnostic imaging findings include cardiomegaly on chest radiography and CT and increased ^{67}Ga uptake on scintigraphy. Positive MRI findings of rejection include increased left ventricle muscle mass attributed to edema; high T2 myocardial signal,[18] especially in the interventricular septum; and marked reductions in the ratio of phosphocreatine and adenosine triphosphate on MR spectroscopy. Functional CT and MRI can show decreased ventricular function. Echocardiography is useful in the diagnosis of moderate rejection. Echocardiography findings include increased wall thickness (sum of interventricular septum and left ventricle posterior wall) and echogenicity, pericardial effusion, more than 20-ms decrease in pressure half-time and isovolumetric relaxation time, more than 10% decrease in left ventricular ejection fraction, and decreased ejection fractions, with reported sensitivity and specificity of 80% and 98.6%.[19] Follow-up ^{111}In studies are of value after the first few postoperative months. Heart-to-lung count density ratio is calculated and correlates with severity of damage seen on endomyocardial biopsy. Chronic rejection can be diagnosed with serial myocardial perfusion scans.

Infections can be manifested as pneumonia, empyema, mediastinitis, abdominal abscess, acute diverticulitis with rupture, sinusitis or mastoiditis, and intracranial abscesses.

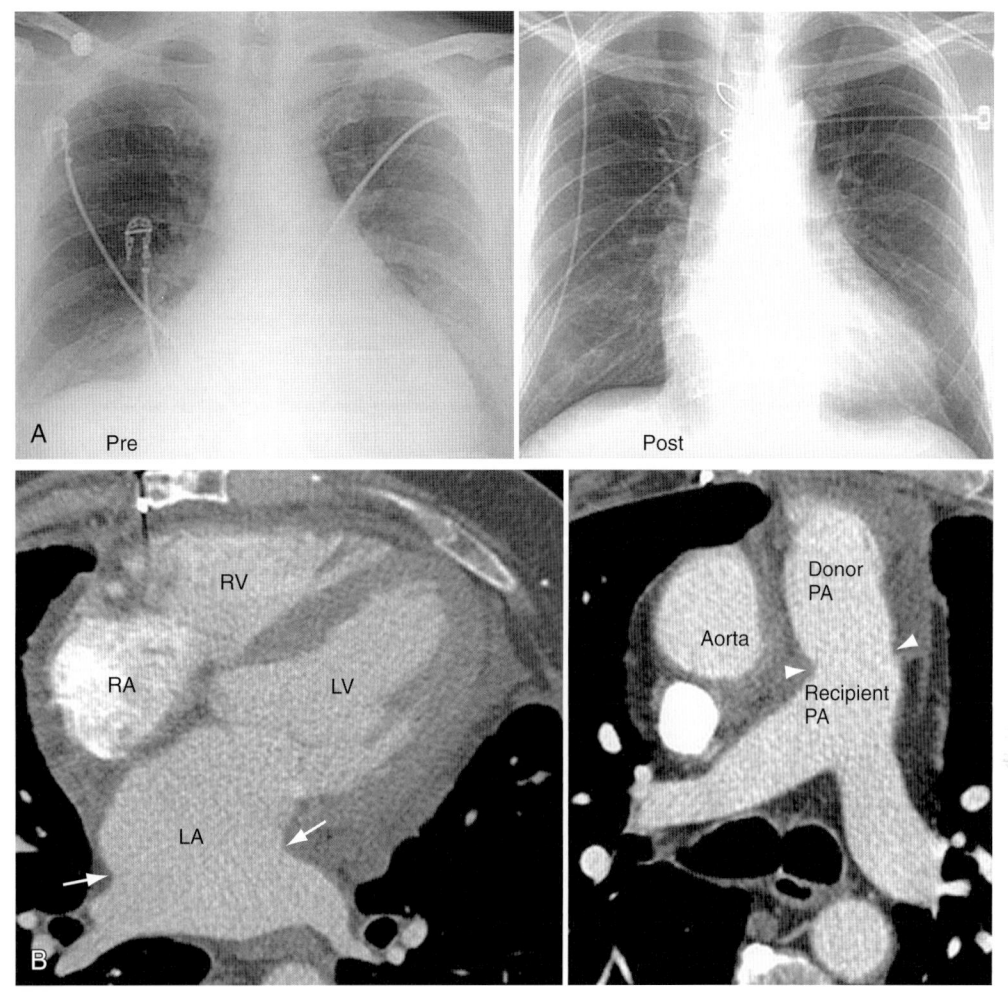

FIGURE 59-6 A 55-year-old patient after heart transplantation for cardiac failure due to ischemic heart disease. **A,** Chest radiograph showing pretransplantation (*left panel*) and post-transplantation (*right panel*) cardiac silhouette. Note cardiomegaly with pulmonary congestion before transplantation (*left panel*) compared with normal cardiac silhouette with clear lung fields after transplantation (*right panel*). **B,** Axial cardiac CT images show normal postoperative appearance of the heart transplant and its anastomoses. Axial image (*left panel*) at the level of four chambers shows typical waist at the junction of the anastomosis (*arrows*) between the anterior part of the donor's left atrium and the posterior part of the recipient's left atrium. Axial image of CTA (*right panel*) shows donor's proximal part of main pulmonary artery anastomosed distally with recipient's main pulmonary artery, resulting in minimal caliber change at this level (*arrowheads*).

Infections caused by *Staphylococcus aureus, Pseudomonas aeruginosa*, and *Klebsiella pneumoniae* can proceed to abscesses and cavitations recognized on radiographs and CT scan. *Aspergillus* infections can be manifested radiographically as isolated or multiple pulmonary nodules with cavitation, predominantly in the upper lobe, or as an invasive type with larger nodular consolidation and a rim of ground-glass opacity (CT halo sign) due to hemorrhage, with or without cavitation (Fig. 59-9).[20] Cerebral aspergillosis can produce bifrontal hypodense cerebral lesions with rim enhancement, sometimes with intralesional hemorrhage.[20] Recipients are susceptible to other infections, such as *Legionella, Pneumocystis carinii,* and *Nocardia* infections. *Nocardia* can produce extensive soft tissue abscesses with an enhancing rim on contrast-enhanced CT. Viral infection with cytomegalovirus results in cytomegaloviral pneumonitis in 9% to 11% of cardiac transplant recipients; death occurs in 14% of affected patients.[9,17] Cytomegalovirus can also cause myocarditis, hepatitis, and gastrointestinal ulceration. Pulmonary radiographic and CT findings include diffuse pulmonary airspace disease, consolidation with multiple nodules smaller than 5 mm, bilateral patchy ground-glass opacities, and multiple centrilobular or subpleural nodules.

Mediastinal infection can lead to weakening of suture lines and aortic dissection and pseudoaneurysm formation.[9] On chest radiography, it is manifested as widening of the mediastinum and an anterior mediastinal mass. Contrast-enhanced CT demonstrates the contrast-filled focal outpouching from the ascending aorta with or without thrombus or intramural hematoma, usually at the cannulation site for cardiopulmonary bypass.[9] Mycotic pseudoaneurysms are manifested with signs of infection and are fatal because of rapid growth. Cerebral infarction or abscess formation can occur, and cerebral infarction will be in respect to vascular territory and will produce less contrast enhancement than abscesses do. Radiologic modalities for diagnosis of coronary allograft vasculopathy or atherosclerosis include invasive coronary angiography, intracoronary ultrasonography, coronary artery CTA with coronary artery calcium screening, and cardiac function MRI with coronary MR angiography. Angiographic findings are typically characterized by diffuse concentric narrowing in the middle to distal coronary arteries with occasional distal vessel obliteration.[21] Specific types of lesions are described as focal and discrete, tubular, multiple, abrupt or gradually occurring long smooth narrowings with obliterated distal vessels, or abruptly terminating narrowed and irregular distal vessels (pruned tree effect).

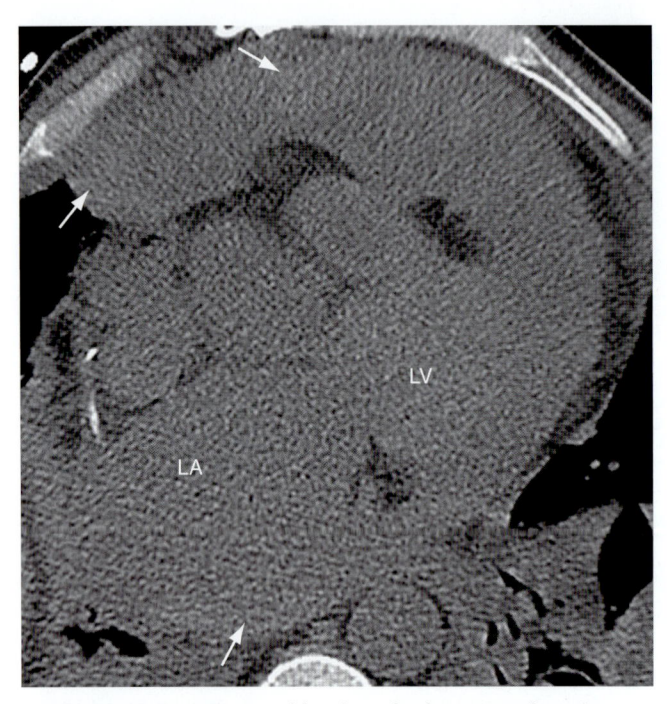

FIGURE 59-7 A 60-year-old patient after heart transplantation. Axial image from unenhanced chest CT shows a relatively high density mediastinal and pericardial collection (*arrows*), consistent with hematoma.

Late enhancement patterns that are seen on magnitude and phase-sensitive inversion recovery MRI sequences include infarct-typical transmural patterns and infarct-atypical patterns (diffuse, spotted, intramural, and localized without association with specific coronary artery vascular territory). Infarct-typical patterns are more common in the mid ventricle and apical levels; infarct-atypical patterns are more common in the basal and mid ventricle levels.[22]

Other diagnostic examinations to assess function and ischemia include dobutamine stress echocardiography, radionuclide scintigraphy, serial myocardial perfusion scans, and exercise electrocardiography. Identification of regional perfusion defects is often difficult because of the balanced ischemia patterns related to the diffuse nature of the distal arterial narrowing. Gated studies can reveal abnormal diastolic function with a small, noncompliant ventricle as well as low ejection fraction.

Dobutamine SPECT thallium study can show elevated lung-to-heart uptake. Contrast-enhanced CT can provide a complete survey of malignant neoplasms associated with heart transplantations, such as lymphomas, acute leukemia, skin cancer, visceral tumors, Kaposi sarcoma, gynecologic cancers, and primary lung carcinoma.[9] Squamous cell cancer accounts for most skin cancers. Post-transplantation lymphoproliferative disorders are commonly of B-cell origin and are associated with Epstein-Barr virus.[9] Lymphomas are usually extramedullary and may be localized or disseminated. They can involve any organ, including lung, liver, kidneys, spleen, gastrointestinal tract, and lymph nodes. Pulmonary involvement is manifested radiographically as solitary or multiple noncavitating nodules with or without adenopathy. Hepatic and splenic findings can include multiple hypoattenuating masses. Gastrointestinal tract involvement can be manifested as bowel wall thickening and intestinal obstruction.[20]

Aortic allograft rejection can produce aortic dehiscence with severe periaortic hematoma. Leukoencephalopathy produces bilateral white matter hypodensities on CT.[20]

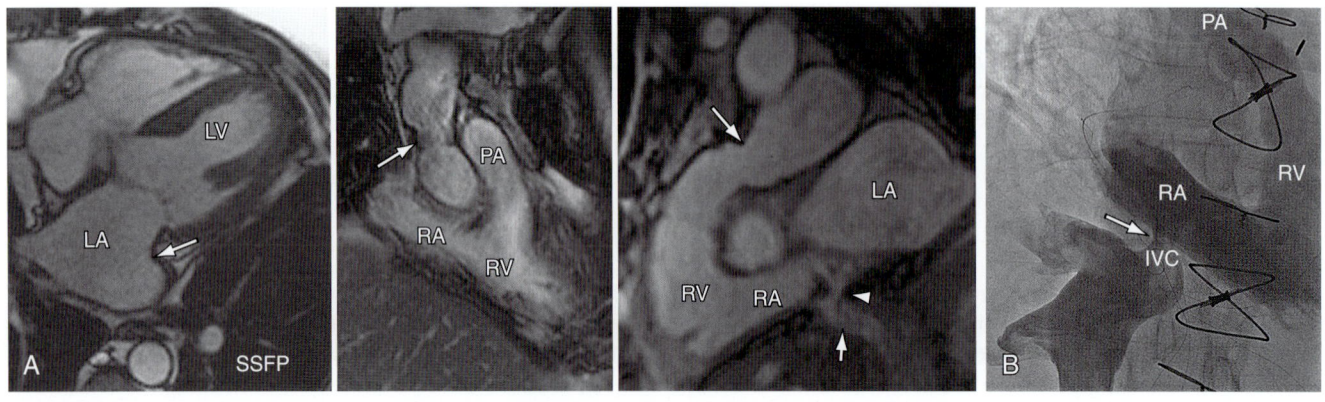

FIGURE 59-8 Adult patient after orthotopic heart transplantation and recent onset of lower extremity edema. **A,** Axial cardiac MR image (*left panel*) shows characteristic appearance of the left atrium with a waist at the level of the anastomosis (*arrow*) between the anteriorly placed donor and posteriorly located recipient left atria. Right ventricular outflow tract cine SSFP MR images (*middle and right panels*) show narrowing of inferior vena cava at the site of anastomosis near the right atrium. Also noted are anastomosis at the thoracic ascending aorta (*arrow*) and anastomosis between the recipient's dilated main pulmonary artery and the donor's normal-caliber main pulmonary artery (*long arrow*)—thus the appearance of a stretched main pulmonary artery. **B,** Digital subtraction angiography in the same patient confirms a moderate to severe narrowing of the inferior vena cava (*arrow*) at the right atrial junction.

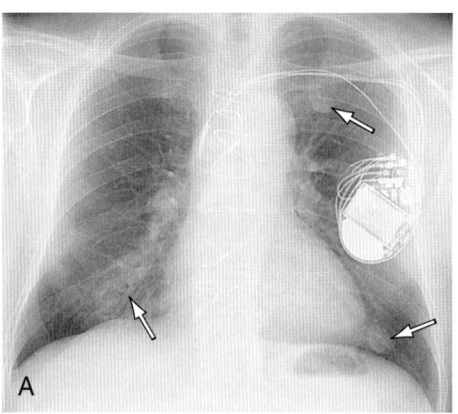

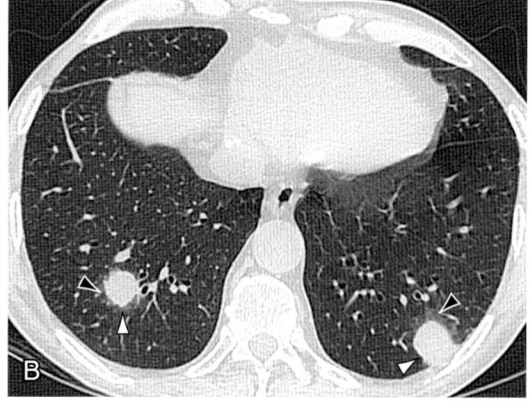

■ **FIGURE 59-9** A 65-year-old man after heart transplantation admitted for recent onset of fever and breathlessness. **A,** Frontal chest radiograph shows multiple ill-defined nodules (*arrows*) in bilateral lungs. **B,** High-resolution chest CT shows dense parenchymal nodules in lower lobes (*white arrowheads*) with surrounding ground-glass attenuation (CT halo sign, *black arrowheads*), findings consistent with invasive aspergillosis.

Postoperative Management

VAD failure, right-sided heart failure, mediastinal bleeding, infection, and thromboembolism are all considered during postoperative management of LVAD patients. Right ventricular failure is supported by phosphodiesterase inhibitors and nitric oxide. Afterload reduction is also important, especially with axial flow devices. Diuresis is necessary because of chronic volume overload status at clinical presentation. Early extubation, enteral feeding, and rehabilitation are desired. Because mediastinal bleeding is not uncommon and often requires reoperation, anticoagulation can be initiated usually by 24 to 36 hours postoperatively after bleeding has subsided with platelet transfusions, fresh frozen plasma, and cryoprecipitate. Aspirin is liberally used for its antiplatelet and anti-inflammatory effects, and the international normalized ratio is maintained between 2.5 and 3.5 with heparin and warfarin; dipyridamole and clopidogrel are also often used to prevent pulmonary and cerebral thromboembolism. Some common infectious agents include *Staphylococcus, Pseudomonas, Enterococcus,* and *Candida;* antibiotics, drainage and débridement, device exchanges, and device removal with transplantation are all considered. Urgent reoperation and parts replacement may be required for device failure. Some devices may have backup support, for example, a pneumatic console on the HeartMate LVAD in case of electrical failure. Patients with VADs have higher frequencies of circulating antiphospholipids and anti–human leukocyte antigen antibodies; these patients are at higher risk for post-transplantation acute rejections. Early intravenous immune globulin therapy and cyclophosphamide therapy are used to reduce alloreactivity before transplantation.[23]

Operative and perioperative mortality, although relatively low, can be encountered in patients undergoing surgical ventricular restoration.[24,25] Mortality is most often related to urgency of surgery and cardiogenic shock. These sick patients are likely being treated with inotropic agents, pressors, and short-term mechanical support, such as intra-aortic balloon pump. Stroke is an adverse outcome, sometimes related to unexpected intraventricular soft thrombus that is undetected preoperatively. Refractory postoperative biventricular failure can be addressed by VADs.[24,25] A common nonfatal morbidity is residual inducible arrhythmia, such as ventricular tachycardia. If intraoperative scar ablation is not done or is unsuccessful, postoperative cardiac electrophysiology consultation with possible implantation of an implantable cardioverter-defibrillator is an option. Postoperative mitral regurgitation can occur with continued ventricular remodeling, despite effective ventricular restoration. An akinetic or poorly functioning inferobasal ventricular wall can contribute to mitral insufficiency. Preoperative mitral insufficiency can be addressed intraoperatively with annuloplasty at the time of a Dor procedure or with a more complex repair if there is progression of postoperative mitral regurgitation. Long-term postoperative care includes maintenance of combinations of diuretics, β blockers, and angiotensin-converting enzyme inhibitors for patients in NYHA class I.[24,25]

Allograft failure and opportunistic infections are the most serious complications in the early postoperative period (Fig. 59-10). Infection is the most common cause of death in the early postoperative period.[26] Transplant rejection may be caused by both cellular and antibody-mediated processes. Antibody-mediated rejection is associated with greater risk of allograft vasculopathy (Fig. 59-11) and more severe hemodynamic compromise at presentation. Cellular rejection involves myocardial infiltration with mononuclear cells. Induction therapy provides more intensive immunosuppression in the initial days after transplantation for highly sensitized patients and renal failure patients.[26] Maintenance immunosuppression includes corticosteroids, calcineurin inhibitors, and an antiproliferative agent.[27] Prednisone, tacrolimus, and mycophenolate mofetil are commonly used agents. Strategies to reduce post-transplantation infections include bacterial and viral prophylaxis, early corticosteroid withdrawal, and use of more effective antifungal agents. Survival of patients with invasive aspergillosis is improved with medications such as caspofungin, voriconazole, and posaconazole. Post-transplantation progression and regression of malignant neoplasms may be pursued with proliferation signal inhibitors such as sirolimus. Management options for transplant graft vasculopathy include statin therapy, sirolimus therapy, percutaneous revascularization, and retransplantation, the only definitive therapy.[27]

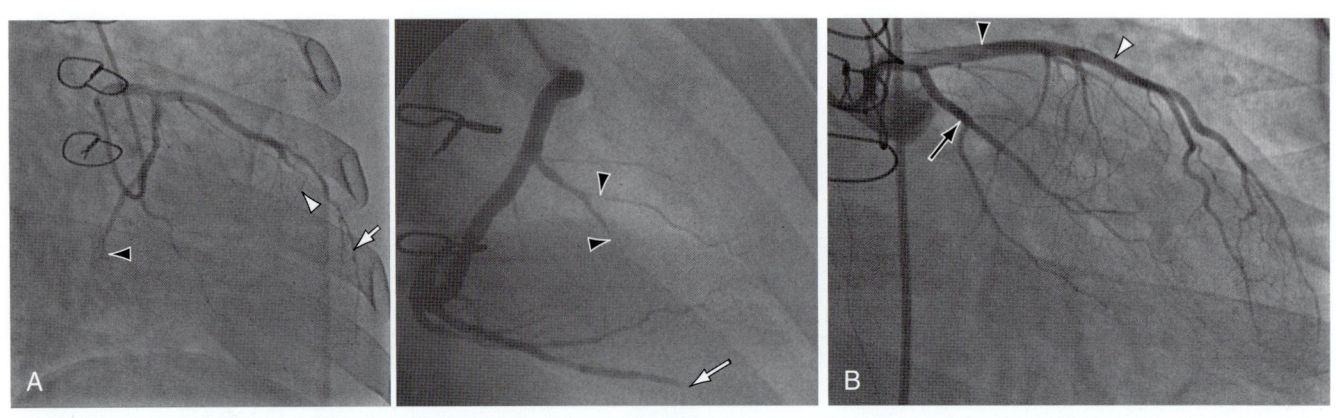

FIGURE 59-10 A 57-year-old man with redo orthotopic heart transplantation due to prior allograft rejection arteriopathy. **A,** Images from digital subtraction angiography of left (*left panel*) and right (*right panel*) coronary arteries 5 years after orthotopic heart transplantation show multiple areas of concentric narrowing, distal pruning, and marked attenuation of mid to distal left anterior descending (*short arrow* [*left panel*]), circumflex (*black arrowhead* [*left panel*]), diagonal (*white arrowhead* [*left panel*]), and acute marginal (*arrowheads* [*right panel*]) and distal right coronary (*arrow* [*right panel*]) arteries. These features are consistent with allograft coronary arteriopathy due to graft rejection. **B,** Digital subtraction angiography of left coronary arteries of the same patient after heart retransplantation shows normal appearance of left main stem (*black arrowhead*), left anterior descending (*white arrowhead*), and circumflex arteries (*arrow*).

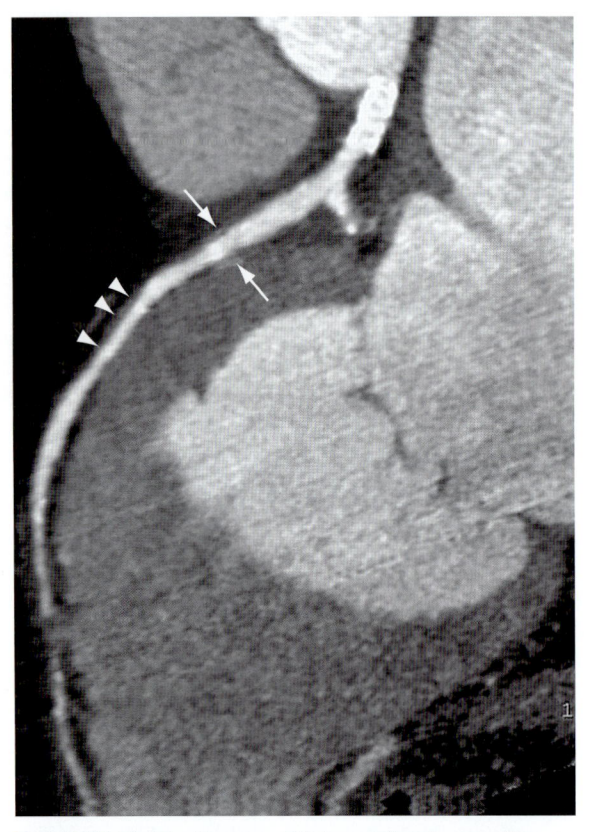

FIGURE 59-11 Coronary CTA in a patient 3 years after orthotopic heart transplantation shows tubular (*arrowheads*) and concentric (*arrows*) narrowing of left anterior descending coronary artery due to noncalcified plaque. This is consistent with transplant coronary vasculopathy. Left main stem stent is also noted. (*Courtesy of Naama Bogot, MD.*)

KEY POINTS

- Common non–coronary artery bypass graft surgical options for ischemic heart disease include cardiac assist device, ventricular restoration procedure (Dor procedure), and heart transplantation.
- The ventricular assist device can provide electromechanical circulatory support for heart failure patients despite maximum medical therapy, and it serves as a bridge to transplantation and also as destination therapy. Imaging, especially contrast-enhanced CT, helps identify the normal course of inflow and outflow conduits and cannulas and complications such as perigraft hematoma, conduit thrombosis, perigraft infection, iatrogenic aortic dissection, or intramural hematoma and pulmonary embolus.
- Surgical left ventricular restoration repair or the Dor procedure may be an option for cardiac failure patients with left ventricle aneurysm and akinetic or dyskinetic myocardial segments. This procedure reduces left ventricular volume and restores the elliptical shape of the ventricle as well. Echocardiography, CT, and MRI are useful tools to evaluate for an expected elliptical shape of the left ventricle, quantification of left ventricular volumes, and intracardiac thrombus.
- Orthotopic cardiac transplantation has emerged as the most reliable long-term treatment option for patients with end-stage heart failure, despite maximum revascularization and medical therapies.
- Infection is the most common cause of death in the early postoperative period. Transplant coronary arteriopathy is the most serious complication in the late period, followed by neoplastic diseases.
- MRI is the best noninvasive imaging modality to assess for rejection of the cardiac transplant. Myocardial delayed hyperenhancement may be seen during the early period due to cellular rejection and also in the late period due to coronary arteriopathy.

SUGGESTED READINGS

Bogot NR, Durst R, Shaham D, Admon D. Cardiac CT of the transplanted heart: indications, technique, appearance, and complications. Radiographics 2007; 27:1297-1309.

Rose EA, Gelijns AC, Moskowitz AJ. Long-term use of a left ventricular assist device for end-stage heart failure. N Engl J Med 2001; 345:1435-1443.

Sartipy U, Albage A, Lindblom D. The Dor procedure for left ventricular reconstruction. Ten-year clinical experience. Eur J Cardiothorac Surg 2005; 27:1005-1010.

REFERENCES

1. Goldstein DJ, Smego D, Michler RE. Surgical aspects of congestive heart failure. Heart Fail Rev 2006; 11:171-192.
2. Rose EA, Gelijns AC, Moskowitz AJ. Long-term use of a left ventricular assist device for end-stage heart failure. N Engl J Med 2001; 345:1435-1443.
3. Athanasuleas CL, Buckberg GD, Stanley AWH. Surgical ventricular restoration in the treatment of congestive heart failure due to postinfarction ventricular dilation. J Am Coll Cardiol 2004; 44:1439-1445.
4. Sartipy U, Albage A, Lindblom D. The Dor procedure for left ventricular reconstruction. Ten-year clinical experience. Eur J Cardiothorac Surg 2005; 27:1005-1010.
5. Menicanti L, Donato M. The Dor procedure: what has changed after fifteen years of clinical practice? J Thorac Cardiovasc Surg 2002; 124:886-890.
6. Blom AS, Acker MA. The surgical treatment of end-stage heart failure. Curr Probl Cardiol 2007; 32:553-599.
7. Bogot NR, Durst R, Shaham D, Admon D. Cardiac CT of the transplanted heart: indications, technique, appearance, and complications. Radiographics 2007; 27:1297-1309.
8. Kuhlman JE. Thoracic imaging in heart transplantation. J Thorac Imaging 2002; 17:113-121.
9. Knisely BL, Mastey LA, Collins J, et al. Imaging of cardiac transplantation complications. Radiographics 1999; 19:321-339.
10. Knisely BL, Collins J, Jahania SA, et al. Imaging of ventricular assist devices and their complications. AJR Am J Roentgenol 1997; 169:385-391.
11. Carmichael BB, Setser RM, Stillman AE, et al. Effects of surgical ventricular restoration on left ventricular function: dynamic MR imaging. Radiology 2006; 241:710-717.
12. Dor V, Sabatier M, Di Donato M, et al. Efficacy of endoventricular patch plasty in large postinfarction akinetic scar and left ventricular dysfunction: comparison with a series of large dyskinetic scars. J Thorac Cardiovasc Surg 1998; 116:50-59.
13. Naftel DC, Brown RN. Survival after heart transplantation. In Kirklin JK, Young JB, McGiffin DC (eds). Heart Transplantation. Philadelphia: Churchill Livingstone; 2002. p 587-614.
14. Shellock FG, Valencerina S. Ventricular assist device implant (AB 5000) prototype cannula: in vitro assessment of MRI issues at 3-Tesla. J Cardiovasc Magn Reson 2008; 10:23.
15. Wu YW, Yen RF, Lee CM, et al. Diagnostic and prognostic value of dobutamine thallium-201 single-photon emission computed tomography after transplantation. J Heart Lung Transplant 2005; 24:544-550.
16. Flotats A, Carrio I. Value of radionuclide studies in cardiac transplantation. Ann Nucl Med 2006; 20:13-21.
17. Henry DA, Corcoran HL, Lewis TD, et al. Orthotopic cardiac transplantation: evaluation with CT. Radiology 1989; 170:343-350.
18. Marie PY, Angioi M, Carteaux JP, et al. Detection and prediction of acute heart transplant rejection with the myocardial T2 determination provided by a black-blood magnetic resonance imaging sequence. J Am Coll Cardiol 2001; 37:825-831.
19. Ciliberto GR, Mascarello M, Gronda E, et al. Acute rejection after heart transplantation: noninvasive echocardiographic evaluation. J Am Coll Cardiol 1994; 23:1156-1161.

20. Knollmann FD, Hummel M, Hetzer R, et al. CT of heart transplant recipients: spectrum of disease. Radiographics 2000; 20:1637-1648.
21. Benza RL, Tallaj J. Cardiac allograft vasculopathy (chronic rejection). In Kirklin JK, Young JB, McGiffin DC (eds). Heart Transplantation. Philadelphia: Churchill Livingstone; 2002. pp 615-665.
22. Steen H, Merten C, Refle S, et al. Prevalence of different gadolinium enhancement patterns after heart transplantation. J Am Coll Cardiol 2008; 52:1160-1167.
23. Aggarwal S, Cheema F, Oz M, et al. Long-term mechanical circulatory support. In Cohn LH (ed). Cardiac Surgery in the Adult, 3rd ed. New York: McGraw-Hill; 2008. pp 1609-1628.
24. Raman J, Dixit A, Bolotin G, et al. Failure modes of left ventricular reconstruction or the Dor procedure: a multi-institutional perspective. Eur J Cardiothorac Surg 2006; 30:347-352.
25. Dor V. Left ventricular reconstruction for ischemic heart failure. In Fang JC, Couper GS (eds). Surgical Management of Congestive Heart Failure. Totowa, NJ: Humana Press; 2005. pp 279-298.
26. Abbara S, Walker G (eds). Diagnostic Imaging: Cardiovascular. Salt Lake City, Utah: Amirsys; 2008. pp I-7, 8-11.
27. Hunt SA, Haddad F. The changing face of heart transplantation. J Am Coll Cardiol 2008; 52:587-598.

PART SEVEN

Valvular Heart Disease

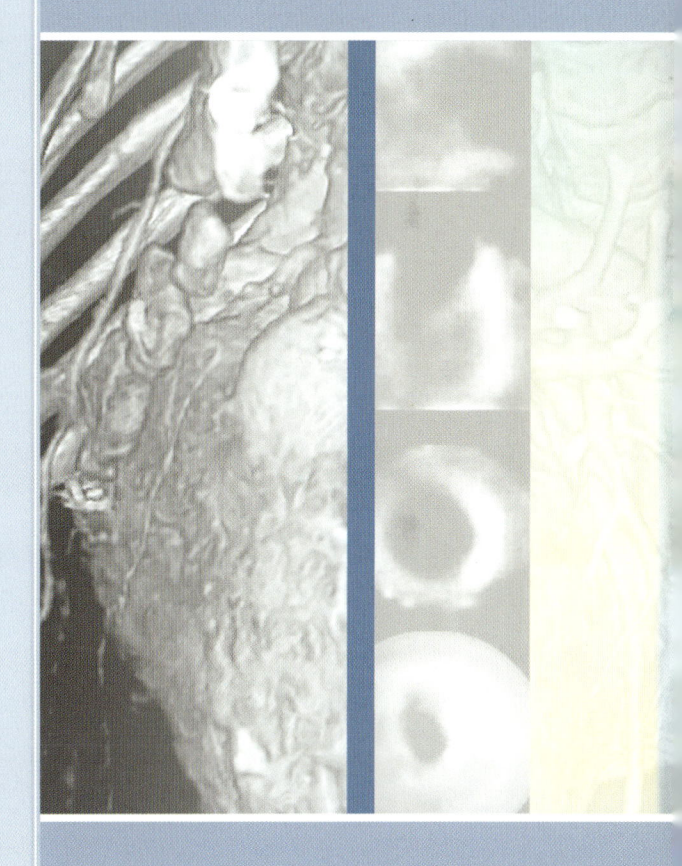

CHAPTER 60

Aortic and Mitral Valvular Disease

Roi Lotan and Jens Vogel-Claussen

For the diagnosis of aortic and mitral valvular disease, a variety of noninvasive techniques are available to assess cardiac valve morphologic features and function, with echocardiography currently being the most widely used modality for this purpose. Technical advances in electrocardiographically gated multidetector row computed tomography (MDCT) and magnetic resonance (MR) imaging allow the noninvasive visualization of the cardiac valves. In this article, we describe noninvasive imaging methods including radiography, echocardiography, and cardiac CT and MRI to assess aortic and mitral valvular disease.

AORTIC STENOSIS

Definition

Aortic stenosis is obstruction to left ventricular outflow at or near the level of the aortic valve. The stenosis can be subvalvular, supravalvular, or valvular. The valvular stenosis is by far the most frequently encountered type in adults, most commonly secondary to calcification of tricuspid or congenitally bicuspid aortic leaflets.[1]

Prevalence

Aortic stenosis has become the most common valvular disease in the Western world, largely because of the increased life expectancy of the population. The prevalence of aortic stenosis in the population older than 65 years is 2% to 7%; aortic sclerosis, the precursor to aortic stenosis in which there is valve thickening but no stenosis, is present in approximately 25% of this age group.[2,3] Whereas aortic stenosis is seen in patients with both tricuspid and bicuspid aortic valves, the patients with bicuspid aortic valves will become symptomatic and present for valve replacement an average of one to two decades earlier in life.[4] Nonatherosclerotic causes of aortic stenosis, such as rheumatic and congenital, are rare in the developed world.[2]

Etiology and Pathophysiology

Aortic stenosis should be considered part of a disease continuum in which initially non–hemodynamically significant valve thickening and calcification eventually progress to heavily calcified, immobile leaflets causing obstruction of left ventricular outflow. The early, asymptomatic portion of this continuum may last several decades; the symptomatic phase is often short and rapidly progressive, with a 2-year survival rate of 50% after onset of symptoms.[4] At that point, only aortic valve replacement can reverse the poor prognosis and offer long-term survival.

Aortic stenosis is associated with several risk factors, the main ones being increased age, male gender, hypertension, smoking, diabetes mellitus, and elevated serum low-density lipoprotein and elevated lipoprotein levels.[1,4] Aortic stenosis is an active disease process that follows a pattern similar to that seen in vascular atherosclerosis—inflammation followed by lipid accumulation and dystrophic calcification.[3] The aortic calcifications tend to accumulate preferentially at the edges of the valve leaflets, which influences valvular function.

Manifestations of Disease

Clinical Presentation

Aortic stenosis in asymptomatic patients is usually identified incidentally during the cardiac auscultation portion of the physical examination, when note is made of a late systolic murmur or a normally split second heart sound. Symptomatic patients can present with angina, syncope, dyspnea on exertion, and eventually symptoms of heart failure.[1] The patient's symptoms are associated with the

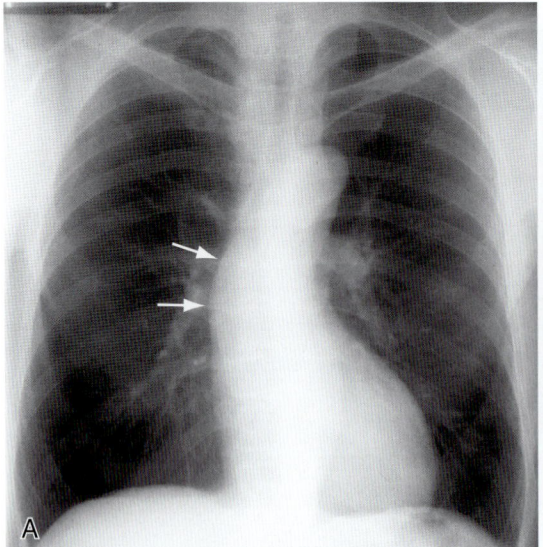

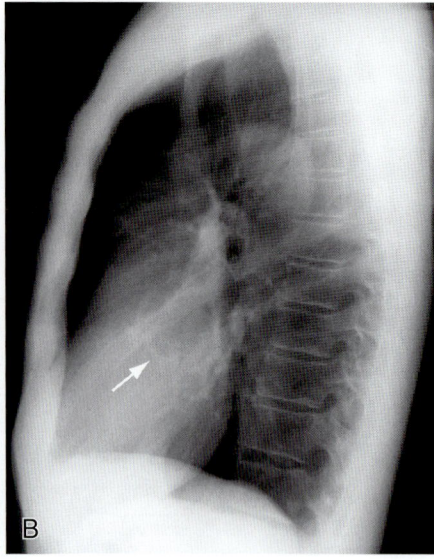

FIGURE 60-1 Aortic stenosis. Posterior-anterior plain film radiograph (**A**) shows dilation of the ascending aorta (*arrows*) due to aortic stenosis. The heart size as seen in this patient is often normal because the left ventricle first responds with concentric hypertrophy to the increased left ventricular pressure. Aortic valve calcifications can also often be seen, usually better assessed on a lateral view (**B**). *(Images courtesy of Dr. William Scott, Johns Hopkins Hospital, Baltimore, Md.)*

degree of stenosis at the level of the aortic valve and with the degree of resulting left ventricular dysfunction. As the stenosis becomes more significant, with a higher pressure gradient across the valve, the left ventricle responds to the systolic pressure overload with concentric hypertrophy. Whereas this increased wall thickness is the expected, appropriate adaptation to increased pressure, it in turn causes a diastolic dysfunction that reduces cardiac output. In addition, hypertrophy may also cause reduced or imbalanced distribution of coronary blood flow, thereby increasing the risk of subendocardial ischemia and worsening the symptoms of heart failure.[1]

Imaging Indications

The grading of aortic stenosis is based on several values—the valvular orifice area, the pressure gradient across the valve, and the stenotic jet velocity—all of which require imaging for measurement. Transthoracic echocardiography is the imaging modality of choice and therefore the gold standard for grading of aortic stenosis severity. The severity of symptoms does not always correlate with the degree of stenosis, and some patients with moderate stenosis become symptomatic, whereas others with severe stenosis by imaging criteria remain without symptoms.[1] The importance of this is underlined by the fact that the timing of therapy depends more on the presence of symptoms than on the grade of aortic stenosis.[2]

Imaging Techniques

Radiography

The most prominent finding on chest radiographs in adults with aortic stenosis is enlargement of the ascending aorta, although extent of dilation does not directly correlate with severity of stenosis (Fig. 60-1).[5] Conversely, the degree of aortic valve calcification does correlate with disease severity. Other, less specific findings, such as pulmonary venous congestion and pulmonary edema, can occur late in the disease process as a result of left ventricular dysfunction.[5]

Echocardiography

As previously noted, echocardiography is the gold standard for evaluation of aortic stenosis. It is the modality of choice for both initial diagnosis and assessment of disease severity as well as for re-evaluation and monitoring of both asymptomatic patients and those in whom symptoms have appeared or are progressing.[1] In general, asymptomatic patients with mild to moderate stenosis are monitored every 1 to 2 years; those with moderate to severe stenosis are evaluated every 6 to 12 months.[4]

In addition to evaluating the valve orifice size and velocity of the stenotic jet, echocardiography can be used to assess the thickness of the left ventricular wall as well as left ventricular size and function. By use of the modified Bernoulli equation ($\Delta P = 4V^2$), the pressure gradient across the valve is calculated by measuring the peak velocity of the flow jet. Whereas a normal aortic valve has a peak jet velocity of 0.9 to 1.8 m/sec, a peak pressure gradient of less than 25 mm Hg, and a valve orifice area of 2.0 to 3.5 cm^2, a severely stenotic valve will have a peak velocity of more than 4.0 m/sec, a peak gradient of more than 64 mm Hg, and a valve area of less than 0.5 cm^2.[4]

Computed Tomography

Although echocardiography will likely continue to be the first-line modality for diagnosis, grading, and monitoring of aortic stenosis, ECG-gated multislice CT can add more information in patients in whom clinical symptoms for some reason do not match the echocardiographic findings

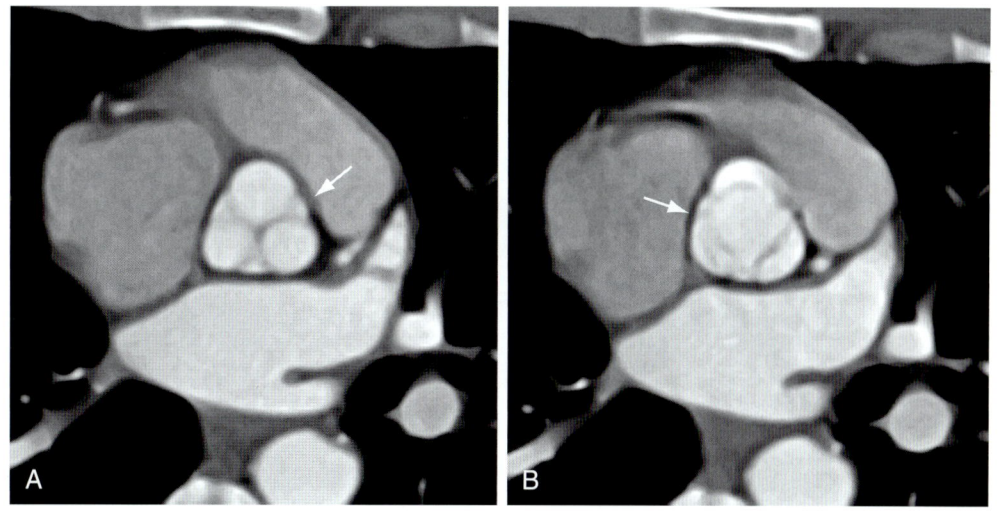

■ **FIGURE 60-2** Normal aortic valve. Maximum intensity projection reformatted images from 64-section MDCT data show a normal aortic valve in diastole (**A**, *arrow*) and systole (**B**, *arrow*). Four-dimensional reconstructions are often reviewed to assess cardiac valve motion throughout the cardiac cycle.

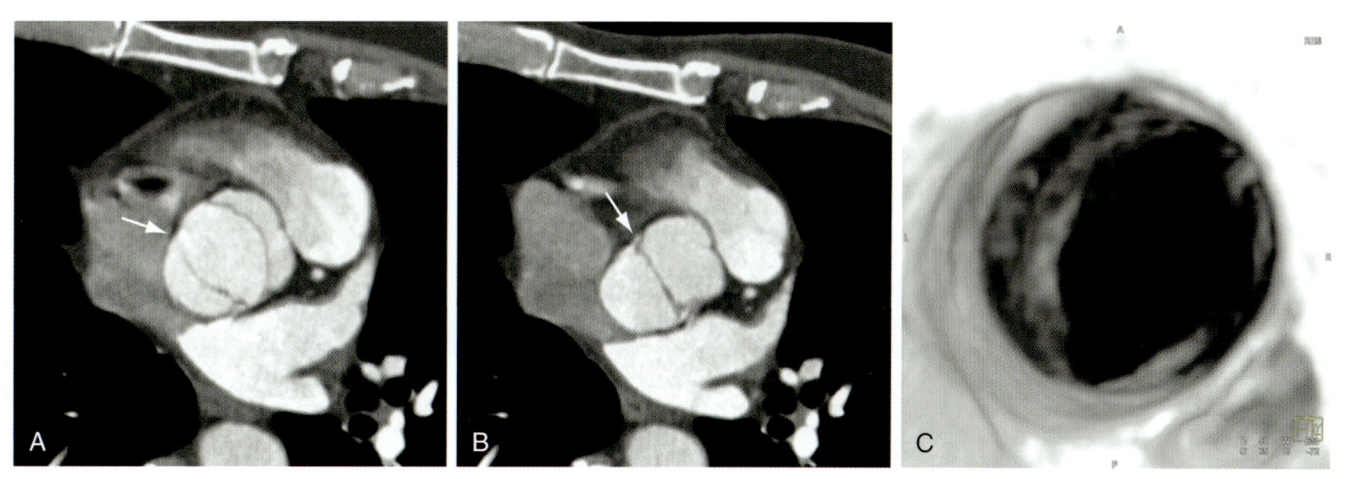

■ **FIGURE 60-3** Bicuspid aortic valve in a 61-year-old man. **A** and **B**, Maximum intensity projection reformatted images from 64-section MDCT data show the aortic valve (*arrow*) in systole (**A**) and diastole (**B**). Endoluminal volume rendering reformatted image from 64-section MDCT data shows a bicuspid aortic valve in open (**C**) position. Bicuspid valves occur in 2% of the population, and half of the affected patients develop at least mild aortic stenosis by the age of 50 years. However, the patient in this case had no significant stenosis or aortic valve calcifications.

or in patients who are technically challenging.[6] The main advantage of CT over transthoracic echocardiography, other than being faster, is the more reliably accurate measurement of valve orifice area by planimetry, which in CT is not limited by hemodynamic factors, such as low cardiac output, as it is in transthoracic echocardiography (Figs. 60-2 and 60-3).[6] In addition, CT can give a reproducible assessment and quantification of valve calcification, a major component of stenosis that correlates with its severity (Figs. 60-4 and 60-5).[7] Newer multidetector CT scanners do not require pretreatment with β blockers for rate control if the heart rate is below 85 beats/min and allow a dynamic display of valve motion throughout the full cardiac cycle.[8] The main disadvantages of CT, in addition to the relatively higher cost and lower availability, are radiation and the need for intravenous administration of contrast material.

Magnetic Resonance

Qualitative assessment of aortic valve stenosis can be performed by steady-state free precession (SSFP) cine MR because of the excellent temporal resolution, which allows highly accurate evaluation of valve motion.[7] A signal void due to spin dephasing representing the stenotic jet is identified projecting from the valve toward the proximal aorta. Adequate quantitative measurements are not possible with the SSFP MR technique. For quantification of aortic stenosis, phase contrast MR imaging is typically used. With this technique, the peak flow of the jet in the ascending aorta can be measured, and as with echocardiography, the pressure gradient can be calculated by the modified Bernoulli equation ($\Delta P = 4V^2$) (Fig. 60-6). A disadvantage of MR in evaluation of aortic stenosis is the poor visualization of leaflet calcification, a major factor in the disease process.

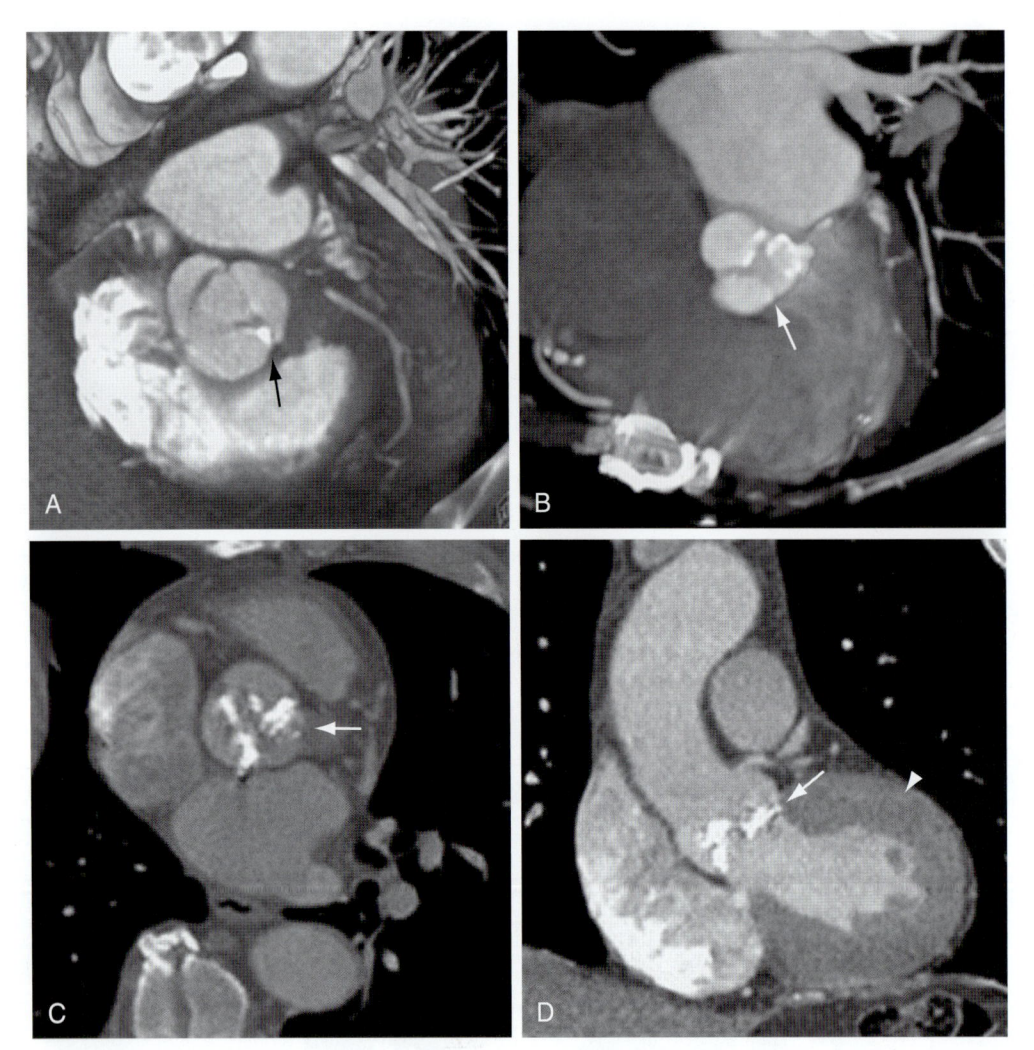

FIGURE 60-4 Aortic valve calcifications. The 64-section MDCT scans show minimal aortic valve calcifications without significant aortic stenosis (*arrow* in **A**), moderate aortic valve calcifications (*arrow* in **B**), and severe aortic valve calcifications causing significant aortic stenosis (*arrow* in **C** and **D**). Note also the concentric left ventricular hypertrophy (*arrowhead* in **D**).

Treatment Options

Medical

The key elements of medical management of asymptomatic patients with aortic stenosis include advising against strenuous exercise in cases of moderate to severe stenosis; antibiotic prophylaxis against endocarditis for dental or other interventional procedures; antihypertensive therapy; and close monitoring both of the severity of stenosis and for appearance of symptoms.[1] The last item is of great importance, both because disease progression tends to be unpredictable and as surgical therapy, namely, aortic valve replacement, is usually indicated once symptoms appear or are thought to be imminent. Recognition of the onset of symptoms can be especially difficult in patients with other comorbidities, and special attention needs to be paid to any change in tolerance of strenuous activity or appearance of chest pain in either rest or stress.[1]

Surgical

As the combined risk of aortic valve replacement (up to 10% mortality in the elderly or in those with severe comorbidities) and complications associated with having a prosthetic valve (2% to 3% per year) is much greater than the risk of sudden cardiac death in the asymptomatic patient, even those with severe stenosis by imaging, surgical therapy is usually not indicated until symptoms appear.[4] The exception to this rule of thumb is if there is significant stenosis-related left ventricular dysfunction or if there has been a substantial increase in peak aortic jet velocity (>0.3 m/sec within 1 year), indicating imminent onset of symptoms.[2]

In terms of surgical techniques, open aortic valve replacement is the conventional surgical therapy, with either a bioprosthesis or a mechanical valve (Fig. 60-7). The mechanical valves have a longer lifespan, but they require permanent anticoagulation and are therefore usually used in younger patients. Aortic balloon valvotomy can sometimes be used to relieve stenosis, although it is usually reserved for young patients without valve calcifications. In older adults, it is used only in cases of palliation in poor surgical candidates or as a temporary bridge to valve replacement in clinically unstable patients.[4]

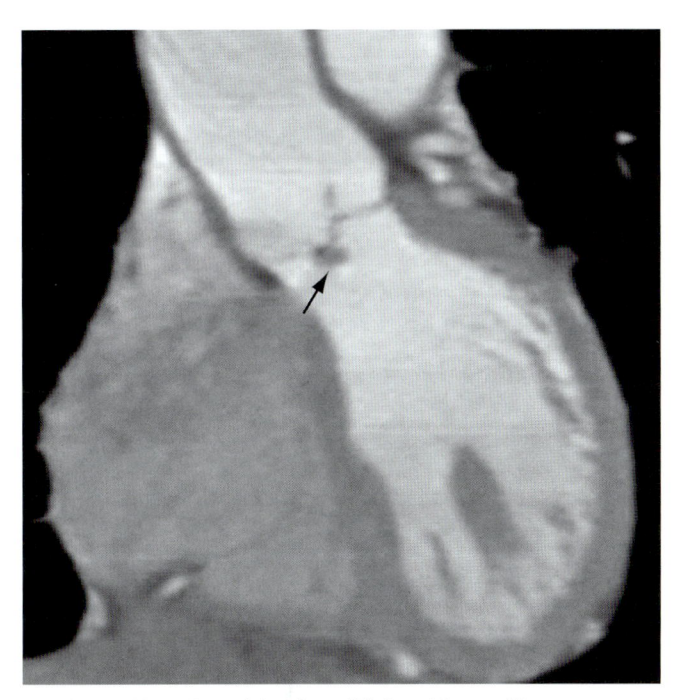

CHAPTER 60 ● *Aortic and Mitral Valvular Disease* 831

FIGURE 60-5 Bacterial endocarditis in a 45-year-old woman. Maximum intensity projection reformatted image from MDCT data shows a vegetation of the aortic valve (*arrow*).

AORTIC REGURGITATION

Definition

Aortic regurgitation is the reflux of blood into the left ventricle during diastole due to failure of the aortic valve to close properly (malcoaptation of the valve cusps). Aortic regurgitation can be categorized by severity (trace, mild, moderate, severe) and chronicity (acute vs. chronic).

Prevalence

Trace or mild chronic aortic regurgitation is relatively common, affecting approximately 13% of men and 8.5% of women.[9] Moderate or severe chronic aortic regurgitation is rare. The main predictors for chronic aortic regurgitation are increased age and male gender.

Etiology and Pathophysiology

Chronic aortic regurgitation is most commonly a result of atherosclerotic degeneration of a normal, tricuspid aortic valve or a congenital abnormality, namely, a bicuspid valve. Aortic valve leaflet structure and closure can also be affected by the diameter of the adjacent aorta, and thus diseases that cause dilation of the aortic root or annulus

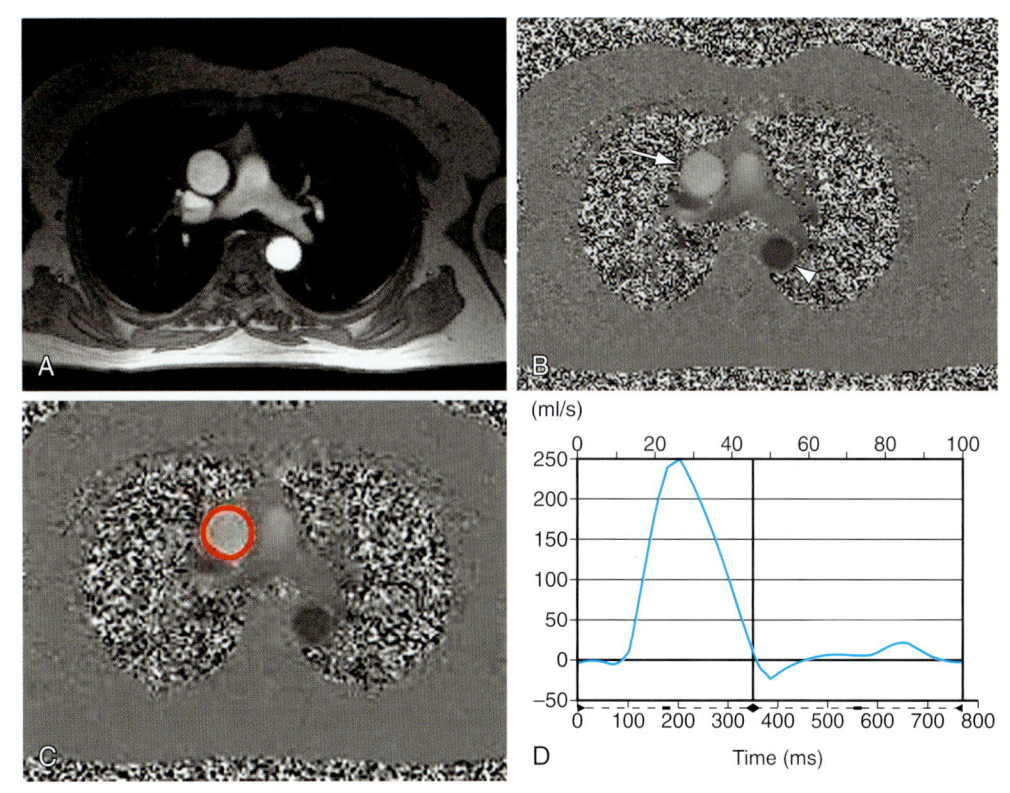

FIGURE 60-6 Normal aortic valve. **A,** Magnitude phase contrast MR image used for anatomic correlation. **B,** On a velocity MR image, the gray-scale value of each voxel represents the velocity value of that voxel. Black areas represent caudal blood flow in the descending aorta (*arrowhead*); white areas represent cephalad flow in the ascending aorta (*arrow*). The thoracic wall demonstrates an intermediate signal intensity that corresponds to no flow. **C,** On a velocity phase contrast MR image, orthogonal measurements of the ascending aorta at the level of the pulmonary bifurcation (*outlined in red*) have been performed. **D,** Flow volume graph of one cardiac cycle illustrates a normal flow curve.

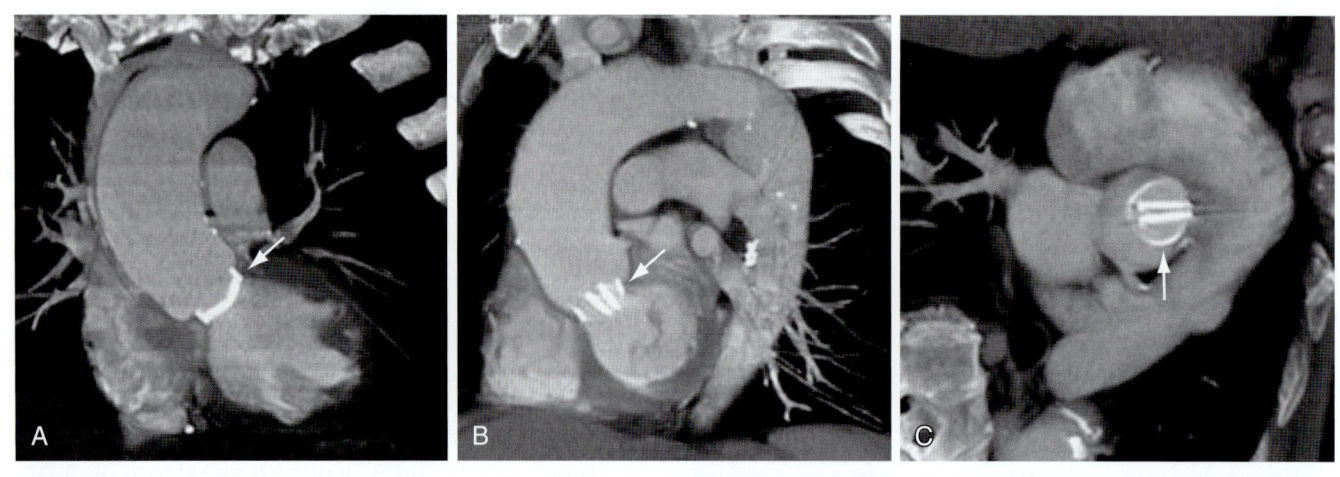

FIGURE 60-7 Aortic valve replacement. The 64-section MDCT scans show a mechanical bileaflet valve (*arrow*) during diastole (**A**) and systole (**B, C**).

can also lead to regurgitation.[1] These include aortic dissection (Stanford A or DeBakey type I), ascending aortic aneurysm, Marfan syndrome, and Ehlers-Danlos syndrome. Acute aortic regurgitation is most commonly a result of bacterial endocarditis, acute dissection, or severe thoracic trauma and usually has a poor prognosis.[9]

As chronic aortic regurgitation progresses from mild to severe, the initial minimal volume overload at end-diastole becomes a significant volume overload with concomitant pressure overload secondary to systolic hypertension. There is progressive dilation of the left ventricle as well as dilation of the aortic root, which in turn exacerbates the regurgitation.[9] This progression parallels the path from a compensated state to a decompensated state and simultaneous development of symptoms.

Manifestations of Disease

Clinical Presentation

Mild chronic aortic regurgitation is usually asymptomatic, but as the left ventricular volume overload eventually leads to both diastolic and systolic dysfunction, the symptoms of heart failure appear. Dyspnea on exertion is the most common symptom.

Imaging Indications

Although transthoracic echocardiography is the most important and widely used diagnostic imaging modality in evaluation of aortic regurgitation, it has inherent limitations, the most prominent being operator dependence, interobserver variability, and susceptibility to a patient's morphologic characteristics.[7] During the last few years, both MDCT and MRI have been increasingly applied to the evaluation of aortic regurgitation.

Imaging Techniques

Radiography

Aortic regurgitation is commonly associated with aortic root disease and eventually, if untreated, causes left ven-

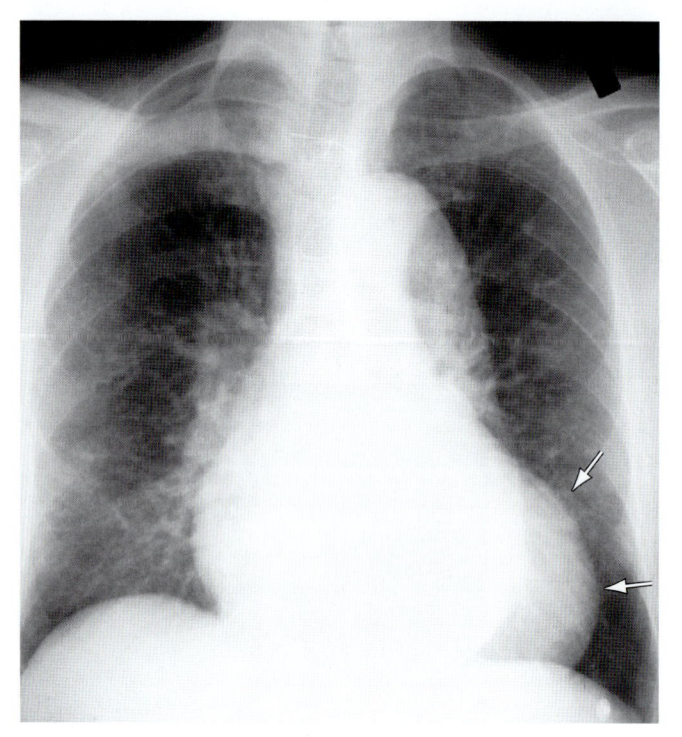

FIGURE 60-8 Aortic regurgitation can cause isolated enlargement of the left ventricle (*arrows*) due to the end-systolic volume overload. (Courtesy of Dr. William Scott, Johns Hopkins Hospital, Baltimore, Md.)

tricular dilation due to the high end-diastolic volume (Fig. 60-8). Findings on plain chest radiography therefore correspond to the severity of the regurgitation; the two most typical findings are cardiomegaly and ascending aortic dilation.[5] Pulmonary venous congestion and edema do not usually occur until late in the natural progression of the disease or in the setting of acute severe regurgitation, such as can be seen with bacterial endocarditis (see Fig. 60-5).[5]

Echocardiography

Transthoracic echocardiography allows evaluation of morphology of both valve leaflets and the aortic root as well as characterization of left ventricular size and function. Doppler color flow mapping can be used to identify the presence of regurgitation initially and to gauge its severity.[9]

Computed Tomography

MDCT can quantify the left ventricular volume and function as well as the aortic root diameter, useful for following the course of aortic regurgitation. The main advantage of MDCT over echocardiography and MR, especially with the advent of the 64-slice scanner, is the excellent spatial resolution, which, as in aortic stenosis, allows better evaluation of valvular anatomy and morphology (see Fig. 60-4).[7] Specifically, planimetric measurement of the regurgitant orifice area can be performed, enabling direct quantification of the area between the cusps that remains open during diastole. The severity of aortic regurgitation corresponds directly to the size of the orifice, and as the regurgitant orifice area increases, so too does the severity of the symptoms. A study has shown a high degree of sensitivity in differentiating between mild, moderate, and severe aortic regurgitation on the basis of the regurgitant orifice area, as determined independently by transthoracic echocardiography.[10] Whereas both echocardiography and MR often measure the valvular dysfunction indirectly, by the regurgitant jet and the left ventricular volume measurements, MDCT can provide direct high-resolution visualization of the valve.[11] The main disadvantage of CT with respect to echocardiography is radiation exposure to the patient (mean of 11 mSv), which is especially important in aortic regurgitation given the high rate of repeated studies needed to closely monitor the disease.[10]

Magnetic Resonance

Cardiac MR can be used to identify aortic regurgitation initially and to monitor its effects on left ventricular volume and function. As in aortic stenosis, SSFP cine MR is used to identify the signal void that represents the regurgitant flow jet, which in aortic regurgitation projects from the closed aortic valve back into the left ventricle during diastole (Fig. 60-9).[5] In addition, actual quantification of the regurgitant volume can be performed by comparing the right and left ventricular volumes and subtracting the left ventricular volume from the right, assuming only one valve is regurgitant.[5] During diastole, there is often observation of anterior motion of the anterior mitral leaflet as a result of turbulent regurgitant flow.[7] Last, cine MR allows quantification of left ventricular volume and function, as these two parameters are crucial for treatment planning.

An additional method of quantification is phase contrast MR, in which a plane perpendicular to the blood flow is chosen at the level of the ascending aorta and main pulmonary artery. This method compares the stroke volumes during systole and can also identify and quantify the retrograde aortic flow during diastole.[5]

Treatment Options

Medical

Treatment options differ according to where the patient is along the spectrum of disease. On one end, the asymp-

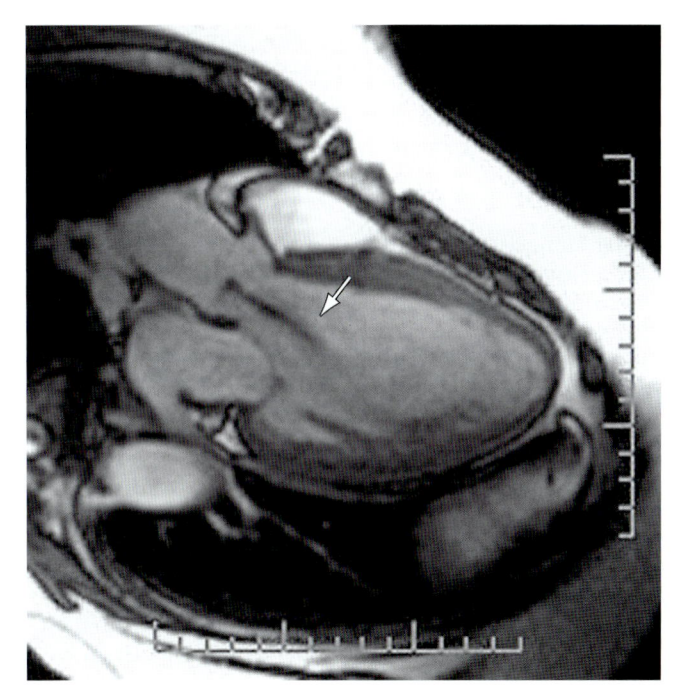

■ **FIGURE 60-9** Aortic regurgitation in a 58-year-old woman. Cine MR image shows a signal void (jet) in the left ventricular outflow tract due to turbulent flow. The *arrow* indicates aortic regurgitation. There was also anterior motion (flutter) of the anterior mitral valve leaflet during diastole due to the turbulent regurgitant flow in the left ventricular outflow tract.

tomatic patients with normal systolic function and left ventricular size are usually monitored for development of symptoms or progressive left ventricular dilation or dysfunction. At the other end of the spectrum, symptomatic patients with chronic severe aortic regurgitation have a mortality rate that is greater than 10% per year and thus need to undergo surgical intervention unless it is contraindicated by severe comorbidities.[9] The key question in terms of treatment is at which point an asymptomatic or minimally symptomatic patient should undergo surgery to prevent irreversible left ventricular function. Multiple studies during the past decade have pointed to better outcomes in patients with left ventricular ejection fractions above 55% or an end-systolic left ventricular diameter of less than 55 mm.[9] This guideline, termed the 55 rule, can be used to select patients for surgery.[9] Medical treatment, namely, the use of antihypertensives to reduce systolic hypertension and to improve left ventricular function, is limited to two groups of patients: those with severe chronic aortic regurgitation who are not surgical candidates; and those who are asymptomatic and in whom surgery might be delayed even longer.[1]

Surgical

As discussed before, aortic valve replacement or repair is usually reserved for symptomatic patients with severe aortic regurgitation or asymptomatic patients with left ventricular dysfunction. In addition, patients with severe aortic regurgitation undergoing planned coronary bypass or other aortic surgery should also undergo valve repair or replacement. Because regurgitation is associated with aortic root dilation in many patients, simultaneous aortic root reconstruction is performed as well.[1]

MITRAL STENOSIS

Definition

Mitral stenosis is defined as obstruction of the left ventricular outflow tract at the level of the mitral valve due to either a structural abnormality of the valve itself or a space-occupying lesion, such as a mass or a thrombus, that effectively prevents proper filling of the left ventricle during diastole.[1]

Prevalence and Epidemiology

With the dramatic decrease in incidence of rheumatic fever in the developed world, mitral stenosis, which is most commonly caused by rheumatic carditis, has become a rare entity in the United States, and most patients today who present with mitral stenosis in this country have in fact emigrated at some point from developing countries.[12] In 2004, approximately 1500 patients in the United States underwent balloon mitral valvotomies, the most common interventional therapy for mitral stenosis, which gives a rough estimate of the prevalence of the severe form of the disease.[12]

Apart from rheumatic fever, mitral stenosis can be caused by congenital anomalies, severe mitral annular calcifications, left atrial myxomas, carcinoid syndrome, and obstructive left atrial thrombus. Although rates of rheumatic fever are equal between the genders, there is a female predominance of nearly 2:1 in presentation of isolated mitral stenosis, a discrepancy thought to be associated with the autoimmune nature of the process in the heart after infection with group A streptococcus.[1]

Etiology and Pathophysiology

The rheumatic process causes inflammation of the heart valves, which leads to thickening and calcification of the valve leaflets as well as to fusion of the valve commissure. This results in progressive narrowing of the valve area, which normally is between 4 and 5 cm^2. Symptoms of mitral stenosis do not usually develop until the valve area has decreased to less than 2.5 cm^2, at which point the free flow of blood between the left atrium and left ventricle is impeded and a pressure gradient develops across the valve.[1] As the pressure gradient increases during diastole, it is transmitted in a retrograde fashion, in turn leading to left atrial enlargement, pulmonary venous hypertension, pulmonary arterial hypertension, and eventually, in severe cases, pulmonary regurgitation and right ventricular dilation. With worsening stenosis, there is also flow restriction causing decreased left ventricular output. The dilation of the left atrium can alter its electrophysiologic properties and can lead to atrial fibrillation, which in turn increases the risk of stroke and other arterial embolization.[12] In most patients with untreated mitral stenosis, mortality is a result of progressive pulmonary and systemic congestion; the majority of the remaining patients die of either systemic or pulmonary embolism.[1]

Manifestations of Disease

Clinical Presentation

As in aortic stenosis or regurgitation, mild disease is often asymptomatic. In many patients, initial symptomatic presentation with mitral stenosis is directly attributable to the increased pressure gradient and lowered left ventricular output, resulting in nonspecific symptoms such as fatigue and dyspnea.[1] In others, the symptoms during initial presentation are due to atrial fibrillation. An increase in heart rate causes a shortened diastole, which, given the hemodynamic obstruction at the level of the mitral valve, in turn leads to decreased left ventricular filling. Therefore, the initial symptoms and clinical manifestations occur during exercise, stress, or pregnancy.[1]

Imaging Indications

As in the evaluation of aortic valve disease, the diagnostic gold standard in identification, evaluation, grading, and monitoring of mitral stenosis remains echocardiography.[12] With technologic advances in both MDCT and MRI, these modalities have also been applied to the evaluation of mitral stenosis.

Imaging Techniques

Radiography

Although understandably limited in utility, plain chest radiography can be a useful tool in initial evaluation of mitral stenosis by roughly assessing its severity, namely, by identifying pulmonary venous hypertension and the extent of left atrial enlargement (Fig. 60-10).[5] The pres-

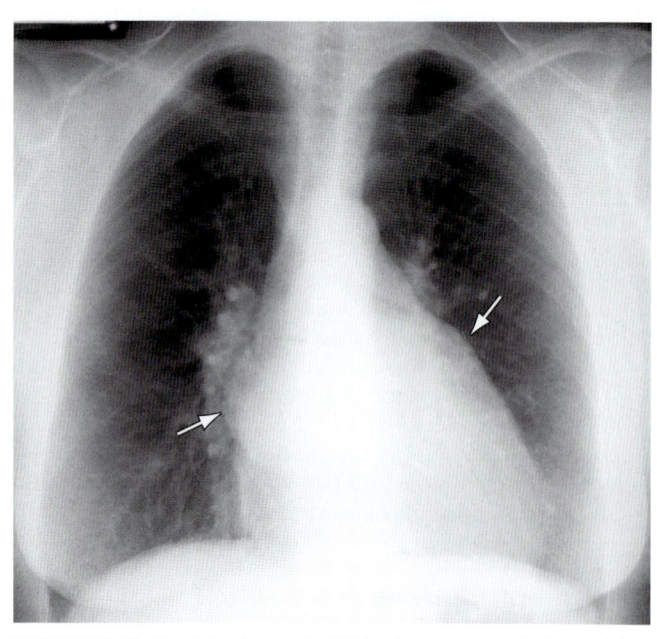

■ **FIGURE 60-10** Mitral stenosis. With obstruction at the level of the mitral valve, there is enlargement of the left atrium (*arrow*) as well as of the left atrial appendage (*arrow*). (*Image courtesy of Dr. William Scott, Johns Hopkins Hospital, Baltimore, Md.*)

CHAPTER 60 • *Aortic and Mitral Valvular Disease* 835

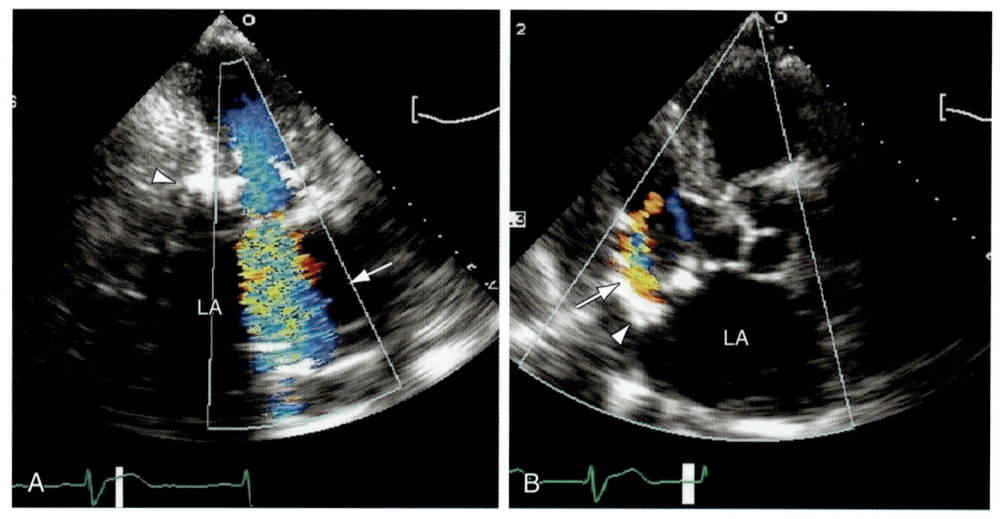

FIGURE 60-11 Mitral regurgitation and stenosis as seen on echocardiography. In regurgitation (**A**), the flow jet is directed back toward the left atrium (LA), whereas in stenosis (**B**), it is directed from the mitral valve (*arrowhead*) into the left ventricle (*arrow*). (*Images courtesy of Dr. Christopher Sibley, Johns Hopkins Hospital, Baltimore, Md.*)

ence of pulmonary edema can also be noted. In addition, signs of concomitant tricuspid or aortic valvular disease can also be identified by evaluating for right-sided heart enlargement or ascending aortic prominence, respectively.[5]

Echocardiography

As noted before, two-dimensional echocardiography is the first-line modality for evaluation of mitral stenosis, given its ability to accurately assess mitral annular structure and function, valve leaflets, chordae tendineae, papillary muscles, and left ventricular size and function.[13] As in other cardiac valvular disease, velocity of blood flow in the stenotic jet is used to quantify the gradient pressure by the modified Bernoulli equation, and mean pressure gradient across the valve and the valve orifice area are used to estimate severity of the disease (Fig. 60-11B).[13]

Computed Tomography

As in the case of aortic valve evaluation, the distinct advantage of MDCT in mitral valve imaging is the excellent spatial resolution it provides.[7] This again allows better characterization of valve anatomy (Fig. 60-12). Evaluation of the valve area by planimetric measurement allows more accurate staging of the stenosis, and close morphologic assessment can help in deciding the type of therapy and its timing. Specifically, the mobility of the leaflets and the presence or absence of commissural calcifications and subvalvular or valvular thickening help assess the suitability of one of the main interventional therapies.[1]

Magnetic Resonance

Just as with aortic valvular disease, the advantage of MR is in its temporal resolution. Cine MR imaging is used to identify the flow jet signal void, which in the case of mitral stenosis is seen projecting into the left ventricle during

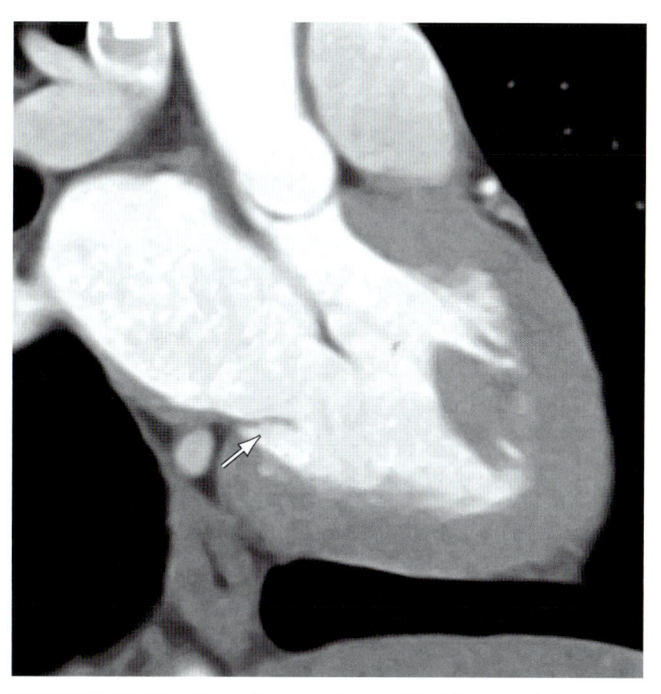

FIGURE 60-12 Normal mitral valve on CT. Reformatted three-dimensional maximum intensity projection image shows normal mitral valve leaflets (*arrow*).

diastole. With phase contrast MR, the peak pressure gradient across the mitral valve can be calculated by measuring the peak velocity of the stenotic jet during diastole and then applying the modified Bernoulli equation. New valve tracking algorithms are currently on the way to account for the significant through-plane motion of the mitral valve during the cardiac cycle, which can affect the phase contrast MR measurements. Whereas there is good correlation between MR and echocardiography in assessing the pressure gradient, MR tends to underestimate the value because of a lower sampling rate.[5]

Treatment Options

Medical

Because mitral stenosis is almost entirely a surgical disease, medical therapy is mostly limited to antibiotic prophylaxis against bacterial endocarditis and to rate control and anticoagulation in cases of atrial fibrillation.[1] Keeping a steady sinus rhythm is key in preventing a shortening of the diastolic left ventricular filling period. Patients are also advised to avoid physical exertion, which has the same effect by raising the heart rate.[1]

Surgical

The goal of surgical therapy in mitral stenosis is to release the mechanical obstruction of blood flow from across the valve. Depending on the morphology of the valve and its supporting structures, this is commonly achieved by one of three types of procedures discussed below.

Balloon Mitral Valvotomy

The least invasive of the procedures, this involves percutaneous placement of a balloon across the mitral valve and inflating it to "fracture" the fused leaflets at the commissures, allowing better opening of the valve during diastole. Balloon mitral valvotomy is most successful in patients with good leaf mobility, limited valve calcification, and mild leaflet thickening. The main contraindication to the procedure is a thrombus in the left atrium.[12]

Open Commissurotomy

Whereas open surgical commissurotomy is more invasive than balloon valvotomy, it enables a direct visual inspection of the valve apparatus and allows a more exact separation of the commissures and debulking of the valvular calcifications.[1] Permitting conservation of the native valve, this procedure can also include simultaneous amputation of the left atrial appendage, which results in a decreased risk of thrombus development. As in balloon mitral valvotomy, suitability of the procedure depends on valvular morphology.[12]

Mitral Valve Replacement

In the presence of severe fibrosis, valvular calcification, and subvalvular disease, the native valve cannot be conserved and replacement is necessary. Because of the inherent intraoperative risk, the usual presence of comorbidities, and the potential short- and long-term complications of having a prosthetic valve, mitral valve replacement is usually performed as the last resort, often after failed attempts at balloon valvotomy or even open commissurotomy. The type of prosthesis depends on the patient's age, the risk of long-term anticoagulation, and the patient's preference.[12]

MITRAL REGURGITATION

Definition

Mitral regurgitation is abnormal flow of blood from the left ventricle to the left atrium during systole due to dysfunction of the mitral valve apparatus or supporting structures. As in aortic regurgitation, a distinction is made between the acute and chronic forms of the disease. In addition, mitral regurgitation can be either primary (i.e., directly associated with leaflet dysfunction) or secondary to ischemic dyskinesia or annular dilation.

Prevalence

Mitral regurgitation is thought to affect approximately 2% of the population in the United States, with no gender predominance. Most patients remain asymptomatic throughout their lives.

Etiology and Pathophysiology

Acute mitral regurgitation is most commonly caused by either endocarditis or rupture of the papillary muscles or chordae tendineae. Chronic mitral regurgitation is most often due to mitral valve prolapse, infective endocarditis, cardiac ischemia, or dilated cardiomyopathy. Formerly a major cause, rheumatic heart disease is now rare in the Western world and if seen is often in patients who, as in cases of mitral stenosis, have migrated from developing countries.

Mitral valve prolapse, in which myxomatous degeneration of the mitral leaflets leads to their ballooning and "billowing" into the left atrium during systole, is quite common, affecting 2.3% of the population, although only a small percentage of these develop significant regurgitation.[14] Secondary mitral regurgitation is seen in approximately 30% of patients with coronary artery disease, although again, the severity is usually mild.[15] Nevertheless, ischemic mitral regurgitation, even if it is mild, worsens prognosis after myocardial infarction.[16] Dilated cardiomyopathy results in a change in the size and shape of the left atrium and ventricle and can also cause dilation of the mitral annulus, all of which lead to poor coaptation of the mitral leaflets.

In acute mitral regurgitation, there is a sudden volume overload on both the left atrium and left ventricle. In the absence of adaptive left ventricular hypertrophy, the cardiac output decreases. In addition, the left atrium is unable to handle the regurgitant volume, and the overload is transferred to the pulmonary veins, resulting in pulmonary vascular congestion.[1] In severe cases, both cardiogenic shock and pulmonary edema are evident. In chronic mitral regurgitation, the patients remain asymptomatic for years, during which there evolves compensatory left ventricular enlargement, which results in increased left ventricular end-diastolic volume that can maintain the increased stroke volume needed to sustain the cardiac output, although eventually there is left ventricular dysfunction as well.[1]

Manifestations of Disease

Clinical Presentation

As previously noted, most patients with chronic mitral regurgitation, including many with severe disease, remain asymptomatic. Some who do present clinically do so with associated entities, such as infective endocarditis and atrial fibrillation, that point to the underlying valvular dysfunction. On physical examination, the classic sign is an apical holosystolic murmur radiating to the axilla.[1] This is then usually confirmed on echocardiography. Patients who eventually progress to symptomatic disease present with the expected findings of left ventricular dysfunction and pulmonary venous congestion, namely, dyspnea, exercise intolerance, and fatigue.

Imaging Indications

As with all cardiac valvular disease, echocardiography is the modality of choice for diagnosis, grading, and monitoring of mitral regurgitation. Clinicians will use the echocardiographic grading or severity, in conjunction with clinical signs and symptoms, to make decisions about the necessity and timing of surgical intervention.[17] Both cardiac MR and MDCT serve as adjunct imaging tools in case the transthoracic echocardiographic examination is technically difficult or if additional anatomic information is needed for surgical planning.

Imaging Techniques

Radiography

With severe acute mitral regurgitation, the characteristic finding on chest radiography is pulmonary edema in the setting of a normal heart size.[16] With long-standing chronic mitral regurgitation, there is enlargement of both the left atrium and ventricle due to chronic volume overload.[5]

Echocardiography

The main goals of echocardiography in mitral regurgitation are to establish an etiology and mechanism for the regurgitation, to grade its severity, and to determine the need for surgical intervention. Compared with evaluation of mitral stenosis, the size and velocity of the regurgitant jet in mitral regurgitation do not correlate well with the clinical severity of the disease. A more important factor is the size of the left ventricle and its systolic function, as measured by the end-systolic diameter and ejection fraction, respectively (see Fig. 60-11A).[13]

Computed Tomography and Magnetic Resonance Imaging

The methods and principles of the mitral regurgitation assessment with CT and MRI are the same as in mitral stenosis discussed earlier (Fig 60-13; see also Fig. 60-12).

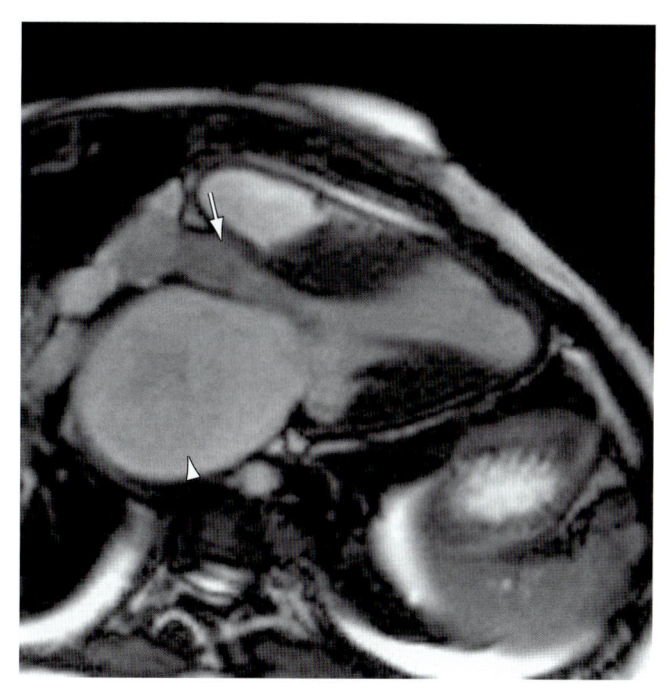

■ **FIGURE 60-13** Mitral regurgitation on MR. Young patient with idiopathic hypertrophic obstructive cardiomyopathy with subaortic stenosis and turbulent left ventricular outlet blood flow (*arrow*). The systolic anterior motion of the anterior mitral leaflet in turn causes mitral regurgitation and moderate to severe dilation of the left atrium (*arrowhead*).

Treatment Options

Medical

As most patients incidentally diagnosed with mitral regurgitation never become symptomatic, the goals of nonsurgical treatment are to monitor the severity of the disease and to prevent associated complications.[14] In mild to moderate mitral regurgitation without left ventricular dysfunction, echocardiography does not need to be performed on a regular basis, and patients are instructed to report any change in exercise tolerance. In moderate to severe mitral regurgitation, echocardiography should be performed on a yearly basis, unless there is a change in physical examination findings or symptoms appear. In addition, for all patients with known mitral regurgitation, antibiotic prophylaxis to prevent endocarditis should be administered before any invasive procedure, including dental work. In patients with atrial fibrillation, rate control and anticoagulation therapy is needed.

Surgical

There is consensus for performing mitral valve repair or replacement for patients with one of three entities: acute mitral regurgitation, symptomatic chronic mitral regurgitation, or asymptomatic chronic mitral regurgitation with a certain level of left ventricular dysfunction as measured by ejection fraction (<60%) and end-systolic left ventricular diameter (>45 mm).[18] In general, surgery in asymptomatic patients should be timed before the development of irreversible systolic dysfunction.[14] Surgical treatment of secondary mitral regurgitation, as in ischemia or dilated cardiomyopathy, is controversial because the problem lies not within the valve itself but rather with the supporting structures.[18] As with mitral stenosis, the choice between repair and replacement depends on the state of the valve leaflets. Repair, if possible, is obviously preferred, given the advantage of avoiding long-term anticoagulation and preserving the continuity of the papillary muscles and mitral annulus. On average, operative mortality for repair is 1% to 2%, compared with 5% to 10% with replacement.[18]

> **KEY POINTS**
> - Doppler ultrasound remains the modality of choice for assessment of aortic and mitral valve disease.
> - As complementary tools, CT and MRI are useful new noninvasive imaging modalities to assess valvular heart disease.

SUGGESTED READINGS

Bonow RO, et al. 2008 focused update incorporated into the ACC/AHA 2006 Guidelines for the Management of Patients With Valvular Heart Disease. A report of the American College of Cardiology/American Heart Association task force on practice guidelines. Circulation 2008; 118:e523-e661.

REFERENCES

1. American College of Cardiology/American Heart Association Task Force on Practice Guidelines; Society of Cardiovascular Anesthesiologists; Society for Cardiovascular Angiography and Interventions; Society of Thoracic Surgeons, Bonow RO, Carabello BA, Kanu C, et al. ACC/AHA 2006 guidelines for the management of patients with valvular heart disease: a report of the American College of Cardiology/American Heart Association Task Force on Practice Guidelines (writing committee to revise the 1998 Guidelines for the Management of Patients With Valvular Heart Disease): developed in collaboration with the Society of Cardiovascular Anesthesiologists: endorsed by the Society for Cardiovascular Angiography and Interventions and the Society of Thoracic Surgeons. Circulation 2006; 114:e84-e231.
2. Baumgartner H. Aortic stenosis: medical and surgical management. Heart 2005; 91:1483-1488.
3. Freeman RV, Otto CM. Spectrum of calcific aortic valve disease: pathogenesis, disease progression, and treatment strategies. Circulation 2005; 111:3316-3326.
4. Cowell SJ, Newby DE, Boon NA, et al. Calcific aortic stenosis: same old story? Age Ageing 2004; 33:538-544.
5. Webb WR, Higgins CB. Thoracic Imaging: Pulmonary and Cardiovascular Radiology. Philadelphia, Lippincott Williams & Wilkins, 2004.
6. Bouvier E, Logeart D, Sablayrolles JL, et al. Diagnosis of aortic valvular stenosis by multislice cardiac computed tomography. Eur Heart J 2006; 27:3033-3038.
7. Vogel-Claussen J, Pannu H, Spevak PJ, et al. Cardiac valve assessment with MR imaging and 64-section multi-detector row CT. Radiographics 2006; 26:1769-1784.
8. Feuchtner GM, Muller S, Bonatti J, et al. Sixty-four slice CT evaluation of aortic stenosis using planimetry of the aortic valve area. AJR Am J Roentgenol 2007; 189:197-203.
9. Bekeredjian R, Grayburn PA. Valvular heart disease: aortic regurgitation. Circulation 2005; 112:125-134.
10. Alkadhi H, Desbiolles L, Husmann L, et al. Aortic regurgitation: assessment with 64-section CT. Radiology 2007; 245:111-121.
11. Gilkeson RC, Markowitz AH, Balgude A, et al. MDCT evaluation of aortic valvular disease. AJR Am J Roentgenol 2006; 186:350-360.
12. Carabello BA. Modern management of mitral stenosis. Circulation 2005; 112:432-437.
13. Mora S, Wu K. Echocardiography in cardiac surgery. In Yuh D, Vricella L, Baumgartner W (eds). The Johns Hopkins Manual of Cardiothoracic Surgery. New York, McGraw-Hill Medical, 2007, p 943.
14. Keeffe BG, Otto CM. Mitral regurgitation. Minerva Cardioangiol 2003; 51:29-39.
15. Levine RA, Schwammenthal E. Ischemic mitral regurgitation on the threshold of a solution: from paradoxes to unifying concepts. Circulation 2005; 112:745-758.
16. Filsoufi F, Salzberg SP, Adams DH. Current management of ischemic mitral regurgitation. Mt Sinai J Med 2005; 72:105-115.
17. Irvine T, Li XK, Sahn DJ, et al. Assessment of mitral regurgitation. Heart 2002; 88(Suppl 4):iv11-iv19.
18. Otto CM. Timing of surgery in mitral regurgitation. Heart 2003; 89:100-105.

CHAPTER 61

Tricuspid and Pulmonary Valvular Disease

Jeffrey C. Hellinger

The right heart functions to receive systemic deoxygenated blood in the atrial chamber and pump it via the ventricular chamber into the pulmonary arterial system for gas exchange. This process is well coordinated. Although the electrical conduction pathways and muscular contraction are fundamental to achieving continuous blood flow through the right heart, equally important are the tricuspid and pulmonary valves that regulate flow between the right atrium and ventricle and right ventricle and pulmonary artery, respectively. These valves ensure appropriate antegrade flow during the cardiac cycle.

The tricuspid and pulmonary valves can fail as a result of disease states, which may lead to stenosis (Figs. 61-1 to 61-3), insufficiency (Figs. 61-4 to 61-6), or a combination of both (Figs. 61-7 to 61-9). Stenosis impedes forward flow, resulting in pressure overload, and insufficiency results in blood flowing backward, leading to volume overload. Tricuspid and pulmonary valvular disease may present in isolation or in conjunction. Clinical presentation, involvement of the cardiac chambers, severity of secondary chamber dysfunction, and impact on systemic and pulmonary vasculature and other viscera depend on which valves are involved, which type of valvular dysfunction predominates, the severity and duration of valvular dysfunction, and the degree of cardiac compensation. Pharmacologic, endovascular, and surgical management for diseased valves relies on accurate and comprehensive noninvasive diagnostic evaluation, using a combination of chest radiography, echocardiography, magnetic resonance imaging (MRI), magnetic resonance angiography (MRA), and computed tomography angiography (CTA). Invasive catheterization is no longer used to diagnose primarily tricuspid and pulmonary valvular disease and should be reserved for cases in which flow dynamics require direct assessment. Noninvasive modalities also form the basis for surveillance imaging.

TRICUSPID REGURGITATION

Anatomy and Normal Function of the Tricuspid Valve

The tricuspid valve is the right-sided atrioventricular valve, situated anterior and slightly apical in relation to the left sided mitral atrioventricular valve. It is aligned vertically, with anterior-left lateral angulation, in plane with the right ventricle and an orifice that is the largest of the four cardiac valves. The tricuspid valve is further distinguished from the mitral valve in that the mitral valve anteroseptal border is continuous with the aortic valve apparatus, whereas the tricuspid valve does not have any direct continuity to the pulmonary arterioventricular valve. Structurally, the tricuspid valve is composed of an annulus, three leaflets, and three commissures, which together with the right ventricle's chordae tendinae, corresponding papillary muscles, and adjacent right atrium and right ventricle myocardium, form the tricuspid valve complex.[1] The major function of the complex is to control leaflet aperture and closure. This process is governed by the pressure gradient between the right atrium and right ventricle, which in turn is regulated by preload, afterload, and myocardial contractility. Tricuspid valve opening occurs during ventricular diastole. It is closed during systole, preventing backflow. Physiologic tricuspid regurgitation occurs during systole; however, it may be found in structurally normal hearts of 17% to 65% of adults[2-6] and 6.3% to 71% of pediatric patients,[6,7] with most regurgitation being trivial to mild.

With regard to the components of the tricuspid valve complex, the annulus anchors the tricuspid valve to the right trigone of the cardiac fibrous skeleton, providing firm support for the entire complex. It is oval in shape and slightly larger than the mitral valve annulus,

Text continued on page 844

840 PART SEVEN • *Valvular Heart Disease*

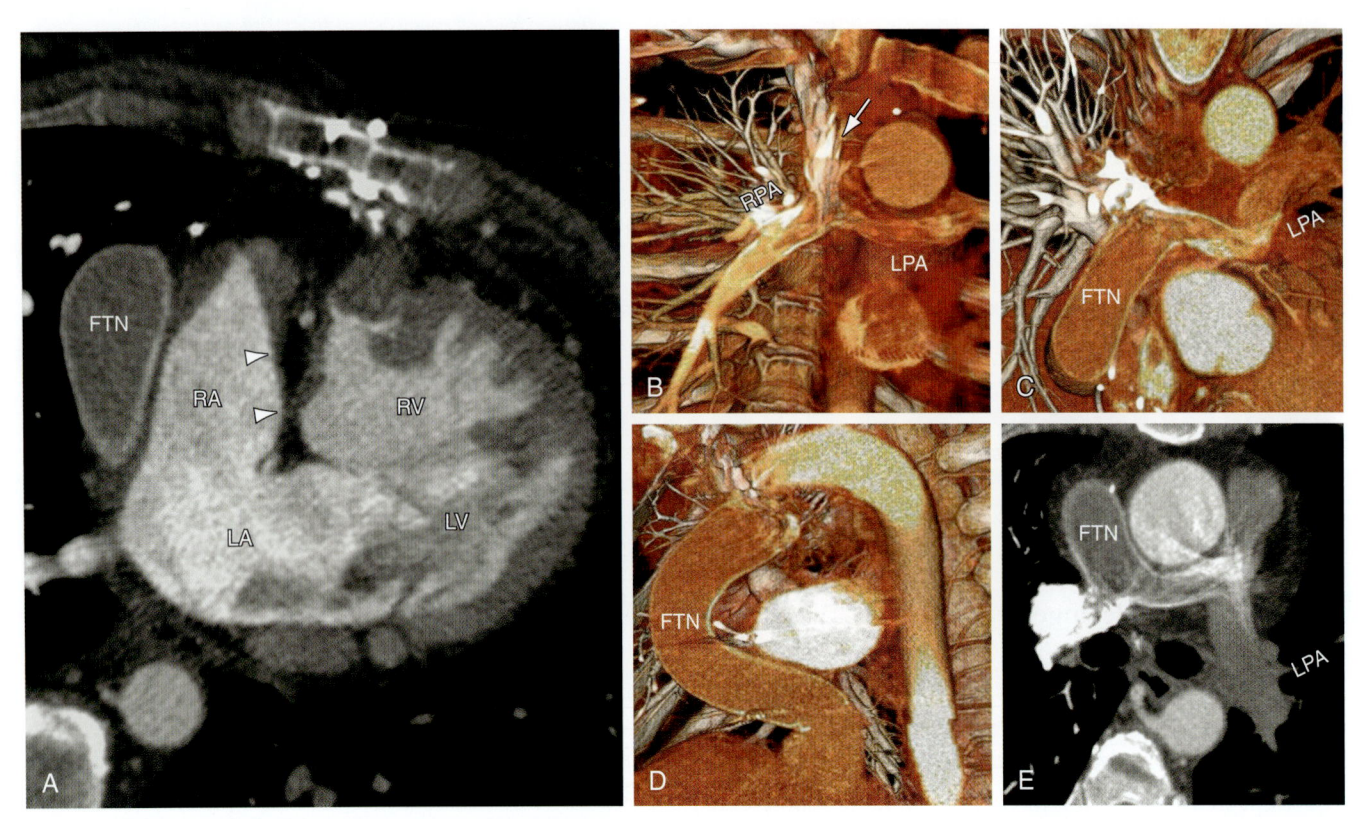

■ **FIGURE 61-1** Tricuspid atresia; 30-year-old patient with tricuspid atresia, now status postcompletion Fontan **A,** Four-chamber CTA projection shows a continuous atrioventricular groove (*arrowheads*) with absent communication between the right atrium (RA) and right ventricle (RV). Note the single-ventricle physiology with a single atrial chamber formed by the RA and left atrium (LA) and wide communication between the RV and left ventricle (LV) across a ventricular septal defect (VSD; bulboventricular foramen). **B-D,** Fontan pathway demonstrates dominant superior vena cava flow (*arrow*) into the right pulmonary artery (RPA). **E,** The extracardiac Fontan conduit (FTN) provides preferential flow into the neo- and native left pulmonary artery (LPA).

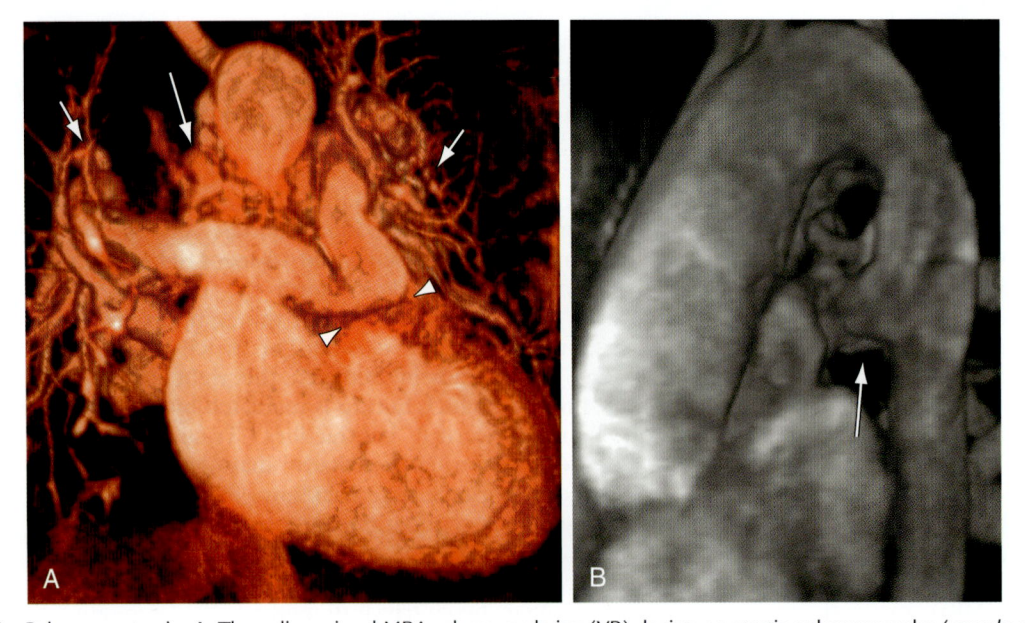

■ **FIGURE 61-2** Pulmonary atresia. **A,** Three-dimensional MRA volume rendering (VR) depicts an atretic pulmonary valve (*arrowheads*). Native pulmonary arteries (*short arrows*) receive blood flow, reconstituted from a dominant single major arterial pulmonary collateral artery (**B,** *long arrow*) off the proximal descending aorta, which then feeds a mediastinal collateral network (**A,** *long arrow*). Blood flows retrograde into the central branch pulmonary arteries.

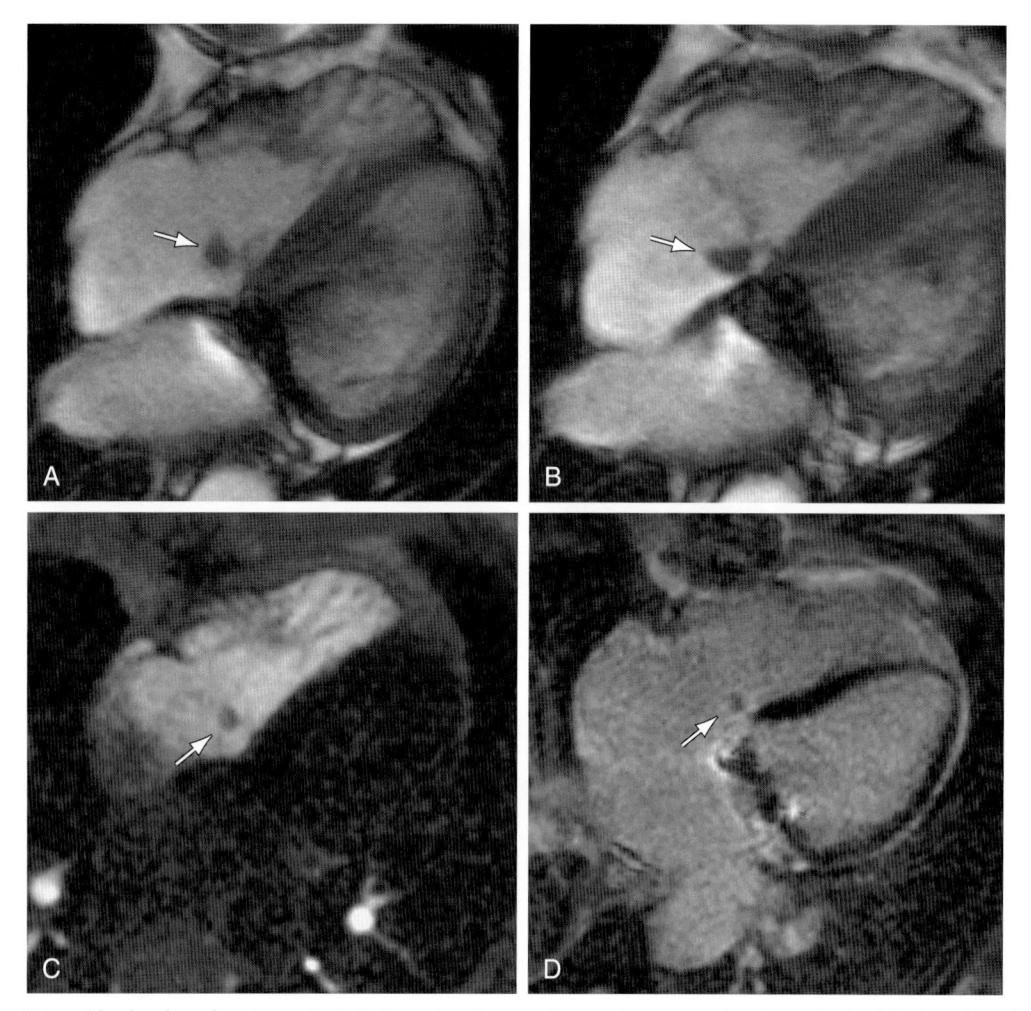

CHAPTER 61 • *Tricuspid and Pulmonary Valvular Disease* 841

■ **FIGURE 61-3** Tricuspid valve thrombus (*arrows*). **A, B,** Four-chamber steady-state free precession views obtained in diastole and systole, respectively. Thrombus is attached to the septal leaflet by a thin stalk. **C, D,** Four-chamber dynamic perfusion and 15-minute delayed imaging reveal no enhancement or hyperenhancement, respectively.

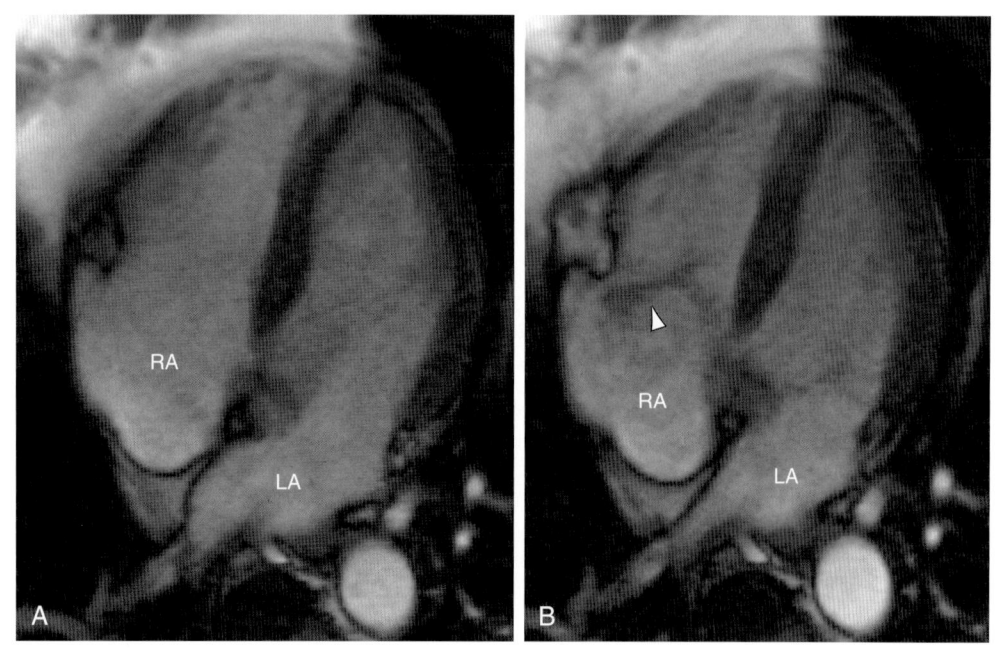

■ **FIGURE 61-4** Tricuspid insufficiency. Four-chamber cine steady-state free precession shows right atrial enlargement in both diastole (**A**) and systole (**B**). Mild tricuspid regurgitation is present at systole (**B,** *arrowhead*).

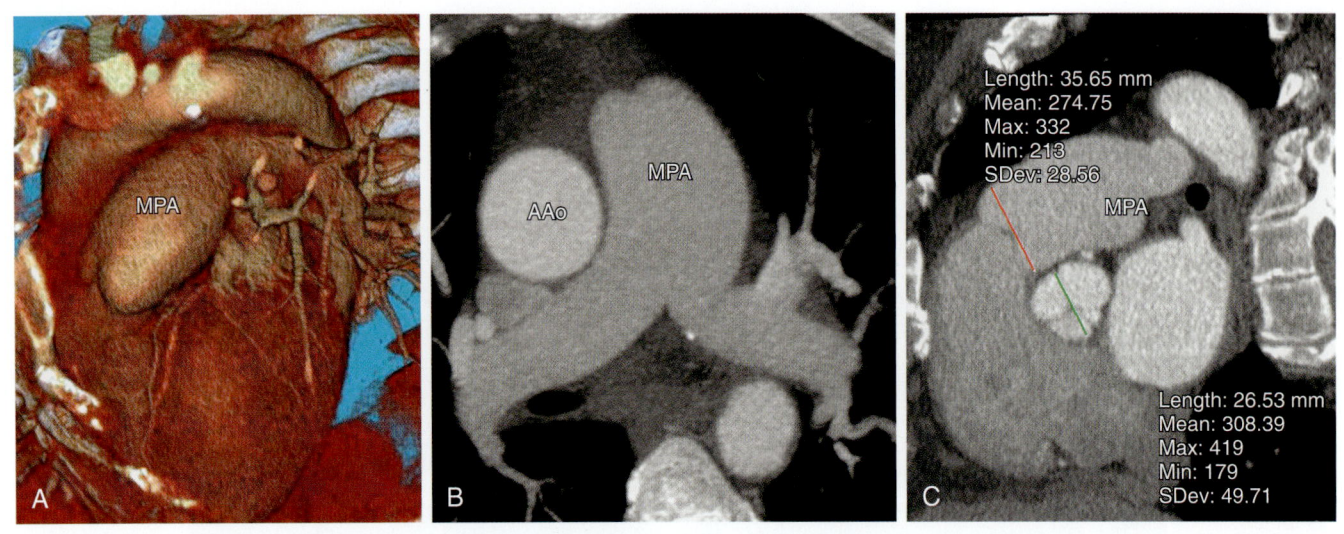

FIGURE 61-5 A-C, Pulmonary insufficiency. CTA was performed in a 50-year-old patient with pulmonary insufficiency. Note the enlarged main pulmonary artery (MPA) relative to the ascending aorta (AAo) by approximately 30%.

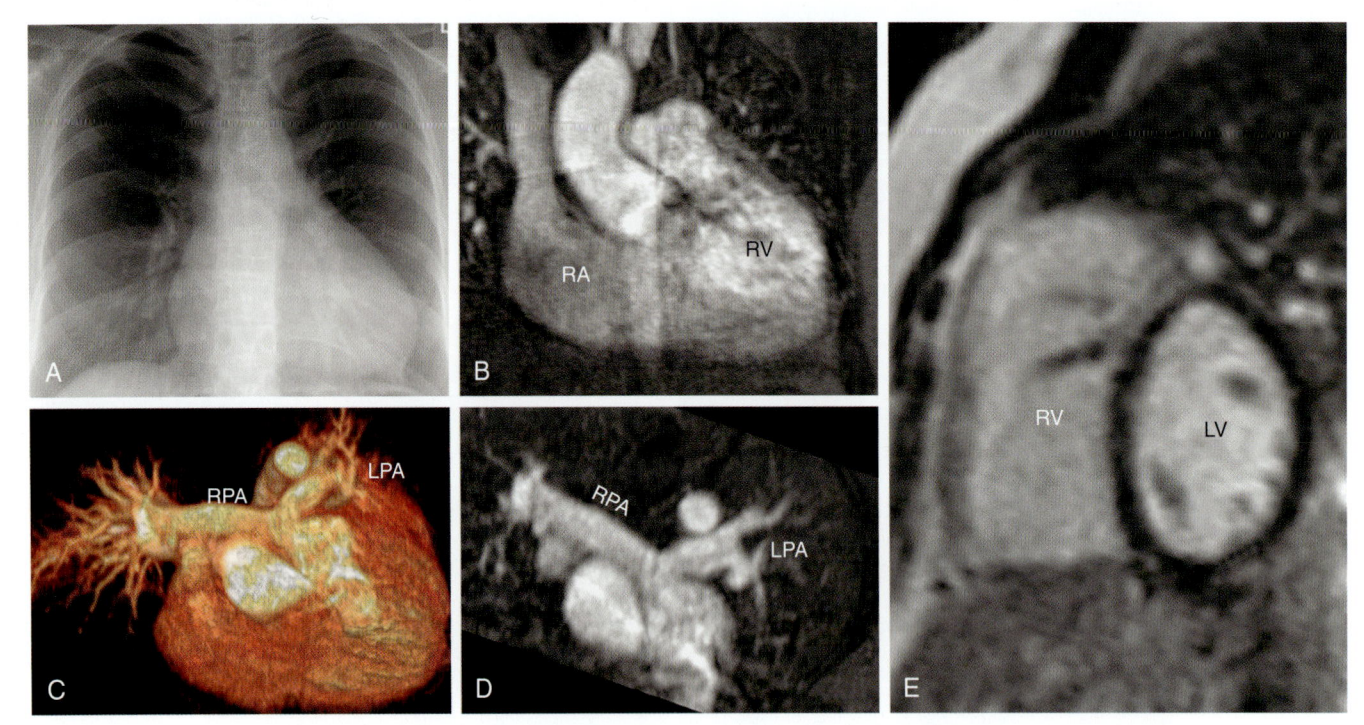

FIGURE 61-6 Pulmonary insufficiency, status post–tetralogy of Fallot repair, determined by MRI and MRA. A, Anteroposterior chest radiograph demonstrates prominent right and left heart borders, corresponding to an enlarged right atrium (RA) and ventricle (RV), respectively, as shown on an MRA coronal reformation (B). The main pulmonary artery is mildly enlarged (A, C, D), whereas the branch pulmonary arteries (RPA, LPA) are normal in caliber. E, RV volume overload, with flattening of the interventricular septum, is also shown in a postgadolinium 15-minute delayed short-axis projection. No RV, septal, or left ventricular hyperenhancement was present.

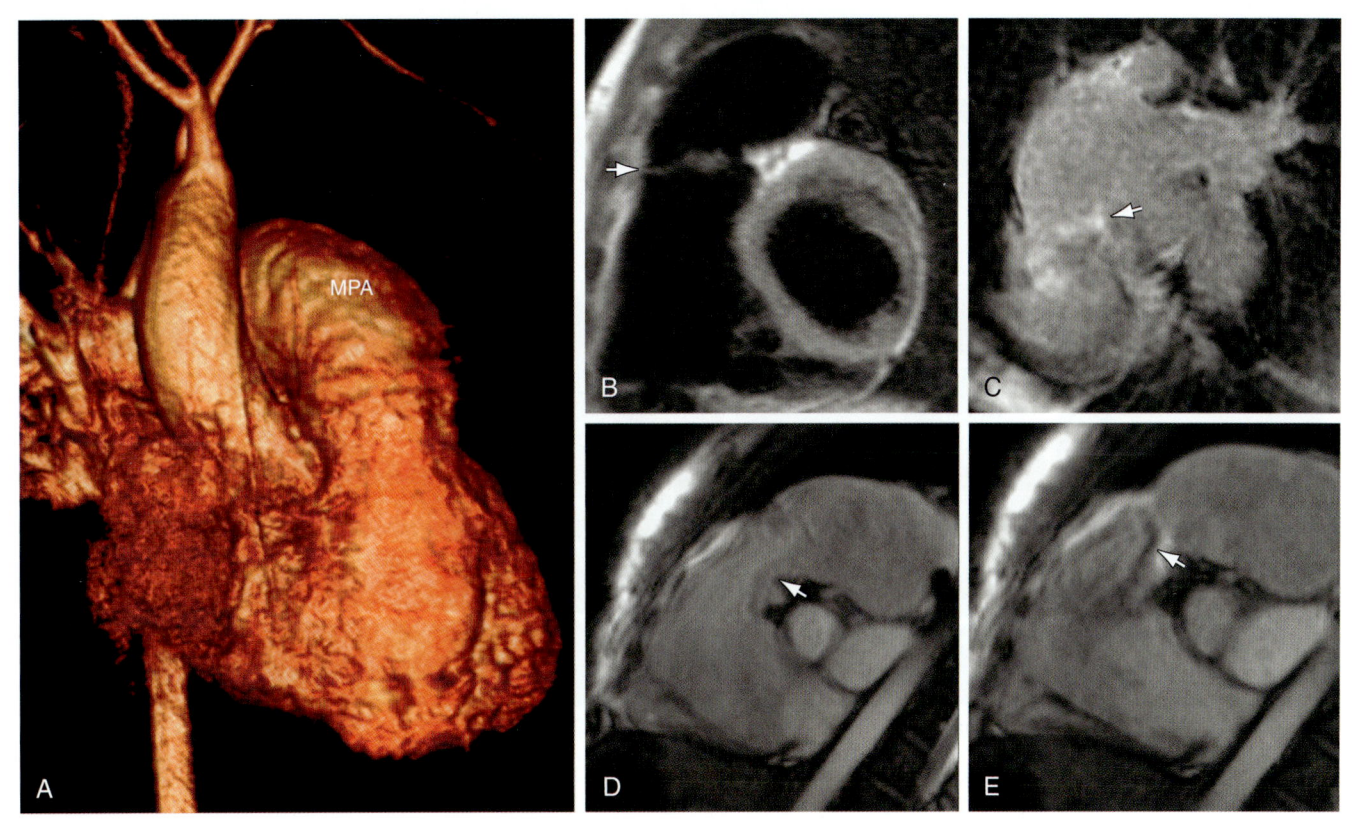

■ **FIGURE 61-7** Pulmonary dysplasia with stenosis and insufficiency. **A**, Three-dimensional MRA volume rendering demonstrates enlargement of the main pulmonary artery (MPA) and the right ventricle (RV). **B**, Short-axis dark blood imaging shows a dysplastic thickened pulmonary valve (*arrow*). **C**, Fibrosis is present in the valve apparatus, evidenced by delayed hyperenhancement (*arrow*). Cine steady-state free precession in systole (**D**) and diastole (**E**) demonstrates both stenosis (turbulent antegrade signal, *arrow*) and insufficiency (retrograde signal), respectively.

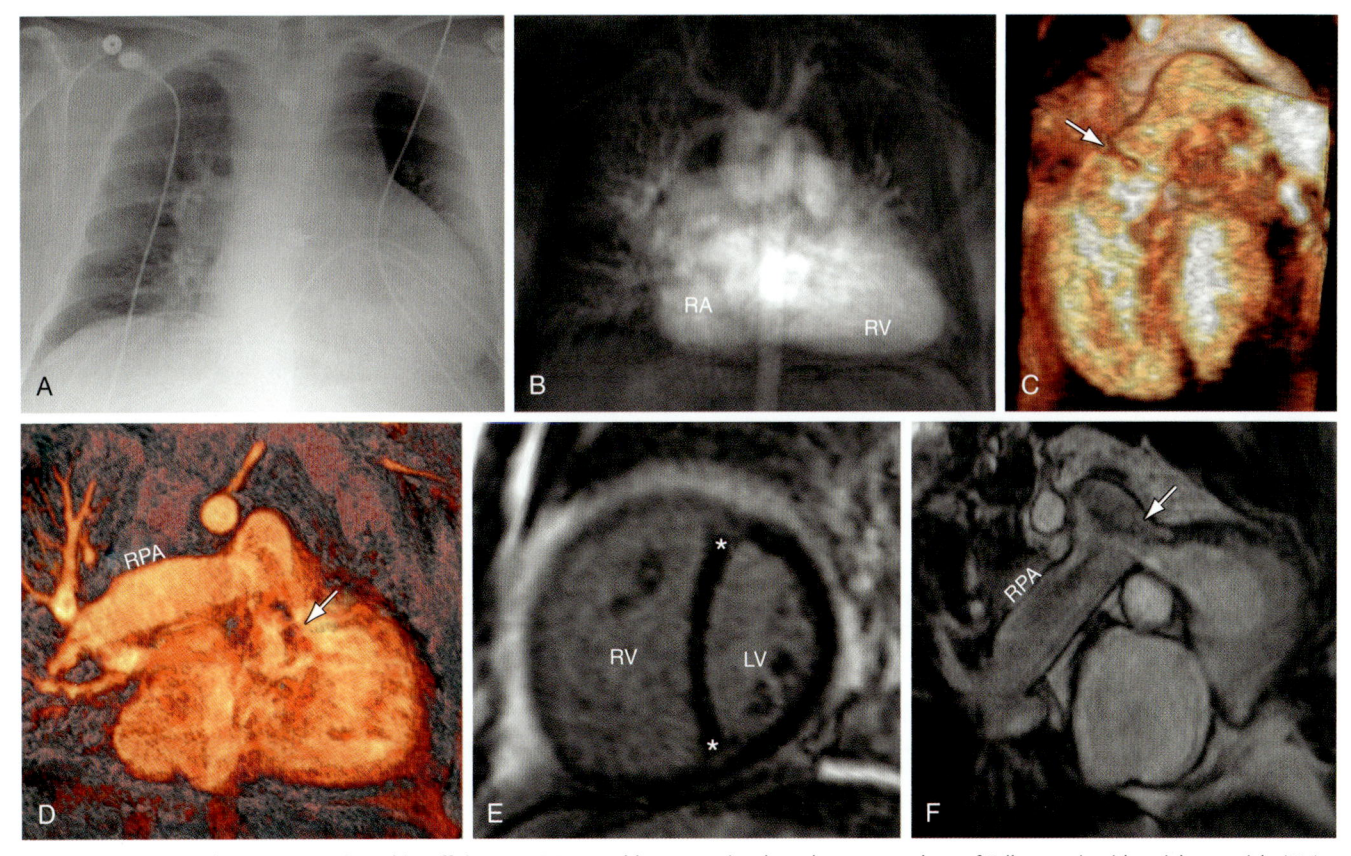

■ **FIGURE 61-8** Pulmonary stenosis and insufficiency. A 35-year-old man previously underwent tetralogy of Fallot repair with a right ventricle (RV) to main pulmonary artery conduit. **A**, Frontal chest radiograph shows right cardiac chamber and right pulmonary artery (RPA) enlargements. **B**, Three-dimensional MRA ray sum frontal projection confirms that this is secondary to right atrium (RA) and RV enlargement. **C, D**, RV enlargement from volume overload is also shown on the three-dimensional MRA volume-rendered images and the 15-minute delayed short-axis projection. Note the mild focal septal hyperenhancement at the RV insertion sites, related to RV strain from both volume and pressure overload. Increased pressure is caused by eccentric conduit stenosis (**C**, *arrow*). Stenosis results in turbulent flow across the conduit into the right pulmonary artery (RPA), with enlargement of the RPA.

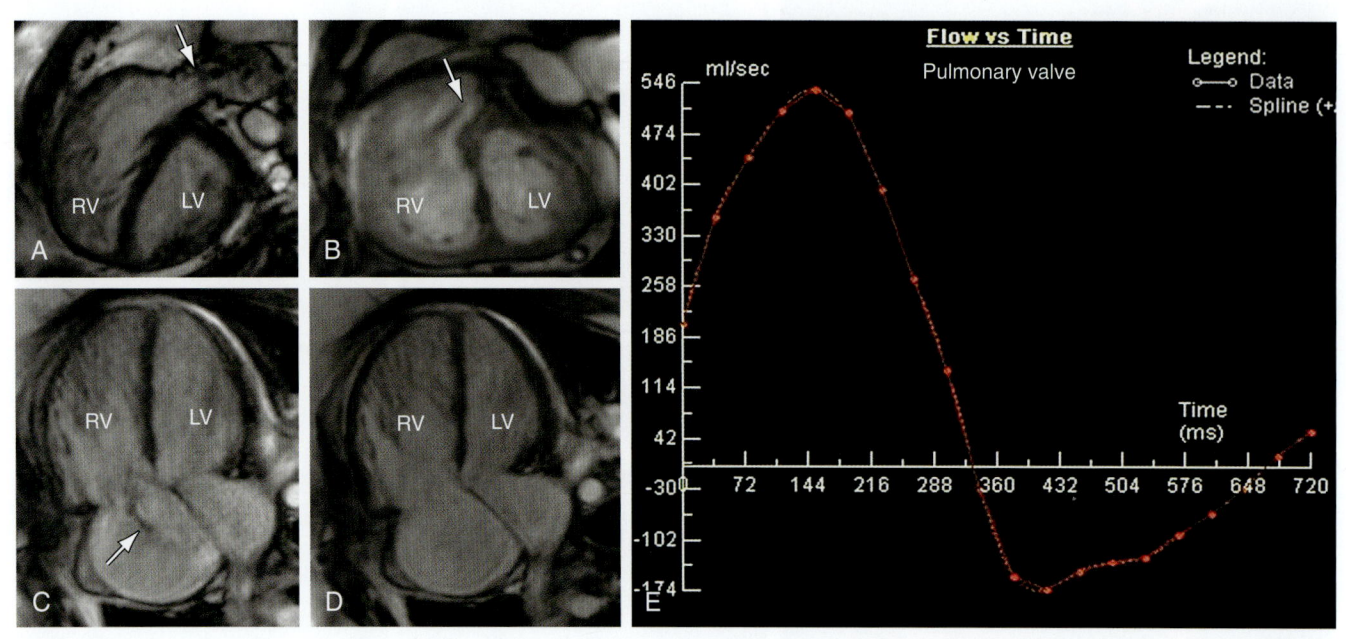

FIGURE 61-9 Pulmonary stenosis and insufficiency with tricuspid insufficiency—functional analysis. Steady-state free precession short-axis and four-chamber projections from the patient shown in Figure 61-8 are shown in systole (**A, C**) and diastole (**B, D**). Turbulent signal (*arrows*) at the pulmonary valve corresponds to stenosis (**A**) and insufficiency (**B**). **C,** Turbulent signal (*arrow*) at the tricuspid valve corresponds to insufficiency. **E,** Quantitative analysis from phase contrast imaging yielded a pulmonary regurgitant fraction of approximately 25%.

demarcating the boundaries of the tricuspid orifice.[8] The annulus contracts during systole and reaches maximum size at end-systole.[9] The mean major diastolic annulus diameter, area, and fractional shortening during three dimensional echocardiography are reported to be 3.9 to 4.3 mm, 10 to 18.4 cm^2, and 18.5% to 26%, respectively,[1,8,10] whereas MRI values are reported to be 4.4 mm, 18.7 cm^2, and 27%, respectively.[8] Two-dimensional echocardiography underestimates annulus diameter and fractional shortening, with reported four-chamber values of 2.9 to 3.3 mm and 13.5% to 19%, respectively.

The three leaflets, labeled as anterior, posterior, and septal, are asymmetric in size, shape, and function.[1] Each is attached to the annulus and separated and supported by the three commissures—anteroposterior, anteroseptal, and posteroseptal. Using three-dimensional echocardiography, Anwar and colleagues[1] have reported the valve area to be 4.8 cm^2 and each commissure to have an approximate width of 5 mm.

The anterior leaflet is the largest and most mobile, with a semicircular shape and an average width of 3.7 cm.[11] It is located anteriorly along the right ventricular free wall, extending from the anterolateral to inferolateral margin. The septal leaflet has a semioval shape, paralleling the interventricular septum, from anteroseptal margin to the posterior right ventricle wall. It is typically smaller than anterior leaflet, but is reported to have a width up to 3.6 cm.[11] The septal leaflet is the least mobile of the three leaflets. The posterior leaflet extends along the posterior margin of the annulus from the inferolateral margin of the right ventricular free wall to the septum. It is variable in size and morphology, containing one or more (up to four) scallops, with an average width up to 2.8 cm.[11]

The chordae tendinae and papillary muscles form the subvalvular apparatus. The apparatus generates opposing tension and functions to prevent leaflet prolapse into the right atrium. There are three groups of papillary muscles, labeled as anteroseptal, anteroposterior, and posteroseptal.[12] The anteroseptal and anteroposterior group may have up to four muscles, whereas the posteroseptal group may have up to five.[12] Each muscle is paired with chordae tendineae which insert onto the leaflets. There are five distinct types of tricuspid valve chordae tendineae, each with variable leaflet distribution and insertion.[11]

Tricuspid regurgitation most commonly is secondary to other diseases such as left heart failure, pulmonary regurgitation or hypertension, or chamber enlargement, which can result in dilation of the valve annulus.[13] Other causes of tricuspid regurgitation include rheumatic heart disease and endocarditis.[14]

Manifestations of Disease

Clinical Presentation

In the setting of tricuspid regurgitation, decreased cardiac output can cause fatigue and decreased exercise tolerance.[15] Right atrial pressure elevation can result in lower extremity edema, hepatic congestion, and abdominal fullness. Chronic severe tricuspid regurgitation can lead to ascites and anasarca.

Patients often have a holosystolic murmur, but this is not common when there is severe regurgitation with equalization of right atrial and ventricular pressures.[16] Jugular venous distention occurs in up to 75% of patients and hepatomegaly in 90%.[15]

Imaging Indications and Algorithm

Standard qualitative and quantitative evaluation of the tricuspid valve includes the annulus, leaflets, commissures, valve area, and degree of aperture and coaptation. Direct and indirect assessment should be made for the presence of tricuspid stenosis and regurgitation. Direct assessment includes leaflet thickening, incomplete aperture, and incomplete coaptation. Real-time echocardiography will show a regurgitant color stream and increased velocity measurement. Assessment should also address the morphology and size of the pulmonary arteries, pulmonary valve, right ventricle (including the right ventricular outflow tract), right atrium, right atrial appendage, superior vena cavae, inferior vena cavae, and central hepatic veins.

Imaging Technique and Findings

Radiography

Radiography demonstrates enlargement of the right side of the heart. Severe tricuspid regurgitation can result in profound cardiomegaly, manifesting as wall to wall heart on the posteroanterior chest radiograph, in which the cardiac silhouette occupies the entire diameter of the thorax.

Ultrasound

Echocardiography is the mainstay of tricuspid valve imaging, allowing the identification of tricuspid regurgitation and evaluation of the severity and cause. Two-dimensional echocardiography is the traditional method of evaluation and can include color Doppler flow mapping. Three-dimensional echocardiography may hold some advantages over the two-dimensional technique because of the complicated three-dimensional structure of the right ventricle.[17] Doppler echocardiography can be used for semiquantitative grading of tricuspid regurgitation or for functional parameters such as change in pressure over time.[18,19]

Magnetic Resonance Imaging

MRI is able to provide accurate quantitative evaluation of regurgitant volumes. Velocity-encoded cine (VEC) phase contrast MRI of the tricuspid valve can be performed. Because of the motion of the valve during the cardiac cycle, direct measurement of valvular regurgitation is challenging. Another approach for quantification of tricuspid regurgitation is to calculate total right ventricular stroke volume using cine steady-state free precession imaging (see Chapter 15) and the antegrade stroke volume using a VEC MRI sequence prescribed in the pulmonary artery. The regurgitant volume is the difference between total right ventricular stroke volume and forward stroke volume.

MRI also has the advantage of yielding highly accurate and reproducible volumes of the right ventricle, whose complex shape limits the usefulness of formulas used for estimation.[20]

PULMONARY STENOSIS

Anatomy and Normal Function of the Pulmonary Valve

The pulmonary valve is the right-sided semilunar, ventriculoarterial valve. It is situated anterior and to the left of the aortic semilunar valve, at a 90-degree posteriorly directed plane. The primary function of the pulmonary valve is to regulate blood flow into the pulmonary arterial system and prevent backflow of blood into the right ventricle. This is achieved by the anatomic integration of three pulmonary root sinuses with three fibrous semilunar cusps, leaflets, and supporting commissures. In distinction to the tricuspid valve complex, chordae tendineae and papillary muscles are not present.

The right ventricular infundibulum and fibrous semilunar cusps provide the core structural support for the pulmonary valve. Each semilunar cusp extends from the sinotubular junction to merge with the circumferential infundibulum. The valve leaflets are incorporated into the cusps, terminating inferiorly at the ventriculoarterial junction, to define the annulus margin. Superiorly, at the sinotubular junction, the commissures provide zones of attachment for the leaflets, which are directed and open toward the main pulmonary artery.[21]

Using three-dimensional echocardiography to evaluate adult patients referred for assessment of congenital heart disease, Anwar and associates[1] have reported the maximum diameters of the right ventricular outflow tract (infundibulum) and pulmonary valve annulus to be 22 and 19.4 mm, respectively. Two-dimensional echocardiography underestimated both regions, with measurements in the long- and short-axis projections to be 19.7 and 16.4 mm and 16.4 and 13.5 mm, respectively.[22]

Similar to tricuspid valve function, pulmonary valvular aperture and coaptation is determined by the relative pressure gradient across the valve, between the right ventricle and pulmonary arterial system. This gradient, in turn, is regulated by right ventricular preload, pulmonary afterload, and right ventricular contractility. The valve is open during ventricular systole when pressure in the right ventricle rises above the pressure in the pulmonary system. The valve closes during ventricular diastole, when right ventricular pressure falls below the pulmonary pressure. Physiologic pulmonary regurgitation during diastole, however, may be found in structurally normal hearts of 5% to 92% of adults[2-6] and 22% to 75% of pediatric patients,[6,7] with most regurgitation being trivial to mild.

More than 95% of the time, pulmonary stenosis is congenital in cause.[15] A common association with pulmonary stenosis (PS) is Noonan syndrome. Acquired causes of valvular pulmonary stenosis include rheumatic heart disease and carcinoid syndrome, but isolated pulmonary valve involvement is rare.

Manifestations of Disease

Clinical Presentation

PS usually causes symptoms only when severe. Symptoms include fatigue and dyspnea, lightheadedness on exertion, or syncope.[15] Right heart failure can occur with long-standing severe PS. On physical examination, patients have a pulmonary ejection murmur.

Imaging Indications and Algorithm

Standard qualitative and quantitative evaluation of the pulmonary valve includes the right ventricular outflow tract, annulus, leaflets, valve area, degree of aperture, and coaptation. Direct and indirect assessment should be made for the presence of pulmonary stenosis and regurgitation. Direct assessment includes leaflet thickening, incomplete aperture, and incomplete coaptation. Assessment should also address the morphology and size of the pulmonary arteries, right ventricle, right atrium, right atrial appendage, the superior vena cavae, inferior vena cavae, and central hepatic veins.

Imaging Technique and Findings

Radiography

Typically, chest radiographs show enlargement of the main pulmonary artery caused by a poststenotic jet. The left pulmonary artery may also be dilated because the flow jet is typically directed toward the left. Diminished pulmonary vascularity may be appreciated when the stenosis is severe.

Ultrasound

Echocardiography is the primary imaging modality for the evaluation of valvular PS. Characteristic findings include thickened valve leaflets and doming of the valve during systole.[23] Continuous-wave Doppler technique can be used to obtain peak velocity. The pressure gradient is derived using the modified Bernoulli equation (see Chapter 17). PS is considered to be mild if the pressure gradient is less than 36 mm Hg, moderate if between 36 and 60 mm Hg, and severe if greater than 60 mm Hg.[23]

Magnetic Resonance Imaging

VEC MRI can be used to interrogate the peak velocity and derive the pressure gradient across the valve. MRI has a limited temporal resolution compared with echocardiography, and measuring the peak velocity may be challenging because of a limited interrogation window and limitations to maximum velocity encoding. Because of the accuracy and reliability of echocardiography, the use of MRI is usually limited to situations in which the echocardiogram is suboptimal or when the pulmonary valve is assessed for another reason, such as coexisting regurgitation.

Synopsis of Treatment Options

Medical Therapy

In mild PS, patients are usually without symptoms, and management is conservative. Approximately 25% of patients with moderate PS will require intervention, especially those with a high peak systolic gradient and diminished cardiac output.[24]

Surgical and Interventional Therapy

Moderate PS with a peak gradient of more than 50 mm Hg and severe PS require intervention.[23] Percutaneous balloon valvuloplasty is the usual treatment, but most patients may develop pulmonary regurgitation after valvuloplasty.[25] Open or percutaneous prosthetic valve placement are therapeutic options but are less commonly used than balloon valvuloplasty.

PULMONARY REGURGITATION

Pulmonary regurgitation (PR) is most commonly secondary to prior intervention, such as surgery for tetralogy of Fallot or valve repair or valvuloplasty for PS.[26,27] Rheumatic heart disease and endocarditis are rare causes of PR.

Manifestations of Disease

Clinical Presentation

PR results in right ventricular enlargement, and chronic severe regurgitation can lead to right ventricular dysfunction, diminished cardiac output, and ultimately heart failure.[15] Arrhythmias and sudden death can also occur.[28] Patients with PR typically have a diastolic murmur.

Imaging Indications and Algorithm

Standard qualitative and quantitative evaluation of the pulmonary valve include the right ventricular outflow tract, annulus, leaflets, valve area, degree of aperture, and coaptation.

Imaging Technique and Findings

Radiography

On chest radiography, findings include cardiomegaly with enlargement of the right-sided chambers and enlargement of the central pulmonary arteries.

Ultrasound

The diagnosis of PR is usually made by echocardiography, which shows regurgitant color stream, increased velocity measurement. Color Doppler technique can be used to evaluate the severity of PR and to assess right ventricular pressure. The degree of PR can be graded on a 1 to 4 scale.[15] Echocardiography can underestimate the degree of PR if the PR is unrestricted and the pulmonary pressure is low.[19]

Magnetic Resonance Imaging

MRI yields accurate quantitative evaluation of regurgitant volumes using the VEC technique. Because echocardiography has the potential to underestimate the severity of PR, MRI has a key role in the quantification of regurgitation, especially after treatment for tetralogy of Fallot.[29]

VEC MRI can be used to interrogate flow in the main pulmonary artery and to determine the regurgitant volume and fraction.[30]

As noted, MRI has the capability of generating highly accurate and reproducible volumes of the right ventricle (see Chapter 15), which is especially important in congenital heart disease, such as tetralogy of Fallot.[20] Information on the severity of PR and right ventricular

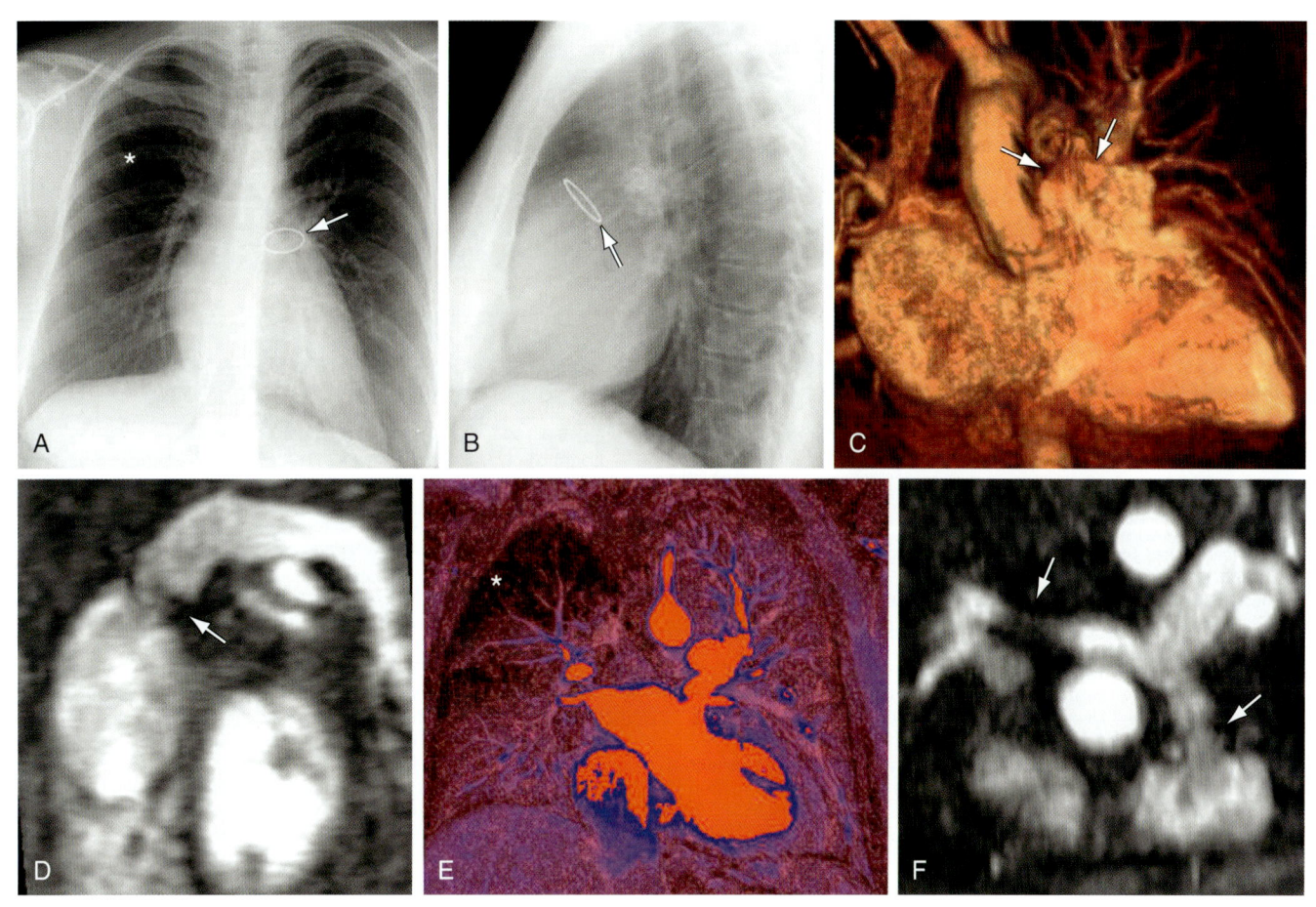

FIGURE 61-10 Pulmonary valve replacement with right pulmonary artery (RPA) stent. **A, B,** Frontal and lateral chest radiographs (*arrows*) demonstrate a pulmonary valve ring prosthesis. **C, D, F,** Three-dimensional MRA volume rendered and maximum intensity projection displays show mild luminal valvular stenosis with turbulent signal (*arrows*). The frontal chest radiograph is also remarkable for mild right upper lobe (RUL) oligemia (**A,** *asterisk*). **E,** A coronal MRA perfusion map confirms mild RUL decreased perfusion (*asterisk*). **F,** The presence of the distal RPA stent (*arrows*) is suggestive for in-stent restenosis.

volumes are used to determine the necessity for pulmonary valve repair.[30,31]

Synopsis of Treatment Options

Medical therapy has not been shown to reduce PR or its effect on the right ventricle.[15] Pulmonary valve replacement (Fig. 61-10) is recommended for PR for several indications, most commonly manifestation of symptoms, including arrhythmia, decreased right ventricular function (ejection fraction <40%, as assessed by MRI), and right ventricular enlargement (MRI end-diastolic volume, 160 mL/m^2).[15]

SUGGESTED READINGS

Altrichter PM, Olson LJ, Edwards WD, et al. Surgical pathology of the pulmonary valve: a study of 116 cases spanning 15 years. Mayo Clin Proc 1989; 64:1352-1360.

Bonow RO, Carabello BA, Chatterjee K, et al. 2008 focused update incorporated into the ACC/AHA 2006 guidelines for the management of patients with valvular heart disease: a report of the American College of Cardiology/American Heart Association Task Force on Practice Guidelines (Writing Committee to Revise the 1998 Guidelines for the Management of Patients With Valvular Heart Disease): endorsed by the Society of Cardiovascular Anesthesiologists, Society for Cardiovascular Angiography and Interventions, and Society of Thoracic Surgeons. Circulation 2008; 188:e523-e661.

Bonow RO, Carabello BA, Kanu C, et al; American College of Cardiology/American Heart Association Task Force on Practice Guidelines: ACC/AHA 2006 guidelines for the management of patients with valvular heart disease: a report of the American College of Cardiology/American Heart Association Task Force on Practice Guidelines (writing committee to revise the 1998 Guidelines for the Management of Patients With Valvular Heart Disease): developed in collaboration with the Society of Cardiovascular Anesthesiologists: endorsed by the Society for Cardiovascular Angiography and Interventions and the Society of Thoracic Surgeons. Circulation 2006; 114:e84-e231.

Hauck AJ, Freeman DP, Ackermann DM, et al. Surgical pathology of the tricuspid valve: a study of 363 cases spanning 25 years. Mayo Clin Proc 1988; 63:851-863.

Jenkins KJ, Correa A, Feinstein JA, et al. Noninherited risk factors and congenital cardiovascular defects: current knowledge: a scientific statement from the American Heart Association Council on Cardiovascular Disease in the Young: endorsed by the American Academy of Pediatrics. Circulation 2007; 115:2995-3014.

Lam YY, Kaya MG, Goktekin O, et al. Restrictive right ventricular physiology: its presence and symptomatic contribution in patients with pulmonary valvular stenosis. J Am Coll Cardiol 2007; 50:1491-1497.

Møller JE, Pellikka PA, Bernheim AM, et al. Prognosis of carcinoid heart disease: analysis of 200 cases over two decades. Circulation 2005; 112:3320-3327.

Ramadan FB, Beanlands DS, Burwash IG. Isolated pulmonic valve endocarditis in healthy hearts: a case report and review of the literature. Can J Cardiol 2000; 16:1282-1288.

REFERENCES

1. Anwar AM, Geleijnse ML, Soliman OI, et al. Assessment of normal tricuspid valve anatomy in adults by real-time three-dimensional echocardiography. Int J Cardiovasc Imaging 2007; 23:717-724.
2. Berger M, Hecht SR, Van Tosh A, et al. Pulsed and continuous wave Doppler echocardiographic assessment of valvular regurgitation in normal subjects. J Am Coll Cardiol 1989; 13:1540-1545.
3. Choong CY, Abascal VM, Weyman J. Prevalence of valvular regurgitation by Doppler echocardiography in patients with structurally normal hearts by two-dimensional echocardiography. Am Heart J 1989; 117:636-642.
4. Kostucki W, Vandenbossche JL, Friart A, et al. Pulsed Doppler regurgitant flow patterns of normal valves. Am J Cardiol 1986; 58:309-313.
5. Klein AL, Burstow DJ, Tajik AJ, et al. Age-related prevalence of valvular regurgitation in normal subjects: a comprehensive color flow examination of 118 volunteers. J Am Soc Echocardiogr 1990; 3:54-63.
6. Yoshida K, Yoshikawa J, Shakudo M, Akasara T, et al. Color Doppler evaluation of valvular regurgitation in normal subjects. Circulation 1988; 78:840-847.
7. Brand A, Dollberg S, Keren A. The prevalence of valvular regurgitation in children with structurally normal hearts: a color Doppler echocardiographic study. Am Heart J 1992; 123:177-180.
8. Anwar AM, Soliman OI, Nemes A, et al. Value of assessment of tricuspid annulus: real-time three-dimensional echocardiography and magnetic resonance imaging. Int J Cardiovasc Imaging 2007; 23:701-705.
9. Tei C, Pilgrim JP, Shah PM, et al. The tricuspid valve annulus: study of size and motion in normal subjects and in patients with tricuspid regurgitation. Circulation 1982; 66:665-671.
10. Anwar AM, Geleijnse ML, Ten Cate FJ, et al. Assessment of tricuspid valve annulus size, shape and function using real-time three-dimensional echocardiography. Interact Cardiovasc Thorac Surg 2006; 5:683-687.
11. Silver MD, Lam JH, Ranganathan N, et al. Morphology of the human tricuspid valve. Circulation 1971; 43:333-348.
12. Joudinaud TM, Flecher EM, Duran CM. Functional terminology for the tricuspid valve. J Heart Valve Dis 2006; 15:382-388.
13. Cohn LH. Tricuspid regurgitation secondary to mitral valve disease: when and how to repair. J Card Surg 1994; 9:237-241.
14. Tang GH, David TE, Singh SK, et al. Tricuspid valve repair with an annuloplasty ring results in improved long-term outcomes. Circulation 2006; 114(suppl):I577-I581.
15. Bruce CJ, Connolly HM. Right-sided valve disease deserves a little more respect. Circulation 2009; 119:2726-2734.
16. Salazar E, Levine H. Rheumatic tricuspid regurgitation. Am J Med 1962; 33:111-129.
17. Lang RM, Bierig M, Devereux RB, et al. Recommendations for chamber quantification: a report from the American Society of Echocardiography's Guidelines and Standards Committee and the Chamber Quantification Writing Group, developed in conjunction with the European Association of Echocardiography, a branch of the European Society of Cardiology. J Am Soc Echocardiogr 2005; 18:1440-1463.
18. Imanishi T, Nakatani S, Yamada S, et al. Validation of continuous wave Doppler-determined right ventricular peak positive and negative dP/dt: effect of right atrial pressure on measurement. J Am Coll Cardiol 1994; 23:1638-1643.
19. Zoghbi WA, Enriquez-Sarano M, Foster E, et al; American Society of Echocardiography. Recommendations for evaluation of the severity of native valvular regurgitation with two-dimensional and Doppler echocardiography. J Am Soc Echocardiogr 2003; 16:777-802.
20. Sechtem U, Pflugfelder PW, Gould RG, et al. Measurement of right and left ventricular volumes in healthy individuals with cine MR imaging. Radiology 1987; 163:697-702.
21. Anderson RH, Freedom RM: Normal and abnormal structure of the ventriculo-arterial junctions. Cardiol Young 15(suppl 1):3-16, 2005.
22. Anwar AM, Soliman OI, ten Cate FJ, et al. True mitral annulus diameter is underestimated by two-dimensional echocardiography as evidenced by real-time three-dimensional echocardiography and magnetic resonance imaging. Int J Cardiovasc Imaging 2007; 23:541-547.
23. Bonow R, Carabello B, Chatterjee K, et al. ACC/AHA 2006 guidelines for the management of patients with valvular heart disease: a report of the American College of Cardiology/American Heart Association Task Force on Practice Guidelines (Writing Committee to Revise the 1998 Guidelines for the Management of Patients With Valvular Heart Disease): developed in collaboration with the Society of Cardiovascular Anesthesiologists: endorsed by the Society for Cardiovascular Angiography and Interventions and the Society of Thoracic Surgeons. Circulation 2006; 114:e84-e231.
24. Hayes C, Gersony W, Driscoll D, et al. Second natural history study of congenital heart defects: results of treatment of patients with pulmonary valvar stenosis. Circulation 1993; 87(suppl):I28-I37.
25. Garty Y, Veldtman G, Lee K, Benson L. Late outcomes after pulmonary valve balloon dilatation in neonates, infants and children. J Invasive Cardiol 2005; 17:18-22.
26. Roos-Hesselink JW, Meijboom FJ, Spitaels SE, et al. Long-term outcome after surgery for pulmonary stenosis (a longitudinal study of 22-33 years). Eur Heart J 2006; 27:482-488.
27. Oechslin E, Harrison D, Harris L, et al. Reoperation in adults with repair of tetralogy of Fallot: indications and outcomes. J Thorac Cardiovasc Surg 1999; 118:245-251.
28. Therrien J, Siu S, Harris L, et al. Impact of pulmonary valve replacement on arrhythmia propensity late after repair of tetralogy of Fallot. Circulation 2001; 103:2489-2494.
29. Rebergen SA, Chin JG, Ottenkamp J, et al. Pulmonary regurgitation in the late postoperative followup of tetralogy of Fallot: volumetric quantitation by NMR velocity mapping. Circulation 1993; 88:2257-2266.
30. Varaprasathan GA, Araoz PA, Higgins CB, Reddy GP. Quantification of flow dynamics in congenital heart disease: applications of velocity-encoded cine MR imaging. Radiographics 2002; 22:895-906.
31. Therrien J, Siu SC, McLaughlin PR, et al. Pulmonary valve replacement in adults late after repair of tetralogy of Fallot: are we operating too late? J Am Coll Cardiol 2000; 36:1670-1675.

PART EIGHT

Cardiomyopathies and Other Myocardial Diseases

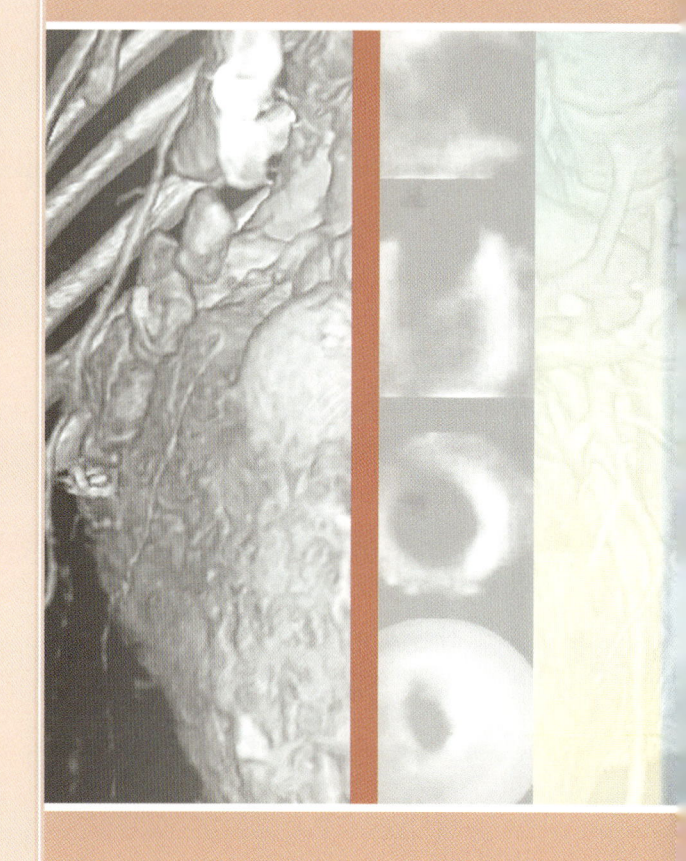

CHAPTER 62

Dilated Cardiomyopathy

James F. Glockner

Dilated cardiomyopathy (DCM) is the most common cardiomyopathy and is responsible for significant morbidity and mortality. The etiology of DCM is quite heterogeneous, and the DCM phenotype likely represents a common final outcome in response to many different myocardial insults; however, it has been recognized more recently that genetic factors probably account for 35% to 50% of all cases of DCM.[1,2] Advances in imaging have provided insight into mechanisms of pathology in DCM, and have allowed more confident noninvasive separation of patients with ischemic DCM from patients with nonischemic DCM.

DEFINITION

DCM is a disease of the myocardium that is characterized by dilation and impaired systolic function of the left ventricle or both ventricles.[3]

PREVALENCE AND EPIDEMIOLOGY

DCM is the most common of the cardiomyopathies, accounting for approximately 55% of cases, and responsible for greater than 90% of cases referred to specialty centers.[3] Idiopathic DCM is the most common cause of congestive heart failure in young patients with an estimated prevalence of 36.5 per 100,000 individuals in the United States, and is responsible for more than 10,000 deaths per year.[4] Depending on the diagnostic criteria applied, the annual incidence in adults is 5 to 8 cases per 100,000 population.[5] The true incidence is likely underestimated because many asymptomatic cases are unrecognized. DCM is responsible for a high proportion of cases of heart failure and sudden cardiac death, and is a leading cause of cardiac transplantation. The mortality rate in the United States owing to cardiomyopathy is greater than 10,000 deaths per year, with DCM the major contributor to this mortality.[6]

ETIOLOGY AND PATHOPHYSIOLOGY

DCM has been linked to many different etiologies, including infection, hypertension, pregnancy, alcohol, autoimmune disease, nutritional deficiency, cardiotoxins (e.g., anthracycline, heavy metals, cocaine, methamphetamines), genetic inheritance (e.g., mitochondrial disorders), or any cardiovascular disease in which the degree of myocardial dysfunction is not explained by the abnormal load conditions (e.g., valvular dysfunction) or the extent of ischemic damage.[3] The World Health Organization definition of DCM excludes patients with enlarged and dysfunctional ventricles secondary to ischemic or valvular dysfunction, which are categorized as their own specific cardiomyopathy (i.e., ischemic cardiomyopathy and valvular cardiomyopathy).[3] Viral myocarditis may be an important etiology in childhood, but in adults the relationship between myocarditis and DCM is less clear, and inconsistent results have been achieved in the attempt to isolate specific disease pathogens.

Family screening has emphasized the importance of inheritance in the etiology of DCM. Genetic transmission is most often autosomal dominant, with a lesser number of autosomal recessive, or X-linked, cases. Echocardiography family screening studies have shown abnormalities in approximately 25% of relatives of patients with DCM, including DCM and isolated left ventricular enlargement. Of individuals with left ventricular enlargement, 10% to 25% develop clinical DCM with symptomatic heart failure, arrhythmias, or thromboembolism within 5 years.[7] These observations suggest that familial DCM is a slowly progressive disorder, and that screening of first-degree relatives of patients with DCM should assume a similar role to that of screening in hypertrophic cardiomyopathy patients, with more well-established genetic linkages.

The autosomal forms of familial DCM can be grouped into forms with a pure DCM phenotype or DCM with cardiac conduction system disease. Genetic heterogeneity is the hallmark of autosomal dominant DCM with 15 loci mapped for pure DCM and 5 for DCM with cardiac conduction system disease. These mutations include genes encoding cardiac actin, desmin, δ-sarcoglycan, β-sarcoglycan, cardiac troponin T, and α-tropomyosin. Most genes identified to date encode either cytoskeletal or sarcomeric proteins. These proteins are important for structural integrity and for force transmission.[2]

X-linked DCM occurs in adolescent boys and young men with rapid progression from congestive heart failure to death or transplantation, and is characterized by mutations in the gene for cardiac dystrophin, a cytoskeletal protein providing structural support to the myocyte and linking it to the sarcolemma. The dystrophin gene is also responsible for Duchenne and Becker muscular dystrophies, which also have DCM as a prominent feature.[8]

Histologic changes associated with DCM are frequently nonspecific, and not all features may be present. DCM is characterized by progressive interstitial fibrosis with a reduced number of functional myocytes and, in advanced stages, relative wall thinning. Although atrophic changes predominate histologically, there is also myocyte elongation with an addition of newly formed sarcomeres, which is the major factor responsible for increased chamber size. Myocyte diameter increases, but is inadequate to preserve a normal ratio of wall thickness to chamber diameter. Myocyte nuclear hypertrophy and pleomorphism may also be seen. There is often an increase in interstitial T lymphocytes and focal accumulation of macrophages associated with individual myocyte death.[8]

MANIFESTATIONS OF DISEASE

Clinical Presentation

The clinical presentation of DCM varies, but typically includes signs and symptoms of left heart failure, including fatigue; dyspnea on exertion; shortness of breath; orthopnea; paroxysmal nocturnal dyspnea; and increasing edema, weight, or abdominal girth. On physical examination, patients may exhibit tachypnea, tachycardia, hypertension, jugular venous distention, and peripheral edema. Many patients have minimal symptoms. Right-sided heart failure is less common and is generally seen in severe cases.

Imaging Indications and Algorithm

Indications for imaging in patients with known or suspected DCM can be grouped into a few broad categories. For initial diagnosis, echocardiography, MRI, or ECG gated contrast-enhanced CT all show dilated ventricular cavities and reduced function characteristic of DCM.

When the diagnosis of DCM is established, the distinction between ischemic and nonischemic DCM needs to be made because treatment options differ. Traditionally, conventional coronary angiography was performed to determine whether or not significant coronary atherosclerosis was present, and this is still a common alternative. More recently, noninvasive alternatives to coronary angiography have become widely available, including stress and rest nuclear perfusion imaging using technetium or thallium agents, positron emission tomography (PET) viability imaging, stress echocardiography, coronary CT angiography (or noncontrast CT for coronary calcium assessment), and contrast-enhanced MRI with myocardial delayed enhancement (MDE) images.

A third set of indications for imaging involves assessing for prognostic factors, such as the presence of significant nonischemic fibrosis on MRI MDE images, and the presence or absence of significant coronary flow reserve or inotropic reserve or both on nuclear medicine stress/rest perfusion images or stress echocardiography. Finally, imaging may be performed to assess for changes in ventricular function after therapeutic intervention.

The optimal imaging technique should be safe, should be noninvasive, should have relatively few contraindications, should be widely available, should be easily interpretable, should be reproducible, and should be able to confirm the diagnosis and provide prognostic information in a single examination. Currently, there is no widely accepted single modality that fulfills these criteria in most patients.

Imaging Technique and Findings

Radiography

Findings on chest x-ray are nonspecific and include cardiomegaly and signs of congestive heart failure, such as pleural effusions, pulmonary vascular congestion, and interstitial edema.

Ultrasonography

Echocardiography reveals a dilated left ventricular cavity with reduced global function. End-systolic and end-diastolic diameter are increased, and ejection fraction, fractional shortening, stroke volume, and cardiac output are decreased (Figs. 62-1 and 62-2).

The left ventricle becomes more spherical, with the sphericity index (long-axis/short-axis dimension) nearing 1 (normal value >1.5). Left ventricular wall thickness varies, but is usually normal; however, left ventricular mass is generally increased.

Secondary features of DCM include dilation of the mitral annulus and incomplete coaptation of mitral valve leaflets with mitral regurgitation and enlarged left atrium. As ventricular size increases and function declines, thrombi may develop, with the ventricular apex a common location. Interventricular conduction delay (left or right bundle branch block) is common and contributes to ventricular dysfunction.

Doppler echocardiography is an important tool for evaluation of patients with DCM and can be used to assess cardiac output, pulmonary artery pressure, mitral inflow patterns, left ventricular filling pressure, and mechanical dyssynchrony. Mitral regurgitation is common in DCM and is related to left ventricular enlargement and remodeling. The mitral leaflets become tented because of apical displacement of papillary muscles with reduced coaptation.

There is a wide range in severity of systolic and diastolic dysfunction. Persistence of restrictive filling after therapy is associated with high mortality; whereas patients

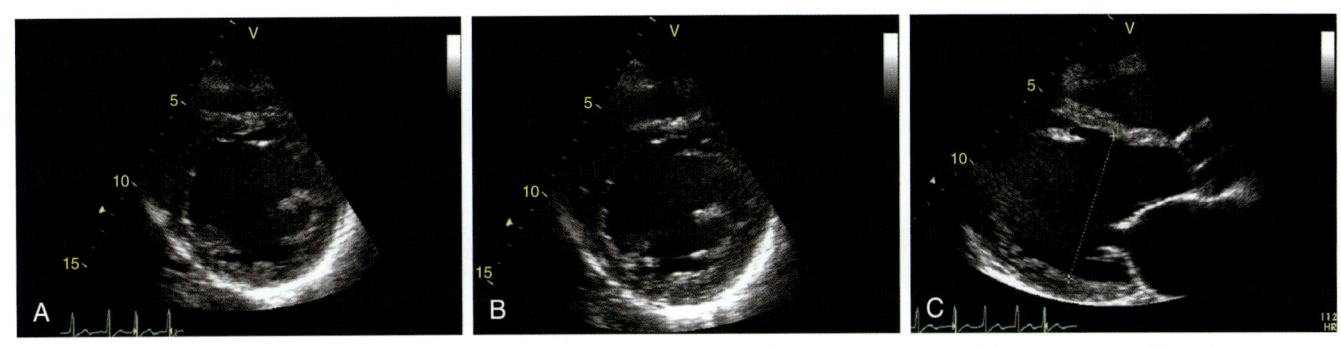

FIGURE 62-1 DCM shown by echocardiography. **A** and **B,** Short-axis end-diastolic (**A**) and end-systolic (**B**) frames reveal a dilated left ventricle with poor function. **C,** Three-chamber view shows left ventricular enlargement with end-diastolic dimension of 73 mm.

with reversible restrictive filling have high probability of clinical improvement and excellent survival. Pulmonary artery pressure can be estimated from the tricuspid valve regurgitant (TR) velocity. Patients with TR velocity greater than 3 m/s have higher mortality and higher incidence of heart failure and more frequent hospitalizations.

Proper timing of diastolic filling is important in optimizing cardiac output. If the P-R interval is prolonged, atrial contraction may occur before early diastolic filling is completed. If the P-R interval is too short, the atrium may contract at the same time as the ventricle. Optimizing the P-R interval with guidance of Doppler echocardiography may improve cardiac output and reduce the severity of symptoms.

Evaluation of right ventricular function is also important. Patients with biventricular dysfunction have a lower New York Heart Association functional class, tend to have more severe left ventricular dysfunction, and have a worse long-term prognosis.[9,10]

Stress echocardiography may also play a role in assessment of patients with DCM. Patients with improvement in ejection fraction greater than 20% during stress echocardiography have a better prognosis. Drozd and colleagues[11] showed that the incidence of cardiac death or transplantation is lower in patients with preserved contractile reserve. Another study assessed the prognostic significance of high-dose dobutamine stress echocardiography, and concluded that the change in wall motion score index is able to identify patients at greater risk for cardiac death during follow-up, and that change in wall motion score index had superior prognostic information to change in ejection fraction.[12]

Stress echocardiography with dipyridamole has also been used to assess coronary flow reserve in patients with DCM. Rigo and colleagues[13] evaluated 129 patients with DCM and found that coronary flow reserve, assessed via Doppler velocity interrogation of the mid left anterior descending coronary artery, was often impaired, and that reduced coronary flow reserve was an independent marker of poor prognosis. Pratali and coworkers[14] performed dobutamine and dipyridamole stress echocardiography in 87 patients with DCM and found that both tests have similar feasibility and prognostic accuracy.

Computed Tomography

Traditional nongated thoracic CT can provide useful but nonspecific information in assessment of patients with DCM. Signs of congestive heart failure, including enlargement of pulmonary vessels, thickening of interlobular septa, pleural effusions, and cardiomegaly, are easily appreciated on CT. CT also allows assessment for alternative or confounding pathologies, such as pulmonary embolus, infectious or inflammatory pulmonary infiltrates, emphysema, and pulmonary fibrosis. Assessment of the cardiac chambers is limited without cardiac gating; however, large ventricular or atrial thrombi can often be seen on contrast-enhanced CT, and significant chamber enlargement can be appreciated.

ECG gated CT, particularly with the advent of 64-row multidetector systems, offers many additional possibilities in the assessment of patients with known or suspected DCM. CT can provide excellent spatial resolution, with isotropic submillimeter voxels and rapid acquisitions

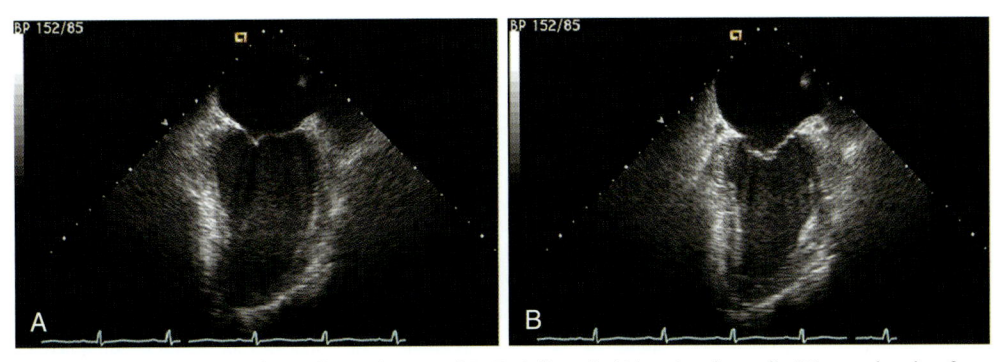

FIGURE 62-2 DCM on transesophageal echocardiography. **A** and **B,** End-diastolic (**A**) and end-systolic (**B**) two-chamber frames reveal dilated left ventricle and atrium with poor ejection fraction.

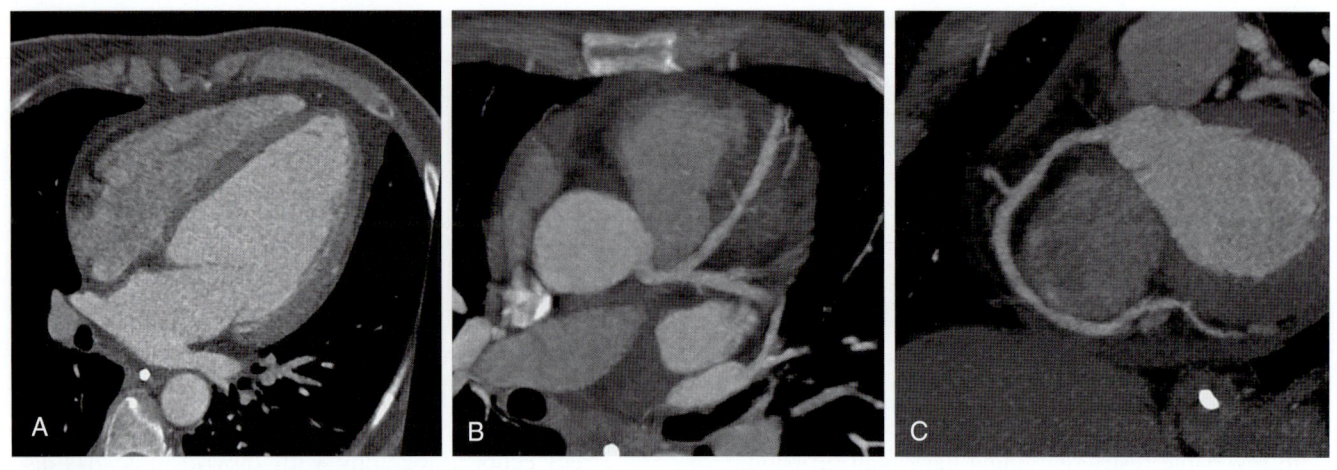

FIGURE 62-3 DCM. **A,** Four-chamber reformatted view from coronary CT angiogram shows dilated left ventricle. **B** and **C,** Subvolume maximum intensity projection images from coronary CT angiography reveals only minimal disease in the left anterior descending and circumflex coronary arteries (**B**) and normal right coronary artery (**C**).

(10 to 20 seconds) and short total examination times. A typical contrast-enhanced ECG gated CT acquisition consists of spiral overlapping data from each detector row obtained over several heartbeats. These data are retrospectively sorted into different spatial and temporal locations, and can generate axial images in an optimal motion-free diastolic time frame and short-axis and long-axis cine images, which can be used to evaluate and quantify ventricular size, function, and mass.

Although MRI is generally considered the gold standard for assessment of ventricular mass and function, preliminary results indicate that CT has similar accuracy and reproducibility. Limitations of CT include temporal resolution, which is typically on the order of 150 ms for single source 64-row MDCT. Dual source CT improves temporal resolution to 70 to 80 ms, which approaches that of MRI. Functional ventricular assessment with CT also requires the use of iodinated contrast material, limiting the application of this technique in patients with renal insufficiency or allergy to iodinated contrast agents. Finally, radiation dose in cardiac CT is significant, even considering the dose reduction algorithms currently employed by most vendors. Ionizing radiation exposure is particularly problematic in pediatric patients, women (with the high radiation dose to the breast), and patients requiring multiple follow-up imaging evaluations.

In addition to assessing ventricular function, myocardial mass, and chamber size, CT can be used to screen for coronary artery disease. A few more recent investigations have compared the accuracy of coronary CT angiography with conventional angiography in assessing patients with ischemic or nonischemic DCM (Fig. 62-3). Andreini and associates[15] studied 61 patients with idiopathic DCM and 139 patients with normal cardiac function and indications for coronary angiography. Using 16-row MDCT, the authors found excellent agreement with angiography, with sensitivity, specificity, and positive and negative predictive values for identification of greater than 50% stenosis of 99%, 96%, 81%, and 99%. Cornily and colleagues[16] achieved similar results with a smaller group of 36 patients with DCM, also using a 16-row system and comparing results with conventional angiography.

It has also been suggested that coronary calcification scoring alone may be adequate for distinguishing ischemic from nonischemic DCM (Fig. 62-4). Budoff and associates[17] assessed 56 patients with cardiomyopathy using

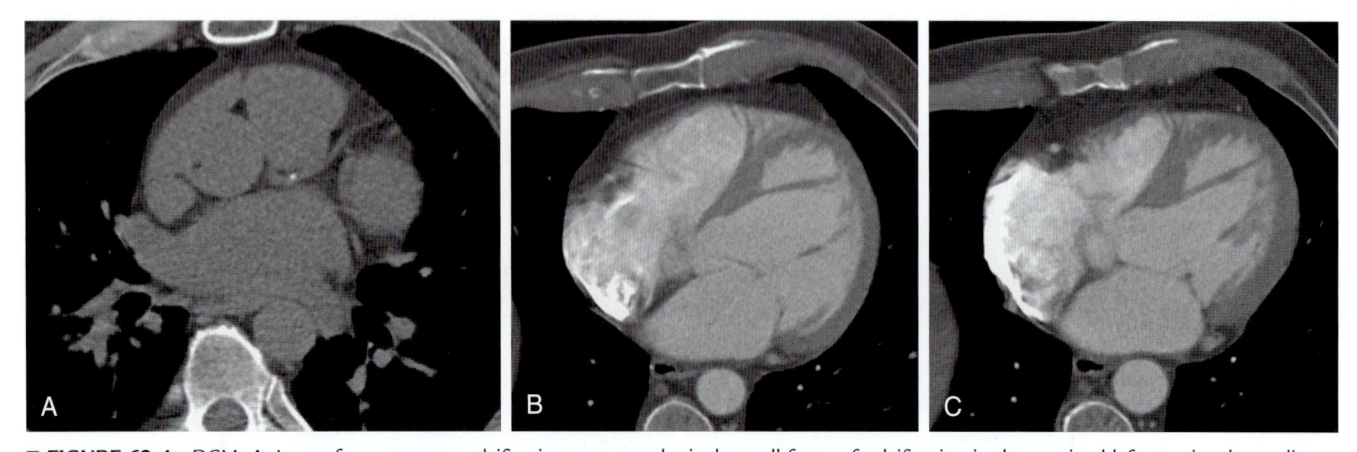

FIGURE 62-4 DCM. **A,** Image from coronary calcification scan reveals single small focus of calcification in the proximal left anterior descending coronary artery. Coronary angiography was also performed and showed no significant coronary artery lesions. **B** and **C,** Axial end-diastolic (**B**) and end-systolic (**C**) images show mildly dilated left ventricle with reduced function.

coronary angiography, nuclear exercise stress testing (Tc 99m sestamibi), and coronary calcification electron-beam CT. Nuclear stress testing had a sensitivity of 97% using the criteria of a reversible or fixed defect, but a low specificity of 18%. Using receiver operating curve analysis, the authors determined that a cutoff coronary calcification score of 100 yielded a sensitivity and specificity of 82%. CT has the potential to reduce or eliminate the use of conventional coronary angiography in distinguishing ischemic from nonischemic DCM. CT also effectively detects complications of DCM, such as atrial or ventricular thrombus.

A major limitation of CT with respect to MRI is in the area of tissue characterization. MDE acquisitions have proved valuable in distinguishing ischemic versus nonischemic DCM, and the presence of mid-wall hyperenhancement on MDE imaging seems to have prognostic implications as well. More recently, delayed contrast enhancement has been described in CT; however, its role in routine clinical practice is uncertain, and the potential diagnostic benefit of this acquisition must be balanced against the additional radiation exposure.

Magnetic Resonance Imaging

MRI is the gold standard for quantification of myocardial size and function. The diagnosis of DCM can be confirmed by obtaining standard gated cine steady-state free precession (SSFP) bright blood images in long-axis and short-axis orientations. End-diastolic and end-systolic frames are traced to obtain end-diastolic and end-systolic volumes, stroke volume, and myocardial mass. Typical findings include left ventricular and atrial enlargement, increased left ventricular mass, reduced stroke volume and ejection fraction, increased end-diastolic and end-systolic volumes, and frequently right-sided chamber enlargement and reduced function.

Much interest in MRI evaluation of patients with DCM more recently has focused on the diagnostic and prognostic implications of hyperenhancement on MDE imaging. MDE images are typically obtained 10 to 20 minutes after an intravenous injection of 0.1 to 0.2 mM/kg of a standard gadolinium-chelate contrast agent. MDE pulse sequences are usually T1-weighted inversion recovery sequences in which the inversion time (TI) is selected to null the signal from normal myocardium. Damaged, scarred, or infarcted myocardium has a larger extravascular volume by virtue of its acellularity or damaged cell membranes, leading to longer wash-in and washout times for standard gadolinium-chelate contrast agents, and retention of contrast agent in these regions (i.e. "hyperenhancement") relative to normal myocardium.

Infarcts on MDE images have a characteristic appearance, showing subendocardial or transmural enhancement in a distribution corresponding to the territory of the affected coronary artery. MDE imaging has a high sensitivity for detection of infarcts, and it has been shown that small infarcts seen using this technique are often missed with nuclear medicine perfusion imaging. MDE imaging is an excellent method for distinguishing nonischemic DCM from ischemic cardiomyopathy (Figs. 62-5 and 62-6). Soriano and colleagues[18] evaluated 71 patients with heart failure and left ventricular systolic dysfunction without a prior history of myocardial infarction with coronary angiography and MDE imaging. Subendocardial or transmural hyperenhancement on MDE imaging characteristic of previous infarction was present in 81% of the angiography-positive group, whereas only 9% of the angiography-negative patients had an ischemic MDE pattern. McCrohon and coworkers[19] evaluated 90 patients with heart failure with MRI and MDE imaging, and compared the results with coronary angiography. All angiography-positive patients showed an ischemic subendocardial or transmural MDE pattern. In the angiography-negative patients, 59% showed no hyperenhancement on MDE imaging, 13% had an ischemic hyperenhancement pattern (i.e., subendocardial or transmural), and 28% had a longitudinal or patchy mid-wall hyperenhancement pattern with subendocardial sparing on MDE imaging that was not restricted to distinct coronary territories.

Although most patients with nonischemic DCM show no late gadolinium enhancement, there is more recent evidence that some patients have nonischemic enhancement patterns, in particular enhancement in the middle of the ventricular myocardium (Fig. 62-7), and that the presence of this late enhancement is an indicator of poor prognosis compared with patients without MDE. Assomull and colleagues[20] evaluated 101 patients with DCM and found a mid-wall fibrosis pattern in 35% of patients. Mid-wall fibrosis was associated with a higher mortality and hospitalization for cardiovascular events and sudden cardiac death and ventricular tachycardia. Park and associates[21] also evaluated 46 patients with nonischemic left ventricular systolic dysfunction with late enhancement MRI and showed that the absence of delayed hyperenhancement had excellent sensitivity and negative predictive value in predicting functional recovery of left ventricular systolic dysfunction.

The mid-wall late myocardial hyperenhancement described in approximately one third of patients is probably not specific for idiopathic nonischemic DCM. Myocarditis and myocardial sarcoid can also exhibit similar hyperenhancement patterns. The distinction between ischemic and nonischemic hyperenhancement is not always obvious, particularly in patients with thin ventricular walls. The prognostic value of mid-wall hyperenhancement on MDE has been described in only a few patients.

MRI has yet unrealized potential with regard to evaluation of patients with DCM. Nuclear and echocardiographic stress testing provides useful prognostic information from estimation of perfusion and inotropic reserve. Pharmacologic MRI stress testing can be performed using first-pass perfusion imaging and vasodilators (typically adenosine) or inotropic agents (dobutamine), and some protocols employ both methods. These techniques are employed routinely in some centers as an alternative to nuclear and echocardiographic stress tests, but little investigation has been performed regarding the use of these techniques in patients with DCM. MRI is also unparalleled in assessment of the right ventricle, and echocardiographic data indicate that assessment of right ventricular function may have an important role in determining prognosis of these patients. MRI tissue tagging pulse sequences

856 PART EIGHT • *Cardiomyopathies and Other Myocardial Diseases*

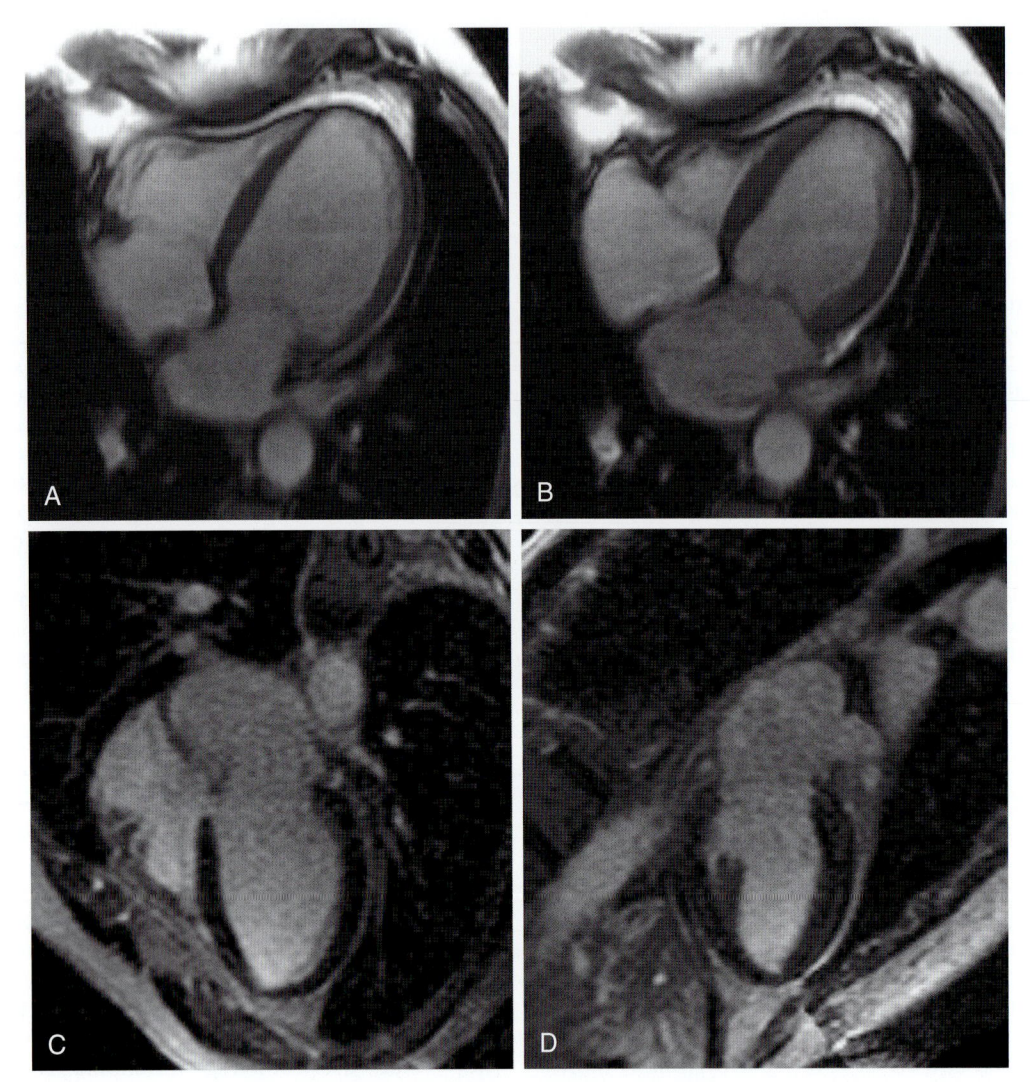

■ FIGURE 62-5 MRI demonstration of DCM. **A** and **B,** End-diastolic (**A**) and end-systolic (**B**) four-chamber SSFP images reveal dilated left ventricle with mildly reduced function. **C** and **D,** Four-chamber (**C**) and two-chamber (**D**) MDE images show no late hyperenhancement, indicating nonischemic etiology.

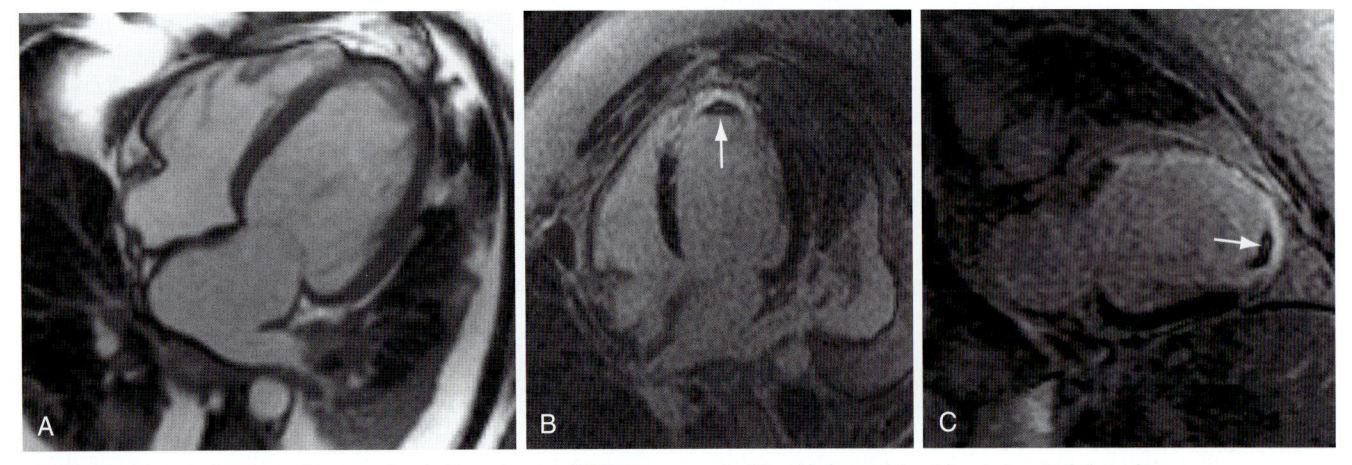

■ FIGURE 62-6 Ischemic cardiomyopathy. **A,** Four-chamber SSFP image reveals dilated left ventricle with subtle apical thrombus. **B** and **C,** Four-chamber (**B**) and two-chamber (**C**) MDE images reveal extensive transmural hyperenhancement in the apex and anterior wall, consistent with a large infarct. Note better visualization of nonenhancing apical thrombus (*arrows*).

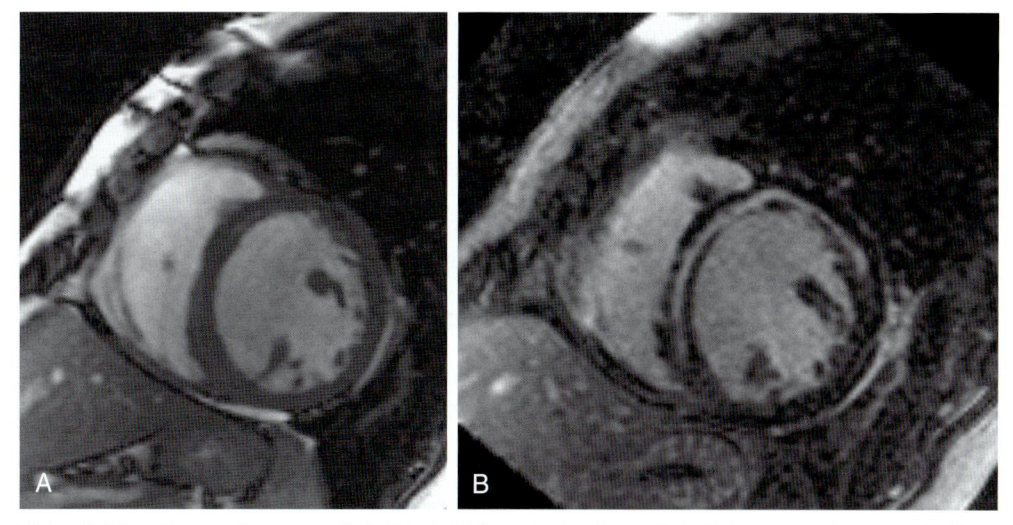

■ **FIGURE 62-7** Mid-wall delayed hyperenhancement in DCM. **A,** Mid-ventricular short-axis SSFP image reveals concentric dilation of the left ventricle. **B,** Corresponding MDE image reveals curvilinear mid-myocardial hyperenhancement of the inferoseptal, anteroseptal, anterior, and anterolateral walls of the left ventricle.

can be used to investigate intrinsic contractile properties of myocardium. The relationship between asynchronous electrical excitation and the onset of mechanical contraction has been investigated with MRI tagging, and these techniques may be useful in understanding the nature of mechanical asynchrony found in some patients with DCM, particularly patients who are candidates for cardiac resynchronization therapy (CRT).

MRI has several general and specific limitations for the investigation of DCM. Patients with pacemakers and defibrillators and other internal electrical devices are currently excluded. Claustrophobia is a relative contraindication. More recent concern regarding nephrogenic systemic fibrosis and gadolinium contrast agents may limit the availability of this technique in patients with severe renal insufficiency. MRI is expensive and is less widely available than most other noninvasive imaging techniques.

Nuclear Medicine

Nuclear medicine techniques have an important role in evaluation of patients with DCM. More recent development of ECG gated single photon emission computed tomography (SPECT) techniques allows assessment of myocardial perfusion and ventricular function, and SPECT would seem to be an ideal tool for distinguishing ischemic and nonischemic DCM (Fig. 62-8). Danias and colleagues[22] assessed 37 patients with severely reduced left ventricular function with exercise Tc 99m sestamibi gated SPECT and found that the summed stress and rest perfusion defect scores were widely separated between the two groups, and completely distinguished ischemic from nonischemic patients. A larger trial from the same group using the same technique assessed 164 patients with ejection fraction less than 40% and without known coronary artery disease.

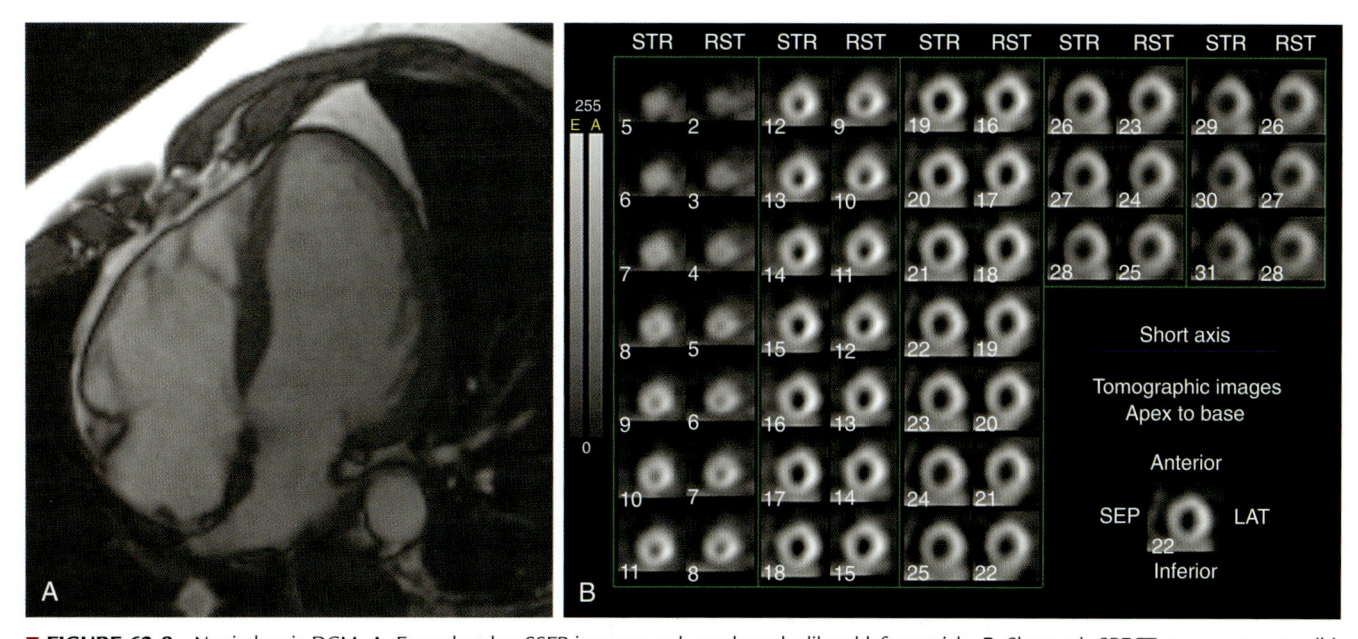

■ **FIGURE 62-8** Nonischemic DCM. **A,** Four-chamber SSFP image reveals moderately dilated left ventricle. **B,** Short-axis SPECT stress-rest sestamibi scan reveals normal resting and stress perfusion images, and no evidence of ischemic etiology.

Using a combined analysis of stress perfusion, reversibility, and regional wall motion deficits, Danias and colleagues[23] achieved a high sensitivity (94%) but relatively low specificity (45%) for detection of ischemic cardiomyopathy. Generally, patients with ischemic cardiomyopathy have more severe perfusion defects than patients with nonischemic cardiomyopathy. Fixed defects are occasionally encountered in nonischemic cardiomyopathy, and may be related to attenuation associated with the severely dilated left ventricular cavity and supine imaging.

Dobutamine stress myocardial perfusion imaging has been used to predict patient response to β blocker therapy in DCM. Kasama and coworkers[24] found that the change in ejection fraction measured by Tc 99m tetrofosmin gated SPECT was significantly higher in patients who responded to therapy than in nonresponders.

PET can also be used to assess DCM patients. O'Neill and colleagues[25] examined 44 patients with PET, echocardiography, and radionuclide ventriculography, and found that myocardial scarring (defined as a matched perfusion and metabolic defect) was very common, occurring in 91% of patients, and that the extent of scar correlated with the QRS duration.

Another group has used PET to assess global and regional myocardial oxygen consumption ($M\dot{V}O_2$) and blood flow in patients with DCM and left bundle branch block.[26] Complete left bundle branch block is a common finding in severe DCM and is a strong predictor of mortality. Global and regional $M\dot{V}O_2$ and myocardial blood flow were assessed using acetate C 11 PET. Patients with severe DCM and left bundle branch block exhibited a significantly lower (impaired) global $M\dot{V}O_2$ and reduced myocardial blood flow at rest than patients with mild or moderate disease without left bundle branch block. Analysis of regional differences in $M\dot{V}O_2$ and blood flow revealed more heterogeneous distribution of $M\dot{V}O_2$ and myocardial blood flow in DCM patients with left bundle branch block.

CRT has been advocated in patients with poor left ventricular function and conduction delays for symptomatic improvement and prolonging survival. Lindner and colleagues[27] studied patients with nonischemic cardiomyopathy before and 4 months after CRT using acetate C 11 PET, and showed that CRT induces changes of $M\dot{V}O_2$ and myocardial blood flow leading to a more uniform distribution with less regional heterogeneity. More novel applications of nuclear medicine include the use of Tc 99m–labeled annexin A5 to identify focal, regional, or global uptake of annexin A5, a marker of cellular apoptosis.[28]

Limitations of nuclear medicine techniques include significant radiation doses, often in the same range as those delivered in CT, and poor spatial resolution compared with echocardiography, CT, and MRI. Examination times are often longer compared with other noninvasive imaging techniques.

Angiography

Conventional coronary angiography has traditionally been used to distinguish ischemic from nonischemic DCM. Although several noninvasive alternatives are available, and have been discussed in this chapter, they all have limitations, and coronary angiography remains the current gold standard.

DIFFERENTIAL DIAGNOSIS

Clinical Presentation

Clinical signs and symptoms are often nonspecific and can result from many different etiologies, including myocardial ischemia and congestive heart failure resulting from other causes. Pulmonary diseases, including infectious and inflammatory disorders and emphysema and pulmonary fibrosis, can mimic or exacerbate signs and symptoms of heart failure.

Imaging Findings

The major differential diagnosis is ischemic DCM, in which case revascularization should be considered. Apical ballooning syndrome, a transient dilation of the left ventricular apex often manifesting with signs and symptoms similar to acute coronary syndrome, can also simulate DCM.

TREATMENT OPTIONS

Medical

Prognosis in DCM is generally poor, and most patients, particularly patients older than 55 years, die within 4 years of the onset of symptoms. Spontaneous improvement or stabilization occurs in about 25% of patients. Death is due to either progressive heart failure or ventricular arrhythmias and sudden cardiac death. Systemic embolization is a concern, and patients with atrial fibrillation or known atrial or ventricular thrombus should be candidates for anticoagulation therapy. Pharmacologic treatment is the mainstay of medical therapy, and may include angiotensin-converting enzyme inhibitors, β blockers, loop diuretics, and aldosterone antagonists.

Surgical/Interventional

Patients with depressed ejection fraction, symptomatic heart failure, and conduction delay manifested by a QRS duration greater than 120 ms may exhibit asynchronous ventricular contraction and are candidates for biventricular pacing or CRT. Consequences of ventricular asynchrony include poor ventricular filling, reduced left ventricular contractility, prolonged duration (and greater severity) of mitral regurgitation, and paradoxical septal wall motion. CRT stimulates both ventricles almost simultaneously, and improves the coordination of ventricular contraction with corresponding reduction in the severity of mitral regurgitation. CRT has been shown to result in a significant reduction in patient mortality and hospitalization, a reversal of left ventricular remodeling, and improved quality of life and exercise capacity. Cardiac transplantation is an option for patients with end-stage or refractory heart failure who meet transplantation criteria.

INFORMATION FOR THE REFERRING PHYSICIAN

The most important information to include in the report is whether DCM is present or absent, and whether the cause is likely ischemic or nonischemic. Additional supporting data, if available, should include left and right ventricular end-systolic and end-diastolic volume, stroke volume, ejection fraction, end-diastolic dimension, and end-systolic dimension—all of which can be indexed to body surface area. Additional findings include atrial enlargement, mitral regurgitation or other valvular disease, and the presence of atrial or ventricular thrombus.

> **KEY POINTS**
> - DCM is the most common cardiomyopathy and is a frequent cause of congestive heart failure.
> - DCM can result from numerous etiologies, but a significant percentage of cases are genetic.
> - A major role for imaging is distinguishing ischemic DCM from nonischemic DCM.

SUGGESTED READINGS

Agricola E, Oppizzi M, Pisani M, et al. Stress echocardiography in heart failure. Cardiovasc Ultrasound 2004; 2:11-25.

Jackson E, Bellenger N, Seddon M, et al. Ischaemic and non-ischaemic cardiomyopathies—cardiac MRI appearances with delayed enhancement. Clin Radiol 2007; 62:395-403.

Kim DH, Choi SI, Chang HJ, et al. Delayed hyperenhancement by contrast-enhanced magnetic resonance imaging: clinical applications for various cardiac diseases. J Comput Assist Tomogr 2006; 30:226-232.

Rochitte CE, Tassi EM, Shiozaki AA. The emerging role of MRI in the diagnosis and management of cardiomyopathies. Curr Cardiol Rep 2006; 8:44-52.

Soler R, Rodriguez E, Remuinan C, et al. Magnetic resonance imaging of primary cardiomyopathies. J Comput Assist Tomogr 2003; 27:724-734.

Thiene G, Basso C, Calabrese F, et al. Twenty years of progress and beckoning frontiers in cardiovascular pathology: cardiomyopathies. Cardiovasc Pathol 2005; 14:165-169.

Wood MJ, Picard MH. Utility of echocardiography in the evaluation of individuals with cardiomyopathy. Heart 2004; 90:707-712.

REFERENCES

1. Murphy RT, Starling RC. Genetics and cardiomyopathy: where are we now? Cleve Clin J Med 2005; 72:465-483.
2. Hughes SE, McKenna WJ. New insights into the pathology of inherited cardiomyopathy. Heart 2005; 91:257-264.
3. Richardson P, McKenna W, Bristow M, et al. Report of the 1995 World Health Organization/International Society and Federation of Cardiology Task Force on the Definition and Classification of Cardiomyopathies. Circulation 1996; 93:841-842.
4. Gillum RF. Idiopathic dilated cardiomyopathy in the United States, 1970-1982. Am Heart J 1986; 111:752-755.
5. Codd MB, Sugrue DD, Gersh BJ, et al. Epidemiology of idiopathic dilated and hypertrophic cardiomyopathy: a population-based study in Olmsted County, Minnesota, 1975-1984. Circulation 1989; 80:564-672.
6. Gillum RF. Idiopathic cardiomyopathy in the United States, 1970-1982. Am Heart J 1986; 111:752-755.
7. Baig MK, Golman JH, Caforio AL, et al. Familial DCM: cardiac abnormalities are common in asymptomatic relatives and may represent early disease. J Am Coll Cardiol 1998; 31:195-201.
8. Towbin JA, Bowles NE. Dilated cardiomyopathy: a tale of cytoskeletal proteins and beyond. J Cardiovasc Electrophysiol 2006; 17:919-926.
9. LaVecchia L, Paccanara M, Bonanno C, et al. Left ventricular versus biventricular dysfunction in idiopathic dilated cardiomyopathy. Am J Cardiol 1999; 83:120-122.
10. La Vecchia L, Varotto L, Zanolla L, et al. Right ventricular function predicts transplant-free survival in idiopathic dilated cardiomyopathy. J Cardiovasc Med 2006; 7:706-710.
11. Drozd J, Krzeminska-Pakula M, Plewka M, et al. Prognostic value of low-dose dobutamine echocardiography in patients with dilated cardiomyopathy. Chest 2002; 121:216-222.
12. Pratali L, Picano E, Otasevic P, et al. Prognostic significance of the dobutamine echocardiography test in idiopathic dilated cardiomyopathy. Am J Cardiol 2001; 88:1374-1378.
13. Rigo F, Gherardi S, Galderisi M, et al. The independent prognostic value of contractile and coronary flow reserve determined by dipyridamole stress echocardiography in patients with idiopathic dilated cardiomyopathy. Am J Cardiol 2007; 99:1154-1158.
14. Pratali L, Otasevic P, Nekovic A, et al. Prognostic value of pharmacologic stress echocardiography in patients with idiopathic dilated cardiomyopathy: a prospective head-to-head comparison between dipyridamole and dobutamine test. J Cardiac Fail 2007; 13:836-842.
15. Andreini D, Pontone G, Pepi M, et al. Diagnostic accuracy of multidetector computed tomography coronary angiography in patients with dilated cardiomyopathy. J Am Coll Cardiol 2007; 49:2044-2050.
16. Cornily JC, Gilard M, Le Gal G, et al. Accuracy of 16-detector multislice spiral computed tomography in the initial evaluation of dilated cardiomyopathy. Eur J Radiol 2007; 61:84-90.
17. Budoff MJ, Jacob B, Rasouli ML, et al. Comparison of electron beam computed tomography and technetium stress testing in differentiating cause of dilated versus ischemic cardiomyopathy. J Comput Assist Tomogr 2005; 29:699-703.
18. Soriano CJ, Ridocci F, Estornell J, et al. Noninvasive diagnosis of coronary artery disease in patients with heart failure and systolic dysfunction of uncertain etiology, using late gadolinium-enhanced cardiovascular magnetic resonance. J Am Coll Cardiol 2005; 45:473-478.
19. McCrohon JA, Moon JC, Prasad SK, et al. Differentiation of heart failure related to dilated cardiomyopathy and coronary artery disease using gadolinium-enhanced cardiovascular magnetic resonance. Circulation 2003; 108:54-59.
20. Assomull RG, Prasad SK, Lyne J, et al. Cardiovascular magnetic resonance, fibrosis, and prognosis in dilated cardiomyopathy. J Am Coll Cardiol 2006; 48:1977-1985.
21. Park S, Choi BW, Rim SJ, et al. Delayed hyperenhancement magnetic resonance imaging is useful in predicting functional recovery of

nonischemic left ventricular systolic dysfunction. J Card Fail 2006; 12:93-99.
22. Danias PG, Ahlberg AW, Clark BA, et al. Combined assessment of myocardial perfusion and left ventricular function with exercise technetium-99m sestamibi gated single-photon emission computed tomography can differentiate between ischemic and nonischemic dilated cardiomyopathy. Am J Cardiol 1998; 82:1253-1258.
23. Danias PG, Papaioannou GI, Ahlberg AW, et al. Usefulness of electrocardiographic-gated stress technetium-99m sestamibi single-photon emission computed tomography to differentiate ischemic from nonischemic cardiomyopathy. Am J Cardiol 2004; 94:14-19.
24. Kasama S, Toyama T, Kumakura H, et al. Dobutamine stress ^{99m}Tc-tetrofosmin quantitative gated SPECT predicts improvement of cardiac function after carvedilol treatment in patients with dilated cardiomyopathy. J Nucl Med 2004; 45:1878-1884.
25. O'Neill JO, McCarthy PM, Brunken RC, et al. PET abnormalities in patients with nonischemic cardiomyopathy. J Card Fail 2004; 10:244-249.
26. Lindner O, Vogt J, Baller D, et al. Global and regional myocardial oxygen consumption and blood flow in severe cardiomyopathy with left bundle branch block. Eur J Heart Fail 2005; 7:225-230.
27. Lindner O, Vogt J, Kammeier A, et al. Effect of cardiac resynchronization therapy on global and regional oxygen consumption and myocardial blood flow in patients with non-ischaemic and ischaemic cardiomyopathy. Eur Heart J 2005; 26:70-76.
28. Kietselaer BL, Reutelingsperger CP, Boersma HH, et al. Noninvasive detection of programmed cell loss with ^{99m}Tc-labeled annexin A5 in heart failure. J Nucl Med 2007; 48:562-567.

CHAPTER 63

Restrictive Cardiomyopathy

James F. Glockner

Restrictive cardiomyopathy (RCM) is the least common cardiomyopathy, and is characterized by diastolic dysfunction with restrictive ventricular filling with normal or near-normal systolic function and wall thickness.[1] RCM may be idiopathic or associated with other infiltrative diseases, such as amyloidosis, endomyocardial disease, sarcoidosis, iron deposition disease, and storage diseases. Numerous other diseases may have a prominent restrictive component. Presentation of RCM is variable, and diagnosis is often difficult. The prognosis for most forms of RCM is poor, and it is important to distinguish RCM from constrictive pericarditis, which may have a similar clinical presentation

CARDIAC AMYLOIDOSIS

Definition

Amyloidosis is an infiltrative disorder in which insoluble proteins known as *amyloid* are deposited in multiple organs, including the heart (cardiac amyloidosis).

Prevalence and Epidemiology

Primary amyloidosis is a rare but devastating disease, with an incidence of 9 per 1 million and mean survival of approximately 13 months after diagnosis.[2] Cardiac involvement in primary amyloidosis is common, with 60% of patients exhibiting ECG or echocardiographic abnormalities. Death is attributed to cardiac causes in at least 50% of patients with primary amyloidosis who die either from heart failure or from a malignant arrhythmia.[2]

Senile amyloidosis predominantly affects men older than 70 years and involves the heart in 25% of individuals older than 80 years.[3] Senile cardiac amyloidosis is often clinically silent; however, extensive amyloid deposition can lead to significant clinical symptoms.

Etiology and Pathophysiology

Amyloidosis can arise from numerous diverse diseases, and 24 heterogeneous proteins have been identified within amyloid deposits. These misfolded proteins result from mutations or excessive production and form a β-pleated sheet that aligns in an antiparallel manner. The sheets form insoluble amyloid fibrils that resist proteolysis, cause mechanical disruption, and generate local oxidative stress in various organs.

Amyloid deposits, regardless of their protein composition, all have a characteristic appearance on light microscopy, staining pink with Congo red dye and exhibiting apple-green birefringence under polarized light microscopy. Nearly all organ systems can be involved, including the kidneys, heart, blood vessels, central and peripheral nervous system, liver, bowel, lungs, eyes, skin, and bones. Cardiac amyloidosis is a devastating progressive process that leads to congestive heart failure, angina, and arrhythmias.[1]

Cardiac amyloidosis is classified by the protein precursor as primary, secondary, senile systemic, hereditary, isolated atrial, and hemodialysis-associated amyloidosis. Primary amyloidosis (AL) is caused by abnormalities of plasma cells that result in production of amyloidogenic immunoglobulin light chain proteins. Secondary amyloidosis (AA) results from accumulation of fibrils formed from an acute-phase reactant, serum amyloid A protein, and may be associated with rheumatoid arthritis, familial Mediterranean fever, chronic infections, and inflammatory bowel disease. Secondary cardiac amyloidosis is most often clinically insignificant, and the major pathology involves the kidney, with development of proteinuria and renal failure.

Senile systemic amyloidosis is an age-related disorder with amyloid deposits formed by wild-type transthyretin TTR, a transport protein synthesized in the liver and choroid plexus. Hereditary amyloidosis is an autosomal dominant disease resulting from mutations in apolipoprotein 1 and TTR. Isolated atrial amyloidosis is also associated with advanced age and results from secretion of atrial natriuretic peptide by atrial myocytes. Hemodialysis-related amyloidosis can develop from accumulation of $β_2$-microglobulin secondary to chronic uremia.

Cardiac amyloidosis causes numerous pathophysiologic consequences. Amyloid filaments deposited within the myocardial interstitial space result in stiffening of the myocardium and diastolic dysfunction with elevated filling pressures. As the disease progresses, the atria dilate in response to increased diastolic filling pressures. Thickening of the ventricles may occur, and eventually systolic function is also affected.

In addition to mechanical effects on myocardial stiffness, amyloid deposition induces oxidative stress that depresses myocyte contractile function. Myocardial ischemia may also result from microvascular disease. Amyloid deposits typically spare the epicardial vessels, whereas involvement of intramyocardial vasculature is seen in more than 90% of patients with AL amyloidosis.[4]

Manifestations of Disease

Clinical Presentation

Symptoms in patients with cardiac amyloidosis are dominated by diastolic heart failure resulting from RCM. Findings of right-sided heart failure, including ascites, elevated jugular pressure, hepatomegaly, and lower extremity edema, are common. Anginal pain secondary to microvascular ischemia may also occur.

Serum biomarkers of cardiac injury or stress are often elevated in cardiac amyloidosis. Cardiac-specific troponin and natriuretic peptide levels may be elevated and portend a poor prognosis. Low-voltage QRS amplitudes in the precordial leads or limb leads, a pseudoinfarction pattern (QS waves in consecutive leads) and conduction delays are common.

Imaging Indications and Algorithm

Cardiac imaging is typically performed in patients with known systemic amyloidosis presenting with cardiac symptoms or signs, or in patients without known amyloidosis, but clinically suspected to have a RCM. In either case, echocardiography is usually the first test performed, on the basis of its wide availability, relatively low cost, and ability to suggest the diagnosis in many cases. Additionally, echocardiography is the noninvasive technique of choice to assess diastolic dysfunction. MRI is also a first-line test in patients with suspected cardiac amyloidosis on the basis of its superior soft tissue characterization, in particular the unique appearance of cardiac amyloidosis on postcontrast myocardial delayed enhancement (MDE) sequences. Both techniques should also detect associated findings and complications (e.g., atrial thrombus) with reasonable accuracy.

Imaging Techniques and Findings

Radiography

Radiography is typically nonspecific for the diagnosis of cardiac amyloidosis. Pericardial and pleural effusions may be seen.

Ultrasonography

Increased wall thickness without dilation of the ventricular cavity and preserved systolic function until relatively

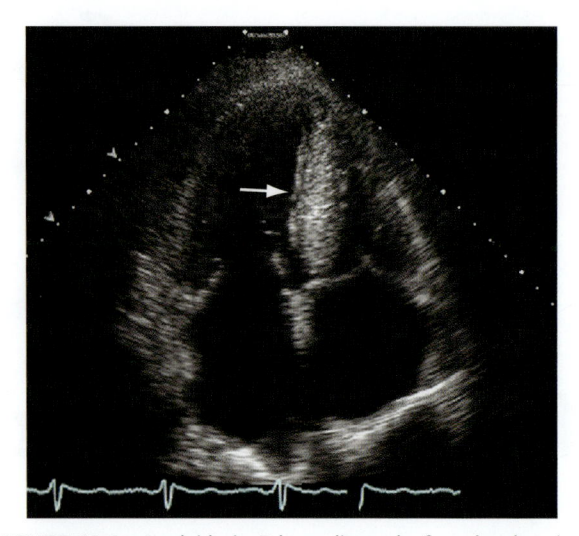

■ **FIGURE 63-1** Amyloidosis. Echocardiography four-chamber view reveals atrial dilation and thickening of the ventricular septum with a granular sparkling appearance (*arrow*).

advanced stages of the disease are hallmarks of cardiac amyloidosis on echocardiography (Fig. 63-1). Amyloid deposits may involve nearly all regions of the heart, including valves, myocardium, interatrial septum, and pericardium, and manifestations of this involvement can be seen as multivalvular regurgitation, thickening of the interatrial septum, atrial dilation, pericardial effusions, and diffuse thickening of the right ventricular and left ventricular (LV) myocardium.[5] A classic finding of myocardial amyloidosis is a granular sparkling pattern on two-dimensional echocardiography. This pattern is not specific for amyloidosis, however, and can be seen in patients with hypertensive cardiomyopathy, glycogen storage disorders, and hypertrophic cardiomyopathy. Atrial and ventricular thrombi are common findings, particularly in advanced disease.

Pulsed wave Doppler echocardiography is helpful in assessing diastolic dysfunction in cardiac amyloidosis. The initial diastolic abnormality is abnormal relaxation (grade 1 diastolic dysfunction) resulting from increased ventricular wall thickness; the pattern becomes restrictive (grades 3 to 4) when progressive amyloid infiltration decreases LV compliance and increases left atrial pressure. The filling pattern may normalize temporarily (pseudonormalization—grade 2 diastolic dysfunction) as a result of combined relaxation abnormality and moderate increase in left atrial filling pressure before becoming frankly restrictive. Deceleration time is an important prognostic variable in cardiac amyloidosis; the average survival for patients with a deceleration time less than 150 ms is less than 1 year versus 3 years for patients with a deceleration time greater than 150 ms.[6] A combination of LV wall thickness greater than 15 mm and fractional shortening of less than 20% (thought to reflect combined systolic and diastolic dysfunction) is associated with a median survival of 4 months.[7] Right ventricular function has also been correlated with poor prognosis in patients with cardiac amyloidosis.[8]

Tissue Doppler imaging (TDI) has emerged more recently as a useful technique in assessment of LV regional

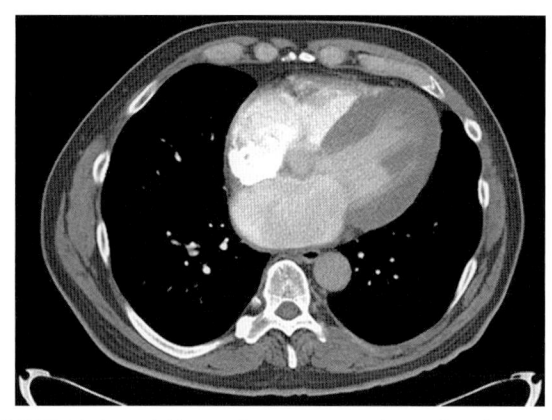

FIGURE 63-2 Axial image from contrast-enhanced CT in a patient with cardiac amyloidosis reveals mild diffuse LV thickening and left atrial enlargement.

wall motion and diastolic dysfunction in patients with cardiac amyloidosis. Koyama and colleagues[9] showed that TDI measurements differentiated patients without from patients with cardiac amyloidosis, and amyloidosis patients with and without heart failure. TDI more clearly documented diastolic function than conventional Doppler-derived indices. Myocardial strain and strain rate imaging have also been investigated in cardiac amyloidosis, and these techniques have documented early impairment in systolic function before the onset of clinical heart failure.[10]

Computed Tomography

ECG gated contrast-enhanced CT reveals many of the findings discussed previously with regard to echocardiography: ventricular thickening with preserved systolic function, enlarged atria, and pericardial and pleural effusions (Fig. 63-2). Little evidence currently available suggests that CT is useful in the initial diagnosis of cardiac amyloidosis or in distinguishing amyloidosis from other causes of RCM.

Magnetic Resonance Imaging

MRI has shown considerable promise in diagnosis and characterization of cardiac amyloidosis.[11-14] Cine steady-state free precession (SSFP) images readily show findings of ventricular thickening with normal chamber size, atrial enlargement, and preserved systolic function (Fig. 63-3). Pleural and pericardial effusions are common and are well depicted on MRI. Impaired diastolic relaxation is often appreciated on cine SSFP images, and mitral inflow measurements can be obtained using cine phase contrast pulse sequences to obtain information analogous to Doppler echocardiography.

After administration of contrast medium, striking abnormalities are often seen on MDE pulse sequences, with patients with cardiac amyloidosis typically showing diffuse irregular hyperenhancement in noncoronary distributions (Fig. 63-4). A circumferential subendocardial hyperenhancement pattern has been described and correlated with predominant amyloid deposition in the subendocardial myocardium; however, in our experience, patterns of hyperenhancement are quite variable. Right ventricular late enhancement is a notable feature of amyloidosis and can help to distinguish this from hypertrophic cardiomyopathy with foci of enhancing fibrotic tissue.

Abnormalities of myocardial nulling are also common in amyloidosis and can help to distinguish this disease from other pathologies. A cine multi-TI inversion recovery sequence, in which each image or phase is acquired with a slightly longer inversion time (TI), is often used to select the optimal TI for the delayed enhancement acquisition. As TI increases, blood and myocardium pass through a null point at which signal is minimized. Generally, the blood pool contains a higher concentration of gadolinium, has a shorter T1 relaxation time, and passes through the null point before myocardium. In many amyloid patients, this progression is reversed, with myocardial tissue reaching the null point before the blood pool (Fig. 63-5).

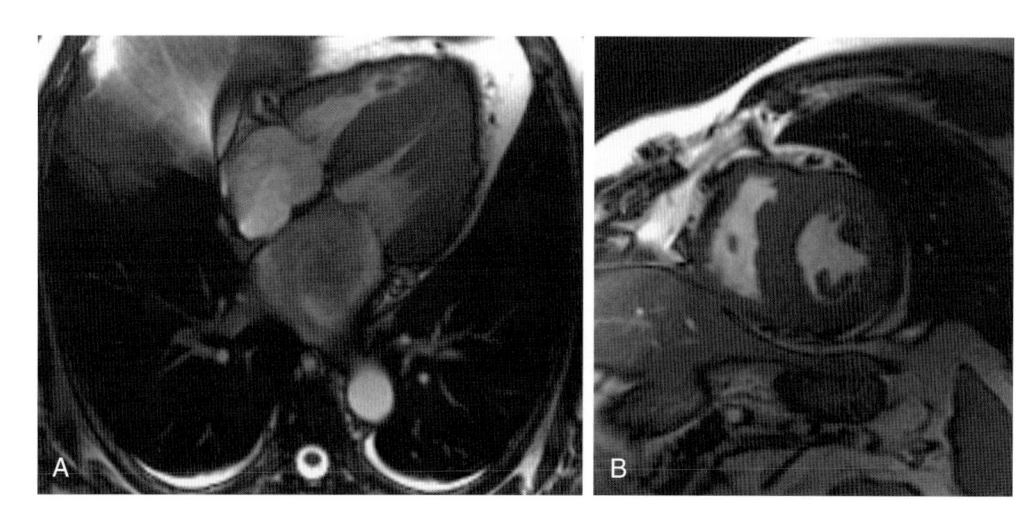

FIGURE 63-3 A and B, Four-chamber (A) and short-axis (B) mid-diastolic SSFP images in a patient with amyloid reveal diffuse LV thickening, biatrial enlargement, and small bilateral pleural effusions.

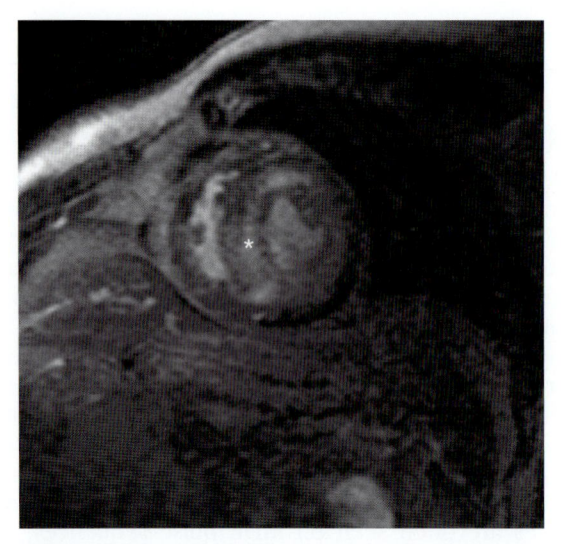

FIGURE 63-4 Short-axis MDE image in a patient with cardiac amyloidosis. Note diffuse enhancement of the left ventricle, most prominently in the septum (*asterisk*).

Nuclear Medicine

Nuclear medicine has generally played a minor role in the diagnosis and characterization of cardiac amyloidosis. Various tracers, mainly phosphonates, have been used to assess patients with suspected cardiac involvement, with heterogeneous results. More recent developments include the use of Tc 99m DPD scintigraphy to distinguish between AL and senile or transthyretin-related cardiac amyloidosis in patients with known cardiac amyloidosis.[15]

Angiography

Coronary angiography is typically normal because involvement of epicardial coronary vessels is rare in amyloidosis. Right heart catheterization with pressure measurements may be performed to verify RCM, showing elevated diastolic ventricular pressures and a dip and plateau or square root sign in the pressure tracing. Right ventricular biopsy may also be required for diagnosis in difficult cases.

EOSINOPHILIC ENDOMYOCARDIAL DISEASE

Definition

The classification of eosinophilic endomyocardial disease includes Löffler endocarditis (or idiopathic hypereosinophilic syndrome [IHES]) and endomyocardial fibrosis.

Prevalence and Epidemiology

It is unclear whether these are two distinct diseases or different manifestations of the same underlying pathologic process. IHES occurs in temperate countries, has a more aggressive and rapidly progressive course, and is related to hypereosinophilia, whereas endomyocardial fibrosis occurs most commonly in equatorial Africa and is not definitely related to hypereosinophilia. Endomyocardial fibrosis occurs mainly in children and adolescents belonging to the poorest groups of the population and is an endemic cause of heart disease in certain tropical areas, such as the coastal regions of Mozambique, where 9% of the population is affected.[16] The etiology of endomyocardial fibrosis is unclear; however, in most cases eosinophilia is seen in the initial inflammatory process, and histologically the endocardial lesions are similar to those seen in IHES. An alternative hypothesis has focused on an animal protein–deficient cassava diet, which has induced endomyocardial fibrosis in an animal model.

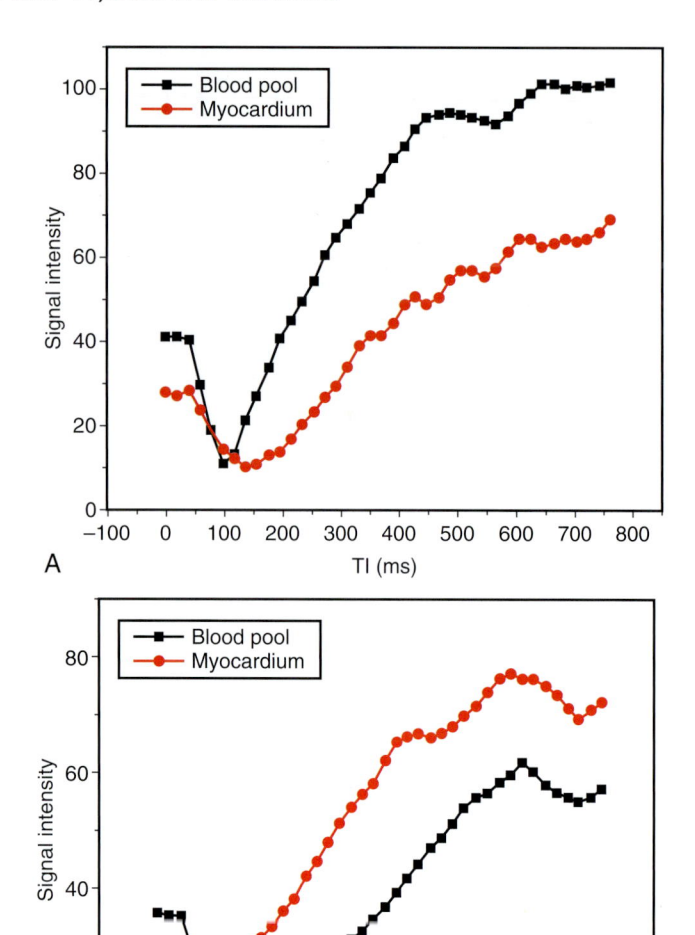

FIGURE 63-5 A and B, Plots of signal intensity versus TI from cine inversion recovery sequence in patients without (A) and with (B) cardiac amyloidosis. The inflection point of the myocardial curve occurs before the blood pool inflection point in the patient with amyloidosis.

Etiology and Pathophysiology

IHES is a rare idiopathic disorder characterized by persistent eosinophilia of greater than $1.5 \times 10^9/L$ for longer than 6 months with evidence of multiorgan dysfunction. The heart is frequently involved, and eosinophil-mediated damage progresses through three stages. An acute necrotic stage, during which the disease is usually clinically silent, is followed by an intermediate phase characterized by thrombus formation, and a final fibrotic stage, in which

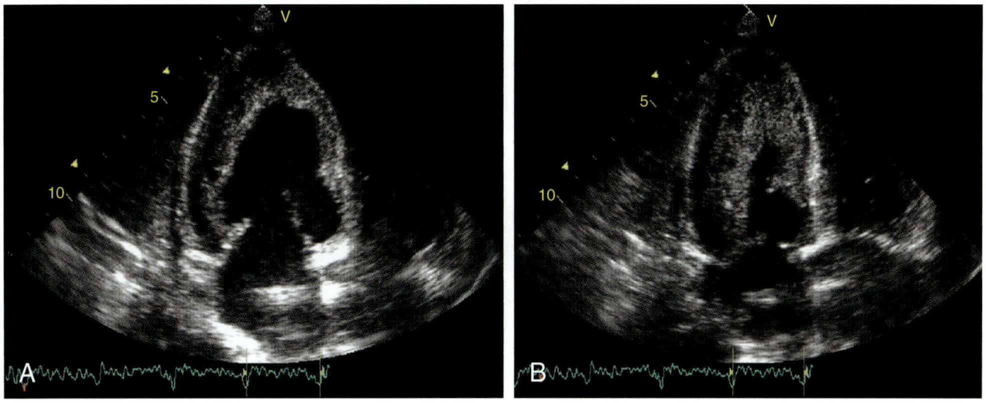

■ **FIGURE 63-6** Eosinophilic endomyocardial disease. **A** and **B,** Two-chamber end-diastolic (**A**) and end-systolic (**B**) views from an echocardiogram reveal a layer of subendocardial echogenic thrombus/fibrosis.

endomyocardial fibrosis is responsible for an RCM. Histologic confirmation of the diagnosis after right ventricular biopsy entails visualizing endomyocardial fibrosis, thrombus, granulation tissue, or chronic inflammation from eosinophilic infiltration.

Essential features of endomyocardial fibrosis are the formation of fibrous tissue on the endocardium and, to a lesser extent, in the myocardium of the inflow tract and apex of one or both ventricles. This fibrous tissue results in endocardial rigidity, atrioventricular valve incompetence secondary to papillary muscle involvement, and progressive reduction of the ventricular cavity with restricted filling and atrial enlargement. The pathophysiology of eosinophilic endomyocardial disease is thought to be related to active damage of the endocardium and myocardium by eosinophils.

Manifestations of Disease

Clinical Presentation

The initial presentation of IHES or endomyocardial fibrosis is often vague, including palpitations, dyspnea, fever, and malaise. During later stages of the disease, heart failure and atrioventricular valvular regurgitation can lead to progressive fatigue and dyspnea with abdominal and lower extremity swelling. When cardiac disease is primarily right-sided, predominant symptoms are peripheral edema, hepatomegaly, ascites, and other signs of right heart failure. Left-sided disease often manifests with signs of severe mitral regurgitation and congestive heart failure. Pulmonary and systemic embolism may also occur, with devastating consequences.

Imaging Indications and Algorithm

Because the etiology is often unsuspected, and patients present with vague symptoms, echocardiography is usually the first examination performed. Echocardiography may often suggest the diagnosis, which can be confirmed with demonstration of peripheral eosinophilia in the appropriate clinical setting. MRI and CT have an important role in this disease; visualization of subendocardial apical thrombus is generally less problematic compared with echocardiography, and either of these techniques may be preferred in cases where the diagnosis is suspected.

Imaging Techniques and Findings

Radiography

Radiographic findings are nonspecific. Cardiomegaly with atrial enlargement and signs of left-sided failure, including pulmonary vascular congestion and pleural effusions, may be seen.

Ultrasonography

Characteristic findings on echocardiography include apical obliteration of the involved ventricle with echogenic material, and thickening and adherence to the ventricular wall of the posterior atrioventricular valvular chordae tendineae cordis and adjacent papillary muscles, with enlargement of the corresponding atrium (Fig. 63-6).[17] Doppler echocardiography may reveal typical findings of restriction, including shortened deceleration time and reduced isovolumetric relaxation time. Contrast-enhanced techniques may aid in visualizing the rim of hypoenhancing thrombus and subendocardial fibrotic tissue.

Computed Tomography

Contrast-enhanced CT may show hypoenhancing thrombus or fibrotic material along the endocardial surface of the myocardium, which should suggest the diagnosis (Fig. 63-7).[18] Atrial enlargement may also be seen.

Magnetic Resonance Imaging

MRI findings of endomyocardial fibrosis typically include subendocardial thrombus and fibrosis, which can be visualized on SSFP, myocardial perfusion, and MDE pulse sequences. First-pass contrast-enhanced perfusion sequences typically reveal perfusion defects along the endocardial margin of the myocardium in the left ventricle and often right ventricle. Hyperenhancing fibrotic granulation tissue may surround a core of nonenhancing thrombus and can be seen on MDE imaging (Fig. 63-8).[19-21]

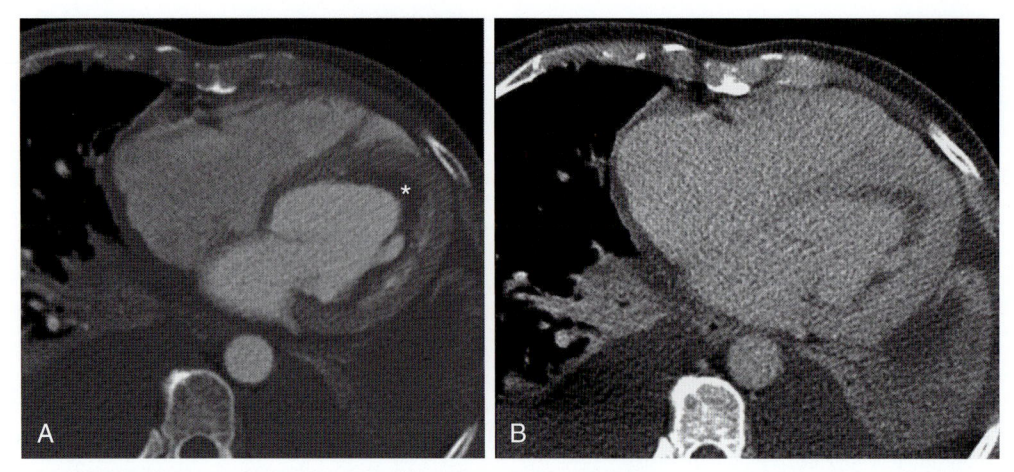

■ FIGURE 63-7 Eosinophilic endomyocardial disease. A and B, Immediate (A) and delayed (B) axial CT images in a patient with IHES reveals a thick layer of subendocardial thrombus (*asterisk*), which persists as a filling defect on the delayed image.

Nuclear Medicine

There is little role for nuclear medicine in diagnosis or assessment of patients with eosinophilic endomyocardial disease.

Angiography

On angiography, there is characteristic obliteration of the apex of the involved ventricle with atrioventricular valve regurgitation.[22] Endomyocardial biopsy can be performed in cases where the diagnosis is uncertain.

SIDEROTIC CARDIOMYOPATHY

Definition

Hemochromatosis/siderotic cardiomyopathy refers to the conditions characterized by excessive iron deposition within the myocardium, leading to progressive diastolic and systolic dysfunction.

Prevalence and Epidemiology

Cardiac failure as a result of transfusional iron overload is the most common cause of death in patients with thalassemia major, with more than 50% of these patients dying before age 35.[23] Sickle cell and other hereditary anemias are also common causes of transfusional iron overload. Primary hemochromatosis is an autosomal recessive disorder affecting approximately 1 in 220 individuals and is an important cause of siderotic cardiomyopathy.[24]

Etiology and Pathophysiology

Iron overload occurs as a result of either excessive absorption or repeated transfusions. In hemochromatosis, iron is deposited in periportal hepatocytes and, in severe disease, the pancreas, heart, and endocrine organs. In thalassemia, iron overload results from overabsorption and transfusional siderosis. Transfusional iron is deposited in reticuloendothelial cells of the spleen, liver, and bone marrow. In severe cases, iron also accumulates in parenchymal

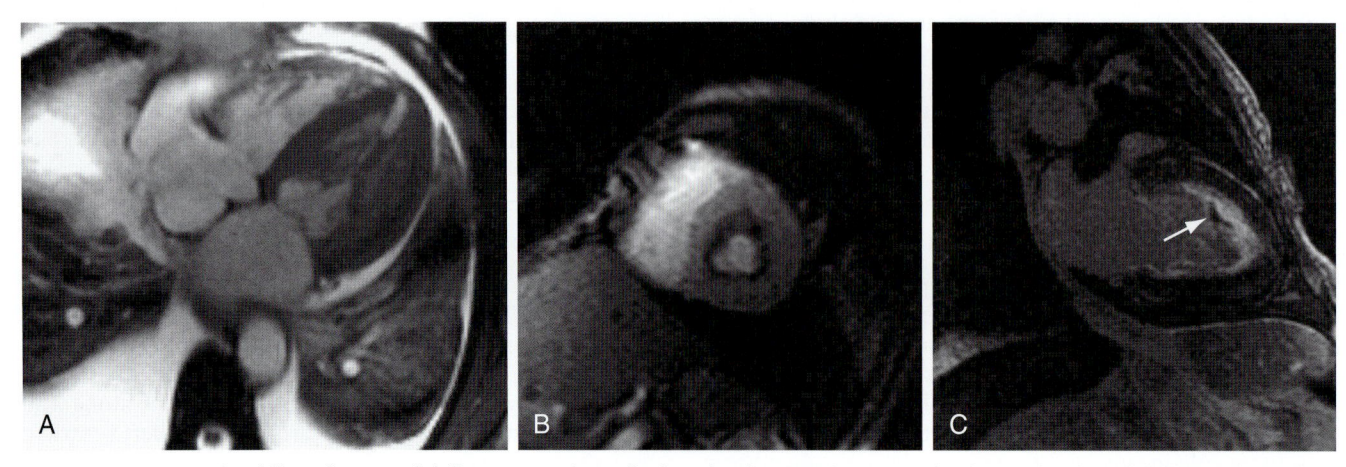

■ FIGURE 63-8 Eosinophilic endomyocardial disease. A, End-systolic, four-chamber SSFP image reveals a large subendocardial filling defect in the left ventricle. B, Short-axis contrast-enhanced perfusion image has a corresponding circumferential subendocardial perfusion defect. C, Two-chamber MDE image reveals enhancing subendocardial fibrosis with nonenhancing thrombus (*arrow*).

cells of the liver, heart, and endocrine organs. At normal body iron levels, plasma iron is bound to transferrin, which prevents catalytic activity and free radical production. When transferrin is fully saturated, surplus iron appears as non–transferrin-bound iron (NTBI), and enters cells where it is stored as ferritin and hemosiderin. NTBI, probably by virtue of its more accessible unpaired electrons, promotes free radical formation and consequent damage to membrane lipids and proteins. As iron accumulates in the heart, there is little effect on function until a threshold is reached where the iron storage capacity is exhausted, and NTBI begins to appear. Excessive iron in myocytes may impair Na^+,K^+-ATPase function, reduce mitochondrial activity, and increase lysosomal fragility.[25]

Manifestations of Disease

Clinical Presentation

Initially, myocardial iron overload is asymptomatic, with a mild increase in LV wall thickness and mild LV dilation. Diastolic dysfunction usually precedes systolic abnormalities and is characterized by a restrictive filling pattern. Classic cardiac abnormalities of excess iron deposition include congestive heart failure and dysrhythmias. ECG abnormalities are present in 35% of symptomatic patients, including ventricular ectopies, supraventricular and ventricular tachycardias, ventricular fibrillation, and heart block.[26]

Imaging Indications and Algorithm

Indications for imaging include assessment of cardiac function and myocardial iron burden in patients with known or suspected siderotic cardiomyopathy. Imaging may also be indicated for assessment of response to therapy. Echocardiography can assess ventricular function and detect focal wall motion abnormalities and diastolic dysfunction. MRI is the gold standard for assessment of cardiac volumes and function, and can estimate the myocardial iron content via measurement of $T2^*$ or $R2^*$.

Imaging Techniques and Findings

Radiography

Findings on radiography in patients with siderotic cardiomyopathy are nonspecific, and may include cardiomegaly and signs of congestive heart failure, including pulmonary vascular congestion, interlobular septal thickening, and pleural effusions.

Ultrasonography

Typical two-dimensional echocardiographic findings in siderotic cardiomyopathy include mild LV dilation, LV systolic dysfunction, normal wall thickness, normal valves, and biatrial enlargement. The LV diastolic filling pattern is usually restrictive.

More recent investigation has shown that assessment of pulmonary venous flow and TDI echocardiographic indices add useful information in assessing patients with hemochromatosis, and that alterations in these parameters may be seen before symptomatic involvement.[27] TDI has also been used to assess thalassemic patients with siderotic cardiomyopathy. Wall motion abnormalities were significantly more common in patients with myocardial iron overload than in patients without overload, and may represent an early sign of cardiac disease in patients with preserved systolic function.[28]

Computed Tomography

Dual-energy CT has been used to assess and quantify iron overload in the liver and other organs. The correlation between iron content and tissue density is weak, with numerous confounding factors, and the technique has not seen widespread clinical application. Increased density may be seen, however, in cases of severe siderotic cardiomyopathy.

Magnetic Resonance Imaging

MRI is an attractive choice for imaging patients with known or suspected siderotic cardiomyopathy because iron can be detected and quantified noninvasively. Iron induces local magnetic field inhomogeneities, which cause significant reduction in $T2^*$, the time constant describing the rate at which the phase coherence of spins in the transverse plane decays after an initial radiofrequency pulse. Although many factors affect intrinsic tissue relaxation times, the presence of large quantities of iron represents the dominant contribution, and measurements of myocardial $T2^*$ or $R2^*$ (relaxivity, or the inverse of $T2^*$) can be related to the tissue concentration of iron.

Several techniques for measuring $T2^*$ are available. Probably the most commonly employed clinical method is an ECG gated multi-echo gradient-echo sequence, which acquires a series of images in the same location with progressively longer echo times (TE). The signal intensity of each image pixel or of a user-drawn region of interest can be plotted versus TE and the resulting curve can be fit to an exponential decay function and solved for $T2^*$ or $R2^*$, which can be related to the tissue iron concentration on the basis of calibration curves constructed from animal models or from human biopsy data (Fig. 63-9). Wood and colleagues[29] used an animal model to show that MRI measurements of $T2$ and $T2^*$ can quantify cardiac and hepatic iron concentrations.

Measurement of myocardial $T2^*$ has been shown to have clinical utility. Anderson and associates[30] showed a progressive decline in myocardial ejection fraction as $T2^*$ decreased in thalassemia patients, and found that all patients with ventricular dysfunction had a myocardial $T2^*$ less than 20 ms. Myocardial $T2^*$ measurements have also been used to follow reversal of siderotic cardiomyopathy with intravenous desferrioxamine.[31]

Even when iron quantification pulse sequences are not used in MRI, the diagnosis of iron deposition disease can often be made on the basis of the striking decrease in signal intensity seen on standard sequences. Because $T2^*$ relaxation rates are greatly increased in the presence of iron, nearly all pulse sequences, but especially

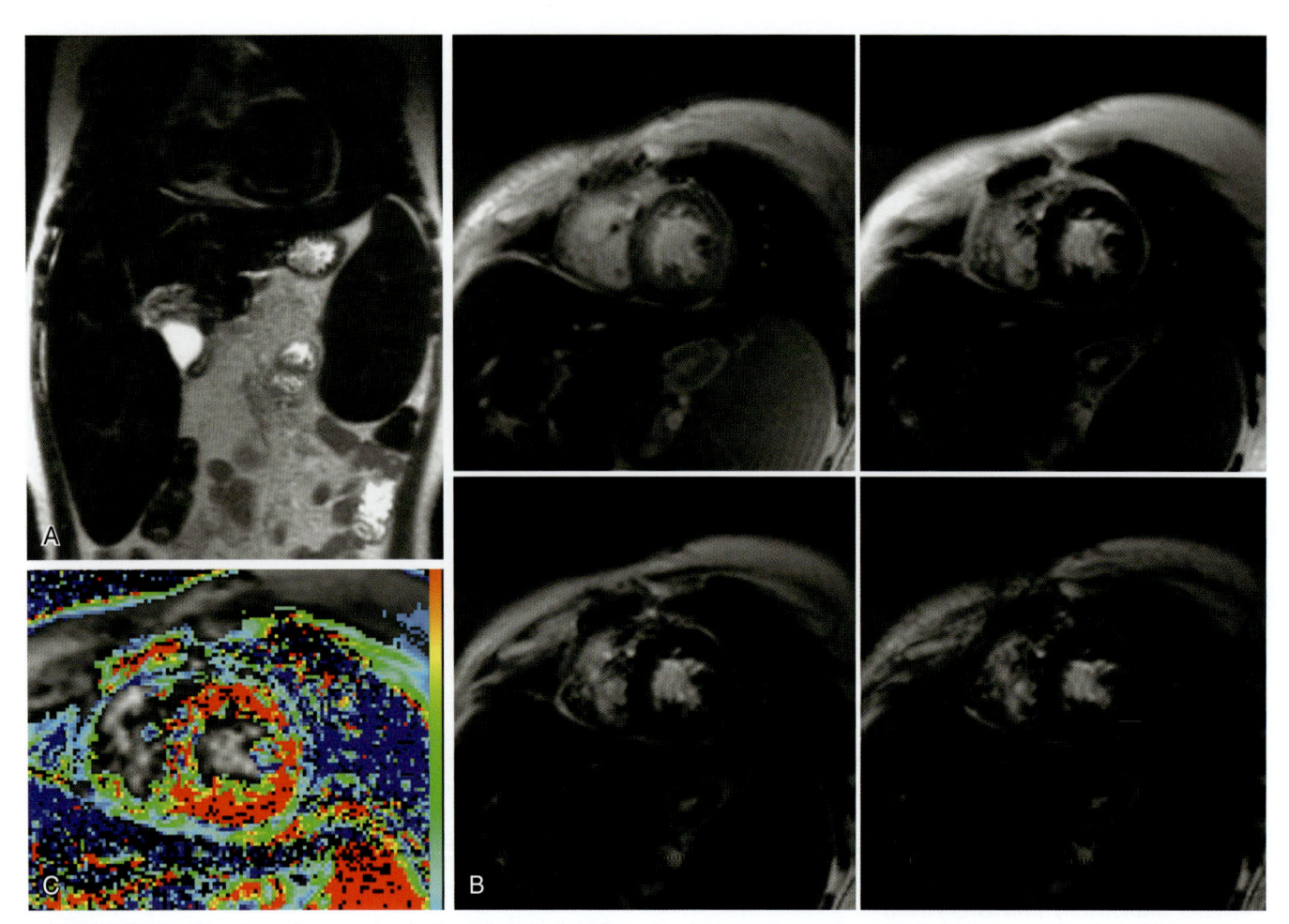

FIGURE 63-9 Siderotic cardiomyopathy. **A,** Coronal single short fast spin-echo image in a patient with thalassemia reveals enlarged liver, spleen, and heart with decreased signal intensity owing to iron deposition. **B,** Frames from multi-echo gradient-echo sequence with increasing TE reveal rapid signal drop-off in heart and liver as TE increases. **C,** Parametric T2* image confirms iron deposition based on data in **B**.

gradient-echo sequences, show much lower signal intensity in the affected tissues.

Nuclear Medicine

Currently, no significant clinical role exists for nuclear medicine in diagnosis or management of patients with siderotic cardiomyopathy.

Angiography

Coronary arteries are typically normal in patients with siderotic cardiomyopathy. Reduced LV ejection fraction, dilation of the LV cavity, and restrictive findings on right heart catheterization may be seen.

CARDIAC SARCOIDOSIS

Definition

Cardiac sarcoidosis refers to myocardial involvement by sarcoidosis, a multisystem disease characterized by the formation of noncaseating granulomas.

Prevalence and Epidemiology

Sarcoidosis is common and affects individuals of both sexes, and almost all ages, races, and geographic locations. There is remarkable diversity in the prevalence of sarcoid among ethnic and racial groups, with a prevalence of 1 to 64 per 100,000 worldwide.[32] The main organ systems targeted are the lungs and lymph nodes of the thorax. The estimated incidence of cardiac involvement is 4% to 5%, although autopsy series have found higher rates of 20% to 25%.[33,34] In Japan, cardiac involvement is present in 58% of patients and is responsible for 85% of deaths from sarcoidosis.[35]

Etiology and Pathophysiology

The etiology of sarcoid is unknown, although numerous infective agents and environmental exposures have been proposed. There may also be a genetic predisposition because familial clusters have been described, and incidence is higher in monozygotic than in dizygotic twins.

Sarcoidosis is defined pathologically by noncaseating (non-necrotizing) granulomas containing epithelioid cells and large multinucleated giant cells. The gold standard for diagnosis of cardiac sarcoidosis is endomyocardial biopsy displaying typical noncaseating granulomas. Myocardial involvement is typically not diffuse, however, and random biopsies have a high sampling error; the overall diagnostic yield of biopsy is less than 25%, and the procedure is associated with considerable risk.

Sarcoid has a predilection to involve the conducting system, and patients can develop various degrees of heart block and tachyarrhythmias, and are liable to sudden cardiac death. A common site for cardiac involvement is the base of the interventricular septum. Mitral valve abnormalities, papillary muscle dysfunction, LV aneurysm formation, pericardial effusions, and dilated cardiomyopathy may also be seen. With severe diffuse involvement, massive infiltration may lead to diffuse myocardial thickening with impaired relaxation and a predominant RCM.

Manifestations of Disease

Clinical Presentation

Various clinical signs and symptoms may occur in cardiac sarcoidosis. Sarcoidosis should be suspected in any young patient presenting with heart block. Patients may also present with congestive heart failure, cor pulmonale, supraventricular and ventricular arrhythmias, conduction disturbances, ventricular aneurysms, pericardial effusions, mitral valve abnormalities, and sudden cardiac death. Extensive cardiac infiltration leads to increased myocardial stiffness, reduced diastolic function, and a predominant RCM.

Prognosis and disease course in sarcoidosis vary greatly. In many cases, granulomas resolve spontaneously. This is particularly true in patients presenting asymptomatically with hilar and mediastinal adenopathy, who are likely to experience spontaneous resolution within 2 years. Patients who are symptomatic at presentation are less likely, however, to experience spontaneous recovery. The prognosis with cardiac involvement is significantly worse, and it is estimated that 5% to 8% of these patients eventually die of their disease.[36]

Imaging Indications and Algorithm

Evaluation of patients with suspected cardiac sarcoidosis may include chest x-ray or thoracic CT scan to evaluate for signs of pulmonary or mediastinal involvement. Echocardiography is useful to assess function and focal wall motion abnormalities in typical locations for sarcoidosis, but is relatively nonspecific. MRI may reveal patterns of delayed hyperenhancement typical of sarcoidosis, although this appearance can be indistinguishable from myocarditis. Imaging with thallium, Tc 99m sestamibi, and gallium and positron emission tomography (PET) all have been useful in assessing patients with suspected cardiac sarcoidosis. Gallium and PET have the additional advantage of detecting extracardiac disease.

Imaging Techniques and Findings

Radiography

Plain radiographs provide no information regarding cardiac sarcoidosis. The presence of typical signs of mediastinal and pulmonary sarcoidosis (bilateral hilar and right paratracheal adenopathy with or without interstitial pulmonary infiltrates) in the setting of cardiac symptoms consistent with sarcoidosis should suggest the diagnosis (Fig. 63-10A).

Ultrasonography

Abnormalities on echocardiography, including increased or decreased wall thickness, ventricular dilation, functional impairment, mitral regurgitation, impaired diastolic relaxation, and pericardial effusion, have been reported in 14% to 40% of patients with sarcoidosis. Echocardiography is usually the first examination performed when the diagnosis is suspected, and may show regional wall motion abnormalities and thickening of the interventricular septum, with bright echoes suggesting infiltration. Alternatively, the ventricles might appear thinned with global dysfunction and aneurysm formation. Diastolic dysfunction may be seen during the initial interstitial inflammatory stage when systolic function is still normal. RCM with dominant diastolic dysfunction may occur with extensive infiltration.[37,38]

Computed Tomography

CT plays a similar role to radiography; however, it is considerably more sensitive than plain radiographs for detecting mediastinal and hilar adenopathy (see Fig. 63-10B). CT is the test of choice for detecting pulmonary involvement in sarcoidosis, including nodules in a subpleural and bronchovascular distribution, pulmonary fibrosis, ground-glass opacities, bronchiectasis, and cystic changes. There is little evidence in the literature to suggest that CT provides information leading to a specific diagnosis of cardiac sarcoidosis.

Magnetic Resonance Imaging

MRI offers many advantages in imaging patients with suspected cardiac sarcoidosis. Acute myocardial inflammation resulting from sarcoid infiltration may be seen as regions of focal thickening with increased signal intensity on T2-weighted black blood images. Perfusion images or early T1-weighted postcontrast images may show increased contrast enhancement of affected myocardium, and MDE images may show epicardial patchy hyperenhancement, reflecting edema and myocardial injury. Focal wall motion abnormalities can be identified on cine SSFP images. Late changes include wall thinning and delayed hyperenhancement thought to reflect chronic scarring (Fig. 63-11). These changes may be difficult to distinguish from chronic infarction, although they tend to be in a noncoronary distribution and may spare the subendocardium. The appearance of cardiac sarcoidosis is very similar to that of myocarditis, and distinguishing between these two entities on the basis of MRI findings alone may be quite difficult.

Several more recent studies have evaluated the efficacy of MRI in detecting cardiac sarcoidosis. Smedema and colleagues[39] assessed 55 patients with pulmonary sarcoidosis who had evaluation for cardiac involvement consisting of

ECG, echocardiography, thallium 201 scintigraphy, and MRI. MRI detected cardiac involvement in an additional six patients compared with the other techniques. The extent of delayed hyperenhancement correlated with disease duration, ventricular function, mitral regurgitation, and presence of ventricular tachycardia. Patel and coworkers[40] assessed 58 sarcoidosis patients without cardiac symptoms and reported a twofold higher rate of cardiac involvement with gadolinium-enhanced MRI compared with evaluation with ECG and echocardiography.

Nuclear Medicine

Thallium 201 scintigraphy myocardial perfusion studies typically show segmental areas of decreased uptake in the ventricular myocardium that disappear or decrease in size during stress or after intravenous dipyridamole administration. This reverse distribution is not specific for sarcoidosis and has been described in other cardiomyopathies. Gallium 67 scintigraphy has also been used to show cardiac and extracardiac disease, for follow-up of active disease, and as a guide for potential sites for biopsy. More recently, Tc 99m sestamibi has been used as a perfusion agent, with a reverse distribution similar to that described in thallium. ^{18}FDG-PET is useful for showing cardiac and extracardiac manifestations of sarcoidosis.

Ohira and associates[41] compared ^{18}FDG-PET and MRI in assessing 21 patients with suspected cardiac sarcoidosis. According to the Japanese guidelines, 8 of 21 patients were diagnosed with cardiac sarcoidosis. PET had sensitivity and specificity of 88% and 38% versus 75% and 77% for MRI. The specificity of ^{18}FDG-PET was lower in this study than in previous trials, and the authors speculated that some of the false-positive results might represent cases in which early subclinical involvement had been detected. ^{18}FDG accumulates in cells with augmented glucose uptake, such as inflammatory cells or ischemic myocardial cells.

Angiography

Coronary angiography is usually normal in patients with cardiac sarcoidosis. Right ventricular biopsy may be per-

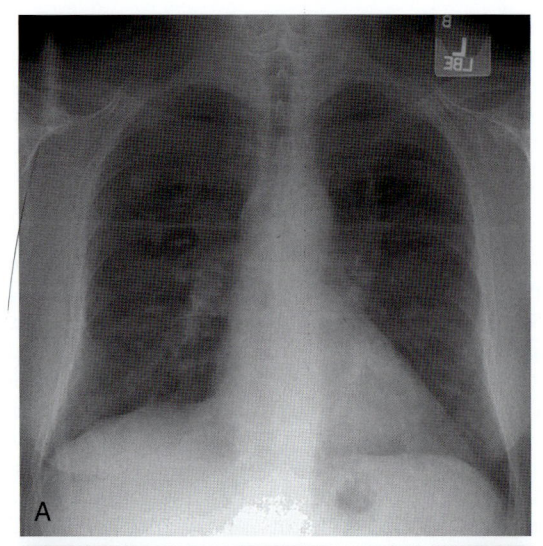

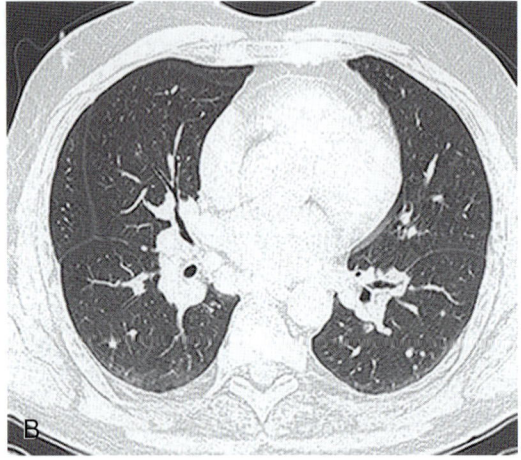

■ **FIGURE 63-10** Pulmonary findings in patient with cardiac sarcoidosis. **A,** Chest x-ray reveals bilateral hilar adenopathy and pulmonary nodules. **B,** Thoracic CT scan shows hilar adenopathy and multiple bilateral pulmonary nodules.

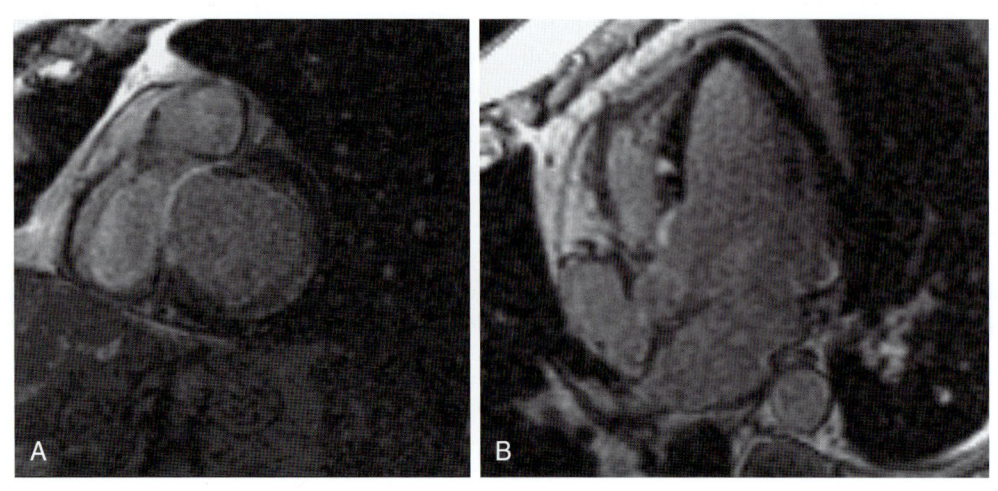

■ **FIGURE 63-11** Cardiac sarcoidosis. **A** and **B,** Short-axis (**A**) and four-chamber (**B**) MDE images reveal thinning and hyperenhancement of the basal septum and lateral wall.

formed in difficult cases; however, the sensitivity of detecting sarcoid granulomas on endomyocardial biopsy specimens is low (20% to 30%) because of the patchy involvement of the myocardium.

ADDITIONAL CAUSES OF RESTRICTIVE CARDIOMYOPATHY

Additional causes of RCM are as follows:

- Cardiac involvement in metabolic storage diseases such as type I or type II glycogenosis, Gaucher disease, Niemann-Pick disease, galactosialidosis, and mucopolysaccharidosis is characterized by LV wall thickening, valvular involvement, and LV diastolic dysfunction with preserved systolic function.
- Patients with diabetes mellitus may develop an RCM with abnormal myocardial relaxation and elevated LV filling pressures. Histologically, these patients have interstitial fibrosis with increased amounts of collagen, glycoprotein, triglycerides, and cholesterol in the myocardial interstitium.
- Radiation-induced myocardial and endocardial fibrosis typically manifest several years after treatment and can result in RCM. Differential diagnosis between constriction and restriction in these patients is particularly difficult because radiation may also induce pericardial fibrosis and constriction.
- Anthracyclines and methysergide have also been reported to cause endomyocardial fibrosis and RCM.
- RCM has been described in a patient with primary hyperoxaluria who had oxalate deposits throughout the myocardium on biopsy specimen.
- Idiopathic RCM can occur sporadically, but may also have a genetic component. Several groups of patients with familial RCM have been described, some in association with Noonan syndrome.

DIFFERENTIAL DIAGNOSIS

Constrictive pericarditis often manifests with signs and symptoms similar to those of RCM and is characterized by abnormal ventricular filling in the setting of normal or near-normal systolic function. Distinguishing between pericardial constriction and RCM is important because the treatment and prognosis are quite different. On imaging, visualization of a thickened pericardium, often with focal distortion of the ventricular contour and atrial enlargement, allows confident diagnosis of constrictive pericarditis. On echocardiography, respiratory-dependent variation in diastolic filling suggests pericardial constriction, and mitral annular velocity is generally normal in pericardial constriction and decreased in RCM.

The absence of pericardial disease on imaging suggests RCM. The imaging findings in RCM may be subtle, and even when a diagnosis of RCM is made, it is often difficult to reach an exact diagnosis. Patients with amyloidosis are occasionally mistakenly thought to have hypertrophic cardiomyopathy, particularly when ventricular thickening is asymmetric, and there is systolic anterior motion of the mitral valve. Common imaging features discussed previously are listed in Table 63-1.

TREATMENT OPTIONS

Medical

The underlying medical treatment options vary based on the underlying cause for the RCM. Cardiac amyloidosis generally has a poor prognosis, with an average survival of 13 months for patients presenting with primary amyloidosis. Medical therapy is provided for symptomatic relief. Oral chemotherapy, including melphalan and prednisone, has shown limited benefits to patients with cardiac involvement. Stem cell transplantation has shown promising results for treatment of primary amyloidosis; however, the mortality associated with transplantation is five times higher in amyloidosis compared with other hematologic malignancies.

Medical therapy for endomyocardial eosinophilic disease includes anticoagulation, diuretics, and digitalis. Corticosteroids, hydroxyurea, cytotoxic drugs, and imatinib all have been employed, with variable results.

Siderotic cardiomyopathy is treated with phlebotomy and chelation therapy. Reduction in myocardial iron content often lags behind the liver.

Sarcoidosis is unique among potential life-threatening disease because many patients do not require treatment. Approximately two thirds of patients experience spontaneous regression.[42] Treatment of cardiac sarcoidosis usually involves corticosteroids, immunosuppressive therapy, or both, although no randomized controlled trials have substantiated their efficacy.

Surgical/Interventional

Surgical treatment is uncommon in RCM. Endocardiectomy has been performed in patients with eosinophilic endomyocardial disease, with relatively high operative mortality. Valve repair or replacement may also be performed in some cases.

INFORMATION FOR THE REFERRING PHYSICIAN

Reports for the referring physician should emphasize the presence or absence of pericardial disease and features suggestive of RCM (see Table 63-1), highlighting the possible etiologies.

KEY POINTS

- RCM is characterized by diastolic dysfunction leading to impairment of ventricular filling caused by stiffening of endocardial, subendocardial, or myocardial tissue.
- RCM is uncommon. Etiologies include amyloidosis, eosinophilic endomyocardial disease, siderotic cardiomyopathy, sarcoidosis, radiation, storage diseases, diabetes, and idiopathic.
- Imaging is helpful to distinguish RCM from constrictive pericarditis.
- The etiology of RCM can sometimes be identified on the basis of a characteristic appearance on imaging; however, findings are often subtle and nonspecific.
- Prognosis for most patients with RCM is poor.

TABLE 63-1 Imaging Features of Restrictive Cardiomyopathies

Disease	Imaging Features
Cardiac amyloidosis	*General*: Ventricular thickening without dilation, dilated atria, pleural and pericardial effusions, diastolic dysfunction with preserved systolic function *Echocardiography*: Granular sparkling myocardium *MRI*: Diffuse circumferential subendocardial enhancement with difficulties achieving suitable myocardial nulling on MDE imaging
Eosinophilic endomyocardial disease	*General*: Apical subendocardial fibrosis and thrombus, atrial enlargement *Echocardiography and angiography*: Apical obliteration *MRI*: Apical subendocardial hyperenhancement with nonenhancing thrombus on MDE
Siderotic cardiomyopathy	*General*: Diffuse diastolic and systolic LV dysfunction *MRI*: Decreased signal intensity on all MRI sequences, but most notably gradient-echo sequences; myocardial iron deposition can be measured using T2 and T2* imaging techniques
Cardiac sarcoidosis	*General*: Mediastinal and hilar adenopathy, regional wall motion abnormalities with involvement of the basal septum *MRI*: Subepicardial hyperenhancement on MDE *Nuclear medicine*: Reverse distribution (resting defects that disappear on stress images) on thallium and sestamibi scintigraphy, focal uptake in cardiac and extracardiac sites with gallium and PET

SUGGESTED READINGS

Dubrey SW, Bell A, Mittal TK. Sarcoid heart disease. Postgrad Med J 2007; 83:618-623.

Hassan W, Al-Sergani H, Mourad W, et al. Amyloid heart disease: new frontiers and insights in pathophysiology, diagnosis, and management. Tex Heart Inst J 2005; 32:178-184.

Shah KB, Inoue Y, Mehra MR. Amyloidosis and the heart. Arch Intern Med 2006; 166:1805-1813.

REFERENCES

1. Richardson P, McKenna W, Bristow M, et al. Report of the 1995 World Health Organization/International Society and Federation of Cardiology Task Force on the Definition and Classification of cardiomyopathies. Circulation 1996; 93:841-842.
2. Kyle RA, Gertz MA. Primary systemic amyloidosis: clinical and laboratory features in 474 cases. Semin Hematol 1995; 32:45-59.
3. Cornwell GG III, Murdoch WL, Kyle RA, et al. Frequency and distribution of senile cardiovascular amyloid: a clinicopathologic correlation. Am J Med 1983; 75:618-623.
4. Hassan W, Al-Sergani H, Mourad W, et al. Amyloid heart disease: new frontiers and insights in pathophysiology, diagnosis, and management. Tex Heart Inst J 2005; 32:178-184.
5. Roberts WC, Waller BF. Cardiac amyloidosis causing cardiac dysfunction: analysis of 54 necropsy patients. Am J Cardiol 1983; 52:137-146.
6. Klein AL, Hatle LK, Taliercio CP, et al. Prognostic significance of Doppler measures of diastolic function in cardiac amyloidosis: a Doppler echocardiography study. Circulation 1991; 83:808-816.
7. Cueto-Garcia L, Roeder GS, Kyle RA, et al. Echocardiographic findings in systemic amyloidosis: spectrum of cardiac involvement and relation to survival. J Am Coll Cardiol 1985; 6:737-743.
8. Ghio S, Perlini S, Palladini G, et al. Importance of the echocardiographic evaluation of right ventricular function in patients with AL amyloidosis. Eur J Heart Fail 2007; 9:808-813.
9. Koyama J, Ray-Sequin PA, Falk RH. Prognostic significance of ultrasound myocardial tissue characterization in patients with cardiac amyloidosis. Circulation 2002; 106:556-561.
10. Bellavia D, Abraham TP, Pellikka PA, et al. Detection of left ventricular systolic dysfunction in cardiac amyloidosis with strain rate echocardiography. J Am Soc Echocardiogr 2007; 20:1194-1202.
11. Celletti F, Fattori R, Napoli G, et al. Assessment of restrictive cardiomyopathy of amyloid or idiopathic etiology by magnetic resonance imaging. Am J Cardiol 1999; 83:798-801.
12. Maceira AM, Joshi J, Prasad SK, et al. Cardiovascular magnetic resonance in cardiac amyloidosis. Circulation 2005; 111:186-193.
13. Krombach GA, Hahn C, Tomars M, et al. Cardiac amyloidosis: MR imaging findings and T1 quantification, comparison with control subjects. J Magn Reson Imaging 2007; 25:1283-1287.
14. Cheng ASH, Banning BP, Mitchell ARJ, et al. Cardiac changes in systemic amyloidosis: visualization by magnetic resonance imaging. Int J Cardiol 2006; 113:e21-e23.
15. Perugini E, Guidalotti PL, Salvi F, et al. Noninvasive etiologic diagnosis of cardiac amyloidosis using 99mTc-3,3-diphosphono-1,2-propanodicarboxylic acid scintigraphy. J Am Coll Cardiol 2005; 46:1076-1084.
16. Marijon E, Ou P. What do we know about endomyocardial fibrosis in children of Africa? Pediatr Cardiol 2006; 27:523-524.
17. Hassan WM, Fawzy ME, Al Helaly S, et al. Pitfalls in diagnosis and clinical, echocardiographic, and hemodynamic findings in endomyocardial fibrosis: a 25-year experience. Chest 2005; 128:3985-3992.
18. Salanitri GC. Endomyocardial fibrosis and intracardiac thrombus occurring in idiopathic hypereosinophilic syndrome. AJR Am J Roentgenol 2005; 184:1432-1433.
19. Syed IS, Martinez MW, Feng DL, et al. Cardiac magnetic resonance imaging of eosinophilic endomyocardial disease. Int J Cardiol 2008; 126:e50-e52.
20. Puvaneswary M, Joshua F, Ratnarajah S. Idiopathic hypereosinophilic syndrome: magnetic resonance imaging findings in endomyocardial fibrosis. Austr Radiol 2001; 45:524-527.
21. Alter P, Maisch B. Endomyocardial fibrosis in Churg-Strauss syndrome assessed by cardiac magnetic resonance imaging. Int J Cardiol 2006; 108:112-113.
22. Namboordiri KK, Bohora S. Images in cardiology: clenched fist appearance in endomyocardial fibrosis. Heart 2006; 92:720.
23. Modell B, Khan M, Darlison M. Survival in beta thalassaemia major in the UK: data from the UK thalassaemia register. Lancet 2000; 355:2051-2052.
24. Hanson EH, Imperatore G, Burke W. HFE gene and hereditary hemochromatosis: a HuGE review. Human Genome Epidemiology. Am J Epidemiol 2001; 154:193-206.

25. Hershko C, Link G, Cabantchik I. Pathophysiology of iron overload. Ann N Y Acad Sci 1998; 850:191-201.
26. Niederau C, Fischer R, Purschel A, et al. Long term survival in patients with hereditary haemochromatosis. Gastroenterology 1996; 110:1107.
27. Palka P, Macdonald G, Lange A, et al. The role of Doppler left ventricular filling indexes and Doppler tissue echocardiography in the assessment of cardiac involvement in hereditary hemochromatosis. J Am Soc Echocardiogr 2002; 15:884-890.
28. Vogel M, Anderson LJ, Holden S, et al. Tissue Doppler echocardiography in patients with thalassaemia detects early myocardial dysfunction related to myocardial iron overload. Eur Heart J 2003; 24:113-119.
29. Wood JC, Otto-Duessel M, Aguilar M, et al. Cardiac iron determines cardiac T2*, T2, and T1 in the gerbil model of iron cardiomyopathy. Circulation 2005; 112:535-543.
30. Anderson LJ, Holden S, Davis B, et al. Cardiovascular T2-star magnetic resonance for the early diagnosis of myocardial iron overload. Eur Heart J 2001; 22:2171-2179.
31. Anderson LJ, Westwood MA, Holden S, et al. Myocardial iron clearance during reversal of siderotic cardiomyopathy with intravenous desferrioxamine: a prospective study using T2* cardiovascular magnetic resonance. Br J Haematol 2004; 127:348-355.
32. Crystal RG. Sarcoidosis. In Kasper DL, Braunwald E, Fauci AS, et al. (eds.) Harrison's Principles of Internal Medicine, 16th ed. New York, McGraw-Hill, 2005, pp 2017-2023.
33. Sharma O, Maheshawari A, Thaler K. Myocardial sarcoidosis. Chest 1993; 103:253-258.
34. Ratner SJ, Fenoglio JJ Jr, Ursell PC. Utility of endomyocardial biopsy in the diagnosis of cardiac sarcoidosis. Chest 1986; 90:528-533.
35. Iwai K, Sekiguti M, Hosoda Y, et al. Racial difference in cardiac sarcoidosis incidence observed at autopsy. Sarcoidosis 1994; 11:26-31.
36. Chestnutt AN. Enigmas in sarcoidosis. West J Med 1995; 162:519-526.
37. Lewin RF, Mor R, Spitzer S, et al. Echocardiographic evaluation of patients with systemic sarcoidosis. Am J Cardiol 1989; 63:478-482.
38. Burstow DJ, Tajik J, Baily KR, et al. Two-dimensional echocardiographic findings in systemic sarcoidosis. Am Heart J 1985; 110:116-122.
39. Smedema JP, Snoep G, van Kroonenburgh MPG, et al. Evaluation of the accuracy of gadolinium-enhanced cardiovascular magnetic resonance in the diagnosis of cardiac sarcoidosis. J Am Coll Cardiol 2005; 45:1683-1690.
40. Patel MR, Cawley PJ, Heitner JF, et al. Delayed enhanced MRI improves the ability to detect cardiac involvement in patients with sarcoidosis (abstract). Circulation 2004; 110(Suppl):2995.
41. Ohira H, Tsujino I, Ishimaru S, et al. Myocardial imaging with 18F FDG positron emission tomography and magnetic resonance imaging in sarcoidosis. Eur J Nucl Med Mol Imaging 2008; 35:933-941.
42. Dubrey SW, Bell A, Mittal TK. Sarcoid heart disease. Postgrad Med J 2007; 83:618-623.

CHAPTER 64

Hypertrophic Cardiomyopathy

Gautham P. Reddy, Matthew J. Sharp, and Karen G. Ordovas

Hypertrophic cardiomyopathy (HCM) is distinguished by hypertrophy of either ventricle in the absence of a known cause, such as hypertension or aortic stenosis. The purpose of this chapter is to discuss the clinical features of HCM and imaging evaluation, with a focus on magnetic resonance imaging (MRI) for morphologic and functional assessment and for monitoring response to therapy.

PREVALENCE AND EPIDEMIOLOGY

The incidence of HCM is reported to be as high as 1/500 individuals, making it the most common genetically inherited cardiovascular disease.[1] Nevertheless, HCM is thought to represent no more than 1% of cardiac outpatients,[1] suggesting that many genetically affected individuals remain asymptomatic for most or all of their lives.

ETIOLOGY AND PATHOPHYSIOLOGY

HCM is inherited as an autosomal dominant trait with variable penetrance. The distribution of hypertrophy in HCM is variable, with septal, right ventricular, left ventricular, septal, apical, midventricular, or concentric patterns. Asymmetric hypertrophy of the ventricular septum is by far the most common.[2] Histologically, HCM is characterized by myofibrillar disarray.[1]

MANIFESTATIONS OF DISEASE

Clinical Presentation

The clinical presentation of HCM varies from asymptomatic to sudden cardiac death, which is the leading cause of mortality in affected patients. HCM is responsible for approximately one third of cases of sudden cardiac death in young athletes.[3] The mechanism for sudden cardiac death is ventricular fibrillation.[4] The 1-year mortality rate for clinically evident HCM is approximately 1% to 4%.[2]

Risk stratification has been advocated to help define those patients who may benefit most from antiarrhythmic therapy or an implantable cardiac defibrillator.[4] Ventricular wall thickness more than 30 mm has been shown to be an independent risk factor for sudden cardiac death.[5] The positive predictive value of hypertrophy more than 30 mm is greatly increased when other risk factors are taken into account.[6] More than 90% of patients with HCM have asymmetric septal hypertrophy. Other distributions of hypertrophy include apical, midventricular, and concentric.

In addition to sudden cardiac death, atrial fibrillation and heart failure represent the major morbidities associated with HCM. Atrial fibrillation is encountered in up to 25% of patients.[1] Heart failure in HCM is most often caused by diastolic dysfunction. In patients with significant septal hypertrophy, heart failure may also be attributed to left ventricular outflow tract obstruction.[2]

Imaging Techniques and Findings

Ultrasound

Patients clinically suspected to have hypertrophic cardiomyopathy are initially referred for echocardiography.[2] Asymmetric septal hypertrophy is the most common finding. Septal thickening of 13 to 15 mm or more and a septal-to-posterior wall ratio of 1.5:1 or higher have been the usual definitions of septal hypertrophy.[7] In general, however, any abnormal hypertrophy noted on echocardiography that is not otherwise explained raises the suspicion of HCM.

Computed Tomography

Computed tomography (CT) has been shown to demonstrate morphologic and functional abnormalities in HCM (Fig. 64-1). Multidetector helical CT allows the acquisition

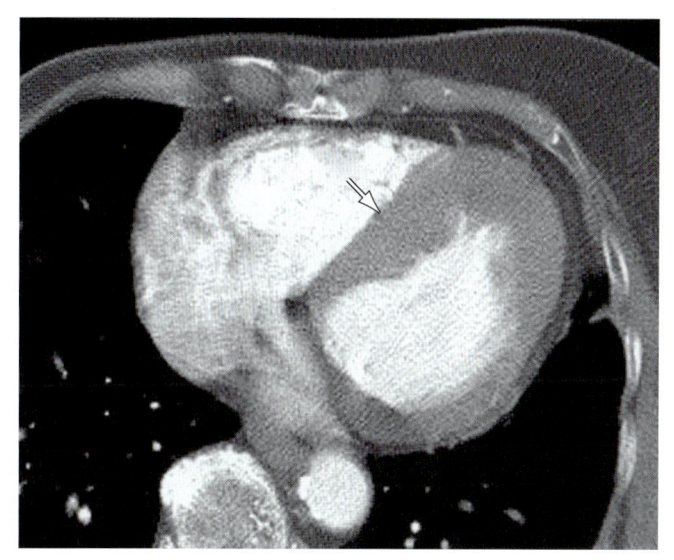

FIGURE 64-1 CT for hypertrophic cardiomyopathy. Contrast-enhanced CT image shows asymmetric septal hypertrophy (*arrow*) in a patient with hypertrophic cardiomyopathy.

TABLE 64-1 Selected Magnetic Resonance Imaging Sequences Used for Hypertrophic Cardiomyopathy

Sequence	Indications and Use	Imaging Plane
Black blood (double-inversion recovery)	Distribution of hypertrophy Identification of intramural cardiac mass	Coronal Axial
Steady-state free precession cine	Cardiac function and wall motion LVOT obstruction (signal void) Mitral valve motion and regurgitation Measurement of myocardial mass	Short axis Long axis (four-chamber view)
First-pass perfusion imaging	Perfusion deficit Perfusion reserve	Short axis
Delayed hyperenhancement imaging	Abnormal or nonviable myocardium Evaluation of alcohol septal wall ablation	Short axis Long axis (four-chamber view)
Velocity-encoded cine	Coronary flow reserve	Orthogonal to coronary sinus

LVOT, left ventricular outflow tract.

of multiphase imaging relatively free of motion, as well as three-dimensional reformations. Reports applying electrocardiographically gated helical CT to the assessment of HCM are encouraging.[8] However, CT has disadvantages, including the use of ionizing radiation and iodinated contrast agent, as well as limited contrast resolution.

Magnetic Resonance Imaging

MRI with electrocardiographic gating provides excellent depictions of cardiac anatomy in hypertrophic cardiomyopathy. MRI can be used for accurate identification of the site and extent of ventricular hypertrophy and subaortic stenosis, and for quantification of myocardial mass.[9] MRI also differentiates septal hypertrophy from septal neoplasm, an important distinction, because the two entities may present with similar symptoms.[10]

MRI can be used for precise and reproducible quantification of left ventricular function, including the measurement of stroke volume, ejection fraction, and mass. MRI can also be used to assess the presence and functional significance of mitral regurgitation and left ventricular outflow tract obstruction.[11] The response of left ventricular outflow tract obstruction to therapy, including septal myectomy and percutaneous transluminal septal wall ablation, has also been demonstrated with MRI.[12] Abnormal systolic wall thickening, a sign of myocardial dysfunction, may be seen in patients with HCM using MRI.[11] In addition, MRI is able to identify associated perfusion abnormalities, such as impaired global perfusion, diminished coronary flow reserve, and isolated perfusion deficits.[13] MRI also may be used to detect abnormal myocardial architecture caused by fibrosis or necrosis.[14]

In patients with suspected HCM not fully assessed by echocardiography, MRI offers improved detection of disease. Specifically, echocardiography is often of limited value in the assessment of the anterior and lateral left ventricular wall and of the ventricular apex.[15] Without the limits of acoustic windows inherent in echocardiography, MRI demonstrates myocardial thickening regardless of location. In addition, the high reproducibility of MRI is an advantage compared with echocardiography in monitoring regression or progression of left ventricular mass in response to therapy.

Morphology

MRI readily shows the location and extent of ventricular hypertrophy. Patients are referred for MRI when echocardiography is nondiagnostic because of a poor acoustic window or when echocardiographic evaluation of myocardial segments is incomplete. End-diastolic ventricular thickness of 1.5 cm or more on MRI scans is a commonly used indicator of HCM in patients without hypertension, aortic stenosis, or other explanations for hypertrophy.[16] Asymmetric hypertrophy is demonstrated by calculating a ratio of wall thickness, such as septal to posterolateral thickness.[16] Electrocardiographically gated black blood and white blood steady-state free precession MRI sequences in the short- and long-axis planes ensure that all myocardial segments are clearly visualized (Table 64-1; Fig. 64-2).[17]

Asymmetric septal hypertrophy is the most common distribution of hypertrophy in HCM.[1] MRI readily demonstrates septal hypertrophy in patients with HCM (Fig. 64-3).[11] Other patterns, such as apical hypertrophy (Fig. 64-4), midventricular hypertrophy, concentric hypertrophy (Fig. 64-5), and right ventricular hypertrophy (Fig. 64-6) are also well visualized by MRI.[15] In particular, the usefulness of MRI for apical HCM has been emphasized.[16] Defining the location of hypertrophy is of clinical importance because some forms of HCM, such as apical HCM, have a more favorable prognosis and because treatment may depend on the distribution of hypertrophy.[2]

Ventricular mass can be used as a predictor of prognosis in patients with HCM.[13] The myocardial mass can be calculated accurately with MRI (Fig. 64-7).[17] Echocardio-

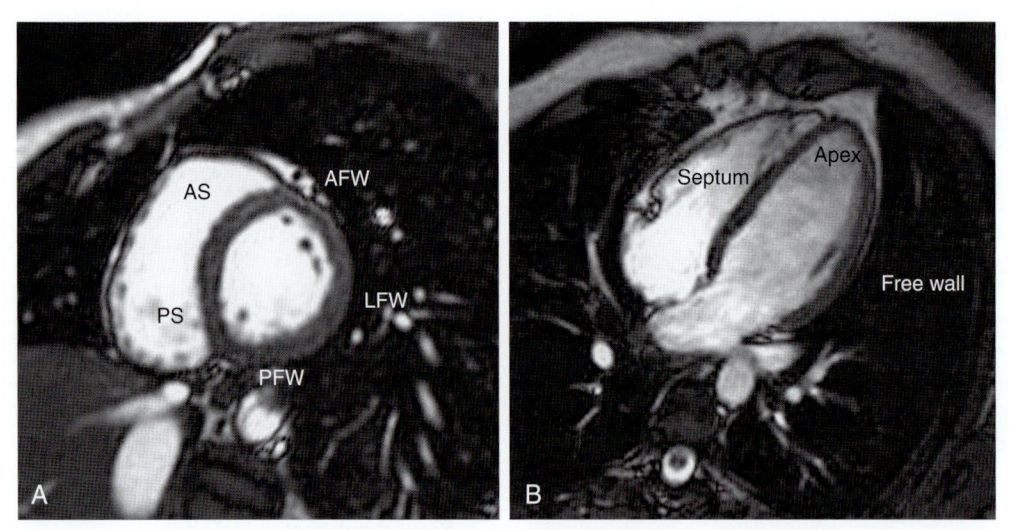

FIGURE 64-2 Normal cardiac anatomy. Steady-state free precession cine MR short-axis and horizontal long-axis images of the heart define the various cardiac regions affected by hypertrophic cardiomyopathy. **A,** Short-axis images. The left ventricle is divided into five equal segments—anteroseptal (AS), posteroseptal (PS), anterior free wall (AFW), lateral free wall (LFW), and posterior free wall (PFW). **B,** Horizontal long-axis images are divided into three segments—septum, apex, and free wall.

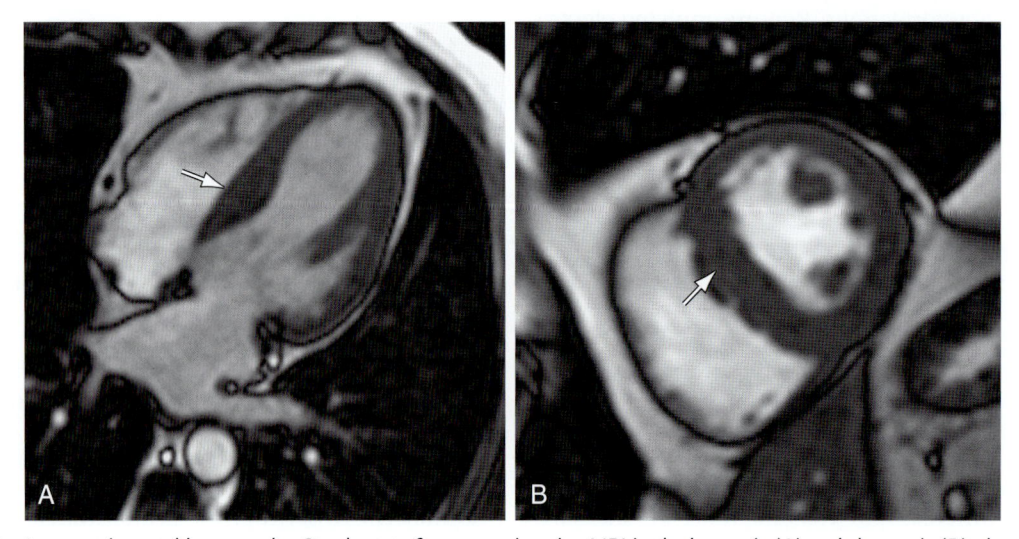

FIGURE 64-3 Asymmetric septal hypertrophy. Steady-state free precession cine MRI in the long-axis (**A**) and short-axis (**B**) planes demonstrate hypertrophy (*arrows*) of the interventricular septum, with a maximal thickness of 1.7 cm and septal-to-posterior wall ratio of 1.8.

graphically derived masses are the product of several measurements entered into a formula that relies on geometric assumptions regarding cardiac morphology. Given the variable nature of hypertrophy encountered with HCM, these assumptions are often incorrect and lead to erroneous mass values.[14] Importantly, the interstudy reproducibility of left ventricular mass measurement with MRI is less than 5%,[18] so MRI is the procedure of choice for monitoring left ventricular mass over time and in response to therapy.

Cardiac Neoplasms

Focal hypertrophic cardiomyopathy can be difficult to distinguish from an intramural cardiac mass on echocardiography. MRI can be used to differentiate HCM from a neoplasm.[10,19] Images obtained using MR tagging can identify active myocardial contraction; whereas focal HCM may exhibit decreased systolic thickening or abnormal wall motion, the absence of identifiable contraction suggests a neoplasm.[19] Gadolinium-enhanced MRI can also distinguish a cardiac mass from HCM (Fig. 64-8).[10]

Cardiac Function

MRI permits the quantitative analysis of cardiac function in patients with HCM. Compared with echocardiography, MRI assessment of cardiac function has the advantages of high reproducibility and operator independence. MRI is therefore ideal for patient monitoring. Stroke volume, ejection fraction, and cardiac output may all be calculated (Fig. 64-9). Although often clinically insignificant, mild diastolic dysfunction is the most common functional abnormality seen in HCM, often with an increased ejection fraction in the setting of decreased stroke volume and cardiac output.[1] Patients with end-stage HCM may exhibit systolic dysfunction caused by progressive myocardial fibrosis, which can cause ventricular wall thinning and dilation.[2]

Abnormal wall motion may be noted in some patients with HCM. MRI scans obtained using myocardial tagging can demonstrate reduced wall motion in areas of hypertrophy and impaired systolic thickening.[20] Cine MR images can also be used to show impaired systolic thickening (Fig. 64-10).[21]

Myocardial Perfusion

MRI can be used to demonstrate impaired myocardial perfusion and perfusion reserve in patients with HCM.[13] First-pass gadolinium MRI allows the direct visualization of impaired perfusion. First-pass images both before and after administration of coronary vasodilator agent are analyzed to determine perfusion reserve. First-pass gadolinium imaging has correlated decreased perfusion reserve to both the site and extent of ventricular hypertrophy.[13]

Viability

Delayed hyperenhancement MRI can be used to differentiate viable myocardial tissue from areas of fibrosis that presumably result from previous ischemia and infarction.[14] Because gadolinium chelate contrast agent cannot cross cell membranes, it accumulates in regions of fibrosis because of slow distribution kinetics and expansion of extracellular space.[22,23] MRI performed 10 to 15 minutes following contrast agent administration may demonstrate this accumulation of gadolinium–diethylenetriamine penta-acetic acid (Gd-DTPA; Fig. 64-11). In HCM, delayed hyperenhancement has been shown in the most hypertrophied areas.[14] Areas of delayed hyperenhancement exhibit reduced systolic wall thickening, an indicator of decreased myocardial function.[24] The presence and severity of

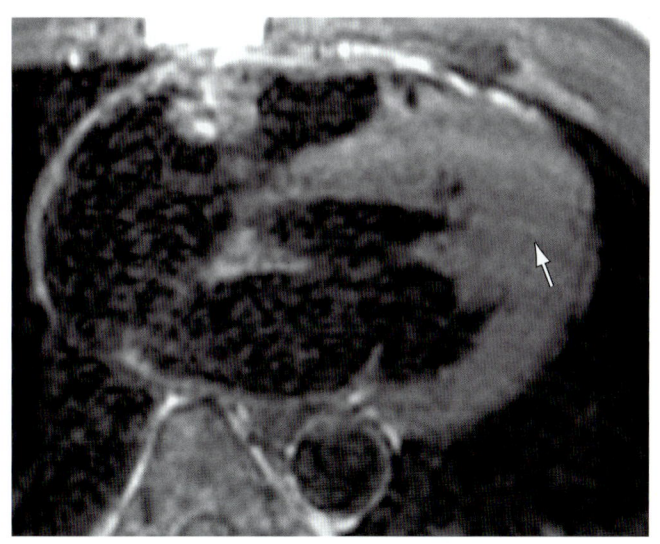

FIGURE 64-4 Apical HCM. This axial black blood image shows hypertrophy of the apical region of the left ventricle, with a maximal thickness of 3.1 cm. A wall thickness of 1.5 cm or more indicates hypertrophy. The septum and free wall are within normal limits.

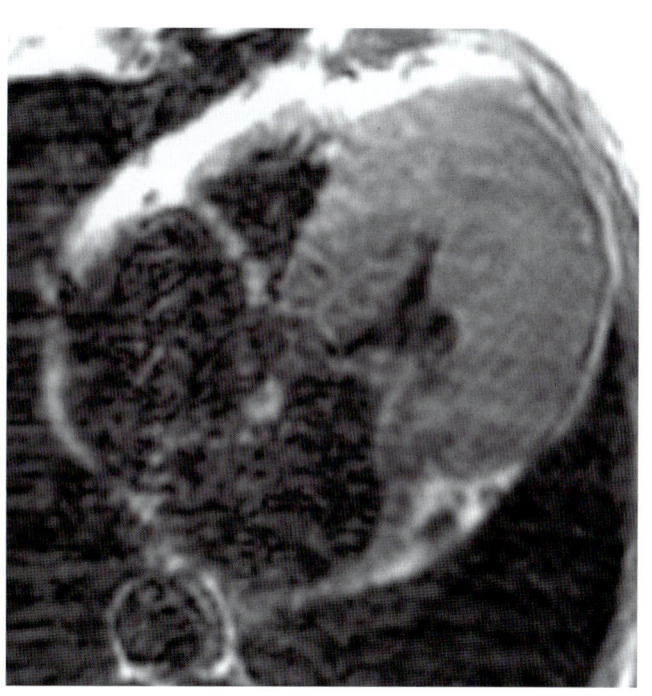

FIGURE 64-5 Concentric hypertrophy. This axial black blood MRI scan reveals hypertrophy of the entire left ventricle, with a septal thickness of 2.3 cm, apical thickness of 3.4 cm, and left ventricular free wall thickness of 2.7 cm.

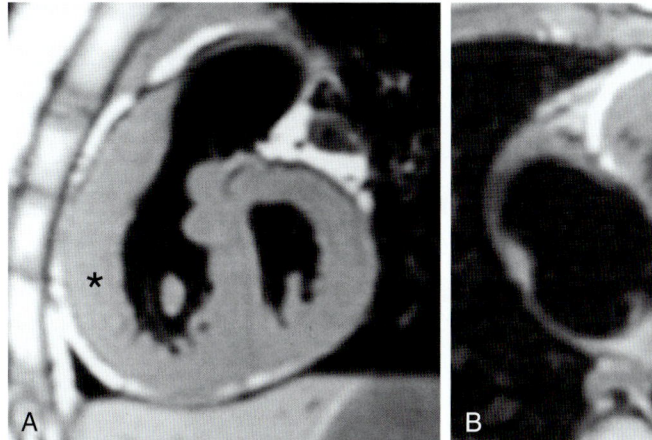

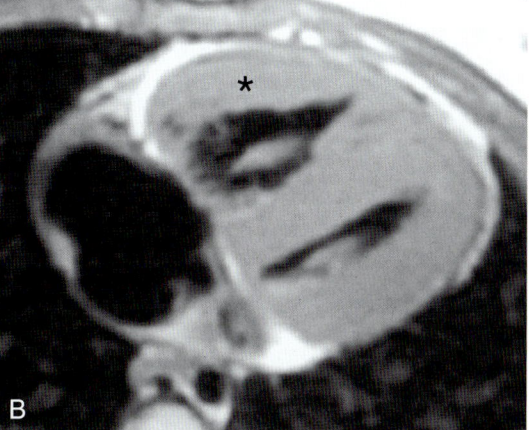

FIGURE 64-6 Right ventricular involvement of HCM. Sagittal (A) and axial black blood (B) MRI scans images show marked RV hypertrophy (*asterisks*) and concentric left ventricular hypertrophy.

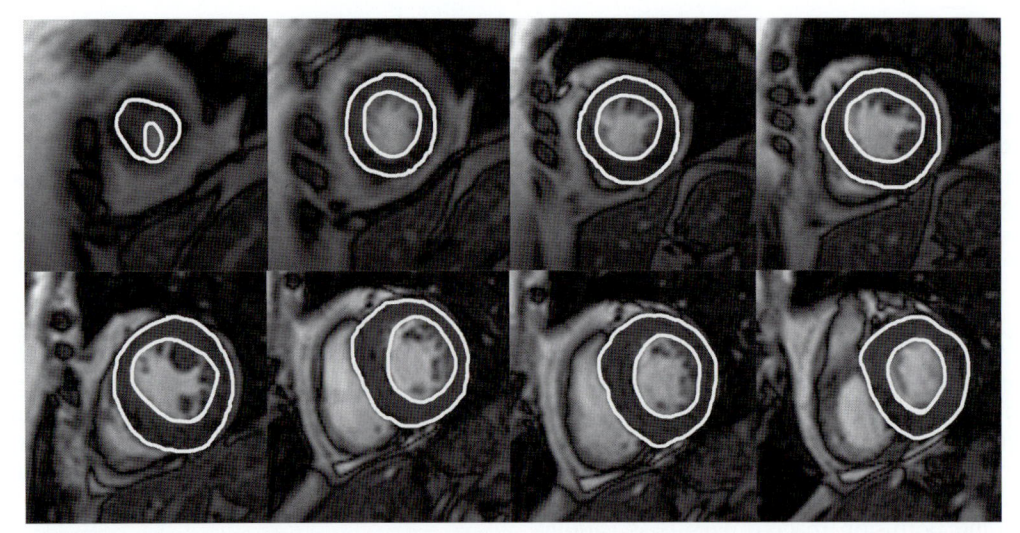

FIGURE 64-7 Quantification of left ventricular mass. Myocardial mass is obtained by multiplying the myocardial volume by the myocardial specific gravity (1.05 g/mL). To estimate the myocardial volume of the left ventricle, cine MR images are selected at end-diastole from the cardiac apex to the cardiac base. The epicardium and endocardium are then outlined on each image. The area enclosed between the epicardium and endocardium is multiplied by the slice thickness, and the values are summed across the entire ventricle, yielding the total left ventricular volume. The normalized left ventricular mass (left ventricular mass index) equals mass divided by body surface area. In this 69-year-old woman, left ventricular mass = 149 g, left ventricular mass index = 55 g/m^2. Normal left ventricular mass index = 78 g/m^2 ± 17 g/m^2 in men and 61 g/m^2 ± 14 g/m^2 in women.

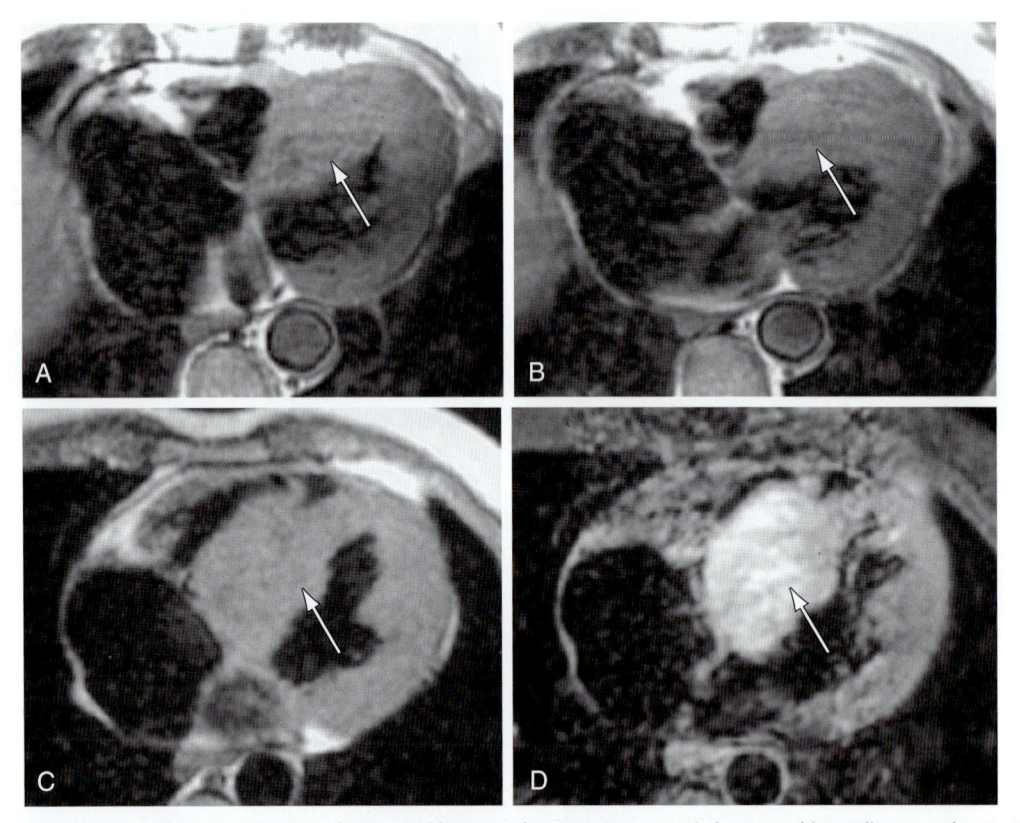

FIGURE 64-8 Differentiation of cardiac neoplasm from septal hypertrophy. **A, B,** Asymmetric hypertrophic cardiomyopathy. **A,** Axial black blood MR image demonstrates septal thickening (*arrow*). **B,** Gadolinium-enhanced axial black blood image shows only mild enhancement of the septal wall (*arrow*), consistent with the diagnosis of hypertrophic cardiomyopathy. **C, D,** Angiosarcoma. **C,** Axial black blood MR image illustrates increased thickness of the septum (*arrow*). **D,** Gadolinium-enhanced axial black blood MR image demonstrates marked septal enhancement (*arrow*), consistent with neoplasm. Endomyocardial biopsy established the diagnosis of angiosarcoma.

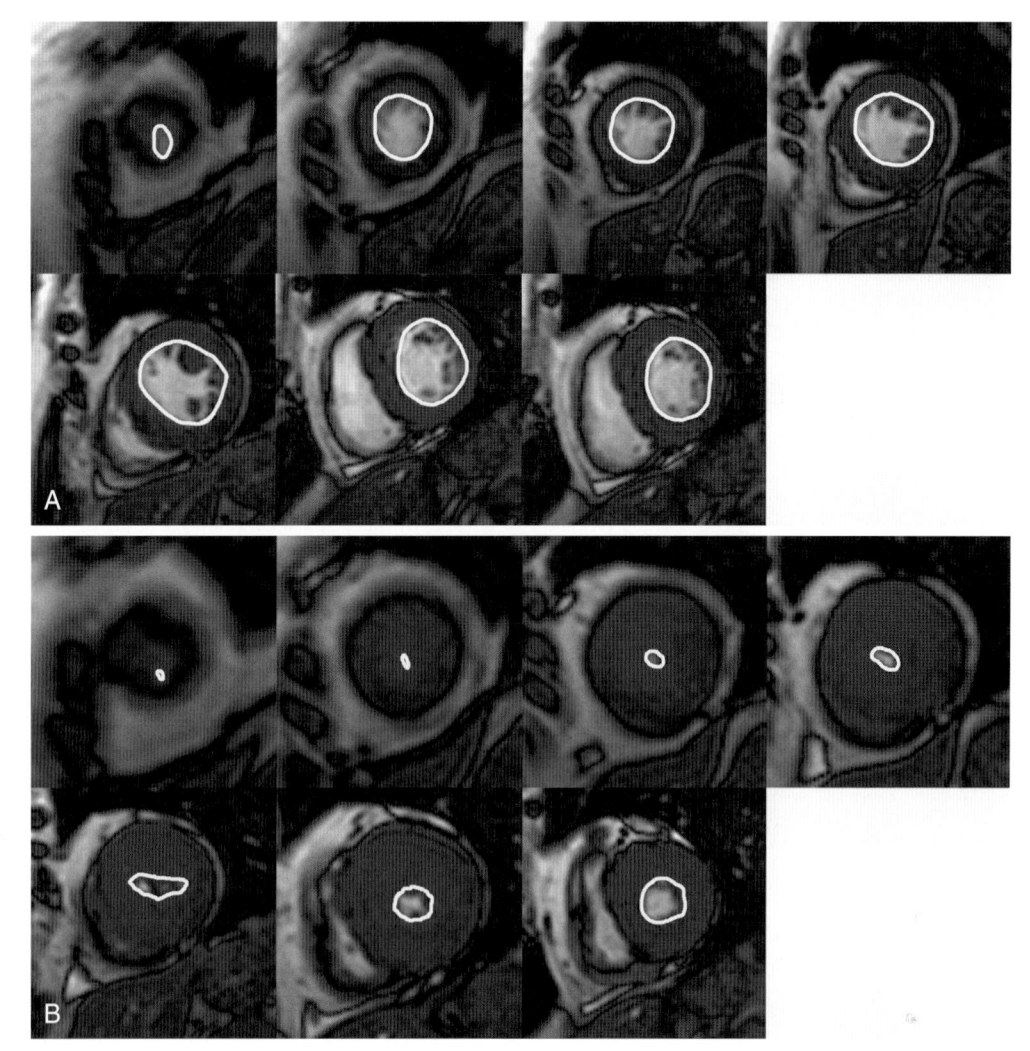

■ **FIGURE 64-9** Calculation of ejection fraction, stroke volume, and cardiac output. Shown are end-diastolic (**A**) and end-systolic (**B**) images from the cardiac apex to the base. These are cine MR images obtained in the short-axis plane. The endocardium is outlined on each image. The area that is outlined is multiplied by the slice thickness and summated across all the slice locations; the sum, from apex to base, yields the total ventricle chamber volume at end-systole and end-diastole. From these values, one can determine the stroke volume (end-diastolic volume minus end-systolic volume), ejection fraction (stroke volume divided by end-diastolic volume), and cardiac output (stroke volume multiplied by heart rate). In this patient, end-diastolic volume = 89 mL and end-systolic volume = 13 mL, stroke volume = 76 mL, ejection fraction = 86%, and cardiac output = 4.6 L/min. Normal ejection fraction for men = 69% and for women = 70%.[29]

delayed hyperenhancement in HCM may be related to a worse prognosis.

Coronary Flow Reserve

Abnormal coronary vasculature and a mismatch between myocardial mass and coronary circulation are thought to be responsible for impaired coronary flow reserve and intermittent myocardial ischemia.[1] The result of these processes is myocyte death, with subsequent fibrosis. The areas of scarring in the setting of acute ischemia, hypotension, or intense physical exertion may be the arrythmogenic substrate responsible for sudden cardiac death by ventricular tachycardia or ventricular fibrillation.[1]

Quantification of coronary flow reserve is possible with MRI.[24] Velocity-encoded cine phase contrast MRI through the coronary sinus permits measurement of coronary flow. Patients with HCM have impairment of coronary flow reserve.[24]

Left Ventricular Outflow Tract Obstruction

In patients with asymmetric septal HCM, left ventricular outflow tract obstruction can result from severe septal hypertrophy or systolic anterior motion of the anterior mitral leaflet. Patients with left ventricular outflow tract obstruction may suffer from angina, dyspnea, or syncope, even on minimal exertion. Identification of left ventricular outflow tract obstruction is an important clinical goal, because patients may benefit from invasive therapy such as septal myectomy or percutaneous septal wall ablation. The severity of outflow tract obstruction is reflected in the pressure gradient across the outflow tract. Surgical or transcathether septal myomectomy is often advocated when the pressure gradient is more than 30 mm Hg.[6]

Because of its high reproducibility and interobserver agreement, MRI is superior to echocardiography for patient monitoring in left ventricular outflow tract obstruction. This is especially true when the feasibility and subsequent efficacy of medical or surgical management must be

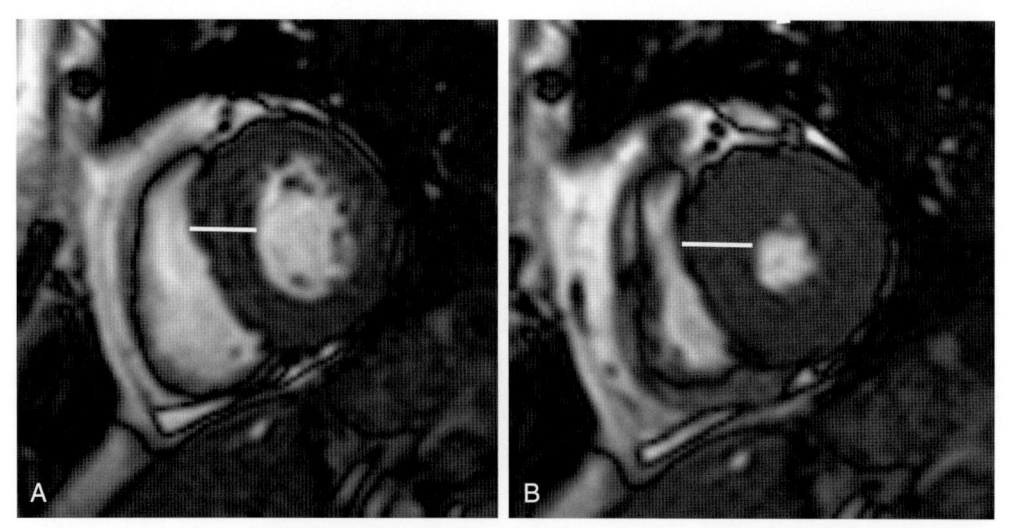

■ **FIGURE 64-10** Impaired systolic thickening in HCM. End-systolic and end-diastolic images are selected at the region of maximal hypertrophy. Systolic thickening can be expressed as fractional thickening (end-systolic thickness/end-systolic thickness) or as a percentage ([end-systolic thickness − end-diastolic thickness]/end-diastolic thickness). End-diastolic **(A)** and end-systolic **(B)** short-axis cine MR images at the cardiac base. **A,** Maximal end-diastolic septal wall thickness is 2.1 cm (*white line*). **B,** Maximal end-systolic septal thickness is 2.2 cm (*white line*). Fractional thickening = 1.1 and percentage thickening = 6%, which is markedly reduced. Normal septal thickening at the cardiac base is approximately 49%.

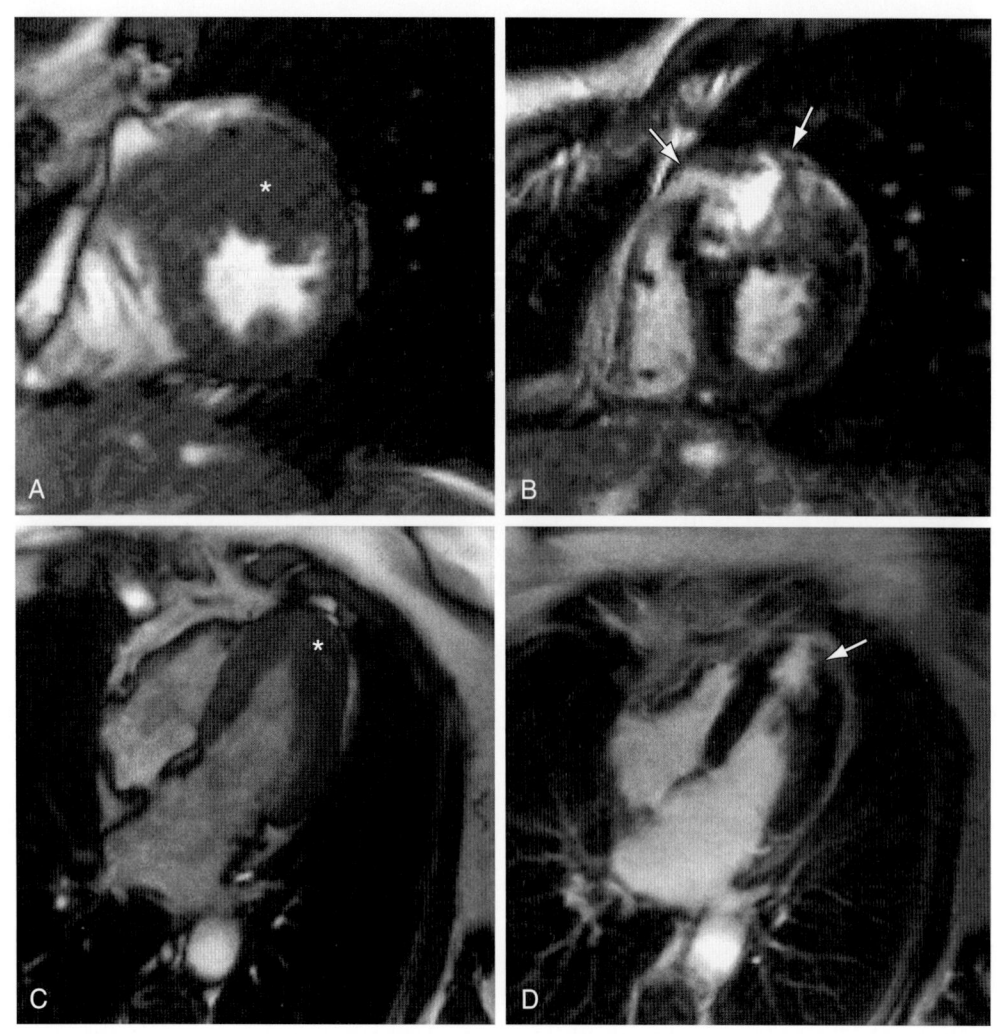

■ **FIGURE 64-11** Delayed hyperenhancement in HCM. Gadolinium chelate contrast agent cannot cross cell membranes and therefore builds up in regions of fibrosis. To demonstrate delayed hyperenhancement, MRI scans are obtained approximately 10 to 15 minutes following the intravenous administration of gadolinium chelate contrast agent. **A, B,** Delayed hyperenhancement in asymmetric septal HCM. **A,** Cine MR image in the cardiac short-axis shows asymmetric septal hypertrophy, with maximum hypertrophy in the anterior interventricular septum and anterior free wall (*asterisk*). **B,** Delayed hyperenhancement image obtained 12 minutes after contrast administration in the same patient demonstrates persistent enhancement in the region of maximal hypertrophy (*arrows*). **C, D,** Delayed hyperenhancement in apical HCM. **C,** MR examination in the horizontal long axis illustrates a patient with apical hypertrophic cardiomyopathy (*asterisk*). **D,** Delayed hyperenhancement MRI scan obtained 10 minutes after contrast administration demonstrates delayed hyperenhancement at the cardiac apex (*arrow*). (*From Bogaert J, Goldstein M, Tannouri F, et al. Late myocardial enhancement in hypertrophic cardiomyopathy with contrast-enhanced MRI. AJR Am J Roentgenol 2003; 180:981-985.*)

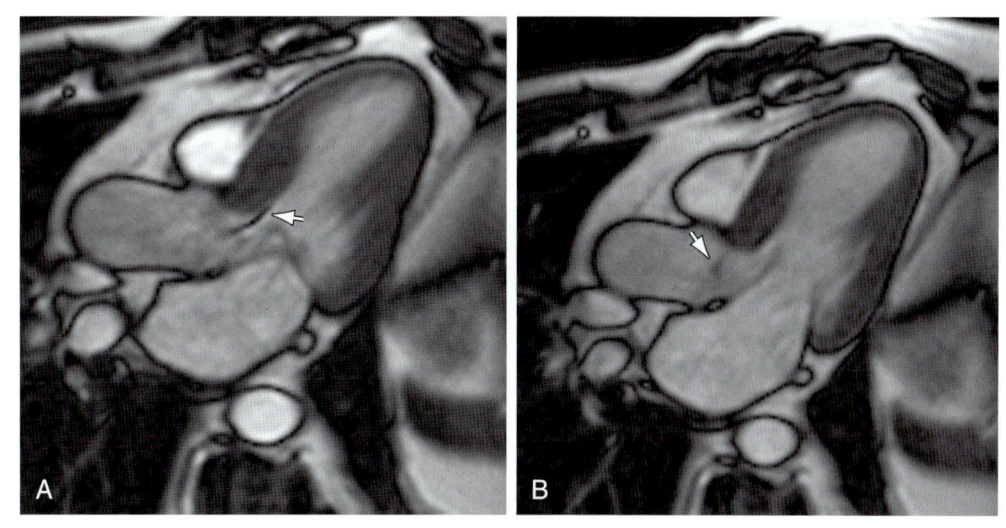

■ **FIGURE 64-12** Left ventricular outflow tract obstruction. Signal void on cine MR images represents a high-velocity jet, implying a flow obstruction or stenosis. The blood in the area of the signal void moves out of the imaging plane too quickly to produce a signal. Asymmetric HCM often causes an obstruction in the left ventricular outflow tract, which causes a signal void on cine MRI scans. **A**, Left ventricular outflow tract cine MR image at late systole demonstrates a signal void (*arrow*) in the left ventricular outflow tract, proximal to the level of the aortic valve. **B**, Early diastolic image at the same level shows the location of the aortic valve (*arrow*).

evaluated. MRI can identify left ventricular outflow tract obstruction in a number of ways. Obstruction is frequently visualized on steady-state free precession cine MR images as a signal void, representing a high-velocity jet in the outflow tract (Fig. 64-12). MRI can directly depict the outflow tract region, and decreased outflow tract area in patients can be quantified.[12]

Systolic anterior motion of the anterior mitral valve leaflet is the most common cause of left ventricular outflow tract obstruction in patients with septal HCM; it also leads to mitral regurgitation. Cine MR images in the horizontal long-axis plane can depict the anterior mitral leaflet adjacent to or near the septum in systole.[21] Mitral regurgitation is visualized with MRI as a systolic signal void emanating from the mitral valve into the left atrium (Fig. 64-13).[17] MRI can be used for qualitative or quantitative characterization of the severity of regurgitation.[25]

Therapy

Invasive therapy for left ventricular outflow tract obstruction is considered when medical management has failed to control symptoms in patients with severe heart failure (NYHA Class III or IV) and a significant outflow tract pressure gradient.[26] Current options include surgical myotomy or myectomy of the septal wall and alcohol septal myocardial ablation.[1,26]

Surgical myotomy or myectomy is a proven technique, with subjective improvement of symptoms in 70% of patients and a mortality of less than 2%. However, there are few centers skilled in these techniques, and many patients are not candidates for surgery given the advanced nature of their disease.[1] Following surgical myotomy or myectomy, MRI can verify improvement of outflow tract obstruction by demonstrating reduction of the signal void in the outflow tract and decrease of the systolic anterior motion of the mitral valve. Moreover, left ventricular function and mass can be measured and compared with pre-surgical values.

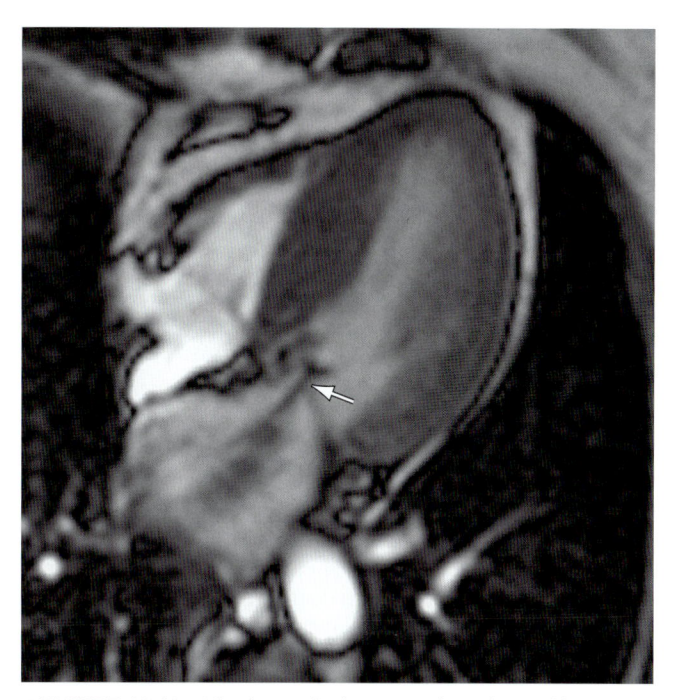

■ **FIGURE 64-13** Mitral regurgitation occurs in patients with asymmetric septal HCM as a consequence of systolic anterior motion of the mitral valve. The presence of mitral regurgitation also implies that a pressure gradient exists in the left ventricular outflow tract. Mitral regurgitation is seen on steady-state free precession cine MRI scans as a signal void that represents a high-velocity jet. In this patient, horizontal long-axis cine MRI scanning in early systole clearly demonstrates a signal void at the level of the mitral valve, extending into the left atrium (*arrow*).

Alcohol septal myocardial ablation is a technique whereby a septal perforator branch of the left anterior descending artery is selectively catheterized and injected with ethanol, causing limited septal infarction.[27] Preliminary studies have shown that this technique has been successful, as judged by a reduction in the pressure gradi-

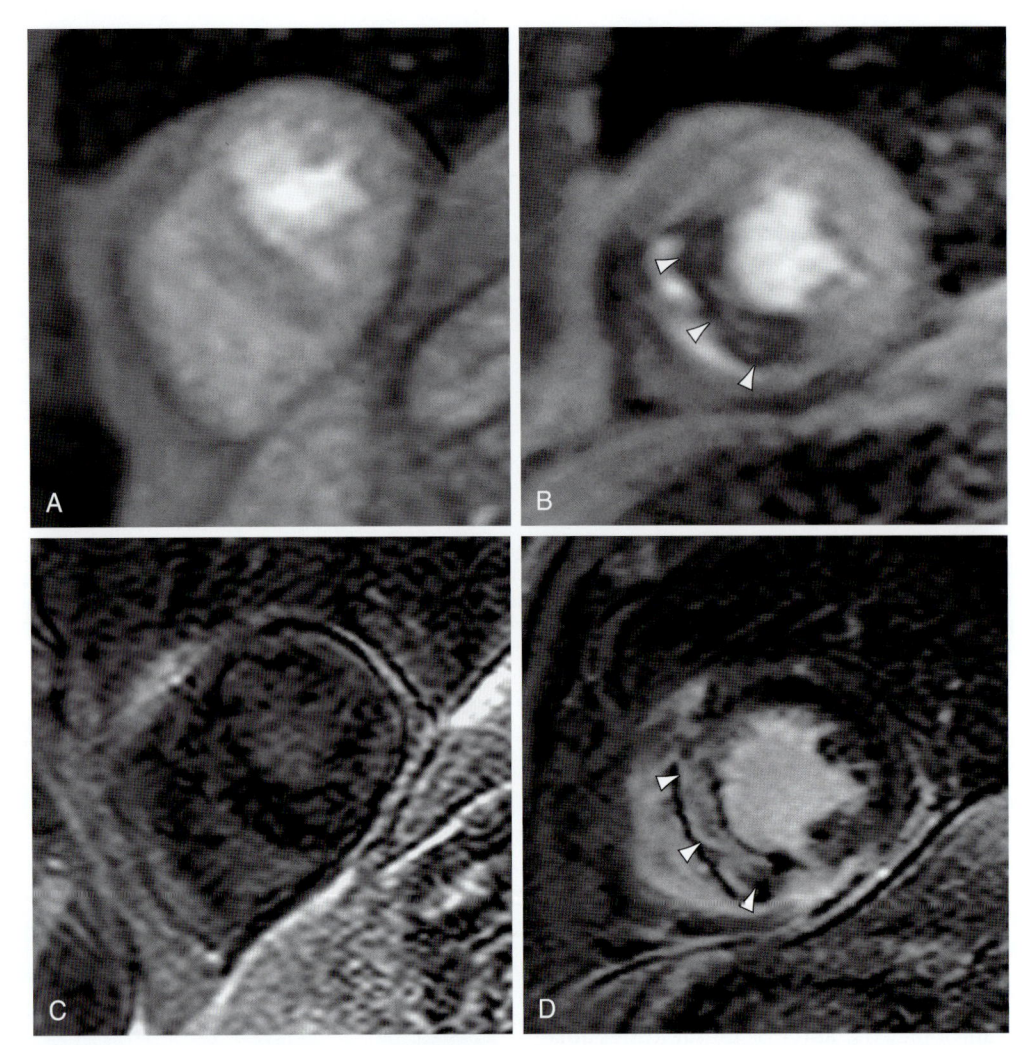

FIGURE 64-14 MR evaluation of alcohol septal myocardial ablation. **A, B,** First-pass MRI. **A,** First-pass perfusion MRI performed before alcohol septal ablation demonstrates normal myocardial perfusion in the septal wall. **B,** Following septal ablation, a significant perfusion deficit is noted in the septal wall (*arrowheads*), depending on patient chosen). **C, D,** Delayed hyperenhancement MRI. **C,** MRI performed 10 minutes after administration of gadolinium chelate demonstrates no areas of enhancement before intervention, implying a normal, viable myocardium. **D,** There is dramatic late hyperenhancement in the septal wall (*arrowheads*) following alcohol septal ablation, indicating nonviable myocardium.

ent across the outflow tract and by symptomatic improvement.[28] MRI offers a useful method to evaluate patients selected for alcohol septal myocardial ablation (Fig. 64-14). A perfusion defect and delayed hyperenhancement are noted after treatment, clearly demonstrating the location and extent of infarcted myocardium. Hypokinesis of the septal wall is readily displayed on cine MR images following intervention.

Angiography

Cardiac catheterization is also performed in cases of HCM, most often to address a particular clinical concern. Catheterization may be performed to determine the magnitude of outflow tract obstruction caused by septal hypertrophy by measuring pressures proximal and distal to the obstruction.[12] Also, catheterization is performed when invasive therapy, such as myectomy or percutaneous transluminal septal wall ablation, is being considered.[13] Angiographic ventriculograms may reveal a characteristic deformity of the left ventricle at end-systole in some forms of HCM, such as the apical form.[1]

SYNOPSIS OF TREATMENT OPTIONS

Surgical and Interventional

In patients with hypertrophic cardiomyopathy, surgical treatment via septal myectomy has traditionally been used.[5] Percutaneous transluminal septal myocardial ablation with ethanol has shown promising success in the treatment of significant outflow obstruction.[9,10]

KEY POINTS

- Echocardiography is the initial imaging modality for the evaluation of HCM
- MRI offers comprehensive assessment of the morphologic and functional characteristics of HCM.
- The ability to delineate uncommon patterns and locations of hypertrophy is an advantage of MRI.
- MRI is capable of delineating myocardial perfusion and viability, coronary flow abnormalities, and pre- and post-treatment evaluation

SUGGESTED READINGS

Hansen MW, Merchant N. MRI of hypertrophic cardiomyopathy: part I, MRI appearances. AJR Am J Roentgenol 2007; 189:1335-1343.

Hansen MW, Merchant N. MRI of hypertrophic cardiomyopathy: part 2, Differential diagnosis, risk stratification, and posttreatment MRI appearances. AJR Am J Roentgenol 2007; 189:1344-1352.

REFERENCES

1. Maron BJ. Hypertrophic cardiomyopathy: a systematic review. JAMA 2002; 287:1308-1320.
2. Wigle ED. Cardiomyopathy: the diagnosis of hypertrophic cardiomyopathy. Heart 2001; 86:709-714.
3. Maron BJ. Sudden death in young athletes. N Engl J Med 2003; 349:1064-1075.
4. McKenna WJ, Behr ER. Hypertrophic cardiomyopathy: management, risk stratification, and prevention of sudden death. Heart 2002; 87:169-176.
5. Spirito P, Bellone P, Harris KM, et al. Magnitude of left ventricular hypertrophy and risk of sudden death in hypertrophic cardiomyopathy. N Engl J Med 2000; 342:1778-1785.
6. Elliott PM, Gimeno Blanes JR, Mahon NG, et al. Relation between severity of left-ventricular hypertrophy and prognosis in patients with hypertrophic cardiomyopathy. Lancet 2001; 357:420-424.
7. Tam JW, Shaikh N, Sutherland E. Echocardiographic assessment of patients with hypertrophic and restrictive cardiomyopathy: imaging and echocardiography. Curr Opin Cardiol 2002; 17:470-477.
8. Funabashi N, Yoshida K, Komuro I. Thinned myocardial fibrosis with thrombus in the dilated form of hypertrophic cardiomyopathy demonstrated by multislice computed tomography. Heart 2003; 89:858.
9. Higgins CB, Byrd BF 3rd, Stark D, et al. Magnetic resonance imaging in hypertrophic cardiomyopathy. Am J Cardiol 1985; 55:1121-1126.
10. Funari M, Fujita N, Peck WW, Higgins CB. Cardiac tumors: assessment with Gd-DTPA enhanced MRI. J Comput Assist Tomogr 1991; 15:953-958.
11. Park JH, Kim YM. MRI of cardiomyopathy. Magn Reson Imaging Clin North Am 1996; 4:269-286.
12. Schulz-Menger J, Strohm O, Waigand J, et al. The value of magnetic resonance imaging of the left ventricular outflow tract in patients with hypertrophic obstructive cardiomyopathy after septal artery embolization. Circulation 2000; 101:1764-1766.
13. Sipola P, Lauerma K, Husso-Saastamoinen M, et al. First-pass MRI in the assessment of perfusion impairment in patients with hypertrophic cardiomyopathy and the Asp175Asn mutation of the alpha-tropomyosin gene. Radiology 2003; 226:129-137.
14. Bogaert J, Goldstein M, Tannouri F, et al. Late myocardial enhancement in hypertrophic cardiomyopathy with contrast-enhanced MRI. AJR Am J Roentgenol 2003; 180:981-985.
15. Devlin AM, Moore NR, Ostman-Smith I. A comparison of MRI and echocardiography in hypertrophic cardiomyopathy. Br J Radiol 1999; 72:258-264.
16. Soler R, Rodriguez E, Rodriguez JA, et al. Magnetic resonance imaging of apical hypertrophic cardiomyopathy. J Thorac Imaging 1997; 12:221-225.
17. Katz J, Milliken MC, Stray-Gundersen J, et al. Estimation of human myocardial mass with MRI. Radiology 1988; 169:495-498.
18. Semelka RC, Tomei E, Wagner S, et al. Interstudy reproducibility of dimensional and functional measurements between cine magnetic resonance studies in the morphologically abnormal left ventricle. Am Heart J 1990; 119:1367-1373.
19. Bergey PD, Axel L. Focal hypertrophic cardiomyopathy simulating a mass: MR tagging for correct diagnosis. AJR Am J Roentgenol 2000; 174:242-244.
20. Dong SJ, MacGregor JH, Crawley AP, et al. Left ventricular wall thickness and regional systolic function in patients with hypertrophic cardiomyopathy. A three-dimensional tagged magnetic resonance imaging study. Circulation 1994; 90:1200-1209.
21. Arrive L, Assayag P, Russ G, et al. MRI and cine MRI of asymmetric septal hypertrophic cardiomyopathy. J Comput Assist Tomogr 1994; 18:376-382.
22. Kim RJ, Chen EL, Lima JA, Judd RM. Myocardial Gd-DTPA kinetics determine MRI contrast enhancement and reflect the extent and severity of myocardial injury after acute reperfused infarction. Circulation 1996; 94:3318-3326.
23. Flacke SJ, Fischer SE, Lorenz CH. Measurement of the gadopentetate dimeglumine partition coefficient in human myocardium in vivo: normal distribution and elevation in acute and chronic infarction. Radiology 2001; 218:703-710.
24. Kawada N, Sakuma H, Yamakado T, et al. Hypertrophic cardiomyopathy: MR measurement of coronary blood flow and vasodilator flow reserve in patients and healthy subjects. Radiology 1999; 211:129-135.
25. Didier D, Ratib O, Lerch R, Friedli B. Detection and quantification of valvular heart disease with dynamic cardiac MRI. Radiographics 2000; 20:1279-1299.
26. Braunwald E, Seidman CE, Sigwart U. Contemporary evaluation and management of hypertrophic cardiomyopathy. Circulation 2002; 106:1312-1316.
27. Seggewiss H, Gleichmann U, Faber L, et al. Percutaneous transluminal septal myocardial ablation in hypertrophic obstructive cardiomyopathy: acute results and 3-month follow-up in 25 patients. J Am Coll Cardiol 1998; 31:252-258.
28. Faber L, Meissner A, Ziemssen P, Seggewiss H. Percutaneous transluminal septal myocardial ablation for hypertrophic obstructive cardiomyopathy: long-term follow-up of the first series of 25 patients. Heart 2000; 83:326-331.
29. Marcus JT, De Waal LK, Gotte MJ, et al. MRI-derived left ventricular function parameters and mass in healthy young adults: relation with gender and body size. Int J Cardiac Imaging 1999; 15:411-419.

CHAPTER 65

Arrhythmogenic Right Ventricular Dysplasia

Aditya Jain, Harikrishna Tandri, Hugh Calkins, and David A. Bluemke

Arrhythmogenic right ventricular dysplasia (ARVD) is a rare, progressive genetic cardiomyopathy that is characterized clinically by ventricular arrhythmias and sudden death, and histologically by fibrofatty infiltration of the right ventricle. Although symptomatic ventricular arrhythmias and sudden death are the most common manifestations of the disease, either right ventricular or biventricular heart failure may be observed. This chapter discusses various aspects of ARVD including etiology and pathogenesis, clinical manifestations, differential diagnosis, and treatment options, with special focus on diagnostic imaging techniques, in particular MRI, which is the current noninvasive diagnostic modality of choice in ARVD.

DEFINITION

ARVD is a genetic cardiomyopathy principally involving the right ventricle that is characterized clinically by ventricular arrhythmias and progressive structural alterations in right ventricular size and function. Fibrofatty replacement of the right ventricular myocardium forms the histopathologic hallmark of this disease. There are three patterns of disease expression: (1) *classic,* characterized by disease limited to the right ventricle with either no or minimal involvement of the left ventricle, which appears late in the course of the disease; (2) *left dominant,* characterized by early or predominant left ventricular involvement; and (3) *biventricular,* characterized by parallel involvement of both ventricles from the beginning of disease process.[1]

PREVALENCE AND EPIDEMIOLOGY

Although the exact incidence of ARVD is unknown, the prevalence has been estimated to be 0.02% of the general population.[2] ARVD reportedly is more prevalent (0.8%) in certain parts of northern Italy (Veneto) and Greece (Naxos Island).[3,4] ARVD most commonly manifests after puberty and before age 50 years.[5,6] ARVD is more common in highly athletic individuals. It is an important cause of sudden cardiac death in young individuals, particularly in athletes, accounting for 5% of sudden deaths in individuals younger than 35 years in the United States, and 25% of deaths in athletes in the Veneto region of Italy.[7] ARVD is believed to be more common than reported because of its frequently asymptomatic clinical course, difficulty in diagnosis using conventional noninvasive methods, and frequent misdiagnosis.

ETIOLOGY AND PATHOPHYSIOLOGY

The exact pathogenesis of ARVD remains speculative, but it is most widely believed to be due to genetic abnormalities mainly affecting cardiac desmosomal structure and function. In the United States, the most common reported genetic abnormality in ARVD is a mutation in plakophilin-2 (PKP2), which is a desmosomal protein and is present in more than one third of patients. Desmosomal mutations are believed to disrupt cell-cell adhesion, which provokes myocyte detachment and death under conditions of high mechanical stress, as suggested by its frequent occurrence in athletics and the thinnest portions of the right ventricle, such as the inferior subtricuspid region, right ventricular apex, and right ventricular infundibulum—together termed the *triangle of dysplasia* (Fig. 65-1).[8] This leads to a compensatory repair process characterized by inflammation and fibrofatty substitution. Familial ARVD accounts for 30% to 80% of cases, and most commonly shows an autosomal dominant inheritance, with age-dependent penetrance and variable clinical expression, which can be attributed to the complex interplay of age, gender effects, and environmental influences such as exposure to viruses and athletic activity with the underlying genetic background in the ultimate disease causation and progression. Mere inheritance of a genetic abnormality does not imply "disease" for the same reason. To date, at least 11 distinct subtypes of autosomal dominant ARVD are known, and at least seven genes have been implicated in ARVD (Table 65-1).[9]

Genetic mutations are also implicated in determining the ventricular predominance in ARVD. Chain-termination mutations causing truncation of the C-terminal domain of desmoplakin can disrupt cytoskeletal integrity, predisposing to predominant left ventricular involvement. Conversely, defects in the N-terminal domain of desmoplakin can result in a primary dysfunction of cell adhesion, leading to predominant right ventricular disease.[8]

In addition to genetic causes, other important proposed etiologic mechanisms of ARVD are (1) apoptosis (programmed cell death), (2) inherited metabolic or ultrastructural defects leading to myocardial dystrophy, and (3) secondary complication of a prior primary right ventricular myocarditis on the basis of frequently found myocardial inflammatory infiltrates and isolation of coxsackie B and enteroviral RNA viruses in some biopsy samples.[10]

Pathologically, ARVD is characterized by gradual myocyte loss and fibrofatty infiltration, which starts in the subepicardial region and gradually involves the endocardium, often sparing the trabecular myocardium. Plexiform arrangement of the residual myocardial fibers, separated by fat and fibrosis, leads to electrical instability and provides a conduit for a reentrant phenomenon. This situation explains the arrhythmogenic propensity characteristic of this disease, which can be worsened further by superimposed myocarditis that occurs frequently in ARVD because of the genetic susceptibility.[11] A myocardial dysplastic process and the associated loss of its strength and integrity are responsible for the varying degrees of structural derangement and functional disturbances of the heart seen in ARVD.

MANIFESTATIONS OF DISEASE

Clinical Presentation

ARVD usually manifests between the second and fifth decades (mean age at diagnosis approximately 30 years). Patients most commonly present with symptomatic ventricular arrhythmias or sudden cardiac death, or may remain asymptomatic, with ARVD discovered only

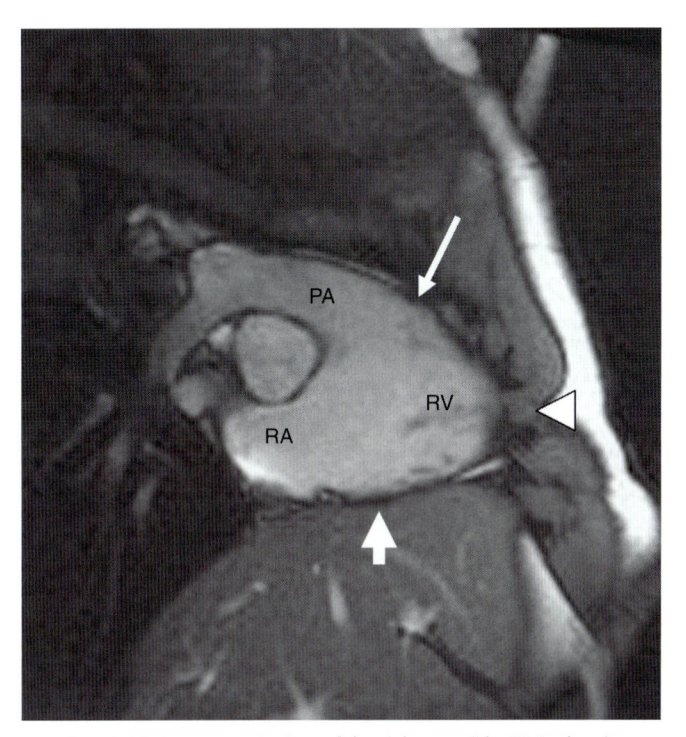

■ FIGURE 65-1 Long-axis view of the right ventricle (RV), showing the triangle of dysplasia, which is formed by the inferior subtricuspid area (*short arrow*), apex (*arrowhead*), and infundibulum (*long arrow*). PA, pulmonary artery; RA, right atrium.

TABLE 65-1	Genetics of Arrhythmogenic Right Ventricular Dysplasia		
ARVD Variant	**Chromosome**	**Gene***	**Characteristics**
Autosomal Dominant			
Type 1	14q24.3	*TGF-β3*	Excessive fibrosis owing to increased expression of TGF-β3
Type 2	1q42	*RYR-2*	Catecholaminergic polymorphic ventricular tachycardia
Type 3	14q11-q12		
Type 4	2q32		Localized involvement of left ventricle and left bundle branch block
Type 5	3p23		
Type 6	10p12-p14		Early onset and high penetrance
Type 7	10q22		Myofibrillar myopathy characterized by skeletal and cardiac muscle weakness and arrhythmias
Type 8	6p24	*DSP*†	Epidermolytic palmoplantar keratoderma, woolly hair, and dilated right ventricle
Type 9	12p11	*PKP2*†	Earlier onset arrhythmias, males more likely to have conduction abnormalities
Type 10	8q12	*DSG2*†	
Type 11	18q21	*DSC2*†	
Autosomal Recessive			Syndromic forms of ARVD that involve skin, hair, and heart
Naxos disease	17q21	*DSC2*	
		JUP†	
Carvajal disease	6p23-24	*DSP*	

*TGF-β3, transforming growth factor β-3; *RYR2*, cardiac ryanodine receptor; *DSP*, desmoplakin; *PKP2*, plakophillin-2; *DSG2*, desmoglein-2; *DSC2*, desmocollin-2; *JUP*, junctional plakoglobin. Various other genes, such as laminin receptor 1 (*LAMR1*), protein tyrosine phosphatase-like gene (*PTPLA*), and desmin (*DES*) are under investigation for a possible etiologic connection with ARVD.
†Genes encoding desmosomal proteins. *JUP* has also been implicated in an autosomal dominant type of ARVD.
From Moric-Janiszewska E, Markiewicz-Loskot G. Review on the genetics of arrhythmogenic right ventricular dysplasia. Europace 2007; 9:259.

TABLE 65-2 Task Force Criteria for the Diagnosis of Arrhythmogenic Right Ventricular Dysplasia

	Major Criteria	Minor Criteria
Global or regional dysfunction and structural alterations*	Severe dilation and reduction of right ventricular ejection fraction with no (or only mild) left ventricular impairment	Mild global right ventricular dilation or ejection fraction reduction with normal left ventricle
	Localized right ventricular aneurysms (akinetic or dyskinetic areas with diastolic bulging)	Mild segmental dilation of right ventricle
	Severe segmental dilation of right ventricle	Regional right ventricular hypokinesia
Tissue characterization of wall	Fibrofatty replacement of myocardium on endomyocardial biopsy specimen	
Repolarization abnormalities		Inverted T waves in right precordial leads (V_2 and V_3) in individuals >12 yr old in absence of right bundle branch block
Depolarization or conduction abnormalities	Epsilon waves or localized prolongation (>110 ms) of the QRS complex in right precordial leads (V_1-V_3)	Late potentials (signal-averaged ECG)
Arrhythmias		Left bundle branch block ventricular tachycardia (sustained and nonsustained) by ECG, Holter, or exercise testing
		Frequent ventricular extrasystoles (>1000/24 hr) (Holter)
Family history	Familial disease confirmed at necropsy or surgery	Family history of premature sudden death (<35 yr old) owing to suspected right ventricular dysplasia
		Familial history (clinical diagnosis based on present criteria)

*Detected by echocardiography, angiography, MRI, or radionuclide scintigraphy.

incidentally on routine examination. The most common symptoms are palpitations, syncope, atypical chest pain, and dyspnea. Ventricular arrhythmias are often precipitated by exercise or stress, and range from isolated ventricular premature beats to sustained monomorphic or polymorphic ventricular tachycardia with left bundle branch block morphology, or abrupt ventricular fibrillation, which is the most common underlying cause of sudden cardiac death in ARVD.[12]

In addition to ventricular arrhythmias, about 25% of patients may also show supraventricular arrhythmias, which include atrial fibrillation, atrial tachycardia, and atrial flutter, in that order of frequency.[13] Left ventricular involvement is associated with an increased incidence of arrhythmic events, more severe right ventricular wall thinning, and heart failure. Frank left-sided heart failure is rare. Figures 65-2, 65-4, and 65-6 illustrate left ventricular involvement in ARVD.

Diagnosis

Diagnosis of ARVD is challenging and is currently based on family history and morphofunctional, ECG, histopathologic, and clinical findings as proposed by the Task Force of Cardiomyopathies in 1994 (Table 65-2).[14] The diagnosis is made in the presence of two major criteria, one major criterion and two minor criteria, or four minor criteria. Various modifications of the existing Task Force criteria are being increasingly proposed and emphasize the increment in the diagnostic sensitivity of these criteria for less severe forms of the disease and asymptomatic first-degree relatives of affected probands. These modifications include more comprehensive characterization of ECG and echocardiographic criteria, inclusion of mutation analysis, and descriptions of left ventricular involvement.[15,16]

As per the standard diagnostic algorithm for ARVD, all patients with clinical suspicion of ARVD first undergo noninvasive testing, which includes a 12-lead ECG, signal-averaged ECG, 24-hour Holter monitor, and cardiac imaging. If the results are consistent with a diagnosis or a high degree of suspicion of ARVD based on the Task Force criteria, at our institution we typically recommend patients to undergo further invasive testing, including right ventricular angiography, endomyocardial biopsy, and electrophysiology testing, for confirmation of the diagnosis and exclusion of other potential etiologies, such as sarcoidosis. The standard of reference for the diagnosis of ARVD has been the histopathologic demonstration of fibrofatty replacement of right ventricular myocardium either on an endomyocardial biopsy specimen or at autopsy. Endomyocardial biopsy carries the risk of perforation of right ventricular free wall, however, and has low sensitivity because of frequent sampling error owing to the segmental, patchy nature of the disease. One particularly important role of endomyocardial biopsy is to distinguish sarcoidosis from ARVD.

Electrocardiogram Evaluation

At least one ECG abnormality (Table 65-3) is detectable in more than 90% of patients with ARVD. A newly proposed marker of delayed right ventricular activation, prolonged S wave upstroke (≥55 ms) in V_1 to V_3, is the most prevalent ECG marker and correlates with disease severity and ventricular tachycardia induction on electrophysiology testing.[17] Signal-averaged ECG is used to detect delayed ventricular activation owing to slowed propagation in the fibrofatty myocardium of ARVD. Late potentials on signal-averaged ECG (two or more of the following: filtered QRS duration ≥114 ms, duration of the low-amplitude signal <40 µV in the terminal portion of filtered QRS (LAS40) ≥38 ms, and root mean square voltage of the terminal 40 ms of filtered QRS (RMS40) <20 µV) form a minor diagnostic criterion for ARVD as per the Task Force

TABLE 65-3 Electrocardiogram Features of Arrhythmogenic Right Ventricular Dysplasia[‡]

T wave inversions in V_1-V_3[*]
QRS duration ≥110 ms in V_1-V_3[†]
Presence of epsilon wave (electrical potentials after the end of the QRS complex or beginning of the ST segment)[†]
Parietal block (QRS duration in leads V_1-V_3 that exceeds the QRS duration in lead V_6 by >25 ms)
Ratio of QRS duration in leads $V_1 + V_2 + V_3/V_4 + V_5 + V_6$ ≥1.2
Pattern of incomplete/complete right bundle branch block
QRS dispersion (≥40 ms) and QT dispersion (>65 ms)
Prolonged S wave upstroke in V_1-V_3 ≥55 ms
Ventricular ectopic beats >1000/day
Ventricular tachycardia with left bundle branch block morphology

[*]Minor Task Force criterion in the absence of right bundle branch block in individuals >12 yr old.
[†]Major Task Force criterion.
[‡]These electrical abnormalities are believed to be caused by intraventricular myocardial defect (parietal block) rather than definite alteration of conduction in the bundle branch (septal block).

TABLE 65-4 Angiographic Features of Arrhythmogenic Right Ventricular Dysplasia

Akinetic/dyskinetic aneurysmal bulges especially in infundibular, apical, and subtricuspid regions
Areas of dilation akinesia with an irregular and mammillated aspect, most often involving inferior wall
Transversely arranged hypertrophic trabeculae (>4 mm)/disarray with deep fissures
Coarse trabeculae in apical region distal to moderator band
Round areas of negative contrast in the trabecular zone or the moderator band or both
Prominent moderator band
Increased end-diastolic and end-systolic volumes
Decreased ejection fraction
Tricuspid valve prolapse, usually associated with mild tricuspid insufficiency and reduced tricuspid annulus plane systolic excursion

---

criteria. Similar to extent of right precordial T wave inversion, late potentials on signal-averaged ECG are correlated with the extent of right ventricular involvement in ARVD. More recently, our group found that using filtered QRS 110 ms or greater identifies ARVD patients with inducible ventricular tachycardia more accurately than does conventional signal-averaged ECG criteria.[18] T wave inversions and signal-averaged ECG abnormalities are more commonly seen in left-sided involvement in ARVD.

Imaging Techniques and Findings

Chest Radiograph

Chest radiographs generally show cardiac enlargement depending on the stage of the disease, with the cardiothoracic ratio generally less than 0.6. The heart can also show a convexity between the aortic knob and the left ventricle, and there is no pulmonary vascular redistribution.[11] Radiographs are not a sensitive modality to diagnose ARVD.

Cine Angiography

Right ventricular cine angiography has been regarded as the traditional gold standard, with high specificity and positive and negative predictive values in ARVD diagnosis. It is performed using two orthogonal views in 30 degrees right anterior oblique and 60 degrees left anterior oblique during sinus rhythm with careful evaluation of structure and function of the right ventricle. Coexistence of subtricuspid and anterior infundibular wall bulging and hypertrophic trabeculae has been shown to have 96% sensitivity and 87.5% specificity in angiographic diagnosis of ARVD.[10] Invasiveness of the procedure, frequent ventricular ectopy during catheter manipulation and contrast injection, and interobserver variability in the visual assessment of right ventricular wall motion abnormalities are important limitations. Because of these limitations, and the availability of other, more quantitative imaging tools such as MRI, right ventricular cine angiography plays only a small role today in the evaluation of patients with suspected ARVD. Table 65-4 lists major angiographic features of ARVD.

Nuclear Ventriculoscintigraphy

Nuclear ventriculoscintigraphy provides information about the size, ejection fraction, contraction pattern of the ventricles, and site of origin of ventricular tachycardia. In most cases of ARVD, the size of the right ventricle is increased, and ejection fraction is diminished. Contraction pattern of the right ventricular wall is asynchronous as a result of the ongoing dysplastic process. Use of specific radionuclide tracers has shown abnormal sympathetic myocardial innervation in ARVD patients, providing a new insight into the arrhythmogenicity of the disease. Myocardial imaging with iodine 123 MIBG and thallium 201 has detected left ventricular involvement early in the course of the disease, suggesting that it may be potentially more sensitive in the diagnosis of ARVD.[19,20] Although nuclear imaging can be used in the evaluation of patients with suspected ARVD, it is rarely employed today.

Echocardiography

Two-dimensional echocardiography is an important first-line imaging tool for diagnosis and follow-up in ARVD because of its noninvasiveness, low cost, wide availability, and ease of performance. Echocardiographic abnormalities associated with the Task Force criteria for ARVD are summarized in Table 65-5. A right ventricular outflow tract long-axis diameter greater than 30 mm on echocardiography has been found to have the highest sensitivity and specificity for the diagnosis of ARVD. Right ventricular dysfunction has been defined as a fractional area contraction less than 32%, or the presence of segmental right ventricular wall motion abnormalities (mostly observed in anterior and apical walls) for the purpose of echocardiographic diagnosis of ARVD.[21]

We evaluated three-dimensional echocardiography, tissue Doppler echocardiography, and strain echocardiography, and found that these imaging modalities show high feasibility and reproducibility in ARVD. Three-dimensional echocardiography measurement of right ventricular

TABLE 65-5 Echocardiography Features Associated with Task Force Criteria for Arrhythmogenic Right Ventricular Dysplasia

Right ventricular regional wall motion abnormality
Right ventricular outflow tract dilation
Right ventricular dilation
Reduced right ventricular global function
Hyper-reflective moderator band
Exaggerated/abnormal trabeculations
Sacculations

volumes and ejection fraction showed close correlation with MRI, the current reference standard, and three-dimensional echocardiography may be potentially more useful in the assessment of right ventricular function and follow-up of patients with ARVD, in contrast to two-dimensional echocardiography. Tissue Doppler echocardiography and strain echocardiography showed higher sensitivity in detection of mild cases of ARVD with normal right ventricle on conventional echocardiography. In our opinion, these new echocardiographic modalities may have a potentially greater diagnostic utility in ARVD than conventional methods.[22,23] Contrast echocardiography using saline injections may outline the right ventricle better, enabling better evaluation of right ventricular volumes and regional and global function.[11]

Computed Tomography

Electron-beam CT and multidetector CT can yield accurate and reliable qualitative and quantitative assessment of the right ventricle at an excellent spatial and temporal resolution. They can also provide tissue characterization of the myocardium and detect fatty changes, similar to MRI. Electron-beam CT can directly assess left ventricular adipose tissue changes and can even detect subclinical cases of ARVD without left ventricular wall motion abnormality.[24] Major abnormalities in ARVD reported on CT include (1) dilated right ventricle, (2) abundant epicardial fatty tissue, (3) intramyocardial fat deposits, (4) scalloped appearance (bulging) of the right ventricular free wall, and (5) conspicuous trabeculae with low attenuation (Figs. 65-2 and 65-3).

CT is less expensive, faster, technologically easier to perform, less operator-dependent, and more reliable in terms of image quality compared with MRI. It is less susceptible to artifacts resulting from respiratory motion and patient movement because of shorter image acquisition times on the order of milliseconds. CT is the diagnostic modality of choice in ARVD patients with claustrophobia and frequent arrhythmic events. Although the presence of an implantable cardioverter defibrillator (ICD) was previously considered to be an indication for a CT scan versus MRI, more recent studies have shown that MRI can be safely performed in patients with ICDs.[25] Limitations of CT include its fixed axial plane for image acquisition, requirement for ionizing radiation exposure, use of nephrotoxic contrast agent, and relatively lower temporal resolution compared with MRI.[7]

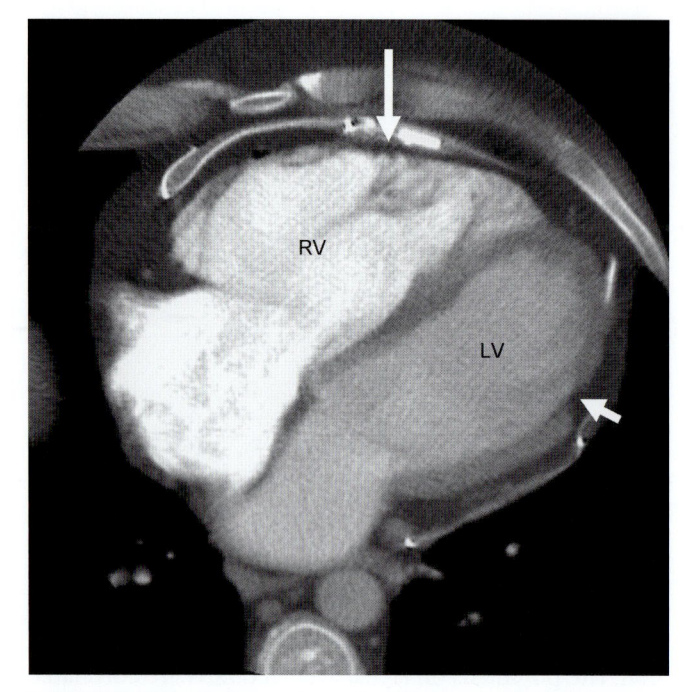

FIGURE 65-2 Contrast-enhanced, multidetector CT image in a patient with ARVD shows right ventricle (RV) (*long arrow*) and left ventricle (LV) (*short arrow*) thinning associated with fat replacement. Note also the dilation of the RV and epicardial pacing lead.

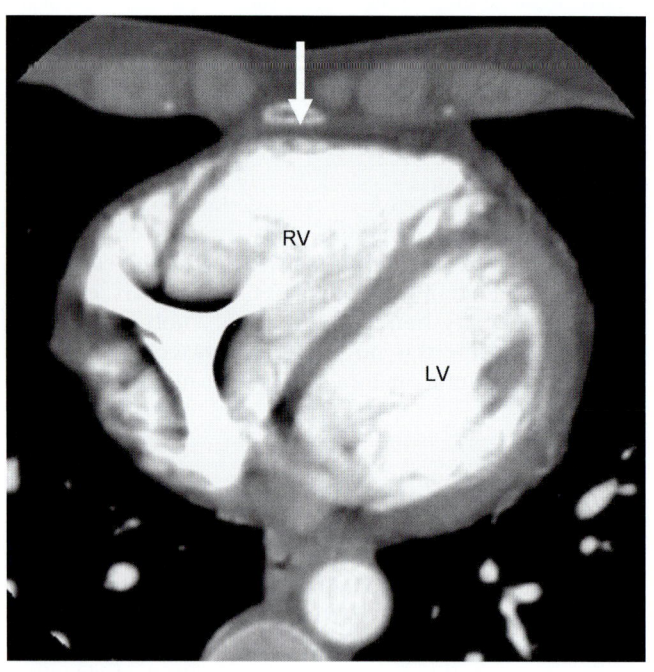

FIGURE 65-3 Contrast-enhanced, multidetector CT image in an ARVD patient shows extreme wall thinning and fat replacement of the right ventricle (RV) (*arrow*) and right ventricular dilation. Note the artifact caused by the ICD lead.

Magnetic Resonance Imaging

MRI has been increasingly recognized as the imaging technique of choice for ARVD. Its three-dimensional, multiplanar visualization of the heart along with excellent spatial and temporal resolution enables highly reproducible assessment of structural morphology and function of the

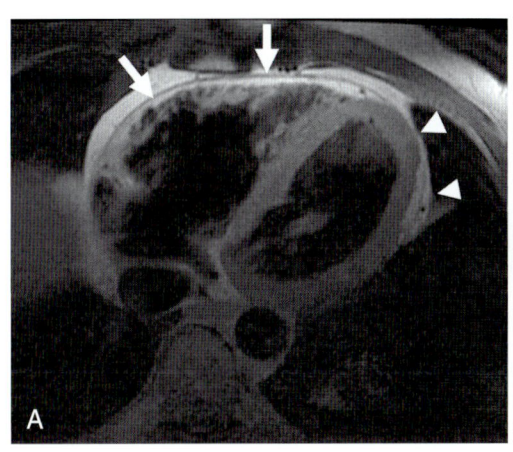

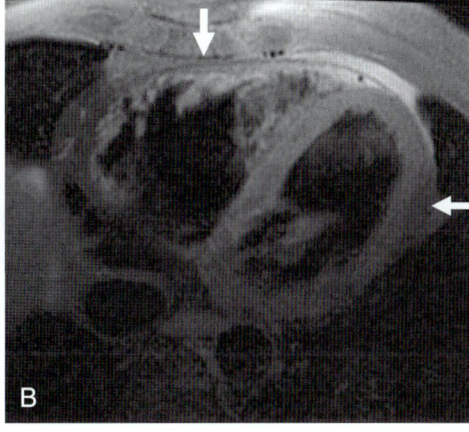

FIGURE 65-4 A, Axial black blood image from a patient with ARVD shows intramyocardial fat infiltration (seen as hyperintense T1 signal) of the right ventricle (*arrows*) and left ventricle (*arrowheads*). B, Axial fat-suppressed image from the same patient at the same slice level shows low signal intensity (owing to fat signal [*arrows*]) corresponding to the areas of high T1 signal in A. The fat suppression images are chemically selective for lipid signal.

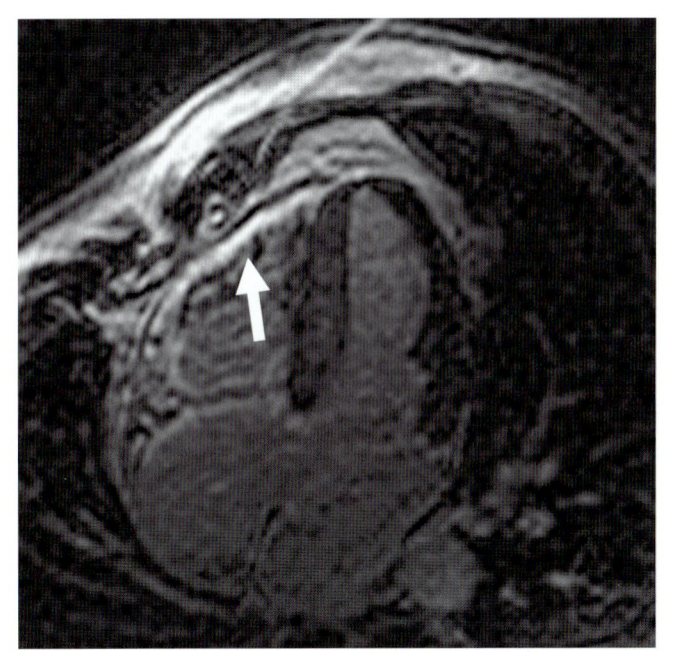

FIGURE 65-5 Delayed-enhancement axial image from a patient with ARVD shows high signal intensity (i.e., hyperenhancement) in the right ventricular free wall (*arrow*). The high signal intensity most commonly correlates with areas of fibrosis in these patients.

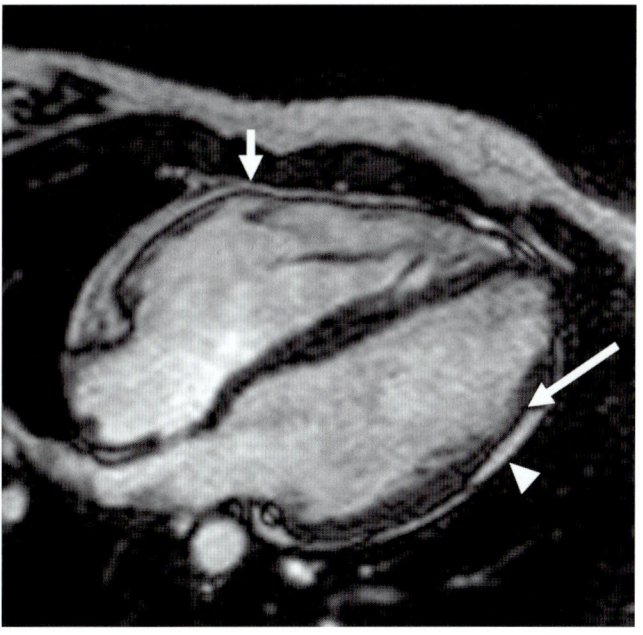

FIGURE 65-6 Axial bright blood image from a patient with ARVD shows thinning of the right ventricular free wall (*short arrow*), and thinning (*long arrow*) and infiltration of fat (*arrowhead*) in the left ventricular lateral wall.

right ventricle without using any geometric assumptions. The improved blood-myocardial image contrast allows optimal visualization of the right ventricle. For myocardial tissue characterization, MRI can specifically locate and quantify intramyocardial adipose infiltration, which forms the pathologic hallmark of the disease (Fig. 65-4).[26] MRI has the potential to visualize fibrous tissue replacement of right ventricular myocardium in ARVD by myocardial delayed enhancement (Fig. 65-5).[27]

MRI can be uniquely applied for the identification of regional and diastolic dysfunction of the right ventricle and minor changes in right ventricular volume over time and other functional details, such as velocity mapping of the tricuspid flow and right ventricular strain measurements using myocardial tagging. MRI also has prognostic significance because of its ability to predict arrhythmia-free survival in ARVD.[28] MRI is noninvasive and devoid of radiation hazards. These features make MRI highly suited and superior to other imaging investigations for the detection and serial follow-up of patients with clinically suspected ARVD.

MRI findings in ARVD can be broadly divided into two groups: (1) *morphologic abnormalities,* including intramyocardial fat infiltration, right ventricular wall thinning (Fig. 65-6), trabecular hypertrophy (Fig. 65-7), and right ventricular outflow tract enlargement (Fig. 65-8), and (2) *functional abnormalities,* including right ventricular wall motion abnormalities, aneurysms (Fig. 65-9), right ventricular dilation (Fig. 65-10), and right atrial enlargement (Fig. 65-11). These findings are listed in Table 65-6.

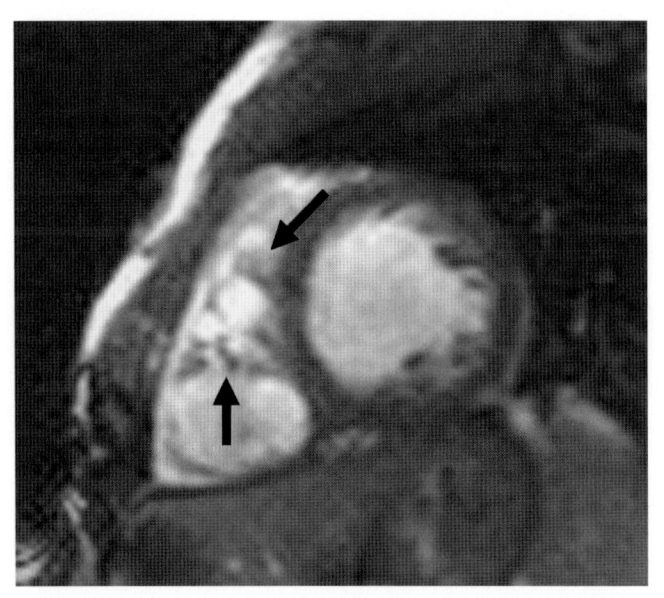

FIGURE 65-7 Short-axis bright blood image from a patient with ARVD shows trabecular hypertrophy and disarray of the right ventricle (*arrows*).

Bright blood cine gradient MRI is the preferred modality for the functional evaluation of the right ventricle. ECG gated steady-state free precession (SSFP) imaging (e.g., FIESTA, true FISP, and balanced fast field echo) is preferred to segmented k-space cine gradient-echo imaging (e.g., fast low-angle shot [FLASH] and fast cardiac-gated gradient-echo [FASTCARD]) because of higher temporal resolution and excellent contrast between myocardium and blood pool, which make it better adapted for assessment of wall motion and volumetric measurement. Also, signal intensity in SSFP is not affected by reduction in blood flow velocity in instances of right ventricular dysfunction compared with gradient-echo imaging.

Black blood breath-hold fast spin-echo MRI (see Figs. 65-4A and 65-8B) with dual magnetization preparation pulse (double inversion recovery) is the preferred modality to detail cardiac morphology. Inversion recovery pulses are used to null (darken) the signal from a tissue of interest to highlight (enhance) the surrounding pathology. Breath-holding reduces motion artifacts and improves overall image quality of myocardial detail. Black blood single-shot spin-echo techniques (e.g., HASTE, turboFLASH, SSFSE)

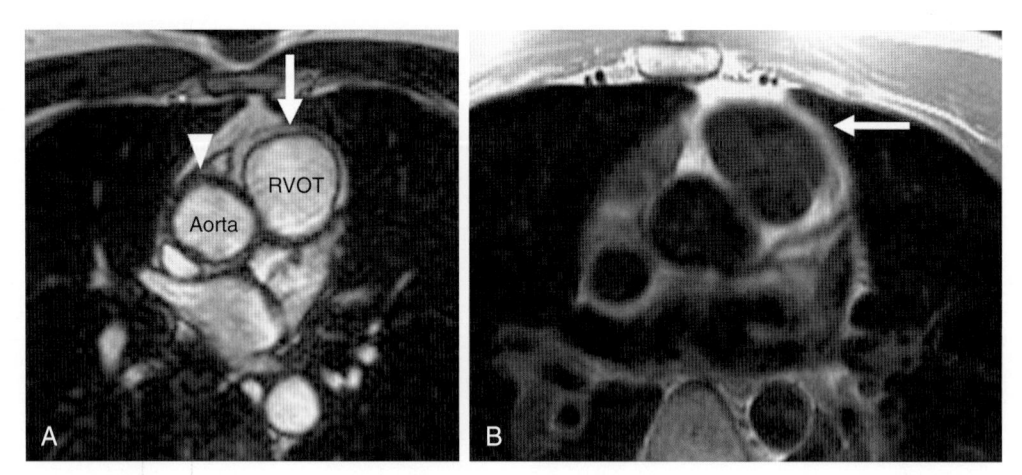

FIGURE 65-8 **A,** Axial bright blood image from a patient with ARVD shows enlarged right ventricular outflow tract (RVOT) (*arrow*) compared with aorta (*arrowhead*). **B,** Axial black blood image from another patient with ARVD shows enlarged and dysmorphic outflow tract (*arrow*).

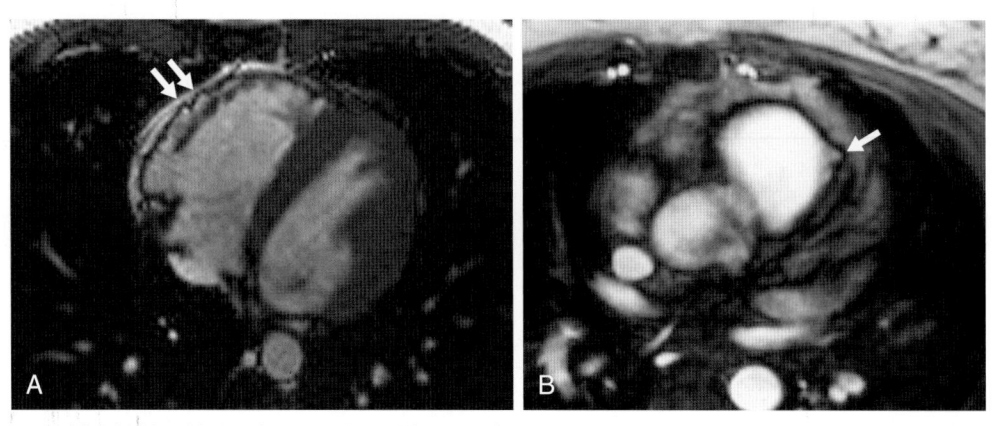

FIGURE 65-9 **A,** Axial bright blood image from a patient with ARVD shows microaneurysms at the right ventricular free mid-wall (*arrows*). **B,** Axial bright blood image from a patient with ARVD shows a microaneurysm in the right ventricular outflow tract (*arrow*).

CHAPTER 65 ● *Arrhythmogenic Right Ventricular Dysplasia* 891

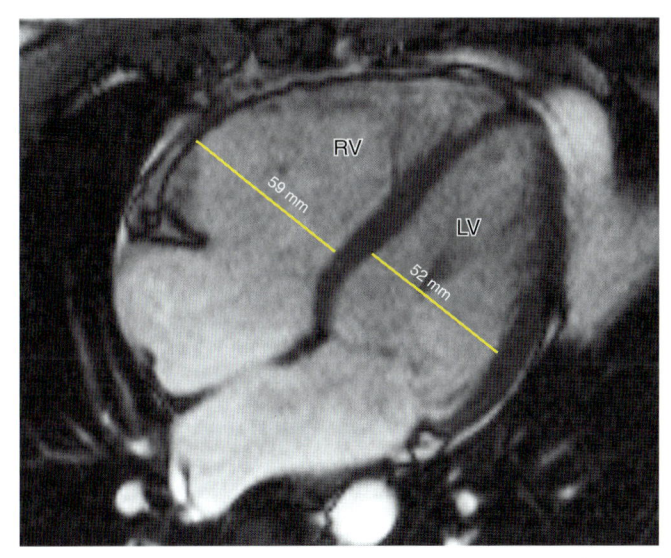

■ **FIGURE 65-10** Axial bright blood image from a patient with ARVD shows dilation of the right ventricle (RV). The end-diastolic diameter of the RV is greater than that of the left ventricle (LV).

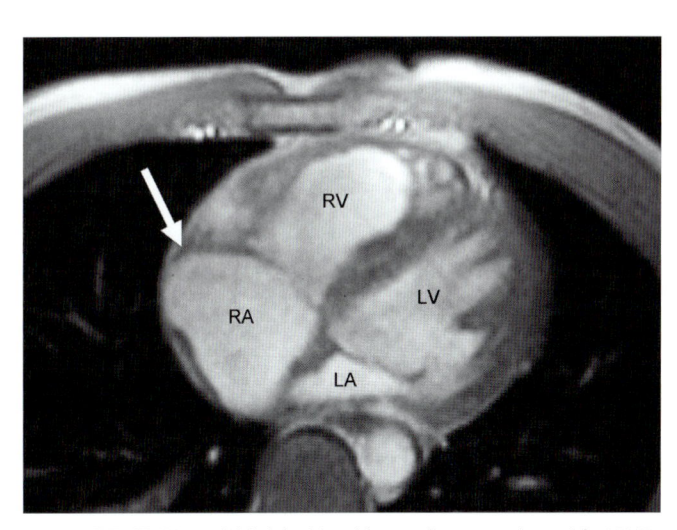

■ **FIGURE 65-11** Axial bright blood image from a patient with ARVD shows enlargement of the right atrium (RA) (*arrow*). LA, left atrium; LV, left ventricle; RV, right ventricle.

TABLE 65-6 Magnetic Resonance Imaging Features of Arrhythmogenic Right Ventricular Dysplasia

Morphologic Abnormalities
Subepicardial intramyocardial fatty infiltration
Focal wall thinning/hypertrophy
Trabecular hypertrophy/disarray
Moderator band hypertrophy
Right ventricular outflow tract ectasia

Functional Abnormalities
Regional wall motion abnormalities
Failure of systolic thickening
Dyskinetic bulges/outpouchings
Right ventricular dilation
Enlargement of the right atrium
Right ventricular diastolic/systolic dysfunction

TABLE 65-7 Magnetic Resonance Imaging Protocol for Arrhythmogenic Right Ventricular Dysplasia

Patient preparation: If the patient is known to have frequent ventricular ectopy, use oral metoprolol, 50 mg, 1 hr before the procedure, provided that the patient has no contraindications. If ventricular arrhythmias are frequent and would have a substantial impact on image quality, the examination should be terminated at this point.

1. Rapid three-plane image localizers
2. Axial black blood images: double inversion recovery fast/turbo spin-echo
3. Axial bright blood cine images: SSFP cine, temporal resolution ≤50 ms
4. Vertical and long-axis cine images (two- or four-chamber view) (same pulse sequence as step 3)
5. Short-axis black blood images (same pulse sequence as step 2)
6. Axial black blood images with fat suppression (optional sequence)

Administer intravenous gadolinium contrast agent, 0.1-0.2 mmol/kg per local protocols

7. Short-axis SSFP cine (same pulse sequence as step 3)
8. TI scout or other method to determine optimal blood suppression
9. Delayed gadolinium short-axis images (10-15 min delay after gadolinium administration)
10. Delayed gadolinium axial axis images

are ultrafast imaging modalities that substantially reduce image acquisition times and motion artifacts, but at the expense of blurring of detail. They are not recommended, unless a severe arrhythmia is present that results in failure of other black blood sequences. Incorporation of fat-suppressed sequences (see Fig. 65-4B) to conventional T1-weighted spin-echo imaging has been found to increase the interobserver agreement and confidence in the diagnosis of intramyocardial fat infiltration.[29,30] Table 65-7 presents a detailed MRI protocol recommended for ARVD.

Right ventricular intramyocardial fat on MRI has a low sensitivity for detection of ARVD compared with other abnormalities, such as regional right ventricular dysfunction. Normal presence of epicardial fat, especially in areas such as the atrioventricular sulcus and anterolateral and apical portions of the right ventricle, sometimes makes distinction from pathologic fat difficult, particularly given the thinness of normal right ventricular wall and limited spatial and contrast resolution achievable by even state-of-the-art MRI protocols.[31] Fat was also found to be the least specific and least reproducible of any of the other parameters in the MRI evaluation of ARVD.[32,33] High intramyocardial T1 signals are not specific for ARVD because isolated fatty infiltration of the right ventricle has also been reported in elderly individuals, obese individuals, patients on long-term steroid therapy, patients with alcohol abuse, patients with idiopathic right ventricular outflow tract tachycardia, and patients with inherited myopathies, and more recently as a separate disorder in itself, clinicopathologically distinct from ARVD.[34] False-positive high signal intensities potentially misconstrued as fat may be produced by various artifacts related to motion, respiration, blood flow, arrhythmia, or truncation band.

The ability of MRI stands out in the diagnosis of early and subtle cases of ARVD because of its potential to detect

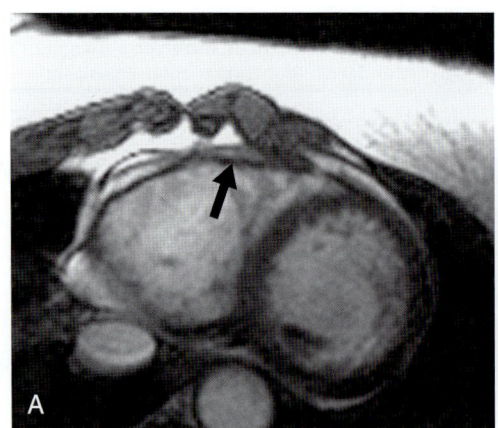

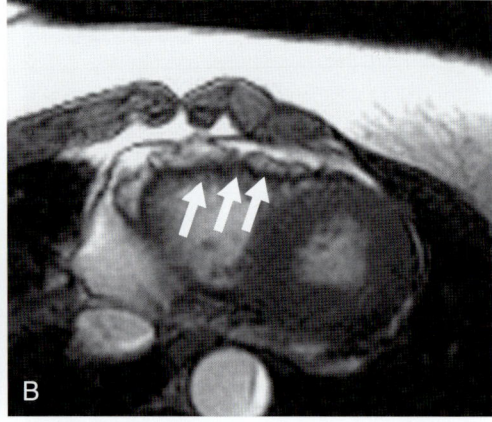

■ **FIGURE 65-12** **A**, End-diastolic axial bright blood image from a patient with ARVD. The right ventricular free wall (*arrow*) appears smooth and regular, with no aneurysms. **B**, End-systolic axial bright blood image from the same patient. Note the focal crinkling of the right ventricle owing to discoordinate contraction (*arrows*).

regional and diastolic ventricular dysfunction, which are thought to precede global and systolic dysfunction during the progressive course of the disease.[35] This capability of MRI can add to the overall sensitivity of diagnosis of ARVD because these patients may otherwise be clinically inapparent and less sensitive to diagnosis by Task Force criteria. In one of our studies, we found that despite preserved systolic function, 37% of patients with early or limited forms of ARVD show focal discoordinate contraction of right ventricular free basal wall on MRI, which was unique in its appearance as focal crinkling of the right ventricular wall in peak systole (Fig. 65-12).

MRI can also have a role in screening of first-degree relatives of ARVD cases. In one of our previous studies, we found that MRI frequently detects mild qualitative and regional functional abnormalities in first-degree relatives of ARVD probands with overall normal chamber sizes and volumes. We also noted focal discoordinate contraction of the right ventricular basal free wall on MRI was found to represent an early phenotypic expression of desmosomal mutation–positive (especially PKP2), asymptomatic first-degree relatives of ARVD probands. This finding showed good correlation with repolarization abnormalities on ECG and inducibility for ventricular arrhythmias.

Despite the diagnostic utility of MRI in ARVD, its specificity and reliability remain in question because of the subjectivity in the interpretation of its findings, dependence on image quality, over-reliance on intramyocardial fat and wall thinning, and lack of standardized protocol and technical and clinical expertise in cardiovascular MRI. Observers without extensive experience in MRI for ARVD can overdiagnose this condition, particularly when the only abnormalities observed are with MRI. MRI can be a low-yield test for the diagnosis of ARVD in children compared with adults. MRI should be considered as only a part of the multidisciplinary diagnostic work-up of the patient, and the final diagnosis of ARVD should be based on an integrated assessment of all noninvasive and invasive testing in reference to Task Force criteria.[35] Follow-up studies, in probands and suspected relatives, can be advantageous—keeping in mind the progressive and evolving nature of the disease.

TABLE 65-8 Differential Diagnosis of Arrhythmogenic Right Ventricular Dysplasia

Related Arrhythmogenic Right Ventricular Cardiomyopathies
Naxos disease
Brugada syndrome
Right ventricular outflow tract tachycardia*
Uhl anomaly

Congenital Heart Disease
Ebstein anomaly
Atrial septal defect
Partial anomalous venous return

Acquired Heart Disease
Isolated myocarditis
Cor adiposum
Idiopathic dilated cardiomyopathy
Pulmonary hypertension
Tricuspid valve disease
Right ventricular infarction
Bundle branch reentrant ventricular tachycardia

Miscellaneous
Sarcoidosis

*Whether right ventricular outflow tract tachycardia represents a form of arrhythmogenic right ventricular cardiomyopathies is still debated.
From Corrado D, Basso C, Thiene G. Arrhythmogenic right ventricular cardiomyopathy: diagnosis, prognosis, and treatment. Heart 2000; 83:588.

DIFFERENTIAL DIAGNOSIS

Numerous clinically diverse conditions can mimic ARVD because of related histologic picture, ventricular tachycardia of right ventricular origin, or right ventricular enlargement and distorted right ventricular anatomy, and must be appropriately excluded (Table 65-8).[11,36] Right ventricular outflow tract tachycardia is one of the most important differential diagnoses from the clinical standpoint (Table 65-9).[37] A few other important conditions are discussed next.

Sarcoidosis

Involvement of the ventricle in cardiac sarcoidosis often can mimic the ECG and structural changes in ARVD.[38]

TABLE 65-9 Differences Between Right Ventricular Outflow Tract (RVOT) Tachycardia and Arrhythmogenic Right Ventricular Dysplasia

Features	RVOT Tachycardia	ARVD
Clinical Presentation		
Family history	No	Frequently yes
Arrhythmias	Premature ventricular contractions, nonsustained ventricular tachycardia, or sustained ventricular tachycardia at rest or with exercise	Same
Sudden cardiac death	Rare	1%/yr
ECG Features		
T wave morphology	T wave upright V_2-V_5	T wave inverted beyond V_1
Parietal block	QRS duration <110 ms in V_1-V_3	QRS duration >110 ms
Epsilon wave V_1-V_3	Absent	Present in one third of cases
Prolonged S wave upstroke	Rarely seen	Usually present
Signal-averaged ECG	Normal	Usually abnormal
Electrophysiology Study		
Presence of more than one ECG morphology during tachycardia	Absent	Seen frequently
Fractionated diastolic potentials during ventricular tachycardia	Absent	Seen frequently
Programmed premature stimulation-induced ventricular tachycardia	Absent	Seen frequently
Imaging Features		
Echocardiogram	Normal	Usually abnormal
Right ventricular ventriculogram	Usually normal	Usually abnormal
MRI	Usually normal	Usually abnormal

From Prakasa KR, Calkins H. Arrhythmogenic right ventricular dysplasia/cardiomyopathy. Curr Treat Options Cardiovasc Med 2005; 7:467.

Presence of hilar lymphadenopathy should alert the physician to consider this diagnosis. MRI may reveal patchy left ventricular delayed hyperenhancement in a noncoronary distribution. Finally, an endomyocardial biopsy specimen of an affected region often reveals noncaseating granulomas, confirming the diagnosis of sarcoidosis.

Idiopathic Dilated Cardiomyopathy

Dilated cardiomyopathy may be mistaken for ARVD, particularly when ARVD is associated with structurally advanced disease involving the left ventricle. In ARVD, left ventricular systolic dysfunction occurs late in the disease, and even the left ventricular involvement is predominantly epicardial—often occurring in the posterobasal left ventricle. This presentation is quite distinct from nonischemic dilated cardiomyopathy, which usually involves the midmyocardial region.

Isolated Myocarditis

Isolated myocarditis may mimic ARVD because both conditions have clinical presentations of arrhythmias, signs and symptoms of heart failure, or sudden cardiac death. The absence of family history and classic ECG findings and biopsy results showing active lymphocytic inflammation should point to the diagnosis of myocarditis.

Cor Adiposum

Cor adiposum is a nonpathologic variant of the normal heart characterized by increased epicardial fat, and is associated with age, obesity, and female gender.

Uhl Anomaly

Uhl anomaly (parchment or paper-thin right ventricle) is an extremely rare anomaly characterized by localized or extensive complete absence of right ventricular myocardial muscle fibers. In contrast to ARVD, Uhl anomaly often initially manifests with congestive heart failure, typically during infancy or childhood and without a major male gender predilection or family history.

Brugada Syndrome

Right ventricular precordial ST segment elevation syndrome, or Brugada syndrome, is characterized by pseudo–right bundle branch block, ST segment elevation in V_1-V_3, and episodes of syncope or sudden cardiac death in patients with a structurally normal heart. Right and left precordial QTc prolongation, right and left precordial right bundle branch block with typical QRS morphology, and right precordial epsilon waves on ajmaline challenge distinguish Brugada syndrome from ARVD.

TREATMENT OPTIONS

All patients with ARVD must avoid athletics, particularly competitive athletics. This recommendation is made because participation in athletics can increase the rate of progression of the disease and may trigger ventricular arrhythmias. Available therapeutic options in ARVD include pharmacologic therapy, catheter ablation, ICD, and surgery. The approach to management is individualized for every patient based on the guidelines discussed in this section.

Medical

The pharmacologic agents commonly used to treat arrhythmias in ARVD include β blockers, calcium channel blockers, and class I and III antiarrhythmic agents. Sotalol and amiodarone (both class III agents) have been found to be the most effective antiarrhythmic drugs in this regard with low proarrhythmogenic risk. Their efficacy in preventing sudden cardiac death is unknown, however. Antiarrhythmic drugs represent a first-line treatment in patients with ARVD. Antiarrhythmic drugs do not prevent sudden cardiac death and are used merely to reduce the frequency of sustained ventricular arrhythmias, and in doing so, they improve quality of life. ARVD patients who have progressed to right ventricular/biventricular failure are treated with the usual regimen, which includes ACE inhibitors, diuretics, β blockers, and digitalis.[12]

Surgical/Interventional

Catheter Ablation

Although it may result in acute procedural success, catheter radiofrequency ablation is seldom effective and is often accompanied by recurrence of ventricular tachycardia in the long-term because of the progressive nature of the disease. Its clinical role is limited as a short-term palliative procedure in cases of (1) ventricular arrhythmia when pharmacologic therapy is ineffectual, and (2) frequent ICD discharges owing to recurrent ventricular tachycardia refractory to antiarrhythmic therapy.[12]

Implantable Cardioverter-Defibrillator

ICD provides a decisive survival benefit in ARVD by effectively terminating life-threatening arrhythmias. We currently advise ICD implantation in all patients who meet the Task Force criteria for ARVD. Although it is well recognized that patients with a prior sustained ventricular arrhythmia are at highest risk, and that patients with syncope or severe disease, or both, are also at increased risk, it is difficult to identify a patient population of ARVD patients who may not benefit from an ICD. The only exceptions are patients who are diagnosed with ARVD based on a family history and have little evidence of structural involvement with ARVD. More information is needed in this particular patient population, and placement of an ICD in this subgroup relies to a great degree on patient preference.

Surgical Treatment

The only currently employed surgical treatment for ARVD is cardiac transplantation. Although right ventricular disarticulation was used in the past, this procedure has been abandoned. Cardiac transplantation is a last resort measure in the wake of associated high morbidity and mortality and limited availability of donors.

FUTURE DIRECTIONS

More research is needed for accurate and reliable characterization of risk factors for sudden cardiac death, which would better define the role and status of ICD intervention in ARVD. Risk stratification in asymptomatic relatives would also help establish the prognostic value of early identification of asymptomatic gene carriers. Natural history of the disease is still not well defined. ARVD in early, preclinical forms is a diagnostic dilemma, and interpretation of Task Force criteria in relatives of known affected probands remains subject to lack of definitive agreement. More complete understanding of the genetic basis of the disease, genetic-environmental interactions, and genotype/phenotype correlation is needed for better diagnosis, prognostication, and therapeutic decision making.

INFORMATION FOR THE REFERRING PHYSICIAN

1. *Global left ventricular structure and function*: end-diastolic volume, end-systolic volume, stroke volume, ejection fraction, corresponding values corrected for body size (body surface area indexed values)
2. *Global right ventricular structure and function*: end-diastolic volume, end-systolic volume, stroke volume, ejection fraction, corresponding values corrected for body size (body surface area indexed values)
3. *Regional wall motion abnormalities*: comment on synchrony of contraction of the right and left ventricles
4. *Myocardial signal abnormalities*: areas of T1 high signal that may correspond to fat
5. *Gadolinium hyperenhancement areas*: restricted to right ventricle versus left ventricle
6. *Other*: pulmonary outflow tract size, pulmonary artery size, mediastinal abnormalities, evidence of shunts or valve disorders, atrial size

---

KEY POINTS

- ARVD is a genetic cardiomyopathy associated with ventricular arrhythmias typically in young individuals.
- The diagnosis of ARVD is based on a set of clinical, electrical, and imaging-based criteria because no single test is diagnostic by itself.
- Echocardiography and MRI are the major noninvasive imaging tests used for ARVD diagnosis.

SUGGESTED READINGS

Ahmad F. The molecular genetics of arrhythmogenic right ventricular dysplasia-cardiomyopathy. Clin Invest Med 2003; 26:167.

Corrado D, Basso C, Thiene G. Arrhythmogenic right ventricular cardiomyopathy: diagnosis, prognosis, and treatment. Heart 2000; 83:588.

Fontaine G, Fontaliran F, Hebert JL, et al. Arrhythmogenic right ventricular dysplasia. Annu Rev Med 1999; 50:17.

Gemayel C, Pelliccia A, Thompson PD. Arrhythmogenic right ventricular cardiomyopathy. J Am Coll Cardiol 2001; 38:1773.

Kayser HW, van der Wall EE, Sivananthan MU, et al. Diagnosis of arrhythmogenic right ventricular dysplasia: a review. RadioGraphics 2002; 22:639.

Moric-Janiszewska E, Markiewicz-Loskot G. Review on the genetics of arrhythmogenic right ventricular dysplasia. Europace 2007; 9:259.

Paul M, Schulze-Bahr E, Breithardt G, et al. Genetics of arrhythmogenic right ventricular cardiomyopathy—status quo and future perspectives. Z Kardiol 2003; 92:128.

Prakasa KR, Calkins H. Arrhythmogenic right ventricular dysplasia/cardiomyopathy. Curr Treat Options Cardiovasc Med 2005; 7:467.

Tandri H, Bomma C, Calkins H, et al. Magnetic resonance and computed tomography imaging of arrhythmogenic right ventricular dysplasia. J Magn Reson Imaging 2004; 19:848.

REFERENCES

1. Sen-Chowdhry S, Syrris P, Ward D, et al. Clinical and genetic characterization of families with arrhythmogenic right ventricular dysplasia/cardiomyopathy provides novel insights into patterns of disease expression. Circulation 2007; 115:1710.
2. Norman MW, McKenna WJ. Arrhythmogenic right ventricular cardiomyopathy: perspectives on disease. Z Kardiol 1999; 88: 550-554.
3. Thiene G, Basso C. Arrhythmogenic right ventricular cardiomyopathy: an update. Cardiovasc Pathol 2001; 10:109-117.
4. Kies P, Bootsma M, Bax J, et al. Arrhythmogenic right ventricular dysplasia/cardiomyopathy: screening, diagnosis, and treatment. Heart Rhythm 2006; 3:225-234.
5. Dalal D, Nasir K, Bomma C, et al. Arrhythmogenic right ventricular dysplasia: a United States experience. Circulation 2005; 112: 3823-3832.
6. Nava A, Bauce B, Basso C, et al. Clinical profile and long-term follow-up of 37 families with arrhythmogenic right ventricular cardiomyopathy. J Am Coll Cardiol 2000; 36:2226-2233.
7. Tandri H, Bomma C, Calkins H, et al. Magnetic resonance and computed tomography imaging of arrhythmogenic right ventricular dysplasia. J Magn Reson Imaging 2004; 19:848.
8. Sen-Chowdhry S, Syrris P, McKenna WJ. Genetics of right ventricular cardiomyopathy. J Cardiovasc Electrophysiol 2005; 16:927.
9. Moric-Janiszewska E, Markiewicz-Loskot G. Review on the genetics of arrhythmogenic right ventricular dysplasia. Europace 2007; 9:259.
10. Gemayel C, Pelliccia A, Thompson PD. Arrhythmogenic right ventricular cardiomyopathy. J Am Coll Cardiol 2001; 38:1773.
11. Fontaine G, Fontaliran F, Hebert JL, et al. Arrhythmogenic right ventricular dysplasia. Annu Rev Med 1999; 50:17.
12. Corrado D, Basso C, Thiene G. Arrhythmogenic right ventricular cardiomyopathy: diagnosis, prognosis, and treatment. Heart 2000; 83:588.
13. Tonet JL, Castro-Miranda R, Iwa T, et al. Frequency of supraventricular tachyarrhythmias in arrhythmogenic right ventricular dysplasia. Am J Cardiol 1991; 67:1153.
14. McKenna WJ, Thiene G, Nava A, et al. Diagnosis of arrhythmogenic right ventricular dysplasia/cardiomyopathy. Task Force of the Working Group Myocardial and Pericardial Disease of the European Society of Cardiology and of the Scientific Council on Cardiomyopathies of the International Society and Federation of Cardiology. Br Heart J 1994; 71:215.
15. Sen-Chowdhry S, Syrris P, McKenna WJ. Desmoplakin disease in arrhythmogenic right ventricular cardiomyopathy: early genotype-phenotype studies. Eur Heart J 2005; 26:1582.
16. Hamid MS, Norman M, Quraishi A, et al. Prospective evaluation of relatives for familial arrhythmogenic right ventricular cardiomyopathy/dysplasia reveals a need to broaden diagnostic criteria. J Am Coll Cardiol 2002; 40:1445.
17. Nasir K, Bomma C, Tandri H, et al. Electrocardiographic features of arrhythmogenic right ventricular dysplasia/cardiomyopathy according to disease severity: a need to broaden diagnostic criteria. Circulation 2004; 110:1527.
18. Nasir K, Tandri H, Rutberg J, et al. Filtered QRS duration on signal-averaged electrocardiography predicts inducibility of ventricular tachycardia in arrhythmogenic right ventricle dysplasia. Pacing Clin Electrophysiol 2003; 26:1955.
19. Takahashi N, Ishida Y, Maeno M, et al. Noninvasive identification of left ventricular involvements in arrhythmogenic right ventricular dysplasia: comparison of 123I-MIBG, 201TlCl, magnetic resonance imaging and ultrafast computed tomography. Ann Nucl Med 1997; 11:233.
20. Lindstrom L, Nylander E, Larsson H, et al. Left ventricular involvement in arrhythmogenic right ventricular cardiomyopathy—a scintigraphic and echocardiographic study. Clin Physiol Funct Imaging 2005; 25:171.
21. Yoerger DM, Marcus F, Sherrill D, et al. Echocardiographic findings in patients meeting task force criteria for arrhythmogenic right ventricular dysplasia: new insights from the multidisciplinary study of right ventricular dysplasia. J Am Coll Cardiol 2005; 45:860.
22. Prakasa KR, Wang J, Tandri H, et al. Utility of tissue Doppler and strain echocardiography in arrhythmogenic right ventricular dysplasia/cardiomyopathy. Am J Cardiol 2007; 100:507.
23. Prakasa KR, Dalal D, Wang J, et al. Feasibility and variability of three dimensional echocardiography in arrhythmogenic right ventricular dysplasia/cardiomyopathy. Am J Cardiol 2006; 97:703.
24. Tada H, Shimizu W, Ohe T, et al. Usefulness of electron-beam computed tomography in arrhythmogenic right ventricular dysplasia: relationship to electrophysiological abnormalities and left ventricular involvement. Circulation 1996; 94:437.
25. Nazarian S, Roguin A, Zviman MM, et al. Clinical utility and safety of a protocol for noncardiac and cardiac magnetic resonance imaging of patients with permanent pacemakers and implantable-cardioverter defibrillators at 1.5 tesla. Circulation 2006; 114:1277.
26. Fattori R, Tricoci P, Russo V, et al. Quantification of fatty tissue mass by magnetic resonance imaging in arrhythmogenic right ventricular dysplasia. J Cardiovasc Electrophysiol 2005; 16:256.
27. Tandri H, Saranathan M, Rodriguez ER, et al. Noninvasive detection of myocardial fibrosis in arrhythmogenic right ventricular cardiomyopathy using delayed-enhancement magnetic resonance imaging. J Am Coll Cardiol 2005; 45:98.
28. Keller DI, Osswald S, Bremerich J, et al. Arrhythmogenic right ventricular cardiomyopathy: diagnostic and prognostic value of the cardiac MRI in relation to arrhythmia-free survival. Int J Cardiovasc Imaging 2003; 19:537.
29. Tandri H, Friedrich MG, Calkins H, et al. MRI of arrhythmogenic right ventricular cardiomyopathy/dysplasia. J Cardiovasc Magn Reson 2004; 6:557.
30. Abbara S, Migrino RQ, Sosnovik DE, et al. Value of fat suppression in the MRI evaluation of suspected arrhythmogenic right ventricular dysplasia. AJR Am J Roentgenol 2004; 182:587.
31. Castillo E, Tandri H, Rodriguez ER, et al. Arrhythmogenic right ventricular dysplasia: ex vivo and in vivo fat detection with black-blood MR imaging. Radiology 2004; 232:38.
32. Tandri H, Castillo E, Ferrari VA, et al. Magnetic resonance imaging of arrhythmogenic right ventricular dysplasia: sensitivity, specificity, and observer variability of fat detection versus functional analysis of the right ventricle. J Am Coll Cardiol 2006; 48:2277.
33. Bluemke DA, Krupinski EA, Ovitt T, et al. MR imaging of arrhythmogenic right ventricular cardiomyopathy: morphologic findings and interobserver reliability. Cardiology 2003; 99:153.
34. Macedo R, Prakasa K, Tichnell C, et al. Marked lipomatous infiltration of the right ventricle: MRI findings in relation to arrhythmogenic right ventricular dysplasia. AJR Am J Roentgenol 2007; 188:W423.
35. Bomma C, Dalal D, Tandri H, et al. Regional differences in systolic and diastolic function in arrhythmogenic right ventricular dysplasia/cardiomyopathy using magnetic resonance imaging. Am J Cardiol 2005; 95:1507.
36. Fontaine G, Fontaliran F, Frank R. Arrhythmogenic right ventricular cardiomyopathies: clinical forms and main differential diagnoses. Circulation 1998; 97:1532.
37. Prakasa KR, Calkins H. Arrhythmogenic right ventricular dysplasia/cardiomyopathy. Curr Treat Options Cardiovasc Med 2005; 7: 467.
38. Ott P, Marcus FI, Sobonya RE, et al. Cardiac sarcoidosis masquerading as right ventricular dysplasia. Pacing Clin Electrophysiol 2003; 26:1498.

CHAPTER 66

Myocarditis

Carol C. Wu and Mayil S. Krishnam

Myocarditis—acute inflammatory syndrome of myocardium—is a rare cause of acute chest pain and an important cause of dilated cardiomyopathy. The most common cause of myocarditis in the Western world is viral infection. The patient presents acutely with chest pain and dyspnea or, rarely, hemodynamic compromise of the fulminant type. Chronic myocarditis usually is manifested with symptoms and signs of dilated cardiomyopathy. Clinical presentations, biochemistry, and echocardiographic findings may overlap with those of myocardial infarction or ischemic heart disease. Imaging is critical in the diagnosis. Currently, cardiac magnetic resonance imaging (MRI) has proved to be the most robust and accurate noninvasive imaging tool, not only in the diagnosis of myocarditis but also in guiding targeted endomyocardial biopsy and in the subsequent follow-up. Treatment of myocarditis is usually supportive. Cardiac transplantation may be considered for patients with deteriorating cardiac function in dilated cardiomyopathy.

Definition

Myocarditis refers to focal or diffuse inflammation of the cardiac muscle associated with myocyte damage or necrosis and lymphocyte infiltration as a result of various infectious, immune, or nonimmune insults in the absence of significant acute or chronic ischemia.[1-3]

Prevalence and Epidemiology

Myocarditis is found in 1% to 10% of postmortem examinations; however, the true prevalence is unknown because of its insidious and variable clinical presentation.[1,2] It accounts for 20% of cardiac causes of sudden deaths in military recruits[1] and 40% of acute presentations of dilated cardiomyopathy.[2] Up to 50% of patients with acquired immunodeficiency syndrome (AIDS) have evidence of myocarditis on biopsy.[2]

Etiology and Pathophysiology

Infections are a major cause of myocarditis. Viruses, such as coxsackieviruses A and B and other enteroviruses, adenovirus, influenza virus, and Epstein-Barr virus, are the most important causes of myocarditis in the United States.[2,4] A wide range of bacteria (*Streptococcus, Chlamydia, Neisseria, Borrelia*) and parasites (*Trypanosoma, Toxoplasma, Trichinella*) can also cause myocarditis. Various medications, such as doxorubicin (Adriamycin) and sulfonamides, and toxins, such as cocaine, have also been associated with myocarditis. Large-vessel vasculitis, such as Takayasu arteritis, and autoimmune diseases, such as systemic lupus erythematosus, sarcoidosis, and Wegener granulomatosis, are also important but rare causes of myocarditis.[2,4]

Manifestations of Disease

Clinical Presentation

The clinical manifestation of myocarditis is variable, ranging from progressive dyspnea and weakness to left ventricular failure to sudden death. Patients may present with influenza-like symptoms, such as fever, fatigue, malaise, and arthralgia.[1-3] Arrhythmia is common.[4] In addition, chest pain with abnormal electrocardiographic (ECG) recordings and serum troponin elevation in patients with myocarditis can mimic acute myocardial infarction.[5] Patients may also present at a late stage with dilated cardiomyopathy.[4]

Imaging Indications and Algorithm

Imaging plays a pivotal role in the diagnosis of myocarditis. In the past, endomyocardial biopsy was once considered the gold standard for diagnosis of myocarditis; however, it has been shown to have low sensitivity due to sampling error related to the patchy nature of the

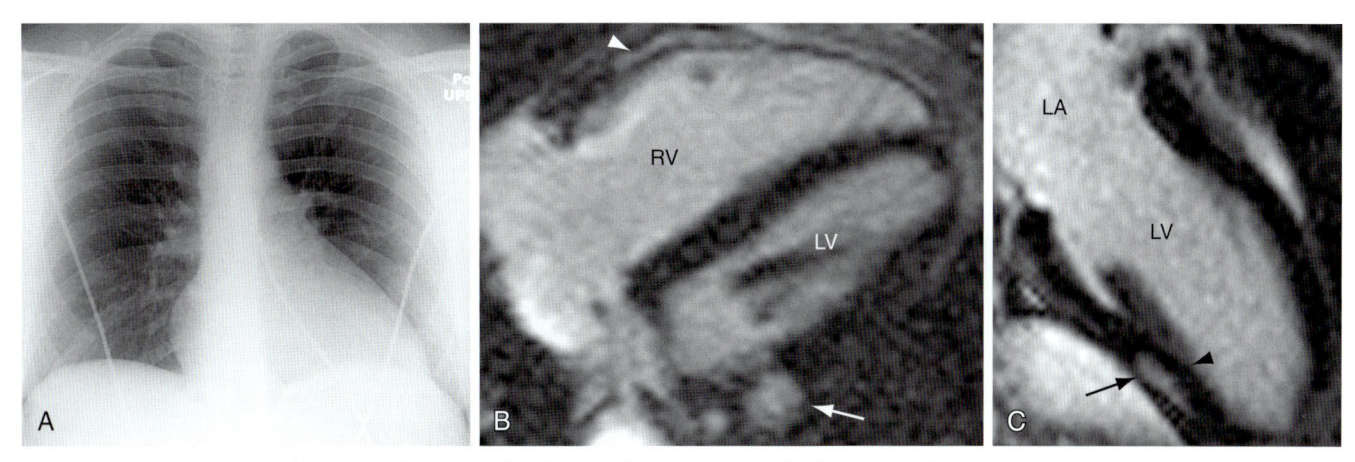

■ **FIGURE 66-1** A 31-year-old patient who presented with acute chest pain, eventually diagnosed with acute myocarditis. **A,** An upright posteroanterior chest radiograph is essentially normal. The cardiac silhouette is at the upper limit of normal in size. There is no evidence of pulmonary edema or pleural effusions. **B,** Horizontal long-axis view of delayed postcontrast T1-weighted gradient-echo sequence shows dilation of the right ventricle (RV) relative to the left ventricle (LV) and linear subepicardial hyperenhancement of the anterior wall of the right ventricle (*arrowhead*). A nodular focus of non-subendocardial delayed hyperenhancement is also noted in the lateral myocardial wall of the left ventricle (*arrow*). **C,** Vertical long-axis view of delayed postcontrast T1-weighted gradient-echo sequence shows a well-defined oval focus of subepicardial delayed hyperenhancement (*arrow*) and subendocardial sparing (*arrowhead*). These features are consistent with acute myocarditis.

disease.[6] Echocardiography and cardiac MRI should be part of the initial diagnostic evaluation in conjunction with ECG and serum troponin evaluation. More selected biopsy, if needed, may be performed with the MRI result as a guide.[5] Coronary computed tomographic angiography (CTA) can be performed in the acute setting to exclude significant coronary arterial stenosis in patients with myocarditis who are presenting with chest pain, raised abnormal cardiac enzymes, and abnormal ECG changes.

Imaging Technique and Findings

Radiography

Chest radiographs may be completely normal in patients with myocarditis, especially acutely (Fig. 66-1). Alternatively, cardiomegaly, interstitial or alveolar pulmonary edema, pleural effusions, and pericardial effusion may be detected as a result of left ventricular failure.[2] Less commonly, right ventricular failure may be manifested by right atrial enlargement, prominent azygos vein, and superior vena cava enlargement.

Ultrasonography

Echocardiographic findings of myocarditis are nonspecific, including segmental wall motion abnormalities and increased left ventricular volume.[7] During the acute phase, transient left ventricular wall thickening can be observed, probably related to interstitial edema.[8,9] The average brightness of the myocardium is also higher in patients with myocarditis than in control patients.[10]

Computed Tomography

Recent literature shows that multidetector computed tomography (MDCT) may play a role in establishing the diagnosis of myocarditis in patients presenting in the acute setting as MDCT is more accessible and less time-consuming than MRI. In addition, ECG-gated MDCT also offers concurrent evaluation of the coronary arteries. However, the amount of iodinated contrast material administered must be considered in patients who may have already undergone conventional coronary arteriography.

On delayed enhanced images, nodular, patchy, band-like enhancement of the mid and epicardial layer of the left ventricular wall can be seen in patients with myocarditis (Fig. 66-2).[11] In a study of 12 consecutive patients with acute chest pain consistent with myocardial ischemia and normal coronary angiogram, delayed enhanced MDCT performed 5 minutes after injection of contrast material demonstrated the same accuracy as MRI in differentiating between myocardial infarction and myocarditis in the acute phase.[12] Similarly, another study also showed good correlation in the extent and location of hyperenhancement at MDCT compared with cardiac MRI in the early phase of suspected acute myocarditis.[13]

Magnetic Resonance

Cardiac MRI has been established as an important imaging tool in the diagnosis of myocarditis. By identifying inflammatory lesions in the myocardium, it helps guide endomyocardial biopsy for histopathologic confirmation of diagnosis. It is also an excellent modality for subsequent assessment of natural regression of inflammation or treatment response in patients already diagnosed with myocarditis.

ECG-triggered segmented cine steady-state free precession imaging may show segmental or global wall motion abnormality, such as hypokinesis or akinesis. Tissue characterization can be performed with ECG-triggered T2-weighted fat-saturated double-inversion recovery turbo spin-echo sequence (or T2 short tau inversion recovery [STIR]) and postcontrast delayed (10 minutes) T1-weighted inversion recovery gradient-echo sequence; the latter is the most important MR pulse

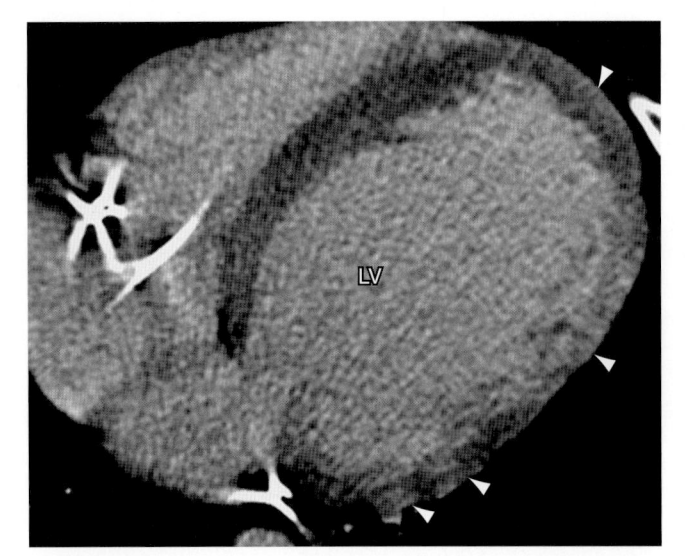

FIGURE 66-2 A 40-year-old man with history of progressive exertional dyspnea for months. Axial view of contrast-enhanced CT scan in the delayed phase shows dilated left ventricle (LV) with patchy areas of subepicardial and transmural delayed hyperenhancement (*arrows*) in a nonvascular distribution involving the lateral wall and apex, consistent with myocarditis.

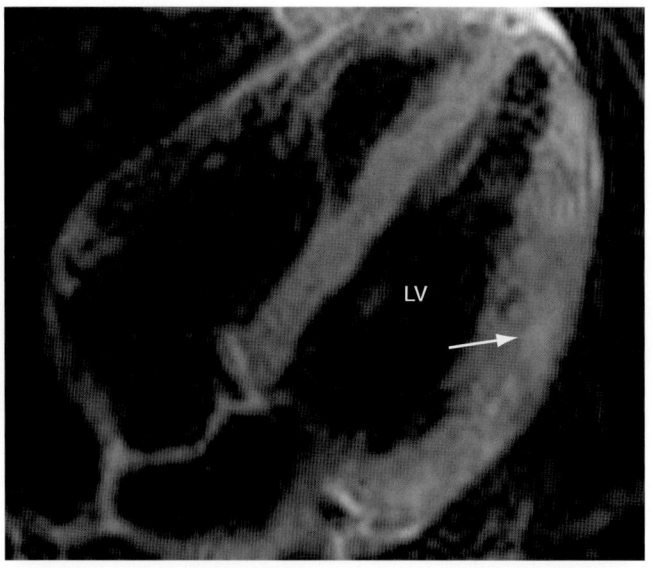

FIGURE 66-3 A 35-year-old woman with clinically suspected acute myocarditis. CT angiography of the chest was negative for pulmonary embolism and acute aortic syndrome. Horizontal long-axis view of T2-weighted dark blood double-inversion recovery sequence shows foci of hyperintensity within the mid-myocardium, more prominent within the lateral myocardium (*arrow*), consistent with focal inflammation related to myocarditis. T1-weighted delayed postcontrast images showed corresponding hyperenhancement of left ventricular myocardium and also pericardial enhancement consistent with myopericarditis.

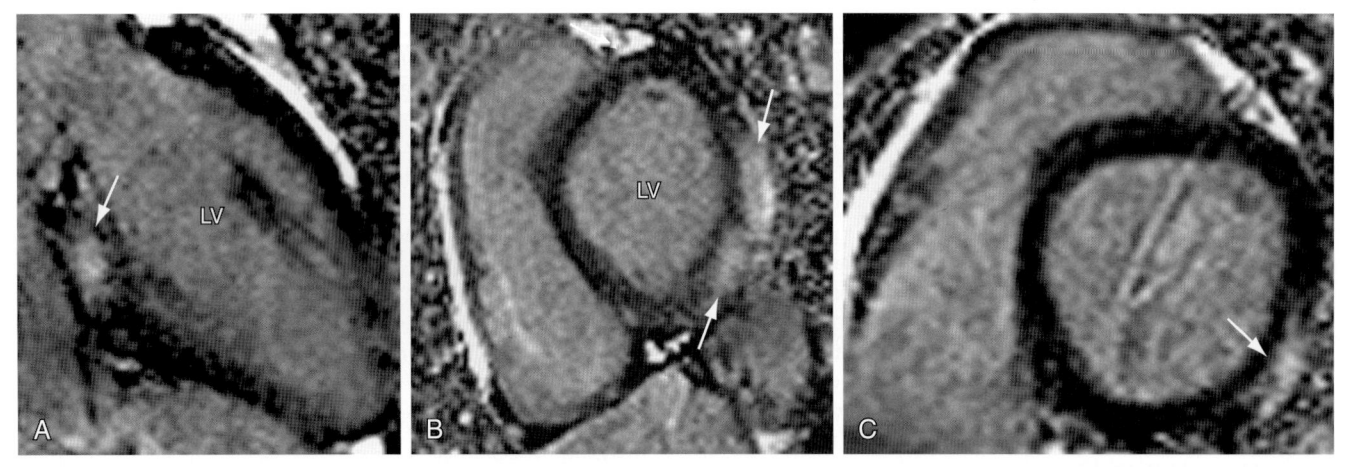

FIGURE 66-4 An 18-year-old man with clinically suspected acute myocarditis. **A,** Vertical long-axis view of delayed postcontrast T1-weighted gradient-echo sequence shows a nodular focus of delayed hyperenhancement (*arrow*) of the basal inferior left ventricular (LV) wall. **B,** Short-axis view of delayed postcontrast T1-weighted gradient-echo sequence shows subepicardial and mid-wall myocardial delayed hyperenhancement (*arrows*) involving the lateral wall of the left ventricle (LV). **C,** Short-axis view of delayed postcontrast T1-weighted gradient-echo sequence performed after 2 months shows interval decrease in the area of delayed hyperenhancement (*arrow*), consistent with resolving myocarditis.

sequence in the diagnosis of myocarditis (Fig. 66-3). T2-weighted images may show patchy areas of increased myocardial signal. Postcontrast T1-weighted gradient-echo images typically demonstrate ovoid or nodular, patchy, epicardial and mid-wall delayed hyperenhancement of myocardium in a nonsegmental vascular territory. Focal delayed hyperenhancement may become diffuse later in the disease process but with eventual regression (Fig. 66-4). Resolution of inflammation may be seen in 3 months. Persistent inflammation may lead to myocardial fibrosis and scar formation, resulting in myocardial thinning and dilated cardiomyopathy in some patients.

A large study showed that areas of delayed hyperenhancement are associated with active inflammation defined by histopathologic examination.[14] In a study that included 44 patients with myocarditis, inferolateral wall delayed hyperenhancement was a common feature, although other segments were also involved. About two thirds of all lesions were subepicardial in location.[15] Another study suggested that the delayed hyperenhancement pattern may be different between myocarditis caused by parvovirus B19 (PVB19) and myocarditis caused by human herpesvirus 6 (HHV6). Patients with PVB19 infection tended to have presentations similar to that of myocardial infarction and had subepicardial delayed hyperenhancement in the lateral wall. Patients with HHV6 or combined PVB19/HHV6 infection presented with new-onset heart failure and had septal delayed hyperenhancement; this group of patients more frequently progressed toward chronic heart failure.[16]

Delayed hyperenhancement detects irreversible myocardial injury but is unable to differentiate acute from chronic myocarditis.[17] The sensitivity may be limited because myocarditis does not always result in irreversible myocardial injury.[18]

Perfusion cardiac MR imaging can also play a role in differentiating acute myocardial infarction from myocarditis in patients with acute chest pain. A prospective study showed that all the patients with acute myocardial infarction had a segmental early subendocardial defect on first-pass perfusion and corresponding segmental subendocardial or transmural delayed hyperenhancement in a predominantly anteroseptal or inferior vascular distribution. All but one of 24 patients with myocarditis had no early perfusion defect and focal or diffuse nonsegmental non-subendocardial delayed hyperenhancement predominantly in the inferolateral location.[19]

T2 imaging has also been used to identify acute myocarditis or edema of the myocardium as part of the acute inflammatory process. Because myocarditis usually results in global, instead of focal, high T2 signal abnormality, the signal intensity of the myocardium is compared with that of skeletal muscle.[17] Areas of high T2 signal intensity have been shown to correlate with serum markers of acute myocardial injury.[20]

In the setting of suspected chronic myocarditis, however, a study of 83 patients showed that increased calculated myocardial global relative enhancement on T1-weighted images and edema ratio on T2-weighted images indicating inflammation were common findings. Delayed hyperenhancement, however, had low sensitivity and accuracy.[21] It was suggested that if MRI is normal in this setting, endomyocardial biopsy may not be necessary.

Nuclear Medicine/Positron Emission Tomography

Gallium Ga 67, an agent used for evaluation of inflammation, has been used to distinguish acute myocarditis from acute myocardial infarction and to identify myocarditis in children with Kawasaki disease.[22,23] The study result is positive when the myocardial uptake is equal to or greater than that in the sternum.

Indium In 111-labeled antimyosin antibodies, which detect myocardial necrosis, have also been used for diagnosis of myocarditis with high sensitivity and negative predictive value.[24]

Angiography

Conventional catheter angiography is performed to exclude coronary artery disease in some patients with myocarditis because of overlapping clinical features of myocardial infarction or ischemia. In myocarditis, coronary arteries are normal without a significant stenosis. Coronary CTA is equally good to exclude significant coronary artery disease, especially in patients with low to intermediate probability of having ischemic heart disease.

Classic Signs

Radiography

Findings on radiography are normal, but cardiomegaly and interstitial edema may be seen.

Computed Tomographic Angiography

CTA is not routinely indicated for myocarditis. Patchy delayed hyperenhancement of the left ventricular myocardium may be seen. Coronary CTA usually shows no significant stenosis.

Magnetic Resonance Imaging

Patchy areas of high signal intensity in the myocardium may be seen on T2-weighted turbo spin-echo sequence (dark blood double-inversion recovery), T2 STIR (dark blood triple-inversion recovery), or HASTE images. Wall motion abnormality may be seen on cine images. Typically, ovoid or nodular epicardial and mid-wall delayed hyperenhancement areas of left ventricular myocardium that are unrelated to arterial distribution may be demonstrated.

Differential Diagnosis

From Clinical Presentation

In patients with ST elevation on ECG and elevated serum cardiac markers, ischemic coronary disease must be strongly considered and excluded by CT or conventional coronary angiography. Cardiac sarcoidosis and idiopathic or ischemic dilated cardiomyopathy should be considered in patients with chronic myocarditis presenting with progressive shortness of breath.

From Imaging Findings

Delayed hyperenhancement is also seen in acute myocardial infarction, sarcoidosis, amyloidosis, and dilated cardiomyopathy. In infarction, segmental, linear, subendocardial delayed hyperenhancement of left ventricular myocardium is seen in typical coronary arterial distribution. The subendocardium is always involved in infarction. In myocarditis, there is patchy, ovoid, epicardial or mid-wall delayed hyperenhancement with no relation to arterial territory. Sarcoid typically causes a nonischemic pattern of hyperenhancement like myocarditis but usually involves mid-wall inferior interventricular septum. Amyloidosis typically causes diffuse subendocardial delayed hyperenhancement. Nonischemic dilated cardiomyopathy can cause mid-wall hyperenhancement.

Synopsis of Treatment Options

Medical

The first line of treatment is largely supportive, including hemodynamic support in patients with severe left ventricular failure. In the subacute or chronic phase, management of systolic dysfunction includes angiotensin-converting enzyme inhibitor and β-adrenergic blocker. Immunosuppressants such as prednisone, cyclosporine, and azathioprine may be helpful in selected patients, particularly those with myocarditis related to autoimmune disease or giant cell myocarditis. Intravenous immune globulin, interferon alfa, and interferon beta have also been shown to be effective in selected patients in early studies.[5]

Surgical/Interventional

Rarely, in patients with heart failure, ventricular assist device or extracorporeal membrane oxygenation may be required until recovery of cardiac function.[5] Cardiac transplantation is an option for patients with irreversible ventricular failure.

Reporting: Information for the Referring Physician

The report to the referring physician includes the presence or absence of delayed hyperenhancement of myocardium.

- If it is present, the exact location within the left ventricular myocardium is described (base, mid, distal, or apex; anterior, lateral, septal, or inferior wall on 17-segment model of the left ventricle).
- Delayed hyperenhancement of right ventricular myocardium is noted if it is present.
- Wall motion abnormality and left ventricular ejection fraction are described. If the right ventricle is involved, its ejection fraction is mentioned.

Short-term follow-up MRI can be recommended in 3 months from the time of acute presentation or initial abnormal scan. Interval changes in size, shape, and location of delayed hyperenhancement should be mentioned (it usually decreases or disappears but rarely progresses to dilated cardiomyopathy).

KEY POINTS

- Myocarditis is focal or diffuse inflammation of the cardiac muscle associated with myocyte damage or necrosis and lymphocyte infiltration.
- Viral infections are the most important causes in North America.
- Patients present with chest pain, dyspnea, heart failure, or sudden death.
- Echocardiography and MR are most commonly used for initial evaluation.
- Patchy areas of high signal intensity in the myocardium are demonstrated on precontrast T2-weighted turbo spin-echo sequence (dark blood double-inversion recovery), T2 STIR (dark blood triple-inversion recovery), or HASTE.
- ECG-gated, delayed contrast-enhanced MR typically shows patchy nodular subepicardial or mid-wall hyperenhancement of left ventricular myocardium in a nonvascular distribution.
- Involvement of the right ventricular wall suggests a poor prognosis; the chance is increased for development of chronic myocarditis and dilated cardiomyopathy.
- Treatment is mostly supportive. Immunosuppressants are given to selected patients. Cardiac transplantation is an option for patients with progressive cardiac dysfunction.

SUGGESTED READINGS

Ellis CR, Di Salvo T. Myocarditis: basic and clinical aspects. Cardiol Rev 2007; 15:170-177.

Magnani JW, Dec GW. Myocarditis: current trends in diagnosis and treatment. Circulation 2006; 113:876-890.

REFERENCES

1. Ellis CR, Di Salvo T. Myocarditis: basic and clinical aspects. Cardiol Rev 2007; 15:170-177.
2. Brady WJ, Ferguson JD, Ullman EA, et al. Myocarditis: emergency department recognition and management. Emerg Med Clin North Am 2004; 22:865-885.
3. Abbara S, Miller SW. Pericardial and myocardial disease. In Miller SW (ed). Cardiac Imaging: The Requisites. Philadelphia, Elsevier Mosby, 2005, pp 280-282.
4. Burns DK, Kumar V. The heart. In Kumar V, Cotran RS, Robbins SL (eds). Basic Pathology. Philadelphia, WB Saunders, 1997, pp 329-330.
5. Magnani JW, Dec GW. Myocarditis: current trends in diagnosis and treatment. Circulation 2006; 113:876-890.
6. Hauck AJ, Kearney DL, Edwards WD. Evaluation of postmortem endomyocardial biopsy specimens from 38 patients with lymphocytic myocarditis: implications for role of sampling error. Mayo Clin Proc 1989; 64:1235-1245.
7. Skouri HN, Dec GW, Friedrich MG, et al. Noninvasive imaging in myocarditis. J Am Coll Cardiol 2006; 48:2085-2093.
8. Hiramitsu S, Morimoto S, Kato S, et al. Transient ventricular wall thickening in acute myocarditis: a serial echocardiographic and histopathologic study. Jpn Circ J 2001; 65:863-866.
9. Nakagawa M, Hamaoka K. Myocardial thickening in children with acute myocarditis. Chest 1993; 104:1676-1678.
10. Lieback E, Hardouin I, Meyer R, et al. Clinical value of echocardiographic tissue characterization in the diagnosis of myocarditis. Eur Heart J 1996; 17:135-142.
11. Brooks MA, Sane DC. CT findings in acute myocarditis: 2 cases. J Thorac Imaging 2007; 22:277-279.
12. Boussel L, Gamondes D, Staat P, et al. Acute chest pain with normal coronary angiogram: role of contrast-enhanced multidetector computed tomography in the differential diagnosis between myocarditis and myocardial infarction. J Comput Assist Tomogr 2008; 32:228-232.

13. Dambrin G, Laissy JP, Serfaty JM, et al. Diagnostic value of ECG-gated multidetector computed tomography in the early phase of suspected acute myocarditis. A preliminary comparative study with cardiac MRI. Eur Radiol 2007; 17:331-338.
14. Mahrholdt H, Goedecke C, Wagner A, et al. Cardiovascular magnetic resonance assessment of human myocarditis: a comparison to histology and molecular pathology. Circulation 2004; 109:1250-1258.
15. Bohl S, Wassmuth R, Abdel-Aty H, et al. Delayed enhancement cardiac magnetic resonance imaging reveals typical patterns of myocardial injury in patients with various forms of non-ischemic heart disease. Int J Cardiovasc Imaging 2008; 24:597-607.
16. Mahrholdt H, Wagner A, Deluigi CC, et al. Presentation, patterns of myocardial damage, and clinical course of viral myocarditis. Circulation 2006; 114:1581-1590.
17. Abdel-Aty H, Simonetti O, Friedrich MG. T2-weighted cardiovascular magnetic resonance imaging. J Magn Reson Imaging 2007; 26:452-459.
18. Aretz HT, Billingham ME, Edwards WD, et al. Myocarditis. A histopathologic definition and classification. Am J Cardiovasc Pathol 1987; 1:3-14.
19. Laissy JP, Hyafil F, Feldman LJ, et al. Differentiating acute myocardial infarction from myocarditis: diagnostic value of early- and delayed-perfusion cardiac MR imaging. Radiology 2005; 237:75-82.
20. Abdel-Aty H, Boye P, Zagrosek A, et al. Diagnostic performance of cardiovascular magnetic resonance in patients with suspected acute myocarditis: comparison of different approaches. J Am Coll Cardiol 2005; 45:1815-1822.
21. Gurberlet M, Spors B, Thoma T, et al. Suspected chronic myocarditis at cardiac MR: diagnostic accuracy and association with immunohistologically detected inflammation and viral persistence. Radiology 2008; 246:401-409.
22. Hung MY, Hung MJ, Cheng CW. Use of gallium 67 scintigraphy to differentiate acute myocarditis from acute myocardial infarction. Tex Heart Inst J 2008; 34:305-309.
23. Matsuura H, Ishikita T, Yamamoto S, et al. Gallium-67 myocardial imaging for the detection of myocarditis in the acute phase of Kawasaki disease (mucocutaneous lymph node syndrome): the usefulness of single photon emission computed tomography. Br Heart J 1987; 58:385-392.
24. Narula J, Malhotra A, Yasuda T, et al. Usefulness of antimyosin antibody imaging for the detection of active rheumatic myocarditis. Am J Cardiol 1999; 84:946-950.

PART NINE

Tumors and Masses

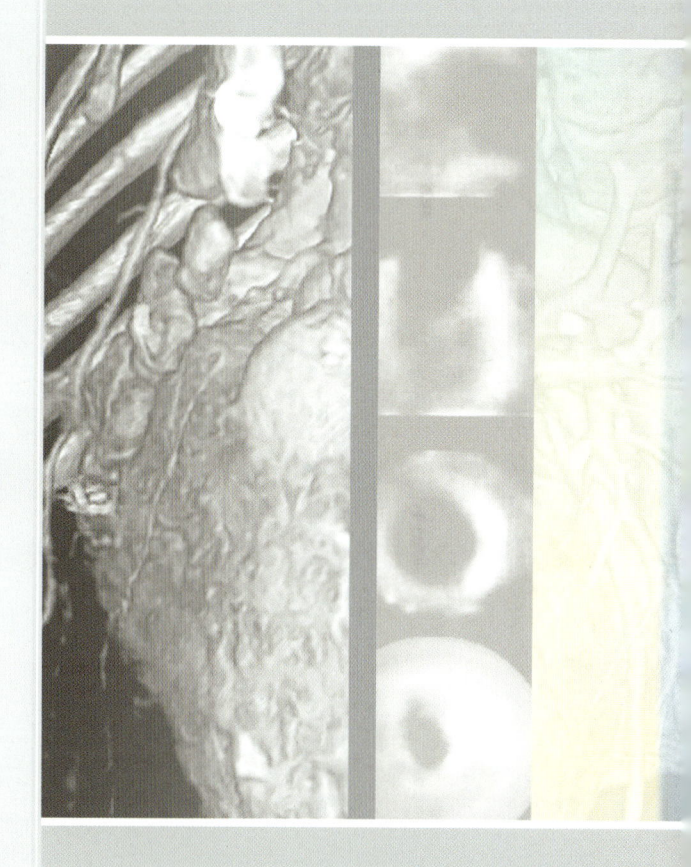

CHAPTER 67

Cardiac Tumors

Aletta Ann Frazier and Rachel Booth Lewis

BENIGN CARDIAC TUMORS

Primary cardiac tumors are uncommon, with incidence at autopsy of 0.02% to 0.05%. Approximately 75% of primary cardiac tumors are benign, but the clinical presentation of benign cardiac neoplasms overlaps considerably with malignant cardiac masses. Heart failure, dysrhythmias, symptoms of tumor or bland thromboembolism, syncope, and sudden cardiac death may occur in the presence of either benign or malignant cardiac neoplasms. To confound the distinction further, primary cardiac sarcomas are largely found in a similar age group to cardiac myxoma, the most common primary benign tumor of the heart.

Imaging features of cardiac masses that suggest benignancy include a left-sided location; a unifocal intracavitary or intramural mass with well-defined margins; and the absence of valvular, pericardial, or extracardiac involvement. Although primary malignant cardiac tumors often cannot be radiologically distinguished, benign cardiac neoplasms tend to show features on imaging that reflect their underlying pathology. Cardiac myxomas are usually left atrial masses and show a narrow base of attachment to the fossa ovalis. Papillary fibroelastomas are subcentimeter, pedunculated valvular masses usually discovered incidentally on an aortic valve leaflet. Cardiac fibromas are generally ventricular in location and often calcified. Rhabdomyomas are also often ventricular in location, but more commonly multiple in number. Lipomas and lipomatous hypertrophy of the interatrial septum (LHIS) may be distinguished by their fat content and location on cross-sectioning imaging. Characteristic features derived from radiologic-pathologic correlation may assist in limiting the differential diagnosis of a primary cardiac neoplasm.

Myxoma

Definition

Cardiac myxomas are benign neoplasms of endocardial origin, most commonly located in the atria.

Prevalence

With an incidence of 0.03%, cardiac myxoma is the most common primary cardiac tumor.[1] It represents approximately 50% of all benign cardiac tumors.[2] Myxomas have been reported in patients of every age, but most frequently patients present with myxomas between the third and sixth decades, with an average age of approximately 50 years.[2,3] There is a higher prevalence in women.[2]

A rare autosomal dominant form of cardiac myxoma is termed the *Carney complex*. Associated features include pigmented skin lesions, cutaneous myxomas, primary pigmented nodular adrenocortical disease, mammary myxoid fibroadenomas, large cell calcifying Sertoli-cell tumors, pituitary adenomas, thyroid tumors, and melanotic schwannomas.[4] Patients with the Carney complex present at an earlier age compared with patients with sporadic cases of cardiac myxoma, with an average age of 26 years.[4] These patients are also more predisposed to develop multiple tumors, documented in 41%[4] compared with 6% of patients with sporadic cardiac myxomas.[5]

Pathology

Cardiac myxomas arise from the endothelial surface by either a narrow or a broad-based pedicle and extend into the cardiac chamber (intracavitary growth) (Fig. 67-1). They range in size from 1 to 15 cm in diameter (average 5 to 6 cm).[2] Approximately 75% originate in the left atrium, 15% to 20% originate in the right atrium, and 5% are biatrial.[1] Myxomas rarely occur within the ventricular chamber or along the atrioventricular valves. Most are smoothly marginated, firm, and fibrotic (Fig. 67-2). The remaining one third to one half are gelatinous and friable with a villous or frondlike surface (Fig. 67-3).[1] This latter type is the morphology typically found in the Carney complex and is more likely to produce embolization.[6] Focal areas of hemorrhage may be evident on the surface of a myxoma.

Histologically, myxomas consist of inflammatory cells and myxoma cells in a myxoid matrix (Fig. 67-4). Myxoma cells are stellate multinucleate cells that form elongated

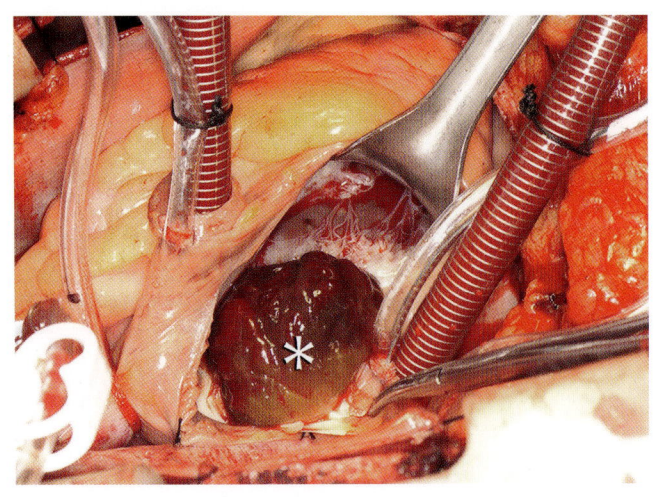

FIGURE 67-1 Gross surface features of cardiac myxoma. Intraoperative photograph of a left atriotomy reveals a lobulated, hemorrhagic mass (*asterisk*) arising from the endothelial surface and extending into the left atrial chamber.

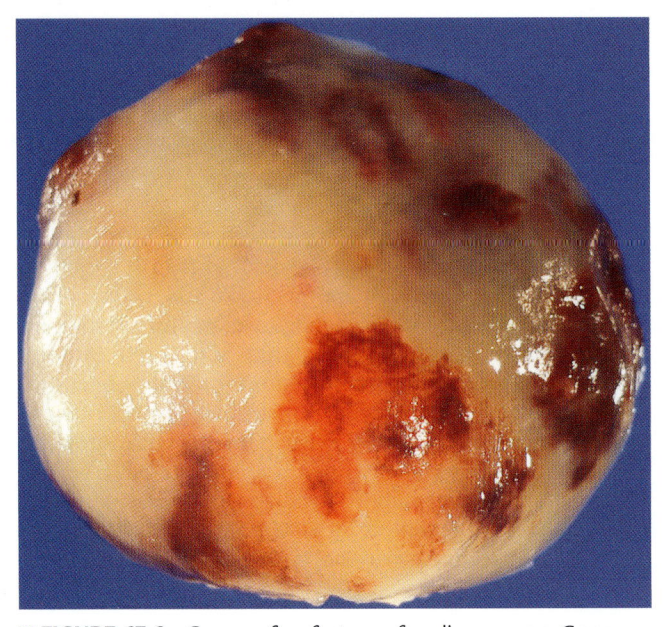

FIGURE 67-2 Gross surface features of cardiac myxoma. Gross specimen shows a glistening, smoothly contoured mass with focal areas of hemorrhage.

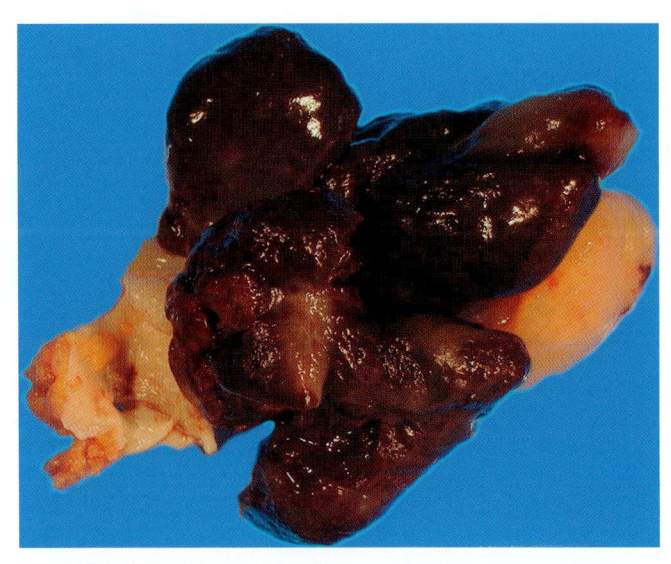

FIGURE 67-3 Gross surface features of cardiac myxoma. Gross specimen of a different myxoma shows an irregular, polypoid surface with multiple frondlike excrescences, predisposing to embolization.

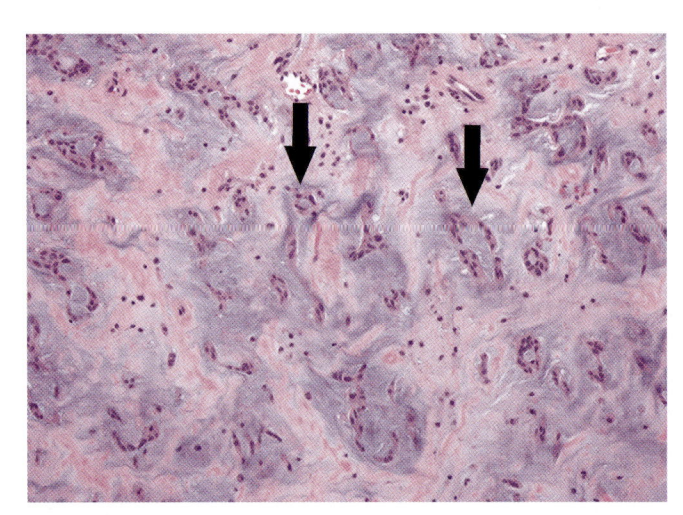

FIGURE 67-4 Intermediate-power photomicrograph shows nests of myxoma cells (*arrows*) embedded in a myxoid matrix (hematoxylin-eosin stain).

cords and rings.[6] They are of uncertain origin, but may arise from residual embryonal multipotential mesenchymal cells of the heart.[2] Myxomas also characteristically contain cysts, hemorrhage, extramedullary hematopoiesis and, rarely, glandular elements.[6] Calcification is common microscopically, and for unknown reasons is more prevalent in lesions on the right side of the heart.[1]

Manifestations of Disease

Clinical Presentation

Clinical presentation is extremely varied and depends on location, morphology, and size of the myxoma. The classic clinical triad is intracardiac obstruction, embolization, and constitutional symptoms.[2] Approximately 20% of patients are asymptomatic.[5] The most common symptoms of cardiac myxomas are secondary to obstruction.[3] Obstruction from left atrial myxomas mimics mitral valve stenosis, causing dyspnea and orthopnea from pulmonary edema. Obstructive right atrial myxomas may produce peripheral edema and syncope. Ventricular myxomas may mimic aortic or pulmonic valve stenosis, causing syncope. Obstruction may be intermittent and positional with pedunculated tumors.[3] Sudden cardiac death is rare, caused by temporary complete obstruction of the mitral or tricuspid valve.[2] Additionally, the motion of pedunculated atrial tumors may cause incomplete closure of, or damage to, the atrioventricular valve apparatus.[2]

Emboli have been reported in 35% of left-sided and 10% of right-sided cardiac myxomas.[3] Most emboli are systemic, originating from left-sided lesions or paradoxical emboli originating from right atrial myxomas. They may

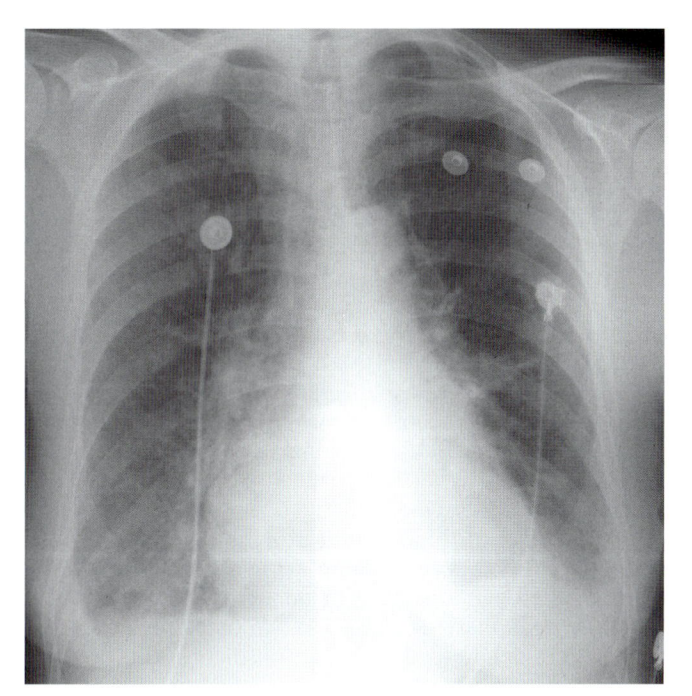

■ **FIGURE 67-5** Frontal chest radiograph in an elderly woman with progressive dyspnea shows vascular congestion, prominent septal (Kerley B) lines, small bilateral pleural effusions, and mild cardiomegaly with left atrial appendage enlargement. Presumptive diagnosis was congestive heart failure, but a left atrial myxoma was discovered by echocardiogram.

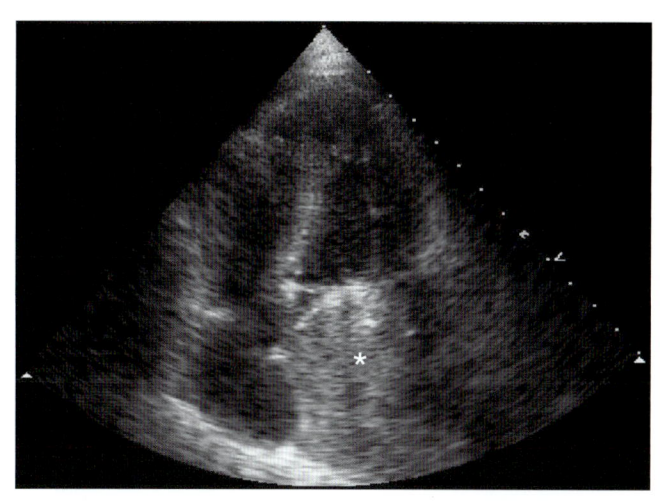

■ **FIGURE 67-6** Two-dimensional transthoracic echocardiogram (four-chamber view) shows an echogenic mass (*asterisk*) filling the left atrium, confirmed intraoperatively as a left atrial myxoma.

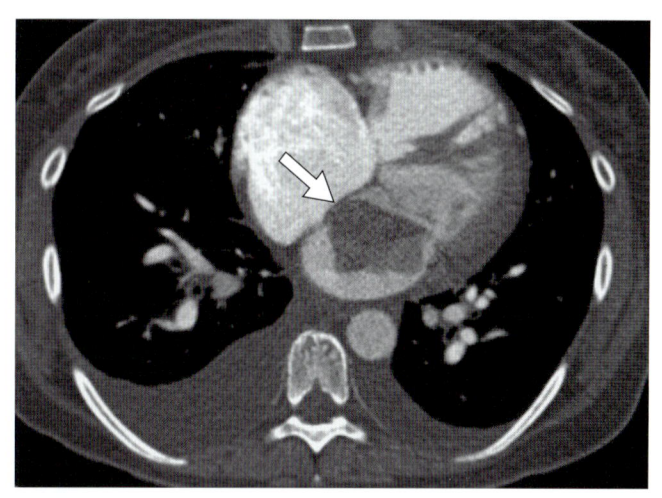

■ **FIGURE 67-7** Contrast-enhanced axial CT image (soft tissue windows) of a left atrial myxoma shows a lobulated, hypodense mass with a narrow base of attachment (*arrow*) to the interatrial septum.

affect the cerebral, visceral, renal, peripheral, or coronary arteries. Clinically evident pulmonary emboli are infrequent, but have been reported in right-sided cardiac myxomas.[2]

Constitutional symptoms, including fever, fatigue, and weight loss, occur in approximately one third of patients.[3] Other reported symptoms include arthralgias, myalgias, rashes, clubbing, cyanosis, and Raynaud phenomenon.[2] Cardiac arrhythmias or palpitations occur in 20% of patients with myxomas.[3] Less common presentations include chest pain, anemia, and sepsis.

Imaging Techniques and Findings

Radiography

Findings on chest radiograph vary with tumor location. Approximately 50% of left atrial myxomas produce findings suggestive of mitral valve obstruction, such as left atrial enlargement, prominence of the left atrial appendage, vascular redistribution, and pulmonary edema (Fig. 67-5).[3] Cardiomegaly and pleural effusions are less frequent findings, but may occur with either right-sided or left-sided myxomas. Radiographically evident calcification is reported in 50% of right atrial myxomas, but is not seen in left atrial myxomas.[3] Approximately one third of chest radiographs are normal.[3]

Ultrasonography

Transesophageal echocardiography may allow for better visualization of atrial tumors compared with the transthoracic approach (Fig. 67-6). Myxomas are pedunculated mobile masses on echocardiography, often apparently attached to the interatrial septum by a narrow stalk.[7] Myxomas may be homogeneous or heterogeneous, with echogenic foci owing to calcification and hypoechoic areas from hemorrhage, necrosis, or cysts.[7] Dynamic prolapse of the mass across the atrioventricular valve is often well visualized on echocardiography.

Computed Tomography

On contrast-enhanced CT, cardiac myxomas appear as intracavitary round or ovoid filling defects with smooth or lobulated contours.[3] Most myxomas are hypodense to myocardium and unopacified blood (Fig. 67-7).[3,5] Myxomas tend to enhance heterogeneously after administration of contrast medium (Fig. 67-8).[3] CT may show a narrow base of attachment to the interatrial septum, although a pedicle is usually not as well seen as with echocardiography.[7] Calcification may be evident, but typically only in right

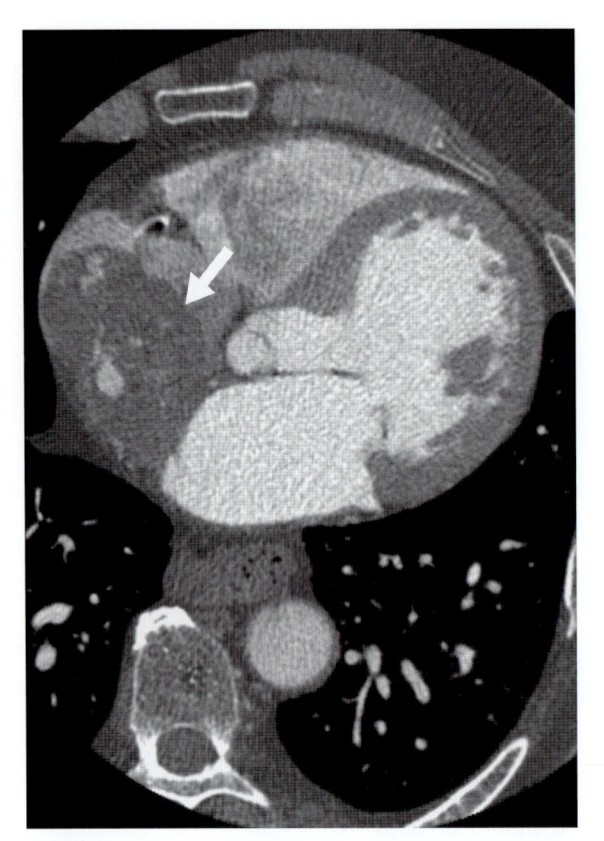

FIGURE 67-8 Coned axial CT image (soft tissue windows; cardiac gated) of a heterogeneously enhancing right atrial myxoma (*arrow*).

Magnetic Resonance Imaging

On MRI, myxomas are usually isointense on T1-weighted sequences and high signal intensity on T2-weighted sequences because of their myxoid stroma composition (Fig. 67-9A and B).[8] Myxomas are typically heterogeneous, likely reflective of varying components of hemorrhage, calcification, cysts, and myxoid or fibrous tissue.[3] Loss of signal intensity occurs with gradient-recalled-echo (GRE) imaging possibly because of magnetic susceptibility from high iron content.[3] Myxomas are usually hypointense to blood pool and hyperintense to myocardium on steady-state free precession (SSFP) sequences, although they may be isointense to blood and possibly missed on this sequence.[9] Myxomas enhance with gadolinium, usually with a heterogeneous pattern on perfusion and delayed enhancement phases (Fig. 67-9C).[10] MRI has been reported to be more accurate than CT in predicting the point of attachment to the wall, which may be best seen on cine images.[3] Cine MRI also may show prolapse of the tumor across a cardiac valve (Fig. 67-10).[10]

Differential Diagnosis

The differential diagnosis of an intracavitary cardiac mass includes thrombus and other neoplasms, such as meta-

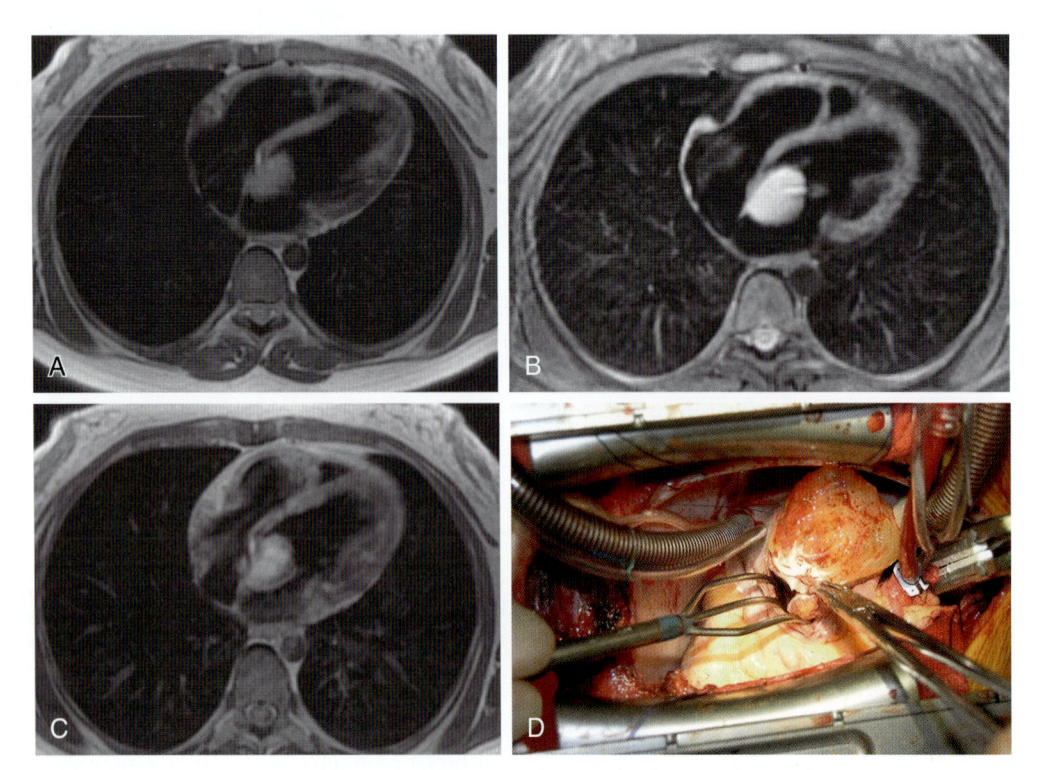

FIGURE 67-9 Left atrial myxoma in a 17-year-old boy. **A** and **B,** On axial T1-weighted MR image (**A**), the lesion is isointense to slightly hyperintense in signal intensity, whereas axial T2-weighted MR image (**B**) shows marked homogeneous high signal intensity. **C,** Postgadolinium axial T1-weighted MR image shows heterogenous enhancement. **D,** Intraoperative view of pedunculated left atrial myxoma. *(Courtesy of Gil Boswell, MD, Naval Medical Center San Diego.)*

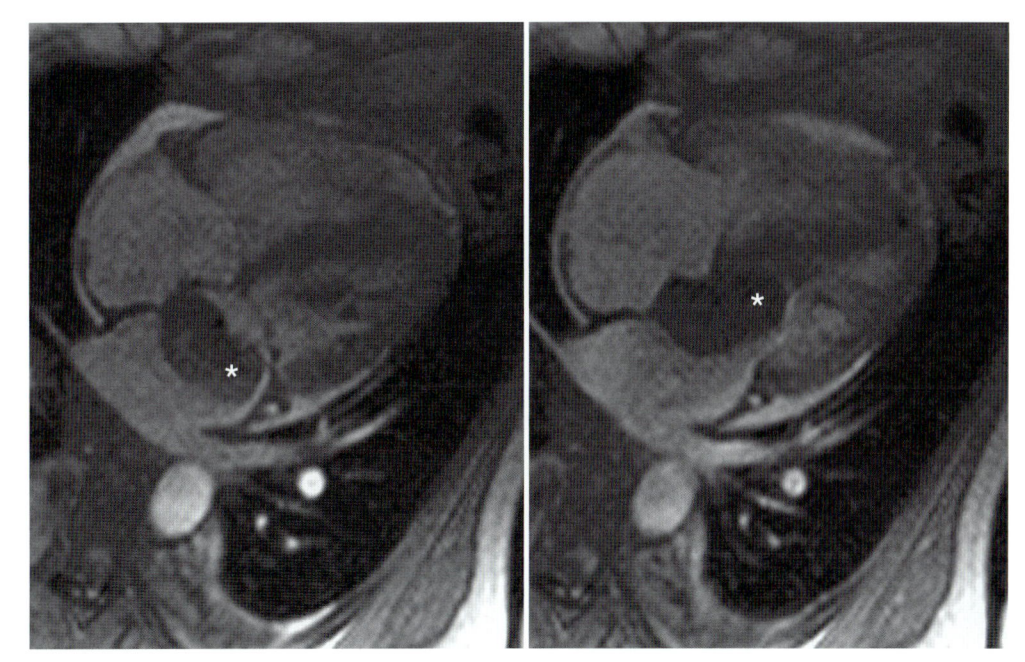

FIGURE 67-10 Horizontal long-axis cine images of a pedunculated left atrial myxoma in systole and diastole show partial prolapse of the lesion (*asterisk*) across the mitral valve plane during diastole.

static disease and sarcoma. As opposed to atrial myxomas, atrial thrombi are found in the setting of atrial fibrillation and mitral valve disease, and are usually located in the atrial appendage or posterior or lateral atrial walls, rather than along the interatrial septum. Additionally, thrombi do not typically show contrast enhancement, a feature best evaluated on MRI. Metastatic disease may occur in any location within the heart, but is most frequent in the right-sided chambers. Sarcomas are generally much more invasive and infiltrative in appearance.

Treatment Options

To prevent complications such as embolization or sudden cardiac death owing to valvular obstruction, the treatment of cardiac myxoma is prompt surgical resection. The stalk and zone of attachment are excised, including the full thickness of the interatrial septum for myxomas that arise in this location. Long-term prognosis is excellent. Recurrence occurs in less than 3% of nonfamilial cases and is considered related to incomplete resection.[2] In patients with the Carney complex, recurrence is 20%, which may be due in part to multifocality of lesions.[2,4]

> **KEY POINTS: MYXOMA**
> - Clinical and radiographic manifestations of cardiac myxomas may mimic valvular disease, particularly mitral stenosis.
> - Typical imaging appearance is an intracavitary, pedunculated mass located in the left atrium arising from the interatrial septum.
> - Contrast-enhanced MRI may help to distinguish between thrombus and myxoma.

Papillary Fibroelastoma

Definition

Papillary fibroelastoma is an endocardial-based mass most commonly found on the aortic valve. It is of uncertain etiology and may be a hamartoma, neoplasm, or reparative process.

Prevalence

Cardiac papillary fibroelastomas are the second most common primary cardiac tumor, representing approximately 10% of benign cardiac tumors.[7] They are the most common tumor of the cardiac valves. Papillary fibroelastomas have been reported in all ages, but are most frequently found in the fourth to eighth decades of life, with a mean age of 60 years.[11] In the largest case analysis, there was a slight male predominance of 55%.[11] This lesion is usually solitary, and no familial cases have been described.

Pathology

Papillary fibroelastomas consist of multiple fronds attached to the endocardium by a short pedicle. When immersed in water or saline, they are described as having the appearance of a sea anemone (Fig. 67-11).[1] The papillary fronds are avascular with an elastic fiber and collagen core surrounded by myxomatous matrix and endothelial cells.[6] Dystrophic calcification has been reported, but is rare.[11] Most lesions are approximately 1 cm in maximum diameter, although lesions up to 7 cm in size have been reported.[11] More than 75% of papillary fibroelastomas are found on the cardiac valves, involving the aortic, mitral, tricuspid, and pulmonary valves in decreasing frequency.[11] Aortic and pulmonary valve papillary fibroelastomas most

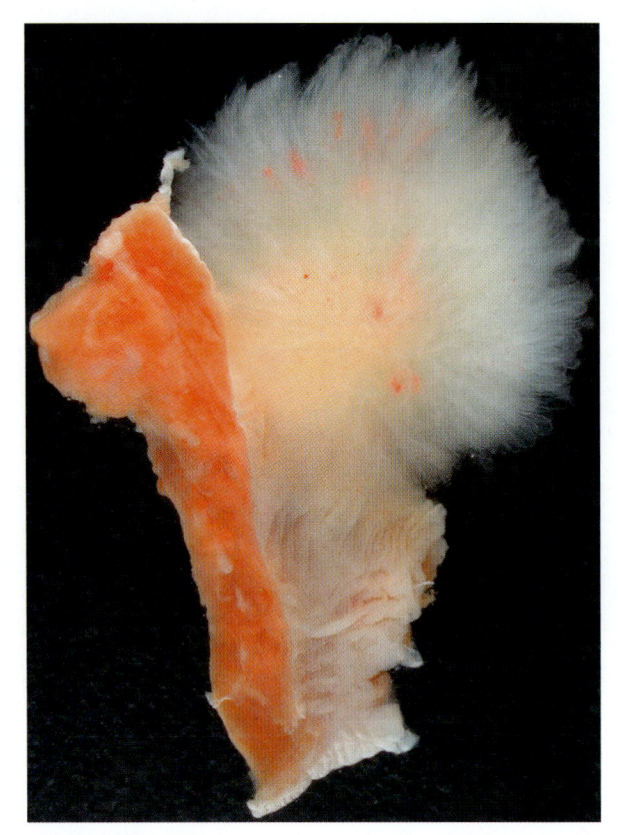

■ **FIGURE 67-11** Immersed in fluid, a papillary fibroelastoma exhibits multiple branching papillary fronds, which create the appearance of a sea anemone.

commonly project into the vascular lumen, whereas papillary fibroelastomas on the atrioventricular valves usually project into the atria.[11] They may also occur along the endocardial surfaces of the atria and ventricles or on the eustachian valve.

Manifestations of Disease

Clinical Presentation

Most papillary fibroelastomas are found incidentally during imaging, cardiac surgery, or autopsy.[11] No longitudinal studies have been performed, and the natural history of these lesions is unknown. The most common clinical manifestation is embolism. Either the tumor itself or associated thrombus may embolize into the cerebral, visceral, renal, peripheral, coronary, or, less frequently, pulmonary arteries.[11] Heart failure, arrhythmia, syncope, and sudden death are less common manifestations.

Imaging Techniques and Findings
Radiography

Because of their small size, papillary fibroelastomas would not be expected to produce any findings on chest radiography. If there is obstruction of the mitral valve, findings of pulmonary venous hypertension may be apparent. Calcification is rarely visible.[11]

Ultrasonography

Most papillary fibroelastomas are found incidentally during echocardiography. They typically appear as small, homogeneous, valvular masses that may be sessile or pedunculated.[5] A stippled pattern may be seen near the edges, reflective of the papillary projections.[11] Almost half of papillary fibroelastomas are mobile with evidence of flutter or prolapse.[11,12]

Computed Tomography

The few studies of the CT appearance of papillary fibroelastomas have used ECG gating. They describe a tiny, well-defined spherical mass attached to a valve leaflet (Fig. 67-12).[13,14]

Magnetic Resonance Imaging

Because of their small size, papillary fibroelastomas are infrequently visualized on MRI. Papillary fibroelastoma is typically a mobile, nodular mass with homogeneous intermediate signal intensity on T1-weighted sequences and intermediate or low signal intensity on T2-weighted sequences.[14,15] It is best appreciated on cine MRI sequences as a small valvular mass with adjacent turbulent blood flow.[10] It is characteristically hypointense to myocardium on GRE sequences.[16] After administration of gadolinium, papillary fibroelastomas show delayed hyperenhancement possibly because of their fibroelastic tissue composition.[15,17]

Differential Diagnosis

The differential diagnosis of a cardiac valvular mass includes vegetation from endocarditis, thrombus, and valvular myxoma. The clinical context of endocarditis differs from papillary fibroelastoma. Additionally, these entities can be differentiated on imaging by the function of the underlying valve. Leaflet destruction and valvular incompetence are usually seen in endocarditis, but normal valve function is preserved in the presence of a papillary fibroelastoma. Valvular thrombus usually is nonmobile and lacks enhancement. Valvular myxomas are usually larger than papillary fibroelastomas and may be differentiated by their heterogeneous and high T2 signal intensity on MRI.

Treatment Options

Treatment is surgical excision, particularly for left-sided lesions, to prevent the consequences of systemic embolization. Recurrence has not been reported.[11] The efficacy of long-term anticoagulation is unknown.

> **KEY POINTS: PAPILLARY FIBROELASTOMA**
>
> ■ Papillary fibroelastoma is the most common cardiac valve tumor.
> ■ It is most frequently located on the aortic or mitral valves, and is a potential source of systemic emboli.

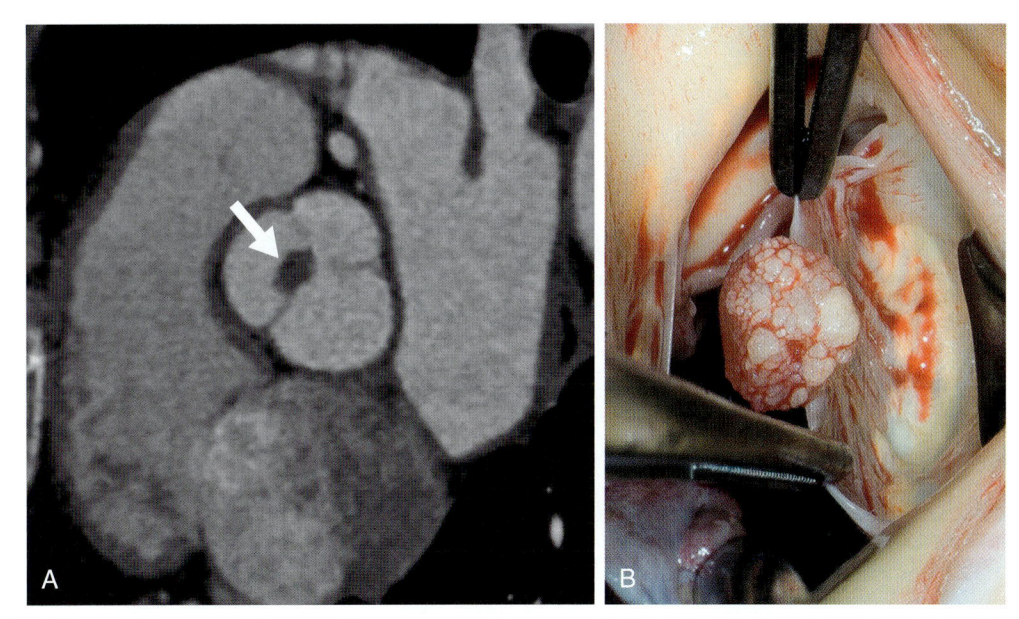

FIGURE 67-12 A 59-year-old woman with new cardiac murmur and 1-cm rounded lesion identified on the aortic valve by echocardiogram. **A,** Contrast-enhanced, cardiac gated CT image (soft tissue windows), reconstructed through the aortic valve plane, shows a 9-mm lesion (*arrow*) attached to the right aortic valve cusp. **B,** Intraoperative photograph reveals a papillary-appearing lesion at the leading edge of the mid–right coronary cusp of the aortic valve.

Fibroma

Definition

Cardiac fibroma is a congenital neoplasm or hamartoma of fibrous tissue that usually manifests in childhood.

Prevalence

Cardiac fibromas are the second most common tumor in childhood after rhabdomyoma. In contrast to rhabdomyomas, they are uniformly solitary.[5] One third of patients present before 1 year of age, although 15% of cardiac fibromas are discovered in adolescence and adulthood.[5] There is no sex predilection.[18] Fibromas are associated with Gorlin syndrome (also known as basal cell nevus syndrome), an autosomal dominant syndrome of multiple basal cell carcinomas, odontogenic keratocysts, skeletal anomalies, and other neoplasms such as medulloblastoma.[8]

Pathology

Fibromas are mural-based whorled masses of white tissue (Fig. 67-13). Mean size is 5 cm (range 2 to 10 cm).[5,7] They are not encapsulated and may have either circumscribed or infiltrating margins. Fibromas are typically located in the interventricular septum or left ventricular free wall.[1,6] Less frequently, they are found in the right ventricle or atria. In newborns and infants, fibromas are highly cellular with numerous fibroblasts. With age, cellularity decreases, and the amount of collagen increases.[6,19] Fibromas contain microscopic calcification in one third of cases; they are otherwise fairly homogeneous on histologic and gross examination.[6]

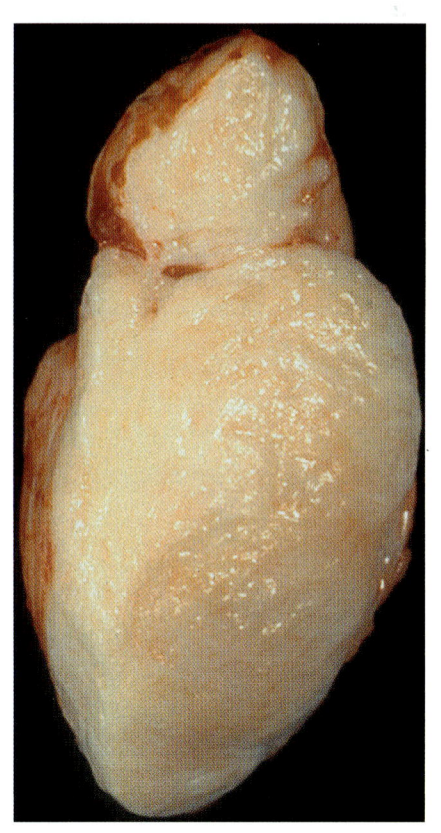

FIGURE 67-13 Gross photo of a ventricular fibroma (cut section) reveals firm, whorled white tissue.

Manifestations of Disease

Clinical Presentation

Fibromas are asymptomatic in one third to one half of cases. Symptoms include heart failure, arrhythmia, chest

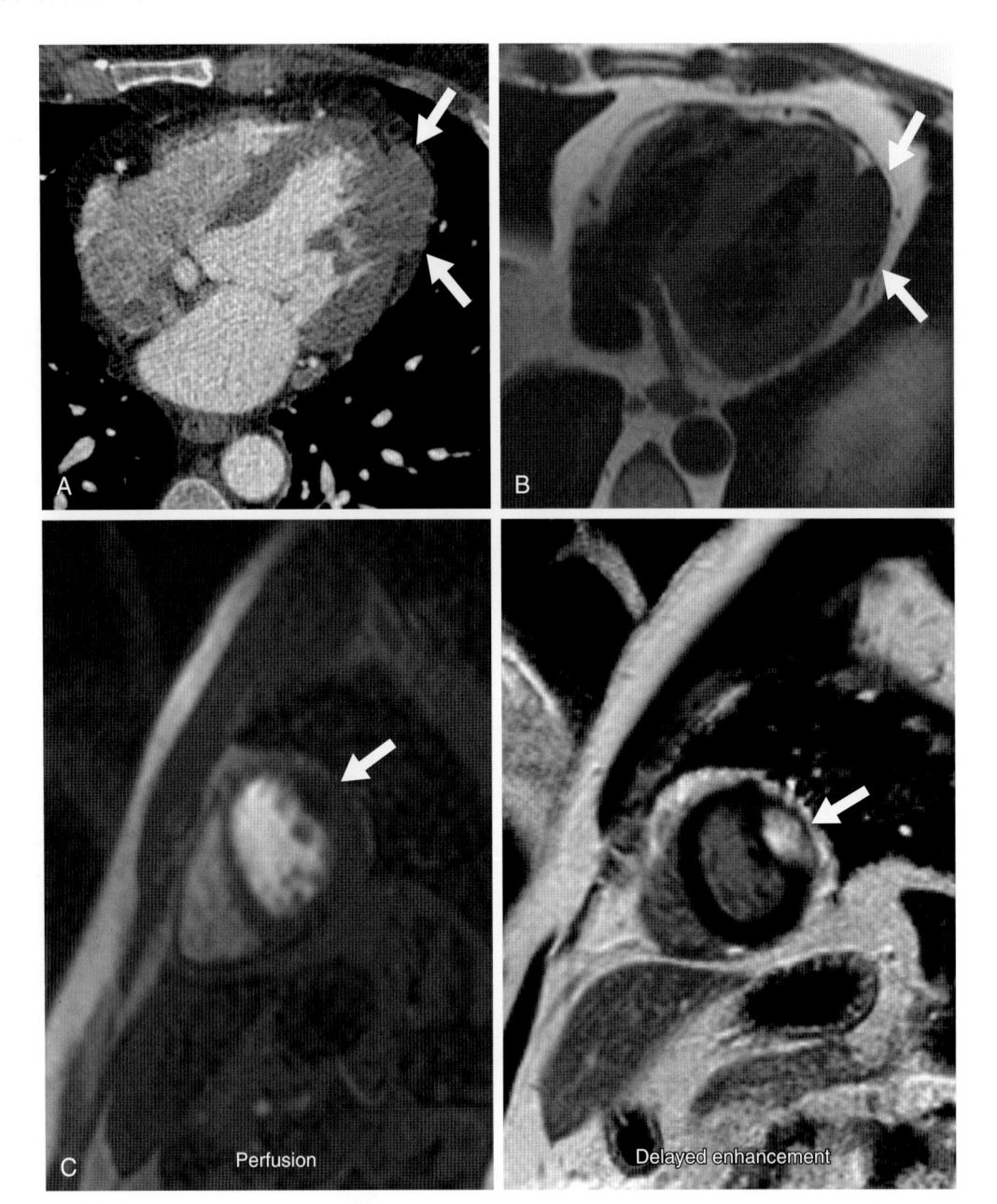

FIGURE 67-14 An asymptomatic 45-year-old man with left ventricular fibroma. **A,** Axial CT angiogram shows an oblong, homogeneous soft tissue mass (*arrows*) in the lateral left ventricle, partly surrounded by epicardial fat. **B,** Axial MR image (double inversion recovery) at similar level to the CT angiogram confirms an oblong, hypointense mass (*arrows*) associated with the left ventricular wall, partly outlined by epicardial fat. **C,** Short-axis MRI perfusion (*left*) and delayed enhancement (*right*) images. Perfusion image shows the lesion (*arrow*) relatively hypointense compared with adjacent myocardium; delayed phase imaging reveals characteristic intense hyperenhancement of the lesion (*arrow*).

pain, syncope, and sudden death.[1,20] In one study of primary cardiac tumors that caused sudden cardiac death, fibroma was the second most common underlying cause (after endodermal heterotopia of the atrioventricular node).[21]

Imaging Techniques and Findings

Radiography

The most common abnormality on chest radiograph is cardiomegaly.[22] A focal bulge of the cardiac contour can also be seen.[19] Calcification overlying the cardiac silhouette is visualized radiographically in approximately one quarter of cases, and may appear dense or amorphous.[5,20]

Ultrasonography

Cardiac fibroma may appear as a discrete mass or a focal area of wall thickening mimicking focal hypertrophic cardiomyopathy on echocardiogram. Fibromas are echogenic and may appear heterogeneous.[5]

Computed Tomography

Fibromas are circumscribed or infiltrative mural-based masses on CT (Fig. 67-14A). They show soft tissue attenuation and often calcification.[8] Enhancement may be either homogeneous or heterogeneous.[5,19]

Magnetic Resonance Imaging

On MRI, a cardiac fibroma appears as an intramural mass or focal myocardial thickening on T1-weighted sequences, where it is isointense or hypointense to myocardium (Fig. 67-14B).[8,23] In contrast to other cardiac tumors, fibromas are characteristically hypointense on T2-weighted and SSFP sequences because of their fibrous tissue composition, which has low water content.[8,23,24] The fibrous tissue is also hypovascular, causing little or no enhancement on perfusion imaging (Fig. 67-14C).[24] On myocardial delayed enhancement MRI, fibromas typically show marked hyperenhancement, however, occasionally with central regions of hypointensity (see Fig. 67-14C).[24] The delayed enhancement is currently attributed to the significant extracellular space for gadolinium accumulation.[24]

Differential Diagnosis

The differential diagnosis of a cardiac mass in an infant or child is rhabdomyoma, fibroma, and rhabdomyosarcoma. Rhabdomyoma is supported by findings of tuberous sclerosis, multiplicity, and lack of calcification. Rhabdomyosarcoma may be discriminated by its heterogeneous appearance, reflecting cystic change and necrosis.

Treatment Options

In contrast to soft tissue fibromatosis, there is little evidence that cardiac fibromas may enlarge, and spontaneous regression has been reported.[1] Treatment for symptomatic patients is complete surgical excision, although partial excision may be performed for more extensive tumors. Postsurgical recurrence is rare.[5]

KEY POINTS: FIBROMA

- Fibroma should be considered in the differential diagnosis of a solitary mural-based mass in a child.
- Characteristic MRI appearances are hypointensity on T2-weighted sequences, minimal enhancement on perfusion images, and marked hyperenhancement on myocardial delayed enhancement imaging.

Rhabdomyoma

Definition

Rhabdomyoma is a congenital hamartoma of altered cardiac myocytes.

Prevalence

Rhabdomyoma is the most common cardiac neoplasm in infants and children, and accounts for 50% to 75% of pediatric cardiac tumors.[10] It occurs equally in boys and girls.[10] Approximately 50% of patients with rhabdomyomas have tuberous sclerosis, an association that increases to 95% in fetuses and neonates with multiple cardiac tumors.[25] Conversely, virtually all infants with tuberous sclerosis have cardiac rhabdomyomas, although this incidence decreases with age because of spontaneous regression.[8] Rhabdomyoma is rarely associated with congenital heart diseases, such as Ebstein anomaly, tetralogy of Fallot, and hypoplastic left heart syndrome.[22]

Pathology

Rhabdomyomas usually consist of circumscribed mural-based nodules that average 1 to 3 cm in size; multiple nodules are present in 70% to 90% of cases.[1] The left ventricle or interventricular septum is the most common location, followed by the right ventricle and atria in decreasing frequency.[26] Rhabdomyomas protrude into the cardiac chambers in 50%,[27] a characteristic observed more often in patients who do not have tuberous sclerosis.[6] Histologically, the rhabdomyoma cell has a distinctive spider-like appearance with vacuolated cytoplasm and radiating myofibers surrounding a central nucleus. The cells stain with periodic acid–Schiff because of their high glycogen content.[5]

Manifestations of Disease

Clinical Presentation

Rhabdomyomas are most commonly diagnosed incidentally on routine second-trimester fetal ultrasound examinations.[27] The most frequent presentation in utero is arrhythmia, including tachycardias and bradycardias.[26] Additional fetal manifestations include hydrops and fetal death. Infants may be asymptomatic or present with arrhythmia, heart failure, or left ventricular outflow obstruction.[26]

Imaging Techniques and Findings

Radiography

Chest radiographs may show cardiomegaly.[22]

Ultrasonography

Prenatal and postnatal echocardiograms show intramural, solid hyperechoic masses typically located in the ventricular myocardium.

Computed Tomography

CT scan may show multiple intramural nodules that appear either hypodense or hyperdense to normal myocardium.[28]

Magnetic Resonance Imaging

Cardiac rhabdomyomas are intramural masses that are isointense on T1-weighted MRI sequences and hyperintense on T2-weighted sequences (Fig. 67-15).[8] They may produce focal abnormalities of contractility.[8] Rhabdo-

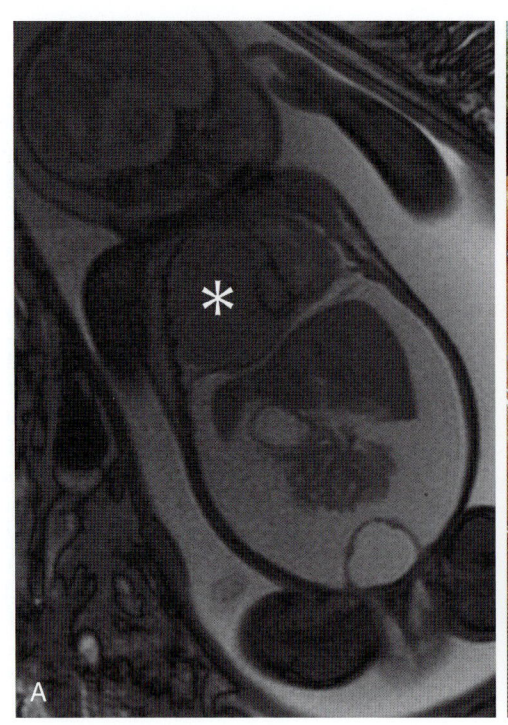

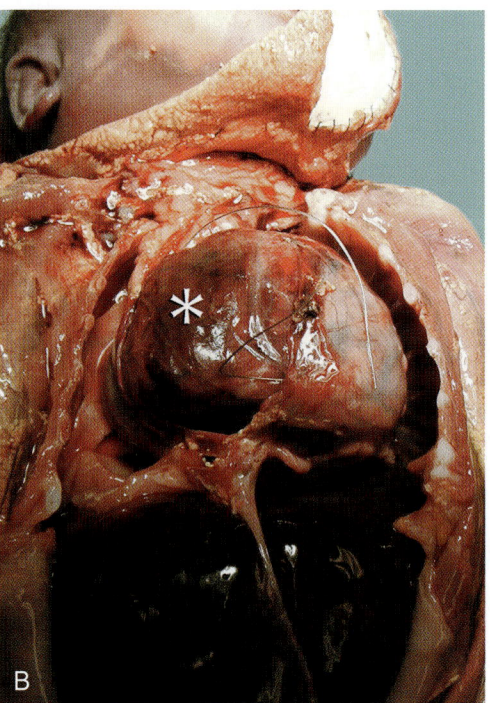

■ **FIGURE 67-15** Obstetric ultrasound examination in a 33-week gestational age fetus showed a large "mediastinal mass." **A,** MR image (SSFP) oriented in the coronal plane of the fetus shows a large mass (*asterisk*) inseparable from the heart, with mass effect on the remainder of the heart and both lungs. Note small pleural effusions, ascites, subcutaneous edema, and polyhydramnios. **B,** Autopsy reveals a large, 7 × 5 × 5 cm left ventricular rhabdomyoma (*asterisk*) that fills the chest cavity and, by mass effect, rotates the heart in an abnormal orientation and causes pulmonary hypoplasia. Note residual pacemaker wires.

myomas enhance homogeneously and intensely with gadolinium.[8,10] Numerous rhabdomyomas less than 1 mm in size, so-called rhabdomyomatosis, may produce diffuse myocardial thickening without a discrete mass.[53]

Differential Diagnosis

The differential diagnosis of a neonatal cardiac mass includes rhabdomyoma, fibroma, teratoma, and rhabdomyosarcoma. Rhabdomyomas are typically multifocal and lack the calcification and T2 hypointensity of fibromas, or the heterogeneity of teratomas and rhabdomyosarcomas.

Treatment Options

Approximately 80% of cardiac rhabdomyomas regress spontaneously during childhood and are not resected, unless life-threatening symptoms are present.[27] They regress less frequently, however, in patients who do not have tuberous sclerosis, more often requiring surgical excision.[8]

KEY POINTS: RHABDOMYOMA

- Rhabdomyoma is the most common cardiac tumor of childhood.
- Half of patients with rhabdomyoma have tuberous sclerosis, and virtually all patients with tuberous sclerosis have cardiac rhabdomyomas.
- The typical imaging appearance is multiple ventricular mural-based masses.

Lipoma

Definition

Lipomas are true neoplastic lesions of mature fat cells.

Prevalence

Lipomas reportedly represent 8% of primary cardiac tumors,[29] although this may be an overestimate because many series do not differentiate lipomas from LHIS. They may manifest at any age, but patients are typically younger than patients with lipomatous hypertrophy.[30] There is no gender prevalence.[29]

Pathology

Lipomas are circumscribed masses of homogeneous yellow fat that may be found within the myocardium, occasionally with extension into the pericardial space or cardiac chambers. The most common sites are the right atrium, left ventricle, and interatrial septum.[29] Half are subendocardial, with the remaining half split between myocardial and subepicardial locations.[29] Histologically, lipomas are encapsulated masses of mature fat cells, without the brown fat or hypertrophic myocytes found in lipomatous hypertrophy.

Manifestations of Disease

Clinical Presentation

Most cardiac lipomas are asymptomatic and are discovered during imaging or autopsy. Occasionally, they may cause obstruction or arrhythmias.[8]

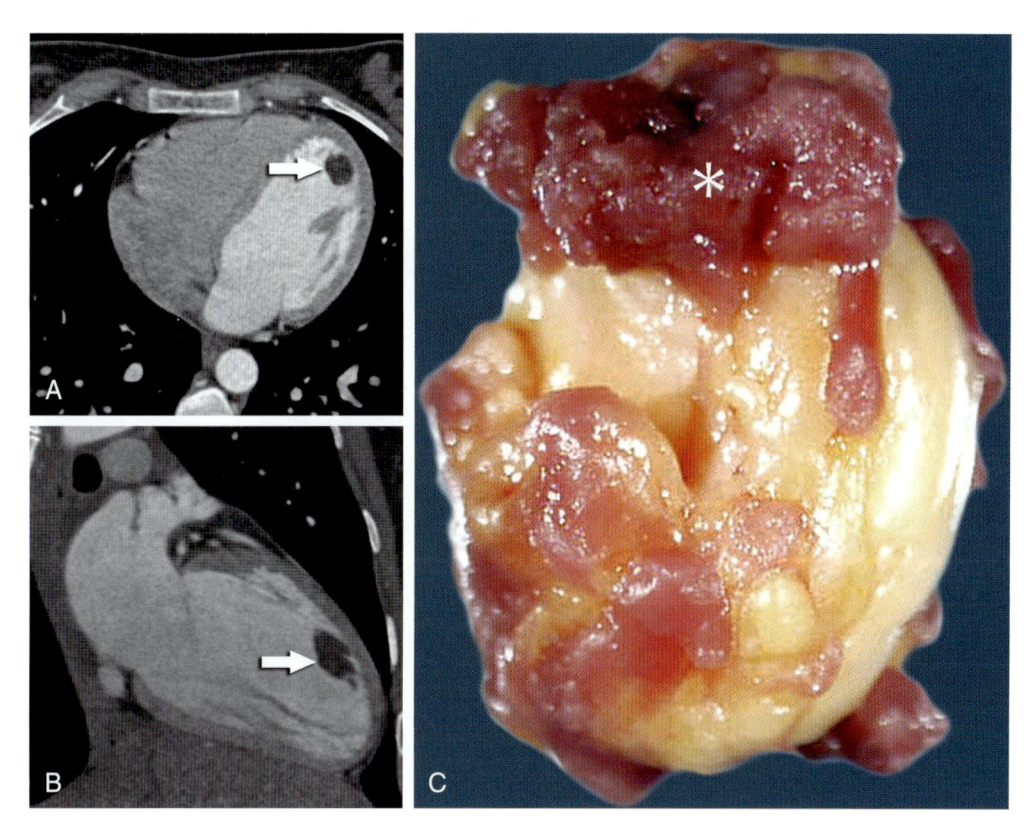

FIGURE 67-16 A 26-year-old woman with palpitations. **A** and **B**, Axial CT slice (**A**) and two-chamber view reformat (**B**) (soft tissue windows) show a rounded filling defect of fat density at the left ventricular apex (*arrows*). **C**, Gross photograph of the left ventricular lipoma with fragments of cardiac muscle (*asterisk*); at surgery, the 2.4 × 1.3 cm lesion was attached to the anterolateral papillary muscle.

Imaging Techniques and Findings

Radiography

Chest radiographs may be normal or show cardiomegaly.[5]

Ultrasonography

Lipomas are nonspecific homogeneous, immobile echogenic masses on echocardiography.[5]

Computed Tomography

CT and MRI have the advantage over echocardiography of being able to characterize the tissue type. Lipomas have homogeneous low attenuation on CT similar to subcutaneous or mediastinal fat, typically less than −50 Hounsfield units (Fig. 67-16). Thin strands of soft tissue attenuation septa may be present without any nodularity. No significant enhancement occurs with administration of contrast medium.

Magnetic Resonance Imaging

On MRI, lipomas are homogeneous, smoothly contoured masses. They show homogeneous fat signal intensity on all sequences, including decreased signal intensity on fat-suppressed sequences, and no enhancement with gadolinium.[8,29] There may be thin septations, but no nodular components. Chemical shift artifact occurs on SSFP sequences at the interface between the lipoma and the myocardium or blood pool, resulting in a low signal intensity margin.[29]

Differential Diagnosis

In the differential diagnosis of a fat-containing cardiac mass, LHIS should be considered for lesions located in the interatrial septum. A true lipoma is more often round or oval instead of bilobed, discovered incidentally in younger patients or in patients with little mediastinal fat. Liposarcoma is also in the differential diagnosis of a fat-containing cardiac mass, although it usually contains significant soft tissue components.

Treatment Options

Surgical resection is performed only for symptomatic cardiac lipomas.

KEY POINTS: LIPOMA

- CT and MRI are diagnostic for lipomas, showing homogeneous fat-containing masses without soft tissue components other than thin septations.
- Lipomas tend to be found in a younger patient population than LHIS.

Lipomatous Hypertrophy of the Interatrial Septum

Definition

LHIS is not a true neoplasm, but rather a benign diffuse thickening (defined as >2 cm) of the normal extension of epicardial fat within the interatrial groove.[30]

Prevalence

LHIS is significantly more common than true cardiac lipomas. In a prospective study of sequential chest CT scans, the incidence was 2.2%.[31] The reported age range is 22 to 91 years, with most patients presenting with LHIS older than 60 years.[30] Associations include age, obesity, pulmonary emphysema, and long-term parenteral nutrition.[31] Some reports suggest a slight female predominance.[30,31]

Pathology

Lipomatous hypertrophy is a misnomer because the lesion actually represents hyperplasia rather than hypertrophy of the normal fat found within the interatrial septum. LHIS is a nonencapsulated, poorly circumscribed thickening of the fat of the interatrial groove that extends from the aortic root caudally to the coronary sinus; it is occasionally contiguous with mediastinal fat. LHIS spares the fossa ovalis, causing a bilobed appearance. In a prospective CT study, the thickness ranged from 2 to 6.2 cm (mean 3.2 cm).[31] A combination of vacuolated brown fat cells, hypertrophic myocytes, and normal mature fat cells is seen on histologic examination.[6]

Manifestations of Disease

Clinical Presentation

Although most often an incidental finding, LHIS can be associated with supraventricular arrhythmias, sudden cardiac death, and heart failure.[31]

Imaging Techniques and Findings

Ultrasonography

Echocardiography shows an echogenic, dumbbell-shaped mass in the interatrial septum sparing the fossa ovalis.[32]

Computed Tomography

CT reveals a homogeneous fatty attenuation mass, shaped like an hourglass or a dumbbell, which shows focal sparing at the fossa ovalis (Fig. 67-17). No significant enhancement occurs with administration of contrast medium. A large amount of concomitant epicardial or mediastinal fat, or both, is often present.[29,31]

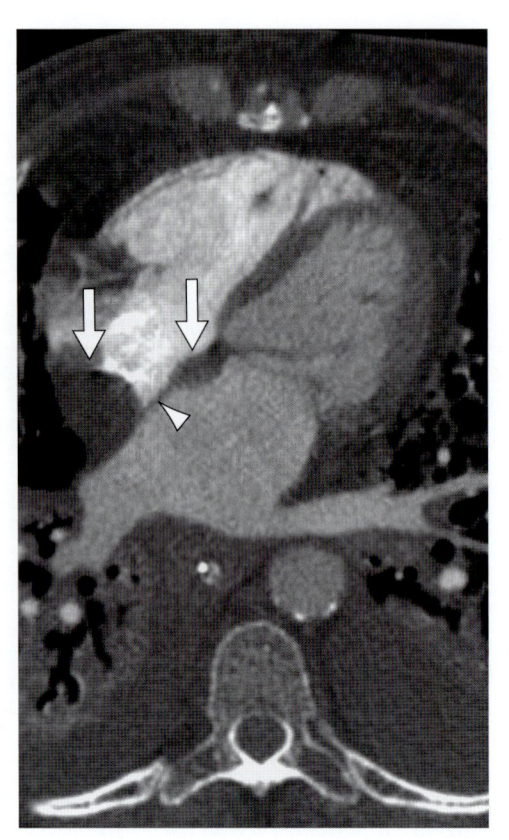

FIGURE 67-17 A 74-year-old woman with LHIS, an incidental finding. Contrast-enhanced coned axial CT image (soft tissue windows) shows a dumbbell shaped, homogeneous lesion of fat density (*arrows*) located in the interatrial septum, with sparing of the fossa ovalis (*arrowhead*). Note prominence of epicardial and mediastinal fat planes.

Magnetic Resonance Imaging

LHIS also has an hourglass shape on MRI. It is homogeneous and similar in signal intensity to subcutaneous or mediastinal fat on all sequences, with signal dropout on fat saturation sequences (Fig. 67-18A).[29] SSFP sequences show central hyperintensity with a low signal intensity margin at the interface with blood or myocardium, presumably from chemical shift artifact (Fig. 67-18B).[29]

Nuclear Medicine

In positron emission tomography (PET) imaging with ^{18}FDG, increased uptake of ^{18}FDG compared with background mediastinum has been reported and is presumably related to the presence of brown fat.[33]

Differential Diagnosis

The differential diagnosis of LHIS includes other fat-containing masses, such as lipoma and liposarcoma. Cardiac lipomas typically do not have a bilobed appearance and can be found in any location within the heart. Cardiac liposarcoma is extremely rare, and nonlipomatous soft tissue components may be expected on imaging.

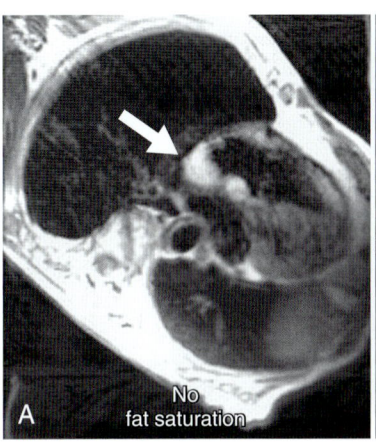

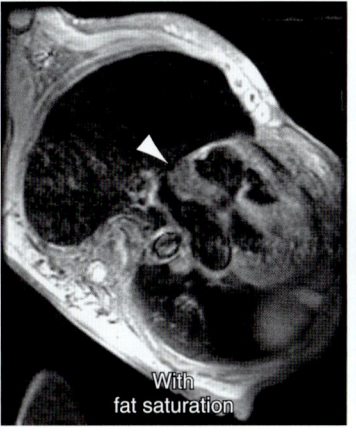

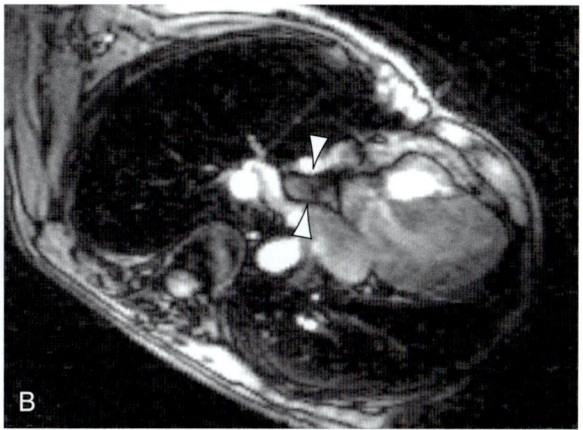

FIGURE 67-18 An 80-year-old woman with an incidental finding. **A,** Horizontal long-axis T1-weighted MR image (without and with fat saturation). Without fat saturation, the bilobed mass (*arrow*) has high signal intensity that matches the subcutaneous fat. With fat saturation, the mass (*arrowhead*) shows decreased signal intensity, which confirms its fatty composition. **B,** Horizontal long-axis cine image shows characteristic low signal intensity margin (*arrowheads*) outlining the lipomatous hypertrophy.

Treatment Options

Surgical resection may be performed in cases causing arrhythmias unresponsive to medical treatment, or in cases with LHIS lesions causing obstruction of the superior vena cava or right atrium.

> **KEY POINTS: LIPOMATOUS HYPERTROPHY OF THE INTERATRIAL SEPTUM**
>
> - Although usually incidental, LHIS is a cause of supraventricular arrhythmias.
> - Imaging appearance is diagnostic, with an hourglass-shaped mass of fat attenuation or fat signal intensity in the interatrial septum.

Paraganglioma

Definition

A cardiac paraganglioma is an extra-adrenal catecholamine-producing tumor derived from chromograffin neuroectodermal cells.

Prevalence

Cardiac paragangliomas are extremely rare. Only 1% to 2% of pheochromocytomas or paragangliomas are found within the thorax, most of which are located in the posterior mediastinum. Cardiac paragangliomas typically manifest in adulthood, with an age range of 18 to 85 years (mean 40 years).[5] Extracardiac paragangliomas occur in about 5% to 10% of patients with a cardiac paraganglioma.[34] Metastatic disease also occurs in 5% to 10% of cases of cardiac paragangliomas, typically involving the skeleton. Cardiac paraganglioma has been described in a patient with the Carney triad, which consists of gastrointestinal stromal tumor, pulmonary chondroma, and extra-adrenal pheochromocytoma.[34] To our knowledge, cardiac paragangliomas have not been reported in patients with multiple endocrine neoplasia syndromes.

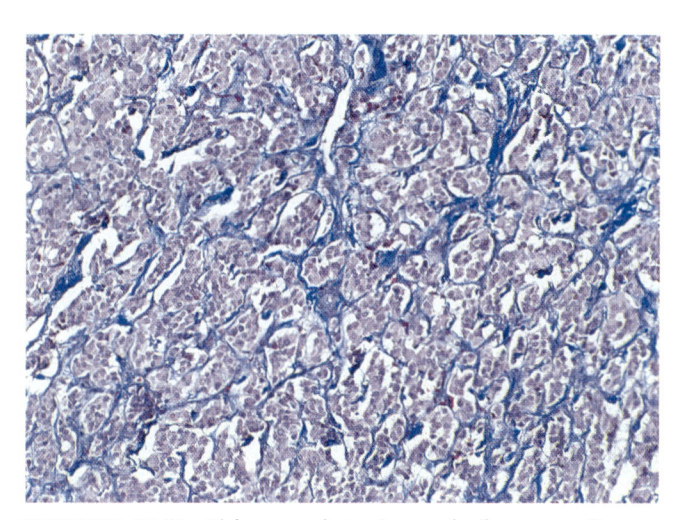

FIGURE 67-19 High-power photomicrograph of a paraganglioma shows the typical nesting (*zellballen*) appearance of paraganglial cells (hematoxylin-eosin stain).

Pathology

Cardiac paragangliomas are usually masses 3 to 8 cm in diameter with encapsulated or infiltrative margins and central necrosis.[8] They follow the distribution of cardiac paraganglia, most involving the left atrium.[34,35] Other reported locations include the interatrial septum, the anterior surface of the heart, the right atrium, the aortic root, and the left ventricle.[35] Cardiac paragangliomas have identical histology to extracardiac paragangliomas, with nests of paraganglial cells, described as *zellballen,* surrounded by sustentacular cells (Fig. 67-19).[5,6]

Manifestations of Disease

Clinical Presentation

Approximately half of paragangliomas are functional, causing hypertension.[6] Additional symptoms of catechol-

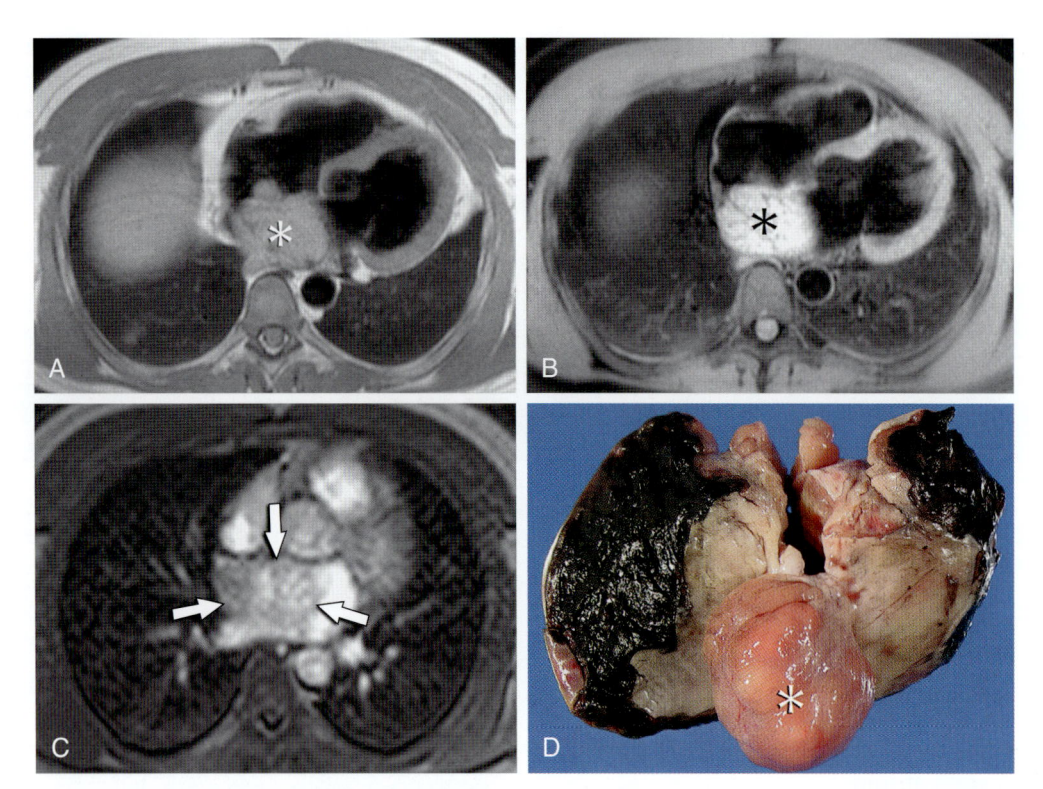

FIGURE 67-20 A 38-year-old man with generalized weakness and left upper extremity paresthesias. **A,** T1-weighted axial MR image shows a multilobulated mass (*asterisk*) centered in the left atrium with extension into the right atrium. At surgery, a 5 × 3 × 4 cm paraganglioma was identified straddling the foramen ovale. **B,** T2-weighted fat-saturated axial MR image shows a slightly heterogeneous mass (*asterisk*) filling the left atrium, which is hyperintense compared with the myocardium. **C,** First-pass perfusion MR image shows rapid enhancement of the mass (*arrows*) compatible with the highly vascular nature of a paraganglioma. **D,** Gross image of resected atrium shows the fleshy pink rounded tumor (*asterisk*).

amine excess include flushing, sweating, palpitations, anxiety, paresthesias, headache, and weight loss. Depending on location and size, mass effect may cause obstruction or compression of adjacent mediastinal structures.[36] Laboratory abnormalities are similar to those of adrenal pheochromocytoma, with elevated urine or blood catecholamines, metanephrine, or vanillylmandelic acid.

Imaging Techniques and Findings

Radiography

In a small series, the most common finding on chest radiographs was a middle mediastinal mass, most splaying the carina.[34]

Ultrasonography

Cardiac paragangliomas are echogenic masses most often involving the left atrium.[7] Echocardiography may show compression of nearby structures, including the superior vena cava.

Computed Tomography

CT reveals a mass typically involving the roof or posterior wall of the left atrium with circumscribed or infiltrative margins.[34] Enhancement is usually intense, with about half of cases showing peripheral enhancement with central low attenuation areas compatible with cystic change or necrosis.[5]

Magnetic Resonance Imaging

Cardiac paragangliomas are isointense or hypointense to myocardium on T1-weighted MRI sequences (Fig. 67-20A), although they may contain areas of hyperintensity from hemorrhage. On T2-weighted sequences, they are generally markedly hyperintense and may appear "light-bulb bright" (Fig. 67-20B), similar to their adrenal counterpart.[8] Paragangliomas often show intense, heterogeneous enhancement with central nonenhancing components attributable to foci of necrosis (Fig. 67-20C).[8]

Nuclear Medicine

Nuclear medicine imaging with iodine 131 or iodine 123 MIBG is often used to localize extra-adrenal paragangliomas. These studies show focal abnormal uptake in almost all cases of cardiac paraganglioma and may show metastatic or multifocal disease.[34]

Differential Diagnosis

The differential diagnosis of a left atrial mass includes myxoma and sarcoma. Clinical and laboratory abnormalities occurring with paragangliomas secondary to catecholamine excess are the most diagnostic findings. On CT and

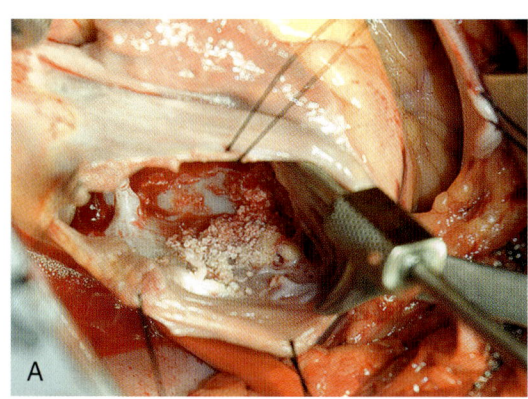

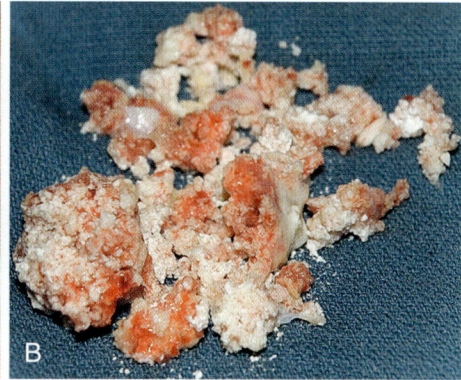

FIGURE 67-21 Calcified amorphous tumor. **A** and **B**, Intraoperative view of opened right atrium (**A**) and specimen photograph (**B**) reveal a glistening white, granular-appearing lesion containing pink tissue.

MRI, heterogeneity and a broad base of attachment favor paraganglioma over myxoma. Imaging findings cannot differentiate paraganglioma from primary cardiac sarcomas.

Treatment Options

Surgical resection with reconstruction is the treatment of choice when feasible. If the lesion is not resectable, heart transplantation and medical management with α and β blockade are options in symptomatic patients.

> **KEY POINTS: PARAGANGLIOMA**
>
> - Paragangliomas are prominently enhancing masses in the left atrial posterior wall or roof.
> - Laboratory abnormalities of elevated catecholamines are diagnostic.

Calcified Amorphous Tumor of the Heart

Definition

Calcified amorphous tumor is a rare, non-neoplastic, diffusely calcified mass of uncertain etiology.

Prevalence

Prevalence of calcified amorphous tumor is extremely low, with very few case reports in the literature. In the largest series of 11 cases, the age range at presentation was 16 to 75 years (mean 52 years).[37]

Pathology

Most cases of calcified amorphous tumor are pedunculated intracavitary masses, although it has also been reported to involve diffusely the myocardium, papillary muscles, and valve chordae.[37,38] The tissue is grossly a yellow-white color (Fig. 67-21). Microscopic analysis shows nodular deposits of calcium within a background of amorphous fibrinous material.[37] One hypothesis for the origin of calcified amorphous tumor is degeneration and organization of intramural thrombus; however, hemosiderin and laminations, usually found in organizing thrombi, are rare within this lesion.[37]

Manifestations of Disease

Clinical Presentation

The clinical presentation of calcified amorphous tumor includes heart failure, syncope, and evidence of embolization.[37]

Imaging Techniques and Findings

Radiography

Chest radiograph may show dense calcification within the cardiac silhouette (Fig. 67-22A).[38]

Ultrasonography

Most lesions evaluated with echocardiography were pedunculated, intracavitary diffusely calcified masses.[37]

Computed Tomography

There is little literature regarding cross-sectional imaging of calcified amorphous tumor of the heart. Two studies that include CT findings describe a pedunculated, calcified right ventricular mass in one case,[39] and diffuse dense calcification of the left ventricle apical, septal, and lateral walls; papillary muscles; and mitral chordal apparatus in the other.[38]

Magnetic Resonance Imaging

A single case report of a calcified amorphous tumor that includes MRI evaluation describes a right ventricular immobile broad-based mass.[40] Signal intensity is low on T1-weighted, T2-weighted, and delayed enhancement MRI sequences (Fig. 67-22B and C).[40]

Differential Diagnosis

The differential diagnosis of a calcified cardiac mass includes neoplasms such as cardiac myxoma, fibroma, and osteosarcoma, and non-neoplastic causes of calcification, such as calcified thrombus, tumoral calcinosis, and prominent mitral annular calcification. Imaging findings are not specific.

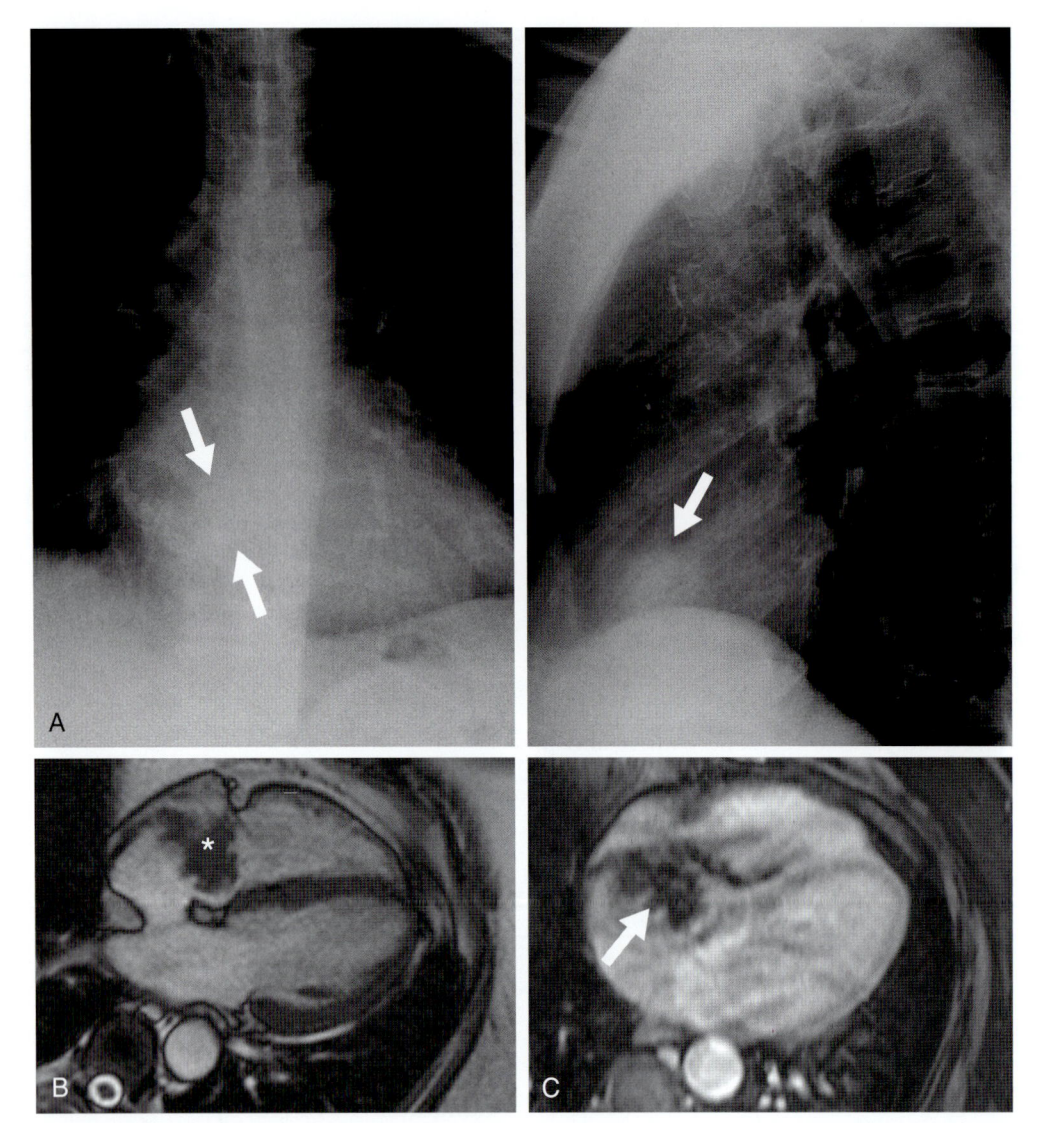

FIGURE 67-22 A 51-year-old asymptomatic woman with calcified amorphous tumor of the right atrium and remote history of breast cancer. **A,** Posteroanterior and lateral chest radiographs (narrow window) coned to the cardiac silhouette show a calcified masslike opacity (*arrows*) located in the right atrium. **B,** MR cine image (four-chamber view) shows a broad-based intracavity right atrial mass (*asterisk*) marginated by multiple, small frondlike projections. **C,** Gadolinium-enhanced T1-weighted axial MR image shows a mass of predominantly low signal intensity (*arrow*) containing a few punctate areas of mild enhancement.

Treatment Options

Treatment is surgical excision or heart transplantation if the infiltration is extensive. Postoperative recurrence has been reported.[38]

> **KEY POINTS: CALCIFIED AMORPHOUS TUMOR OF THE HEART**
>
> - Calcified amorphous tumor is an extremely rare cause of a diffusely calcified cardiac mass.

MALIGNANT CARDIAC TUMORS

Metastatic disease to the heart is 20 to 40 times more frequent than all primary cardiac tumors. Only one quarter of primary cardiac tumors are malignant, and almost all are sarcomas. Angiosarcoma is the most common cardiac sarcoma with a definable histologic subtype, followed by smaller (and variably reported) numbers of malignant fibrous histiocytoma (MFH), leiomyosarcoma, osteosarcoma, rhabdomyosarcoma, fibrosarcoma, myxosarcoma, synovial sarcoma, and liposarcoma. Primary cardiac lymphoma (PCL) is even rarer than cardiac sarcomas and is characteristically found in immunocompromised individuals.

Although it is often difficult to distinguish a particular subtype of primary cardiac sarcoma radiologically, it is more important to recognize its aggressive biologic behav-

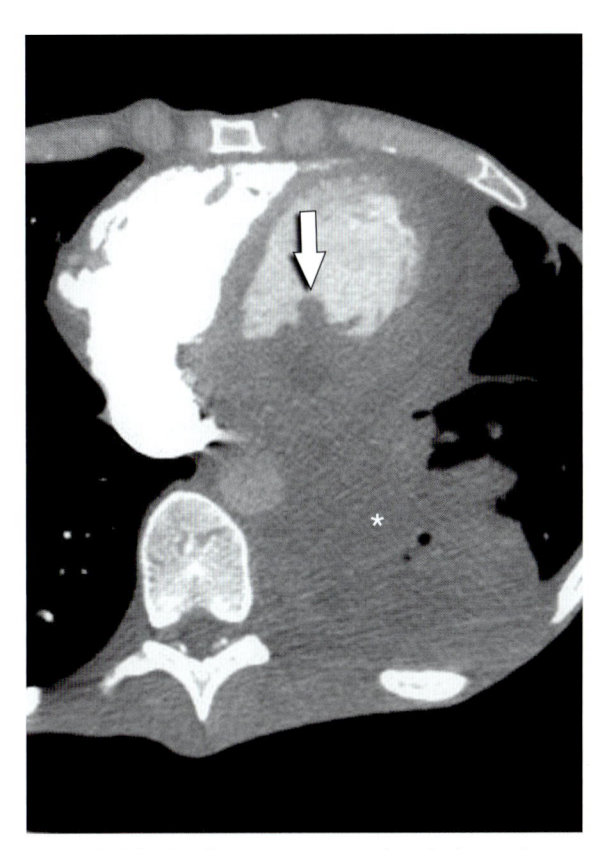

■ **FIGURE 67-23** Contiguous tumor spread to the heart. Contrast-enhanced coned axial CT image (soft tissue windows) reveals an aggressive left lower lobe lung cancer (*asterisk*) directly invading pericardium and myocardium, with nodular intracavitary extension into the left ventricular chamber (*arrow*).

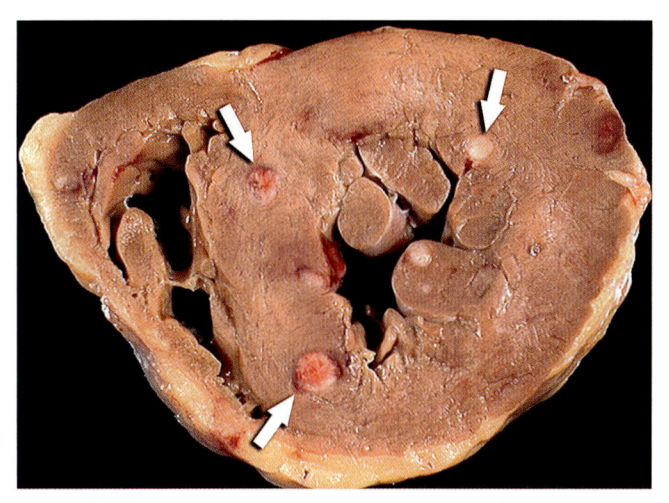

■ **FIGURE 67-24** Hematogeneous tumor spread to the heart. Gross section through the ventricles from a patient with metastatic melanoma reveals multiple intramural nodules (*arrows*), many showing hemorrhagic features, compatible with hematogenous metastases to the left ventricular myocardium.

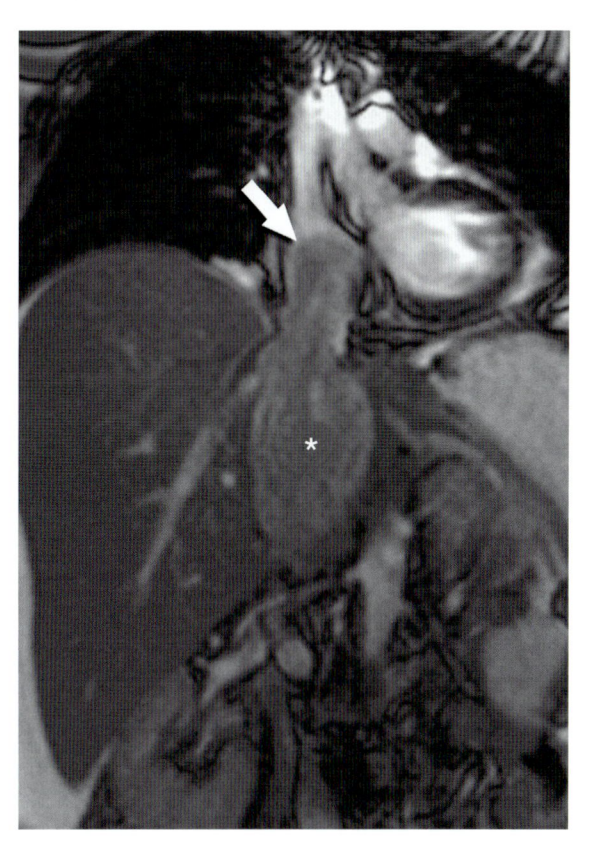

■ **FIGURE 67-25** Endovascular tumor spread to the heart. Coronal MR image (SSFP) of a leiomyosarcoma (*asterisk*) extending superiorly via the inferior vena cava to fill the right atrial chamber (*arrow*).

ior. Imaging features that suggest malignancy are location on the right side of the heart; single or multiple, poorly marginated intramural or broad-based intracavitary masses; internal heterogeneity (suggesting necrosis); contiguous valvular involvement; invasion of regional veins or coronary arteries; and pericardial thickening, nodularity, or significant effusion. Multifocal intracardiac lesions are further evidence of malignancy, particularly in metastatic disease to the heart, rhabdomyosarcoma, and cardiac lymphoma. Lung metastases may reflect the presence of either an extracardiac primary tumor or a right-sided cardiac malignancy with tumor embolization (e.g., angiosarcoma).

Metastases

Definition

Cardiac metastases are malignancies that involve the myocardium, endocardium, epicardium, or pericardium secondarily. The pathways of spread include direct extension from a mediastinal or thoracic tumor, hematogenous spread, lymphatic spread, and intracavitary extension via the inferior vena cava or pulmonary veins (Figs. 67-23 through 67-26). Lung carcinoma, breast carcinoma, mesothelioma, and other thoracic malignancies may directly invade the heart and pericardium by contiguous growth. Melanoma, sarcomas, leukemia, and renal cell carcinoma tend to deposit neoplastic cells hematogenously within the myocardium. Epithelial malignancies, such as lung or breast carcinoma, tend to metastasize to the heart via lymphatic channels; regional lymphadenopathy and pericardial involvement often accompany superficial myocardial infiltration in these cases. Endovascular spread to the right heart via systemic venous drainage is characteristic

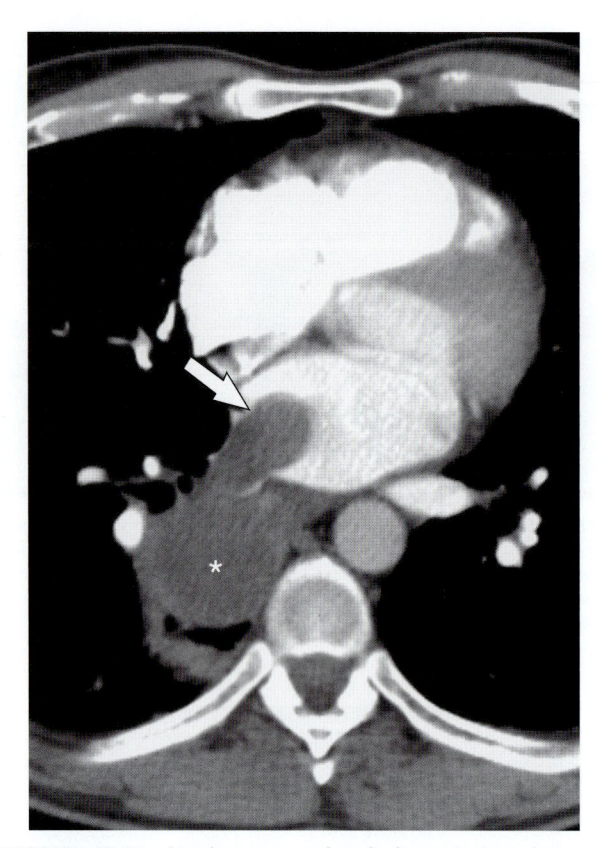

FIGURE 67-26 Contiguous spread to the heart via the pulmonary vein. Contrast-enhanced coned axial CT image (soft tissue windows) shows a right lower lobe lung cancer (*asterisk*) invading the left atrium via the right inferior pulmonary vein (*arrow*).

of melanoma and renal, adrenal, hepatic, and uterine tumors. Lung neoplasms may invade the left atrium via a pulmonary vein. Lymphomas and leukemias secondarily involve the heart via any of the above-described pathways, typically affecting pericardium, epicardium, and myocardium diffusely.[1]

Prevalence

Cardiac metastases are far more common than primary cardiac tumors. The incidence of cardiac metastases, largely based on autopsy studies, is 2% to 18% (vs. postmortem rates of primary cardiac tumors, which range from 0.001% to 0.28%).[41] The following tumors have a particularly high rate (>15%) of cardiac metastases: leukemia, melanoma, thyroid carcinoma, extracardiac sarcomas, lymphomas, renal cell carcinomas, lung carcinomas, and breast carcinomas. In order of decreasing incidence, the most common malignancies to produce secondary cardiac involvement are lung carcinomas, lymphomas, breast carcinomas, leukemia, gastric carcinomas, melanoma, hepatocellular carcinoma, and colon carcinoma.[1] According to one large review, the male and female incidences of cardiac metastases are equivalent.[41]

Melanoma produces the largest tumor burden of any metastatic malignancy in the heart, and the myocardium is involved in almost all cases.[1] In one autopsy series, 64% of melanoma cases metastasized to the heart.[42] Cardiac metastases in melanoma are also typically accompanied by metastases to several other sites.[42]

Lymphomas typically show secondary involvement of the heart and pericardium later in the disease course, with median onset 20 months after diagnosis. One autopsy series revealed cardiac involvement in 16% of disseminated Hodgkin and 18% of disseminated non-Hodgkin lymphoma patients.[42]

Pericardial metastases are overall the most common manifestation of cardiac metastatic disease.[41,42] Myocardial metastases are less common and develop in the right heart in 20% to 30% of cases, the left heart 10% to 33% of cases, and both sides in 30% to 35% of cases. Endocardial or intracavitary metastases are unusual (5%), and the valves are almost always spared.[1,41] More recent analysis suggests that invasion via the heart's lymphatic networks represents the major route of cardiac metastases, most often originating from involved mediastinal lymph nodes.[41]

Pathology

On gross inspection, metastatic deposits in the heart vary in appearance and may be multinodular, diffusely infiltrative, or, less likely, a single mass. Tumor deposits may be evident on the pericardial surface. Mediastinal nodal enlargement is reported in 80% of cases. On histologic examination, metastatic foci in the heart tend to show features that identify the primary extracardiac malignancy. Sarcomatous deposits from an extracardiac tumor may be difficult to discern, however, from a primary cardiac sarcoma with intracardiac spread of disease. Extracardiac sarcomas that metastasize to the heart include osteosarcoma, liposarcoma, leiomyosarcoma, rhabdomyosarcoma, neurofibrosarcoma, synovial sarcoma, and MFH. In some instances, immunohistochemical markers may help to make the distinction between an extracardiac sarcoma and a primary cardiac sarcoma.[1]

Manifestations of Disease

Clinical Presentation

Cardiac metastases are often clinically undetected and discovered postmortem.[41] Depending on their location, however, metastatic deposits in the heart may produce valvular or ventricular outflow obstruction, interruption of conduction pathways, decreased myocardial contractility, coronary artery invasion, or malignant pericardial disease.[1] Clinically, patients may experience a range of signs and symptoms, including syncope or right-sided heart failure, dysrhythmias, complete atrioventricular block, diastolic dysfunction with congestive heart failure, myocardial infarction, or pericardial effusion.[1,41] ECG abnormalities are common.[41] Impaired cardiac function reportedly occurs in 30% of patients, most often attributable to a significant pericardial effusion.[42] The typical clinical scenario is pericardial tamponade from neoplastic effusion, producing symptoms including chest pain, dyspnea, hypotension, and tachycardia.[41] Contiguous endovascular invasion of the right atrium via the inferior vena cava (e.g., metastatic hepatocellular, renal, adrenal, and uterine carcinomas) may produce obstructive pathophysiology, including

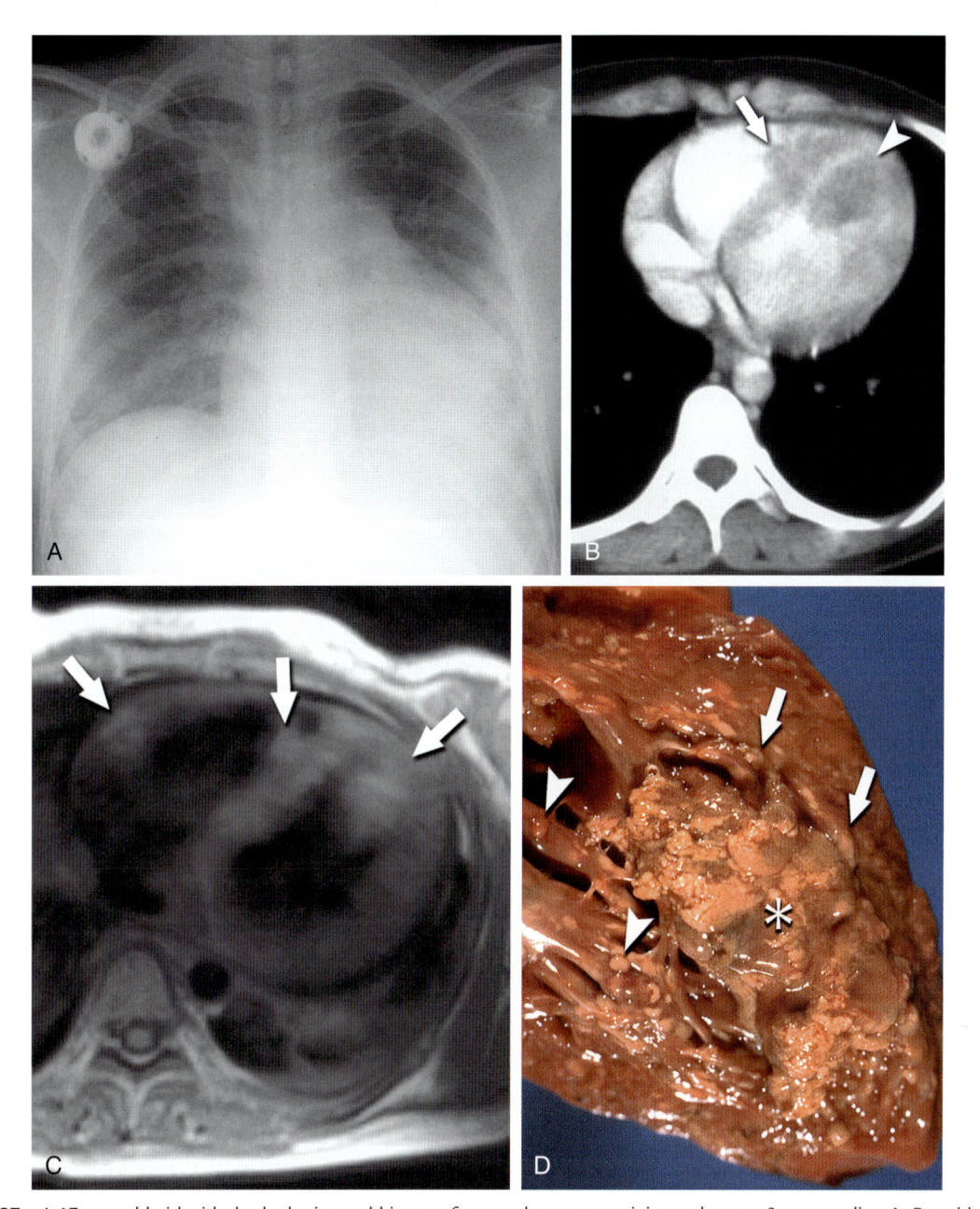

■ FIGURE 67-27 A 17-year-old girl with dysrhythmias and history of resected nevus containing melanoma 2 years earlier. **A,** Portable chest radiograph shows congestive heart failure with enlarged cardiomediastinal silhouette, diffuse ground-glass opacities, and prominent vasculature. **B,** Contrast-enhanced coned axial CT image (soft tissue windows) shows slightly hypodense lobulated masses centered in the interventricular septum (*arrow*) and left ventricle (*arrowhead*). **C,** T1-weighted axial MR image reveals multifocal, hyperintense masses (*arrows*) within the interventricular septum and the left and right ventricular walls. High T1 signal is compatible with metastatic melanoma. **D,** Gross autopsy specimen photograph (coned to the left ventricle) reveals a bulky, infiltrative mass (*asterisk*) located within the wall of the left ventricle and interventricular septum, which was histologically confirmed as melanoma. There are additional widespread tumor nodules studding the pericardium (*arrows*) and endocardium (*arrowheads*).

peripheral edema, tumor emboli, cor pulmonale, and pulmonary arterial hypertension.[1,41,43,44]

Imaging Techniques and Findings

Radiography

The chest radiograph is often unremarkable in cardiac metastatic disease. It may show global enlargement of the cardiac silhouette, however, if a large pericardial effusion is present (Fig. 67-27A). Pulmonary or mediastinal neoplasm, lymphadenopathy, or underlying metastatic disease in the lungs may be evident radiographically in some cases.

Ultrasonography

Transthoracic echocardiography in cardiac metastatic disease may show pericardial effusion or intracavitary, nonmobile and nonpedunculated masses, or both. Cardiac

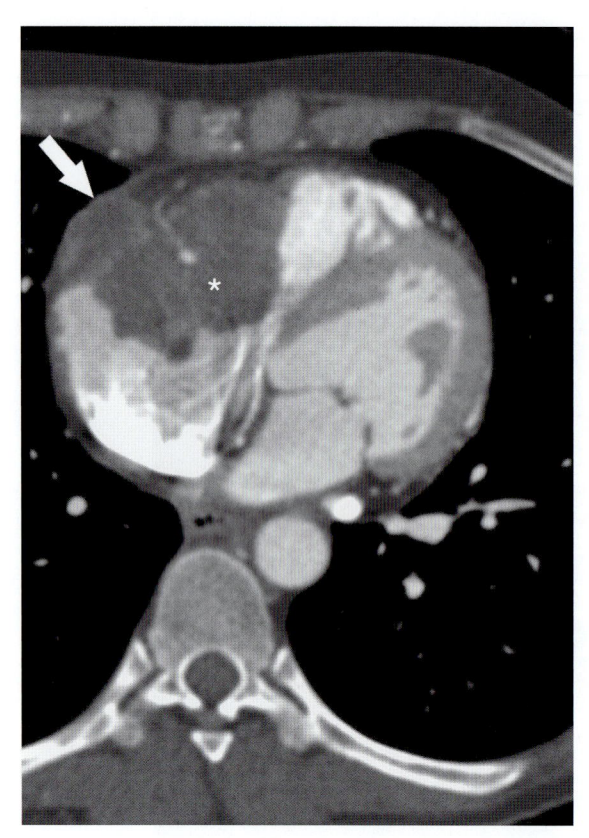

FIGURE 67-28 A 42-year-old woman with progressive dyspnea and history of metastatic cervical carcinoma. Cardiac gated, contrast-enhanced axial CT image (soft tissue windows) shows an aggressive appearing infiltrative, multilobulated soft tissue mass (*asterisk*) involving right atrial and ventricular chambers with involvement of the tricuspid valve and contiguous spread to the pericardium (*arrow*).

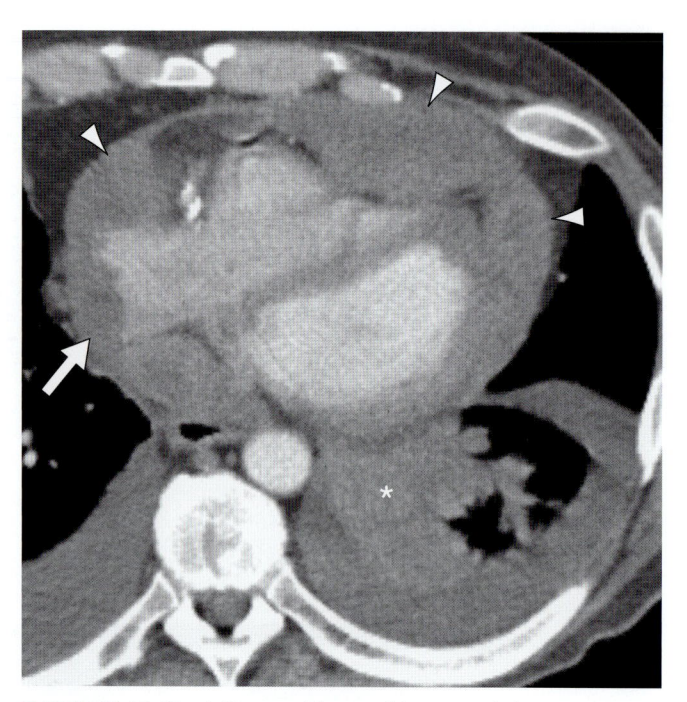

FIGURE 67-29 A 53-year-old man with metastatic lung carcinoma. Contrast-enhanced coned axial CT image (soft tissue windows) reveals a left lower lobe mass (*asterisk*), intramural nodules in the right atrial wall (*arrow*), and nodular thickening and irregular enhancement (*arrowheads*) of the pericardium. Note also bowing of the interventricular septum and encasement of the ventricles, which support the diagnosis of cardiac tamponade. (*Courtesy of Tan-Lucien Mohammed, MD, Cleveland Clinic.*)

geometry and function may be assessed with parameters of possible obstruction, chamber dilation, compromised valve movement, hypokinesis, and elevated pressure gradients at ventricular outflow tracts.[45,46]

Computed Tomography

CT provides a more detailed picture of intrathoracic anatomy, potentially revealing a lung carcinoma, pleural-based tumor (e.g., mesothelioma), or mediastinal mass (e.g., lymphoma) with contiguous cardiac invasion. CT may also identify a primary neoplasm or underlying metastatic disease, or both, elsewhere in the chest or upper abdomen. Intramural metastatic tumor deposits in the heart may be evident as myocardial-based nodules or masses (Fig. 67-27B). CT may show aggressive features, including multichamber involvement, intracavitary or intravascular tumor extension, engulfment of the cardiac valves, and pericardial infiltration (Fig. 67-28).[42,47] A moderate or large pericardial effusion may be evident and, in advanced cases, accompanied by pericardial thickening or nodularity (Fig. 67-29).

Magnetic Resonance Imaging

MRI allows for the differentiation between tumor, cardiac anatomy (myocardium), thrombus, and blood flow artifact. Most cardiac neoplasms are of low signal intensity on T1-weighted images and are brighter on T2-weighted images; they also tend to enhance after intravenous contrast medium administration.[42] In the case of metastatic melanoma, intramural nodular deposits characteristically appear bright on T1-weighted and T2-weighted MR images because of the presence of paramagnetic metals bound by melanin (see Fig. 67-27C and D).[42] Cine MRI may be helpful to confirm the presence of intravascular or valvular tumor extension (Fig. 67-30). Gadolinium-enhanced MR images may help to distinguish intracavitary tumor from thrombus; enhancement and neovascularity are characteristic of most neoplasms, but not typical of thrombus.[42] Changes in cardiac function, including compromised cardiac wall motion and myocardial viability, may also be viewed on MRI.[48] It may be difficult to discern benign from malignant cardiac masses based on either CT or MRI; it may not be obvious that the lesion is a metastatic versus a primary cardiac neoplasm unless other evidence exists to suggest the diagnosis.

Differential Diagnosis

Significant pericardial effusion in a patient with underlying malignancy may represent not only advanced neoplastic disease, but also concomitant infectious, drug-induced, radiation-induced, or idiopathic pericarditis.[42] An intracardiac mass with multiple myocardial components may represent metastasis, but the differential diagnosis includes unusual primary cardiac neoplasms such as leiomyosarcoma, rhabdomyosarcoma (in children and young adults),

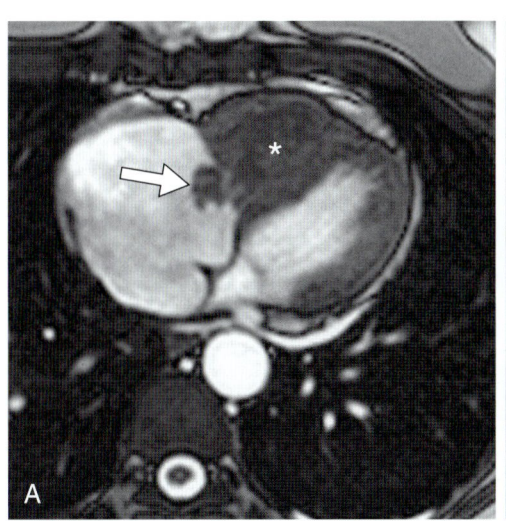

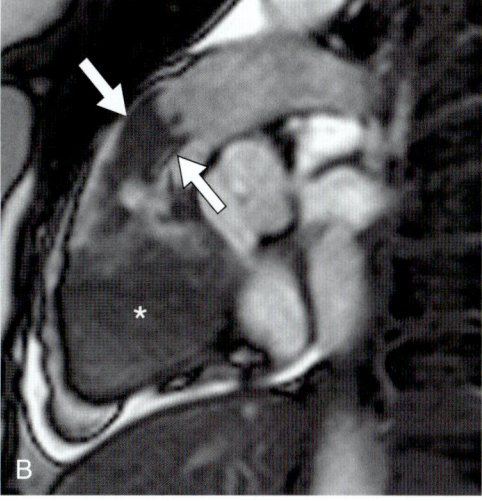

FIGURE 67-30 A 57-year-old woman with cough, progressive dyspnea, and metastatic cervical carcinoma. **A,** Axial SSFP MR image shows a mass filling the right ventricular chamber (*asterisk*) with nodular extension through the tricuspid valve (*arrow*) into the right atrium. **B,** Sagittal SSFP MR image shows the right ventricular mass (*asterisk*) extending across the pulmonary valve (*arrows*).

rhabdomyoma (in infants), and PCL (in immunosuppressed patients).

Treatment Options

Metastatic tumors in the heart are surgically resected for palliation rather than cure. The clinical goal is at least temporary improvement of cardiac function. Long-term prognosis is poor.[1]

> ### KEY POINTS: METASTASES
> - Metastases to the heart are far more common than primary cardiac malignancies.
> - Malignancies most likely to involve the heart secondarily are lung and breast carcinomas, lymphomas, melanoma, and leukemias.
> - Malignant pericardial effusion is often the first clinical expression of cardiac metastatic disease.
> - Right atrial masses may reflect contiguous endovascular invasion by hepatic, renal, adrenal, or uterine malignancy.

Angiosarcoma

Definition

Cardiac sarcomas arise from pleuropotential mesenchymal cells within the cardiac muscle.[1] In contrast to most other histologic subtypes of cardiac sarcomas (which typically arise in the left atrium), angiosarcomas are located in the right atrium in greater than 90% of cases. Angiosarcomas often infiltrate the pericardium, leading to malignant pericardial effusion.

Prevalence

Primary cardiac sarcomas as a group are rare (<25% of primary cardiac tumors). Angiosarcomas are the most common differentiated histologic subtype (37% of cardiac sarcomas), but the unclassifiable cardiac sarcomas seem to occur with equal frequency.[1,49] Mean age at presentation is approximately 40 years (range 3 months to 80 years) with a male predilection (2.5:1).[21]

Pathology

On gross inspection, angiosarcomas are multinodular, hemorrhagic masses centered in the right atrial wall, often with sheetlike pericardial invasion and thickening (Fig. 67-31). There may be contiguous involvement of the venae cavae and tricuspid valve. Histologic features include anastomosing vascular channels lined by malignant endothelial cells that may occasionally form atypical papillary tufts. Vacuoles containing red blood cells may be seen, and most lesions contain areas of necrosis.[1,21] Findings of high mitotic rate and necrosis are important predictors of poor patient survival.[1]

Manifestations of Disease

Clinical Presentation

Clinical presentation is often the consequence of a malignant, often hemorrhagic pericardial effusion producing pericardial tamponade, pericardial restriction, or right ventricular outflow obstruction.[21] Signs and symptoms include chest pain, dyspnea, syncope, fever, and lower extremity swelling.[1] If the tumor causes valvular obstruction or conduction disturbance, cardiac arrest may result. Cardiac rupture owing to loss of myocardial integrity has been reported. Right-sided cardiac tumors such as angiosarcoma may also produce pulmonary emboli.[49]

Metastatic disease at clinical presentation is found more often in angiosarcoma than in other cardiac sarcomas; 66% to 89% of patients have metastases within the lung (most commonly), bone, liver, adrenal glands, or spleen.[21] Survival is poor for all cardiac sarcomas, regardless of histologic subtype.[1] Mean survival for angiosarcoma is 3 months to 2 years after diagnosis.[21] Death is frequently due to complications of local recurrence or metastatic disease.

Imaging Techniques and Findings

Radiography

At diagnosis, approximately 30% of patients with cardiac angiosarcoma have pulmonary nodules on the initial chest radiograph compatible with metastases.[1] Enlargement of the cardiac silhouette may reflect an underlying malignant pericardial effusion.

Ultrasonography

Echocardiography may reveal a broad-based, chiefly intramural right atrial mass located near the inferior vena cava. Pericardial effusion or contiguous tumor extension into the pericardium, endocardium, and left atrial chamber may be identified.[27]

Computed Tomography

CT often shows a fairly well-defined, enhancing right atrial mass. In many cases, associated pericardial thickening, nodularity, and effusion are present (Fig. 67-32).[49] Pulmonary metastases may be evident, occasionally framed by halos of ground glass because of their hemorrhagic character (Fig. 67-33).

Magnetic Resonance Imaging

Angiosarcomas are typically infiltrative masses in the right atrial myocardium that when compared with myocardium are isointense with higher signal intensity areas (owing to focal hemorrhage) on T1-weighted MRI, isointense on T2-weighted sequences, and heterogeneous with areas of high intensity on cine MRI (Fig. 67-34). These tumors tend to show strong, heterogeneous enhancement after contrast administration; this is termed a "sunray" appearance if pericardial tumor infiltration also enhances.[8,10]

Differential Diagnosis

The differential diagnosis of a right atrial mass includes thrombus, metastatic disease, liposarcoma, angiosarcoma, an unusual right-sided cardiac myxoma or fibroma (both

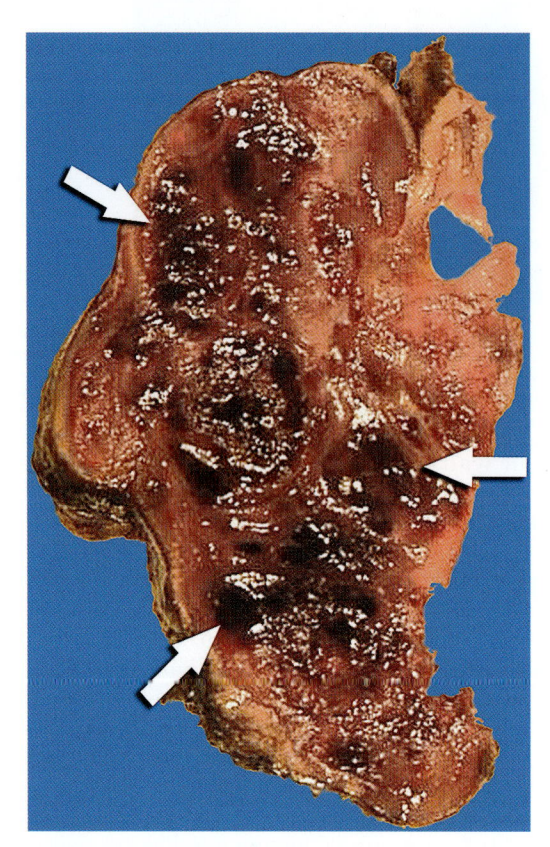

■ **FIGURE 67-31** Gross specimen photograph of a cardiac angiosarcoma reveals an infiltrative mass with multiple vacuoles containing hemorrhagic material (*arrows*).

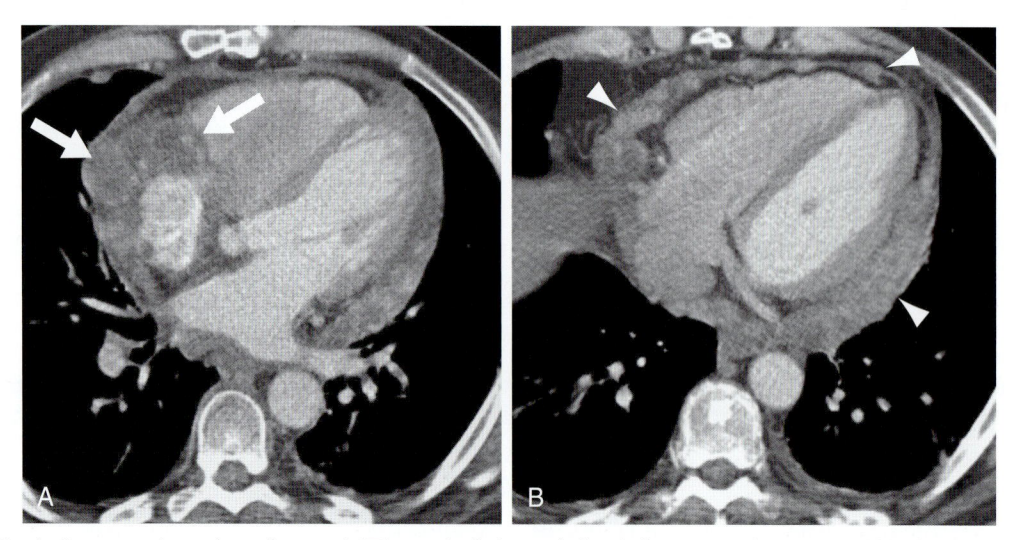

■ **FIGURE 67-32 A,** Contrast-enhanced, cardiac gated CT image (soft tissue windows) shows an angiosarcoma within the right atrial myocardium (*arrows*), which contains punctate areas of marked enhancement compatible with highly vascular tumor components. **B,** There is neoplastic involvement of the pericardium, which is studded by multiple, prominently enhancing nodules (*arrowheads*) and contains pericardial effusion. *(Courtesy of Tan-Lucien Mohammed, MD, Cleveland Clinic.)*

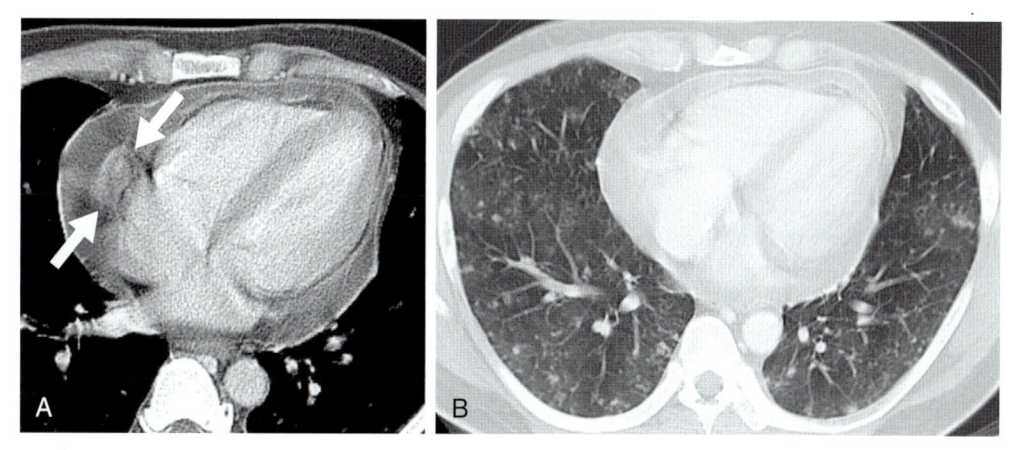

FIGURE 67-33 Angiosarcoma in a 33-year-old man with a 1-month history of hemoptysis and dyspnea. **A,** Contrast-enhanced coned CT image (soft tissue windows) shows an enhancing, oblong mass within the right atrial wall (*arrows*). Note diffuse enhancement of the pericardium surrounding a moderate pericardial effusion. **B,** Axial CT image (lung windows) reveals widespread pulmonary nodules with halos of ground-glass density, compatible with hemorrhagic metastases.

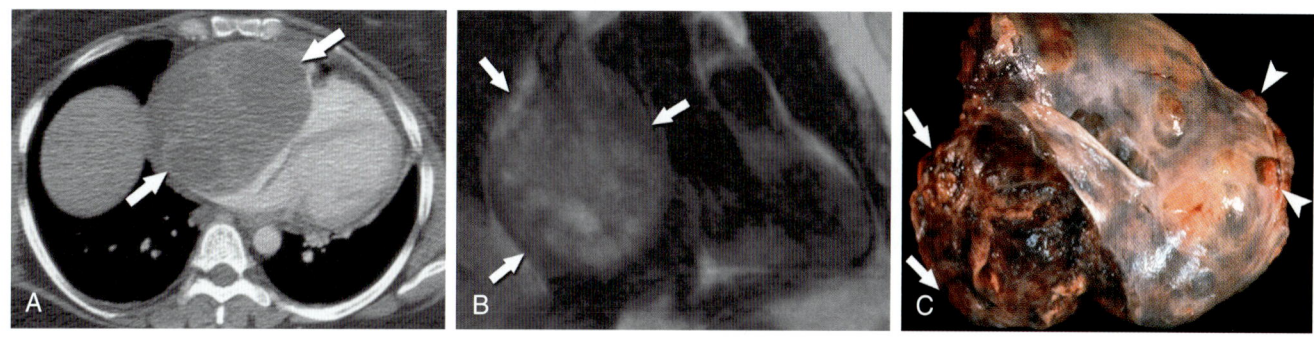

FIGURE 67-34 Right atrial angiosarcoma in a 35-year-old woman. **A,** Contrast-enhanced axial CT scan (soft tissue windows) shows a large, heterogeneously enhancing mass (*arrows*) filling the right atrial chamber. **B,** Coronal T1-weighted MR image shows multiple areas of high signal intensity within the mass (*arrows*), consistent with hemorrhagic foci. **C,** Gross specimen photograph shows the mass (*arrows*) in identical orientation to B. There are several areas of purple hemorrhagic material within the tumor. Note nodular metastatic deposits within the pericardium (*arrowheads*).

tend to calcify), and PCL.[50] Aggressive features, such as a broad-based or intramural tumor configuration, infiltration of the pericardium, involvement of cardiac valves, and pulmonary metastases, all argue in favor of a malignant rather than a benign etiology. The presence of a hemorrhagic pericardial effusion is particularly supportive evidence of angiosarcoma.

Treatment Options

Surgery for cardiac sarcomas may be performed, but depends on tumor location, degree of local invasion, and presence of metastases at presentation. Surgical intervention ranges from open biopsy to palliative debulking to wide surgical resection.[49] Cardiac transplantation may be considered if the lesion is considered unresectable, excluding the presence of extracardiac metastases.[51] Transplantation is not commonly done because of the high risk of local recurrence and immunosuppression-induced lymphoma (2% to 13% in cardiac allograft recipients).[49] Adjuvant chemotherapy or radiation therapy may provide limited benefit and may be used in patients with advanced (nonsurgical) disease, local tumor recurrence, or resections with positive tumor margins.[49,51]

> **KEY POINTS: ANGIOSARCOMA**
>
> - Cardiac angiosarcoma must be suspected in the setting of a right atrial mass with pericardial effusion, especially if the pericardial effusion is high attenuation (hemopericardium).
> - Cardiac angiosarcoma is the only differentiated cardiac sarcoma that chiefly arises in the right atrium (90%). Other cardiac sarcomas tend to arise in the left atrium, or do not have a site predilection.
> - Characteristic MRI features include focal high intensity areas on T1 (corresponding to areas of hemorrhage) and strong postcontrast enhancement (reflecting tumor vascularity).

Leiomyosarcoma

Definition

Leiomyosarcomas account for 8% to 10% of cardiac sarcomas and are chiefly located in the posterior wall of the left atrium. Some tumors may represent the atrial extension of sarcomas arising within the pulmonary veins or venae cavae.[1,49] In 30% of cases, leiomyosarcomas are multifocal.[8]

Prevalence

Approximately 75% to 80% of cardiac leiomyosarcomas arise in the left atrium.[1] The male-to-female ratio is variably reported (4:2 vs. 5:7), and sexual predilection cannot be stated with certainty.[1] The mean age at presentation has been reported to be 37 years (range 20 to 61 years).[1]

Pathology

Histologic features of cardiac leiomyosarcoma include intracytoplasmic glycogen, perinuclear vacuoles, blunt-end nuclei, fascicular growth at right angles, and cytoplasmic fuchsinophilia. The distinction between leiomyosarcoma and MFH at microscopic inspection may be difficult.[1]

Manifestations of Disease

Clinical Presentation

As an aggressive left atrial mass, leiomyosarcomas may produce clinical signs and symptoms of compromised pulmonary venous drainage (including pulmonary edema) or mitral valve obstruction or both.[8,10] Prognosis is poor. Mean survival after diagnosis is 7 to 9 months.[1] Patients with the unusual form of right-sided cardiac leiomyosarcoma may have Budd-Chiari syndrome.[6]

Imaging Techniques and Findings

Radiography

Although no specific reports are available concerning radiographic manifestations of leiomyosarcoma, the most common radiographic abnormality in cardiac sarcomas overall is cardiomegaly.[5] In situations of significantly compromised pulmonary venous drainage resulting from an enlarging left atrial mass, features of prominent septal lines and vascular congestion may develop on chest radiographs.

Ultrasonography

No reports are available at this time concerning specific echocardiographic manifestations of leiomyosarcoma.

Computed Tomography

Similar to primary cardiac osteosarcomas, these tumors typically arise in the left atrium as lobulated, low-density lesions that mimic atrial myxoma. Helpful differentiating features of osteosarcoma from myxoma include a broad base of attachment and signs of aggressive behavior including involvement of regional veins, pericardium, and mitral valve.[8,49]

Magnetic Resonance Imaging

Leiomyosarcomas are reported as isointense on T1-weighted MR images and hyperintense on T2-weighted MR images. They may enhance after contrast medium administration.[8,49]

Differential Diagnosis

The differential diagnosis of a left atrial mass includes myxoma, thrombus, pulmonary venous extension of lung malignancy, leiomyosarcoma, osteosarcoma, MFH, and very rarely, paraganglioma.

Treatment Options

Surgical excision of the neoplasm may be attempted, ranging from debulking to attempted wide resection. Cardiac transplantation may be considered in advanced disease except when distal metastases are present.[51] Adjuvant chemotherapy or radiation therapy may provide some benefit and is indicated in patients with advanced (nonsurgical) disease, local tumor recurrence, or resections with positive tumor margins.[49,51]

> **KEY POINTS: LEIOMYOSARCOMA**
> - Cardiac leiomyosarcomas typically (80%) arise in the left atrium, similar to osteosarcoma and MFH, and may mimic an atrial myxoma.
> - Almost one third of cardiac leiomyosarcomas are multifocal in the heart.

Osteosarcoma

Definition

Cardiac sarcomas with osteosarcomatous differentiation arise almost exclusively (>95%) in the left atrium.[1,10] Osteosarcomas commonly involve the mitral valve.[8]

Prevalence

Osteosarcomas account for 3% to 10% of cardiac sarcomas.[1]

Pathology

Grossly, cardiac osteosarcomas are typically large tumors (4 to 10 cm) almost uniformly located within the posterior left atrial wall.[10] On cut section, they have a pale mucoid or gelatinous appearance with gritty components.[6] Microscopic features include osteoid material and atypical osteocytes indistinguishable from skeletal osteosarcomas. Notably, these tumors are often pleomorphic and may contain areas of fibrosarcoma, chondrosarcoma, or giant cell tumor.[6]

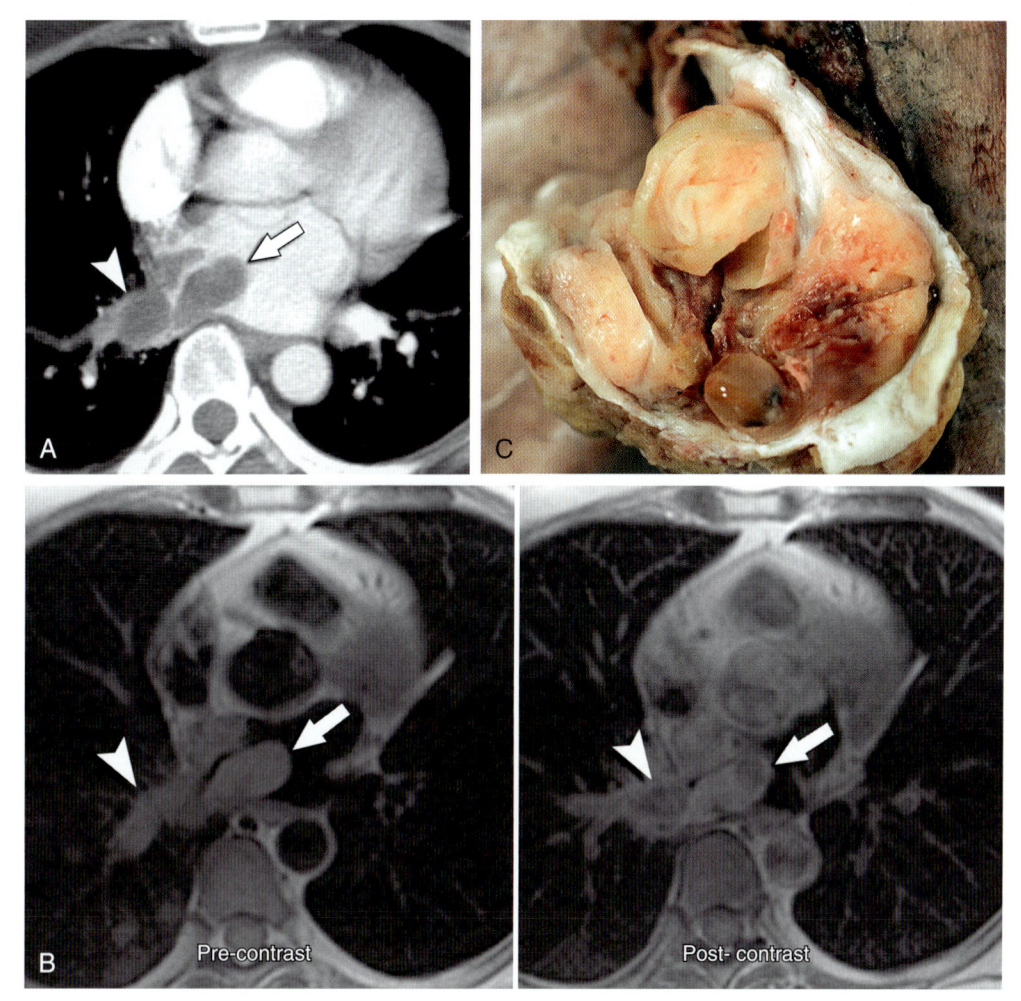

FIGURE 67-35 Osteosarcoma in a 50-year-old woman who presented with chronic cough. **A,** Contrast-enhanced axial CT scan (soft tissue windows) shows a lobulated mass (*arrow*) in the left atrium with extension into, and expansion of, the right inferior pulmonary vein (*arrowhead*). **B,** T1-weighted axial MR images, before and after administration of gadolinium, show a lobulated left atrial mass (*arrow*) and pulmonary venous extension (*arrowhead*) with heterogeneous enhancement. **C,** Surgical specimen of opened left atrium shows a polypoid mass occupying the chamber with components of necrosis, hemorrhage, and cystic change.

Manifestations of Disease

Clinical Presentation

Clinical presentation includes symptoms of dyspnea, congestive heart failure, mitral valve obstruction, pulmonary hypertension, and syncope.[6] Metastatic disease has been reported in lymph nodes, thyroid, skin, lung, and thoracotomy incisions.[6] Prognosis is poor.[8]

Imaging Techniques and Findings

Radiography

No reports are available concerning specific radiographic manifestations of osteosarcoma, but the most common radiographic abnormality in cardiac sarcomas overall is cardiomegaly.[5] In situations of significantly compromised pulmonary venous drainage, features of prominent septal lines and vascular congestion may develop on chest radiographs.

Ultrasonography

No reports are available concerning echocardiographic depiction of a cardiac osteosarcoma.

Computed Tomography

Calcification may be evident on CT images, but this is not a consistent feature of cardiac osteosarcoma.[8] This neoplasm mimics a left atrial myxoma, but discerning features include invasion of adjacent structures, a broad base of attachment to the atrial wall, and lack of association with the fossa ovalis (Fig. 67-35A).[8]

Magnetic Resonance Imaging

Osteosarcomas are reported as heterogeneous and isointense when compared with myocardium on T1-weighted MR images, heterogeneous and hyperintense on T2-weighted MR images, and largely hyperintense on cine MRI. There is no consistent postcontrast appearance (Fig. 67-35B).[8]

Differential Diagnosis

The differential diagnosis of a left atrial mass includes myxoma, lung tumor invasion via a pulmonary vein, leiomyosarcoma, MFH, osteosarcoma, and rarely paraganglioma.

Treatment Options

Excision of the neoplasm should be attempted, ranging from palliative debulking to wide surgical resection. Cardiac transplantation may be considered, but is not indicated when distal metastases are present.[51] Adjuvant chemotherapy or radiation therapy may provide some benefit and is indicated in patients with advanced (nonsurgical) disease, local tumor recurrence, or resections with positive tumor margins.[49,51]

KEY POINTS: OSTEOSARCOMA

- Cardiac osteosarcomas arise almost exclusively (>95%) in the left atrium.
- Cardiac osteosarcomas only variably show calcification on radiologic imaging.
- Histologic appearance of the tumor is essentially indistinguishable from cardiac metastasis of skeletal osteosarcoma, but metastatic osteosarcoma is usually deposited in the right atrium, whereas primary cardiac osteosarcoma arises in the left atrium.

Rhabdomyosarcoma

Definition

Rhabdomyosarcoma is the most common subtype of cardiac sarcoma in children and young adults.[1,8] In contrast to other cardiac sarcomas, rhabdomyosarcoma shows no chamber predilection and does not tend to involve the pericardium.[1,27] This tumor is multifocal in 60% of patients, and is more likely than other sarcomas to involve a cardiac valve.[8,52]

Prevalence

Rhabdomyosarcomas account for 4% to 7% of cardiac sarcomas. Mean age at presentation ranges from 14 to 30 years, which is decades younger than other sarcomas. Sexual predilection (male-to-female) is contradicted in separate case series (2:4 or 3:2) and is inconclusive.[1]

Pathology

On gross examination, these tumors are located within the myocardium and tend to exhibit necrotic areas.[8] Cardiac rhabdomyosarcomas are embryonal; the diagnostic feature on histologic examination is the presence of rhabdomyoblasts, best identified by periodic acid–Schiff positivity.[6] Immunohistochemical staining to identify cells with muscle antigens (desmin and myoglobin) is necessary for diagnosis.[1]

Manifestations of Disease

Clinical Presentation

Clinical presentation varies because the tumor may arise in any part of the heart, extend into the nearest chamber, and ultimately cause valvular obstruction.[22] Infants present with cyanosis, heart murmur, dysrhythmias, or congestive heart failure.[22] Older children and young adults present with nonspecific symptoms of fever, weight loss, and malaise.[27] Prognosis is poor, and survival is often less than 5 months from diagnosis.[1]

Imaging Techniques and Findings

Radiography

There are no specific manifestations of rhabdomyosarcoma described on chest radiography. Cardiomegaly is the most common radiographic feature of cardiac sarcomas.[5] In situations of significantly compromised pulmonary venous drainage owing to tumor mass effect, features of prominent septal lines and vascular congestion may develop on chest radiographs.

Ultrasonography

Transesophageal or transthoracic echocardiography may reveal intramural involvement by rhabdomyosarcoma (solitary or multifocal), intracavitary extension, and the impact on an adjacent cardiac valve.[53]

Computed Tomography

On CT, rhabdomyosarcomas are shown as solitary or multifocal intramural masses, often lower in density than normal myocardium.[49]

Magnetic Resonance Imaging

Rhabdomyosarcomas are reported as isointense to myocardium on T1-weighted MRI, isointense or heterogeneous on T2-weighted sequences, and isointense on cine MRI (Fig. 67-36). These tumors tend to enhance heterogeneously after contrast medium administration, with focal nonenhancement in necrotic areas.[8,49]

Differential Diagnosis

Primary cardiac rhabdomyosarcoma has no particular site predilection in the heart. The differential diagnosis includes right-sided and left-sided cardiac masses and tumors that may arise in multiple intracardiac sites such as metastatic disease, rhabdomyoma (in infants), leiomyosarcoma, and PCL in addition to rhabdomyosarcoma (in children and young adults).

Treatment Options

Excision of the neoplasm may be attempted, ranging from palliative debulking to wide surgical resection. In most patients, the tumor is advanced at presentation.[52]

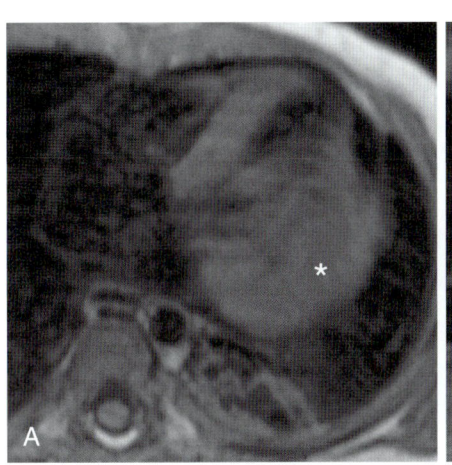

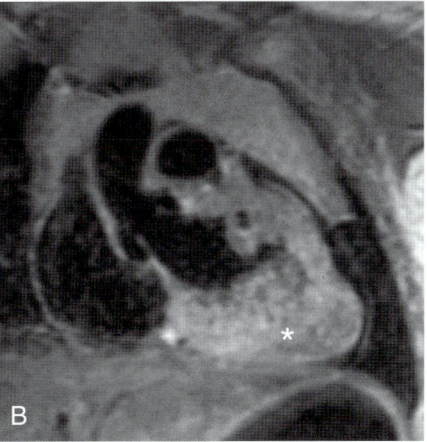

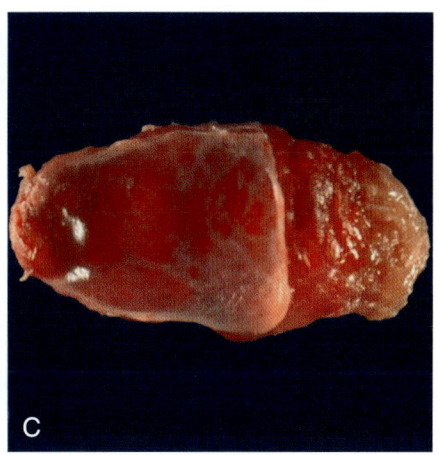

FIGURE 67-36 Rhabdomyosarcoma of the left ventricle in a 6-month-old girl status post resuscitation from cardiac arrest. **A** and **B**, T1-weighted axial (**A**) and coronal (**B**) MR images show a slightly hyperintense mass (*asterisk*) arising from the left ventricular myocardium. **C**, Resected specimen has the gross appearance of muscular tissue.

Cardiac transplantation may be considered, but is excluded when distal metastases are present.[51] This malignancy shows poor response to adjuvant radiation or chemotherapy.[52]

> **KEY POINTS:**
> **RHABDOMYOSARCOMA**
>
> - Rhabdomyosarcoma is the most common primary cardiac sarcoma in children and young adults.
> - Rhabdomyosarcoma has no site predilection in the heart and may be multifocal at presentation (60% of cases).
> - In contrast to most other primary cardiac sarcomas, pericardial involvement by rhabdomyosarcoma is unusual, but valvular invasion is common.

Liposarcoma

Definition

Liposarcoma is a rare histologic subtype of cardiac sarcoma and tends to arise in the right side of the heart.[49]

Prevalence

Primary cardiac liposarcomas account for less than 1% of cardiac sarcomas. A liposarcoma metastatic to the heart occurs much more frequently than primary cardiac liposarcoma.[30]

Pathology

Grossly, the tumor has a yellow, soft, and smooth surface with ill-defined margins often bulging into the right atrial or ventricular chamber.[30] Histologic features include atypical fat cells with malignant lipoblasts invading the adjacent myocardium.[1,30] On microscopic examination, liposarcomas may be easily confused with LHIS and pleomorphic MFH.[1]

Manifestations of Disease

Clinical Presentation

Similar to other right-sided cardiac masses, liposarcoma may produce the signs and symptoms of valvular dysfunction, right ventricular outflow obstruction, pulmonary embolism, or dysrhythmias.[54]

Imaging Techniques and Findings
Radiography

Chest radiography may be unremarkable, or the cardiac silhouette may be enlarged.[54]

Ultrasonography

Echocardiography may show an echo-free space compatible with a fat-containing tissue mass, with or without intracavitary extension.[54]

Computed Tomography

Foci of fat density may be evident on CT images (Fig. 67-37), but liposarcomas are also described as soft tissue masses without fat components.[8] Areas of low-density necrosis or hemorrhage may be present within the tumor. CT may delineate myocardial, intracavitary, intravascular, or pericardial extension of tumor, and involvement of a cardiac valve (see Fig. 67-37).[54] Metastases to the lungs, bone, or brain may also be identified.[30]

Magnetic Resonance Imaging

Reports describe a heterogeneous appearance on MRI.[8] In contrast to cardiac lipoma or LHIS, fat saturation sequences are not particularly helpful in diagnosing a cardiac liposarcoma.[30]

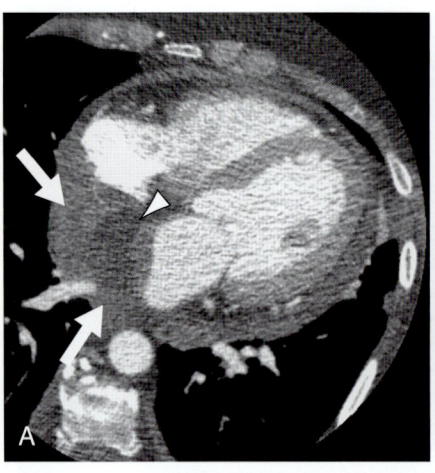

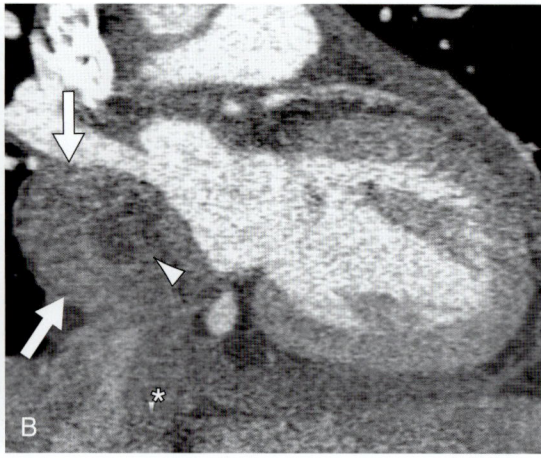

FIGURE 67-37 Primary cardiac liposarcoma in a 53-year-old woman with back pain. **A** and **B**, Cardiac gated contrast-enhanced axial (**A**) and coronal reformat (**B**) CT images show an infiltrative mass (*arrows*) within walls of the right and left atria that contains fat density (*arrowhead*). There is invasion of the inferior vena cava (*asterisk*). Note associated pericardial effusion.

Differential Diagnosis

The differential diagnosis of fat-containing lesions in the heart includes lipoma, LHIS (typically dumbbell-shaped and limited to the interatrial septum), and liposarcoma (which may have soft tissue components and features of local invasion). Right-sided cardiac masses that show aggressive features of intramural or intracavitary extension include metastatic disease, angiosarcoma, liposarcoma, and PCL.

Treatment Options

Excision of the neoplasm may be attempted, ranging from palliative debulking to wide surgical resection. Cardiac transplantation may be considered, but is not indicated when distal metastases are present.[51] Adjuvant chemotherapy or radiation therapy may provide some benefit, and is indicated in patients with advanced (nonsurgical) disease, local tumor recurrence, or resections with positive tumor margins.[49,51]

KEY POINTS: LIPOSARCOMA

- Cardiac liposarcomas tend to arise in the right atrium.
- Fat density is not always appreciated on radiologic imaging of cardiac liposarcoma, which may manifest as a heterogeneous soft tissue mass.
- Metastatic liposarcoma to the heart is much more common than primary cardiac liposarcoma (<1% of cardiac sarcomas).

Primary Cardiac Lymphoma

Definition

PCL is defined as an aggressive non-Hodgkin lymphoma involving exclusively the heart or pericardium or both, or a non-Hodgkin lymphoma with most of the tumor located within the heart.[49] PCL tends to develop in immunocompromised patients.[49]

Prevalence

PCL is rare, with an incidence of 0.056% in one large autopsy series.[55] PCL represents 1.3% of primary cardiac tumors and 0.5% of extranodal lymphomas.[55] Approximately 50% of reported cases are in immunocompromised patients, including patients with human immunodeficiency virus (HIV) infection or allograft transplant.[1] There is a slight male predominance.[10]

Pathology

On gross examination, PCL appears as multiple firm, whitish nodular lesions centered in the myocardium or epicardium, often with pericardial infiltration. The right atrium and ventricle are both involved in 75% of cases.[10] PCL is less likely than a cardiac sarcoma to show necrotic zones, or valvular or intracavitary invasion.[1,8] Virtually all PCLs are high-grade B cell lymphomas.[1,6] Immunohistochemical staining is typically positive for common leukocyte and L26 antigens (specific for B cell lymphoma).[49] Most PCLs in immunocompromised patients contain Epstein-Barr virus DNA.[1,6] Cytology of the pericardial fluid is diagnostic for PCL in 67% of cases.

Manifestations of Disease

Clinical Presentation

In immunocompetent patients presenting with PCL, the average age at presentation is 58 years (range 13 to 80 years).[6,10] The most common clinical presentation is congestive heart failure; additional signs and symptoms include dyspnea, dysrhythmias, complete heart block, chest pain, superior vena cava syndrome, or cardiac tamponade owing to a large pericardial effusion.[49]

Imaging Techniques and Findings

Radiography

Cardiomegaly and signs of pulmonary edema may be evident when a pericardial effusion is present (Fig. 67-38).[5,56]

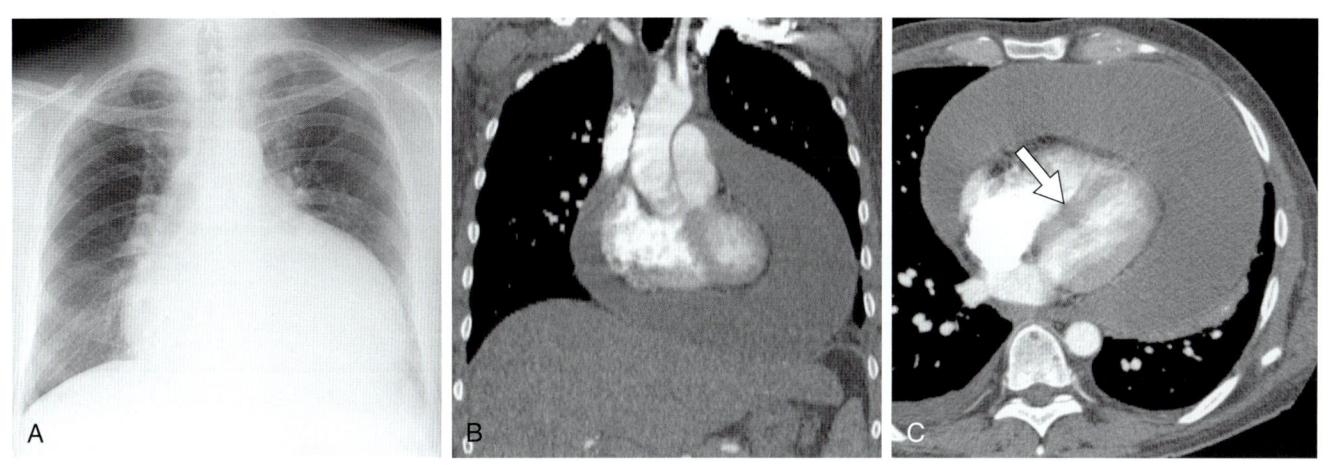

FIGURE 67-38 A 47-year-old HIV-positive man with cardiac tamponade. Pericardiocentesis confirmed non-Hodgkin lymphoma. **A,** Frontal chest radiograph shows enlargement of the cardiac silhouette. **B** and **C,** Coronal reformat (**B**) and axial (**C**) contrast-enhanced CT images show a large pericardial effusion exerting critical mass effect on the heart, including bowing of the interventricular septum (*arrow*), consistent with tamponade.

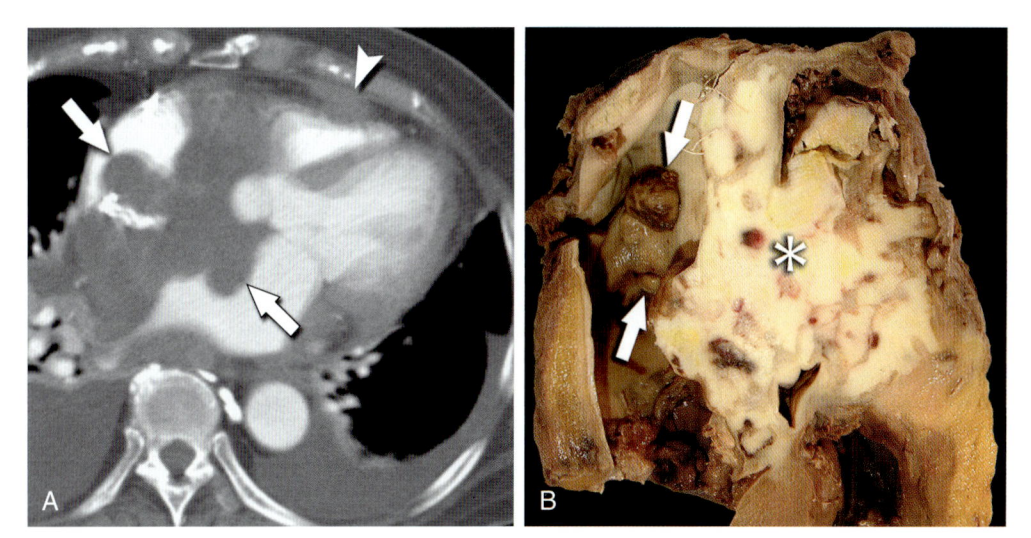

FIGURE 67-39 PCL (large B cell) in a 73-year-old woman who presented with a 2-month history of fatigue and anasarca. **A,** Contrast-enhanced coned axial CT image shows a multilobulated soft tissue mass infiltrating the interatrial septum and atrioventricular septum. Note polypoid intracavitary extension (*arrows*) and pericardial involvement (*arrowhead*). **B,** Gross autopsy photograph confirms expansion of the interatrial septum by an infiltrative, pale yellow soft tissue mass (*asterisk*). Note the polypoid projections into the left atrial chamber (*arrows*).

Ultrasonography

Echocardiography may reveal hypoechoic masses of the right atrium and ventricle, pericardial effusion, and, occasionally, diastolic collapse of the right heart chambers when cardiac tamponade is present.[5,56]

Computed Tomography

PCLs are multinodular, intramural masses located in the right atrium and ventricle, characteristically with pericardial thickening, nodularity, or effusion (Figs. 67-39 and 67-40).[10,49] The pericardial effusion may be quite large.[10]

Magnetic Resonance Imaging

PCLs manifest as nodular or infiltrative lesions that are isointense or hypointense on T1-weighted MRI and hyper-intense on T2-weighted sequences (Fig. 67-41). Postcontrast images may show homogeneous or heterogeneous tumor enhancement.[8,49] Delayed enhancement imaging (with inversion times to null myocardium) may improve delineation of the tumor.[10]

Differential Diagnosis

The differential diagnosis of multifocal cardiac masses (with or without pericardial effusion) includes metastatic disease to the heart (including leukemia and secondary cardiac lymphoma), leiomyosarcoma, rhabdomyoma/rhabdomyosarcoma (in younger patients), and PCL.

Treatment Options

When superior vena caval obstruction develops because of tumor bulk, it may be treated surgically or with metallic stents. In contrast to other cardiac malignancies, gross resection is not indicated in most cases of PCL.[49] Randomized trials have shown prolonged survival and reduction of cardiac symptoms with the use of chemotherapy (including anthracycline-based agents), either alone or followed by field radiation.[55]

KEY POINTS: PRIMARY CARDIAC LYMPHOMA

- PCL is a B cell lymphoma limited to the heart or pericardium or both, and is even rarer than primary cardiac sarcomas.
- PCL is associated with immunosuppressed conditions (including HIV-positive or post-transplant patients).
- PCL tends to arise in multiple sites and often manifests clinically as congestive heart failure with significant pericardial effusion.

SUMMARY

The spectrum of cardiac neoplasia includes benign, malignant, and secondary metastatic tumors to the heart. Primary cardiac tumors are far less common than metastatic disease, and most are benign histologically. Any cardiac tumor may produce, however, life-threatening cardiac rhythm disturbances, valvular entrapment, pulmonary or systemic embolization, heart failure, or sudden cardiac death. With rare exception (e.g., lymphoma), prompt surgical intervention, whether palliative or curative, is the cornerstone of therapy. Radiologic detection, localization, morphologic assessment, and tissue characterization are crucial for the differential diagnosis and treatment planning of a cardiac mass. Important considerations include patient age, lesion location, mobility, and internal components (including calcium, fat, and necrosis). Past medical history may provide clues such as known extracardiac malignancy, underlying genetic predisposition, HIV positivity, or prior organ transplantation.

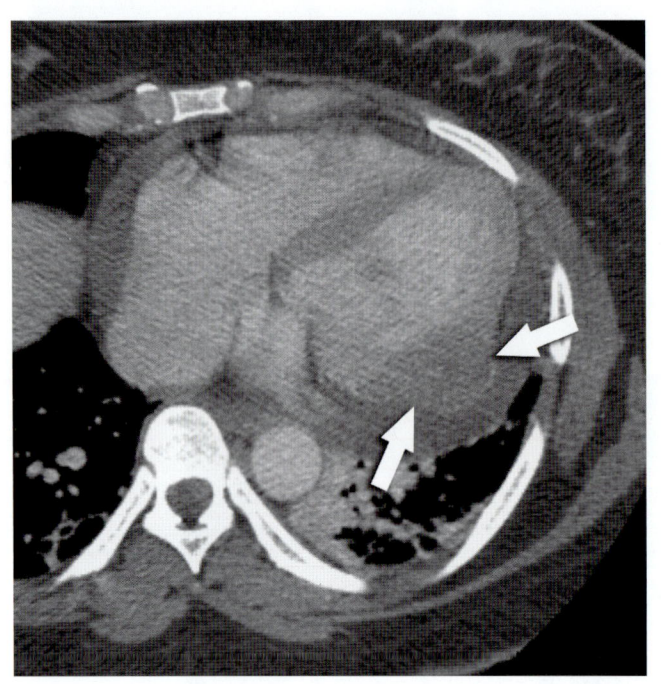

■ **FIGURE 67-40** PCL (anaplastic large cell lymphoma) in a 29-year-old pregnant woman with chest pain. Contrast-enhanced axial CT image shows a homogeneous oval mass arising from the posterior left ventricular wall (*arrows*) and a moderate-sized pericardial effusion. Autopsy confirmed extensive nodularity of the pericardium compatible with contiguous lymphomatous involvement.

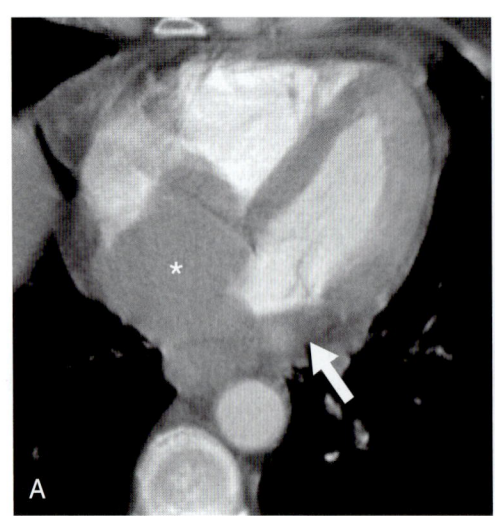

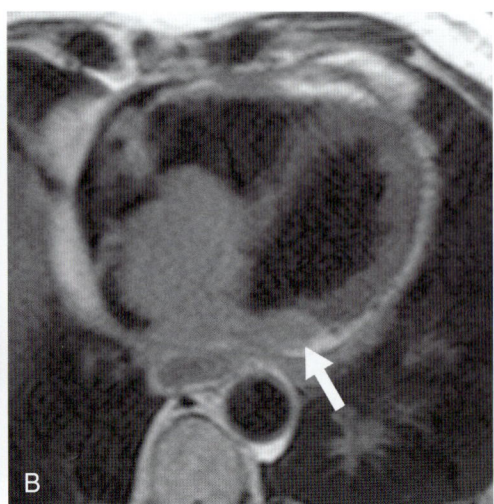

■ **FIGURE 67-41** PCL (non-Hodgkin) in a 74-year-old man with pericardial effusion. **A**, Contrast-enhanced axial CT image shows wide-based right atrial mass (*asterisk*) with probable extension into the posterior left atrial wall (*arrow*). **B**, T2-weighted axial MR image more clearly delineates hyperintense intramural tumor extending within the left atrial wall (*arrow*).

TABLE 67-1 Differential Diagnosis of Cardiac Tumors*

Right Atrial Mass
Thrombus
Metastasis
Endovascular tumor extension via inferior vena cava (hepatic, renal, adrenal, uterine malignancies)
Angiosarcoma (± hemorrhagic pericardial effusion)
Liposarcoma (may contain fat)
PCL (may be multifocal; necrosis unusual)
Myxoma (may contain calcification)

Left Atrial Mass
Thrombus (left atrial appendage location; ± mitral valve disease)
Metastasis
Myxoma (narrow septal attachment near fossa ovalis)
Pulmonary venous extension of tumor from the lung
Leiomyosarcoma
Osteosarcoma (variably calcified)
MFH
Paraganglioma (50% produce symptoms owing to elevated catecholamines)

Left Ventricular Mass
Thrombus
Metastasis
Fibroma
Rhabdomyoma (infants)

Valvular Mass
Vegetation
Thrombus
Papillary fibroelastoma (aortic or mitral)
Myxoma (unusual form)

Multiple Intracardiac Masses
Metastases
Rhabdomyoma (infants)
Rhabdomyosarcoma (children, young adults)
Leiomyosarcoma (30% of cases)
PCL (immunocompromised patients)

Cardiac Mass in an Infant or Child
Rhabdomyoma (multifocal, homogeneous, noncalcified, ± tuberous sclerosis)
Fibroma (marked T2 hypointensity to myocardium; often calcify)
Teratoma (heterogeneity on imaging)
Rhabdomyosarcoma (single or multiple; heterogeneity; valvular involvement)

Fat-containing Cardiac Masses
Lipoma
LHIS (interatrial septum location; dumbbell-shaped)
Liposarcoma (contains soft tissue components; aggressive features)

Calcified Cardiac Masses
Calcified thrombus
Fibroma
Myxoma (if right atrial)
Osteosarcoma (variably calcifies)
Calcified amorphous tumor of the heart (rare)
Tumoral calcinosis
Mitral annular calcification (may mimic a mass)

*Helpful differentiating features provided in parentheses.

Although there are exceptions, one must also recognize the potentially distinguishing imaging features of benign versus malignant cardiac tumor. Findings suggestive of benignancy include left-sided location, well-defined lesion margins, pedunculated mural attachment (when intracavitary), and lack of associated pericardial effusion or thickening. Features suspicious for malignancy are right-sided heart location; ill-defined tumor margins; wide-based mural attachment (when intracavitary); heterogeneity (necrosis); and, most importantly, the invasion of regional structures including valves, pericardium, regional vessels, or mediastinum. Multifocal intracardiac lesions and pulmonary metastases also suggest an underlying malignant etiology. A simplified approach to the differential diagnosis of cardiac tumors is provided in Table 67-1 with helpful differentiating features listed in parentheses.

SUGGESTED READINGS

Araoz PA, Mulvagh SL, Tazelaar HD, et al. CT and MR imaging of benign primary cardiac neoplasms with echocardiographic correlation. RadioGraphics 2000; 20:1303-1319.

Grebenc ML, Rosado de Christenson ML, Burke AP, et al. Primary cardiac and pericardial neoplasms: radiologic-pathologic correlation. RadioGraphics 2000; 20:1073-1103; quiz 1110-1071, 1112.

Grebenc ML, Rosado de Christenson ML, Green CE, et al. Cardiac myxoma: imaging features in 83 patients. RadioGraphics 2002; 22:673-689.

Grizzard JD, Ang GB. Magnetic resonance imaging of pericardial disease and cardiac masses. Magn Reson Imaging Clin N Am 2007; 15: 579-607.

Sparrow PJ, Kurian JB, Jones TR, et al. MR imaging of cardiac tumors. RadioGraphics 2005; 25:1255-1276.

Syed IS, Feng D, Harris SR, et al. MR imaging of cardiac masses. Magn Reson Imaging Clin N Am 2008; 16:137-164.

Uzun O, Wilson DG, Vujanic GM, et al. Cardiac tumours in children. Orphanet J Rare Dis 2007; 2:11.

Virmani R, Burke A, Farb A. Atlas of Cardiovascular Pathology. Philadelphia, Saunders, 1996.

Virmani R, Burke A, Farb A, et al. Cardiovascular Pathology. Philadelphia, Saunders, 2001.

REFERENCES

1. Virmani R, Burke A, Farb A, et al. Cardiovascular Pathology. Philadelphia, Saunders, 2001.
2. Reynen K. Cardiac myxomas. N Engl J Med 1995; 333:1610-1617.
3. Grebenc ML, Rosado de Christenson ML, Green CE, et al. Cardiac myxoma: imaging features in 83 patients. RadioGraphics 2002; 22:673-689.
4. Edwards A, Bermudez C, Piwonka G, et al. Carney's syndrome: complex myxomas: report of four cases and review of the literature. Cardiovasc Surg 2002; 10:264-275.
5. Grebenc ML, Rosado de Christenson ML, Burke AP, et al. Primary cardiac and pericardial neoplasms: radiologic-pathologic correlation. RadioGraphics 2000; 20:1073-1103; quiz 1110-1071, 1112.
6. Virmani R, Burke A, Farb A. Atlas of Cardiovascular Pathology. Philadelphia, Saunders, 1996.
7. Araoz PA, Mulvagh SL, Tazelaar HD, et al. CT and MR imaging of benign primary cardiac neoplasms with echocardiographic correlation. RadioGraphics 2000; 20:1303-1319.
8. Syed IS, Feng D, Harris SR, et al. MR imaging of cardiac masses. Magn Reson Imaging Clin N Am 2008; 16:137-164.
9. Sparrow PJ, Kurian JB, Jones TR, et al. MR imaging of cardiac tumors. RadioGraphics 2005; 25:1255-1276.
10. Grizzard JD, Ang GB. Magnetic resonance imaging of pericardial disease and cardiac masses. Magn Reson Imaging Clin N Am 2007; 15:579-607.
11. Gowda RM, Khan IA, Nair CK, et al. Cardiac papillary fibroelastoma: a comprehensive analysis of 725 cases. Am Heart J 2003; 146:404-410.
12. Sun JP, Asher CR, Yang XS, et al. Clinical and echocardiographic characteristics of papillary fibroelastomas: a retrospective and prospective study in 162 patients. Circulation 2001; 103:2687-2693.
13. Bootsveld A, Puetz J, Grube E. Incidental finding of a papillary fibroelastoma on the aortic valve in 16 slice multi-detector row computed tomography. Heart 2004; 90:e35.
14. Lembcke A, Meyer R, Kivelitz D, et al. Images in cardiovascular medicine: papillary fibroelastoma of the aortic valve: appearance in 64-slice spiral computed tomography, magnetic resonance imaging, and echocardiography. Circulation 2007; 115:e3-e6.
15. Luna A, Ribes R, Caro P, et al. Evaluation of cardiac tumors with magnetic resonance imaging. Eur Radiol 2005; 15:1446-1455.
16. Shiraishi J, Tagawa M, Yamada T, et al. Papillary fibroelastoma of the aortic valve: evaluation with transesophageal echocardiography and magnetic resonance imaging. Jpn Heart J 2003; 44:799-803.
17. Kelle S, Chiribiri A, Meyer R, et al. Images in cardiovascular medicine: papillary fibroelastoma of the tricuspid valve seen on magnetic resonance imaging. Circulation 2008; 117:e190-e191.
18. Butany J, Nair V, Naseemuddin A, et al. Cardiac tumours: diagnosis and management. Lancet Oncol 2005; 6:219-228.
19. Burke AP, Rosado de Christenson M, Templeton PA, et al. Cardiac fibroma: clinicopathologic correlates and surgical treatment. J Thorac Cardiovasc Surg 1994; 108:862-870.
20. Iqbal MB, Stavri G, Mittal T, et al. A calcified cardiac mass. Int J Cardiol 2007; 115:e126-e128.
21. Cina SJ, Smialek JE, Burke AP, et al. Primary cardiac tumors causing sudden death: a review of the literature. Am J Forensic Med Pathol 1996; 17:271-281.
22. Isaacs H Jr. Fetal and neonatal cardiac tumors. Pediatr Cardiol 2004; 25:252-273.
23. Yan AT, Coffey DM, Li Y, et al. Images in cardiovascular medicine: myocardial fibroma in Gorlin syndrome by cardiac magnetic resonance imaging. Circulation 2006; 114:e376-e379.
24. De Cobelli F, Esposito A, Mellone R, et al. Images in cardiovascular medicine: late enhancement of a left ventricular cardiac fibroma assessed with gadolinium-enhanced cardiovascular magnetic resonance. Circulation 2005; 112:e242-e243.
25. Tworetzky W, McElhinney DB, Margossian R, et al. Association between cardiac tumors and tuberous sclerosis in the fetus and neonate. Am J Cardiol 2003; 92:487-489.
26. Bader RS, Chitayat D, Kelly E, et al. Fetal rhabdomyoma: prenatal diagnosis, clinical outcome, and incidence of associated tuberous sclerosis complex. J Pediatr 2003; 143:620-624.
27. Uzun O, Wilson DG, Vujanic GM, et al. Cardiac tumours in children. Orphanet J Rare Dis 2007; 2:11.
28. Burke A, Jeudy J Jr, Virmani R. Cardiac tumours: an update. Heart 2008; 94:117-123.
29. Salanitri JC, Pereles FS. Cardiac lipoma and lipomatous hypertrophy of the interatrial septum: cardiac magnetic resonance imaging findings. J Comput Assist Tomogr 2004; 28:852-856.
30. Cunningham KS, Veinot JP, Feindel CM, et al. Fatty lesions of the atria and interatrial septum. Hum Pathol 2006; 37:1245-1251.
31. Heyer CM, Kagel T, Lemburg SP, et al. Lipomatous hypertrophy of the interatrial septum: a prospective study of incidence, imaging findings, and clinical symptoms. Chest 2003; 124:2068-2073.
32. O'Connor S, Recavarren R, Nichols LC, et al. Lipomatous hypertrophy of the interatrial septum: an overview. Arch Pathol Lab Med 2006; 130:397-399.
33. Fan CM, Fischman AJ, Kwek BH, et al. Lipomatous hypertrophy of the interatrial septum: increased uptake on FDG PET. AJR Am J Roentgenol 2005; 184:339-342.
34. Hamilton BH, Francis IR, Gross BH, et al. Intrapericardial paragangliomas (pheochromocytomas): imaging features. AJR Am J Roentgenol 1997; 168:109-113.
35. Mandak JS, Benoit CH, Starkey RH, et al. Echocardiography in the evaluation of cardiac pheochromocytoma. Am Heart J 1996; 132:1063-1066.
36. Lupinski RW, Shankar S, Agasthian T, et al. Primary cardiac paraganglioma. Ann Thorac Surg 2004; 78:e43-e44.
37. Reynolds C, Tazelaar HD, Edwards WD. Calcified amorphous tumor of the heart (cardiac CAT). Hum Pathol 1997; 28:601-606.
38. Ho HH, Min JK, Lin F, et al. Images in cardiovascular medicine: calcified amorphous tumor of the heart. Circulation 2008; 117:e171-e172.
39. Fealey ME, Edwards WD, Reynolds CA, et al. Recurrent cardiac calcific amorphous tumor: the CAT had a kitten. Cardiovasc Pathol 2007; 16:115-118.
40. Lewin M, Nazarian S, Marine JE, et al. Fatal outcome of a calcified amorphous tumor of the heart (cardiac CAT). Cardiovasc Pathol 2006; 15:299-302.
41. Bussani R, De Giorgio F, Abbate A, et al. Cardiac metastases. J Clin Pathol 2007; 60:27-34.

42. Chiles C, Woodard PK, Gutierrez FR, et al. Metastatic involvement of the heart and pericardium: CT and MR imaging. RadioGraphics 2001; 21:439-449.
43. Odeh M, Oliven A, Misselevitch I, et al. Acute cor pulmonale due to tumor cell microemboli. Respiration 1997; 64:384-387.
44. Borsaru AD, Lau KK, Solin P. Cardiac metastasis: a cause of recurrent pulmonary emboli. Br J Radiol 2007; 80:e50-e53.
45. Poh KK, Avelar E, Hua L, et al. Cardiac metastases from malignant melanoma. Clin Cardiol 2007; 30:359-360.
46. Ozyuncu N, Sahin M, Altin T, et al. Cardiac metastasis of malignant melanoma: a rare cause of complete atrioventricular block. Europace 2006; 8:545-548.
47. Khan N, Golzar J, Smith NL, et al. Intracardiac extension of a large cell undifferentiated carcinoma of lung. Heart 2005; 91:512.
48. Salanitri J. Cardiac metastases: ante-mortem diagnosis with cardiac magnetic resonance imaging. Intern Med J 2005; 35:303-304.
49. Shanmugam G. Primary cardiac sarcoma. Eur J Cardiothorac Surg 2006; 29:925-932.
50. Kucukarslan N, Kirilmaz A, Ulusoy E, et al. Eleven-year experience in diagnosis and surgical therapy of right atrial masses. J Card Surg 2007; 22:39-42.
51. Vander Salm TJ. Unusual primary tumors of the heart. Semin Thorac Cardiovasc Surg 2000; 12:89-100.
52. Neragi-Miandoab S, Kim J, Vlahakes GJ. Malignant tumours of the heart: a review of tumour type, diagnosis and therapy. Clin Oncol (R Coll Radiol) 2007; 19:748-756.
53. Skopin II, Serov RA, Makushin AA, et al. Primary rhabdomyosarcoma of the right atrium. Interact Cardiovasc Thorac Surg 2003; 2:316-318.
54. Uemura S, Watanabe M, Iwama H, et al. Extensive primary cardiac liposarcoma with multiple functional complications. Heart 2004; 90:e48.
55. Rockwell L, Hetzel P, Freeman JK, et al. Cardiac involvement in malignancies, case 3: primary cardiac lymphoma. J Clin Oncol 2004; 22:2744-2745.
56. Nakakuki T, Masuoka H, Ishikura K, et al. A case of primary cardiac lymphoma located in the pericardial effusion. Heart Vessels 2004; 19:199-202.

PART TEN

Pericardial Disease

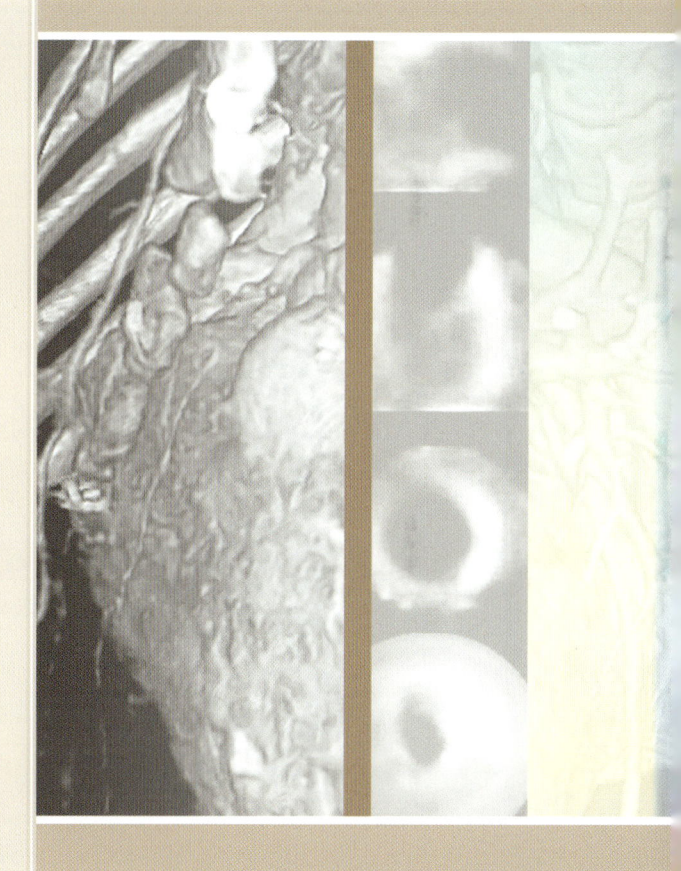

CHAPTER 68

Pericardial Effusion

Lynn S. Broderick

Pericardial effusion can occur from various causes, including infection, trauma, and systemic disease. Infectious causes of pericardial effusion are described in more detail in Chapter 69. This chapter focuses on pericardial effusion secondary to systemic disease.

DEFINITION

Pericardial effusion refers to the abnormal accumulation of fluid within the pericardial space. The pericardial fluid may be a transudate, may be an exudate, or may be hemorrhagic.

PREVALENCE AND EPIDEMIOLOGY

The prevalence of pericardial effusion depends on the underlying cause. Pericardial effusion detectable by echocardiography may be present in 50% of patients with rheumatoid arthritis. Pericardial effusion is also common in patients with systemic lupus erythematosus and scleroderma.

ETIOLOGY AND PATHOPHYSIOLOGY

Pericardial effusion is an abnormal accumulation of fluid within the pericardial space. In the absence of acute inflammation, clinical symptoms depend on the size of the effusion, the rate of accumulation, and the ability of the pericardium to expand. Cardiac tamponade occurs when the intrapericardial pressure is high enough to impede cardiac filling. The pericardial fluid may be a transudate, an exudate, or hemorrhagic. Pericardial effusion is common in some diseases, such as chronic renal disease and heart failure. Pericardial effusion can occur in any collagen vascular disease, but is particularly common in patients with lupus erythematosus and rheumatoid arthritis (Fig. 68-1).

Pericardial effusion can occur in patients with acute myocardial infarction, particularly if the infarction is large in size. It can also occur in a delayed manner after myocardial infarction or surgery (Dressler syndrome). Metastatic disease involving the pericardium results in pericardial effusion, often without detectable pericardial nodules or thickening. Pericardial disease is frequent in patients with rheumatoid arthritis, particularly in patients with active disease. Patients are typically asymptomatic, however. Rheumatoid pericardial disease may manifest as serous or serosanguineous fluid. Pericardial fluid can be present in patients with rheumatic fever, although this is an uncommon entity in the United States. In patients with pericardial effusion secondary to rheumatic fever, there is usually a classic presentation of acute pericarditis that occurs 1 week or so after the initial onset of fever.

MANIFESTATIONS OF DISEASE

Clinical Presentation

Pericardial effusion in the absence of acute pericarditis may be clinically silent, unless tamponade physiology is present. The clinical symptoms of cardiac tamponade are related to the resulting decrease in cardiac output and include hypotension and tachycardia. Jugular venous distention is present on physical examination. A decrease in systemic blood pressure by more than 10 mm Hg during inspiration is diagnostic of pulsus paradoxus. Pulsus paradoxus was originally described as the disappearance of the radial pulse during inspiration. Pulsus paradoxus is actually an exaggeration of the normal decrease in systemic blood pressure during inspiration.[1]

Imaging Indications and Algorithm

Asymptomatic pericardial effusion may be discovered incidentally. When pericardial effusion is suspected, echocardiography is the imaging modality of choice to document the effusion and to determine if there is evidence of tamponade.

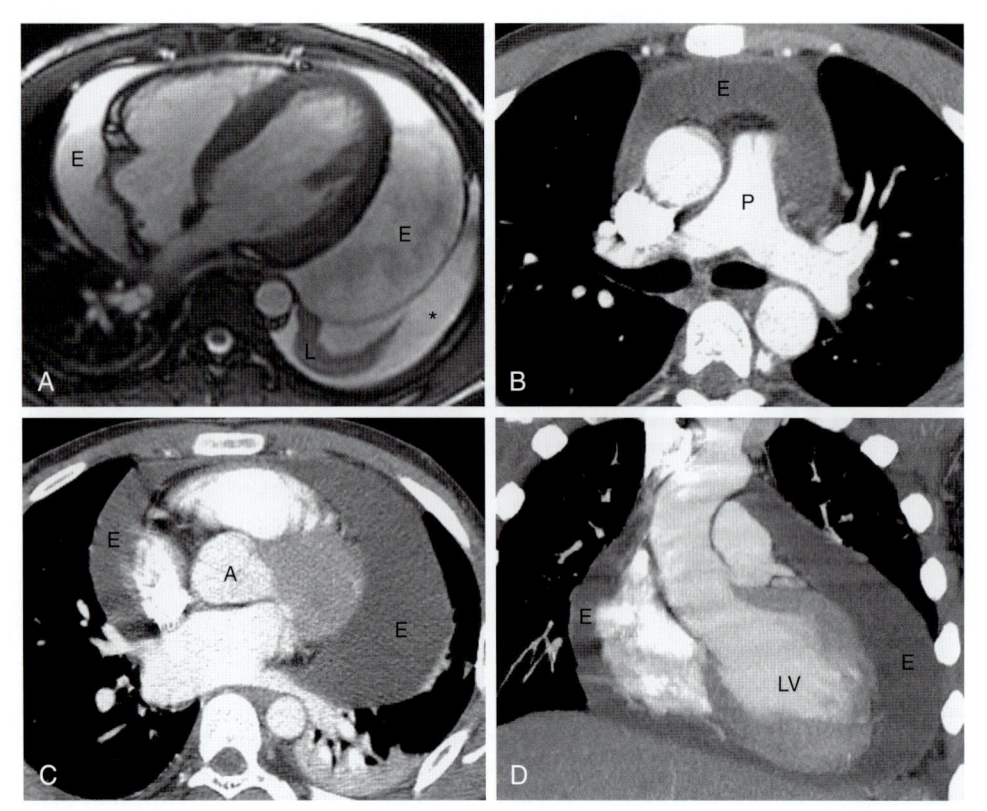

FIGURE 68-1 A 19-year-old man with systemic lupus erythematosus presented with increasingly severe left-sided chest pain, which worsened on inspiration and with movement. CT scan with intravenous contrast medium was performed to evaluate for possible pulmonary embolism. **A,** Bright blood axial MR image shows a large pericardial effusion (E) and a left pleural effusion (*asterisk*) causing passive atelectasis of the left lower lobe (L). **B-D,** Contrast-enhanced axial CT images at the level of the pulmonary artery (P) (**B**) and at the level of the aortic valve (A) (**C**), and a coronal reconstructed image (**D**) show a large pericardial effusion (E). Echocardiography (not shown) showed minimal collapse of the right ventricle during diastole. Pericardiocentesis was performed, and the patient's symptoms resolved. LV, left ventricle.

Imaging Techniques and Findings

Radiography

Chest radiographs may show interval enlargement of the cardiac silhouette. Pericardial effusion should be suspected when cardiac enlargement occurs over a short period of time (Fig. 68-2). The classic "water flask" appearance of the cardiac silhouette in pericardial effusion can also be seen in patients with dilated cardiomyopathy. In patients with dilated cardiomyopathy, the hilar structures are displaced laterally as the heart enlarges. In patients with large pericardial effusion, the hila may become obscured because the pericardial reflections extend to cover the proximal portions of the great vessels.[2] If there is sufficient subepicardial fat, and the fat is oriented such that it is visible on radiographs, widening of the pericardial line, indicative of pericardial effusion, can be detected on chest radiograph—the epicardial fat pad sign (see Fig. 68-2).[3,4]

Ultrasonography

On echocardiography, uncomplicated pericardial fluid is hypoechoic and is found diffusely throughout the pericardial space. The size of the effusion is quantified as small when the space between the visceral and parietal pericardium measures less than 5 mm, moderate when the space measures between 5 mm and 2 cm, and large when the space measures more than 2 cm.[5] Loculated fluid and intrapericardial stranding may be present. Echocardiographic findings of pericardial tamponade in the presence of a pericardial effusion include collapse of the right atrium during systole lasting more than a third of the systolic interval, collapse of the right ventricular free wall during diastole, and abnormal septal motion toward the left ventricle.

Computed Tomography

CT may be requested to evaluate further pericardial effusion identified on echocardiography if there is suspicion for loculation or associated pericardial thickening. Pericardial effusion is more frequently an incidental finding on CT examinations obtained for evaluation of other disease entities. When pericardial fluid is identified in patients with neoplasm, the pericardium should be carefully inspected to determine if there is nodular thickening that would indicate metastatic disease as the cause of the effusion. In patients with recent cardiac surgery or instrumentation, the density of the fluid should be evaluated to assess for possible hemopericardium. ECG gated sequences can be used to detect abnormal wall and septal motion indicative of pericardial tamponade. When ECG gating has not been used, compression of the cardiac chambers may be an indication of elevated intrapericardial pressure.

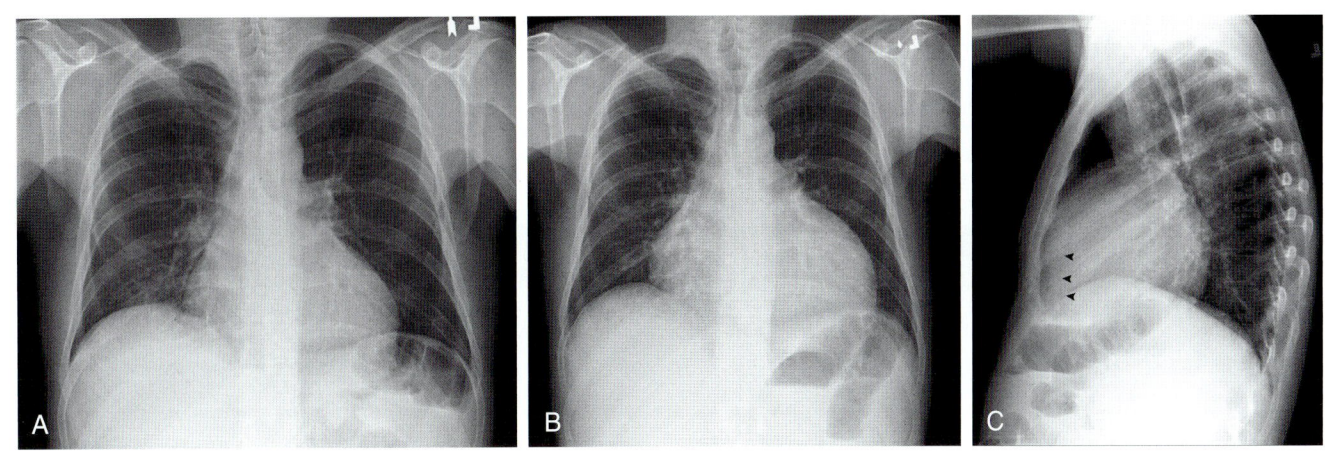

■ **FIGURE 68-2** A 42-year-old man with acquired immunodeficiency syndrome (AIDS) who had been treated for cryptococcal infection in the past presented with fatigue. **A,** Baseline chest radiograph from June shows a normal cardiac silhouette. **B,** Posteroanterior chest radiograph obtained in October shows interval cardiac enlargement. **C,** Lateral chest radiograph obtained in October shows posterior displacement of the subepicardial fat (*arrowheads*), consistent with pericardial effusion. Pericardial effusion was confirmed by echocardiography. *Cryptococcus* was cultured from the pericardiocentesis sample.

Magnetic Resonance Imaging

ECG gated MRI sequences can be used to detect abnormal wall and septal motion indicative of pericardial tamponade. MRI is better able to distinguish small pericardial effusion from pericardial thickening compared with CT. Pericardial effusion may be found incidentally on MRI.

DIFFERENTIAL DIAGNOSIS
Clinical Presentation

Pericardial effusion may be clinically silent. In the setting of cardiac tamponade, other causes of hypotension, shock, and elevated jugular venous distention, such as heart failure, pulmonary embolism, and myocardial infarction of the right ventricle, should also be considered.[6]

Imaging Findings

If the amount of pericardial fluid is very small, it may be difficult to distinguish pericardial effusion from pericardial thickening on CT scans.

TREATMENT OPTIONS
Medical

Treatment of patients with pericardial effusion is primarily directed at the underlying cause because the effusion is a manifestation of the systemic disease.

Surgical/Interventional

Emergent pericardiotomy is indicated in patients with evidence of pericardial tamponade. Pericardiotomy or pericardiectomy may be indicated in patients with metastatic pericardial disease. Surgical intervention may also be required for patients with unexpected postoperative hemopericardium.

INFORMATION FOR THE REFERRING PHYSICIAN

The imaging report should include an indication of the size of the pericardial effusion; whether there is pericardial thickening, nodularity, or loculation; and any finding associated with pericardial tamponade, if present.

KEY POINTS

- Congestive heart failure is the most common cause of small to moderate-sized pericardial effusion.
- Enlarging cardiac silhouette over a short time or in the postoperative setting should raise suspicion of the presence of pericardial fluid.

SUGGESTED READING

Spodick DH. Pericarditis in systemic diseases. Cardiol Clin 1990; 8:709-716.

REFERENCES

1. Spodick DH. Pulsus paradoxus. In Spodick DH (ed). The Pericardium. New York, Marcel Dekker, 1997, pp 191-199.
2. Baron MG. Pericardial effusion. Circulation 1971; 44:294-299.
3. Lane EJ, Carsky EW. Epicardial fat: lateral plain film analysis in normals and in pericardial effusion. Radiology 1968; 91:1-5.
4. Carsky EW, Mauceri RA, Azimi F. The epicardial fat pad sign. Radiology 1980; 137:303-308.
5. Otto CM. Pericardial disease: two-dimensional echocardiographic and Doppler findings. In Otto CM (ed). Textbook of Clinical Echocardiography. Philadelphia, Saunders, 2000, pp 213-228.
6. LeWinter MM, Kabbani S. Pericardial diseases. In Zipes DP, Libby P, Bonow RO, et al (eds). Braunwald's Heart Disease: A Textbook of Cardiovascular Medicine. 7th ed. Philadelphia, Saunders, 2005, pp 1757-1780.

CHAPTER 69

Acute Pericarditis

Lynn S. Broderick

Acute pericarditis may result in fibrinous exudate, pericardial effusion, or cardiac tamponade. Various systemic diseases may result in acute pericarditis or pericardial effusion (see Chapter 68). In many cases, the cause of the acute pericarditis is unknown, however.

DEFINITION

Acute pericarditis is a symptomatic inflammation of the pericardium of sudden onset with symptoms of less than 2 weeks' duration. Acute pericarditis may result in fibrinous secretions or the development of a pericardial effusion.

PREVALENCE AND EPIDEMIOLOGY

The true prevalence of acute pericarditis is unknown, but it may account for 1% of all emergency department visits for chest pain.[1]

ETIOLOGY AND PATHOPHYSIOLOGY

There are many causes of acute pericarditis (Table 69-1).[2-6] The specific etiology is often unknown, thereby resulting in the diagnosis of idiopathic pericarditis. The use of a systematic approach to the diagnosis of the cause of acute pericarditis, including a detailed history, blood cultures, antibody testing, and viral testing, can reduce the number of "idiopathic" diagnoses.[7] Viral infection is the most common cause of acute pericarditis in the United States, and is probably the etiology in patients with idiopathic pericarditis.[8,9] The most common viral agents causing acute pericarditis are coxsackievirus group B and echovirus.[8] Viral pericarditis is usually preceded by upper respiratory infection symptoms, and typically is a self-limited disease that can be diagnosed by serologic testing of antiviral titers. Numerous systemic diseases can also result in acute pericarditis and pericardial effusion. These diseases are discussed in Chapter 70. It is difficult to distinguish cases of acute pericarditis from cases of pericardial effusion in the literature because the presence of pericardial fluid is sometimes seen as an indicator of the presence of pericarditis.

MANIFESTATIONS OF DISEASE

Clinical Presentation

The fibrous portion of the parietal pericardium contains pain fibers, which account for the symptoms associated with acute pericarditis. The proximity of the parietal pericardium to the pleura, esophagus, and phrenic nerves accounts for differing pain symptoms. The pain associated with acute pericarditis is typically sudden in onset and sharp in nature. Similar to the pain associated with myocardial ischemia, pain associated with acute pericarditis may radiate into the left neck and arm, owing to inflammation of the phrenic nerve. In contrast to anginal pain, pain secondary to acute pericarditis is not relieved by nitroglycerin. Pain associated with acute pericarditis may also be pleuritic in nature, accentuated by respiratory motion and change in position. An occasional characteristic of acute pericarditis is pain accentuated by swallowing because of inflammation affecting the adjacent esophagus.

On physical examination, the patient typically appears distressed and often is leaning forward when sitting because this position helps to alleviate the pain. Fever may be present and typically follows the onset of pain. In 85% of patients, a triphasic pericardial friction rub, often characterized as the sound of leather squeaking against leather, is heard on auscultation, although this finding may be intermittent. The intensity of the rub can vary with the position of the patient. Characteristic ECG changes also are associated with acute pericarditis. Early in the disease, there is ST segment elevation in a nonanatomic distribution. The triad of characteristic pain, pericardial friction rub, and characteristic ECG changes is diagnostic of acute pericarditis. Laboratory abnormalities associated with acute viral or idiopathic pericarditis include elevation of the erythrocyte sedimentation rate and C-reactive protein, and early leukocytosis followed by development of lym-

TABLE 69-1	Etiology of Acute Pericarditis

Infectious Causes
  Viral
    Coxsackievirus (particularly group B)
    Echovirus
    Adenovirus
    Influenza virus
    Infectious mononucleosis
    Varicella
    Mumps
    Human immunodeficiency virus
  Bacterial
    Streptococcus
    Staphylococcus
    Francisella tularensis
    Rickettsia
    Actinomyces
    Nocardia
    Mycobacterium tuberculosis
  Fungal
    Histoplasma
    Coccidioides
    Blastomyces
    Aspergillus
Noninfectious Causes
  Connective tissue diseases and vasculitides
    Rheumatoid arthritis
    Systemic lupus erythematosus
    Scleroderma
    Sjögren syndrome
    Wegener granulomatosis
    Dermatomyositis
    Churg-Strauss syndrome
  Neoplasm
    Primary mesothelioma and other mesenchymal tumors
    Metastatic disease
  Metabolic
    Uremia
    Dialysis-related pericarditis
    Myxedema
  Trauma
    Blunt or penetrating trauma
    Postsurgical or postinstrumentation
  Radiation
  Cardiopulmonary processes
    Acute myocardial infarction
    Dressler syndrome
    Pneumonia
  Idiopathic

phocytosis. Serum enzymes, such as creatine phosphokinase, and troponin levels may be elevated in patients with acute pericarditis because of a concomitant superficial myocarditis (also called *myopericarditis*).[10]

Imaging Indications and Algorithm

Typically, the diagnosis of acute pericarditis is based on presenting signs and symptoms. Echocardiography is often employed to assess for pericardial effusion and any associated complications. If the clinical presentation makes the diagnosis less certain, patients may undergo CT to evaluate for possible pulmonary embolism, aortic dissection, or other causes of chest pain.

Imaging Techniques and Findings

Radiography

Typically, because of the acute onset of symptoms, the chest radiograph is normal in appearance. Depending on the amount of pericardial fluid, there may be an increase in the size of the cardiac silhouette. The chest radiograph can also be assessed for absence of findings associated with other disease entities that result in chest pain, such as pneumonia or pneumothorax.

Ultrasonography

Echocardiography may be performed to assess for the presence of pericardial effusion, to assess for evidence of cardiac tamponade, or to establish a baseline appearance of the pericardial space. The echocardiographic findings of acute pericarditis include a normal examination, pericardial thickening with or without pericardial effusion, and pericardial effusion without pericardial thickening.[11] Depending on the echocardiographic findings, assessment can be made for tamponade or constrictive physiology.

Computed Tomography

Contrast-enhanced CT scans may be performed in patients in whom the clinical presentation is unclear or to exclude other potential causes of chest pain. Typical findings of acute pericarditis on CT scans include enhancement of smooth, uniformly thickened pericardium and pericardial effusion (Fig. 69-1).[12]

Magnetic Resonance Imaging

Although not frequently performed for the evaluation of acute pericarditis, MRI can show a pericardial effusion, thickening, and enhancement.

Nuclear Medicine

Nuclear medicine studies are usually not performed for assessment of patients with acute pericarditis.

Angiography

Angiography is usually not performed for assessment of patients with acute pericarditis.

Classic Signs

The typical appearance of acute pericarditis in patients who undergo CT is enhancing, smooth, and regularly thickened pericardium with a small to moderate-sized pericardial effusion.

DIFFERENTIAL DIAGNOSIS

Clinical Presentation

Patients with angina pectoris, aortic dissection, community-acquired pneumonia, and pulmonary embolism all can

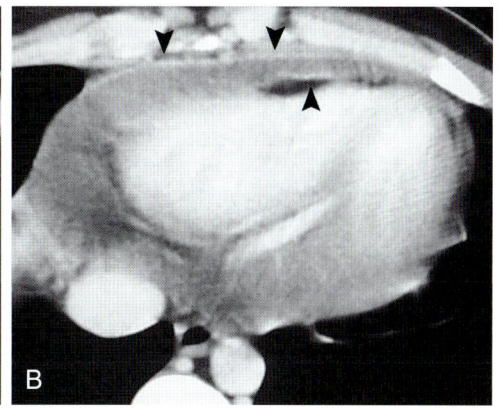

FIGURE 69-1 A 19-year-old man presented with a 3-week history of chest pain. The chest pain was sharp in nature and radiated to his throat and left trapezius muscle. The pain worsened when lying flat and relieved on sitting upright and leaning forward. **A** and **B,** Contrast-enhanced CT scan of the chest was performed and shows a small to moderate-sized pericardial effusion with smoothly thickened, enhancing pericardium (*arrowheads*). The patient was initially thought to have viral pericarditis. On further testing, the diagnosis of adult-onset Still disease was made.

present with chest pain. The chest pain that occurs in patients with angina pectoris is typically severe but not sharp in nature, does not change with patient position, and has ECG changes typical of ischemia. The chest pain that occurs in patients with dissecting aortic aneurysm is typically severe, radiating to the back, without alteration of pain with change of position. Patients with aortic dissection do not have the characteristic pericardial rub or ECG changes. Patients with pulmonary emboli can also present with chest pain, but do not have the characteristic ECG changes or pericardial rub. Pleuritic chest pain can also be seen in patients with pneumonia. If dysphagia is present, esophageal disease is included in the differential diagnosis. Because the pain associated with acute pericarditis may localize to the epigastrium, intra-abdominal pathology, such as peptic ulcer disease and cholecystitis, may be suspected.

Imaging Findings

Pericardial thickening in patients with constrictive pericarditis may be calcified and is often irregular. Early enhancement of the pericardium is seen in patients with acute pericarditis studied with CT or MRI. If perfusion MRI is performed, there is typically delayed enhancement of the pericardium in patients with constrictive pericarditis, a feature that is absent in patients with acute pericarditis. The typical morphologic changes associated with constrictive pericarditis (see Chapter 70) are absent in patients with acute pericarditis.

TREATMENT OPTIONS

Medical

For viral or idiopathic pericarditis, ibuprofen is the preferred nonsteroidal anti-inflammatory drug. It is used to prevent recurrence of pericarditis.[2,10,13] Antibiotic therapy is indicated when specific organisms are cultured.

Surgical/Interventional

If cardiac tamponade is present, if the infectious agent is bacterial (Fig. 69-2), or if neoplastic involvement is suspected, pericardiotomy is indicated.[2,10,13] In cases of neoplasm or granulomatous disease, pericardial biopsy may be necessary to establish the diagnosis.

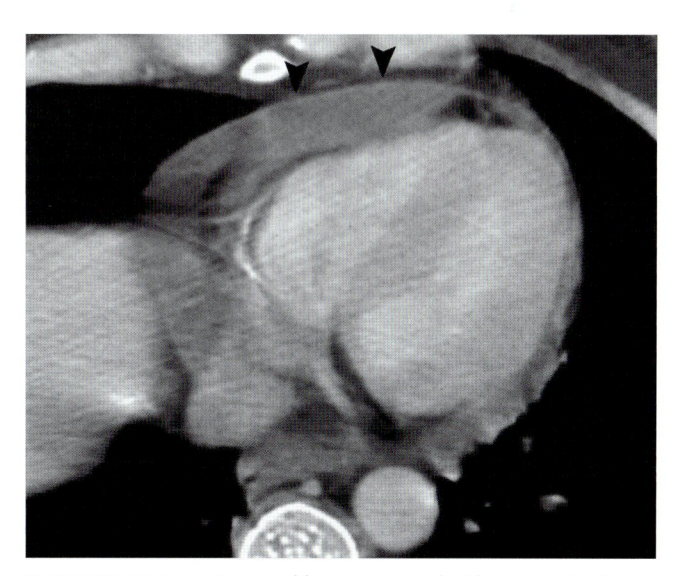

FIGURE 69-2 A 61-year-old man presented with a 2-month history of progressive soft tissue infection involving the right shoulder that had not been treated. CT scan was performed to evaluate the extent of the infection and to assess for involvement of the chest and mediastinum. Contrast-enhanced CT scan shows a moderate-sized pericardial effusion with enhancement of the visceral and parietal pericardium (*arrowheads*) consistent with acute pericarditis. Pericardial window was performed, and *Staphylococcus aureus* was cultured from the pericardial fluid.

INFORMATION FOR THE REFERRING PHYSICIAN

Chest radiograph and CT scan should be assessed for associated findings such as pleural effusion or any other findings that may provide clues as to the etiology. If there are erosive changes at the distal ends of the clavicle, consideration can be given to rheumatoid arthritis as the possible etiology.

KEY POINTS

- Acute pericarditis is a clinical diagnosis.
- Characteristic imaging findings may be present in patients undergoing CT to evaluate for pulmonary emboli, aortic dissection, or coronary artery disease.
- Idiopathic pericarditis is usually caused by a virus. Because the pericarditis usually occurs 1 to 3 weeks after initial viral infection, the virus is often not recovered.

SUGGESTED READING

Axel L. Assessment of pericardial disease by magnetic resonance and computed tomography. J Magn Reson Imaging 2004; 19:816-826.

REFERENCES

1. Zayas R, Anguita M, Torres F, et al. Incidence of specific etiology and role of methods for specific etiologic diagnosis of primary acute pericarditis. Am J Cardiol 1995; 75:378-382.
2. Lange RA, Hillis LD. Acute pericarditis. N Engl J Med 2004; 351:2195-2202.
3. Spodick DH. Pericarditis in systemic diseases. Cardiol Clin 1990; 8:709-716.
4. Troughton RW, Asher CR, Klein AL. Pericarditis. Lancet 2004; 363:712-727.
5. Lorbar M, Spodick DH. "Idiopathic" pericarditis—the clinician's challenge (nothing is idiopathic). Int J Clin Pract 2007; 91:138-142.
6. Ariyarajah V, Spodick DH. Acute pericarditis: diagnostic cues and common electrocardiographic manifestations. Cardiol Rev 2007; 15:24-30.
7. Levy PY, Corey R, Berger P, et al. Etiologic diagnosis of 204 pericardial effusions. Medicine (Baltimore) 2003; 82:385-391.
8. Shabetai R. Acute pericarditis. Cardiol Clin 1990; 8:639-644.
9. Little WC, Freeman GL. Pericardial disease. Circulation 2006; 113:1622-1632.
10. Spodick DH. Acute pericarditis: current concepts and practice. JAMA 2003; 289:1150-1153.
11. Otto CM. Pericardial disease: two-dimensional echocardiographic and Doppler findings. In Otto CM (ed). Textbook of Clinical Echocardiography. Philadelphia, Saunders, 2000, pp 213-228.
12. Rienmuller R, Groll R, Lipton MJ. CT and MR imaging of pericardial disease. Radiol Clin North Am 2004; 42:587-601.
13. Maisch B, Seferovic PM, Ristic AD, et al. Guidelines on the diagnosis and management of pericardial diseases executive summary: the Task Force on the Diagnosis and Management of Pericardial Diseases of the European Society of Cardiology. Eur Heart J 2004; 25:587-610.

CHAPTER 70

Constrictive Pericarditis

Lynn S. Broderick

In constrictive pericarditis, the interpreting physician is consulted to establish the presence or absence of pericardial thickening or calcification or both. Documentation of abnormal pericardial thickening or calcification and characteristic alterations of cardiac structures, coupled with the appropriate hemodynamic changes, establishes the diagnosis of constrictive pericarditis in most cases.

DEFINITION

Constrictive pericarditis is a disease state in which previous insult to the pericardium results in pericardial scarring leading to constriction and compression of the underlying cardiac chambers.

PREVALENCE AND EPIDEMIOLOGY

Constrictive pericarditis is uncommon. It is more commonly seen in patients with a preexisting episode of pericarditis, prior surgery, or prior radiation therapy, although many patients have no documented antecedent pericardial disease. In a prospective assessment of the outcome of acute pericarditis, 56% of patients with tuberculous pericarditis, 35% of patients with purulent pericarditis, and 17% of patients with neoplastic pericardial disease developed constrictive pericarditis.[1] Only 1% of patients with idiopathic pericarditis developed constrictive pericarditis in this series. In contrast, transient constrictive pericarditis (see later) was more commonly seen in patients with idiopathic pericarditis, occurring in approximately 20% of cases.[2]

ETIOLOGY AND PATHOPHYSIOLOGY

In the United States, the most common causes of constrictive pericarditis are idiopathic or postviral pericarditis, prior cardiac surgery, and radiation therapy (Table 70-1). The scarred pericardium inhibits the ability of the cardiac chambers to dilate during diastolic filling, acting as a cage covering the heart. As a result of the inability to dilate, the intracardiac pressures of each chamber are elevated and equalized. This elevated pressure is transmitted to the pulmonary and systemic veins. Because the atrial pressures are elevated, there is rapid filling of the ventricles early in ventricular diastole. This ventricular filling rapidly ceases when the ventricle can no longer expand to accept the incoming volume. Systemic venous hypertension results in hepatomegaly, ascites, and peripheral edema.

MANIFESTATIONS OF DISEASE

Clinical Presentation

Patients with constrictive pericarditis present with signs and symptoms of right heart failure. Patients may complain of dyspnea, orthopnea, and paroxysmal nocturnal dyspnea, abdominal fullness secondary to ascites, and pedal edema. On physical examination, there is distention of the neck veins, peripheral edema, and hepatomegaly. In a patient without pericardial constriction, there is a decrease in jugular venous pressure during inspiration because of decrease in intrathoracic pressure. In patients with constrictive pericarditis, because the intrapericardial pressure is dissociated from the intrathoracic pressure, there is an increase in jugular venous pressure during inspiration (Kussmaul sign).[3] A pericardial knock, which corresponds to the rapid cessation of ventricular filling, can be heard along the cardiac apex and left sternal border.

Imaging Indications and Algorithm

Patients suspected to have constrictive pericarditis based on history, physical examination, and echocardiographic findings are referred for CT or MRI to evaluate for thickening or calcification within the pericardium.

Imaging Techniques and Findings

Radiography

If pericardial calcification is present, it may be visible on chest radiograph. Pericardial calcification is usually best

TABLE 70-1	Etiologies of Constrictive Pericarditis
Idiopathic or viral	
Postsurgical (e.g., coronary artery bypass graft surgery, valvular surgery)	
Radiation therapy	
Miscellaneous causes (tuberculosis, connective tissue disease, bacterial pericarditis, Wegener granulomatosis, blunt chest trauma, neoplasm)	

Data from Bertog SC, Thambidorai SK, Parakh K, et al. Constrictive pericarditis: etiology and cause-specific survival after pericardiectomy. J Am Coll Cardiol 2004; 43:1445-1452.

seen on lateral view, where it is often located anteriorly and along the diaphragmatic surface. Bilateral pleural effusion may be present. Signs of pulmonary edema are typically absent, however.

Ultrasonography

The classic finding of constrictive pericarditis is the equalization of the end-diastolic pressure in all four cardiac chambers with early rapid diastolic filling. Paradoxical motion of the interventricular septum may also be seen. Pericardial thickening may be missed on transthoracic echocardiography, particularly if it is located in the near field, or if there is localized involvement.[4,5] Transesophageal echocardiography has been found to be more sensitive in detecting pericardial thickening compared with transthoracic echocardiography.[6] Dilation of the atria, inferior vena cava, and hepatic veins may be noted.

Computed Tomography

CT is able to document the presence of pericardial thickening or calcification or both. The pericardium normally measures 2 mm or less, and can be reliably identified only when surrounded by mediastinal and subepicardial fat. Pericardial thickening may involve most of the pericardial surface or may be localized, either unilateral or affecting the atrioventricular groove preferentially. The effect of the pericardial thickening on the cardiac chambers and mediastinal structures can also be assessed by CT. Global or unilateral pericardial thickening in the setting of constrictive pericarditis causes a tubelike narrowing of the ventricles (Fig. 70-1). If there is involvement of the pericardium covering the atrioventricular groove, waistlike narrowing can be seen. The atria and superior and inferior venae cavae may be enlarged reflecting the increased pressure limiting inflow of blood into the ventricles. The interventricular septum is often straightened or sinusoidal in appearance. Pleural effusions and ascites are frequently identified as well.

A subset of patients with constrictive physiology may have no detectable pericardial thickening yet would benefit from pericardiectomy.[7,8] In a series of 26 patients who underwent pericardiectomy despite the absence of pericardial thickening or calcification, on pathologic examination, all showed areas of either focal fibrosis or calcification.[7] In these patients without demonstrable pericardial thickening, the constrictive physiology is thought to be the result of pericardial adhesions.[5] If ECG gated images are obtained, abnormal septal motion can be evaluated. The myocardium can also be assessed for myocardial thinning because this finding has been associated with increased mortality after pericardiectomy.[9]

Magnetic Resonance Imaging

Although it cannot differentiate between calcified and thickened pericardium, MRI can be used to detect pericardial thickening and the associated cardiac deformities typically seen in patients with constrictive pericarditis (Fig. 70-2). MRI is better than CT in distinguishing small pericardial effusions from pericardial thickening. In patients who have constrictive pericarditis without associated pericardial thickening, myocardial tagging techniques

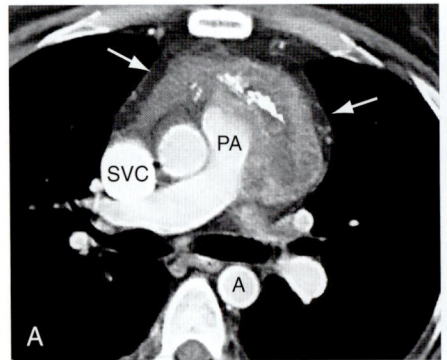

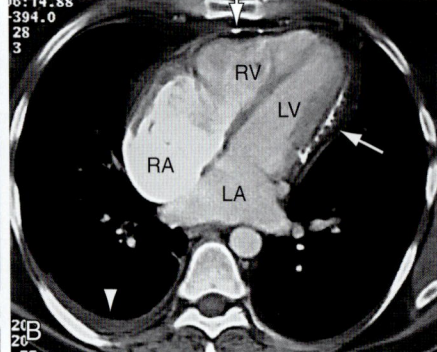

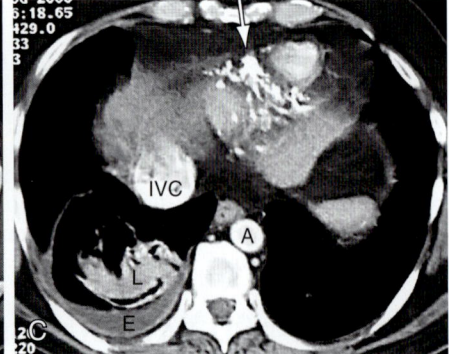

FIGURE 70-1 Contrast-enhanced CT scan of a 42-year-old man with alcoholic cirrhosis. The patient underwent a CT scan at an outside institution for symptoms of orthopnea and paroxysmal nocturnal dyspnea. **A,** CT image at the level of the pulmonary artery (PA) shows abnormal soft tissue and calcification in the pericardium. The superior vena cava (SVC) is larger than the descending aorta (A). **B,** CT image at the level of the right and left ventricles (RV and LV) shows calcification of the pericardium (*arrows*). Note the tubelike configuration of the ventricles. The right atrium (RA) is enlarged. A small right pleural effusion (*arrowhead*) is present. LA, left atrium. **C,** CT image at the inferior margin of the pericardium shows pericardial calcification (*arrow*). The inferior vena cava (IVC) is more than twice the size of the descending aorta (A). Note the pleural effusion (E) with an adjacent area of rounded atelectasis (L).

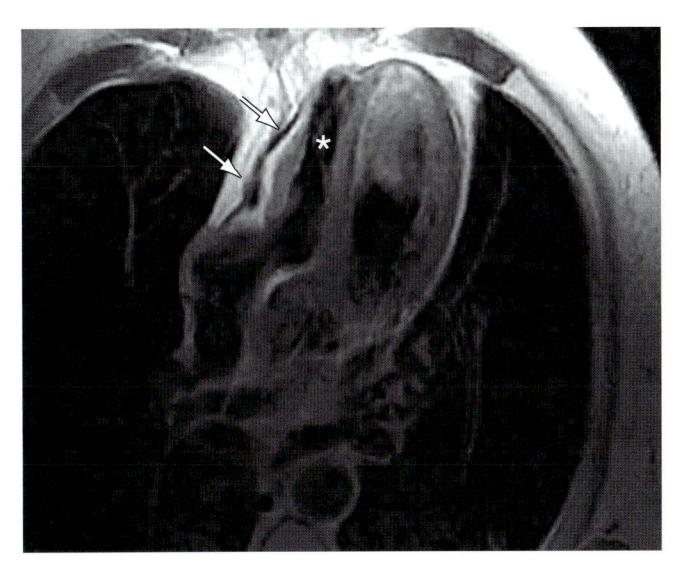

FIGURE 70-2 A 49-year-old man with a history of diabetes and status post renal transplant presented with worsening dyspnea on exertion and lower extremity edema. Double inversion recovery MR image of the heart shows abnormal pericardial thickening (*arrows*) with tubelike compression of the right ventricle (*asterisk*). Increased signal in the left ventricular apex is secondary to artifact from slow flow. The patient underwent pericardiectomy. The cause of the constrictive pericarditis was unknown.

can be used to document the lack of normal movement between the myocardium and pericardium.[10] Just as pericardial thickening can exist without constrictive pericarditis, pericardial adhesions identified with myocardial tagging can also occur in the absence of constrictive physiology. Septal motion can be evaluated using cine MRI sequences. As with echocardiography, paradoxical diastolic motion ("septal bounce") may be present.[11] The myocardium can also be assessed for myocardial thinning because this finding has been associated with increased mortality after pericardiectomy.[9]

Classic Signs

Classic signs include the following:

- Thickened or calcified pericardium
- Tubelike configuration of the ventricles
- Waistlike narrowing of the atrioventricular groove
- Atrial and caval enlargement

DIFFERENTIAL DIAGNOSIS
Clinical Presentation

Constrictive pericarditis must be distinguished from other causes of right heart failure. In patients with ascites and evidence of hepatic cirrhosis, it is important to assess for cardiac causes of cirrhosis because this may be a secondary abnormality.

Imaging Findings

Left ventricular calcification secondary to prior myocardial infarction can be distinguished from pericardial calcification based on location. On posteroanterior radiograph, left ventricular calcification is typically located at the cardiac apex. Pericardial calcification on posteroanterior radiograph is best seen in the juxtadiaphragmatic pericardium, and typically is more obvious on lateral radiograph. On lateral radiograph, pericardial calcification is typically located anteriorly and along the juxtadiaphragmatic pericardium, and is typically thicker and more irregular than calcification of the left ventricle. Calcification of the left ventricular apex is located over the mid-anterior aspect of the heart on lateral radiograph, corresponding to its anatomic location behind the right ventricle.

The physiologic changes of constrictive pericarditis identified by echocardiography can also be seen in patients with restrictive cardiomyopathy. CT and MRI are used to distinguish between constrictive pericarditis and restrictive cardiomyopathy based on the appearance of the pericardium. The presence of pericardial thickening or calcification in patients with appropriate physiologic findings confirms the diagnosis of constrictive pericarditis. Patients with constrictive pericarditis may not have pericardial thickening or calcification, yet improve after pericardiectomy. The absence of pericardial thickening does not exclude the possibility of constrictive pericarditis. In difficult cases, myocardial biopsy may be performed to exclude the diagnosis of restrictive cardiomyopathy. Pericardial calcification and thickening can also occur in the absence of constrictive pericarditis.

TREATMENT OPTIONS
Medical

Transient constrictive pericarditis can acutely follow acute pericarditis. In these cases, constrictive physiology is present on echocardiography and persists after pericardiocentesis. This constrictive physiology occurs in a relative subacute phase and differs from chronic cases of constrictive pericarditis that tend to develop some time after the initial insult. Patients who develop signs related to constrictive pericarditis shortly after being diagnosed with acute pericarditis can receive conservative medical therapy, and their symptoms may resolve. If resolution does not occur over time, pericardiectomy can be considered.[12,13]

Surgical/Interventional

For chronic cases of constrictive pericarditis, radical pericardiectomy is the preferred treatment, although the mortality rate is significant. In a series of 163 patients undergoing pericardiectomy for constrictive pericarditis, the overall mortality rate was 6.1%, although mortality was 21.4% for patients in whom the constrictive pericarditis was caused by prior radiation therapy.[14] In one series, there was a 100% mortality rate in patients with evidence of myocardial atrophy or fibrosis on CT or MRI who subsequently underwent pericardiectomy.[9]

INFORMATION FOR THE REFERRING PHYSICIAN

Cross-sectional imaging reports should include the location, distribution, and measurement of the abnormally thickened pericardium; the presence of pericardial fluid, if any; and a description of the associated alteration of the cardiac chambers and whether myocardial atrophy or fibrosis is suspected. The location of pericardial abnormality is important in determining the surgical approach.

KEY POINTS

- The diagnosis of constrictive pericarditis is based primarily on physiologic abnormalities.
- Constrictive pericarditis has been reported in the absence of appreciable thickening or calcification of the pericardium.
- Calcification and thickening of the pericardium are not pathognomonic for constrictive pericarditis, and the physiologic abnormalities must be present to confirm the diagnosis.
- The diameter of the superior vena cava is normally less than the diameter of the descending aorta. The diameter of the inferior vena cava is normally less than two times the diameter of the descending aorta.

SUGGESTED READINGS

Kim JS, Kim HH, Yoon Y. Imaging of pericardial diseases. Clin Radiol 2007; 62:626-631.

Rienmüller R, Gröll R, Lipton MJ. CT and MR imaging of pericardial disease. Radiol Clin North Am 2004; 42:587-601.

Wang ZJ, Reddy GP, Gotway MB, et al. CT and MR imaging of pericardial disease. RadioGraphics 2003; 23:S167-S180.

REFERENCES

1. Permanyer-Miralda G, Sagristá-Sauled J, Soler-Soler J. Primary acute pericardial disease: a prospective series of 231 consecutive patients. Am J Cardiol 1985; 56:623-630.
2. Sagristá-Sauled J. Pericardial constriction: uncommon patterns. Heart 2004; 90:257-258.
3. Talreja DR, Nishimura RA, Oh JK, et al. Constrictive pericarditis in the modern era: novel criteria for diagnosis in the cardiac catheterization laboratory. J Am Coll Cardiol 2008; 51:315-319.
4. Otto CM. Pericardial disease: two-dimensional echocardiographic and Doppler findings. In Otto CM (ed). Textbook of Clinical Echocardiography. Philadelphia, Saunders, 2000, pp 213-228.
5. Goldstein JA. Cardiac tamponade, constrictive pericarditis, and restrictive cardiomyopathy. Curr Probl Cardiol 2004; 29:503-567.
6. Ling LH, Oh JK, Tei C, et al. Pericardial thickness measured with transesophageal echocardiography: feasibility and potential clinical usefulness. J Am Coll Cardiol 1997; 29:1317-1323.
7. Talreja DR, Edwards WD, Danielson GK, et al. Constrictive pericarditis in 26 patients with histologically normal pericardial thickness. Circulation 2003; 108:1852-1857.
8. Oh KY, Shimzu M, Edwards WD, et al. Surgical pathology of the parietal pericardium: a study of 344 cases (1993-1999). Cardiovasc Pathol 2001; 10:157-168.
9. Rienmüller R, Gürgan M, Erdmann E, et al. CT and MR evaluation of pericardial constriction: a new diagnostic and therapeutic concept. J Thorac Imaging 1993; 8:108-121.
10. Kojima S, Yamada N, Goto Y. Diagnosis of constrictive pericarditis by tagged cine magnetic resonance imaging. N Engl J Med 1999; 341:373-374.
11. Spodick DH. Acute pericarditis: current concepts and practice. JAMA 2003; 289:1150-1153.
12. Haley JH, Tajik AJ, Danielson GK, et al. Transient constrictive pericarditis: causes and natural history. J Am Coll Cardiol 2004; 43:271-275.
13. Sagristá-Sauled J, Permanyer-Miralda G, Candell-Riera J, et al. Transient cardiac constriction: an unrecognized pattern of evolution in effusive acute idiopathic pericarditis. Am J Cardiol 1987; 59:961-966.
14. Bertog SC, Thambidorai SK, Parakh K, et al. Constrictive pericarditis: etiology and cause-specific survival after pericardiectomy. J Am Coll Cardiol 2004; 43:1445-1452.

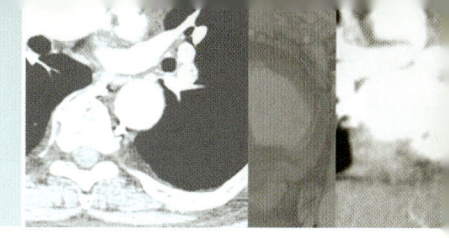

Index

A

A number, 270, 271t
Abdomen
  arterial anatomy of, 969-977. *See also named artery, e.g.*, Abdominal aorta.
  CT angiography of, 1061t, 1065-1068
    aorta in, 1065-1066, 1067f
    hepatic vasculature in, 1066, 1068f
    mesenteric vasculature in, 1066-1068, 1069f
    pancreas in, 1066, 1067f
    renal vasculature in, 1066, 1067f-1068f
  vascular disorders of, MR imaging of, 1451-1470. *See also under specific disorder.*
    gadolinium use and safety in, 1453
    methodology in, 1451
    of arteries, 1451-1452
    of veins and soft tissue, 1452-1453
  venous anatomy of
    portal circulation in, 1005-1009, 1006f-1007f
      differential considerations of, 1008-1009, 1008f, 1008t
      variants of, 1008
    systemic circulation in, 1009-1012, 1009f-1010f
      differential considerations of, 1011-1012, 1011f-1012f
      variants of, 1010-1011
Abdominal aorta, 969-976
  acute occlusion of, 1410-1411, 1411f-1413f
  anatomy of
    descriptions in, 969, 970f
    differential considerations of, 975, 976f
    normal variants in, 970-975
    pertinent imaging considerations and, 975-976
    specific areas in, 970-976
  aneurysm of. *See* Abdominal aortic aneurysm.
  aortography of, 1158-1159
  descending, 955-956
  dissection of, 1416-1417, 1416f
  imaging of
    contrast media in, 1398-1399
      dosage of, 1399
    CT angiography in, 1065-1066, 1067f
      protocol parameters for, 1061t
    CT scans in, technique of, 1397
    Doppler ultrasound in, anatomic considerations in, 1508, 1508f-1509f
    MR scans in
      coil choice for, 1398
      patient position for, 1397-1398
      pulse sequences in, 1398, 1398f
      technique of, 1397-1398
      techniques of, 1397-1398

Abdominal aorta *(Continued)*
  major branches of, 971t, 973f
  traumatic injury of, 1409-1410, 1410f
Abdominal aortic aneurysm, 1399-1404
  atherosclerotic disease causing, 1194, 1199
  clinical manifestations of, 1400
  differential diagnosis of, 1207t, 1402
  endovascular repair of, 1420, 1421f
    aneurysm sac (endoleak) after, 1426, 1428t
    clinical presentation after, 1426
    complication(s) of
      arterial dissection as, 1436
      colon necrosis as, 1435-1436
      endoleaks as, 1431-1434, 1431f-1434f
      graft infection as, 1434
      graft kinking as, 1434
      graft occlusion as, 1434-1435
      graft thrombosis as, 1434, 1434f-1436f
      hematoma at arteriotomy site as, 1436
      shower embolism as, 1435
    death during, 1426
    goal of, 1420
    graft placement in, 1422-1423, 1424f-1426f
      surgical conversion after, 1423-1424, 1427f, 1440, 1441t
    imaging of
      indications and algorithm for, 1426-1429
      techniques and findings in, 1429-1436, 1429f-1430f, 1430t
    postoperative assessment of, 1420-1436, 1423f-1428f
    postoperative management after, 1436-1437
    preprocedural interventions and, 1422-1423, 1423f
    success of, 1422
      anatomic appearance after, 1426, 1428f
    vs. open surgical repair, 1424-1426
  etiology and pathophysiology of, 1399-1400
  hybrid repair procedures in, 1181-1182, 1183f-1184f
  imaging of
    FDG-PET, 1402
    indications and algorithm for, 1400, 1400t
    MRA scan in, 1205-1206, 1401, 1402f
    radiography in, 1400, 1400f
    ultrasound in, 1400-1401, 1401f
  prevalence and epidemiology of, 1399
  rupture of, 1420
    signs of, 1401-1402, 1402f-1404f
  screening for, 1200
  surgical repair of, 1179-1180, 1211
    clinical presentation after, 1440-1441
      anastomotic pseudoaneurysms, 1441, 1447, 1449f
      postoperative management of, 1449

Abdominal aortic aneurysm *(Continued)*
      aortic graft infection, 1441, 1443-1447, 1446f-1447f
        postoperative management of, 1449
      aortocaval fistula, 1441, 1443
      aortoenteric fistula, 1441, 1445-1447, 1448f
        postoperative management of, 1447
      aortoiliac occlusive disease, 1441, 1447, 1448f
      renal infarction, 1447, 1449f
    complications of
      early postoperative, 1439-1440
      late postoperative, 1440
    contraindications to, 1180
    conversion from endovascular repair to, 1440, 1441t
    imaging after
      indications and algorithm for, 1441-1442
      techniques and findings in, 1442-1443, 1443f-1445f
    imaging findings in, 1180-1181, 1181f-1182f
    indications for, 1180
    mortality and survival after, 1440
    outcomes and complications of, 1176f, 1180
    postoperative assessment of, 1439-1447
    postoperative management of, 1447-1449
    vs. endovascular repair, 1424-1426
  treatment options for, 1402-1404
Abdominal trauma, vascular, 1468-1469, 1469f
AbiRahma criteria, in diagnosis of carotid stenosis, 1173, 1174t
Ablation procedures
  for arrhythmogenic right ventricular dysplasia, 894
  for atrial fibrillation, 445-446, 446f
  for left ventricular outflow tract obstruction, 881-882
Above-knee amputation, for chronic limb ischemia, 1583-1584
Above-knee femoropopliteal graft, patency of, 1590, 1590f
Abscess, embolization and, 1170
Acceleration index (AI), in Doppler imaging, 1045, 1513
Acceleration time (AT), in Doppler imaging, 1045, 1513
Acipimox, in ^{18}FDG imaging, 332-333
Acoustic noise, of MRI scanners, 267
Acoustic power, in Doppler ultrasonography, 1040

Acquisition protocols, for myocardial perfusion imaging with SPECT, 745-746
  dual isotope, 746
  same-day rest-stress Tc 99m radiotracer protocol, 746
  stress-redistribution thallium 201 protocol, 746
  two-day rest-stress Tc 99m radiotracer protocol, 746
Acute aortic syndrome, 1288-1305
  dissection as, 1288-1296
  intramural hematoma as, 1296-1299
  penetrating atherosclerotic ulcer as, 1299-1302
  ruptured aneurysm as, 1302-1303, 1303f
Acute coronary syndrome, 715-725
  angiography of, 722
  classic signs of, 722
  clinical presentation of, 716
  CT imaging of, 717-721, 718f-720f
    protocol parameters for, 720t
    University of Maryland triage studies in, 721t
  definition of, 715
  differential diagnosis of, 723
  etiology and pathophysiology of, 715-716
  imaging of
    indications and algorithm for, 716
    technique and findings in, 716-722
  MR imaging of, 721, 721f
  myocardial perfusion imaging of, 742
  nuclear imaging of, 722, 722f
  percutaneous coronary interventions for, 402, 723
  plaque rupture and, 61
  prevalence and epidemiology of, 715
  radiography of, 716, 717f
  reporting of, 723
  treatment options for, 723
  ultrasonography of, 716-717
Acute limb ischemia. See Limb ischemia, acute.
Acute lung injury, 1376
Acyanotic congenital heart disease. See Congenital heart disease (CHD), acyanotic.
Adaptive detector, in multislice CT, 1053-1054, 1053f
Adenocarcinoma, pancreatic. See Pancreatic adenocarcinoma.
Adenosine, 353
  chemical structure of, 284f
  in cardiac MRI stress testing, 267
  infusion of, in MR imaging, 733-734
  mechanism of action of, 354f
  perfusion imaging protocol with, 353, 355f
    contraindications to, 205, 206t
    exercise and, 357
    in PET, 316
    in SPECT, 284-285, 744-745
  side effects of, 353, 354t
Adrenal artery, 973
Adrenocortical carcinoma, inferior vena cava invasion by, 1530
Adson's maneuver, for thoracic outlet syndrome, 1669
Adult, congenital heart disease in, radiographic studies of, 89, 91f-92f
Adult respiratory distress syndrome (ARDS), 1376-1377
  causes of, 1377b
  histopathologic abnormalities in, 1376-1377
  imaging findings in
    during exudative phase, 1377-1378, 1378f
    during proliferative phase, 1378, 1378f
  stages of, 1377b

Adventitial cystic disease, 987, 1600
  imaging of, 1604, 1605f
Agatson score, 459
Age, advanced, atherosclerosis and, 1196
Air accumulation, in ischemic heart disease, 813
Air space (alveolar) edema, 1375f, 1376
Akinesia, definition of, 232
Alcohol, as embolic agent, 1168
Alcohol septal myocardial ablation, for left ventricular outflow tract obstruction, 881-882
Aliasing, in Doppler ultrasonography, 1041, 1041t
Allergy, contrast, as contraindication to CT angiography, 1614
Allograft(s), kidney
  Doppler ultrasonography of, 1519, 1519f-1520f
  segmental infarction in, 1520, 1521f
Allograft rejection
  after cardiac transplantation, 812
  aortic, 820
  diagnosis of, 818
  postoperative management of, 821-823, 822f
  renal, 1519, 1520f
Allograft renal vessels
  parameters in, normal values of, 1519b
  stenosis of, criteria for, 1519b
  thrombosis of, pitfalls in sonography of, 1513
Alpha particles, 272, 272t
Alveolar damage, diffuse
  permeability edema with, 1376-1378. See also Pulmonary edema, permeability.
  permeability edema without, 1379
Alveolar (air space) edema, 85-87, 1375f, 1376
Alveolar hemorrhage, diffuse, 1383-1384, 1391
Ambiguity, directional, in Doppler ultrasonography, 1042, 1042f
American College of Rheumatology classification, of Takayasu arteritis, 1315t
American College of Rheumatology criteria, for giant cell arteritis, 1320t
American Heart Association (AHA) recommendations, for coronary artery bypass graft surgery, 416t
Ammonia N 13
  in PET imaging
    for identifying myocardial viability, 799-800
    myocardial perfusion imaging with, 749-750
  in PET/CT imaging, 325-326, 339-340, 340f, 340t
Ampere-Maxwell law, 263
Amplatz vascular plug, as embolic agent, 1168
Amplitude, in Doppler imaging, 1043
Amputations, for chronic limb ischemia, 1583-1584
Amyloid deposits, 861
  characteristics of, 861
Amyloidosis
  clinical presentation of, 862
  definition of, 861
  etiology and pathophysiology of, 861-862
  imaging of
    echocardiographic, 115-116, 116f
    indications and algorithm for, 862
    technique and findings in, 862-864, 862f-864f, 872t
  prevalence and epidemiology of, 861
Analgesia, intravenous, for acute coronary syndrome, 723

Anastomosis
  microvascular, in coronary artery bypass graft surgery, 413, 415f-416f
  piggy-back technique of, in hepatic transplantation, 1534-1535, 1534f-1535f
Anastomotic pseudoaneurysm, 1441, 1447, 1449f
  after abdominal aortic aneurysm repair, 1180
  postoperative management of, 1449
Aneurysm
  aortic. See Aortic aneurysm.
  arterial, lower extremity. See Lower extremity aneurysm.
  bypass graft, after CABG surgery, 525
  coronary artery. See Coronary artery aneurysm.
  Doppler imaging of, 1044
  ductus, vs. patent ductus arteriosus, 590-591, 591f
  false, 1271, 1277, 1277f. See also Pseudoaneurysm.
    delayed hyperenhancement MR imaging of, 209-210
  formation of, after surgical repair of coarctation of aorta, 539-540, 540f
  iliac artery. See Iliac artery aneurysm.
  nontraumatic, vs. patent ductus arteriosus, 592-594, 594f
  popliteal artery. See Popliteal artery aneurysm.
  post–myocardial infarction, 94
  renal artery, Doppler ultrasound diagnosis of, 1515
  splanchnic artery, 1462-1463, 1463f-1464f
  true, 1271, 1277
  venous, after liver transplantation, 1551, 1554f
Aneurysm sac, opacification of, after stent graft insertion. See Endoleak(s).
Angina
  stable, 715-716
    percutaneous coronary interventions for, 402
  typical, definition of, 61-62
  unstable, percutaneous coronary interventions for, 402
Angiography, 1157-1161
  cerebral, 1159
  cine, of arrhythmogenic right ventricular dysplasia, 887, 887t
  computed tomographic. See Computed tomographic angiography (CTA).
  contraindications to, 1160
  contrast agents in, choice of, 1158
  digital subtraction. See Digital subtraction angiography (DSA).
  first-pass radionuclide, of ventricular function
    data acquisition in, 776-778, 779f
    image interpretation in, 778-779
    indications for, 775-776
  hepatic, 1159
  indications for, 1159-1160
  mesenteric, 1159
  multiple overlapping thin slab, 1094, 1094f
  of abdominal aorta, 1158-1159
  of acute coronary syndrome, 722
  of amyloidosis, 864
  of aortic aneurysm
    abdominal, 1442
    thoracic, 1282
  of aortic arch, 1158, 1158f
  of aortic dissection, 1294, 1294f
  of aortic trauma, thoracic, 1310-1311

Angiography *(Continued)*
 of arteriovenous fistula failure, 1680-1682, 1682f-1683f
 of atherosclerosis, 1206-1207, 1207f
 of atrial septal defect, 568-569
 of cardiomyopathy
  dilated, 858
  hypertrophic, 882
  siderotic, 868
 of carotid arteries, 1159
 of carotid stenosis, 1219-1220, 1219f-1220f
 of chronic thromboembolic pulmonary hypertension, 1349-1350, 1367
  differential diagnosis in, 1350, 1351f
 of coarctation of aorta, 537
  during and after repair, 373, 376f
 of cor triatriatum, 633
 of coronary arteries, 412, 413f
 of coronary atherosclerosis, 708
 of double-outlet right ventricle, 684
 of eosinophilic endomyocardial disease, 866
 of giant cell arteritis, 1321, 1322f, 1414
 of inferior vena cava anomalies, 1529
 of inferior vena cava stenosis, after hepatic transplantation, 1535, 1536f-1537f
 of inferior vena cava tumors, 1531-1532
 of intramural hematoma of aorta, 1297-1298
 of ischemic heart disease, postoperative, 815
 of limb ischemia
  acute, 1577
  chronic, 1583
 of mycotic aortic aneurysm, 1407
 of myocarditis, 899
 of patent ductus arteriosus
  postoperative, 370, 374f
  preoperative, 370, 371f-374f
 of penetrating atherosclerotic ulcer, 1300-1301
 of peripheral artery disease, 1634
 of pulmonary artery stenosis, 375-377, 377f
  postoperative, 377, 379f
 of pulmonary hypertension
  chronic thromboembolic, 1349-1350, 1367
   differential diagnosis in, 1350, 1351f
  idiopathic, 1359
  with unclear multifactorial mechanisms, 1371
 of pulmonary insufficiency, 380-381, 380f-381f
 of pulmonary venous connections
  partial anomalous, 628
  total anomalous, 636, 637f
 of renal artery stenosis, 1502f, 1505
  in transplant recipient, 1564
 of renal vasculature, in living kidney donor, 1568
 of sarcoidosis, 870-871
 of single ventricle, 677, 678f
 of subclavian steal syndrome, 1329, 1330f
 of Takayasu arteritis, 1319f, 1389-1390, 1389f, 1414
 of tetralogy of Fallot, 646-647, 662
 of transposition of great arteries, 660
 of truncus arteriosus, 666
 of upper limb, 1159, 1159f
 of upper limb medium and small vessel disease, 1651-1652, 1658f
 of ventricular septal defect, 577-579, 580f
 outcomes and complications of, 1160
 pelvic, 1159
 postprocedural surveillance after, 1161
 preprocedural planning in, 1160-1161

Angiography *(Continued)*
 pulmonary, 1159f, 1336
  contraindications to, 1337b
 renal, 1159, 1160f
 specific regions of interest in, 1158-1159, 1158f-1160f
 three-dimensional
  optimal, 1131-1133, 1134f-1135f
  simulating, 1133, 1135f
 vascular access for, 1157-1158
Angiomyolipoma, renal, 1533, 1533f
Angioplasty, 1161-1163, 1161f
 and stent placement, in lower extremity revascularization, 1591-1592, 1592f-1593f
 for mesenteric atherosclerotic disease, 1212
 for Takayasu arteritis, 1318
 imaging findings in, 1162-1163
 indications for and contraindications to, 1162, 1163f
 outcomes and complications of, 1162
 percutaneous balloon, for coarctation of aorta, 539
 percutaneous transluminal, for peripheral artery disease, 1210-1211, 1210t
 percutaneous transluminal coronary. *See* Percutaneous transluminal coronary angioplasty (PTCA).
 special considerations in, 1162
Angiosarcoma
 definition of, 925
 differential diagnosis of, 926-927
 echocardiography of, 116
 manifestations of disease in, 925-926, 926f-927f
 pathology of, 925, 926f
 prevalence of, 925
 treatment options for, 927
Angiotensin-converting enzyme (ACE) inhibitor(s)
 for cerebrovascular atherosclerotic disease, 1208
 for peripheral artery disease, 1208-1209
 radiolabeled, 805, 806f
Angiotensin-converting enzyme inhibitor (ACEI) scintigraphy, of renal arteries
 captopril administration in, 1493
 contraindications to, 1492-1493
 enalaprilat administration in, 1493
 indications for, 1492
 pitfalls and solutions in, 1494
 postprocessing of, 1494
 procedure in, 1493-1494
 protocol for
  1-day, 1493
  2-day, 1493-1494
 reporting of, 1492, 1495f
 ^{99m}Tc-DTPA in, 1494
 ^{99m}Tc-MAG3 in, 1494
 technical requirements for, 1492
Angle of correction, in Doppler ultrasonography, 1040
Angle of insonation, in Doppler ultrasonography, 1039-1040, 1040f
 plaque evaluation and, 1229-1231, 1231f
Ankle-brachial index (ABI)
 in intermittent claudication, 1580-1581
 in peripheral artery disease, 1194
 ultrasound measurement of, 1202
Anomalous origin of left coronary artery from pulmonary artery (ALCAPA), 470, 606-607
 myocardial ischemia in, 470-471
 surgical treatment for, 471

Anomalous pulmonary venous connections, 10
 partial, 625-628. *See also* Partial anomalous pulmonary venous connections (PAPVC).
 total, 634-638. *See also* Total anomalous pulmonary venous connections (TAPVC).
Antecubital vein, median, 1020
Anterior interventricular vein (AIV), 51, 54f
Anticoagulants, for inferior vena cava thrombosis, 1539
Antihypertensive agents
 for cerebrovascular atherosclerotic disease, 1208
 for peripheral artery disease, 1208-1209
Antiplatelet therapy
 for cerebrovascular atherosclerotic disease, 1208
 for ischemic stroke or transient ischemic attack, 1222
 for peripheral artery disease, 1209
 preprocedural, for carotid artery stenting, 1224
Aorta
 abdominal. *See* Abdominal aorta.
 anatomy of, 549, 556, 556f
 aneurysm of. *See* Aortic aneurysm.
 ascending, post-stenotic dilation of, 1275, 1276f
 calcification of, 89, 90f
 coarctation of. *See* Coarctation of aorta.
 descending, mild bulging of, 1273, 1275f
 dissection of. *See* Aortic dissection.
 elastic lamina of, 549, 550f
 elasticity of
  MR imaging of, 556, 557f-558f
  reduced, 550
 in Marfan syndrome, 550-551, 551f
 intramural hematoma of, 1296-1299. *See also* Intramural hematoma, aortic.
 malposition of, 18, 20f
 MR imaging of, technique and protocol in, 555-556, 555t, 556f-558f
 occlusion of, balloon catheter embolectomy for, 1578
 penetrating atherosclerotic ulcer of
  definition of, 1299
  differential diagnosis of, 1301
  etiology and pathophysiology of, 1299
  manifestations of, 1299-1301, 1299f-1301f
  prevalence and epidemiology of, 1299
  reporting of, 1302
  treatment options for, 1301-1302
 post-traumatic pseudoaneurysm of, 592, 593f
 pseudocoarctation of, 539, 539f
 thoracic
  ascending. *See* Thoracic aorta, ascending.
  descending, 955-956
 traumatic injury of, vs. patent ductus arteriosus, 592, 593f
 wall of, intrinsic abnormalities of, 549
Aortic aneurysm, 434
 abdominal. *See* Abdominal aortic aneurysm.
 ascending, 1276
 endovascular repair of, endoleaks after, 1407-1409
  etiology and pathophysiology of, 1408, 1408f, 1408t
  imaging of
   indications and algorithm for, 1408
   techniques and findings in, 1408-1409, 1409f
  prevalence and epidemiology of, 1407
  treatment options for, 1409

Aortic aneurysm *(Continued)*
  inflammatory, 1404-1406
    clinical manifestations of, 1404
    definition of, 1404
    differential diagnosis of, 1405
    etiology and pathophysiology of, 1404
    imaging of, 1405, 1405f-1406f
    prevalence and epidemiology of, 1404
    treatment options for, 1405-1406
  mycotic (infectious), 594, 594f, 1406-1407, 1407f
  rupture of
    definition of, 1302
    etiology and pathophysiology of, 1302
    manifestations of, 1302-1303, 1303f
    treatment options for, 1303
  thoracic. See Thoracic aortic aneurysm.
  thoracoabdominal
    Crawford classification of, 1176-1177, 1177f, 1276, 1277f
    repair of, 1176-1178
Aortic arch
  anatomy of, 955, 957f-958f
  anomalous position of, 960-961, 961f
  aortography of, 1158, 1158f
  defined, 955
  development of, 10-11, 12f
    pathology in, 11
  double, 11, 544, 544f-545f, 958, 959f
  embryonic development of, 957, 958f
  interruption of
    vs. coarctation of aorta, 537-538, 539f
    vs. patent ductus arteriosus, 595, 595f
  left, with aberrant right subclavian artery, 544, 546f, 959-960, 960f
  radiography of, 72-73, 73f
  right
    subtypes of, 959, 959f
    with aberrant left subclavian artery, 11, 72, 73f, 544, 545f-546f, 959, 960f
    with mirror image branching, 11
Aortic atherosclerotic disease. *See also* Atherosclerosis.
  medical treatment of, 1209
  presenting findings in, 1198t
  prevalence and epidemiology of, 1194
  surgical/interventional treatment of, 1211
Aortic balloon valvotomy, 407f, 408-409
Aortic bifurcation, lesions involving, MR angiography of, 1635-1636
Aortic border, radiography of, ascending aorta in, 75-76
Aortic bypass graft, for Takayasu arteritis, 1318-1319, 1319f
Aortic dissection, 433-434, 434f
  abdominal, 1416-1417, 1416f
  aneurysmal, 1273, 1275f
  angiography of, 1294, 1294f
  chest radiography of, 1290, 1290f
  classic signs of, 1294, 1294f-1295f
  classification of, 434, 434f, 1289, 1289f
  clinical presentation of, 1289, 1289f
  CT imaging of, 1291, 1292f-1293f
  differential diagnosis of, 1294
  echocardiography of, 117, 118f
  etiology and pathophysiology of, 1288-1289, 1289f
  imaging of, indications and algorithm for, 1289-1290
  medical treatment of, 1295
  MR imaging of, 1291-1294, 1293f
  prevalence and epidemiology of, 1288
  repair of, surveillance studies after, 420f, 437
  reporting of, 1296

Aortic dissection *(Continued)*
  risk factors for, 433-434, 434t
  surgical/interventional treatment of
    for type A (ascending) dissection, 1295
    for type B (descending) dissection, 1295-1296, 1296f
  ultrasonography of, 1290-1291, 1290f
Aortic graft infection, 1441, 1443-1447, 1446f-1447f
  postoperative management of, 1449
Aortic isthmus
  other vascular entities at, vs. patent ductus arteriosus, 588-595, 590f
  traumatic injury to, 1306, 1308f
Aortic neck dilation, after abdominal aortic aneurysm repair, 1440
Aortic root
  anatomy of, 955, 956f
  dilation and regurgitation of, in tetralogy of Fallot, 641
Aortic root–to–right heart shunt, in acyanotic congenital heart disease, 384, 385t
Aortic sac, 3-4
Aortic spindle, vs. patent ductus arteriosus, 588, 590f
Aortic valve
  anatomy of, 35-36, 36f, 417, 417f
  bicuspid, 7
    MR imaging of, 66f, 552, 552f
    pathophysiology of, 551-552
    prevalence and epidemiology of, 551
  calcifications in, 87, 88f
    patterns of, 87
  prosthetic
    mechanical bileaflet, 420, 420f
    tissue, 420, 421f
      advantage of, 421
  replacement of, 418-419, 418f-419f
  velocity-encoded MR imaging of, 556
Aortic valve disease, surgery for, 417-422
  anatomic considerations in, 417-419, 417f-419f
  contraindications to, 420
  indications for, 419-420, 419t-420t
  outcomes and complications of, 418f, 420-421, 420f-421f
  postoperative surveillance after, 416
  preoperative imaging in, 421-422, 422f-423f
Aortic valve insufficiency
  severity of, classification of, 419t
  surgical intervention for, 389
Aortic valve regurgitation
  after arterial switch operation, 555
  clinical presentation of, 832
  definition of, 831
  etiology of, 831-832
  imaging of
    echocardiographic, 110, 832-833
    indications for, 832
    radiographic, 92-93
    techniques of, 832-833, 832f-833f
  medical treatment of, 833
  pathophysiology of, 418, 831-832
  prevalence of, 831
  quantification of, 241, 243f
  surgical treatment of, 833-834
    indications for, 420t
Aortic valve stenosis, 65
  catheter-based intervention for, 389
  clinical presentation of, 827-828
  critical, vs. coarctation of aorta, 538-539
  definition of, 827
  etiology of, 827

Aortic valve stenosis *(Continued)*
  imaging of
    echocardiographic, 109, 828
    indications for, 828
    radiographic, 92
    techniques of, 828-829, 828f-831f
  medical treatment of, 830
  pathophysiology of, 417-418, 827
  prevalence of, 827
  severity of, classification of, 419t
  surgical treatment of, 830, 832f. *See also* Prosthetic aortic valve.
    indications for, 419t
    success of, 421, 422f
Aorticopulmonary window, 72-73
Aortitis, 1314-1325. *See also* Giant cell arteritis; Takayasu arteritis.
  classification of, 1314, 1315t
  infected, 1275
  syphilitic, 1322-1324, 1322t, 1323f
  thoracic, differential diagnosis of, 1323-1324, 1324f
Aortobifemoral bypass, 1182
  contraindications to, 1182-1184
  imaging findings in, 1184-1185, 1184f-1185f
  indications for, 1182
  outcomes and complications of, 1184
Aortocaval fistula, 1441, 1443
Aortoduodenal fistula, after abdominal aortic aneurysm repair, 1180
Aortoenteric fistula, 1415-1416, 1416f, 1441, 1445-1447, 1448f
  postoperative management of, 1447
Aortography
  abdominal, 1158-1159
  arch, 1158, 1158f
Aortoiliac occlusive disease, 1441, 1447, 1448f
  hybrid procedures for, 1188-1189, 1188f
Aortoplasty, for aortic coarctation, 539
Aortopulmonary window, vs. patent ductus arteriosus, 588
Aortopulmonary-level shunt, in acyanotic congenital heart disease, 384, 385t
Apical thinning, myocardial perfusion imaging and, 748
Apolipoprotein E *(APOE)* gene, lipid abnormalities associated with, 1196
Apoptosis, 792
  targeting, 805
Arc of Buehler, 975
Arc of Riolan, 975, 976f
Arcuate artery, Doppler ultrasonography of, anatomic considerations in, 1507
Area-length method, of global left ventricular function, 231
Arrhythmias. *See also specific arrhythmia.*
  in arrhythmogenic right ventricular dysplasia, 885-886
Arrhythmogenic right ventricular cardiomyopathy (ARVC), 113, 237, 237f
Arrhythmogenic right ventricular dysplasia (ARVD), 884-895
  chest radiography of, 887
  cine angiography of, 887, 887t
  clinical presentation of, 885-892, 888f-889f
  CT imaging of, 888, 888f
  definition of, 884
  diagnosis of, 886, 886t
  differential diagnosis of, 890f, 892-893, 892t
  echocardiographic evaluation of, 113, 887-888, 888t
  electrocardiographic evaluation of, 886-887, 887t
  etiology and pathophysiology of, 884-885, 885f

Arrhythmogenic right ventricular dysplasia (ARVD) *(Continued)*
  future directions for, 894
  genetics of, 885, 885t
  MR imaging of, 888-892, 889f-892f, 891t
  nuclear ventriculoscintigraphy of, 887
  patterns of disease in, 884
  prevalence and epidemiology of, 884
  reporting of, 894
  treatment options for, 893-894
Arterial dynamics, contrast media–enhanced, 160-161, 160f
  basic rules of, 161
Arterial embolic occlusion. *See also* Embolus (embolism).
  site of, in acute limb ischemia, 1574-1575, 1574f
Arterial mapping, left, contrast media injection protocol for, 164t-165t
Arterial stenosis, Doppler imaging of, 1044
Arterial switch procedure
  aortic regurgitation after, 555
  for transposition of great arteries, 554-555, 608, 608f-609f
    cardiac-gated CTA after, 612, 612f
    surgical outcome of, 608-609, 609f
Arterial thrombosis. *See* Thrombosis, arterial.
Arteriography. *See* Angiography.
Arterioles, pulmonary, 1353
Arterioportal shunting, MR imaging of, 1455-1456, 1456f
Arteriotomy site, hematoma at, after endovascular aneurysm repair, 1436
Arteriovenous fistula, 1600-1601, 1601f, 1672-1685
  after renal transplantation, 1520-1521, 1521f
  dysfunction of
    classic signs in, 1682
    differential diagnosis of, 1683
    treatment options for, 1683
  in hemodialysis patient
    creation of, 1672, 1673f
    role of imaging of, 1673
    use of, 1672-1673
    vascular evaluation of
      angiography in, 1680-1682, 1682f-1683f
      CT angiography in, 1676-1677, 1677f-1678f
      indications and algorithm for, 1674
      MR angiography in, 1677-1680, 1679f-1681f
      ultrasound in, 1675-1676, 1675f
  in renal transplant recipient, 1520-1521, 1521f
  vascular evaluation of, 1564-1566
    clinical presentation of, 1565
    etiology and pathophysiology of, 1564-1565
    imaging of
      indications and algorithm for, 1565
      technique and findings in, 1565, 1565f-1566f
    prevalence and epidemiology of, 1564
    treatment options for, 1565-1566, 1566f
  involving carotid arteries, Doppler imaging of, 1244, 1246f
  management of, 1601
    endovascular exclusion procedures in, 1603
Arteriovenous graft, 1672
Arteriovenous malformations
  hepatic, 1468
  splenic, 1468
Arteriovenous shunts, Doppler imaging of, 1044

Arteritis
  giant cell. *See* Giant cell arteritis.
  Takayasu. *See* Takayasu arteritis.
Artery(ies). *See named artery.*
Artifact(s). *See also specific artifact.*
  in cardiac CT imaging, 147, 147f-148f
  in coronary CT angiography, 495-500, 495t, 496f
  in Doppler ultrasonography, 1041-1043, 1041t
Aspirin
  for acute coronary syndrome, 723
  for cerebrovascular atherosclerotic disease, 1208
  for ischemic stroke or transient ischemic attack, 1222
  preprocedural, for carotid artery stenting, 1224
Asplenia complex, 18
ASTRAL trial, 1480
Asymmetric septal hypertrophy, in cardiomyopathy, MR imaging of, 875, 876f-877f
Asymptomatic Carotid Atherosclerosis Study (ACST), 1172, 1210
Atherectomy, 1156-1157, 1167
  devices for, 1156-1157
  in lower extremity revascularization, 1592, 1593f-1594f
  percutaneous transluminal coronary rotational, 400, 401f
Atheroembolus, 1575. *See also* Embolus (embolism).
Atheroma, 705
  thin cap, and vulnerable plaque, 706
Atherosclerosis
  aortic, 1194
    medical treatment of, 1209
    presenting findings in, 1198t
    prevalence and epidemiology of, 1194
    surgical/interventional treatment of, 1211
  cerebrovascular, 1194
    medical treatment of, 1208
    surgical/interventional treatment of, 1210
  clinical presentation of, 1198-1199, 1198t
  coronary, 59-62, 60f-61f. *See also* Coronary artery disease (CAD), atherosclerotic.
    calcium associated with, 457. *See also* Coronary artery calcium (CAC).
  definition of, 1193
  differential diagnosis of, 1207-1208, 1207t
  etiology and pathophysiology of, 1195-1196
  extracellular matrix formation in, 1195
  fibrous cap in, 1195, 1196f
  Glagov phenomenon in, 1195, 1195f
  imaging of
    angiographic, 1206-1207, 1207f
    CT angiography of, 1203-1204, 1203f
    indications and algorithm for, 1199-1200, 1200f
    MR angiography of, 1204-1206, 1205f
    PET scan, 1206
    radiographic, 1201
    technique and findings in, 1201-1207, 1201t
    ultrasound, 1201-1203, 1202f
  injury hypothesis of, response to, 1195
  mesenteric, 1194
    medical treatment of, 1210
    surgical/interventional treatment of, 1212
  oxidation hypothesis of, 1195
  peripheral, 1194. *See also* Peripheral arterial disease.

Atherosclerosis *(Continued)*
    medical treatment of, 1208-1209
    surgical/interventional treatment of, 1210-1211, 1210t
  physical examination of, 1199
  plaque in. *See* Plaque, atherosclerotic.
  prevalence and epidemiology of, 1193-1194
  primary stages of, 1195
  progression of, to clinical significance, 1195-1196, 1195f-1196f
  renal. *See* Renal atherosclerotic disease.
  reporting of, 1212
  risk factors for, 1196-1198, 1197t
    modifiable, 1196-1198, 1197f
    non-modifiable, 1196
    novel, 1198
  thoracic aortic aneurysm caused by, 1271, 1272f
  treatment options for
    medical, 1208-1210
    surgical/interventional, 1210-1212, 1210t
  vascular biology of, 60-61, 60f-61f
Atherosclerotic ulcer, penetrating
  definition of, 1299
  differential diagnosis of, 1301
  etiology and pathophysiology of, 1299
  manifestations of, 1299-1301, 1299f-1301f
  prevalence and epidemiology of, 1299
  reporting of, 1302
  treatment options for, 1301-1302
Atoll sign, in Wegener's granulomatosis, 1385, 1386f
Atom, structure of, 270, 271f
Atresia, premature, of pulmonary vein, 1001-1002
Atrial amyloidosis, isolated, 861. *See also* Amyloidosis.
Atrial baffle leak, after atrial switch procedure, 612
Atrial border, left, radiography of, 74, 74f-75f
  in lateral projection, 77
Atrial fibrillation
  clinical presentation of, 443
  clinically relevant anatomy in, 443-444, 443f-445f
  definition of, 442
  epidemiology of, 442
  lone, 442
  pathophysiology of, 442-443
  prevalence of, 442
  reporting of, 451-452
  treatment of, 444-451
    ablation procedure in, 445-446, 446f
    imaging techniques in, 446-450
      image fusion, 449-450, 450f
      MRI scans, 449, 450f
      multidetector CT, 447-449, 447f-449f
    postprocedural imaging after, 450-451
      atrioesophageal fistula in, 451, 451f
      pulmonary venous stenosis in, 450-451, 451f
      recurrent atrial fibrillation in, 451
    Wolf mini-Maze procedure in, 445, 446f
Atrial isthmus, left, implication of, in recurrent atrial fibrillation, 451
Atrial kick, 57, 59
Atrial myxoma, 906. *See also* Myxoma.
Atrial septal defect (ASD), 363-366
  angiography of, 568-569
  clinical presentation of, 564
  considerations regarding, 383, 385t
  coronary sinus, 563, 567f
  CT imaging of, 566, 568f
  definition of, 563

Atrial septal defect (ASD) (Continued)
  device closure for, 363
    contraindications to, 363-364
    indications for, 363
    outcomes and complications of, 364
    postoperative surveillance after, 365-366, 367f-368f
    preoperative imaging and, 364-365, 364f-366f
  differential diagnosis of, 570
  etiology and pathophysiology of, 563-564
  imaging of
    indications and algorithm for, 564
    technique and findings in, 564-569
  medical treatment of, 570
  MR imaging of, 566-567, 568f-569f
  nuclear imaging of, 567-568, 569f
  ostium primum, 8, 563, 566f
  ostium secundum, 8, 363, 563-564
    radiography of, 90, 91f
  prevalence and epidemiology of, 563
  radiography of, 564-565, 565f-566f
  reporting of, 570
  sinus venosus, 563, 567f
  surgical/interventional treatment of, 570
  types of, 563
  ultrasonography of, 117-118, 565-566, 566f-567f
  vs. partial anomalous pulmonary venous connections, 628
Atrial septum
  anatomy of, 33
  anomalies associated with, evaluation of, 24, 26f
  developmental pathology of, 8
  formation of, 7-8, 9f
Atrial situs ambiguous, 16, 17f
Atrial switch procedure
  atrial baffle leak after, 612
  for transposition of great arteries, 389, 609-610, 609f-610f
  imaging after, 612
Atrial tumors
  left, 432, 433f
  right, 432, 433f
Atrial-level shunt, in acyanotic congenital heart disease, 383, 385t
Atrioesophageal fistula, after ablation for atrial fibrillation, 451, 451f
Atrioventricular canal, developmental pathology of, 5
Atrioventricular connection(s)
  biventricular, types of, 19-20, 22f
  twisted, 20, 24f
  univentricular, 119, 119f
    types of, 20, 23f
Atrioventricular groove, 39-40, 40f
Atrioventricular junction
  first connecting segment of, 19-20, 22f-24f
  second connecting segment of, 22-24, 25f
Atrioventricular node
  abnormal development in, congenitally corrected transposition of great arteries, 606
  in cardiac electrophysiology, 57
Atrioventricular septal defect
  multiple-level shunts in, 386
  surgical treatment of, 386, 387f
Atrioventricular sulcus, 3-4
Atrium (atria). See also Atrial entries.
  identification of, 13-14, 14f
  left
    accessory appendage of, 32-33, 32f, 443, 443f. See also Left atrial appendage.

Atrium (atria) (Continued)
  anatomy of, 32-33, 32f, 443-444, 443f
  diastolic filling patterns in, 103, 106f
  echocardiographic imaging of, 103, 104f-105f
  formation of, 10, 11f
  morphologic, features of, 14, 14f
  oblique vein of, 53-55
  venous component of, 443-444, 444f-445f
  vestibular component of, 443
  primitive, paired, 3-4
  right
    anatomy of, 30-31, 32f
    formation of, 8-10, 10f
    morphologic, features of, 13-14, 14f
  third, 632. See also Cor triatriatum.
Attenuation, in photon-matter interactions, 276
Attenuation correction, in PET imaging, 308
  protocols for, 311-312
  placement of, 312
Attenuation event, in PET imaging, 306, 306f-307f
Attenuation maps, in PET imaging, and conversion to CT images, 308-309, 309f
Attenuation mismatch, in PET imaging, 309-311
  patient motion causing, 309, 310f
  respiratory and contractile cardiac motion causing, 309-310, 311f
  thoracic cavity drift causing, 310-311, 311f
Auger electron, 271-272, 272f
Autocorrelation, in Doppler ultrasonography, 1035-1036
Autonomic innervation, targeting, 805-807, 806f
Autoregulation, of coronary blood flow, 352
Autosomal dilated cardiomyopathy, 851-852. See also Cardiomyopathy, dilated.
Autosomal dominant inheritance, of arrhythmogenic right ventricular dysplasia, 884-885, 885t
Autosomal dominant myxoma, 905. See also Myxoma.
Autosomal recessive inheritance, of arrhythmogenic right ventricular dysplasia, 884-885, 885t
Axial images
  in cardiac CT imaging, 168-169
  in coronary CT angiography, 500
  in phase contrast MR angiography, 1096, 1097f
Axial resolution, in CT angiography, 1056
Axillary artery, 989-990, 990f
Axillary vein, 1661, 1662f
Axillary-femoral bypass graft, 981-982, 982f
Axillofemoral bypass graft, 1586-1588, 1587f
Azygos vein
  anatomy of, 1000, 1000f-1001f
  variations in, 1000, 1002f
  continuation of, in inferior vena cava anomaly, 1525, 1526f
  radiography of, 76-77

B

Back pain, postoperative new-onset, ischemic heart disease and, 813
Balloon(s)
  as embolic agent, 1168
  compliant and noncompliant, 1156
  in percutaneous vascular interventions, 1156

Balloon angioplasty
  cryoplasty, 1156
  cutting, 1156
  in lower extremity revascularization, 1593
  percutaneous, for coarctation of aorta, 539
Balloon catheter embolectomy, for saddle embolus, 1578
Balloon dilation, for pulmonary artery stenosis, 375. See also Pulmonary artery stenosis, balloon dilation for.
Balloon pump placement, intra-aortic, carotid Doppler waveform pattern after, 1244-1245, 1247f
Balloon thrombectomy, for iliac occlusion, 1578, 1578f
Balloon valvotomy
  aortic, 407f, 408-409, 830
  mitral, 407f, 408, 836
  pulmonic, 408f, 409
Balloon valvuloplasty, mitral, percutaneous, 427, 428t
Balloon-mounted stents, 1157
Banding artifacts, in CT angiography, 1070
Bare metal stent, 515, 516f
  risk of thrombosis in, 516, 517f
Baseline shift, in Doppler ultrasonography, 1041
Basilic vein, in upper extremity, 1020-1022, 1021f-1022f
Bat-wing appearance, of pulmonary edema, 86
Beak sign, in type B aortic dissection, 1294, 1294f
Beam(s), ultrasound, 1033, 1034f
Beam filtration, increased, to reduce radiation in CT imaging, 153-154
Beam hardening artifacts, in coronary CT angiography, 495-496, 495t, 496f
Beam pitch, increased, to reduce radiation in CT imaging, 153
Beam-hardening artifact, in CT angiography, 1070
Beer's law, 1047
Behçet syndrome, 1387, 1388f
Below-knee amputation, for chronic limb ischemia, 1583-1584
Below-knee femoropopliteal graft, patency of, 1590, 1590t
Bernoulli equation, modified, estimation of pressure gradients by, 99, 240, 241f
Beta particle emission, 272, 272t, 273f
Beta-blockers
  for aortic dissection, 1295
  for peripheral artery disease, 1208-1209
  used in cardiac imaging, 156
    contraindications to, 158t
    effects mediated by, 157t
    protocols for, 143-144, 156-157, 158t
B-flow image, in ultrasonography, 1034, 1037
Bidirectional superior cavopulmonary connection (BSCC), in single ventricle repair, 671-672
  MR imaging after, 674-675
Bile duct injury, 1468
Binding energy, 271
Bipolar gradients, in phase contrast MR angiography, 1095, 1096f
Black blood imaging, 1099-1100, 1100f
  of cardiac anatomy, 182-184
    acquisition parameters in, 183-184, 184f
    blood suppression achievement in, 183, 183f
Blalock-Taussig shunt
  for decreased pulmonary blood flow, 391
  modified, for tetralogy of Fallot, 648

Bleed localization scan, GI. *See*
  Gastrointestinal bleed localization scan.
Bleeding. *See* Hemorrhage.
Blood flow
  in Doppler imaging
    quantification of, 1045
    turbulent, 1043, 1043t
  MR evaluation of, 239-250
    flow-encoding axes in, 239-240, 241f
    indications for, 240
    limitations and pitfalls in, 240, 242f
    phase contrast imaging in, 239-240, 240f
    technical requirements for, 239-240, 240f-242f
    techniques for, 240-249
      in coarctation of aorta, 242-243, 244f
      in pulmonary flow evaluation, 244-249, 246f-248f
      in shunting, 243-244, 245f
      in valvular heart disease, 241-242, 243f
    velocity encoding in, 240, 242f
  pulmonary, anatomy and physiology of, 1353
Blood vessels. *See also named artery or vein.*
  in three-dimensional image
    automated extraction of, 1129
    automated pathline detection of, 1135-1136, 1136f
    validation of, 1136, 1136t
    bifurcation of, projection overlap in, 1133, 1135f
    lumen analysis of, 1134
    presegmentation of, 1129, 1130f
    segmentation of, 1131-1132, 1133f
      lumen, 1136-1137, 1137f-1138f
      validation of, 1137, 1139f, 1139t
    stenosis of, quantification of, 1131
    wall morphology of, assessment of, 1137-1138, 1139f-1140f
  wall of
    CT angiography of, 488-489, 489f-490f
    layers of, 60, 60f
Blooming artifact
  in coronary CT angiography, 495t, 496, 496f-497f
  in Doppler evaluation of plaque, 1228-1229, 1230f
Blunt trauma
  aortic, 1306, 1307f. *See also* Thoracic aortic trauma.
    acute injury due to, 592, 593f
    with deceleration mechanism injury, 1273
  upper extremity, 1644
Blurring artifacts, in coronary CT angiography, 495t, 496-499, 498f-499f
B-mode ultrasonography, 1034. *See also* Ultrasonography.
  image in, 1034, 1037
Bohr atom, 270, 271f
Bolus
  in contrast-enhanced CT angiography
    testing of, 1059-1060, 1062, 1399
    tracking of, 1058-1060, 1062
  in contrast-enhanced MR angiography, timing of, 1086-1087, 1088f, 1399
Bolus-triggering technique, of contrast media injection, 161-162, 1399
Bony pelvis. *See also* Pelvis.
  venous origin outside, 1012, 1013f-1014f
Bovine arch, 957, 958f
Bovine jugular venous valve, in pulmonary insufficiency repair, 379, 379f
Bovine xenograft, in vascular bypass surgery, 1586, 1587f

Brachial artery
  anatomy of
    normal, 991-994, 992f-993f
    variants of, 994
  angiographic access via, 1158
Brachial artery reactivity testing, 1202
Brachial vein, anatomy of, 1023, 1023f, 1661, 1662f
Brachiocephalic vein, anatomy of, 1023, 1023f, 1661, 1662f
  variant, 999
Brain perfusion tomography
  image interpretation of, 1149-1150, 1150f
  indications and contraindications to, 1148, 1149f
  pitfalls and solutions in, 1148-1149
Breath-hold technique
  used in cardiac CT imaging, 144
  used in MR imaging, 1398, 1398f
    cardiac, 202
Breathing, sleep-disordered, 1365-1366
Bremsstrahlung, 274-275
Bronchial artery, 965
Brugada syndrome, vs. arrhythmogenic right ventricular dysplasia, 893
Bruit, in carotid stenosis, 1218-1219
Budd-Chiari syndrome, 1011, 1011f, 1529
  clinical presentation of, 1461
  definition of, 1461
  differential diagnosis of, 1462
  etiology and pathophysiology of, 1461
  MR imaging of, 1461, 1462f
  treatment options for, 1462
Buerger disease (thromboangiitis obliterans), 1645, 1651-1652, 1658f. *See also* Upper extremity, medium and small vessel disease of.
  etiology and pathophysiology of, 1646
  incidence of, 1646
Bulboventricular looping, of primitive heart tube, 4, 5f
Bulbus cordis, 3-4
Bundle of His, in cardiac electrophysiology, 57-58
Butterfly appearance, of pulmonary edema, 86
N-Butyl cyanoacrylate, as embolic agent, 1168
Bypass graft(s)
  aneurysm of, after CABG surgery, 525
  arterial, 981-982. *See also specific bypass graft, e.g.,* Coronary artery bypass graft (CABG) *entries.*
  choice of conduit for, 522
  extra-anatomic, in vascular bypass surgery, 1586-1588, 1587f-1589f
  thrombosis and occlusion of, after CABG surgery, 524-525, 527f-529f
  thrombosis of, 1573

C

^{11}C-acetate, in PET imaging, 343-344
Cadaveric hepatic transplantation. *See also* Hepatic transplantation.
  surgical anatomy of, 1546-1547, 1547f
Calcification(s)
  aortic aneurysm, 1279
  atherosclerosis associated with, 60-61, 457, 707. *See also* Plaque, atherosclerotic.
  coronary. *See* Coronary artery calcium (CAC).
  femoral artery, 1188, 1188f
  great vessel, 89, 90f

Calcification(s) *(Continued)*
  heavy, in coronary CT angiography, 479-481, 483f-484f
  myocardial, 87, 87f
  pericardial, 82, 82f
  valvular, 87, 88f
Calcified amorphous cardiac tumor, 919-920, 919f-920f
Calcified stenosis, angioplasty and, 1162
Calcium channel blockers, used in cardiac imaging, 157, 158t
  contraindications to, 158t
Camera
  gamma
    components of, 276, 276f
    used in SPECT, 739
  PET, 304-305
Cancer. *See at anatomic site; specific neoplasm.*
Captopril, oral administration of, in ACEI renal scintigraphy, 1493
^{15}O-Carbon monoxide, 340
Cardiac. *See also* Heart *entries.*
Cardiac amyloidosis. *See* Amyloidosis.
Cardiac anomalies. *See specific anomaly.*
Cardiac catheterization
  for hypertrophic cardiomyopathy, 882
  in diagnosis and treatment of heart defects, 383
  standard projection views for, 416t
Cardiac cycle, abnormal Doppler waveform patterns involving, 1242-1245
  arteriovenous fistula, 1244, 1246f
  carotid dissection, 1243, 1245f
  carotid pseudoaneurysm, 1243, 1246f
  intra-aortic balloon pump, 1244-1245, 1247f
Cardiac devices, as MRI safety issue, 264-266
Cardiac electrophysiology, 57-58, 58f
Cardiac embryology, 3-25, 4f-27f. *See also specific components of heart.*
Cardiac events, coronary artery calcium as predictor of, 461-462
Cardiac function analysis, in hypertrophic cardiomyopathy, MR imaging of, 876-877, 879f-880f
Cardiac myocytes. *See* Myocytes.
Cardiac pacemakers, as MRI safety issue, 264-265
Cardiac resynchronization therapy (CRT), for dilated cardiomyopathy, 858
Cardiac rupture, post-myocardial, 94
Cardiac sarcoidosis. *See* Sarcoidosis.
Cardiac segment(s), major
  first: visceroatrial situs, 16-18, 17f-19f
  second: ventricular loop, 18, 19f
  third: great arterial relationship, 18, 20f
  analysis of, 16-18
  identification of, 13-16
Cardiac surgery, coronary CT angiography in, 486-487, 488f
Cardiac tamponade. *See* Tamponade.
Cardiac tumors, 905-937
  benign, 905-920. *See also named tumor, e.g.,* Myxoma.
  differential diagnosis of, 935t
  in hypertrophic cardiomyopathy, MR imaging of, 876, 878f
  malignant, 920-934. *See also named tumor, e.g.,* Angiosarcoma.
  metastatic, 921-922
  summary of, 934-935
Cardiac vein(s)
  anatomy of, 36
  anterior, 55
  great, 51-52, 54f

Cardiac vein(s) (Continued)
    middle, 52-53, 54f
    small, 53, 54f
Cardiac wall motion
    abnormalities of, 216-217
        during dobutamine infusion, 218, 220f
    MR assessment of, 188-190, 189f-190f
Cardiac wall thickness, end-diastolic, 782
Cardiomegaly
    in Ebstein anomaly, 653, 654f
    with decreased pulmonary vascularity, 651-653, 652f
Cardiomyopathy
    arrhythmogenic right ventricular, 237, 237f
    dilated
        clinical presentation of, 852
        definition of, 851
        differential diagnosis of, 858
        etiology and pathophysiology of, 851-852
        imaging of
            angiographic, 858
            CT scans in, 853-855, 854f
            indications and algorithm for, 852
            MR scans in, 855-857, 856f-857f
            nuclear medicine, 857-858, 857f
            radiographic, 852
            ultrasound, 110, 852-853, 853f
        medical treatment of, 858
        prevalence and epidemiology of, 851
        reporting of, 859
        surgical/interventional treatment of, 858
        vs. arrhythmogenic right ventricular dysplasia, 893
    hypertrophic, 63, 874-883
        asymmetric septal, MR imaging of, 875, 876f-877f
        cardiac function analysis in, MR imaging of, 876-877, 879f-880f
        cardiac neoplasms in, MR imaging of, 876, 878f
        clinical presentation of, 874
        coronary reserve flow in, MR imaging of, 879
        etiology and pathophysiology of, 874
        imaging of
            angiographic, 882
            CT, 874-875, 875f
            MRI scans in, 875-882
                morphology in, 875-876, 875t, 876f-878f
            radiographic, 94
            ultrasound, 110-113, 874
        impaired myocardial perfusion in, MR imaging of, 877
        left ventricular outflow tract obstruction in
            MR imaging of, 879-882, 881f
            treatment of, 881-882
        myocardial viability in, MR imaging of, 877-879, 880f
        prevalence and epidemiology of, 874
        surgical/interventional treatment of, 882
        ventricular mass in, MR imaging of, 875-876, 878f
    ischemic, 62
    noncompaction, echocardiography of, 113, 114f-115f
    restrictive, 861
        additional causes of, 871
        amyloidosis associated with, 861-864
        differential diagnosis of, 871
        eosinophilic endomyocardial disease associated with, 864-866

Cardiomyopathy (Continued)
        imaging features of, 872t
            echocardiographic, 113
            radiographic, 94
        reporting of, 871
        sarcoidosis associated with, 868-871
        treatment options for, 871
    siderotic
        clinical presentation of, 867
        definition of, 866
        etiology and pathophysiology of, 866-867
        imaging of
            indications and algorithm for, 867
            technique and findings in, 867-868, 868f, 872t
        medical treatment of, 871
        prevalence and epidemiology of, 866
    tako-tsubo, 107
Cardiopulmonary bypass, in coronary artery bypass graft surgery, 412-413, 414f
Cardiovascular disease, syphilitic manifestations in, 1322t
Cardioverter-defibrillators, implantable
    as MRI safety issue, 264-265
    as PET image artifact, 321-322, 322f
    for arrhythmogenic right ventricular dysplasia, 894
Carney complex, 905
Carotid artery
    anatomy of, 961-963, 961f-963f
        variations in, 962-963, 963f-964f
    angiography of, 1159
    bifurcation of, 961-962, 961f
        disease at, risk factors for, 1227
        variability of, 962
    common
        division of, 961
        normal Doppler tracing of, 1231-1232, 1232f. See also Doppler ultrasonography, of carotid arteries.
    CT angiography of, 1060, 1062f, 1260-1267. See also Computed tomographic angiography (CTA), carotid.
        protocol parameters for, 1061t
    dissection of, 1242-1243
        CT angiography of, 1262, 1263f
        Doppler imaging of, 1243, 1245f
    external, 961, 961f-962f
        normal Doppler tracing of, 1231-1232, 1232f. See also Doppler ultrasonography, of carotid arteries.
        variations of, 963, 963f
        vs. internal carotid artery, 1232, 1233f
    internal, 961-962, 961f-962f
        normal Doppler tracing of, 1231-1232, 1232f. See also Doppler ultrasonography, of carotid arteries.
        stenosis of. See also Carotid artery stenosis.
            caliper measurements of
                direct, 1258, 1259f
                multiplanar reformations in, 1258, 1259f
            grading of, 1227, 1228f, 1233, 1234f-1235f
            in contralateral side, 1236-1237, 1238f
            measuring and reporting of, 1258-1259
            vs. external carotid artery, 1232, 1233f
        MR angiography of, 1252-1259. See also Magnetic resonance angiography (MRA), contrast-enhanced, of carotid arteries.

Carotid artery (Continued)
    occlusive disease of, 1217-1226. See also Carotid artery stenosis.
    pseudoaneurysm of, Doppler imaging of, 1243, 1246f
    stenting of, status and patency in, CT angiographic evaluation of, 1261-1262, 1262f
    tortuous, peak systolic velocity in, 1235, 1236f
    ulceration of, CTA detection of, 1266-1267
    ultrasound evaluation of, 1227-1250. See also Doppler ultrasonography, of carotid arteries.
Carotid artery stenosis, 1217-1225. See also Stroke.
    asymptomatic, treatment of, 1222
    clinical presentation of, 1218-1219
    definition of, 1217
    differential diagnosis of, 1221
    etiology of, 1218
    imaging of
        angiographic, 1219-1220, 1219f-1220f
        CT angiography in, 1220
        indications and algorithm for, 1219
        MR angiography in, 1220
        ultrasound, 1220, 1220f
    internal
        caliper measurements of
            direct, 1258, 1259f
            multiplanar reformations in, 1258, 1259f
        grading of, 1227, 1228f, 1233, 1234f-1235f
        in contralateral side, 1236-1237, 1238f
        measuring and reporting of, 1258-1259
    pathophysiology of, 1218, 1218f
    plaque in, morphology of, 1220-1221, 1221f
    prevalence and epidemiology of, 1217-1218
    reporting of, 1224-1225
    symptomatic, treatment of, 1222
    treatment option(s) for
        carotid artery stenting as, 1222-1224
            procedure for, 1224, 1224f
        carotid endarterectomy as, 1222, 1223f. See also Carotid endarterectomy.
        current indications in, 1224
        for asymptomatic carotid stenosis, 1222
        for symptomatic carotid stenosis, 1222
        medical, 1222
        synopsis of, 1221-1224
Carotid artery stenting, 1222-1224
    procedure for, 1224, 1224f
    recommendations for, 1224
    status and patency in, CT angiographic evaluation of, 1261-1262, 1262f
Carotid coils, dedicated, in contrast-enhanced MR angiography, 1253-1254
Carotid endarterectomy, 1172-1175, 1222, 1223f
    contraindications to, 1172-1173
    for cerebrovascular atherosclerotic disease, 1210
    imaging findings in
        postoperative surveillance and, 1174-1175
        preoperative assessment and, 1173-1174, 1173f-1175f, 1174t
        preoperative planning and, 1174
    indications for, 1172
    outcomes and complications of, 1173
Carotid intimal-medial thickness (CIMT), ultrasound measurement of, 1199-1202, 1202f
Carotid Revascularization Endarterectomy versus Stent Trial (CREST), 1222-1223

Carotid triangle, 961-962, 963f
Carotid-subclavian bypass, 1175
  contraindications to, 1175
  imaging findings in, 1175-1176, 1175f-1176f
  indications for, 1175
Carrel patch, 1546
Catecholamines, radiolabeled, in PET/SPECT imaging, 806, 806f
Catheter(s), 1155-1156
  central venous, deep vein thrombosis associated with, 1662, 1663f
  Fogarty embolectomy, 1577-1578, 1577f
Catheter ablation, for arrhythmogenic right ventricular dysplasia, 894
Caudate lobe vein, 1010
Celiac stenosis, CT angiography of, 1066-1068
Celiac trunk, branches of, 970-972, 971f, 973f
Cell death
  after myocardial ischemia, 792
  programmed, 792
    targeting, 805
Cell survival, programmed, 792
Central venous catheter, deep vein thrombosis associated with, 1662, 1663f
Cephalic vein, in upper extremity, 1020-1022, 1021f-1022f
Cerebral angiography, 1159
Cerebral artery, fetal origin of, 963, 964f
Cerebral embolism, in infective endocarditis, 429, 429f
Cerebrovascular atherosclerotic disease. See also Atherosclerosis.
  differential diagnosis of, 1207t
  medical treatment of, 1208
  presenting findings in, 1198t
  prevalence and epidemiology of, 1194
  surgical/interventional treatment of, 1210
Cervicoaxillary compression syndrome, 1644
CHARGE syndrome, 640
Chelation therapy, for peripheral artery disease, 1209
Chest pain
  acute, 715. See also Acute coronary syndrome.
  clinical classification of, 482t
  in emergency department setting
    coronary artery calcium assessment and, 462
    CT angiographic evaluation of, 485-486, 487f
  sudden-onset, postoperative, ischemic heart disease and, 813
Chest radiography. See also Radiography.
  in intensive care, 94-96, 95f, 95t
  of acute coronary syndrome, 716, 717f
  of amyloidosis, 862
  of angiosarcoma, 926
  of aortic aneurysm
    ruptured, 1302
    thoracic, 1279-1280, 1280f
  of aortic dissection, 1290, 1290f
  of aortic regurgitation, 92-93, 832, 832f
  of aortic stenosis, 92, 828, 828f
  of aortic trauma, thoracic, 1306-1307, 1308f
  of aortitis, syphilitic, 1323, 1323f
  of arrhythmogenic right ventricular dysplasia, 887
  of atherosclerotic ulcer, penetrating, 1300
  of atrial septal defect, 564-565, 565f-566f
    ostium secundum, 90, 91f
    postoperative, 365-366, 368f
  of Behçet syndrome, 1387, 1388f
  of cardiac borders, 71-97
    aortic arch and, 72-73, 73f
    aortic border in, ascending, 75-76

Chest radiography (Continued)
  atrial border in, left, 74, 74f-75f
    in lateral projection, 77
  azygos vein and, 76-77
  in left anterior oblique projection, 77-78, 80f
  in right anterior oblique projection, 77, 79f
  left ventricle in, lateral projection of, 77
  measurement of heart size by, 78-80
  mediastinal border in
    left, 72, 72f-73f
    right, 75, 76f
  normal and abnormal, 71-78
  pulmonary artery border in, 74, 74f
  ventricular border in
    left, 74-75, 75f-76f
    right, 75
  of cardiac metastases, 923, 923f
  of cardiac tumor, calcified amorphous, 919, 920f
  of cardiomyopathy
    dilated, 852
    hypertrophic, 94
    restrictive, 94
    siderotic, 867
  of Churg-Strauss syndrome, 1390, 1390f
  of coarctation of aorta, 536
    classic signs in, 537, 537f
    thoracic, 89-90, 91f
  of congenital heart disease, in adult, 89, 91f-92f
  of cor triatriatum, 632, 633f
  of coronary artery calcification, 88, 89f
  of diffuse alveolar hemorrhage, 1384
  of double-outlet right ventricle, 682, 682f
  of Ebstein anomaly, 653, 654f
  of eosinophilic endomyocardial disease, 865
  of fibroma, 912
  of Goodpasture syndrome, 1393
  of great vessel calcification, 89, 90f
  of intramural hematoma of aorta, 1296-1297
  of ischemic heart disease, postoperative, 813
  of leiomyosarcoma, 928
  of lipoma, 915
  of mitral regurgitation, 93-94, 837
  of mitral stenosis, 93, 93f, 834-835, 834f
  of myocardial calcification, 87, 87f
  of myocarditis, 897, 897f
  of myxoma, 907, 907f
  of nonthrombotic embolization, 1369
  of osteosarcoma, 929
  of papillary fibroelastoma, 910
  of paraganglioma, 918
  of patent ductus arteriosus, 585, 586f
  of pericardial calcification, 82, 82f
  of pericardial constriction, 80-82
  of pericardial cyst, 82, 83f
  of pericardial effusion, 80, 81f, 942, 943f
  of pericarditis
    acute, 946
    constrictive, 949-950
  of pericardium, 80-82
    normal, 80, 81f
  of pneumothorax, postoperative, 96
  of primary cardiac lymphoma, 932, 933f
  of pulmonary capillary hemangiomatosis, 1363
  of pulmonary edema, 85-87, 86f
    hydrostatic, 1373-1374, 1374b, 1375f
    neurogenic, 1379, 1379f
    permeability, 86-87, 1377-1378
    postoperative, 96
    re-expansion, 1380, 1380f

Chest radiography (Continued)
  of pulmonary embolism, 1333-1334, 1333f-1334f
  of pulmonary hemosiderosis, idiopathic, 1392
  of pulmonary hypertension, 1356, 1357f
    arterial, 84-87, 85f
    caused by lung disease/hypoxia, 1366
    chronic thromboembolic, 1345, 1346f-1348f, 1367
    idiopathic, 1358
    related to associated conditions, 1360, 1361f
    venous, 85
    with left heart disease (venous), 1364, 1364f
    with unclear multifactorial mechanisms, 1371
  of pulmonary valve regurgitation, 846
  of pulmonary valve stenosis, 92, 92f, 846
  of pulmonary vasculature, 82-89
    abnormal blood flow in, 84, 84f-85f
    normal anatomy in, 82-84, 83f-84f
  of pulmonary veno-occlusive disease, 1362, 1362f
  of pulmonary venous connections
    partial anomalous, 626, 627f
    total anomalous, 635, 635f
  of rhabdomyoma, 913
  of rhabdomyosarcoma, 930
  of sarcoid granulomatosis, necrotizing, 1392
  of sarcoidosis, 869, 870f
  of single ventricle, 672, 673f
  of sinus venous defect, 629, 630f
  of subaortic stenosis, 92-94
  of Takayasu arteritis, 1316
  of tetralogy of Fallot, 641-647, 641f-642f, 660, 661f
  of thorax, lateral view in, 77, 78f
  of transposition of great arteries, 657, 658f
    complete, 611-612, 612f
  of tricuspid valve regurgitation, 845
  of truncus arteriosus, 664
  of valvular calcification, 87, 88f
  of vascular rings, 543
  of ventricular septal defect, 574, 574f-575f
  of Wegener's granulomatosis, 1385, 1385f
  postoperative, early, 96
Chest trauma, blunt, aortic, 1306, 1307f. See also Thoracic aortic trauma.
  acute injury due to, 592, 593f
  with deceleration mechanism injury, 1273
Chest wall
  arteries of, 964-965
  venous drainage of, 999, 1000f
Child-Turcotte-Pugh score, 1453
Cholangiocarcinoma, intrahepatic, 1458-1459
Cholesterol ester transfer protein (CETP) gene, lipid abnormalities associated with, 1196
Chronic kidney disease (CKD), 403
  classification of, 1673t
  clinical presentation of, 1674
  definition of, 1673-1674
  etiology and pathophysiology of, 1674
  hemodialysis for, 1672. See also Arteriovenous fistula, in hemodialysis patient; Arteriovenous graft.
  in patients with coronary artery disease, 403
  prevalence and epidemiology of, 1674

Chronic kidney disease (CKD) *(Continued)*
vascular imaging in
angiography in, 1680-1682, 1682f-1683f
CT angiography in, 1676-1677, 1677f-1678f
indications and algorithm for, 1674
MR angiography in, 1677-1680, 1679f-1681f
ultrasound in, 1675-1676, 1675f
Chronic limb ischemia. *See* Limb ischemia, chronic.
Chronic obstructive pulmonary disease (COPD)
definition of, 1365
etiology and pathophysiology of, 1365
manifestations of, 1366-1367
prevalence and epidemiology of, 1365
pulmonary hypertension caused by, 1365
Chronic thromboembolic pulmonary hypertension (CTPH), 1344-1351, 1366-1368. *See also* Pulmonary hypertension.
classic signs of, 1350
clinical presentation of, 1345, 1366-1367
definition of, 1366
differential diagnosis of, 1350, 1351f
etiology and pathophysiology of, 1344, 1366
imaging of
indications and algorithm for, 1345
technique and findings in, 1345-1350, 1346f-1350f, 1367
medical treatment of, 1350-1351, 1367-1368
prevalence and epidemiology of, 1344
reporting of, 1351
surgical/interventional treatment of, 1351, 1368
Churg-Strauss syndrome, 1390, 1390f
diagnostic criteria for, 1391b
Cilostazol, for peripheral artery disease, 1209
Circle of Willis, 1217
Circulation. *See* Blood flow.
Circumferential-longitudinal shear angle, of left ventricle, 234-235
Cirrhosis
clinical presentation of, 1453
definition of, 1453
differential diagnosis of, 1456-1457
etiology and pathophysiology of, 1453
imaging of
indications and algorithm for, 1454, 1454f
technique and findings in, 1454-1456
treatment options for, 1457
Claudication, intermittent, 1578-1581, 1579f
differential diagnosis of, 1583
in peripheral artery disease, 1628. *See also* Peripheral arterial disease (PAD).
Clopidogrel
for ischemic stroke or transient ischemic attack, 1222
for peripheral artery disease, 1209
preprocedural, for carotid artery stenting, 1224
Clopidogrel versus Aspirin in Patients at Risk of Ischemic Events (CAPRIE) trials, 1208
Clubbing, in Eisenmenger syndrome, 585
Coarctation of aorta, 371-373, 535, 536f
blood flow in
abnormal, 248f
MR evaluation of, 242-243, 244f
classic signs of, 537, 537f-538f
clinical manifestations of, 535-537
definition of, 535
differential diagnosis of
from clinical presentation, 537-539, 539f
from imaging findings, 539, 539f

Coarctation of aorta *(Continued)*
etiology and pathophysiology of, 535
imaging studies of, 535
in pediatric patients, 536
postoperative, 697-698, 698f-699f
medical treatment of, 539
pathophysiology of, 552-553
prevalence and epidemiology of, 535, 552
surgical repair of, 371-372, 539-540, 540f
abnormal circular-type flow after, 248f
considerations regarding, 373, 388, 388t
contraindications to, 373
indications for, 372-373
mortality rate from, 539-540
outcomes and complications of, 373
postoperative management after, 698, 698f-699f
postoperative surveillance after, 373, 376f-377f, 552-553, 553f
preoperative imaging in, 373, 375f-376f
thoracic, radiography of, 89-90, 91f
vs. patent ductus arteriosus, 594, 594f
Cobweb sign, in type B aortic dissection, 1294, 1295f
Coeur en sabot sign, in tetralogy of Fallot, 647
Coils. *See* Gradient coils.
COL3A1 gene, in Ehlers-Danlos syndrome, 1273
Colchicine, for pericarditis, 947
Colic vein, 1006, 1006f-1007f
Collateral pathways, of lower extremity arteries, 985-986, 986f-987f
Collett and Edwards classification, of truncus arteriosus, 616, 617f
Collimator(s)
in SPECT, 276-277, 277f-278f
low energy all purpose, 277
Colon necrosis, after endovascular aneurysm repair, 1435-1436
Color and spectrum invert, in Doppler ultrasonography, 1041
Color Doppler ultrasonography, 1036. *See also* Doppler ultrasonography.
Color flash artifact, in Doppler ultrasonography, 1043
Color flow imaging, in Doppler ultrasonography, 98-100, 101f
Color gain
in Doppler ultrasonography, 1040, 1040f
setting of, 1042
incorrect, in carotid artery Doppler ultrasonography, 1234
Commissurotomy, open, for mitral stenosis, 836
Compartment pressure, measurement of, 1575-1576
Complementary *spatial modulation* of *magnetization* (C-SPAMM) technique, for quantifying myocardial motion, 230
Complete transposition of great arteries, 601. *See also* Transposition of great arteries (TGA), complete.
Compliance index, 1512
Compliant balloons, in vascular interventions, 1156
Compression syndrome, cervicoaxillary, 1644
Compton scatter
in PET imaging, 306
in photon-matter interactions, 275, 275f, 1047
Computed tomographic angiography (CTA), 1055-1077
abdominal, 1065-1068
of aorta, 1065-1066, 1067f
of hepatic vasculature, 1066, 1068f

Computed tomographic angiography (CTA) *(Continued)*
of mesenteric vasculature, 1066-1068, 1069f
of pancreas, 1066, 1067f
of renal vasculature, 1066, 1067f-1068f
advantages of, 1055-1056, 1064f-1065f
carotid, 1060, 1062f, 1260-1267
contraindications to, 1262-1263
detection of ulceration in, 1266-1267
image interpretation of, 1264-1267
imaging parameters for, 1263-1264, 1264t
indications for, 1260-1262, 1260f-1263f
pitfalls and solutions in, 1264
postprocessing of, 1264-1266, 1265f
reporting of, 1266f, 1267
technical requirements for, 1260
technique of, 1263-1264, 1264t
cerebral, 1060, 1061f
contrast media in
administration of, 145
bolus tracking of, 1058-1059
concentration of, 1059
detection and administration of, 1058-1060
dual-head power injectors for, 1059-1060
fixed scan delay and, 1058
test bolus of, 1059
coronary, 123-132
after arterial switch procedure, 612, 612f
after pulmonary artery banding, 611f, 612
after Rastelli procedure, 612-613, 613f
angiographic views in, 124-126, 124f-127f
artifact(s) in, 495-500, 495t, 496f
beam hardening, 495-496, 496f
blooming (partial volume), 496, 496f-497f
blurring (patient motion), 496-499, 498f-499f
incomplete coverage, 499-500
noise-induced, 499
poor vessel enhancement, 499
stair-step, 499, 500f-501f
streaks (metallic materials), 496, 497f-498f
contraindications to, 123, 494
contrast media in, injection protocol for, 164t-165t
emerging applications of, 485-489
in cardiac surgery, 486-487, 488f
in chest pain evaluation, 485-486, 487f
in noncardiac surgery, 486
in vessel wall imaging, 488-489, 489f-490f
estimation of cardiovascular risk and pretest probability for CAD with, 482t-483t
image interpretation of, 127-131, 127f-131f, 500-504
plaque characterization in, 503-504
postprocessing, 500-502
axial images in, 500
maximum intensity projection in, 502
multiplanar reformation in, 500, 502f
volume rendering in, 502
stenosis assessment in, 502-503, 503f
indications for, 123, 478, 479f-482f, 494
in asymptomatic patients, 478
of aneurysms, 510f-513f, 513
overview of evidence and trends in, 477-478

Computed tomographic angiography (CTA) (*Continued*)
  patient-related consideration(s) in, 479-485
    heart rate and heart rate variability as, 481-482, 485f
    heavy calcifications as, 479-481, 483f-484f
    obesity as, 484-485, 485f-486f
    renal insufficiency as, 485
  pitfalls and solutions in, 126
  procedure-related risks associated with, 489-490
  radiation exposure associated with, 346-347, 346f
    dose reduction in, 348-350, 349f-350f
  reporting of, 504-507, 504f-506f, 506t
  role of, in context of other noninvasive tests, 479
  segment-based and patient-based analysis in, 478-485
  technical requirements in, 123, 493-494
  technique of, 123-124, 494-507, 1061t, 1063-1064
  detectors in, 1056-1057
  dual-energy mode of, 1057
  ECG dose modulation in, 1058
  image acquisition in, 1057-1058
  image interpretation in, 1073-1075
  image quality in, 1056
  of aortic aneurysm
    abdominal, 1181, 1181f, 1441-1442
    thoracic, 1178-1179, 1178f-1179f
  of aortic occlusion, 1411, 1412f-1413f
  of arteriovenous fistula failure, 1676-1677, 1677f-1678f
  of atherosclerosis, 1203-1204, 1203f
  of atherosclerotic ulcer, penetrating, 1299-1300, 1299f, 1301f
  of carotid stenosis, 1220
  of celiac artery thrombosis, 1548-1549, 1549f
  of chronic thromboembolic pulmonary hypertension, 1348, 1348f
  of coarctation of aorta, 536
  of cor triatriatum, 632-633
  of graft infection, after lower extremity bypass, 1185-1186, 1186f
  of hepatic artery stenosis, 1550, 1552f-1553f
  of hepatic artery thrombosis, 1548-1549, 1549f-1551f
  of inferior vena cava stenosis, 1553-1554, 1555f-1556f
  of limb ischemia
    acute, 1576
    chronic, 1582-1583
  of lower extremities, 1610-1627
    contraindications to, 1611-1614, 1614f
    contrast bolus considerations in, 1617-1619
      bolus tracking technique, 1618-1619, 1618f-1619f
      test bolus technique, 1619
    image acquisition in, 1614-1617
      field of view and, 1614, 1615f
      reconstruction parameters and, 1617, 1617f-1618f
      scanning protocols and, 1614-1617, 1615t-1616t
    image interpretation in, 1622-1627
      maximum intensity projection, 1622, 1624f-1625f
      multiplanar reformation, 1622, 1623f
      reporting of, 1625-1627, 1626f
      thin slab or thick slab, 1622-1625
      volume rendering, 1622, 1625f

Computed tomographic angiography (CTA) (*Continued*)
  indications for, 1611, 1611f-1613f
  pitfalls and considerations in, 1619-1622
    acquisition considerations, 1619-1620, 1620f-1621f
    inherent limitations, 1621-1622
    interpretation considerations, 1620-1621, 1621f
  technical requirements for, 1610
  of lower extremity vasculature, 1068-1069, 1069f-1072f
  of portal vein thrombosis, 1551, 1553f-1554f
  of pulmonary venous connections
    partial anomalous, 627
    total anomalous, 636, 636f
  of renal arteries, 1066, 1067f-1068f
    contraindications to, 1485
    image interpretation in, 1488-1490, 1489f-1490f
    pitfalls and solutions in, 1488
    reporting of, 1490
    technique of, 1485-1486, 1485t, 1486f
  of renal artery stenosis, 1475, 1475f-1476f
  of subclavian artery occlusion, 1176, 1176f
  of thoracic outlet syndrome, 1669
  of thoracic vasculature, 1060-1062, 1063f-1064f
  pitfalls and solutions in, 1069-1073
  postprocessing in, 1073-1074
    limits of, 1074-1075
  preoperative
    of carotid artery stenosis, 1174, 1174f
    of thoracoabdominal aortic aneurysm, 1177-1178
  prestent and poststent protocol for, 1429, 1430t
  prospective gating in, 1057-1058
  pulmonary, 1062-1063, 1064f-1065f
  radiation and dosage in, 1070-1073
  reconstruction techniques in, 1058
  retrospective gating in, 1057
  scanner design in, 1056
  scanner noise in, 1056
  technical components and design in, 1056-1057
  techniques of, 1060-1075, 1061t
  three-dimensional postprocessing in, basic, 1120-1127. *See also* Three-dimensional postprocessing, in CTA and MRA.
Computed tomographic venography (CTV), of pulmonary embolism, 1340
Computed tomography (CT). *See also* CT entries; PET/CT imaging systems.
  after surgical repair of truncus arteriosus, 622-623, 622f
  cardiac
    artifacts in, 147, 147f-148f
    clinical techniques of, 143-149
    contrast media in, 159
      administration of, 145-146, 145f
      early arterial dynamics of, 160-161, 160f
      injection of, 161
        clinical protocols for, 163-165, 164t-165t
      timing of, 161-162, 162f
      safety issues of, 159-160
      saline flushing and, 163, 163f
    dual-source, 140
    ECG-synchronized, 134, 135f
    goals of, definition of, 133

Computed tomography (CT) (*Continued*)
  imaging processing in, 167-179, 168f-171f
    axial images in, 168-169
    coronal and sagittal images in, 170-171, 172f
    curved planar reconstruction in, 171-173, 173f-175f
    maximum intensity projection in, 173-176
    technical requirements for, 167-168
    volume rendering technique of, 176-178, 177f
  imaging reconstruction techniques in, 134
  imaging requirements in, 133
  in myocardial perfusion studies, 326
  medications for, 156-159, 157f, 157t-158t. *See also specific medication.*
  new developments in, 140-141
  patient preparation for, 143-144, 144f
  physics of, 133-142
  postprocedural considerations in, 146-147
    pitfalls and solutions in, 147, 147f-148f
  radiation dose reduction in, 348-350, 349f-350f
    increased beam filtration technique for, 153-154
    increased beam pitch technique for, 153
    increased reconstructed slice thickness technique for, 154, 154f
    reduced tube current technique for, 150-152, 151f
    reduced tube voltage technique for, 152-153
    shortened scan length technique for, 153
    technical requirements for, 150
    tubal modulation for, 146
  radiation exposure associated with, 346-347, 346f, 347t
  scanning technique of, 144-146
    contrast administration in, 145-146, 145f
    image quality in, 144-145
    minimizing radiation dose in, tubal modulation to, 146
  technical principle(s) of, 134-140
    ECG tube current modulation, 138-140, 139f
    multisegment image reconstruction, 136-137, 138f-139f
    optimal reconstruction phase, 137
    prospective triggering, 134-136, 135f
    retrospective gating, 136, 137f
    with volume detectors, 140-141
  dual-source, technology of, 1057
  electron-beam
    of coronary artery calcium, vs. multidetector CT imaging, 460
    technology of, 1056
  high-resolution
    of ARDS during exudative phase, 1377, 1378f
    of ARDS during proliferative phase, 1378, 1378f
  multidetector, 1055
    of atrial fibrillation, 447-449, 447f-449f
    of coronary artery calcium, 459
      vs. electron-beam CT imaging, 460
    of pulmonary embolism, 1339-1340, 1339t
      limitations of, 1339-1340
    of thoracic aortic trauma, 1307-1308

Computed tomography (CT) *(Continued)*
  of acute coronary syndrome, 717-721, 718f-720f
    protocol parameters for, 720t
    University of Maryland triage studies in, 721t
  of amyloidosis, 863, 863f
  of angiosarcoma, 926, 926f-927f
  of aortic aneurysm
    abdominal, 1441-1442
    inflammatory, 1405, 1405f-1406f
    mycotic, 1407, 1407f
    ruptured, 1302-1303, 1303f
    thoracic, 1280-1281, 1281f
  of aortic dissection, 1291, 1292f-1293f
  of aortic regurgitation, 833
  of aortic stenosis, 828-829, 829f-831f
  of aortic trauma
    abdominal, 1410, 1410f
    thoracic, 1307-1309
      aortic pseudoaneurysm in, 1308, 1309f
      contour abnormality in, 1308
      contrast agent extravasation in, 1309
      intimal flap in, 1308
      multidetector technique of, 1307-1308
      periaortic mediastinal hemorrhage in, 1309, 1309f
  of aortitis, syphilitic, 1323, 1323f
  of aortoenteric fistula, 1415-1416, 1416f
  of arrhythmogenic right ventricular dysplasia, 888, 888f
  of atherosclerotic plaque, ulcerated, 1299-1300, 1300f
  of atrial septal defect, 566, 568f
  of atrium
    left, 32-33, 32f
    right, 30-31, 32f
  of Behçet syndrome, 1387, 1388f
  of cardiac function, 758, 759f
    during stress, 769
    left ventricular, 761
    regional, 766-767
    right ventricular, 762-763
  of cardiac lymphoma, primary, 933, 933f-934f
  of cardiac metastases, 921f-924f, 924
  of cardiac tumor, calcified amorphous, 919
  of cardiomyopathy
    dilated, 853-855, 854f
    hypertrophic, 874-875, 875f
    sideritic, 867
  of chronic thromboembolic pulmonary hypertension, 1345-1349, 1346f-1349f, 1367
  of coarctation of aorta, 536
    classic signs in, 537, 538f
    repaired, 373, 377f
  of coronary anomalies, congenital, 467
  of coronary artery bypass graft, 523, 523f
  of coronary atherosclerosis, 710, 710f-711f
  of diffuse alveolar hemorrhage, 1384, 1384f, 1391
  of double-outlet right ventricle, 683-684
  of endoleaks, 1409
  of eosinophilic endomyocardial disease, 865, 866f
  of fibroma, 912-913, 912f
  of giant cell arteritis, 1320-1321, 1321f, 1391, 1391f, 1414, 1415f
  of Goodpasture syndrome, 1393-1394, 1393f
  of inferior vena cava anomalies, 1528
  of inferior vena cava thrombosis, 1537, 1538f
  of inferior vena cava tumors, 1530
    findings in, 1530-1531, 1531f-1533f

Computed tomography (CT) *(Continued)*
  of in-stent restenosis and thrombosis, 518-519, 519f
  of intramural hematoma, 1297, 1297f
  of ischemic heart disease, 755, 756t
    postoperative, 814
  of leiomyosarcoma, 928
  of lipoma, 915, 915f
  of lipomatous hypertrophy of interatrial septum, 916, 916f
  of liposarcoma, 931, 932f
  of mitral regurgitation, 837
  of mitral stenosis, 835, 835f
  of myocardial perfusion, 326, 730-733
    animal studies in, 730-731, 731t
    contraindications to, 733
    human studies in, 731-733, 732t
    image interpretation in, 735
    indications for, 733
    pitfalls and solutions in, 734
    reporting of, 735-736
    stress multidetector, 733
    technique of, 734
  of myocardial viability, 784-787, 787f
    limitations of, 787-788
  of myocarditis, 897-899, 898f
  of myxoma, 907-909, 907f-908f
  of nonthrombotic embolization, 1369, 1369f-1370f
  of osteosarcoma, 929, 929f
  of papillary fibroelastoma, 910, 911f
  of paraganglioma, 918
  of patent ductus arteriosus, 585-586, 587f
  of pericardial effusion, 942
  of pericarditis
    acute, 946, 947f
    constrictive, 950, 950f
  of peripheral artery disease, 1630
  of pulmonary capillary hemangiomatosis, 1363, 1363f
  of pulmonary edema, hydrostatic, 1374, 1374b, 1375f
  of pulmonary embolism, 1337-1339
    benefits and accuracy of, 1338
    classic findings in, 1337-1338, 1338f
    limitations of, 1338-1339
    multidetector, 1339-1340, 1339t
      limitations of, 1339-1340
    technical considerations in, 1337
  of pulmonary hemosiderosis, idiopathic, 1392, 1393f
  of pulmonary hypertension, 1356-1357, 1357f
    caused by lung disease/hypoxia, 1366
    chronic thromboembolic, 1345-1349, 1346f-1349f, 1367
    idiopathic, 1358, 1358f-1359f
    related to associated conditions, 1360
    with left heart disease (venous), 1364, 1365f
    with unclear multifactorial mechanisms, 1371
  of pulmonary veno-occlusive disease, 1362
  of renal vasculature, in living kidney donor, 1568
  of rhabdomyoma, 913
  of rhabdomyosarcoma, 930
  of sarcoidosis, 869, 870f
  of single ventricle, 673
  of sinus venous defect, 630
  of subclavian steal syndrome, 1328, 1328f
  of Takayasu arteritis, 1316, 1316f, 1388-1389, 1389f
  of tetralogy of Fallot, 643, 644f

Computed tomography (CT) *(Continued)*
  of transposition of great arteries, 658
    levo-, 679-680
  of truncus arteriosus, 664-665, 665f-666f
  of upper extremity medium and small vessel disease, 1648-1649, 1648f-1650f
  of vascular anatomy, in pancreas transplant recipient, 1569
  of vascular rings, 544
  of ventricular septal defect, 574-575, 577f-578f
  of Wegener's granulomatosis, 1385-1386, 1386f
  postoperative, of occluded aortobifemoral bypass limb, 1185, 1185f
  radionuclides in, 325-326. *See also* Radionuclide(s).
  x-ray
    fundamentals of, 1047, 1048f
    important performance parameters in, 1047-1051, 1048f-1051f
    multislice, 1053-1054, 1053f
    physics of, 1047-1054
    step-and-shoot vs. helical (spiral), 1051-1053, 1051f-1052f
Conal septum, in double-outlet right ventricle physiology, 682
Conduction system, of heart, 57-58, 58f
Conduit(s), in vascular bypass surgery
  autogenous saphenous vein as, 1585-1586
  definition of, 1585
  extra-anatomic bypass grafts as, 1586-1588, 1587f-1589f
  prosthetic, 1586
  xenografts as, 1586, 1587f
Congenital heart disease (CHD). *See also specific cardiac defect, e.g., Tetralogy of Fallot.*
  acyanotic
    with shunt, 383-387, 385f, 385t
      surgery for
        contraindications to, 386
        indications for, 386, 387f
        outcomes and complications of, 386
        postoperative surveillance after, 387
        preoperative imaging in, 386-387
    without shunt, 387-389, 388t
      surgery for
        indications for and contraindications to, 388-389
        postoperative surveillance after, 389
  adult, in general population, 383, 384t
  complex, 656
  cyanotic
    evaluation of patient with, 651-653, 652f
    with decreased pulmonary blood flow, 390-392, 391t
      surgery for, 391-392
    with increased pulmonary blood flow, 389-390, 389t
      surgery for, 390
  diagnosis and management of, segmental approach to, 12-13, 13f
  echocardiography of, 117-118
  in adult, 89, 91f-92f
  incidence of, 651
  postoperative evaluation of
    coronary artery imaging, perfusion imaging, and myocardial viability in, 693-694, 693f-694f
    gadolinium-enhanced three-dimensional MR angiography in, 693, 693f
    MR imaging of, 689-701
      cine imaging, 690-691, 690f-691f
      clinical presentation indicating, 694

Congenital heart disease (CHD) *(Continued)*
    indications and algorithm for, 694
    spin-echo imaging, 691, 691f
    technique and findings in, 694-700, 695f-699f
    velocity-encoded cine sequences, 691-693, 692f
  relative frequency of, 383, 384t
Congenital venolobar syndrome, 625, 626f-627f
  repair of, baffle obstruction after, 628, 629f
Congenitally corrected transposition of great arteries, 601. *See also* Transposition of great arteries (TGA), congenitally corrected.
Connective tissue disease, 1391
  pulmonary hypertension associated with, 1359
Conotruncus, development of, 22-24, 25f
Constrictive pericarditis. *See* Pericarditis, constrictive.
Continuous wave Doppler ultrasonography, 98-99, 1036-1037. *See also* Doppler ultrasonography.
Contour abnormality(ies), in thoracic aortic trauma, 1308
Contractile cardiac motion, causing attenuation mismatch, in PET imaging, 309-310, 311f
Contrast agents, 1398-1399. *See also specific agent entries, e.g.*, Gadolinium.
  allergy to, as contraindication to CT angiography, 1614
  clinical injection protocols for, 163-165, 164t-165t
  dosage of, 1399
  extravasation of, in thoracic aortic trauma, 1309
  in angiography, choice of, 1158
  in contrast-enhanced MR angiography. *See also* Magnetic resonance angiography (MRA), contrast-enhanced.
    injection protocols for, 1633
    novel, 1633
  in CT angiography
    administration of, 145
    bolus tracking of, 1058-1059
    concentration of, 1059
    detection and administration of, 1058-1060
    dual-head power injectors for, 1059-1060
    fixed scan delay and, 1058
    test bolus of, 1059
  in CT imaging, 159
    administration of, 145-146, 145f
    early arterial dynamics of, 160-161, 160f
    injection of, 161
      clinical protocols for, 163-165, 164t-165t
      timing of, 161-162, 162f
    safety issues of, 159-160
    saline flushing and, 163, 163f
  in MR imaging, 251-260
    classification of, 255-259, 255f, 257t-258t
    cost of, 255
    development of, 251
    pharmacovigilance of, 253
    regulatory label of, 251-252
    safety issues of, 252-253, 266
  in perfusion imaging, dosing range of, 206
Contrast bolus, in CT angiography
  of abdominal aorta
    detection/triggering methods of, 1399
    timing techniques of, 1399

Contrast bolus, in CT angiography *(Continued)*
  of lower extremities, 1617-1619
    bolus tracking technique and, 1618-1619, 1618f-1619f
    test bolus technique and, 1619
Contrast-enhanced harmonic imaging, in ultrasonography, 1037
Contrast-induced nephropathy (CIN), 159
Contrast-to-noise ratio, in contrast-enhanced MR angiography, 1258
Conus branch, of right coronary artery, 40, 42f
Conus cordis, 3-4
Cor adiposum, vs. arrhythmogenic right ventricular dysplasia, 893
Cor triatriatum
  clinical presentation of, 632
  definition of, 632
  differential diagnosis of, 633
  etiology and pathophysiology of, 632
  imaging technique and findings in, 632-633, 633f
  incidence of, 632
  reporting of, 634
  treatment options for, 634
CORAL trial, 1480
Coronal images, in cardiac CT imaging, 170-171, 172f
Coronary allograft vasculopathy, after cardiac transplantation, 813
  angiography of, 815
Coronary angioplasty, percutaneous transluminal. *See* Percutaneous transluminal coronary angioplasty (PTCA).
Coronary artery(ies), 38-56
  anatomy of
    normal, 39-48, 39f
    segmental, 48f, 49-50
  calcium in. *See* Coronary artery calcium (CAC).
  congenital anomalies of
    classification of, 467t
    CT imaging of, 467
    definition of, 466
    differential diagnosis of, 468-473
    etiology and pathophysiology of, 466-467
    manifestation of disease in, 467
    MR imaging of, 467
    of intrinsic anatomy, 472-473, 473f-474f
    of origin and course, 468-472, 468f-473f
      duplication in, 48-49, 471-472, 472f
      from noncoronary sinus, 471, 471f
      from opposite sinus of Valsalva, 468-469, 468f-470f
      from pulmonary artery, 470-471
      high arterial origin, 471, 471f
      multiple ostia in, 471, 472f
      single artery, 472, 473f
    of termination: fistula, 473, 474f
    prevalence and epidemiology of, 466
  diagnostic computed angiography of, 123-132. *See also* Computed tomographic angiography (CTA), coronary.
  diseased, evaluation of collateral flow to, 129-131, 130f-131f, 130t
  dissection of, 129, 129f
  duplication of, 48-49, 471-472
  intramuscular, prevalence of, 49
  left, anatomy of, 43-44, 43f-44f, 413f
  left anomalous, diagnosis of, 386

Coronary artery(ies) *(Continued)*
  left anterior descending, 44-46, 44f-45f, 412, 413f
    aneurysm of, 509, 510f
    duplication of, 471-472, 472f
  left circumflex, 46, 46f-47f, 413f
    aneurysm of, 509, 510f
  MR imaging of, 190-191, 191f
    in postoperative congenital heart disease patients, 693-694, 693f-694f
    respiratory-navigator techniques of, 190-191, 191f
    short breath-hold three-dimensional techniques of, 190
  narrowing of
    diffuse, 128, 128f
    discreet, 127-128, 128f
  network of, 38
  percutaneous transluminal coronary angioplasty of. *See* Coronary artery disease (CAD), percutaneous coronary intervention for.
  ramus intermedius, 46, 47f
  right
    aneurysm of, 509, 510f, 513f
    branches of, 39-41, 40f-42f, 413f
    dominance of, 46-48, 48f
  single, anomalous, 472, 473f
  stenosis of
    calcification as indicator of, 461, 461t
    CT assessment of, 502-503, 503f
  stenting of. *See* Coronary stents.
  thrombus in, during angioplasty intervention, 129, 129f
  variations in
    definitions of, 38-39
    normal, 48-49, 48f-50f
Coronary artery aneurysm, 128-129, 128f-129f
  angiography of, 513
  atherosclerotic, 509
  clinical presentation of, 509-512
  congenital, 472, 473f
  CT angiography of, 510f-513f, 513
  definition of, 509
  differential diagnosis of, 513
  epidemiology of, 509, 510f-513f
  etiology and pathophysiology of, 509
  incidence of, 509
  medical treatment of, 513
  radiographic imaging of, 512-513
  surgical treatment of, 513, 514f
Coronary artery bypass graft (CABG), computed angiography of, contrast media injection protocol for, 164t-165t
Coronary artery bypass graft (CABG) surgery, 412-417
  anatomic considerations in, 412-413, 413f
  arterial grafts in, 522
  assessment of, 522-530
    background in, 522
    CT imaging in, 523, 523f
    MR imaging in, 523-524
  cardiopulmonary bypass in, 412-413, 414f
  choice of conduits in, 522
  complication(s) of, 524-525
    graft aneurysm as, 525
    graft thrombosis and occlusion as, 524-525, 527f-529f
  contraindications to, 413-414, 416t
  for coronary atherosclerosis, 713
  goals of, 412, 413f
  indications for, 413, 416t
  internal mammary artery grafts in, 522
  microvascular anastomoses in, 413, 415f-416f

Coronary artery bypass graft (CABG) surgery *(Continued)*
  outcomes and complications of, 414-415
  postoperative evaluation of, 524, 525f-526f
  postoperative surveillance after, 417
  preoperative imaging for, 413, 416f, 416t
  preoperative planning in, 524
  preoperative risk factors for, 416t
  saphenous vein grafts in, 522
  technique of, 412
Coronary artery calcium (CAC)
  as indicator of stenosis, 461, 461t
  as predictor of cardiac events, 461-462
  assessment of, in elderly populations, 462-463
  imaging of, 458-460, 458f
    clinical importance of, 461-462
    electron-beam CT in, 458-459
    interscan reproducibility in, 460
    multidetector CT in, 459
      vs. electron-beam CT imaging, 460
    radiation dosage in, 460
    radiographic, 88, 89f
    standardization of, 459-460, 460f
  in asymptomatic individuals, risk assessment of, 462
  in patients with chest pain, presenting to emergency departments, 462
  in plaque formation, 457-458. *See also* Plaque, atherosclerotic.
  in specialized populations, 462-463
  pathophysiology of, 457-458
  prevalence of, in renal failure, 463
  screening for
    in diabetic patients, 463
    with treadmill and nuclear stress imaging, 463
Coronary artery calcium (CAC) score, 331, 331f
  progression of, 463
    effect of statins on, 463-464
  relationship between race and, 462
  reporting of, 459
  zero, value of, 461
Coronary artery disease (CAD)
  atherosclerotic. *See also* Atherosclerosis; Plaque, atherosclerotic.
    angiography of, 708
    biology of, 60-61, 60f-61f
    calcium associated with, 457. *See also* Coronary artery calcium (CAC).
    clinical presentation of, 708
    CT imaging of, 710, 710f-711f
    definition of, 705
    differential diagnosis of, 712-713
    etiology and pathophysiology of, 705-707, 706f-707f
    imaging of
      indications and algorithm for, 708
      investigational catheter-based techniques of, 712, 712f
      technique and findings in, 708-712
    MR imaging of, 710-711
    nuclear imaging of, 711-712
    prevalence and epidemiology of, 705
    treatment options for, 713
    ultrasonography of, 107, 708-709, 709f
  chronic, 61-62
  CT angiography of, 1063
    protocol parameters for, 1061t
  evaluation of, prognostic approach to, 281, 282f
  lifetime risk of, 790
  multivessel, evaluation of, 329, 329f-330f

Coronary artery disease (CAD) *(Continued)*
  obstructive
    CT angiography of. *See also* Computed tomographic angiography (CTA), coronary.
      image interpretation of, 127-131, 127f-131f, 500-504
        plaque characterization in, 503-504
        postprocessing, 500-502
          axial images in, 500
          maximum intensity projection in, 502
          multiplanar reformation in, 500, 502f
          volume rendering in, 502
        stenosis assessment in, 502-503, 503f
      reporting of, 504-507, 504f-506f, 506t
    definition of, 477
    percutaneous coronary intervention for, 394-403
      adverse periprocedural events in, 405, 405f-406f
      after saphenous vein bypass graft, 394-395, 396f
      chronic total occlusion and, 395-397, 398f
      contraindications to, 402
      in stent era, 403-405, 404f
        restenosis and, 404, 405f
      indications for, 401-402
      of bifurcation-type lesions, 394, 395f
      of complex, angulated, and lesions distal to proximal vessel tortuosity, 395, 396f-397f, 397
      of left main artery stenosis, 397, 398f-399f
      of long lesions and diffuse disease, 397, 398f
      of specific lesion subsets, catheter modification in, 400, 401f
      outcomes and complications of, 402-403
      ST segment elevation myocardial infarction and, 399, 400f
      stent thrombosis and, 399, 400f
    perfusion imaging of
      diagnostic accuracy of, 342t
      myocardial, 739, 741f-743f
        accuracy of, 749
        pharmacologic stress agents in, 356-357
      pretest probability of, according to age and sex, 483t
    surgery for, 412-417. *See also* Coronary artery bypass graft (CABG) surgery.
    ultrasonography of, 107, 108f-109f
Coronary artery fistula, 473, 474f
Coronary blood flow, 352-353
  at rest vs. hyperemia, 354f
Coronary collateral pathways, common, 130t
Coronary flow reserve, 352-353, 353f
  and radiotracer uptake, 353, 354f
Coronary ostia
  congenital stenosis of, 472, 473f
  location of, 39, 39f
  multiple, anomalous origin of coronary artery from, 471, 472f
  number of, 39
Coronary reserve flow, in hypertrophic cardiomyopathy, MR imaging of, 879
Coronary reverse flow, 61-62
Coronary sinus, 50-51, 53f
  formation of, 8-10, 10f
  tributaries of, 51-52

Coronary stents, 403-405
  for atherosclerosis, 713
  in-stent restenosis and thrombosis
    clinical presentation of, 516-517
    etiology, prevalence, and pathophysiology of, 515-516, 516f-517f
    imaging of, 517-522
      analysis of, 519-520, 520f-521f
      CT scans in, 518-519, 519f
      MR scans in, 518
      radiography in, 517
      ultrasound in, 517-518
    percutaneous coronary intervention for, 399, 400f, 520
    reporting of, 520
    treatment options for, 520
  noninvasive evaluation of, 515-522, 516f
Coronary syndrome, acute. *See* Acute coronary syndrome.
Coronary vein(s)
  anatomy of, 50-55, 53f-54f
  mapping of, contrast media injection protocol for, 164t-165t
Corticosteroids, for Takayasu arteritis, 1318
Costocervical trunk, 989, 990f
Count density, in PET/CT imaging, 327-328
Cox Maze procedure, for atrial fibrillation, 445
^{11}C-palmitate, in PET imaging, 343-344
Crawford classification, of thoracoabdominal aortic aneurysm, 1176-1177, 1177f, 1276, 1277f
C-reactive protein, increased levels of, 1197-1198
Crescent sign, in intramural hematoma of aorta, 1298
CREST syndrome, 1645, 1658f
  pulmonary hypertension associated with, 1359
Crista terminalis, 8-10
Critical limb ischemia, 1579, 1580f-1582f, 1581. *See also* Limb ischemia.
  differential diagnosis of, 1583
Cryogens, as MRI safety issue, 264
Cryoplasty, in lower extremity revascularization, 1592, 1595f
Cryoplasty balloons, 1156
Crystals, scintillation, in SPECT, 277, 278t
CT. *See also* Computed tomography (CT).
CT number
  accuracy of, CT scanner and, 1049-1050
  equation defining, 1049
  in water phantom, 1049, 1050f
CT scanner
  320-slice, 1057
  CT number accuracy of, 1049-1050
Current, x-ray tube, in computed tomography, reduction of, 150-152, 151f
Curved multiplanar reformatted (CMPR) image, 1129, 1130f
  contour detection of, 1129-1131, 1131f-1132f
Curved planar reconstruction (CPR)
  in cardiac CT imaging, 171-173, 173f-175f
  in carotid CT angiography, 1265
Cutting balloon(s), 1156
Cutting balloon angioplasty, in lower extremity revascularization, 1593
Cyanosis, in Eisenmenger syndrome, 585
Cyanotic congenital heart disease. *See* Congenital heart disease (CHD), cyanotic.
Cyst(s), pericardial, radiography of, 82, 83f
Cystic disease, adventitial, 987, 1600
  imaging of, 1604

Cystic medial necrosis, thoracic aortic aneurysm caused by, 1272-1273, 1273f-1274f
Cystic vein, 1008

D

Damus-Kaye-Stansel procedure
 for single-ventricle defects, 390
 for transposition of great arteries, 611, 611f
Dana Point classification, of pulmonary hypertension, 1354-1356, 1356b
Data
 acquisition of, in MR angiography, 1078-1081
 reconstruction and display of, in PET imaging, 318-319
Data processing, three-dimensional, in CTA and MRA, 1120-1127. *See also* Three-dimensional postprocessing, in CT and MRA.
David's and Yacoub's surgical technique, for type A aortic dissection, 1295
D-Dimer assay, sensitivity and specificity of, 1333t
D-Dimer levels, in pulmonary embolism, 1333
Death
 during endovascular aneurysm repair, 1426
 sudden, arrhythmogenic right ventricular dysplasia and, 884
DeBakey classification, of aortic dissection, 434, 434f, 1289, 1289f
Decay constant, of radionuclide, 273-274
Deep vein(s). *See also named vein.*
 of lower extremity, 1027-1029
 of upper extremity, 1022-1023, 1023f
Deep vein thrombosis (DVT)
 ultrasound detection of, 1334-1335
 upper extremity, 1661
  clinical presentation of, 1663
  complications of, 1663
  etiology of, 1661
  imaging of, 1663-1664
   findings in, 1664-1666, 1664f-1668f
   pitfalls in, 1666, 1668f-1669f
  ultrasound, 1647, 1648f
  prevalence, etiology, and risk factors for, 1661-1663, 1663f
Delayed hyperenhancement magnetic resonance imaging (DE-MRI)
 description of, 210-211, 211f
 indications for, 207-210, 208f-210f
 pitfalls and solutions in, 212, 212f
 reporting of, 212-213, 213f
Detector(s)
 in CT angiography, 1056-1057
 in PET, material properties of, 306-308, 308t
Dextrotransposition of great arteries, 601. *See also* Transposition of great arteries (TGA).
Diabetes mellitus
 atherosclerosis associated with, 1197, 1197f
 coronary artery calcium screening in, 463
 in patients with coronary artery disease, 403
 peripheral artery disease associated with, 1197
 restrictive cardiomyopathy associated with, 871
Diastole
 MRI in assessment of, 218, 219f
 physiology of, 63
 ventricular, 59
Diastolic filling ration, early-to-late, 754

Diastolic flow abnormalities, waveform analysis of, in carotid arteries, 1241-1242, 1241f-1244f
Diastolic function
 echocardiography of, 103, 104f-106f
 left ventricular, image interpretation of, 235, 235f
 right ventricular, image interpretation of, 237
Dietary restriction protocols, for PET imaging, 316
Diffuse alveolar hemorrhage, 1383-1384, 1391
Digital subtraction angiography (DSA), 1055, 1060
 of aortic occlusion, 1184, 1184f
 of aortitis, syphilitic, 1323, 1323f
 of arteriovenous fistula failure, 1680-1682, 1683f
 of carotid artery stenosis, 1251
 of femoral artery calcifications, 1188, 1188f
 of graft thrombosis, after lower extremity bypass, 1185-1186, 1186f
 of peripheral artery disease, 1206, 1207f
 of renal artery stenosis, 1478, 1479f-1480f
 of stenosis, after vascular bypass surgery, 1589, 1590f
 of subclavian artery occlusion, 1176, 1176f
 preoperative
  of carotid artery stenosis, 1174, 1175f
  to assessment of inflow, outflow, and runoff, before bypass, 1186-1187, 1188f
Digital vein(s), dorsal
 of lower extremity, 1024-1026, 1026f
 of upper extremity, 1019, 1020f
Dilated cardiomyopathy, 851-860. *See also* Cardiomyopathy, dilated.
Dilators, vascular, 1156
Dipyridamole, 353-355
 chemical structure of, 284f
 mechanism of action of, 354f
 perfusion imaging protocol with, 355, 355f
 in PET, 316
 in SPECT, 284-285, 745
 side effects of, 354t, 355
Directional ambiguity, in Doppler ultrasonography, 1042, 1042f
Displacement encoding with stimulated echoes (DENSE), for quantifying myocardial motion, 230-231, 230t, 765, 765f
Dissection(s)
 aortic. *See* Aortic dissection.
 arterial, after endovascular aneurysm repair, 1436
 carotid artery, 1242-1243
  CT angiography of, 1262, 1263f
  Doppler imaging of, 1243, 1245f
 coronary artery, 129, 129f
 during angioplasty, 1162
Diverticulum of Kommerell, vs. patent ductus arteriosus, 591-592, 591f-592f
Dobutamine, 356
 chemical structure of, 285f
 for MR stress imaging, 267-268
 MR assessment of cardiac function with, 218-223, 767-768
  diagnostic criteria and, 768, 769f
  myocardial ischemia and, 218-221, 220t, 221f
  myocardial viability and, 221-222, 222f, 782
  patient prognosis and, 222-223, 223f
  physiology and safety profile of, 218, 220f

Dobutamine *(Continued)*
 protocols for, 768
 sensitivity and specificity of, 220t
 myocardial viability assessment with, 358
 perfusion imaging protocol with, 355f, 356
  contraindications to, 205, 206t
  in SPECT, 285, 745
  vs. echocardiography, 357-358, 357f
 side effects of, 354t, 356
Dobutamine stress echocardiography (DSE). *See also* Echocardiography.
 vs. dobutamine MR imaging, 218-219
Döhle-Heller syndrome, 1323
Doppler angle, incorrect choice of, in carotid artery ultrasonography, 1233-1234, 1235f
Doppler frequency shift, 1034-1035, 1035f, 1039-1040
 choice of, 1038
 formula for, 1035
Doppler indices, 1045, 1045t
Doppler signal, 1041, 1041t
Doppler spectrum, 1043, 1043f
Doppler ultrasonography. *See also* Echocardiography; Ultrasonography.
 artifacts, pitfalls, and solutions in, 1041-1043, 1041t
 color, 1036
 color flow imaging in, 98-100, 101f
 continuous wave, 98-99, 1036-1037
 contraindications to, 1038
 historical perspective on, 1034-1036, 1035f
 image interpretation in, 1043-1044, 1043f-1044f
 indications for, 1037
 of amyloidosis, 862
 of carotid arteries, 1227-1250
  assessment of plaque in, 1237-1240, 1238f-1239f
  complex waveform pattern in, 1248f, 1249
  components of, 1228
  contraindications to, 1228
  grading of stenosis in, 1233, 1234f-1235f
  indications for, 1228
  normal findings in, 1231-1232, 1232f-1233f
  pitfalls in
   pathological, 1235-1237, 1236f-1238f
   technical, 1233-1234, 1235f
  protocol for, 1231
  technical requirements in, 1227-1237
  technique of, 1228-1231, 1229f-1231f
  waveform analysis in, 1240-1245
   abnormal patterns involving cardiac cycle and, 1242-1245
    arteriovenous fistula, 1244, 1246f
    carotid dissection, 1243, 1245f
    carotid pseudoaneurysm, 1243, 1246f
    intra-aortic balloon pump, 1244-1245, 1247f
    diastolic flow abnormalities in, 1241-1242, 1241f-1244f
    systolic peak abnormality(ies) in, 1240-1241
     parvus tardus waveform, 1240, 1240f
     pulsus alternans waveform, 1241, 1241f
     pulsus bisferiens waveform, 1241, 1241f
 of dilated cardiomyopathy, 852
  anatomic considerations in, 1505-1509
  functional assessment in, 1509, 1510f
  of abdominal aorta, 1508, 1508f-1509f

Doppler ultrasonography *(Continued)*
    of renal arteries, 1505-1507, 1507f-1508f
    of renal veins, 1507-1508, 1508f
    of segmental, interlobar, and arcuate arteries, 1507, 1508f
  fibromuscular dysplasia and, 1498, 1503f
  image interpretation in, 1513-1522
    diagnosis of renal artery aneurysm, 1515
    diagnosis of renal artery stenosis, 1513
      direct criteria for, 1513, 1513b, 1514f
      indirect criteria for, 1513, 1513b, 1515f
    diagnosis of renal artery thrombosis, 1515
    diagnosis of renal vein thrombosis, 1515-1519, 1518f
    diagnostic accuracy of, 1513
    postangioplasty renal artery assessment and, 1514-1515, 1516f-1518f
    renal transplants and, vascular evaluation of, 1519-1522, 1519b, 1519f-1522f
  indications for, 1498b
  pitfalls and solutions in, 1512-1513
    allograft renal vein thrombosis and, 1513
    renal artery stenosis and, 1497-1498
      atherosclerotic, 1497-1498, 1499f-1502f
    renal artery thrombosis and, 1498-1505, 1505f
    renal transplant assessment in, 1505
    renal vein thrombosis and, 1505, 1506f
    Takayasu arteritis and, 1498, 1503f-1504f
  technical considerations in, 1509-1512
    of intrarenal arteries, 1511, 1512f
    of renal arteries, 1509-1511, 1510f-1511f
    of renal morphology, 1511-1512
  technical requirements for, 1497
  techniques of, 1497-1505
    description of, 1505-1512
  of subclavian steal syndrome, 1247-1249, 1247f-1248f
  of thoracic outlet syndrome, 1669
  of upper extremity arteries, 1647-1648, 1648f
  of upper extremity deep vein thrombosis, 1663-1664
    findings in, 1664-1666, 1664f-1668f
    limitations of, 1666, 1668f-1669f
  of vertebral artery, 1246-1249
  postprocessing in, 1044-1045, 1045t
  power, 1036-1037
  pulsed wave, 1036-1037
  reporting of, 1045
  spectral, 1037
  technique of, 1037-1045
    acoustic power in, 1040
    angle of correction in, 1040
    angle of insonation in, 1039-1040, 1040f
    baseline shift in, 1041
    choice of instrumentation in, 1038
    choice of probe and frequency in, 1038
    choice of pulse repetition frequency/velocity scale in, 1038, 1039f
    color and spectrum invert in, 1041
    dwell time in, 1041
    focal zone in, 1041
    gain in, 1040, 1040f
    high-pass filter in, 1040-1041
    sample volume in, 1038, 1039f

Dor procedure, for ischemic heart disease, 811
  postoperative appearance of, 817, 818f
  postoperative complications of, 812
  imaging of, 817-818
Dorsal veins
  digital
    of lower extremity, 1024-1026, 1026f
    of upper extremity, 1019, 1020f
  of penis, 1014
Dorsal venous plexus, upper extremity, 1019-1020, 1021f
Dorsalis pedis artery, 984-985, 985f
Dose modulation, radiation, in CT angiography, 1058
Dosimetry, PET, 319
Double aortic arch, 544, 544f-545f, 958, 959f. *See also* Aortic arch.
Double-outlet right ventricle (DORV), 680-684
  clinical presentation of, 682-684
  definition of, 680
  differential diagnosis of, 607, 608f, 684-685
  etiology and pathophysiology of, 682
  imaging of
    indications and algorithm for, 682
    technique and findings in, 682, 682f-685f
  incidence and epidemiology of, 680-682
  medical treatment of, 685-686
  pathology of, 7
  surgical/interventional treatment of, 686-687
DRASTIC trial, 1480
Dressler syndrome, 94
Drug(s). *See also* named drug or drug group; Pharmacologic stress agent(s).
  as risk factor for pulmonary hypertension, 1359b
  illicit, ventricular septal defect risk associated with, 572-573
  in cardiac MRI stress testing, 267-268
  in CT imaging, 156-159, 157f, 157t-158t
Drug-eluting stents, 515, 517f, 1157
  effectiveness of, 515-516
  repeat stenting with, 520
  risk of thrombosis in, 516, 517f
Dual-energy mode
  in CT angiography, 1057
  of CT angiography, 1057
Dual-head power injectors, of contrast, in CT angiography, 1059-1060
Dual-isotope imaging protocols, with thallium 201 and Tc 99m, for SPECT, 282-283, 746
Ductus aneurysm
  definition of, 590-591
  vs. patent ductus arteriosus, 590-591, 591f
Ductus arteriosus
  patent. *See* Patent ductus arteriosus (PDA).
  physiologic closure of, 583, 584f
    mechanism of, 583
    schematic of, 584f
Ductus bump, vs. patent ductus arteriosus, 588, 590f
Ductus diverticulum
  definition of, 588-590
  vs. patent ductus arteriosus, 588-590, 590f
  vs. traumatic aortic pseudoaneurysm, 1311, 1311f
Duplex ultrasonography. *See also* Ultrasonography.
  of atherosclerotic carotid plaque, 1220-1221, 1221f
  of atherosclerotic disease, 1202-1203
  of carotid and vertebral arteries, in subclavian steal syndrome, 1175, 1175f
  of carotid stenosis, 1220, 1220f

Duplex ultrasonography *(Continued)*
  of limb ischemia
    acute, 1576
    chronic, 1582
  of lower extremity bypass, 1187, 1188f
  of peripheral artery disease, 1629
  of renal artery stenosis, 1473-1475, 1474f
  preoperative, of carotid artery stenosis, 1173-1174, 1173f, 1174t
Duplication(s)
  coronary artery, 48-49
  inferior vena cava, 1525, 1525f
    with retroaortic left renal vein and azygos continuation, 1527
    with retroaortic right renal vein and hemiazygos continuation, 1526-1527
  superior vena cava, 998, 998f
Dwell time, in Doppler ultrasonography, 1041
Dynamic (multiframe) imaging protocol, in emission scanning, 326-327
Dyskinesia, definition of, 232

E

Ebstein anomaly, 653-654, 654f
  considerations regarding, 388, 388t, 391, 391t
  echocardiography of, 119, 653-654
ECG. *See also* Electrocardiography (ECG).
ECG dose modulation, in CT angiography, 1058
ECG gated imaging protocol, in emission scanning, 326-327
ECG gating, in MR angiography, 1103
ECG triggering, prospective, in CT imaging, 134-136, 135f
ECG tube current modulation, in CT imaging, 138-140, 139f
ECG-based reduction, in x-ray tube current, 151
  pitfalls and solutions for, 151-152
ECG-gated reconstruction, retrospective, in CT imaging, 136, 137f
Echocardiography, 98-122. *See also* Ultrasonography.
  contrast, 107
  dobutamine stress, vs. dobutamine MR imaging, 218-219
  Doppler. *See* Doppler ultrasonography.
  fundamental image in, 98
  harmonic image in, 98
  intracardiac, 101-110
    indications for, 101-110
  M mode, 98, 99f
  of amyloidosis, 115-116, 116f
  of aortic aneurysms, thoracic, 1280
  of aortic dissection, 117, 118f
  of aortic regurgitation, 110, 832-833
  of aortic stenosis, 109, 828
  of arrhythmogenic right ventricular dysplasia, 113, 887-888, 888t
  of atrial septal defect, 117-118
  of cardiomyopathy, 110-113
    dilated, 110
    hypertrophic, 110-113
    noncompaction, 113, 114f-115f
    restrictive, 113
  of congenital heart disease, 117-118
  of coronary artery disease, 107, 108f-109f
  of cyanotic heart lesions, 651
  of diastolic function, 103, 104f-106f
  of Ebstein anomaly, 119, 653-654
  of endocarditis, 110, 113f

Echocardiography *(Continued)*
  of fibroma, 116
  of ischemic heart disease, postoperative, 813-814
  of malignant tumors, 116
  of mitral regurgitation, 110, 837
  of mitral stenosis, 109-110, 111f-112f, 835, 835f
  of myxoma, 116, 117f
  of papillary fibroelastoma, 116
  of patent ductus arteriosus, 118
  of pericardial diseases, 113-115
  of pericarditis, constrictive, 115, 116f
  of prosthetic valves, 110
  of pulmonary hypertension, 105, 106f, 1356
    chronic thromboembolic, 1345
    with left heart disease (venous), 1364
  of pulmonary insufficiency, 381, 381f
  of pulmonary valve stenosis, 846
  of pulmonary venous connections, anomalous, 118
  of rhabdomyoma, 116
  of systemic veins, anomalous, 118
  of systolic function and quantification, 103, 104f-105f
  of tamponade, 113
  of tetralogy of Fallot, 119, 642
    postnatal, 642-643, 643f
  of transposition of great arteries
    complete, 119, 611-612
      after atrial switch procedure, 612
    congenitally corrected, 119
  of tricuspid valve regurgitation, 845
  of univentricular atrioventricular connection, 119, 119f
  of valvular heart disease, 65-66, 107
  of ventricular outflow tract obstruction, 118
  of ventricular septal defect, 118
  stress
    of acute coronary syndrome, 717
    of coronary artery disease, 107
    of dilated cardiomyopathy, 853
  technical requirements in, 98-110
  three-dimensional, 101
  tissue velocities and strain imaging in, 119-122, 120f-121f
  transesophageal. *See* Transesophageal echocardiography (TEE).
  transtracheal. *See* Transtracheal echocardiography (TTE).
  two-dimensional, 98, 100f
  vs. dobutamine stress perfusion imaging, 357-358, 357f
Echo-planar imaging (EPI) technique, of MR imaging, 228-229, 228t
Edema, pulmonary. *See* Pulmonary edema.
Edge artifact, in Doppler ultrasonography, 1043
Edwards hypothetical double aortic arch, 542, 543f
Effective orifice area (EOA), patient-prosthetic mismatch due to, 421
Effective orifice area (EOA) index, 421
Effusion
  pericardial. *See* Pericardial effusion.
  pleural, postoperative, radiographic features of, 96
Effusive pericarditis, 438, 438f. *See also* Pericarditis.
Ehlers-Danlos syndrome, 1601, 1603f
  vascular, 1273
Eisenmenger syndrome, 573, 577, 584, 1359
  cyanosis and clubbing in, 585

Ejection fraction (EF), 58
  left ventricular
    ^{99m}Tc-sestamibi imaging of, 286f
    calculation of, 103, 106f
    change in, after revascularization, 335t
    coronary artery disease and, 329, 329f-330f
    MR assessment of, 216
    Simpson's rule in, 215
Elastic recoil
  contributing to coronary restenosis, 515, 516f
  in angioplasty, 1162
Elbow, brachial artery at, 993, 993f
Elderly populations, coronary artery calcium assessment in, 462-463
Electrical impulse, conduction of, 57
Electricity, as MRI safety issue, 263
Electrocardiography (ECG). *See also* ECG entries.
  abnormal, in arrhythmogenic right ventricular dysplasia, 886-887, 887t
  during gated MPI acquisition, in ventricular function assessment, 772
  monitoring of, during exercise or pharmacologic stress imaging, 358-359
  normal appearance of, 57, 58f
  synchronization of, with computed tomography, 134, 135f
Electromagnetic energy, in radiation, 270
Electron(s)
  Auger, 271-272, 272f
  physics of, 270, 271f
  recoil, 275
Electron capture, 272-273, 272t, 273f
Electron shells, 270, 271f
Electron transition, mechanisms of, 271-272, 272f
Embolectomy, balloon catheter, for saddle embolus, 1578
Embolic agents, 1167-1169
  liquid, 1168-1169
  particulate, 1167-1168
Embolization, 1167-1170
  for arteriovenous fistula and pseudoaneurysm, in renal transplant recipient, 1565-1566, 1566f
  imaging findings in, 1170
  indications for and contraindications to, 1170
  liquid agents for, 1168-1169, 1169f
  mechanical occlusion devices for, 1168
  nontarget, 1170
  nonthrombotic, 1368-1370
    clinical presentation of, 1369
    etiology and pathophysiology of, 1368
    imaging technique and findings in, 1369-1370, 1369f-1370f
  outcomes and complications of, 1170
  particulate agents for, 1167-1168
  principles of, 1169-1170
Embolus (embolism)
  cerebral, in infective endocarditis, 429, 429f
  coronary artery, 129
  in myxomas, 906-907
  pulmonary. *See* Pulmonary embolism.
  shower, after endovascular aneurysm repair, 1435
  sites of, in acute limb ischemia, 1574-1575, 1574f
Embryogenesis, of inferior vena cava, 1527
Emission scans, in myocardial perfusion studies, 326-327
Enalaprilat, IV administration of, in ACEI renal scintigraphy, 1493

Endarterectomy, carotid. *See* Carotid endarterectomy.
Endarterectomy versus Angioplasty in patients with Symptomatic Severe Carotid Stenosis (EVA-3S) trial, 1223
End-diastolic velocity (EDV), effect of heart rate on, 1235-1236
Endocardial cushion defect, 5
Endocarditis
  infective. *See* Infective endocarditis.
  Löffler, 864-866. *See also* Eosinophilic endomyocardial disease.
Endograft(s). *See also* Stent(s).
  aneurysm repair with, 1420, 1421f
    clinical presentation after, 1426
    complication(s) of
      arterial dissection as, 1436
      colon necrosis as, 1435-1436
      endoleaks as, 1431-1434, 1431f-1434f
      graft infection as, 1434
      graft kinking as, 1434
      graft occlusion as, 1434-1435
      graft thrombosis as, 1434, 1434f-1436f
      hematoma at arteriotomy site as, 1436
      shower embolism as, 1435
    death during, 1426
    endoleak after, 1426, 1428t
    goal of, 1420
    graft placement in, 1422-1423, 1424f-1426f
      surgical conversion after, 1423-1424, 1427f, 1440, 1443f
    imaging of
      indications and algorithm for, 1426-1429
      techniques and findings in, 1429-1436, 1429f-1430f, 1430t
    postoperative assessment of, 1420-1436, 1423f-1428f
    postoperative management after, 1436-1437
    preprocedural interventions and, 1422-1423, 1423f
    success of, 1422
      anatomic appearance after, 1426, 1428f
    vs. open surgical repair, 1424-1426
  classification of, 1408t
  percutaneous placement of, for aortic atherosclerotic disease, 1195-1196
Endoleak(s)
  after endovascular aneurysm repair, 1407-1409, 1431-1434
  classification of, 1426, 1428t
  etiology and pathophysiology of, 1408, 1408f, 1408t
  imaging of
    indications and algorithm for, 1408
    techniques and findings in, 1408-1409, 1409f
  prevalence and epidemiology of, 1407
  treatment options for, 1409
  Type I, 1431-1434, 1431f-1432f, 1436
  Type II, 1431-1434, 1432f-1433f, 1436-1437
  Type III, 1431-1434, 1434f, 1437
  Type IV, 1437
  definition of, 1436
  postoperative management of, 1436-1437
  primary and secondary, 1436
  recurrent, 1436
Endomyocardial fibrosis, 864-866. *See also* Eosinophilic endomyocardial disease.
  radiation-induced, 871

Endovascular aortic aneurysm repair (EVAR), 1181-1182, 1183f-1184f
  complications of, 1407-1409. See also Endoleak(s).
Endovascular Aortic Aneurysm Repair (EVAR) trial, 1420-1422
Endovascular procedure(s)
  exclusion or occlusion, for lower extremity aneurysm, 1604-1608. See also Lower extremity aneurysm, endovascular exclusion procedures for.
  for abdominal aortic aneurysm. See Abdominal aortic aneurysm, endovascular repair of.
  for penetrating atherosclerotic ulcer, 1301-1302
  for thoracic aortic trauma, 1312-1313, 1312f
  for type B aortic dissection, 1295-1296, 1296f
  lower extremity, 1591-1598
    anatomic considerations in, 1591-1594, 1592f-1595f
    angioplasty and stent placement as, 1591-1592, 1592f-1593f
    atherectomy as, 1592, 1593f-1594f
    contraindications to, 1596
    cryoplasty as, 1592, 1595f
    cutting balloon angioplasty as, 1593
    imaging findings in, 1597-1598, 1597f
    indications for, 1594-1596, 1595t, 1596f
    outcomes and complications of, 1596-1597
Endovascular stents, 1157
End-stage renal disease, 1673-1674
Energy discrimination, in SPECT, 278
Energy metabolism, alterations of, in hibernating myocardium, 792
Enzyme-linked immunosorbent assay (ELISA), sensitivity and specificity of, 1333, 1333t
Eosinophilic endomyocardial disease
  clinical presentation of, 865
  definition of, 864
  etiology and pathophysiology of, 864-865
  imaging of
    indications and algorithm for, 865
    technique and findings in, 865-866, 865f-866f, 872t
  medical treatment of, 871
  prevalence and epidemiology of, 864
Epigastric artery
  inferior, 978, 979f
  thoracoabdominal arterial anastomosis through, 985, 986f
Equilibrium gated blood pool imaging, of ventricular function
  indications for, 773
  technique of, 773-775, 774f-778f
Esophageal varices, from portal hypertension, 1008-1009, 1008f
  MR imaging of, 1454-1455, 1455f
Esophagus, CT imaging of, 447-448, 448f
Ethylene-vinyl alcohol copolymer, as embolic agent, 1168-1169, 1169f
EUROSTAR registry, of endoleaks, 1407
Evian classification, of pulmonary hypertension, 1354, 1354b
Excitation, of transferred energy, 271
Exclusion procedure(s), lower extremity
  endovascular methods as, 1604-1608
  surgical excision and vascular bypass as, 1600-1604
Exercise
  for peripheral artery disease, 1209
  MR assessment of cardiac function with, 223-224, 223f, 767

Exercise stress protocols
  in SPECT, 283, 283t, 744
  vs. pharmacologic stress protocols, 358-359, 359t, 744
Extracellular matrix formation, in atherosclerosis, 1195
Extremity
  lower. See Lower extremity.
  upper. See Upper extremity.

F

False aneurysm, 1271, 1277, 1277f. See also Pseudoaneurysm.
  delayed hyperenhancement MR imaging of, 209-210
Faraday's law, 263
Fast low-angle shot (FLASH) technique
  comparison of left ventricular volume by, vs. steady-state free precession, 231-232
  of MR imaging, 227, 228t
Fast pulse sequences, in accelerated MR imaging, 194-195, 194f
Fast-field echo (FFE) technique, of MR imaging, 227, 228t
Fat pad sign, epicardial, in pericardial effusion, 942
Fatty acid radiotracers, in PET/SPECT imaging, 800-801, 801f-802f
Fatty streaks, in atherosclerosis, 60
FBN1 gene, in Marfan syndrome, 550
Femoral artery
  calcifications in, digital subtraction angiography of, 1188, 1188f
  common, 978, 979f, 983
    angiographic access via, 1157-1158
  superficial, 983, 983f, 987f
Femoral vein, deep, 1028
Femoral-femoral bypass graft, 981-982, 982f
  right-to-left, 1586-1588, 1588f
Femoral-popliteal bypass graft, 981-982, 982f
Femoropopliteal artery(ies), occlusion of, MR angiography of, 1636, 1637f
Femoropopliteal bypass graft
  above-knee, 1590, 1590t
  below-knee, 1590, 1590t
Ferucarbotran (SHU555), 258t, 259
Feruglose (NC100150), 258t, 259
Ferumoxide (AMI 25), 258t, 259
Ferumoxtran (AMI 227), 258t, 259
Fever, postoperative, ischemic heart disease and, 813
Fibrillation, atrial. See Atrial fibrillation.
Fibroatheroma, 457-458
Fibroelastoma, papillary, 116, 909-910, 910f-911f
Fibroma
  differential diagnosis of, 913
  echocardiography of, 116
  manifestations of disease in, 911-913, 912f
  pathology of, 911, 911f
  prevalence of, 911
  treatment options for, 913
Fibromuscular dysplasia
  arterial narrowing or aneurysm caused by, 975, 976f
  Doppler ultrasonography of, 1498, 1503f
  renal artery stenosis caused by, 1471
  prevalence and epidemiology of, 1471-1472
Fibrosing mediastinitis
  clinical presentation of, 1371
  etiology and pathophysiology of, 1370-1371
  imaging of, 1371

Fibrosis, nephrogenic systemic, 253-255
  as contraindication to contrast-enhanced MR angiography, 1255-1257
  causes of, 254
  in chronic kidney disease, 1673
  risk of, gadolinium-containing contrast agents and, 254, 1453
Fibrous cap, in atherosclerosis, 1195, 1196f
Field of view
  in contrast-enhanced MR angiography, 1254-1255, 1255f-1256f
  in CT angiography of lower extremities, 1614, 1615f
Field strength, in MR angiography, 1102
Filter
  in Doppler ultrasonography
    high-pass, 1040-1041
    wall, setting of, 1041-1042
  inferior vena caval, 1540, 1540f
Filtered back projection (FBP) approach
  to PET reconstruction, 313
  to SPECT reconstruction, 279
Fistula
  aortocaval, 1441, 1443
  aortoduodenal, after abdominal aortic aneurysm repair, 1180
  aortoenteric, 1415-1416, 1416f, 1441, 1445-1447, 1448f
    postoperative management of, 1447
  arteriovenous. See Arteriovenous fistula.
  atrioesophageal, after ablation for atrial fibrillation, 451, 451f
  coronary artery, 473, 474f
  hemodialysis, 1672-1685. See also Arteriovenous fistula, in hemodialyis patient; Arteriovenous graft.
Fixed scan delay, in CT angiography, 1058
Fleischner lines, 1334
Flow direction artifact, in Doppler ultrasonography, 1042, 1042f
Flow-encoding axes, in MR evaluation of blood flow, 239-240, 241f
Fluorodeoxyglucose (FDG)
  in PET imaging, 801
    protocol(s) in, 801-803
      hyperinsulinemic-euglycemic clamping, 803
      intravenous glucose loading, 803
      nicotinic acid derivative, 803
      oral glucose loading, 802-803
  in PET/CT imaging, 326, 342-343, 342f-343f
    of myocardial perfusion, 333-334, 333f-334f
    patient preparation for, 332-333, 333f
  in SPECT imaging, 805
  kinetics of, 315
Focal neurologic deficits, postoperative, ischemic heart disease and, 813
Focal zone, in Doppler ultrasonography, 1041
Fogarty embolectomy catheter, 1577-1578, 1577f
Fontaine stages, of peripheral artery disease, of limbs, 1578, 1579t
Fontan procedure
  MR imaging after, 675-676, 676f-677f, 699-700
  variant of, for single-ventricle defects, 390
  postoperative management after, 699-700
Food and Drug Administration (FDA)
  regulatory approval, of contrast agents, 251-252
Foot amputation, for chronic limb ischemia, 1583-1584

Foramen ovale
  anatomy of, 443
  patent. See Patent foramen ovale.
Fourier transform scanning, two-dimensional, 1080, 1080f-1081f
  gradient pulse echo sequence for, 1080, 1080f
Fracture, rib, 1306-1307
Frequency shift, Doppler, 1034-1035, 1035f, 1039-1040
  choice of, 1038
  formula for, 1035
Frequency-encoding gradient, in MR angiography, 1080
Friction rub, in pericarditis, 945-946
Fusobacterium necrophorum, in Lemierre's syndrome, 1670

G

Gadobenate, 256, 257t
Gadobuterol, 256, 257t
Gadodiamide, 256, 257t
Gadolinium agents
  pharmacovigilance of, 253
  physiochemical characteristics of, 257t
  standard nonprotein interacting, 256
  use and safety of, in MR imaging of abdominal vascular disorders, 1453
  with macromolecular structures, 253-254
  with strong protein interaction, 256-258
  with weak protein interaction, 256
Gadopentate dimeglumine, 256, 257t
Gadotexetate disodium, 256, 257t
Gadoversetamide, 256, 257t
Gamma camera
  components of, 276, 276f
  used in SPECT, 739
Gamma ray(s), 270
  emission of, 272t, 273
Gangrene
  lower limb, 1581
  wet, 1581
Gastric artery, 970, 973f
Gastric vein, 1006f-1007f, 1007-1008
Gastroduodenal artery, 972, 973f
Gastroduodenal pseudoaneurysm, 1463, 1464f, 1469f
Gastroepiploic vein
  left, 1006-1007, 1006f-1007f
  right, 1006, 1006f-1007f
Gastrointestinal bleed localization scan
  image interpretation of, 1146
  indications and contraindications to, 1144-1146
  pitfalls and solutions in, 1146, 1147t
Gated blood pool (GBP) imaging, of ventricular function
  indications for, 773
  technique of, 773-775, 774f-778f
Gating
  in cardiac MR imaging, 201-202
    electrocardiographic, 201-202
    navigator echo technique of, 202, 203f
  in CT angiography
    prospective, 1057-1058
    retrospective, 1057
Gauss' law, 263
Gelfoam, as embolic agent, 1167
Gender, role of, in atherosclerosis, 1196
Generalized autocalibrating partially parallel acquisitions (GRAPPA), in parallel imaging, 195

Genetic mutations, in arrhythmogenic right ventricular dysplasia, 884-885, 885t
Genetic predisposition, to atherosclerosis, 1196
Genetic screening
  for dilated cardiomyopathy, 851
  for truncus arteriosus, 618
Giant cell arteritis, 1390-1391, 1414-1415
  aneurysm dilation due to, 1275
  clinical presentation of, 1320, 1391
  definition of, 1320
  diagnosis of, American College of Rheumatology criteria for, 1320t
  differential diagnosis of, 1414
  etiology and pathophysiology of, 1320, 1414
  imaging of
    indications and algorithm for, 1320, 1414
    technique and findings in, 1320-1321, 1321f-1322f, 1391, 1391f, 1414, 1415f
  incidence of, 1644
  prevalence and epidemiology of, 1320, 1414
  treatment options for, 1322, 1415
  upper extremity affected by, 1643-1644
  vs. Takayasu arteritis, 1319t
Glagov phenomenon, in atherosclerosis, 1195, 1195f
Glucocorticoids, for giant cell arteritis, 1322
Glucose loading
  in ^{18}FDG-PET imaging, 332-333
    intravenous, 803
    oral, 802-803
  principle of, 316
Gluteal artery, inferior, 978-981, 980f
Gluteal vein, 1012, 1013f-1014f
Gonadal artery, 975, 981
Goodpasture syndrome, 1393-1394, 1393f
Gorlin syndrome, fibromas associated with, 911
Gradient coils
  as embolic agents, 1168
  in MR angiography, 1084, 1084f
    birdcage, 1083
    contrast-enhanced, dedicated, 1253-1254
    gradient, 1102
    phased-array surface, 1102-1103
    RF field detection by, 1083
Gradient system, magnetic field
  as MRI safety issue, 263
  in MR angiography, 1083
Gradient-recalled-echo (GRE) techniques, of MR imaging, 181
  three-dimensional, 1452
Graft(s). See also Allograft(s); Bypass graft(s); Prosthetic graft(s); Xenograft(s).
  arteriovenous, 1672
  failure of, focal lesion causing, 1591
  placement of, in endovascular aneurysm repair, 1422-1423, 1424f-1426f
  success of, 1423-1424, 1427f
Graft aneurysm, after CABG surgery, 525
Graft infection
  after abdominal aortic aneurysm repair, 1180, 1180f
  after endovascular aneurysm repair, 1434
  after lower extremity bypass, 1185-1186, 1186f
  after vascular bypass surgery, 1589
  aortic, 1441, 1443-1447, 1446f-1447f
  postoperative management of, 1449
Graft kinking, after aneurysm repair, 1434
  endovascular, 1434

Graft occlusion
  after CABG surgery, 524-525, 527f-529f
  after endovascular aneurysm repair, 1434-1435
Graft patency
  femoropopliteal
    above-knee, 1590, 1590t
    below-knee, 1590, 1590t
  in revascularization procedures, 1589
  infrapopliteal, 1590, 1591t
Graft thrombosis
  after endovascular aneurysm repair, 1434, 1434f-1436f
  after lower extremity bypass, 1185-1186, 1186f
Granulomatosis
  necrotizing sarcoid, 1392
  Wegener's. See Wegener's granulomatosis.
Grating artifact, in Doppler ultrasonography, 1042
Great arteries. See also Aorta; Pulmonary artery(ies).
  identification of, 16, 16f
  relationship of, 18, 20f
  transposition of. See Transposition of great arteries (TGA).
Grey-Turner sign, in abdominal aortic aneurysm, 1440
Ground-glass opacity
  in Wegener's granulomatosis, 1385, 1386f
  of lung, 1376
Guide wires, 1156

H

Half-Fourier acquisition single-shot turbo spin-echo (HASTE) imaging, 204
Hampton hump sign, in pulmonary embolism, 1334, 1334f
Hand
  arch variations in, 994f
  arterial anatomy of, 993f
  superficial veins of, 1019-1020, 1020f-1021f
Harmonic imaging, contrast-enhanced, in ultrasonography, 1037
Hazards, associated with MR imaging, 261-262
Head and neck
  arterial blood supply to, 1217
  venous drainage of, 999
Hearing protection, for MR imaging, 267
Heart. See also Cardiac; Cardio-; Myocardial entries.
  anatomy of, 30-37, 31f-36f
  boot-shaped, in tetralogy of Fallot, 641-642, 642f
  chambers of. See also Atrial entries; Atrium (atria); Ventricle(s); Ventricular entries.
    anatomy of, 30, 31f
    blood flow through, 58-59, 59f
    contraction of, 57
    identification of, 13
  conduction system of, 57-58, 58f
  coronary arteries of, 412, 413f. See also Coronary artery(ies).
  CT imaging of, 133-142. See also Computed tomography (CT), cardiac.
  echocardiography of, 98-122. See also under Echocardiography.
  hypertrophy of, 63
  left-sided lesions of, extreme forms of, 388, 388t

Heart (Continued)
    MR imaging of, 180-200, 215-226. See also
        Magnetic resonance imaging (MRI),
        cardiac.
    physiology of, 57-68
    radiology of, 71-97. See also Chest
        radiography.
        normal and abnormal cardiac borders in,
            71-78. See also Chest radiography, of
            cardiac borders.
    right-sided lesions of, 388, 388t
    size of, radiographic measurement of, 78-80
    types of, different, 19-25, 21f
Heart disease
    congenital. See Congenital heart disease
        (CHD).
    ischemic. See Ischemic heart disease (IHD).
    segmental approach to, 3
        case study in, 27f, 28
        embryologic basis for, 11-12
        evaluation of function in, 24-25, 27f
    valvular
        catheter-based management of, 405-409,
            407f-408f
        MR evaluation of blood flow in, 241-242,
            243f
        radiographic studies of, 92-94, 93f
Heart failure
    congestive, 810
    hyperadrenergic state of, 805
    mortality rates associated with, 790
Heart murmur, holosystolic, in ventricular
    septal defect, 573
Heart rate
    effect of, on peak systolic velocity and
        end-diastolic velocity, 1235-1236, 1236f
    in three-dimensional steady-state free
        precession MR angiography, 1107
    variability of, in coronary CT angiography,
        481-482, 485f
Heart rhythm, in three-dimensional steady-
    state free precession MR angiography,
    1107
Heart sounds, S_2, in atrial septal defect, 564
Heart transplantation
    for arrhythmogenic right ventricular
        dysplasia, 894
    for ischemic heart disease, 811-812
        postoperative appearance of, 818,
            819f-820f
        postoperative complications of, 812-813
            imaging of, 818-820, 821f
Heart tube
    components of, 3-4, 4f
    formation of, 3-13
Heart valves. See also named valve.
    anatomy of, 34-36, 35f-36f
    function of, 58-59
    insufficiency or stenosis of, 64-66. See also
        under specific valve.
        imaging assessment of, 65-66, 66f
    prosthetic. See Prosthetic heart valve.
Heart-to-blood pool count ratio, in PET/CT
    imaging, 327-328
Heath-Edwards grading system, of pulmonary
    hypertension, 1359-1360
Helical (spiral) computed tomography. See
    also Computed tomography (CT).
    vs. step-and-shoot CT, 1051-1053,
        1051f-1052f
Helical pitch (h)
    definition of, 1051-1052
    increased helical artifacts with, 1052, 1052f
    selection of, 1053
Helium, liquid, used in MRI scanners, 264

Hemangiomatosis, pulmonary capillary,
    1362-1363, 1363f
Hematoma
    at arteriotomy site, after endovascular
        aneurysm repair, 1436
    intramural
        CT imaging of, 816-817, 817f
        of aorta, 1296-1299. See also Intramural
            hematoma, aortic.
Hemiazygos vein, anatomy of, 1000,
    1001f
Hemitruncus, 621
Hemodialysis, for chronic kidney disease,
    1672
    access fistulas in, 1672, 1673f. See also
        Arteriovenous fistula, in hemodialysis
        patient; Arteriovenous graft.
Hemodialysis-associated amyloidosis, 861.
    See also Amyloidosis.
Hemolytic anemia, chronic, pulmonary
    hypertension associated with, 1360
Hemorrhage
    after vascular bypass surgery, 1589
    diffuse alveolar, 1383-1384, 1391
    mediastinal, postoperative, radiographic
        features of, 96
    periaortic mediastinal, in thoracic aortic
        trauma, 1309, 1309f
    perioperative
        in operative field, 816, 817f
        ischemic heart disease and, 813
    pulmonary, differential diagnosis of, 1384t
Hemorrhagic telangiectasia, hereditary, 1468
Hemosiderosis, idiopathic pulmonary,
    1392-1393, 1393f
Heparin
    for inferior vena cava thrombosis, 1539
    preprocedural, for carotid artery stenting,
        1224
Hepatic. See also Liver entries.
Hepatic angiography, 1159
Hepatic arteriovenous malformations, 1468
Hepatic artery, 971-972, 972f
    anatomy of
        CT angiography of, 1545, 1545f-1546f
        Michel classification of, 1545, 1546t
    variant donor, 1546, 1546f
Hepatic artery pseudoaneurysm, after liver
    transplantation, 1551, 1553f
Hepatic artery stenosis, after liver
    transplantation, 1550, 1552f-1553f
Hepatic artery thrombosis
    after liver transplantation, 1548-1551,
        1548f-1552f
    MR imaging of, 1460-1461, 1460f
Hepatic transplantation, 1544-1558
    cadaveric, surgical anatomy of, 1546-1547,
        1547f
    complication(s) after, 1547-1554
        hepatic artery pseudoaneurysm as, 1551,
            1553f
        hepatic artery stenosis as, 1550,
            1552f-1553f
        hepatic artery thrombosis as, 1548-1551,
            1548f-1552f
        inferior vena cava stenosis as, 1534-1535,
            1553-1554, 1555f-1556f
            clinical presentation of, 1534
            definition of, 1534
            differential diagnosis of, 1535
            imaging of, 1534-1535, 1534f-1537f
            prevalence and epidemiology of, 1534
            treatment options for, 1535
        portal vein stenosis as, 1551-1553,
            1554f-1555f

Hepatic transplantation (Continued)
        portal vein thrombosis as, 1551,
            1553f-1554f
        venous aneurysms as, 1551,
            1554f
    contraindications to, 1544
    imaging prior to
        indications and algorithm for,
            1459-1460
        technique and findings in, 1460-1461,
            1460f-1461f
    indications for, 1544
    manifestations of disease prior to, 1459
    pretransplant work-up for, 1544-1546
        imaging of liver transplant recipients in,
            1544-1545
        imaging of potential living donors for,
            1545-1546, 1545f-1546f, 1546t
    prevalence and epidemiology of, 1459
Hepatic vasculature, CT angiography of, 1066,
    1068f
Hepatic vein, anatomy of, 1010, 1010f,
    1545-1546
    variations of, 1010-1011
Hepatic veno-occlusive disease, vs. Budd-
    Chiari syndrome, 1461, 1462f
Hepatocellular carcinoma
    inferior vena cava invasion by, 1530-1531,
        1533f
    MR imaging of, 1458-1459, 1459f
    vs. arterioportal shunts, 1457
Hereditary amyloidosis, 861. See also
    Amyloidosis.
Hereditary hemorrhagic telangiectasia,
    1468
Heterotaxy
    definition of, 16-18
    syndromic approach to, 18, 18f-19f
High-altitude pulmonary edema, 1381-1382
High-attenuation object, as contraindication to
    CT angiography, 1614, 1614f
High-pass filter, in Doppler ultrasonography,
    1040-1041
Holosystolic murmur, in ventricular septal
    defect, 573
Human herpes virus 6, in myocarditis,
    898-899
Human immunodeficiency virus (HIV)
    infection, pulmonary hypertension
    associated with, 1359-1360
Hunter's canal, 983
Hybrid devices, for valvular heart disease,
    409
Hybrid procedures
    for aortoiliac and lower extremity occlusive
        disease, 1188-1189, 1188f
    in abdominal aortic aneurysm repair,
        1181-1182, 1183f-1184f
    in thoracic aortic aneurysm repair,
        1178-1179, 1178f-1179f
Hypercoagulability, in deep vein thrombosis,
    1663
Hyperenhancement
    delayed, in cardiac MR imaging
        description of, 210-211, 211f
        indications for, 207-210, 208f-210f
        pitfalls and solutions in, 212, 212f
        reporting of, 212-213, 213f
    of myocardial viability, MR imaging of,
        782-784, 783f-786f
Hyperinsulinemic-euglycemic clamping,
    332-333
    in ^{18}FDG-PET imaging, 803
Hyperperfusion syndrome, after carotid
    endarterectomy, 1173

Hypertension
  atherosclerosis associated with, 1196-1197
  portal. See also Portal hypertension.
  pulmonary, 1353-1358. See also Pulmonary hypertension.
  renovascular
    ACEI scintigraphy of. See Angiotensin-converting enzyme inhibitor (ACEI) scintigraphy, of renal arteries.
    secondary to renal artery stenosis, 1471, 1492
Hypertrophic cardiomyopathy, 63, 874-883. See also Cardiomyopathy, hypertrophic.
Hypoplastic left heart syndrome (HLHS), 8
  etiology and pathophysiology of, 671-672
  Norwood procedure for, 389, 672
  prevalence and epidemiology of, 671
  vs. coarctation of aorta, 538
Hypothenar hammer syndrome, 1645
  incidence of, 1646
Hypoxia, pulmonary hypertension caused by, 1365-1366

I

Ibuprofen, for pericarditis, 947
Idiopathic hypereosinophilic syndrome (IHES), 864-866. See also Eosinophilic endomyocardial disease.
Idiopathic pulmonary hemosiderosis, 1392-1393, 1393f
Idiopathic pulmonary hypertension, 1358-1359, 1358f-1359f. See also Pulmonary hypertension.
  definition of, 1358
Ileal vein, anatomy of, 1005, 1006f
Ileocolic vein, anatomy of, 1006, 1006f
Iliac artery
  circumflex, deep and superficial, 978, 979f
  common, 975, 978, 979f, 1028-1029
  external, 978, 979f, 1028-1029
  internal, 978
    anterior division of, 978-981, 980f
    posterior division of, 978, 980f
    variations of, 981
  lesions involving, MR angiography of, 1635-1636, 1636f
Iliac artery aneurysm
  definition of, 1019
  endovascular repair of, 1420, 1422f. See also Endograft(s), aneurysm repair with.
  goal of, 1420
Iliac occlusion, balloon thrombectomy for, 1578, 1578f
Iliac vein
  common, 1012
  external, 1012, 1013f
  internal, 1012-1014, 1013f-1014f
Iliac vein compression syndrome (IVCS), 1015, 1015f, 1535
Iliolumbar artery, 978, 980f
Illicit drug use, ventricular septal defect risk associated with, 572-573
Image acquisition
  in CT angiography, 1057-1058
  in MR imaging, 227-229
Image aliasing artifact, in MR imaging, 1397
Image encoding, in MR angiography, 1079-1081, 1080f-1082f
Image generation, in SPECT, 279

Image interpretation
  of brain perfusion tomography, 1148-1150
  of CT angiography, 1073-1075
    coronary, 127-131, 127f-131f, 500-504
  of GI bleed localization scan, 1146
  of Meckel diverticulum scan, 1148
  of SPECT, 285-296, 286f-296f
  of three-dimensional contrast-enhanced MR angiography, 1116-1118
  of three-dimensional steady-state free precession MR angiography, 1108-1109, 1108f
  of time-of-flight MR angiography, 1105
  of TR MR angiography, 1112
Image quality
  in cardiac CT imaging, 144-145
  in CT angiography, 1056
  in PET/CT systems, 320-322
    elevated activity in inferior wall at stress and, 322, 323f
    metal implants and, 321-322, 322f
    prompt gamma correction and, 321, 321f
    streaking and lateral wall overcorrection and, 321, 321f
    truncation and, 322, 323f
Image reconstruction
  in MR angiography, 1078-1081
  in PET imaging, 313-314, 314f
Imaging modalities. See specific modality.
Imaging processing, in computed tomography, 168-171, 172f
Imaging times, prolonged, in time-of-flight MR angiography, 1105
Implantable cardioverter-defibrillators (ICDs)
  as MRI safety issue, 264-265
  as PET image artifact, 321-322, 322f
  for arrhythmogenic right ventricular dysplasia, 894
Implants, metallic, as contraindication to contrast-enhanced MR angiography, 1257
Infarction
  myocardial. See Myocardial infarction.
  renal, 1447, 1449f
  segmental, in renal allograft, 1520, 1521f
  splenic, 1466-1467, 1467f
Infection
  after cardiac transplantation
    imaging of, 818-819, 821f
    mediastinal, 812-813, 819-820
    postoperative management of, 821-823
  aortic aneurysm after, 594, 594f
    thoracic, 1275, 1276f
  aortic graft, 1441, 1443-1447, 1446f-1447f
    postoperative management of, 1449
  graft
    after endovascular aneurysm repair, 1434
    after lower extremity bypass, 1185-1186, 1186f
  prosthetic graft, 1284-1285
Infectious agents
  causing acute pericarditis, 945, 946t
  causing myocarditis, 896
Infective endocarditis, 429-432
  clinical manifestations of, 429, 429f-430f, 430t
  echocardiography of, 110, 113f
  surgery for
    contraindications to, 430-431
    goals of, 430, 430f
    indications for, 430, 430t-431t
    outcomes and complications of, 431
    postoperative surveillance after, 431-432, 432f
    preoperative imaging in, 431-432, 432f-433f

Inferior vena cava
  anastomosis of, 1547, 1547f
  anatomy of, 998-999
    normal, 1524, 1525f
    variations in, 998-999, 999f, 1014-1015
  azygos continuation of, 1525, 1526f
  circumaortic left renal vein anomaly of, 1525, 1527f
  circumcaval ureter anomaly of, 1526
  congenital anomalies of, 1524-1527, 1525f-1527f
    clinical presentation of, 1527-1528
    etiology and pathophysiology of, 1527
    imaging of
      indications and algorithm for, 1528
      technique and findings in, 1528-1529
    prevalence and epidemiology of, 1527
    reporting of, 1529
  duplicated right renal vein anomaly of, 1526
  duplication of, 1525, 1525f
    with retroaortic left renal vein and azygos continuation, 1527
    with retroaortic right renal vein and hemiazygos continuation, 1526-1527
  embryogenesis of, 1527
  formation of, 1009, 1009f
  inflow to, 1009-1010, 1010f
  left-sided anomaly of, 1525
  partial/complete absence of, 1526
  retroaortic left renal vein anomaly of, 1525
  tumors of, 1529-1532
    clinical presentation of, 1529
    differential diagnosis of, 1532-1533, 1533f
    etiology and pathophysiology of, 1529
    imaging of
      indications and algorithm for, 1529-1530
      technique and findings in, 1530-1532, 1531f-1533f
    prevalence and epidemiology of, 1529
    reporting of, 1533
    treatment options for, 1533
Inferior vena cava interventions
  definition of, 1540
  filters, 1540, 1540f
  shunts, 1540-1541, 1541f
  stents, 1541-1542, 1541f
Inferior vena cava obstruction syndrome, 1529
Inferior vena cava stenosis, after liver transplantation, 1534-1535, 1553-1554, 1555f-1556f
  clinical presentation of, 1534
  definition of, 1534
  differential diagnosis of, 1535
  imaging of, 1534-1535, 1534f-1537f
  prevalence and epidemiology of, 1534
  treatment options for, 1535
Inferior vena cava thrombosis, 1535-1540
  clinical presentation of, 1536-1539
  definition of, 1535
  differential diagnosis of, 1539-1540
  etiology and pathophysiology of, 1536, 1537t
  imaging of
    CT scan in, 1537, 1538f
    indications and algorithm for, 1536
    MR scan in, 1537-1539, 1539f
    nuclear medicine, 1539
    ultrasound, 1536
  prevalence and epidemiology of, 1536
  reporting of, 1540
  treatment options for, 1539
Infrapopliteal bypass graft, 1590, 1591t

Injection, of contrast media, 161
    clinical protocols for, 163-165, 164t-165t
    MR power-controlled, 1085, 1086f
    timing of, 161-162, 162f
Injection duration (ID), of contrast media, 160-161
Injury hypothesis, of atherosclerosis, response to, 1195
Innominate artery, tracheal compression of, 544, 547f
Inotropic agents, 355-356
    mechanism of action of, 355-356, 355f
    perfusion imaging protocol for, in SPECT, 285, 285f
Insertable loop recorders (ILRs), as MRI safety issue, 265
Instrumentation
    in Doppler ultrasonography, choice of, 1038
    in positron emission tomography, 319-320
    in single-photon emission computed tomography, 276-279, 276f. See also Single-photon emission computed tomography (SPECT), instrumentation in.
Integrins, 58
Intensive care unit (ICU), chest radiography in, 94-96, 95f, 95t
Interatrial septum
    developmental pathology of, 8
    formation of, 7-8, 9f
    lipomatous hypertrophy of, 916-917, 916f-917f
Interlobar artery, Doppler ultrasonography of, anatomic considerations in, 1507
Interlobular septal thickening, from hydrostatic pulmonary edema, 1374-1375, 1375f
Intermittent claudication, 1578-1581, 1579f
    differential diagnosis of, 1583
    in peripheral artery disease, 1628. See also Peripheral arterial disease (PAD).
Intermuscular veins, of lower extremity, 1028
Internal conversion, radioactive, 272t, 273, 273f
Internal mammary artery bypass graft, 522
    postoperative evaluation of, 524
Interpolation, in image reconstruction, 1120-1121, 1123f
Interposition graft, for penetrating atherosclerotic ulcer, 1301-1302
Interstitial edema, 85-87, 1374
Interventricular septum
    anatomy of, 34, 34f
    developmental pathology of, 4
    formation of, 4, 5f-6f
Interventricular sulcus, 3-4
Intima, of blood vessels, 60, 60f
Intimal flap, in thoracic aortic trauma, 1311
    CT imaging of, 1308
Intimal tear, with pseudoaneurysm, 1311, 1311f
Intra-aortic balloon pump, placement of, carotid Doppler waveform pattern after, 1244-1245, 1247f
Intracranial vascular disease, CT angiography of, 1060, 1061f
    protocol parameters for, 1061t
Intramural hematoma, aortic
    classic signs of, 1298
    definition of, 1296
    differential diagnosis of, 1298
    etiology and pathophysiology of, 1296
    imaging of
        indications and algorithm for, 1296
        technique and findings in, 1296-1298, 1297f-1298f

Intramural hematoma, aortic (Continued)
    medical treatment of, 1298
    prevalence and epidemiology of, 1296
    reporting of, 1299
    surgical/interventional treatment of, 1298-1299
Intramuscular veins, of lower extremity, 1028
Intrarenal artery(ies), Doppler ultrasonography of
    anatomic considerations in, 1507, 1508f
    technical considerations in, 1511, 1512f
Intravenous glucose loading protocol, in ^{18}FDG-PET imaging, 803
Intravoxal dephasing, in time-of-flight MR angiography, 1105
Inversion-recovery turbo field-echo (IF-TFE) sequences, in cardiac MR imaging, 211
Ionization, 271
Iron oxide contrast agents
    physiochemical characteristics of, 258t
    superparamagnetic, 254
Ischemic cardiomyopathy, 62. See also Cardiomyopathy.
Ischemic heart disease (IHD), 726. See also specific ischemic process.
    algorithm for management of, 726-727, 727f
    cardiac transplantation for, 811-812
        postoperative appearance of, 818, 819f-820f
        postoperative complications of, 812-813
            imaging of, 818-820, 821f
    clinical presentation of, postoperative, 813
    evaluation of
        CT imaging in, 755, 756t
        MRI scans in, 755, 755t
    postoperative assessment of, 812-813
        angiography in, 815
        CT imaging in, 814
        echocardiography in, 813-814
        MRI scans in, 814
        nuclear imaging in, 814-815
        PET scans in, 814-815
        radiography in, 813
        specific, 812-813
        surgery-related complications in, 812
    postoperative management of, 821-823, 822f
    prevalence, epidemiology, and background of, 810-812
    surgical ventricular restoration for: Dor procedure, 811
        postoperative appearance of, 817, 818f
        postoperative complications of, 812
            imaging of, 817-818
    ventricular assist device for, 810-811
        postoperative appearance of, 815, 816f
        postoperative complications of, 812
            imaging of, 816-817, 817f
        preoperative and perioperative assessment of, 815
Isobar, 271t
Isomer, 271t
Isometric transition, 273
Isotone, 271t
Isotope, 271t
Iterative reconstruction, of SPECT images, 279
Iterative reconstruction method, of PET image reconstruction, 313-314, 314f

J

Jejunal vein, 1005, 1006f
Judkins' technique, of coronary angiography, 123-124

Jugular vein(s)
    head and neck drainage via, 999
    internal, anatomy of, 1661, 1662f
Jugular venous valve, bovine, in pulmonary insufficiency repair, 379, 379f

K

Kawasaki's disease, aneurysm dilation in, 509, 511f-512f
Kerley A lines, 1374-1375
Kerley B lines, 1374-1375
Kidney. See Nephro-; Renal entries.
Kinetic energy, in radiation, 270
Kinetics, tracer, 314-315
Knee, arteries in
    collateral pathways of, 985-986, 987f
    pathologies of, 986
Knuckle sign, in pulmonary embolism, 1334
K-space, in contrast-enhanced MR angiography, 1088-1089, 1089f, 1399
K-space filling, triggering of
    in three-dimensional contrast-enhanced MR angiography, 1115-1116
    in three-dimensional steady-state free precession MR angiography, 1107
K-t methods, of accelerated MR imaging, 195-197
Kussmaul sign, in constrictive pericarditis, 949

L

Large vessel occlusive disease, of upper extremity, 1643-1645
    cause and pathophysiology of, 1644
    clinical presentation of, 1644-1645
    imaging indications and algorithm for, 1645
    prevalence and epidemiology of, 1644
Larmor equation, 1078-1079
LDL receptor gene, mutations of, 1196
Lecompte maneuver, for tetralogy of Fallot with absent pulmonary valve, 648, 649f
Left anterior descending (LAD) artery
    anatomy of, 44-46, 44f-45f
        segmental, 49
    aneurysm of, 509, 510f
    duplication of, 471-472, 472f
    subtypes of, 48-49, 48f
Left anterior oblique (LAO) projection, in chest radiography, 77-78, 80f
Left atrial appendage, 32-33, 32f, 443. See also Atrial entries.
    thrombus in, 443, 443f
        CT imaging of, 447, 447f-448f
Left bundle branch block (LBBB), 58
    myocardial perfusion imaging and, 358, 748
Left circumflex (LCX) artery
    anatomy of, 46, 46f-47f
        segmental, 49
    aneurysm of, 509, 510f
Left ventricle. See Ventricle(s), left.
Left ventricular assist device (LVAD), temporary percutaneous, 811
Left ventricular border, radiography of, 74-75, 75f-76f
Left ventricular function. See also Ventricular function.
    CT assessment of, 761
    diastolic, 235, 235f
Left ventricular mass, image interpretation of, 232

Left ventricular outflow tract (LVOT)
  obstruction, in hypertrophic
    cardiomyopathy
      MR imaging of, 879-882, 881f
      treatment of, 881-882
Left-to-right shunt
  in acyanotic heart defects, surgical
    intervention for, 386
  in patent ductus arteriosus, 584
  in ventricular septal defect, 573, 577-579
  quantification of, 243-244, 245f
Leiomyosarcoma, 927-928
  inferior vena cava invasion by
    extraluminal, 1530
    intraluminal, 1530, 1531f
Lemierre's syndrome, 1670, 1670f
Lenz effect, 265
Leriche syndrome, 1635-1636, 1636f
Lethargy, postoperative, ischemic heart
  disease and, 813
Levotransposition of great arteries, 602,
  677-680. *See also* Transposition of great
  arteries (TGA).
    clinical presentation of, 678-680
    definition of, 677
    etiology and pathophysiology of, 678
    imaging of
      indications and algorithm for, 678
      technique and findings in, 678-680,
        679f-681f
    incidence and epidemiology of, 677-678
Life cycling, of atherosclerotic plaque, 707
Lifestyle changes, for peripheral artery disease,
  1209
Limb ischemia
  acute, 1573-1578
    clinical presentation of, 1573-1577,
      1574f
    critical categorization of, 1575-1576,
      1575t, 1576f, 1598, 1598t
    definition of, 1573
    differential diagnosis of, 1577
    etiology and pathophysiology of, 1573,
      1574t
    imaging of
      indications and algorithm for, 1576
      technique and findings in, 1576-1577
    medical treatment of, 1577
    prevalence and epidemiology of, 1573,
      1574t
    surgical/interventional treatment of,
      1577-1578, 1577f-1578f
  chronic, 1578-1584
    clinical presentation of, 1580-1581
      critical, 1579, 1580f-1582f, 1581
    definition of, 1578, 1579t
    differential diagnosis of, 1583
    etiology and pathophysiology of,
      1579-1580
    imaging of
      indications and algorithm for,
        1581-1582
      technique and findings in, 1582-1583
    intermittent claudication in, 1578-1581,
      1579f
    medical treatment of, 1583
    prevalence and epidemiology of,
      1578-1579, 1579f-1580f
    Rutherford categorization of, 1578, 1579t,
      1588, 1589t
    surgical/interventional treatment of,
      1583-1584
Linear attenuation coefficient (μ), 276
Linear interpolation, in image reconstruction,
  1121

Lipid abnormalities
  genes promoting, 1196
  in atherosclerotic process, 1197
Lipid-lowering therapy
  for cerebrovascular atherosclerotic disease,
    1208
  for peripheral artery disease, 1209
Lipomatous hypertrophy, 916
Lipomatous hypertrophy of interatrial septum
  (LHIS), 916-917, 916f-917f
Liposarcoma, 931-932, 932f
Liquid embolic agents, 1168-1169
Liquid helium, used in MRI scanners, 264
List mode imaging protocol, in emission
  scanning, 326-327
Liver. *See also* Hepatic *entries*.
Liver cancer, 1458-1459. *See also*
  Cholangiocarcinoma; Hepatocellular
  carcinoma.
    endovascular treatment of, 975-976
Liver disease
  cirrhotic. *See* Cirrhosis.
  pulmonary hypertension associated with,
    1360
Liver transplant recipients. *See also* Hepatic
  transplantation.
    manifestations of disease in, 1459
    pretransplant imaging of, 1544-1545
      indications and algorithm for, 1459-1460
      MR scans in, 1460
Living donors
  for hepatic transplantation
    pretransplant imaging of, 1545-1546,
      1545f-1546f, 1546t
    split-liver, 1534
  for renal transplantation, vascular evaluation
    of, 1567-1568
Loeys-Dietz syndrome, 1273, 1274f
Löffler endocarditis, 864-866. *See also*
  Eosinophilic endomyocardial disease.
Long-segment stenosis, of carotid arteries,
  Doppler ultrasonography of, 1236,
    1237f
Low contrast detectability (LCD), in CT
  systems, 1050, 1050f-1051f
Low-density lipoprotein (LDL), oxidation of,
  1195
Lower extremity
  arterial anatomy of, 983-988. *See also*
    named artery, *e.g.*, Femoral artery.
    collateral pathways in, 985-986, 986f-987f
    differential considerations in, 986-987
    general description of, 983-985, 983f-985f
    normal variants of, 985-986
    pertinent imaging considerations in,
      987-988
  CT angiography of, 1610-1627. *See also*
    Computed tomographic angiography
    (CTA), of lower extremities.
  exclusion procedure(s) for. *See also specific
    procedure*.
      endovascular methods, 1604-1608
      surgical excision and vascular bypass,
        1600-1604
  occlusive disease of
    bypass procedures for. *See* Lower
      extremity bypass.
    hybrid procedures for, 1188-1189, 1188f
    pulse volume recordings identifying,
      1186, 1187f
    revascularization procedure(s) for. *See also
      specific procedure*.
        catheter-directed or pharmacomechanical
          thrombolysis, 1597f, 1599-1600
        endovascular methods, 1591-1598

Lower extremity *(Continued)*
  surgical thromboembolectomy, 1598-
    1599, 1598t
  vascular bypass surgery, 1585-1591
  thrombosis in, ultrasound detection of,
    1334-1335
  vasculature of, CT angiography of,
    1068-1069, 1069f-1072f
    protocol parameters for, 1061t
  venous anatomy of, 1023-1029, 1024f-1025f.
    See also named vein.
      deep veins in, 1027-1029
      perforator veins in, 1029
      superficial veins in, 1024-1027,
        1026f-1028f
Lower extremity aneurysm
  endovascular exclusion procedures for,
    1604-1608
    anatomic considerations in, 1604
    contraindications to, 1605
    imaging findings in, 1606-1608,
      1606f-1607f
    indications for, 1605
    outcomes and complications of,
      1605-1606
  surgical excision and vascular bypass of
    anatomic considerations in, 1600-1601,
      1601f
    contraindications to, 1601-1602
    imaging findings in, 1603-1604,
      1604f-1605f
    indications for, 1601, 1602f-1603f
    outcomes and complications of,
      1602-1603
Lower extremity bypass, 1185
  contraindications to, 1185
  imaging findings in
    postoperative surveillance and, 1187, 1188f
    preoperative assessment and, 1186,
      1186t-1187t, 1187f
    preoperative planning and, 1186-1187,
      1188f
  indications for, 1185
  outcomes and complications of, 1185-1186,
    1186f, 1186t
Lumber artery, 975
Lumber vein, 1009, 1010f
Lung(s). *See also* Pulmonary; Respiratory
  entries.
    ground-glass opacity of, 1376
Lung disease
  chronic obstructive. *See* Chronic obstructive
    pulmonary disease (COPD).
  pulmonary hypertension caused by,
    1365-1366
  thromboembolic, 1332-1343. *See also*
    Pulmonary embolism.
    definition of, 1332
Lung injury
  acute, 1376
  direct and indirect, 1377b
Lymphoma
  metastatic to heart, 922
  primary cardiac
    definition of, 932
    manifestations of disease in, 932-933,
      933f-934f
    pathology of, 932
    prevalence of, 932

M

M mode, in echocardiography, 98, 99f
Macrophages, lipid-laden, 60, 60f

Magnetic fields
  as MRI safety issue
    gradient, 263
    static, 263, 263t
  in MR angiography, gradient, 1083
Magnetic resonance angiography (MRA)
  after surgical repair of truncus arteriosus, 622-623, 623f
  black blood, 1099-1100, 1100f
  contrast-enhanced, 1086-1091, 1087f, 1398-1399
    agent dosage in, 1399
    k-space view ordering in, 1088-1089, 1089f, 1399
    mask mode subtraction in, 1091, 1091f
  of carotid arteries, 1252-1255, 1253f
    contraindication(s) to
      metallic implants as, 1257
      nephrogenic systemic fibrosis as, 1255-1257
    dedicated carotid coils in, 1253-1254
    field of view in, 1254-1255, 1255f-1256f
    image interpretation of, 1258-1259, 1259f
    imaging parameters for, 1257, 1257t
    indications for, 1252
    parallel imaging in, 1253, 1254f
    pitfalls and solutions in, 1258
    spatial resolution in, 1252-1253
    technical requirement for, 1252
    technique of, 1257-1258, 1257t
  of coarctation of aorta, 373, 375f, 536-537
  of coronary atherosclerosis, 711
  of penetrating atherosclerotic ulcer, 1300, 1301f
  of peripheral artery disease, 1630-1634
    contrast media and injection protocols in, 1633
    novel contrast media in, 1633
    resolution requirements in, 1632-1633
    strategies to decrease venous enhancement in, 1631-1632
    strategies to optimize vessel to background contrast in, 1631
    three-dimensional, with contrast arrival, 1630-1631
    vascular anatomy considerations in, 1630
  of renal arteries, 1487-1488
  of tetralogy of Fallot, 643-645, 645f-646f
  overall scan time in, 1087-1088, 1089f
  preoperative, of carotid artery stenosis, 1174
  techniques of, 1086-1100, 1087f
  three-dimensional, 1112-1118
    contraindications to, 1115
    indications for, 1113-1115, 1113f-1118f
    of arterial system, 1451
    of venous system and soft tissue, 1452
    pitfalls and solutions in, 1115-1116
    postprocessing of, 1116-1117
    reporting of, 1117-1118
    time-resolved, 1089-1091, 1090f-1091f
  data acquisition in, 1078-1081
  ECG gating in, 1103
  field strength in, 1102
  gadolinium-enhanced three-dimensional, of postoperative congenital heart disease patients, 693, 693f
  gradient coils in, 1102
  image encoding in, 1078, 1080f-1082f
  image reconstruction in, 1078-1081, 1079f
  new developments in, 1487-1488
  nonenhanced, of peripheral artery disease, 1634

Magnetic resonance angiography (MRA) (Continued)
  of abdominal aortic aneurysm, 1205-1206, 1401, 1402f, 1442
  of aortic dissection, 1292, 1293f
  of arteriovenous fistula and pseudoaneurysm, in renal transplant recipient, 1565, 1566f
  of arteriovenous fistula failure, 1677-1680, 1679f-1681f
  of atrium, right, 30-31, 32f
  of carotid stenosis, 1220
  of cyanotic heart lesions, 652
  of heart valves, 34-36, 35f-36f
  of inferior vena cava stenosis, 1553-1554, 1556f
  of interventricular septum, 34, 34f
  of limb ischemia
    acute, 1576
    chronic, 1583
  of pericardium, 30, 31f
  of portal vein stenosis, 1551-1553, 1554f-1555f
  of pulmonary hypertension, related to associated conditions, 1361, 1361f
  of renal arteries, 1485, 1487-1488
    contraindications to, 1485
    contrast-enhanced, 1487-1488
    image interpretation in, 1488-1490, 1488f
    indications for, 1483-1485, 1484f
    pitfalls and solutions in, 1488
    reporting of, 1490
    technical requirements for, 1483
    technique of, 1486-1487, 1486t
  of renal artery stenosis, 1475-1477, 1477f-1478f, 1483-1484, 1484f
    in transplant recipient, 1561-1564, 1563f
      accuracy of, 1562t
  of renal artery thrombosis, in transplant recipient, 1567
  of renal donor, 1484-1485, 1484f
  of renal vasculature, in living kidney donor, 1568
  of renal vein thrombosis, in transplant recipient, 1567
  of subclavian steal syndrome, 1328-1329, 1328f-1330f
  of thoracic outlet syndrome, 1669
  of vascular anatomy, in pancreas transplant recipient, 1569
  of ventricle
    left, 33-34, 34f
    right, 33, 33f
  parallel imaging techniques in, 1102-1103
  patient preparation for, 1103
  phase contrast, 1094-1098, 1095f-1097f, 1105-1106
    intravoxel dephasing in, 1096
    postprocessing in, 1096-1098, 1097f-1098f
  phased-array surface coils in, 1102-1103
  steady-state free precession, 1098-1099, 1099f
  three-dimensional, 1106-1109, 1107f-1108f
    contraindications to, 1106
    image interpretation in, 1108-1109, 1108f
    indications for, 1106
    pitfalls and solutions in, 1107-1108
  technical requirements in, 1081-1085, 1102-1103
    gradient system and, 1083
    magnetic resonance scanner and, 1082-1083, 1082f

Magnetic resonance angiography (MRA) (Continued)
  parallel imaging and, 1084, 1085f
  patient monitoring and, 1084-1085
  power injector and, 1085, 1086f
  radiofrequency system and, 1083-1084, 1083f-1084f
  three-dimensional postprocessing in, basic, 1120-1127. See also Three-dimensional postprocessing, in CTA and MRA.
  time-of-flight, 1091-1094, 1092f, 1103-1105, 1104f
    contraindications to, 1103-1105
    image interpretation in, 1105
    indications for, 1103
    of carotid artery stenosis, 1252
    pitfalls and solutions in, 1105
    three-dimensional, 1093
    sequential, 1094, 1094f
    two-dimensional, 1092-1093, 1092f-1093f
  time-resolved, 1109-1112, 1109f
    contraindications to, 1110-1111
    contrast-enhanced, 1089-1091, 1090f-1091f
    image interpretation in, 1112
    indications for, 1109-1110, 1110f-1111f, 1112t
    pitfalls and solutions in, 1111
Magnetic resonance imaging (MRI). See also MRI entries.
  cardiac, 180-200, 215-226
    accelerated, 192-198
      fast pulse sequences in, 194-195, 194f
      k-t methods of, 195-197
      parallel imaging in, 195, 196f
      real time, 197-198
    anatomic overview in, 203-205, 204f
    application-specific methods of, 181-192
    black blood imaging used in, 182-184, 183f-184f
    cardiovascular protocol for, 555t
    clinical applications of, 180
    clinical techniques of, 201-214
    delayed hyperenhancement in
      description of, 210-211, 211f
      indications for, 207-210, 208f-210f
      pitfalls and solutions in, 212, 212f
      reporting of, 212-213, 213f
    determining global measures in, 215-216
    diastolic function and, 218, 219f
    dynamic left ventricular function and
      with dobutamine, 218-223, 220f-223f, 220t
      with exercise, 223-224, 223f
    image acquisition technique(s) for, 227-229
      echo-planar imaging, 228-229, 228t
      in assessing quantitative analysis of myocardial motion, 229-231, 229f, 230f
      sensitivity encoding parallel imaging, 228t, 229
      spoiled gradient echo, 227, 228t
    interpretation of, 231-237
      left ventricular volume and function and, 231-235, 231f-232f, 233t, 234f-235f
      right ventricular volume and function and, 235-237, 236t, 237f
    motion compensation in, 201-203, 202f-203f
    perfusion in
      contraindications to, 205, 206t
      description of, 205-207

Magnetic resonance imaging (MRI) *(Continued)*
    indications for, 205, 205f
    pitfalls and solutions in, 207
    reporting of, 207
  phase contrast images in, 192, 192f-194f
  resting regional wall motion abnormalities and, 216-217
  right ventricular function and, 217, 217f
  spatial resolution in, 180-181
  technical requirements for, 215
  temporal resolution in, 180-181
  contrast agents in, 251-260, 1398-1399
    classification of, 255-259, 255f, 257t-258t
    cost of, 255
    development of, 251
    dosage of, 1399
    pharmacovigilance of, 253
    regulatory label of, 251-252
    safety of, 252-253, 266
  of acute coronary syndrome, 721, 721f
  of amyloidosis, 863, 863f-864f
  of angiosarcoma, 926, 927f
  of aorta, 555-556, 555t, 556f-558f
  of aortic aneurysm
    abdominal, 1442
    inflammatory, 1405, 1406f
    ruptured, 1303
    thoracic, 1281-1282
  of aortic dissection, 1291-1294, 1293f
  of aortic regurgitation, 833, 833f
  of aortic stenosis, 829, 831f
  of aortic trauma, thoracic, 1309-1310, 1310f
  of arrhythmogenic right ventricular dysplasia, 888-892, 889f-892f, 891t
    black blood breath-hold fast spin-echo, 890-891
    bright blood cine gradient, 890
    functional abnormalities in, 889, 890f-891f, 891t
    morphologic abnormalities in, 889, 889f-890f, 891t
    right ventricular intramyocardial fat on, 891
    screening role of, 892
  of atherosclerosis, 1204-1206, 1205f
  of atherosclerotic carotid plaque, 1220-1221, 1221f
  of atrial fibrillation, 449, 450f
  of atrial septal defect, 566-567, 568f-569f
    postoperative, 365-366, 368f
    preoperative, 364, 365f-366f
  of blood flow, 239-250
    flow-encoding axes in, 239-240, 241f
    indications for, 240
    limitations and pitfalls in, 240, 242f
    phase contrast, 239-240, 240f
    technical requirements in, 239-240, 240f-242f
    techniques for, 240-249
      in coarctation of aorta, 242-243, 244f
      in pulmonary flow evaluation, 244-249, 246f-248f
      in shunting, 243-244, 245f
      in valvular disease, 241-242, 243f
    velocity encoding in, 240, 242f
  of Budd-Chiari syndrome, 1461, 1462f
  of cardiac function, 756-757
    anatomic planning and standard views in, 756
    during stress, 218-223, 767-768
      diagnostic criteria and, 768, 769f
      exercise, 223-224, 223f, 767

Magnetic resonance imaging (MRI) *(Continued)*
      pharmacologic agents in, 767-768. *See also specific agent. e.g.,* Dobutamine.
      protocols for, 768
    image analysis in, 757, 758f
    left ventricular, 556, 733-734, 758-759, 760t-761t
    regional, 764-766, 765f-767f
      image interpretation of, 232-235, 233t, 234f-235f, 237, 237f
    right ventricular, 217, 217f, 761-762, 762t-763t
    sequences in, 756-757
  of cardiac lymphoma, primary, 933, 934f
  of cardiac metastases, 921f, 923f, 924, 925f
  of cardiac tumor, calcified amorphous, 919, 920f
  of cardiomyopathy
    dilated, 855-857, 856f-857f
    hypertrophic, 875-882
      morphology in, 875-876, 875t, 876f-878f
    siderotic, 867-868, 868f
  of coarctation of aorta, 373, 376f, 536-537
    classic signs in, 537, 538f
  of congenital heart disease, postoperative evaluation in, 689-701
    cine imaging, 690-691, 690f-691f
    clinical presentation indicating, 694
    indications and algorithm for, 694
    spin-echo imaging, 691, 691f
    technique and findings in, 694-700, 695f-699f
    velocity-encoded cine sequences, 691-693, 692f
  of cor triatriatum, 633
  of coronary anomalies, congenital, 467
  of coronary arteries, 190-191, 191f
  of coronary artery bypass graft, 523-524
  of coronary atherosclerosis, 710-711
  of cyanotic heart lesions, 652
  of double-outlet right ventricle, 684, 685f
  of endoleaks, 1409, 1409f
  of eosinophilic endomyocardial disease, 865, 866f
  of fibroma, 912f, 913
  of giant cell arteritis, 1321, 1321f-1322f
  of hereditary hemorrhagic telangiectasia, 1468
  of inferior vena cava anomalies, 1528-1529
  of inferior vena cava thrombosis, 1537-1539, 1539f
  of inferior vena cava tumors, 1531
  of in-stent restenosis and thrombosis, 518
  of intramural hematoma of aorta, 1297, 1298f
  of ischemic heart disease
    advantages and disadvantages of, 756t
    indications for and applications of, 755, 755t
    postoperative, 814
  of leiomyosarcoma, 928
  of lipoma, 915
  of lipomatous hypertrophy of interatrial septum, 916, 917f
  of liposarcoma, 931
  of mitral regurgitation, 837, 837f
  of mitral stenosis, 835
  of myocardial perfusion, 184-185, 185f-187f, 728-730
    contraindications to, 733
    image interpretation in, 734-735, 735f
    indications for, 733

Magnetic resonance imaging (MRI) *(Continued)*
    pitfalls and solutions in, 734
    preclinical and clinical evaluation in, 728-730, 728f-729f, 730t
    reporting of, 735-736
    technique of, 733-734
  of myocardial viability, 185-188, 187f-189f
    contraindications to, 787
    hyperenhancement on, 782-784, 783f-786f
    in postoperative congenital heart disease patients, 693-694, 693f-694f
    wall thickness in, 782
    with dobutamine, 221-222, 222f, 782
  of myocarditis, 897-899, 898f
  of myxoma, 908, 908f-909f
  of osteosarcoma, 929, 929f
  of pancreatic adenocarcinoma, 1465-1466, 1465f-1466f
  of papillary fibroelastoma, 910
  of paraganglioma, 918, 918f
  of patent ductus arteriosus, 586-588, 587f-589f
  of pericardial effusion, 943
  of pericarditis
    acute, 946
    constrictive, 950-951, 951f
  of polyarteritis nodosa, 1468
  of pulmonary artery stenosis, 377, 378f
  of pulmonary embolism, 1340
  of pulmonary hypertension, 1357-1358
    chronic thromboembolic, 1349, 1367
    with left heart disease (venous), 1364
    with unclear multifactorial mechanisms, 1371
  of pulmonary insufficiency, 380-381, 380f
  of pulmonary valve regurgitation, 846-847
  of pulmonary valve stenosis, 846
  of pulmonary venous connections
    partial anomalous, 627
    total anomalous, 636, 637f
  of rhabdomyoma, 913-914, 914f
  of rhabdomyosarcoma, 930, 931f
  of sarcoidosis, 869-870, 870f
  of single ventricle, 673-676
    after bidirectional superior cavopulmonary connection, 674-675
    after Fontan procedure, 675-676, 676f-677f
    after stage I, 674
    in native state, 674
  of sinus venosus defect, 630, 631f
  of splanchnic artery aneurysm, 1463, 1464f
  of splenic infarcts, 1467, 1467f
  of tagging and wall motion, 188-190, 189f-190f, 764-765, 765f
  of Takayasu arteritis, 1316-1317, 1317f-1318f, 1389, 1389f
  of tetralogy of Fallot, 643-646, 645f-647f, 661, 662f-663f
  of transposition of great arteries, 658-660, 659f
  of tricuspid valve regurgitation, 845
  of truncus arteriosus, 665-666, 667f-670f
  of upper extremity medium and small vessel disease, 1649-1650, 1651f-1654f
  of valvular disease, 66, 66f
  of vascular rings, 544
  of ventricular function, 181-182, 181f-182f
    left, 556, 733-734, 758-759, 760t-761t
    right, 217, 217f, 761-762, 762t-763t
  of ventricular septal defect, 575-577, 578f-579f

Magnetic resonance imaging (MRI) (Continued)
  repetition time in, 181-182
  safety of, 261-269, 262b
    acoustic noise and, 267
    future issues in, 268
    general concerns regarding, 261-264
      cryogens and, 264
      electricity and magnetism and, 263
      gradient magnetic fields and, 263
      hazards and, 261-262
      MRI clinic and, 262-263, 262f
      radiofrequency fields and, 263-264
      static magnetic field strength and, 263, 263t
    hearing protection and, 267
    insertable loop recorders and, 265
    pacemakers, implantable cardioverter-defibrillators, other devices and, 264-265
    prosthetic heart valves and, 265
    sedation and, 266-267, 266t
    stents and, 265-266
    stress testing and, 267-268
    terminology issues and, 264, 264t-265t
  steady-state free precession, 181, 228, 228t, 1398, 1398f
  dilated cardiomyopathy diagnosis with, 855, 856f
  evaluation of cardiac function in, 756-757
  image acquisition techniques for, 228, 228t
  localization of heart in, 733-734
Magnetic resonance scanner, in MR angiography, 1082-1083, 1082f
Magnetism, as MRI safety issue, 263
Malignancy. See also Metastases; specific neoplasm.
  as risk factor in deep vein thrombosis, 1662-1663
  renal vein thrombosis associated with, 1518-1519, 1518f
Marfan syndrome, cystic medial necrosis in, 1272-1273, 1273f-1274f
  pathophysiology and follow-up of, 550-551, 551f
  prevalence and epidemiology of, 550
Marginal artery of Drummond, 975
Marginal veins
  cardiac, 52
  lower extremity, 1024-1026, 1027f
Mask mode subtraction, in contrast-enhanced MR angiography, 1091, 1091f
Matrix detector, in multislice CT, 1053-1054, 1053f
Matter, radiation interactions with, 274-276, 275f-276f
Maximum intensity projection (MIP)
  in CT angiography, 1074, 1121-1123, 1123f-1124f
    carotid, 1265-1266
    coronary, 502
    lower extremity, 1622, 1624f-1625f
    renal, 1489, 1489f
  in CT imaging, cardiac, 173-176
  in MR angiography, 1488, 1488f
    contrast-enhanced, 1258, 1259f
    time-of-flight, 1105
  sliding, 173-176
May-Thurner syndrome, 1015, 1015f, 1535
Mechanical occlusion devices, as embolic agents, 1168
Meckel diverticulum scan, 1146-1148

Mediastinal border, radiography of
  left, 72, 72f-73f
  right, 75, 76f
Mediastinal hemorrhage
  periaortic, in thoracic aortic trauma, 1309, 1309f
  postoperative, radiographic features of, 96
Mediastinal infection, after cardiac transplantation, 812-813, 819-820
Mediastinal widening, in thoracic aortic trauma, 1311
Mediastinitis
  fibrosing
    clinical presentation of, 1371
    etiology and pathophysiology of, 1370-1371
    imaging of, 1371
  postoperative, ischemic heart disease and, 813
Medium vessel disease, of upper extremity, 1645-1652. See also Upper extremity, medium and small vessel disease of.
Melanoma, metastatic, to heart, 922
Mesenteric angiography, 1159
Mesenteric artery
  inferior, 972, 973f-974f
  superior, 972, 973f-974f
Mesenteric atherosclerotic disease. See also Atherosclerosis.
  clinical presentation of, 1198t, 1199
  CT angiography of, 1203-1204
  differential diagnosis of, 1207t
  medical treatment of, 1210
  prevalence and epidemiology of, 1194
  screening for, 1200
  surgical/interventional treatment of, 1212
Mesenteric ischemia
  angiography of, 1207
  MR angiography of, 1205
Mesenteric vasculature, CT angiography of, 1066-1068, 1069f
Mesenteric vein
  inferior, 1006f-1007f, 1007
    variations of, 1008
  superior, 1005-1006, 1006f-1007f
    variations of, 1008
  thrombosis of, 1457-1458
Mesocaval shunt, inferior vena cava, 1541
Metabolic agents, radionuclide. See also specific radionuclide.
  in PET imaging, 342-344, 342f-343f
Metabolic storage diseases, restrictive cardiomyopathy associated with, 871
Metacarpal veins, 1024-1026, 1026f
123-Metaiodobenzylguanidine, radiolabeled, in PET/SPECT imaging, 806, 806f
Metallic components, implantable, as PET image artifact, 321-322, 322f
Metallic implants, as contraindication to contrast-enhanced MR angiography, 1257
Metallic material artifacts, in coronary CT angiography, 496, 497f-498f
Metastases
  cardiac
    clinical presentation of, 922-923
    definition of, 921-922, 921f-922f
    differential diagnosis of, 924-925
    imaging technique and findings in, 923-924, 923f-925f
    pathology of, 922
    prevalence of, 922-925
    treatment options for, 925

Metastases (Continued)
  myocardial, 922
  pericardial, 922
  pericardial effusion in, 941
Metoprolol
  used in cardiac imaging, 144
  used in CTA examination, 1064
Michel classification, of hepatic artery anatomy, 1545, 1546t
Microscopic polyangiitis, 1386-1387
Mirror image artifact, in Doppler ultrasonography, 1042
Mitral annulus velocities, 103
Mitral balloon valvotomy, 407f, 408, 836
Mitral balloon valvuloplasty, percutaneous, indications for, 427, 428t
Mitral inflow velocities, 103
Mitral valve
  anatomy of, 34, 35f, 422-424, 423f-424f
  calcifications in, 87, 88f
  formation of, 5
Mitral valve disease, surgery for, 417-429
  anatomic considerations in, 422-426, 423f-427f
  contraindications to, 427-428
  indications for, 426-427, 427t-428t
  outcomes and complications of, 424f, 426f, 428
  postoperative surveillance after, 415
  preoperative imaging in, 428-429
Mitral valve insufficiency, 64-65
Mitral valve regurgitation
  clinical presentation of, 837
  definition of, 836
  etiology of, 836
  imaging of
    echocardiographic, 110, 837
    indications for, 837
    radiographic, 93-94
    techniques of, 837, 837f
  medical treatment of, 837
  pathophysiology of, 424, 425f, 836
  prevalence of, 836
  quantification of, 241-242
  surgical treatment of, 837-838
    considerations regarding, 387-388, 388t
    indications for, 426-427, 427t
Mitral valve stenosis, 65
  clinical presentation of, 834
  definition of, 834
  etiology of, 834
  imaging of
    echocardiographic, 109-110, 111f-112f, 835, 835f
    indications for, 834
    radiographic, 93, 93f
    techniques of, 834-835, 834f-835f
  medical treatment of, 424-425, 836
  pathophysiology of, 424, 834
  percutaneous balloon valvuloplasty for, indications for, 427, 428t
  prevalence and epidemiology of, 834
  surgical treatment of, 426f-427f, 836
    indications for, 427, 428t
Mitral valve vegetation, in infective endocarditis, 429f-430f
Mixed edema, 1379, 1379b
Modulation transfer function (MTF), of CT systems, 1048-1049
Morphine, intravenous, for acute coronary syndrome, 723
Mortality rate
  for abdominal aortic aneurysm repair, 1440
  for heart failure, 790
  for infective endocarditis, 431

Mortality rate *(Continued)*
  for mitral valve repair, 428
  for thoracic aortic repair, 436
MRI. *See also* Magnetic resonance imaging (MRI).
MRI clinic, zones of, 262-263, 262f
MRI compatible, definition of, 263t-264t, 264
MRI safe, definition of, 263t-264t, 264
MRI scanners, acoustic noise of, 267
MRI suite, rapid evacuation of, emergency procedures for, 267
MRI unsafe, definition of, 264, 264t
MR-IMPACT trial, 730
Multi-Ethnic Study of Atherosclerosis (MESA) trial, 460
Multiframe (dynamic) imaging protocol, in emission scanning, 326-327
Multiplanar (reconstruction) reformation (MPR)
  in contrast-enhanced MR angiography, 1258, 1259f
  in CT angiography, 1073-1074, 1120-1121, 1121f-1122f
    carotid, 1264-1265
    coronary, 500, 502f
    lower extremity, 1622, 1623f
  in steady-state free precession MR angiography, 1108
  interpolation in, 1120-1121, 1123f
  linear interpolation in, 1121
Multiple overlapping thin slab angiography (MOTSA), 1094, 1094f
Multiple-level shunt, in acyanotic congenital heart disease, 385t, 386
Multisegment image reconstruction, in CT imaging, 136-137, 138f-139f
Muscle tissue deficits, in acute limb ischemia, 1574
Muscular septum, long/short, myocardial perfusion imaging and, 748
Mustard and Stenning procedure, for transposition of great arteries, 389
Mycotic aortic aneurysm, 594, 594f, 1406-1407, 1407f
Myectomy, for left ventricular outflow tract obstruction, 881
Myocardial bridging, of coronary arteries, 49, 49f-50f, 472-473, 474f
Myocardial calcification, radiography of, 87, 87f
Myocardial contractility, evaluation of, MRI scans in, 757
Myocardial delayed enhancement (MDE) imaging, 734
  hyperenhancement on, 782-784, 783f-786f
Myocardial function
  assessment of, 756-767
    CT imaging in, 758, 759f
      during stress, 769
      of left ventricle, 761
      of right ventricle, 762-763
    MR imaging in, 756-757
      anatomic planning and standard views in, 756
      during stress, 218-223, 767-768
        diagnostic criteria and, 768, 769f
        exercise, 223-224, 223f, 767
        pharmacologic agents for, 767-768. *See also specific agent, e.g.,* Dobutamine.
      protocols for, 768
      image analysis in, 757, 758f
      of left ventricle, 758-759, 760t-761t
      of right ventricle, 761-762, 762t-763t
      sequences in, 756-757
  disorders of, systolic, 62

Myocardial function *(Continued)*
  regional
    CT assessment of, 766-767
    MRI assessment of, 764-766, 765t-767t
    nomenclature for, 763, 764f
Myocardial hibernation, 62, 331
  definition of, 781, 790
  energy metabolism alterations in, 792
  phenomenon of, 792, 792f
  schematic of, 791f
Myocardial infarction
  chronic coronary artery disease and, 62
  complications of, 94
  definition of, 61
  imaging after, 357-358
    delayed hyperenhancement MR, 208, 209f
  non–ST segment elevation, 715
    percutaneous coronary interventions for, 402, 723
  pericardial effusion in, 941
  prognosis after, 754
  ST segment elevation, 715
    percutaneous coronary interventions for, 399, 400f, 723
Myocardial ischemia
  causes of, 726
  definition of, 792, 792f
  dobutamine MRI and, 218-221, 220t, 221f
  identification of, stress multidetector CT in, 733
  injury resulting from, categorization of, 792, 793f
Myocardial metabolism, 800-805
  ^{18}FDG PET imaging of, 801
    protocol(s) in, 801-803
      hyperinsulinemic-euglycemic clamping, 803
      intravenous glucose loading, 803
      nicotinic acid derivative, 803
      oral glucose loading, 802-803
  fatty acid radiotracer PET/SPECT imaging of, 800-801, 801f-802f
Myocardial metastases, 922
Myocardial motion
  causing attenuation mismatch, in PET imaging, 309-310, 311f
  compensation for, during MR imaging, 201-203, 202f-203f
  MRI quantitative analysis of, 229-231
    displacement encoding with stimulated echoes in, 230-231, 230t
    phase-contrast velocity mapping in, 230, 230t
    tagged imaging in, 229-230, 229f, 230t
Myocardial perfusion
  assessment of, 326-331, 727-728
    CT imaging in, 326, 730-733
      animal studies of, 730-731, 731t
      contraindications to, 733
      human studies of, 731-733, 732t
      image interpretation of, 735
      indications for, 733
      pitfalls and solutions in, 734
      reporting of, 735-736
      stress multidetector, 733
      technique of, 734
    emission scans in, 326-327
    MR imaging in, 184-185, 185f-187f, 205-207, 728-730
      contraindications to, 205, 206t, 733
      image interpretation of, 734-735, 735f
      indications for, 205, 205f, 733
      pitfalls and solutions in, 207, 734
      preclinical and clinical evaluation of, 728-730, 728f-729f, 730t

Myocardial perfusion *(Continued)*
    reporting of, 207, 735-736
    technique of, 733-734
  PET/CT imaging in, 326-331
    diagnostic accuracy of, 328-329, 329t
    evaluation of coronary artery disease and, 329, 329f-330f
    glucose-loaded ^{18}FDG patterns in, 333-334, 333f-334f
    imaging protocols for, 326-327, 327f
    quality assurance for, 327-328, 328f
    risk stratification and, 329-331, 331f
  defects in, ^{99m}Tc-sestamibi imaging of, 285-296, 287f-296f
  functional recovery of, after revascularization, 334-335, 335t
  impaired, in hypertrophic cardiomyopathy, MR imaging of, 877
Myocardial perfusion imaging (MPI)
  with gated SPECT, of ventricular function, 771-773
    data processing, reconstruction, and analysis of, 772-773
    electrogram gated acquisition in, 772
    pitfalls and solutions in, 773
    technique(s) of, 773-779
      equilibrium gated blood pool imaging, 773-775, 774f-778f
      first-pass radionuclide angiography, 775-779, 779f
  with PET, 749-751
    clinical indications for, 749, 750f
    future directions of, 751-752
    image acquisition data in, 750-751
    myocardial viability and, 751, 752f
    pitfalls and solutions in, 751
    radiotracers in, 749-750
    stress protocols for, 750
    technical aspects of, 749-750
    technique and protocols for, 750-751, 750f
  with SPECT, 738-749. *See also under* Single-photon emission computed tomography (SPECT).
    description of technique and protocols in, 744-746
    image interpretation of, 746-749, 747f-748f
    technical aspects of, 738-739
    techniques of, 739-744, 741f-743f
Myocardial scarring, 331
Myocardial strain, 764
Myocardial stunning, 62, 331, 721
  definition of, 781, 790
  phenomenon of, 792, 792f
  schematic of, 791f
Myocardial tagging, MR imaging of, 188-190, 189f-190f, 764-765, 765f
Myocardial torsion, 764
Myocardial twist, 764
Myocardial viability, 62-63
  assessment of, 331-336
    CT imaging in, 784-787, 787f
    limitations of, 787-788
    hibernation vs. stunning in, 331-332
    impact of, on patient outcomes, 335-336, 336f, 336t
    PET/CT imaging protocols in, 332-333, 332f
      accuracy of, predicting functional recovery, 334-335, 335t
      myocardial perfusion and glucose-loaded ^{18}FDG patterns in, 333-334, 333f-334f
      patient preparation for, 332-333, 333f
    with dobutamine, 358

Myocardial viability (Continued)
  definitions of, 781-782, 790-794
  identification of, nuclear imaging
    technique(s) in, 794-800. See also
    under specific imaging modality.
    fatty acid radiotracers in, 800-801,
      801f-802f
    18FDG, 801
    18FDG-PET mismatch and match patterns,
      803-804
      functional recovery in, 803, 804f
      prognosis of, 803-804, 804f
    18FDG-PET protocols, 801-803
    18FDG-SPECT, 805
    future opportunities for, 805-807, 806f
    PET, 799-800, 799f-800f
    SPECT, 794-797, 795f-798f
  in hypertrophic cardiomyopathy, MR
    imaging of, 877-879, 880f
  MR imaging of, 185-188, 187f-189f, 782-784
    contraindications to, 787
    hyperenhancement on, 208, 209f,
      782-784, 783f-786f
    in postoperative congenital heart disease
      patients, 693-694, 693f-694f
    wall thickness in, 782
    with dobutamine, 221-222, 222f, 782
  studies of, end points used in, 792-794,
    794f
  201Tl-labeled SPECT imaging showing,
    299-300, 300f
  accuracy of, 749
Myocarditis, 896-901
  classic signs in, 899
  clinical presentation of, 896
  definition of, 896
  differential diagnosis of, 899
  etiology and pathophysiology of, 896
  imaging of
    indications and algorithm for, 896-897
    technique and findings in, 897, 897f-898f
  isolated, vs. arrhythmogenic right
    ventricular dysplasia, 893
  prevalence and epidemiology of, 896
  reporting of, 900
  treatment options for, 900
Myocytes
  contraction of, 58, 59f
  glucose and fatty acid pathways in, 342,
    342f
  necrosis of, 61
Myopericarditis, 945-946
Myotomy, for left ventricular outflow tract
  obstruction, 881
Myxoma
  clinical presentation of, 906-907
  definition of, 905
  differential diagnosis of, 908-909
  imaging of
    echocardiographic, 116, 117f
    technique and findings in, 907-908,
      907f-909f
  pathology of, 905-906, 906f
  prevalence of, 905
  surgery for, 432-433, 432f-433f, 909
Myxoma cells, 905-906, 906f

N

Naked aorta sign, 1207
National Electronic Manufacturers Association
  (NEMA) procedures, 319
Native artery thrombosis, 1573
Navier-Stokes equations, 245-249

Navigator band location, in three-dimensional
  steady-state free precession MR
  angiography, 1107
Navigator echo gating, motion compensation
  with, in cardiac MR imaging, 202, 203f
Near-infrared spectroscopy (NIRS), of coronary
  arteries, 712, 712f
Necrosis, colon, after endovascular aneurysm
  repair, 1435-1436
Necrotizing sarcoid granulomatosis, 1392
Negative remodeling mechanism, contributing
  to coronary restenosis, 515, 516f
Neointimal proliferation, contributing to
  coronary restenosis, 515, 516f
Neonate, respiratory distress in, cyanotic heart
  lesions causing, 652, 652f
Nephrogenic systemic fibrosis, 253-255
  as contraindication to contrast-enhanced MR
    angiography, 1255-1257
  causes of, 254
  in chronic kidney disease, 1673
  risk of, gadolinium-containing contrast
    agents and, 254, 1453
Nephropathy, contrast-induced, 159
Nerve tissue deficits, in acute limb ischemia,
  1574
Neurohormonal agents, radiotracer in PET
  imaging, 344, 344t
Neutron(s), physics of, 270
New York University Renal CTA Protocol,
  1485t
New York University Renal MRA Protocol,
  1486t
Nicotinic acid derivative protocol, 18FDG-PET
  imaging, 803
Nitroglycerin
  sublingual, for acute coronary syndrome,
    723
  used in cardiac imaging, 144, 157-159, 158t
  contraindications to, 158t, 159
Noise
  acoustic, of MRI scanners, 267
  of CTA scanners, 1056
Noise-induced artifacts, in coronary CT
  angiography, 499
Noncardiac surgery, coronary CT angiography
  in, 486
Noncompliant balloons, in vascular
  interventions, 1156
Non–ST segment elevation myocardial
  infarction (NSTEMI), 715
  percutaneous coronary interventions for,
    402, 723
Nonthrombotic embolization, 1368-1370
  clinical presentation of, 1369
  etiology and pathophysiology of, 1368
  imaging technique and findings in,
    1369-1370, 1369f-1370f
North American Symptomatic Carotid
  Endarterectomy Trial (NASCET), 1172,
  1210, 1227
Norwood procedure, for hypoplastic left heart
  syndrome, 389, 672
Nubbin sign, in graft occlusion, 524-525, 528f
Nuclear medicine imaging
  extrathoracic, 1144-1151
    bleeding studies in, 1144, 1145f
    brain perfusion tomography, 1148-1150,
      1149f-1150f
    gastrointestinal bleed localization scan,
      1144-1146, 1147t
    Meckel diverticulum scan, 1146-1148
    technical requirements in, 1144
  of acute coronary syndrome, 722, 722f
  of amyloidosis, 864

Nuclear medicine imaging (Continued)
  of aortic aneurysm
    mycotic, 1407
    thoracic, 1282
  of arrhythmogenic right ventricular
    dysplasia, 887
  of atrial septal defect, 567-568, 569f
  of coronary atherosclerosis, 711-712
  of dilated cardiomyopathy, 857-858, 857f
  of double-outlet right ventricle, 684
  of inferior vena cava thrombosis, 1539
  of inferior vena cava tumors, 1531
  of ischemic heart disease, postoperative,
    814-815
  of myocarditis, 899
  of paraganglioma, 918
  of pulmonary capillary hemangiomatosis,
    1363
  of pulmonary venous connections, partial
    anomalous, 628
  of renal artery stenosis, 1477-1478, 1479f
    in transplant patient, 1564
  of sarcoidosis, 870
  of single ventricle, 677
  of tetralogy of Fallot, 661
  of transposition of great arteries, 660
  of truncus arteriosus, 666
  of ventricular septal defect, 577
  stress, coronary artery calcium screening
    with, 463
  technique(s) of, for identifying myocardial
    viability, 794-800
    fatty acid radiotracers in, 800-801,
      801f-802f
    18FDG, 801
    18FDG-PET mismatch and match patterns,
      803-804
      functional recovery in, 803, 804f
      prognosis of, 803-804, 804f
    18FDG-PET protocols, 801-803
    18FDG-SPECT, 805
    future opportunities for, 805-807, 806f
    PET, 799-800, 799f-800f
    SPECT, 794-797, 795f-798f
  ventilation-perfusion (V/Q)
    of pulmonary embolism, 1335,
      1335f-1336f
    of pulmonary hypertension
      chronic thromboembolic, 1349, 1350f,
        1367
      idiopathic, 1358-1359
      with unclear multifactorial mechanisms,
        1371
    of pulmonary veno-occlusive disease,
      1362
    of tumor embolization, 1370
Nuclear nomenclature, 270, 271t
Nuclear pulmonary flow scan, of stenosis,
  before and after repair, 375-377,
  378f
Nuclear transformation, 272
Nucleus
  electrons orbiting, 270, 271f
  proton:neutron ratio in, 270, 271f
Nuclide, 271t. See also Radionuclide(s).
Nutcracker syndrome, 1011-1012, 1012f

O

Obesity
  and accuracy of coronary CT angiography,
    484-485, 485f-486f
  definition of, 484-485
Oblique vein of Marshall, 53-55

Obturator artery, 978-981, 980f
Obturator bypass, 1586-1588, 1589f
Obturator vein, 1012, 1013f
Occlusion. See also at anatomic site.
  bypass graft, after CABG surgery, 524-525, 527f-529f
  chronic, angioplasty and, 1162
Occlusion devices, mechanical, as embolic agents, 1168
Oculostenotic reflex, 127
One-day ^{99m}Tc labeled imaging protocol, for SPECT, 282
Optical coherence tomography (OCT), of coronary arteries, 712
Oral glucose loading protocol, in ^{18}FDG-PET imaging, 802-803
Orthopedic hardware, as contraindication to CT angiography, 1614
Osler-Weber-Rendu disease, 1468
Osteosarcoma, 928-930, 929f
  echocardiography of, 116
Ostial stenosis, congenital, in coronary arteries, 472, 473f
Ostium (ostia), coronary
  location of, 39, 39f
  multiple, anomalous origin of coronary artery from, 471, 472f
  number of, 39
Ostium primum, in atrial septal defect, 8, 563, 566f
Ostium secundum, in atrial septal defect, 8, 363, 563-564
  radiography of, 90, 91f
Ovarian vein, 1010, 1010f
Oxidation, of low-density lipoprotein, 1195
Oxidation hypothesis, of atherosclerosis, 1195
Oxygen 15–carbon monoxide, 340
Oxygen 15–water, in PET imaging, 340, 340t
  of myocardial viability, 800, 800f
Oxygen tension measurements, transcutaneous, in wound healing, 1186, 1187t
Oxygen therapy, for acute coronary syndrome, 723

P

Pacemaker(s), as MRI safety issue, 264-265
Pacemaker leads, as MRI safety issue, 265
PAD Awareness, Risk, and Treatment: New Resources for Survival (PARTNERS) study, 1194
Pain
  back, 813
  chest. See Chest pain.
Pair production, in photon-matter interactions, 275, 275f
Palmar arch, 1022
  variants of, 994f-995f, 995
Palmar vein, 1020
Pancreas, CT angiography of, 1066, 1067f
Pancreas transplant recipients, vascular evaluation of, 1568-1569
Pancreatic adenocarcinoma
  clinical presentation of, 1464
  definition of, 1464
  differential diagnosis of, 1466
  etiology and pathophysiology of, 1464
  imaging of
    indications and algorithm for, 1464-1465
    technique and findings in, 1465-1466, 1465f-1466f

Pancreatic adenocarcinoma (Continued)
  staging of, multiphasic CT in, 1066
  treatment options for, 1466
Pancreatic vein, 1007
Pancreaticoduodenal artery, 972, 973f
Pancreaticoduodenal vein, 1006, 1006f-1007f
Papillary fibroelastoma, 116, 909-910, 910f-911f
Papillary muscle rupture, post-myocardial, 94
Paraesophageal varices, from portal hypertension, MR imaging of, 1454-1455, 1455f
Paraganglioma
  differential diagnosis of, 918-919
  manifestations of disease in, 917-918, 918f
  pathology of, 917, 917f
  prevalence of, 917
  treatment options for, 919
Parallel imaging
  in accelerated MR imaging, 195, 196f
  in MR angiography, 1084, 1085f, 1102-1103
    contrast-enhanced, 1253, 1254f
Paraplegia
  after aortic aneurysm rupture repair, 1303
  after thoracic aortic aneurysm repair, with prosthetic graft, 1285, 1285f
Parasitic embolization
  clinical presentation of, 1369
  etiology and pathophysiology of, 1368
  imaging technique and findings in, 1369
Paraumbilical vein, 1005
PARR-2 study, 336
Partial anomalous pulmonary venous connections (PAPVC), 625-628
  classic signs of, 628
  clinical presentation of, 625-626
  definition of, 625
  differential diagnosis of, 628
  etiology and pathophysiology of, 625, 626f
  imaging of
    indications and algorithm for, 626
    technique and findings in, 626-628, 627f
  medical treatment of, 628
  prevalence and epidemiology of, 625
  reporting of, 625
  surgical/interventional treatment of, 628, 629f
Partial anomalous pulmonary venous return, 1001-1002, 1003f
Particulate embolic agents, 1167-1168
Particulate embolization
  etiology and pathophysiology of, 1368
  imaging technique and findings in, 1369
Parvovirus B19, in myocarditis, 898-899
Parvus tardus waveform, 1240, 1240f
Patch aortoplasty, for aortic coarctation, 539
Patent ductus arteriosus (PDA), 366-369
  clinical presentation of, 585-588
  complications of, 585
  CT imaging of, 585-586, 587f
  definition of, 583
  device closure for, 369-370
    contraindications to, 370
    indications for, 370
    outcomes and complications of, 370-371
    postoperative surveillance after, 370-371, 374f
    preoperative imaging for, 370, 371f-374f
  differential diagnosis of, 588-595
  echocardiography of, 118
  etiology and pathophysiology of, 584-585
  grading of, 585
  imaging of, technique and findings in, 585-588
  medical treatment of, 596

Patent ductus arteriosus (PDA) (Continued)
  MR imaging of, 586-588, 587f-589f
  prevalence and epidemiology of, 583-584
  radiography of, 585, 586f
  surgical/interventional treatment of, 596-597, 596f. See also Patent ductus arteriosus, device closure of.
  ultrasonography of, 585, 586f
  vs. aortic spindle or ductus bump, 588, 590f
  vs. aortopulmonary window, 588
  vs. coarctation of aorta, 594, 594f
  vs. diverticulum of Kommerell, 591-592, 591f-592f
  vs. ductus aneurysm, 590-591, 591f
  vs. ductus diverticulum, 588-590, 590f
  vs. interrupted aortic arch, 595, 595f
  vs. nontraumatic aneurysm and pseudoaneurysm, 592-594, 594f
  vs. other vascular entities at aortic isthmus, 588-595, 590f
  vs. traumatic aortic injury, 592, 593f
Patent foramen ovale, 366-369, 368f
  CT imaging of, 447, 448f
  device closure of, 366
    contraindications to, 368
    indications for, 367-368
    outcomes and complications of, 368
    postoperative surveillance after, 369
    preoperative imaging for, 369, 369f
Patient monitoring, in MR angiography, 1084-1085
Patient motion
  causing attenuation mismatch, in PET imaging, 309, 310f
  in three-dimensional steady-state free precession MR angiography, 1107-1108
Patient positioning
  in MR imaging, 1397-1398
  in PET protocols, 316
Patient preparation
  for cardiac computed tomography, 143-144, 144f
  for MR angiography, 1103
  PET protocols of, 316
Patient prognosis, dobutamine MRI and, 222-223, 223f
Patient-prosthetic mismatch, in aortic valve surgery, 421
Pauli exclusion principle, 270
Peak filling rate (PFR), 754
Peak systolic velocity (PSV)
  effect of Doppler angle on, 1233-1234, 1235f
  effect of heart rate on, 1235-1236, 1236f
  in carotid artery stenosis, 1233, 1234f-1235f
    effect of contralateral occlusion on, 1236-1237, 1238f
  in renal artery stenosis, 1513
  in tortuous carotid arteries, 1235, 1236f
  increased, in vertebral artery, 1246
Pedal artery(ies), occlusion of, MR angiography of, 1636-1638, 1637f-1638f
Pediatric cardiology. See also Congenital heart disease (CHD).
  impact of prostaglandins on, 383
  milestones in, 383, 384t
Pelvic angiography, 1159
Pelvic congestion syndrome, 1015-1016, 1016f
Pelvis
  arterial anatomy of, 978-983
    differential considerations in, 981-983, 982f
    general descriptions of, 978-981, 979f-980f

Pelvis *(Continued)*
  normal variants in, 981, 981f
  pertinent imaging considerations in, 983
  venous anatomy of, 1012-1016
    differential considerations in, 1015-1016, 1015f-1016f
    of specific veins, 1012-1014, 1013f-1014f
    pertinent imaging considerations in, 1016, 1017f
    variants in, 1014-1015
Penetrating atherosclerotic ulcer, of aorta. *See* Aorta, penetrating atherosclerotic ulcer of.
Penetrating trauma, upper extremity, 1644
Penicillin, for syphilitic aortitis, 1323
Penis, dorsal veins of, 1014
Pentoxifylline, for peripheral artery disease, 1209
Percutaneous coronary intervention (PCI), for coronary artery disease. *See* Coronary artery disease (CAD), percutaneous intervention for.
Percutaneous transluminal angioplasty (PTA)
  for peripheral artery disease, 1210-1211, 1210t
  for transplant renal artery stenosis, 1564
Percutaneous transluminal coronary angioplasty (PTCA)
  historical aspects of, 393, 394f, 515
  of coronary arteries. *See also* Coronary artery disease (CAD), percutaneous coronary intervention for.
    anatomic considerations regarding, 394-400, 395f-401f
    contraindications to, 402
    in stent area, 403-405, 404f-406f, 520
    indications for, 401-402
    outcomes and complications of, 402-403
Percutaneous transluminal coronary rotational atherectomy, 400, 401f
Percutaneous vascular interventions, 1155-1171. *See also specific intervention, e.g.,* Angiography.
  equipment and tools used in, 1155-1157
Perforator veins, of lower extremity, 1029
Perfusion, myocardial. *See* Myocardial perfusion.
Perfusion agents
  contraindications to, 206t
  radiotracer. *See also specific radionuclide.*
    diagnostic accuracy of, 342, 342t
    in PET imaging, 339-342, 340f-341f, 340t
Perfusion imaging protocols
  for MR imaging, 205-207, 206t
  for PET, 317-318, 317f-318f
Periaortic mediastinal hemorrhage, in thoracic aortic trauma, 1309, 1309f
Peribronchial cuffing, 1375, 1375f
Pericardial calcification, radiography of, 82, 82f
Pericardial constriction, radiography of, 80-82
Pericardial cyst, radiography of, 82, 83f
Pericardial disease, 63-64, 437-440
  disorders associated with, 438t
  echocardiography of, 113-115
  rheumatoid, 941
Pericardial effusion
  clinical presentation of, 941
  definition of, 941, 942f
  differential diagnosis of, 943
  etiology and pathophysiology of, 941
  imaging of
    indications and algorithm for, 941
    radiographic, 80, 81f, 439, 440f
    technique and findings in, 942-943, 943f

Pericardial effusion *(Continued)*
  prevalence and epidemiology of, 941
  reporting of, 943
  treatment options for, 943
  with tamponade, 941
  without tamponade, 64f
Pericardial metastases, 922
Pericardiectomy
  radical, for constrictive pericarditis, 951
  technique of, 438, 439f
Pericardiotomy
  for pericardial effusion, 943
  for pericarditis, 947
Pericarditis
  acute
    classic signs of, 946
    clinical presentation of, 945-946
    definition of, 945
    differential diagnosis of, 946-947
    etiology and pathophysiology of, 945, 946t
    imaging of
      indications and algorithm for, 946
      technique and findings in, 946, 947f
    medical treatment of, 947
    prevalence and epidemiology of, 945
    reporting of, 948
    surgical treatment of, 438-439, 947, 947f
  chronic, surgical treatment of, 438-439
  constrictive, 64, 65f, 65t, 437-438, 438t
    causes of, 64t
    classic signs of, 951
    clinical presentation of, 949
    definition of, 949
    differential diagnosis of, 951
    etiology and pathophysiology of, 949, 950t
    imaging of
      echocardiographic, 115, 116f
      indications and algorithm for, 949
      technique and findings in, 949-951, 950f-951f
    medical treatment of, 951
    prevalence and epidemiology of, 949
    reporting of, 952
    surgical treatment of, 438-439, 439f, 951
      indications for and contraindications to, 439
      outcomes and complications of, 439
      postoperative surveillance after, 439-440
      preoperative imaging in, 439, 440f
  effusive, 438, 438f
Pericardium
  anatomy of, 30, 31f, 63, 63f, 437, 437f
  normal, radiography of, 80, 81f
Perihilar haze, 1375, 1375f
Peripheral arterial bypass grafts, imaging and evaluation of, postinterventional, 1638-1639, 1638f-1639f
Peripheral artery disease (PAD), 1573-1584. *See also specific disorder, e.g.,* Limb ischemia.
  classic signs of, 1634, 1634f
  clinical presentation of, 1198t, 1199, 1628-1634
  diagnostic algorithm for, 1200f
  differential diagnosis of, 1207t, 1634-1635, 1635f
  etiology and pathophysiology of, 1628
  imaging of
    angiography in, 1634
    CT angiography in, 1203
    CT scans in, 1630

Peripheral artery disease (PAD) *(Continued)*
  digital subtraction angiography in, 1206, 1207f
  indications and algorithm for, 1629
  MR angiography in, 1206, 1630-1634. *See also* Magnetic resonance angiography (MRA), contrast-enhanced, of peripheral artery disease.
  radiography in, 1629
  technique and findings in, 1629-1634
  ultrasound in, 1629
  increased risk of, pathologic mechanisms for, 1197
  medical treatment of, 1208-1209
  prevalence and epidemiology of, 1194, 1628
  reporting of, 1635-1639
    in aorta and iliac arteries, 1635-1636, 1636f
    in femoropopliteal arteries, 1636, 1637f
    in lower leg and pedal arteries, 1636-1638, 1637f-1638f
  screening for, 1200
  surgical/interventional treatment of, 1210-1211, 1210t
Peripheral vascular ischemia, sudden-onset, postoperative, ischemic heart disease and, 813
Peritoneal dialysis, for chronic kidney disease, 1673
Peroneal artery, 984, 984f
  occluded, 987f
Peroneal vein, 1028
Persistent truncus arteriosus, 618. *See also* Truncus arteriosus.
PET/CT imaging systems. *See also* Computed tomography (CT); Positron emission tomography (PET).
  cardiac
    accuracy of, 334-335, 335t
      diagnostic, 328-329, 329t
    future directions of, 336-337
    imaging protocols for, 332-333, 333f
    quality assurance for, 327-328, 328f
    risk stratification in, 330
  of upper extremity medium and small vessel disease, 1650-1651, 1655f-1657f
Pharmacologic stress agent(s), 352-360. *See also specific agent.*
  in MR imaging, 767-768
  in PET imaging, 316-317
  in SPECT
    protocols for, 283-285, 284f-285f, 744-745
    vs. echocardiography, 357-358, 357f
  inotropic, 355-356
    mechanism of action of, 355-356, 355f
    utility of, in coronary artery disease, 356-357
  vasodilator, 352-355
    side effects of, 354t
  vs. exercise stress protocols, 358-359, 359t
Pharmacomechanical thrombolysis, 1599-1600
Pharmacovigilance, of MR contrast agents, 253
Phase contrast images, in cardiac MR imaging, 192, 192f-194f
Phase contrast magnetic resonance angiography, 1094-1098, 1095f-1097f, 1105-1106. *See also* Magnetic resonance angiography (MRA).
  postprocessing in, 1096-1098, 1097f-1098f
Phase shift, in Doppler ultrasonography, 1035-1036
Phase-contrast velocity mapping, for quantifying myocardial motion, 230, 230t

Phased-array surface coils, in MR angiography, 1102-1103
Phase-encoding gradient, in MR angiography, 1080, 1080f
Photoelectric effect, in photon-matter interactions, 275, 275f, 1047
Photomultiplier tubes, in SPECT, 277-278, 279f
Photon(s)
  energy transmitted by, 271
  matter interactions with, 274-276, 275f
    probability of, 275-276, 276f
  physics of, 270
  x-ray, 1047
Photon attenuation, in PET imaging, 306, 307f
Phrenic artery, inferior, 973-975, 975t
Phrenic vein, inferior, 1009, 1010f
Picture archiving and communication system (PACS), 1128
Pink tetralogy, 641
Pixels, ultrasound, 1033
Plantar artery, 984, 985f
Plantar vein
  deep, 1027-1028
  superficial, 1026
Plaque, atherosclerotic
  accumulation of, 60, 61f
  calcification in, 60-61, 707
  CTA image interpretation of, 503-504
  development of, 457-458
  Doppler ultrasound assessment of, 1228-1229, 1230f, 1237-1240, 1238f-1239f
  echotexture of, 1228, 1229f
  erosion of, 707, 707f
  fibrointimal thickening and, 1237-1240, 1239f
  histologic evaluation of, 1218, 1218f
  hypoechoic, 1237, 1238f
  irregular, 1237, 1239f
  life cycling of, 707
  morphology of, 1220-1221, 1221f
  progression of
    atheromatous, 706, 706f
    nonatheromatous, 707, 707f
    stages of, 706
  rupture of, 61, 458
    and acute coronary syndromes, 61
  surface contour of, 1228, 1230f
  three-dimensional image assessment of, 1140-1142, 1140f-1141f, 1140t
  ulcerated, 1237, 1239f
    CT imaging of, 1299-1300, 1300f
    vs. penetrating atherosclerotic ulcer, 1299-1300, 1299f
  vulnerable, thin cap atheroma and, 706
Pleural effusion, postoperative, radiographic features of, 96
Plexogenic pulmonary arteriopathy, 1354
Pneumothorax, radiography of, 96
Point spread function (PSF), in contrast-enhanced MR angiography, 1254-1255
PolarCath angioplasty system, 1156
Polyangiitis, microscopic, 1386-1387
Polyarteritis nodosa, 1467-1468
Polysplenia complex, 18
Polyvinyl alcohol, as embolic agent, 1167-1168
Poor vessel enhancement artifact, in coronary CT angiography, 495t, 499
Popliteal artery, 983, 984f
  adventitial cystic disease of, 987
  angiographic access via, 1158
  division of, 985

Popliteal artery aneurysm, 987
  repair of, indications for, 1601, 1602f
  with limb ischemia, 1578
Popliteal artery entrapment syndrome (PAES), 986, 1600
  classification of, 986-987
  surgical treatment of, 1601
Popliteal vein, 1028
Porta hepatis, 971-972
Portal hypertension, 1008-1009, 1008f, 1008t
  clinical presentation of, 1453
  definition of, 1453
  differential diagnosis of, 1456-1457
  etiology and pathophysiology of, 1453, 1454f
  imaging of
    indications and algorithm for, 1454, 1454f
    technique and findings in, 1454-1456, 1455f-1456f
  treatment options for, 1457
Portal vein
  anastomosis of, 1546
  anatomy of, 1005, 1006f-1007f
  imaging of, 1545, 1546f
  variations in, 1008
Portal vein stenosis, after liver transplantation, 1551-1553, 1554f-1555f
Portal vein thrombosis, 1457-1458, 1457f
  after liver transplantation, 1551, 1553f-1554f
Portal venous circulation
  anatomy of, 1005-1008
    in specific veins, 1005-1008, 1006f-1007f
  variants of, 1008
  differential considerations of, 1008-1009, 1008f, 1008t
Portosystemic gradient (PSG), 1008
Portosystemic shunting, intrahepatic, MR imaging of, 1454-1455, 1456f
Positron emission, 272, 272t, 273f
Positron emission tomography (PET). *See also* PET/CT imaging systems.
  and CT coregistration, 312
  attenuation correction in, 308
    protocols for, 311-312
    placement of, 312
  attenuation event in, 306, 306f-307f
  attenuation maps in, conversion of CT images to, 308-309, 309f
  attenuation mismatch in, 309-311
    patient motion causing, 309, 310f
    respiratory and contractile cardiac motion causing, 309-310, 311f
    thoracic cavity drift causing, 310-311, 311f
  detectors in, 306-308, 308t
  dilated cardiomyopathy assessment with, 858
  dosimetry in, 319
  fatty acid radiotracers in, of myocardial metabolism, 800-801, 801f-802f
  FDG-labeled
    mismatch and match patterns in, 803-804, 804f, 806f
    of abdominal aortic aneurysm, 1402
    of giant cell arteritis, 1414
    of lipomatous hypertrophy of interatrial septum, 916
    of myocardial metabolism, 801
    protocol(s) in, 801-803
      hyperinsulinemic-euglycemic clamping, 803
      intravenous glucose loading, 803
      nicotinic acid derivative, 803
      oral glucose loading, 802-803

Positron emission tomography (PET) *(Continued)*
  of sarcoidosis, 870
  of Takayasu arteritis, 1317, 1318f, 1414
  for identifying myocardial viability, 799-800, 799f-800f
    ammonia N 13 as radiotracer in, 799-800
    rubidium 82 as radiotracer in, 799, 799f
  image reconstruction in, 313-314, 314f
  myocardial perfusion imaging with, 749-751
    clinical indications for, 749, 750f
    future directions of, 751-752
    image acquisition data in, 750-751
    myocardial viability and, 751, 752f
    pitfalls and solutions in, 751
    radiotracers in, 749-750
    stress protocols for, 750
    technical aspects of, 749-750
    technique and protocols for, 750-751, 750f
  myocardial perfusion studies with, 326-331
    coronary artery disease evaluation in, 329, 329f-330f
    diagnostic accuracy of, 328-329, 329t
    imaging protocols for, 326-327, 327f
    quality assurance for, 327-328, 328f
    risk stratification and, 329-331, 331f
  myocardial viability assessment with, 331-336
    accuracy of, 328f-329f, 334-335, 751
    hibernation vs. stunning and, 331-332
    imaging protocols for, 332-333, 332f-333f
    impact of, on patient outcome, 330f, 335-336, 336f
    perfusion and glucose-loaded ^{18}FDG patterns in, 333-334, 333f-334f
  of atherosclerosis, 1206
    coronary, 712
  of giant cell arteritis, 1321
  of ischemic heart disease, postoperative, 814-815
  of myocarditis, 899
  of thoracic aortic aneurysms, 1282
  prompt gamma event in, 306, 307f
  protocol(s) in, 315-319
    data reconstruction and display, 318-319
    dietary restriction, 316
    patient preparation and positioning, 316
    pharmacologic stress, 316-317
    rest-stress, 317-318, 317f-318f
    viability, 318, 318f
  quality control in, 319-322
    image, 320-322, 321f-323f
    PET/CT systems, 319-320
    ^{82}Rb generator, 320
  radiation exposure associated with, 347-348, 348f
  dose reduction in, 348-350, 349f
  radionuclides in, 325-326, 339-344. *See also* Radionuclide(s).
    metabolic agents, 342-344, 342f-343f
    neurohormonal agents, 344, 344t
    perfusion agents, 339-342, 340f-341f, 340t
      diagnostic accuracy of, 342, 342t
  scanner physics in, 304-314, 305f
  scatter correction in, 312-313
  scatter event in, 306, 307f
  tracer kinetics in, 314-315
    fluorodeoxyglucose, 315
    rubidium 82, 314-315
  vs. SPECT, 328-329
Postembolization syndrome, 1170
Posterior descending artery, coronary, 39-41, 41f-42f
Posterior lateral ventricular vein, 52, 54f

Posterolateral ventricular branch, of coronary artery, 39-41, 41f-42f
Post-infarct imaging, 357-358
Post-stenotic dilation, of ascending aorta, 1275, 1276f
Potential energy, 271
Potts shunt, for decreased pulmonary blood flow, 391
Power Doppler ultrasonography, 1036-1037. *See also* Doppler ultrasonography.
Power injector
　dual-head, in CT angiography, 1059-1060
　in MR angiography, 1085, 1086f
Pravastatin, for cerebrovascular atherosclerotic disease, 1208
Precapillary vs. postcapillary etiology classification, of pulmonary hypertension, 1354, 1355b
Premature atresia, of pulmonary vein, 1001-1002
Pressure gradients, estimation of, modified Bernoulli equation in, 99, 240, 241f
Pressure overload, 63
Primary amyloidosis, 861. *See also* Amyloidosis.
Primary cardiac lymphoma
　definition of, 932
　manifestations of disease in, 932-933, 933f-934f
　pathology of, 932
　prevalence of, 932
Probe, in Doppler ultrasonography, choice of, 1038
Profunda femoral artery, 983, 983f
　variants of, 985
Programmed cell death, 792
　targeting, 805
Programmed cell survival, 792
Prompt gamma event, in PET imaging, 306, 307f
　failure to correct, 321, 321f
Prospective gating, in CT angiography, 1057-1058
Prospective Investigation of Pulmonary Embolism Disorders (PIOPED) I study, 1333-1334
　V/Q scan in, 1335
Prospective Investigation of Pulmonary Embolism Disorders (PIOPED) II study, 1339
　diagnostic reference standard for, 1339t
　limitations of, 1339
Prostacyclin, and patent ductus arteriosus, 583
Prostaglandin(s), impact of, on pediatric cardiology, 383
Prostaglandin E_2, and patent ductus arteriosus, 583
Prosthetic graft(s)
　complications of, 1284-1285, 1285f
　for thoracic aortic aneurysm, 1284, 1284f
　used in vascular bypass surgery, 1586
Prosthetic heart valve
　as MRI safety issue, 265
　echocardiography of, 110
　for aortic regurgitation, 833-834
　　indications for, 420t
　for aortic stenosis, 830, 832f
　　indications for, 419t
　　success of, 421, 422f
　mechanical bileaflet, 420, 420f
　tissue, 420, 421f
　　advantage of, 421
Prosthetic valve endocarditis, 429. *See also* Infective endocarditis.
　surgery for, indications for, 431t

Proton, 270
Pseudoaneurysm, 1271, 1277, 1277f. *See also* Aneurysm.
　anastomotic, 1441, 1447, 1449f
　　after abdominal aortic aneurysm repair, 1180
　　postoperative management of, 1449
　aortic, post-traumatic, 592, 593f
　carotid artery
　　Doppler imaging of, 1243, 1246f
　　traumatic dissection with, 1262, 1263f
　chronic calcified, 1312, 1312f
　Doppler imaging of, 1044
　gastroduodenal, 1463, 1464f, 1469f
　hepatic artery, after transplantation, 1551, 1553f
　in renal transplant recipient, vascular evaluation of, 1564-1566
　　clinical presentation of, 1565
　　etiology and pathophysiology of, 1564-1565
　　imaging of
　　　indications and algorithm for, 1565
　　　technique and findings in, 1565, 1565f-1566f
　　prevalence and epidemiology of, 1564
　　treatment options for, 1565-1566, 1566f
　in thoracic aortic trauma, 1311
　CT imaging of, 1308, 1309f
　lower extremity
　　post-catheterization, imaging of, 1603-1604, 1604f
　　repair of, 1600
　　　contraindications to, 1601-1602
　　　indications for, 1601
　nontraumatic, vs. patent ductus arteriosus, 592-594, 594f
Pseudoartifact, in Doppler ultrasonography, 1043
Pseudocoarctation of aorta, 539, 539f. *See also* Coarctation of aorta.
Pseudofilling defects, in three-dimensional contrast-enhanced MR angiography, 1115-1116
Pseudohypocalcemia, after gadolinium-enhanced MR angiography, 252-253
Pseudothrombus artifact, 1537
Pseudotruncus, 621
Pudendal artery, internal, 978-981, 980f
Pudendal plexus, 1014
Pudendal vein, 1012, 1013f-1014f
Pulmonary. *See also* Lung *entries*.
Pulmonary angiography, 1159, 1336
　contraindications to, 1337b
　CT, 1337-1340
　　single-detector helical, 1337
　　　accuracy of, 1337
Pulmonary arterioles, 1353
Pulmonary arteriopathy, plexogenic, 1354
Pulmonary artery(ies)
　anatomy of, 965-966, 965f
　　variations in, 966, 967f
　anomalous origin of coronary artery from, 470-471
　calcification of, 89
　flow in
　　decreased, radiographic evaluation of, 84, 85f
　　increased, radiographic evaluation of, 84, 84f
　　MR evaluation of, 244-249, 246f
　　　secondary parameters in, 245-249
　　　time-resolved, three-dimensional phase contrast, 244-249, 247f-248f
　involvement of, in Takayasu arteritis, 1315

Pulmonary artery(ies) *(Continued)*
　left, 965, 965f
　　anomalous, 545, 547f
　　lower lobe, 966, 967f
　　radiography of, 74
　　upper lobe, 966, 967f
　main, radiography of, 74, 74f
　right, 965, 965f
　　lower lobe, 966, 967f
　　upper lobe, 966, 966f
　segmental, 966
Pulmonary artery banding, CT angiography of, 611f
Pulmonary artery pressure, increased, pulmonary embolism and, 1332
Pulmonary artery sling, 545, 547f, 966
Pulmonary artery stenosis, 375-377
　balloon dilation for, 375
　　contraindications to, 375
　　indications for, 375
　　outcomes and complications of, 375
　　postoperative surveillance after, 377, 378f-379f
　　preoperative imaging for, 375-377, 377f-378f
Pulmonary balloon valvotomy, 408f, 409
Pulmonary blood flow
　decreased, cyanotic congenital heart disease with, 390-392, 391t, 651-653, 652f
　　surgery for, 391-392
　increased, cyanotic congenital heart disease with, 389-390, 389t
　　surgery for, 390
Pulmonary capillary hemangiomatosis, 1362-1363, 1363f
Pulmonary circulation, anatomy and physiology of, 1353
Pulmonary edema, 1373-1382
　air space (alveolar), 85-87, 1376
　high-altitude, 1381-1382
　hydrostatic, 1373-1376
　　classic signs of, 1374-1376
　　course and clearing of, 1373
　　CT imaging of, 1374, 1375f
　　distribution of, 1376, 1376b
　　etiology and pathophysiology of, 1373
　　radiographic findings in, 1373-1374, 1374b, 1375f
　interstitial, 85-87, 1374
　mixed, 1379, 1379b
　neurogenic, 1379, 1379f
　permeability, 86-87, 1376-1378
　　clinical presentation of, 1376-1377, 1377b
　　differential diagnosis of, 1379, 1379b
　　etiology and pathophysiology of, 1376
　　imaging findings in
　　　during ARDS exudative phase, 1377-1378, 1378f
　　　during ARDS proliferative phase, 1378, 1378f
　postoperative, radiography of, 96
　re-expansion, 1379-1381, 1380f
　subpleural, 1375-1376
　types of, radiographic differentiation of, 1381-1382, 1381b
Pulmonary embolism
　angiography of, 1336, 1337b
　chest radiography of, 1333-1334, 1333f-1334f
　chronic, 1344-1351. *See also* Chronic thromboembolic pulmonary hypertension (CTPH).
　definition of, 1344
　clinical presentation of, 1333, 1333t
　consequences of, 1332

Pulmonary embolism (Continued)
  CT imaging of, 1337-1339
    benefits and accuracy of, 1338
    classic findings in, 1337-1338, 1338f
    limitations of, 1338-1339
    multidetector, 1339-1340, 1339t
      limitations of, 1339-1340
    technical considerations in, 1337
  CT venography of, 1340
  definition of, 1332
  differential diagnosis of, 1340-1341
  etiology and pathophysiology of, 1332
  imaging techniques and findings in, 1333-1340
  inferior vena cava tumors causing, 1529
  MR imaging of, 1340
  prevalence and epidemiology of, 1332
  treatment options for, 1341
  ultrasonography of, in lower and upper extremity, 1334-1335
  upper extremity DVT associated with, 1663
  V/Q scintigraphy of, 1335, 1335f-1336f
  V/Q SPECT of, 1335-1336, 1336f
  Wells clinical decision rule for, 1333t
Pulmonary hemorrhage, differential diagnosis of, 1384t
Pulmonary hemosiderosis, idiopathic, 1392-1393, 1393f
Pulmonary hypertension, 1353-1358. See also Chronic thromboembolic pulmonary hypertension (CTPH).
  arterial, radiographic evaluation of, 84-87, 85f
  caused by lung disease/hypoxia, 1365-1366
  classification of, 1354-1356
    Dana Point, 1354-1356, 1356b
    Evian, 1354, 1354b
    precapillary vs. postcapillary etiologies in, 1354, 1355b
    Venice-revised WHO, 1354, 1355b
  definition of, 1344, 1353
  etiology and pathophysiology of, 1353
  idiopathic, 1358-1359, 1358f-1359f
    definition of, 1358
  manifestations of
    echocardiographic, 105, 106f, 1356
    imaging technique and findings in, 1356-1358, 1357f
  pathogenesis of, 1353
  primary, 1358
  related to associated conditions, 1359-1361, 1359b
    clinical presentation of, 1360
    definition of, 1359
    etiology and pathophysiology of, 1359-1360
    imaging technique and findings in, 1360-1361, 1361f
  secondary, 1358
  venous, radiographic evaluation of, 85, 86f
  with left heart disease (venous)
    definition of, 1363
    etiology and pathophysiology of, 1364
    manifestations of, 1364, 1364f-1365f
    treatment options for, 1355
  with unclear multifactorial mechanisms
    definition of, 1370
    etiology and pathophysiology of, 1370-1371
    manifestations of, 1371
Pulmonary infundibulum spasm, in tetralogy of Fallot, 641
Pulmonary thromboembolism. See also Pulmonary embolism.
  definition of, 1332

Pulmonary valve
  anatomy of, 36, 36f, 845
  failure of, disease causing, 839, 840f, 842f-844f
  normal function of, 845
Pulmonary valve atresia, 840f
Pulmonary valve insufficiency, 375-381, 842f-844f
  valve implantation for, 377
    contraindications to, 379, 379f
    indications for, 379
    outcomes and complications of, 379
    postoperative surveillance after, 381, 381f
    preoperative imaging for, 380-381, 380f-381f
Pulmonary valve regurgitation
  clinical presentation of, 846
  imaging of, 846
  quantification of, 241
  treatment options for, 847, 847f
Pulmonary valve stenosis, 843f-844f
  clinical presentation of, 845
  imaging of
    indications and algorithm for, 845-846
    radiographic, 92, 92f
    technique and findings in, 846
  interventional catheterization for, 389
  treatment options for, 846
Pulmonary vasculature. See also Pulmonary artery(ies); Pulmonary vein(s).
  CT angiography of, 1062-1063, 1064f-1065f
    protocol parameters for, 1061t
  radiography of, 82-89
    abnormal blood flow in, 84, 84f-85f
    normal anatomy in, 82-84, 83f-84f
Pulmonary vasculitis, 1384, 1385t
Pulmonary vein(s)
  anatomy of, 1001, 1002f
    variations in, 1001-1004, 1003f
  developmental pathology of, 10
  flow velocities in, 103
  formation of, 10, 11f
Pulmonary veno-occlusive disease
  definition of, 1361
  etiology and pathophysiology of, 1361
  manifestations of, 1362, 1362f
Pulmonary venous connections, anomalous, 10
  echocardiography of, 118
  partial, 625-628. See also Partial anomalous pulmonary venous connections (PAPVC).
  total, 634-638. See also Total anomalous pulmonary venous connections (TAPVC).
Pulmonary venous return, anomalous, 10
  partial, 1001-1002, 1003f
  total, 1002-1004, 1003f
  infracardiac, 1008
Pulmonary venous stenosis, after ablation for atrial fibrillation, 450-451, 451f
Pulsatility index (PI), in Doppler imaging, 1513
Pulsation artifacts, in CT angiography, 1070
Pulse repetition frequency, in Doppler ultrasonography, 1036
  choice of, 1038, 1039f
Pulse sequences, MR, 1398
Pulse volume recordings, in location of arterial occlusive disease, 1581, 1582f
Pulse wave velocity, calculation of, for aortic arch and descending aorta, 556, 558f
Pulsed wave Doppler ultrasonography, 1036-1037. See also Doppler ultrasonography.

Pulsus alternans waveform, 1241, 1241f
Pulsus bisferiens waveform, 1241, 1241f
Pulsus paradoxus, 63-64

Q

Qp:Qs ratio, 243
  in atrial septal defect, 565, 568-569
  in partial anomalous pulmonary venous connections, 628
  measurement of, 243-244, 245f
  in single ventricle, 674-675
Quadrilateral space syndrome, 991, 991f
Quality assurance (QA) program
  for gamma camera SPECT operation, 743-744
  for PET/CT systems, 327-328, 328f
Quality control
  image. See Image quality.
  of CT instrumentation, 320
  of PET instrumentation, 319-320
  of PET/CT systems, 319-320
  of SPECT instrumentation, 279

R

Race, CAC score and, 462
Radial artery
  anatomy of, 994-995
  angiographic access via, 1158
  branches of, 993-994
Radial vein, 1022-1023, 1023f
Radiation
  exposure to, ^{201}Tl-labeled SPECT imaging and, 300-301, 300t, 301f
  interactions of, with matter, 274-276, 275f-276f
  ionizing
    in CT angiography, 1070-1073
      dose modulation of, 1058
    in PET/CT systems, 344-345, 345f, 345t
      dose reduction in, 348-350, 349f-350f
      for CT portion of examination, 346-347, 346f, 347t
      for PET portion of examination, 347-348, 348f
  physics of, 270-271
Radiation dose, effective, in CT imaging of coronary calcium, 460
Radiation reduction strategy(ies), 1073
  in computed tomography, 150-155
    increased beam filtration technique, 153-154
    increased beam pitch technique, 153
    increased reconstructed slice thickness technique, 154, 154f
    reduced tube current technique, 150-152, 151f
    reduced tube voltage technique, 152-153
    shortened scan length technique, 153
    technical requirements for, 150
    tubal modulation, 146
Radiation-sensitive population, as contraindication to CT angiography, 1614
Radioactive decay, 273-274
  types of, 272t
Radioactivity, 270-273, 272f-273f
Radioembolization, using yttrium 90, 975-976
Radiofrequence system, in MR angiography, 1083-1084, 1083f-1084f
Radiofrequency ablation, for atrial fibrillation, 445-446

Radiofrequency coils, in carotid MR angiography, 1252
Radiofrequency excitations, in MR angiography, 1079
Radiofrequency fields
  as MRI safety issue, 263-264
  in MR angiography, 1078-1079
Radiography
  chest. See Chest radiography.
  of abdominal aortic aneurysm, 1400, 1400f
  of calcifications, in atherosclerosis, 1201
  of endoleaks, 1408-1409
  of inferior vena cava anomalies, 1528
  of inferior vena cava tumors, 1530
  of in-stent restenosis and thrombosis, 517
  of peripheral artery disease, 1629
  of transplant renal artery stenosis, 1560
  of ulcer or gangrenous wounds, in limb ischemia, 1582
  of upper extremity medium and small vessel disease, 1647, 1647f
Radionuclide(s). See also specific radionuclide.
  half-life of, 273-274
  in PET imaging, 325-326, 339-344
    metabolic agents, 342-344, 342f-343f
    neurohormonal agents, 344, 344t
    perfusion agents, 339-342, 340f-341f, 340t
      diagnostic accuracy of, 342, 342t
  in PET/CT imaging, 325-326
    ammonia N 13, 325-326
    fluorodeoxyglucose 18, 326
    rubidium 82, 325
  in SPECT imaging, 298-303
    technetium 99m labeled, 301
    technetium 99m-N-NOET, 302
    technetium 99m sestamibi, 301, 739, 740f-741f
    technetium 99m-teboroxime, 302
    technetium 99m-tetrofosmin, 301-302, 739
    thallium 201, 298-301, 299f-301f, 738-739
  manufacture of, 274
  photons released from, 271
  specific activity of, 274
Radionuclide angiography, first-pass, of ventricular function
  data acquisition in, 776-778, 779f
  image interpretation in, 778-779
  indications for, 775-776
Radionuclide medicine imaging. See Nuclear medicine imaging.
Radiotracer(s). See Radionuclide(s).
Ramipril, for peripheral artery disease, 1208-1209
Ramus intermedius (RI) artery, anatomy of, 46, 47f
Rastelli procedure, 390
  for complete transposition of great arteries, 610-611, 610f
  imaging after, 612-613, 613f
Rayleigh scattering, 1047
Raynaud's complex, 1646
Raynaud's phenomenon, 1645-1647. See also Upper extremity, medium and small vessel disease of.
Recoil electron, 275
Reconstruction parameters, for CT angiography of lower extremities, 1617, 1617f-1618f
Reconstruction phase, optimal, in CT imaging, 137
Rectal venous plexus, 1013, 1014f
Redistribution phenomenon, in ^{201}Tl cardiac imaging, 796

Reflex, oculostenotic, 127
Regadenoson protocol, for PET imaging, 317
Relative velocity, in Doppler ultrasonography, 1034, 1035f
Renal allograft
  Doppler ultrasonography of, 1519, 1519f-1520f
  rejection of, 1519, 1520f
  segmental infarction in, 1520, 1521f
Renal angiography, 1159, 1160f
Renal angiomyolipoma, 1533, 1533f
Renal artery(ies), 972-973, 1483-1491
  ACEI scintigraphy of
    captopril administration in, 1493
    contraindications to, 1492-1493
    1-day protocol for, 1493
    2-day protocol for, 1493-1494
    enalaprilat administration in, 1493
    indications for, 1492
    pitfalls and solutions in, 1494
    postprocessing of, 1494
    procedure in, 1493-1494
    reporting of, 1492, 1495f
    ^{99m}Tc-DTPA in, 1494
    ^{99m}Tc-MAG3 in, 1494
    technical requirements for, 1492
  aneurysm of, Doppler ultrasound diagnosis of, 1515
  CT angiography of, 1066, 1067f-1068f
    contraindications to, 1485
    image interpretation in, 1488-1490, 1489f-1490f
    pitfalls and solutions in, 1488
    reporting of, 1490
    technique of, 1485-1486, 1485t, 1486f
  Doppler ultrasonography of
    anatomic considerations in, 1505-1507, 1507f-1508f
    technical considerations in, 1509-1511, 1510f-1511f
  fibromuscular disease affecting, 975, 976f, 1471
    Doppler ultrasonography of, 1498, 1503f
    prevalence and epidemiology of, 1471-1472
  MR angiography of
    contraindications to, 1485
    contrast-enhanced, 1487-1488
    image interpretation in, 1488-1490, 1488f
    indications for, 1483-1485, 1484f
    pitfalls and solutions in, 1488
    reporting of, 1490
    technical requirements for, 1483
    technique of, 1486-1487, 1486t
  postangioplasty, Doppler assessment of, 1514-1515, 1516f-1518f
Renal artery stenosis, 1471
  atherosclerotic. See Renal atherosclerotic disease.
  classic signs of, 1478
  clinical presentation of, 1472
  differential diagnosis of, 1478-1480
  Doppler ultrasonography of, 1497-1498
    image interpretation in, 1513
      direct criteria for, 1513, 1513b, 1514f
      indirect criteria for, 1513, 1513b, 1515f
  etiology and pathophysiology of, 1472
  imaging of
    indications and algorithm for, 1472, 1473f
    technique and findings in, 1473-1478, 1474f-1480f
  in allograft vessels, criteria for, 1519b
  in transplant patient, 1519-1520, 1520f
  MR angiography of, 1483-1484, 1484f
  prevalence and epidemiology of, 1471-1472

Renal artery stenosis (Continued)
  renovascular hypertension caused by, 1471, 1492
  reporting of, 1480-1481
  transplant, 1559-1564. See also Transplant renal artery stenosis (TRAS).
  treatment options for, 1480
Renal artery thrombosis
  Doppler ultrasonography of, 1498-1505, 1505f
  image interpretation in, 1515
  in renal allograft, 1520, 1521f, 1566-1567
Renal atherosclerotic disease, 1471. See also Atherosclerosis.
  conventional angiography of, 1206
  differential diagnosis of, 1207t
  Doppler ultrasonography of, 1497-1498, 1499f-1502f
  medical treatment of, 1209
  MR angiographic assessment of, 1205, 1205f
  presenting findings in, 1198t
  prevalence and epidemiology of, 1194, 1471
  screening for, 1200
  surgical/interventional treatment of, 1211-1212
Renal cell carcinoma, inferior vena cava invasion by, 1530, 1532f
Renal disease
  chronic. See Chronic kidney disease (CKD).
  end-stage, 1673-1674
Renal donor, evaluation of, MR angiography in, 1484-1485, 1484f
Renal failure
  after ruptured aortic aneurysm repair, 1303
  as contraindication to CT angiography, 1262-1263
  coronary artery calcium and, 463
Renal impairment, as contraindication to CT angiography, 1611-1614
Renal infarction, 1447, 1449f
Renal insufficiency, CT angiography and, 485
Renal morphology, Doppler ultrasonography of, technical considerations in, 1511-1512
Renal transplantation
  Doppler ultrasound assessment of, 1505
  living donor for, vascular evaluation of, 1567-1568
  vascular evaluation of, 1559-1568
    arteriovenous fistula and pseudoaneurysm in, 1564-1566
      clinical presentation of, 1565
      etiology and pathophysiology of, 1564-1565
      imaging of
        indications and algorithm for, 1565
        technique and findings in, 1565, 1565f-1566f
      prevalence and epidemiology of, 1564
      treatment options for, 1565-1566, 1566f
    Doppler ultrasound assessment in, 1519-1522, 1519b, 1519f-1522f
    transplant renal artery and vein thrombosis in, 1566-1567
    transplant renal artery stenosis in, 1559-1564. See also Transplant renal artery stenosis (TRAS).
Renal tumor, imaging evaluation of, 1485
Renal vein(s), 1009, 1010f
  Doppler ultrasonography of, anatomic considerations in, 1507-1508, 1508f
  left
    circumaortic, 1525, 1527f
    retroaortic, 1525

Renal vein(s) *(Continued)*
  right, duplicated, 1526
  variants of, 1011
    reporting of, 1529
Renal vein thrombosis
  Doppler ultrasonography of, 1505, 1506f
    image interpretation in, 1515-1519, 1518f
  in renal allograft, 1521, 1522f, 1566-1567
  pitfalls of sonography of, 1513
Renal-aortic ratio (RAR)
  calculation of, 1509
  in renal artery stenosis, 1513
Renin-angiotensin system, targeting, 805, 806f
Renovascular hypertension
  ACEI scintigraphy of. *See* Angiotensin-converting enzyme inhibitor (ACEI) scintigraphy, of renal arteries.
  secondary to renal artery stenosis, 1471, 1492
Resistive index (RI), in Doppler imaging, 1512-1513
Resolution phantoms, of CT systems, 1048, 1048f
Resolution testing patterns, of CT systems, 1048, 1048f
Respiratory acceptance window, in three-dimensional steady-state free precession MR angiography, 1107
Respiratory artifacts, in cardiac CT imaging, 147, 147f
Respiratory distress, neonatal, cyanotic heart lesions causing, 652, 652f
Respiratory distress syndrome. *See* Adult respiratory distress syndrome (ARDS).
Respiratory rhythm, in three-dimensional steady-state free precession MR angiography, 1107
Rest and stress perfusion, multidetector CT
  animal studies of, 730-731, 731t
  human studies of, 731-733, 732t
Rest pain, ischemic, 1581
Restenosis
  after angioplasty, 1162
  in-stent. *See* Coronary stents, in-stent restenosis and thrombosis.
  recurrent, after carotid endarterectomy, 1173
Resting perfusion
  CT sequence of, 734
  MRI sequence of, 733-734
  PET sequence of, 750
Restrictive cardiomyopathy, 861-873. *See also* Cardiomyopathy, restrictive.
Rest-stress protocols
  for PET imaging, 317-318, 317f-318f
  for SPECT
    same-day Tc 99m radiotracer, 746
    two-day Tc 99m radiotracer, 746
Retrospective gating, in CT angiography, 1057
Revascularization procedure(s). *See also specific procedure, e.g.,* Coronary artery bypass graft (CABG) surgery.
  for peripheral artery disease, 1210-1211, 1210t
  for renal atherosclerotic disease, 1211-1212
  lower extremity
    catheter-directed or pharmacomechanical thrombolysis, 1597f, 1599-1600
    endovascular methods, 1591-1598
    surgical thromboembolectomy, 1598-1599, 1598t
    vascular bypass surgery, 1585-1591
  with stents, 1163-1164, 1164f
Rhabdomyolysis, in acute limb ischemia, 1576
Rhabdomyoma, 116, 913-914, 914f

Rhabdomyosarcoma, 930-931, 931f
  echocardiography of, 116
Rheumatoid arthritis, atherosclerosis associated with, 1196
Rib fracture, 1306-1307
Rib notching, bilateral symmetrical, 89
Right anterior oblique (RAO) projection, in chest radiography, 77, 79f
Right ventricle. *See also* Ventricle(s); Ventricular *entries*.
  double-outlet. *See* Double-outlet right ventricle (DORV).
  normal values of, 65t
Right ventricular border, radiography of, 75
Right ventricular cardiomyopathy, arrhythmogenic, 237, 237f
Right ventricular dysplasia, arrhythmogenic, 884-895. *See also* Arrhythmogenic right ventricular dysplasia (ARVD).
Right ventricular function. *See* Ventricular function, right.
Right ventricular outflow tract (RVOT), vs. arrhythmogenic right ventricular dysplasia, 893t
Roger disease, 580
Roof ablation line, 446
Ross procedure, for aortic valve disease, 389
Rubidium 82 (^{82}Rb)
  decay of, in prompt gamma, 306, 307f
  generator activity of, 320
  in myocardial perfusion imaging with PET, 750
  in PET imaging, 799, 799f
  in PET/CT imaging, 325, 340t, 341-342, 341f
  kinetics of, 314-315
  manufacture of, 274
Rutherford categorization
  of acute limb ischemia, 1575, 1575t
  of chronic limb ischemia, 1578, 1579t, 1588, 1589t

S

S_2 heart sounds, in atrial septal defect, 564
Saccular aneurysm. *See* Pseudoaneurysm.
Sacral artery
  lateral, 978, 980f
  median, 975
Sacral vein, lateral, 1012
Saddle embolus, 1575. *See also* Embolus (embolism).
  balloon catheter embolectomy for, 1578
Safety
  of contrast agents, 159-160, 252-253
  of MR imaging, 261-269, 262b. *See also* Magnetic resonance imaging (MRI), safety issues of.
Safety profile, of dobutamine MRI, 218, 220f
Sagittal images, in cardiac CT imaging, 170-171, 172f
Saline flushing, contrast media and, 163, 163f
Same-day ^{99m}Tc radiotracer protocol, for SPECT, 746
Sample volume, in Doppler ultrasonography, 1038, 1039f
Saperstein principle, 298
Saphenous vein
  great, 1024-1027, 1026f, 1028f
    in vascular bypass surgery, 1585-1586
  small, 1027, 1027f
Saphenous vein bypass graft, 522
  aneurysm of, 509, 511f
Sarcoid granulomatosis, necrotizing, 1392

Sarcoidosis
  cardiac involvement in, delayed hyperenhancement MR imaging of, 209, 210f
  clinical presentation of, 869
  definition of, 868
  etiology and pathophysiology of, 868-869
  imaging of
    indications and algorithm for, 869
    technique and findings in, 869-871, 870f, 872t
  medical treatment of, 871
  prevalence and epidemiology of, 868
  vs. arrhythmogenic right ventricular dysplasia, 892-893
Sarcomas, echocardiography of, 116
Saturation, in time-of-flight MR angiography, 1105
Scan delay, fixed, in CT angiography, 1058
Scan length, shortened, to reduce radiation in CT imaging, 153
Scan time, in MR angiography, 1087-1088, 1089f
Scanner
  CTA
    16-detector, protocol for, 1615t-1616t
    design of, 1056
  PET, 304-314, 305f
    events recorded in
      multiple, 306, 306f
      types of, 305, 305f
Scanning protocols
  for cardiac computed tomography, 144-146, 145f
  for CT angiography of lower extremities, 1614-1617, 1615t-1616t
Scatter correction, in PET imaging, 312-313
Scatter event, in PET imaging, 306, 307f
Schistosomiasis, pulmonary, 1368
  hypertension associated with, 1360
Sciatic artery, persistent, 981, 981f
  clinical importance of, 982
Scimitar sign, in partial anomalous pulmonary venous connections, 628
Scimitar syndrome, 625, 626f-627f
  repair of, baffle obstruction after, 628, 629f
Scintigraphy. *See* Nuclear medicine imaging.
  ACEI. *See* Angiotensin-converting enzyme inhibitor (ACEI) scintigraphy.
Scintillation crystals, in SPECT, 277, 278t
Scintillation detector, in PET scanners, 304, 305f
Scintillation event, 277
  localization of, in SPECT, 278
Secondary amyloidosis, 861. *See also* Amyloidosis.
Sedation
  depth of, four levels of, 266, 266t
  in MR imaging, safety issues of, 266-267
Segmental artery(ies), Doppler ultrasonography of, anatomic considerations in, 1507, 1508f
Self-expanding stents, 1157
Senile systemic amyloidosis, 861. *See also* Amyloidosis.
Sensitivity encoding (SENSE)
  in parallel MR angiography, 1084, 1085f
  in parallel MR imaging, 195, 228t, 229
Septal defect(s)
  asymmetric, in hypertrophic cardiomyopathy, MR imaging of, 875, 876f-877f
  atrial. *See* Atrial septal defect (ASD).
  atrioventricular
    multiple-level shunts in, 386
    surgical treatment of, 386, 387f

Septal defect(s) *(Continued)*
  ventricular. *See* Ventricular septal defect (VSD).
Septal thickening, interlobular, from hydrostatic pulmonary edema, 1374-1375, 1375f
Septum primum, 7-8, 9f
Septum secundum, 7-8, 9f
Shaded surface display, in CT angiography, 1074
Sheaths, vascular, 1156
Shower embolism, after endovascular aneurysm repair, 1435
Shunt(s). *See also specific type of shunt.*
  acyanotic congenital heart disease with, surgery for, 383-387, 385f, 385t, 387f
  acyanotic congenital heart disease without, surgery for, 387-389, 388t
  arterioportal, MR imaging of, 1455-1456, 1456f
  arteriovenous, Doppler imaging of, 1044
  inferior vena cava, 1540-1541
    mesocaval, 1541
    side-to-side portacaval, 1541, 1541f
    veno-venous (intrahepatic), MR imaging of, 1454-1455, 1456f
Sickle cell disease, pulmonary hypertension associated with, 1360
Side-lobe artifact, in Doppler ultrasonography, 1042
Siderotic cardiomyopathy, 866-868. *See also* Cardiomyopathy, siderotic.
Side-to-side portacaval shunt, inferior vena cava, 1541, 1541f
Signal-to-noise ratio
  in MR angiography, 1081, 1102, 1252-1253
    contrast enhanced, 1258
  in MR imaging, 1398
Simpson's rule
  in MRI assessment of ejection fraction, 215
  in MRI determinants of left ventricular volume, 215
  multislice, of global left ventricular function, 231, 231f-232f
Simultaneous acquisition of spatial harmonics (SMASH), in parallel imaging, 195, 1084
Simvastatin, for cerebrovascular atherosclerotic disease, 1208
Single-detector helical CT pulmonary angiography, 1337
  accuracy of, 1337
Single-photon emission computed tomography (SPECT)
  fatty acid radiotracers in, of myocardial metabolism, 800-801, 801f-802f
  [18]FDG-labeled, 805
  for identifying myocardial viability, 794-797
    Tc 99m labeled radiotracers in, 794-795, 795f
    Tc 99m labeled radiotracers with nitrate administration in, 795-796, 796f
    thallium 201 in, 796-797
      protocols for, 797, 797f-798f
  gated, 283
  image interpretation in, 285-296, 286f-296f
  instrumentation in, 276-279, 276f
    advances in, 279
    collimators, 276-277, 277f-278f
    energy discrimination and, 278
    image generation and, 279
    photomultiplier tubes, 277-278, 279f
    quality control of, 279
    scintillation crystals, 277, 278t
    scintillation event localization and, 278

Single-photon emission computed tomography (SPECT) *(Continued)*
  myocardial perfusion imaging with, 738-749
    acquisition protocols for, 745-746
      dual isotope, 746
      same-day rest-stress Tc 99m radiotracer protocol, 746
      stress-redistribution thallium 201 protocol, 746
      two-day rest-stress Tc 99m radiotracer protocol, 746
    artifacts and normal variants in, 748-749
    contraindications to, 743
    exercise protocols for, 744
    image interpretation in, 747-748, 747f-748f
    indications for, 739-743, 741f-743f
    instrumentation in, 739
    pharmacologic protocols for
      adenosine, 744-745
      dipyridamole, 745
      dobutamine, 745
    pitfalls and solutions in, 743-744
    postprocessing in, 746-747
    quality assurance of, 743-744
    radionuclide imaging protocols for, 744-745
    radiotracer in, 738-739, 740f-741f
      characteristics of, 298
      technetium 99m labeled, 301, 739, 740f-741f
      thallium 201 labeled, 298-301, 738-739
    stress protocols for, 744
    technical aspects of, 738-739
    techniques of, 739-744
    test accuracy of, 749
  of acute coronary syndrome, 722
  of coronary atherosclerosis, 712
  of dilated cardiomyopathy, 857-858, 857f
  physics of, 270-276
    anatomic structure in, 270, 271f, 271t
    interactions of matter in, 274-276, 275f-276f
    radioactive decay in, 273-274
    radioactivity and, 270-273, 272f-273f, 272t
    radionuclide manufacture and, 274, 274f
  radiotracer imaging agent(s) in. *See also specific radionuclide.*
    technetium 99m labeled, 301
    technetium 99m–N-NOET, 302
    technetium 99m–sestamibi, 301
    technetium 99m–teboroxime, 302
    technetium 99m–tetrofosmin, 301-302
    thallium 201, 298-301, 299f-301f
  stress protocols for, 283-285
    exercise, 283, 283t
    pharmacologic, 283-285, 284f-285f
  ^{99m}Tc-labeled imaging protocol(s) for, 282-283
    dual-isotope protocol, 282-283
    one-day protocol, 282
    two-day protocol, 282
  technical requirements for, 281-283
    description of, 298-302
  [201]Tl imaging protocols for, 281-282
  ventilation-perfusion (V/Q), of pulmonary embolism, 1335-1336, 1336f
  vs. PET imaging, 328-329
Sinoatrial nodal artery, 40-41, 42f
Sinoatrial node
  anatomy of, 444, 445f
  depolarization initiated by, 57, 58f
  electrical impulses originating in, 57

Sinus of Valsalva
  aneurysms of, imaging of, 1279-1280
  coronary arteries arising from, 39, 39f-40f, 956f, 957-961
  noncoronary cusp of, 39
  opposite, anomalous origin of coronary arteries from, 468-469, 468f-470f
Sinus venarum, 8-10
Sinus venosus, formation of, 3-4
Sinus venous defect
  clinical presentation of, 629
  definition of, 628-629
  differential diagnosis of, 631
  etiology and pathophysiology of, 629
  imaging of, technique and findings in, 629-631, 630f-631f
  prevalence and epidemiology of, 629
  reporting of, 632
  surgical/interventional treatment of, 631-632
Situs inversus, visceral, 16, 17f
Situs solitus, visceral, 16, 17f
  in Ebstein anomaly, 653
Sized-based reduction, in x-ray tube current, 151, 151f
  pitfalls and solutions for, 152
Sleep-disordered breathing, 1365-1366
Slice thickness, increased, CT radiation reduction and, 154, 154f
Small vessel disease, of upper extremity, 1645-1652. *See also* Upper extremity, medium and small vessel disease of.
Snowman sign, in pulmonary venous connections
  partial anomalous, 628
  total anomalous, 636
Sodium tetradecyl, as embolic agent, 1160
Soft tissue, abdominal, MR imaging of, 1452-1453
Sones' technique, of coronary angiography, 123-124
Spasm, pulmonary infundibulum, in tetralogy of Fallot, 641
Spatial encoding, in MR angiography, 1079-1080
*Spa*tial *m*odulation of *m*agnetization (SPAMM) technique, for quantifying myocardial motion, 229-230
Spatial resolution
  in cardiac MR imaging, 180-181
  in contrast-enhanced MR angiography, 1252-1253
    while minimizing imaging time and motion artifact, 1258
  in CT angiography, 1049, 1049f, 1056
Specialized populations, coronary artery calcium in, 462-463
Specific absorption rate (SAR), of MRI scanners, FDA recommendations for, 263-264
Specific activity, of nuclide, 274
Spectral broadening artifact, in Doppler ultrasonography, 1042
Spectral Doppler ultrasonography, 1037. *See also* Doppler ultrasonography.
Spectral gain
  in Doppler ultrasonography, 1040, 1040f
  incorrect, in carotid artery Doppler ultrasonography, 1234
Spectral window, in Doppler imaging, 1043, 1043t
Splanchnic artery aneurysm, 1462-1463, 1463f-1464f
Splenic arteriovenous malformations, 1468
Splenic artery, 970-971, 973f

Splenic infarction, 1466-1467, 1467f
Splenic trauma, 1468
Splenic vein, 1006-1007, 1006f-1007f
Spoiled gradient echo technique, of MR imaging, 227, 228t
ST segment elevation myocardial infarction (STEMI), 715
　percutaneous coronary interventions for, 399, 400f, 723
Stable coronary disease, percutaneous coronary interventions for, 402
Stair-step artifact
　in CT angiography, 1070
　　coronary, 495t, 499, 500f-501f
　in CT imaging, cardiac, 147, 147f
Stanford classification, of aortic dissection, 434, 434f, 1289, 1289f
Stanford protocol, for medications used in cardiac imaging, 156-157, 158t
Static magnetic field strength, as MRI safety issue, 263, 263t
Statins
　effect of, on progression of CAC score, 463-464
　for coronary atherosclerosis, 713
Steady-state free precession (SSFP) technique
　comparison of left ventricular volume by, vs. FLASH, 231-232
　of MR angiography, 1098-1099, 1099f
　　three-dimensional, 1106-1109, 1107f-1108f
　　　contraindications to, 1106
　　　image interpretation in, 1108-1109, 1108f
　　　indications for, 1106
　　　pitfalls and solutions in, 1107-1108
　of MR imaging, 181, 228, 228t, 1398, 1398f
　　dilated cardiomyopathy diagnosis with, 855, 856f
　　evaluation of cardiac function in, 756-757
　　localization of heart in, 733-734
Steal phenomenon, Doppler imaging of, 1044
Stenosis. See under anatomy.
Stent(s). See also Endograft(s).
　as MRI safety issue, 265-266
　balloon-mounted, 1157
　bare metal, 515, 516f
　　risk of thrombosis in, 516, 517f
　carotid, 1222-1224
　　procedure for, 1224, 1224f
　　recommendations for, 1224
　　status and patency of, CT angiographic evaluation of, 1261-1262, 1262f
　coronary, 403-405. See also Coronary stents.
　drug-eluting, 515, 517f, 1157
　　effectiveness of, 515-516
　　repeat stenting with, 520
　　risk of thrombosis in, 516, 517f
　endovascular, 1157
　　for thoracic aortic aneurysm, 1283, 1284f
　　for thoracic aortic injury, 1312-1313, 1312f
　　for type B aortic dissection, 1295-1296, 1296f
　　inferior vena caval, 1541-1542, 1541f
　　placement of, angioplasty and, in lower extremity revascularization, 1591-1592, 1592f-1593f
　　revascularization with, 1163-1164, 1164f
　　self-expanding, 1157
Stent graft(s), 1157
　revascularization with, 1163-1164, 1164f
Stent-Protected Angioplasty versus Carotid Endarterectomy (SPACE) trial, 1223

Step-and-shoot computed tomography. See also Computed tomography (CT).
　vs. helical (spiral) CT, 1051-1053, 1051f-1052f
Storage diseases, metabolic, restrictive cardiomyopathy associated with, 871
Strain, in Doppler imaging, 119-122
Strain rate, 120
Strandness criteria, in diagnosis of carotid stenosis, 1173, 1174t
Streak artifacts, in CT angiography, 1069
　coronary, 496, 497f-498f
Streptokinase, for inferior vena cava thrombosis, 1539
Stress, evaluation of cardiac function during, 767-769
　CT imaging in, 769
　MR imaging in, 767-768
　　diagnostic criteria in, 768, 769f
　　dobutamine stress protocol and, 768
　　pharmacologic stress agents and, 767-768
Stress perfusion, CT, 322, 323f, 734
Stress protocols
　for MR imaging, dobutamine, 768
　for PET imaging, 750
　for SPECT, 283-285, 744
　　exercise, 283, 283t, 744
　　pharmacologic, 283-285, 284f-285f, 744-745. See also Pharmacologic stress agent(s).
Stress test(ing)
　in MRI setting, 267-268
　selection of, 359t
Stress-perfusion MRI studies, diagnostic accuracy of, 729, 730t
Stress-redistribution thallium 201 protocol, in SPECT, 746
Stroke
　antiplatelet therapy for, 1222
　causes of, 1227
　CT angiography of, 1060
　etiology of, 1217
　prevalence of, 1217
　probability of, noninvasive testing and, sensitivity and specificity of, 1251, 1252f
　risk factors for, 1218
　risk reduction of, carotid endarterectomy in, 1172
Stroke volume, definition of, 58
Subaortic conus, development of, 22-24, 25f
Subaortic stenosis, radiography of, 92-94
Subclavian artery
　aberrant
　　associated with tetralogy of Fallot, 640
　　left, right aortic arch with, 11, 72, 73f, 544, 545f-546f, 959, 960f
　　right
　　　aneurysmal origin of, 591-592. See also Diverticulum of Kommerell.
　　　left aortic arch with, 544, 546f, 959-960, 960f
　anatomy of
　　normal, 989-991, 990f
　　variants of, 990-991
　aneurysm of, CT imaging of, 1648-1649, 1649f
　differential considerations of, 991, 991f
　involvement of, in Takayasu arteritis, 1315
　stenosis of, 1326. See also Subclavian steal syndrome.
　　carotid-subclavian bypass for, 1175-1176, 1175f-1176f
　MR imaging of, 1650, 1651f-1653f

Subclavian flap aortoplasty, for aortic coarctation, 539
Subclavian steal syndrome, 1326-1331
　carotid-subclavian bypass for, 1175, 1175f-1176f
　clinical presentation of, 1326-1327, 1645
　definition of, 1326
　differential diagnosis of, 1329
　etiology and pathophysiology of, 1326
　imaging of
　　angiographic, 1329, 1330f
　　CT scans in, 1328, 1328f
　　indications and algorithm for, 1327
　　MR scans in, 1328-1329, 1328f-1330f
　　ultrasound, 1327-1328, 1327f
　　　Doppler, 1247-1249, 1247f-1248f
　prevalence and epidemiology of, 1326
　treatment options for, 1329-1330
　　surgical and interventional, 1330
Subclavian vein
　anatomy of, 1661, 1662f
　upper extremity drainage via, 999
Subpleural edema, 1375-1376
Subpulmonary conus, development of, 22-24, 25f
Sudden death, arrhythmogenic right ventricular dysplasia and, 884
Superficial veins
　of lower extremity, 1024-1027, 1026f-1028f
　of upper extremity, 1019-1022, 1020f-1022f. See also named vein.
Superior vena cava, anatomy of, 996-998, 997f
　variations in, 997-998, 997f-998f
Supraduodenal artery, 972
Suprarenal vein, 1010, 1010f
Surgical excision, of lower extremity aneurysm
　anatomic considerations in, 1600-1601, 1601f
　contraindications to, 1601-1602
　imaging findings in, 1603-1604, 1604f-1605f
　indications for, 1601, 1602f-1603f
　outcomes and complications of, 1602-1603
Surgical ligation, for patent ductus arteriosus, 596-597
Surgical thrombolectomy, lower extremity, 1598-1599, 1598t
Surgical ventricular restoration (Dor procedure), for ischemic heart disease, 811
　postoperative appearance of, 817, 818f
　postoperative complications of, 812
　imaging of, 817-818
Sympathetic nervous system, neurohormonal PET imaging of, 344, 344t
Syphilitic aortitis, 1322-1324, 1322t, 1323f
Systemic fibrosis, nephrogenic, as contraindication to contrast-enhanced MR angiography, 1255-1257
Systemic lupus erythematosus, 1391
　atherosclerosis associated with, 1196
Systemic veins
　anomalous, echocardiography of, 118
　formation of, 8-10, 10f
Systolic function
　disorders of, etiologies of, 790
　echocardiography of, 103, 104f-105f
　global, 756-758
　left ventricular, image interpretation of, 232-235, 233t, 234f
Systolic peak, abnormality(ies) of, carotid vessel stenosis causing, 1240-1241
　parvus tardus waveform, 1240, 1240f
　pulsus alternans waveform, 1241, 1241f
　pulsus bisferiens waveform, 1241, 1241f

T

T lymphocytes, activation of, in atherosclerosis, 1195-1196
Tagged imaging, for quantifying myocardial motion, 229-230, 229f, 230t
Takayasu arteritis, 1411-1414
  aneurysm dilation in, 509, 511f, 1275
  arteriography of, 1414
  classification of, 1315t
  clinical presentation of, 1314-1315, 1315f, 1388
  CT and MR scans of, 1413, 1413f
  definition of, 1314
  diagnostic criteria for, 1388t
  differential diagnosis of, 1390, 1413
  Doppler ultrasonography of, 1498, 1503f-1504f
  etiology and pathophysiology of, 1314, 1388, 1411, 1644
  FDG-PET scan of, 1414
  imaging of
    indications and algorithm for, 1315-1316, 1413-1414
    technique and findings in, 1316-1318, 1316f-1319f, 1388-1390, 1389f
  incidence of, 1644
  prevalence and epidemiology of, 1314, 1388
  treatment options for, 1318-1319, 1319f, 1414
  upper extremity affected by, 1643-1644
  vs. giant cell arteritis, 1319t
Tako-tsubo cardiomyopathy, 107
Tamponade, 63-64, 64f
  causes of, 64t
  echocardiography of, 113
  pericardial effusion with, 941
Technetium 99m (^{99m}Tc), manufacture of, 274
Technetium 99m (^{99m}Tc) erythrocyte scan
  of gastrointestinal bleed, 1144-1146
  pitfall of, 1146
  report of, 1146
Technetium 99m (^{99m}Tc) labeled radiotracer, 301
  in ACEI renal scintigraphy, 1494
  in SPECT
    for identifying myocardial viability, 794-795, 795f
    with nitrate administration, 795-796, 796f
    imaging protocol(s) of, 282-283
      dual-isotope, 282-283
        with thallium 201 and, 282-283, 746
      one-day, 282
      two-day protocol, 282
Technetium 99m (^{99m}Tc)-pertechnetate scan, of Meckel diverticulum, 1146-1148
Technetium 99m (^{99m}Tc) radiotracer
  protocol(s), rest-stress
    same-day, 282, 746
    two-day, 282, 746
Technetium 99m-N-NOET radiotracer, in SPECT, 302
Technetium 99m-sestamibi radiotracer, in SPECT, 301, 739, 740f-741f, 750f
Technetium 99m-teboroxime radiotracer, in SPECT, 302
Technetium 99m-tetrofosmin radiotracer, in SPECT, 301-302, 739
Telangiectasia, hereditary hemorrhagic, 1468
Temporal artery biopsy, for giant cell arteritis, 1322
Temporal resolution, in cardiac MR imaging, 180-181

Terminology issues, in MRI safety, 264, 264t-265t
Test bolus, in contrast CT angiography, 1059-1060, 1062
Test bolus injection, of contrast media, 161-162
Testicular vein, 1010, 1010f
Tet spells, treatment of, 648
Tetralogy, pink, 641
Tetralogy of Fallot, 640-650
  angiography of, 646-647, 662
  classic signs of, 647
  clinical presentation of, 641, 660
  considerations regarding, 390, 391t
  coronary artery anomalies associated with, 640
  CT imaging of, 643, 644f, 661
  definition of, 640, 660
  differential diagnosis of, 647-648
  etiology and pathophysiology of, 640-641, 660
  imaging of
    indications and algorithm for, 641, 660
    technique and findings in, 641-647, 660-662
  medical treatment of, 648
  MR imaging of, 643-646, 645f-647f, 661, 662f-663f
    postoperative, 694-695, 695f
  nuclear imaging of, 661
  pathology of, 7
  pathophysiology and follow-up of, 554, 554f
  prevalence and epidemiology of, 553-554, 640, 660
  radiography of, 641-647, 641f-642f, 660, 661f
  reporting of, 648-649
  surgical repair of, 391, 648, 649f
    postoperative management after, 694-695, 695f
  ultrasonography of, 119, 642-643, 643f, 660-661, 661f-662f
    postnatal, 642-643, 643f
  vs. double-outlet right ventricle, 684
Thallium 201 (^{201}Tl)
  in SPECT, 298-301, 738-739
    dosage and image quality of, 301
    dual-isotope imaging protocol with Tc 99m and, 282-283, 746
    extraction and biodistribution of, 299, 299f
    for identifying myocardial viability, 796-797
    protocols for, 797, 797f-798f
    imaging protocols for, 281-282, 746
    radiation exposure to, 300-301, 300t, 301f
    redistribution of, 299, 299f
    showing myocardial viability, 299-300, 300f
  manufacture of, 274
  physical properties of, 298
  washout of, necrotic myocardial tissue and, 796
Thienopyridines, for cerebrovascular atherosclerotic disease, 1208
Thigh arteries, collateral pathways of, 985
Thoracic aorta. See also Aorta; Aortic entries.
  anatomy of
    normal, 955-961, 956f-958f
    variant, 957-961, 958f-961f
  ascending
    anatomy of, 955, 956f
    pathologic conditions of, 433. See also Aortic aneurysm; Aortic dissection.

Thoracic aorta (Continued)
  surgical repair of, 433-437
    anatomic considerations in, 435, 435f
    contraindications to, 436
    indications for, 436
    outcomes and complications of, 436
    postoperative surveillance after, 437, 437t
    preoperative imaging in, 436-437, 436f
  descending, 955-956
  injury to. See Thoracic aortic trauma.
Thoracic aortic aneurysm, 1271-1286
  asymptomatic, 1277
  causes of, 1271
  clinical presentation of, 1277-1278
  definition of, 1271
  differential diagnosis of, 1282
  etiology and pathophysiology of, 1271-1277
    atherosclerosis in, 1271, 1272f
    cystic medial necrosis in, 1272-1273, 1273f-1274f
    dissection in, 1273, 1275f
    increased aortic flow in, 1276
    infection and inflammation in, 1275, 1276f
    post-stenotic dilation in, 1275, 1276f
    trauma in, 1273, 1275f
  false, 1277, 1277f
  imaging of
    echocardiographic, 1280
    indications and algorithm for, 1278-1279, 1278f
    technique and findings in, 1279-1282, 1280f-1281f
  prevalence and epidemiology of, 1271, 1272f
  reporting of, 1285-1286
  rupture of, 1278
  symptomatic, 1278
  treatment option(s) for, 1282-1285
    hybrid procedures in, 1178-1179, 1178f-1179f
    medical, 1282-1283
    prosthetic graft as, 1284, 1284f
      complications of, 1284-1285, 1285f
    stent graft as, 1283, 1284f
  true, 1277
Thoracic aortic trauma
  angiography of, 1310-1311
  classic signs of, 1311
  clinical presentation of, 1306
  CT imaging of, 1307-1309
    aortic pseudoaneurysm in, 1308, 1309f
    contour abnormality in, 1308
    contrast agent extravasation in, 1309
    intimal flap in, 1308
    periaortic mediastinal hemorrhage in, 1309, 1309f
    technique of, 1307-1308
  differential diagnosis of, 1311, 1311f
  etiology and pathophysiology of, 1306-1313, 1307f-1308f
  imaging of, indications and algorithm for, 1306
  medical treatment of, 1312, 1312f
  MR imaging of, 1309-1310, 1310f
  radiography of, 1306-1307, 1308f
  reporting of, 1313
  surgical/interventional treatment of, 1312-1313, 1312f
  ultrasonography of, 1307
Thoracic aortitis, 1314-1325. See also Giant cell arteritis; Takayasu arteritis.
  differential diagnosis of, 1323-1324, 1324f
Thoracic artery, internal, 964-965, 989, 990f

Thoracic cavity drift, causing attenuation mismatch, in PET imaging, 310-311, 311f
Thoracic outlet, anatomy of, 1666-1667, 1669f
Thoracic outlet syndrome, 991, 991f, 1644, 1666-1669
　definition of, 1666
　imaging of, 1669
　incidence of, 1644
　tests for, 1669
Thoracic vasculature, CT angiography of, 1060-1062, 1063f-1064f
　protocol parameters for, 1061t
Thoracic vein, 996
Thoracoabdominal aortic aneurysm
　Crawford classification of, 1176-1177, 1177f, 1276, 1277f
　repair of, 1176-1178
Thoracotomy, for thoracic aortic injury, 1312
Thorax
　arterial anatomy of, 955-968. *See also named artery, e.g.,* Thoracic aorta.
　radiography of. *See also* Chest radiography.
　　lateral view of, 77, 78f
　venous anatomy of, 996-1004. *See also named vein, e.g.,* Superior vena cava.
　　azygos and hemiazygos systems in, 1000
　　chest wall drainage via, 999, 1000f
　　normal, 996
　　pulmonary veins and, 1001-1004
　　upper extremity and head drainage via, 999
　　venae cavae and, 996-999
Three-dimensional echocardiography, 101. *See also* Echocardiography.
Three-dimensional postprocessing, in CTA and MRA
　advanced, 1128-1143
　　accurate assessment of, 1133-1134
　　application of x-ray angiographic planning purposes in, 1131
　　automated vessel extraction in, 1129
　　automated vessel lumen analysis from, 1134
　　automated vessel lumen segmentation in, 1136-1137, 1137f-1138f
　　　validation of, 1137, 1139f, 1139t
　　automated vessel pathline detection in, 1135-1136, 1136f
　　　validation of, 1136, 1136t
　　centerline detection in, 1129, 1130f
　　contour detection in, 1129-1131, 1131f-1132f
　　coronary vessel presegmentation in, 1129
　　curved multiplanar reformatting in, 1129, 1130f
　　introduction to, 1128-1142
　　optimal angiographic view in, 1133, 1135f
　　plaque assessment in, 1140-1142, 1140f-1141f, 1140t
　　projection overlap in, 1133, 1134f
　　region of interest in, 1132, 1134f
　　segmentation steps in, 1131-1132, 1133f
　　simulating angiographic views in, 1133, 1135f
　　stenosis quantification in, 1131
　　technical requirements for, 1129-1131
　　user interaction in, 1134-1135
　　vessel wall morphology in, automated assessment of, 1137-1138, 1139f-1140f
　basic, 1120-1127
　　maximum intensity projection in, 1121-1123, 1123f-1124f

Three-dimensional postprocessing, in CTA and MRA *(Continued)*
　　multiplanar reformation in, 1120-1121, 1121f-1122f
　　　interpolation in, 1120-1121, 1123f
　　　linear interpolation in, 1121
　　of arterial system, 1451
　　of venous system and soft tissue, 1452
　　volume rendering in, 1122f, 1123-1125, 1124f-1126f
Thrombectomy
　balloon, for iliac occlusion, 1578, 1578f
　mechanical, 1599
Thrombin, as embolic agent, 1169
Thromboangiitis obliterans (Buerger disease), 1645, 1651-1652, 1658f. *See also* Upper extremity, medium and small vessel disease of.
　etiology and pathophysiology of, 1646
　incidence of, 1646
Thrombolectomy, surgical, lower extremity, 1598-1599, 1598t
Thrombolysis, 1164-1167
　agents in, 1599
　catheter-directed, 1597f, 1599-1600
　　for acute limb ischemia, 1577
　contraindications to, 1166
　for acute coronary syndrome, 723
　for inferior vena cava thrombosis, 1539
　for mesenteric atherosclerotic disease, 1210
　imaging findings in, 1166-1167
　indications for, 1165-1166
　outcomes and complications of, 1166
　pharmacomechanical, 1599-1600
　special considerations in, 1165, 1166f
Thrombosis
　arterial
　　coronary, during angioplasty intervention, 129, 129f
　　hepatic
　　　after liver transplantation, 1548-1551, 1548f-1552f
　　　MR imaging of, 1460-1461, 1460f
　　native, 1573
　　renal. *See* Renal artery thrombosis.
　during angioplasty, 1162
　extremity, ultrasound detection of, 1334-1335
　graft, 1573
　　after CABG surgery, 524-525, 527f-529f
　　after endovascular aneurysm repair, 1434, 1434f-1436f
　　after lower extremity bypass, 1185-1186, 1186f
　in-stent. *See* Coronary stents, in-stent restenosis and thrombosis.
　venous
　　deep. *See* Deep vein thrombosis (DVT).
　　Doppler imaging of, 1044
　　inferior vena cava, 1535-1540, 1537t, 1538f-1539f
　　mesenteric, 1457-1458
　　portal, 1457-1458, 1457f
　　　after liver transplantation, 1551, 1553f-1554f
　　renal. *See* Renal vein thrombosis.
Thrombus
　in left atrial appendage, 443, 443f
　　CT imaging of, 447, 447f-448f
　intracardiac, delayed hyperenhancement MR imaging of, 210, 210f
　tricuspid valve, 841f
　tumor, 1458
Thyrocervical trunk, 989, 990f

Tibial artery
　anterior, 983, 984f
　posterior, 984, 984f
Tibial vein
　anterior, 1028
　posterior, 1028
Ticlopidine Aspirin Stroke Study (TASS), 1208
Time to peak filling rate to R-R interval (tPFR/RR), 754
Time-of-flight (TOF) magnetic resonance angiography, 1091-1094, 1092f, 1103-1105, 1104f. *See also* Magnetic resonance angiography (MRA).
　contraindications to, 1103-1105
　image interpretation in, 1105
　indications for, 1103
　of carotid artery stenosis, 1252
　pitfalls and solutions in, 1105
　three-dimensional, 1093
　sequential, 1094, 1094f
　two-dimensional, 1092-1093, 1092f-1093f
Time-resolved imaging of contrast kinetics (TRICKS), three-dimensional, 1090-1091
Time-resolved (TR) magnetic resonance angiography, 1109-1112, 1109f. *See also* Magnetic resonance imaging (MRA).
　contraindications to, 1110-1111
　contrast-enhanced, 1089-1091, 1090f-1091f
　image interpretation in, 1112
　indications for, 1109-1110, 1110f-1111f, 1112t
　pitfalls and solutions in, 1111
Tissue Doppler imaging (TDI), 119-122, 120f-121f, 230
　of amyloidosis, 862-863
Tissue phase mapping (TPM), for quantifying myocardial motion, 230, 230t
Tissue plasminogen activator (tPA), for inferior vena cava thrombosis, 1539
Tissue-weighting factors, in irradiation, 1070-1071
Tobacco use
　atherosclerosis associated with, 1197, 1197f
　Buerger disease associated with, 1646
Toe amputation, for chronic limb ischemia, 1583-1584
Torsion, renal transplant, 1521-1522
Total anomalous pulmonary venous connections (TAPVC)
　classic signs of, 636
　clinical presentation of, 635-636
　definition of, 634
　differential diagnosis of, 636-637
　etiology and pathophysiology of, 634-635
　imaging of
　　indications and algorithm for, 635
　　technique and findings in, 635-636, 635f
　medical treatment of, 637
　prevalence and epidemiology of, 634
　reporting of, 638
　surgical/interventional treatment of, 638
Total anomalous pulmonary venous return (TAPVR), 1002-1004, 1003f
　infracardiac, 1008
Toxin(s), as risk factor for pulmonary hypertension, 1359b
Tracer kinetics, 314-315
　fluorodeoxyglucose 18, 315
　rubidium 82, 314-315
Tracheal compression, of innominate artery, 544, 547f

I-40 Index

TransAtlantic Inter-Society Consensus (TASC) Working Group classification, of aortoiliac and infrainguinal occlusive disease, 1594, 1595t
Transcatheter intravascular ultrasonography, of in-stent restenosis and thrombosis, 517-518
Transcatheter occlusion, for patent ductus arteriosus, 596, 596f
Transcutaneous oxygen tension measurements, in wound healing, 1186, 1187t
Transducers, ultrasound, 1033
 types of, 1034f
Transesophageal echocardiography (TEE), 101, 102f. See also Echocardiography.
 contraindications to, 120
 dobutamine, vs. dobutamine MRI, 221-222
 of aortic dissection, 1290-1291, 1290f
 of atrial septal defect, 564-565, 566f-567f
  postoperative, 365-366, 367f
  preoperative, 364, 364f-365f
 of intramural hematoma of aorta, 1297
 of patent foramen ovale, 369, 369f
 of penetrating atherosclerotic ulcer, 1300
 of thoracic aortic trauma, 1307
 of ventricular septal defect, 576f
 pitfalls and solutions in, 120-122
Transient ischemic attack (TIA). See also Stroke.
 antiplatelet therapy for, 1222
Transient ischemic dilation (TID), 359
Transit time (TT), of contrast media, 160
Transmission-emission misalignment, in PET/CT imaging, 327-328, 328f
Transplant renal artery stenosis (TRAS), 1559-1564
 clinical presentation of, 1559-1560
 differential diagnosis of, 1564
 etiology and pathophysiology of, 1559, 1560f
 imaging of
  angiographic, 1564
  indications and algorithm for, 1560
  MR angiographic, 1561-1564, 1562t, 1563f
  nuclear medicine, 1564
  radiographic, 1560
  ultrasound, 1560-1561, 1560f-1561f
 prevalence and epidemiology of, 1559
 treatment options for, 1564
Transplantation
 heart. See Heart transplantation.
 liver. See Hepatic transplantation.
 pancreas, vascular evaluation of recipient of, 1568-1569
 renal. See Renal transplantation.
Transposition of great arteries (TGA), 389t, 601-615
 cardiac anomalies associated with, 604-605, 604f-605f
 classifications of, 601-602, 602f
 clinical manifestations of, 605-606, 606f, 657
 complete, 601
  cardiac anomalies associated with, 604, 604f-605f
  clinical presentation of, 603
  definition of, 601
  embryology of, 603-604
  imaging of, 611-612
   echocardiographic, 119

Transposition of great arteries (TGA) (Continued)
  surgery for, 607-611, 608f-611f. See also specific procedure, e.g., Arterial switch procedure.
  imaging after, 611-613, 612f-613f
  vs. double-outlet right ventricle, 607, 608f
 congenitally corrected, 601
  abnormal AV node development in, 606
  cardiac anomalies associated with, 604-605, 605f
  definition of, 602
  embryology of, 604
  imaging of, 613-614
   echocardiographic, 119
  late complications of, 606, 606f
  physiology and natural history of, 606
  surgery for, 611
 definition of, 601-602, 656
 dextro-, 601, 656-657
 differential diagnosis of, 606-607, 607f-608f
 epidemiology of, 603
 etiology and pathophysiology of, 603-605, 604f-605f, 657
 genetics of, 603
 imaging of
  indications and algorithm for, 611-613, 657
  postoperative, 695-697, 696f-697f
  technique and findings in, 657-660, 658f-659f
 levo-, 602, 677-680. See also Levotransposition of great arteries.
 medical treatment of, 607
 pathology of, 7
 pathophysiology of, 555
 prevalence and epidemiology of, 554-555, 656-657
 surgical treatment of, 389-390, 607-611, 608f-610f
  follow-up after, 555, 555f
  postoperative management after, 696-697, 696f-697f
 three-letter scheme categorizing, 602, 603f
 vs. double-outlet right ventricle, 684
Transthoracic echocardiography (TTE). See also Echocardiography.
 of atrial septal defect, 564, 566f-567f
 of cardiac metastases, 923-924
 of ventricular septal defect, 574, 576f
Trauma. See at specific anatomic site.
Treadmill stress testing, coronary artery calcium screening with, 463
Triangle of dysplasia, in arrhythmogenic right ventricular dysplasia, 884-885, 885f
Tricuspid valve
 anatomy of, 839-844
 anomalies of, 388, 388t
 failure of, disease causing, 839, 840f-841f
 formation of, 5
 normal function of, 839-844
Tricuspid valve atresia, 840f
 single-ventricle palliation pathway for, 391-392
Tricuspid valve insufficiency, 841f
Tricuspid valve regurgitation
 clinical presentation of, 844
 echocardiography of, 845
 imaging of
  indications and algorithm for, 844-845
  technique and findings in, 845
Tricuspid valve thrombus, 841f
Trigeminal artery, persistent, 963, 964f
Trigger delay, in cardiac MR imaging, 201, 202f

Trig window, in MR imaging, 181-182
Trisacryl gelatin microspheres, as embolic agent, 1168
True aneurysm, 1271, 1277. See also Aneurysm.
Truncal valve
 tricuspid, 619, 619f
 ventricular septal defect and, 618-619, 618f
Truncation, of CT image, 322, 323f
Truncus arteriosus, 3-4, 616-624
 angiography of, 666
 cardiac anomalies associated with, 618-620, 618f-619f
 classification of, 616-618, 617f, 662-663
 clinical presentation of, 620, 620f, 664
 CT imaging of, 664-665, 665f-666f
 definition of, 616, 662-663
 differential diagnosis of, 621
 embryology of, 618
 epidemiology of, 618
 etiology and pathophysiology of, 618-620, 663-664
 genetic screening for, 618
 imaging of
  indications and algorithm for, 664
  technique and findings in, 664-666, 665f-670f
 MR imaging of, 665-666, 667f-670f
 nuclear imaging of, 666
 pathology of, 7
 persistent, 618
 radiography of, 664
 septation of, 6-7, 7f-8f
 surgical treatment of, 621, 621f
  imaging after, 622-623, 622f-623f
  prognosis after, 621-622,
  ultrasonography of, 664, 665f
 vs. double-outlet right ventricle, 684-685
Tubal modulation, radiation dose minimization with, in cardiac CT imaging, 146
Tumor(s). See named tumor; at anatomic site.
Tumor embolization
 clinical presentation of, 1369
 etiology and pathophysiology of, 1368
 imaging technique and findings in, 1369-1370
Tumor thrombus, 1458
Tunica adventia, of blood vessels, 60, 60f
Tunica media, of blood vessels, 60, 60f
Turbo spin-echo (TSE) sequences, in cardiac MR imaging, 204, 204f
Turbulent flow, in Doppler imaging, 1043, 1043t
Twinkle artifact, in Doppler ultrasonography, 1043
Two-day ^{99m}Tc radiotracer protocol, for SPECT, 282, 746
Two-dimensional echocardiography, 98. See also Echocardiography.

U

Uhl anomaly, vs. arrhythmogenic right ventricular dysplasia, 893
Ulcer (ulceration)
 atherosclerotic, penetrating. See Atherosclerotic ulcer, penetrating.
 carotid artery, detection of, 1266-1267
 lower limb, 1581, 1581f
Ulnar artery
 anatomy of, 994-995
 at elbow, 993f, 994
 branches of, 994
 CT angiography of, 1648-1649, 1649f-1650f

Ulnar vein, 1022-1023, 1023f
Ultrasonography. See also Echocardiography.
  aortic trauma, thoracic, 1307
  B-mode, 1033-1034
    image in, 1034, 1037
  contrast-enhanced harmonic imaging in, 1037
  Doppler. See Doppler ultrasonography.
  duplex. See Duplex ultrasonography.
  lower and upper extremity, for pulmonary embolism, 1334-1335
  of acute coronary syndrome, 716-717
  of amyloidosis, 862-863, 862f
  of angiosarcoma, 926
  of aortic aneurysm
    abdominal, 1180, 1400-1401, 1401f, 1441
    inflammatory, 1405
    thoracic, 1280
  of aortic dissection, 1290-1291, 1290f
  of aortic occlusion, acute, 1411, 1411f
  of arteriovenous fistula and pseudoaneurysm, in renal transplant recipient, 1565, 1565f
  of arteriovenous fistula failure, 1675-1676, 1675f
  of atherosclerosis, 1201-1203, 1202f
  of atrial septal defect, 565-566, 566f-567f
  of cardiomyopathy
    dilated, 852-853, 853f
    hypertrophic, 874
    sideritic, 867
  of carotid stenosis, 1220, 1220f
  of chronic thromboembolic pulmonary hypertension, 1345
  of coarctation of aorta, 536
  of cor triatriatum, 632, 633f
  of coronary atherosclerosis, 708-709, 709f
  of double-outlet right ventricle, 682, 683f-684f
  of endoleaks, 1409
  of eosinophilic endomyocardial disease, 865, 865f
  of fibroma, 912
  of giant cell arteritis, 1320
  of inferior vena cava anomalies, 1528
  of inferior vena cava stenosis, after hepatic transplantation, 1534-1535, 1534f-1535f
  of inferior vena cava thrombosis, 1536
  of inferior vena cava tumors, 1530
  of in-stent restenosis and thrombosis, 517-518
  of intramural hematoma of aorta, 1297
  of lipoma, 915
  of lipomatous hypertrophy of interatrial septum, 916
  of liposarcoma, 931
  of myocarditis, 897
  of myxoma, 907, 907f
  of papillary fibroelastoma, 910
  of paraganglioma, 918
  of patent ductus arteriosus, 585, 586f
  of penetrating atherosclerotic ulcer, 1300
  of pericardial effusion, 942
  of pericarditis
    acute, 946
    constrictive, 950
  of primary cardiac lymphoma, 933
  of pulmonary valve regurgitation, 846
  of pulmonary venous connections
    partial anomalous, 626-627
    total anomalous, 635-636
  of renal artery and vein thrombosis, in transplant recipient, 1567

Ultrasonography (Continued)
  of renal artery stenosis, in transplant recipient, 1560-1561, 1560f-1561f
  of rhabdomyoma, 913
  of rhabdomyosarcoma, 930
  of sarcoidosis, 869
  of single ventricle, 672, 674f-675f
  of sinus venous defect, 629-630, 630f
  of subclavian steal syndrome, 1327-1328, 1327f
  of Takayasu arteritis, 1316, 1316f
  of tetralogy of Fallot, 642-643, 643f, 660-661, 661f-662f
  of transposition of great arteries, 657-658, 658f
  of truncus arteriosus, 664, 665f
  of upper extremity medium and small vessel disease, 1647-1648, 1648f
  of vascular anatomy, in pancreas transplant recipient, 1569
  of vascular rings, 543
  of ventricular septal defect, 574, 576f
  vascular
    physical principles and instrumentation in, 1033-1037, 1034f-1035f
    techniques of, 1037-1045. See also Doppler ultrasonography.
Unaliasing by Fournier-encoding overlaps using temporal dimension (UNFOLD), in parallel imaging, 197
University of Maryland triage, for cardiac multidetector CT studies, 721t
Unstable angina/non–ST segment elevation myocardial infarction, percutaneous coronary interventions for, 402
Upper extremity
  angiography of, 1159, 1159f
  arterial anatomy of, 989-995. See also named artery, e.g., Subclavian artery.
  large vessel disease of, 1643-1645
    cause and pathophysiology of, 1644
    clinical presentation of, 1644-1645
    imaging indications and algorithm for, 1645
    prevalence and epidemiology of, 1644
  medium and small vessel disease of, 1645-1652
    classic signs in, 1652
    clinical presentation of, 1646-1647
    differential diagnosis of, 1652
    etiology and pathophysiology of, 1646
    imaging of
      angiographic, 1651-1652, 1658f
      CT scan in, 1648-1649, 1648f-1650f
      indications and algorithm for, 1647
      MR scan in, 1649-1650, 1651f-1654f
      PET-CT, 1650-1651, 1655f-1657f
      radiographic, 1647, 1647f
      ultrasound, 1647-1648, 1648f
    prevalence and epidemiology of, 1646
    reporting of, 1658-1659
    treatment options for, 1652-1658
  thrombosis in
    deep vein. See Deep vein thrombosis (DVT), upper extremity.
    ultrasound detection of, 1334-1335
  venous anatomy of, 1019-1023, 1661, 1662f
    deep veins in, 1022-1023, 1023f
    superficial veins in, 1019-1022, 1020f-1022f
  venous drainage of, 999
Ureter(s), circumcaval (retrocaval), 1526
Urokinase, for inferior vena cava thrombosis, 1539

Uterine artery, 980f, 981
Uterine plexus, 1014

V

VACTERL syndrome, 640
Vaginal artery, 981
Valve implantation, for pulmonary insufficiency, 377. See also Pulmonary insufficiency, valve implantation for.
Valve replacement
  for aortic regurgitation, 833-834
    indications for, 420t
  for aortic stenosis, 830, 832f
    indications for, 419t
  for mitral stenosis, 836
Valvotomy, balloon. See Balloon valvotomy.
Valvular calcification, radiography of, 87, 88f
Valvular heart disease
  catheter-based management of, 405-409, 407f-408f
  echocardiography of, 65-66, 107
  MR evaluation of blood flow in, 241-242, 243f
  radiographic studies of, 92-94, 93f
Valvuloplasty, balloon. See Balloon valvuloplasty.
Van Praagh and Van Praagh classification, of truncus arteriosus, 616, 617f, 662-663
Van Praagh's types, of human heart, 19, 21f
Varices, esophageal, from portal hypertension, 1008-1009, 1008f
  MR imaging of, 1454-1455, 1455f
Vascular access, in angiography, 1157-1158
Vascular bypass surgery, lower extremity, 1585-1591
  anatomic considerations in, 1585-1588, 1586f-1589f
  conduits in
    autogenous saphenous vein as, 1585-1586
    definition of, 1585
    extra-anatomic bypass grafts as, 1586-1588, 1587f-1589f
    prosthetic, 1586
    xenografts as, 1586, 1587f
  contraindications to, 1588-1589
  imaging of
    postoperative surveillance with, 1591
    preoperative planning with, 1591
  indications for, 1588, 1589t
Vascular dilators, 1156
Vascular disorders, of abdomen, MR imaging of, 1451-1470. See also under specific disorder.
  gadolinium use and safety in, 1453
  methodology in, 1451
  of arteries, 1451-1452
  of veins and soft tissue, 1452-1453
Vascular indistinctness, in pulmonary edema, 1375
Vascular interventions, percutaneous, 1155-1171. See also specific intervention, e.g., Angiography.
  equipment and tools used in, 1155-1157
Vascular plug, Amplatz, as embolic agent, 1168
Vascular rings, 542
  classic sign(s) of, 544-545
    anomalous left pulmonary artery, 545, 547f
    double aortic arch, 544, 544f-545f
    innominate artery compression, 544, 547f

Vascular rings *(Continued)*
    left aortic arch with aberrant right subclavian artery, 544, 546f
    right aortic arch with aberrant left subclavian artery, 544, 545f-546f
  clinical presentation of, 542-543
  complete, 542
  definition of, 542
  differential diagnosis of, 545-546
  etiology and pathophysiology of, 542, 543f
  formation of, 11
  imaging studies of, 543-544
  incomplete, 542
  prevalence and epidemiology of, 542
  surgical/interventional treatment of, 546-547
Vascular sheaths, 1156
Vascular slings, 542
Vascular trauma, abdominal, 1468-1469, 1469f
Vasculitis. *See also specific type, e.g.*, Takayasu arteritis.
  definition of, 1643-1644
  pulmonary, 1384, 1385t
  upper extremity, 1643-1644
Vasodilator agents, 352-355. *See also specific vasodilator.*
  in SPECT
    contraindications to, 745
    protocol for, 284-285, 284f
Vein(s), abdominal, MR imaging of, 1452-1453
Velocity encoding (VENC)
  in MR evaluation of blood flow, 240, 242f
  in phase contrast MR angiography, 1094-1095, 1095f-1096f, 1105
Velocity scale, in Doppler ultrasonography, choice of, 1038, 1039f
Vena cava. *See* Inferior vena cava; Superior vena cava.
Vena cordia parva, 53, 54f
Venice-revised WHO classification, of pulmonary hypertension, 1354, 1355b
Venography
  CO_2, of arteriovenous fistula failure, 1682, 1682f
  CT, of pulmonary embolism, 1340
  x-ray, of upper extremity deep vein thrombosis, 1663
Veno-occlusive disease, hepatic, vs. Budd-Chiari syndrome, 1461, 1462f
Venous aneurysms, after liver transplantation, 1551, 1554f
Venous flow, in Doppler imaging, 1043-1044
Venous obstruction, Doppler imaging of, 1044
Venous plexus, dorsal, upper extremity, 1019-1020, 1021f
Venous thrombosis. *See* Thrombosis, venous.
  deep. *See* Deep vein thrombosis (DVT).
Veno-venous shunt, intrahepatic, MR imaging of, 1454-1455, 1456f
Ventilation-perfusion (V/Q) scintigraphy. *See* Nuclear medicine imaging, ventilation-perfusion (V/Q).
Ventricle(s)
  developmental pathology of, 4
  formation of, 4, 5f-6f
  identification of, 15-16, 15f-16f
  left
    anatomy of, 33-34, 34f
    circumferential-longitudinal shear angle of, 234-235
    dysfunction of
      associated with coronary artery disease, 403
      management of, 62
    ejection fraction of. *See* Ejection fraction, left ventricular.

Ventricle(s) *(Continued)*
    normal values of, 65t
    pressure-volume relationships in, 58-59, 59f
    radiography of, of cardiac borders, in lateral projection, 77
    segmentation of, 49-50, 51f-52f
    ^{99m}Tc-sestamibi imaging of, 286f
    two-dimensional echocardiographic imaging of, 103
  primitive, 3-4
  right
    anatomy of, 33, 33f
    double-outlet. *See* Double-outlet right ventricle (DORV).
    echocardiographic imaging of, 103
    normal values of, 65t
  single, 671-677
    angiography of, 677, 678f
    clinical presentation of, 672
    CT imaging of, 673
    defects of, 389-390, 389t
      repair of, 390
    definition of, 671
    etiology of, 671
    imaging of
      indications and algorithm for, 672
      technique and findings in, 672-677
    MR imaging of, 673-676
      after bidirectional superior cavopulmonary connection, 674-675
      after Fontan procedure, 675-676, 676f-677f, 699-700
      after stage I, 674
      in native state, 674
    nuclear imaging of, 677
    pathophysiology of, 671-672
    prevalence and epidemiology of, 671
    radiography of, 672, 673f
    ultrasonography of, 672, 674f-675f
Ventricular assist device (VAD)
  for ischemic heart disease, 810-811
    postoperative appearance of, 815, 816f
    postoperative complications of, 812
      imaging of, 816-817, 817f
    preoperative and perioperative assessment of, 815
  long-term, 811
  temporary percutaneous, 811
Ventricular border, radiography of
  left, 74-75, 75f-76f
  right, 75
Ventricular cardiomyopathy, right, arrhythmogenic, 237, 237f
Ventricular dysplasia, right, arrhythmogenic, 884-895. *See also* Arrhythmogenic right ventricular dysplasia (ARVD).
Ventricular function
  gated MPI assessment of, 771-773
    data processing, reconstruction, and analysis of, 772-773
    electrogram gated acquisition in, 772
    pitfalls and solutions in, 773
    technique(s) of, 773-779
      equilibrium gated blood pool imaging, 773-775, 774f-778f
      first-pass radionuclide angiography, 775-779, 779f
  global, image interpretation of, 231-232, 231f-232f
  left
    CT assessment of, 761
    diastolic, 235, 235f

Ventricular function *(Continued)*
    MRI assessment of, 181-182, 181f-182f, 556, 733-734, 758-759, 760t-761t
    using dobutamine, 218-223
      contraindications to, 223
      image interpretation in, 223
      indications and clinical utility for, 218-223, 220f-223f, 220t
      pitfalls and solutions in, 223
    using exercise, 223-224, 223f
  normal values of, in healthy persons, 233t
  regional, image interpretation of, 232-235, 233t, 234f-235f
  right
    CT assessment of, 762-763
    diastolic, 237
    global, image interpretation of, 235, 236t
    MRI assessment of, 217, 217f, 761-762, 762t-763t
    normal values of, in healthy persons, 236t
    regional, image interpretation of, 237, 237f
  systolic, 232-235, 233t, 234f
Ventricular loop, analysis of, 18, 19f
Ventricular mass
  in hypertrophic cardiomyopathy, MR imaging of, 875-876, 878f
  left, image interpretation of, 232
Ventricular myxoma, 906. *See also* Myxoma.
Ventricular outflow tract(s)
  developmental pathology of, 7, 8f
  formation of, 6-7, 7f-8f
  right, vs. arrhythmogenic right ventricular dysplasia, 893t
Ventricular outflow tract obstruction
  echocardiography of, 118
  left, in hypertrophic cardiomyopathy
    MR imaging of, 879-882, 881f
    treatment of, 881-882
Ventricular septal defect (VSD)
  angiography of, 577-579, 580f
  associated with d-TGA, 657
  clinical presentation of, 573
  considerations regarding, 383, 385f, 385t
  CT imaging of, 574-575, 577f-578f
  definition of, 572
  developmental pathology of, 4
  differential diagnosis of, 579-580
  etiology and pathophysiology of, 572-573
  imaging of
    indications and algorithm for, 573
    technique and findings in, 574
  medical treatment of, 580
  MR imaging of, 575-577, 578f-579f
  nuclear imaging of, 577
  prevalence and epidemiology of, 572
  radiography of, 574, 574f-575f
  reporting of, 581
  subtruncal, 618-619, 618f
    surgical repair of, 621, 621f
  surgical/interventional treatment of, 386, 580-581
  type I, 572
  type II, 572
  type III, 572
  type IV, 572
  ultrasonography of, 118, 574, 576f
Ventricular septum
  anatomy of, 34, 34f
  anomalies associated with, evaluation of, 24, 26f
  developmental pathology of, 4
  formation of, 4, 5f-6f
Ventricular strain, left, 234-235, 235f

Ventricular volume
  left
    MRI determination of, Simpson's rule in, 215
    quantification of, FLASH vs. steady-state free precession in, 231-232
  right, image interpretation of, 235-237
Ventricular-level shunt, in acyanotic congenital heart disease, 383, 385t
Ventriculoarterial (VA) discordance, in levotransposition of great arteries, 677
Ventriculoscintigraphy, of arrhythmogenic right ventricular dysplasia, 887
Vertebral artery, 989, 990f
  Doppler ultrasonography of, 1246-1249
    normal tracing in, 1231-1232, 1232f
  pre-steal waveform of, 1247-1249, 1247f
Vesical artery, inferior, 981
Vesical venous plexus, 1014
Viability protocols, for PET imaging, 318, 318f
Visceral plexus(es), venous origin in, 1013-1014, 1014f
Visceral situs solitus, in Ebstein anomaly, 653
Visceroatrial situs, analysis of, 16-18, 17f-19f
Voltage, x-ray tube, in computed tomography, reduction of, 152-153
Volume detectors, in CT imaging, 140-141
Volume overload, 63
Volume rendering technique (VRT)
  equation for, 1124
  of CT angiography, 1074, 1122f, 1123-1125, 1124f-1126f
    carotid, 1266
    coronary, 502
    lower extremity, 1622, 1625f
    renal, 1489, 1490f
  of CT imaging, cardiac, 176-178, 177f
Voxel, volume flow rate through, calculation of, 1097

W

Walking adenosine protocol, 357. *See also* Adenosine.
Warfarin, for inferior vena cava thrombosis, 1539
  of myocardial viability, 800, 800f
Water flask silhouette, in pericardial effusion, 942
Water phantom, in CT systems, 1049, 1050f
Waterston shunt, for decreased pulmonary blood flow, 391
Waveform, in Doppler imaging, 1043
Waveform analysis, Doppler, of carotid arteries, 1240-1245
  abnormal patterns involving cardiac cycle, 1242-1245
    arteriovenous fistula, 1244, 1246f
    carotid dissection, 1243, 1245f
    carotid pseudoaneurysm, 1243, 1246f
    intra-aortic balloon pump, 1244-1245, 1247f
  diastolic flow abnormalities in, 1241-1242, 1241f-1244f
  systolic peak abnormality(ies) in, 1240-1241
    parvus tardus waveform, 1240, 1240f
    pulsus alternans waveform, 1241, 1241f
    pulsus bisferiens waveform, 1241, 1241f
WaveProp algorithm, 1129
Wegener's granulomatosis, 1384-1386
  clinical manifestations of, 1385
  differential diagnosis of, 1386
  imaging of, 1385-1386, 1385f-1386f
  limited, 1386
  prevalence and epidemiology of, 1385
Wells clinical decision rule, for pulmonary embolism, 1333t
Westermark sign, in pulmonary embolism, 1333f, 1334
Wet aneurysm, 1591
Winiwarter-Buerger disease, 1645
Wires, guide, 1156
Wolf mini-Maze procedure, for atrial fibrillation, 445, 446f
Wolff-Parkinson-White syndrome, 606
Wooden shoe sign, in tetralogy of Fallot, 647

X

Xenograft(s), bovine, in vascular bypass surgery, 1586, 1587f
X-linked dilated cardiomyopathy, 852. *See also* Cardiomyopathy, dilated.
X-ray(s), 270
  characteristic, 271, 272f
X-ray photons, 1047
X-ray physics, fundamentals of, 1047, 1048f
X-ray tube current, in CT imaging
  ECG-based reduction of, 151
    pitfalls and solutions for, 151-152
  size-based reduction of, 151, 151f
    pitfalls and solutions for, 152
X-ray tube voltage, in CT imaging, reduction of, 152-153

Y

Yttrium 90, radioembolization using, 975-976

Z

Z number, 270, 271t
Zellaballen, 917, 917f